Neonatology:
Clinical Practice
and Procedures

Neonatology: Clinical Practice and Procedures

David K. Stevenson, MD
Professor of Pediatrics
Stanford University School of Medicine
Stanford, California

Ronald S. Cohen, MD
Clinical Professor of Pediatrics
Stanford University School of Medicine
Stanford, California

Philip Sunshine, MD
Professor Emeritus of Pediatrics
Stanford University School of Medicine
Stanford, California

New York   Chicago   San Francisco   Athens   London   Madrid   Mexico City
Milan   New Delhi   Singapore   Sydney   Toronto

Neonatology: Clinical Practice and Procedures

Copyright © 2015 by McGraw-Hill Education. All rights reserved. Printed in the United States of America. Except as permitted under the United States Copyright Act of 1976, no part of this publication may be reproduced or distributed in any form or by any means, or stored in a database or retrieval system, without the prior written permission of the publisher.

1 2 3 4 5 6 7 8 9 0   DOW/DOW   19 18 17 16 15

ISBN 978-0-07-176376-9
MHID 0-07-176376-7

This book was set in Plantin by Cenveo® Publisher Services.
The editors were Alyssa K. Fried and Christina M. Thomas.
The production supervisor was Catherine Saggese.
Project management was provided by Vastavikta Sharma, Cenveo Publisher Services.
RR Donnelley was printer and binder.

This book is printed on acid-free paper.

Library of Congress Cataloging-in-Publication Data

Neonatology (Stevenson)
  Neonatology : clinical practice and procedures / [edited by] David K. Stevenson, Philip Sunshine, Ronald S. Cohen.
    p. ; cm.
  Includes bibliographical references and index.
  ISBN 978-0-07-176376-9 (hardcover : alk. paper)—ISBN 0-07-176376-7
  I. Stevenson, David K. (David Kendal), 1949-, editor.   II. Sunshine, Philip, 1930-, editor.
III. Cohen, Ronald S., editor.   IV. Title.
  [DNLM: 1. Infant, Newborn, Diseases.   WS 421]
  RJ254
  618.92'01—dc23
                                                                                    2014027202

McGraw-Hill Education books are available at special quantity discounts to use as premiums and sales promotions, or for use in corporate training programs. To contact a representative, please visit the Contact Us pages at www.mhprofessional.com.

Dedication

To our own children and all others to whom we owe a better future than the one we had once dreamed for ourselves.

Contents

I INTRODUCTION

II ORGAN SYSTEMS

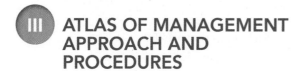

III ATLAS OF MANAGEMENT APPROACH AND PROCEDURES

Contributors

Alexandra Abrams, MD
Pediatric Hematology/Oncology Fellow
Division of Pediatric Hematology/Oncology/Stem Cell
  Transplantation
Stanford University School of Medicine
Palo Alto, California

David H. Adamkin, MD
Professor of Pediatrics
University of Louisville
Louisville, Kentucky

Winifred Adams, MD
Pediatric Urology Fellow
Department of Urology
Stanford University School of Medicine
Stanford, California

Pankaj B. Agrawal, MD, MBBS
Program in Genomics and the Manton Center for Orphan
  Disease Research
Division of Neonatology and Department of Pediatrics
Children's Hospital Boston and Harvard Medical School
Boston, Massachusetts

Vishnu Priya Akula, MD
Post-doctoral fellow in Neonatology
Division of Neonatal and Developmental Medicine
Stanford University School of Medicine
Palo Alto, California

Jennifer Andrews, MD, MSc
Clinical Assistant Professor of Pathology
  (Transfusion Medicine) and Pediatrics
  (Hematology/Oncology)
Stanford Hospital & Clinics and Lucile Packard
  Children's Hospital
Palo Alto, California

David M. Axelrod, MD
Clinical Assistant Professor, Pediatrics
Division of Pediatric Cardiology
Department of Pediatrics
Lucile Packard Children's Hospital
Stanford University Medical Center
Stanford University School of Medicine
Palo Alto, California

Natali Aziz, MD, MS
Assistant Clinic Professor
Director of Perinatal Infectious Diseases
Division of Maternal-Fetal Medicine
Department of Obstetrics and Gynecology
Stanford University School of Medicine
Stanford, California

Jay Michael S. Balagtas, MD
Assistant Clinical Professor
Section of Pediatric Hematology/Oncology
University of California
Davis Medical Center
Sacramento, California

M. Bethany Ball, CCRC
Neonatology Research Coordinator
Division of Neonatal and Developmental Medicine
Stanford University School of Medicine
Palo Alto, California

Richard Barth, MD
Professor of Radiology
Chief of Pediatric Radiology
Stanford University School of Medicine;
Director of Pediatric Imaging and Radiologist in Chief
Lucile Packard Children's Hospital
Palo Alto, California

Mark L. Batshaw, MD
Children's Research Institute
Children's National Medical Center;
Department of Pediatrics
George Washington University School of Medicine and
  Health Sciences
Washington, DC

Alan H. Beggs, PhD
Program in Genomics and the Manton Center for Orphan
  Disease Research
Children's Hospital Boston and Harvard Medical School
Boston, Massachusetts

Latanya T. Benjamin, MD
Assistant Clinical Professor of Dermatology and Pediatrics
Lucile Packard Children's Hospital
Stanford University School of Medicine
Palo Alto, California

Daniel Bernstein, MD
Alfred Woodley Salter and Mabel Smith Salter Endowed
    Professor in Pediatrics
Department of Pediatrics-Cardiology
Stanford University School of Medicine
Palo Alto, California

William Berquist, MD
Professor of Pediatric Gastroenterology
Pediatric Gastroenterology
Lucile Packard Children's Hospital at Stanford
Palo Alto, California

Vinod K. Bhutani, MD, FAAP
Stanford University
Lucile Packard Children's Hospital
Palo Alto, California

Nader Bishara, MD
Attending Neonatologist
Huntington Memorial Hospital
Pasadena, California

Charlotte M. Boney, MD
Associate Professor of Pediatrics
Rhode Island Hospital/The Warren Alpert Medical School
    of Brown University
Providence, Rhode Island

Kenneth Boyer, MD
Woman's Board Professor and Chairperson
Department of Pediatrics
Rush University Medical Center
Chicago, Illinois

William J. Britt, MD
Charles Alford Chair of Pediatrics
Division of Infectious Diseases
Departments of Pediatrics, Microbiology, and Neurobiology
University of Alabama School of Medicine
Birmingham, Alabama

Ruben Bromiker, MD
Department of Neonatology
Shaare Zedek Medical Center
Faculty of Medicine of the Hebrew University
Jerusalem, Israel

Anna L. Bruckner, MD
University of Colorado School of Medicine
Departments of Dermatology and Pediatrics
Children's Hospital Colorado
Aurora, Colorado

Matias Bruzoni, MD
Assistant Professor
Division of Pediatric Surgery
Lucile Packard Children's Hospital
Department of Surgery
Stanford University
Palo Alto, California

Bruce Buckingham, MD
Professor of Pediatric Endocrinology
Department of Pediatrics-Endocrinology
Stanford University School of Medicine
Palo Alto, California

Jennifer Burgis, MD
Division of Pediatric Gastroenterology
Hepatology and Nutrition
Stanford University
Palo Alto, California

Waldemar A. Carlo, MD
Professor of Pediatrics
Director, Division of Neonatology
Director, Newborn Nurseries
Department of Pediatrics
UAB School of Medicine
University of Alabama at Birmingham
Birmingham, Alabama

Kimberly Chapman, MD, PhD
Children's National Medical Center
Genetics and Metabolism
Washington, DC

Abanti Chaudhuri, MD
Lucile Packard Children's Hospital
Stanford University Medical Center
Stanford, California

Dennis Chia, MD
Associate Professor of Pediatrics
Icahn School of Medicine at Mount Sinai
New York, New York

Valerie Y. Chock, MD
Clinical Associate Professor of Pediatrics
Division of Neonatal and Developmental Medicine
Stanford University School of Medicine
Palo Alto, California

Jane Chueh, MD
Professor of Obstetrics and Gynecology
Division of Maternal Fetal Medicine
Stanford University School of Medicine;
Director, Perinatal Diagnostic Center
Lucile Packard Children's Hospital
Palo Alto, California

Curtis J. Clark, MD
Clinical Instructor
Northeast Ohio Medical University
Children's Hospital Medical Center of Akron
Ohio, Ohio

Fatima Clouser
Toxoplasmosis Study Coordinator
University of Chicago
Ophthalmology and Visual Science
Chicago, Illinois

Ronald S. Cohen, MD
Clinical Professor of Pediatrics
Division of Neonatal and Developmental Medicine
Stanford University School of Medicine
Palo Alto, California

Christopher E. Colby, MD
Assistant Professor of Pediatrics
Mayo Clinic
Rochester, Minnesota

Waldo Concepcion, MD
Professor of Surgery
Chief of Clinical Transplantation
Chief of Pediatric Kidney Transplantation
Division of Transplantation
Stanford University School of Medicine
Palo Alto, California

Robert B. Cotton, MD
Professor, Department of Pediatrics
Monroe Carrell Jr. Children's Hospital at Vanderbilt
Vanderbilt University Medical Center
Nashville, Tennessee

Alexa Craig, MD
Neonatal Neurology Fellow
Washington University
St. Louis, Missouri

Christopher Cunniff, MD
Professor of Pediatrics
Chief, Section of Medical and Molecular Genetics
The University of Arizona College of Medicine
Tucson, Arizona

Robert A. Darnall, MD
Professor of Pediatrics, and of Physiology and Neurobiology
Dartmouth Medical School and the Children's Hospital at Dartmouth
Lebanon, New Hampshire

Alexis S. Davis, MD, MS Epi
Clinical Assistant Professor
Division of Neonatal and Developmental Medicine
Department of Pediatrics
Stanford University School of Medicine
Palo Alto, California

Romano T. DeMarco, MD
Associate Professor
Division of Pediatric Urology
Departments of Surgery and Pediatrics
Sanford School of Medicine of the University of South Dakota
Sanford Children's Hospital
Sioux Falls, South Dakota

Yaser A. Diab, MBBS
Division of Hematology
Center for Cancer and Blood Disorders
Children's National Medical Center
George Washington School of Medicine and Health Sciences
Washington, DC

Reed Dimmitt
Director, UAB Division of Pediatric Gastroenterology and Nutrition
Professor of Pediatrics and Surgery
Divisions of Neonatology and Pediatric GI/Nutrition
University of Alabama at Birmingham
Birmingham, Alabama

Anne M. Dubin, MD
Division of Pediatric Cardiology
Department of Pediatrics
Stanford University
Palo Alto, California

Jennifer M. Duchon, MDCM, MPH
Assistant Professor of Clinical Pediatrics
Department of Pediatrics, Division of Neonatology
Columbia University Medical Center
New York, New York

Sanjeev Dutta, MD, FRCS(C), FACS
Associate Professor
Division of Pediatric Surgery
Lucile Packard Children's Hospital
Department of Surgery
Stanford University
Palo Alto, California

Jonathan A. Dyer, MD
Departments of Dermatology and Child Health
University of Missouri
Columbia, Missouri

Karen E. Effinger, MD
Pediatric Hematology/Oncology Fellow
Division of Pediatric Hematology/Oncology/Stem Cell Transplantation
Stanford University School of Medicine
Palo Alto, California

Donna M. Ferriero, MD
W.H. and Marie Wattis Distinguished Professor & Chair Department of Pediatrics
Physician-in-Chief, UCSF Benioff Children's Hospital
University of California
San Francisco, California

Magali Fontaine, MD, PhD
Associate Professor of Pathology and Medicine
Department of Pathology
University of Maryland School of Medicine
Baltimore, Maryland

Björn Frenckner, MD, PhD
Professor of Pediatric Surgery
Karolinska University Hospital, Solna
Stockholm, Sweden

Bertil Glader MD, PhD
Professor of Pediatrics and Pathology
Stanford University
Stanford, CA;
Professor, Pediatric Hematology-Oncology
Lucile Packard Children's Hospital
Stanford University
Palo Alto, California

Michael Goldberg, MD
Chief, Skeletal Dysplasia Clinic
Clinical Professor
Seattle Children's Hospital
Seattle, Washington

Evan Graber, DO
Fellow, Division of Pediatric Endocrinology and Diabetes
Icahn School of Medicine at Mount Sinai
New York, New York

Elizabeth A. Greene, MD
Pediatric Cardiologist
Children's National Health System
Washington, DC

Paul Grimm, MD
Department of Pediatrics
Division of Nephrology
Stanford University Medical Center
Lucile Packard Children's Hospital
Stanford, California

Arun Gupta, MD
Clinical Assistant Professor
Department of Pediatrics, Division of Neonatology
Stanford University
Stanford, California

Kathleen Gutierrez, MD
Associate Professor of Pediatric Infectious Disease
Stanford University School of Medicine
Lucile Packard Children's Hospital
Stanford, California

Jin S. Hahn, MD
Professor of Neurology, of Pediatrics
Stanford University School of Medicine
Palo Alto, California

Louis P. Halamek, MD, FAAP
Professor
Division of Neonatal and Developmental Medicine
Department of Pediatrics
Stanford University
Palo Alto, California

Cathy Hammerman, MD
Department of Neonatology
Shaare Zedek Medical Center
Faculty of Medicine of the Hebrew University
Jerusalem, Israel

George Van Hare, MD
Lewis Larrick Ward Professor, PediatricsDirector, David Goldring Division of Pediatric CardiologyDirector, Pediatric Arrhythmia Service
St Louis Children's Hospital
St. Louis, Missouri

Gary E. Hartman, MD, MBA
Clinical Professor of Surgery
Stanford University School of Medicine
Stanford, California

Anne Hilgendorff, MD
Neonatology
Perinatal Center Grosshadern
Dr. von Haunersches Children's Hospital
Ludwig-Maximilians University Munich
Munich, Germany

Susan Hintz, MD, MS Epi
Associate Professor of Pediatrics
Division of Neonatology
Stanford University School of Medicine;
Director, The Center for Fetal and Maternal Health
Lucile Packard Children's Hospital
Palo Alto, California

Seth Hollander, MD
Clinical Assistant Professor
Associate Section Chief of Heart Failure and Transplantation
Department of Pediatrics-Cardiology
Stanford University School of Medicine
Palo Alto, California

H. Eugene Hoyme, MD
Chief Academic Officer, Sanford Health
President, Sanford Research/USD
Professor of Pediatrics
Sanford School of Medicine of the University of South Dakota
The Sanford Center
Sioux Falls, South Dakota

Christopher H. Hsu, MD, PhD
Pediatric Hematology/Oncology Fellow
Division of Pediatric Hematology/Oncology/Stem Cell Transplantation
Stanford University School of Medicine
Palo Alto, California

Louanne Hudgins, MD
Professor of Pediatrics
Chief, Division of Medical Genetics
Stanford University School of Medicine;
Director of Perinatal Genetics
Lucile Packard Children's Hospital
Palo Alto, California

Melissa Hurwitz, MD
Division of Pediatric Gastroenterology
Hepatology and Nutrition
Stanford University
Palo Alto, California

Meghan N. Imrie, MD
Clinical Assistant Professor
Pediatric Orthopaedics
Lucile Packard Children's Hospital
Stanford, California

Amanda Jacobson, PhD
Division of Pediatric Immunology and Allergy
Stanford University
Stanford, California

Lucky Jain, MD, MBA
Richard W Blumberg Professor
Executive Vice Chairman
Department of Pediatrics
Emory University School of Medicine
Medical Director, Emory-Children's Center
Emory Children's Center
Atlanta, Georgia

Michael R. Jeng, MD
Associate Professor of Pediatrics
Division of Pediatric Hematology/Oncology/Stem Cell
    Transplantation
Stanford University School of Medicine
Palo Alto, California

Jennifer Jenks, MD, PhD
Division of Immunology and Allergy
Stanford University
Stanford, California

Thomas Jinguji
Alan H. Jobe, MD, PhD
Cincinnati Children's Hospital
Division of Pulmonary Biology
Cincinnati, Ohio

Peter B. Kang, MD
Program in Genomics and the Manton Center for Orphan
    Disease Research
Department of Neurology
Children's Hospital Boston and Harvard Medical School
Boston, Massachusetts

Michael Kaplan, MB, ChB
Department of Neonatology
Shaare Zedek Medical Center
Faculty of Medicine of the Hebrew University
Jerusalem, Israel

Zachary Kastenberg, MD
Surgical Resident
Department of Surgery
Stanford University
Stanford, California

Sarah Keene, MD
Assistant Professor of Pediatrics
Division of Neonatology
Emory University School of Medicine
Atlanta, Georgia

William A. Kennedy II, MD, FAAP
Associate Professor of Urology
Department of Urology
Stanford University School of Medicine
Chief, Pediatric Urology
Lucile Packard Children's Hospital at Stanford
Stanford, California

John Kerner, MD
Professor of Pediatrics & Director of Nutrition
Division of Pediatric Gastroenterology, Hepatology, and
    Nutrition
Lucile Packard Children's Hospital/Stanford University
    Medical Center
Palo Alto, California

Uta Lichter-Konecki, MD
Children's Research Institute
Children's National Medical Center;
Department of Pediatrics
George Washington University School of Medicine and
    Health Sciences
Washington, DC

Rajiv Kumar, MD
Medical Director of Mobile Health, Lucile Packard
    Children's Hospital
Clinical Assistant Professor of Pediatrics, Division of
    Pediatric Endocrinology & Diabetes
Stanford University, Stanford Children's Health and the
    California Pacific Medical Center
Palo Alto, California

Norman Lacayo, MD
Assistant Professor
Division of Pediatric Hematology/Oncology
Lucile Packard Children's Hospital & Stanford Cancer
    Institute
Stanford University School of Medicine
Palo Alto, California

Alfred T. Lane, MD
Professor of Dermatology and Pediatrics
Stanford University School of Medicine
Lucile Packard Children's Hospital at Stanford
Stanford, California

Brendan Lanpher, MD
Children's Research Institute
Children's National Medical Center;
Department of Pediatrics
George Washington University School of Medicine and
  Health Sciences
Washington, DC

John D. Lantos, MD
Professor of Pediatric, University of Missouri
Director, Children's Mercy Bioethics Center
Children's Mercy Hospital
Kansas City, Missouri

Abbot R. Laptook, MD
Professor of Pediatrics
The Warren Alpert Medical School of Brown University
Medical Director, Neonatal Intensive Care Unit
Women & Infants Hospital of Rhode Island
Providence, Rhode Island

Yu-Lung Lau, MD
Department of Paediatrics and Adolescent Medicine
Queen Mary Hospital
Li Ka Shing Faculty of Medicine
The University of Hong Kong
Hong Kong

Jean Baptiste Le Pichon, MD, PhD
Associate Professor of Pediatrics
Program Director for the Child Neurology Residency
Children's Mercy Hospitals and Clinics
Kansas City, Missouri

Pamela Lee, MBBS
Department of Paediatrics and Adolescent Medicine
Queen Mary Hospital
Li Ka Shing Faculty of Medicine
The University of Hong Kong
Hong Kong

Daniel Lee
Clinical Coordinator, National Collaborative Toxoplasmosis
  Study
The University of Chicago
Chicago, Illinois

Henry C. Lee, MD
Assistant Professor
Department of Pediatrics, Division of Neonatology
Stanford University
Stanford, California

Amy Lightner, MD
UCLA General Surgery Resident
Stanford Postdoctoral Fellow
Stanford University School of Medicine
Stanford, California

Clara Y. Lo, MD
Instructor, Pediatric Hematology-Oncology
Lucile Packard Children's Hospital
Stanford University
Palo Alto, California

Naomi L.C. Luban, MD
Division of Hematology
Center for Cancer and Blood Disorders and Division of
  Laboratory Medicine;
Children's National Medical Center
Washington, DC;
George Washington School of Medicine and Health
  Sciences
Washington, DC

Katsuhide Maeda, MD
Assistant Professor of Cardiothoracic Surgery
Lucile Packard Children's Hospital
Stanford University
Palo Alto, California

Yvonne A. Maldonado, MD
Department of Pediatrics
Stanford University School of Medicine
Palo Alto, California

Melanie Manning, MD
Clinical Assistant Professor, Pathology and Pediatrics
Division of Medical Genetics
Department of Pediatrics
Stanford University School of Medicine
Stanford, California

Katherine McCallie, MD
Clinical Instructor
Division of Neonatal and Developmental Medicine
Department of Pediatrics
Stanford University School of Medicine
Palo Alto, California

Rebecca McEachern, MD
Department of Pediatrics
Warren Alpert School of Medicine at Brown University
Providence, Rhode Island

Thomas J. McIntee, MD
University of Colorado School of Medicine
Department of Dermatology
Children's Hospital Colorado
Aurora, Colorado

Rima McLeod, MD
Professor
The University of Chicago
Chicago, Illinois

William L. Meadow, MD, PhD
Professor of Pediatrics University of Chicago
Co-Section Chief, Section of Neonatology
Assistant Director, MacLean Center for Clinical Medical
    Ethics
Chicago, Illinois

Ram Menon
Professor of Pediatric Endocrinology
Division of Pediatric Endocrinology, Diabetes, and
    Metabolism
C.S. Mott Children's Hospital
University of Michigan Health System
Ann Arbor, Michigan

Krisa Van Meurs, MD
Rosemarie Hess Professor of Pediatrics
Division of Neonatal and Developmental Medicine
Stanford University School of Medicine
Palo Alto, California

Nick Mickas, MD
Attending Neonatologist
John Muir Medical Center
Walnut Creek, California

Vladana Milisavljevic, MD, MS
Associate Clinical Professor
Department of Pediatrics
David Geffen School of Medicine at UCLA
Associate Director, NICU
Cedars-Sinai Medical Center
Los Angeles, California

Christina Y. Miyake, MD
Division of Pediatric Cardiology
Department of Pediatrics
Stanford University
Palo Alto, California

R. Lawrence Moss, MD
Surgeon-in-Chief
Nationwide Children's Hospital
E. Thomas Boles Jr., Professor of Surgery
The Ohio State University, College of Medicine
Columbus, Ohio

Kari Nadeau, MD, PhD
Division of Immunology and Allergy
Stanford University
Stanford, California

Josef Neu, MD
Professor of Pediatrics
Pediatrics/Neonatology
University of Florida
Gainesville, Florida

Anna-Kaisa Niemi, MD, PhD
Clinical Life Science Research Associate
Department of Pediatrics, Division of Medical Genetics
Stanford University
Stanford, California

Shahab Noori, MD
Associate Professor of Pediatrics
Center for Fetal and Neonatal Medicine
USC Division of Neonatal Medicine
Children's Hospital Los Angeles and the LAC+USC
    Medical Center
Keck School of Medicine
University of Southern California
Los Angeles, California

Mary E. Norton, MD
Professor
Director of Perinatal Research
Division of Maternal-Fetal Medicine
Department of Obstetrics and Gynecology
Stanford University School of Medicine
Stanford, California

Gia Oh, MD
Department of Pediatrics
Division of Nephrology
Stanford University Medical Center
Lucile Packard Children's Hospital
Stanford, California

Robin K. Ohls, MD
Professor of Pediatrics
University of New Mexico
Albuquerque, New Mexico

Donald M. Olson, MD
Department of Neurology
Stanford University School of Medicine
Palo Alto, California

Kristina Cusmano-Ozog, MD
Children's National Medical Center
Genetics and Metabolism
Washington, DC

Lu-Ann Papile, MD
Professor of Pediatrics
Indiana University School of Medicine
Department of Pediatrics
Neonatal-Perinatal Medicine
James Whitcomb Riley Hospital for Children
Indianapolis, Indiana

Parul Patel, MD
Pediatric Endocrinologist
Stanford University School of Medicine
Palo Alto, California

Robert P. Payne, MD, FRCSC
John and Tasha Morgidge Postdoctorate Fellow
Department of Urology
Stanford University School of Medicine
Stanford, California

Johann Peterson, MD
Assistant Professor of Pediatrics (Gastroenterology)
University of California, Davis
Sacramento, California

Alistair G.S. Philip, MD, FRCPE
Emeritus Professor of Pediatrics
Division of Neonatal and Developmental Medicine
Stanford University School of Medicine
Palo Alto, California

Kevin Pieroni, MD
Division of Pediatric Gastroenterology, Hepatology, and
    Nutrition
Lucile Packard Children's Hospital/Stanford University
    Medical Center
Palo Alto, California

Rajesh Punn, MD
Clinical Assistant Professor
Division of Pediatric Cardiology
Lucile Packard Children's Hospital
Stanford University
Palo Alto, California

Jose Bernardo Quintos, MD
Assistant Professor of Pediatrics (Clinical)
Rhode Island Hospital/The Warren Alpert Medical School
    of Brown University
Providence, Rhode Island

Robert Rapaport, MD
Professor of Pediatrics
Emma Elizabeth Sullivan Professor
Director, Division of Pediatric Endocrinology and Diabetes
Icahn School of Medicine at Mount Sinai
New York, New York

V. Mohan Reddy, MD
Professor of Cardiothoracic Surgery and Pediatrics
Director of Pediatric Cardiac Surgery
Lucile Packard Children's Hospital
Stanford University
Palo Alto, California

Jeff Reese, MD
Associate Professor
Departments of Pediatrics and Cell and Developmental
    Biology
Vanderbilt University Medical Center
Nashville, Tennessee

Molly O. Regelmann, MD
Clinical Instructor, Division of Pediatric Endocrinology and
    Diabetes
Icahn School of Medicine at Mount Sinai
New York, New York

Stacie Rohovit, RN, MS, NNP-BS
Neonatal Nurse Practitioner
Lucile Packard Children's Hospital
Palo Alto, California

Juan C. Roig, MD
Assistant Professor
Pediatrics/Neonatology
University of Florida
Gainesville, Florida

Amanda Roof, MD
Department of Orthopaedics and Sports Medicine
University of Washington
Seattle, Washington

Stephen J. Roth, MD, MPH
Professor, Pediatrics
Chief, Division of Pediatric Cardiology
Department of Pediatrics
Lucile Packard Children's Hospital
Stanford University Medical Center
Stanford University School of Medicine
Palo Alto, California

Rakesh Sahni, MBBS
Professor of Clinical Pediatrics
Columbia University College of Physicians and Surgeons
New York, New York

Lisa Saiman, MD, MPH
Professor of Clinical Pediatrics
Department of Pediatrics, Division of Pediatric Infectious
    Diseases
Columbia University Medical Center;
Hospital Epidemiologist, Morgan Stanley Children's
    Hospital of New York-Presbyterian
Department of Infection Prevention & Control
New York-Presbyterian Hospital
New York, New York

Professor Ravi Savariraya, MD, BS, FRACP, ARCPA
Victorian Clinical Genetic Services
Murdoch Children's Research Institute
Victoria, Australia

Istvan Seri, MD, PhD
Professor of Pediatrics
Center for Fetal and Neonatal Medicine
USC Division of Neonatal Medicine
Children's Hospital Los Angeles and the LAC+USC
	Medical Center
Keck School of Medicine
University of Southern California
Los Angeles, California

Sejal Shah, MD
Fellow, Pediatric Endocrinology & Diabetes
Stanford University
Stanford California

Steven M. Shapiro, MD, MSHA
Division Director, Neurology
Children's Mercy Hospital & Clinics
Professor of Pediatrics, University of Missouri-Kansas City
Professor of Neurology and Pediatrics, University of Kansas
	Medical Center
Kansas City, Missouri

Gary M. Shaw, DrPH
Professor
Department of Pediatrics
Division of Neonatal & Developmental Medicine
Stanford University
Stanford, California

Arlene Sheehan, NNP
Lucile Salter Packard Children's Hospital
Neonatal Intensive Care Nursery
Palo Alto, California

Kareem Shehab, MD
Fellow, Pediatric Infectious Disease
Stanford University School of Medicine
Stanford, California

Avinash K. Shetty, MD
Department of Pediatrics
Wake Forest School of Medicine
Winston-Salem, North Carolina

Masako Shimamura, MD
Division of Infectious Diseases
Department of Pediatrics
University of Alabama School of Medicine
Birmingham, Alabama

Erik D. Skarsgard, MD, FRCSC, FACS, FAAP
Professor of Surgery
Surgeon in Chief
BC Children's Hospital
The University of British Columbia
Vancouver, BC, Canada

Jonathan L. Slaughter, MD, MPH
Assistant Professor of Pediatrics
Division of Neonatology
Center for Perinatal Research, The Research Institute at
	Nationwide Children's Hospital
Nationwide Children's Hospital/The Ohio State University
Columbus, Ohio

Mark A. Sperling, MD
Professor, Chair Emeritus,
Department of Pediatrics
University of Pittsburgh
Pittsburgh, Pennsylvania

Elaine B. St. John, MD
Associate Professor of Pediatrics
Division of Neonatology
Department of Pediatrics
University of Alabama at Birmingham
Women and Infants Center
Birmingham, Alabama

Robin H. Steinhorn, MD
Professor and Chair
Department of Pediatrics
UC Davis Medical Center
Sacramento, California

Marshall Summar, MD
Children's Research Institute
Children's National Medical Center;
Department of Pediatrics
George Washington University School of Medicine and
	Health Sciences
Washington, DC

Scott M. Sutherland, MD
Lucile Packard Children's Hospital
Stanford University Medical Center
Stanford, California

Juliet Taylor, MBChB
Victorian Clinical Genetic Services
Murdoch Children's Research Institute
Victoria, Australia

Megha M. Tollefson, MD
Roberto Murgas Torrazza, MD
Neonatology-Perinatology Fellow
University of Florida
Gainesville, Florida

Valencia P. Walker, MD
Assistant Clinical Professor
Department of Pediatrics
David Geffen School of Medicine at UCLA;
Associate Director, Newborn Nursery
Mattel Children's Hospital UCLA
Ronald Reagan UCLA Medical Center
Los Angeles, California

Michele C. Walsh, MD, MSE
Professor, Pediatrics
Case Western Reserve University
Chief, Division of Neonatology
Rainbow Babies & Children's Hospital
Cleveland, Ohio

Aviva E. Weinberg, MD
Urology Resident
Department of Urology
Stanford University School of Medicine
Stanford, California

Klane K. White, MD, MSc
Pediatric Orthopedic Surgeon
Seattle Children's Hospital
Associate Professor—Orthopaedic Surgery
University of Washington
Seattle, Washington

Mary Williams, MD
Departments of Dermatology and Pediatrics
University of California
San Francisco, California

Yael Wilnai, MD
Medical Genetics Resident
Division of Medical Genetics
Department of Pediatrics
Stanford University School of Medicine
Stanford, California

Wendy Wong, MD
Clinical Associate Professor of Pediatrics
Stanford University
Stanford, California

Jen-Tien Wung, MD, FCCM
Professor of Clinical Pediatrics
Columbia University College of Physicians and
    Surgeons
Neonatal Intensive Care Unit
New York, New York

Ann Ming Yeh, MD
Fellow in Gastroenterology
Hepatology and Nutrition
Pediatric Gastroenterology
Lucile Packard Children's Hospital at Stanford
Palo Alto, California

Neda Zadeh, MD
Division of Medical Genetics
Children's Hospital of Orange County
Orange, California

Preface/Introduction

The diagnosis and management of acute problems of the newborn are common in the daily clinical practice of neonatologists and pediatricians as well as other health care professionals involved in the care of babies after birth. A variety of comprehensive neonatology textbooks exists addressing both acute and chronic problems of the newborn. These texts typically contain limited specific details about management approaches or procedures relevant to the topical areas. On the other hand, there are a number of manuals for clinical care or procedures that provide more detail but do not provide much in the way of comprehensive topical reviews. The goal of the current book is to combine the knowledge content feature of a comprehensive neonatology textbook with the practical nature of an atlas. This practical aspect of the book should make it more useful to the practitioner on a day-to-day basis as well as provide the knowledge content needed for ensuring a more fundamental understanding of the selected topics. To make the book manageable and based on the experiences of the editors, we decided to focus on what we would describe as essential neonatology and concentrate on selected acute problems of the newborn. Thus, our book has a practical orientation to the topics, and the last section covers detailed information about management approaches and procedures that would complement the various topical areas of the text. Finally, the book is intended to be useful to all physicians involved in the diagnosis and management of newborn infants after birth. In one book, we offer comprehensive reviews of selected topics and comprehensive advice about management approaches and procedures based on the highest level of evidence available in each case. Our goal is to provide an authoritative practical medical resource for neonatologists, pediatricians, and other health care providers dealing with newborns after birth.

Acknowledgments

We thank our wives, Joan, Aileen, and Sara, for their support, understanding, and patience with our lifelong commitment to the care of babies. We further thank our colleagues, who have agreed to share their knowledge and experience and have helped to ensure that there will be others like them who will know even more than they do and will be better able to apply what they know. Finally, we thank Lisa, Cele, and Ana for their careful scrutiny of our editorial efforts and all things administrative, and we also thank our many residents and fellows, whose intellect and enthusiasm have continued to inspire us.

Section I Introduction

1 Epidemiology of Structural Birth Defects and Preterm Birth

Gary M. Shaw

EPIDEMIOLOGIC CONCEPTS

Epidemiology is the study of the distributions and the etiologic factors of diseases in human populations. Epidemiologists employ a variety of designs and statistical procedures to identify and assess potential etiologic factors. Unless a particular exposure (procedure) is beneficial, most studies cannot ethically be experimental in design, such as randomized clinical trials. Therefore, epidemiologists are typically relegated to conducting *observational* studies of populations. As a contrast, in experimental studies, the investigator has much more "control" over the many exposures study subjects may encounter, whereas in observational studies, the investigator is relegated to being an "observer" of the exposure of subjects in a study population. In some instances, such exposures may not be known or cannot be adequately controlled for. Thus, observational epidemiology studies provide us with associations and do not "establish" causation.

The 2 primary types of observational studies that epidemiologists utilize are *cohort* or *case-control* studies. The cohort study approach, sometimes referred to as a prospective study design, starts with one group of individuals in a defined population exposed to a particular agent and compares the risk of disease/outcome in that group to a second group of individuals from the population not exposed to the same agent. These studies tend to involve large populations or long periods of follow-up time to establish the risk of disease/outcome reliably between the 2 groups. The second main type of study design—case-control studies (sometimes referred to as a retrospective study design)—is

the reverse of the cohort approach. That is, the epidemiologist identifies a group of individuals from the population with the disease/outcome of interest and compares the frequency of the desired exposure/factor in that group to a second group of individuals from the population who do not have the disease/outcome. This design receives the moniker of retrospective because it starts with the disease and looks "backward" for factors that affect risk. Case-control studies, compared to cohort studies, tend to be more economical because one does not have to enroll large numbers of individuals, many of whom will never develop the disease/outcome that is of interest for study.

Associations in these studies are assessed by calculating "risk estimates." The typical measure calculated in cohort studies to estimate how large an association is between a factor of interest and a disease/outcome of interest is known as the *relative risk*. A relative risk of 1.0 indicates that risk of disease in the group exposed to the risk factor is the same as the risk of disease in the group not exposed. Relative risks more than 1.0 indicate that risks are higher in the exposed group, whereas relative risks less than 1.0 indicate that risks are lower in the exposed group when compared to the unexposed. The typical measure used in case-control studies to estimate how large an association is between a factor of interest and a disease/outcome of interest is known as the odds ratio. Similar to the relative risk measure, an odds ratio of 1.0 indicates no association between factor and disease, an odds ratio greater than 1.0 indicates an increased risk association, and an odds ratio less than 1.0 indicates a decreased risk association. Confidence intervals are a measure of statistical precision of the relative risk or the odds ratio. Confidence intervals that contain 1.0 indicate that relative risk or odds ratio estimates do not differ statistically from the null (no effect) value of 1.0.

Conducting epidemiologic studies of *structural birth defects* or *preterm birth* requires attention to several methodologic issues specific to these conditions. These issues include the granularity of "case" definitions, completeness of condition ascertainment, completeness and narrowness of timing associated with exposure assessment, choice of comparison groups, analytic control of potential covariates, and evaluation of potential biases that could have influenced observed results.

STRUCTURAL BIRTH DEFECTS: EPIDEMIOLOGIC OBSERVATIONS

Birth defects, also known as congenital anomalies, are abnormalities of structures that are present at birth. Birth defects were recognized more than 5000 years ago, as evidenced by Egyptian wall paintings of structural abnormalities, including clubfoot and achondroplasia.[1] The study of birth defects and their causes is known as *teratology*.

Birth defects are a global problem; they affect approximately 6% of births worldwide.[2] Around the globe, at least 3.3 million children younger than 5 years die each year because of a birth defect.[2] In the United States, 3 of every 100 babies—more than 100,000 babies/year—are born with a major birth defect; for the majority, the unsatisfying message communicated to parents will be: We do not know what caused your baby to be born with this condition. Birth defects are often associated with physical or mental disability and are the leading cause of infant mortality in the United States.[3,4] Birth defects in the United States are the leading cause of pediatric hospitalizations.[5,6] The medical, economic, social, and family implications of birth defects are tremendous. For example, it was estimated almost 2 decades ago that the cost of just 18 of the most common birth defects accounted for $8 billion in annual US expenditures.[7]

The scientific community has stated for several decades that as many as 75% of birth defects have an unknown cause, and only a small percentage of causes can currently be attributed to known environmental (in the broad sense) exposures or genetic effects. There are some known teratogenic exposures. These include rubella, thalidomide, valproic acid, and isotretinoin; such exposures have been associated with specific types of birth defects and not all birth defects combined.[8] Further, not all women exposed to such recognized teratogens appear to deliver malformed offspring. It is commonly posited that many, if not most,

structural birth defects are caused by the combined effects of environmental exposures and their interaction of genetic factors.[9] However, despite this prevailing idea, efforts to comprehensively examine the role of common genetic variation and the interaction of these genetic variants with environmental/lifestyle factors in the etiologies of birth defects have been insufficient, particularly in comparison to other diseases, such as cancer and cardiovascular disease.

Most human structures are complete in their development by approximately 12 weeks postconception. The period of greatest sensitivity to teratogenesis is likely from weeks 3–8 postconception.[10] Human birth defects are not one disease entity. That is, birth defects affect many different developmental systems and structures. These differences likely reflect manifold differences in underlying etiologies. It is widely accepted in the field that agents that cause birth defects—teratogens—do not tend to increase risks of all birth defects but rather fairly specific birth defects.[11] There are numerous environmental factors (eg, smoking, alcohol use, medications) and genetic factors (eg, microdeletion 22q11, Stickler syndrome) that have been identified to increase the risk of one phenotype or several birth defect phenotypes. With the exception of supplemental folic acid intake, which has been shown to decrease the risk for a number of different birth defects, the exogenous factors identified thus far explain only a small fraction of the population burden of birth defects. Similarly, genetic factors such as single-gene disorders, chromosomal abnormalities, or gene polymorphisms, in general, have not yet been identified as contributing to a *substantial* proportion of the etiology of overall birth defects.[12] Surprisingly, little is known about the etiologies of most structural birth defects.

Given that birth defects are a composite of many different developmental systems and structures, corresponding to the many variations in underlying pathogeneses and etiologies, a discussion of overall birth defects as a composite is generally uninformative for purposes of understanding etiologies. The following sections highlight the epidemiologic features of some of the more commonly occurring or commonly studied birth defect phenotypes (heart defects, orofacial clefts, neural tube defects [NTDs], gastroschisis, and hypospadias). These sections are meant to be illustrative of current knowledge; a comprehensive treatise of these areas is beyond the purposes of this textbook.

Congenital Heart Defects

As a group, congenital heart defects are the most frequently occurring human birth defects, affecting nearly 1 in 100 births and therefore representing about one-third of all birth defects.[13–15] Within the overall group of heart defects, defects of the ventricular or atrial septa are the most frequent subphenotypes. Despite their sizable population burden on child morbidity and infant mortality, the etiologies of the majority of congenital heart defects remain unknown. The various subphenotypes that make up all structural defects of the heart are likely to be etiologically heterogeneous, resulting from cytogenetic, Mendelian, and environmental contributions. For example, conotruncal defects, one more commonly studied subphenotype of the larger heart defect grouping, appear to have a higher recurrence risk than other cardiac defects, suggesting the importance of monogenic inheritance.[16] This group of defects may also be associated with chromosomal abnormalities,[17-21] especially microdeletion 22q11[22] and Mendelian disorders.[23,24] But, individually, each suspected genetic "cause" is rare.

The fetal heart develops during weeks 2–7 of gestation[25]; therefore, the time period for focus of exposures that could influence the risk of heart defect phenotypes is generally the first trimester of pregnancy or the month or two preceding conception. Several maternal conditions or exposures have been shown to influence the risk of heart defects. Pregestational diabetes has been associated with several heart defect phenotypes, including septal defects, conotruncal defects, and hypoplastic left heart syndrome, with observed risks of more than 3-fold.[26-28] Other conditions that have been implicated include phenylketonuria, with observed risks of more than 6-fold[29]; influenza or febrile illness, with risks in the range of 2-fold[30]; epilepsy, with risks in the range of 3–6 fold[28]; and maternal prepregnant obesity, with risks in the range of 1.5-fold for selected heart defects (eg, hypoplastic left heart syndrome).[31-33]

A sizable number of environmental/lifestyle exposures have been studied as risk factors for selected heart defects; there were varying levels of certainty regarding conclusions about the presence or absence of an association.[26,28] For example, studies investigated numerous medications (eg, lithium, antibiotics, angiotensin-converting enzyme [ACE] inhibitors, oral contraceptives); maternal cigarette smoking[34]; alcohol consumption[35]; life event stressors[36]; marijuana use[30]; drinking water contaminants[37]; proximity to waste sites[38]; air pollution[39]; and pesticides.[40]

One factor that has been studied to have the potential of *reducing* the risk of heart defects is the vitamin folic acid. Since the mid-1990s, a fair amount of evidence has emerged that periconceptional folic acid supplementation reduces the risk of both first occurrence and recurrence of certain birth defects, including heart defects. The evidence pertaining to heart defects shows risk reductions for conotruncal heart defects,[41-44] ventricular septal defects,[42,44] atrial septal defects,[44] and coarctation of aorta.[44] Not all studies have shown an association,[45,46] and most studies that did find an association could only do so for multivitamin supplements overall; that is, they could not disentangle folic acid effects from the overall composite multivitamin effects. However, Hernandez-Diaz and her colleagues[47] did show that periconceptional intake of medications that act as folate antagonists, such as carbamazepine or trimethoprim, could substantially increase the risk of women delivering babies with heart defects and that the increased risks associated with folate antagonists were attenuated by supplementation by folic acid intake. More recently, several studies have investigated the potential contribution of genetic variation of folate transport and metabolism genes to risk of heart defects.[48-50] Beyond the evidence that folic acid intake is associated with reduced risks of heart defects, there is evidence that alterations in serum folate status via elevated homocysteine, lower B_{12}, and lower methionine may be predictive of risk[51-53] as well.

Orofacial Clefts

Orofacially, cleft lip and cleft palate are common congenital anomalies with reported prevalences of 1–2 per 1000 live births.[54] In addition to the anguish experienced by parents and relatives, babies born with these conditions have difficulty feeding as infants, suffer from more frequent speech problems and ear infections, and must undergo a series of corrective surgeries in the first year of life that frequently require subsequent surgical revisions. There are long-term orthodontic and dental problems as well. Surgical closure of a cleft palate at a young age may induce later growth disturbances as a result of scar formation on the palate.[55]

Although their causes are largely unknown, orofacial clefts are suspected of being etiologically heterogeneous.[56] Clinical observations have long indicated that orofacial clefts should be classified into at least 2 distinct phenotypic groups: cleft lip with or without cleft palate and cleft palate alone.[57] A number of characteristics are unique to these phenotypes. For example, cleft lip with or without cleft palate is more common among males, whereas cleft palate is more common among females[6,54]; both phenotypes are more common among Asians and less common among African Americans.[58] Both appear to be more common among children born to women over the age of 35.[6]

Many genetic syndromes include orofacial clefts as a feature.[59] Recognized syndromic associations include chromosomal abnormalities and Mendelian disorders, but each is individually rare.[59] Several genes, including *IRF6, FGFR1, MSX1, PVRL1,* and *TBX22,* known to be associated with syndromic forms of cleft lip with or without cleft palate also contribute to the etiology of nonsyndromic clefts. For instance, variants in the *IRF6* (*interferon regulatory factor 6*) gene, reported to cause autosomal dominant van der Woude syndrome,[60] were recently found to be associated with nonsyndromic cleft lip with or without cleft palate.[61,62] Studies have shown an association between genetic variation at the transforming growth factor-alpha locus,[63] in genes associated with xenobiotic metabolism,[64] and in nutrient metabolism.[65] Most recently, a genome-wide association study (GWAS) identified risk variants near *MAFB* and *ABCA4* genes in addition to the known regions at chromosome 8q24 and IRF6.[66] These studies, however, explained only a small fraction of the population burden of these human birth defects.

Epidemiologic observations indicated that environmental risk factors might contribute to orofacial cleft phenotypes.[67] Maternal smoking during pregnancy has been observed to be a substantial risk for cleft lip with or without cleft palate; however, less-consistent findings have emerged for cleft palate.[68] Gene-environment interactions have been investigated between maternal smoking and a variety of genes, including xenobiotic metabolism genes such as *NOS3*.[69] Maternal nutrition has been suggested to play a role in orofacial clefts. Maternal use of multivitamin supplements containing folic acid in early pregnancy has been associated with decreased risk of orofacial cleft phenotypes.[70]

Importantly, a sizable proportion of risk reduction may also be associated with intakes of nutrients other than folate. Although there is little information about nutritional factors as potential risks of orofacial clefts, several other factors have been suggested to influence clefting risk, including B vitamins and zinc.[71–73]

Other suggested factors that have been associated with clefting risk include maternal alcohol consumption,[74] maternal occupational exposure to organic solvents,[75] parental exposure to agricultural chemicals,[76,77] and maternal exposure to anticonvulsant drugs[78] and corticosteroids.[79]

Neural Tube Defects

The NTDs are complex malformations of the central nervous system. Anencephaly and spina bifida are the most common and severe forms of NTDs. The development and closure of the neural tube is usually completed within 28 days postconception. It has been proposed that in humans, as in mice, closure of the neural tube occurs at several discontinuous sites, and that the clinical types of NTD differ depending on the site at which closure fails to take place normally.[80] Infants with anencephaly are stillborn or die shortly after birth, whereas many infants with spina bifida survive. Infants with spina bifida who survive are likely to have severe, lifelong disabilities and are at risk for psychosocial maladjustment.

The birth prevalence of NTDs has varied over time and currently varies widely based on geography,

race/ethnic background, and antenatal screening. For example, the prevalence of NTDs in the United States is approximately 0.5/1000 and in Mexico is many times higher.[2] Within the United States, several studies have shown that Hispanics have higher prevalences of NTDs,[81] and blacks have lower prevalences.[82] Epidemiologic studies have long suggested that both environmental and genetic factors contribute to NTDs.[83]

From the environmental vantage point, studied factors have included organic solvents,[84] pesticides,[85] ambient air pollution,[86] indoor air pollution,[87] hyperthermia,[88] maternal infections and illnesses,[89] stress,[36,90] alcohol use,[35] cigarette use,[35] and low socioeconomic status.[91] However, none of these factors appears to explain a significant proportion of the population burden of NTDs.

One factor that has substantially contributed to the etiology of NTDs is folic acid. More than 30 years ago, seminal work by Smithells and colleagues demonstrated that diets and postpartum blood levels of women who had a fetus with an NTD were low for selected micronutrients, especially folate.[92] A substantial amount of research, including observational studies and randomized trials, has since provided considerable evidence for the ability of folic acid to reduce the risk of NTD-affected pregnancies.[93] The fortification of the US food supply in 1998 led to a reduction in prevalence of NTDs.[94] Of note, however, the underlying mechanisms by which folic acid contributes to reduction in NTD risks remain unknown.[93] Also unknown is why a substantial proportion of women who take folic acid supplements in the periconceptional period still deliver offspring with NTDs. Recent investigations have not only explored genetic variation in folate transport and metabolism, but given emerging evidence that maternal immunological responses can have substantive impact on embryonic development, investigations also have explored autoantibodies to the folate receptor.[95]

Beyond folic acid, other nutrients and nutrition-related factors appear to contribute to risk of NTDs. Notable factors here include diabetes,[27] prepregnant obesity,[96] elevated glycemic load/index,[97] lower methionine intake,[98] lower serum levels of vitamin B_{12},[99] lower zinc intake,[100] lower vitamin C levels,[101] and lower serum choline levels.[102]

In terms of genetic underpinnings, monozygotic twinning and single-gene disorders have long been associated with NTDs.[83] Since the mid-2000s, numerous studies have explored a variety of candidate gene pathways.[103] Studies have investigated genetic variants associated with the folate/1-methyl carbon metabolic pathway,[104–106] glucose metabolism/transport,[103] DNA repair,[107] oxidative stress pathway,[103] retinoic acid receptors,[108] and various other genetic candidates, such as polymorphisms in *WNT* signaling believed to be fundamental to embryonic pattern development.[109]

Gastroschisis

Gastroschisis is a severe malformation in which an infant is delivered with a portion of intestines and sometimes other abdominal organs extruding through a defect in the abdominal wall, usually to the right of the umbilicus.[110] The embryonic timing of this defect is believed to be between gestational weeks 5 and 10. The underlying pathogenesis is unknown, but several hypotheses have been put forward, some of which focus on vascular disruption in development.[111] The prevalence of gastroschisis in the United States is approximately 3–4/10,000 births.[112] There are 2 notable features of the epidemiology of gastroschisis. First, its prevalence has been increasing substantially (4-fold or more) in the United States and worldwide since the 1980s.[113–115] The reasons for the increasing prevalence are unknown; both true risk factors and artifacts owing to variable ascertainment have been suggested contributors to the increase. Second, the most consistently identified risk factor for gastroschisis has been young maternal age at delivery.[116] For example, teenaged women have more than 5 times the risk of gastroschisis compared to women aged 25–29 years.[113,115]

Several other factors have been suggested for gastroschisis risk. These factors include genetic contributors such as increased sibling recurrence risk, higher frequency in monozygotic twins, and associations with single-gene disorders and chromosomal anomalies.[116] Nongenetic factors as contributors to gastroschisis risk have included maternal smoking and recreational drug use,[117] use of decongestants,[118] low body mass index,[96] low intake of antioxidant nutrients,[119] change in paternity,[120] and possible viral infections.[121]

Hypospadias

Hypospadias is a congenital malformation in which the urethral opening is on the ventral side of the penis. Normal closure of the urethral meatus occurs during the 10th to 16th week of gestation. Hypospadias affects about 5 per 1000 male births.[122–124] Hypospadias ranges in severity from a urethral meatus that is slightly off center to a meatus in the perineal area. About 70% of cases are considered "mild," that is, the meatus is at or distal to the coronal sulcus. Its public health impact is significant, given that it usually involves surgical correction, and individuals with hypospadias may experience impaired sexual function and psychosocial difficulties related to sexuality and sexual activity.[125,126]

Some hypospadias cases (<10%) have been associated with known underlying genetic causes or syndromes, but most are idiopathic.[127] Heritability of hypospadias is high, approximately 75%, and risk is estimated to be 12- to 20-fold among first-degree relatives.[128,129] Evidence from family-based studies points toward multifactorial inheritance, suggesting that many genes and environmental factors likely act in concert to affect risk.[129] Genetic studies have been small and have largely focused on genes related to genital tubercle development and sex steroid metabolism. A GWAS found a 2-fold increased risk for hypospadias with the *DGKK* gene, but the mechanism underlying this association is as yet unknown.[130]

Hypospadias tends to be more common among babies born to women who are non-Hispanic white, have higher education, and are older and nulliparous, and babies with hypospadias are more likely to be small for gestational age.[127] Experimental evidence suggests that endocrine disruptors (defined broadly as exogenous substances that interfere with hormones) can cause hypospadias.[131,132] Actual evidence in humans, however, is mixed at best. Other factors that may be associated with hypospadias include progestins used to become pregnant or prevent pregnancy complications[133] as well as subfertility or fertility-related procedures.[134,135] Factors such as maternal smoking and intake of multivitamin/mineral supplements do not appear to be strongly associated with hypospadias.[136,137]

METHODOLOGIC CONSIDERATIONS FOR STUDIES OF BIRTH DEFECTS

Conducting epidemiologic studies of *structural birth defects* requires attention to several methodologic issues specific to these conditions. Such issues include the granularity of "case" definitions, completeness of condition ascertainment, and choice of comparison (control) groups.

With regard to granularity of case definitions, human birth defects are not one disease entity. That is, birth defects comprise many different developmental systems and structures. These differences reflect manifold differences in underlying etiologies. Known teratogens do not tend to increase risks of all birth defects but rather fairly specific birth defects.[11] Many investigators have also pointed out that various anatomical defects, such as "heart defects," are themselves heterogeneous in anatomy, development, and epidemiologic factors.[16,26] Thus, we would not expect a single exposure to be associated with a broad range of heart defect phenotypes because heart defects vary in their embryology. For example, some specific heart defects, such as conotruncal defects, derive from neural crest cells and have been studied as a limited group for a variety of exposures. It has been suggested that even the component defects that comprise conotruncal defects may not be appropriately grouped.[138]

If we want to know whether a particular exposure causes a specific birth defect, say a specific heart defect, we would narrow our case definition to be specific because we know from a sizable amount of past research that not all defects of the heart will be caused by the same pathogenic processes. The practice of "lumping" all birth defects together may be appropriate for defining and explaining public policy or for generating hypotheses for further study, but such a broad grouping cannot inform an inference of causal association regarding a specific birth defect. Yoon and colleagues[5] noted in 1997 that lumping of birth defect types is a valid approach only if the birth defects being lumped have an underlying pathogenesis that is similar.

Regarding completeness of ascertainment, some birth defects are more easily ascertained, for example, NTDs, limb defects, and severe heart defects such as hypoplastic left heart syndrome or d-transposition of the great arteries. However, less clinically obvious or less-severe birth defects such as some septal defects and some pulmonary valve stenoses are much more difficult to ascertain uniformly in a population because they may be asymptomatic in early life. Thus, a study of less-severe heart defects needs to be particularly concerned about ascertainment influences associated with detection because ascertainment influences can lead to bias and potentially wrong conclusions. Further, ascertainment influences can arise based on length of follow-up postbirth. If follow-up includes only defects observed in the newborn period, the less-severe birth defects (eg, septal defects) are less likely to be included than in a study that has follow-up extending to 1 or more years postdelivery. That is, the detection of certain less-severe structural defects will be augmented based on more pediatric visits over time. Moreover, if clinical scrutiny for a particular defect is associated with some other exposure or condition, the subsequent investigation of the defect will be artifactually associated with that exposure or condition.

For most studies of birth defects, the most appropriate control or comparison population is a random sample of mothers/babies who had the same opportunity to have the exposure of interest but did not and did not have another birth defect. Because of the low prevalence of specific birth defects, studies of such outcomes usually have a case-control design. This retrospective approach relies on recall of early pregnancy experiences. Differential error in exposure reporting by case and control status, which has alternatively been referred to as "recall bias" and "reporting bias," may result in biased effect measures. Some investigators attempt to avoid reporting bias by comparing exposures between 2 malformed groups rather than between cases and nonmalformed controls.

This approach, however, may introduce its own bias, which is a form of selection bias.[139]

PRETERM BIRTH: EPIDEMIOLOGIC OBSERVATIONS

Preterm birth involves deliveries before 37 weeks' gestation. Approximately 13 million babies are born preterm every year in the world, with a global prevalence approximating 10%.[140] Recent data indicated that the overall prevalence of preterm birth in the United States is approximately 13% overall and approximately 11% among singleton births.[141] That is, 1 in every 8 or 9 babies is born before 37 weeks—a significant public health problem. The prevalence is substantially higher for African American babies, with more than 18% born before 37 weeks' gestation.[141] The frequency of preterm birth in the United States is higher than observed in other industrialized countries (eg, frequency in Canada is 7% and in France is 6%).[142] Despite medical advances in obstetrics and newborn intensive care, the frequency of preterm birth has increased in the United States for decades.[143]

Babies born preterm have a greater risk of death. An estimated 29% of the 4 million annual neonatal deaths in the world are caused by preterm birth.[140] The survival for most babies born preterm has improved considerably, with morbidity inversely correlated with gestational length.[144] Nevertheless, surviving preterm babies remain at increased risk for a variety of neurodevelopmental, gastrointestinal, and respiratory complications, many of which extend well beyond the neonatal period and indeed contribute to lifelong challenges for individuals and their families, as well as to burdensome economic costs to society.[144]

There are a number of iatrogenic causes of preterm delivery, most of which can be attributed to maternal or fetal conditions requiring medical or surgical intervention to facilitate preterm birth. Some of these are more easily addressed, like multiple gestations arising from the use of assisted reproductive technologies and purely elective cesarean section without assessment of fetal maturity. Despite their iatrogenic nature, many others are more difficult to address, such as preeclampsia or fetal distress.

Risk factors and possible causes of *spontaneous* preterm birth, however, remain largely mysterious. Factors associated with the increased risk of spontaneous preterm birth have been reviewed previously, with leading candidates including racial disparities, infection, stress, and genetics.[145] Despite our knowledge about such associations, effective interventions to prevent or treat preterm labor or have a measurable impact on the preterm birth prevalence in the United States have not been forthcoming. Even the most recent findings about the use of progesterone supplementation for women with a previous preterm delivery or a short cervix will not be widely applicable to most of circumstances of preterm birth encountered in the population at large.[146]

Similar to birth defects, preterm birth is a complex phenomenon and not well understood as a singular condition defined simply by the arbitrary dichotomy of birth at less than 37 completed weeks of gestation (versus more than 37 weeks).[147] This classification has been argued to be too simplistic for etiologic studies owing to the heterogeneity that has been observed with this outcome.[148] Indeed, more detailed phenotypic classifications have even been suggested for extremely early (<28 weeks' gestation) preterm birth.[149] In general, one finds the following definitions in the literature: less than 28 weeks, extremely preterm; 28–31 weeks, very preterm; and 32–36 weeks, moderately preterm.

The following sections briefly highlight the epidemiologic features of some of the more commonly studied factors as potential contributors to the etiologies of preterm birth. Excellent comprehensive reviews can be found elsewhere.[143,145,147,150]

Demographic Factors

African Americans have approximately double the risk of preterm birth compared to non-Hispanic whites, and such an increased risk has been observed irrespective of socioeconomic class.[151] The risk is approximately 3-fold for African Americans compared to non-Hispanic whites for preterm birth before 28 weeks.[141] In contrast, Hispanic whites and Asians appear to have lowered risks of preterm birth relative to non-Hispanic whites. The racial gap in risk between African Americans and non-Hispanic whites has not been sufficiently explained by myriad sociodemographic factors, behavioral factors, or underlying biomedical conditions.[152] Interestingly, a 2011 study showed a sizable neighborhood component to racial disparities in risk that extended beyond individual-level socioeconomic factors.[153] Nativity (country of origin) and length of time in the United States are additional factors that appear to influence the risk of preterm birth.[154]

Younger maternal age (<20 years) and older maternal age (>35 years) have been suggested as risk factors for preterm birth. Multifetal pregnancy is associated with an increased risk of preterm birth, and it contributes to approximately 15% of preterm births.[143] Among preterm infants, there is an excess of males.[155]

Behavioral Factors

Although cigarette smoking has been associated with several outcomes of pregnancy (eg, reduced birth weight), the relationship of cigarette smoking to preterm birth is modest (relative risks of 1.3–2.0) and not consistent.[147] Similarly, use of alcohol, caffeine, and marijuana has not revealed consistent associations for risk of preterm birth. The use of cocaine during pregnancy has shown consistent evidence of approximately a 2-fold increased risk of preterm birth.[147]

Nutritional Factors

Several studies have investigated whether folic acid influences the occurrence of preterm delivery. These studies have varied in the exposure of interest; some have examined folic acid sources from supplements or diet; some have measured folate in serum; and others have been trend analyses based on folic acid fortification of the US food supply.[156] Consequently, results have been mixed, with many studies finding an inverse association between exposure to folic acid and risk of preterm delivery, but not all have found such an association. Other nutritional aspects that have been variably observed to increase risk for preterm birth include low prepregnancy body mass index[157] and insufficient levels of the nutrients iron, zinc, omega-3, omega-6, vitamin D, calcium, and magnesium.[158] Higher levels of antioxidants such as carotenoids have been associated with a reduced risk of preterm birth.[159] Some findings in 2011 indicated that probiotic dairy product intake might be associated with a reduced risk of preterm birth.[160]

Stress Factors

Indicators of both biologic and psychosocial stress have been studied for their contribution to risk of preterm birth. The motivation to study such indicators rests on the observation that placental corticotrophin-releasing hormone levels peak at the time of delivery.[161] Corticotrophin-releasing hormone, cortisol, other biomarkers of stress, as well as a variety of indicators of perceived stress (eg, life events) have been measured. The approaches employed thus far have produced what many investigators conclude are mixed results. In a recent well-conducted study in Montreal, Kramer, and colleagues[162] investigated a sizable number of stress indicators and measures of psychological distress as predictors of spontaneous preterm birth. Only women's reported pregnancy-related anxiety (odds ratio = 1.8) was observed to be associated with preterm birth. A 2009 study that measured urinary catecholamines (dopamine, epinephrine, and norepinephrine) (ie, biomarkers of stress) showed a 2- to 4-fold elevation for preterm birth among those with the highest urinary levels in midpregnancy.[163]

Environmental Toxicants

Several studies have explored a variety of air pollutants as contributors to risks of preterm birth. Elevated levels of fine particulate matter, ozone, carbon monoxide, sulfur dioxide, nitrogen dioxide, and lead, also known as criteria pollutants, have been associated with risks of preterm birth.[164] Exposures to various pesticide compounds have also been explored as risk factors for preterm birth.[164,165] Other potential putative exposures in the environment, such as waste sites and water constituents (eg, trihalomethanes and nitrate), have been investigated as well.[166]

Infection Factors

Host immune and microbial factors have been implicated in the risk of preterm birth. Identified infections thus far have tended to be bacterial. Intrauterine infections, lower genital tract infections, maternal systemic infections, and periodontal infections have all been implicated as risk factors for preterm birth.[147] Intrauterine infections have been estimated to contribute to a substantial proportion of preterm birth, particularly early preterm birth.[167] Investigations reported in 2008 employing molecular methods nicely showed that previously unrecognized intra-amniotic infections caused by cultivation-resistant microbes may also play a role in preterm birth.[168] Although the downstream mechanism is unknown, bacterial vaginosis has been associated with preterm birth. Further, bacterial vaginosis has specifically been implicated as a contributor to the higher frequency of preterm birth observed among African Americans.[169,170] Maternal periodontal disease appears to be an infectious stimulus for preterm birth through a mechanism that is unknown. However, 2010 trial data demonstrated that treatment of periodontal disease during pregnancy did not appear to reduce preterm birth risk.[171]

Genetic Factors

Host susceptibility clearly plays a role in the risk of preterm birth, evidenced, for example, by variability across population subgroups and individuals' responses to stressors and infections. Moreover, mothers, sisters, and daughters appear to share risks for preterm birth. The emerging evidence for genetic involvement in signaling parturition points toward the mother's genome and maternally transmitted genes acting in the fetus.[172] Paternally inherited genes appear not to contribute to the risk of preterm birth.[173] Familial aggregation of preterm birth has been observed and inferred through a coefficient of kinship to have a genetic component.[174] Numerous gene variants have been investigated involving genes in biologically relevant pathways, including inflammation and infection (eg, tumor necrosis factor-alpha); uterine contraction (eg, β_2-adrenergic receptor); placental function (eg, vascular endothelial growth factor); connective tissue remodeling (eg, matrix

metalloproteinase 1); biotransformation of toxicants (eg, glutathione transferases); and 1-methyl carbon metabolism (eg, methyltetrahydrofolate reductase). There are many inconsistencies and gaps in our understanding of this body of literature—all of which have been nicely summarized by Plunkett and Muglia.[175] There are currently several genome-wide investigations of preterm birth (ie, GWAS). The initial unpublished reports of findings from these efforts have not revealed any strong genetic candidates. However, the extent that genetic background contributes to variability in risk of preterm birth will certainly become more disentangled in the next few years as our tool kit of genetic technologies has already substantially increased.

CONCLUSION

Interestingly, birth defects and preterm birth have some overlapping features. First, they co-occur; that is, fetuses with birth defects are more likely to be born prematurely, and among premature infants, the prevalence of birth defects is substantially higher than among term infants.[176] Second, risk factors may be common to both some birth defects and preterm birth (eg, assisted reproductive techniques, low folate, and smoking).

As can be readily gleaned from this chapter, birth defects and preterm birth do not have single or likely simple etiologies. There is a growing understanding that such reproductive events have their etiologic roots in complex gene-environment interactions. Thus, a concomitant consideration of biologic, genetic, behavioral, social, and physical environmental risk factors is fundamental to unraveling complex etiologies.

Our nascent understanding of potential causes, including factors that may reduce the risk of birth defects or preterm birth, is at an important juncture given the rapidly advancing technologies and experience gained by scientific communities investigating genomics. Thoughtful use of multiple new laboratory and analytical technologies undoubtedly will overcome barriers that for decades made the search for causes, especially genetic ones, elusive.[177]

Despite substantial enthusiasm and intellectual capacity among scientists who have complementary expertise in multiple basic and applied sciences to discover new etiologies, new ways to investigate complex interactions between genetically distinct individuals and the social and physical environments in which they reside most likely will be required to mitigate the problem of birth defects and preterm birth. This will require entirely new investigative approaches to research on such outcomes and the assembly of investigators from diverse disciplines, sharing databases rich in information about the human condition and including biologic specimens or samples, all linked in a way that would make possible an understanding of complex phenotypes (Stevenson et al.).[178]

Birth defects and babies born preterm plague our most vulnerable members of society. Results from epidemiologic studies can make important contributions toward establishing risks. However, it is critical to consider that epidemiologic results reflect the experience of a population group's experience; therefore, such a group's experience may not translate directly to an individual's experience for establishing risk. Thus, in establishing risk for an individual patient, epidemiologic information as well as specific patient information need to be considered to establish or infer an individual's risk.

REFERENCES

1. Barrow MV. A brief history of teratology to the early 20th century. *Teratology*. 1971;4:119–129.
2. Christianson A, Howson CP, Modell B. *March of Dimes Global Report on Birth Defects*. White Plains, NY: March of Dimes Birth Defects Foundation; 2006.
3. Heron M. Deaths: leading causes for 2004. *Natl Vital Stat Rep*. 2007;56:1–95.
4. Malcoe LH, Shaw GM, Lammer EJ. Congenital anomalies and mortality risk in white and black infants. *Am J Pub Health*. 1999;89:887–892.
5. Yoon PW, Olney RS, Khoury MJ, et al. Contribution of birth defects to and genetic disease to pediatric hospitalizations. A population-based study. *Arch Pediatr Adolesc Med*. 1997;151:1096–1103.
6. Shaw GM, Croen LA, Curry CJ, . Oral cleft malformations: associations with maternal and infant characteristics in a California population. *Teratology*.. 1991;43:225–228.
7. Centers for Disease Control and Prevention (CDC). Economic costs of birth defects and cerebral palsy—United States, 1992. *MMWR Morb Mortal Wkly Rep*. 1995;44:694–699.
8. Obican S, Scialli AR. Teratogenic exposures. *Am J Med Genet*. 2011;157:150–169.
9. Wlodarczyk BJ, Palacios AM, Chapa CJ, Zhu H, George TM, Finnell RH. Genetic basis of susceptibility to teratogen induced birth defects. *Am J Med Genet*. 2011;157:215–226.
10. Sadler TW. *Langman's Medical Embryology*. 10th ed. Baltimore, MD: Lippincott Williams and Wilkins; 2006.
11. Mitchell AA. Studies of drug induced birth defects. In: Strom BL, ed. *Pharmacoepidemiology*. 4th ed. New York, NY: Wiley; 2005:501–514.
12. Turnpenny P, Ellard S, eds. *Emery's Elements of Medical Genetics*. 12th ed. Edinburgh, UK: Elsevier Churchill Livingston; 2005.
13. Botto LD, Correa A, Erickson JD. Racial and temporal variations in the prevalence of heart defects. *Pediatrics*. 2001;107:E32.
14. Botto LD, Correa A. Decreasing the burden of congenital heart anomalies: an epidemiologic evaluation of risk factors and survival. *Prog Ped Cardiol*. 2003;18:111–121.
15. Reller MD, Strickland MJ, Riehle-Colarusso T, Mahle WT, Correa A. Prevalence of congenital heart defects in metropolitan Atlanta, 1998–2005. *J Pediatr*. 2008;153:807–813.

16. Pierpont ME, Basson CT, Benson DW, et al. Genetic basis for congenital heart defects: current knowledge. *Circulation*. 2007;115:3015–3038.
17. Johnson MC, Hing A, Wood, MK, et al. Chromosome abnormalities in congenital heart disease. *Am J Med Genet*. 1997;70:292–298.
18. Giglio S, Graw SL, Gimelli G, et al. Deletion of a 5-cM region at chromosome 8p23 is associated with a spectrum of congenital heart defects. *Circulation*. 2000;102:432–437.
19. Schuffenhauer S, Lichtner P, Peykar-Derakhshandeh P, et al. Deletion mapping on chromosome 10p and definition of a critical region for the second DiGeorge syndrome locus (DGS2). *Eur J Hum Genet*. 1998;63:213–225.
20. Ferencz C, Neill CA, Boughman JA, et al. Congenital cardiovascular malformations associated with chromosome abnormalities: an epidemiologic study. *J Pediatr*. 1989;114:79–86.
21. Lammer EJ, Chak JS, Iovannisci DM, et al. Chromosomal abnormalities among children born with conotruncal cardiac defects. *Birth Defects Res A Clin Mol Teratol*. 2009;85:30–35.
22. Goldmuntz E, Clark BJ, Mitchell LE, et al. Frequency of 22q11 deletions in patients with conotruncal defects. *J Am Coll Cardiol*. 1998;322:492–498.
23. Debrus S, Berger G, de Meeus A, et al. Familial non-syndromic conotruncal defects not associated with a 22q11 microdeletion. *Hum Genet*. 1996;97:138–144.
24. Lammer EJ, Scholes T, Abrams L. Autosomal recessive tetralogy of Fallot, unusual facies, communicating hydrocephalus, and delayed language development: a new syndrome? *Clin Dysmorphol*. 2001;10:9–13.
25. Srivastava D. Genetic assembly of the heart: implications for congenital heart disease. *Annu Rev Physiol*. 2001;63:451–469.
26. Jenkins KJ, Correa A, Feinstein JA, et al. Noninherited risk factors and congenital cardiovascular defects: current knowledge. *Circulation*. 2007;115:2995–3014.
27. Becerra JE, Khoury MJ, Cordero JF, Erickson JD. Diabetes mellitus during pregnancy and the risks for specific birth defects: a population-based case-control study. *Pediatrics*. 1990;85:1–9.
28. Ferencz C, et al. Defects of laterality and looping. In: Ferencz C, Loffredo CA, Correa-Villasenor, Wilson PD, eds. *Genetic and Environmental Risk Factors for Major Cardiovascular Malformations: The Baltimore Washington Infant Study*. Armonk, NY: Futura; 1997:41–58.
29. Levy HL, Guldberg P, Güttler F, et al. Congenital heart disease in maternal phenylketonuria: report from the Maternal PKU Collaborative Study. *Pediatr Res*. 2001;49:636–642.
30. Adams MM, Mulinare J, Dooley K. Risk factors for conotruncal cardiac defects in Atlanta. *J Am Coll Cardiol*. 1989;14:432–442.
31. Mills JL, Troendle J, Conley MR, Carter T, Druschel CM. Maternal obesity and congenital heart defects: a population-based study. *Am J Clin Nutr*. 2010;91:1543–1549.
32. Blomberg ML, Kallen B. Maternal obesity and morbid obesity: the risk for birth defects in the offspring. *Birth Def Res A*. 2010:88;35–40.
33. Gilboa SM, Correa A, Botto LD, et al. Association between prepregnancy body mass index and congenital heart defects. *Am J Obstet Gynecol*. 2010;202:e1–e10.
34. Wasserman CR, Shaw GM, O'Malley CD, et al. Parental cigarette smoking and risk for congenital anomalies of the heart, neural tube, and limb. *Teratology*. 1996;53:261–267.
35. Grewal J, Carmichael SL, Ma C, Lammer EJ, Shaw GM. Maternal periconceptional smoking and alcohol consumption and risk for select congenital anomalies. *Birth Defects Res A Clin Mol Teratol*. 2008;82:519–526.
36. Carmichael SL, Shaw GM. Maternal life event stress and congenital anomalies. *Epidemiology*. 2000;11:30–35.

37. Shaw GM, Ranatunga D, Quach T, et al. Trihalomethane exposures from municipal water supplies and risks of selected congenital malformations in California. *Epidemiology*. 2003;14:191–199.

38. Croen LA, Shaw GM, Sanbonmatsu L, Selvin S, Buffler PA. Maternal residential proximity to hazardous waste sites and risk for selected congenital malformations. *Epidemiology*. 1997;8:347–354.

39. Gilboa SM, Mendola P, Olshan AF, et al. Relation between ambient air quality and selected birth defects, seven county study, Texas, 1997–2000. *Am J Epidemiol*. 2005;162:238–252.

40. Shaw GM, Wasserman CR, O'Malley CD, et al. Maternal pesticide exposures as risk factors for selected congenital anomalies. *Epidemiology*. 1999;10:60–66.

41. Shaw GM, O'Malley CD, Wasserman CR, et al. Maternal periconceptional use of multivitamins and reduced risk for conotruncal heart defects and limb deficiencies among offspring. *Am J Med Genet*. 1995;59:536–545.

42. Czeizel AE. Prevention of urinary tract and cardiovascular defects by periconceptional multivitamin supplementation. *Am J Med Genet*. 1996;62:179–183.

43. Botto LD, Khoury MJ, Mulinare J, Erickson JD. Periconceptional multivitamin use and the occurrence of conotruncal heart defects: results from a population-based, case-control study. *Pediatrics*. 1996;98:911–917.

44. Botto LD, Mulinare J, Erickson JD. Occurrence of congenital heart defects in relation to maternal multivitamin use. *Am J Epidemiol*. 2000;151:878–884.

45. Scanlon KS, Ferencz C, Loffredo CA, et al. Preconceptional folate intake and malformations of the cardiac outflow tract. *Epidemiology*. 1998;9:95–98.

46. Werler MM, Hayes C, Louik C, et al. Multivitamin supplementation and risk of birth defects. *Am J Epidemiol*. 1999;150:675–682.

47. Hernandez-Diaz S, Werler MM, Walker AM, et al. Folic acid antagonists during pregnancy and risk of birth defects. *N Engl J Med*. 2000;343:1608–1614.

48. Shaw GM, Iovannisci DM, Yang W, et al. Risks of human conotruncal heart defects associated with 32 single nucleotide polymorphisms of selected cardiovascular disease-related genes. *Am J Med Genet*. 2005;138:21–26.

49. Hobbs CA, James SJ, Parsian A, et al. Congenital heart defects and genetic variants in the methylenetetrahydrofolate reductase gene. *J Med Genet*. 2006;43:162–166.

50. Pei L, Zhu H, Zhu J, et al. Genetic variation of infant reduced folate carrier (A80G) and risk of orofacial defects and congenital heart defects in China. *Ann Epidemiol*. 2006;16:352–356.

51. Kapusta L, Haagmans ML, Steegers EA, et al. Congenital heart defects and maternal derangement of homocysteine metabolism. *J Pediatr*. 1999;135:773–774.

52. Hobbs CA, Cleves MA, Melnyk S, et al. Congenital heart defects and abnormal maternal biomarkers of methionine and homocysteine metabolism. *Am J Clin Nutr*. 2005;81:147–153.

53. Hobbs CA, Malik S, Zhao W, et al. Maternal homocysteine and congenital heart defects. *J Am Coll Cardiol*. 2006;47:683–685.

54. Genisca AE, Frías JL, Broussard CS, et al.; National Birth Defects Prevention Study. Orofacial clefts in the National Birth Defects Prevention Study, 1997–2004. *Am J Med Genet A*. 2009;149A:1149–1158.

55. van Beurden HE, Von den Hoff JW, Torensma R, Maltha JC, Kuijpers-Jagtman AM. Myofibroblasts in palatal wound healing: prospects for the reduction of wound contraction after cleft palate repair. J Dent Res. 2005;84:871–880.

56. Dixon MJ, Marazita ML, Beaty TH, Murray JC. Cleft lip and palate: understanding genetic and environmental influences. *Nat Rev Genet*. 2011;12:167–177.

57. Fogh-Anderson P. Genetic and non-genetic factors in the etiology of facial clefts. *Scand J Plastic Reconstr Surg*. 1967;1:22–29.

58. Khoury MJ, Erickson JD, James LM. Maternal factors in cleft lip with or without palate: evidence from interracial crosses in the United States. *Teratology*. 1983;27:351–357.

59. Gorlin RJ, Cohen MM, Levin LS. *Syndromes of the Head and Neck*. 3rd ed. New York, NY: Oxford University Press; 1990.

60. Kondo S, Schutte BC, Richardson RJ, et al. Mutations in IRF6 cause Van der Woude and popliteal pterygium syndromes. *Nat Genet*. 2002;32:285–289.

61. Scapoli L, Palmieri A, Martinelli M, et al. Strong evidence of linkage disequilibrium between polymorphisms at the IRF6 locus and nonsyndromic cleft lip with or without cleft palate, in an Italian population. *Am J Hum Genet*. 2005;76:180–183.

62. Zucchero TM, Cooper ME, Maher BS, et al. Interferon regulatory factor 6 (IRF6) gene variants and the risk of isolated cleft lip or palate. *N Engl J Med*. 2004;351:769–780.

63. Vieira AR. Association between the transforming growth factor alpha gene and nonsyndromic oral clefts: a HuGE review. *Am J Epidemiol*. 2006;163:790–810.

64. Lammer EJ, Shaw GM, Iovannisci DM, Finnell RH. Maternal smoking, genetic variation of glutathione s-transferases, and risk for orofacial clefts. *Epidemiology*. 2005;16:698–701.

65. Vieira AR, Murray JC, Trembath D, et al. Studies of reduced folate carrier 1 (RFC1) A80G and 5,10-methylenetetrahydrofolate reductase (MTHFR) C677T polymorphisms with neural tube and orofacial cleft defects. *Am J Med Genet A*. 2005;135:220–223.

66. Beaty TH, Murray JC, Marazita ML, et al. A genome-wide association study of cleft lip with and without cleft palate identifies risk variants near MAFB and ABCA4. *Nat Genet*. 2010;42:525–529.

67. Mossey PA, Little J, Munger RG, Dixon MJ, Shaw WC. Cleft lip and palate. *Lancet*. 2009;374:1773–1785.

68. Little J, Cardy A, Munger RG. Tobacco smoking and oral clefts: a meta-analysis. *Bull World Health Organ*. 2004;82:213–218.

69. Shaw GM, Iovannisci DM, Yang W, et al. Endothelial nitric oxide synthase (NOS3) genetic variants, maternal smoking, vitamin use, and risk of human orofacial clefts. *Am J Epidemiol*. 2005;162:1207–1214.

70. Wilcox AJ, Lie RT, Solvoll K, et al. Folic acid supplements and risk of facial clefts: national population based case-control study. *BMJ*. 2007;334:464.

71. Shaw GM, Carmichael SL, Laurent C, Rasmussen SA. Maternal nutrient intakes and risk of orofacial clefts. *Epidemiology*. 2006;17:285–291.

72. Munger RG, Sauberlich HE, Corcoran C, et al. Maternal vitamin B-6 and folate status and risk of oral cleft birth defects in the Philippines. *Birth Def Res A*. 2004;70:464–471.

73. Krapels IPC, van Rooij IALM, MC Ocke, et al. Maternal dietary B vitamin intake, other than folate, and the association with orofacial cleft in the offspring. *Eur J Nutr*. 2004;43:7–14.

74. Boyles AL, DeRoo LA, Lie RT, et al. Maternal alcohol consumption, alcohol metabolism genes, and the risk of oral clefts: a population-based case-control study in Norway, 1996–2001. *Am J Epidemiol*. 2010;172:924–931.

75. Garlantézec R, Monfort C, Rouget F, Cordier S. Maternal occupational exposure to solvents and congenital malformations: a prospective study in the general population. *Occup Environ Med*. 2009;66:456–463.

76. Gordon JE, Shy CM. Agricultural chemical use and congenital cleft lip and/or palate. *Arch Environ Health*. 1981;36:213–221.

77. García AM, Fletcher T, Benavides FG, Orts E. Parental agricultural work and selected congenital malformations. *Am J Epidemiol*. 1999;149:64–74.

78. Dansky LV, Finnell RH. Parental epilepsy, anticonvulsant drugs, and reproductive outcome: epidemiologic and experimental findings spanning three decades; 2: human studies. *Reprod Toxicol.* 1991;5:301–335.

79. Park-Wyllie L, Mazzotta P, Pastuszak A, et al. Birth defects after maternal exposure to corticosteroids: prospective cohort study and meta-analysis of epidemiological studies. *Teratology.* 2000;62:385–392.

80. O'Rahilly R, Müller F. The two sites of fusion of the neural folds and the two neuropores in the human embryo. *Teratology.* 2002;65:162–170.

81. Canfield MA, Ramadhani TA, Shaw GM, et al. Anencephaly and spina bifida among Hispanics: maternal, sociodemographic, and acculturation factors in National Birth Defects Prevention Study. *Birth Defects Res A Clin Mol Teratol.* 2009;85:637–646.

82. Cragan JD, Roberts HE, Edmonds LD, et al. Surveillance for anencephaly and spina bifida and the impact of prenatal diagnosis—United States, 1985–1994. *MMWR CDC Surveill Summ.* 1995;44:1–13.

83. Hall JG, Friedman JM, Kenna BA, Popkin J, Jawanda M, Arnold W. Clinical, genetic, and epidemiological factors in neural tube defects. *Am J Hum Genet.* 1988;43:827–837.

84. Cordier S, Bergeret A, Goulard J, et al. Congenital malformations and maternal exposure to glycol ethers. *Epidemiology.* 1997;8:355–363.

85. Brender JD, Felkner M, Suarez L, Canfield MA, Henry JP. Maternal pesticide exposure and neural tube defects in Mexican Americans. *Ann Epidemiol.* 2010;20:16–22.

86. Lupo PJ, Symanski E, Waller DK, et al. Maternal exposure to ambient levels of benzene and neural tube defects among offspring: Texas, 1999–2004. *Environ Health Perspect.* 2011;119:397–402.

87. Li Z, Zhang L, Ye R, et al. Indoor air pollution from coal combustion and the risk of neural tube defects in a rural population in Shanxi Province, China. *Am J Epidemiol.* 2011;174:451–458.

88. Moretti ME, Bar-Oz B, Fried S, Koren G. Maternal hyperthermia and the risk for neural tube defects in offspring: systematic review and meta-analysis. *Epidemiology.* 2005;16:216–219.

89. Shaw GM, Todoroff K, Velie EM, et al. Maternal illness, including fever, and medication use as risk factors for neural tube defects. *Teratology.* 1998;57:1–7.

90. Suarez L, Cardarelli K, Hendricks K. Maternal stress, social support, and risk of neural tube defects among Mexican Americans. *Epidemiology.* 2003;14:612–616.

91. Wasserman CR, Shaw GM, Selvin S, et al. Socioeconomic status, neighborhood social conditions and neural tube defects. *Am J Public Health.* 1998;88:1674–1680.

92. Smithells RW, Sheppard S, Schorah CJ. Vitamin deficiencies and neural tube defects. *Arch Dis Child.* 1976;51:944–950.

93. Obican SG, Finnell RH, Mills JL, Shaw GM, Scialli AR. Folic acid in early pregnancy: a public health success story. *FASEB J.* 2010;24:4167–4174.

94. Canfield MA, Collins JS, Botto LD, et al.; National Birth Defects Prevention Network. Changes in the birth prevalence of selected birth defects after grain fortification with folic acid in the United States: findings from a multi-state population-based study. *Birth Defects Res A Clin Mol Teratol.* 2005;73:679–689.

95. Cabrera RM, Shaw GM, Ballard JL, et al. Autoantibodies to folate receptor during pregnancy and neural tube defect risk. *J Reprod Immunol.* 2008;79:85–92.

96. Waller DK, Shaw GM, Rasmussen SA, et al. National Birth Defects Prevention Study. Prepregnancy obesity as a risk factor for structural birth defects. *Arch Pediatr Adolesc Med.* 2007;161:745–750.

97. Yazdy MM, Mitchell AA, Liu S, Werler MM. Maternal dietary glycaemic intake during pregnancy and the risk of birth defects. *Paediatr Perinat Epidemiol.* 2011;25:340–346.

98. Shaw GM, Velie EM, Schaffer DM. Is dietary intake of methionine associated with a reduction in risk for neural tube defect-affected pregnancies? *Teratology.* 1997;56:295–299.

99. Ray JG, Blom HJ. Vitamin B_{12} insufficiency and the risk of fetal neural tube defects. *QJM.* 2003;96:289–295.

100. Velie EM, Block G, Shaw GM, Samuels SJ, Schaffer DM, Kulldorff M. Maternal supplemental and dietary zinc intake and the occurrence of neural tube defects in California. *Am J Epidemiol.* 1999;150:605–616.

101. Schorah CJ, Wild J, Hartley R, Sheppard S, Smithells RW. The effect of periconceptional supplementation on blood vitamin concentrations in women at recurrence risk for neural tube defect. *Br J Nutr.* 1983;49:203–211.

102. Shaw GM, Finnell RH, Blom HJ, et al. Choline and risk of neural tube defects in a folate-fortified population. *Epidemiology.* 2009;20:714–719.

103. Au KS, Ashley-Koch A, Northrup H. Epidemiologic and genetic aspects of spina bifida and other neural tube defects. *Dev Disabil Res Rev.* 2010;16:6–15.

104. Shaw GM, Lu W, Zhu H, et al. 118 SNPs of folate-related genes and risks of spina bifida and conotruncal heart defects. *BMC Med Genet.* 2009;10:49.

105. Molloy AM, Brody LC, Mills JL, Scott JM, Kirke PN. The search for genetic polymorphisms in the homocysteine/folate pathway that contribute to the etiology of human neural tube defects. *Birth Defects Res A Clin Mol Teratol.* 2009;85:285–294.

106. Boyles AL, Billups AV, Deak KL, et al.; NTD Collaborative Group. Neural tube defects and folate pathway genes: family-based association tests of gene-gene and gene-environment interactions. *Environ Health Perspect.* 2006;114:1547–1552.

107. Olshan AF, Shaw GM, Millikan RC, Laurent C, Finnell RH. Polymorphisms in DNA repair genes as risk factors for spina bifida and orofacial clefts. *Am J Med Genet A.* 2005; 135:268–273.

108. Tran PX, Au KS, Morrison AC, et al. Association of retinoic acid receptor genes with meningomyelocele. *Birth Defects Res A Clin Mol Teratol.* 2011;91:39–43.

109. Wen S, Zhu H, Lu W, et al. Planar cell polarity pathway genes and risk for spina bifida. *Am J Med Genet A.* 2010;152A: 299–304.

110. Lammer EJ, Iovannisci DM, Tom L, Schultz K, Shaw GM. Gastroschisis: a gene-environment model involving the VEGF-NOS3 pathway. *Am J Med Genet C Semin Med Genet.* 2008;148C:213–218.

111. Sadler TW, Rasmussen SA. Examining the evidence for vascular pathogenesis of selected birth defects. *Am J Med Genet A.* 2010;152A:2426–2436.

112. Canfield MA, Honein MA, Yuskiv N, et al. National estimates and race/ethnic-specific variation of selected birth defects in the United States, 1999–2001. *Birth Defects Res A Clin Mol Teratol.* 2006;76:747–756.

113. Vu LT, Nobuhara KK, Laurent C, Shaw GM. Increasing prevalence of gastroschisis: population-based study in California. *J Pediatr.* 2008;152:807–811.

114. Kazaura MR, Lie RT, Irgens LM, et al. Increasing risk of gastroschisis in Norway: an age-period-cohort analysis. *Am J Epidemiol.* 2004;159:358–363.

115. Castilla EE, Mastroiacovo P, Orioli IM. Gastroschisis: international epidemiology and public health perspectives. *Am J Med Genet C Semin Med Genet.* 2008;148C:162–179.

116. Rasmussen SA, Frías JL. Non-genetic risk factors for gastroschisis. *Am J Med Genet C Semin Med Genet.* 2008;148C:199–212.

117. Draper ES, Rankin J, Tonks AM, et al. Recreational drug use: a major risk factor for gastroschisis? *Am J Epidemiol.* 2008;167:485–491.

118. Werler MM, Mitchell AA, Shapiro S. First trimester maternal medication use in relation to gastroschisis. *Teratology.* 1992;45:361–367.

119. Torfs CP, Lam PK, Schaffer DM, Brand RJ. Association between mothers' nutrient intake and their offspring's risk of gastroschisis. *Teratology*. 1998;58:241–250.

120. Chambers CD, Chen BH, Kalla K, Jernigan L, Jones KL. Novel risk factor in gastroschisis: change of paternity. *Am J Med Genet A*. 2007;143:653–659.

121. Werler MM. Hypothesis: could Epstein-Barr virus play a role in the development of gastroschisis? *Birth Defects Res A Clin Mol Teratol*. 2010;88:71–75.

122. Paulozzi LJ, Erickson JD, Jackson RJ. Hypospadias trends in two US surveillance systems. *Pediatrics*. 1997;100:831–834.

123. Paulozzi LJ. International trends in rates of hypospadias and cryptorchidism. *Environ Health Perspect*. 1999;107:297–302.

124. Dolk H, Vrijheid M, Scott JE, et al. Toward the effective surveillance of hypospadias. *Environ Health Perspect*. 2004;112:398–402.

125. Mieusset R, Soulie M. Hypospadias: psychosocial, sexual, and reproductive consequences in adult life. *J Androl*. 2005;26:163–168.

126. Jugenburg I, Kipikasa A. Fertility in patients with hypospadias. *Acta Chir Plast*. 1988;30:86–93.

127. Manson JM, Carr MC. Molecular epidemiology of hypospadias: review of genetic and environmental risk factors. *Birth Defects Res A Clin Mol Teratol*. 2003;67:825–836.

128. Schnack TH, Zdravkovic S, Myrup C, Westergaard T, Christensen K, Wohlfahrt J, et al. Familial aggregation of hypospadias: a cohort study. *Am J Epidemiol*. 2008;167:251–256.

129. Harris EL. Genetic epidemiology of hypospadias. *Epidemiol Rev*. 1990;12:29–40.

130. van der Zanden LF, van Rooij IA, Feitz WF, Knight J, Donders AR, Renkema KY, et al. Common variants in DGKK are strongly associated with risk of hypospadias. *Nat Genet*. 2010;43:48–50.

131. Gray LE Jr, Ostby J, Furr J, et al. Toxicant-induced hypospadias in the male rat. *Adv Exp Med Biol*. 2004;545:217–241.

132. Noriega NC, Ostby J, Lambright C, Wilson VS, Gray LE Jr. Late gestational exposure to the fungicide prochloraz delays the onset of parturition and causes reproductive malformations in male but not female rat offspring. *Biol Reprod*. 2005;72:1324–1335.

133. Carmichael SL, Shaw GM, Laurent C, et al. Maternal progestin intake and risk of hypospadias. *Arch Pediatr Adolesc Med* 2005;159:957–962.

134. Ericson A, Kallen B. Congenital malformations in infants born after IVF: a population-based study. *Hum Reprod*. 2001;16:504–509.

135. Sorensen HT, Pedersen L, Skriver MV, Norgaard M, Norgard B, Hatch EE. Use of clomifene during early pregnancy and risk of hypospadias: population based case-control study. *BMJ*. 2005;330:126–127.

136. Carmichael SL, Shaw GM, Laurent C, Lammer EJ, Olney RS. National Birth Defects Prevention Study. Hypospadias and maternal exposures to cigarette smoke. *Paediatr Perinat Epidemiol*. 2005;19:406–412.

137. Carmichael SL, Yang W, Correa A, Olney RS, Shaw GM. National Birth Defects Prevention Study. Hypospadias and intake of nutrients related to one-carbon metabolism. *J Urol*. 2009;181:315–321.

138. Harris JA, Francannet C, Pradat P, Robert E. The epidemiology of cardiovascular defects, part 2: a study based on data from three large registries of congenital malformations. *Pediatr Cardiol*. 2003;24:222–235.

139. Swan SH, Shaw GM, Schulman J. Reporting and selection bias in case-control studies of congenital malformations. *Epidemiology*. 1992;3:356–363.

140. March of Dimes. *White Paper on Preterm Birth: The Global and Regional Toll*. White Plains, NY: March of Dimes Foundation; 2009.

141. Martin JA, Kung HC, Mathews TJ, et al. Annual summary of vital statistics: 2006. *Pediatrics*. 2008;121:788–801.

142. Blondel B, Kogan MD, Alexander GR, et al. The impact of the increasing number of multiple births on the rates of preterm birth and low birthweight: an international study. *Am J Public Health*. 2002;92:1323–1330.

143. Goldenberg RL, Culhane JF, Iams JD, Romero R. Epidemiology and causes of preterm birth. *Lancet*. 2008;371:75–84.

144. Saigal S, Doyle LW. An overview of mortality and sequelae of preterm birth from infancy to adulthood. *Lancet*. 2008;371: 261–269.

145. Muglia LJ, Katz M. The enigma of spontaneous birth. *N Engl J Med*. 2010;362:529–535.

146. Hassan SS, Romero R, Vidyadhari D, et al.; for the PREGNANT Trial. Vaginal progesterone reduces the rate of preterm birth in women with a sonographic short cervix: a multicenter, randomized, double-blind, placebo-controlled trial. *Ultrasound Obstet Gynecol*. 2011 Apr 6. Epub ahead of print.

147. Behrman RE, Butler AS, eds. *Preterm Birth: Causes, Consequences, and Prevention*. Institute of Medicine of the National Academies of Science. Washington, DC: National Academy Press; 2007.

148. Zhang J, Savitz DA. Duration of gestation and timing of birth. In: Buck Louis GM, Platt RW, eds. *Reproductive and Perinatal Epidemiology*. New York, NY: Oxford University Press; 2011:152–167.

149. McElrath TF, Hecht JL, Dammann O, et al. Pregnancy disorders that lead to delivery before the 28th week of gestation: an epidemiologic approach to classification. *Am J Epidemiol*. 2008;168:980–999.

150. Slattery MM, Morrison JJ. Preterm delivery. *Lancet*. 2002;360:1489–1497.

151. McGrady GA, Sung JF, Rowley DL, Hogue CJ, Preterm delivery and low birth weight among first-born infants of black and white college graduates. *Am J Epidemiol*. 1992;136:266–276.

152. Culhane JF, Goldenberg RL. Racial disparities in preterm birth. *Semin Perinatol*. 2011;35:234–239.

153. Schempf AH, Kaufman JS, Messer LC, Mendola P. The neighborhood contribution to black-white perinatal disparities: an example from two North Carolina counties, 1999–2001. *Am J Epidemiol*. 2011;174:744–752.

154. Collins JW, David RJ, Mendivil NA, Wu SY. Intergenerational birth weights among the direct female descendants of US-born and Mexican-born Mexican-American women in Illinois: An exploratory study. *Ethn Dis*. 2006;16:166–171.

155. Murphy DJ. Epidemiology and environmental factors in preterm labour. *Clin Obstet Gynecol*. 2007;21:773–789.

156. Shaw GM, Carmichael SL, Yang W, Siega-Riz AM. Periconceptional intake of folic acid and food folate and risks of preterm delivery. *Am J Perinatol*. 2011;28:247–252.

157. Hendler I, Goldenberg RL, Mercer BM, et al. The Preterm Prediction Study: association between maternal body mass index and spontaneous and indicated preterm birth. *Am J Obstet Gynecol*. 2005;192:882–886.

158. Dunlop AL, Kramer M, Hogue CJ, Menon R, Ramakrishan U. Racial disparities in preterm birth: an overview of the potential role of nutrient deficiencies. *Acta Obstet Gynecol Scand*. 2011;90:1332–1341.

159. Kramer MS, Kahn SR, Platt RW, et al. Antioxidant vitamins, long-chain fatty acids, and spontaneous preterm birth. *Epidemiology*. 2009;20:707–713.

160. Myhre R, Brantsæter AL, Myking S, et al. Intake of probiotic food and risk of spontaneous preterm delivery. *Am J Clin Nutr*. 2011;93:151–157.

161. Smith R. Parturition. *N Engl J Med*. 2007;356:271–283.

162. Kramer MS, Lydon J, Séguin L, et al. Stress pathways to spontaneous preterm birth: the role of stressors, psychological distress, and stress hormones. *Am J Epidemiol.* 2009;169: 1319–1326.

163. Holzman C, Senagore P, Tian Y, et al. Maternal catecholamine levels in midpregnancy and risk of preterm delivery. *Am J Epidemiol.* 2009;170:1014–1024.

164. Stillerman KP, Mattison DR, Giudice LC, Woodruff TJ. Environmental exposures and adverse pregnancy outcomes: a review of the science. *Reprod Sci.* 2008;15:631–650.

165. Harley KG, Huen K, Schall RA, et al. Association of organophosphate pesticide exposure and paraoxonase with birth outcome in Mexican-American women. *PLOS One.* 2011;6:e23923. Epub 2011 Aug 31.

166. Wigle DT, Arbuckle TE, Turner MC, et al. Epidemiologic evidence of relationships between reproductive and child health outcomes and environmental chemical contaminants. *J Toxicol Environ Health B Crit Rev.* 2008;11:373–517.

167. Andrews WW, Hauth JC, Goldenberg RL. Infection and preterm birth. *Am J Perinatol.* 2000;17:357–365.

168. DiGiulio DB, Romero R, Amogan HP, et al. Microbial prevalence, diversity and abundance in amniotic fluid during preterm labor: a molecular and culture-based investigation. *PLOS One.* 2008;3:e3056.

169. Goldenberg RL, Klebanoff MA, Nugent R, Krohn MA, Hillier S, Andrews WW. Bacterial colonization of the vagina during pregnancy in four ethnic groups. Vaginal Infections and Prematurity Study Group. *Am J Obstet Gynecol.* 1996; 174:1618–1621.

170. Fiscella K. Racial disparities in preterm births. The role of urogenital infections. *Public Health Rep.* 1996;111:104–113.

171. Boggess KA. Treatment of localized periodontal disease in pregnancy does not reduce the occurrence of preterm birth: results from the Periodontal Infections and Prematurity Study (PIPS). *Am J Obstet Gynecol.* 2010;202:101–102.

172. Plunkett J, Feitosa MF, Trusgnich M, et al. Mother's genome or maternally-inherited genes acting in the fetus influence gestational age in familial preterm birth. *Hum Hered.* 2009;68:209–219.

173. Wilcox AJ, Skjaerven R, Lie RT. Familial patterns of preterm delivery: maternal and fetal contributions. *Am J Epidemiol.* 2008;167:474–479.

174. Ward K, Argyle V, Meade M, Nelson L. The heritability of preterm delivery. *Obstet Gynecol.* 2005;106:1235–1239.

175. Plunkett J, Muglia LJ. Genetic contributions to preterm birth: implications from epidemiological and genetic association studies. *Ann Med.* 2008;40:167–195.

176. Dolan SM, Callaghan WM, Rasmussen SA. Birth defects and preterm birth: overlapping outcomes with a shared strategy for research and prevention. *Birth Defects Res A.* 2009;85:874–878.

177. Olshan AF, Hobbs CA, Shaw GM. Discovery of genetic susceptibility factors for human birth defects: an opportunity for a national agenda. *Am J Med Genet.* 2011;154A:1794–1797. Epub 2011 Jul 7.

178. Stevenson DK, Shaw GM, Wise PH, Norton ME, Druzin ML Valantine HA, McFarland DA. Transdisciplinary translational science and the case of preterm birth. *J Perinatol.* 2013;33(4):251–258.

Ethics, Epidemiology, Prognostication, and Legal Issues in the NICU

2

John D. Lantos and William L. Meadow

INTRODUCTION

Clinical ethics in the NICU, unlike clinical ethics in most other contexts, does not consider the values, preferences, or wishes of the patient. The neonatal patient is unable to participate in decisions. Parents have the legal right to make decisions for their child, but only if those decisions are judged by doctors or (if challenged) judges to be reasonable decisions in the circumstances. Often, this is called the "best-interest" standard, but that term has been thoughtfully critiqued. Parents do not always have to do what is the absolute best thing for the neonate without regard to the interests of others. But, they may only do what is reasonable in the circumstances, considering the current and future interests of the neonate as well as the interests of other family members.

Because future interests loom large, one important basis for judging the acceptability of a proposed treatment choice is the accuracy of prognostication. What will the child's life be like if treatment is provided? What will it be like if treatment is withheld? The better the prognosis for intact survival is, the more difficult it becomes to justify withholding or withdrawing life-sustaining treatment. The lower the likelihood of survival, or the higher the likelihood that survival will be accompanied by major impairment, the more justifiable it becomes to withhold life-sustaining treatment.

The problem with prognostication is that it is uncertain and probabilistic and changes over time with advances in treatment. So, estimating the likelihood that any given baby in any given neonatal intensive care unit (NICU) today will survive with or without severe impairment is necessarily an inexact science. Yet, such prognostications drive the ethics of neonatal decisions.

The uncertainty is greatest for a relatively small group of infants in the NICU. NICU care is virtually futile for babies born before 23 weeks of gestation. Outcomes are predictably good for babies born at 26 weeks or more of gestation. Most congenital anomalies can be treated with satisfactory outcomes. So, the real dilemmas are for babies born at 23–25 weeks of gestation or babies with complex congenital anomalies for which treatment is nonvalidated and the outcomes are ambiguous or uncertain. For such babies, the burdens of treatment are real, immediate, long term, and nontrivial (months of painful procedures like intubation, ventilation, intravenous catheterization, to name just a few, plus, of course, whatever permanent sequelae might ensue), while the benefits of NICU interventions are distant, statistical, and nonpredictable.

How, then, should doctors use evidence to improve ethical decision making in the NICU? We begin by discussing this at the level of the individual patient. At the end of this chapter, we discuss whether economic considerations should be considered in developing policies about the treatment of classes of patients.

CLINICAL ETHICS FOR INDIVIDUAL PATIENTS

Parents want to know the answer to two questions: Is my baby going to survive? If so, how healthy will the baby be when ready to go home? These questions are central to any assessment of the ethics of informed consent for parents. If it turned out that caretakers were clueless about which infants were doomed to die in the NICU, which would survive impaired, and which would survive relatively unimpaired, then informed consent would be impossible, decisions about which babies to treat would be random, and it would be impossible to judge one decision as better than another. Of course, doctors and nurses are not clueless, but neither are they perfect. We know a lot, now, about just how good the decisions are, so we can put fairly precise margins of error around prognostic estimate.

We have studied two different approaches used by doctors and nurses to arrive at predictions about how babies will do in the NICU. One uses objective data to develop prognostic algorithms. The other measures the accuracy of something much more difficult to quantify: the clinical intuitions of experienced doctors and nurses.

Objective illness severity scores measure physiologic stability. This algorithmic approach to NICU prognostication was originated by Richardson and colleagues and has been dubbed SNAP (Score for Acute Neonatal Physiology). The higher the score, the more deranged the physiology is and the more likely the baby is to die. SNAP scores are most useful in differentiating babies who will survive from those who will die on their first day of life. Over the course of NICU treatment, SNAP scores are less and less able to differentiate survivors from those who will die. Thus, with every passing day, illness severity is less likely, not more likely, to distinguish babies who are doomed to die in the NICU from those who will go home to their families.

How can this possibly be? Two phenomena are at work here. First, NICU doctors and nurses are good at what they do, and what they do is fix physiologic derangements. So, low blood pressure is raised, metabolic acid is neutralized, electrolytes become balanced, and SNAP scores go down, even for sick kids (especially for sick kids, whose scores were particularly high at the beginning). Second, the sickest kids, with the highest SNAP scores, die soonest. They are then no longer in the population of babies still alive on day 4. Therefore, the scores for babies who will go on to survive and those who will go on to die look more alike with each passing day.

What about intuitions? Perhaps serial algorithms cannot take into account all of the intangible factors that allow an experienced clinician to predict whether a baby will live or die. If so, then the intuitions of health professionals who watch babies over hours and days might be better at predicting which babies will live or die.

We have tested this hypothesis in the NICU at the University of Chicago. On every day, we asked caretakers of every baby who was on mechanical ventilation whether they thought the baby was going to survive to discharge or die in the NICU. Then, we correlated the intuitions with outcomes.[1]

We have studied nearly 2000 infants with this protocol. The findings have powerful implications for neonatal ethics. First, for the vast majority of ventilated NICU babies, the doctors and nurses all agreed on the prognosis, and they were usually correct. About 70% of the time, everybody predicted that the baby would survive—and the baby did survive. About 5% of the time, everyone knew the baby was going to die—and they did die. So, the entire phenomenon of ethical dilemma in the NICU turns out to be restricted to at most one-quarter of the ventilated patients. What can we say about these?

Approximately 25% of ventilated NICU infants were predicted by at least 1 doctor or nurse to be heading for death. Of these babies, 40% survived to discharge nonetheless. Prognostications were a little more accurate when more than 1 professional predicted death. When every professional predicted that a baby would die, the chance of dying was 80%. That means, of course, that 20% of such babies survived to leave the NICU.

Recently, we combined objective measures of physiologic derangement with clinical intuitions. Lagatta and colleagues demonstrated that prognostic accuracy increases significantly when health care professionals' predictions that a baby will die are combined with abnormal head ultrasounds (grade II, III, or IV Intraventricular hemorrhage [IVH] or periventricular leukomalacia [PVL]).[2] Of the babies who have both a professional prediction of death and an abnormal head ultrasound, 96% either die or, if they survive, are severely impaired, with a mental development index/ physical development index (MDI/PDI) less than 70 at 2 years of age. In other words, if a ventilated infant has both a prediction of "die while in the NICU" and an abnormal head ultrasound, the likelihood of being alive and neurologically normal at 2 years of age is about 4 in 100.

Even more interesting, Lagatta et al showed that the predictive power of the combination of head ultrasounds and clinical intuitions is independent of gestational age (at least in the study population of babies who were on ventilators). That is, babies born at 25 weeks are more likely to survive than babies born at 23 weeks. But among the survivors, 23 weekers are not more likely to be cognitively impaired than 25 weekers. This finding, from Lagatta's data, is also true in larger data sets. Data from the National Institute of Child Health and Development (NICHD) network website (http://www .nichd.nih.gov/about/org/cdbpm/pp/prog_epbo/epbo _case.cfm) and from the EPICure study in Britain,[3] both converge on the fact that the big difference between being born at 23 vs 25 weeks gestation is the likelihood of survival to discharge from the NICU. There is not much difference in MDI, PDI, or percentage impairment (no matter how impairment is defined) comparing neurologic outcomes for babies born at 23–24 weeks who survive compared to those born at 25 or 26 weeks.

OPERATIONALIZING EPIDEMIOLOGY TO ACHIEVE BETTER ETHICS

A combination of objective data such as need for mechanical ventilation and head ultrasound results and subjective data such as a clinician's intuition that a baby will die can accurately predict either death or MDI/PDI less than 70 with more than 95% positive predictive value. One problem with this type of data is that it is not available at the time of birth. Treatment must be initiated to allow the clinician time to form a clinical judgment and to obtain a head ultrasound. For most babies, this takes at least a few days and up to a week. Using such data, then, to decide which babies should receive NICU care and life support requires a willingness on the part of parents and doctors to (1) initiate treatment on babies who are known to be at high risk of a bad outcome and (2) be willing to withdraw life support if things look bad. Both requirements are difficult.

Much work in trying to refine prognostic estimations focuses on factors that are known (or knowable) in the delivery room at the time of birth. For example, Tyson and colleagues developed prognostic algorithms based on birth weight, gestational age, gender, whether antenatal steroids were given, and singleton status vs multiple gestations. These can be used to allow a decision about whether to initiate treatment in the delivery room.

Similarly, many hospital policies and national guidelines use gestational age alone to guide decisions about whether to initiate treatment.

Part of the reason for these approaches is that it is emotionally easier not to start treatment than it is to stop treatment. The ethical dilemma, however, is that a trial of therapy with a willingness to withdraw treatment will provide much more accurate individualized decision making than a process that requires these decisions to be made before birth.

THE "QUALITY-OF-LIFE" DILEMMA

Even if our skill at prognostication improves, we will still have to face the decision about what threshold of anticipated quality of life or neurocognitive impairment should be used to decide that a baby's life will be so miserable that it would be preferable to let him or her die. Standard measures of quality of life consider such impairments as cerebral palsy, mental retardation, blindness, and deafness. Advocates for people with disabilities have criticized each and all of these as discriminatory judgments about the quality of life for people with disabilities. Recent work on self-assessed quality of life among NICU survivors, and on parental assessments of their children's quality of life, suggest that concerns about discrimination are warranted.[4] Most parents, and most people with disabilities, rate their own quality of life higher than it is rated by their doctors. That is, doctors (and nurses) tend to think that physical or cognitive impairments of one sort or another are worse than death. Parents of children with disabilities—and people with disabilities themselves—do not share these bleak views.

We are also refining our understanding of the way different impairments and disabilities change over time. Johnson and colleagues assessed functional disability among preemies born at or before 25 weeks gestation at 11 years of age.[5] These results were from a cohort that had previous developmental assessments at 2.5 and 6 years of age.[6] The prevalence of serious disability was found to be stable between 6 and 11 years of age. Their study suggests that follow-up to 6 years of age may be adequate to predict prevalence of continued impairment through middle childhood.

The Johnson et al study reported higher prevalence of functional and cognitive impairment, 40% and 45%, respectively, than other similar population-based cohort studies. In addition to the possibility of differing study methodologies, the authors highlighted the fact that they compared their cohort directly with classroom peers of the same age rather than standardized test norms. When using traditional standardized norms, their prevalence of functional and cognitive impairment drop to 14% and 22%, respectively—figures much more in line with previous studies. These differences suggest that adequate counseling of parents regarding long-term disabilities should include not only the statistics but also some of the subtleties.

Included in these subtleties is an understanding of the varied definitions of impairment held by individuals. Some would argue that impairments are imposed by society and that without society there can be no impairment. Under such a view, an infant who is blind because of severe retinopathy of prematurity (ROP) is impaired only because the structure of our society places him or her at a disadvantage compared to those with normal vision. On the other hand, it has been said that a disabling condition is defined as one that "is harmful to the person in that condition and that consequently that person has a strong rational preference not to be in such a condition."[7] Following that logic, the infant with ROP may be impaired. When counseling parents regarding potential outcomes, it is essential to understand the meaning of such outcomes from the family's perspective and from the perspective of people who live with such disabilities.

Researchers have been examining the correlation between objective measures of disability or neurocognitive impairment and subjective assessments of quality of life. The results may surprise many doctors.

A recent European study evaluated 1174 children aged 8–12 years with cerebral palsy to learn more about their self-reported quality of life.[8] The children were from diverse areas covering six European countries (France, Ireland, Sweden, England, Denmark, and Italy). Self-reported quality of life was assessed with a new European questionnaire (KIDSCREEN).

Six of the KIDSCREEN domains of quality of life were similar among children with cerebral palsy and their peers, including psychological well-being, self-perception, social support, school environment, financial resources, and social acceptance. Certain specific impairments were associated with decreased quality of life in four other domains: Those less ambulatory had poorer physical well-being; those with intellectual impairment had lower moods and emotions and less autonomy; and those with speech difficulty had poorer relationships with their parents. Despite these differences in specific circumstances, most of the studied patients with cerebral palsy had similar overall quality-of-life scores as their peers. This study is particularly intriguing in that the quality-of-life measures were reported by the patients themselves, rather than parents or other proxies. This fact also limits the study. Of those studied, 39% were excluded from the study because they could not adequately self-report. It is possible that among those too impaired to self-report, the results would have been different.

When making best-interest determinations near the borderline of viability, it would be irresponsible to ignore the real risks of long-term neurologic impairment. Still, quality-of-life studies suggest that survivors who subsequently develop impairment may live happier lives than doctors imagine.

COST, RESOURCE ALLOCATION, AND DISTRIBUTIVE JUSTICE

Clinical ethics and individualized decision making lead us toward an approach that would allow a trial of therapy for every baby born at 23 weeks and above. Some have criticized this approach as too costly. In this section, we examine the data on the costs and the cost-effectiveness of NICU care.

In the United States, about 4 million babies are born each year. Of these, roughly 1 in 10 (or 400,000/y) is premature (<37 weeks gestation) or low birth weight (<2500 g). Many of these babies go to NICUs. Almost all survive without significant impairments. Without NICU care, many would die or survive with impairments. NICU care is clearly cost-effective for these babies.

Approximately 1 baby in 50 (80,000/y) is a baby with a "very low birth weight" (VLBW; < 1.5 kg or 3.3 pounds) or an extremely low gestational age

neonate (ELGAN; < 32 weeks gestation). All of these babies are admitted to NICUs. Almost all survive and do well.

Only 1% of babies (40,000/y) are born with an "extremely low birth weight" (ELBW; < 1.0 kg or 2.2 pounds). All go to the NICU, and about two-thirds survive.

Finally, 1 baby in 500 (8000/y) is born alive with a birth weight less than 1 pound (~450 g; < 23 weeks gestation)—some go to NICUs, almost all die.

The "gray zone" of NICU ethics, then, is for babies between 500 g and 1 kg. Above 1 kg, survival is so good (well over 90%) that, absent other medical anomalies, the ethical principle of "best interests of the baby" requires intervention, overriding any arguments for comfort care, made either by the parents or physicians. Below 500 g, survival rates are so low that most doctors are comfortable acceding to parental requests to withhold intensive intervention and providing comfort care. More important, for arguments about cost-effectiveness, the absolute number of such babies is relatively small. There are no more than 30,000 babies per year born in the gray zone in the United States. This is about 1% of the number of adults who either die or are critically ill in intensive care units (ICUs) each year. So, among all intensive care delivered in the United States, NICUs account for a small fraction of total expenditures.

Another feature of NICU care is relevant to arguments about cost-effectiveness. Most infants who do not survive also do not live long. The babies who die are the smallest and the sickest babies, and they tend to die in the first few days of life. This observation has an important economic implication. Because most babies who do not survive die quickly, most of the bed-days in the NICU are taken up by babies who ultimately survive. As a result, NICU care is surprisingly cost-effective, even for babies born at the borderline of viability.

Doyle and colleagues studied this in NICUs in Australia. They showed no difference in the overall dollars per quality-adjusted life-year (QALY) comparing babies born at 500 g and those born at 1000 g. Furthermore, the absolute dollars/QALY was remarkably low—between $3000 and $5000/QALY. This compares favorably with every other form of ICU care and for common lifesaving interventions like renal dialysis or bypass surgery.

The most expensive NICU babies are those who have complex chronic problems, who stay in the NICU for a long time, and who survive with chronic health problems or neurocognitive impairments that require lifelong interventions. But, the absolute number of such babies is so relatively small that, although each case is tragic, the overall impact of such cases on national health expenditures is relatively small. Furthermore, as shown in the previous discussion, it is difficult to predict which babies will ultimately fall into that group.

The prognostic uncertainty, combined with the overall cost-effectiveness of NICU care, suggests that rationing of NICU care as a way of maximizing distributive justice is indefensible. Instead, if such rationing is necessary, it ought to be based on objective measures of cost-effectiveness that would dictate that care for critically ill adults would save much more money with a far lower cost in terms of years of life lost.

LEGAL ISSUES

We conclude this chapter with a discussion of some legal issues in neonatology. We discuss malpractice cases and recent legislation that may have an impact on neonatal decisions.

Malpractice

Neonatologists in the United States are sued for medical negligence roughly once every 10 years, and the average US neonatologist will be sued more than once in his or her practice lifetime.[9] Other than case-specific failures or oversights, are there any overarching themes that have arisen from medical malpractice cases in the NICU?

In the United States, most malpractice allegations are state based, as opposed to federal cases. Consequently, the decisions of lower state courts, or even state supreme courts, are not binding in any other state. But, of course, they may be informative. For the purposes of our discussion, the first important legal NICU case in the United States was *Miller v HCA*.[10] In 1990, Mrs. Miller came to a Hospital Corporation of America (HCA) hospital in Texas in labor at 23 weeks gestation. The fetus was estimated to weigh between 500 and 600 g. No baby born that size had ever survived at that hospital. Mrs. Miller, her husband, and the attending physicians agreed that the baby was pre-viable and that no intervention was indicated. The baby was born, a different doctor resuscitated, the infant survived with brain damage, and the Millers sued the hospital corporation for a breach of informed consent. They were awarded $50 million by a trial jury. The case wound its way to the Texas Supreme Court, which dismissed the verdict and articulated an "emergency exception" for physicians—that is, if a Texas doctor finds himself or herself in the emergency position of needing to resuscitate a patient or the patient will die, right there, right then, the doctor may try to resuscitate without being obligated to obtain consent from anyone. Whether it would be OK for a doctor not to resuscitate in an emergency was left unarticulated by the Texas court.

The case of *Montalvo v Borkovec*,[11] in Wisconsin, took the legal obligations of neonatologists and parents to a different place. *Montalvo* derived from the

resuscitation of a male infant born between 23 weeks and 4 days and 24 weeks and 7 days gestation, weighing 679 g. The parents claimed a violation of informed consent, arguing that the decision to use "extraordinary measures" should have been relegated to the parents. The Wisconsin Appellate Court disagreed, holding that "in the absence of a persistent vegetative state, the right of a parent to withhold life-sustaining treatment from a child does not exist." Because virtually no preemie is born in persistent vegetative state (PVS), this decision would apparently eliminate, in Wisconsin, the ethical possibility of a gray zone of parental discretion. No other jurisdiction in the United States has adopted this position. The Wisconsin Appellate Court in *Montalvo*, like the Texas Supreme Court in *Miller*, was silent on whether doctors have discretion not to resuscitate. However, in Texas and Wisconsin, doctors are apparently immunized if they choose to do so.

A number of other state courts have addressed issues of treatment or nontreatment. In general, they are permissive of doctors who resuscitate babies. They err on the side of life. If courts are asked to sanction decisions to allow babies to die, most will do so only if there is consensus among doctors and parents, and, at times, ethics committees. Courts are not eager to punish doctors who treat babies over parental objections or to empower doctors to stop treatment when parents want it to continue. However, an open question for jurisdictions outside Texas and Wisconsin is whether "informed consent" need be obtained from parents before resuscitative efforts are initiated or continued.

Baby Doe Regulations

The "Baby Doe regulations" were one of the first attempts to codify, and impose, a federal vision of appropriate ethical behavior in the NICU. The regulations followed care in which a baby with Down syndrome and esophageal atresia was born in Bloomington, Indiana, in 1982. Baby Doe's parents refused to consent to surgery and chose palliative care instead. His pediatrician alerted the state child protection agency, which investigated the case. At a court hearing, the parents claimed that they were following the advice not of their pediatrician but of their obstetrician. The court opined that parents only had to follow the advice of a licensed physician and that, because they were doing that, they were not neglectful. The doctor and hospital appealed. The Indiana Supreme Court refused to hear the appeal. The baby died at 8 days of age.[12]

This case led to a national controversy that eventually reached the Oval Office. The Reagan administration claimed that nontreatment of babies with Down syndrome or other congenital anomalies was discrimination against people with disabilities and ordered all hospitals to post signs in NICUs defining such non-treatment as a violation of federal civil rights laws. These regulations were challenged and eventually struck down by the US Supreme Court.[13]

A watered-down version of the original Baby Doe guidelines was eventually incorporated into the federal Child Abuse and Treatment Act.[14,15] That act, however, is primarily a funding mechanism to channel federal funds to state child protection agencies, not a regulation that can be enforced for doctors or hospitals. For all practical purposes, the Baby Doe regulations do not exist today and have not existed since 1984. Nevertheless, some of the policies that they advocated have been widely adopted. For babies with trisomy 21, or those whose outcomes are likely to be similar to those seen in trisomy 21, it is no longer permissible to withhold life-sustaining treatment.

Born-Again Infant Protection Act

In 2002, the US Congress passed a law called the Born Alive Infant Protection Act (BAIPA).[16] BAIPA, like the discredited Baby Doe regulations, was an attempt to insert federal values into doctor/infant/parent deliberations. There are some interesting similarities and distinctions between Baby Doe and BAIPA. To be blunt, Baby Doe was about disability, whereas BAIPA is about abortion. BAIPA declares that "for the purposes of Federal law, the words 'person', 'human being', 'child', and 'individual' shall include every infant who is born alive at any stage of development." As Sayeed noted, "The agency arguably substitutes a nonprofessional's presumed sagacious assessment of survivability for reasonable medical judgment."[20] It is difficult to know exactly what the implications of this law might be. On the one hand, all infants born alive prior to BAIPA were also treated as human beings. That did not necessarily mean that they received all available life support and resuscitation. After all, human beings can have do not resuscitate (DNR) orders or receive palliative care rather than intensive care. Still, the purpose of BAIPA seemed to be less about the treatment of babies and more about restrictions on abortion. Although some authors have expressed concern that BAIPA's influence may transform neonatal care of infants born at, or even below, the threshold of viability, it appears to have had little measurable impact to date. Partridge and colleagues surveyed neonatologists in California and found that they were concerned about the implications of BAIPA. They wrote, "If this legislation were enforced, respondents predicted more aggressive resuscitation potentially increasing risks of disability or delayed death."[17]

There have been no cases to date in which BAIPA has been invoked or in which doctors and hospitals have been found in violation of BAIPA's requirements.

FUTURE DIRECTIONS

What is coming? As Yogi Berra is reputed to have said, "Prediction is hard, especially about the future." A few intuitions seem clear. There is no new technology "in the pipeline" that appears likely to have a significant impact on outcomes. Consequently, for infants who receive resuscitation in the delivery room, birth-weight-specific mortality and morbidity are unlikely to change much in the near future. Nonetheless, two developments may change the way we think about newborns and consequently shift the terrain of neonatal bioethics.

High-Risk Maternal-Fetal Medicine Centers

Many children's hospitals are now developing high-risk maternal-fetal medicine centers. The goal of these centers is to identify fetuses at risk—particularly those with congenital anomalies—and to care for those fetuses and their mothers in centers where there is expertise in fetal diagnosis and therapy as well as in neonatal care. The hope is that such centers will allow more timely, and therefore more effective, intervention for babies with congenital heart disease, congenital diaphragmatic hernia, or other anomalies.

The medical effectiveness of fetal centers will depend on two distinct developments. First, on a population basis, these centers will only be as effective as fetal screening and diagnosis. The existence of these centers will, almost certainly, create an expectation and a demand for better fetal screening. Such screening is likely to include both better imaging and better screening tests that can be done on maternal blood. Both will lead to earlier diagnosis of fetal anomalies. This will create dilemmas that are more complex for perinatologists and parents, who will need to decide, in any particular case, whether to terminate pregnancy, whether to offer fetal therapy, or whether to offer either palliative care or interventions after birth. Ironically, available studies show that better fetal diagnosis increases the likelihood of pregnancy termination, even if postnatal treatment is possible, such as hypoplastic left heart syndrome.

Second, the effectiveness of fetal centers will depend on the effectiveness of fetal interventions. Perhaps surprisingly, other than in utero transfusion for Rh disease or vascular ablation for twin-twin transfusion syndromes (neither of which is particularly new and neither of which is performed by pediatric surgeons or pediatricians), there is little evidence that any fetal intervention has had any impact on any neonatal outcome. This lack of demonstrated effectiveness has, thus far, not suppressed the proliferation of fetal intervention centers. Other factors, including institutional prestige, finances, and recruitment of "desirable" patients, may be in play.

Expanded Newborn Screening

In recent years, the number of diseases and conditions that can be diagnosed through newborn screening has expanded dramatically. Such screening is under the purview of states, rather than the federal government, and there is wide variation in the number of tests that are done. In 1995, the average number of tests done per state was 5 (range 0–8 disorders). Between 1995 and 2005, most states added tests,[18] so that the average number of screening tests done by 2005 was 24. Expansion of newborn screening raises three problems. First, even the most accurate test has false positives. For rare conditions, the percentage of positive tests that are false positives is increased. Thus, the more conditions that are rare that are added to a newborn screening panel, the more false positives there will be. False positives are associated with considerable parental anxiety and may also lead to potentially dangerous and unnecessary diagnostic procedures or treatments. Second, expanded newborn screening costs money. Interestingly, the tests themselves are astoundingly inexpensive, and that is why policy makers are tempted to add more and more to the panels. However, the follow-up counseling and testing after positive tests is expensive, and without such follow-up, the screening programs will not work. The Centers for Disease Control and Prevention (CDC) has recently expressed concern about these costs.[19] Finally, there is the potential for discrimination against patients when documented heterozygous carrier status conveys no recognized medical infirmity, but social (insurance/employment) or psychological stigma may be real. There is little money anywhere to assist or counsel these patients.

CONCLUSION

Ethical philosophy is a place to start, not a place to finish. Data are relatively easy to acquire and agree on. Policy is intriguingly insensitive to data, but that may well reflect social/political realities that exist beyond the NICU—perceptions of disability, abortion politics, individual-vs-communitarian emphasis, fascination with technology, discrimination, publicity, financial constraints—so that an ethical course of action in one country, one city, or even one family might seem perverse elsewhere. The central question—now and in the future—is how much ethical diversity we can tolerate. Which diagnostic tests or treatments should be considered obligatory for all babies everywhere, which should be prohibited for any baby anywhere, and which should be provided only with parental informed consent and parental discretion? The answer to that question is a constantly moving target that reflects advances in technology, the availability of societal resources, and shifting cultural norms.

REFERENCES

1. Meadow W, Lagatta J, Andrews B, et al. Just, in time: ethical implications of serial predictions of death and morbidity for ventilated premature infants. *Pediatrics*. 2008;121:732–740.
2. Lagatta J, Andrews B, Caldarelli L. Early neonatal intensive care unit therapy improves predictive power for the outcomes of ventilated extremely low birth weight infants. *J Pediatr*. 2011;159:384–391.e1.
3. Wood NS, Costeloe K, Gibson AT, et al. The EPICure study: associations and antecedents of neurological and developmental disability at 30 months of age following extremely preterm birth. *Arch Dis Child Fetal Neonatal Ed*. 2005;90:F134–F140.
4. Payot A, Barrington KJ. The quality of life of young children and infants with chronic medical problems: review of the literature. *Curr Probl Pediatr Adolesc Health Care*. 2011;41:91–101.
5. Johnson S, Fawke J, Hennessy E, et al. Neurodevelopmental disability through 11 years of age in children born before 26 weeks of gestation. *Pediatrics*. 2009;124;e249–e257.
6. Wood N, Marlow N, Costeloe K, Gibson A, Wilkinson A. Neurologic and developmental disability after extremely preterm birth. *N Engl J Med*. 2000;343(6):378–384.
7. Harris J. Is there a coherent social conception of disability? *J Med Ethics*. 2000;26:95–100.
8. Ravens-Sieberer U, Gosch A, Rajmil L, et al. KIDSCREEN-52 quality-of-life measure for children and adolescents. *Expert Rev Pharmacoecon Outcomes Res* 2005;5:353–364.
9. Meadow W, Bell A, Lantos J. Physicians' experience with allegations of medical malpractice in the neonatal intensive care unit. *Pediatrics*. 1997;99(5):E10.
10. *Miller v HCA, Inc*, 118 S.W. 3d 758, 771 (Texas 2003).
11. *Montalvo v Borkovec*, 647 N.W. 2d 413 (Wis.App. 2002).
12. Lantos J. Baby Doe five years later. Implications for child health. *N Engl J Med*. 1987;317(7):444–447.
13. Annas GJ. The Baby Doe regulations: governmental intervention in neonatal rescue medicine. *Am J Public Health*. 1984;74:618–620.
14. Annas GJ. Checkmating the Baby Doe regulations. *Hastings Cent Rep*. 1986;16(4):29–31.
15. Kopelman LM. The second Baby Doe rule. *JAMA*. 1988;259:843–844.
16. Born-Alive Infants Protection Act of 2001, report together with additional and dissenting views of the House Committee on the Judiciary, 107th Congress, 1st Session (2001), August 2, 2001. 1–38, 3. (Purpose and Summary.)
17. Partridge JC, Sendowski MD, Drey EA, Martinez AM. Resuscitation of likely nonviable newborns: would neonatology practices in California change if the Born-Alive Infants Protection Act were enforced? *Pediatrics*. 2009;123(4):1088–1094.
18. Tarini BA, Christakis DA, Welch HG. State newborn screening in the tandem mass spectrometry era: more tests, more false-positive results. *Pediatrics*. 2006;118(2):448–456.
19. Centers for Disease Control and Prevention (CDC). Impact of expanded newborn screening—United States, 2006. *MMWR Morb Mortal Wkly Rep*. 2008;57(37):1012–1015.
20. Sayeed SA. Baby doe redux? The Department of Health and Human Services and the Born-Alive Infants Protection Act of 2002: a cautionary note on normative neonatal practice. *Pediatrics*. 2005;116(4):e576–585, p. 580.

Considerations in NICU Design

3

Michele C. Walsh

Many neonatologists have assumed that the optimal design for a neonatal intensive care unit (NICU) is one that successfully merges high technology with a supportive "womb-like" environment. In the 1970s, NICUs were sterile, technology-filled dormitories with bombarding visual and auditory stimuli. From the late 1980s forward, efforts have focused on reducing stimulation. Initial attempts led to reduced-light environments, which were thought to simulate the in utero environment. Subsequent randomized trials failed to confirm the protective effects of reduced light on retinopathy of prematurity.[1] Other studies demonstrated the importance of cycled lighting on the development of circadian rhythms.[2] The application of studies to health care design has been termed evidence-based design. This process, led by architects at the Center for Health Design, has strengthened the evidence base for architectural practices. The field of neonatology has been an early adopter of this principle, with a robust and enthusiastic team that has contributed to ongoing innovations.[3,4]

When the NICU is appreciated as a place where crucial brain growth and development occur over a period of weeks or months, it becomes apparent that the sensory environment has comparable importance to the provision of direct medical care. This is even more evident when one realizes that the physical environment can affect the physical and mental health and performance of the caregivers as well as parental involvement and satisfaction. Thus, proper design should provide the best technological and environmental support possible to three constituencies: infants, families, and caregivers. The goal is difficult to achieve, not only because of space and financial limitations common to almost all construction projects, but also because some of these needs are in conflict with one another, as illustrated briefly in the previous discussion of circadian biology.

ADJACENCIES

In an ideal setting, the NICU is located in close proximity to the high-risk delivery rooms—in some NICUs, close enough to use a pass-through window. In hospitals with large maternity services or in children's hospitals, however, the NICU may be on a separate floor or in a different building. In this case, a stabilization area must be provided within or adjacent to the high-risk delivery area where the infant can be stabilized before transfer to the NICU. Transfer should be on a neonatal transport device with appropriate monitoring and respiratory support, proceed through nonpublic areas as much as possible, and use dedicated or controlled-access elevators.

Adjacencies to other support services in the hospital, including operating rooms, imaging, laboratories, and pharmacies, should be carefully considered. One must carefully evaluate traffic patterns for families to reach the NICU and the areas they need to use for eating, sleeping, personal needs, and interacting with other families. While making access convenient for families, good design also minimizes traffic congestion of NICU visitors or staff for both safety and aesthetic reasons. Public access should be limited to provide infant safety and prevent infant abductions.

CHAPTER 3

SINGLE-FAMILY ROOMS VERSUS MULTIPLE-PATIENT ROOMS

Private rooms have now become the standard for new construction in all inpatient areas in the hospital except for the NICU, where the benefits and downsides of this concept are still debated. Many of these factors are summarized in Table 3-1. For some hospitals with limited space available, this is not an option because single-family room design requires at least 600, and preferably 800, gross square feet per bed (total available floor space divided by the number of beds) when the relatively fixed needs for support space are considered as well. Even for hospitals with sufficient space and funding, however, there are concerns about single-family room design: Is it safe? Will it require more staff? Will the additional up-front cost be offset by savings elsewhere? Enough hospitals have now built single-family rooms for some or all of their NICU beds and have conducted studies to answer many of these questions.

Domanico and colleagues documented that infants cared for in a single-family-room NICU, compared to those in a multiple-patient room, had fewer apneic spells, reduced nosocomial sepsis, and earlier transition to enteral nutrition.[5] Other studies demonstrated that substantial modifications to NICU operations are needed to maximize efficiencies of nursing staff and address the concerns of staff concerning isolation.[6–8]

DESIGN STANDARDS

A committee organized by the American Academy of Pediatrics (AAP) Perinatal Section, in collaboration with the Gravens Institute of the University of South Florida, has periodically released detailed standards for the physical requirements for NICU design.[3] Key recommendations are summarized in Table 3-2 and explored in more detail in the following sections.

Lighting in the NICU

There has been a great deal of attention to the lighting conditions in intensive care units. Lighting is one area that involves tensions between meeting the needs of the adult caregivers and the needs of the individual infants. Adults need bright, focused light to conduct procedural and other focused tasks, such as medication preparation and administration. Adequate light has been shown to decrease errors in these areas.[9] Adequate light intensity has also been linked to levels of alertness, particularly in workers who may alternate between day and night shifts. In contrast, it has been believed that the optimal environment for preterm infants is an environment that duplicates the low-light

Table 3-1 Benefits of Single-Family and Multiple-Patient Rooms

Feature	Single-Family Room	Multiple-Patient Room
Privacy	Maximal	Easily compromised but can be provided to some degree
Light and sound	Individualized	Generally targeted to most acutely ill infant
Parental role	Easily supported	Must be actively facilitated
Staff needs: communication	Must be accomplished by electronic means as well as with a central station	Visualization of and collaboration with other team members is generally easier
Infection control	Reduced risk of cross-contamination by staff	More ability to monitor family's adherence to infection control measures
Patient safety	Attentive design permits direct visualization; increased technology required	Permits some degree of direct visualization of the patient area at all times
Cost	Construction costs higher and may require more staffing in some cases	In theory, may have higher infection rates and impaired neurodevelopment because of environmental factors

Adapted with permission from Fanaroff RJ, Martin AA, Walsh MC. Fanaroff and Martin's Neonatal-Perinatal M. St. Louis, MO: Elsevier/Mosby; 2011.

levels found in the womb. Although older facilities still use round-the-clock bright lighting designed to better meet the caregivers' needs, modern NICUs cycle their lighting in a day/night cycle and keep lighting levels as low as possible. Incubators may be kept covered in an effort to duplicate the dark conditions of the womb.

Work by McMahon and colleagues has found that exposure to constant light in a newborn rat model disrupted the development of the internal master clock responsible for sleep-wake cycles.[10] This supports the idea that cycled lighting may be better than constant lighting for premature babies from the perspective of developing their internal clocks. Indeed, the finding

Table 3-2 Key Factors in Designing the Intensive Care Nursery

Location • Close proximity or controlled access to delivery and transport areas • Controlled access and egress for patient and staff safety	**Lighting** • Ambient lighting levels adjustable through a range of 10 to 600 lux • No direct ambient lighting in patient care areas • Light sources with suitable spectrum to permit accurate color rendering • Procedure lighting capable of providing at least 2000 lux at the bed surface and adjustable in both location and intensity • Daylighting for adult work areas, with appropriate shading and insulation
Space allocation • Minimum of 120 ft^2 per bed space, excluding sinks and aisles (150 ft^2 minimum for single-patient rooms) • Adequate and easily accessible storage (30 ft^2 per bed) for supplies and equipment	**Acoustics** • Noise control measures to maintain the combination of background and operation sound below a mean level of 45 dB
Access • At least 4-ft aisles in multibed rooms • At least 8-ft corridors outside private rooms	**Heating, ventilation, and air conditioning** • Ambient temperature of 22°C to 26°C (72°F to 78°F) • Relative humidity of 30% to 60% • Minimum of 6 air exchanges per hour with appropriate filtering; two changes should be with outside air • Exhaust vents situated to minimize drafts near patient beds and appropriately sized and constructed to minimize noise from airflow
Privacy • Minimum of 8 ft between beds, with provisions for family and speech privacy	**Family support** • Adequate and welcoming directional and informational signage • Lounge, refreshments, restrooms, storage, library, telephones • Overnight rooms—at least 1 per 5 patient beds • Consultation/grieving room • Lactation area (if sufficient privacy is not available at the bedside) • Dedicated area at the bedside for infant care, work, and rest
Headwall • Twenty simultaneously accessible electrical outlets, divided between normal and emergency power circuits • Three each of compressed air, oxygen, and vacuum outlets, all simultaneously accessible • Data transmission port	**Staff Support** • Lockers, lounge, restrooms, on-call rooms • Adequate and comfortable charting/work area at each bedside • Clerical/work areas away from, but easily accessible to, each bedside • Office/desk space for all disciplines that routinely provide care
Hand hygiene • Large sinks with hands-free controls in each patient care room and within 20 ft of every bed • Sinks designed to accommodate children and persons in wheelchairs • Appropriate provision for soap, towel dispensers, and receptacles for trash, recyclables, and biohazardous waste	**Sustainable design** • Use of materials that are free of substances known to be teratogenic, mutagenic, carcinogenic, or otherwise harmful to human health • Designs and materials that reduce consumption of energy, fluids, and nonrenewable resources
Surfaces • Floors: easily cleanable, durable, glare free, and cushioned in patient care areas • Walls: easily cleanable and durable; attractive visual accents and sound-absorbent materials can be used where they can be protected from damage • Ceilings: washable, highly sound-absorbent acoustical tile wherever feasible	

that exposure to constant light disrupts the developing biological clock in baby mice provides an underlying mechanism that helps explain the results of several previous clinical studies. One found that infants from neonatal units with cyclic lighting tended to begin sleeping through the night more quickly than those from units with constant lighting.[11] In contrast, a study performed in convalescent preterm infants found no effect of cycled lighting on the development of sleep cycles.[2]

The optimal lighting environment in the NICU is still not known but must accommodate the needs of both the adults and the babies. The predominant evidence suggests bright task lighting in a natural light spectrum combined with reduced, but cycled, lighting may be the best compromise. Temporary increases in illumination necessary to evaluate a baby or to perform a procedure should be possible without increasing lighting levels for other babies in the same room. All lighting should be out of the direct line of sight of the infant.

Sound Environment in the NICU

The acoustic environment is a function of both the building (eg, noise from mechanical systems and equipment, sound containment by doors and walls, and sound absorption by surface finishes) and operations (eg, the activities of people and medical equipment).

The acoustic conditions of the NICU must support optimal communication without raised voices by minimizing background noise and auditory distractions. These conditions will ensure that speech is intelligible, which may reduce medical errors, provide privacy for staff and parents, and promote uninterrupted sleep and physiologic stability in infants. During design, specific attention to the acoustic environment must be accomplished if this goal is to be achieved. The project may benefit from early consultation with an acoustics engineer as the specifics needed may exceed the services of typical architectural services. Early engagement may prevent later costly retrofits.[12]

It is recommended that the permissible noise criteria is an hourly Leq of 45 dB (a weighted, slow response) in infant rooms and adult sleep areas. Focused efforts and specific product purchasing of major mechanical systems, such as those for heating and cooling, are required to achieve this low level of background noise (equivalent to a soft conversation).[3]

Acoustically absorptive surfaces reduce reverberation and therefore sound levels at a distance from the sound source. Glass, which will reflect all sounds, should be limited to the area actually required for visualization to leave wall surface available for absorptive

surface treatment. Although a variety of flooring will limit impact noise somewhat, specialized flooring with acoustical dampening or carpet offers the most protection. The type of water supply and faucets in infant areas should be selected to minimize noise and should provide instant warm water to minimize time "on."

Thoughtful consideration must be given to the adjacencies of unit support spaces. Some functions that generate significant noise should be isolated from the infant care areas. Examples include unit clerk areas, supply carts, conference rooms, and workstations. Equipment should be acoustically isolated from the infant area. Vibration isolation pads are recommended under leveling feet of permanent equipment and appliances in noise-sensitive areas or areas in open or frequent communication with them.

REFERENCES

1. Morag I, Ohlsson A. Cycled light in the intensive care unit for preterm and low birth weight infants. *Cochrane Database Syst Rev.* 2011;(1):CD006982. doi:10.1002/14651858.CD006982. pub2.
2. Mirmiran M, Baldwin RB, Ariagno RL. Circadian and sleep development in preterm infants occurs independently from the influences of environmental lighting. *Pediatr Res.* 2003;53(6):933–938.
3. White RD. Recommended standards for the newborn ICU. *J Perinatol.* 2007;27(suppl 2):S4–S19.
4. Harrell JW, Moon RG. Designs for the delicate: a look at evolving NICU design standard. *Health Facil Manag.* 2008;21(12):45–48.
5. Domanico R, Davis DK, Coleman F, Davis BO. Documenting the NICU design dilemma: comparative patient progress in open-ward and single family room units. *J Perinatol.* 2011;31(4):281–288.
6. Smith TJ, Schoenbeck K, Clayton S. Staff perceptions of work quality of a neonatal intensive care unit before and after transition from an open bay to a private room design. *Work.* 2009;33(2):211–227.
7. Carlson B, Walsh S, Wergin T, Schwarzkopf K, Ecklund S. Challenges in design and transition to a private room model in the neonatal intensive care unit. *Adv Neonatal Care.* 2006;6(5):271–280.
8. Walsh WF, McCullough KL, White RD. Room for improvement: nurses' perceptions of providing care in a single room newborn intensive care setting. *Adv Neonatal Care.* 2006;6(5):261–270.
9. Mahmood A, Chaudhury H, Valente M. Nurses' perceptions of how physical environment affects medication errors in acute care settings. *Appl Nurs Res.* 2011;24(4):229–237.
10. Ohta H, Mitchell AC, McMahon DG. Constant light disrupts the developing mouse biological clock. *Pediatr Res.* 2006;60(3):304–308.
11. Rivkees S, Rivkees SA, Mayes L, Jacobs H, Gross I. Rest and activity patterns of preterm infants are regulated by cycled lighting. *Pediatrics.* 2004;113(4):833–839.
12. Gray L, Philbin MK. Effects of the neonatal intensive care unit on auditory attention and distraction. *Clin Perinatol.* 2004;31(2):243–260.

Temperature Control and Environment

Robert A. Darnall

INTRODUCTION

Maintaining an adequate thermal environment for the premature infant is one of the most fundamental principles of newborn intensive care. The failure of the premature infant to adequately respond to a cold stress was perhaps the earliest historically recognized distinguishable characteristic (other than size) of the premature infant. This characteristic formed the rationale for the history and origins of incubators.[1] From the earliest experience of Pierre-Constant Budin, a student of Etienne Tarnier in Paris around 1900, it became apparent that survival of the premature infant is dependent on providing an adequate thermal environment.[2,3] In the present day, hypothermia continues to be an independent risk factor for death.[4] Indeed, thermal care has become routine in the neonatal intensive care unit (NICU).

Although all NICUs have routines for providing an appropriate thermal environment, there have been numerous changes in practice that may have introduced subtle, sometimes-unrecognized, influences on the thermal environment. A thorough understanding of the physiology of thermoregulation is necessary to maintain vigilance with respect to how subtle changes in practice might put the very immature infant at thermal risk. Much of the systems physiology of thermoregulation in the human newborn infant was thoroughly investigated in the 1960s and 1970s and continues to provide a basis of our current practice. However, the care or the extremely low birth weight infant, the introduction of developmental care, a variety of incubator designs, and changes in respiratory care practices potentially affect the nature or consistency of the thermal environment. Moreover, since the early 2000s, there have been major advances in our knowledge of the neural pathways involved in the afferent and efferent limbs of the mammalian thermoregulatory control system that have led to a reexamination of our overall concepts of thermoregulatory control.

The purpose of this chapter is to review the current state of knowledge with respect to the neural control of thermoregulation and concepts of thermal control, to review the principles of systems physiology that remain applicable to current practice, and to provide a snapshot of current practice, highlighting some areas that have received little emphasis.

PHYSIOLOGY

Fetus

The fetus has little control over its thermal environment. Fetuses are metabolically active, and thermal balance is achieved by heat transfer to the mother largely via the placenta. Thus, fetal temperature closely tracks maternal temperature and is on average 0.5°C higher. The fetus has limited capacity to increase heat production because nonshivering thermogenesis is largely inhibited secondary to reduced oxygen availability[5] and the inability to respond to catecholamines[6,7] and thyroid hormones[8] and because of placental inhibitory factors, including adenosine and prostaglandin E_2 (PGE2).[9–12] Thus, when umbilical blood flow is interrupted, fetal temperature increases.[13–15]

When body temperature is elevated just after delivery, one must therefore consider maternal temperature as well as impaired placental function in the differential diagnosis. Indeed, in clinical practice, these causes are far more common than infection.

Newborn

The newly born infant must rapidly adapt to a new thermal environment, which in almost all climates consists of a "cold" challenge. The universal response is an increase in metabolic rate, even in the premature infant. Although the mechanisms to increase heat production and reduce heat loss are present, newborn infants cannot maintain their temperature without some external "help" in reducing heat loss. In the full-term infant, this can usually be accomplished with external clothing. However, the premature infant has decreased capabilities to both produce heat and reduce heat loss through vasoconstriction, large surface-area-to-mass ratio, and limited insulation, underlying the rationale for practices and devices designed to reduce excessive heat loss. In addition, there are important interactions between hypoxia and thermoregulation that have meaningful implications for the thermal management of the sick premature infant.

Models of Thermoregulatory Control

A simple model of thermoregulatory control includes sensors located in critical locations to allow responses to changes in the external and internal environmental temperature, an integrating mechanism that receives sensory information and coordinates effector activity, and efficient balanced effector mechanisms designed to counteract any deviations from the controlled body temperature. Figure 4-1 illustrates the general organization of the thermoregulatory system.[16] The process of thermoregulation can be described as a controlled system in which body temperature is determined by metabolic heat production and heat transfer to the environment.

The traditional concept that deep body temperature is controlled by a system with a single controller has recently been challenged. Instead, it has been postulated that body temperature is regulated by independent thermoeffector loops, each having overlapping, but distinct, afferent and efferent pathways.[17] In this model, the activity of each effector system is triggered by a unique combination of surface and core temperatures. Thermal stimulation of sensory neurons leads to the activation (or inhibition) of neurons in the corresponding thermoeffector loop, resulting in a thermoeffector response. Therefore, it is not necessary to

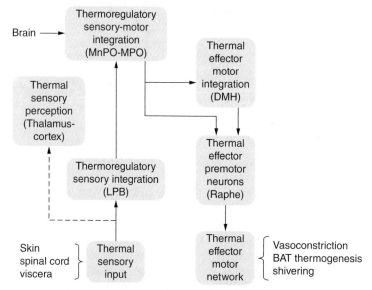

FIGURE 4-1 General organization of the thermoregulatory control system. Relevant rodent brain regions are in parentheses. Thermal sensory input from the skin, spinal cord, and viscera are integrated (perhaps in the lateral parabrachial nucleus [LPB]) before ascending to the preoptic area (POA) of the hypothalamus, where sensorimotor integration occurs within circuits involving the median preoptic nucleus (MnPO) and medial preoptic nucleus (MPO), including sensing local brain temperature. A separate pathway ascends via the thalamus to the sensory cortex important for thermal sensory perception. Descending effector information is transmitted to thermal effector premotor neurons located in the medullary raphe and spinal cord. Some descending motor information is integrated in the dorsomedial hypothalamus (DMH) before descending to the medullary raphe. BAT, brown adipose tissue. (Adapted from Morrison and Nakamura.[16])

calculate an integrated body temperature and compare it to a "set point." Coordination between thermoeffector loops is achieved through their common controlled variable, body temperature. The use of the term *set point*, however, continues to be controversial and is used with different meanings. In this review, the term *set point* is used simply to designate a "regulated level of body temperature."

Neural Control of Thermoregulation and Mechanisms of Heat Loss and Production

Our knowledge about the neural pathways involved in the control of body temperature has increased dramatically since the early 2000s. A full discussion of all of the recent advancements is beyond the scope of this chapter, and a review has been recently published.[16] Different neural pathways sense changes in cutaneous, visceral, spinal cord, and brain temperature and ultimately activate effector mechanisms to protect against changes in the temperature of the brain and other critical organs. Many mechanisms involved in the defense against cooling or heating are common to all mammals, including the human infant. The effector responses to *cooling* include those to reduce heat loss, including changes in behavior and cutaneous vasoconstriction, and those to produce heat, including nonshivering thermogenesis of brown adipose tissue (BAT), shivering thermogenesis, and generalized movement. Responses to *warming* are focused on increasing heat loss and include behavioral changes, cutaneous vasodilation, sweating, and, in some species, panting. Many of the neural pathways that sense and respond to cooling, warming, and fever have been worked out in the rodent using sophisticated track tracing and neurochemical activating and lesioning techniques. Figure 4-2 illustrates a functional neuroanatomical and neurotransmitter model for the pathways providing thermoregulatory control in response to cutaneous cooling and fever.[16] Although the exact nuclei involved may vary by species, it is likely that afferent and efferent limbs are similar in the human.

Thermosensation and Afferent Thermoregulatory Pathways

Sensory nerve endings in the skin detect changes in environmental temperature and transmit this information to the *preoptic area* (POA), a sensorimotor integration region of the hypothalamus.[16] The transient receptor potential (TRP) family of cation channels are thought to mediate cold (TRPM8, TRPA1) and warm (TRPV3, TRPV4) sensation across a broad physiological range of skin temperatures[17,18] (see Figure 4-3). Cutaneous thermal sensation is transmitted from lamina I neurons in the dorsal horn of the spinal cord either to the thalamus in the spinothalamocortical pathway, where neurons project to regions in the sensory cortex important for perception and discrimination of cutaneous temperature,[19,20] or to the *lateral parabrachial nucleus* (LPB) in the pons, where separate subgroups of neurons receive cutaneous cool and warm information.[21-24] Glutamatergic neurons in the LPB then project to the *median preoptive nucleus* (MnPO) of the POA.

Temperature-sensing mechanisms also exist in the brain, spinal cord, and abdomen. Neurons in the *medial* POA (MPO) sense changes in brain temperature. Information from cold and warm receptors in the abdominal viscera travels in the splanchnic and vagus nerves, but the specific pathways that carry information to the POA are unknown. The thermoregulatory responses to visceral temperature sensation are similar to those of cutaneous sensation,[25,26] suggesting that integration may occur in the LPB before being transmitted to the POA, an important region for integration of many homeostatic functions. The activity of neurons in the POA is also influenced by spinal cord temperature.[27] Because the temperature of centrally located organs is less susceptible to changes in environmental temperature, it is likely that, under normal circumstances, central temperature sensation contributes mostly when cutaneous stimulation has failed to produce an adequate thermal response.

Integrative Function of the POA

The MPO contains warm-sensitive neurons that are continuously active; cutaneous cooling both decreases their firing rate and increases their sensitivity to preoptic temperature.[28] Both cutaneous and local POA cooling promote nonshivering and shivering thermogenesis, suggesting that this region integrates peripheral and central temperature. The integrative function of the POA likely depends on a local circuit between the MnPO and the MPO, which contains continuously active inhibitory neurons that project to the caudal medullary raphe (CMR), either directly or via the *dorsomedial hypothalamus* (DMH). The CMR contains neurons involved in BAT thermogenesis, shivering, and peripheral vasoconstriction (see Figure 4-2). The interaction between neurons in the MnPO and MPO may be responsible for the apparent balance or set point, which is influenced by both local and peripheral temperature.

The POA is also important in the development of fever, a "controlled" increase in body temperature. During an infection, endogenous pyrogens, including interleukin (IL) 1β, IL-1α, IL-6, and other cytokines are released into the circulation, where they migrate to the circumventricular regions of the brain and bind with endothelial receptors or interact with glia,

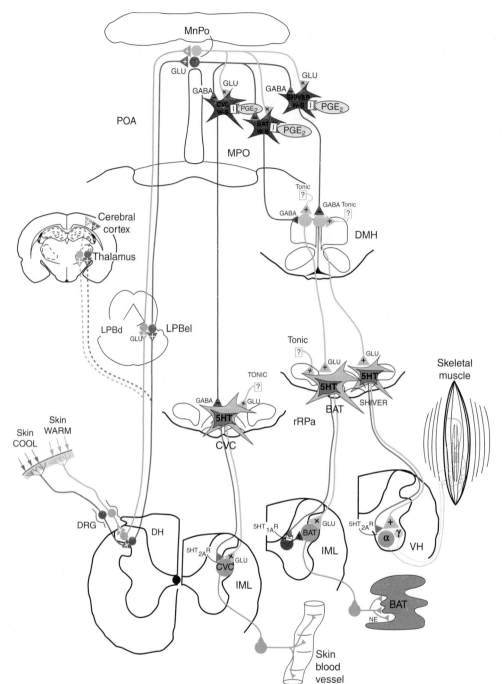

FIGURE 4-2 Neuroanatomical and neurotransmitter model for thermoregulatory pathways, including cutaneous temperature sensation, cutaneous vasoconstriction, brown adipose tissue (BAT) thermogenesis, and shivering. Information from the skin is transmitted to the dorsal horn of the spinal cord, ascends either to the lateral parabrachial nucleus (LPB) or to the thalamus. Glutamatergic neurons in the LPB project to the median preoptic nucleus of the hypothalamus (MnPO), where they synapse either on glutamatergic neurons (red) (warming) or GABAergic neurons (green) (cooling). Glutamatergic and GABAergic neurons in the MnPO project to the medial preoptic nucleus of the hypothalamus (MPO), where they synapse on tonically active, warm-sensitive γ-aminobutyric acid-mediated (GABAergic) neurons, which project either directly to the medullary raphe (mostly nucleus raphe pallitus [nRPa]) or to the dorsomedial hypothalamus (DMH). These warm-sensitive neurons in the MPO are also responsive to local brain temperature. Those that project directly to the nRPa tonically inhibit glutamatergic and serotonergic (5-HT) neurons involved in vasoconstriction. Those that project to the DMH tonically inhibit glutamatergic neurons, which then project to glutaminergic and 5-HT neurons in the medullary raphe or adjacent nucleus paragigantocellularis lateralis (PGCL) controlling BAT thermogenesis and shivering. Separate groups of raphe glutamatergic and 5-HT neurons project to sympathetic motor neurons in the interomediolateral region of the spinal cord (IML), which modulate thermoregulatory sympathetic outflow to peripheral vessels and BAT, or to α-motor neurons in the ventral horn involved in shivering. As this diagram illustrates, there are separate neuronal circuits involved in cutaneous vasoconstriction, BAT thermogenesis, and shivering. (From Morrison and Nakamura.[16])

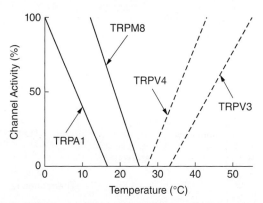

FIGURE 4-3 Schematic representation of the active temperature ranges of selected transient receptor potential (TRP) channels. TRPA1 and TRPM8, candidates for cold reception, demonstrate increasing channel activity with decreasing temperatures, whereas TRPV3 and TRPV4, candidates for warm reception, increase channel activity with increasing temperature. The thresholds of activation and temperatures of maximal activation are based on the activity of the channels in heterologous systems; some of the thresholds are means of values obtained in several studies. (Adapted from Romanovsky.[17])

activating the arachidonic acid pathway to produce PGE_2. PGE_2 binds to EP3 inhibitory receptors in the POA to produce fever. Neurons in the MPO that are activated by PGE_2 are largely inhibitory (GABAergic) and project either directly or via the DMH to the CMR. Those that project directly to the CMR are involved in cutaneous vasoconstriction (CVC), and those that travel through the DMH and then to the CMR are involved in BAT thermogenesis and shivering.

Thermoregulatory Effector Mechanisms

The thermoregulatory effector mechanisms include heat production and behaviors that decrease or increase heat transfer from the body to the environment (behavior, CVC, and vasodilation).

Behavioral Changes include huddling in the cold or spreading the limbs in the heat or moving to a *"preferred"* environment. The human infant has also been observed to flex extremities when cooled and extend them when warmed.[29] Some nonshivering behaviors can also generate heat. For example, in the newborn human infant, generalized increases in body movements often accompany cooling and contribute to the increase in metabolism observed in these conditions.[30]

Cutaneous Blood Flow carries heat to the body surface, where it can be transferred to the environment. Presympathetic neurons responsible for CVC are located in the intermediolateral (IML) region of the spinal cord and receive inputs from glutamatergic and serotonergic neurons located in the CMR. Neurons in

the CMR that receive direct input from the MPO that are involved in CVC are separate from those (mostly in the raphe pallidus) that receive inputs from the MPO via the DMH that are involved in BAT thermogenesis and shivering (see Figure 4-2). In humans, sympathetic outflow from the IML mediates both CVC during cooling and vasodilation during warming.[31-33] Although the subject of some debate, evidence supports a role for both acetylcholine and norepinephrine in peripheral vasodilation, depending on whether stimulated by whole-body or local warming. Prostanoids are involved in cholinergic mechanisms, and nitric oxide is associated with norepinephrine-mediated vasodilation. In addition, in both humans and rodents, heating-evoked vasodilation is accompanied by visceral vasoconstriction mediated by angiotensin.[34] In several species, including humans and rodents, there is a moderate level of CVC even at thermoneutrality. In human infants, it is thought that changes in CVC are responsible for the maintenance of a "flat" core body temperature over the thermal neutral zone.

Sweating increases heat loss by evaporative cooling. Although active sweating is rarely observed in newborn infants, sweating can occur, particularly on the forehead, when core body temperature exceeds about 37.2°C.[35] Sweat glands start to appear on the palms during the third or fourth month of fetal life and shortly thereafter on the forehead[36]; there is a full complement of sweat glands, some with lumens, by the seventh month of gestation.[35] Whether sweat glands are functional in the very immature infant is unknown. Sweat glands are innervated by sympathetic cholinergic fibers and may be linked to cutaneous vasodilation. Indices of "emotional" sweating, such as changes in skin conductance, can be detected as early as 29 weeks gestational age, even perhaps within hours of birth,[37] and at least by 10 days of age.[38] Sweating occurs most commonly on the forehead, followed by the chest, upper arm, and cheek.[35] The number of sites that exhibit simultaneous sweating also increases with maturity. Thus, for the preterm infant, sweating is not an efficient "programmed" way to lose heat. Evaporative cooling, however, without active sweating, is a major source of heat loss, especially immediately after birth.

BAT Thermogenesis. Thermogenesis is the primary function of BAT and is achieved by a significant proton leak across the mitochondrial membranes facilitated by the high expression of uncoupling protein 1 (UCP-1)[39] (see Figure 4-4). BAT thermogenesis is an oxidative process and depends on sympathetically mediated norepinephrine release. BAT plays an important role in thermal control in infant and adult rodents and in newborn human infants. Recent evidence now confirms that BAT can also be recruited in adult humans,

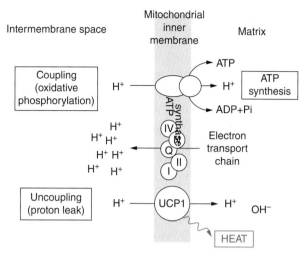

FIGURE 4-4 Simplified illustration of the action of uncoupling protein (UCP) in brown adipose tissue. Heat is produced when protons "leak" across the inner mitochondrial membrane (uncoupling) without being incorporated into adenosine triphosphate (ATP) synthesis (coupling). ADP, adenosine diphosphate.

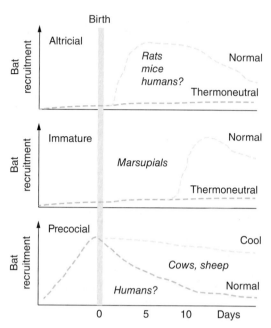

FIGURE 4-5 Brown adipose tissue (BAT) recruitment patterns in different species. With respect to BAT development, human infants are similar to precocial animals in that BAT is present at birth. In other respects, human are more like altricial animals in that they require considerable maternal care with respect to the thermal environment. (Adapted from Cannon and Nedergaard.[39])

particularly when chronically exposed to cold environments.[40] Moreover, there is an increasing focus on the important link between BAT and obesity.[41] The sympathetic outflow to BAT originates from presympathetic neurons in the IML of the thoracic spinal cord, which receive glutamatergic and serotonergic inputs from the CMR nuclei, which are in turn driven by glutamatergic inputs from the DMH. Thus, both cutaneous or body cooling and fever result in the disinhibition of DMH neurons, resulting in increased excitation of CMR and then IML presympathetic neurons to stimulate BAT metabolism (see Figure 4-2).

The development of BAT varies among animal species. In *altricial* animals, including the rat and mouse, very little BAT is present at birth, but under normal thermal environmental conditions, recruitment occurs early. In *immature* animals, including Siberian hamsters and most marsupials, BAT is recruited only after leaving the pouch. *Precocial* animals, including lambs, calves, and guinea pigs, develop BAT during fetal life and are born with considerable amounts of BAT and thermal insulation (hair). Human infants resemble both *altricial* and *precocial* animals. Like *altricial* animals, human newborns have only minimal amounts of thermal insulation and require considerable maternal care, including the provision of an adequate thermal environment. However, with respect to BAT development, they more resemble *precocial* animals. Human infants, even those born prematurely, have considerable amounts of BAT at birth and exhibit some degree of nonshivering thermogenesis within hours of delivery.[42]

Figure 4-5 shows the patterns of BAT development in various species, including the human infant.

The classic report from Aherne and Hull described the location and microscopic description of BAT in the newborn infant, emphasizing the intrascapular and neck regions and suprarenal locations in the abdomen[43] (see Figure 4-6). The function of BAT is also highly dependent on thermal history.[44] For example, rat pups

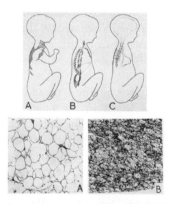

FIGURE 4-6 Location and microscopic description of brown adipose tissue (BAT) in the human infant from the classic 1964 description of Aherne and Hull.[43] In the upper panel, A and B represent the distribution of BAT and C represents the venous drainage from the interscapular pad. In the lower panel, A represents a micrograph (×170) of unilocular white adipose tissue and B multilocular brown adipose tissue. Note the dense appearance of BAT compared to white adipose tissue.

reared at thermoneutrality fail to recruit BAT and use shivering exclusively. Although in the human infant the amount of BAT diminishes and the capability for shivering increases over the first year of life,[45] little is known about the ability of the very small premature infant to recruit BAT. There is some evidence that infants nursed in cooler environments are more resistant to a subsequent cold exposure, suggesting BAT recruitment.[46] On the other hand, we make major efforts to maintain thermoneutrality, potentially inhibiting the recruitment of BAT in the very premature infant.

Shivering Thermogenesis involves production of heat by rapid repeated skeletal muscle contractions that result in inefficient energy utilization. Shivering is the last cold-defense mechanism to be activated and has a lower thermal threshold than CVC or BAT thermogenesis, suggesting that there is a separate subpopulation of warm-sensitive neurons in the MPO responsible for shivering. Although the general afferent and efferent pathways for shivering are similar to those that activate BAT and CVC, projections from the CMR are to the anterior horn of the spinal cord. Muscle contractions during shivering result from rhythmic bursts of activity in the α-motoneurons innervating skeletal muscle fibers. Newborn infants can shiver when body temperature falls significantly and when the combination of BAT thermogenesis and heat conservation mechanisms have been insufficient to maintain body temperature.

Increases in Heart Rate (HR) accompany thermoregulatory responses and are mediated by neurons in the CMR that project to the IML of the spinal cord, resulting in an increase in sympathetic outflow to cardiovascular regions controlling HR. An increase in HR is thought to ensure adequate blood flow to BAT and skeletal muscles and help distribute heat produced by BAT and shivering thermogenesis to other parts of the body.

Systems Physiology in the Human Infant

Systems physiology in the human infant involves heat loss, heat production, heat balance, the concept of thermoneutrality, and the metabolic responses to cooling.

Heat Loss

The infant loses heat to its environment by *conduction*, *convection*, *radiation*, and *evaporation*. Depending on the route of heat loss, heat transfer to the environment will be determined by the temperature difference between the infant's skin and the environment (convection and evaporation for air, conduction by surface in contact with the skin, radiation by a remote radiant surface),

the velocity of air moving across the skin (convection, evaporation, the water content of the surrounding air via evaporation, and the exposed surface area for exchange via convection, conduction, evaporation, radiation). In thermoneutral conditions and depending on the amount of clothing and the methods used to provide a thermal environment, heat transfer will occur mainly by convection, radiation, and evaporation. In most clinical conditions, heat loss by conduction accounts for only a small fraction of total heat loss. Evaporation becomes increasingly important with decreasing gestational age and weight. In addition, heat can be gained by convection, conduction, and radiation. For example, for an infant cared for under a radiant warmer, heat gained by radiation balances large losses by convection and evaporation. A warming blanket or mattress can result in a reduction of heat losses or even heat gain by conduction. For example, after delivery, exothermic mattresses have been shown to help prevent hypothermia in small premature infants.[47,48]

Care must also be taken to consider respiratory heat losses.[49] In small infants managed in incubators that provide humidity, heat losses from the respiratory tract are relatively low but can increase dramatically with certain respiratory care practices. In term infants at 50% relative humidity, the water loss from the skin and respiratory tract are roughly equivalent. Decreasing gestational age is associated with decreasing respiratory-to-skin water loss ratios. As relative humidity increases, water loss from the skin decreases more than that from the respiratory tract. For example, if relative humidity is increased from 50% to 80%, water loss from the skin decreases from about 9 to about 2 g/kg/24 hours, and water loss from the respiratory tract decreases from about 9 to about 5 g/kg/24 hours. Heat loss from the respiratory tract is dependent on minute ventilation (V_E) and activity such that in infants from 27 to 37 weeks gestational age measured within a few days after birth, a change in respiratory rate from 40 to 100 beats/minute results in about a 150% increase in respiratory water loss.[49]

Respiratory heat loss has convective and evaporative components; evaporation accounts for about 6 times more heat loss than convection. Heated and humidified breathing gas in ventilated infants and those receiving nasal continuous positive airway pressure (CPAP) greatly reduce respiratory water losses. However, cold and unhumidified oxygen/air continues to be used in many delivery rooms for initial resuscitation and in NICUs for nasal cannula oxygen delivery systems and can result in considerable heat loss. The use of humidified and heated air during stabilization in the delivery room has been shown to significantly improve temperature on arrival to the NICU.[50] The use of heated humidified high-flow nasal cannula (HHHFNC) therapy, although not an efficient way to provide CPAP, can significantly reduce respiratory heat losses.[51] With some assumptions, the convective and evaporative components of respiratory water loss can be calculated.[49] We have estimated, using these calculations, that the use of HHHFNC compared to using standard nasal prong oxygen delivery can reduce heat loss as much as 12 kcal/kg/24 hours.

Heat Production

Because the infant in the NICU is receiving either intravenous nutrition or frequent enteral feedings, thinking about "fasting" or "basal" metabolic rate is not practical. Rather, it is more useful to think about "resting" metabolic rate when the infant is quiet, or preferably asleep. Heat production in small animals and newborn human infants is commonly measured as oxygen consumption (VO_2) using indirect calorimetry in the form of flow-through respirometry. In its simplest form, where the animal or infant is in a chamber provided with a constant flow of breathing gas, VO_2 is calculated from the difference in fractional O_2 concentration of gas entering and leaving the chamber multiplied by the gas flow rate and is usually expressed as milliliters per minute of oxygen consumed normalized to body weight (ml/kg/min). To be accurate, one must also take into account the amount of CO_2 and water vapor produced. Detailed discussions of the mathematics of metabolic rate measurements using indirect calorimetry are beyond the scope of this chapter, and excellent discussions have been published elsewhere.[52] Recent studies in very small premature infants using these techniques in modern incubators with added humidity have confirmed that resting metabolic rate varies with postmenstrual age (PMA) and energy intake.[53] Figure 4-7 shows resting metabolic rate in infants less than 30 weeks gestation referenced to age, weight, and energy intake.

Heat Balance

The control of heat loss is a fundamental requirement of all homeotherms. The general equation describing the thermal balance with the environment has been described by Hardy et al,[54]: $Q_{tot} = Q_{loss} + Q_{storage}$, where Q_{tot} is the heat produced by metabolism per unit of time, Q_{loss} is the total heat losses per unit of time, and $Q_{storage}$ is the total heat stored per unit of time. In a thermal steady state, heat storage is zero, and total heat loss (from all sources) equals total metabolic heat production. If heat loss exceeds heat production, the decreased storage is manifested by a fall in body temperature. Conversely, when heat loss is less than heat production, an increase in heat storage is manifest by an increase in body temperature.

Thermoneutrality

For the neonatal care provider, the concept of thermoneutrality has been complicated by definitions of

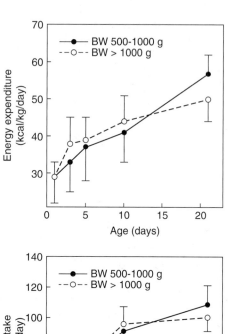

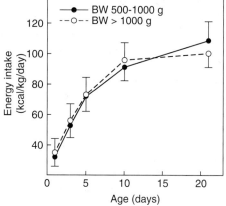

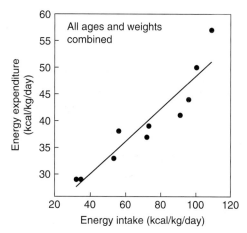

FIGURE 4-7 Resting metabolic rate in infants less than 30 weeks gestational age at birth is related to age and energy intake. Top: Energy expenditure vs age in days for infants 500–1000 g and larger than 1000 g. Middle: Energy intake vs age for infants 500–1000 g and larger than 1000 g. Bottom: Energy intake vs energy expenditure (derived from data in top and middle panels). BW, body weight. (Graphs created from data in Bauer et al.[53])

overlapping terms, including the "thermoregulatory range" and the "thermal neutral zone." These terms are often used interchangeably to define the optimal thermal environment for the newborn infant.

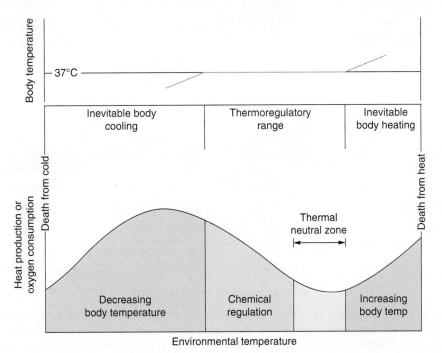

FIGURE 4-8 The concept of thermoneutrality. The *thermoregulatory range* is the region where body temperature can be maintained constant. Within this range, no extra heat production is necessary when in the *thermal neutral zone*. Within this narrow range, heat balance is achieved by adjustments in cutaneous blood flow alone. At environmental temperatures below the thermal neutral zone, body temperature can be maintained by producing additional heat with both shivering and nonshivering thermogenesis. As environmental temperature decreases further, body temperature starts to fall when heat production can no longer keep up with heat losses. (Adapted with permission from Klaus MH, Fanaroff AA, eds. Care of the high risk neonate, 6th ed. Philadelphia, PA: Saunders; 2013.)

The narrowest range is the *thermal neutral zone*, in which there is a thermal steady state, metabolic rate is minimal, and thermoregulation occurs by a nonevaporative physical process alone (changes in cutaneous blood flow). The *thermoregulatory range* is the wider range and includes the environmental temperature range over which thermoregulation (both physical and chemical) occurs and body temperature can be maintained. Moreover, because infants are always losing water, and thus heat, through the skin, evaporative heat loss is always present. Thus, a practical definition of the neutral thermal zone is that environment (usually a range of air temperatures or abdominal skin temperature in an incubator, or abdominal skin temperatures under a radiant warmer) in which the infant, when quiet or asleep, is not required to increase heat production above 'resting' levels to maintain body temperature. Figure 4-8 illustrates the concept of thermoneutrality.

From a historical perspective, traditional studies defining thermoneutrality were done in incubators using ambient or "operant" temperatures as an index of the environment. Currently, combinations of traditional incubators, radiant warmers, and incubators capable of providing high levels of humidity are commonly used to provide a thermal environment for premature infants. It is important to keep in mind that,

during a steady state, resting heat production or gain is balanced by total energy losses rather than loss by one route alone. For example, in an incubator, thermoneutrality can be achieved by several combinations of air, incubator wall (radiant) temperatures, and levels of humidity. Because heat storage can occur under radiant warmers, despite large convective and evaporative losses, it is likely that there is a level of radiant warmer output at which thermal equilibrium occurs.[56,57]

Metabolic Responses to Cooling

Most of our information about early responses to cooling comes from the older literature. There are few studies from the modern era of neonatal care. From the older studies, it is evident that the lower critical temperature (lower end of the *thermal neutral zone*) and the slope of the oxygen consumption response to cooling vary with gestational age and chronological age. It appears that nonshivering thermogenesis not only is active within minutes after birth (reflecting the presence of BAT at birth) but also becomes more effective with age, starting in the first 24 hours.[42] The results of the classic studies of Hey are shown in Figure 4-9.[30] Note that the resting VO_2 was similar in infants weighing more than 2.5 kg and those weighing 1–2 kg at 4–12 hours of age, but rose more slowly with age in

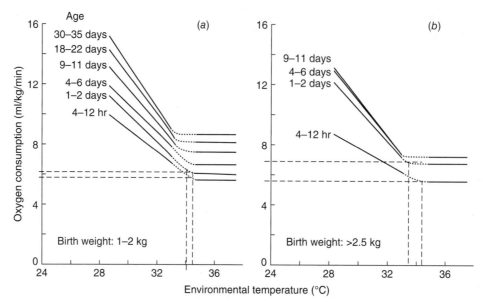

FIGURE 4-9 Lower critical temperatures and the oxygen consumption (VO$_2$) response to changes in environmental temperature (T$_E$) at different ages and weights from the classic studies in 1969 by Hey.[30] A, Data from infants weighing 1–2 kg; B, data from infants weighing more than 2.5 kg. Resting VO$_2$ (horizontal dashed lines) and lower critical temperatures (vertical dashed lines) are shown for studies done at 4–12 hours and 1–2 days of age. Note that resting VO$_2$ increased and the lower critical temperature decreased more in the first 1–2 days of life in the larger (more mature) infants. The slope of the VO$_2$/T$_E$ also became "steeper" with age in both weight groups. In these studies, naked infants were studied in a metabolic chamber with plexiglass walls surrounded by a water jacket. Thus, the wall and air temperature was controlled. The environmental temperature was calculated using the relationship T$_E$ = 0.4T$_A$ + 0.6T$_W$. Each infant was studied at 5–8 different values of T$_E$. VO$_2$ was calculated as the mean of 10–20 minutes of measurements at each T$_E$.

the smaller infants. Similarly, the slopes (VO$_2$/°C) were similar at 4–12 hours but became steeper with age. The results of studies investigating the metabolic response to cooling also clearly showed that the increase in VO$_2$ during cooling is accomplished by BAT thermogenesis and generalized movement, both components of "nonshivering" thermogenesis.

It is sometimes not recognized that cooling of certain areas of the body, even when abdominal skin and core temperature are normal, can produce dramatic increases in metabolic rate. For example, the trigeminal area of the face is exquisitely sensitive to changes in temperature,[58,59] and differential cooling of the face can result in increases in oxygen consumption without any changes in either abdominal skin or core temperature. Figure 4-10 illustrates the metabolic consequences of cooling the abdominal skin, even when core temperature is normal, and cooling

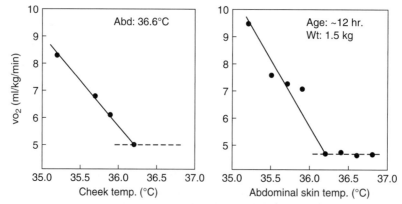

FIGURE 4-10 Effects of changing abdominal and cheek skin temperature on oxygen consumption (VO$_2$). Left: VO$_2$ was measured as the cheek temperature was altered by covering the face under a radiant warmer. Abdominal skin temperature was servo controlled to 36.6°C. Right: Radiant warmer was adjusted to servo control skin temperature from 35.2°C to 36.3°C. VO$_2$ was measured for approximately 10 minutes at each temperature. Rectal temperature did not change during these experiments. VO$_2$ was measured using respirometry as described previously.[56,68]

the face with normal abdominal skin and core temperatures. In these experiments, the infant was nursed under a radiant warmer with abdominal skin temperature servo controlled. Face cooling was induced by simply covering the face.[60] Cooling of the facial skin can occur easily in an intensive care setting, and when using a radiant warmer, one must be cautious about blocking the radiant heat source illuminating the face. Most modern incubators have double walls that serve to decrease radiant heat loss, but some nurseries may elect to use plastic heat shields in an incubator. Some have advocated introducing "warm" humidified air under the shield. When directed over the face, such practices can also inadvertently cool the face (because the air introduced is rarely 37°C or higher) and potentially result in an increase in metabolic rate.

Hypoxia and Thermoregulation

Small premature infants who require oxygen are increasingly maintained at low levels of PaO_2 to reduce the incidence and severity of retinopathy of prematurity (ROP).[61] These same infants require considerable effort to maintain thermoneutrality. It is well known, starting with early studies in both animals[62] and humans,[63] that thermoregulatory heat production is inhibited during even mild hypoxemia. Studies in rodents have recently shown that stimulation of peripheral chemoreceptors with hypoxia directly inhibits sympathetic outflow to BAT through an excitatory amino-acid-mediated activation of secondary neurons in the nucleus tractus solitarius (NTS).[64] It is therefore possible that very immature infants, purposely kept relatively hypoxic, will lose their already-limited ability to respond to a cold stress.

Sleep and Thermoregulation

In most small mammals, active thermoregulation, including BAT thermogenesis, shivering, panting, and vasoconstriction, is greatly diminished or even abolished during rapid eye movement (REM) or active sleep.[65,66] The premature infant spends up to 70% of sleep time in active sleep, and a suspension of thermoregulation might put the infant at further risk. However, the human infant appears to be different from small mammals of most species and can increase metabolic rate in response to a cold stress even during active sleep.[67,68]

CLINICAL MANAGEMENT OF THE THERMAL ENVIRONMENT

Measurement of Core Temperature

The best location to measure core temperature in the sick premature infant remains controversial. Esophageal, rectal, axillary, and tympanic membrane temperature have all been used. Axillary temperature measurement has become standard in most NICUs, and there are good correlations between rectal, axillary, and tympanic temperatures.[69] Routine rectal temperature measurement is not recommended. Esophageal temperatures are commonly monitored during therapeutic cooling for hypoxic-ischemic brain injury. Core temperature measurement using axillary, rectal, or tympanic measurements are intermittent, whereas esophageal temperature measurement can be continuous. Continuous measurements, particularly when displayed along with other vital sign measurements, would be advantageous particularly with changing thermal environments associated with care practices such as kangaroo care and procedures. There appears to be some interest in developing a feeding tube with embedded thermal sensors that could be used in the smallest preterm infants. When obtaining axillary temperatures, it is important to completely cover the temperature probe with the arm. Temperature could be underestimated if exposed to the incubator air or overestimated if exposed to a radiant warmer heat source.

Care in the Delivery Room

Although heat loss in the delivery room has always been a challenge, interest has recently been redirected at this old problem. How does one maintain the temperature of the smallest newborn infant immediately after birth and during stabilization? This is clearly most important for the smallest and most immature infants. Rapid decreases in skin and core body temperature will occur immediately after birth unless appropriate measures are used to reduce heat loss from evaporation and convection. The core (and skin) temperature of the fetus is normally about 0.5°C warmer than maternal temperature and in most delivery room configurations can rapidly fall into the hypothermic range within minutes if left unattended.

The classic study by Dahm et al., although carried out in full-term infants, illustrated 2 major interventions that can be used to prevent hypothermia in the delivery room.[70] Adequately drying the infant and using a radiant warmer with skin temperature servo controlled between 36.5°C and 37.0°C can almost completely eliminate the fall in skin temperature and thus core temperature in all but the smallest infants (see Figure 4-11). It is important to emphasize again that the mammalian thermoregulatory system is designed to respond primarily to changes in skin temperature. As long as skin temperature is not allowed to fall and maintained to at least 36°C, decreases in core temperature can be minimized. For most infants larger than 1500 g, removing any wet blankets, prewarming any contact surfaces, eliminating drafts, and maximizing delivery room temperature should be employed

CHAPTER 4

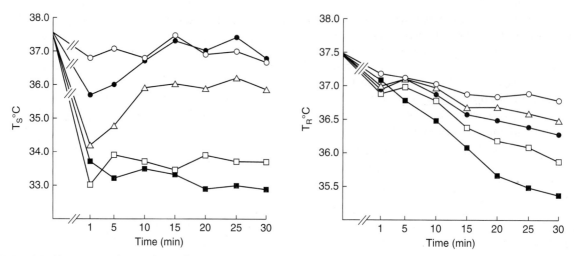

FIGURE 4-11 Changes in skin and rectal temperature after birth in full-term infants. Left: Decreases in mean abdominal skin temperature during the first 30 minutes of life with different treatments. Right: Decreases in rectal temperature during the first 30 minutes of life with different treatments. Symbols: ■ no intervention, □ drying alone, △ drying plus blankets, ○ radiant warmer alone, ● drying plus radiant warmer. (From Dahm and James.[70])

along with providing radiant heat. In healthy full-term infants, skin-to-skin care can also be employed and used successfully to eliminate decreases in skin temperature.

The very small infant less than 1500 g presents a special problem in that, despite most routine measures, skin temperature cannot be easily maintained. One of the major impediments is that the majority of these infants require some level of resuscitation and procedures, with the radiant heat source often blocked by drapes and clinical personnel. In addition, many radiant warmers may have insufficient output to warm the very small preterm infant under normal delivery room conditions.[71] Prewarming the delivery room to 26°C,[72] covering the baby in plastic wrapping,[73,74] and putting the baby on an exothermic mattress[48] and under a radiant warmer[75] are all recommended practices aimed at reducing heat loss and are included in the 2010 American Heart Association (AHA) guidelines.[47] A woolen hat may also decrease heat losses[76]; tube-stocking hats are not effective, but other materials are currently being tested. In addition, as mentioned previously, under a radiant warmer, care must be taken not to cover the face. In addition, using heated and humidified air-oxygen mixtures may further reduce heat losses in the delivery room.[50]

Maintaining a Neutral Thermal Environment

There are 2 major goals of providing a neutral thermal environment. The first is maintaining normal core and skin temperature in infants who cannot mount a metabolic response to cooling as occurs in the very immature infants in the first hours and perhaps days of life or in those infants who are hypoxemic or otherwise sick. The second goal is to prevent increases in metabolic rate for the purpose of maintaining body temperature. Because we do not continuously measure metabolic rate, we are limited in knowing for sure, at any given time, whether the metabolic rate is minimal. Early studies showed, however, that if abdominal skin temperature is maintained in the normal range (36°C to 37°C) either under a radiant warmer or in an incubator, and core temperature is normal and not increasing or decreasing, it is likely that a thermoneutral environment has been achieved. Under a radiant warmer, heat balance is achieved at the expense of increased evaporative and convective heat losses. In modern incubators that can provide high humidity, a combination of skin and air temperature and a level of humidity can be chosen to optimize heat reduction while maintaining skin and core temperature in the normal range. There are a number of Web-based tools that can suggest settings based on weight, gestational age, age, room temperature, need for mechanical ventilation and phototherapy, and type of incubator used. One website from Dräger (http://www.babyfirst.com/heatbalance/#stepper), although designed for use with Dräger incubators, illustrates the changes in heat balance resulting from changes in room and incubator air temperature, percentage humidity, or the addition of mechanical ventilation or phototherapy.

Recent practices introduced into neonatal care may result in subtle changes in the thermal environment. The addition of added insulation, in the form of "nesting" or other clothing, will change the relationships between VO₂ and environmental temperature such that the *lower critical temperature* will decrease and the slope of the VO₂/temperature function will

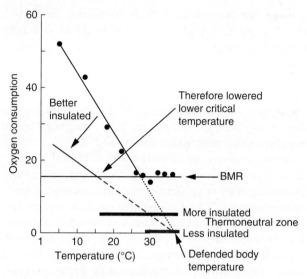

FIGURE 4-12 **Effects of added insulation of the lower critical temperature and slope of the VO$_2$/environmental temperature (T$_E$) relationship. Schematic diagram showing that added insulation lowers the lower critical temperature and "flattens" the slope of the VO$_2$/T$_E$ relationship . BMR: basal metabolic rate.** (From Cannon and Nedergaard.[44])

become less steep. Figure 4-12 shows the general effect of added insulation on the relationship between VO$_2$ and environmental temperature. Using a substantial hat will have a similar effect, as will the natural addition of tissue insulation with growth.

Small premature infants are frequently taken out of their thermal environment for "kangaroo care." Although there is no doubt that this increases parent satisfaction, the potential thermal risks of changing environments in very small immature infants have not been fully evaluated. One must consider not only the environment when "skin-to-skin" care is established, but also the transition from the incubator to the site of kangaroo care and the transition back to the incubator. Many nurseries routinely completely cover incubators with materials of various thicknesses and thermal conductivity. This will change the radiant loss to the wall of the incubator, thus changing thermal balance. Theoretically, servo controlling skin temperature should accommodate for changes in both insulation or radiant heat flux, but in our experience, small reductions in servo skin temperature may need to be made to avoid overheating, especially in high-humidity environments.

Incubators, Radiant Warmers, and Humidity

Modern incubators allow the operator to choose whether to servo control air or skin temperature. Controlling air temperature allows skin and body temperature to vary, thus making it easier to detect

decreases in temperature that might occur with a developing infection. Commonly, a range of temperatures is chosen according to the weight and age of the infant. Alternatively, one can first servo control abdominal skin temperature to determine the correct air temperature and then switch to air temperature mode. There are some disadvantages of maintaining a constant air temperature. After caregiving, infant temperature tends to decrease when air is servo controlled and remains relatively constant if skin is controlled, associated with an increase in air temperature.[77] If there is an addition of a radiant heat source, such as that of phototherapy, without reducing air temperature, skin temperature will increase, resulting in increases in insensible water loss. In practice, increases in insensible water loss from the skin with the use of phototherapy can be greatly reduced by servo controlling skin temperature.

In newer incubators that provide high levels of humidity, servo controlling air temperature may result in overheating the infant. In a recent Cochrane review, a meta-analysis of 2 older studies that compared maintaining abdominal skin temperature at 36°C to a constant air temperature of 31.8°C found that in infants (800–1599 g), in the first week of life, servo controlling abdominal skin temperature to at least 36°C improved survival compared to keeping incubator air temperature constant (relative risk 0.72; 95% CI, 0.54–0.97; risk difference −12.7%; 95% CI, −1.6 to −23.9).[78] Although this review is based on 2 studies done in the 1960s with technology not used commonly today, it seems prudent to servo control abdominal skin temperature, especially when providing high levels of humidity.

Humidified incubators have been used over the years to reduce evaporative losses, enhance skin integrity, and improve fluid and electrolyte balance during the first few days or weeks of life when transepidermal water loss is at its greatest.[49] The smallest infants may require as much as 80% humidity to adequately reduce insensible water losses. There are some safety concerns associated with using high humidity, including the risk for nosocomial infection. Although modern incubators that use high humidity are designed to reduce the risk of sepsis, the association has yet to be tested. Despite the increasing use of high humidity in the care of the very low birth weight infant, there remains wide variation in humidification practices.[79,80] The optimum length of time to use high humidity is also not known, but for the smallest infants most recommend that incubator humidity gradually be reduced over the first 2 weeks to below 50%.

When providing a thermal environment using servo control, whether in an incubator or under a radiant warmer, particular attention must be paid to probe placement. It is important to remember that the warmer is designed to keep the probe at a desired temperature. It is *assumed* that the probe temperature and skin temperature are equivalent. The probe position should be checked frequently to ensure that it is pressed flat on the skin and covered with a reflective shield. If the probe lifts off the skin, the warmer will continue to keep the probe warm, resulting in overheating. In addition, the probe should be placed so that it "sees" the radiant heat source and in an incubator is not covered by nesting materials or clothing. When the infant is supine, the best place to place the probe is over the abdomen. When prone, the probe should be placed on the back, avoiding the intrascapular area where the location of BAT is most concentrated. In most instances, overheating when providing skin servo control is related to probe attachment or position.

Infants must be able to maintain their temperature in an open crib before discharge. Weaning from an incubator can usually be done when the infant achieves a weight between 1600 and 1800 g. It is usual practice to slowly reduce the environmental temperature over several days prior to weaning. One should anticipate that some cooling will occur after transition to a crib, resulting in an increase in metabolic rate if the infant can mount a response. One recent report noted an 18% increase (increased caloric needs by 17 kcal/d).[81] Thus, the ability to wean from an isolette may depend on the ability to institute BAT thermogenesis. The amount of effective BAT would be dependent on the amount of BAT present at birth and the amount of BAT recruited since birth, which would in turn be dependent on some exposure to cooling, including the effectiveness of an "adaptation" period prior to weaning. After moving to a crib, using a hat and extra clothing for a short period may be necessary until the temperature becomes stable and the infant can be managed without excessive clothing. If the infant has reached 32 weeks PMA and is otherwise stable, every effort should be made to ensure safe sleep practices (supine sleeping, remove extra blankets and other soft materials).[82] A recent Cochrane review found that medically stable preterm infants can be transferred to an unheated open crib at 1600 g without adverse effects on temperature stability or weight gain. However, earlier weaning does not necessarily result in earlier discharge.[83]

Hypothermia, Hyperthermia, and Fever

Both hypo- and hyperthermia are common occurrences in the NICU. Hypothermia most commonly occurs soon after birth and is associated with delivery room care. Cold stress (core temperature < 36.5°C) can be associated with mottled or pale skin, increased capillary refill time, increased oxygen requirements, metabolic acidosis, tachycardia, hypoglycemia, and apnea. Small infants are best initially warmed under a radiant warmer. Abdominal skin temperature should be set between 36.5°C and 37°C, with higher temperatures

chosen for the smaller infants. Ventilator or oxygen delivery gases should be warmed to 37°C and fully humidified. After skin temperature reaches the desired temperature and axillary temperature is greater than 36.5°C, the infant can be placed in an incubator (or the incubator closed in the case of the Giraffe®) with continued skin servo control. When the temperature has been stable for at least an hour, humidity at the recommended percentage can be added.

In some cases, particularly when increased environmental air temperature is used for warming, respiratory instability with apnea can occur with increasing body temperatures.[84,85] In our experience, this occurs less often when a radiant heat source is used for warming. Under stable thermal conditions, when managed with servo control, hypothermia secondary to infection will not be evident. Instead, the incubator air temperature will increase in an attempt to maintain the controlled skin temperature. It is therefore important to monitor air temperature frequently as well as skin and axillary temperature. When the infant is removed from the incubator, as for kangaroo care, the incubator should be switched to air-servo and the air temperature kept at the temperature that existed before removal of the infant. If the incubator is opened for procedures and a radiant heat source is not integrated into the incubator (such as is the case with the Giraffe), a portable radiant heater should be used to maintain skin temperature. Intentional cooling can also be performed in cases of hypoxic-ischemic encephalopathy, associated with its own unique challenges. This topic is discussed elsewhere in this volume.

Overheating when skin is servo controlled is almost always iatrogenic and can result in hyperpyrexia. This is usually indicated by an axillary temperature that is above 37.3°C and rising, tachycardia, tachypnea, restlessness, and sometimes forehead sweating. Usually, the skin is very pink, consistent with maximal vasodilation. If this occurs, any nesting or clothing materials should be removed and the probe attachment and location should be checked and corrected. In most cases, it is best to note the incubator air temperature, discontinue skin servo control, and reduce air temperature by 1°C every 15–30 minutes, closely monitoring abdominal skin and axillary temperature. When axillary temperature has reached 37°C and abdominal skin temperature reaches 36°C, servo control can be reinstituted and increased gradually as necessary to maintain axillary temperature.

Infants in the NICU will sometimes become febrile. There is an increase in axillary temperature, and many of the symptoms and signs of overheating may be present. However, infants may be lethargic instead of restless, and the skin often becomes pale with increase in capillary refill times associated with peripheral vasoconstriction, a normal response to a higher controlled temperature.

Noting whether an infant's skin is very pink or pale is one simple way to clinically distinguish between fever and overheating. Note that the thermoregulatory responses to fever are the same as those associated with cooling, including peripheral vasoconstriction to conserve heat and BAT and even shivering thermogenesis. Similar to overheating, skin servo control can be discontinued and the air temperature range gradually lowered in 0.5°C to 1°C increments to lower body temperature. True fever is rare in preterm infants, particularly in the first few days of life. If overheating has been ruled out, one should consider infection, particularly a viral infection. For example, one should consider the diagnosis of herpes simplex virus (HSV) in an infant in the first few days of life with signs of pneumonia and fever.

Oxygen Delivery Systems

Every effort should be made to ensure that all breathing gases are heated and humidified, especially for the very low birth weight preterm infant. HHHFNC devices can safely deliver air-oxygen mixtures at rates as low as 0.3 L/min and should be used until the infant is ready to be weaned from the incubator. When used at low-flow rates, care should be taken not to have any "dead" sections of tubing (those without a heating wire) in the circuit to prevent "rain out." It is important to remember that significant energy must be expended to heat and humidify room temperature and unhumidified breathing gas to 37°C at 100% relative humidity. By calculation, it is estimated that an extra 12 kcal/kg/d would be needed when using cold and unhumidified vs heated and humidified air-oxygen mixtures.

Anesthesia and Thermoregulation

Because body temperature can rapidly fall in anesthetized newborns and infants, it has been assumed that anesthetics and paralytic agents suppress nonshivering thermogenesis and peripheral vasoconstriction. The current consensus is that there is not a single mechanism by which anesthetic agents suppress thermoregulation, rather that there are selective modes of action for different types of anesthetic agents.[86] Experiments in isolated BAT suggest that suppression of BAT thermogenesis is most prominent with the volatile anesthetics, including halothane, isoflurane, and enflurane, and is less of a problem with nonvolatile agents.[86] Propofol, for example, used commonly in preterm infants, does not inhibit BAT thermogenesis[86] but appears to inhibit peripheral vasoconstriction.[87] Muscle relaxants will inhibit shivering and generalized muscle activity, leaving BAT thermogenesis as the only means of producing thermoregulatory heat. Thus, the inability to maintain body temperature is most likely a combination of

impaired vasoconstriction, BAT and shivering thermogenesis, and perhaps a lowering of the controlled temperature. To maintain body temperature during surgery, both active and passive methods can be used to reduce heat loss, including heating mattresses, radiant heaters, forced-air warming, and increasing operating room temperatures. When infants are returned to the NICU, particular care must be taken both during the transport from the operating room and during the initial period in the NICU to maintain temperature. If the infant is cold, using a radiant heat source is probably the best way to initially restore body temperature. The effects of some anesthetic or paralytic agents may be prolonged, and particular attention must be paid to maintaining an adequate thermal environment until the effects of anesthesia are no longer present.

SUMMARY AND CONCLUSIONS

This review has focused on new information about the neural control of thermoregulation, reviewed the basic concepts of clinical thermoregulatory physiology, and discussed relevant clinical issues, including care in the delivery room, maintenance of a thermoneutral environment, care in incubators and radiant warmers, and the management of hypothermia, hyperthermia, and fever. We have also discussed some issues not commonly considered, including the risks of differential skin cooling, the use of cold unhumidified breathing gas both in the delivery room and in the NICU, and the effects of recently introduced practices on the thermal environment. One of the most challenging tasks is to ensure that the NICU and delivery room are designed to reduce the risks of hypothermia by avoiding drafts, "cold spots," and large, cold radiant surfaces and achieving consistent and appropriate air temperatures.

REFERENCES

1. Stern L. Thermoregulation in the newborn infant: historical, physiological and clinical considerations. In: Smith GF, Vidyasagar D, eds. *Historical Review and Recent Advances in Neonatal and Perinatal Medicine*. Glenview, IL: Mead Johnson Nutritional Division; 1980:chap 3.
2. Buetow KC, Klein SW. Effect of maintenance of "normal" skin temperature on survival of infants of low birth weight. *Pediatrics*. 1964;34:163–170.
3. Day RL, Caliguiri L, Kamenski C, Ehrlich F. Body temperature and survival of premature infants. *Pediatrics*. 1964;34:171–181.
4. Costeloe K, Hennessy E, Gibson AT, Marlow N, Wilkinson AR. The EPICure study: outcomes to discharge from hospital for infants born at the threshold of viability. *Pediatrics*. 2000;106(4):659–671.
5. Frappell PB, Leon-Velarde F, Aguero L, Mortola JP. Response to cooling temperature in infants born at an altitude of 4,330 meters. *Am J Respir Crit Care Med*. 1998;158(6):1751–1756.

6. Irestedt L, Lagercrantz H, Hjemdahl P, Hagnevik K, Belfrage P. Fetal and maternal plasma catecholamine levels at elective cesarean section under general or epidural anesthesia versus vaginal delivery. *Am J Obstet Gynecol.* 1982;142(8):1004–1010.

7. Clarke L, Heasman L, Firth K, Symonds ME. Influence of route of delivery and ambient temperature on thermoregulation in newborn lambs. *Am J Physiol.* 1997;272(6 Pt 2):R1931–R1939.

8. Heasman L, Clarke L, Symonds ME. Influence of thyrotrophin-releasing hormone on thermoregulatory adaptation after birth in near-term lambs delivered by caesarean section. *Exp Physiol.* 1999;84(5):979–987.

9. Gunn TR, Ball KT, Gluckman PD. Withdrawal of placental prostaglandins permits thermogenic responses in fetal sheep brown adipose tissue. *J Appl Physiol.* 1993;74(3):998–1004.

10. Gunn TR, Ball KT, Gluckman PD. Reversible umbilical cord occlusion: effects on thermogenesis in utero. *Pediatr Res.* 1991;30(6):513–517.

11. Sack J, Beaudry M, DeLamater PV, Oh W, Fisher DA. Umbilical cord cutting triggers hypertriiodothyroninemia and non-shivering thermogenesis in the newborn lamb. *Pediatr Res.* 1976;10(3):169.

12. Sawa R, Asakura H, Power GG. Changes in plasma adenosine during simulated birth of fetal sheep. *J Appl Physiol.* 1991;70:1524–1528.

13. Morishima HO, Yeh MN, Niemann WH, James LS. Temperature gradient between fetus and mother as an index for assessing intrauterine fetal condition. *Am J Obstet Gynecol.* 1977;129(4):443–448.

14. Power GG, Kawamura T, Dale PS, Schroder H, Gilbert RD. Temperature responses following ventilation of the fetal sheep in utero. *J Dev Physiol.* 1986;8(6):477–484.

15. Schroder HJ, Power GG. Increase of fetal arterial blood temperature by reduction of umbilical blood flow in chronically instrumented fetal sheep. *Pfluegers Arch.* 1994;427(1–2):190–192.

16. Morrison SF, Nakamura K. Central neural pathways for thermoregulation. *Front Biosci.* 2011;16:74–104.

17. Romanovsky AA. Thermoregulation: some concepts have changed. Functional architecture of the thermoregulatory system. *Am J Physiol Regul Integr Comp Physiol.* 2007;292(1):R37–R46.

18. McKemy DD, Neuhausser WM, Julius D. Identification of a cold receptor reveals a general role for TRP channels in thermosensation. *Nature.* 2002;416(6876):52–58.

19. Craig AD. How do you feel? Interoception: the sense of the physiological condition of the body. *Nat Rev Neurosci.* 2002;3:655–666.

20. Craig AD, Bushnell MC, Zhang ET, Blomqvist A. A thalamic nucleus specific for pain and temperature sensation. *Nature.* 1994;372:770–773.

21. Li J, Xiong K, Y. P, Dong Y, Kaneko T, Mizuno N. Medullary dorsal horn neurons providing axons to both the parabracheal nucleus and thalamus. *J Comp Neurol.* 2006;498:539–551.

22. Hylden JL, Anton F, Nahin RL. Spinal lamina I projection neurons in the rat: collateral innervation of parabrachial area and thalamus. *Neuroscience.* 1989;28:27–37.

23. Nakamura K, Morrison SF. A thermosensory pathway mediating heat defense responses. *Proc Natl Acad Sci USA.* 2010;107:8848–8853.

24. Nakamura K, Morrison SF. A thermosensory pathway that controls body temperature. *Nat Neurosci.* 2008;11:62–71.

25. Gupta BN, Nier K, Hensel H. Cold-sensitive afferents from the abdomen. *Pflueger Arch.* 1979;380:203–204.

26. Riedel W. Warm receptors in the dorsal abdominal wall of the rabbit. Pflueger Archives 1976;361:205–206.

27. Guieu JD, Hardy JD. Effects of heating and cooling of the spinal cord on preoptic unit activity. *J Appl Physiol.* 1970;29:675–683.

28. Boulant JA, Hardy JD. The effect of spinal and skin temperatures on the firing rate and thermosensitivity of preoptic neurones. *J Physiol.* 1974;240(3):639–660.

29. Thomas KA. Back to basics: thermoregulation in neonates. *Neonatal Netw.* 1994;13(2):15–22.

30. Hey EN. The relation between environmental temperature and oxygen consumption in the new-born baby. *J Physiol.* 1969;200:589–603.

31. Wallin BG, Charkoudian N. Sympathetic neural control of integrated cardiovascular function: insights from measurement of human sympathetic nerve activity. *Muscle Nerve.* 2007;36(5):595–614.

32. Hodges GJ, Jackson DN, Mattar L, Johnson JM, Shoemaker JK. Neuropeptide Y and neurovascular control in skeletal muscle and skin. *Am J Physiol Regul Integr Comp Physiol.* 2009;297(3):R546–R555.

33. Hodges GJ, Kosiba WA, Zhao K, Johnson JM. The involvement of norepinephrine, neuropeptide Y, and nitric oxide in the cutaneous vasodilator response to local heating in humans. *J Appl Physiol.* 2008;105(1):233–240.

34. Escourrou P, Freund PR, Rowell LB, Johnson DG. Splanchnic vasoconstriction in heat-stressed men: role of renin-angiotensin system. *J Appl Physiol.* 1982;52(6):1438–1443.

35. Harpin VA, Rutter N. Sweating in preterm babies. *J Pediatr.* 1982;100(4):614–619.

36. Dubowitz LM, Dubowitz V, Goldberg C. Clinical assessment of gestational age in the newborn infant. *J Pediatr.* 1970;77(1):1–10.

37. Salavitabar A, Haidet KK, Adkins CS, Susman EJ, Palmer C, Storm H. Preterm infants' sympathetic arousal and associated behavioral responses to sound stimuli in the neonatal intensive care unit. *Adv Neonatal Care.* 2010;10(3):158–166.

38. Storm H. Development of emotional sweating in preterms measured by skin conductance changes. *Early Hum Dev.* 2001;62(2):149–158.

39. Cannon B, Nedergaard J. Brown adipose tissue: function and physiological significance. *Physiol Rev.* 2004;84(1):277–359.

40. Saito M, Okamatsu-Ogura Y, Matsushita M, et al. High incidence of metabolically active brown adipose tissue in healthy adult humans: effects of cold exposure and adiposity. *Diabetes.* 2009;58(7):1526–1531.

41. Himms-Hagen J. Does brown adipose tissue (BAT) have a role in the physiology or treatment of human obesity? *Rev Endocr Metab Disord.* 2001;2(4):395–401.

42. Smales OR, Kime R. Thermoregulation in babies immediately after birth. *Arch Dis Child.* 1978;53(1):58–61.

43. Aherne W, Hull D. The site of heat production in the newborn infant. *Proc R Soc Med.* 1964;57:1172–1173.

44. Cannon B, Nedergaard J. Nonshivering thermogenesis and its adequate measurement in metabolic studies. *J Exp Biol.* 2011;214(Pt 2):242–253.

45. Hull D, Smales ORC. Heat production in the newborn. In: Sinclair JC, ed. *Temperature Regulation and Energy Metabolism in the Newborn.* New York, NY: Grune & Stratton; 1978:129–156.

46. Glass L, Silverman WA, Sinclair JC. Effect of the thermal environment on cold resistance and growth of small infants after the first week of life. *Pediatrics.* 1968;41(6):1033–1046.

47. Kattwinkel J, Perlman JM, Aziz K, et al. Neonatal resuscitation: 2010 American Heart Association Guidelines for cardiopulmonary resuscitation and emergency cardiovascular care. *Pediatrics.* 2010;126(5):e1400–e1413.

48. Singh A, Duckett J, Newton T, Watkinson M. Improving neonatal unit admission temperatures in preterm babies: exothermic mattresses, polythene bags or a traditional approach? *J Perinatol.* 2010;30(1):45–49.

49. Sedin G. Physics and physiology of human neonatal incubation. In: Polin RA, Fox WW, Abman SH, eds. *Fetal and Neonatal Physiology*. Philadelphia, PA: Saunders; 2004;chap 57.

50. te Pas AB, Lopriore E, Dito I, Morley CJ, Walther FJ. Humidified and heated air during stabilization at birth improves temperature in preterm infants. *Pediatrics*. 2010;125(6):e1427–e1432.

51. Kubicka ZJ, Limauro J, Darnall RA. Heated, humidified high-flow nasal cannula therapy: yet another way to deliver continuous positive airway pressure? *Pediatrics*. 2008;121(1):82–88.

52. Lighton JRB. *Measuring Metabolic Rates: A Manual for Scientists*. New York, NY: Oxford University Press; 2008.

53. Bauer K, Laurenz M, Ketteler J, Versmold H. Longitudinal study of energy expenditure in preterm neonates < 30 weeks' gestation during the first three postnatal weeks. *J Pediatr*. 2003;142(4):390–396.

54. Hardy JD, Gagge AP, Rapp GM. Proposed standard system of symbols for thermal physiology. *J Appl Physiol*. 1969;27:439–446.

55. Klaus MH, Fanaroff AA. The physical environment. In: Klaus MH, Fanaroff AA, eds. *Care of the High Risk Neonate*. 5th ed. Philadelphia, PA: Saunders; 2001:130–146.

56. Darnall RA Jr, Ariagno RL. Minimal oxygen consumption in infants cared for under overhead radiant warmers compared with conventional incubators. *J Pediatr*. 1978;93(2):283–287.

57. Flenady VJ, Woodgate PG. Radiant warmers versus incubators for regulating body temperature in newborn infants. *Cochrane Database Syst Rev*. 2003(4):CD000435.

58. Mestyan J, Jarai I, Bata G, Fekete M. The significance of facial skin temperature in the chemical heat regulation of premature infants. *Biol Neonat*. 1964;7:243–254.

59. Mestyan J, Jarai I, Bata G, Fekete M. Surface temperature versus deep body temperature and the metabolic response to cold of hypothermic premature infants. Biol Neonat 1964;7:230–242.

60. Darnall RA. The role of CO_2 and central chemoreception in the control of breathing in the fetus and the neonate. *Respir Physiol Neurobiol*. 2010;173(3):201–212.

61. Askie LM, Henderson-Smart DJ, Ko H. Restricted versus liberal oxygen exposure for preventing morbidity and mortality in preterm or low birth weight infants. *Cochrane Database Syst Rev*. 2009(1):CD001077.

62. Hill JR. The oxygen consumption of new-born and adult mammals. Its dependence on the oxygen tension in the inspired air and on the environmental temperature. *J Physiol*. 1959(149):346–373.

63. Ceruti E. Chemoreceptor reflexes in the newborn infant: effect of cooling on the response to hypoxia. *Pediatrics*. 1966;37(4):556–564.

64. Madden CJ, Morrison SF. Hypoxic activation of arterial chemoreceptors inhibits sympathetic outflow to brown adipose tissue in rats. *J Physiol*. 2005;566(Pt 2):559–573.

65. Parmeggiani PL, Rabini C. Shivering and panting during sleep. *Brain Res*. 1967;6(4):789–791.

66. Parmeggiani PL, Zamboni G, Cianci T, Calasso M. Absence of thermoregulatory vasomotor responses during fast wave sleep in cats. *Electroencephalogr Clin Neurophysiol*. 1977;42(3):372–380.

67. Stothers JK, Warner RM. Oxygen consumption of the newborn infant in a cool environment, measured within regard to sleep state. *J Physiol*. 1977;273:16.

68. Darnall RA, Ariagno RL. The effect of sleep state on active thermoregulation in the premature infant. *Pediatr Res*. 1982;16:512–514.

69. Uslu S, Ozdemir H, Bulbul A, et al. A comparison of different methods of temperature measurements in sick newborns. *J Trop Pediatr*. 2011;57(6):418–423.

70. Dahm LS, James LS. Newborn temperature and calculated heat loss in the delivery room. *Pediatrics*. 1972;49(4):504–513.

71. Watkinson M. Temperature control of premature infants in the delivery room. *Clin Perinatol*. 2006;33(1):43–53, vi.

72. Kent AL, Williams J. Increasing ambient operating theatre temperature and wrapping in polyethylene improves admission temperature in premature infants. *J Paediatr Child Health*. 2008;44(6):325–331.

73. Vohra S, Frent G, Campbell V, Abbott M, Whyte R. Effect of polyethylene occlusive skin wrapping on heat loss in very low birth weight infants at delivery: a randomized trial. *J Pediatr*. 1999;134(5):547–551.

74. Vohra S, Roberts RS, Zhang B, Janes M, Schmidt B. Heat Loss Prevention (HeLP) in the delivery room: a randomized controlled trial of polyethylene occlusive skin wrapping in very preterm infants. *J Pediatr*. 2004;145(6):750–753.

75. Meyer MP, Bold GT. Admission temperatures following radiant warmer or incubator transport for preterm infants < 28 weeks: a randomised study. *Arch Dis Child Fetal Neonatal Ed*. 2007;92(4): F295–F297.

76. Stothers JK. Head insulation and heat loss in the newborn. *Arch Dis Child*. 1981;56:530–534.

77. Thomas KA. Preterm infant thermal responses to caregiving differ by incubator control mode. *J Perinatol*. 2003;23(8):640–645.

78. Sinclair JC. Servo-control for maintaining abdominal skin temperature at 36°C in low birth weight infants. *Cochrane Database Syst Rev*. 2002(1):CD001074.

79. Sinclair L, Crisp J, Sinn J. Variability in incubator humidity practices in the management of preterm infants. *J Paediatr Child Health*. 2009;45(9):535–540.

80. Sinclair L, Sinn JKH. Higher versus lower humidity for the prevention of morbidity and mortality in preterm infants in incubators. Cochrane Database Syst Rev 2007;(2):CD006472. doi:10.1002/14651858.

81. Dollberg S, Mimouni FB, Weintraub V. Energy expenditure in infants weaned from a convective incubator. *Am J Perinatol*. 2004;21(5):253–256.

82. Moon RY, Darnall RA, Goodstein MH, Hauck FR, Willinger M, Shapiro-Mendoza CK. SIDS and other sleep-related infant deaths: expansions for recommendations for a safe infant sleeping environment. *Pediatrics*. 2011;128(5):1030–1039.

83. New K, Flenady V, Davies MW. Transfer of preterm infants from incubator to open cot at lower versus higher body weight. *Cochrane Database Syst Rev*. 2011;9:CD004214.

84. Daily WJ, Klaus M, Meyer HB. Apnea in premature infants: monitoring, incidence, heart rate changes, and an effect of environmental temperature. *Pediatrics*. 1969;43:510–518.

85. Perlstein PH, Edwards NK, Sutherland JM. Apnea in premature infants and incubator-air-temperature changes. *N Engl J Med*. 1970;282(9):461–466.

86. Ohlson KB, Lindahl SG, Cannon B, Nedergaard J. Thermogenesis inhibition in brown adipocytes is a specific property of volatile anesthetics. *Anesthesiology*. 2003;98(2):437–448.

87. Leslie K, Sessler DI, Bjorksten AR, et al. Propofol causes a dose-dependent decrease in the thermoregulatory threshold for vasoconstriction but has little effect on sweating. *Anesthesiology*. 1994;81(2):353–360.

Monitoring Devices

Valerie Y. Chock

IDEAL BEDSIDE NEWBORN INTENSIVE CARE UNIT MONITORING

Goals

Accuracy: Validation against gold standard measurements is needed. Accuracy of measurements must also span gestational age and birth weight differences of all patients in a newborn intensive care unit (NICU) setting. Movement of neonates should not significantly interfere with measurements. Fluctuation in temperature and humidity should also not affect monitoring.

Reliability: Application, data acquisition, and removal of monitoring devices should not be affected by differences in caregivers. Measurements should demonstrate minimal variation with respect to time of monitoring, caregiver, and infant position.

Feasibility: Devices should be minimally invasive, inexpensive, and easy to apply and remove for widespread use in a NICU setting. Minimal interference with patient care is essential, for example, with smaller-size neonatal sensors or with portable or wireless devices. Data would ideally be continuously recordable, easy to interpret, and compatible with simultaneous monitoring of other physiologic parameters. Real-time data collection would also allow personnel to respond to an event at the same time the data are being displayed.

Patient safety: Sensors, leads, or other methods of acquiring data must be safe for patient use. Considerations of skin sensitivity have led to the development of smaller-size hydrocolloid sensors. Risk of infection is typically minimized by disposable equipment or limiting duration

of patient exposure to monitoring device interfaces. Signal interference between different modes of monitoring and electromagnetic radiation shielding must be considered for neonatal use of any monitoring device.

CARDIAC MONITORING

Electrocardiogram

Description: An electrocardiogram (EKG or ECG) provides measurement of electrical signals generated by cardiac cell potentials by a surface electrode. The most common type of electrode for EKG monitoring is a silver-silver chloride, foil-based electrode. Instead of requiring a separate electrolyte solution to be applied to the patient, most EKG monitoring electrodes now come packaged in sets of three with an adhesive electrolyte gel backing (hydrogel) that serves as the electrolyte interface solution as well as an adhesive. An approaching excitation wave to a surface lead is recorded as a positive potential and represented on the EKG as an upward deflection. Typical lead placement and EKG module diagram are shown in Figure 5-1.

Indications: The EKG is used for measurement of heart rate for conditions potentially leading to cardiac instability. Basic arrhythmias and abnormal waveforms may be detectable. However, for complete evaluation of arrhythmias, a 12-lead EKG is recommended rather than the typical 3-lead EKG used for continuous-monitoring purposes.

Accuracy/Reliability: Accuracy is dependent on skill level and experience of the interpreter. Computer-assisted interpretation should not be relied on for accuracy.

47

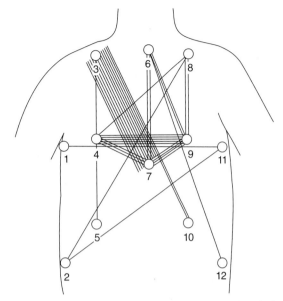

FIGURE 5-1 Optimal electrocardiogram (EKG) lead placement. (Adapted with permission from Baird TM, et al. Optimal electrode location for monitoring the ECG and breathing in neonates. *Pediatr Pulmonol.* 1992;12(4):247–250.)

Reliability for measuring heart rate is good, and signal is acquired more readily than pulse oximetry.

Limitations:

1. Artifacts: Computer-based cardiac monitoring systems now have more sophisticated filtering components to reduce noise and artifact. However, artifacts may still be generated by poor contact between skin and electrode or improper placement of leads. Electrical interference from other equipment may be problematic. Problems with cable connections, cables, or internal hardware or software failure of the EKG module may also contribute to artifact.

2. Skin fragility: In extremely preterm infants, removal of adhesive EKG leads has been associated with stripping of the stratum corneum, with the potential increased risk of infection[1] and increased transepidermal water losses.[2]

3. Difficulties with lead placement: A limited flat thoracic surface, especially in a preterm infant, may cause difficulties with lead placement, resulting in more artifact generation.

4. Electrical safety: Allowable current level for flow through any patient-connected lead is established at 10 mA.[3]

Cardiac Output Monitoring

Impedance Electrical Cardiometry

Description: Impedance electrical cardiometry is a noninvasive assessment of beat-to-beat cardiac output by measuring changes in thoracic electrical bioimpedance of aortic blood flow during the cardiac cycle with 4 adhesive skin sensors. The related concept of electrical velocimetry is based on the assumption that conductivity of blood in the aorta changes during the cardiac cycle. A random orientation of erythrocytes occurs during periods of no flow across the aortic valve (lower conductivity), followed by alignment of erythrocytes in parallel with blood flow during pulsatile flow across the aortic valve (higher conductivity). Impedance is the reciprocal of conductivity; thus, impedance waveforms are measured with this technology to calculate stroke volume and cardiac output[4]: SV (mL) × HR (1/min) = CO (mL/min) (Figure 5-2).

Indications: This is potentially useful for monitoring of cardiac output in neonates with circulatory compromise. Infants with congenital heart disease, hypotension requiring pressors, infection, or other conditions contributing to hemodynamic instability may benefit from noninvasive cardiac output monitoring.

Accuracy/Reliability: This method was compared in adults to cardiac catheterization and thermodilution techniques employing the Fick principle for measurement of cardiac output as well as echocardiographic measurements of stroke volume and cardiac output.[5-7] It was found that estimates of cardiac output from electrical cardiometry were highly correlated with both thermodilution techniques (precision of ± 0.46 L/min)[7] and transesophageal Doppler echocardiographic measurements of cardiac output ($r^2 = 0.86$).[5] However, validation studies in the pediatric population are limited,[8] and no data are currently available for the neonatal population.

Limitations: This procedure requires additional validation for use in neonatal patients. Because of varying degrees of ductal shunting in a neonate, measurements may not be accurate. Placement of sensors on the face, neck, and chest of a neonate may also not be feasible for some extremely small or preterm infants with skin sensitivity. An accurate weight must be input by the user to calculate stroke volume.

Continuous-Wave Doppler Ultrasound

Description: Compact continuous-wave Doppler ultrasound devices can be used for noninvasive serial measurements of cardiac output after acquiring a Doppler waveform of transvalvar flow.

Indications: Indications for use are conditions of hemodynamic instability or circulatory compromise as listed previously for which cardiac output measurements may be useful to assess response to treatment and time.

Accuracy/Reliability: Reliability of measurements largely is dependent on the experience of the user. Conflicting studies of preterm and term neonates using

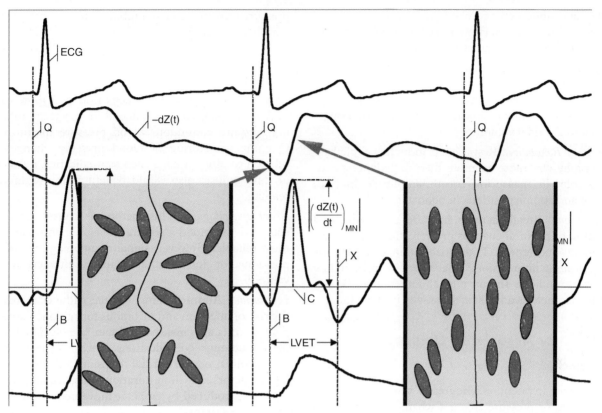

FIGURE 5-2 Parallel readings of electrocardiogram (EKG), impedance waveforms, and pulse plethysmogram. (Used with permission from Cardiotronic, Inc.)

a continuous-wave Doppler ultrasound (USCOM; Coffs Harbour, NSW, Australia) found good interrater correlation (0.93)[9] but poor correlation with conventional echocardiography measurements.[10] When compared to the gold standard thermodilution method, a continuous-wave Doppler ultrasound device underestimated cardiac output during states of high cardiac output[11] and showed poor agreement in children.[12]

Limitations: Currently, this technique is not ideal for continuous monitoring as the device must be held in place by the user. This requires training and experience to acquire appropriate images for accurate assessment of cardiac output. Difficulties in reliably measuring cardiac output require additional clinical research with this modality.[9,10]

RESPIRATORY MONITORING

Surface Monitoring

Transthoracic Impedance Pneumography

Description: Transthoracic impedance pneumography measures electrical impedance changes between two electrodes on the thorax during respiration. Change in impedance from breathing activity is separated from baseline impedance of the thorax, and then the signal is filtered by a microprocessor. Most devices utilize the same leads as used for EKG measurement.

Indications: This method is used for measurement of respiratory rate, especially during conditions associated with tachypnea, or for detection of apneic events.

Accuracy/Reliability: Measurement of breath amplitude by impedance pneumography had poor correlation with tidal volume, with higher values during supine positioning compared to prone positioning.[13] This type of respiratory monitoring also frequently underestimated breath amplitude.[14] Impedance monitors may also miss obstructive apneic events and misinterpret cardiac artifact as a breath.[15]

Limitations: Introduction of artifact is common because of improper lead placement, poor skin contact, or patient movement. Changes in impedance may also be introduced by changes in thoracic blood volume unrelated to respirations. The technique is less accurate for detection of obstructive apnea. Skin irritation from the electrodes may be a limitation, especially in preterm neonates.

Inductance Plethysmography

Description: In inductance plethysmography, a band containing an electrical wire coil is placed around the chest and abdomen of an infant. The inductance is measured and is proportional to changes in the area of the thorax and abdomen as the patient breathes.

Indications: This is another indirect monitor of respiration for infants requiring monitoring of respiratory rate or to detect apnea. Also, it is useful for estimates of lung tidal volumes because the signal is proportional to the tidal volume.

Accuracy/Reliability: Respiratory inductance plethysmography was more accurate than impedance pneumography in measuring breath amplitude in both prone and supine positions in neonates.[14]

Limitations: Breath activity may be underestimated because of postural changes or overestimated because of infant movement. Thoracoabdominal asynchrony may result in imprecision.[16] Placement of an encircling band around the thorax and abdomen may be too cumbersome or lead to skin sensitivity in some infants.

Ventilator-Associated Devices

Pneumotachography

Description: In pneumotachography, sensors detect airflow, heat, or pressure changes when placed in series with the airway.

Indications: Mechanically ventilated patients requiring real-time monitoring of respirations, pressure waves, flow waves, and volumes to assist in adjustment of ventilation when patient lung compliance or resistance changes.

Accuracy/Reliability: Accuracy of measurements from a pneumotachograph when compared to spirometry-measured flows and volumes is largely dependent on the type of flow sensor, placement, and calibration techniques that are used.[17]

Limitations: This method is limited by the degree of air leakage around the endotracheal tube, which will make measurements inaccurate.

New Cardiorespiratory-Monitoring Devices

Several newer types of cardiorespiratory-monitoring devices are currently under development to eliminate the need for traditional EKG leads. One type uses a piezoelectric transducer sensor placed under an infant to detect an acoustic cardiorespiratory signal.[18]

BLOOD PRESSURE MONITORING

Continuous Blood Pressure

Description: Continuous blood pressure monitoring is obtained from an indwelling arterial line by a catheter

pressure transducer in an umbilical arterial catheter or peripheral arterial catheter. Blood flow deflects a diaphragm, which is relayed into an electrical signal after adjustment for parameters such as viscous drag factor and stiffness of the transducer.

Indication: The need for recognition of hypotension or hypertension in critically ill or preterm infants may require continuous blood pressure monitoring. Ongoing monitoring of blood pressure changes in relation to interventions such as medication infusions or fluid boluses also would benefit from continuous reading.

Accuracy/Reliability: This method is considered gold standard for blood pressure measurements and the most reliable. However, signal dampening from malpositioned or clotted catheters may result in erroneous values.[19]

Limitations: An in-dwelling vascular catheter increases the risk of infection and thrombus formation. Catheter placement is also invasive and can be associated with life-threatening complications, such as necrotizing enterocolitis or pericardial effusions, if misplaced. These factors may limit duration of use. Artifacts may also be introduced by catheter movement or air bubbles in the system.

Indirect (Noninvasive) Blood Pressure Monitoring

Description: An occlusive device typically consisting of a cuff with an inflatable bladder is placed around an extremity to cause occlusion of arterial flow distal to the cuff. Measurements of systolic and diastolic pressure are obtained noninvasively during cuff deflation using the oscillometric method, which detects small pulsations in the artery through a pressure sensor (Figure 5-3). Different algorithms exist to convert these oscillatory signals into systolic and diastolic

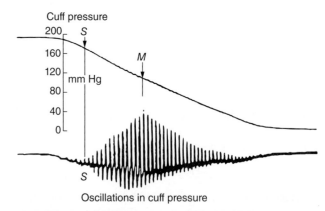

FIGURE 5-3 Oscillometric method of blood pressure monitoring. (Reproduced with permission from Geddes LA. Cardiovascular devices and their applications. New York, NY: John Wiley & Sons; 1984.)

pressure readings. Cuff placement on the upper arm or calf in preterm infants has not shown significant differences in pressure measurements.[20]

Indications: Indirect measurements reflect the need for monitoring of blood pressure when an indwelling arterial catheter is not available or infeasible.

Accuracy/Reliability: The differences between the oscillometric method and continuous blood pressure monitoring by a catheter transducer are minimal in newborns, including preterm extremely low birth weight infants.[21] However, poor correlation between readings has been noted in *hypotensive* preterm infants, for whom oscillometric measurements read higher than continuous blood pressure measurements.[21,22] Cuff size is also important for the accuracy of noninvasive measurements, with the most accurate measurements associated with a ratio of cuff width to arm circumference of 0.44–0.55.[23] Small cuff sizes are associated with overestimated blood pressure measurements.

Limitations: This monitoring does not provide continuous measurement. Accuracy is also less certain with severe hypotension. Measurements are sensitive to patient movement and are dependent on selection of cuff size in comparison to infant limb size.

PULSE OXIMETRY

Description: A pulse oximeter utilizes a sensor with two light-emitting diodes placed over the skin of a well-perfused capillary bed to measure the percentage of oxygen saturation of hemoglobin available for oxygen transport. The amount of light absorbed is proportional to the amount of oxygenated and deoxygenated hemoglobin present in the underlying tissue, although background absorption must be subtracted from pulsatile changes in absorption with each heartbeat to reflect arterial oxygen saturation. Figure 5-4 shows an oxyhemoglobin dissociation curve for neonates; the curve is corrected for fetal hemoglobin. The normal oxyhemoglobin dissociation curve in a term infant is shifted to the left in comparison to an adult curve because of the increased presence of fetal hemoglobin. The curve shifts to the right with increased acidosis and increasing temperature.

Indications: Pulse oximetry provides noninvasive, continuous measurement of oxygen saturation levels, particularly in infants at risk for poor oxygen delivery. Recommendations have also been made for use of pulse oximetry in the delivery room to assist with neonatal resuscitation efforts.[24]

Accuracy/Reliability: Performance differences between oximeters are considerable because of differences in signal-processing software and calibration curves.[25]

Inaccuracy of pulse oximetry occurs at upper and lower extremes of values. Saturations greater than 95% do not allow for precise estimation of PaO_2.[26] Saturations below 70% are also less precise and highly variable between devices, partly because of the minimal amount of calibration data available for these low-saturation states.[27] The pulse oximeter will also measure other hemoglobin fractions (eg, methemoglobin or carboxyhemoglobin), leading to falsely high values.

Limitations:

1. Poor correlation between SpO_2 and PaO_2 occurs at both upper and lower extremes of values. Pulse oximetry values at these extremes may require correlation with arterial blood gas values.

2. Conditions associated with poor perfusion and loss of pulsatility (eg, septic shock) will result in loss of signal or inaccurately low readings.

3. Patient movement, excessive external lighting, or electrical interference may cause artifacts, although newer signal-processing algorithms may minimize these effects.

4. Abnormal hemoglobin (eg, methemoglobin) will affect values.

TISSUE OXIMETRY

Near-Infrared Spectroscopy

Description: In near-infrared spectroscopy (NIRS), monitoring of regional tissue oxygenation is accomplished through the transmission and subsequent detection of near-infrared light by an adhesive-backed sensor placed on the skin. Cerebral, renal, and mesenteric regional saturations are most commonly measured with sensor placement on the forehead, flank, and abdomen, respectively. With spatially resolved spectroscopy, differential absorption of near-infrared light by oxygenated and deoxygenated hemoglobin in the underlying tissue allows for calculation of a regional tissue oxygen saturation, which reflects a weighted average of both venous and arterial blood. Regional saturation levels (rSO_2) reflect a regional balance between oxygen supply and demand.

Indications: NIRS is used for monitoring of cerebral oxygenation in the context of impaired cerebral blood flow as may be seen with conditions such as hypoxic ischemic encephalopathy, congenital heart disease, intraventricular hemorrhage, and veno-venous extracorporeal membrane oxygenation (ECMO). Use of NIRS to indirectly measure cerebral autoregulation has also been described[28,29] and is depicted in Figure 5-5. Measuring somatic saturations may reflect earlier hemodynamic compromise.[30] Monitoring of mesenteric oxygenation

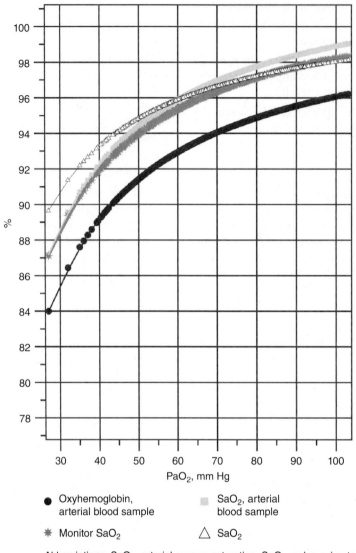

● Oxyhemoglobin,   SaO₂, arterial
   arterial blood sample   blood sample

✳ Monitor SaO₂   △ SaO₂

Abbreviations: SaO₂, arterial oxygen saturation; SaO₂, pulse oximetry oxygen saturation.

FIGURE 5-4 Neonatal hemoglobin oxygen dissociation curve. (With permission from Shiao SY, Ou CN. Validation of oxygen saturation monitoring in neonates. *Am J Crit Care.* 2007;16(2):168–178.)

to detect early necrotizing enterocolitis is also under investigation.[31]

Accuracy/Reliability: Accuracy and reliability are validated with internal jugular venous bulb saturation measurements ($r^2 = 0.9$).[32]

Limitations:

1. Depth of signal penetration limits measurement of deeper-tissue structures.

2. Absolute values may differ significantly between patients depending on location of sensor placement, and reference values are still being studied in different populations. NIRS devices are better for monitoring trends in tissue saturation and changes over time or with interventions in an individual patient.

3. NIRS values must be interpreted in the context of other factors that influence oxygen delivery and extraction, such as anemia, hypotension, hypocarbia, and metabolic rate.

Visible Light Spectroscopy

Description: Also known as reflectance spectrophotometry, visible light spectroscopy (VLS) utilizes visible light to noninvasively measure hemoglobin oxygen saturation in mucosal tissues. A fiber-optic sensor emits and then detects white light, which is transmitted to underlying tissues and differentially absorbed by oxygenated hemoglobin. VLS measures small, superficial tissue depths compared to NIRS and is better for use on thin mucosal surfaces like oral, esophageal, or rectal

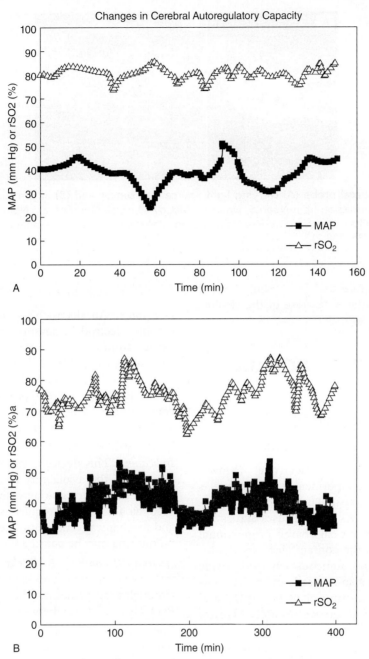

FIGURE 5-5 Examples of near-infrared spectroscopy (NIRS) monitoring to measure cerebral autoregulation. (With permission from Chock VY, Ramamoorthy C, Van Meurs KP. Cerebral autoregulation in neonates with a hemodynamically significant patent ductus arteriosus. *J Pediatr.* 2012;160(6):936–942.) A, Simultaneous rSO_2 (cerebral oxygenation) and mean arterial pressure (MAP) tracing from a 26-week gestation infant. Despite fluctuations in MAP, rSO_2 remains relatively stable, indicating intact cerebral autoregulation ($r = 0.43$). B, The same preterm infant now demonstrates concordance between MAP and rSO_2, indicating a loss of cerebral autoregulation ($r = 0.82$).

mucosa (Figure 5-6). StO_2 (mucosal tissue oxygenation) can also be measured under conditions of poor perfusion.

Indications: Settings of tissue ischemia may be useful for real-time VLS monitoring, including monitoring of neonates with congenital heart disease or hypotension and during ECMO.

Accuracy/Reliability: Although validated in animal and adult human subjects, neonatal studies are limited. Buccal StO_2 had a weak correlation with left ventricular output ($r = 0.37$) but no correlation with middle cerebral artery flow.[33]

Limitations: VLS is still predominantly a research tool at present and will require additional validation and

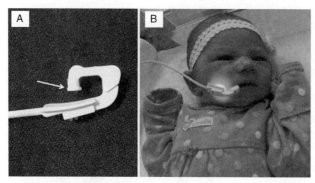

FIGURE 5-6 Neonatal buccal probe (A) carrying light source and sensor and (B) in use for monitoring buccal tissue saturations. (With permission from Noori S, Drabu B, McCoy M, et al. Noori et. al.: Non-invasive measurement of local tissue perfusion and its correlation with hemodynamic indices during the early postnatal period in term neonates. *J Perinatol.* 2011; 31(12):785–788.[33])

feasibility studies for future use. It is mainly limited to use over mucosal surfaces because of the shallow depth of light penetration.

ALTERNATIVES TO BLOOD GAS MONITORING

Transcutaneous Monitoring

Transcutaneous Carbon Dioxide Monitoring

Description: A pH-sensitive electrode (Stowe-Severinghaus) with a semipermeable membrane is applied to the skin for transcutaneous carbon dioxide monitoring (tcP_{CO_2}). As CO_2 diffuses across the skin, it generates an electrical charge proportional to the change in pH of the contact electrolyte solution. A combined transcutaneous carbon dioxide and oxygen sensor can also be used, and newer sensors also combine monitoring of pCO_2, SpO_2, and pulse from a single optoelectrode (Sentec, Medical Dynamics, Inc.).

Indications: This method is used for conditions requiring close monitoring of CO_2 levels, such as infants who are mechanically ventilated, recently extubated, or are otherwise at risk for significant hypercarbia or hypocarbia and for whom frequent blood gas sampling or end-tidal CO_2 monitoring is unavailable or infeasible.

Accuracy/reliability: Different systems have different accuracy levels, but detection of hypercarbia has better sensitivity and specificity than detection of hypocarbia.[34]

Limitations: The need for daily recalibration and relocation to different skin sites is a limitation. Extremely preterm infants with fragile skin may be at risk for irritation from the electrode. Poor perfusion may result in inaccurately high measurements.

Transcutaneous Oxygen Monitoring

Description: An electrochemical sensor (Clark polarographic electrode) measures the partial pressure of oxygen from the skin surface for transcutaneous oxygen monitoring (tcP_{O_2}). The oxygen from the skin reacts with the platinum/silver chloride sensor to create an electrical current proportional to the oxygen concentration. This requires heating the electrode to 43°C–44°C for better arterialization of the capillary bed prior to sensor placement.

Indications: This device is less frequently utilized now because of the availability of newer technologies. In conditions requiring noninvasive monitoring of PaO_2, such as for infants requiring supplemental oxygen and mechanical ventilation, the use of transcutaneous monitoring may be considered.

Accuracy/Reliability: A linear relationship between tcP_{O_2} measurements and PaO_2 values has been found, although these values may be discrepant at high or low PaO_2 levels and vary between different instruments.[34]

Limitations: The need for frequent recalibration and repositioning of the electrode to different skin sites is limiting. Similarly, there is a risk for skin irritation and thermal burns from the electrode, particularly in preterm infants with sensitive skin. Poor skin perfusion or edema may also reduce the accuracy of measurements.

Capnography

Description: Capnography involves continuous measurement of the partial pressure of expired respiratory gases (Pet_{CO_2}). Most commonly, it uses infrared (IR) spectroscopy in a module attached to the patient's breathing circuit. IR light absorption is proportional to the concentration of CO_2 in the gas stream. Disposable colorimetric devices for CO_2 detection are also widely available and utilize an indicator dye that changes color after a threshold carbon dioxide level (eg, > 2%) is reached.

Indications: Colorimetric CO_2 detectors may be utilized to assist with confirmation of endotracheal intubation in the delivery room or NICU setting. In-line capnography may be useful as a trending device to monitor for hypercarbia or hypocarbia and to adjust ventilator support.

Accuracy/Reliability: Pet_{CO_2} typically underestimates $PaCO_2$ values and is less accurate among patients with primary pulmonary disease.[35] Low tidal volumes and high respiratory rates of neonates may result in falsely low Pet_{CO_2} levels.[36] However, several studies still demonstrated a strong correlation between $PaCO_2$ and Pet_{CO_2} ($r = 0.8$).[35]

Limitations: Continuous capnography cannot be used in nonintubated patients. Water vapor may absorb IR light and interfere with the accuracy of measurements. As pulmonary function worsens, capnography may be less accurate. Newer capnographic monitoring devices contribute less to dead space in the ventilator circuit, but endotracheal tube leaks will affect data acquisition.

Continuous Blood Gas Monitoring

Description: Intravascular sensors for blood gas analysis allow for real-time, continuous measurements of blood gases without patient blood loss. Several types of continuous-monitoring systems exist. Most utilize several sensors placed within an umbilical artery catheter. Another type of blood gas-monitoring system uses a closed-loop system whereby a reversible pump withdraws blood from an arterial line into a sensor cell with electrodes and then returns the blood to the patient with a heparinized flush solution.

Indication: Infants requiring frequent blood gas monitoring because of respiratory compromise, hemodynamic instability, or metabolic disorders may benefit from this type of monitoring to reduce blood loss.

Accuracy/Reliability: Initial studies in the adult population have revealed good correlation[37] with in vitro blood gas measurements, and initial studies in the neonatal population have shown minimal infection risk and good precision.[38]

Limitations: This method must use a proprietary catheter and still requires calibration with traditional blood gas analysis. Further evaluation of feasibility of use in the neonatal population is ongoing.

ELECTROENCEPHALOGRAPHY

Description: Electroencephalography (EEG) continuously records electrical activity of the brain after the placement of reference electrodes on the scalp.

Amplitude-integrated electroencephalography (aEEG) utilizes fewer electrodes and then filters and time compresses data. The resulting patterns are more easily interpreted.

Indication: aEEG may be indicated in infants with clinical suspicion of seizure activity. Infants at risk for neurologic injury, including those with hypoxic-ischemic encephalopathy, intracranial hemorrhage, metabolic disorders, central nervous system malformations, chromosomal abnormalities, or developmental delay may benefit from EEG studies. It has been increasingly used for monitoring changes in brain activity in neonates with hypoxic-ischemic encephalopathy in response to therapeutic hypothermia.[39]

Accuracy: Comparison with standard EEG for seizure detection found 80% sensitivity and 50% specificity with an overdiagnosis of seizures by aEEG.[40] Others have found that seizures that are brief, infrequent, or low amplitude are missed in more than 50% of aEEG recordings.[41] Confirmation of seizure activity with a conventional EEG is recommended.

Reliability: Tests of interobserver variability showed good agreement for assessment of amplitude (κ statistic = 0.85) and for detection of seizures (κ statistic = 0.76).[42]

Limitations:

1. Brief seizures and those originating from the frontal or occipital regions may be missed because of time compression and fewer channel recordings.

2. Artifacts from movement, electrical interference, poor electrode contact, or use of sedating medication may affect EEG tracings.

FUTURE DIRECTIONS

1. A continued focus on minimizing size and invasiveness of current monitors will be important, particularly to enhance the family-centered-care initiatives in many NICU environments and to address space constraints.

2. Addressing additional monitoring needs will be necessary. For example, metabolic monitoring of glucose, lactate, and electrolyte levels in a noninvasive manner would be useful.[43]

3. Multimodality monitoring and integration of various streams of data will also be extremely important for future medical devices (Figure 5-7). Current patient bedside monitors display typical vital signs, but how to deal with the large amounts of data generated through compatible platforms and enhanced interpretation of such combined data will be key to future research with monitoring devices.

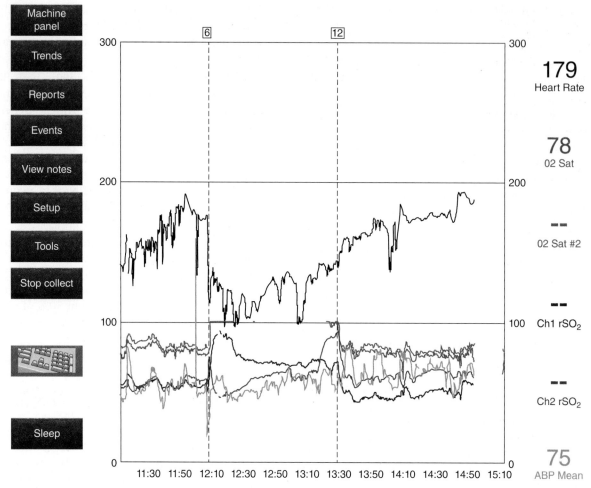

FIGURE 5-7 Multiple simultaneous monitoring of heart rate, blood pressure, systemic oxygen saturation, and regional oxygen saturation levels.

REFERENCES

1. Harpin VA, Rutter N. Barrier properties of the newborn infant's skin. *J Pediatr.* 1983;102(3):419–425.
2. Cartlidge PH, Rutter N. Karaya gum electrocardiographic electrodes for preterm infants. *Arch Dis Child.* 1987;62(12):1281–1282.
3. Watson AB, Wright JS, Loughman J. Electrical thresholds for ventricular fibrillation in man. *Med J Aust.* 1973;1(24):1179–1182.
4. Cardiotronic I. Electrical Cardiometry. 2009.
5. Schmidt C, Theilmeier G, Van Aken H, et al. Comparison of electrical velocimetry and transoesophageal Doppler echocardiography for measuring stroke volume and cardiac output. *Br J Anaesth.* 2005;95(5):603–610.
6. Suttner S, Schollhorn T, Boldt J, et al. Noninvasive assessment of cardiac output using thoracic electrical bioimpedance in hemodynamically stable and unstable patients after cardiac surgery: a comparison with pulmonary artery thermodilution. *Intensive Care Med.* 2006;32(12):2053–2058.
7. Zoremba N, Bickenbach J, Krauss B, et al. Comparison of electrical velocimetry and thermodilution techniques for the measurement of cardiac output. *Acta Anaesthesiol Scand.* 2007;51(10):1314–1319.
8. Norozi K, Beck C, Osthaus WA, et al. Electrical velocimetry for measuring cardiac output in children with congenital heart disease. *Br J Anaesth.* 2008;100(1):88–94.
9. Meyer S, Todd D, Shadboldt B. Assessment of portable continuous wave Doppler ultrasound (ultrasonic cardiac output monitor) for cardiac output measurements in neonates. *J Paediatr Child Health.* 2009;45(7–8):464–468.
10. Patel N, Dodsworth M, Mills JF. Cardiac output measurement in newborn infants using the ultrasonic cardiac output monitor: an assessment of agreement with conventional echocardiography, repeatability and new user experience. *Arch Dis Child Fetal Neonatal Ed.* 2011;96(3):F206–F211.
11. Tan HL, Pinder M, Parsons R, et al. Clinical evaluation of USCOM ultrasonic cardiac output monitor in cardiac surgical patients in intensive care unit. *Br J Anaesth.* 2005;94(3):287–291.
12. Knirsch W, Kretschmar O, Tomaske M, et al. Cardiac output measurement in children: comparison of the Ultrasound Cardiac Output Monitor with thermodilution cardiac output measurement. *Intensive Care Med.* 2008;34(6):1060–1064.
13. Baird TM, Neuman MR. Effect of infant position on breath amplitude measured by transthoracic impedance and strain gauges. *Pediatr Pulmonol.* 1991;10(1):52–56.
14. Adams JA, Zabaleta IA, Stroh D, et al. Measurement of breath amplitudes: comparison of three noninvasive respiratory monitors to integrated pneumotachograph. *Pediatr Pulmonol.* 1993;16(4):254–258.
15. Brouillette RT, Morrow AS, Weese-Mayer DE, et al. Comparison of respiratory inductive plethysmography and thoracic impedance for apnea monitoring. *J Pediatr.* 1987;111(3):377–383.

16. Emeriaud G, Eberhard A, Benchetrit G, et al. Calibration of respiratory inductance plethysmograph in preterm infants with different respiratory conditions. *Pediatr Pulmonol.* 2008;43(11): 1135–1141.

17. Kreit JW, Sciurba FC. The accuracy of pneumotachograph measurements during mechanical ventilation. *Am J Respir Crit Care Med.* 1996;154(4 Pt 1):913–917.

18. Sato S, Ishida-Nakajima W, Ishida A, et al. Assessment of a new piezoelectric transducer sensor for noninvasive cardiorespiratory monitoring of newborn infants in the NICU. *Neonatology.* 2010; 98(2):179–190.

19. Weindling AM. Blood pressure monitoring in the newborn. *Arch Dis Child.* 1989;64(4 Spec No):444–447.

20. Kunk R, McCain GC. Comparison of upper arm and calf oscillometric blood pressure measurement in preterm infants. *J Perinatol.* 1996;16(2 Pt 1):89–92.

21. Takci S, Yigit S, Korkmaz A, et al. Comparison between oscillometric and invasive blood pressure measurements in critically ill premature infants. *Acta Paediatr.* 2011;101(2):132–135.

22. Diprose GK, Evans DH, Archer LN, et al. Dinamap fails to detect hypotension in very low birthweight infants. *Arch Dis Child.* 1986;61(8):771–773.

23. Sonesson SE, Broberger U. Arterial blood pressure in the very low birthweight neonate. Evaluation of an automatic oscillometric technique. *Acta Paediatr Scand.* 1987;76(2):338–341.

24. Kattwinkel J, Perlman JM, Aziz K, et al. Part 15: neonatal resuscitation: 2010 American Heart Association Guidelines for Cardiopulmonary Resuscitation and Emergency Cardiovascular Care. *Circulation.* 2010;122(18 Suppl 3):S909–S919.

25. Praud JP, Carofilis A, Bridey F, et al. Accuracy of two wavelength pulse oximetry in neonates and infants. *Pediatr Pulmonol.* 1989;6(3):180–182.

26. Hay WW Jr, Brockway JM, Eyzaguirre M. Neonatal pulse oximetry: accuracy and reliability. *Pediatrics.* 1989;83(5):717–722.

27. Fanconi S. Reliability of pulse oximetry in hypoxic infants. *J Pediatr.* 1988;112(3):424–427.

28. Gilmore MM, Stone BS, Shepard JA, et al. Relationship between cerebrovascular dysautoregulation and arterial blood pressure in the premature infant. *J Perinatol.* 2011;31(11):722–729.

29. Tsuji M, Saul JP, du Plessis A, et al. Cerebral intravascular oxygenation correlates with mean arterial pressure in critically ill premature infants. *Pediatrics.* 2000;106(4):625–632.

30. Hoffman GM, Ghanayem NS, Tweddell JS. Noninvasive assessment of cardiac output. *Semin Thorac Cardiovasc Surg Pediatr Card Surg Annu.* 2005:12–21.

31. Cortez J, Gupta M, Amaram A, et al. Noninvasive evaluation of splanchnic tissue oxygenation using near-infrared spectroscopy in preterm neonates. *J Matern Fetal Neonatal Med.* 2011;24(4): 574–582.

32. Benni PB, Chen B, Dykes FD, et al. Validation of the CAS neonatal NIRS system by monitoring vv-ECMO patients: preliminary results. *Adv Exp Med Biol.* 2005;566:195–201.

33. Noori S, Drabu B, McCoy M, et al. Non-invasive measurement of local tissue perfusion and its correlation with hemodynamic indices during the early postnatal period in term neonates. *J Perinatol.* 2011;31(12):785–788.

34. Carter B, Hochmann M, Osborne A, et al. A comparison of two transcutaneous monitors for the measurement of arterial PO_2 and PCO_2 in neonates. *Anaesth Intensive Care.* 1995;23(6):708–714.

35. Wu CH, Chou HC, Hsieh WS, et al. Good estimation of arterial carbon dioxide by end-tidal carbon dioxide monitoring in the neonatal intensive care unit. *Pediatr Pulmonol.* 2003;35(4):292–295.

36. Kirpalani H, Kechagias S, Lerman J. Technical and clinical aspects of capnography in neonates. *J Med Eng Technol.* 1991;15(4–5):154–161.

37. Menzel M, Soukup J, Henze D, et al. Experiences with continuous intra-arterial blood gas monitoring: precision and drift of a pure optode-system. *Intensive Care Med.* 2003;29(12):2180–2186.

38. Coule LW, Truemper EJ, Steinhart CM, et al. Accuracy and utility of a continuous intra-arterial blood gas monitoring system in pediatric patients. *Crit Care Med.* 2001;29(2):420–426.

39. Toet MC, Lemmers PM, van Schelven LJ, et al. Cerebral oxygenation and electrical activity after birth asphyxia: their relation to outcome. *Pediatrics.* 2006;117(2):333–339.

40. Evans E, Koh S, Lerner J, et al. Accuracy of amplitude integrated EEG in a neonatal cohort. *Arch Dis Child Fetal Neonatal Ed.* 2010;95(3):F169–F173.

41. Shellhaas RA, Soaita AI, Clancy RR. Sensitivity of amplitude-integrated electroencephalography for neonatal seizure detection. *Pediatrics.* 2007;120(4):770–777.

42. al Naqeeb N, Edwards AD, Cowan FM, et al. Assessment of neonatal encephalopathy by amplitude-integrated electroencephalography. *Pediatrics.* 1999;103(6 Pt 1):1263–1271.

43. Raju TN, Stevenson DK, Higgins RD, et al. Safe and effective devices and instruments for use in the neonatal intensive care units: NICHD Workshop summary. *Biomed Instrum Technol.* 2009;43(5):408–418.

Principles of Infection Control

Jennifer M. Duchon and Lisa Saiman

INTRODUCTION

An ounce of prevention is worth a pound of cure.

The importance of appropriate and sustained infection prevention and control (IP&C) practices in the neonatal intensive care unit (NICU) cannot be overstated as infants in the NICU are extremely vulnerable to health-care-acquired infections (HAIs). This chapter introduces the basic components of an IP&C program, including the roles of workforce health and safety and the clinical microbiology laboratory. In addition, strategies to reduce HAIs in the NICU, including staff education, transmission precautions, and bundle practices to reduce central-line-associated bloodstream infections (CLABSIs) and ventilator-associated pneumonia (VAP) are described. Reduction of HAIs must be accompanied by effective surveillance for HAIs and multidrug-resistant organisms (MDROs). This is particularly important in an era of mandatory reporting. Finally, this chapter describes evidence-based antimicrobial stewardship interventions.

Throughout the chapter, citations are provided from the Centers for Disease Control and Prevention (CDC) Healthcare Infection Control Practices Advisory Committee (HICPAC) authoritative guidelines on prevention strategies for HAIs. This federal advisory board has infection control experts from the Society for Healthcare Epidemiology of America (SHEA), Infectious Disease Society of America (IDSA), and the American Academy of Pediatrics (AAP).[1] In addition, the CDC provides guidelines and tools through the National Healthcare Safety Network (NHSN) system to assist hospitals to develop surveillance, analysis, and reporting systems for HAIs that can enable interventions, when necessary (http://www.cdc.gov/nhsn/).

Discussion of the pathophysiology and treatment of bacterial and viral pathogens, including MDROs, is beyond the scope of this chapter; these topics are addressed in other chapters in this guide.

COMPONENTS OF INFECTION PREVENTION AND CONTROL PROGRAMS

Administrative Support

Administrative support is crucial to secure the resources and infrastructure needed to provide an effective IP&C program to serve the NICU. As NICUs are part of larger hospitals and health care systems and may be the only pediatric unit within some hospitals, the administrative leadership should be educated by the IP&C program and NICU leadership about the unique needs of the neonatal population. Elements of education should include the types of HAIs that neonates can acquire; the morbidity associated with these infections (ie, increased length of stay, health care costs, and potential mortality); preventive strategies and the cost of such strategies, including maintaining adequate bedside nurse staffing; reporting requirements to institutional committees, local health departments, and other regulatory bodies; relevant Joint Commission patient safety goals and priorities; the potential impact of HAIs on hospital reputation; and the role of families and visitors.

Support for IP&C efforts must be provided by NICU medical and nursing leadership as well as the bedside health care professionals and ancillary caregivers (eg, respiratory therapists, radiology technicians, phlebotomists, and environmental service workers). Regular presentations should be made to the administrative leadership and the NICU team by the IP&C staff, who should serve on the NICU quality council. These presentations should describe the results of both *process measures* to prevent HAIs and *outcome measures* of HAI rates as described in this chapter.

Infection Prevention and Control Staff

There is no universally accepted staffing requirement for IP&C, but a Delphi panel suggested a ratio of 0.8 to 1.0 infection preventionists per 100 occupied acute care beds based on time estimates for infection control functions.[2] However, experts emphasized that more research is needed to identify effective staffing levels that consider the expanding surveillance and reporting responsibilities of IP&C staff.[3] Given the high rates of HAIs in NICUs, dedicated IP&C staff should serve the NICU and measures be taken to ensure appropriate

resources for effective education, surveillance, mandatory reporting, and implementation of preventive strategies.

Additional IP&C program requirements include a director (generally a physician trained in infectious diseases and IP&C), data manager/analyst, and administrative assistant. In addition, close collaborations with the workforce (employee) health service (WHS), clinical microbiology laboratory, and pharmacy are critical (see the following discussion). Infection control liaisons (eg, staff members from nursing units) are helpful in facilitating implementation of IP&C strategies.

Workforce (Employee) Health Service

The WHS is an integral part of IP&C and is charged with preventing transmission of potential pathogens from staff to patients and from patients to staff. Strategies to prevent transmission include primary prevention through vaccination (see Table 6-1 for 2011 Advisory Committee on Immunization Practices [ACIP] recommendations for health care workers)[4]; screening for latent tuberculosis infection; banning artificial nails and promoting skin care[5,6]; and policies to prevent staff from working ill. Mandatory vaccination requirements

Table 6-1 Current Recommendations for Vaccinations for Health Care Providers in the United States[a]

Vaccination	Strategy	Comments
Hepatitis B	3-dose series	Obtain anti-hepatitis B surface antigen testing 1–2 months after third dose Anti-HBs testing not routinely recommended for previously vaccinated health care providers
Influenza	Annual vaccination recommended Intramuscular or intranasal formulations available	Education, providing vaccines in the workplace, and signed declinations have not improved vaccination rates for health care providers Mandatory vaccination policies have improved vaccination rates

Measles	2-dose series of measles, mumps, rubella (MMR) vaccine
	Immunity documented by one of following:
	    Two documented measles vaccinations
	    Positive measles serology
	    Documented measles infection
		Commercial serologic assays may have low sensitivity and specificity
		Note: Birth before 1957 is not considered acceptable evidence for health care providers

Mumps	MMR	
Pertussis	Use of 1-time dose of Tdap recommended for health care professionals	No interval required between Tdap and other tetanus toxoid-containing vaccines
Rubella	MMR	

Varicella	2-dose series varicella zoster vaccine (VZV)
	Immunity documented by one of following:
	    Documentation of 2 doses of VZV
	    Laboratory evidence of immunity
	    History of varicella disease (primary or zoster) by health care provider
		Commercial serologic assays may have low sensitivity and specificity
		Zoster vaccine as per recommendations for non-health-care professionals

[a]Data from Advisory Committee on Immunization Practices (ACIP), 2011.

vary from state to state, and compliance is reviewed by the Joint Commission, which is currently recommending that facilities increase annual influenza vaccination rates. As recommended by the ACIP, health care professionals should have documented evidence of presumptive immunity to hepatitis B, measles, mumps, rubella, and varicella. Health care professionals should be vaccinated annually for influenza and receive a single dose of Tdap as soon as feasible.[4]

The WHS must have *written* policies (crafted with the IP&C Department and human resources) for furloughing, paying, and returning to work staff who are infected or colonized with potentially communicable pathogens. Policies should be developed for vaccine-preventable illnesses as well as methicillin-resistant *Staphylococcus aureus* (MRSA), influenza-like illness, gastrointestinal tract illness, herpes stomatitis, and varicella zoster, to name a few.

Clinical Microbiology Laboratory

The clinical microbiology laboratory contributes greatly to preventing transmission of infectious diseases in the NICU because the laboratory is responsible for identifying epidemiologically important microorganisms (see the section on surveillance that follows), detecting changes in resistance patterns, and implementing rapid diagnostic testing for viruses. The clinical microbiology laboratories that serve NICUs may be on-site hospital laboratories that serve several patient populations or off-site contract laboratories. Nonetheless, laboratories should be able to support the IP&C Department and provide the frequency of specific pathogens in the NICU (eg, MRSA); antibiograms (ie, aggregate reports of susceptibility to specific agents); and assist in outbreak investigations, including the ability to save isolates, perform surveillance cultures, and arrange for molecular typing of selected isolates, when needed.

Policy and Procedures for Devices, Supplies, and Equipment

Policies and procedures must be developed for use of all devices, including insertion strategies, maintenance practices, and disinfection/sterilization, when appropriate. It is not uncommon for the NICU team to consider a new product (eg, catheter hub, Y connector) or new piece of equipment (eg, isolette, glucose monitor). Although staff satisfaction is clearly important when considering a change, infection control implications must also be considered. For example, how is the product cleaned, disinfected, or sterilized? Has the product been associated with an increased risk of malfunction or HAIs? Are single-use medications available because multiuse vials can become contaminated?

STRATEGIES TO PREVENT HAIS IN THE NICU

Education

Education of health care professionals as well as families and visitors is crucial to promote appropriate IP&C in the NICU. The optimal methods of education are actually unknown, but posted signs, electronic learning sites, small-group huddles, interactive audience response systems, and didactic lectures can be used. Mandatory education can be used as a component to demonstrate competencies. Notably, health care professionals should receive "booster" education at regular intervals to reinforce IP&C principles and practices. Education about hand hygiene, the rationale for different transmission precautions, respiratory hygiene/cough etiquette, and vaccinations should be provided to families and visitors as well.

However, education alone cannot improve practices. Practices are improved by a combination of education, strategies to improve adherence such as checklists or observations of desired practices (*process measures*) with feedback to staff, and providing HAI rates (*outcome measures*) to key stakeholders. In addition, during the past decade there has been increasing attention to creating a culture of safety and quality in health care.

Hand Hygiene

For over 150 years, hand hygiene has been recognized as the most effective way to prevent HAIs. Despite the relative ease and low cost of this intervention, adherence rates by health care professionals have been less than 50% in many studies, and physicians generally have lower rates than nurses.[7] Both the CDC and the World Health Organization (WHO) have developed guidelines for hand hygiene that include how and when to perform hand hygiene.[8] The WHO's 5 Moments for Hand Hygiene (representing 5 fingers) are shown in Table 6-2. A WHO video, *SAVE LIVES: Clean Your Hands*, is available for the education of health care professionals (http://www.who.int/gpsc/5may/video/en/index.html).

When compared to soap and water, alcohol-based hand rubs are preferred; this method is less costly, less time consuming, less damaging to skin, and effective against gram-negative and gram-positive pathogens as well as yeast and most viruses. Hands should be washed with soap and water when visibly soiled with blood or body fluids or visibly dirty. Other aspects of hand hygiene include minimal-to-no-jewelry; short, well-groomed nails; no artificial nails or nail enhancements; and maintenance of good skin health (ie, avoiding contact with solutions in the non-health care environment that can dry hands, applying moisturizer frequently outside the NICU, and seeking prompt medical

Table 6-2 World Health Organization's Five Moments for Hand Hygiene[a]

Moment	Activity[b]	Comment/Rationale
1	Before touching a patient	Hands become contaminated with microorganisms during previous activities, which can result in patient-to-patient transmission of pathogens.
2	Before clean/aseptic procedure	Hands become contaminated with microorganisms, which can cause infection following high-risk procedures.
3	After body fluid exposure risk	Includes contact with patients' mucous membranes, nonintact skin, wound dressings, which can be colonized with potential pathogens. One body site (eg, endotracheal tube) can be colonized and subsequently colonize/infect another body site (eg, catheter hub) if hand hygiene not performed between tasks.
4	After touching a patient	Hands become contaminated with microorganisms during patient care and may contaminate the environment or be transmitted to another patient.
5	After touching patient care environment	Includes inanimate surfaces and objects in patient care environment (eg, knobs, bedside rails, linens), which become contaminated with microorganisms colonizing/infecting patients.

[a]From WHO 5 Moments for Hand Hygiene.[8]
[b]Hand hygiene must be performed even if gloves are worn.

attention for dermatitis or other skin or nail lesions, eg, paronychia, whitlow, onychomycosis).

Adherence to hand hygiene should be monitored and rates shared with staff. Adherence can be greatly facilitated by having the NICU team participate in the selection of products and by ensuring adequate hand hygiene supplies. NICU staff should also participate in selecting the locations where the dispensers are located. If wall space is limited, additional dispensers can be placed at the bedside. All visitors to the NICU, including siblings, should practice hand hygiene before and after visiting their infant. Bedside staff are responsible for teaching appropriate use of alcohol hand rub material and observing the practice to ensure proper use.

Transmission Precautions

Two recent evidence-based guidelines from HICPAC address prevention of transmission of MDROs[9] and transmission precautions.[10] Standard precautions and contact precautions are the most frequently used transmission precautions in the NICU; droplet and airborne precautions are rarely implemented, but nonetheless should be understood by NICU staff. The personal protective equipment (PPE) worn by health care professionals caring for patients on transmission precautions and examples of specific pathogens for different types of precautions are shown in Table 6-3. NICUs should ensure that an adequate supply of gowns and gloves (in different sizes) is available and that restocking and appropriate disposal of PPE waste occur often. Hand hygiene is always performed before and after gloves are donned.

The terms and concepts for standard precautions have replaced the former term universal precautions. The principles underlying standard precautions are the foundation of prevention of transmission of infectious pathogens during patient care and include appropriate use of PPE, respiratory hygiene/cough etiquette, and safe handling of blood and body fluids, including phlebotomy practices. The rationale for standard precautions is that any patient could be harboring a potential pathogen that could be transmitted to another patient or to a health care professional during care. Thus, in addition to hand hygiene, gloves should be worn by all health care providers for all patients when touching blood, body fluids, secretions, excretions, mucous membranes, nonintact skin, and contaminated items. Gowns should be worn when contact of clothing or exposed skin with blood, body fluids, secretions, or excretions is anticipated. Surgical masks and eye protection (goggles or face shield) should be worn during procedures or care activities that may generate splashes or sprays of blood, body fluids, or secretions (eg, during intubation). Masks should also be worn when performing a sterile technique (eg, placement of a central venous catheter [CVC]) to protect patients from exposure to infectious agents present in a health care worker's nose or mouth. Observations of standard precautions are desirable as adherence may be suboptimal.

VISITOR POLICIES

Although the CDC guidelines did not address the use of PPE (eg, gowns and gloves) by family members visiting their infants, many NICUs are no longer requiring that

Table 6-3 Implementation of Transmission Precautions in the Neonatal Intensive Care Unit[a]

Type of Precaution	Mode of Transmission	Pathogens or Conditions	Personal Protective Equipment	Comments
Standard	See following material for contact and droplet	Necrotizing enterocolitis, viral or gram-negative meningitis or pneumonia if not caused by MDRO	Guided by type of interaction	Policies for PPE use for common procedures (eg, intubation, open suctioning if used, surgical dressing changes) should be developed to ensure standard practice.
Contact	*Direct* transfer of microorganisms from infected person to another *Indirect* transfer of microorganisms by contaminated intermediate object or person (including hands)	Colonization or infection with MRSA, VRE, MDR-GNB, RSV, rotavirus, herpes simplex, staphylococcal scalded skin syndrome	Gowns and gloves	Each institution must develop own definition for MDR-GNB based on local epidemiology and experience.
Droplet	Respiratory droplets of microorganisms travel from infectious person to susceptible mucosal surfaces (ie, nasal mucosa, mouth, conjunctiva) of another person within ~ 3–6 feet	Influenza, adenovirus, pertussis, *Neisseria meningitidis*	Surgical mask	Eyes may be a portal of entry for infectious droplets; use eye shields or goggles if spray or splash with respiratory tract secretions anticipated (eg, during intubation, extubation, or suctioning).
Airborne	Dissemination of droplet nuclei from infectious person that are inhaled by susceptible individual and may remain infectious over time and space	Tuberculosis, varicella, measles	Respirator (eg, N95)	This requires special air-handling and ventilation systems. Potentially infectious infants include those born to mothers who develop chickenpox 2 days prior to delivery to 5 days after delivery.

Abbreviations: GNB, gram-negative bacilli; MDR, multidrug resistant; MDRO, multidrug-resistant organism; PPE, personal protective equipment; RSV, respiratory syncytial virus; VRE, vancomycin-resistant enterococci.
[a]From Siegel JD, Rhinehart E, Jackson M, Chiarello L, and the Healthcare Infection Control Practices Advisory Committee. *2007 Guideline for Isolation Precautions: Preventing Transmission of Infectious Agents in Healthcare Settings.* http://www.cdc.gov/hicpac/pdf/isolation/Isolation2007.pdf.

visitors wear gowns or gloves except for family members of infants in multiple gestations. However, it is critical that hand hygiene be emphasized. The rationale for the use of gowns and gloves for multiple gestations is that if one twin is on contact precautions, for example, for MRSA, visitors could inadvertently transmit MRSA to the other twin unless adhering to contact precautions. Bedside staff are responsible for providing education to family members and observing practice to ensure appropriate use of PPE, including discarding gowns and gloves.

In an era of family-centered care, families, including siblings, are encouraged to visit infants hospitalized in the NICU and sometimes may even participate in care practices. Family-centered care is safe provided there are sound policies to prevent visitors with potentially infectious illnesses from entering the NICU. Thus, no visitors with respiratory tract symptoms, gastro-intestinal symptoms, fever, or rash are permitted into the NICU. The challenge of such policies is ensuring compliance, which can be aided by providing written policies to families, signage, and screening tools for staff to administer. Mothers who are infected with potentially transmissible pathogens should not visit their infants until no longer infectious. On a case-by-case basis, mothers who are colonized with MDROs may be able to visit their infants provided they are instructed in effective hand hygiene and the use of gowns and gloves. The department of IP&C must be alerted about such instances and ensure that visitation complies with institutional policies.

Environmental Services

The inanimate health care environment may serve as a reservoir for potential pathogens and has been implicated in transmission.[10] HICPAC has published guidelines for disinfection and sterilization in health care facilities.[11] Thus, environmental service workers (housekeeping service) are another key group that participates in prevention of HAIs. Adequate training and documentation of effective cleaning and disinfection of environmental surfaces and equipment, including the use of checklists and observations, should be implemented for every NICU. In the NICU, crowding and high rates of device and equipment use can make cleaning challenging.

PREVENTION OF DEVICE-RELATED HAIS

Critically ill neonates often require indwelling devices to meet their ongoing need for nutrition and ventilation. Unfortunately, these necessary support devices may also be portals of entry for microorganisms that cause HAIs. The following sections provide guidelines for prevention of the most common device-related infections in the NICU population. More in-depth discussions of the management of nosocomial infections can be found in Chapter 53.

Central Line-Associated Bloodstream Infections

The CLABSIs contribute to substantial morbidity and potential mortality in the neonate. Very low birth weight (VLBW) infants afflicted by a CLABSI have increased risk for death and neurodevelopmental disability.[12] A hospital-acquired bloodstream infection (BSI) may increase both the length of hospital stay and the cost (attributable cost as high as $12,500 per CLABSI).[13]

Pathogenesis

The pathogenesis of CLABSIs has been well studied and informs preventive strategies. The most common mechanism of infection results from contamination of the catheter by colonizing skin flora at the insertion site. Infection may also be caused by contamination or colonization of the catheter at the hub, contaminated infusions of fluid or blood products, or hematogenous seeding of the catheter by bacteria from distal sites of infection. Bacterial species, especially coagulase-negative staphylococci (CONS) can adhere to and multiply on synthetic catheter surfaces. Many strains produce a glycocalyx biofilm, which further stimulates adherence to intravascular catheters, as well as protects the organisms from host defense mechanisms and the action of antibiotics.[14]

The most common pathogens causing CLABSIs are predominantly gram-positive organisms, including CONS, *Staphylococcus aureus*, and enterococcal species. *Escherichia coli* and *Klebsiella* spp. are the most common gram-negative organisms recovered. Rates of CLABSIs caused by fungal pathogens, primarily *Candida* spp., vary widely across NICUs.[15]

CLABSI Case Definition

Much effort has been put into standardizing case definitions for CLABSIs to ensure interrater reliability, promote accurate rate data, and stratify by risk (ie, birth weight). The NHSN case definition for CLABSIs is shown in Table 6-4. This case definition excludes a single positive blood culture for common contaminants, as positive blood cultures may represent skin

Table 6-4 Centers for Disease Control and Prevention National Healthcare Safety Network Case Definition for Central Line-Associated Bloodstream Infections[a]

Definition of a bloodstream infection (BSI) associated with a central line (CLABSI) is a primary bloodstream infection in a patient with a central line[b] present *within*[c] the 48-hour period before the development of the BSI.	
Specific Criteria	**Comments**
A recognized pathogen is cultured from ≥ **1** blood cultures **AND** The organism(s) cultured **not** related to an infection at another site	Common skin contaminants, such as coagulase-negative staphylococci, are cultured from ≥ **2** blood cultures drawn on separate occasions within 48 hours (eg, 2 peripheral cultures drawn 24 hours apart) **OR** 1 peripheral culture and central line culture
Fever (>38°C rectally), hypothermia (<37°C rectally), apnea, or bradycardia are present **AND** Clinical signs and symptoms **not** related to an infection at another site	At least 1 of the clinical signs must be present Hypotension and chills, if present, are sufficient but not necessary

[a]Data from Centers for Disease Control and Prevention. Central line-associated blood stream infection (CLABSI) event. January 24. http://www.cdc.gov/nhsn/PDFs/pscManual/4PSC_CLABScurrent.pdf.
[b]A central line (CL) is defined as a vascular infusion device that terminates at or close to the heart or great vessels. In the newborn intensive care unit (NICU) population, the CLs include both umbilical artery and umbilical venous catheters.
[c]There is no minimum time period that a CL must be in place for the BSI to be considered a CLABSI.

flora from inadequately disinfected skin, contamination in the microbiology laboratory, or contamination from inadequately disinfected central line (CL) hubs. It also excludes secondary BSIs that could arise from other types of infections (eg, necrotizing enterocolitis or urosepsis). Notably, more than 2 positive blood cultures are required to define a CLABSI caused by skin flora (eg, *Staphylococcus epidermidis*). Thus, 2 blood cultures are highly desirable, but achieving an adequate blood volume (ie, 0.5 to 1 mL per bottle) can be challenging in the NICU population.

CLABSI Preventive Strategies

Much effort has focused on methods to prevent CLABSIs. Bundles, defined as evidence-based practices essential for effective and safe patient care that, when implemented together, result in greater improvements in patient outcomes, can reduce the rate of CLABSIs in the NICU population.[15,16] Bundled intervention strategies for both insertion and maintenance of CVCs[15,17] are shown in Table 6-5. Physician and nursing leadership, along with IP&C staff, should participate in interdisciplinary efforts committed to reducing CLABSIs in the NICU population. Family education describing these efforts should also be provided.

Skin Preparation

The CDC recommends use of a greater than 0.5% chlorhexidine gluconate (CHG) and alcohol-containing solution for skin preparation at CVC insertion in adults, children, and infants aged greater than 2 months.[18] CHG has not yet been approved by the US Food and Drug Administration (FDA) for use in infants less than 2 months of age because of concerns about potential toxicity. Hexachlorophene, an antiseptic used in bathing solutions in the past, was found to be percutaneously absorbed and to cause neurotoxicity in preterm infants.[19] Recent experimental and observational data with CHG has demonstrated that most adverse reactions were related to skin integrity in term and preterm neonates, with little evidence of systemic absorption in amounts that are thought to be neurotoxic.[20-22] A survey of 100 neonatal program directors found that most NICUs with fellowship training programs use CHG-containing products for CVC insertion or maintenance care.[22]

Central Line Insertion

Recent evidence supports the use of a core group of personnel trained in the insertion of CLs (ie, "PICC [peripherally inserted central catheter] line teams") to reduce the incidence of CLASBIs.[23] At minimum, health care professionals who insert CLs should have formal training in the bundles strategies and be observed inserting CLs to document competence before attempting the procedure independently. In addition, the use of checklists can facilitate adherence to the bundle strategies and reduce CLABSIs.[18] Competence and adherence to guidelines for insertion

Table 6-5 Bundle Strategies for Insertion and Maintenance of Central Lines[a,b]

Insertion Bundle	1. Create standardized central line kit containing all items necessary for central line insertion. 2. Perform hand hygiene with alcohol-based product or antiseptic-containing soap before and after inserting central line. 3. Use maximal barrier precautions (sterile gown, sterile gloves, surgical mask, hat, and large sterile drape) during central line insertion. 4. All central line insertions should be a two-person procedure. 5. Disinfect skin with appropriate antiseptic (eg, 2% chlorhexidine, 70% alcohol) before central line insertion. 6. Reapply skin antisepsis after insertion is complete, before applying sterile dressing to insertion site. 7. Use sterile transparent semipermeable dressing to cover insertion site.
Maintenance Bundle	1. Assess central line insertion site daily for signs of infection or breaches in dressing integrity. 2. Perform hand hygiene with alcohol-based product or antiseptic-containing soap before and after accessing a catheter or before and after changing dressing. 3. If dressing is damp, soiled, or loose, change dressing aseptically, using an appropriate antiseptic to disinfect the skin around insertion site and appropriate barrier precautions. 4. Develop and use standardized intravenous tubing setup and changes. 5. Maintain aseptic technique when changing intravenous tubing and when entering central line (ie, "scrub the hub").

[a]Data from http://www.cdc.gov/hicpac/pdf/guidelines/bsi-guidelines-2011.[19]
[b]From Schulman J et al.[15,17]

and maintenance should be reassessed periodically for personnel who insert and care for CVCs.

Central Line Maintenance

Maintenance bundles for CLs are as critical to prevent CLABSIs as insertion, as CLs remain in infants for weeks (Table 6-5).[15,17] Maintenance strategies to reduce CLABSIs should include nursing education and empowerment to recognize and report sites in need of attention. The integrity of the CL dressing is important because the insertion site is the main portal of entry of potential pathogens from infants' skin. Routine dressing changes at a minimum of every 7 days are recommended for adult populations, but catheter dislodgment or damage or injury to fragile skin preclude evidence-based recommendations for routine dressing changes in neonates. Reduction of overall CL usage is an integral component of CLABSI reduction efforts. Strategies to promote removal as soon as possible include daily assessments of the need for a CL and checklists to document line necessity. Efforts should also include development of standardized feeding protocols, which include early introduction and advancement of feeds and the volume of enteral feeding for which CL removal can occur.

Other strategies to reduce CLASBIs that are used in adult populations are not feasible or recommended for the NICU population and include antibiotic-impregnated catheters and antimicrobial catheter locks or flushes.

Routine replacement of CLs is not currently recommended, although duration of use greater than 1 month may be an independent risk factor for CLABSIs.[24] The use of prophylactic systemic antimicrobial agents to reduce CLABSIs is strongly discouraged. Although studies do show a reduction in infections with prophylactic antibiotics,[25] the risk of toxicity and emergence of resistance outweigh potential benefits of this practice.

Ventilator-Associated Pneumonia

Ventilator-associated pneumonia may be the second-most-common HAI in the NICU population, and the incidence is estimated to be as high as 28% in the low birth weight and preterm population.[26] However, the rates vary greatly between institutions, likely because of different patient populations, ventilatory strategies, or the complexity and lack of interrater reliability of VAP case definitions.[27,28] Although the attributable cost of VAP has not been reported for the NICU population, the attributable cost of VAP in the pediatric ICU has been estimated to be as high as $50,000, incurred primarily through increased length of stay.[29,30]

VAP Pathogenesis

Most commonly, VAP is caused by invasion of the lower respiratory tract by bacterial pathogens, although viral and fungal pathogens can cause VAP. The endotracheal tube provides a conduit for microorganisms between the oral cavity and upper and lower airway and promotes formation of a biofilm in which potential pathogens are embedded that have been acquired from exogenous sources, such as staff hands or the ventilatory circuit.[29,31,32] Host factors also predispose to VAP, which include immunologic immaturity; more permeable and friable respiratory tract mucosa that provides a less-effective barrier defense; and altered, abnormal endogenous microbial colonization, often caused by selective pressure from antimicrobial therapy. The most common causes of VAP include gram-negative bacilli (*Klebsiella pneumoniae*, *Pseudomonas aeruginosa*) and staphylococcal species.[26,33] However, it is often difficult to determine if positive clinical cultures reflect colonizing flora from the upper airway, the gastrointestinal tract, or the endotracheal tube or represent pathogens causing VAP. In older children and adults, quantitative bronchoalveolar lavage (BAL) has been used to facilitate interpretation of positive cultures; greater than 10^4 colony forming units per milliliter of BAL fluid is thought to be consistent with VAP.[34] However, this strategy is not feasible in infants.

VAP Case Definitions

The CDC defines VAP as pneumonia that develops more than 48 hours after the patient has been placed on mechanical ventilation. The diagnosis of VAP for infants less than 1 year of age includes clinical signs and symptoms, laboratory data, and radiographic findings, as shown in Table 6-6. Unfortunately, these criteria are generally nonspecific and can be associated with other conditions, such as bronchopulmonary dysplasia, respiratory distress syndrome, heart failure, and neonatal sepsis. Furthermore, some diagnostic criteria may be relatively subjective, such as changes in respiratory tract secretions or radiographic findings. The CDC is currently exploring alternative case definitions for VAP in adults in an attempt to use criteria that are more objective (eg, duration and changes in ventilator settings),[35] but such efforts have not been explored for neonates.

VAP Preventive Strategies

Compared with efforts for CLABSIs, preventive strategies and risk factors for VAP are not as well studied in neonates. Nonetheless, intervention strategies have targeted reducing entry of contaminated secretions into the lower respiratory tract during patient care or from contaminated equipment and decreasing abnormal colonization of the aerodigestive tract.

Table 6-6 Centers for Disease Control and Prevention Criteria for Ventilator-Associated Pneumonia in Infants Less than 1 Year of Age[a]

Clinical and Laboratory Data	Worsening gas exchange as evidence by 1. Increased desaturation episodes, O_2 demand, or need for ventilatory support AND 3 of the following: 1. Temperature instability 2. Leukopenia or leukocytosis and left shift 3. Change in quality or quantity of sputum, increased need for suctioning 4. Apnea, tachypnea, nasal flaring, grunting, or chest wall retractions 5. Wheeze, rales, or rhonchi 6. Vital sign instability (tachycardia or bradycardia)
Radiographic Data	>2 serial x-rays in patients *with* underlying disease (eg, bronchopulmonary dysplasia) or > 1 serial x-ray in patients *without* underlying pulmonary disease AND 1 of the following: 1. New or progressive AND persistent infiltrate 2. Consolidation 3. Cavitation 4. Pneumatocoeles

[a]Adapted from http://www.cdc.gov/nhsn/pdfs/pscmanual/6pscvapcurrent.pdf.

Table 6-7 shows potential VAP prevention strategies.[36] However, these guidelines should be extrapolated with caution to neonates. For example, multiple episodes of daily oral care with an antiseptic solution (eg, CHG) are recommended to reduce the bacterial burden in the oropharynx of adults, but the risks and benefits of this preventive strategy have not been explored in neonates. Cuffed endotracheal tubes are rarely used in neonates. Elevation of the head of the bed greater than 30° has also been recommended to reduce aspiration in adult intensive care unit patients, but this has not been validated as safe and effective in neonates. Of note, a randomized clinical trial of neonates ventilated in the lateral recumbent position demonstrated a reduction in positive tracheal cultures, but this trial did not assess the impact on VAP.[37] Ulcer prophylaxis is also a component of VAP prevention bundles, but the use of H_2 blockers or other pharmacologic agents to increase pH of gastric secretions in neonates has been linked to candidemia, necrotizing enterocolitis, and development of abnormal colonizing intestinal flora.[38,39]

Closed endotracheal suctioning systems are widely used in the NICU because they may help prevent

Table 6-7 Proposed Bundle Strategies for Prevention of Ventilator-Associated Pneumonia[a]

Strategy	Intervention	Comment
Infection control	Standard precautions Hand hygiene Staff education	Should be employed as part of general strategy to reduce health-care-acquired infections (HAIs)
Oral care	Use of antiseptic solution General oral care (ie, sterile water swabs, oral suctioning)	Chlorhexidine gluconate (CHG) not approved for use in neonates; may have increased systemic absorption when used on mucous membranes
Suctioning	Closed suctioning systems	May reintroduce contaminated secretions with repeated-use suction catheters
Reduce bacterial load	Avoid use of H_2 blockers or proton pump inhibitors	Reduces the development and density of abnormal colonizing gastrointestinal flora
Positioning	Head of bed > 30° Lateral recumbent position	May reduce aspiration of oral secretions
Equipment care	Ventilator circuit maintenance and cleaning	Change circuit material only when mechanically malfunctioning or visibly soiled Remove condensate from ventilatory circuits

[a]Data from Coffin SE et al.[36]

physiologic derangements that occur when an infant is disconnected from the ventilator and allow frequent suctioning during special techniques, such as high-frequency oscillatory ventilation. Furthermore, these systems may reduce environmental contamination that occurs with frequent disconnection and manipulation of the ventilatory apparatus. However, such systems may increase the likelihood of reintroduction of contaminated secretions on the multiuse suction catheter into the lower respiratory tract. Despite their widespread use, the impact of closed suctioning systems on VAP in the neonate has not been adequately studied.[40,41]

Finally, the noninvasive ventilation strategy of early use of nasal continuous positive airway pressure (NCPAP) has been shown to be a safe and effective strategy to ventilate preterm neonates in randomized controlled trials.[42,43] Reducing the duration or avoiding intubation and mechanical ventilation may be one of the best strategies to reduce VAP.[44]

Surgical Site Infections

Few data describe the epidemiology of surgical site infections (SSIs) in the NICU population. Rates of SSIs following cardiac surgery range from 3% to 10%.[45–48] Potential risk factors for SSIs in the NICU population have been described and include relative immunosuppression; severity of underlying cardiac disease; previous infections; intraoperative surgical factors, including the environment of care; and microbial factors such as colonization with endogenous flora and microbial virulence factors.

SSI Case Definitions

The NHSN[49] classifies SSIs as superficial incisional, deep incisional, and organ space infections as shown in Table 6-8, and these definitions appear to be relevant for neonates.[50] The NHSN recommends SSI surveillance for 1 month for superficial infections and for 90 days for deep and organ space infections if an implant is in place.

SSI Preventive Strategies

Evidence-based guidelines are available to prevent SSIs in adult populations.[49,51] Although no evidence-based guidelines exist specifically for the NICU population, several pre-, intra-, and postoperative strategies to prevent SSIs are relevant for infants, as shown in Table 6-9. Much attention has focused on appropriate use of perioperative antimicrobial prophylaxis. These strategies include correct drug, correct dose, correct timing, intraoperative redosing (if appropriate for prolonged surgery), and prompt discontinuation of postoperative antibiotics (24 hours for noncardiac and 48 for cardiac surgery). Patients undergoing cardiothoracic surgery often require chest tubes, pacing wires, and catheters placed intraoperatively, which can remain in place for several days postoperatively. In adults, continuing antibiotics until the chest tubes are removed does not reduce SSIs.[52] Although data are limited on this topic in children and neonates, the CDC does not recommend prolonged prophylaxis of indwelling surgical lines and tubes beyond the 24–48 hours of routine postoperative antimicrobial prophylaxis.[52]

SURVEILLANCE

Although surveillance is the responsibility of the department of IP&C, the NICU staff is often the first to identify epidemiologically significant pathogens and potential outbreaks. In addition, the clinical

Table 6-8 National Healthcare Surveillance Network Criteria for Surgical Site Infections[a]

Type of Surgical Site Infection	Timing	Extent of Infection	Examples of Signs and Symptoms
Superficial incisional	Within 30 days of surgery	Skin or subcutaneous tissue	Purulent drainage, pathogen from aseptically obtained culture, pain or tenderness, swelling, erythema, surgeon diagnosis
Deep incisional	Within 30 days of surgery if no implant or within 1 year if implant in place	Deep soft tissues such as fascia and muscle layers	Purulent drainage, wound dehiscence, fever, pain, tenderness, abscess, surgeon diagnosis
Organ space	Within 30 days of surgery if no implant or within 1 year if implant in place	Organ(s)/space(s) opened or manipulated during surgery	Purulent drainage, pathogen aseptically obtained from organ/space, abscess involving organ/space, surgeon diagnosis

[a]Adapted from Mangram AJ et al.[51]

Table 6-9 Potential Preventive Strategies for Surgical Site Infections in the Newborn Intensive Care Unit Population[a]

Timing of Strategy	Type of Strategy	Comments
Preoperative	Maximize nutrition Minimize devices	Device may be potential portal of entry for pathogens
Intraoperative	Appropriate perioperative antimicrobial prophylaxis Appropriate intraoperative redosing for prolonged cases	Cover skin flora for cardiac surgery Cover gastrointestinal tract flora for intestinal surgery Know local epidemiology of pathogens causing surgical site infections
Postoperative	Avoid hypothermia Discontinue postoperative antimicrobial prophylaxis Observe standard precautions when performing dressing changes Maintain nutrition	Discontinue 24 hours (48 hours for cardiac surgery) following first intraoperative dose Don clean gloves for dressing changes

[a]Data from Anderson et al.[49]

microbiology laboratory should have a set of surveillance "panic values" that prompt notification of the department of IP&C.

Epidemiologically Significant Pathogens

Surveillance for epidemiologically significant pathogens should be conducted in real time. Surveillance for both colonized and infected infants is relevant as colonized infants may serve as reservoirs for potential pathogens for other infants. Epidemiologically significant pathogens include MDROs such as vancomycin-resistant enterococci, MRSA, and antimicrobial-resistant gram-negative bacilli. Studies have suggested that detection of MDROs should prompt surveillance cultures of neighboring infants, who may be colonized as well,[53] and early detection of MDROs and initiation of contact precautions can prevent further transmission. Surveillance for antimicrobial-resistant gram-negative bacilli should be guided by local epidemiology.

The ability to perform rapid viral diagnostic testing for viral pathogens is critical. Although relatively rare, gastrointestinal (eg, rotavirus and norovirus)[54,55] and respiratory viral pathogens (eg, influenza, respiratory syncytial virus, and parainfluenza)[56] can cause devastating outbreaks in the NICU. Thus, strategies to prevent transmission to other infants, staff, and visitors must be implemented immediately following identification of a single infected infant.

NICUs should also perform surveillance for *Candida* species. Rates of candidemia should be stratified by birth weight so that a NICU can determine if fluconazole is an appropriate preventive strategy.

Detection of *Aspergillus* should prompt immediate investigation for an environmental source, such as a leak or dust-generating renovation that was not appropriately contained.

Surveillance for MDROs in Infants Transferred from Other NICUs

Many institutions have surveillance and isolation policies for infants transferred from other institutions. Surveillance strategies vary by the organisms targeted (eg, MRSA only); the screening methods used (eg, polymerase chain reaction or culture); and the characteristics of the infants (eg, age) selected for surveillance cultures. Evidence suggests that infants are unlikely to be colonized with an MDRO within the first 3 days of life,[57,58] but the risk of MDRO colonization increases for older infants. NICUs should assess the yield of surveillance cultures to determine their effectiveness.

Mandatory Reporting

Outcome Measures

There are numerous statewide initiatives mandating public reporting of HAIs, including those in the NICU population. To date, CLABSIs are most commonly reported using the CDC NHSN case definitions (Table 6-4) and stratified by birth weight categories: less than 750, 750 to less than 1000, 1000 to less than 1500, 1500–2500, and more than 2500 g. Surveillance for CLABSIs is performed by IP&C staff rather than NICU staff to minimize reporting bias. Electronic surveillance should not be used exclusively because of the lack of specificity as electronic sources may miss alternative sites of infection. Some states have initiated surveillance for other HAIs, such as VAP.

Process Measures

Process measures of preventive strategies for HAIs are increasingly Joint Commission National Patient Safety Goals or Center for Medicare and Medicaid Service mandates. These include hand hygiene rates, checklists to measure adherence to insertion and maintenance policies for CLs, and the Surgical Care Improvement Project (SCIP). Although SCIP is currently limited to adult populations, it is likely that measures to prevent SSIs in pediatric populations will soon be monitored.

ANTIMICROBIAL STEWARDSHIP

Antimicrobial stewardship seeks to optimize the selection of antimicrobial agents to maximize clinical outcomes while minimizing toxicity, the emergence of resistance, and health care costs. Efforts to reduce inappropriate antibiotic use are urgently needed as infections with MDROs are increasing and are associated with increased morbidity and mortality in the NICU, including increased length of stay.[59,60] A multicenter point prevalence survey found that as many as 43% of all infants in the NICU were receiving one or more antimicrobial agents on a given day, often for a presumed HAI.[61] Furthermore, a multicenter study found that about 28% of courses and 25% of antibiotic days were inappropriate based on the CDC's guidelines for appropriate antimicrobial usage; failure to target the pathogen was the most common reason for inappropriate use.[62]

Antimicrobial Stewardship Strategies

Strategies to improve antimicrobial stewardship are often interdisciplinary. Antimicrobial stewardship programs are being increasingly recognized as an important mechanism to curtail antimicrobial resistance and improve quality of care. The CDC, IDSA, and SHEA have developed numerous educational tools for clinicians as well as evidence-based recommendations to decrease inappropriate antibiotic use in specific patient groups, including pediatrics, as shown in Table 6-10.[63] These recommendations were developed for hospitalized adults and older children but can be extrapolated to NICU patients. Recent guidelines have been crafted on implementing a stewardship program that includes an interdisciplinary team with members from IP&C, the pharmacy,

Table 6-10 Antimicrobial Stewardship Recommendations for the Neonatal Population[a]

Core Strategies	Practice	Example
Audit and feedback: Individual or aggregate feedback to providers about	• Spectrum of antibiotic • Excess duration of antibiotic therapy for a particular disease process • Redundant or unnecessary antibiotic coverage	• Narrow coverage for culture-proven pathogens • Mean duration of therapy for culture-negative sepsis • Excess days of prophylaxis of surgical procedures • Continued use of coverage for gram-negative organisms when treating a gram-positive organism and vice versa
Formulary restriction	• Formulary limitation • Preauthorization	• Stewardship committee evaluates antibiotics for inclusion on hospital formulary • Infectious disease service or antimicrobial stewardship staff approval for vancomycin, third-generation cephalosporins
Supplementary Strategies		
Education	• Didactic lectures	• Education of providers involved in audit and feedback to clinical practice guidelines
Computerized order entry/ decision support	• Computer surveillance and decision support system related to antimicrobial prescribing	• Computer-based antimicrobial prescribing linked to electronic medical records, which integrates culture data, treatment recommendations, and warnings regarding drug-drug interactions, dosing regimens, and duration
Guidelines	• Clinical practice guidelines	• Development of evidence-based protocols for perioperative antibiotic prophylaxis

[a]Data from Dellit et al.[63]

information technology, clinical microbiology, and infectious diseases.[64]

The 2 core strategies of antimicrobial stewardship are prospective audit with feedback and antimicrobial restriction and preauthorization for certain broad-spectrum antimicrobial agents. Antimicrobial restriction can be implemented by limiting the available formulary or by requiring preauthorization following justification by treating clinicians for the use of restricted agents. Typical drugs that are targeted include vancomycin, second- and third-generation cephalosporin agents, and carbapenem agents. Restriction can produce immediate reduction in the use of these drugs, although subsequent reduction in resistance is more difficult to assess. Prospective audit with feedback reviews the use of selected antibiotics and provides feedback to clinicians on their prescribing practices within a predetermined time. Feedback may be given to an individual clinician or to a group of prescribers. Feedback may be face to face or via written report. The interval between feedback actions should be appropriately timed to allow for meaningful changes in practices while preserving momentum. Examples of prescribing practices that could be audited are shown in Table 6-10.

Another mechanism to optimize the implementation of practice guidelines involves the use of health care information technology. Computerized physician order entry (CPOE) and clinical decision support (CDS) can improve antimicrobial practices through incorporating microbiology data (eg, cultures and susceptibilities), renal function, and possible medication interactions. Antimicrobial prescribing in the neonate can be complex and often requires both dose and interval adjustments based on birth weight, current weight, gestational age, and postmenstrual age. Although it can be challenging to develop and integrate recommendations within a cohesive CDS and CPOE system, stewardship bundles that have included CPOE and CDS have improved outcome measures in children, including the reduction of excessive antibiotic days and adverse drug events.[65-69]

REFERENCES

1. Centers for Disease Control and Prevention (CDC). Healthcare Infection Control Practices Advisory Committee (HICPAC). 2012.
2. O'Boyle C, Jackson M, Henly SJ. Staffing requirements for infection control programs in US health care facilities: Delphi project. *Am J Infect Control*. 2002;30:321–333.
3. Stone PW, Dick A, Pogorzelska M, Horan TC, Furuya EY, Larson E. Staffing and structure of infection prevention and control programs. *Am J Infect Control*. 2009;37:351–357.
4. Advisory Committee on Immunization Practices, Centers for Disease Control and Prevention. Immunization of health-care personnel: recommendations of the Advisory Committee on Immunization Practices (ACIP). *MMWR Morb Mortal Wkly Rep*. 2011;60(RR-7):1–65.
5. Boyce JM, Pittete D. Guideline for hand hygiene in healthcare settings: recommendations of the Healthcare Infection Control Practices Advisory Committee and the HICPAC/SHEA/APIC/IDSA hand hygiene task force. *MMWR Morb Mortal Wkly Rep*. 2002;51:1–45.
6. Pittet D, Allegranzi B, Boyce J. The World Health Organization guidelines on hand hygiene in health care and their consensus recommendations. *Infect Control Hosp Epidemiol*. 2009;30(7):611–622.
7. Guideline for Hand Hygiene in Health Care Settings: Recommendations of the Healthcare Infection Control Practices Advisory Committee and the HICPAC/SHEA/APIC/IDSA Hand Hygiene Task Force. 2002 October;51:1–56.
8. World Health Organization. *WHO Guidelines on Hand Hygiene in Health Care*. Geneva, Switzerland: World Health Organization; 2009:270.
9. Siegel J, Rhinehart E, Jackson M, Chiarello L, Healthcare Infection Control Practices Advisory Committee. Multidrug-resistant organisms in healthcare settings, 2006. *Am J Infect Control*. 2007;35(10 Suppl 2):S165–S193.
10. Siegel J, Rhinehart E, Jackson M, Chiarello L, Healthcare Infection Control Practices Advisory Committee. 2007 guidelines for isolation precautions: preventing transmission of infectious agents in healthcare settings. *Am J Infect Control*. 2007;35(10 Suppl 2):S65–S164.
11. Rutala WA, Weber DJ, Committee tHICPA. Guideline for disinfection and sterilization in healthcare facilities, 2008. http://www.cdc.gov/hicpac/pdf/guidelines/Disinfection_Nov_2008.pdf.
12. Stoll BJ, Hansen N, Fanaroff AA, et al. Late-onset sepsis in very low birth weight neonates: the experience of the NICHD Neonatal Research Network. *Pediatrics*. 2002;110:285–291.
13. Payne NR, Carpenter JH, Badger GJ, Horbar JD, Rogowski J. Marginal increase in cost and excess length of stay associated with nosocomial bloodstream infections in surviving very low birth weight infants. *Pediatrics*. 2004;114:348–355.
14. Safdar N, Maki DG. The pathogenesis of catheter-related bloodstream infection with noncuffed short-term central venous catheters. *Intensive Care Med*. 2004;30:62–67.
15. Schulman J, Stricof R, Stevens TP, et al. Statewide NICU central-line-associated bloodstream infection rates decline after bundles and checklists. *Pediatrics*. 2011;127:436–444.
16. Bizzarro MJ, Jiang Y, Hussain N, Gruen JR, Bhandari V, Zhang H. The impact of environmental and genetic factors on neonatal late-onset sepsis. *J Pediatr*. 2011;158:234–238 e1.
17. Schulman J, Stricof RL, Stevens TP, et al. Development of a statewide collaborative to decrease NICU central line-associated bloodstream infections. *J Perinatol*. 2009;29:591–599.
18. O'Grady NP, Alexander M, Burns LA, et al. Healthcare Infection Control Practices Advisory Committee (HICPAC). *Clin Infect Dis*. 2011;52(19):e162–e193.
19. Powell H, Swarner O, Gluck L, Lampert P. Hexachlorophene myelinopathy in premature infants. *J Pediatr*. 1973;82:976–981.
20. Mullany LC, Darmstadt GL, Tielsch JM. Safety and impact of chlorhexidine antisepsis interventions for improving neonatal health in developing countries. *Pediatr Infect Dis J*. 2006;25:665–675.
21. Chapman AK, Aucott SW, Milstone AM. Safety of chlorhexidine gluconate used for skin antisepsis in the preterm infant. *J Perinatol*. 2012;32:4–9.
22. Tamma PD, Aucott SW, Milstone AM. Chlorhexidine use in the neonatal intensive care unit: results from a national survey. *Infect Control Hosp Epidemiol*. 2010;31:846–849.
23. Taylor T, Massaro A, Williams L, et al. Effect of a dedicated percutaneously inserted central catheter team on neonatal catheter-related bloodstream infection. *Adv Neonatal Care*. 2011;11:122–128.
24. Sengupta A, Lehmann C, Diener-West M, Perl TM, Milstone AM. Catheter duration and risk of CLA-BSI in neonates with PICCs. *Pediatrics*. 2010;125:648–653.

25. Jardine LA, Inglis GD, Davies MW. Prophylactic systemic antibiotics to reduce morbidity and mortality in neonates with central venous catheters. *Cochrane Database Syst Rev.* 2008:CD006179.

26. Apisarnthanarak A, Holzmann-Pazgal G, Hamvas A, Olsen M, Fraser V. Ventilator-associated pneumonia in extremely preterm neonates in a neonatal intensive care unit: characteristics, risk factors, and outcomes. *Pediatrics.* 2003;112(6 Pt 1):1283–1289.

27. Cordero L, Ayers LW, Miller RR, Seguin JH, Coley BD. Surveillance of ventilator-associated pneumonia in very-low-birth-weight infants. *Am J Infect Control.* 2002;30:32–39.

28. Bradley JS. Considerations unique to pediatrics for clinical trial design in hospital-acquired pneumonia and ventilator-associated pneumonia. *Clin Infect Dis.* 2010;51(Suppl 1):S136–S143.

29. Foglia E, Meier MD, Elward A. Ventilator-associated pneumonia in neonatal and pediatric intensive care unit patients. *Clin Microbiol Rev* 2007;20:409–425, table of contents.

30. Brilli RJ, Sparling KW, Lake MR, et al. The business case for preventing ventilator-associated pneumonia in pediatric intensive care unit patients. *Jt Comm J Qual Patient Saf.* 2008;34:629–638.

31. Garland JS. Strategies to prevent ventilator-associated pneumonia in neonates. *Clin Perinatol.* 2010;37:629–643.

32. Goodwin SR, Graves SA, Haberkern CM. Aspiration in intubated premature infants. *Pediatrics.* 1985;75:85–88.

33. Yuan TM, Chen LH, Yu HM. Risk factors and outcomes for ventilator-associated pneumonia in neonatal intensive care unit patients. *J Perinat Med.* 2007;35:334–338.

34. Chastre J, Fagon JY, Bornet-Lecso M, et al. Evaluation of bronchoscopic techniques for the diagnosis of nosocomial pneumonia. *Am J Respir Crit Care Med.* 1995;152:231–240.

35. Klompas M. Multicenter evaluation of a novel surveillance paradigm for complications of mechanical ventilation. CDC Prevention Epicenters Program. *PLOS One.* 2011 Mar 22;6:e18062.

36. Coffin SE, Klompas M, Classen D, et al. Strategies to prevent ventilator-associated pneumonia in acute care hospitals. *Infect Control Hosp Epidemiol.* 2008;29(Suppl 1):S31–S40.

37. Aly H, Badawy M, El-Kholy A, Nabil R, Mohamed A. Randomized, controlled trial on tracheal colonization of ventilated infants: can gravity prevent ventilator-associated pneumonia? *Pediatrics.* 2008;122:770–774.

38. Deng C, Li X, Zou Y, et al. Risk factors and pathogen profile of ventilator-associated pneumonia in a neonatal intensive care unit in China. *Pediatr Int.* 2011;53:332–337.

39. Feja KN, Wu F, Roberts K, et al. Risk factors for candidemia in critically ill infants: a matched case-control study. *J Pediatr.* 2005;147:156–161.

40. Cordero L, Sananes M, Ayers LW. Comparison of a closed (Trach Care MAC) with an open endotracheal suction system in small premature infants. *J Perinatol.* 2000;20:151–156.

41. Taylor J, Hawley G, Flenady V, Woodgate P. Tracheal suctioning without disconnection in intubated ventilated neonates. *Cochrane Database Syst Rev.* 2011;(12):CD003065. doi:10.1002/14651858.CD003065.pub2.

42. Morley CJ, Davis PG, Doyle LW, Brion LP, Hascoet JM, Carlin JB. Nasal CPAP or intubation at birth for very preterm infants. *N Engl J Med.* 2008;358:700–708.

43. Finer NN, Carlo WA, Walsh MC, et al. Early CPAP versus surfactant in extremely preterm infants. *N Engl J Med.* 2010;362:1970–1979.

44. Hentschel J, Brungger B, Studi K, Muhlemann K. Prospective surveillance of nosocomial infections in a Swiss NICU: low risk of pneumonia on nasal continuous positive airway pressure? *Infection.* 2005;33:350–355.

45. Levy I, Ovadia B, Erez E, et al. Nosocomial infections after cardiac surgery in infants and children: incidence and risk factors. *J Hosp Infect.* 2003;53:111–116.

46. Pollock EM, Ford-Jones EL, Rebeyka I, et al. Early nosocomial infections in pediatric cardiovascular surgery patients. *Crit Care Med.* 1990;18:378–384.

47. Sarvikivi E, Lyytikainen O, Nieminen H, Sairanen H, Saxen H. Nosocomial infections after pediatric cardiac surgery. *Am J Infect Control.* 2008;36:564–569.

48. Valera M, Scolfaro C, Cappello N, et al. Nosocomial infections in pediatric cardiac surgery, Italy. *Infect Control Hosp Epidemiol.* 2001;22:771–775.

49. Anderson DJ, Kaye KS, Classen D, et al. Strategies to prevent surgical site infections in acute care hospitals. *Infect Control Hosp Epidemiol.* 2008;29(Suppl 1):S51–S61.

50. Kagen J, Bilker WB, Lautenbach E, et al. Risk adjustment for surgical site infection after median sternotomy in children. *Infect Control Hosp Epidemiol.* 2007;28:398–405.

51. Mangram AJ, Horan TC, Pearson ML, Silver LC, Jarvis WR. Guideline for prevention of surgical site infection, 1999. Hospital Infection Control Practices Advisory Committee. *Infect Control Hosp Epidemiol.* 1999;20:250–278.

52. Anderson DJ, Podgorny K, Berrios-Torres SI, . et al. Strategies to prevent surgical site infections in acute care hospitals: 2014 Update. *Infect Control Hosp Epidemiol.* 2014;35:605–627.

53. Carey AJ, Duchon J, Della-Latta P, Saiman L. The epidemiology of methicillin-susceptible and methicillin-resistant *Staphylococcus aureus* in a neonatal intensive care unit, 2000–2007. *J Perinatol.* 2010;30:135–139.

54. Rotbart HA, Nelson WL, Glode MP, et al. Neonatal rotavirus-associated necrotizing enterocolitis: case control study and prospective surveillance during an outbreak. *J Pediatr.* 1988;112:87–93.

55. Stuart RL, Tan K, Mahar JE, et al. An outbreak of necrotizing enterocolitis associated with norovirus genotype GII.3. *Pediatr Infect Dis J.* 2010;29:644–647.

56. Kilani RA. Respiratory syncytial virus (RSV) outbreak in the NICU: description of eight cases. *J Trop Pediatr.* 2002;48:118–122.

57. Gregory ML, Eichenwald EC, Puopolo KM. Seven-year experience with a surveillance program to reduce methicillin-resistant *Staphylococcus aureus* colonization in a neonatal intensive care unit. *Pediatrics.* 2009;123:e790–e796.

58. Myers PJ, Marcinak J, David MZ, et al. Universal admission screening for methicillin-resistant *Staphylococcus aureus* in a level IIID neonatal intensive care unit: the first 9 months. *Infect Control Hosp Epidemiol.* 2011;32:398–400.

59. Stone PW, Gupta A, Loughrey M, et al. Attributable costs and length of stay of an extended-spectrum beta-lactamase-producing Klebsiella pneumoniae outbreak in a neonatal intensive care unit. *Infect Control Hosp Epidemiol.* 2003;24:601–606.

60. Gupta A, Della-Latta P, Todd B, et al. Outbreak of extended-spectrum beta-lactamase-producing *Klebsiella pneumoniae* in a neonatal intensive care unit linked to artificial nails. *Infect Control Hosp Epidemiol.* 2004;25:210–215.

61. Grohskopf LA, Huskins WC, Sinkowitz-Cochran RL, Levine GL, Goldmann DA, Jarvis WR. Use of antimicrobial agents in United States neonatal and pediatric intensive care patients. *Pediatr Infect Dis J.* 2005;24:766–773.

62. Patel SJ, Oshodi A, Prasad P, et al. Antibiotic use in neonatal intensive care units and adherence with Centers for Disease Control and Prevention 12 Step Campaign to Prevent Antimicrobial Resistance. *Pediatr Infect Dis J.* 2009;28:1047–1051.

63. Dellit TH, Owens RC, McGowan JE Jr, et al. Infectious Diseases Society of America and the Society for Healthcare Epidemiology of America guidelines for developing an institutional program to enhance antimicrobial stewardship. *Clin Infect Dis.* 2007;44:159–177.

64. Society for Healthcare Epidemiology of America, Pediatric Infectious Diseases Society, and Infectious Diseases Society

of America. Policy statement on antimicrobial stewardship by the Society for Healthcare Epidemiology of America (SHEA), the Infectious Diseases Society of America (IDSA), and the Pediatric Infectious Diseases Society (PIDS). *Infect Control Hosp Epidemiol.* 2012;33:322–327.

65. Di Pentima MC, Chan S, Hossain J. Benefits of a pediatric antimicrobial stewardship program at a children's hospital. *Pediatrics.* 2011;128:1062–1070.

66. Di Pentima MC, Chan S. Impact of antimicrobial stewardship program on vancomycin use in a pediatric teaching hospital. *Pediatr Infect Dis J.* 2010;29:707–711.

67. Kazemi A, Ellenius J, Pourasghar F, et al. The effect of computerized physician order entry and decision support system on medication errors in the neonatal ward: experiences from an Iranian teaching hospital. *J Med Syst.* 2011;35:25–37.

68. Taylor JA, Loan LA, Kamara J, Blackburn S, Whitney D. Medication administration variances before and after implementation of computerized physician order entry in a neonatal intensive care unit. *Pediatrics.* 2008;121:123–128.

69. Cordero L, Kuehn L, Kumar RR, Mekhjian HS. Impact of computerized physician order entry on clinical practice in a newborn intensive care unit. *J Perinatol.* 2004;24:88–93.

Prenatal Diagnosis and Consultation

Susan Hintz, Jane Chueh, Richard Barth, Christopher Cunniff, and Louanne Hudgins

THE INCREASINGLY COMPLEX LANDSCAPE OF PRENATAL DIAGNOSIS AND CONSULTATION

Advances in prenatal diagnosis, imaging, and prenatal maternal-fetal and postnatal neonatal care have led to dramatically expanded opportunities and challenges for fetal management and prenatal counseling. Over the recent decades, medical and surgical treatment options for newborns with even the most complex congenital anomalies have substantially increased. Concurrently, prenatal screening and diagnostic capabilities have expanded, leading to early diagnosis of fetal problems. Maternal and family anxiety have been shown to be significantly reduced after antenatal consultation by an experienced, specialized staff.[1,2] Nevertheless, depending on the specific fetal finding, the physician and family may still be left with significant uncertainty regarding outcomes. If the pregnancy is continued, management strategies for the expectant mother and fetus range from those narrowly focused on maternal or fetal well-being to pursuing prenatal interventions, which may now be offered for some fetal indications. How these strategies are presented, and by whom, may strongly affect an expectant mother's decisions.[3,4] Furthermore, incomplete communication and collaboration among medical and surgical subspecialists in complex fetal cases may lead to incorrect information dissemination, confused message framing for the family, and a muddied picture of maternal, fetal, and neonatal risk-benefit and outcomes.[5] Finally, learning that an eagerly awaited child may be born with congenital anomalies can be the most emotionally stressful and difficult period in the life of an expectant mother or father; for some, the experience constitutes a true psychiatric trauma.[6] Therefore, experienced personnel in support services, including medical social services, palliative care, and biomedical ethics, must be available for expectant mothers and families in these circumstances.

For all of these reasons, a multidisciplinary approach to complex fetal diagnosis, management, intervention, and family consultation is critical to presenting as balanced and accurate a view as possible and to protect the interests of both mother and fetus.[7] The expertise and input of each member is crucial to inform plans for the pregnancy management, delivery mode and venue, and immediate postdelivery neonatal requirements. The team composition in a multidisciplinary fetal center may vary depending on the cases evaluated and managed at a particular institution. Genetics, maternal-fetal medicine, fetal and pediatric diagnostic imaging, and neonatology expertise, as well as a range of medical and surgical subspecialists and social service support, are important for building a strong foundation in complex fetal care and prenatal counseling.

This chapter is too brief to provide a comprehensive presentation of all aspects of prenatal diagnosis and counseling. We therefore focus on fundamental principles of three areas: genetic prenatal screening and diagnosis; imaging of fetal anomalies; and the benefits of a prenatal consultation by a neonatologist in complex fetal cases.

GENETIC PRENATAL SCREENING AND DIAGNOSIS

Over the last quarter century, prenatal genetic screening and diagnosis have become mainstays of the medical care of women who are pregnant or contemplating pregnancy. Maternal serum α-fetoprotein (AFP) measurement and fetal ultrasound examination make it possible to identify neural tube defects (NTDs) in up to 95% of affected pregnancies.[8] First- and second-trimester screening for aneuploidies such as trisomy 21 and 18 detect 65%–90% of these disorders.[9] Improvements in the acceptability, availability, and reliability of such testing have resulted in substantial changes in obstetric and pediatric practice. New technology has improved the sensitivity and positive predictive value of screening tests, as well as the safety and accuracy of tests used for prenatal diagnosis. These tests have the potential to be highly beneficial for prospective parents, and pediatricians and others caring for children need to be aware of the significance of the results.

Screening for Neural Tube Defects

Neural tube defects, including spina bifida and anencephaly, represent some of the most common birth defects in humans, occurring in 1–2/1000 pregnancies. When isolated, the etiology is considered to be multifactorial, involving a combination of genetic predisposition and environmental influences. One such environmental influence is folic acid, which prevents both occurrence and recurrence of NTDs.

In 1977, Wald et al reported on the efficacy of measuring the concentration of AFP in the serum of pregnant women to screen for the presence of NTDs.[10] Maternal serum AFP alone detects 75%–90% of open NTDs and more than 95% of anencephaly, with a false-positive rate of 5% or less. Currently, maternal serum AFP testing is offered to all pregnant women between 15 and 20 weeks gestation. When ultrasound examination is performed in conjunction with maternal serum AFP measurement, the detection rate is further improved, although some pregnancies require evaluation of amniotic fluid AFP and acetylcholinesterase levels for confirmation.[8]

Elevated maternal serum AFP is associated with other conditions, including abdominal wall defects such as gastroschisis and omphalocele,[11] supporting the role of ultrasound as a first-line evaluation in screen-positive cases. Adverse pregnancy outcomes, including fetal loss, preterm delivery, intrauterine growth restriction, and placental abruption are also associated with elevated maternal serum AFP.[12]

First-Trimester Screening for Aneuploidy

First-trimester screening uses a combination of maternal serum analytes and ultrasound measurement of fetal nuchal translucency (NT) to provide an age-adjusted risk for trisomy 21 and 18. The maternal serum markers pregnancy-associated plasma protein A (PAPP-A) and human chorionic gonadotrophin (hCG) are measured at 9 to 14 weeks gestational age, and NT is measured at 11 to 14 weeks gestational age. Using such a protocol, about 80%–90% of Down syndrome pregnancies are detected at a 5% screen-positive rate.[9,13,14] The detection rate for trisomy 18 is slightly lower. PAPP-A levels are decreased and hCG levels are increased in trisomy 21; levels of both analytes are decreased in trisomy 18.

Nuchal translucency is present in virtually all fetuses and consists of a space of varying size behind the fetal neck. The size of the NT is correlated with fetal size as measured by crown-rump length. NT alone detects up to 70% of trisomy 21 pregnancies and a similar proportion of those with other chromosomal abnormalities, such as trisomy 13, trisomy 18, and 45,X,[15] but is not used as a stand-alone test. Some researchers, however, suggest that an NT of 4.0 mm or greater should serve as an indication for invasive diagnostic testing because the use of serum markers offers little in the way of further risk adjustment for trisomy 21.[16,17] In addition to its utility in detecting aneuploidy, increased NT size is associated with a wide range of other fetal abnormalities, such as cardiac defects, diaphragmatic hernia, and a number of single-gene disorders, including skeletal dysplasias.[18,19] In general, the risk for an adverse outcome is positively correlated with the size of the NT. The American College of Obstetricians and Gynecologists (ACOG) recommends that in pregnancies with a NT measurement of 3.5 mm or greater, fetal echocardiography and targeted ultrasound examination should be offered for detection of specific malformations or malformation syndromes.[20]

Second-Trimester Screening for Aneuploidy

Multiple maternal serum markers are used to assess the risk for trisomy 21 and trisomy 18 in the second trimester, usually at about 15–20 weeks gestational age. The most effective strategy uses maternal serum AFP, hCG, unconjugated estriol (uE3), and inhibin A. Often called the "quad screen," this test detects about 75% of trisomy 21 pregnancies at a 5% screen-positive rate.[9] Typically, the AFP and uE3 levels are lower and the hCG and inhibin A levels are higher in trisomy 21 pregnancies. The detection rate for trisomy 18 is slightly lower. In most screening programs, the quad screen has replaced the triple screen, which uses only AFP, hCG, and uE3. The quad screen detects about 10% more cases of trisomy 21 than the triple screen, with a similar screen-positive rate. Second-trimester screening does not generally detect other aneuploidies, such as trisomy 13, Klinefelter syndrome (47,XXY), or Turner syndrome (45,X).

Combined First-Trimester and Second-Trimester Screening for Aneuploidy

Protocols for use of varying combinations of first-trimester and second-trimester screening have been investigated. Integrated screening provides a single adjusted risk estimate after all testing is completed and detects about 95% of trisomy 21 fetuses.[9] This method requires that first-trimester results be withheld until completion of second-trimester screening. To mitigate this problem, 2 sequential screening strategies have been developed to provide first-trimester risk information. Stepwise screening discloses results of first-trimester screening for high-risk pregnancies and defers those at lower risk for final risk assessment after the second-trimester results have been received.[21] Contingency screening uses first-trimester screening results to offer invasive testing for women at high risk, to defer risk assessment until completion of second-trimester screening for women at intermediate risk, and to suggest no further testing for women at low risk.[22] Each of these strategies detects about 90% of trisomy 21 fetuses, but their complexity makes them more difficult to implement than either first- or second-trimester screening alone.[23]

Fetal Renal Pelvis Dilation

As described in the next section, prenatal ultrasound may identify fetal markers of unknown clinical significance such as renal pelvis dilation (RPD) or short femurs. Communication with the neonatologist or pediatrician is important, as he or she will need to be aware of the implications of the prenatal findings, perform newborn and follow-up examinations, and decide if postnatal evaluation is warranted. Although most cases of RPD either resolve or remain stable and require no active treatment,[24] when the RPD is greater than 15 mm, the risk of serious renal disease is high. There is no consensus on how best to evaluate and treat those with mild or moderate dilation. Many follow-up protocols recommend that a single postnatal ultrasound examination demonstrating RPD less than 15 mm does not require follow-up studies, although in practice it appears common to perform at least one additional ultrasound examination to confirm resolution.[25] These and other authors have questioned the need for invasive studies such as voiding cystourethrogram (VCUG) in this group of patients.[26]

Prenatal Diagnosis by Amniocentesis

Amniocentesis for diagnosis of chromosome abnormalities has been performed since the 1960s and is usually carried out between 15 and 18 weeks gestation. Using ultrasound guidance, amniocentesis has a procedure-related pregnancy loss rate of about 1 in 300 to 600.[27,28] In the recent past, amniocentesis was offered only to women who had an increased risk for fetal aneuploidy based on abnormal screening results or to women more than 35 years of age based on the rationale that the risk for having a child with a chromosomal abnormality approached the procedure-related pregnancy loss rate. However, current guidelines from the American College of Medical Genetics (ACMG) and ACOG call for amniocentesis or chorionic villus sampling (CVS) to be made available to all pregnant women, after appropriate counseling regarding its risks and benefits, and that maternal age should no longer be used as a threshold to determine who is offered invasive testing.[27,29] In addition to diagnosis of fetal aneuploidy, amniocentesis is also a useful procedure for diagnosis of many single-gene disorders, either by mutation analysis of cultured amniocytes or through biochemical analysis of analytes diagnostic of inborn errors of metabolism. Amniocentesis may also be performed to measure amniotic fluid AFP levels and acetylcholinesterase for confirmation of open NTDs.

Prenatal Diagnosis by Chorionic Villus Sampling

Chorionic villus sampling gained acceptance in the United States in the 1980s and 1990s as an alternative to amniocentesis and is usually performed from 10 to 13 weeks gestation. The pregnancy loss rate after CVS is greater than the rate for midtrimester amniocentesis, but much of this increase may be related to an increased background loss rate between 10 and 16 weeks gestation.[20] The major advantage of CVS over amniocentesis is that it can be performed earlier in pregnancy and provide earlier reassurance, earlier knowledge of a fetal abnormality and a longer period of preparation for care and management of an affected infant, or an opportunity for an earlier pregnancy termination, which may be associated with fewer maternal complications. Like amniocentesis, CVS is also a useful procedure for obtaining fetal tissue that can be used for mutation analysis for diagnosis of a known genetic disorder. Because amniotic fluid is not collected by CVS, measurement of analytes that can diagnose inborn errors of metabolism or confirm the diagnosis of open NTDs is not possible. Therefore, maternal serum AFP screening between 15 and 20 weeks gestation is still recommended. Also, because fetal anatomy is not well visualized at 10–12 weeks gestation, a high-resolution ultrasound examination is recommended between 16 and 18 weeks gestation.

Chromosome Analysis: Cytogenetic analysis versus Array-Based Comparative Genomic Hybridization

Conventional cytogenetic analysis is used to detect fetal chromosome abnormalities after amniocentesis or CVS. In pediatric practice, array-based comparative genomic hybridization (aCGH), also known as chromosomal microarray (CMA), is now recommended as the first-tier clinical diagnostic test for individuals with developmental disabilities or congenital anomalies.[30] The utility of aCGH for prenatal diagnosis has been investigated in several large case series and found to have some benefits over conventional karyotyping,[31,32] but concerns about its high cost, its inability to detect unbalanced chromosome rearrangements, and its detection of copy number variants of unknown clinical significance has led the ACOG to recommend against its routine use in prenatal diagnosis at present.[33]

Cell-Free Fetal DNA in Maternal Plasma

Approximately 5% of cell-free DNA in maternal blood is of fetal origin, and massively parallel shotgun sequencing (MPSS) has been used to detect trisomy 21 prenatally. One recent study of high-risk pregnant women identified Down syndrome with a 98.6% detection rate, a 0.2% false-positive rate, and a 0.8% false-negative rate.[34] This technology shows promise in improving screening for trisomy 21 as well as other aneuploidies; however, validation studies in non-high-risk populations is necessary before this technique will be considered standard of care.

Imaging of Fetal Anomalies

Fetal imaging with high-resolution ultrasound and rapid acquisition magnetic resonance imaging (MRI) is central to accurate diagnosis of congenital anomalies. Imaging has enhanced our understanding of the natural history of many prenatally diagnosed fetal anomalies, allowed for improved prediction of outcome and counseling and for pregnancy planning and newborn management. Communication of the prenatal findings to the postnatal caregivers is critical to ensure that the newborn is optimally managed, with appropriate postnatal imaging studies and correct treatment protocols.[35]

Ultrasound is the primary imaging modality for the diagnosis of most fetal anomalies. MRI can provide incremental information compared with ultrasound by defining lesion extent or detecting additional abnormalities. Studies have shown that ultrasound and MRI can

be powerful, effecting a change or adding a diagnosis in 57% of cases.[36] MRI has advantages over ultrasound when the position of the fetal head is low in the pelvis or is difficult to see because large maternal body habitus, oligohydramnios, or the presence of another fetus precludes detailed examination (Figure 7-1). Furthermore, MRI provides a large field of view in three spatial planes—axial, sagittal, and coronal—which is helpful for understanding anatomic relationships of larger anomalies (Figure 7-2). A thorough discussion of fetal anomaly imaging is beyond the scope of this chapter. We discuss the role of imaging for fetal anomalies, focusing on chest and central nervous system (CNS) findings.

Fetal Brain Anomalies

The majority of fetal brain MRIs are performed to further evaluate ventriculomegaly, a posterior fossa cyst, or absence of the cavum septum pellucidum (CSP) diagnosed on ultrasound. Associated diseases identified with MRI and not detected with ultrasound are for the most part abnormalities of the cerebral/cerebellar parenchyma, such as neuronal migration disorders, delayed sulcation and gyration, small periventricular cysts, and intraparenchymal hemorrhagic foci.[37,86] (Figure 7-3). In a study of 145 fetuses with fetal central nervous system abnormalities diagnosed on ultrasound, Levine et al noted that MRI led to a change in diagnosis in 32%, a change in counseling in 50%, and a change in management in 19% of cases.

Fetal ventriculomegaly is a relatively common abnormality identified in approximately 1/1000 births and often represents a counseling dilemma for predicting outcome.[38] Ventriculomegaly is a nonspecific dilation of the lateral ventricles, which can result from many different types of brain abnormalities or insults. Prognosis for ventriculomegaly depends on the severity and the presence or absence of associated cerebral or extracerebral anomalies. Ventriculomegaly is usually categorized as mild (atrial diameter 11–15 mm) or severe (atrial diameter > 15 mm). The most guarded outcomes occur in cases of ventriculomegaly associated with abnormal karyotype or additional anomalies by fetal imaging.[38,39] Several studies have reported an increased detection rate by MRI compared with ultrasound for both CNS and non-CNS anomalies associated with ventriculomegaly.[40] However in a subset of isolated mild ventriculomegaly (10-12 mm), MRI provided additional findings to ultrasound in 19.5% of cases, and changed the clinical prognosis in 1.1% of cases.[40]

Beeghly et al reported only 60% live delivery and survival through the neonatal period in fetuses with ventriculomegaly associated with other CNS findings.[39] Approximately 60% of ventriculomegaly cases are classified as isolated on ultrasound and present a counseling dilemma because of heterogeneous outcome. Up to 23%

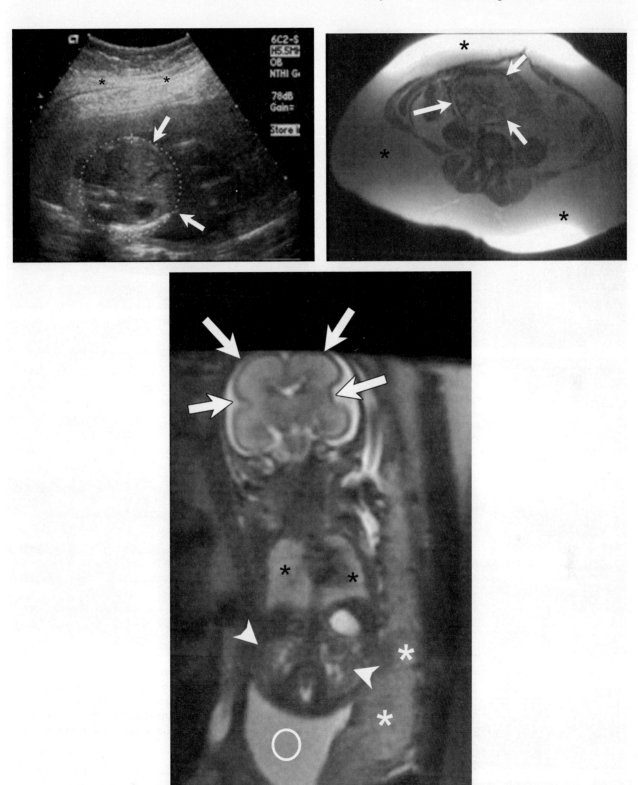

FIGURE 7-1 Expectant mother carrying fetus at 23 weeks gestational age. A, Axial plane sonogram through the fetal abdomen shows severe image degradation secondary to maternal body habitus (asterisks = subcutaneous fat; arrows = fetal abdomen). B, Axial magnetic resonance imaging (MRI) through the maternal pelvis shows a large amount of maternal subcutaneous fat (asterisks = fat; arrows = fetus). C, Coronal plane MRI of the fetus shows no significant image degradation despite maternal obesity (arrows = fetal brain; black asterisks = fetal lungs; arrowheads = fetal kidneys; white asterisks = placenta; circle = amniotic fluid).

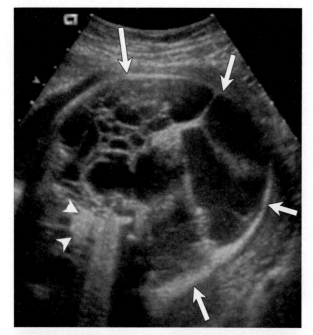

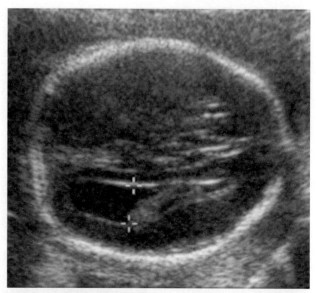

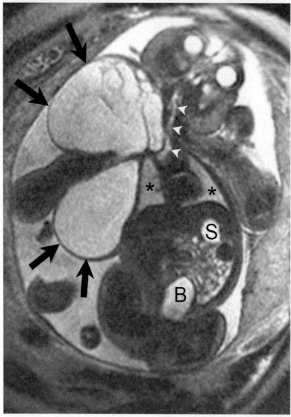

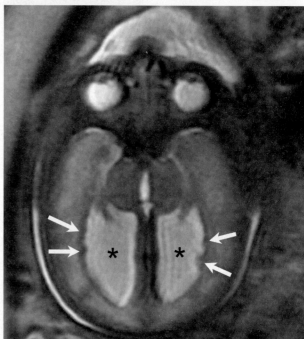

FIGURE 7-3 Cortical heterotopia. A, Axial sonogram demonstrates mild dilation of the lateral ventricle (calipers = 12 mm). B, Axial plane magnetic resonance imaging (MRI) confirms mild ventriculomegaly (asterisks) and subependymal nodularity (arrows), consistent with cortical heterotopia.

FIGURE 7-2 Lymphatic malformation involving fetal neck and chest. A, Axial sonogram through the lower fetal neck shows a large multicystic mass (arrows = lymphatic malformation; arrowheads = fetal spine). B, Coronal plane magnetic resonance imaging (MRI) depicts anatomic relationship of the lymphatic malformation (large arrows) to the fetal neck, chest, and airway (arrowheads) (asterisks = fetal lungs; S, stomach; B, bladder). Fetal neck mass deviates fetal neck to the left, but there is no evidence for airway compromise.

of isolated mild ventriculomegaly cases are reported to have an abnormal outcome because of associated cerebral malformations, infection, or aneuploidy.[41] When a fetal patient has isolated mild ventriculomegaly diagnosed on ultrasound and MRI shows no additional cerebral or extracerebral malformations, the prognosis is very good; greater than 90% have been reported to have a normal outcome (Figure 7-4).[38] Mild asymmetrical ventriculomegaly diagnosed on ultrasound and confirmed on MRI has also been reported to be associated with neurodevelopmental delay.[42,43]

Sonographic diagnosis of a posterior fossa cyst raises concern for the Dandy Walker spectrum: mega cisterna magna, inferior vermian dysgenesis, and Dandy Walker malformation. Fetal MRI can differentiate between these entities and search for additional associated brain or extracerebral anomalies. The distinction is important because isolated mega cisterna magna is associated with an excellent clinical outcome, whereas inferior vermian dysgenesis and Dandy Walker malformation may have more guarded outcomes (Figures 7-5 and 7-6).[44,45] The vermis undergoes rapid development prior to 22 weeks gestational age, and the inferior vermis in particular may lag in development, which may lead to overdiagnosis of vermian hypoplasia on MRI.

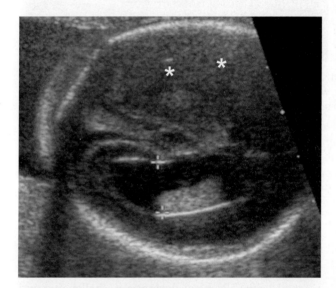

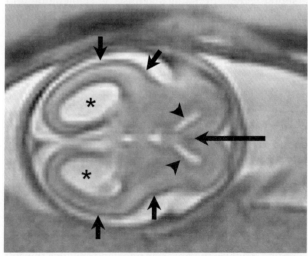

FIGURE 7-4 Mild ventriculomegaly on ultrasound with normal postnatal outcome (20 weeks gestational age). A, Axial ultrasound demonstrates mild ventriculomegaly (calipers = 12 mm). Brain parenchyma (asterisks), particularly in the near field, was difficult to visualize. B, Axial magnetic resonance imaging (MRI) confirms mild ventriculomegaly (asterisks) but otherwise normal brain parenchyma, including the frontal horns (arrowheads), anterior corpus callosum (long arrow), and brain mantle (short arrows).

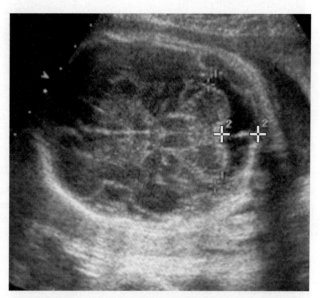

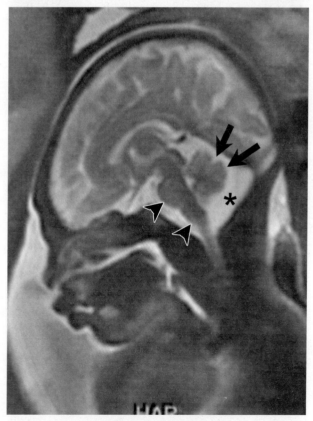

FIGURE 7-5 Mega cisterna magna (29 weeks gestational age) with normal postnatal outcome. A, Axial sonogram shows enlargement of the cisterna magna (calipers = 12 mm). B, Sagittal plane magnetic resonance imaging (MRI) confirms normal cerebellar vermis (arrows) and brain stem (arrowheads) (asterisk = enlarged cisterna magna).

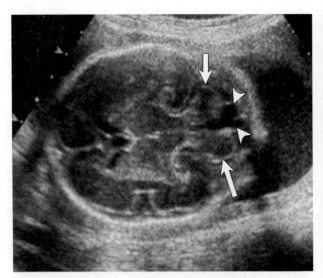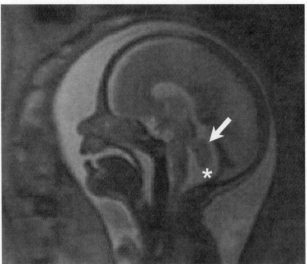

FIGURE 7-6 Inferior vermian dysgenesis (25 weeks gestational age). A, Axial sonogram demonstrates 12-mm posterior fossa cyst (arrowheads) (short arrows = cerebellar vermis). B, Vermian hypoplasia. Sagittal plane magnetic resonance imaging (MRI) confirms normal superior vermis (arrow) but under development of the inferior vermis (asterisk = cisterna magna).

The CSP is a normal midline structure that separates the anterior horns of the lateral ventricles, and its presence has a high correlation with normal midline brain formation. The CPS should be identified on all second- and third-trimester fetal ultrasound examinations. Absence or abnormal configuration of the CSP is associated with agenesis of the corpus callosum, holoprosencephaly, and septo-optic dysplasia (SOD). The corpus callosum represents the fiber tracks that connect the two hemispheres of the brain. The corpus callosum may be partially or completely absent (agenesis), which can occur as an isolated finding or in combination with other cerebral abnormalities. Partial or complete agenesis of the corpus callosum can be diagnosed by ultrasound by demonstrating separation of the frontal horns of the lateral ventricles on a coronal view of the brain or colpocephaly, often associated with a teardrop configuration to the posterior lateral ventricles. MRI is useful in confirming the diagnosis in equivocal cases on ultrasound and in evaluating for associated anomalies (Figure 7-7). Absence or partial agenesis to corpus callosum has been reported as an incidental or isolated finding, which can have a normal neurologic outcome; however, associated abnormal CNS or extracerebral findings are associated with substantially increased risk for neurodevelopmental impairment.[46]

Holoprosencephaly is a heterogeneous entity caused by impaired midline cleavage of the embryonic forebrain. Most children with holoprosencephaly are afflicted with seizures, cognitive disorders, and developmental delay. Approximately 50% of cases are associated with chromosomal abnormalities, including trisomy 13. Holoprosencephaly is often classified into lobar, semilobar, or alobar types, which correspond to increasing severity of forebrain fusion. Similarly, the clinical manifestations and neurologic sequelae are most severe in the alobar type of holoprosencephaly. Most cases of holoprosencephaly are readily detected by ultrasound.

Septo-optic dysplasia is a rare disorder characterized by abnormal development of the optic disk, pituitary deficiencies, and often absence of the CSP or of a septal leaflet. Prenatal diagnosis is challenging and may be missed on fetal MRI given the small size of the optic nerves and chiasm.[47]

Fetal Neck Masses

A fetal neck mass should always raise a high level of concern for potential airway compromise, which can result in perinatal asphyxia. Teratomas are the most common neonatal tumor, and approximately 10% are located in the head and neck region. In the presonographic era, a very high mortality rate was noted, with overall mortality rate of 30% for cervical teratomas and 21% for oropharyngeal teratomas.[48] Cystic hygromas (lymphatic malformations) usually are located in the posterolateral neck, but a subset of these malformations involves the anterior neck and invades the soft tissue planes into the oral cavity and superior mediastinum. Lymphatic malformations may also result in airway compromise, however, to a lesser extent than teratomas. Steigman et al reported that 67% of teratomas vs 11% of lymphatic malformations require neonatal airway intervention.[49]

The majority of fetal neck masses are detected by ultrasound; however, visualization may be limited by shadowing from the fetal facial bones, which impedes

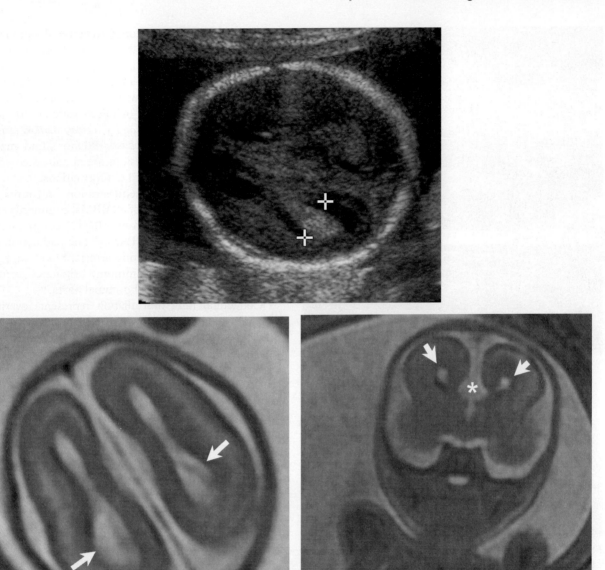

FIGURE 7-7 Agenesis of the corpus callosum (22 weeks gestational age). A, Axial sonogram shows borderline ventriculomegaly (calipers = 10 mm). B, Axial plane magnetic resonance imaging (MRI) demonstrates colpocephaly (arrows) (dilation of the posterior body of the lateral ventricles) and parallel orientation of the ventricles. C, Coronal plane MRI through the region of the frontal horns shows absence of the anterior corpus callosum and a prominent interhemispheric fissure (asterisk) extending inferiorly (short arrows = frontal horns).

visualization of the fetal airway (Figure 7-8). On ultrasound, teratomas are usually complex solid and cystic masses, which frequently contain calcification. Fetal MRI image quality is not degraded by the fetal facial bones or skull, and assessment of airway patency is usually possible. This additional information may enhance counseling and delivery planning decisions in selected cases (Figure 7-8). The airway-compromised fetus is a candidate for the *ex utero* intrapartum treatment (EXIT) procedure, a specialized surgical

delivery procedure. During the EXIT procedure, a hysterotomy is performed, followed by the delivery of the fetal head and neck. The fetus is maintained on placental circulation as an airway is secured by neonatology, otolaryngology, pediatric anesthesia, or pediatric surgery via intubation or tracheostomy. If an airway cannot be secured during an EXIT procedure, surgical resection of the mass or placing the infant on extracorporeal membrane oxygenation (ECMO) may be considered.

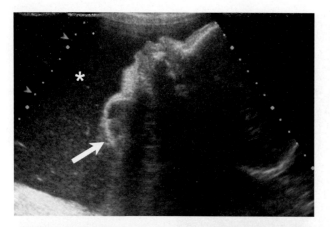

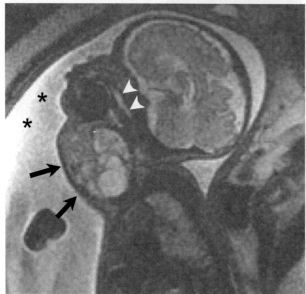

FIGURE 7-8 Anterior neck teratoma compromising fetal airway (35 weeks gestational age). A, Sagittal plane sonogram demonstrates an anterior neck mass (arrow). Airway was not visualized secondary to acoustic shadowing from the fetal facial bones and skull (asterisk = polyhydramnios). B, Sagittal plane magnetic resonance imaging (MRI) demonstrates anterior neck mass (arrows) and compromise of the airway (arrowheads) which is not visualized below the level of the nasopharynx (asterisks = amniotic fluid).

Fetal Chest Masses

Bronchopulmonary Malformations

Congenital bronchopulmonary malformations (BPMs) represent a spectrum of lung anomalies that include congenital pulmonary airway malformation (CPAM), bronchopulmonary sequestration (BPS), and congenital lobar overinflation (CLO).[50–52] Our understanding of the natural history of congenital airway malformations has significantly improved via prenatal imaging, which now plays a key role in management decisions and family counseling regarding likely outcomes. BPMs are usually detected as an incidental finding on prenatal ultrasound (Figure 7-9).

CPAMs are the most common cause of a prenatally diagnosed BPM, accounting for approximately half of all lesions.[53] CPAMs result from early airway maldevelopment and represent a benign hamartoma or dysplastic tumor, which is usually characterized by the presence of macroscopic or microcystic components. The term *congenital pulmonary airway malformation* is preferable to congenital cystic adenomatoid malformation (CCAM) as the lesions are not always cystic or comprised of adenomatoid malformations.

Bronchopulmonary sequestration accounts for approximately one-third of all BPMs, commonly existing as hybrid lesions with histological components of both sequestration and CPAM.[53] The pathognomonic finding of BPS is a systemic arterial blood supply to the mass, which most commonly originates from the lower thoracic or upper abdominal aorta.[54]

Congenital lung overinflation represents overinflation of a lung segment or lobe, which on microscopic analysis is characterized by air space enlargement without maldevelopment. Therefore, the term *overinflation* is preferred to that of *emphysema* (Figure 7-9).

Bronchopulmonary malformations appear as cystic, solid, or complex masses on ultrasound. On MRI, the normal fetal lungs demonstrate increasing signal intensity as the pregnancy progresses, which correlates with intrapulmonary fluid accumulation during fetal lung development.[55,56] Most fetal lung malformations appear as higher signal masses compared to the normal fetal lung on MRI.[57] Combined with ultrasound, MRI has been reported to be highly accurate in the diagnosis of the specific type of BPM as correlated with postnatal pathology or imaging.[58] In addition, MRI provides alternative or additional diagnoses compared with ultrasound in 38%–50% of fetuses.[55,59]

The majority of fetuses with an isolated BPM have an excellent prognosis and usually are asymptomatic at birth. A small subset of fetuses with large masses will develop fetal hydrops, with a mortality approaching 100% without intervention.[60] For CPAMs, the sonographic measurement of a CPAM volume ratio (CVR) is useful in prognosis and management, with CVR greater than 1.6 predicting an 80% risk for developing fetal hydrops.[60] An MRI derived lung mass volume ratio has also been reported to predict fetal complications of hydrops and mortality and postnatal morbidity including respiratory distress, intubation, and need for neonatal surgery in fetuses with congenital lung masses.[87] Maternal antenatal steroid treatment has been reported to be associated with decreased fetal mass size, reduction in risk for hydrops, and improved survival.[61,62] Some investigators have also reported in utero open fetal surgical resection in cases of large fetal lung mass with hydrops prior to 32 weeks estimated gestational age (EGA); this approach requires appropriate personnel and resources and carries risk to mother and fetus.[63] Cass et al. have reported EXIT

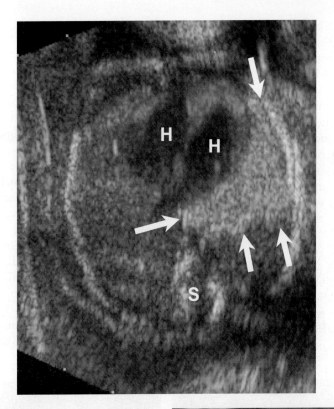

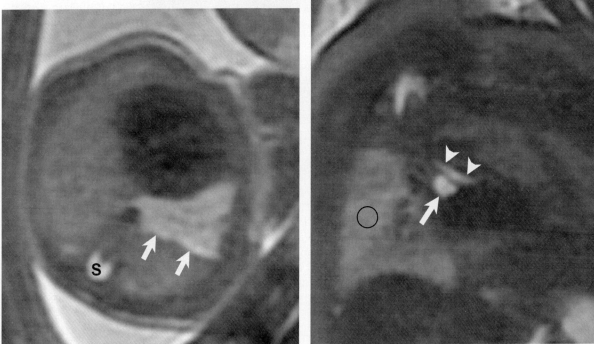

FIGURE 7-9 Congenital lobar overinflation secondary to bronchogenic cyst (22 weeks gestational age). A, Axial sonogram demonstrates a hyperechogenic mass (arrows) in the left lingula (S = spine; H = heart). B, Axial plane magnetic resonance imaging (MRI) through the fetal chest demonstrates high signal mass (arrows) with normal branching vascular pattern consistent with lobar overinflation (S = spine). C, Coronal plane MRI demonstrates subcarinal bronchogenic cyst (arrow) as the cause for the lobar hyperinflation (arrowheads = left main stem bronchus; circle = right lung).

to resection for fetuses with large lung masses and persistent mediastinal compression near term to reduce neonatal morbidity and mortality.[88]

The assessment of a BPM during the third trimester is helpful in planning delivery location. In our program, delivery venue recommendations are made after multidisciplinary review and consultation, including maternal fetal medicine specialists (MFM), pediatric surgery, neonatology, and radiology. When the malformation is small and unassociated with mass effect, patients can be delivered in their local community, with outpatient follow-up with pediatric surgery. In our experience, MRI plays an important role in optimizing the postnatal imaging algorithm. The historical imaging algorithm for an asymptomatic newborn with a prenatally diagnosed intrathoracic mass was a chest x-ray followed by chest computed tomography (CT) to confirm and characterize the mass.[64] Third-trimester fetal MRI shows a high correlation with newborn CT for the size and type of lesion, thereby negating the need for an early CT in asymptomatic newborns.[65]

Congenital Diaphragmatic Hernia

Congenital diaphragmatic hernia (CDH) occurs secondary to a developmental defect in the diaphragm, which results in intrathoracic herniation of abdominal contents. The herniated contents may include the fetal stomach, small intestine, colon, or liver and interferes with normal lung development. Prognosis depends on the severity of pulmonary hypoplasia, pulmonary hypertension, and the presence of associated anomalies or genetic abnormalities. CDH occurs more frequently on the left side than the right (85% vs 15%).[66] There is no clear evidence that MRI is superior to ultrasound for detecting additional anomalies, but MRI may be considered complimentary to ultrasound, particularly when the findings are equivocal.[67]

Both ultrasound and MRI accurately diagnose CDH by visualizing the stomach, small bowel, colon, or liver within the chest (Figure 7-10). For left-sided CDH, liver position and ultrasound-measured lung-to-head ratio (LHR) when the liver is above the level of the

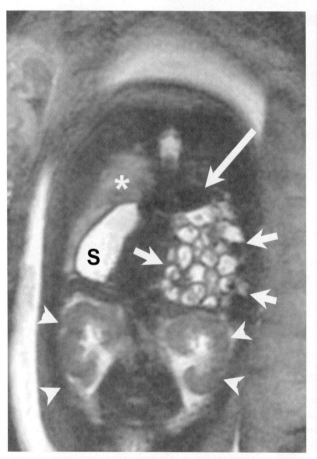 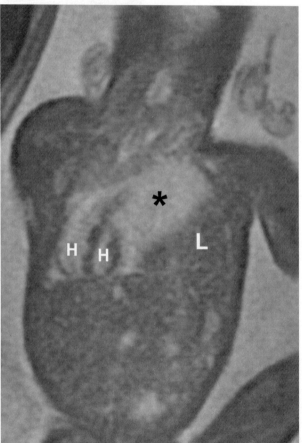

FIGURE 7-10 Congenital diaphragmatic hernia. A, 30 weeks gestational age. Coronal plane magnetic resonance imaging (MRI) demonstrates left-sided congenital diaphragmatic hernia comprised of small bowel (arrows), stomach (S), and colon (long arrow) (asterisk = right lung; arrowheads = intra-abdominal kidneys). B, 22 weeks gestational age. Coronal plane MRI demonstrates a left-sided congenital diaphragmatic hernia containing herniated liver (L) and a moderate amount of residual ipsilateral lung (asterisk), which was not seen on the prenatal ultrasound (H = heart). The infant survived without need for extracorporeal membrane oxygenation (ECMO).

diaphragm have been reported to be useful in predicting neonatal mortality or need for ECMO. The most consistent prenatal imaging indicator for postnatal outcome is the position of the liver.[68–70] Measurement of fetal lung volumes by MRI as a predictor for postnatal survival or morbidity has received much attention in the literature. MRI can be used to measure normal fetal lung volumes[71] and may provide complimentary information regarding severity of predicted pulmonary hypoplasia and postnatal outcome in fetuses with CDH; however, several studies have reported overlap in the lung volumes of CDH survivors vs nonsurvivors.[72] Futhermore, fetuses with adequate measured lung volumes may still experience significant morbidity related to significant pulmonary hypertension.[89] Although it would be highly desirable to accurately and reliably predict neonatal mortality and morbidity because of CDH from early prenatal measures, it is important to understand that the pathophysiology of CDH is complex. In addition, prenatal technology and measures and postnatal management strategies have evolved and continue to evolve, making neonatal outcome prediction in the current era challenging. Ultimately, the best prognostic approach will likely involve a combination of fetal findings from ultrasound, MRI, and fetal echocardiogram, which may include current and evolving predictors such as percentage predicted lung volume (PPLV)[73] and prenatal pulmonary hypertension index (PPHI)[74] (Figure 7-11).

THE BENEFITS OF A PRENATAL CONSULTATION BY A NEONATOLOGIST

Routine involvement of a neonatologist in complex fetal case consultations is a relatively recent phenomenon. Traditionally, because care of both the expectant mother and the fetus is the purview of the obstetrician and perinatologist, they have had the primary responsibility for conveying screening and diagnostic imaging results to families and for discussing their significance. But, given the rapidly changing options for postnatal treatment of even the most complex medical and surgical problems, involvement by neonatologists and other pediatric specialists as part of a multidisciplinary team approach can be important to help families integrate a sometimes-enormous volume of diagnostic data, to provide information about short-term and long-term implications of the findings, and to coordinate immediate neonatal care and follow-up. There clearly can be hurdles to routinely integrating a neonatologist into the prenatal consultation process and even more to creating a robust team approach to complex maternal-fetal evaluations and consultations. For some institutions, the physical organization and location of delivery units, neonatal intensive care units (NICUs), and other

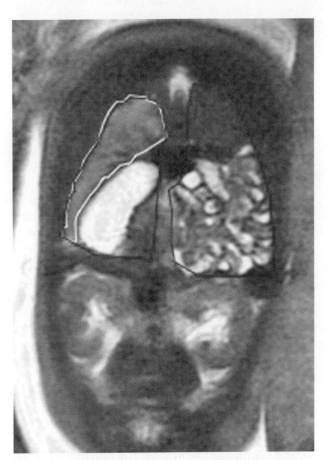

FIGURE 7-11 Severe congenital diaphragmatic hernia. Fetal lung volume, measured on coronal plane magnetic resonance imaging (MRI; region of interest in white) compared with expected lung volume (region of interest in red) was estimated to be less than 15%.

pediatric medical and surgical subspecialty care do not lend themselves easily to team creation. Furthermore, there may be frankly conflicting goals and recommendations for pregnancy management, delivery, and postnatal care reflected by the differing interests of medical and surgical specialists, social service personnel, and ethicists—from a focus on the current and future reproductive health of the expectant mother, to an emphasis on the fetus as a distinct patient.[5,75,76] These disagreements can be further intensified when fetal intervention is under consideration.[7,77,78] However, embedded within these disparities and challenges lies the opportunity for a multidisciplinary team to openly evaluate the evidence supporting differing approaches to management and to integrate the goals and wishes of the expectant mother and family.

In cases of relatively minor fetal findings, the neonatologist's input may be limited to a discussion of required neonatal imaging or follow-up care and ensuring communication of the team's recommendation to the pediatrician. However, for cases in which significant complex fetal anomalies are expected and neonatal intensive care will be required, the neonatologist can be a crucial point of continuity of care for fetus and infant and for the family. Although many pediatric medical and surgical subspecialists may be important members of the prenatal and postnatal care team, the neonatologist can be considered the "primary care provider" to the most vulnerable and critically ill infants. The neonatologist has unique insight into moment-to-moment bedside care; the technologies, diagnostic testing, and therapeutic interventions the infant is most likely to experience; and the uncertainties of the NICU course. Neonatologists in high-level intensive care environments have significant experience in confronting difficult diagnoses and decisions with parents and families. Balancing the goals of providing information, describing treatment options and potential outcomes, framing a message in an unbiased fashion, and attempting to understand the needs of the family is an ethical challenge faced by neonatologists on a daily basis.[79–81] Neonatologists who care for complex patients also are experienced in assimilating input from multiple services and multiple diagnostic tests to present to families.

In the following section, we highlight key aspects of the neonatologist's role in prenatal consultations and the process of communication and difficult decision making in the prenatal setting. This is not meant to be a comprehensive or definitive description of the neonatologist's preferred strategy; rather, it is a starting point toward developing a cohesive approach to integrating neonatal prenatal consultations within a multidisciplinary framework.

HOW CAN A NEONATOLOGIST CONTRIBUTE TO FETAL CARE?

Components of a Prenatal Consultation with a Neonatologist

The elements, complexity, and length of the prenatal visit may vary significantly depending on the reasons for the consultation.[82] The following outlines the basic components of the visit:

- Introduction and role of the neonatologist:
  - The family may have met many individuals prior to meeting with the neonatologist and may meet many more as their journey continues. They should be introduced to the role of the neonatologist in the delivery and NICU, as well as in the multidisciplinary fetal care approach. The family should understand that a neonatologist will be directing the comprehensive care of the infant in the NICU, be coordinating consultations and diagnostic tests, and be the point of

communication for the family in the NICU. In addition, the neonatologist should clarify the roles of other subspecialists that the expectant mother has met and is scheduled to meet.
- Review fetal findings:
  - For some families, there is great anxiety about the appearance of expected fetal findings. It may be useful for some families to have pictures available for specific anomalies (eg, gastroschisis) or access to fetal imaging.
- Discuss implications for delivery room scenario and immediate postnatal plan:
  - The neonatologist should describe the likely series of events in the delivery room: who will be in attendance, how many will be there; whether the mother be able to hold the baby; whether the baby will be able to spend the usual bonding period with the family in the delivery room. The answers to these questions are, of course, specific to the fetal findings and expected neonatal clinical presentation. The neonatologist should also discuss the immediate plan for postnatal care: Will the baby need to be admitted to the NICU or be allowed to room in with the mother (eg, for minor findings)? If the baby goes to the NICU, will a family member be able to accompany the team to the NICU? Will the severity of the fetal problem necessitate immediate intervention or diagnostic procedures?
- Present the possibilities for unexpected or different findings as appropriate:
  - Acknowledging uncertainty in diagnosis, clinical presentation and immediate intensive care needs, or interventions after delivery is important to prepare the family for what may be a challenging time.
- Discuss interventions that may be required or plans for feeding and nutrition:
  - Depending on the findings and problems anticipated, the infant may require a range of interventions, including intubation, intravenous access, and arterial access. The infant may not be fed enterally initially but rather will receive nutrition parenterally. Families may not have understood or integrated these facts prior to the consultation with a neonatologist.
- Describe the expected course of events for diagnostic workup, medical and surgical treatment, and expected outcomes:
  - This should include the general order and timing of diagnostic and therapeutic events, potential further information that could be revealed, and discussion of outcomes, acknowledging uncertainty.
- Discuss the tenets of family-centered care and the critical importance of the mother and family in the care process:
  - Encourage the family to ask questions during the prenatal and postnatal periods, share concerns

with the medical or surgical team, and take an active role.

- Assess the need for other resources:
  - Depending on the needs of the family and the resources of the program, the neonatologist can help to facilitate connections between the family and medical social workers, parent mentors and volunteers, lactation consultants, and nursing representatives for the neonatal unit in which the infant is expected to receive care. Access and communications with these important services and staff may help to ease anxiety greatly and underscore the collaborative approach for the care of the expectant mother and infant.
- Provide a tour of the labor and delivery unit, NICU, or other infant care units as appropriate to the case:
  - Many expectant mothers and family members have enormous apprehension about the NICU. But, for many, the fear of the unknown and abstract intensive care environment is more substantial than the reality. The neonatologist should familiarize the expectant mother and family with the delivery and neonatal care units and other team members who will be caring for the infant, which often greatly alleviates anxiety.
- Assure the family of continued communication among all members of the multidisciplinary prenatal and postnatal care team members.

Reasons to Involve a Neonatologist in Prenatal Consultation and Care

- A complex fetal anomaly is found or suspected:
  - For complex and clear fetal anomalies, the benefits for prenatal neonatology involvement are apparent and are further outlined in the following material. However, even in mild or moderate anomalies (eg, renal pelviectasis or unilateral hydronephrosis with normal amniotic fluid), it may be useful for a neonatologist to become involved to help determine whether and which subspecialists should see the expectant mother or make recommendations regarding need for postnatal diagnostic imaging to clarify the findings and outpatient follow-up with pediatric subspecialists. In many minor cases, the neonatologist may also be able to ameliorate anxiety for the family, discussing the findings and helping to put a postnatal plan in place.
- Helping to determine the best delivery venue:
  - As noted, many fetal anomalies do not result in a need for complex delivery planning, neonatal resuscitation, or a stay in the NICU. In these situations, as long as follow-up for the baby is in place if needed, the neonatologist can partner with the perinatologist to help guide discussions to allow delivery by the expectant mother's obstetrician at

an appropriate hospital close to the family. Some persistent fetal findings may not be associated with complications for the mother or fetus and are not expected to result in immediate and profound neonatal clinical decompensation (eg, fetal bowel obstruction pattern without polyhydramnios) but may nonetheless require diagnostic evaluation by a skilled pediatric radiologist within hours or days, monitoring and treatment in a NICU, and possibly other involvement of other subspecialists (eg, pediatric surgery). Depending on the level of care provided in NICUs in a community, this care may or may not be achievable at the expectant mother's local hospital. The neonatologist providing the prenatal consultation can help to determine these needs and the resources.

- Fetal intervention is anticipated:
  - A neonatologist should be consulted and ideally included early as part of any medical and surgical team discussion of fetal intervention. The neonatologist's perspective may add significantly to the understanding of postnatal complications and may provide an additional perspective for weighing the risks and benefits for the fetus, mother, and baby. Furthermore, increased risk for premature delivery has been reported in association after both open fetal surgery and fetoscopic approaches.[83,84] Therefore, a neonatologist should be consulted to advise and prepare the expectant mother and family regarding the potential morbidities associated with prematurity.
- Admission to the NICU is required:
  - The NICU can be an overwhelming and confusing environment for parents. Although it is never possible to "fully" prepare a family for this experience, the neonatologist can explain the series of events that will likely happen in the first minutes, hours, and days of hospitalization, including intubation, monitoring, line placement, diagnostic tests, medications needed, and subspecialist consultations that will occur. If a surgical intervention is anticipated, the neonatologist can discuss likely timing, personnel, and preparation for the surgery. It is also important to underscore and acknowledge the uncertainties that are inherent to any NICU course, particularly if a long and complex hospitalization is anticipated. If appropriate to the case, the neonatologist should also begin the discussions regarding likely need for blood products and the risks and benefits of transfusions and advise the family of the potential for directed blood donations but not in cases of emergent need.
  - Of great importance, the neonatologist can show the expectant mother and family to the physical space of the NICU, showing them the equipment likely to be utilized for their infant and familiarizing

them with the policies and practices of the NICU. The neonatologist can point out that families are at the bedside with their babies; some are holding and touching their infants, which is incredibly reassuring to families, who may have imagined the NICU in a very different way. The tour is also a good opportunity to introduce the family to other NICU care providers and support services—nurses, nurse practitioners, other neonatologists, and medical social workers—which demonstrates to the family that the coordination and communication in place during the pregnancy will continue through the delivery and throughout the neonatal course. It can be difficult for families to approach the NICU, but they are often enormously relieved after their visits, recognizing that the NICU is a part of the continuum of care, and both the infant and family are valued.

- Complex delivery room scenario is planned:
  - In some cases, a complex delivery plan is required because of the need for multidisciplinary involvement in the delivery room (eg, pediatric otolaryngologist required for potential airway anomaly); immediate surgical or other interventions for the newborn in the delivery room (eg, EXIT procedure required; severe hydrops resuscitation with need for multiple interventions simultaneously); or rapid transfer to another operating room likely for intervention (eg, to cardiac catheterization or cardiac operating room for severely restrictive atrial septal defect in hypoplastic left heart syndrome; to cardiac operating room for pacer wire placement for severe fetal bradycardia). The neonatologist plays a central role in coordination and planning in these cases. Along with the perinatologist and other specialists who may be involved, the neonatologist ensures that the appropriate personnel and resources are available.
  - The organization and team meetings for such cases should begin as early as possible, ideally resulting in written protocols and procedures so that everyone is literally on "the same page," and that preparation for future cases need not be duplicative. In addition, after each such complex delivery scenario, it is important for the team to have at least one debriefing to learn from challenges encountered and refine and improve the approach for the future. The neonatologist can provide unique insight in preparing the expectant mother and families for what can be expected during or immediately after these delivery room scenarios: when family members can expect updates, when they are likely to see the baby, or how the baby will look after a surgical procedure. During prenatal consultations, the neonatologist and multidisciplinary team should emphasize

the complexities and uncertainties of these challenging cases. If appropriate to the case, the team should discuss maternal risks that may be inherent, and that neonatal outcome may not be altered by the interventions.

- Diagnosis clear and severe; or diagnosis unclear and prognosis uncertain:
  - In the NICU, as in complex prenatal consultations, the neonatologist is often in the position of integrating many pieces of complex information and of presenting as complete a picture as possible to the family in words they can understand.[85] The neonatologist should recognize that the expectant mother and family have likely been through a rapid series of diagnostic tests and consultations focused on fetal-specific organ systems or problems. They may have not heard or absorbed all the information together; if there are multiple problems or findings, the severity of the complete situation and significance of the implications may not have been recognized by the expectant mother and family. It is important for the medical team to discuss reasonable and well-considered care options to the family; it is the responsibility of the medical team to evaluate the totality of the findings, consider the therapeutic and management strategies that are possible, and present options that are appropriate. In framing the discussions, the team should acknowledge that uncertainty does exist in many complex situations, both in terms of the etiology of findings and the short- and long-term outcomes implied by those findings.

It is critical during this process to establish a therapeutic alliance with the family, seeking to understand their goals for their baby and recognizing that families have different goals and expectations and are willing to accept different levels of risk in terms of outcomes; for the neonatologist, as the team member who will provide primary continuity from fetal to neonatal care, this partnership and understanding are particularly important. The expectant mother and family should understand that the choices and direction for the baby and family may evolve. For instance, faced with uncertainty about findings and outcomes, the best first direction for a family may be to provide full intensive care support. But, as further postdelivery evaluation is carried out, additional findings may definitively change the direction of care that is appropriate for the goals of the family for their child. The neonatologist should assure the family that frequent discussions will occur in the NICU. Finally, in extremely complex and severe situations when comfort care support is determined by the family to be the most appropriate direction, the neonatologist and other team members must underscore their continued commitment and reiterate their dedication to providing outstanding and coordinated care for the expectant mother, family, fetal patient, and infant.

REFERENCES

1. Aite L, Zaccara A, Trucchi A, et al. When uncertainty generates more anxiety than severity: the prenatal experience with cystic adenomatoid malformation of the lung. *J Perinatol.* 2009;37(5): 539–542.

2. Kemp J, Davenport M, Pernet A. Antenatally diagnosed surgical anomalies: the psychological effect of parental antenatal counseling. *J Pediatr Surg.* 1998;33(9):1376–1379.

3. Strong C. Fetal anomalies: ethical and legal considerations in screening, detection, and management. *Clin Perinatol.* 2003;20:113–126.

4. Brown SD, Truog RD, Johnson JA, Ecker JL. Do differences in the AAP and ACOG positions on the ethics of maternal-fetal interventions reflect subtly divergent professional sensitivities to pregnant women and fetuses. *Pediatrics.* 2006;117:1382–1387.

5. Brown SD, Lyerly AD, Little MO, Lantos JD. Pediatrics-based fetal care: unanswered ethical questions. *Acta Paediatrica.* 2008;97:1617–1619.

6. Aite L, Zaccaro A, Mirante N, et al. Antenatal diagnosis of congenital anomaly: a really traumatic experience? *J Perinatol.* 2011. doi:10.1038/jp.2011.22.

7. American College of Obstetricians and Gynecologists Committee on Ethics, and American Academy of Pediatrics Committee on Bioethics. Committee opinion: maternal-fetal intervention and fetal care centers. *Obstet Gynecol.* 2011;118:405–410.

8. Norem CT, Schoen EJ, Walton DL, Krieger RC, O'Keefe J, To TT, Ray GT. Routine ultrasonography compared with maternal serum alpha-fetoprotein for neural tube defect screening. *Obstet Gynecol.* 2005;106:747–752.

9. Malone FD, Canick JA, Ball RH, et al. First- and Second-Trimester Evaluation of Risk (FASTER) Research Consortium. First-trimester or second-trimester screening, or both, for Down's syndrome. *N Engl J Med.* 2005;353:2001–2011.

10. Wald NJ, Cucckle HS, Brock JH, Peto R, Polani PE, Woodford FP. Maternal serum alpha-fetoprotein measurement in antenatal screening for anencephaly and spina bifid in early pregnancy. Report of the UK Collaborative Study on alpha-fetoprotein in relation to neural tube defects. *Lancet.* 1977;1:1323–1332.

11. Milunsky A. Maternal serum screening for neural tube and other defects. In: Milunsky A, ed. *Genetic Disorders and the Fetus: Diagnosis, Prevention and Treatment.* 4th ed. Baltimore, MD: Johns Hopkins University Press; 1998:635–701.

12. Dugoff L, Society for Maternal-Fetal Medicine. First- and second-trimester maternal serum markers for aneuploidy and adverse obstetric outcomes. *Obstet Gynecol.* 2010;115:1052–1061.

13. Wald NJ, Rodeck C, Hackshaw AK, et al. SURUSS Research Group. First and second trimester antenatal screening for Down's syndrome: the results of the Serum Urine and Ultrasound Screening Study (SURUSS) [erratum in *J Med Screen.* 2006;13:51–52]. *Health Technol Assess.* 2003;7:1–77.

14. Wapner R, Thom E, Simpson JL, et al. First trimester maternal serum biochemistry and fetal nuchal translucency screening (BUN) study group. First-trimester screening for trisomies 21 and 18. *N Engl J Med.* 2003;349:1405–1413.

15. Breathnach FM, Malone FD, Lambert-Messerlian G, et al. First and second trimester evaluation of risk (FASTER) Research Consortium. First- and second-trimester screening: detection of aneuploidies other than Down syndrome. *Obstet Gynecol.* 2007;110:651–657.

16. Comstock CH, Malone FD, Ball RH, et al. FASTER Research Consortium. Is there a nuchal translucency millimeter measurement above which there is no added benefit from first trimester screening? *Am J Obstet Gynecol.* 2006;195:843–847.

17. Malone FD, Ball RH, Nyberg DA, et al. FASTER Trial Research Consortium. First-trimester septated cystic hygroma: prevalence, natural history, and pediatric outcome. *Obstet Gynecol.* 2005;106:288–294.

18. Souka AP, Von Kaisenberg CS, Hyett JA, Sonek JD, Nicolaides KH. Increased nuchal translucency with normal karyotype [published erratum appears in *Am J Obstet Gynecol.* 2005;192:2096]. *Am J Obstet Gynecol.* 2005;192:1005–1021.

19. Makrydimas G, Sotiriadis A, Huggon JC, et al. Nuchal translucency and fetal cardiac defects: a pooled analysis of major fetal echocardiography centers. *Am J Obstet Gynecol.* 2005;192:89–95.

20. ACOG Committee on Practice Bulletin. ACOG Practice Bulletin Number 77: screening for fetal chromosomal abnormalities. *Obstet Gynecol.* 2007;109:217–227.

21. Platt LD, Greene N, Johnson A, et al; First Trimester Maternal Serum Biochemistry and Fetal Nuchal Translucency Screening (BUN) Study Group. Sequential pathways of testing after first-trimester screening for trisomy 21. *Obstet Gynecol.* 2004;104:661–666.

22. Wright D, Bradley L, Benn P, Cuckle H, Ritchie K. Contingent screening for Down syndrome is an efficient alternative to non-disclosure sequential screening. *Prenatal Diagn.* 2004;24:762–766.

23. Weisz B, Pandya P, Chitty L, et al. Practical issues drawn from the implementation of the integrated test for Down syndrome screening into routine clinical practice. *BJOG.* 2007;114:493–497.

24. Morin L, Cendron M, Crombleholme TM, Garmel SH, Klauber GT, D'Alton ME. Minimal hydronephrosis in the fetus: clinical significance and implications for management. *J Urol.* 1996;155:2047–2049.

25. Yiee J, Wilcox D. Management of fetal hydronephrosis. *Pediatr Nephrol.* 2008;23:347–353.

26. Hothi DK, Wade AS, Gilbert R, Winyard PJD. Mild fetal renal pelvis dilatation—much ado about nothing? *Clin J Am Soc Nephrol.* 2009;4:168–177.

27. ACOG Committee on Practice Bulletins-Obstetrics and the Committee on Genetics. Practice Bulletin Number 88: Invasive prenatal testing for aneuploidy. *Obstet Gynecol.* 2007;110(6): 1459–1467.

28. Eddelman KA, Malone FD, Sullivan L, et al. Pregnancy loss rates after midtrimester amniocentesis. *Obstet Gynecol.* 2006;108: 1067–1072.

29. Driscoll DA, Gross SJ. Screening for fetal aneuploidy and neural tube defects. *Genet Med.* 2009;11:818–821.

30. Manning M, Hudgins L. Array-based technology and recommendations for utilization in medical genetics practice for detection of chromosomal abnormalities. *Genet Med.* 2010;12(11): 742–745.

31. Le Caignec C, Boceno M, Saugier-Veber P, et al. Detection of genomic imbalances by array based comparative genomic hybridisation in fetuses with multiple malformations. *J Med Genet.* 2005;42:121–128.

32. Van den Veyver IB, Patel A, Shaw CA, et al. Clinical use of array comparative genomic hybridization (aCGH) for prenatal diagnosis in 300 cases. *Prenat Diagn.* 2009;29:29–39.

33. ACOG Committee on Genetics. ACOG Committee Opinion. Number 446. Array comparative genomic hybridization in prenatal diagnosis. *Obstet Gynecol.* 2009;114:1161–1163.

34. Palomaki GE, Kloza EM, Lambert-Messerlian GM, et al. DNA sequencing of maternal plasma to detect Down syndrome: an international clinical validation study. *Genet Med.* 2011;13(11):913–920.

35. Dacher JN, Mandell J, Lebowitz RL. Urinary tract infection in infants in spite of prenatal diagnosis of hydronephrosis. *Pediatr Radiol.* 1992;22(6):401–404; discussion 404–405.

36. Santos XM, Papanna R, Johnson A, et al. The use of combined ultrasound and magnetic resonance imaging in the detection of fetal anomalies. *Prenat Diagn.* 2010;30(5):402–407.

37. Levine D, Barnes PD, Robertson RR, et al. What does magnetic resonance imaging add to the prenatal sonographic diagnosis of ventriculomegaly? *J Ultrasound Med.* 2007;26:1513–1522.

38. Falip C, Blanc N, Maes E, et al. Postnatal clinical and imaging follow-up of infants with prenatal isolated mild ventriculomegaly: a series of 101 cases. *Pediatr Radiol.* 2007;37(10):981–989.

39. Beeghly M, Ware J, Soul J, et al. Neurodevelopmental outcome of fetuses referred for ventriculomegaly. *Ultrasound Obstet Gynecol.* 2010;35(4):405–416.

40. Parazzini C, Righini A, Doneda C, et al. Is fetal magnetic resonance imaging indicated when ultrasound isolated mild ventriculomegaly is present in pregnancies with no risk factors? *Prenatal Diagnosis.* 2012;32:752–757.

41. Pilu G, Falco P, Gabrielli S, et al. The clinical significance of fetal isolated cerebral borderline ventriculomegaly: report of 31 cases and review of the literature. *Ultrasound Obstet Gynecol.* 1999;14(5):320–326.

42. Jokhi RP, Whitby EH. Magnetic resonance imaging of the fetus. *Dev Med Child Neurol.* 2011;53(1):18–28.

43. Melchiorre K, Bhide A, Gika AD, et al. Counseling in isolated mild fetal ventriculomegaly. *Ultrasound Obstet Gynecol.* 2009;34(2):212–224.

44. Chang MC, Russell SA, Callen PW, et al. Sonographic detection of inferior vermian agenesis in Dandy-Walker malformations: prognostic implications. *Radiology.* 1994;193(3):765–770.

45. Limperopoulos C, Robertson RL, Estroff JA, et al. Diagnosis of inferior vermian hypoplasia by fetal magnetic resonance imaging: potential pitfalls and neurodevelopmental outcome. *Am J Obstet Gynecol.* 2006;194(4):1070–1076.

46. Goodyear PW, Bannister CM, Russell S, et al. Outcome in prenatally diagnosed fetal agenesis of the corpus callosum. *Fetal Diagn Ther.* 2001;16(3):139–145.

47. Damaj L, Bruneau B, Ferry M, et al. Pediatric outcome of children with the prenatal diagnosis of isolated septal agenesis. *Prenat Diagn.* 2010;30(12–13):1143–1150.

48. Zerella JT, Finberg FJ. Obstruction of the neonatal airway from teratomas. *Surg Gynecol Obstet.* 1990;170(2):126–131.

49. Steigman SA, Nemes L, Barnewolt CE, et al. Differential risk for neonatal surgical airway intervention in prenatally diagnosed neck masses. *J Pediatr Surg.* 2009;44(1):76–79.

50. Kunisaki SM, Fauza DO, Nemes LP, et al. Bronchial atresia: the hidden pathology within a spectrum of prenatally diagnosed lung masses. *J Pediatr Surg.* 2006;41(1):61–65; discussion 61–65.

51. Langston C. New concepts in the pathology of congenital lung malformations. *Semin Pediatr Surg.* 2003;12(1):17–37.

52. Riedlinger WF, Vargas SO, Jennings RW, et al. Bronchial atresia is common to extralobar sequestration, intralobar sequestration, congenital cystic adenomatoid malformation, and lobar emphysema. *Pediatr Dev Pathol.* 2006;9(5):361–373.

53. Epelman M, Kreiger PA, Servaes S, et al. Current imaging of prenatally diagnosed congenital lung lesions. *Semin Ultrasound CT MR.* 2010;31(2):141–157.

54. Adzick NS. Management of fetal lung lesions. *Clin Perinatol.* 2003;30(3):481–492.

55. Levine D, Barnewolt CE, Mehta TS, et al. Fetal thoracic abnormalities: MR imaging. *Radiology.* 2003;228(2):379–388.

56. Kasprian G, Balassy C, Brugger PC, et al. MRI of normal and pathological fetal lung development. *Eur J Radiol.* 2006;57(2):261–270.

57. Barth RA. Imaging of fetal chest masses. *Pediatr Radiol.* 2012;42(Suppl 1):S62–S73.

58. Pacharn P, Kline-Fath B, Calvo-Garcia M, et al. Congenital lung lesions: comparison between prenatal magnetic resonance imaging (MRI) and postnatal findings. Paper presented at the Radiological Society of North America 95th Scientific Assembly and Annual Meeting, McCormick Place, Chicago, IL, 2009.

59. Hubbard AM, Adzick NS, Crombleholme TM, et al. Congenital chest lesions: diagnosis and characterization with prenatal MR imaging. *Radiology.* 1999;212(1):43–48.

60. Crombleholme TM, Coleman B, Hedrick H, et al. Cystic adenomatoid malformation volume ratio predicts outcome in prenatally diagnosed cystic adenomatoid malformation of the lung. *J Pediatr Surg.* 2002;37(3):331–338.

61. Peranteau WH, Wilson RD, Liechty KW, et al. Effect of maternal betamethasone administration on prenatal congenital cystic adenomatoid malformation growth and fetal survival. *Fetal Diagnos Ther.* 2007;22:365–371.

62. Curran PF, Jelin EB, Rand L, et al. Prenatal steroids for microcystic congenital cystic adenomatoid malformations. *J Pediatr Surg.* 2010;45(1):145–150.

63. Adzick NS. Management of fetal lung lesions. *Clin Perinatol.* 2009;36:363–376.

64. Winters WD, Effmann EL. Congenital masses of the lung: prenatal and postnatal imaging evaluation. *J Thorac Imaging.* 2001;16(4):196–206.

65. Rubesova E, Bammer S, Chueh J, et al. Third trimester fetal MRI: can we replace the postnatal imaging? Society for Pediatric Radiology Annual Meeting and Postgraduate Course, Miami, FL, 2007.

66. Graziano JN. Cardiac anomalies in patients with congenital diaphragmatic hernia and their prognosis: a report from the Congenital Diaphragmatic Hernia Study Group. *J Pediatr Surg.* 2005;40(6):1045–1049; discussion 1049–1050.

67. Claus F, Sandaite I, DeKoninck P, et al. Prenatal anatomical imaging in fetuses with congenital diaphragmatic hernia. *Fetal Diagn Ther.* 2011;29(1):88–100.

68. Hedrick HL, Danzer E, Merchant A, et al. Liver position and lung-to-head ratio for prediction of extracorporeal membrane oxygenation and survival in isolated left congenital diaphragmatic hernia. *Am J Obstet Gynecol.* 2007;197(4):422; e421–e424.

69. Kilian AK, Schaible T, Hofmann V, et al. Congenital diaphragmatic hernia: predictive value of MRI relative lung-to-head ratio compared with MRI fetal lung volume and sonographic lung-to-head ratio. *AJR Am J Roentgenol.* 2009;192(1):153–158.

70. Jani J, Keller RL, Benachi A, et al. Prenatal prediction of survival in isolated left-sided diaphragmatic hernia. *Ultrasound Obstet Gynecol.* 2006;27(1):18–22.

71. Rypens F, Metens T, Rocourt N, et al. Fetal lung volume: estimation at MR imaging-initial results. *Radiology.* 2001;219(1):236–241.

72. Busing KA, Kilian AK, Schaible T, et al. Reliability and validity of MR image lung volume measurement in fetuses with congenital diaphragmatic hernia and in vitro lung models. *Radiology.* 2008;246(2):553–561.

73. Barnewolt CE, Kunisaki SM, Fauza DO, et al. Percent predicted lung volumes as measured on fetal magnetic resonance imaging: a useful biometric parameter for risk stratification in congenital diaphragmatic hernia. *J Pediatr Surg.* 2007;42(1):193–197.

74. Vuletin JF, Lim F-Y, Cnota J, et al. Prenatal pulmonary hypertension index: novel prenatal predictor of severe postnatal pulmonary artery hypertension in antenatally diagnosed congenital diaphragmatic hernia. *J Pediatr Surg.* 2010;45:703–708.

75. Chervenak FA, McCullough LB. Ethical issues in perinatal genetics. *Semin Fetal Neonat Med.* 2011;16:70–73.

76. Carnevale A, Lisker R, Villa AR, Casanueva E, Alonso E. Counseling following diagnosis of a fetal abnormality: comparison of different clinical specialists in Mexico. *Am J Med Genet.* 1997;69:23–28.

77. Watanabe M, Flake AW. Fetal surgery: Progress and perspectives. *Adv Pediatr.* 2010;57:353–372.

78. Lyerly AD, Mitchell LM, Armstrong EM, et al. Risk and the pregnancy body. *Hastings Cent Rep.* 2009;39:34–42.

79. Paris JJ, Graham N, Schreiber MD, Goodwin M. Approaches to end-of-life decision-making in the NICU: insights from Dostoevsky's *The Grand Inquisitor. J Perinatol.* 2006;26:389–391.

80. Ahluwalia J, Lees C, Paris JJ. Decisions for life made in the perinatal period: who decides and on which standards? *Arch Dis Child Fetal Neonatal Ed.* 2008;93:F332–F334.

81. Haward MF, Murphy RO, Lorenz JM. Message framing and perinatal decisions. *Pediatrics.* 2008;122:109–118.

82. Halamek LP. The advantages of a prenatal consultation by a neonatologist. *J Perinatol.* 2001;21:116–120.

83. Adzick NS, Thom EA, Spong CY, et al. A randomized trial of prenatal versus postnatal repair of myelomeningocele. *N Engl J Med.* 2011;364:993–1004.

84. Kohl T, Gembruch U. Current status and prospects of fetoscopic surgery for spina bifida in human fetuses. *Fetal Diagn Ther.* 2008;24:318–320.

85. Benitz WE. A paradigm for making difficult choices in the intensive care nursery. *Camb Q Healthc Ethics.* 1993;2:281–294.

86. Manganaro L, Savelli S, Francioso A, et al. Role of fetal MRI in the diagnosis of cerebral ventriculomegaly assessed by ultrasonography *Radiol Med.* 2009;114:1013–1023.

87. Zamora IJ, Sheikh , Cassady CI, et al. *J Pediar Surg.* 2014;49:853–858.

88. Cass DL, Olutoye OO, Cassady CI, et al. EXIT to resection for fetuses with large lung masses and persistent mediastinal compression near birth. *J Pediatr Surg.* 2013;48:138–144.

89. Danzer E, Hedrick HL. Controversies in the management of severe congenital diaphragmatic hernia *Seminars in fetal and neonatal medicine.* 2014;19:376–384.

8 Delivery Room Resuscitation of the Newborn

Louis P. Halamek

BACKGROUND

Resuscitation is derived from the Latin word *resuscitare,* meaning "to revive."[1] Although the majority of births involve no or little intervention on behalf of the neonate, approximately 10% of newborns need some form of resuscitation, and 1% require extensive maneuvers, such as endotracheal intubation, intravascular access, and drug delivery in the delivery room (DR).[2] The transition from fetus to neonate requires a number of physiologic changes, most of which must happen immediately in the seconds and minutes after birth. When these transitions fail to occur, or the fetus has been compromised because of intrinsic disease or utero events, resuscitation is necessary to optimize the chances of a normal outcome.

This chapter focuses on resuscitation of the neonate, not of the fetus or of the mother. Similarly, it does not cover topics more appropriate to stabilization, such as management of glucose homeostasis and electrolyte disorders. Although limited in scope to neonatal resuscitation within the context of the first minutes of life immediately after birth, many of the concepts covered in the chapter are also applicable to neonatal resuscitation in other environments and at later points in the life of the infant. This chapter does not attempt to replicate the definitive resource on neonatal resuscitation, the *Textbook of Neonatal Resuscitation* published by the American Academy of Pediatrics (AAP) and the American Heart Association (AHA) as the reference work for the Neonatal Resuscitation Program (NRP).[3] Rather, seeks to provide an overview of neonatal resuscitation, discussing not only the current state of the

scientific evidence and clinical guidelines but also the gaps in present knowledge and the developments likely to occur in the future.

DEVELOPMENT OF NEONATAL RESUSCITATION GUIDELINES

The management of neonates in the DR may have far-reaching consequences, not only on their subsequent neonatal course but also on their long-term outcome. Ideally, all of the interventions undertaken in the DR should be based on the best-available scientific evidence. However, prospective, sufficiently powered, randomized controlled trials (RCTs) of interventions undertaken during neonatal resuscitation are uncommon. Neonatal resuscitation involving more than drying, warming, stimulation, suctioning, and brief positive-pressure ventilation (PPV) is a low-frequency event; in addition, it is hard to anticipate, making RCTs with or without informed consent difficult to undertake. So, how are guidelines for neonatal resuscitation developed?

The development of neonatal resuscitation guidelines involves 2 distinct processes, each carried out on a quinquennial basis. To determine the best-available evidence on which to base recommendations for clinical care, a review of the published science is undertaken by members of the neonatal delegations to the International Liaison Committee on Resuscitation (ILCOR). ILCOR is an international body of health care professionals (HCPs) from resuscitation councils in the United States, Canada, South America,

Europe, Australia, New Zealand, South Africa, and other countries and areas of the world whose members volunteer literally thousands of hours in pursuit of thorough, objective review of the scientific literature on resuscitation.[4,5] This international activity results in consensus regarding what the current science reveals on a particular topic pertinent to resuscitation.[6,7] To achieve accuracy and objectivity in interpretation of the literature as well as uniformity in the process itself, a number of strategies are employed. Only published manuscripts are reviewed, and only primary data are reported; although review articles may occasionally be examined, the original manuscripts are always reviewed and referenced. The results of each manuscript are rated concerning the level of the evidence (eg, RCTs are rated more highly than retrospective case series) and the quality of the methodology. Strict procedures are in place to encourage transparency and minimize any potential for reviewer bias.

Whereas the goal of the review of the published science is international agreement about what the science says about a particular topic, the process of generation of clinical guidelines is a regional or national activity focused on the pragmatic application of the science to patient care based on available local resources. Because the resources available to HCPs in a developed country exceed those present in the developing world, clinical guidelines may differ substantially between regions of the world. For example, the availability of oxygen raises the issue of how much should be used during various stages of resuscitation; in locations where oxygen is not available, there is no debate, and room air (21% oxygen) is used. In the United States, clinical guidelines are the responsibility of the members of and liaisons and consultants to the NRP Steering Committee (NRPSC).[8] Whereas established, accepted practices will remain in the guidelines unless evidence of possible harm or proven ineffectiveness exists, the only new interventions that are added are those that are supported by the evidence review process. In generating clinical guidelines, the NRPSC must consider what is practical not only in levels III–IV neonatal intensive care units (NICUs) but also in any facility in which newborns are delivered. Because every guideline carries potential legal, financial, and ethical implications, the NRPSC carefully debates and scrutinizes each one. These guidelines serve as the de facto national standard of care for newborns in US DRs.

Although the ILCOR process for review of the science readily enables achieving international consensus and generation of clinical guidelines by the NRPSC ensures that such guidelines carefully reflect what is both evidence-based and practical, it nevertheless is far from a nimble activity capable of rapidly incorporating new evidence as it becomes available. The veracity of the evidence evaluation could be enhanced by inviting the original authors of pertinent manuscripts to discuss, pool, and reinterpret their original data, similar to how such reviews are carried out in other domains within health care. New communication technologies and social media may allow for more timely interaction and updating of clinical guidelines (perhaps via an online secure peer-reviewed wiki) while maintaining the meticulous character of the current scientific review process. By constantly reexamining how to enhance this productive but at times tedious and time-consuming process, the care of neonates in the DR will be steadily improved.

IMPLEMENTATION OF NEONATAL RESUSCITATION GUIDELINES

NRP Algorithm Overview

The first steps in resuscitation consist of drying, warming, tactile stimulation, and proper positioning to allow opening of the airway (see Figure 8-1). Neonates should be positioned with the neck slightly extended; this "sniffing" position aligns the posterior pharynx, larynx, and trachea so that air may pass easily through those structures. If, after proper positioning, obstruction of the airway is suspected by the presence of retractions or obvious respiratory effort without evidence of air entry into the lungs, use a bulb syringe or suction catheter to first suction the mouth, then the nose, to remove any large particulate matter or thick secretions. Similarly, suctioning may be undertaken in preparation for PPV. Routine suctioning, however, is not indicated, and neonates who are breathing effectively should simply be dried and warmed.[9–12] Vigorous, repetitive, or deep (posterior pharyngeal and gastric) suctioning should be avoided to minimize the risk of vagal stimulation, resultant bradycardia, and direct trauma to the airway. Only when gastric dilation is so significant that it is likely to be impeding diaphragmatic movement and thereby impairing the neonate's ability to breathe should gastric suctioning be undertaken.

Pulmonary Resuscitation

Assisted Breathing

Unlike the pediatric and adult populations, the vast majority of neonates in need of resuscitation do not have an underlying cardiac etiology for their physiologic compromise and thus will respond to interventions that facilitate adequate gas exchange. Perinatal depression may be caused by in utero events, such as inadequate gas exchange at the placental level or postnatal conditions secondary to obstruction of the airways, pulmonary diseases such as surfactant deficiency, and central nervous system disorders causing

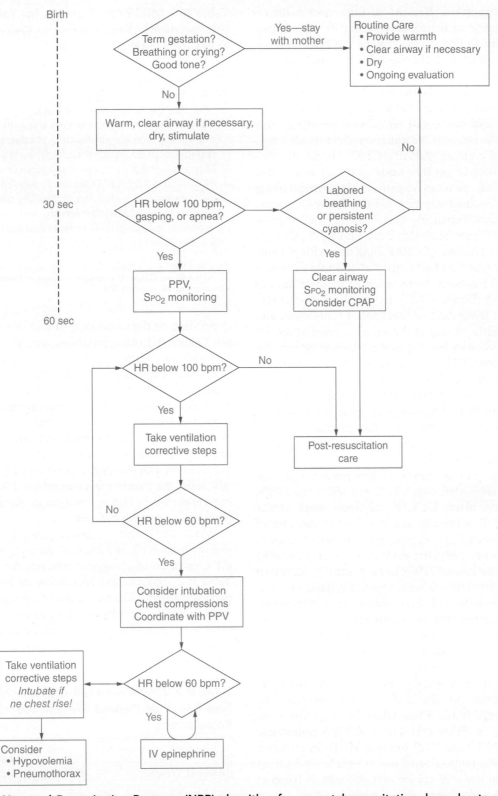

FIGURE 8-1 Neonatal Resuscitation Program (NRP) algorithm for neonatal resuscitation. bpm, beats per minute; CPAP, continuous positive airway pressure; HR, heart rate; PPV, positive-pressure ventilation. (Reproduced with permission from Kattwinkel J, Perlman JM, Aziz K, Colby C, et al. Part 15: neonatal resuscitation: 2010. American Heart Association Guidelines for Cardiopulmonary Resuscitation and Emergency Cardiovascular Care. *Circulation.* 2010;122 (18 Suppl 3):S909–S919.)

apnea or hypopnea. Because of this, most neonates who are apneic or manifesting ineffective respirations will respond to the initial steps of the NRP resuscitation algorithm without the need for more invasive measures such as PPV or intubation.

If, after the initial maneuvers described previously are completed, the neonate has labored breathing (eg, substernal and intercostal retractions, grunting), it is reasonable to consider the initiation of continuous positive airway pressure (CPAP). CPAP provides a continuous source of gas flow under pressure as a means of improving alveolar expansion and maintaining functional residual capacity (FRC), thereby decreasing atelectasis, enhancing surfactant release, improving the ventilation/perfusion ratio, and facilitating gas exchange.[13] The use of CPAP (together with permissive hypercapnea and avoidance of episodes of hyperventilation) has been shown to result in lower rates of chronic lung disease (CLD), less need for supplemental oxygen, fewer days of mechanical ventilation, and shorter lengths of stay in the preterm population.[14–18] This body of work has led to the recommendation by the NRP that CPAP be considered prior to intubation in all spontaneously breathing neonates manifesting respiratory distress. CPAP may be delivered via endotracheal tube (ETT), nasal prongs, or face mask; at the time this chapter was prepared, the optimal method of CPAP delivery as well as range of pressures was yet to be determined.

Neonates who are apneic or hypopneic will not be able to be supported with CPAP and will require PPV delivered via mask, ETT, or laryngeal mask airway (LMA). PPV is initially administered at the rate of 40 to 60 breaths per minute. If the patient begins to breathe in a more effective manner and heart rate (HR) increases, the rate of PPV can be gradually decreased and the patient transitioned to room air, nasal cannula, or CPAP as indicated. Face masks come in different sizes and shapes, and it is important that the mask chosen for a particular neonate cover the patient's nose and mouth without applying pressure to the eyes; this will result in a proper seal, minimize air leakage, and reduce the risk of vagally induced bradycardia.[19–23]

An inability to effectively deliver gas into the patient's lungs should prompt the following steps in the order listed in Table 8-1: The MRSOPA mnemonic is advocated by the NRP to assist HCPs in ensuring that lack of attention to relatively simple issues does not result in unnecessary invasive procedures (such as intubation) and adverse patient outcomes.[3]

The optimal inspiratory times (T_Is) for use during initiation of PPV are unknown. Historically, relatively short initial T_Is (0.3–0.5 seconds) have been advocated, but recent studies indicated a benefit of longer (1–3 seconds) T_Is on achieving FRC, optimal lung inflation, and adequate HR.[24–28] Optimal peak inspiratory pressures (PIPs) vary from patient to patient

Table 8-1 MRSOPA: Prompts for Technical Interventions When Unable to Deliver Positive-Pressure Breaths[a]

M: Adjust the **mask** on the face.
R: **Reposition** the head to ensure an open airway.
S: **Suction** the mouth then the nose.
O: **Open** the mouth and perform a jaw lift.
P: Gradually increase **pressure** until bilateral breath sounds are auscultated and chest rise is visible, keeping in mind that peak inspiratory pressures (PIPs) above 40 cm H_2O are rarely required and likely indicate serious underlying pulmonary pathology.
A: Consider an **alternative airway,** such as an endotracheal tube (ETT) or laryngeal mask airway (LMA).

[a]Data from Kattwinkel J, Bloom RS, et al: Textbook of Neonatal Resuscitation. 6th ed. Elk Grove Village, IL: American Academy of Pediatrics and the American Heart Association; 2010.

depending on the underlying pulmonary anatomy and physiology and other variables, such as T_I. Because of the fluid-filled nature of the fetal lung and the presence of disease states such as surfactant deficiency, PIPs as high as 30 to 40 cm H_2O may need to be delivered initially to establish the FRC. Grunting on auscultation is caused by the neonate exhaling against a partially closed glottis and acts to create end-expiratory pressure to maintain lung inflation. When PPV is delivered, the provision of positive end-expiratory pressure (PEEP) will assist the neonate in establishing FRC and limiting atelectasis.[29] The optimal range for PEEP in the neonate is yet to be defined.

When PPV with a mask is unsuccessful, intubation with an ETT is indicated. As with the mask, the ETT must be of an appropriate size for the neonate. Table 8-2 indicates the correlation of ETT size with neonatal weight. The technique of neonatal intubation is illustrated beautifully in color photos in the *Textbook of Neonatal Resuscitation*[3] and in video in the accompanying multimedia DVD. Intubation is a technical skill

Table 8-2 Recommended Endotracheal Tube Size Based on Patient Weight: Neonatal Population[a]

Patient Weight	ETT Size	Length of Tube at Lip
<1 kg, <28 wk EGA	2.5	6–7 cm
1–2 kg, 28–34 wk EGA	3.0	7–8 cm
2–3 kg, 34–38 wk EGA	3.5	8–9 cm
3–4 kg, >38 wk EGA	3.5–4.0	9–10 cm

Abbreviations: EGA, estimated gestational age; ETT, endotracheal tube. Data from Kattwinkel J, Bloom RS, et al: Textbook of Neonatal Resuscitation. 6th ed. Elk Grove Village, IL: American Academy of Pediatrics and the American Heart Association; 2010.

that is not possessed by all HCPs who attend to newborns in the DR. Because of the difficulty in acquiring and maintaining appropriate skill in intubation, interest in the use of the LMA has grown in recent years.[30–34] The advantage of the LMA is in its relative simplicity of insertion and use. The technique of LMA insertion is also illustrated in the *Textbook of Neonatal Resuscitation* and the accompanying DVD. Currently, there is only one size LMA (size 1) that is available for the neonatal population; it is meant to be used in neonates greater than 2 kg or older than 34 weeks estimated gestational age (EGA). It is especially useful in providing PPV in patients with micrognathia (such as in Pierre Robin sequence) and other craniofacial/airway anomalies that make opening the mouth for placement of a laryngoscope and manipulation of an ETT difficult.

Positive-pressure ventilation (via mask, ETT, or LMA) may be administered using a flow-inflating bag, self-inflating bag, or T-piece resuscitator.[35–37] Resuscitation bags have been in use for decades, and each has its own advantages and disadvantages, as noted in Table 8-3. A flow-inflating bag requires a continuous source of compressed gas to function; compression of the bag provides tactile cues that allow the experienced user to sense the compliance of the neonate's lungs with each breath. Unlike the flow-inflating bag, the self-inflating bag refills spontaneously without the need for a compressed gas source but does not provide the same type of tactile cues. The T-piece resuscitator allows the user to deliver a preset PIP and PEEP and vary the T_I and rate of ventilation. A comparison of the flow-inflating bag, self-inflating bag, and T-piece resuscitator in a neonatal mannequin revealed that the T-piece resuscitator delivered a more

Table 8-3 Advantages and Disadvantages of Self- and Flow-Inflating Bags and T-Piece Resuscitators

Device	Major Advantages	Major Disadvantages
Self-inflating bag	Does NOT require gas source	Requires reservoir to achieve FIO$_2$ = 90%–100%
	Pop-off valve helps avoid excessive PIP	Inconsistent inspiratory time, PIP, PEEP
Flow-inflating bag	Predictable FIO$_2$	Requires gas source to function
		Inconsistent inspiratory time, PIP, PEEP
T-piece resuscitator	Predictable FIO$_2$	Requires gas source to function

Abbreviations: PIP, positive inspiratory pressure; PEEP, positive end-expiratory pressure.

consistent PIP and together with the flow-inflating bag was found to be more effective at generating a consistent PEEP than the self-inflating bag.[38] The subjects in the study described the T-piece resuscitator as requiring the least amount of practice and technical skill to operate in an effective manner.

Dosing of Oxygen

Historically, oxygen has been used liberally during resuscitation; until recently, the NRP recommended the use of a 100% fraction of inspired oxygen (FIO$_2$) any time a neonate required respiratory assistance. This dogma began to evolve in the past decade as a number of studies raised questions regarding both the effectiveness of oxygen and its assumed lack of sequelae.[39–42] A 2005 meta-analysis by Saugstad et al revealed a more rapid increase in HR, shorter time to first breath, and a 5% reduction in mortality for neonates resuscitated with 21% as opposed to 100% FIO$_2$.[43,44] This was followed in 2007 by another meta-analysis, this one by Rabi and colleagues, examining depressed newborns who were resuscitated with 21% vs 100% FIO$_2$; this indicated a lower 1-week and 1-month mortality rate in neonates resuscitated with 21% FIO$_2$.[45] The use of oxygen in premature neonates has raised questions that are even more serious because these patients are at higher risk for oxygen toxicity given their diminished ability to mount an adequate antioxidant defense.[46,47]

Hyperoxia is associated with morbidities like CLD, retinopathy of prematurity (ROP), and necrotizing enterocolitis (NEC). Wang et al performed a prospective, randomized trial of the use of 21% vs 100% FIO$_2$ in preterm neonates at 23–32 weeks gestation and found that all those who were resuscitated with 21% FIO$_2$ failed to achieve predetermined target pulse oximetry (SpO$_2$) levels despite 3 minutes of PPV.[48] Escrig et al compared the use of 30% vs 90% FIO$_2$ in neonates less than 28 weeks EGA and determined that a target SpO$_2$ level of 85% at 10 minutes of life could be achieved using 30% FiO$_2$.[49] The work of these investigators and others has led the NRP to change its recommendation on the use of oxygen during resuscitation.[3] In *term* neonates, the NRP's 2010 recommendations are as follows:

1. Begin PPV with 21% FIO$_2$.
2. Adjust FIO$_2$ to maintain a hemoglobin oxygen saturation by pulse oximetry (SpO$_2$) that mimics that of uncompromised term newborns in the first 10 minutes of life (see Table 8-4).
3. Use a pulse oximeter and oxygen blender to titrate FIO$_2$.
4. Increase FIO$_2$ to 100% whenever chest compressions (CCs) are initiated.

Table 8-4 SpO$_2$ Normal Ranges in the First 10 Minutes of Life

Minute of Life	Target SpO$_2$ (Preductal)
1 min	60%–65%
2 min	65%–70%
3 min	70%–75%
4 min	75%–80%
5 min	80%–85%
10 min	85%–90%

Data from Kattwinkel J, Bloom RS, et al: Textbook of Neonatal Resuscitation. 6th ed. Elk Grove Village, IL: American Academy of Pediatrics and the American Heart Association; 2010.

The 2010 NRP guidelines for the use of oxygen in the *premature* neonate are as follows:

1. When anticipating and planning for a preterm delivery, set up a pulse oximeter and oxygen blender.
2. Begin PPV with an FIO$_2$ somewhat higher than 21% (eg, 30%–40%).
3. Adjust FIO$_2$ to maintain a hemoglobin oxygen saturation by SpO$_2$ that mimics that of uncompromised term newborns in the first 10 minutes of life.
4. Increase FIO$_2$ to 100% whenever CCs are initiated.

Monitoring Oxygen Levels

With the understanding that oxygen should be used in the same manner as any drug and therefore its dose titrated to achieve effect, a means of measuring that effect becomes paramount to delivering appropriate care. Numerous studies have shown that assessment of skin color is an unreliable means of diagnosing cyanosis in the newborn. Detection of abnormal hemoglobin oxygen saturation is best achieved with the use of a pulse oximeter attached via a probe placed on the neonate's right hand or wrist.[50-55] This preductal SpO$_2$ will reflect the hemoglobin oxygen saturation of blood that is perfusing the brain and heart. Pulse oximetry should be used whenever resuscitation is anticipated (as in a preterm delivery); central (lips, tongue, central thorax) cyanosis is persistent; oxygen is in use more than briefly; or PPV is in progress.

Monitoring Carbon Dioxide Levels

The use of end tidal carbon dioxide (ETCO$_2$) detection devices is now recommended by the NRP as a primary means of confirming proper ETT placement. ETCO$_2$ monitoring can be achieved by using colorimetric devices that change color (purple to yellow) in the presence of carbon dioxide (CO$_2$) and capnographs that continuously measure and display CO$_2$ levels via

an electrode placed at the connection between the ventilator circuit and the ETT.[56-62] Whereas colorimetric devices provide a simple yes/no to the presence of CO$_2$, capnographs will present a continuous measurement of the concentration of exhaled CO$_2$. Despite their utility, it is important for HCPs charged with resuscitating neonates to understand that both devices will give false-negative readings when pulmonary blood flow is low (as in severe bradycardia or asystole). In these situations, other indicators of proper ETT placement, such as auscultation of bilateral breath sounds and visualization of symmetric chest rise, should also be used.

Management of the Meconium-Stained Neonate

Meconium-stained amniotic fluid (MSAF) is encountered in approximately 7%–20% of live births, with 2%–9% of those resulting in meconium aspiration syndrome (MAS). MAS refers to the pulmonary dysfunction in the neonate that may accompany the presence of MSAF in the lungs; it is characterized by impaired oxygenation and ventilation caused by obstruction of the larger airways, with resultant under- and overinflation of the alveoli, a generalized pulmonary inflammatory response, and ventilation-perfusion mismatching, all of which act to limit gas exchange. The relative consistency of the meconium does not influence the rate or severity of MAS. Until recently, the standard approach to the neonate with MSAF consisted of aggressive suctioning of the oro- and nasopharynx while the neonate's head was on the perineum prior to delivery of the body, followed by intubation and suctioning of the trachea.[63-65] Much effort was made to accomplish all of this suctioning prior to the first breath to "prevent" meconium present in the trachea from being aspirated deeper into the tracheobronchial tree and increasing the risk of MAS.

Better imaging of fetal activity indicated that fetal breathing movements occur in utero, effectively moving amniotic fluid in and out the lungs; it also was recognized that fetuses in distress will both pass meconium and manifest gasping in utero, thus creating a mechanism whereby meconium passed into the amniotic fluid as a reaction to fetal stress may be aspirated into the tracheobronchial tree prior to labor and birth.[66] Coupled with case reports of stillborn neonates (who obviously never took a breath outside the uterus) with meconium present in their airways on postmortem examination, the conclusion was that not all meconium aspiration occurred during delivery and therefore was preventable.[67-69]

These observations led to several studies that critically examined the dogma surrounding management of the meconium-stained neonate. In 2000, Wiswell et al found that intubation and suctioning of vigorous neonates with MSAF produced no benefit.[70] Halliday's review in 2001 reaffirmed that no significant improvement in the rate of MAS occurs with intubation and tracheal suctioning.[71] Subsequently, Vain and colleagues conducted a study of oropharyngeal suctioning on the perineum of neonates born through MSAF and found no reduction in the incidence of MAS, need for intubation, or mortality in affected neonates.[72] The current recommendations by the NRP for management of the neonate born through MSAF are as follows[3]:

1. If the newborn is vigorous (effective respiratory effort, adequate muscle tone or active movement, HR above 100 beats per minute [BPM]), clear the mouth and nose of secretions and dry, warm, and stimulate the infant.

2. If the newborn is NOT vigorous (absent respirations or gasping, floppy or poor muscle tone, HR below 100 BPM):
   a. Suction the mouth using a 12- or 14-French suction catheter.
   b. Intubate the trachea with an appropriate size ETT.
   c. Connect the hub of the ETT to suction using a meconium aspirator.
   d. Apply suction and slowly withdraw the ETT.
   e. Repeat intubation as necessary until either the amount of meconium returned is greatly reduced or the neonate's HR falls to a level indicating additional steps in resuscitation should be carried out.

Although the studies to date indicated that depressed infants born through MSAF are at risk of developing MAS, no prospective, randomized, controlled, sufficiently powered study of endotracheal intubation and suctioning in depressed infants born through MSAF was completed at the time that this chapter was prepared.[73] Thus, the optimal treatment of the neonate born through MSAF remains unknown.

Naloxone for Opioid-Induced Respiratory Depression

Naloxone is an opioid antagonist that can be administered intravenously, intramuscularly, or intratracheally. Indications for its use include respiratory depression in a neonate exposed to opioids less than 4 hours prior to delivery and born to a mother without a history of narcotic dependency. Despite this indication, there are many reasons why naloxone has been removed by the NRPSC from the short list of medications to be used for neonatal resuscitation in the DR.[74,75] There is no way to ensure that the maternal history is accurate regarding use/abuse of licit/illicit substances; therefore, the neonate's in utero exposure to narcotics cannot be

unequivocally ascertained. Delivery of naloxone may initiate signs of withdrawal, including seizures in neonates who have been chronically exposed to opioids in utero.[76] Because the half-life of naloxone is relatively short (approximately 60 minutes) compared to most narcotics, it is possible that as naloxone is metabolized postnatally the effects of the narcotic may once again produce respiratory depression and require repeat resuscitation.[77]

Respiratory depression has many causes and naloxone may not be indicated; therefore, delivery of naloxone may distract the team from performing other needed interventions and considering/treating other causes. Persistent respiratory depression should be treated with PPV to maintain the HR in the normal range, and the patient should be monitored continuously (eg, with an oximeter and frequent checks by a clinician) for a period of 24 to 48 hours after consistent spontaneous respirations return.

Cardiac Resuscitation

Bradycardia

Bradycardia is the most common dysrhythmia in the neonatal period. It is defined as a HR less than 100 BPM, although some healthy, full-term neonates may have resting HRs in the 70- to 100-BPM range with normal perfusion and hemoglobin oxygen saturation levels, especially at rest or during sleep. As a primary cardiac problem, it is seen in cases of congenital heart disease where the conduction fibers may be malformed or aberrant (as in atrioventricular septal defects, ventricular inversion, or heterotaxy syndromes) and in maternal autoimmune diseases, such as lupus, for which maternal autoantibodies cross the placenta and damage the fetal cardiac conduction system. However, the most common cause of neonatal bradycardia is hypoxia and the resultant acidosis caused by inadequate oxygen content and oxygen delivery; this may occur in utero or postnatally. In these instances, establishing adequate oxygen delivery to the myocardium is the primary goal.

HR should be assessed at 30 seconds of life; if less than 100 BPM, PPV is initiated, and the HR should be rechecked at 1 minute of life (see Figure 8-1). If at any time after PPV has been initiated the HR is found to be less than 60 BPM, CC should be initiated to augment the intrinsic cardiac output. The chest should be compressed to one-third the depth in the anteroposterior diameter using the 2-handed technique. With this technique, HCPs encircle the newborn's thorax with both hands, thumbs side by side on the lower half of the sternum and the other 8 fingers interwoven underneath the patient's back.[78-83] The thumbs should never be completely lifted off the chest during compressions to avoid subsequent misplacement. CC and PPV are to be coordinated, delivered in a ratio of 3 compressions to 1 breath every 2 seconds for a total of 4 interventions every 2 seconds.[84] If the underlying etiology of the bradycardia is felt to be cardiac rather than pulmonary in nature, a compression-to-breath ratio of 15:2 may be used.

When neonatal bradycardia is unresponsive to PPV and CC, epinephrine (EPI) is administered. EPI is an inotropic and chronotropic agent, producing increased myocardial contractility and increased HR, resulting in improved coronary artery perfusion pressure, better blood flow to the myocardium, and enhanced odds for the return of spontaneous circulation.[85] EPI comes in 2 concentrations, 1:10,000 (1 g/10,000 mL = 0.1 mg/mL) and 1:1000 (1 g/1000 mL = 1 mg/mL); the 1:10,000 concentration is recommended for use in the neonatal population. The intravenous (IV) route is preferred, and achieving intravenous access should be a priority for any neonate requiring EPI; this is typically achieved in an emergency situation in the DR by inserting a catheter 2 to 4 cm into the umbilical vein or via the intraosseous (IO) route using an intraosseous needle or mechanical drill.[86-88] The recommended intravenous/intraosseous dose is 0.1–0.3 mL/kg (0.01–0.03 mg/kg) of 1:10,000 EPI given every 3 to 5 minutes. If intravenous access is delayed, it is reasonable to deliver intratracheal (IT) EPI at a dose of 0.5–1 mL/kg (0.05–0.1 mg/kg) of 1:10,000 EPI. The efficacy of intratracheal EPI is dubious, likely limited by dilution in alveolar fluid, inadequate absorption because of poor/absent pulmonary blood flow during bradycardia/asystole, and pulmonary vasoconstriction secondary to acidosis.[89-92]

The use of volume (crystalloid and colloid solutions) in the newborn in the DR should in general be restricted to when clinical signs consistent with hypovolemia (pallor, diminished pulses, poor perfusion), possibly accompanied by a history of likely fetal blood loss (eg, cord laceration), are seen in a neonate who is unresponsive to other resuscitative measures.[3] Delivery of volume without clinical indication is to be avoided to minimize the risk of a decrease in stroke volume as left ventricular end-diastolic pressure rises based on the Frank-Starling mechanism. The choice of volume should be based on overall effectiveness at reestablishing circulating intravascular volume, risk of infectious or immune-mediated sequelae, cost, and general availability.

Because of these factors, crystalloid solutions (normal saline, lactated Ringer's) are used most frequently in emergency situations in the DR.[93-99] Isotonic crystalloid solutions are equivalent to colloid solutions (whole blood, packed red blood cells, fresh frozen plasma, human serum albumin) in terms of their ability to produce short-term increases in intravascular volume and blood pressure. The recommended dose is 10 mL/kg, repeated as necessary to achieve adequate perfusion.[3] Once perfusion and blood pressure are normalized, blood products can be given to treat specific deficits, such as anemia. If fetal blood loss is felt to be likely (as indicated by a sinusoidal fetal HR tracing), non-crossmatched type O Rh-negative packed red blood cells may be ordered so that they can be infused in the DR.

Tachycardia

Neonatal tachycardia is most commonly seen in the context of maternal fever and chorioamnionitis or neonatal sepsis; treatment is not directed at the heart but rather consists of performing an appropriate workup for sepsis and initiation of antibiotic therapy. Tachycardia may also be caused by anemia secondary to acute or chronic causes; associated signs include pallor, poor perfusion, and hypotension. Once again, therapy is directed not at the heart but at volume replacement with crystalloid or colloid. Tachycardic dysrhythmias secondary to intrinsic cardiac disease are typically supraventricular in nature. The resuscitation team will need to determine whether cardiac output is compromised to the extent that such a dysrhythmia requires immediate treatment in the DR at the time of birth or can await a comprehensive evaluation (electrocardiogram [ECG], echocardiogram, and consultation with a pediatric cardiologist) and targeted therapy in the NICU.

An example of a condition that may require extensive treatment immediately after birth is long-standing (weeks to months) fetal tachycardia resulting in hydrops fetalis. Initial therapy is directed at achieving adequate oxygenation and ventilation with PPV; drainage of any pleural effusions, ascites, or pericardial effusions that compromise cardiopulmonary function; and establishing intravenous access for drug and volume delivery. Therapy with vagal maneuvers, medication such as adenosine, or cardioversion may then be indicated.

Monitoring Heart Rate

Studies performed in the real clinical environment and those completed in highly realistic simulated environments raise serious questions about the ability of HCPs (even those who are highly experienced) to accurately determine HR in a neonate at the time of birth, regardless of technique (auscultation of the precordium or palpation of umbilical artery pulsations at the umbilical stump).[100,101] In addition, it has been shown that inaccuracy in HR determination results in errors of commission (performing interventions not indicated) and errors of omission (lack of indicated interventions) that may result in patient harm.[102]

Oximetry provides an indication of pulse rate in addition to SpO_2, but it often requires a minute or more to display its first signal and fails to produce a signal when perfusion is poor or nonexistent.[103,104] ECG leads provide the quickest, most accurate, and most reliable means of determining neonatal HR in the DR and are likely to be used with increasing frequency, especially in low birth weight neonates, when accuracy of HR detection is a high priority.

Special Resuscitation Situations in the Delivery Room

There are a number of neonatal disease states presenting at birth that may complicate efforts at resuscitation and reduce the chance for a good clinical outcome (see Table 8-5). Although a detailed discussion of each of these conditions is beyond the scope of this chapter, it can be stated that, despite their unique nature, a general approach focusing on establishing an adequate airway, initiating effective breathing, and ensuring adequate cardiac output is indicated.

One special resuscitation situation that deserves mention is thermoregulation in the premature neonate. Premature neonates have a significantly reduced ability to maintain a normal body core temperature (defined as 37.0°C + 0.5°C) because of high body surface area/mass ratio, lack of subcutaneous fat, and immature neurologic and endocrine systems. Many premature neonates become hypothermic when exposed to ambient air in the DR and remain hypothermic despite placement on a servo-controlled radiant warmer. Because of this, extra measures not necessary for full-term neonates must be undertaken in the seconds and minutes after the birth of a premature neonate. Newborns delivered at less than 28 weeks EGA should not be dried but rather immediately placed in polyethylene wraps or bags.[105–107]

Exothermic mattresses may also be used, although this increases the risk of hyperthermia (which should also be avoided).[108,109] In addition to these measures, the DR should be maintained at an ambient temperature of at least 26°C whenever the delivery of a neonate less than 28 weeks EGA is anticipated; once the newborn is resuscitated and measures to enhance thermoregulatory mechanisms are in place, the temperature of the DR may be decreased for the comfort of the obstetric team members.[110–112] Transport of the newborn to the nursery in an enclosed neonatal transport unit (as opposed to a radiant warmer open to the ambient air and operating on battery power) may also help to maintain a normal body temperature.[113]

Historically, the focus of resuscitation has been on cardiopulmonary resuscitation (CPR); although the heart and lungs are absolutely critical to survival, the brain is vital to *neurologically intact* survival. Cerebral resuscitation will become an increasingly important component of neonatal resuscitation as more and more evidence-based therapies become available. Head and whole-body cooling strategies to induce hypothermia have been shown to improve outcomes in certain populations of neonates with perinatal depression. Therapeutic hypothermia and cerebral resuscitation are covered elsewhere in this text.[114,115]

Table 8-5 Special Resuscitation Situations in the Delivery Room

Airway
  Pierre Robin sequence
  Oropharyngeal tumors
  Nuchal/thoracic lymphangiomas
Thorax
  Pneumothorax
  Congenital diaphragmatic hernia
  Tracheobronchial malformations
  Cystic pulmonary diseases
  Congenital heart disease
  Ectopia cordis/pentalogy of Cantrell
Abdomen/pelvis
  Gastroschisis
  Omphalocele
  Bladder extrophy
Central nervous system
  Myelomeningocele
  Massive hydrocephalus
  Hydrolethalus syndrome
Miscellaneous malformations
  Hydrops fetalis

Noninitiation and Discontinuation of Resuscitative Efforts

Noninitiation of resuscitative efforts in the DR should be considered and discussed whenever the fetal/neonatal prognosis indicates that survival is highly unlikely, even with aggressive resuscitation and intensive care, or the morbidity associated with survival is excessive as interpreted by the parent(s) or the HCPs delivering care. This may arise in situations involving inherited diseases, malformations, or extreme prematurity. The decision to forgo resuscitation and immediately institute comfort care after birth or to attempt resuscitation with agreed-on criteria by which resuscitative efforts would be judged to be ineffective and therefore no longer indicated ideally involves agreement among all of the HCPs involved as well as the parents, who are informed of the potential outcomes. Of course, this is possible only when there is sufficient time prior to delivery for such conversations to take place.[116,117] When time does allow, thorough counseling of the pregnant woman not only by her obstetrician but also, more importantly, by a knowledgeable pediatrician or neonatologist regarding the likely short-term problems and long-term outcomes is mandatory.

The birth of a neonate at the limits of viability (generally defined as 22–23 weeks EGA) is one of the most challenging situations in modern medicine.[118–120] A useful tool for providing objective information to the pregnant woman about possible outcomes of neonates with characteristics similar to the fetus that she is carrying is found on the National Institute of Child Health and Human Development (NICHD) website.[121] The data provided are derived from births at NICHD Neonatal Network centers as described in 2008 by Tyson et al.[122] It is prefaced with several disclaimers: (1) "It is not intended to be the only information that care decisions are based on, nor is it intended to be a definitive means of predicting infant outcomes. Users should keep in mind that every infant is an individual, and that factors beyond those used to formulate these standardized assessments may influence an infant's outcomes." (2) "If you choose to use these data to determine possible outcomes, please remember that the information provided is not intended to be the sole basis for care decisions, nor is it intended to be a definitive prediction of outcomes if intensive care is provided. Users should keep in mind that every infant is an individual, and that factors beyond those used to formulate these standardized assessments may influence an infant's outcomes."

The HCP using this tool enters the best obstetric estimate (in weeks) of gestational age, birth weight (between 401 and 1000 g), gender, whether this is a singleton birth, and if antenatal corticosteroids were administered within 7 days of delivery. Calculated outcomes include the percentage of neonates who experience survival, survival without profound neurodevelopmental impairment, survival without moderate-to-severe neurodevelopmental impairment, death, death or profound neurodevelopmental impairment, and death or moderate-to-severe neurodevelopmental impairment. Outcomes for all patients as well as patients who receive mechanical ventilation are available. Despite the disclaimers, the data and calculations inherent in this tool can be translated into objective outcome information useful to HCPs attempting to communicate the gravity of the situation being faced by the fetus/neonate and his or her parent(s).

Discontinuation of resuscitative efforts should also be considered and discussed whenever the newborn has been asystolic for 10 minutes or longer. Although newer therapies may ultimately yield different results, historical data indicate that survival in such situations is extremely unlikely and, when it occurs, is associated with significant neurodevelopmental impairment.[123,124] More detailed discussion of the many neonatal, parental, medical, and social issues inherent in noninitiation and discontinuation of intensive care support is beyond the scope of this chapter and is covered elsewhere in this book.

NEONATAL RESUSCITATION TRAINING AND ASSESSMENT

Teaching, Learning, and Skill Sets

There is a distinct difference between teaching and learning: Whereas teaching is something that is done to trainees by instructors, learning is something that requires active participation by both instructors and trainees.[125] The skill sets that must be learned (and maintained) for safe and effective resuscitation include cognitive skills or content knowledge (what we know in our brains), technical or procedural skills (what we do with our hands), and behavioral skills (what we use to employ the first 2 skill sets while caring for patients while working under time pressure). In 2004, the Joint Commission (JC; formerly the Joint Commission for the Accreditation of Healthcare Organizations) published a Sentinel Event Alert that indicated almost three-quarters of the cases of neonatal mortality or severe neonatal morbidity reported to that agency involved ineffective communication.[126] In that alert, the JC recommended that all health care organizations where newborns are delivered incorporate behavioral skills into training and conduct clinical drills and constructive debriefings on a regular basis. Because behavioral skills such as teamwork, leadership, and effective communication (Table 8-6) are critical to successful outcomes in patients undergoing CPR, the most recent iteration of NRP highlights the importance of these skills when optimal human performance is desired.

Evolution of the NRP

The concept of a standardized approach to neonatal resuscitation, based on the best-available evidence, was revolutionary in 1987 when the NRP was initiated.

Table 8-6 Behavioral Skills

1. Know your environment.
2. Anticipate and plan.
3. Assume the leadership role.
4. Communicate effectively.
5. Delegate workload optimally.
6. Allocate attention wisely.
7. Use all available information.
8. Use all available resources.
9. Call for help when needed.
10. Maintain professional behavior.

From the Center for Advanced Pediatric and Perinatal Education, Packard Children's Hospital at Stanford.

The NRP grew out of the pioneering work of Ronald Bloom, MD, and Catherine Cropley, RN, MN, who received a grant from the National Institutes of Health to create a standardized approach to resuscitation of the newborn. Errol Alden, MD, at the AAP and Leon Chameides, MD, at the AHA facilitated expert review of the content of the program and developed a strategy for its dissemination. Since that time, the NRP has set a national standard and international example for training in neonatal resuscitation. The guiding principles that have driven the formation and evolution include use of the best-available evidence to guide the crafting of practice recommendations (via ILCOR), identification of the key skills necessary for successful neonatal resuscitation, emphasis on self-education for the adult learner, adequate preparation of instructors, and regionalization of training whereby NRP instructors are not limited to a specific facility or training center, allowing wider dissemination of its content and methodology. These principles have resulted in a program that can claim over 3 million trainees taught by more than 27,000 instructors in the United States, translation into 25 different languages, and delivery in more than 125 different countries around the world.[127] Because it has continued to incorporate not only the most current science but also effective adult learning strategies, it remains one of the most successful educational interventions in health care.[128]

What NRP Is—and Is Not

Successful completion of NRP provider training requires achieving the minimum passing score on an online multiple-choice examination of content knowledge, demonstration of pertinent technical skills on task trainers, and participation in simulation-based scenarios pertinent to the trainee's level of experience. It is important to note that the *Textbook of Neonatal Resuscitation* states, "Completion of the program does not imply that an individual has the competence to perform neonatal resuscitation. Each hospital is responsible for determining the level of competence and qualifications required for someone to assume clinical responsibility for neonatal resuscitation."[3] The NRPSC makes no claim that an individual who has successfully completed the program is competent to resuscitate real newborns at the time of delivery. Nevertheless, it is not uncommon for phrases such as "certified in NRP" or "NRP certified" to be used by individuals and organizations outside the NRPSC and its staff and liaisons. The NRP is not a measure of HCP competency and should not be used as such. Despite this fact, many hospitals in the United States have policies mandating successful completion of the NRP and possession of an active NRP provider card as a condition for employment for those assuming direct

care of newborns. Such a focus on compliance rather than learning and assessment of skills appropriate to the level of one's experience is inappropriate.

The continued evolution of the NRP will lead to a career-long learning program highly relevant to HCPs from multiple disciplines at all levels of experience. This transition to a career-long learning model requiring regular review of the many aspects of neonatal resuscitation using multiple learning methodologies will stimulate development of new learning materials accessible via the Internet from any location in the world. The incorporation of simulation-based learning and assessment methodologies will foster development of challenging immersive experiences by which human and system weaknesses are identified and then remediated.[129-135] Pioneering work in simulation-based training in neonatal resuscitation has been accomplished at the Center for Advanced Pediatric Education (CAPE) at Packard Children's Hospital at Stanford (Stanford, CA) and has served as the basis for many of the recent developments within NRP.[136]

To improve the safety, efficacy, and efficiency of the delivery of care, HCPs in neonatal-perinatal medicine will need to adopt the methods of training and selection of resuscitation team personnel that have proven to be effective in other industries where the risk to human life is high. Frequent, objective assessment and ongoing simulation-based training will need to become the standard for skill acquisition and maintenance.[137] Human and system weaknesses will be identified through objective evaluation of real-life performance and subsequently remediated via highly realistic simulations designed to replicate these weaknesses and constructive debriefings conducted to optimize learning and retention.[138-143] In addition, combined team training during scenarios involving both obstetric and pediatric HCPs will become the norm.[144]

GAPS IN KNOWLEDGE

Despite tremendous progress in the understanding of the basic science characterizing the transitional physiology between fetal and neonatal states as well as a highly circumspect approach reviewing published evidence relating to interventions undertaken during resuscitation, many gaps in knowledge remain.[145] At the end of each ILCOR cycle of evidence review and guideline development, members of the ILCOR Neonatal Task Force list the areas where the science is inconclusive (or nonexistent) and craft specific questions designed to stimulate research that will ultimately provide conclusive answers. The questions that were most recently identified as keys to advancing the science of neonatal resuscitation are listed in Table 8-7.

Table 8-7 Gaps in Current Knowledge in Neonatal Resuscitation

Meconium-stained neonate

Does intubation and suctioning of the trachea at the time of delivery in full-term nonvigorous neonates delivered through meconium-stained amniotic fluid, compared to no suctioning, affect mortality or the rate of complications?

Supplemental oxygen

In neonates not responding to 30–45 seconds of effective ventilation as manifest by a persistent HR less than 60 BPM, how much supplemental oxygen should be used?

What is the effect of the administration of 21% vs higher concentrations of oxygen during circulatory arrest on cerebral blood flow and subsequent brain injury?

What is the optimal hemoglobin oxygen saturation target in nonhealthy newborns?

Should hemoglobin oxygen saturation targets be different in the preterm and term populations?

Establishing functional residual capacity

In the apneic neonate with a HR less than 100 BPM despite PPV with a conventional T_I (0.35 seconds), does the use of PEEP compared to no PEEP affect duration of bradycardia, requirement for oxygen supplementation, and length of stay?

In the apneic neonate with a HR less than 100 BPM, does the use of a prolonged T_I compared to a conventional T_I (0.35 seconds) affect the duration of bradycardia and requirement for oxygen supplementation?

Delivery of breaths

When administering face-mask ventilation, should volume or pressure be measured, and if so, what is the optimal volume to deliver over what time period as compliance changes?

When administering face-mask ventilation, what sizes and types of masks facilitate effective ventilation?

What is the optimal device for delivering PEEP and CPAP?

What is the efficacy of an LMA in delivering desired tidal volume, particularly as compliance changes or in cases of airway obstruction?

Will measurement of inflation pressure, volume of gas delivered per breath, mask leak, and $ETCO_2$ affect the clinical outcomes of neonates and therefore should they be measured during resuscitation?

Temperature regulation

Does the use of a polyethylene wrap and an exothermic mattress as compared to a polyethylene wrap alone maintain temperature in the normal range and affect mortality and length of stay?

How rapidly should a VLBW infant with an initial temperature less than 35°C be rewarmed?

Does the ambient temperature of the DR affect the initial temperature of the neonate?

Will raising the ambient temperature of the DR produce adverse maternal consequences?

In VLBW neonates whose temperature on nursery admission is below normal, what are the causes and timing of death?

What are the consequences of an elevated temperature during labor in terms of initiation of spontaneous respirations, development of neonatal encephalopathy, occurrence of seizures, and mortality?

Will lowering an elevated maternal temperature during labor reduce the occurrence of neonatal depression, neonatal encephalopathy, and mortality?

Bradycardia

In the neonate with persistent bradycardia less than 60 BPM unresponsive to PPV, will administration of epinephrine (to improve diastolic blood pressure and coronary artery blood flow) before initiating chest compressions increase the heart rate to greater than 100 BPM more rapidly and be associated with less supplemental oxygen, encephalopathy, or intraventricular hemorrhage?

In the neonate with persistent bradycardia less than 60 BPM, can the pulse waveform on an oximeter be used to determine adequacy of compressions?

What is the etiology of bradycardia less than 60 BPM that persists despite adequate ventilation?

Noninitiation or discontinuation of resuscitation

Can the data from the large randomized studies of therapeutic hypothermia be used to determine whether efforts should be discontinued in neonates with a HR 0–59 BPM after 10 minutes of resuscitation?

Can the limits of viability be objectively defined to provide clear guidelines regarding when resuscitation should not be attempted?

Abbreviations: BPM, beats per minute; CPAP, continuous positive airway pressure; DR, delivery room; $ETCO_2$, end tidal carbon dioxide; HR, heart rate; LMA, laryngeal mask airway; PEEP, positive end-expiratory pressure; PPV, positive-pressure ventilation; VLBW, very low birth weight.

FUTURE ISSUES

The typical DR in the United States is designed for the comfort of the pregnant woman and the ease of operation of the obstetric team; often, there is insufficient space for the neonatal resuscitation team to carry out routine procedures, let alone the more extensive interventions required during full resuscitations. In a space designed to optimize the performance of both the obstetric and neonatal teams in caring for both mother and her newborn(s), there will be sufficient square footage to carry out all of the interventions necessary for both fetal and neonatal resuscitation. In addition, this space will be equipped with extensive capabilities for acquiring real-time physiologic data and displaying these data in a manner that facilitates easy recognition and interpretation.[146,147] Because technologic advances will continue to allow monitoring of an ever-increasing number of physiologic variables during neonatal resuscitation, it must be understood that simply adding more data streams to the resuscitation environment without addressing the human factors issues pertaining to the facilitation of that conversion of data to useful information will not result in improved care.[148–151] All of these developments will lead to the creation of a resuscitation environment that is similar to a NICU, where more, rather than fewer, procedures will be performed in an effort to stabilize and definitively treat the newborn prior to transport to the actual nursery. Transfer to the nursery (or to a referral center) will then be accomplished with less risk of decompensation and iatrogenic injury. Thus, the standard in the near future will be a fetal/neonatal resuscitation and transition suite that allows for resuscitation and stabilization of the newborn, including interventions such as intubation and placement on a ventilator, catheterization of umbilical vessels, delivery of surfactant and other medications, and radiographic confirmation of the proper positioning of all instrumentation.[152]

SUMMARY

With its emphasis on evidence-based practice, the field of neonatal-perinatal medicine is increasingly characterized as one in which dogma is being challenged. This is certainly true of resuscitation science and practice, for which organizations such as ILCOR and the NRPSC seek a firm foundation for every action undertaken on behalf of newborns in the DR. Compared to previous versions, the current guidelines for neonatal resuscitation recommend less suctioning, less oxygen, less inspiratory pressure, less intubation, less intervention for patients with meconium staining, and less interruption in compressions once CPR has been initiated. The objectivity of the ILCOR process for achieving international consensus on the science not only will ensure that clinical guidelines are based on the best-available evidence but also will stimulate investigation into areas still characterized by gaps in knowledge. This will be complemented by an increasing reliance on human factors to guide the design of the technologies and physical environments used for neonatal resuscitation and the incorporation of modern adult learning theory into training programs that facilitate the acquisition and maintenance of all of the skills necessary to promote effective and safe resuscitation of the newborn.

List of Abbreviations

AAP	Academy of Pediatrics
AHA	American Heart Association
BPM	beats per minute
CO_2	carbon dioxide
CC	chest compressions
CLD	chronic lung disease
cm	centimeter
CPAP	continuous positive airway pressure
CPR	cardiopulmonary resuscitation
DR	delivery room
EPI	epinephrine
EGA	estimated gestational age
$ETCO_2$	end tidal carbon dioxide
ETT	endotracheal tube
FIO_2	fraction of inspired oxygen
FRC	functional residual capacity
g	gram
HCP	health care professional
HR	heart rate
ILCOR	International Liaison Committee on Resuscitation
IO	intraosseous
IT	intratracheal
IV	intravenous
JC	Joint Commission
kg	kilogram
LMA	laryngeal mask airway
MAS	meconium aspiration syndrome
mL	milliliter
MRSOPA	Mask, Reposition, Suction, Open, Pressure, Alternative Airway
MSAF	meconium-stained amniotic fluid
NEC	necrotizing enterocolitis
NICHD	National Institute of Child Health and Human Development
NICU	neonatal intensive care unit
NRP	Neonatal Resuscitation Program

NRPSC	NRP Steering Committee
PEEP	positive end-expiratory pressure
PIP	peak inspiratory pressure
PPV	positive-pressure ventilation
RCT	randomized controlled trial
ROP	retinopathy of prematurity
SpO$_2$	pulse oximetry
T$_I$	inspiratory time

REFERENCES

1. Dorland. *Dorland's Illustrated Medical Dictionary*. 31st ed. Philadelphia, PA: Saunders; 2007.
2. Perlman JM, Risser R. Cardiopulmonary resuscitation in the delivery room: associated clinical events. *Arch Pediatr Adolesc Med*. 1995;149:20–25.
3. American Academy of Pediatrics and the American Heart Association. *Textbook of Neonatal Resuscitation*. 6th ed. Elk Grove Village, IL: American Academy of Pediatrics; 2010.
4. Chamberlain D. The International Liaison Committee on Resuscitation (ILCOR)—past and present: compiled by the founding members of the International Liaison Committee on Resuscitation. *Resuscitation*. 2005;67(2–3):157–161.
5. http://www.ilcor.org/about-ilcor/about-ilcor/ (accessed September 22, 2014).
6. Perlman JM, Wyllie J, Kattwinkel J, et al. Neonatal resuscitation: 2010 international consensus on cardiopulmonary resuscitation and emergency cardiovascular care science with treatment recommendations. *Pediatrics*. 2010;126(5):e1319–e1344.
7. Soar J, Mancini ME, Bhanji F, et al. Part 12: education, implementation and teams: 2010 international consensus on cardiopulmonary resuscitation and emergency cardiovascular care science with treatment recommendations. *Resuscitation*. 2010;81(Suppl 1):e288–e330.
8. Kattwinkel J, Perlman JM, Aziz K, et al. Neonatal resuscitation: 2010 American Heart Association guidelines for cardiopulmonary resuscitation and emergency cardiovascular care. *Pediatrics*. 2010;126(5):e1400–e1413.
9. Gungor S, Kurt E, Teksoz E, Goktolga U, Ceyhan T, Baser I. Oronasopharyngeal suction versus no suction in normal and term infants delivered by elective cesarean section: a prospective randomized controlled trial. *Gynecol Obstet Invest*. 2006;61:9–14.
10. Prendiville A, Thomson A, Silverman M. Effect of tracheobronchial suction on respiratory resistance in intubated preterm babies. *Arch Dis Child*. 1986;61:1178–1183.
11. Perlman JM, Volpe JJ. Suctioning in the preterm infant: effects on cerebral blood flow velocity, intracranial pressure, and arterial blood pressure. *Pediatrics*. 1983;72:329–334.
12. Simbruner G, Coradello H, Fodor M, Havelec L, Lubec G, Pollak A. Effect of tracheal suction on oxygenation, circulation, and lung mechanics in newborn infants. *Arch Dis Child*. 1981;56:326–330.
13. Halamek LP, Morley C. Continuous positive airway pressure. *Clin Perinatol*. 2006;33(1):83–98.
14. Roehr CC, Proquitté H, Hammer H, Wauer RR, Morley CJ, Schmalisch G. Positive effects of early continuous positive airway pressure on pulmonary function in extremely premature infants: Results of a subgroup analysis of the COIN trial. *Arch Dis Child Fetal Neonatal Ed*. 2011;96(5):F371–F373.
15. Morley CJ, Davis PG, Doyle LW, Brion LP, Hascoet JM, Carlin JB: Nasal CPAP or intubation at birth for very preterm infants [erratum in *N Engl J Med*. 2008;358(14):1529]. *N Engl J Med*. 2008;358:700–708.
16. Hascoet JM, Espagne S, Hamon I. CPAP and the preterm infant: lessons from the COIN trial and other studies. *Early Hum Dev*. 2008;84(12):791–793.
17. Finer NN, Carlo WA, Duara S, et al. Delivery room continuous positive airway pressure/positive end-expiratory pressure in extremely low birth weight infants: a feasibility trial. *Pediatrics*. 2004;114:651–657.
18. Lindner W, Vossbeck S, Hummler H, Pohlandt F. Delivery room management of extremely low birth weight infants: spontaneous breathing or intubation? *Pediatrics*. 1999;103:961–967.
19. Finer NN, Rich W, Wang C, Leone T. Airway obstruction during mask ventilation of very low birth weight infants during neonatal resuscitation. *Pediatrics*. 2009;123:865–869.
20. Wood FE, Morley CJ, Dawson JA, et al. Assessing the effectiveness of two round neonatal resuscitation masks: Study 1. *Arch Dis Child Fetal Neonatal Ed*. 2008;93:F235–F237.
21. Wood FE, Morley CJ, Dawson JA, et al. Improved techniques reduce face mask leak during simulated neonatal resuscitation: Study 2. *Arch Dis Child Fetal Neonatal Ed*. 2008;93:F230–F234.
22. O'Donnell CP, Davis PG, Lau R, Dargaville PA, Doyle LW, Morley CJ. Neonatal resuscitation 2: an evaluation of manual ventilation devices and face masks. *Arch Dis Child Fetal Neonatal Ed*. 2005;90:F392–F396.
23. Palme C, Nystrom B, Tunell R. An evaluation of the efficiency of face masks in the resuscitation of newborn infants. *Lancet*. 1985;1:207–210.
24. Te Pas AB, Walther FJ. A randomized, controlled trial of delivery-room respiratory management in very preterm infants. *Pediatrics*. 2007;120:322–329.
25. Lindner W, Hogel J, Pohlandt F. Sustained pressure-controlled inflation or intermittent mandatory ventilation in preterm infants in the delivery room? A randomized, controlled trial on initial respiratory support via nasopharyngeal tube. *Acta Paediatr*. 2005;94:303–309.
26. Harling AE, Beresford MW, Vince GS, Bates M, Yoxall CW. Does sustained lung inflation at resuscitation reduce lung injury in the preterm infant? *Arch Dis Child Fetal Neonatal Ed*. 2005;90:F406–F410.
27. Vyas H, Field D, Milner AD, Hopkin IE. Determinants of the first inspiratory volume and functional residual capacity at birth. *Pediatr Pulmonol*. 1986;2:189–193.
28. Vyas H, Milner AD, Hopkin IE, Boon AW. Physiologic responses to prolonged and slow-rise inflation in the resuscitation of the asphyxiated newborn infant. *J Pediatr*. 1981;99: 635–639.
29. Morley CJ, Dawson JA, Stewart MJ, Hussain F, Davis PG. The effect of a PEEP valve on a Laerdal neonatal self-inflating resuscitation bag. *J Paediatr Child Health*. 2010;46(1–2):51–56.
30. Singh R. Controlled trial to evaluate the use of LMA for neonatal resuscitation. *J Anaesth Clin Pharmacol*. 2005;21:303–306.
31. Trevisanuto D, Micaglio M, Pitton M, Magarotto M, Piva D, Zanardo V. Laryngeal mask airway: is the management of neonates requiring positive pressure ventilation at birth changing? *Resuscitation*. 2004;62:151–157.
32. Zanardo V, Simbi AK, Savio V, Micaglio M, Trevisanuto D. Neonatal resuscitation by laryngeal mask airway after elective cesarean section. *Fetal Diagn Ther*. 2004;19:228–231.
33. Esmail N, Saleh M, Hussein S, et al. Laryngeal mask airway versus endotracheal intubation for Apgar score improvement in neonatal resuscitation. *Egypt J Anesthesiol*. 2002;18:115–121.
34. Gandini D, Brimacombe JR. Neonatal resuscitation with the laryngeal mask airway in normal and low birth weight infants. *Anesth Analg*. 1999;89:642–643.
35. Oddie S, Wyllie J, Scally A. Use of self-inflating bags for neonatal resuscitation. *Resuscitation*. 2005;67:109–112.

36. Bennett S, Finer NN, Rich W, Vaucher Y. A comparison of three neonatal resuscitation devices. *Resuscitation.* 2005;67:113–118.

37. Finer NN, Rich W, Craft A, Henderson C. Comparison of methods of bag and mask ventilation for neonatal resuscitation. *Resuscitation.* 2001;49:299–305.

38. Hussey SG, Ryan CA, Murphy BP. Comparison of three manual ventilation devices using an intubated mannequin. *Arch Dis Child Fetal Neonatal Ed.* 2004;89:F490–F493.

39. Davis PG, Tan A, O'Donnell CP, Schulze A. Resuscitation of newborn infants with 100% oxygen or air: a systematic review and meta-analysis. *Lancet.* 2004;364:1329–1333.

40. Saugstad OD, Ramji S, Irani SF, et al. Resuscitation of newborn infants with 21% or 100% oxygen: follow-up at 18 to 24 months. *Pediatrics.* 2003;112(2):296–300.

41. Vento M, Asensi M, Sastre J, Garcia-Sala F, Pallardo FV, Vina J. Resuscitation with room air instead of 100% oxygen prevents oxidative stress in moderately asphyxiated term neonates. *Pediatrics.* 2001;107:642–647.

42. Saugstad OD, Rootwelt T, Aalen O. Resuscitation of asphyxiated newborn infants with room air or oxygen: an international controlled trial: the RESAIR 2 study. *Pediatrics.* 1998;102:e1.

43. Saugstad OD, Ramji S, Vento M. Resuscitation of depressed newborn infants with ambient air or pure oxygen: a meta-analysis. *Biol Neonate.* 2005;87(1):27–34.

44. Saugstad OD. Room air resuscitation-two decades of neonatal research. *Early Hum Dev.* 2005;81(1):111–116.

45. Rabi Y, Rabi D, Yee W. Room air resuscitation of the depressed newborn: a systematic review and meta-analysis. *Resuscitation.* 2007;72:353–363.

46. Solberg R, Andresen JH, Escrig R, Vento M, Saugstad OD. Resuscitation of hypoxic newborn piglets with oxygen induces a dose-dependent increase in markers of oxidation. *Pediatr Res.* 2007;62:559–563.

47. Solas AB, Kutzsche S, Vinje M, Saugstad OD. Cerebral hypoxemia-ischemia and reoxygenation with 21% or 100% oxygen in newborn piglets: effects on extracellular levels of excitatory amino acids and microcirculation. *Pediatr Crit Care Med.* 2001;2:340–345.

48. Wang CL, Anderson C, Leone TA, Rich W, Govindaswami B, Finer NN. Resuscitation of preterm neonates by using room air or 100% oxygen. *Pediatrics.* 2008;121:1083–1089.

49. Escrig R, Arruza L, Izquierdo I, et al. Achievement of targeted saturation values in extremely low gestational age neonates resuscitated with low or high oxygen concentrations: a prospective, randomized trial. *Pediatrics.* 2008;121:875–881.

50. Dawson JA, Kamlin CO, Wong C, et al. Oxygen saturation and heart rate during delivery room resuscitation of infants < 30 weeks' gestation with air or 100% oxygen. *Arch Dis Child Fetal Neonatal Ed.* 2009;94:F87–F91.

51. Altuncu E, Ozek E, Bilgen H, Topuzoglu A, Kavuncuoglu S. Percentiles of oxygen saturations in healthy term newborns in the first minutes of life. *Eur J Pediatr.* 2008;167:687–688.

52. Kamlin CO, O'Donnell CP, Davis PG, Morley CJ. Oxygen saturation in healthy infants immediately after birth. *J Pediatr.* 2006;148:585–589.

53. Rabi Y, Yee W, Chen SY, Singhal N. Oxygen saturation trends immediately after birth. *J Pediatr.* 2006;148:590–594.

54. O'Donnell CP, Kamlin CO, Davis PG, Morley CJ. Obtaining pulse oximetry data in neonates: a randomised crossover study of sensor application techniques. *Arch Dis Child Fetal Neonatal Ed.* 2005;90:F84–F85.

55. Toth B, Becker A, Seelbach-Gobel B. Oxygen saturation in healthy newborn infants immediately after birth measured by pulse oximetry. *Arch Gynecol Obstet.* 2002;266:105–107.

56. Hosono S, Inami I, Fujita H, Minato M, Takahashi S, Mugishima H. The role of end-tidal CO_2 monitoring for assessment of tracheal intubations in very low birth weight infants during neonatal resuscitation at birth. *J Perinat Med.* 2009;37:79–84.

57. Garey DM, Ward R, Rich W, Heldt G, Leone T, Finer NN. Tidal volume threshold for colorimetric carbon dioxide detectors available for use in neonates. *Pediatrics.* 2008;121:e1524–e1527.

58. Hughes SM, Blake BL, Woods SL, Lehmann CU. False-positive results on colorimetric carbon dioxide analysis in neonatal resuscitation: potential for serious patient harm. *J Perinatol.* 2007;27:800–801.

59. Leone TA, Lange A, Rich W, Finer NN. Disposable colorimetric carbon dioxide detector use as an indicator of a patent airway during noninvasive mask ventilation. *Pediatrics.* 2006;118:e202–e204.

60. Repetto JE, Donohue P-CP, Baker SF, Kelly L, Nogee LM. Use of capnography in the delivery room for assessment of endotracheal tube placement. *J Perinatol.* 2001;21:284–287.

61. Aziz HF, Martin JB, Moore JJ. The pediatric disposable end-tidal carbon dioxide detector role in endotracheal intubation in newborns. *J Perinatol.* 1999;19:110–113.

62. Roberts WA, Maniscalco WM, Cohen AR, Litman RS, Chhibber A. The use of capnography for recognition of esophageal intubation in the neonatal intensive care unit. *Pediatr Pulmonol.* 1995;19:262–268.

63. Carson BS, Losey RW, Bowes WA Jr, Simemons MA. Combined obstetric and pediatric approach to prevent meconium aspiration syndrome. *Am J Obstet Gynecol.* 1976;126:712–715.

64. Ting P, Brady JP. Tracheal suction in meconium aspiration. *Am J Obstet Gynecol.* 1975;122:767–771.

65. Gregory GA, Gooding CA, Phibbs RH, Tooley WH. Meconium aspiration in infants—a prospective study. *J Pediatr.* 1974;85:848–852.

66. Dooley SL, Pesavento DJ, Depp R, Socol ML, Tamura RK, Wiringa KS. Meconium below the vocal cords at delivery: correlation with intrapartum events. *Am J Obstet Gynecol.* 1985;153(7):767–770.

67. Houlihan CM, Knuppel RA. Meconium-stained amniotic fluid. Current controversies. *J Reprod Med.* 1994;39(11):888–898.

68. Brown BL, Gleicher N. Intrauterine meconium aspiration. *Obstet Gynecol.* 1981;57:26–29.

69. Manning FA, Schreiber J, Turkel SB. Fatal meconium aspiration "in utero": a case report. *Am J Obstet Gynecol.* 1978;132:111–113.

70. Wiswell TE, Gannon CM, Jacob J, et al. Delivery room management of the apparently vigorous meconium-stained neonate: results of the multicenter, international collaborative trial. *Pediatrics.* 2000;105(1):1–7.

71. Halliday HL, Sweet DG. Endotracheal intubation at birth for preventing morbidity and mortality in vigorous, meconium-stained infants born at term. *Cochrane Database Syst Rev.* 2001;(1):CD000500.

72. Vain NE, Szyld EG, Prudent LM, Wiswell TE, Aguilar AM, Vivas NI. Oropharyngeal and nasopharyngeal suctioning of meconium-stained neonates before delivery of their shoulders: a multicentre, randomised controlled trial. *Lancet.* 2004;364:597–602.

73. Velaphi S, Vidyasagar D. The pros and cons of suctioning at the perineum (intrapartum) and post-delivery with and without meconium. *Semin Fetal Neonatal Med.* 2008;13(6):375–382.

74. Guinsburg R, Wyckoff M. Naloxone during neonatal resuscitation: acknowledging the unknown. *Clin Perinatol.* 2006;33:121–132.

75. McGuire W, Fowlie PW. Naloxone for narcotic-exposed newborn infants. *Cochrane Database Syst Rev.* 2002;(4):CD003483.

76. Gibbs J, Newson T, Williams J, Davidson DC. Naloxone hazard in infant of opioid abuser. *Lancet.* 1989;2:159–160.

77. Berkowitz BA. The relationship of pharmacokinetics to pharmacological activity: morphine, methadone and naloxone. *Clin Pharmacokinet.* 1976;1(3):219–230.

78. Christman C, Hemway RJ, Wyckoff MH, Perlman JM. The two-thumb is superior to the two-finger method for administering chest compressions in a manikin model of neonatal resuscitation. *Arch Dis Child Fetal Neonatal Ed.* 2011;96(2):F99–F101.

79. Wyckoff MH, Berg RA. Optimizing chest compressions during delivery-room resuscitation. *Semin Fetal Neonatal Med.* 2008;13(6):410–415.

80. Whitelaw CC, Slywka B, Goldsmith LJ. Comparison of a two-finger versus two-thumb method for chest compressions by healthcare providers in an infant mechanical model. *Resuscitation.* 2000;43:213–216.

81. Houri PK, Frank LR, Menegazzi JJ, Taylor R. A randomized, controlled trial of two-thumb vs two-finger chest compression in a swine infant model of cardiac arrest. *Prehosp Emerg Care.* 1997;1:65–67.

82. Menegazzi JJ, Auble TE, Nicklas KA, Hosack GM, Rack L, Goode JS. Two-thumb versus two-finger chest compression during CPR in a swine infant model of cardiac arrest. *Ann Emerg Med.* 1993;22:240–243.

83. Orlowski JP. Optimum position for external cardiac compression in infants and young children. *Ann Emerg Med.* 1986;15:667–673.

84. Kinney SB, Tibballs J. An analysis of the efficacy of bag-valve-mask ventilation and chest compression during different compression-ventilation ratios in manikin-simulated paediatric resuscitation. *Resuscitation.* 2000;43:115–120.

85. Wyckoff MH, Perlman J, Niermeyer S. Medications during resuscitation—what is the evidence? *Semin Neonatol.* 2001;6(3):251–259.

86. Rajani AK, Chitkara R, Oehlert J, Halamek LP. Comparison of umbilical venous and intraosseous access during simulated neonatal resuscitation. *Pediatrics.* 2011;128(4):e954–e958.

87. Abe KK, Blum GT, Yamamoto LG. Intraosseous is faster and easier than umbilical venous catheterization in newborn emergency vascular access models. *Am J Emerg Med.* 2000; 18(2):126–129.

88. Ellemunter H, Simma B, Trawoger R, Maurer H. Intraosseous lines in preterm and full term neonates. *Arch Dis Child Fetal Neonatal Ed.* 1999;80:F74–F75.

89. Barber CA, Wyckoff MH. Use and efficacy of endotracheal versus intravenous epinephrine during neonatal cardiopulmonary resuscitation in the delivery room. *Pediatrics.* 2006;118: 1028–1034.

90. Mielke LL, Frank C, Lanzinger MJ, et al. Plasma catecholamine levels following tracheal and intravenous epinephrine administration in swine. *Resuscitation.* 1998;36:187–192.

91. Roberts JR, Greenberg MI, Knaub MA, Kendrick ZV, Baskin SI. Blood levels following intravenous and endotracheal epinephrine administration. *JACEP.* 1979;8:53–56.

92. Hornchen U, Schuttler J, Stoeckel H, Eichelkraut W, Hahn N. Endobronchial instillation of epinephrine during cardiopulmonary resuscitation. *Crit Care Med.* 1987;15:1037–1039.

93. Murat I, Humblot A, Girault L, Piana F. Neonatal fluid management. *Best Pract Res Clin Anaesthesiol.* 2010;24(3):365–374.

94. Tabbers MM, Boluyt N, Offringa M. Implementation of an evidence-based guideline on fluid resuscitation: lessons learnt for future guidelines. *Eur J Pediatr.* 2010;169(6):749–758.

95. Boluyt N, Bollen CW, Bos AP, Kok JH, Offringa M. Fluid resuscitation in neonatal and pediatric hypovolemic shock: a Dutch Pediatric Society evidence-based clinical practice guideline. *Intensive Care Med.* 2006;32(7):995–1003.

96. Niermeyer S. Volume resuscitation: crystalloid versus colloid. *Clin Perinatol.* 2006;33:133–140.

97. Wilkes MM, Navickis RJ, Wyckoff MH, Perlman JM, Laptook AR. Use of volume expansion during delivery room resuscitation in near-term and term infants. *Pediatrics.* 2005;115:950–955.

98. So KW, Fok TF, Ng PC, et al. Randomised controlled trial of colloid or crystalloid in hypotensive preterm infants. *Arch Dis Child.* 1997;76:F43–F46.

99. Emery EF, Greenough A, Gamsu HR. Randomised controlled trial of colloid infusions in hypotensive preterm infants. *Arch Dis Child.* 1992;67:1185–1188.

100. Voogdt KG, Morrison AC, Wood FE, van Elburg RM, Wyllie JP. A randomised, simulated study assessing auscultation of heart rate at birth. *Resuscitation.* 2010;81(8):1000–1003.

101. Kamlin CO, O'Donnell CP, Everest NJ, Davis PG, Morley CJ. Accuracy of clinical assessment of infant heart rate in the delivery room. *Resuscitation.* 2006;71(3):319–321.

102. Chitkara R, Rajani AK, Oehlert JW, Lee HC, Halamek LP. The accuracy of human senses in the detection of neonatal heart rate during standardized simulated resuscitation: implications for delivery of care, training and technology design. *Resuscitation.* 2013;84(3):369–372.

103. Hay WW, Rodden DJ, Collins SM, Melara DL, Hale KA, Fashaw LM. Reliability of conventional and new pulse oximetry in neonatal patients. *J Perinatol.* 2002;22:360–366.

104. O'Donnell CP, Kamlin CO, Davis PG, Morley CJ. Feasibility of and delay in obtaining pulse oximetry during neonatal resuscitation. *J Pediatr.* 2005;147:698–699.

105. Cramer K, Wiebe N, Hartling L, Crumley E, Vohra S. Heat loss prevention: a systematic review of occlusive skin wrap for premature neonates. *J Perinatol.* 2005;25:763–769.

106. Vohra S, Roberts RS, Zhang B, Janes M, Schmidt B. Heat loss prevention (HELP) in the delivery room: a randomized controlled trial of polyethylene occlusive skin wrapping in very preterm infants. *J Pediatr.* 2004;145:750–753.

107. Vohra S, Frent G, Campbell V, Abbott M, Whyte R. Effect of polyethylene occlusive skin wrapping on heat loss in very low birth weight infants at delivery: a randomized trial. *J Pediatr.* 1999;134:547–551.

108. Singh A, Duckett J, Newton T, Watkinson M. Improving neonatal unit admission temperatures in preterm babies: exothermic mattresses, polythene bags or a traditional approach? *J Perinatol.* 2010;30:45–49.

109. Almeida PG, Chandley J, Davis J, Harrigan RC. Use of the heated gel mattress and its impact on admission temperature of very low birth-weight infants. *Adv Neonatal Care.* 2009;9:34–39.

110. Kent AL, Williams J. Increasing ambient operating theatre temperature and wrapping in polyethylene improves admission temperature in premature infants. *J Paediatr Child Health.* 2008;44:325–331.

111. Knobel RB, Wimmer JE Jr, Holbert D. Heat loss prevention for preterm infants in the delivery room. *J Perinatol.* 2005;25:304–308.

112. Laptook AR, Salhab W, Bhaskar B. Admission temperature of low birth weight infants: predictors and associated morbidities. *Pediatrics.* 2007;119:e643–e649.

113. Meyer MP, Bold GT. Admission temperatures following radiant warmer or incubator transport for preterm infants < 28 weeks: a randomised study. *Arch Dis Child Fetal Neonatal Ed.* 2007; 92:F295–F297.

114. Perlman J, Davis P, Wyllie J, Kattwinkel J. Therapeutic hypothermia following intrapartum hypoxia ischemia an advisory statement from the Neonatal Task Force of the International Liaison Committee on Resuscitation. *Resuscitation.* 2010;81:1459–1461.

115. Papile LA, Baley JE, Benitz W, Cummings J, Carlo WA, Eichenwald E Kumar P, Polin RA, Tan RC, Wang KS. Hypothermia and neonatal encephalopathy. *Pediatrics.* 2014 Jun;133(6):1146–1150.

116. Halamek LP. Prenatal consultation at the limits of viability. *NeoReviews.* 2003;4:e153–e156.

117. Halamek LP. The advantages of prenatal consultation by a neonatologist. *J Perinatol*. 2001;21:116–120.

118. Paris JJ. What standards apply to resuscitation at the borderline of gestational age? *J Perinatol*. 2005;25:683–684.

119. De Leeuw R, Cuttini M, Nadai M, et al. Treatment choices for extremely preterm infants: an international perspective. *J Pediatr*. 2000;137:608–616.

120. Sanders MR, Donohue PK, Oberdorf MA, Rosenkrantz TS, Allen MC. Perceptions of the limit of viability: neonatologists' attitudes toward extremely preterm infants. *J Perinatol*. 1995;15:494–502.

121. NICHD Neonatal Research Network (NRN). Extremely preterm birth outcome data. 2012. http://www.nichd.nih.gov/about/org/cdbpm/pp/prog_epbo/epbo_case.cfm (accessed September 30, 2012).

122. Tyson JE, Parikh NA, Langer J, Green C, Higgins RD. Intensive care for extreme prematurity: moving beyond gestational age. *N Engl J Med*. 2008;358:1672–1681.

123. Laptook AR, Shankaran S, Ambalavanan N, et al. Outcome of term infants using Apgar scores at 10 minutes following hypoxic-ischemic encephalopathy. *Pediatrics*. 2009;124:1619–1626.

124. Chamnanvanakij S, Perlman JM. Outcome following cardio-pulmonary resuscitation in the neonate requiring ventilatory assistance. *Resuscitation*. 2000;45:173–180.

125. Halamek LP. Teaching versus learning and the role of simulation-based training in pediatrics. *J Pediatr*. 2007; 151(4):329–330.

126. http://www.jointcommission.org/sentinel_event_alert_issue_30_ preventing_infant_death_and_injury_during_delivery/ (accessed September 22, 2014).

127. Kattwinkel J, Perlman J. The Neonatal Resuscitation Program: the evidence evaluation process and anticipating edition 6. *NeoReviews*. 2010;11(12):e673–e680.

128. Halamek LP. The genesis, adaptation, and evolution of the Neonatal Resuscitation Program. *NeoReviews*. 2008;9(4):e142–e149.

129. Lee MO, Brown LL, Bender J, Machan JT, Overly FL. A medical simulation-based educational intervention for emergency medicine residents in neonatal resuscitation. *Acad Emerg Med*. 2012;19(5):577–585.

130. Sawyer T, Sierocka-Castaneda A, Chan D, Berg B, Lustik M, Thompson M. Deliberate practice using simulation improves neonatal resuscitation performance. *Simul Healthc*. 2011;6(6):327–336.

131. Wayne DB, Didwania A, Feinglass J, Fudala MJ, Barsuk JH, McGaghie WC. Simulation-based education improves quality of care during cardiac arrest team responses at an academic teaching hospital: a case-control study. *Chest*. 2008;133:56–61.

132. Kory PD, Eisen LA, Adachi M, Ribaudo VA, Rosenthal ME, Mayo PH. Initial airway management skills of senior residents: simulation training compared with traditional training. *Chest*. 2007;132:1927–1931.

133. Savoldelli GL, Naik VN, Park J, Joo HS, Chow R, Hamstra SJ. Value of debriefing during simulated crisis management: oral versus video-assisted oral feedback. *Anesthesiology*. 2006;105:279–285.

134. Wayne DB, Butter J, Siddall VJ, et al. Simulation-based training of internal medicine residents in advanced cardiac life support protocols: a randomized trial. *Teach Learn Med*. 2005;17:210–216.

135. Shapiro MJ, Morey JC, Small SD, et al. Simulation based teamwork training for emergency department staff: does it improve clinical team performance when added to an existing didactic teamwork curriculum? *Qual Saf Health Care*. 2004;13:417–421.

136. Halamek LP, Kaegi DM, Gaba DM, et al. Time for a new paradigm in pediatric medical education: teaching neonatal resuscitation in a simulated delivery room environment. *Pediatrics*. 2000;106(4):e45. http://www.pediatrics.org/cgi/content/full/106/4/e45 (accessed September 30, 2012).

137. Carbine DN, Finer NN, Knodel E, et al. Video recording as a means of evaluating neonatal resuscitation performance. *Pediatrics*. 2000;106(4):654–658.

138. Edelson DP, Litzinger B, Arora V, et al. Improving in-hospital cardiac arrest process and outcomes with performance debriefing. *Arch Intern Med*. 2008;168:1063–1069.

139. Halamek LP. The simulated delivery room environment as the future modality for acquiring and maintaining skills in fetal and neonatal resuscitation. *Semin Fetal Neonatal Med*. 2008;13:448–453.

140. Clay AS, Que L, Petrusa ER, Sebastian M, Govert J. Debriefing in the intensive care unit: a feedback tool to facilitate bedside teaching. *Crit Care Med*. 2007;35:738–754.

141. Savoldelli GL, Naik VN, Park J, Joo HS, Chow R, Hamstra SJ. Value of debriefing during simulated crisis management: oral versus video-assisted oral feedback. *Anesthesiology*. 2006;105:279–285.

142. DeVita MA, Schaefer J, Lutz J, Wang H, Dongilli T. Improving medical emergency team (MET) performance using a novel curriculum and a computerized human patient simulator. *Qual Saf Health Care*. 2005;14:326–331.

143. Murphy AM, Halamek LP. Simulation-based training in neonatal resuscitation. *NeoReviews*. 2005;6(11):e489–e492.

144. Lipman SS, Daniels KI, Arafeh J, Halamek LP. The case for OBLS: a simulation-based obstetric resuscitation curriculum. *Sem Perinatol*. 2011;35:74–79.

145. Perlman J, Kattwinkel J, Wyllie J, et al. Neonatal resuscitation: in pursuit of evidence gaps in knowledge. *Resuscitation*. 2012;83(5):545–550.

146. Schmolzer GM, Kamlin OC, Dawson JA, et al. Respiratory monitoring of neonatal resuscitation. *Arch Dis Child Fetal Neonatal Ed*. 2010;95(4):F295–F303.

147. Kattwinkel J, Stewart C, Walsh B, Gurka M, Paget-Brown A. Responding to compliance changes in a lung model during manual ventilation: perhaps volume, rather than pressure, should be displayed. *Pediatrics*. 2009;123:e465–e470.

148. Hunt EA, Nelson KL, Shilkofski NA. Simulation in medicine: addressing patient safety and improving the interface between healthcare providers and medical technology. *Biomed Instrum Technol*. 2006;40:399–404.

149. Gawron VJ, Drury CG, Fairbanks RJ, et al. Medical error and human factors engineering: where are we now? *Am J Med Qual*. 2006;21:57–67.

150. Walsh T, Beatty PCW. Human factors errors and patient monitoring. *Physiol Meas*. 2002;23:R111–R132.

151. Gosbee J. Human factors engineering and patient safety. *Qual Saf Health Care*. 2002;11:352–354.

152. Finer NN, Rich W, Halamek LP, Leone TA. The delivery room of the future: The fetal/neonatal resuscitation and transition suite. *Clin Perinatol*. 2012;39(4):931–939.

Fluid Requirements in the Newborn Infant

R. S. Cohen

One of the very first issues that must be dealt with when a newborn infant is admitted to intensive care is that of fluid management. The vast majority of newborn intensive care unit (NICU) patients will need intravenous (IV) fluids initially, and certainly almost all very low birth weight (VLBW) ones will. Thus, the question of how much fluid a baby needs must be answered on the admission orders for most NICU patients.

With rare exceptions, neonates are born well hydrated. Indeed, total body water for neonates is higher than older children and adults. Total body water changes with maturation from up to 85%–90% in the very preterm infant, decreasing to about 75% at term, and eventually becoming about 65% in older children and adults.[1] Total body water includes different compartments—intracellular and extracellular. The extracellular water can also be subdivided into interstitial and plasma fluid volume. The drop in weight over the first few days postpartum is almost entirely caused by loss of excess extracellular water. For well term infants, this increased extracellular water acts as a reserve to prevent dehydration during the first days of life until maternal milk production increases and provides an adequate fluid intake.

Particularly for preterm infants, this loss of water is both physiologic and necessary. Many studies have shown that, for premature infants, delayed water loss results in a worse outcome, specifically an increased incidence of chronic lung disease and persistent patency of the ductus arteriosus.[2-4] Therefore, initial fluid intake for premature infants should be restricted to the least fluid necessary. The degree of fluid restriction is limited by the need to use intravenous fluids to deliver other necessities to the patient. For example, because preterm infants are at risk for hypoglycemia and cannot take adequate nutrition by mouth initially, intravenous dextrose is used as a glucose source. Extrapolating from studies of hepatic glucose production in lambs, a rate of about 4 to 6 mg/kg per minute was estimated for term infants.[5] To provide this rate of dextrose delivery, most NICUs restrict premature infants initially to about 60 to 80 mL/kg IV daily of D10W (10% dextrose by volume in water); 60 mL/kg of D10W provides 4.167 mg/kg per minute of dextrose, and 80 mL/kg of D10W provides 5.56 mg/kg per minute of dextrose. Remember that hydrous dextrose is not equivalent to anhydrous glucose; the conversion factor is simplified as 0.91. Thus, more accurately, intravenous D10W at 60 or 80 mL/kg daily is the equivalent of a glucose infusion rate of about 3.8 or 5.05 mg/kg per minute of glucose, respectively.

Because hepatic glucose production may continue in extremely low gestational age neonates (ELGANs) despite the infusion of intravenous dextrose, some of these patients will become hyperglycemic on this regimen. This may require slowing the infusion rate further or decreasing the dextrose concentration. Most units will not go below a dextrose concentration of about 3% to avoid using overly hypotonic solutions. Occasionally, an insulin infusion may be needed to control this hyperglycemia. This is generally a last resort because premature infants are relatively insulin resistant.

Assuming the initial intravenous rate results in euglycemia, further adjustments of intravenous fluid intake over the first few days of life are then determined by changes in weight, urine output, and serum chemistries. Excessive intravenous fluid administration during the immediate postpartum period will result in either weight gain or inadequate weight loss. Furthermore, a drop in serum sodium levels will often accompany this. Overly restricting fluid intake at this time will result in too much weight loss and a rise in serum sodium. Kidneys of very premature infants have a limited ability to compensate and will neither fully excrete a fluid overload nor be able to decrease obligate free water losses adequately if overly restricted. Thus, it is imperative to monitor weight and serum electrolytes closely over the first few days of life in premature infants and increase or decrease the intravenous fluid rate accordingly.

There are known predictable causes of increased fluid requirements for NICU patients. One is the marked increase in transepidermal water loss (TEWL) seen in ELGANs, generally those born at about 26 weeks gestation or earlier, with very immature skin. Usually, this can be recognized on physical exam because of the shiny red translucent appearance of the skin. These infants can have TEWL as much as 15 times that of term infants,[6,7] which if untreated can rapidly result in hypernatremic dehydration. Much higher intravenous rates are needed for these ELGANs, commonly 2–3 times as high or more, which places them at great risk for hyperglycemia or hyponatremia and requires great vigilance.

Attempts to limit the TEWL have focused on 2 different approaches. One is to use humidified incubators to decrease evaporative water losses. Acceptance of this approach has been hindered by the risk of bacterial or fungal contamination of the water supply, resulting in increased infections, and the lack of convincing evidence of improved long-term outcome.[8,9] However, newer technologies for incubator humidification may have eliminated the risk of waterborne infection and resulted in improved outcomes.[10,11] It appears that neonatology is arriving at a point at which knowledge and technology have advanced to allow us to know how to safely start and modulate humidification for ELGANs. Starting at a high relative humidity of about 85% and then weaning over the first few weeks of life allows for the advantages of decreased TEWL initially while avoiding the increased risk of infection seen with earlier technology and supporting appropriate epidermal maturation.[7]

The other approach to decreasing TEWL has been to use various skin coverings. Many barriers, including semipermeable membranes and ointments, have been tried. Although decreased TEWL has been reported with ointments,[12,13] concerns remain about possible increased skin infection.[14] Wraps have been shown to decrease TEWL.[15–17] They also decrease the incidence of hypothermia, but their impact on long-term outcome is unclear.[18]

Other causes of increased TEWL include phototherapy, which can increase TEWL by over 20%,[19,20] and for ELGAN infants, total intravenous fluid rates should be increased accordingly. TEWL may be increased in disorders of epithelial development, such as "collodion baby" ichthyosis, epidermolysis bullosa, harlequin ichthyosis, and more. Abdominal wall defects (gastroschisis, omphalocele) and spina bifida can also result in an increased insensible water loss that must be compensated.

After the diuresis of extracellular fluid during the first few days of life, fluid administration is advanced slowly to support adequate renal function and provide nutrition. How much to advance is critical given the concerns about fluid overload and the possible adverse consequences thereof.[4] Minimal maintenance fluids are in the 100- to 120-mL/kg daily range, and growth usually requires somewhat more intake. Intake in the 130- to 140-mL/kg daily range seems to allow ductal closure,[21,22] and higher intravenous rates in the range of 170 mL/kg daily are associated with an increased risk for prolonged patency.[3] It seems reasonable therefore to provide a fluid rate that allows for an adequate urine output and maintains normal serum sodium levels, provides adequate nutrition, and remains below 170 mL/kg daily until ductal patency is no longer an issue.

ELECTROLYTE REQUIREMENTS IN THE NEWBORN INFANT

Sodium

Except in extremely unusual situations, fetal serum electrolyte levels reflect maternal levels, and this certainly is true for sodium. Because the fetus and neonate have an increased extracellular fluid volume and normal serum sodium levels, by logical extension, they must also have increased total body sodium. Furthermore, because the newborn must diurese the increased extracellular fluid volume with its concomitant sodium load, there is no need to provide sodium initially. Indeed, providing sodium immediately after birth results in delayed natriuresis and fluid elimination, with resultant slower weight loss and prolonged oxygen requirement.[23] A recent report suggested that increased sodium intake in the first few days of life may increase the risk of intraventricular hemorrhage.[24] Therefore, for the first few days of life, both fluid and sodium restriction are the norm. During this period, a low serum sodium level usually is caused by inadequate free-water restriction rather than inadequate sodium intake. Unless associated with profound weight loss or severe renal dysfunction (eg, polyuric renal failure), further decreasing the intravenous rate is the appropriate treatment for this hyponatremia, rather than giving more sodium. It is also worth noting that there can be a significant inadvertent obligate sodium load provided by other medications.[25] Thus, no sodium should be added to the intravenous dextrose solution while restricting fluids for the first few days until appropriate weight loss (5%–10%) is seen.[23]

Once the initial diuresis has occurred, maintenance sodium needs to be provided. This is usually begun with about 2–3 mEq/kg sodium daily in more mature neonates. However, careful monitoring is necessary with ELGANs because determining the exact degree of fluid restriction can be tricky, and very immature kidneys have increased obligate sodium losses. This may be in the range 8–10 mEq/kg daily or more in the most immature infants.[26] Excessive weight loss in these babies needs replacement with both sodium and water to prevent marked swings in serum sodium levels. On occasion, measuring urine sodium levels can be useful to determine if there is ongoing high urinary sodium loss associated with hyponatremia.

Once feeding, sodium maintenance can continue to be a problem because human milk is a relatively low-sodium diet,[27] and premature kidneys have decreased sodium resorption. Thus, mild hyponatremia is seen fairly commonly in milk-fed premature infants. If mild and stable, this can be monitored, but if progressive or significant (serum sodium less than 130 mEq/L), oral sodium supplementation may be indicated (2–6 mEq/kg daily in divided aliquots) because more severe hyponatremia can have long-term sequelæ, and serum sodium levels less than 120 mEq/L are associated with increased mortality.[28] On the other hand, some women, commonly those with difficulty establishing good lactation, may have elevated concentrations of sodium in their milk. Although rare,[29] this might result in hypernatremia in infants fed their own mothers' milk.[30]

Potassium

Similar to the situation described for sodium, neonates generally are born with adequate potassium stores. In addition to the reasons indicated for withholding sodium initially, potassium is not added to intravenous fluids at first until there is clear demonstration of good urine output and adequate renal function to avoid any risk of iatrogenic hyperkalemia. With normal renal function, urinary potassium losses remain fairly low and stable for most neonates across broad gestational age ranges. Thus, the usual potassium requirement is about 2–5 mEq/kg daily. Again, given concerns about the risks of inadvertent hyperkalemia, it is recommended

to begin adding potassium to intravenous fluids at the lower range, 2–3 mEq/kg daily, and only after normal urine output and serum creatinine have been documented. Hypokalemia in this situation can first be dealt with by incremental increases in potassium administration, but if more than the amount described is needed, a determination of urinary potassium levels and evaluation of renal function would be indicated. On the other hand, hyperkalemia with such low-level potassium administration should be concerning and raises questions about possible tissue breakdown, severe hemolysis, large intraventricular hemorrhage, renal failure, adrenal dysfunction, and so on.

Nonoliguric hyperkalemia in ELGANs remains a major problem with an uncertain pathophysiology and controversy regarding the best treatment.[31] There are some data suggesting that increased amino acid intake with early hyperalimentation may decrease the incidence of nonoliguric hyperkalemia.[32] Given the risks associated with both hyperkalemia and the possible treatments for this, potassium administration should be minimal initially and advanced with caution.

Calcium

Calcium is the most common mineral in the body, with about 99% of it found in bone[33]; this is true of the newborn as well as older patients. During the third trimester, between 90 and 120 mg/kg of calcium are transported across the placenta into the fetus daily. About 80% of the calcium of the term fetus is amassed during the third trimester. This transfer of calcium across the placenta is minimally affected by parathyroid hormone (PTH) or vitamin D, if at all.[34] At birth, this large flux of calcium, about 150 mg/kg daily, stops abruptly. This acute drop in calcium flux results in falling serum calcium levels and an increase in PTH from the very low levels seen in the fetus. If inadequate calcium is provided, this results in hypocalcemia and mobilization of bone calcium stores. Thus, as soon as possible after birth, the goal is to provide up to 120 mg/kg of calcium daily. However, it is difficult to provide this amount of calcium safely and effectively given the limits of solubility of calcium salts in various intravenous solutions.[35] Because of the need to restrict total fluid intake initially, solutions with a high calcium concentration may be needed. Running high-calcium concentrations in intravenous solutions increases the risk of clotting and extravasations, which can result in serious chemical burns to soft tissues. Therefore, if high concentrations are needed, it is recommended to infuse them through central venous catheters. Of course, these lines have their own attendant risks that need to be considered. It is much better and safer to provide calcium orally, which is an added incentive to begin enteral nutrition sooner than later.

REFERENCES

1. Friis-Hanson B. Body water compartments in children: changes during growth and related changes in body composition. *Pediatrics.* 1961;28:169–181.
2. Wadhawan R, Oh W, Perritt R, et al. Association between early postnatal weight loss and death or BPD in small and appropriate for gestational age extremely low-birth-weight infants. *J Perinatol.* 2007;27:35–64.
3. Stephens BE, Gargus RA, Walden RV, et al. Fluid regimens in the first week of life may increase risk of patent ductus arteriosus in extremely low birth weight infants. *J Perinatol.* 2008;28:123–128.
4. Bell EF, Acarregui MJ. Restricted versus liberal water intake for preventing morbidity and mortality in preterm infants. *Cochrane Database Syst Rev.* 2008; 1:CD000503. doi:10.1002/14651858. CD000503.pub2.
5. Mitanchez D. Glucose regulation in preterm newborn infants. *Horm Res.* 2007;68:265–271.
6. Chiou YB, Blume-Peytavi U. Stratum corneum maturation. *Skin Pharmacol Physiol.* 2004;17:57–66.
7. Ågren J, Sjörs G, Sedin G. Ambient humidity influences the rate of skin barrier maturation in extremely preterm infants. *J Pediatr.* 2006;148:613–617.
8. Sinclair L, Crisp J, Sinn J. Variability in incubator humidity practices in the management of preterm infants. *J Pædiatr Child Health.* 2009;45:535–540.
9. Flenady V, Woodgate PG. Radiant warmers versus incubators for regulating body temperature in newborn infants. *Cochrane Database Syst Rev.* 2003;4:CD000435. doi:10.1002/14651858. CD000435.
10. Antonucci R, Porcella A, Fanos V. The infant incubator in the neonatal intensive care unit: unresolved issues and future developments. *J Perinat Med.* 2009;37:587–598.
11. Kim SM, Lee EY, Chen J, Ringer SA. Improved care and growth outcomes by using hybrid humidified incubators in very preterm infants. *Pediatrics.* 2010;125:137–145.
12. Nopper AJ, Horii KA, Sookdeo-Drost S, Wang TH, Mancini AJ, Lane AT. Topical ointment therapy benefits premature infants. *J Pediatr.* 1996;128:660–669.
13. Brandon DH, Coe K, Hudson-Barr D, Oliver T, Landerman LR. Effectiveness of No-Sting skin protectant and Aquaphor on water loss and skin integrity in premature infants. *J Perinatol.* 2010;30:414–419.
14. Conner JM, Soll RF, Edwards WH. Topical ointment for preventing infection in preterm infants. *Cochrane Database Syst Rev.* 2004;1:CD001150. doi:10.1002/14651858.CD001150.pub2.
15. Mancini AJ, Sookdeo-Drost S, Madison KC, Smoller BR, Lane AT. Semipermeable dressings improve epidermal barrier function in premature infants. *Pediatr Res.* 1994;36:306–314.
16. Bhandari V, Brodsky N, Porat R. Improved outcome of extremely low birth weight infants with Tegaderm® application to skin. *J Perinatol.* 2005;25:276–281.
17. Kaushal M, Agarwal R, Aggarwal R, et al. Cling wrap, an innovative intervention for temperature maintenance and reduction of insensible water loss in very low-birthweight babies nursed under radiant warmers: a randomized, controlled trial. *Ann Trop Pædiatr.* 2005;25:111–118.
18. McCall EM, Alderdice F, Halliday HL, Jenkins JG, Vohra S. Interventions to prevent hypothermia at birth in preterm and/or low birthweight infants. *Cochrane Database Syst Rev.* 2010;3:CD004210. doi:10.1002/14651858.CD004210.pub4.
19. Maayan-Metzger A, Yosipovitch G, Hadad E, Sirota L. Transepidermal water loss and skin hydration in preterm infants during phototherapy. *Am J Perinatol.* 2001;18:393–396.
20. Grünhagen DJ, De Boer MG, De Beaufort AJ, Walther FJ. Transepidermal water loss during halogen spotlight phototherapy in preterm infants. *Pediatr Res.* 2002;51:402–405.
21. Vanhaesebrouck S, Zonnenberg I, Vandervoort P, Bruneel E, Van Hoestenberghe MR, Theyskens C. Conservative treatment for patent ductus arteriosus in the preterm. *Arch Dis Child Fetal Neonatal Ed.* 2007;92:F244–F247.
22. Kaempf JW, Wu YX, Kaempf AJ, Kaempf AM, Wang L, Grunkemeier G. What happens when the patent ductus arteriosus is treated less aggressively in very low birth weight infants? *J Perinatol.* 2011 Aug 4. doi:10.1038/jp.2011.102.
23. Hartnoll G, Bétrémieux P, Modi N. Randomised controlled trial of postnatal sodium supplementation on oxygen dependency and body weight in 25–30 week gestational age infants. *Arch Dis Child Fetal Neonatal Ed.* 2000;82:F19–F23.
24. Barnette AR, Myers BJ, Berg CS, Inder TE. Sodium intake and intraventricular hemorrhage in the preterm infant. *Ann Neurol.* 2010;67:817–823.
25. Bhatia J. Fluid and electrolyte management in the very low birth weight neonate. *J Perinatol.* 2006;26:S19–S21.
26. Delgado MM, Rohatgi R, Khan S, Holzman IR, Satlin LM. Sodium and potassium clearances by the maturing kidney: clinical-molecular correlates. *Pediatr Nephrol.* 2003;18:759–767. Epub 2003 Jun 17.
27. Manganaro R, Marseglia L, Mami C, et al. Breast milk sodium concentration, sodium intake and weight loss in breast-feeding newborn infants. *Br J Nutr.* 2007;97:344–348.
28. Guarner J, Hochman J, Kurbatova J, Mullins R. Study of outcomes associated with hyponatremia and hypernatremia in children. *Pediatr Dev Pathol.* 2011;14(2):117–123. Epub 2010 Oct 6.
29. Laing IA, Wong CM. Hypernatraemia in the first few days: is the incidence rising? *Arch Dis Child Fetal Neonatal Ed.* 2002;87:F158–F162.
30. Morton JA. The clinical usefulness of breast milk sodium in the assessment of lactogenesis. *Pediatrics.* 1994;93:802–806.
31. Vemgal P, Ohlsson A. Interventions for non-oliguric hyperkalaemia in preterm neonates. *Cochrane Database Syst Rev.* 2007;1:CD005257. doi:10.1002/14651858.CD005257.pub2.
32. Iacobelli S, Bonsante F, Vintéjoux A, Gouyon J. Standardized parenteral nutrition in preterm infants: early impact on fluid and electrolyte balance. *Neonatology.* 2010;98:84–90.
33. Demarini S. Calcium and phosphorus nutrition in preterm infants. *Acta Pædiatr.* 2005;94(Suppl 449):87–92.
34. Mitchell DM, Jüppner H. Regulation of calcium homeostasis and bone metabolism in the fetus and neonate. *Curr Opin Endocrinol Diabetes Obes.* 2010;17:25–30.
35. Pereira-Da-Silva L, Costa AB, Pereira L, et al. Early high calcium and phosphorus intake by parenteral nutrition prevents short-term bone strength decline in preterm infants. *J Pediatr Gastroenterol Nutr.* 2011;52:203–209.

10 Parenteral Nutrition

David H. Adamkin

TOTAL PARENTERAL NUTRITION

Total parenteral nutrition (TPN) as used today in the neonatal intensive care unit (NICU) became a part of modern medicine in the late 1960s. Dudrick et al, in groundbreaking work, first demonstrated in beagle puppies the technique for parenterally administering nutrients.[1] Shortly thereafter, Wilmore and Dudrick[2] reported the use of this technique in an infant who had virtually no remaining small intestine and was totally dependent on these parenterally delivered nutrients of glucose, fibrin hydrolysate, minerals, and vitamins. There were no intravenous fat emulsions available, so plasma was given in small aliquots to provide some essential fatty acids (EFAs) and trace elements.[2] Although this historic patient did not survive, normal growth and development was maintained for several months solely on this primitive solution. By the early 1970s, the technique was being used extensively in infants and children with congenital or acquired surgically correctable lesions of the gastrointestinal tract[3,4] and in infants with intractable diarrhea.[4,5] Use in the low birth weight infant soon followed.[4,6,7]

Today, TPN is a firmly established strategy in modern neonatal intensive care. The extremely low birth weight (ELBW) infant (<1000 g birth weight) with limited endogenous stores of nutrients and an increased rate of resting energy expenditure is at risk for rapid development of malnutrition or even actual starvation.[8] The pioneering work of Dudrick and Wilmore has led to the current practice of early amino acids as the first infusate within hours of life in a 500-g infant. This chapter focuses on the use of TPN in very low birth weight (VLBW) infants (<1500 g birth weight).

The ELBW infants have unique nutritional requirements characterized by high metabolic rate, high protein turnover, and high glucose utilization. The ELBW infant has endogenous energy reserves of about 200 kcal, only enough energy to last days without exogenous sources. The 23-week infant has reserves that will be exhausted within hours. These infants are extremely vulnerable to inadequate nutrition.

Nutrient intakes provided to ELBW infants parenterally are much lower than what the fetus receives in utero. This intake deficit may persist throughout the infants' stay in the NICU and even after discharge.[9] These suboptimal nutrient intakes are critical in explaining the poor growth these infants often experience. The early growth deficit has long-lasting effects, including short stature and poor neurodevelopmental outcomes.[10,11] Therefore, the observation of postnatal growth failure is a "surrogate" for inadequate nutrition and the likelihood of adverse neurodevelopmental outcome. Early aggressive TPN theoretically allows the transition from fetal to extrauterine life to occur with minimal interruption of growth and development and has been a successful strategy to improve growth and prevent inadequate nutrition.[12,13]

EARLY AGGRESSIVE AMINO ACID ADMINISTRATION

Immaturity of the gastrointestinal tract and critical illness in ELBW infants precludes substantive nutritional support from enteral nutrition the first days or even weeks of life; thus, nearly all of these infants are supported parenterally. Large amounts of amino acids are available to the fetus in utero, which are utilized not only for protein synthesis but also as a fuel source. It seems logical to supply a neonate with adequate amounts of amino acids for energy, as well as a growth substrate, to promote protein accretion for ongoing development.

Understanding fetal nutrition has been helpful in designing postnatal strategies for ELBW infants. At 70% of gestation, there is little fat uptake. Fetal energy metabolism is not dependent on fat until early in the third trimester, and then it increases only gradually toward term. Glucose is delivered to the fetus from the mother at low fetal insulin concentrations, generally at a rate that matches fetal energy expenditure. The human placenta actively transports amino acids into the fetus, and animal studies indicate that fetal amino acid uptake greatly exceeds protein accretion requirements. Approximately 50% of the amino acids taken up by the fetus are oxidized and serve as a significant energy source. Urea production is a by-product of amino acid oxidation. Relatively high rates of fetal urea production are seen in human and animal fetuses compared with the term neonate and adult, suggesting high protein turnover and oxidation rates in the fetus. Therefore, a rise in BUN (serum urea nitrogen), which is often observed after the start of TPN, is not in and of itself an adverse effect or sign of toxicity. Rather, an increase in urea nitrogen is a normal accompaniment of metabolizing amino acids.

Providing early parenteral amino acids prevents metabolic shock. Concentrations of key amino acids begin to decline in the VLBW infant at the time the cord is cut. This metabolic shock may trigger the starvation response, of which endogenous glucose production is a prominent feature. Irrepressible, glucose production may be a cause of so-called glucose intolerance that often limits the amount of energy that can be administered to the ELBW infant. It makes sense to ease the metabolic transition from fetal to extrauterine life. Withholding TPN for days, or even hours, sends the infant unnecessarily into a metabolic emergency. Thus, the need for TPN may never be more acute than right after birth.

It is noteworthy that 3 separate studies measuring glucose tolerance, including one that measured insulin activity, confirmed that glucose tolerance was improved in the infants receiving early, higher-dose amino acids.[13-15] Therefore, early amino acids may stimulate insulin secretion. This is consistent with the notion that forestalling the starvation response improves glucose tolerance. Clinically, this improved glucose tolerance safely allows the provision of more nonprotein energy while avoiding hyperglycemia.

This relationship between early amino acids and insulin secretion is shown on Figure 10.1. This metabolic benefit prevents 2 morbidities—hyperglycemia and nonoliguric hyperkalemia—that make the provision of nutrition difficult. The mechanism may be that, without initiation of early parenteral amino acids, plasma concentrations of certain amino acids (eg, arginine and leucine) decrease. Secretion of insulin depends on the plasma concentrations of these amino acids as well as that of glucose. A shortage of amino acids limits the secretion and activity of insulin. Finally, glucose transport and energy metabolism are adversely affected by a reduction in insulin and insulin-like growth factors. This scenario leads to a downregulation

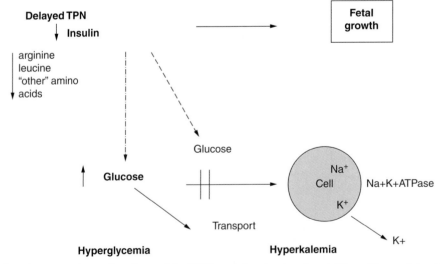

FIGURE 10-1 Early administration of amino acids. TPN, total parenteral nutrition. (From Adamkin DH. *Nutritional Strategies for the Very Low Birth Weight Infant*. Cambridge, UK: Cambridge University Press; 2009.)

of glucose transporters at the cellular level, resulting in intracellular energy failure via a decrease in Na^+, K^+-ATPase (sodium-potassium adenosine triphosphatase) activity. This directly contributes to leakage of intracellular potassium and is associated with nonoliguric hyperkalemia. Early TPN with amino acids minimizes the abrupt postnatal deprivation of amino acid supply and provides the following benefits:

- Prevention of protein catabolism
- Maintenance of growth-regulating factors such as insulin
- Prevention of hyperglycemia and nonoliguric hyperkalemia

Figure 10.2 shows protein loss that occurs in infants that are mechanically ventilated at 26 week of gestation and approximately 900 g birth weight at 2 days of age who were receiving glucose alone.[16] Also shown are clinically stable 32-week gestation premature infants and normal term infants for comparison. It is clear that there is a significant effect of gestation on protein metabolism as the rate of protein loss in ELBW infants is 2-fold higher than in normal term infants.[16]

The impact of this rate of protein loss is shown in Figure 10.3. At 26 weeks of gestation, a 1000-g birth weight infant begins with body stores of approximately 88 g. Without exogenous provision, the infant loses over 1.5% of body protein per day.[16] Contrast this with the normal fetus, who would be accumulating body protein at over 2% per day. Obviously, significant body protein deficits can accumulate rapidly in ELBW infants not receiving early amino acid administration.

The first studies of early TPN used doses between 1.0 and 1.5 g/kg/d, an amount that will replace

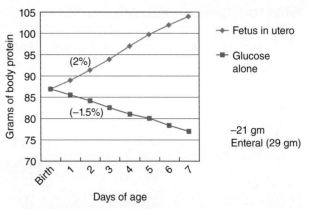

FIGURE 10-3 **Change in body protein stores in a theoretical 26-weeks gestation, 1000-g premature infant receiving glucose alone as compared with a fetus in utero.** (From Denne SC. Protein and energy requirements in preterm infants. *Semin Neonatol.* 2001;6(5):377–382.)

ongoing losses. More recent studies support dosages of 3.0 g/kg/d initiated within hours of birth. Ultimately, amino acid intake should be 3.0 g/kg/d; however, one can consider intakes of 3.5 to 4.0 g/kg/d for infants weighing less 1200 g if enteral feeds are withheld for prolonged periods. Growth benefits associated with parenteral amino acid infusions should be associated with less-extreme postnatal weight loss and an earlier return to birth weight. An earlier return to birth weight means the VLBW infant will be less likely to develop extrauterine growth restriction.

We recently published an 8-year experience developing an early amino acid strategy paying particular attention to clinical and metabolic responses.[13] Table 10.1 shows the benefits of early amino acids, which include a decrease in postnatal weight loss and age at return to birth weight, especially with earlier initiation of amino acids within hours of birth and amino acid dosage over the first 5 days of life at 3.0 g/kg/d.[13] Prevention of extrauterine growth retardation (EUGR) by weight was seen with higher dose and earlier initiation.[13] We also confirmed that there is no demonstrable relationship between the preceding day's amino acid intake and BUN.[13] This is because BUN is related not only to amino acid intake but also renal function, hydration, acuity of illness, as well as degree of prematurity.[13] Therefore, in most situations a modest rise in BUN (a major earlier concern) is consistent with the utilization of amino acids as a source of energy.[17]

Another nutritional benefit in our study showed early intravenous amino acids not only improved energy intakes but also at the same time allowed for more conservative fluid management, which may benefit ELBW infants in prevention of chronic lung disease.[13]

In assessing potential toxicity with amino acid intakes of 3.0–4.0 g/kg/d shortly after birth, a study

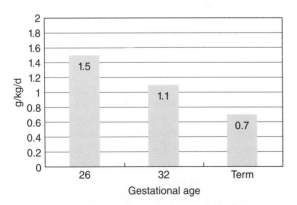

FIGURE 10-2 **Protein losses measured in three groups of infants receiving glucose alone at 2–3 days of age. Protein losses are calculated from measured rates of phenylalanine catabolism.** (From Denne SC. Protein and energy requirements in preterm infants. *Semin Neonatol.* 2001;6(5):377–382.)

Table 10-1 Outcome data (mean ± SD)

	Epoch1 2000–2001	Epoch2 2002–2004	Epoch3 2006–2007	P
Age at TPNi	22.4±22.3	9.5±12.2	4.6±6.3	<0.001(a)
Days of TPN	25.8±12.4	31.5±26.9	25.2±21.3	NS
Age at weight nadir	4.9±3.4	4.4±6.2	2.9±3.2	0.044 (b)
Return to BW	13.9±6.3	10.7±5.7	8.3±5.0	≤0.001 (bc)
Survival (%)	90%	90%	95%	NS
LOS	83.3±24.9	105.2±55.5	83.4±28.8	0.003 (c)
GA at d/c	38.3±2.7	40.9±7.4	38.1±3.4	0.008 (c)
Weight at d/c	2168±436	2799±966	2541±573	<0.001(c)
HC at d/c	32.4±2.2	33.9±2.9	32.1±3.5	<0.015 (cd)
EUGRw at d/c (e)	57.1%	34.7%	25.0%	0.005 (c)
EUGRhc at d/c (e)	10.0%	6.1%	10.0%	NS

Abbreviations: BW, birth weight; dBR, direct bilirubin; d/c, discharge; EUGR, extrauterine growth restriction (<35 percentile for GA); EUGRhc, HC <35 percentile for GA; EUGRw, weight <35 percentile for GA; GA, gestational age; LOS, length of stay; Max, maximum; NS, not significant; TPN, total parental nutrition; TPNi, TPN initiation.
(a)=All epochs, (b)=Epoch 1 vs 3, (c)=Epoch 1 vs 2, (d)=Epoch 2 vs 3, (e)=EUGR: weight for HC, < 35 percentile for GA.
[a]Adapted from Radmacher, Lewis, and Adamkin.[13]

comparing 1 g/kg/d vs 4 g/kg/d showed no significant differences between groups in the amount of sodium bicarbonate administered, the degree of metabolic acidosis, or the BUN concentration.[15] When compared with plasma amino acid concentrations of normally growing second- and third-trimester human fetuses (sampled by cordocentesis), fetal amino acid concentrations for both essential and nonessential amino acids matched well to those in the group receiving 3.0 g/kg/d (except for threonine and lysine, which were significantly lower than seen in fetuses). Concentrations in the group at 1 g/kg/d were about 50% lower compared to fetal levels. Efficacy was significantly lower in the 1-g/kg/d group by nitrogen balance determined using leucine stable isotope methods.[15]

Whether plasma concentrations of amino acids of the fetus should be duplicated in the VLBW infants is unknown. Crystalline amino acid solutions designed for infants promote nitrogen balance and yield "safer" aminograms than the adult mixtures used before the pediatric solutions became available.[18] However, these solutions do not provide sufficient threonine and lysine, both essential amino acids that may at least theoretically increase nitrogen and protein balance.[19] Also, cysteine and tyrosine, considered indispensable amino acids for the infant, are not included in the mixtures[20] because both are insoluble. VLBW infants have been known to have lower plasma concentrations of cysteine and tyrosine. Greater intakes of the precursors of those 2 amino acids, methionine and phenylalanine, respectively, do not necessarily result in greater plasma levels of the desired amino acids, although plasma levels of the 2 precursors do increase.[21] Cysteine hydrochloride can be provided as a supplement to TPN; however,

trials of cysteine addition have not shown consistent clinical benefits.[22] Pediatric amino acid solutions may contain soluble N-acetyl-L-tyrosine, but its efficacy for enhancing tyrosine metabolism is questionable as much of the dipeptide appears to be excreted into the urine.[20] Therefore, both tyrosine and cysteine remain problematic.

Like tyrosine, taurine, and cysteine, glutamine may also be a conditionally essential amino acid in preterm infants.[23] Glutamine is unstable in aqueous solution and therefore is not in any TPN mixture. A review of studies in VLBW infants looking at glutamine supplementation to attenuate gut atrophy, prevent infection, or decrease mortality showed no significant effect on sepsis, necrotizing enterocolitis (NEC), mortality, or long-term development.[24] Although the pediatric amino acid solutions have added safety and efficacy to TPN in VLBW infants, there may be opportunities for "designer" dipeptides or formulation changes to improve outcomes.

INTRAVENOUS CARBOHYDRATES

Intravenous glucose administration is often limited by intolerance in the first days in ELBW infants who are not receiving early amino acids. Hyperglycemia has been reported in 20%–85% of such infants.[25]

The glucose infusion rate (GIR) should be adjusted to maintain euglycemia. Glucose intolerance is defined as inability to maintain euglycemia at glucose administration rates less than 6 mg/kg/min. The plasma glucose concentration should be kept below 130 mg/dL. Hyperglycemia in ELBW infants may occur in combination with nonoliguric hyperkalemia. As discussed, these comorbidities may be prevented with early use of TPN.

Endogenous glucose production is elevated in VLBW infants compared with term infants and adults. High glucose production rates are found in VLBW infants who received only glucose compared to those receiving glucose plus amino acids or lipids. Clinical experience with hyperglycemia suggests that administration of glucose alone does not always suppress glucose production in VLBW infants. It appears that persistent glucose overproduction is the main cause of hyperglycemia and is fueled by ongoing proteolysis that is not suppressed by physiologic concentrations of insulin. Abnormally low peripheral glucose utilization may also contribute to hyperglycemia. Therefore, a 5% glucose concentration instead of the standard 10% concentration of glucose may have to be used in more immature ELBW infants (<750 g). However, this severely limits the provision of energy.

Glucose intolerance can limit delivery of energy to the infant to a fraction of the resting energy expenditure, resulting in negative energy balance. Several strategies can be used to manage this early hyperglycemia in ELBW infants as well as to increase energy intake:

1. Decreasing glucose administration until hyperglycemia resolves (unless the hyperglycemia is so severe that this strategy would require infusion of a hypotonic solution)

2. Administering intravenous amino acids, which decrease serum glucose concentrations in ELBW infants, presumably by enhancing endogenous insulin secretion

3. Initiation of exogenous insulin therapy at rates to control hyperglycemia (plasma glucose > 130 mg/dL at GIR < 6 mg/kg/min)

4. Using exogenous insulin to increase energy intake

The first and third strategies do not promote nutritional intake, and the safety of the last has been questioned in this population because of the possible development of lactic acidemia. Another concern with hyperglycemia is related to studies involving adults and children being treated in intensive care units that indicate glucose control may influence survival.[26–28]

Stress-induced hyperglycemia is associated with increased mortality and morbidity in critically ill adults,[26] children,[27] and preterm infants.[28] Tight blood glucose control with the use of intensive insulin therapy has been reported to reduce mortality and morbidity in patients admitted to adult surgical and medical intensive care units.[28,29,30] The Neonatal Insulin Replacement Therapy in Europe (NIRTURE)[31] trial investigated the effects of a fixed-dose insulin (0.05 U/kg/h and glucose [20% dextrose]) infusion as compared to usual care in VLBW infants. It reduced hyperglycemia but increased hypoglycemia. The study was discontinued by the data and safety monitoring board before complete enrollment because of safety concerns (eg, an excess of dilation of the cerebral ventricles and parenchymal lesions seen on cranial ultrasound images and a trend toward more deaths in the early insulin group).

In the NIRTURE trial, the median values of the mean daily protein intakes at 1 week (1.12 g/kg in the early insulin group and 1.24 g/kg in the control group) are modest vs most NICUs in the United States, where recommended targets for TPN protein are reached in a few hours or days. As discussed previously, insulin activity is influenced by earlier initiation and higher doses of amino acids. Dosage of TPN amino acids is critical in any discussion of hyperglycemia in VLBW infants.[13–15]

The nutritional dilemma for the glucose-intolerant ELBW infant is energy inadequacy. Three studies demonstrated a linkage between energy in the first weeks of life and head circumference, somatic growth, and neurodevelopmental outcome at 18 months.[32–34] Therefore, early nutrition has an impact on outcome. For example, an ELBW infant receiving D10W (10% dextrose by volume in water) at 80–100 mL/k/d has a GIR of 6 to 8 mg/kg/min and receives 27–34 cal/kg of glucose energy. If switched to D5W (5% dextrose by volume in water) because of glucose intolerance, the GIR becomes 2.8 to 3.5 mg/kg/min and energy received of 13 to 17 kcal/kg; therefore, improving energy intakes while allowing for more conservative fluid management is an important benefit with early amino acids.

INTRAVENOUS LIPIDS

Lipids are essential components of parenteral nutrition for preterm infants to provide EFAs and to meet high-energy needs. Parenteral lipids are an attractive source of nutrition in the first postnatal days because of their high energy density, energy efficiency, isotonicity with plasma, and suitability for administration through a peripheral vein. Parenteral lipid emulsions enable the delivery of fat-soluble vitamins.

Parenteral lipid emulsions containing either soybean oil or a mixture of safflower and soybean oils have been used in the United States (Table 10.2). The VLBW neonate is especially susceptible to the development of EFA deficiency because tissue stores of linoleic acid are small and requirements for EFAs are large as a result of rapid growth. The human fetus depends entirely on placental transfer of EFAs. A VLBW infant with limited nonprotein caloric reserve must mobilize fatty acids for energy when receiving intravenous nutrition devoid of lipid. Studies in these infants showed essential fatty acid deficiency (EFAD)

Table 10-2 Composition of Intravenous Lipid Emulsions

Product	Oil Base	Linoleic Acid (%)	Linolenic Acid (%)	Glycerin (%)	Osmolarity (mOsm/L)
Intralipid[a]	100% soybean	50	9	2.25	260
Nutralipid[b]	100% soybean	49–60	6–9	2.21	315
Soyacal[c]	100% soybean	49–60	6–9	2.21	315
Liposyn III[d]	100% soybean	54.5	8.3	2.5	292

[a]KabiVitrum, Almeda, CA.
[b]McGaw, Inc., Irvine, CA.
[c]Alpha Therapeutic, Los Angeles, CA.
[d]Abbott Laboratories, Abbott Park, IL.

can develop in the VLBW infant during the first week of life on lipid-free regimens.[35,36]

The importance of long-chain polyunsaturated fatty acids (LC-PUFAs) for the development of the brain and the retina has been recognized.[37,38] Infants are not capable of forming sufficient quantities of LC-PUFAs from the respective precursor fatty acids (linoleic and α-linolenic acids) and thus need an exogenous source of LC-PUFAs. Intravenous lipid emulsions contain small amounts of these fatty acids as part of the egg phospholipid used as a stabilizer.

Intravenous lipid intakes should be targeted to prevent EFAD (ie, deficiency of linoleic and linolenic acids and their by-products), which can be done with as little as 0.5 g/kg/d of lipid. Because most intravenous lipid emulsions are richer in Ω-6 rather than Ω-3 EFAs, there is the potential for higher doses of intravenous lipid infusion to lead to greater amounts of vasoactive, prostaglandin-derived products from Ω-6 homologues and lesser amounts of critical central nervous system membrane products derived from Ω-3 fatty acids.[39] This issue needs further study and is also discussed further here with regard to intravenous lipids and pulmonary complications.

Clinically, it should be noted that infusion of 20% rather than 10% lipid emulsion results in a lower plasma concentration of phospholipid, cholesterol, and triglycerides.[40] The 20% solutions contain a lower phospholipid emulsifier/triglyceride ratio than the standard 10% lipid emulsions. The excess phospholipids are converted into liposomes, which accumulate cholesterol and phospholipid. These phospholipids may also inhibit lipoprotein, which is responsible for hydrolysis of the lipid solution[41] (Figure 10.4).

Clearance of lipid emulsions from the blood depends on the activity of lipoprotein lipase. Postheparin lipoprotein lipase activity[35] can be increased by relatively high doses of heparin; heparin does not improve utilization of intravenous lipids. Therefore, the increase in lipase activity by heparin leads to an increase in fatty acids, which may exceed the infant's ability to clear the products of lipolysis. The premature infant can clear 0.15 to 0.2 g/kg/h of lipids. However, infants who are small for gestational age and infants with sepsis may

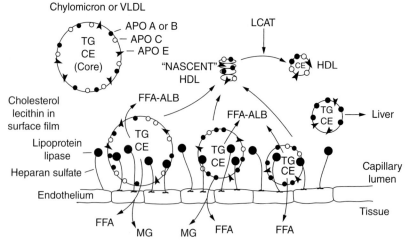

FIGURE 10-4 Hydrolysis of intravenous lipids. APO A, approtein A; APO B, approtein B; APO C, approtein C; CE, cholesterol ester; FFA-ALB, free fatty acid-albumin; HDL, high-density lipoprotein; LCAT, lecichin-cholesterol-acyl-transferase; MG, mono glycerol; TG, triglyceride; VLDL, very low density lipoprotein. (Reproduced with permission from Hamosh M, Hamosh P. Lipoprotein lipase: its physiological and clinical significance. *Mol Aspects Med.* 1983;6(3):199–289.)

not be able to clear standard doses of intravenous lipids and demonstrate hypertriglyceridemia.[42]

Intravenous lipid dosage above that to prevent EFAD is controversial and has resulted in different lipid administration strategies among NICUs. Early initiation or rapid advancement of lipid emulsions has been taken cautiously by clinicians because of several possible complications. Hazards most pertinent to the ventilated VLBW infant include adverse effects on gas exchange and displacement of bilirubin from albumin. Both Brans et al[43] and Adamkin and coworkers[44] found no difference in oxygenation between infants randomly assigned to various lipid doses (including controls without lipids) when using lower rates and longer infusion times of intravenous lipids. The displacement of bilirubin from binding sites on serum albumin may occur even with adequate metabolism of infused lipid. In vitro, displacement of albumin-bound bilirubin by free fatty acids (FFAs) depends on the relative concentrations of all 3 compounds. If the molar FFA/albumin ratio is less than 6, an in vivo study has shown that no free bilirubin is generated.[45] Data with lipid initiation at 0.5 g/kg/d of lipid in VLBW infants on assisted ventilation with respiratory distress syndrome showed a mean FFA/albumin ratio of less than 1; no individual patient value exceeded a ratio of 3 when daily doses were increased to 2.5 g/kg/d (in increments of 0.5 g/kg/d) over an 18-hour infusion time.[46] Other investigators found no adverse effect on bilirubin binding when lipid emulsion was infused at a dose of 2 g/kg/d over either 15 or 24 hours.[45] Proper use includes slow infusion rates (≤0.15 g/kg/h), slow increases in dosage, and avoidance of unduly high doses (eg, > 3.0 g/k/d).

Concerns have been raised regarding the possible adverse effects of intravenous lipids on pulmonary function and pulmonary outcomes. Use of early (<5 days) vs "late" (>5 days of age) initiation of intravenous lipid included 5 studies with 397 neonates and demonstrated no significant statistical differences between groups in the primary outcomes of growth rates, death, and chronic lung disease or the secondary outcomes, which included several pulmonary disorders.[47]

A randomized trial including 110 appropriate-for-gestational-age (AGA) infants demonstrated that a higher dose of intravenous lipid (2.0 g/kg/d) vs controls (0.5 g/kg/d) initiated on the first day of TPN and advanced in both groups to 3.0 g/kg/d in increments of 0.5 g/kg/d was tolerated during the first week of life without significant adverse events.[48] The infants receiving larger amounts of intravenous fat during the 4 weeks had improved energy intake and lower rates of NEC and retinopathy of prematurity and more often maintained their AGA status at discharge.[48] There was no difference in chronic lung disease.[48] These observations suggest 2.0 g/kg/d may be safely administered beginning on the first day of life but must be confirmed in a larger multicenter trial. Modest infusion rates of 0.5 to 1.0 g/kg/d that are commonly initiated today are well tolerated.[19]

For the late preterm infant with increased pulmonary vascular resistance (PVR) and respiratory disease, it appears a more prudent approach with intravenous lipids should be taken. Significant concerns have been raised because of the high PUFA content of lipid emulsions, as excessive omega-6 (linoleic acid, 18:2Ω6) acids are required substrates for arachidonic acid pathways, which lead to synthesizing prostaglandins and leukotrienes (Figure 10.5).[49] It is speculated the intravenous lipid emulsion may enhance thromboxane synthesis activity, which increases thromboxane production.[50] The prostaglandins may cause changes in vasomotor tone with resultant hypoxia.[51] In addition, the production of hydroperoxides in the lipid emulsion might contribute to untoward effects by increasing prostaglandin levels.[51-53]

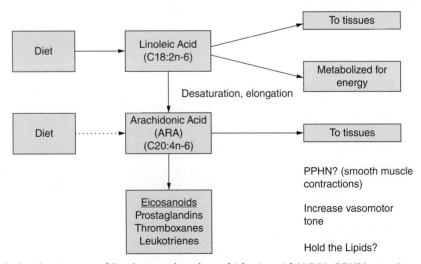

FIGURE 10-5 Metabolic derivatives of linoleic acid and arachidonic acid (ARA). PPHN, persistent pulmonary hypertension. (From Adamkin DH. Feeding problems in the late preterm infant. *Clin Perinatol.* 2006;33(4):831–837.)

Although there is no firm evidence of adverse effects of lipid emulsions in infants with severe acute respiratory failure with or without pulmonary hypertension, it appears prudent to avoid high doses in these patients. For infants with respiratory diseases without increased PVR, one can provide intravenous lipids at a dosage to prevent EFA deficiency. For those with elements of persistent pulmonary hypertension (PPHN), avoidance of lipids during the greatest labile and critical stages of their illness should be considered. Once patient is more stable, intravenous lipids at a modest dosage can be initiated.

Carnitine is an essential cofactor required for transport of long-chain fatty acids (LCFAs) across the mitochondrial membrane for β-oxidation. Because the preterm infant is born with limited carnitine reserves and low plasma carnitine levels develop when parenteral nutrition is not supplemented with carnitine, several investigators have suggested adding carnitine to parenteral nutrition with lipids for preterm infants.[54,55] Addition of supplemental carnitine does increase oxidation of fat and circulating ketone body levels and results in increased tolerance to intravenous lipids. However, data on increase in weight gain and nitrogen retention are not as convincing.[56] Therefore, carnitine is recommended only for ELBW infants who require prolonged (over 2 to 3 weeks) parenteral nutrition. Intravenous carnitine dosage has been used at 8–10 mg/kg without any observable side effects.[57]

REFERENCES

1. Oudrick SJ, Wilmore DW, Vars HM, Rhoads JE. Long term parenteral nutrition with growth, development, and positive nitrogen balance. *Surgery.* 1968;64:134–142.
2. Wilmore DM, Dudrick SJ. Growth and development of an infant receiving all nutrients by vein. *JAMA.* 1968;203:860–864.
3. Filler RM, Eraklis AJ, Rubin VG, Das JB. Long-term parenteral nutrition in infants. *N Engl J Med.* 1969;281:589–594.
4. Heird WC, Winters RW. Total parenteral nutrition: the state of the art. *J Pediatr.* 1975;86:2–16.
5. Keating JP, Ternberg JL. Amino acid-hypertonic glucose treatment for intractable diarrhea in infants. *Am J Dis Child.* 1971;122:226–228.
6. Driscoll JM, Heird WC, Schullinger JN, Gongaware RD, Winters RW. Total intravenous alimentations in low birth weight infants: a preliminary report. *J Pediatr.* 1972;81:145–153.
7. Peden VH, Karpel JT. Total parenteral nutrition in premature infants. *J Pediatr.* 1972;81:137–144.
8. Heird WC. Nutritional support of the pediatric patient. In: Winters RW, Greene HL, eds. *Nutritional Support of the Seriously Ill Patient.* New York, NY: Academic Press; 1983:157–179.
9. Carver JD, Wu PYK, Hall RT, et al. Growth of preterm infants fed nutrient-enriched or term formula after hospital discharge. *Pediatrics.* 2001;107(4):683–689.
10. Lucas A, Morley R, Cole TJ, et al. Early diet in preterm babies and developmental status at 18 months. *Lancet.* 1990;335(8704):1477–1481.
11. Lucas A, Morley R, Cole TJ, et al. Early diet in preterm babies and developmental status in infancy. *Arch Dis Child.* 1989;64(11):1570–1578.
12. Dinerstein A, Neito RM, Solana CL, et al. Early and aggressive nutritional strategy parenteral and enteral decreases postnatal growth failure in VLBW infants. *J Perinatol.* 2000;26:436–442.
13. Radmacher PG, Lewis SL, Adamkin DH. Early amino acids and the metabolic response of ELBW infants (<1000 g) in three time periods. *J Perinatol.* 2009;29:433–437.
14. Rivera A Jr, Bell EF, Bier DM. Effect of intravenous amino acids on protein metabolism of preterm infants during the first three days of life. *Pediatr Res.* 1993;33:106–111.
15. Thureen PJ, Melara D, Fennessey PV, Hay WWJ. Effects of low versus high intravenous amino acid intake on VLBW infants in the early neonatal period. *Pediatr Res.* 2003;53:24–32.
16. Denne SC, Karn CA, Ahlrichs JA, et al. Proteolysis and phenylalanine hydroxylation in response to parenteral nutrition in extremely premature and normal newborns. *J Clin Invest.* 1996;97:746.
17. Neu J, ed. Is it time to stop starving premature infants? *J Perinatol.* 2009;29:399–400.
18. Heird WC, Hay WW Jr, Helms RA, et al. Pediatric parenteral amino acid mixture in low birth weight infants. *Pediatrics.* 1988;81:41–50.
19. Thureen PJ, Hay WW. *Neonatal Nutrition and Metabolism.* New York, NY: Cambridge University Press; 2006.
20. Roberts SA, Ball RO, Filler RM, Moore AM, Pencharz PB. Phenylalanine and tyrosine metabolism in neonates receiving parenteral nutrition differing in pattern of amino acids. *Pediatr Res.* 1998;44:907–914.
21. Wykes KJ, House JD, Ball RO, Pencharz PB. Aromatic amino acid metabolism of neonatal piglets receiving TPN: effect of tyrosine precursors. *Am J Physiol.* 1994; 267:E672–E679.
22. Zlotkin SH, Bryan MK, Anderson GH. Cysteine supplementation to cysteine-free intravenous feeding regimens in newborn infants. *Am J Clin Nutr.* 1981;34:914–923.
23. Parimi PS, Kalhan SC. Glutamine supplementation in the newborn infant. *Semin Fetal Neonatal Med.* 2007;12:19–25.
24. Tubman TRJ, Thompson SW, McGuire W. Glutamine supplementation to prevent morbidity and mortality in preterm infants. *Cochran Database Syst Rev.* 2005;(1):CD001457.
25. Cowett RM, Farrag HM. Selected principles of perinatal-neonatal glucose metabolism. *Semin Neonatol.* 2004;9:37–47.
26. Krinsley JS. Association between hyperglycemia and increased hospital mortality in a heterogeneous population of critically ill patients. *Mayo Clin Proc.* 2003;78:1471–1478.
27. Srinivasan V, Spinella PC, Drott HR, Roth CL, Helfaer MA, Nadkarni V. Association of timing, duration, and intensity of hyperglycemia with intensive care unit mortality in critically ill children. *Pediatr Crit Care Med.* 2004;5:329–336.
28. Hays SP, Smith EO, Sunehag AL. Hyperglycemia is a risk factor for early death and morbidity in extremely low birthweight infants. *Pediatrics.* 2006;118:1811–1818.
29. van den Berghe G, Wouters P, Weekers F, et al. Intensive insulin therapy in critically ill patients. *N Engl J Med.* 2001;345:1359–1367.
30. van den Berghe G, Wilmer A, Hermans G, et al. Intensive insulin therapy in the medical ICU. *N Engl J Med.* 2006;354:449–461.
31. Beardsall K, Vanhaesebrouck S, Ogilvy-Stuart AL, et al. Early insulin therapy in very-low-birth-weight infants. *N Engl J Med.* 2008;359:1873–1884.
32. Poindexter BB, Langer JC, Dusick AM, Ehrenkranz RA. Early provision of parenteral amino acids in extremely low birth weight infants: relation to growth and neurodevelopmental outcome. *J Pediatr.* 2006;148(3):300–305.

33. Stephens BE, Walden RV, Gargus RA, et al. First-week protein and energy intakes are associated with 18-month developmental outcomes in ELBW infants. *Pediatrics*. 2009;123(5):1337–1343.

34. Ehrenkranz RA, Das A, Wrage LA, et al. Early nutrition mediates the influence of severity of illness on extremely LBW infants. *Pediatr Res*. 2011:69(6):522–530.

35. Heird WC. Lipid metabolism in parenteral nutrition. In: Fomon SJ, Heird WC, eds. *Energy and Protein Needs During Infancy*. New York, NY: Academic Press; 1968:215–229.

36. Carlson SE. Docosahexaenoic acid and arachidonic acid in infant development. *Semin Neonatol*. 2001;6:437–444.

37. Uauy RD, Birch DG, Birch EE, et al. Effect of dietary omega-3 fatty acids on retinal function of very-low-birthweight neonates. *Pediatr Res*. 1990;28:485.

38. Uauy R, Mena P. Lipids and neurodevelopment. *Nutr Rev*. 2001;59:S34.

39. Sellmayer A, Koletzko B. Long-chain polyunsaturated fatty acids and eicosanoids in infants—physiological and pathosphysiological aspects and open questions. *Lipids*. 1999;34:199–205.

40. Haumont D, Deckelbaum RJ, Richelle M, et al. Plasma lipid and plasma lipoprotein concentrations in low-birth-weight infants given parenteral nutrition with 20% compared to 10% intralipid. *J Pediatr*. 1989;115:787–793.

41. Fielding CJ. Human lipoprotein lipase inhibition of activity by cholesterol. *Biochem Biophys Acta*. 1970; 218:221–226.

42. Andrew G, Chan G, Schiff D. Lipid metabolism in the neonate. I. The effect of intralipid infusion on plasma triglyceride and free fatty acid concentrations in the neonate. *J Pediatr*. 1976;88:273–278.

43. Brans YW, Dutton EB, Drew DS, et al. Fat emulsion tolerance in very low birthweight neonates: effect on diffusion of oxygen in the lungs and on blood pH. *Pediatrics*. 1986;78:79.

44. Adamkin DH, Gelke KN, Wilkerson SA. Clinical and laboratory observations: influence of intravenous fat therapy on tracheal effluent phospholipids and oxygenation in severe respiratory distress syndrome. *J Pediatr*. 1985;106:122.

45. Andrew G, Chan G, Schiff D. Lipid metabolism in the neonate. II. The effect of intralipid on bilirubin binding in vitro and in vivo. *J Pediatr*. 1976;88:279.

46. Adamkin DH, Radmacher PG, Klingbeil RK. Use of intravenous lipid and hyperbilirubinemia. *J Pediatr Gastroenterol Nutr*. 1992;14:135.

47. Simmer K, Rao SC. Early introduction of lipids to parenterally-fed preterm infants. *Cochrane Database Syst Rev*. 2005;(2):CD005256.

48. Drenckpohl D, McConnell C, Gaffney S, Niehaus M, Macwam KS. Randomized trial of very low birth weight infants receiving higher rates of infusion of intravenous fat emulsions during the first week of life. *Pediatrics*. 2008;122(4):743–751.

49. Hunt CE, Pachman LM, Hageman JR, et al. Lipsyn infusion increases prostaglandin concentrations. *Pediatr Pulmonol*. 1986;2(3):154–158.

50. Hammerman C, Aramburo MJ, Hill V. Intravenous lipids in newborn lungs thromboxane-medicated effects. *Crit Care Med*. 1989;17:430.

51. Lavoic JC, Chessex P. The increase in vasomotor tone induced by a parenteral lipid emulsion is linked to an inhibition of prostacyclin production. *Free Radic Biol Med*. 1994;16:795.

52. Helbock HJ, Motchnik PA, Ames BN. Toxic hydroperoxide in intravenous lipid emulsions used in preterm infants. *Pediatrics*. 1993;91:83.

53. Pitkanen O, Hallman M, Anderson S. Generation of free radicals in lipid emulsion used in parenteral nutrition. *Pediatr Res*. 1991;29:56.

54. Bonner CM, DeBrie KL, Hug G, et al. Effects of parenteral L-carnitine supplementation on fat metabolism and nutrition in premature neonates. *J Pediatr*. 1995;126:287.

55. Shortland GJ, Walter JH, Stroud C, et al. Randomised controlled trial of L-carnitine as a nutritional supplement in preterm infants. *Arch Dis Child Fetal Neonatal Ed*. 1998;78:F185.

56. Shulman RJ, Phillips S. Parenteral nutrition in infants and children. *J Pediatr Gastroenterol Nutr*. 2003;36:557.

57. Sapsford AL. Parenteral nutrition: energy, carbohydrate, protein and fat. In: Groh-Wargo S, Thompson M, Cox JH, eds. *Nutritional Care for High-Risk Newborns*. 3rd ed. Chicago, IL: Precept Press; 2000:119–149.

11 Enteral Nutrition

Roberto Murgas Torrazza, Juan Carlos Roig, and Josef Neu

INTRODUCTION

The enteral route is the most physiologic and natural way of administering nutrients to humans, and attaining full enteral feedings can often be challenging to clinicians who care for preterm infants. Establishing enteral feedings should be one of the most important goals, especially in very low birth weight (VLBW) infants. The utilization of the gastrointestinal tract provides these patients with multiple benefits, which include enhanced growth and neurodevelopment, improved immunologic functions with decreased infections, and acceleration of intestinal adaptation and maturation with a subsequent increase in the absorption of nutrients. Despite the numerous advances made to date in the area of nutrition for preterm infants, such as the use of parenteral solutions with more proteins, the majority of these infants are discharged weighing less than the 10th percentile for age.[1,2] The early initiation of parenteral nutritional support in preterm infants is a trend now widely supported by neonatologists, but often, enteral nutrition is underutilized, delayed, or totally withheld for prolonged times because of concerns of feeding intolerance or the fear for the development of necrotizing enterocolitis (NEC), which remains the most common devastating gastrointestinal complication of the preterm infant. The principles that should be considered to prevent "metabolic shock" and to optimize nutrition in the preterm infant should include the following:

1. Clinicians should be aware that metabolic and nutritional requirements do not stop with birth.

2. That hours, not days, are the longest periods this group of infants should be allowed to face without receiving either enteral or parenteral nutrition (PN).

3. That the metabolic and nutritional requirements of the newborn are equal to or greater than those of the fetus.

In this chapter, we review characteristics of the developing intestine as they relate to enteral nutritional strategies for the preterm infant.

The Developing Intestine

The intestine not only serves as a nutrient digestive absorptive organ but also is one of the largest immune organs of the body and serves a significant endocrine and exocrine role in humans. The intestine has neural tissue in amounts equivalent to that of the entire spinal cord. As the fetal intestine develops, the increase in its total surface area is significant, largely because of the villus and microvillus growth during this period of development.

In many neonatal intensive care units (NICUs), because of concerns of feeding intolerance and NEC, the gastrointestinal tract of the critically ill, low birth weight infant either is not exposed to nutrients at all for prolonged periods after birth or is provided only "minimal enteral nutrition," and most nutrients are only provided parenterally. The PN solutions are lifesaving nutritional medical interventions in the preterm infant, but ideally, the approach should be to provide most of the nutrients via the enteral route as

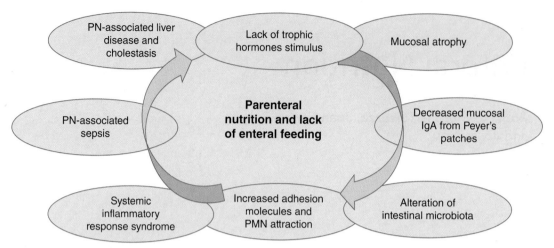

FIGURE 11-1 Detrimental effects of parenteral nutrition (PN) use and lack of enteral nutrition. Vicious cycle of lack of feeding and perpetuation of negative effects at the intestinal, immunological, and liver function levels. IgA, immunoglobulin A; PMN, polymorphonuclear cells.

soon as safely possible to promote intestinal growth and normal physiology. As illustrated in Figure 11-1, the lack or absence of luminal nutrients will result in mucosal atrophy, a decrease in the stimulation of trophic hormones, alterations in the microbiota, increased polymorphonuclear attraction, and an increased likelihood of development of the systemic inflammatory response syndrome, translocation of intestinal microbes, and sepsis. Because of the higher nutritional requirements needed for intestinal growth during the neonatal period, the lack of luminal nutrients may likely be of even more significance in these infants than in adults.

The newborn deprivation of enteral nutrients can be deleterious. These effects have been demonstrated by studies in which neonatal pigs were suckled and subsequently gained 42% of their weight in the first 24 hours after birth. In contrast, such growth did not occur in the unsuckled animals.[3] Using piglets, other researchers have demonstrated not only major differences in intestinal mucosal growth with enteral feeding compared with PN, but also increases in hepatic and superior mesenteric artery blood flow with feedings.[4] Studies have also suggested that enteral feedings increase superior mesenteric blood flow and could thus be a predictor for increased tolerance to enteral feedings in preterm infants.[5] Another study showed that enteral feedings increased mesenteric flow in anemic neonates, but that these responses were blunted in infants receiving blood transfusions.[6] This further suggests that enteral feedings may represent a protective mechanism in counteracting gut ischemia. Studies in animals using near-infrared spectroscopy measurement as an indicator of intestinal blood flow suggested correlations to NEC in premature piglets.[7] Early enteral nutrition also provides trophic benefits

and promotes hormonal secretion by nutrient stimulation to the gut and should preclude the need for using prolonged PN.[8,9]

Immature mucosal barrier function, immature immune response, and alterations of the intestinal microbiota are believed to make preterm neonates particularly susceptible to intestinal inflammation, injury, and bacterial translocation. Late-onset sepsis (LOS), a complication commonly seen in preterm infants, is associated with prolonged use of intravenous catheters for PN because of delays in achieving full enteral feeds or the need for central lines for administration of medications. The likelihood that LOS is at least partially caused by the lack of enteral feedings rather than a catheter-related infection is supported by studies that Wildhaber and colleagues conducted using rodents. These studies showed a combination of enteral feeding and a central line resulted in a much lower incidence of intestinal bacterial translocation than the presence of a PN line without receiving enteral nutrition.[10] In fact, a reduction in incidence of bacteremia was observed in VLBW neonates who achieved full enteral nutrition before the second week of life.[11]

There is a strong correlation between overall size of the intestine and its surface area. In term infants, the length of the small intestine can reach approximately 275 cm. Consequently, the inherent characteristics of the villi and microvilli represent an extensive amount of exposed surface area. Half of the growth in length of the intestine occurs during the last trimester of gestation.[12] During this time, the fetus is known to swallow approximately 400 mL of amniotic fluid per day. This is a physiologic process that may play an important role in the development of the gastrointestinal tract. This process is suddenly interrupted with preterm birth.

It is important to be aware of some of the developmental processes that occur during this time so that enteral nutrition may be optimized.

PROTEIN DIGESTION AND ABSORPTION

General

The composition of proteins ingested by neonates largely reflects that of either the mother's milk or the commercial formulas given. The protein content and composition of human breast milk change throughout the lactation period. For instance, at the beginning of lactation, the protein content is about 2 g/dL with a whey to casein ratio of about 80:20; this changes to a protein content of about 1 g/dL with an about 60:40 whey to casein ratio in the following weeks with the evolution of more mature milk. Most preterm infant formulas are formulated to reflect the latter whey to casein ratio. These different proteins have different amino acid profiles and different digestibility given the concept of "fast" and "slow" proteins. Whey proteins will produce a rapid, high but transient increase in circulating insulin and aminoacidemia, whereas casein proteins produce more gradual, and relatively lower, but more sustained increase in insulin and amino acids.[13]

Several studies have evaluated the metabolic and clinical benefits of enteral amino acid supplementation.[14-17] The postprandial rise in amino acids and insulin stimulates protein synthesis in the neonate and therefore growth.[18,19] Among the individual amino acids that have specific roles in regulating protein synthesis and immune function are leucine, glutamine, and arginine. Leucine is the key amino acid that triggers the stimulation of protein synthesis.[20,21] Using neonatal pig models, studies have shown that enteral or parenteral leucine will stimulate protein synthesis in the muscle and visceral tissue of the neonate even if formulas with low protein milk were used.[22,23] The stimulation of protein synthesis by leucine is through the activation of the mammalian target of rapamycin (mTOR), a nutrient sensor protein kinase, which integrates the input from upstream pathways, including insulin, growth factor, and amino acids.[21-23]

Arginine is an essential amino acid that in the neonate is exclusively synthesized in gut epithelial cells from amino acid precursors such as citrulline, glutamine, and glutamate. Arginine is also a precursor of nitric oxide (NO), a potent vasodilator, and will therefore increase intestinal blood flow.[24,25] Clinical studies have shown that low levels or a deficiency of arginine in preterm infants is associated with an increased incidence of NEC.[26,27] Randomized controlled trials have shown that when arginine supplementation with quantities as low as 1.5 mmol/kg/d are given to premature infants, a reduced incidence of NEC results.[15]

Another amino acid of importance is glutamine; although nonessential, it is not sufficiently synthesized in catabolic states. Several human and animal studies have suggested that glutamine supplementation in the critically ill patient has some benefits as an immunomodulator nutrient.[28-31] Glutamine in the intestine acts as an energy substrate, a precursor to gluthathione, and a nitrogen donor for other amino acids and nucleotides. Despite the attributed benefits of glutamine, studies of enteral supplementation with glutamine in VLBW infants failed to show reduction in nosocomial sepsis. However, on secondary analysis, the neonates who received glutamine supplementation had less gastrointestinal dysfunction and lower intraventricular hemorrhages.[14] A Cochrane review of 7 highly heterogeneous randomized controlled trials of glutamine supplementation in preterm infants failed to demonstrate any statistically significant effect on mortality or other neonatal morbidities.[32]

The digestion of proteins begins in the acidic environment of the stomach and continues in the small intestine under the influence of pancreatic proteases and peptidases. Most dietary proteins in human infants must first be digested into amino acids or di- and tripeptides. Proteolytic enzymes are secreted into the lumen of the upper digestive tube from 2 primary sources: (1) The chief cells of the stomach secrete pepsinogen, which is then converted to the active protease pepsin by the action of acid, and (2) the pancreas secretes a group of potent proteases, among them trypsin, chymotrypsin, and carboxypeptidases, which require activation by enterokinase. Through the action of these gastric and pancreatic proteases, dietary proteins will be hydrolyzed within the lumen of the small intestine predominantly into medium and small peptides (oligopeptides).

Subsequently, small peptides, primarily di- and tripeptides, are absorbed into the small intestinal epithelial cell by cotransport with H^+ ions.[33,34] Once inside the enterocyte, the vast bulk of the absorbed di- and tripeptides is hydrolyzed into single amino acids by cytoplasmic peptidases and exported from the cell into blood. Only a few of these small peptides enter blood intact.

Absorption of amino acids is dependent on the electrochemical gradient of sodium across the epithelium in the small intestine. Further, absorption of amino acids, like that of monosaccharides, contributes to generating the osmotic gradient that drives water absorption. The basolateral membrane of the enterocyte contains additional transporters that export amino acids from the cell into blood; these are not dependent on sodium gradients.

The contribution of the microflora to gastrointestinal amino acid metabolism may be nutritionally important. Studies have indicated that essential amino acids are synthesized and absorbed by the gastrointestinal flora.[35]

Developmental Aspects of Protein Digestion and Absorption

Digestion

Gastric Acidity

When comparing full-term and premature infants, hydrochloric acid secretion was found to be much lower in premature infants than in full-term infants.[36] Of significance, however, is that both basal and pentagastrin-stimulated acid secretion were noted to double from the first to fourth week of postnatal life in preterm infants.[37] The actual pH of the stomach contents in infants is influenced substantially by food intake. The entry of milk into the infant's stomach causes a sharp increase in the pH of the gastric contents and a slower return to lower pH values than in older children and adults.[38]

Pancreatic Proteolytic Activity

The protease cascade in the small intestine is catalyzed by food-stimulated secretion of enterokinase from the upper small intestinal epithelium. However, even though enterokinase is detectable at 24 weeks' gestation, its concentration is relatively low and reaches only 25% of adult activity at term.[39] This theoretically can be limiting to protein digestion and may be responsible for an increased capability of larger antigens or microorganisms to pass into the intestine without breakdown by luminal enzymes.

Pancreatic secretion of proteolytic enzymes starts at the beginning of the fifth month of gestation. Levels of trypsin concentration encountered during the first 2 years of life are reached by the age of 3 months.[40] From birth onward, the concentration of chymotrypsin (after pancreozymin-secretin stimulation) increases approximately 3-fold and reaches adult levels in 3-year-old children.[40] Serial measurement of fecal chymotrypsin concentrations in preterm infants (23 to 32 weeks' gestation) during the first 4 weeks of life demonstrated values generally similar to those found in term infants.[40]

Absorption

For a few days after birth, the "leakiness" of the neonatal gut has the ability to absorb intact proteins. This ability, which is rapidly lost in a process called closure, is of importance because it allows the newborn to acquire passive immunity by absorbing immunoglobulins in colostral milk. Thus, the ability of the gastrointestinal tract to exclude antigenically intact food proteins increases with gestational age, and that gut closure occurs normally before birth.[41]

Proteolytic and Peptidase Activity

In one study, brush border and intracellular proteolytic enzyme activities were measured in fetuses (8–22 weeks' gestation), children (7 months to 14 years), and adults. The peptidase activities in all 3 groups were comparable, suggesting that the small intestine of the term and preterm newborn should be able to efficiently digest peptides.[42]

Clinical Correlations

The fetus accretes about 2.2 g/kg/d of protein at 26 weeks' gestation, and it declines to about 0.9 g/kg/d in the term infant. The placenta supplies up to 3.5 g/kg/d of amino acids to the developing fetus, and preterm delivery will abruptly interrupt this amino acid supply and any further protein accretion. Herein lies the importance of starting nutrition immediately after birth, especially in the preterm infant. Early parenteral and enteral nutrition has been shown to be safe and to decrease morbidity.[8,43] Amino acids supplied in excess of those needed for protein accretion are oxidized and contribute to energy production. Certain patients have a transient increase in the blood serum nitrogen (BUN) levels that usually does not exceed 60 mg/dL.[44] In the absence of an inborn error of metabolism, this is of no clinical significance, and preterm infants normally tolerate it well without risk of encephalopathy.

The limited capacity of premature infants to secrete acid should be considered when using histamine 2 (H_2) blockers or proton pump inhibitors, which are widely prescribed in many NICUs, especially for the treatment of symptomatic gastric reflux. Some studies suggest that critically ill premature infants treated with H_2 blockers have a higher incidence of nosocomial sepsis and NEC.[45,46] Therefore, the use of H_2 blockers should be undertaken with caution and perhaps only in infants that have failed other interventions. Although speculative, it is possible that with the already-limited hydrogen ion production in the stomach of the premature infant, additional blockage further diminishes the acid barrier to microorganisms and allows for a higher load of bacteria in the more distal regions of the intestine.

Despite the digestive limitations and decreased enzymatic capabilities of premature infants, no significant data have been offered to demonstrate benefits or advantages of using a formula of hydrolyzed protein fractions over whole-protein formulas,[45,47] and studies have yet to demonstrate any benefit for choosing a hydrolyzed protein formula over human milk.

CARBOHYDRATE DIGESTION AND ABSORPTION

General

The predominant carbohydrate in human milk and of most infant formulas is lactose. Lactase intestinal activity is limited in the preterm infant when compared to term infants. Interestingly, lactose intolerance is rarely seen in the preterm infant.

Starches and complex carbohydrates must first be hydrolyzed to oligosaccharides by digestive processes in the mouth, stomach, and intestinal lumen. This is accomplished primarily via salivary and pancreatic amylases. Oligosaccharides must then be hydrolyzed in the intestinal epithelial brush border into monosaccharides prior to their absorption. The catalysts required for this process to proceed are the brush border hydrolases, namely, maltase, lactase, and sucrase. Dietary lactose, sucrose, and maltose come in contact with the absorptive surface of the epithelial cells covering the intestinal villi, where they engage with brush border hydrolases: maltase, sucrase, and lactase.

Developmental Aspects of Carbohydrate Digestion and Absorption

Carbohydrate Digestion

Pancreatic amylase activity has been demonstrated in amniotic fluid and pancreatic tissue from 14- to 16-week-old fetuses.[48,49] Although salivary amylase activity rapidly increases shortly after term birth, pancreatic amylase remains low until 3 months of age and does not reach adult levels until nearly 2 years.[50]

Carbohydrate Absorption

Although lactase activity in the small intestine of preterms is thought to be limited, suggesting a limited capacity for lactose hydrolysis, colonic fermentation activity is adequate for colonic salvage of lactose even during the second week of life. Using a stable isotope method for serial assessment of lactose carbon assimilation, Kien and associates[51] demonstrated efficient absorption of lactose in premature infants (30 to 32 weeks' gestation and 11 to 36 days of age). The predominant carbohydrate found in human milk is lactose, and human milk is usually tolerated better than formulas in low birth weight infants.

A study in premature infants was designed to ascertain whether the timing of feeding initiation affected the development of intestinal lactase activity and whether there are clinical ramifications of lower lactase activity.[52] Early feeding increased intestinal lactase

activity in preterm infants. Lactase activity is a marker of intestinal maturity and may influence clinical outcomes. Whether the effects of milk on lactase activity were because of the greater concentration of lactose in human milk compared with that in formula has not yet been determined.[52]

The finding of low lactase activities in the intestines of fetuses has led to the notion that premature babies cannot tolerate lactose.[39] The presence of a high lactose concentration in human milk should not preclude its use in the VLBW infant. Microbial salvage pathways that convert nonabsorbed lactose to short-chain fatty acids that can then be absorbed and utilized for energy production are functional in these infants.[51] Furthermore, feedings for VLBW infants rarely are initiated at levels intended to meet the infants' entire nutritional requirements and usually are advanced slowly. The rationale for using a lactose-free formula instead of human milk or even a commercial lactose-containing formula is weak and theoretically may be harmful.

LIPID DIGESTION AND ABSORPTION

The key mediators of lipid digestion are bile acids and lipases. Bile acids promote lipid emulsification and have both hydrophilic and hydrophobic domains (ie, they are amphipathic). On exposure to a large aggregate of triglyceride, the hydrophobic portions of bile acids intercalate into the lipid, with the hydrophilic domains remaining at the surface. This coating with bile acids aids in breakdown of large aggregates or droplets into increasingly smaller droplets. For a given volume of lipid, the smaller the droplet size, the greater the surface area will be, which will in turn provides a greater surface area for its interaction with lipase. Hydrolysis of triglyceride into monoglyceride and free fatty acids is accomplished predominantly by pancreatic lipase. The function of this enzyme is to cleave the fatty acids at positions 1 and 3 of the triglyceride, creating 2 free fatty acids and a 2-monoglyceride. The major products of lipid digestion (fatty acids and 2-monoglycerides) enter the enterocyte by simple diffusion across the plasma membrane.

After entry into the cell, medium-chain triglycerides, which also require minimal emulsification by bile acids, undergo a relatively simple process of assimilation in which they are not reesterified to partake in chylomicron formation, unlike the long-chain lipids. Medium-chain triglycerides are taken directly into the portal venous system, and chylomicrons formed from long-chain fats enter the lymphatics. In conditions that result in or lead to obstruction of the lymphatics, feeding formulas containing primarily medium-chain triglycerides rather than long-chain triglycerides is recommended.

Because bile acids play a key role in efficient fat digestion and absorption in humans, consideration needs to be given to the fact that in preterm infants, enteral fat absorption may be limited. In VLBW infants, the duodenal concentration of bile acids is reduced because of lower synthesis and ileal reabsorption.[53,54] Lower micellar solubilization leads to inefficient cell-mucosal interaction and subsequently lower absorption of the molecules at the mucosal-cell surface interface. When supplementing the premature infant with enteral lipids, medium-chain fatty acids may be preferred because long-chain fatty acids and not medium-chain fatty acids depend on bile acids for solubilization and thus are most likely to be inefficiently absorbed.

Bile Salt–Stimulated Lipase

Human milk contains lipase activity, and lipase is not detectable in bovine milk.[55] It has been shown that the digestion of long-chain triglycerides can take place only in the presence of bile salts and the enzyme bile salt–stimulated lipase (BSSL), which is present in human colostrum and in preterm and term milk.[56-58] The significance of the presence of BSSL for the digestion of milk lipids is supported by studies on low birth weight preterm infants (3 to 6 weeks old) fed raw or heat-treated (pasteurized or boiled) human milk. Fat from the first was absorbed more (74%) than the last 2 (54% and 46%, respectively).[59]

Pancreatic Lipases

In adults, pancreatic juice lipases are active against neutral lipids. Generally, lipases are at their lowest levels after birth.[60] The increase toward adult values occurs toward the completion of the first 6 months of life. In comparison, the process for amylase takes even longer. Premature and VLBW infants have lower values of amylase/lipase than full-term neonates.[61] During the first week of life, lipase activity increases about 4-fold in premature infants.[60] In healthy preterm infants between days 3 and 40 postnatally, this activity increases linearly (in infants at both gestational age 29 to 32 and 33 to 36 weeks).[53] At 1 month of age, values reach 35% of the values found in 2- to 6-week-old babies.

Despite physiologic evidence suggesting that supplementing with medium-chain triglycerides may be nutritionally advantageous in comparison to using long-chain fats, some studies have shown the latter may be absorbed just as readily. The mechanism may partly be because of the greater gastric lipolytic activity of the longer-chain lipids.[62] This finding is also supported by a Cochrane review that showed no differences in growth, NEC, or other morbidities

in babies fed primarily medium- versus long-chain triglycerides.[63]

Most essential fatty acids provided to neonates are derived from the omega-6 family (linoleic acid). This is because much of the lipid derived from formulas or intravenous lipid solutions is from vegetable oil, which is rich in the omega-6 but not the omega-3 fraction. Soybean oil lipid and plant-derived oil solutions that are rich in omega-6 fatty acids and phytosterols are thought to be the main cause for PN-associated liver disease with an increase in conjugated bilirubin and liver enzymes that could lead to liver failure and to the need for liver transplantation.[64-66]

Fish oil, which is rich in omega-3 fatty acids (specifically docosahexaenoic acid [DHA]), has emerged as a solution for this problem.[67] Omega-3 fatty acids (DHA), which are critical for retinal, brain, and other neural tissue development, have been shown to have anti-inflammatory properties as well as being hepatoprotective in animal and in human studies.[68-71] Despite this, a meta-analysis demonstrated no improvement in visual acuity or neurodevelopment.[72] This is an area that is currently under investigation.

ENTERAL FEEDING RECOMMENDATIONS IN THE PRETERM INFANT

Enteral feeds should be initiated as soon after birth as possible in newborns. Human milk is the first choice for feeding unless known contraindications for its use clearly exist, such as with galactosemia, maternal human immunodeficiency virus (HIV), and miliary tuberculosis. Maternal substance abuse is a relative contraindication, and most neonates can have the benefits of breast milk feeds. The best evidence of the benefit of the use of breast milk in premature infants, especially VLBW infants, is the reduced incidence of NEC.[73]

Basic principles of nutrition should be followed in the newborn (Table 11-1). All preterm infants will benefit from early initiation of nutrition, either parenteral or enteral, in the first hour of life. In our unit, we attempt to start the preterm infant with a stock solution of PN within the first 20 minutes of life. This stock solution provides at least 3 g/kg/d of protein at a rate of 80 mL/kg/d. Enteral feeds should not be withheld for more than 24 hours waiting for breast milk availability. Most preterm infants will tolerate initiation of feeds at rates between 10 and 20 mL/kg/d with advancement of feeds at 20 mL/kg/d. In specific situations when intestinal perfusion or critical clinical condition warrants caution, feeds may be withheld for longer periods or started and advanced at lower volumes (5–10 mL/kg/d). Enteral feedings in the preterm infant have multiple benefits, even when minimal

Table 11-1 Nutrition Principles in the Preterm Infant

Preterm infants have higher metabolic and nutritional requirements.
Parenteral or enteral nutrition should be started within the first hour of life—the "golden hour."
Breast milk is the best milk for all newborns, and enteral feeds should be started as soon as possible.
Use the gastrointestinal tract whenever possible. If the gut works, use it!

enteral volumes are used for nutrition, as in those for "gut priming." The benefits include trophic signaling with subsequent maturation and release of hormones that stimulate intestinal villous growth, improve feeding tolerance, and decrease the time required to reach full PN, therefore potentially reducing the risk of PN-related cholestasis.

Table 11-2 highlights some of the specific goals that should be set in hopes of establishing optimal enteral nutrition in preterm infants. Studies have shown that when a standardized feeding regimen is followed, the outcomes improve and the incidence of NEC in preterm infants is substantially reduced.[74] When breast milk is not available for use in preterm infants, we use preterm formulas with 22–24 kcal/oz. These formulas have been developed to meet the nutritional needs of preterm infants. Preterm formulas are whey predominant, contain reduced amounts of lactose, and have higher contents of calories, calcium, and phosphorus when compared to term formulas.

There are 3 phases in the enteral nutrition of the preterm infant:

Minimal or trophic enteral nutrition phase: In this phase, the goal is to provide the minimal amount of nutrients required to stimulate the gut and to prevent its atrophy and other complications, such as sepsis and NEC.

Advancing phase: In the advancing phase, the goal is to safely increase milk volumes in a manner

Table 11-2 Enteral Nutrition Goals in the Preterm Infant

Weight gain aim of 15–20 g/d.
Minimized prolonged period of nothing by mouth or slow advancement of feeds
Rapid attainment of full feeds more than 150 mL/kg/d and caloric intake greater than 110 kcal/d
Achievement of oral feedings as soon as sucking and swallowing coordination are appropriate

that minimizes the risks for feeding intolerance and NEC and allow a rapid progression toward achieving full feedings to decrease the need of PN and reduce the incidence of catheter-related infections and PN-associated cholestasis.

Fine-tuning phase: In fine-tuning, the goal is to optimize growth. The infant is already receiving full feedings and is tolerating them well. During this phase, we want to maximize weight gain.

Supplementation of the breast milk or infant formulas is also an alternative for those infants who are not meeting growth goals. Human milk fortifiers (HMFs) are available, and the recommendation is to start supplementation with HMFs once the feeding volume approximates 100 mL/kg/d. Iron supplementation is recommended for infants who are being breast-fed or in the group of preterm infants for whom additional iron is needed because of anemia of prematurity. Breast-fed infants also need vitamin D supplementation; the recommended dose is 400 IU per day. Most newborns receive daily multivitamins, although no clear benefit has been attributed to this practice. Supplementation of other products, such as medium chain triglycerides (MCT) oil, polycose, or corn oil, should be considered on a case-by-case basis and are generally used to increase the caloric intake of the preterm infant.

FEEDING CONTROVERSIES (IF THE GUT WORKS, USE IT)

Enteral Feeds and Indomethacin

There is no evidence suggesting that feeding is contraindicated when the infant is receiving indomethacin. We recommend continuing feeding during indomethacin administration if there is no other contraindication. The use of indomethacin together with dexamethasone or hydrocortisone is contraindicated because studies showed a high incidence of spontaneous perforation with these combinations.[75]

Holding Feeds for Gastric Residuals

There is no evidence suggesting holding the feedings because of the presence of gastric residuals is advantageous in preventing complications such as NEC.[76] We recommend continuing feeding if the residuals are nonbilious and if there is no other manifestation of severe intolerance.

Mode of Feeding

When considering whether to bolus feed an infant versus using a continuous or drip mode, there is no evidence to support either the continuous or the drip mode of feeding as superior to bolus feeding or vice versa.[77] Certain patients may benefit from continuous feeding in cases of severe intolerance or severe gastrointestinal reflux disease (GERD). The preferred mode of feeding is to bolus feed intermittently because it is thought to stimulate the patient's gastrointestinal tract in a more physiologic fashion, thus promoting gastrointestinal motility as well as the secretion of intestinal hormones and enzymes.

Transfusion and Feeding Intolerance

Some investigators have suggested a possible association between red blood cell (RBC) transfusion and NEC in premature neonates.[78] Infants who developed NEC had frequently received RBC transfusions in the 48 to 72 hours prior to developing NEC.[79] Randomized controlled trials continue to be necessary to elucidate if blood transfusions cause NEC. Currently, there is not enough evidence to withhold feeds during blood transfusion, but precautions should be taken when feeding infants who are hemodynamically unstable and are receiving blood transfusions.

Prebiotics and Probiotics

Prospective randomized trials have evaluated the effects of different probiotics on the prevention of NEC.[80] A recent multicenter trial of probiotic suggested a beneficial preventive effect against NEC yet no decrease in NEC-related mortality.

However, there was a trend for a higher incidence of sepsis in infants receiving probiotics,[81] especially in those with a birth weight less than 750 g, but the composite outcome of sepsis or death rate did not differ significantly between groups. Despite encouraging data of the beneficial effects of some probiotics and the recent recommendations for their routine use based on a meta-analysis of the current data,[82] routine use is not indicated.[83]

Effects of No Enteral Feeding

The lack of a substantial volume of milk supplied in the intestinal lumen during the first several weeks coincides with provision of a low amount of anti-inflammatory fatty acids and certain immune-active amino acids, such as glutamine, arginine, and cysteine. It is becoming increasingly clear that PN cholestasis, a complication commonly seen in preterm infants with prolonged used of PN, partially results from the lack of enteral nutrients and the exposure to soybean oil lipid and plant-derived oil solutions rich in omega-6 fatty acids and phytosterols. This was supported by studies by Wang and associates, which demonstrated marked pathology in the livers of piglets after only 7 days of PN administration compared with piglets receiving enteral feedings only.[84] Figure 11-2 illustrates the beneficial effects of enteral feeds and the specific effects of different nutrients.

Abnormally high permeability of the intestinal mucosal barrier or mucosal "leakiness" appears to play a role in intestine-derived systemic inflammation. A series of studies in low birth weight infants by Schanler and Schulman and colleagues showed that early enteral feeding is associated with decreased intestinal permeability and improved motility, as evidenced by less retention time of the marker carmine red.[85]

Studies of feeding tolerance and NEC in infants fed early while having indwelling umbilical artery catheters versus infants who were not enterally fed until after the catheters were removed demonstrated no difference in feeding tolerance or occurrence of NEC between the groups. However, the infants who were fed enterally with the catheters in place had fewer sepsis evaluations, central lines, and days with nothing by mouth when compared to the group that did not receive feedings until after catheter removal.[86]

The frequent use of indomethacin, its association with non-NEC isolated intestinal perforations, and its possible mediation of decreased intestinal blood flow have prompted many neonatologists to have infants receive nothing by mouth while indomethacin is infused. Currently, no evidence exists to support a causal relationship between feeding during indomethacin usage and NEC (or spontaneous intestinal perforations). The increase in intestinal blood flow associated with receiving enteral feedings may actually counteract any detrimental hemodynamic effects that indomethacin may induce. A study conducted by Bellander and colleagues showed no difference between infants receiving indomethacin compared with controls in terms of tolerance of feedings or NEC in babies whose average gestational age was 29 weeks and who were advanced to approximately 70 mL/kg/d of feeding by 7 days of age.[87]

Figure 11-3 shows different preterm infants who will require special care and nutritional support. We also show some of the different nutrition modalities that are available to provide the nutrients necessary for these infants to grow. Cup feeding has been used in an attempt to improve breastfeeding rates. In a Cochrane review, the authors concluded that cup feeding cannot be recommended over bottle feeding as a supplement to breastfeeding.[88]

In summary, PN, although necessary, is fraught with hazards. In contrast, early careful use of enteral feeding is associated with innumerable benefits to clinicians and their patients.

Specific nutrients benefits and proposed effects in the preterm infant

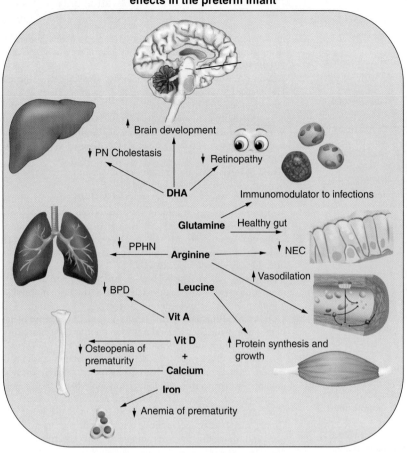

FIGURE 11-2 Specific nutrients and proposed beneficial effects in the preterm infant and newborn in general. Amino acids such as arginine, glutamine, and leucine and long-chain fatty acids such as docosahexaenoic acid (DHA or omega-3); vitamins A and D, calcium, and iron among the minerals that can be supplemented and offer tremendous benefits to the preterm infant. BPD, bronchopulmonary dysplasia; NEC, necrotizing enterocolitis; PN, parenteral nutrition; PPHN, persistent pulmonary hypertension of the newborn.

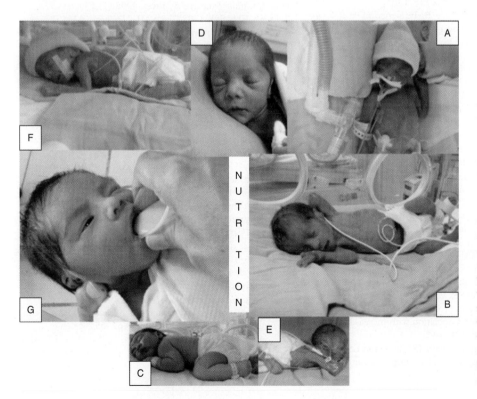

FIGURE 11-3 Nutrition of the preterm infant is an integral and most important part in the care of the newborn, especially in the preterm infant. Very sick baby on mechanical ventilator (A), preterm infants/intrauterine growth retardation (IUGR) infants (B), and infants of diabetic mother (C) all require special care and special nutritional support to obtain the best outcome possible. Different modes of feeding and interactions are available and used in the care of the infant. Breast feeding, kangaroo care while feeding (D), parenteral feeding through a peripherally inserted central catheter (PICC) line (E), enteral feeding via nasogastric (NG) tube (F), cup feeding (G).

REFERENCES

1. Ehrenkranz RA, Younes N, Lemons JA, et al. Longitudinal growth of hospitalized very low birth weight infants. *Pediatrics.* 1999;104:280–289.
2. Martin CR, Brown YF, Ehrenkranz RA, et al. Nutritional practices and growth velocity in the first month of life in extremely premature infants. *Pediatrics.* 2009;124:649–657.
3. Ashwell M. Elsie Widdowson (1906–2000). *Nature.* 2000; 406:844.
4. Stephens J, Stoll B, Cottrell J, Chang X, Helmrath M, Burrin DG. Glucagon-like peptide-2 acutely increases proximal small intestinal blood flow in TPN-fed neonatal piglets. *Am J Physiol Regul Integr Comp Physiol.* 2006;290:R283–R289.
5. Fang S, Kempley ST, Gamsu HR. Prediction of early tolerance to enteral feeding in preterm infants by measurement of superior mesenteric artery blood flow velocity. *Arch Dis Child Fetal Neonatal Ed.* 2001;85:F42–F45.
6. Krimmel GA, Baker R, Yanowitz TD. Blood transfusion alters the superior mesenteric artery blood flow velocity response to feeding in premature infants. *Am J Perinatol.* 2009;26:99–105.
7. Gay AN, Lazar DA, Stoll B, et al. Near-infrared spectroscopy measurement of abdominal tissue oxygenation is a useful indicator of intestinal blood flow and necrotizing enterocolitis in premature piglets. *J Pediatr Surg.* 2011;46:1034–1040.
8. Thureen PJ. Early aggressive nutrition in very preterm infants. *Nestle Nutr Workshop Ser Pediatr Program.* 2007;59:193–204. discussion 204–2008.
9. Adamkin DH. Pragmatic approach to in-hospital nutrition in high-risk neonates. *J Perinatol.* 2005;25(Suppl 2):S7–S11.
10. Wildhaber BE, Yang H, Spencer AU, Drongowski RA, Teitelbaum DH. Lack of enteral nutrition—effects on the intestinal immune system. *J Surg Res.* 2005;123:8–16.
11. Lavoie PM. Earlier initiation of enteral nutrition is associated with lower risk of late-onset bacteremia only in most mature very low birth weight infants. *J Perinatol.* 2009;29:448–454.
12. Weaver L, Austin S, Cole TJ. Small intestinal length: a factor essential for gut adaptation. *Gut.* 1991;32:1321–1323.
13. Dangin M, Boirie Y, Guillet C, Beaufrere B. Influence of the protein digestion rate on protein turnover in young and elderly subjects. *J Nutr.* 2002;132:3228S–3233S.
14. Vaughn P, Thomas P, Clark R, Neu J. Enteral glutamine supplementation and morbidity in low birth weight infants. *J Pediatr.* 2003;142:662–668.
15. Amin HJ, Zamora SA, McMillan DD, et al. Arginine supplementation prevents necrotizing enterocolitis in the premature infant. *J Pediatr.* 2002;140:425–431.
16. Roig JC, Meetze WH, Auestad N, et al. Enteral glutamine supplementation for the very low birthweight infant: plasma amino acid concentrations. *J Nutr.* 1996;126:1115S–1120S.
17. Wilmore D. Enteral and parenteral arginine supplementation to improve medical outcomes in hospitalized patients. *J Nutr* 2004;134:2863S–2867S.; discussion 2895S.
18. O'Connor PM, Kimball SR, Suryawan A, et al. Regulation of neonatal liver protein synthesis by insulin and amino acids in pigs. *Am J Physiol Endocrinol Metab.* 2004;286:E994–E1003.
19. Davis TA, Suryawan A, Orellana RA, Fiorotto ML, Burrin DG. Amino acids and insulin are regulators of muscle protein synthesis in neonatal pigs. *Animal.* 2010;4:1790–1796.
20. Anthony JC, Anthony TG, Kimball SR, Vary TC, Jefferson LS. Orally administered leucine stimulates protein synthesis in skeletal muscle of postabsorptive rats in association with increased eIF4F formation. *J Nutr.* 2000;130:139–145.
21. Anthony JC, Yoshizawa F, Anthony TG, Vary TC, Jefferson LS, Kimball SR. Leucine stimulates translation initiation in skeletal muscle of postabsorptive rats via a rapamycin-sensitive pathway. *J Nutr.* 2000;130:2413–2419.
22. Murgas Torrazza R, Suryawan A, Gazzaneo MC, et al. Leucine supplementation of a low-protein meal increases skeletal muscle and visceral tissue protein synthesis in neonatal pigs by stimulating mTOR-dependent translation initiation. *J Nutr.* 2010;140:2145–2152.
23. Wilson FA, Suryawan A, Gazzaneo MC, Orellana RA, Nguyen HV, Davis TA. Stimulation of muscle protein synthesis by prolonged parenteral infusion of leucine is dependent on amino acid availability in neonatal pigs. *J Nutr.* 2010;140:264–270.
24. Wu G, Bazer FW, Davis TA, et al. Arginine metabolism and nutrition in growth, health and disease. *Amino Acids.* 2009;37:153–168.
25. Wu G, Morris SM, Jr. Arginine metabolism: nitric oxide and beyond. *Biochem J.* 1998;336(Pt 1):1–17.
26. Becker RM, Wu G, Galanko JA, et al. Reduced serum amino acid concentrations in infants with necrotizing enterocolitis. *J Pediatr.* 2000;137:785–793.
27. Zamora SA, Amin HJ, McMillan DD, et al. Plasma L-arginine concentrations in premature infants with necrotizing enterocolitis. *J Pediatr.* 1997;131:226–232.
28. Neu J, Roig JC, Meetze WH, et al. Enteral glutamine supplementation for very low birth weight infants decreases morbidity. *J Pediatr.* 1997;131:691–699.
29. Houdijk AP, Rijnsburger ER, Jansen J, et al. Randomised trial of glutamine-enriched enteral nutrition on infectious morbidity in patients with multiple trauma. *Lancet.* 1998;352:772–776.
30. Wischmeyer PE, Lynch J, Liedel J, et al. Glutamine administration reduces gram-negative bacteremia in severely burned patients: a prospective, randomized, double-blind trial versus isonitrogenous control. *Crit Care Med.* 2001;29:2075–2080.
31. Wischmeyer PE, Kahana M, Wolfson R, Ren H, Musch MM, Chang EB. Glutamine reduces cytokine release, organ damage, and mortality in a rat model of endotoxemia. *Shock.* 2001;16:398–402.
32. Tubman TR, Thompson SW, McGuire W. Glutamine supplementation to prevent morbidity and mortality in preterm infants. *Cochrane Database Syst Rev.* 2008;(1):CD001457.
33. Fairclough PD, Silk DB, Clark ML, Dawson AM. Proceedings: new evidence for intact di- and tripeptide absorption. *Gut.* 1975;6:843.
34. Adibi SA, Morse EL, Masilamani SS, Amin PM. Evidence for two different modes of tripeptide disappearance in human intestine. Uptake by peptide carrier systems and hydrolysis by peptide hydrolases. *J Clin Invest.* 1975;56:1355–1363.
35. Torrallardona D, Harris CI, Fuller MF. Lysine synthesized by the gastrointestinal microflora of pigs is absorbed, mostly in the small intestine. *Am J Physiol Endocrinol Metab.* 2003;284:E1177–E1180.
36. Mignone F, Castello D. Research on gastric secretion of hydrochloric acid in the premature infant. *Minerva Pediatr.* 1961;13:1098–1030.
37. Hyman PE, Clarke DD, Everett SL, et al. Gastric acid secretory function in preterm infants. *J Pediatr.* 1985;106:467–471.
38. Harries JT, Fraser AJ. The acidity of the gastric contents of premature babies during the first fourteen days of life. *Biol Neonat.* 1968;12:186–103.
39. Antonowicz I, Lebenthal E. Developmental pattern of small intestinal enterokinase and disaccharidase activities in the human fetus. *Gastroenterology.* 1977;72:1299–1303.
40. McClean P, Weaver LT. Ontogeny of human pancreatic exocrine function. *Arch Dis Child.* 1993;68:62–65.
41. Roberton DM, Paganelli R, Dinwiddie R, Levinsky RJ. Milk antigen absorption in the preterm and term neonate. *Arch Dis Child.* 1982;57:369–372.

42. Auricchio S, Stellato A, De Vizia B. Development of brush border peptidases in human and rat small intestine during fetal and neonatal life. *Pediatr Res.* 1981;15:991–995.

43. Ehrenkranz RA, Das A, Wrage LA, et al. Early nutrition mediates the influence of severity of illness on extremely LBW infants. *Pediatr Res.* 2011;69:522–529.

44. Ridout E, Melara D, Rottinghaus S, Thureen PJ. Blood urea nitrogen concentration as a marker of amino-acid intolerance in neonates with birthweight less than 1250 g. *J Perinatol.* 2005;25:130–133.

45. Beck-Sague CM, Azimi P, Fonseca SN, et al. Bloodstream infections in neonatal intensive care unit patients: results of a multicenter study. *Pediatr Infect Dis J.* 1994;13:1110–1116.

46. Guillet R, Stoll BJ, Cotten CM, et al. for members of the National Institute of Child Health and Human Development Neonatal Research Network. Association of H2-blocker therapy and higher incidence of necrotizing enterocolitis in very low birth weight infants. *Pediatrics.* 2006;117:e137–e142.

47. Mihatsch WA, Franz AR, Hogel J, Pohlandt F. Hydrolyzed protein accelerates feeding advancement in very low birth weight infants. *Pediatrics.* 2002;110:1199–1203.

48. Davis MM, Hodes ME, Munsick RA, Ulbright TM, Goldstein DJ. Pancreatic amylase expression in human pancreatic development. *Hybridoma.* 1986;5:137–145.

49. Wolf RO, Taussig LM. Human amniotic fluid isoamylases. Functional development of fetal pancreas and salivary glands. *Obstet Gynecol.* 1973;41:337–342.

50. McClean P, Weaver LT. Ontogeny of human pancreatic exocrine function. *Arch Dis Child.* 1993;68:62–65.

51. Kien CL. Digestion, absorption, and fermentation of carbohydrates in the newborn. *Clin Perinatol.* 1996;23:211–228.

52. Shulman RJ, Schanler RJ, Lau C, Heitkemper M, Ou CN, Smith E. Early feeding, feeding tolerance, and lactase activity in preterm infants. *J Pediatr.* 1998;133:645–649.

53. Boehm G, Braun W, Moro G, Minoli I. Bile acid concentrations in serum and duodenal aspirates of healthy preterm infants: effects of gestational and postnatal age. *Biol Neonate.* 1997;71:207–214.

54. Suchy FJ, Balistreri WF, Heubi JE, Searcy JE, Levin RS. Physiologic cholestasis: elevation of the primary serum bile acid concentrations in normal infants. *Gastroenterology.* 1981;80:1037–1041.

55. Tarassuk NP, Nickerson TA, Yaguchi M. Lipase action in human milk. *Nature.* 1964;201:298–299.

56. Freed LM, York CM, Hamosh P, Mehta NR, Hamosh M. Bile salt-stimulated lipase of human milk: characteristics of the enzyme in the milk of mothers of premature and full-term infants. *J Pediatr Gastroenterol Nutr.* 1987;6:598–604.

57. Hernell O, Bläckberg L. Molecular aspects of fat digestion in the newborn. *Acta Paediatr Suppl.* 1994;405:65–69.

58. Hall B, Muller DP. Studies on the bile salt stimulated lipolytic activity of human milk using whole milk as source of both substrate and enzyme. I. Nutritional implications. *Pediatr Res.* 1982l;16:251–255.

59. Williamson S, Finucane E, Ellis H, Gamsu HR. Effect of heat treatment of human milk on absorption of nitrogen, fat, sodium, calcium, and phosphorus by preterm infants. *Arch Dis Child.* 1978;53:555–563.

60. Zoppi G, Andreotti G, Pajno-Ferrara F, Njai DM, Gaburro D. Exocrine pancreas function in premature and full term neonates. *Pediatr Res.* 1972;6:880–886.

61. Katz L, Hamilton JR. Fat absorption in infants of birth weight less than 1,300 grams. *J Pediatr.* 1975;85:608.

62. Hamosh M, Bitman J, Liao TH, et al. Gastric lipolysis and fat absorption in preterm infants: effect of medium-chain triglyceride or long-chain triglyceride-containing formulas. *Pediatrics.* 1989;83:86–92.

63. Klenoff-Brumberg HL, Genen LH. High versus low medium chain triglyceride content of formula for promoting short term growth of preterm infants. *Cochrane Database Syst Rev.* 2003;(1):CD002777.

64. Carter BA, Taylor OA, Prendergast DR, et al. Stigmasterol, a soy lipid-derived phytosterol, is an antagonist of the bile acid nuclear receptor FXR. *Pediatr Res.* 2007;62:301–306.

65. Clayton PT, Bowron A, Mills KA, Massoud A, Casteels M, Milla PJ. Phytosterolemia in children with parenteral nutrition-associated cholestatic liver disease. *Gastroenterology.* 1993;105:1806–1813.

66. Clayton PT, Whitfield P, Iyer K. The role of phytosterols in the pathogenesis of liver complications of pediatric parenteral nutrition. *Nutrition.* 1998;14:158–164.

67. Gura K, Strijbosch R, Arnold S, McPherson C, Puder M. The role of an intravenous fat emulsion composed of fish oil in a parenteral nutrition-dependent patient with hypertriglyceridemia. *Nutr Clin Pract.* 2007;22:664–672.

68. Pawlik D, Lauterbach R, Turyk E. Fish-oil fat emulsion supplementation may reduce the risk of severe retinopathy in VLBW infants. *Pediatrics.* 2011;127:223–228.

69. Yeh SL, Chang KY, Huang PC, Chen WJ. Effects of n-3 and n-6 fatty acids on plasma eicosanoids and liver antioxidant enzymes in rats receiving total parenteral nutrition. *Nutrition.* 1997;13:32–36.

70. Clandinin MT, Van Aerde JE, Merkel KL, et al. Growth and development of preterm infants fed infant formulas containing docosahexaenoic acid and arachidonic acid. *J Pediatr.* 2005;146:461–468.

71. Makrides M, Gibson RA, McPhee AJ, et al. Neurodevelopmental outcomes of preterm infants fed high-dose docosahexaenoic acid: a randomized controlled trial. *JAMA.* 2009;301:175–182.

72. Simmer K, Patole SK, Rao SC. Longchain polyunsaturated fatty acid supplementation in infants born at term. *Cochrane Database Syst Rev.* 2008;(1):CD000376.

73. Sullivan S, Schanler RJ, Kim JH, et al. An exclusively human milk-based diet is associated with a lower rate of necrotizing enterocolitis than a diet of human milk and bovine milk-based products. *J Pediatr.* 2010;156:562–567.e1.

74. Patole SK, de Klerk N. Impact of standardised feeding regimens on incidence of neonatal necrotising enterocolitis: a systematic review and meta-analysis of observational studies. *Arch Dis Child Fetal Neonatal Ed.* 2005;90:F147–F151.

75. Paquette L, Friedlich P, Ramanathan R, Seri I. Concurrent use of indomethacin and dexamethasone increases the risk of spontaneous intestinal perforation in very low birth weight neonates. *J Perinatol.* 2006;26:486–492.

76. Mihatsch WA, von Schoenaich P, Fahnenstich H, et al. The significance of gastric residuals in the early enteral feeding advancement of extremely low birth weight infants. *Pediatrics.* 2002;109:457–459.

77. Premji S, Chessell L. Continuous nasogastric milk feeding versus intermittent bolus milk feeding for premature infants less than 1500 grams. *Cochrane Database Syst Rev.* 2003;(1):CD001819.

78. El-Dib M, Narang S, Lee E, Massaro AN, Aly H. Red blood cell transfusion, feeding and necrotizing enterocolitis in preterm infants. *J Perinatol.* 2011;31:183–187.

79. Singh R, Visintainer PF, Frantz ID, 3rd, et al. Association of necrotizing enterocolitis with anemia and packed red blood cell transfusions in preterm infants. *J Perinatol.* 2011;31:176–182.

80. Bin-Nun A, Bromiker R, Wilschanski M, et al. Oral probiotics prevent necrotizing enterocolitis in very low birth weight neonates. *J Pediatr.* 2005;147:192–196.

81. Lin HC, Hsu CH, Chen HL, et al. Oral probiotics prevent necrotizing enterocolitis in very low birth weight preterm infants: a multicenter, randomized, controlled trial. *Pediatrics.* 2008;122:693–700.

82. Deshpande G, Rao S, Patole S, Bulsara M. Updated meta-analysis of probiotics for preventing necrotizing enterocolitis in preterm neonates. *Pediatrics.* 2010;125:921–930.

83. Neu J. Routine probiotics for premature infants: let's be careful! *J Pediatr.* 2011;158:672–674.

84. Wang H, Khaoustov VI, Krishnan B, et al. Total parenteral nutrition induces liver steatosis and apoptosis in neonatal piglets. *J Nutr.* 2006;136:2547–2552.

85. Shulman RJ, Schanler RJ, Lau C, Heitkemper M, Ou CN, Smith EO. Early feeding, antenatal glucocorticoids, and human milk decrease intestinal permeability in preterm infants. *Pediatr Res.* 1998;44:519–523.

86. Havranek T, Johanboeke P, Madramootoo C, Carver JD. Umbilical artery catheters do not affect intestinal blood flow responses to minimal enteral feedings. *J Perinatol.* 2007;27:375–379.

87. Bellander M, Ley D, Polberger S, Hellstrom-Westas L. Tolerance to early human milk feeding is not compromised by indomethacin in preterm infants with persistent ductus arteriosus. *Acta Paediatr.* 2003;92:1074–1078.

88. Flint A, New K, Davies MW. Cup feeding versus other forms of supplemental enteral feeding for newborn infants unable to fully breastfeed. *Cochrane Database Syst Rev.* 2007;(2):CD005092.

Section II

Organ Systems

CHAPTER 12

CHAPTER 12

Part A: Nervous System

Neonatal Encephalopathy

Abbot R. Laptook

INTRODUCTION

Neonatal encephalopathy is an important clinical condition with which all providers of newborn care should be familiar. It is a condition that is defined and characterized by the findings on physical examination and includes combinations of abnormalities in level of consciousness, muscle tone, activity, reflexes, brainstem function/breathing patterns, seizures, and ability to feed. In the past, these findings have been equated with hypoxia-ischemia or asphyxia as an etiology; however, more comprehensive assessments of neonatal encephalopathy indicated that a casual relationship between encephalopathy and hypoxia-ischemia is not as common as previously thought. What has emerged is the concept that neonatal encephalopathy is a phenotype for a broad array of potential diagnoses in the neonatal period and is without any preconceived implications regarding the timing of events that precipitate neonatal encephalopathy. The term neonatal rather than newborn encephalopathy is more appropriate because this is a condition that may be present at birth or develop at some time after birth. Thus, the objectives of this chapter are to provide an overview of

1. Epidemiology of neonatal encephalopathy
2. Outcome of infants with neonatal encephalopathy
3. Spectrum of diagnoses that may be associated with neonatal encephalopathy

INCIDENCE OF NEONATAL ENCEPHALOPATHY

Meaningful information regarding the incidence of neonatal encephalopathy can only be derived from population-based studies. This type of study avoids referral bias because hospital-based (even tertiary hospitals) studies represent referral centers. Other methodological considerations include case ascertainment (retrospective reviews without clear definitions vs prospective data collection with a priori definitions) and use of the appropriate denominator of infants at risk for neonatal encephalopathy.[1] Estimates of the incidence of neonatal encephalopathy prior to the mid-1990s have been limited to small studies that were not population based and focused on intrapartum events to determine the presence or absence of hypoxia-ischemia. Since that time, there have been 3 population-based studies to examine the epidemiology of neonatal encephalopathy, but all represent work from more than 10 years ago.

A population-based, unmatched, case-control study was performed between 1993 and 1995 of infants with encephalopathy born in Western Australia around the metropolitan area of Perth.[2] All cases of moderate or severe encephalopathy were referred to 1 of 2 tertiary neonatal intensive care units. This investigation focused on term infants in the first week of life using predetermined inclusion criteria of encephalopathy. Inclusion criteria were purposefully broad and included any 2 of specific variables, which needed to last more than 24 hours (abnormal consciousness, difficulty maintaining respirations of a presumed central origin, difficulty feeding, or abnormal tone and reflexes) or seizures alone. Deaths in the first week of life were reviewed to avoid exclusion of infants dying prior to transfer with evidence of encephalopathy. During the study interval, 164 cases of neonatal encephalopathy were identified. The incidence of neonatal encephalopathy was 3.8 per 1000 live term births (95% confidence interval, 3.2–4.4).

During the same years, 1993–1995, a population-based assessment of neonatal encephalopathy was conducted in the Thames region of the United Kingdom.[3] Term infants were identified if they fulfilled deliberately overinclusive criteria similar to those of Badawi et al.[2] Infants with trisomy 21 were excluded unless they fulfilled inclusion criteria that could not be attributable to trisomy 21; although this presumably represents a small number of infants, it is unclear how it was determined if infants with trisomy 21 were excluded. There were 150 cases of neonatal encephalopathy identified during a study period with 57,159 term births, including 97 term stillbirths. Based on these data, the incidence of neonatal encephalopathy was 2.62 per 1000 term births (95% confidence interval, 2.20–3.04). A subsequent observational population-based study was conducted in 2000 from the North Pas-de-Calais area of France.[4] This region is well organized for perinatal services, and the study was planned with input from individuals from all level II and III centers. Cases were term infants in the first week of life who fulfilled inclusion criteria of Badawi et al.[2] Infants with chromosomal abnormalities recognizable at birth, open neural tube defects, or neonatal abstinence syndrome were excluded. Deaths caused by medical termination of pregnancy and deaths occurring in the peripartum period or the first week of life were reviewed. There were 90 infants who fulfilled the inclusion criteria for neonatal encephalopathy, which led to an incidence of 1.64 per 1000 term live births (95% confidence interval, 1.30–1.98). Medical terminations of pregnancy were performed in 23 pregnancies, and if all infants were assumed to have survived and developed encephalopathy, the incidence would be 2.06 per 1000 term live births (95% confidence interval, 1.68–2.44).

None of the studies mentioned provided any information on mild encephalopathy and only focused on cases recognizable at birth or shortly thereafter (first week of life). The available data indicate that even among population-based studies there is a broad range of incidence for moderate and severe neonatal encephalopathy that spans from 1.64 to 3.8 per 1000 term births. Differences in case ascertainment and exclusion criteria may contribute to the differences, but it is unclear whether other factors may be of importance. Other considerations include population differences (eg, genetic susceptibility/resistance to hypoxia-ischemia) and access/quality of the obstetric care, assuming that at least some causes of neonatal encephalopathy are modifiable (see below). Temporal trends in the incidence of neonatal encephalopathy that may reflect population characteristics, care practices, or environmental exposures may also contribute.

A major gap in knowledge is the lack of information regarding risk factors and incidence of neonatal encephalopathy in preterm infants. The neurologic findings that are used to characterize encephalopathy pose a challenge for preterm infants compared to term counterparts. Preterm infants have systematic developmental differences in level of alertness, primitive reflexes, tone, and posture that modify the neurological examination compared to a term infant. Specifically, hypotonia is common to preterm infants and is expected for infants less than 30 weeks' gestation,[5] pupil reaction to light begins to appear at 30 weeks' gestation but is not present consistently until approximately 32 to 35 weeks,[6] and the Moro reflex displays gradual incorporation of all its components (extension and abduction of the upper extremities, followed by adduction at the shoulder) when comparing extreme, moderate, and late preterm infants.[5] Neurological findings characteristic of healthy preterm infants may represent abnormalities in term infants. In addition, some neurological findings (eg, tone, level of alertness) may be influenced by common morbidities of prematurity, such as respiratory distress syndrome. Systematic evaluations of the neurological examination among preterm infants who are thought to have evidence of encephalopathy have not been performed. Even reports that focused on hypoxic-ischemic encephalopathy in preterm infants have not addressed the neurological examination findings.[7]

RISK FACTORS FOR NEONATAL ENCEPHALOPATHY

Enrollment of 400 control term infants (enrolled without matching) from the Perth region population study of neonatal encephalopathy allowed comparison with cases of encephalopathy and provided insight into risk factors associated with this condition.[2] Multiple variables were examined from before conception, the antepartum and intrapartum periods, and infant characteristics. Variables with the strongest association with neonatal encephalopathy (adjusted odds ratio > 5) included older maternal age (30–34 and ≥ 35 years of age), late or no antenatal care, maternal thyroid disease, severe preeclampsia, postdates (gestational age of 42 weeks), and severe growth restriction (birth weight < 3%). A wide number of other sociodemographic and antepartum variables were associated with newborn encephalopathy but with lower odds ratios. Biologically plausible pathways that culminate with encephalopathy could be postulated to incorporate many of these risk factors. For example, older maternal age, severe preeclampsia, and maternal thyroid disease could be associated with placental pathology and associated intrauterine growth restriction. The growth-restricted infant may in turn have poor tolerance of the stress of labor.

Based on these associations, the same authors postulated a number of different pathways to the development of neonatal encephalopathy.[8] Risk factors present in the antepartum period support a potential two-hit hypothesis by which vulnerability of the fetus is increased secondary to the risk factors and, when combined with an intrapartum insult, may result in encephalopathy. Alternatively, a catastrophic/sentinel event during the intrapartum interval (acute abruptio placenta, ruptured uterus) may be sufficient to result in encephalopathy. A third but less-common possibility is that antepartum risk factors result in brain injury remote from the intrapartum period and result in encephalopathy.

OUTCOME OF INFANTS WITH NEONATAL ENCEPHALOPATHY

The same methodological issues that have an impact on the incidence of neonatal encephalopathy have similar relevance and importance for determining an unbiased estimate of its outcome. The largest and most comprehensive follow-up study was performed in Western Australia and included infants from the population-based incidence study from the Perth region[2] but was extended[9] from 1993 to 1996. This study enrolled 276 term infants with moderate and severe encephalopathy and 564 unmatched term control infants. Assessments were performed at an average age of 16 months and included the Griffiths Mental Developmental Scales and determinations of cerebral palsy. Encephalopathy was graded as moderate or severe based on Sarnat scoring.[10] The results are summarized in Table 12-1; of the 276 cases of encephalopathy, 34 died prior to follow-up, and 81% of eligible infants were assessed developmentally. Of the 564 control infants, 1 infant died, and 79% were assessed developmentally. Overall, 39% of infants with encephalopathy had a poor outcome as defined by death, cerebral palsy, or a developmental delay compared with 2.7% of the control subjects. As expected among infants with encephalopathy, a poor outcome was more frequent with severe (62%) compared to moderate (25%) encephalopathy. Data provided in this report represent a group outcome and are irrespective of the cause of encephalopathy.

Table 12-1 Outcome Following Neonatal Encephalopathy[a]

	Cases (%)	Controls (%)
Died	14	0.2
Cerebral palsy, then died	3	0
Cerebral palsy surviving	10	0
Below Griffiths cutoff	11	2.5
Alternative assessment abnormal	1	0
Normal Griffiths	61	97.3

Outcomes were assessed at a median of 16 months for infants of a population-based case-control study from Western Australia.[9] The Griffiths General Quotient (GQ) score data for the control subjects were normally distributed. The mean and standard deviation were calculated for the control subjects, and a cutoff of 2 standard deviations was used to identify subjects in both groups with developmental delay.
[a]Adapted from Figure 3 of Dixon et al.[9]

Follow-up of infants from the population study conducted in France indicated similar outcomes for infants with encephalopathy. Specifically, 27% of the infants died, and there was a 42% overall incidence of death or a severe disability at 2 years of age.[4] Loss to follow-up was minimal at 4.4%. However, follow-up evaluations were not as systematic as the Western Australian study and included standard clinical and neurological evaluations until 2 years of age without formal testing of cognitive functions. Disability was ascertained from registries for the region, which included all handicapped children requiring special education. Similarly, follow-up from the Thames region of the United Kingdom reported that death or disability (cerebral palsy or other impairments) occurred in 34% of infants with neonatal encephalopathy.[3] Follow-up information was obtained from the records of pediatricians; infants who were lost to follow-up per the pediatrician or were seen at less than 15 months ($n = 32$) were presumed to be normal for this report.

Characterization of the outcome of neonatal encephalopathy by the putative underlying etiology is a complex of issues leading to a mix of approaches in the literature. Results from Western Australia did not present defined causative groups but rather classified risk factors into preconceptional, antepartum, and intrapartum periods.[9] Of note, only 4% of encephalopathy cases were associated solely with intrapartum risk factors (factors with odds ratios ≥ 3 included occipito-posterior position, maternal pyrexia, cord prolapse, shoulder dystocia, and acute intrapartum events [avulsed cord, ruptured uterus, hemorrhage, maternal seizures]). In contrast, 29% of encephalopathy cases had both antepartum risk factors and intrapartum markers, supporting the notion of the two-hit hypothesis discussed previously. Thus, almost 70% of encephalopathy cases had no evidence of intrapartum hypoxia; these results question prevalent thinking that most risk factors for newborn encephalopathy occur in the intrapartum period. This approach acknowledges the difficulty in assigning cause to an infant with encephalopathy. Consider the infant born by emergent cesarean section for a nonreassuring fetal heart pattern after a labor complicated by chorioamnionitis and fever; if this infant has poor respiratory effort and muscle tone and bradycardia at birth, requires resuscitation, has a mixed acidemia at birth (metabolic and respiratory abnormalities), and demonstrates encephalopathy in the immediate newborn period, is the etiology infection, inflammation, or hypoxia-ischemia? If infection leads to inflammation, which in turn increases the vulnerability of the fetus to hypoxia-ischemia during labor, what is the correct assignment of causation? Based on these considerations, many investigators have made cogent arguments for using the term *neonatal encephalopathy* and avoiding hypoxic-ischemic encephalopathy.[11]

In contrast to the approach discussed, some follow-up reports have attempted to assign a cause for encephalopathy.[4] For example, in the population study conducted in France, the most common etiology of encephalopathy was perinatal hypoxia-ischemia occurring in the intrapartum period.[4] This was causative in 52% of encephalopathy cases (isolated in 77%, associated with another diagnosis in 17%, and with intrauterine growth retardation [IUGR] in 6%). Other etiologies included infection, intracranial hemorrhage, structural brain defects, genetic syndromes, inborn errors of metabolism, and other poorly defined causes.

RATIONALE FOR ESTABLISHING THE ETIOLOGY OF NEWBORN ENCEPHALOPATHY

Assignment of cause for cases of encephalopathy is controversial, and much of this stems from the challenges of making a diagnosis of perinatal asphyxia. Given the last concerns, is it important to determine the underlying etiology for cases of encephalopathy? Determination of etiology is critical only if there are potential modifiable causes of encephalopathy. There are many causes of newborn encephalopathy (Table 12-2), and some have specific treatments that alter outcome. The importance of establishing a cause for encephalopathy is best appreciated for infants with encephalopathy presumed to be of hypoxic-ischemic origin because there is an available therapy. Hypothermia is a proven therapy for late preterm and term infants with this condition, and its use is associated with a reduction in the composite outcome of death or disability assessed at 18–22 months.[12] The clinical evidence to support

Table 12-2 Causes of Newborn Encephalopathy

Hypoxia-ischemia
Stroke
Sepsis/inflammatory response syndrome
Intracranial hemorrhage
Inborn errors of metabolism
Structural brain abnormalities
Bilirubin toxicity
Drug effects

the efficacy of therapeutic hypothermia culminated approximately 20 years of investigative work spanning the original laboratory observations in adult rodents,[13] confirmation of similar observations in perinatal animals,[14–16] and ultimately pilot studies followed by efficacy trials as summarized in a recent meta-analysis.[17]

Estimates for the number of infants who could be potential candidates for therapeutic hypothermia can be derived from available statistics. If one uses 4 million births per year in the United States and assumes that 88% are greater than or equal to 36 weeks' gestation, there would be 3.52 million births. A population-based incidence of newborn encephalopathy in the United States is unknown, but using the range available in the literature (1.6–3.8/1000 term births[2,4]), there could be approximately 5600–13,400 infants with encephalopathy. If one applies an etiologic fraction for hypoxia-ischemia between 30% and 50% among newborns with encephalopathy, there will be a minimum of 1690 to a maximum of 6700 infants as potential candidates for therapy. Although this number of infants may appear small compared to the burden of other morbidities emanating from the neonatal period (eg, bronchopulmonary dysplasia), this group of infants may have lifelong medical care needs and frequent access to subspecialty health care providers.

Given the importance of ensuring that modifiable causes of encephalopathy are or are not a concern shortly after birth, the following sections provide brief overviews of specific causes for newborn encephalopathy.

SPECIFIC ETIOLOGIES OF NEONATAL ENCEPHALOPATHY

Encephalopathy of Hypoxic-Ischemic Origin

Establishing a diagnosis of encephalopathy associated with hypoxia-ischemia shortly after birth can be challenging. Terminology is important because hypoxia-ischemia is used interchangeably with perinatal asphyxia in clinical practice. Hypoxia is a low content of oxygen in the blood; ischemia represents a reduction in blood flow to tissues. Ischemia in turn can be partial or complete in extent and can be focal or global with regard to regional brain involvement. Hypoxia and ischemia are used together because each component may result in the other. In contrast, asphyxia indicates an impairment of gas exchange and is characterized by anoxia and extremes of hypercapnia. In the clinical setting, asphyxia is more commonly partial in severity, resulting in hypoxia with more moderate increases in CO_2 tension and, if prolonged or acutely severe, can result in ischemia. The potential modulating effects of hypercapnia are frequently overshadowed by hypoxia and ischemia.[18,19] Translating this potential broad range of physiological perturbations into robust, easily applied, clinical criteria that accurately predict brain injury later in childhood has been the subject of intense perinatal research. In clinical practice, we do not have tools to readily assess blood flow to the brain or rapid insights into the integrity of the brain tissue after an apparent hypoxic-ischemic or asphyxia episode.

The clinician is left with examining clinical history, signs or symptoms, laboratory markers, and imaging that support a recent event and its impact on the newborn. An approach to diagnose encephalopathy of hypoxic-ischemic origin has emerged and includes identification of an event that can impair fetal gas exchange or evidence of altered fetal gas exchange. The newborn in turn needs to demonstrate biologic effects consistent with impaired gas exchange. Thus, a sequence needs to be established of a predisposing event; impairment of gas exchange (or markers of such events); depression at birth, usually with the need for resuscitation; abnormalities of the neurological examination; evidence of organ system involvement

not related to the central nervous system (CNS); and the absence of other etiologies for the sequence of events. A number of different scoring systems with or without modification have been widely used in the literature[5,10,20] to characterize the neurological exam of infants with encephalopathy thought to be of hypoxic-ischemic origin. None of these scoring systems is specific for hypoxia-ischemia, and infants with other etiologies may have similar examination findings but without other supporting data. Challenges to clinicians trying to establish a diagnosis shortly after birth are that the neurological examination often changes during the early hours following birth, reflecting the effects of transient birth-associated physiological changes or the effects of maternal anesthesia and analgesia.

The recent randomized trials of therapeutic hypothermia provided valuable information on the outcome of infants with moderate to severe encephalopathy of a hypoxic-ischemic origin. There have been 6 large trials performed in late preterm (typically $\geq$ 36 weeks' gestation) or term infants with encephalopathy recognized within 6 hours of birth.[21-26] Although the criteria to establish encephalopathy of hypoxic-ischemic origin was not the same in each study, all employed an exposure-response sequence with markers of placental gas exchange combined with depression at birth usually requiring resuscitation and followed by evidence of encephalopathy. All of the studies used a similar primary outcome, which was the composite of death or neurodevelopmental disability, assessed typically at 18 months of age. The noncooled comparison group provided estimates of the outcome for moderate or severe encephalopathy in the absence of therapeutic hypothermia; results are summarized in Table 12-3.

Some caution is needed in comparing results among these trials because there are differences in specific inclusion criteria and adjunctive therapies

Table 12-3 Outcome of Noncooled Control Infants from Randomized Trials of Hypothermia

Trial	Author	Year	Noncooled, n	Death or Disability, n (%)	Death, n (%)	Survive with Disability, n (%)	Unimpaired, n (%)
CoolCap	Gluckman[21]	2005	118	73/110 (66%)	42/110 (38%)	21/68 (31%)	—
NICHD	Shankaran[22]	2005	106	64/103 (62%)	38/103 (37%)	25/65 (38%)	22/103 (21%)
TOBY	Azzopardi[23]	2009	102	86/162 (53%)	44/162 (27%)	42/117 (36%)	45/162 (28%)
nEuro	Simbruner[24]	2010	63	48/58 (83%)	33/58 (57%)	15/25 (60%)	—
Chinese	Zhou[25]	2010	94	46/94 (49%)	27/94 (29%)	19/67 (28%)	—
ICE	Jacobs[26]	2011	111	67/109 (66%)	42/109 (39%)	25/59 (42%)	22/97 (23%)

Abbreviation: NICHD, National Institute of Child Health and Human Development.

(eg, morphine for sedation and temperature control). Furthermore, none of these studies was population based. In spite of these differences, the composite primary outcome of death or severe disability for non-cooled infants spans a reasonably narrow range of 49% to 66% except for one outlier[24] (83%). The limitations of criteria to identify infants with a high certainty of brain injury[27] are illustrated by the 3 studies in which 21% to 28% of infants were assessed as without neurological impairment.

Neonatal Stroke

Strokes in the newborn period are commonly discussed in the differential of encephalopathy. The incidence of a vascular occlusive event, termed *ischemic perinatal stroke*, is estimated to range from 1 in 2300 to 1 in 5000 births and represents an important etiology for the development of neurological sequelae such as cerebral palsy.[28] Strokes can affect the newborn with manifestations in the in utero (fetal imaging required) period, neonatal period, or after 28 days of age. However, the timing of when strokes occur remains an important unresolved issue because clinically silent strokes may not become apparent until developmental deficits are observed later in childhood. Ischemic perinatal stroke can be arterial or venous sinus in origin, although the former is more common. The primary etiological hypothesis for arterial lesions is a cerebral embolic event originating from the placenta and passing through the patent foramen ovale into the aorta, where the branching of the left common carotid artery provides the most aligned anatomic path to the brain.[29]

Risk factors associated with stroke after adjustment for covariates include infertility, preeclampsia, prolonged rupture of membranes, and chorioamnionitis and were derived from a case-control study nested within a cohort of almost 200,000 infants born between 1997 and 2002 in the Kaiser Permanente Medical Program.[30] The risk of perinatal ischemic stroke increased with multiple risk factors. How these risk factors affect the placenta and fetus/newborn and link to ischemic perinatal stroke remains unclear.

The majority of infants with arterial ischemic strokes present acutely during the early neonatal period.[30] The presenting symptom is most commonly seizures (90%), frequently focal in type (74%) and often repetitive, with some infants progressing to status epilepticus based on 100 term infants with arterial ischemic stroke.[31] Other manifestations are recurrent apnea or desaturation events. Newborns who present soon after birth with arterial ischemic strokes commonly appear well and often have been triaged to a newborn nursery in spite of associated intrapartum events.[30,31] In contrast, there were 6 infants with acute focal stroke among the 124 infants examined in a prospective cohort of newborns with encephalopathy.[32] All 6 infants required resuscitation at birth and had clinical seizures on day 1 of life as the presenting manifestation. Magnetic resonance imaging (MRI) indicated arterial ischemic lesions in the distribution of the middle cerebral artery in 5 and venous thrombosis in 1. Unfortunately, there is limited description of the neurologic assessment between birth and the onset of seizures. More commonly, the distribution of injury helps distinguish a perinatal ischemic stroke from hypoxic-ischemic encephalopathy; strokes are usually unilateral in the distribution of a major cerebral artery,[33,34] and hypoxic-ischemic encephalopathy is typically bilateral with involvement of the deep gray matter and watershed injury.[35] However, it appears that both stroke and hypoxia-ischemia can be present in the same infant; it is unclear if this solely reflects a continuum of an ischemic lesion.

Sepsis and the Inflammatory Response Syndrome

Recognition of sepsis and its attendant encephalopathy is critical because it represents another modifiable cause of encephalopathy. Sepsis at birth occurs in approximately 1 per 1000 live births and is termed early-onset infection (blood culture positive occurring at < 72 hours of age[36]). In a cohort of almost 400,000 infants, rates for early-onset sepsis were higher in low birth weight infants (11/1000 live births) compared to infants with a birth weight greater than 2500 g (0.6/1000 live births). However, the absolute number of infected infants was greater among late preterm and term infants compared to preterm infants because of the larger number of births at mature gestations. Late-onset sepsis (culture-proven bloodstream infection after 3 days) is a problem encountered more frequently in low birth weight infants. In a cohort of 6215 very low birth weight infants in the National Institute of Child Health and Human Development (NICHD) Neonatal Research Network, late-onset sepsis occurred in 21% of infants with a birth weight below 1500 g.[37] The vast majority of neonatal infections are bacterial in origin, but herpes simplex and candida infections occur with lower frequency.

Both preterm and term infants presenting with symptoms of early-onset sepsis often manifest with respiratory distress. Respiratory distress is one of the most frequent manifestations of disease in the neonatal period and can be difficult to distinguish from noninfectious etiologies. Systemic activation of the innate immune system leads to hemodynamic instability, multiorgan system involvement, and higher morbidity and mortality than in the absence of this response. Activation of the immune response was originally described in adults as the systemic inflammatory response syndrome (SIRS[38]) and has subsequently been identified in the fetus (fetal inflammatory response syndrome, FIRS) with manifestations as part of early-onset sepsis.[39] Encephalopathy may complicate the clinical manifestations of early-onset sepsis but is frequently overlooked by the systemic inflammatory response and consequent cardiopulmonary instability.[40] In contrast, encephalopathy associated with late-onset sepsis is more easily identified because baseline knowledge of the infant's activity pattern is familiar to bedside providers; the initial manifestations of late-onset sepsis are often insidious, and lethargy, decreased activity, poor feeding, temperature instability, and new onset or exacerbation of apnea are often presenting manifestations.

Sepsis-associated encephalopathy represents diffuse cerebral dysfunction; however, the pathological events initiating the alterations in neurological state remain poorly defined. In the absence of meningitis, it is widely presumed that sepsis-associated encephalopathy is a consequence of a systemic inflammatory response to an infection that may have an impact on the brain by activation of cerebral endothelial cells, consequent changes in blood-brain barrier permeability, and ultimately actions of inflammatory cells in brain tissue.[40,41] Sepsis itself and its associated encephalopathy are modifiable by the use of antibiotics appropriate for the specific infection. However, specific therapy for sepsis is a time-sensitive intervention. For low-virulence bacteria such as *Staphylococcus epidermidis* causing late-onset infections in preterm infants, timely antibiotic therapy is usually sufficient to reverse the encephalopathy. However, the appropriate antibiotic for infections that are more fulminant may be insufficient even if initiated in a timely manner if the anti-inflammatory response is inadequate; such is the case with immune-compromised patients such as newborns and even more so with premature infants. Sepsis therefore is a modifiable cause of encephalopathy but with many caveats.

Intracranial Hemorrhage

The incidence of intracranial hemorrhage is well characterized in premature infants, in whom the bleeding arises from the germinal matrix and may extend into the ventricular system.[42] There has been increasing recognition that cerebellar hemorrhage may be more common in preterm infants than previously appreciated.[43] In contrast, the incidence or prevalence of intracranial hemorrhage in late preterm or term infants is not known. Unlike the preterm infant, the most common form of intracranial hemorrhage in the term infant is a subarachnoid hemorrhage. When intraventricular hemorrhages occur in term infants, they originate most commonly from the choroid plexus or as an

extension of thalamic hemorrhages.[44] Other forms of intracranial hemorrhage that occur in term infants are subdural hemorrhage and less commonly intraparenchymal hemorrhage.

Both preterm and term infants may not have any clinical symptoms of an intracranial hemorrhage even with moderate or severe extents of bleeding. With larger hemorrhages, the absence of symptoms is less common in term infants. Common symptoms of an intracranial hemorrhage are features of encephalopathy and include decreased level of consciousness, generalized hypotonia, apnea, and seizures. Apnea in a term newborn is highly suggestive of intracranial hemorrhage but may also be seen after strokes and as a manifestation of hypoxia-ischemia. Neurological manifestations of an intracranial hemorrhage may be apparent at birth or at an interval after birth, making it challenging to distinguish from hypoxia-ischemia or infection. The most important risk factor for intracranial hemorrhage is lower gestational age. When focusing on term infants, risk factors are broad and range from maternal conditions (eg, autoimmune disorders, cocaine exposure, etc); events related to labor and delivery (eg, prolonged labor, instrumented deliveries, etc); and newborn factors (eg, vascular malformations, vitamin K status, thrombocytopenia, bleeding disorders). Intracranial hemorrhage may be seen in infants with hypoxia-ischemia.[45] In an imaging study nested within the Total Body Hypothermia Trial, there were 131 infants with MRI images, and 47 (36%) had evidence of hemorrhage. The hemorrhage was subdural in 39 and was mild in extent in 29 and moderate in 10. Hemorrhage may also be a complication of infection, such as neonatal herpes encephalitis (Figure 12-1). In these cases, it is difficult to attribute an encephalopathy to either the underlying etiology or the secondary intracranial hemorrhage.

Inborn Errors of Metabolism

Inborn errors of metabolism are rare causes of neonatal encephalopathy, but a high index of suspicion is critical to make a diagnosis because intervention may have a large impact on prognosis. Acute encephalopathy caused by inborn errors of metabolism often manifest because of an accumulation of toxic metabolites or the absence of a specific product downfield from the metabolic defect. Metabolites that accumulate in the newborn frequently cross the placenta; thus, manifestations of encephalopathy will not be apparent at birth but occur at some later time, typically after buildup of a toxic metabolite, often in the first week of life.

Defects of protein metabolism are classic examples of inborn errors of metabolism and present after feedings have been established with sufficient protein intake. Ammonia is a normal biochemical product of protein

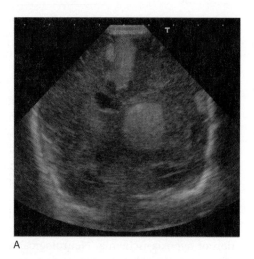 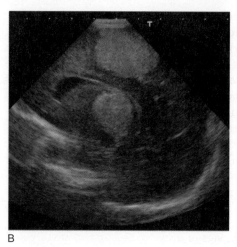

FIGURE 12-1 Coronal (panel A) and sagittal (panel B) views of a cranial ultrasound from a 30-day-old former 27³-week infant who was born to a 17-year-old primigavida mother after an uncomplicated pregnancy until rupture of membranes (11 hours duration) and cesarean delivery for nonreassuring fetal heart tones. The infant was intubated in the delivery room, had respiratory distress syndrome after birth, was extubated by day 3 of life, and received antibiotics for 48 hours following birth. On day of life 20, the infant developed increased apnea and bradycardia; evaluation confirmed herpes simplex encephalitis. This was complicated by increased echogenicity in the paramedian region of the left frontal parietal area and in the left thalamus. Subsequent magnetic resonance imaging confirmed that the regions of increased echogenicity were areas of hemorrhage.

catabolism, but in the presence of urea cycle defects and organic acidemias, hyperammonemia will occur. The mechanism by which hyperammonemia results in encephalopathy is not completely understood, but the target of elevated ammonia concentrations in the brain appears to be astrocytes.[46] A high concentration of ammonia promotes the conversion of glutamate to glutamine in astrocytes, reflecting the almost-exclusive localization of glutamine synthetase to this cell type; high concentrations of glutamine are associated with dysregulation of cell volume and cytotoxic edema, but causal relationships remain suspect.[47] Ammonia also induces oxidative stress and can generate free radicals.

An important consequence of oxidative stress is the induction of the mitochondrial permeability transition.[46] This is a calcium-dependent process associated with collapse of the inner mitochondrial membrane potential caused by opening of the permeability transition pore. Opening of the pores promotes mitochondrial dysfunction with increased free radical production and energy failure, both of which contribute to cytotoxic edema. Prolonged exposure to hyperammonemic encephalopathy is associated with impaired intellectual function; therefore, early diagnosis and therapy are critical.[48]

Other examples of inborn errors of metabolism that manifest with encephalopathy include lactic acidosis associated with either mitochondrial defects or defects in pryruvate metabolism, organic acidemias (eg, methymalonic, proprionic acidemia) secondary to branched-chain amino acid metabolism, and nonketotic hyperglycinemia, which presents with intractable seizures and progressive obtundation.[49] Hypoglycemia is common in the neonatal period; it may be asymptomatic or have nonspecific findings such as jitteriness, hypotonia, or lethargy; and if very severe or prolonged, seizures and encephalopathy may manifest. Hypoglycemia has diverse etiologies, some of which represent inborn errors of metabolism such as gluconeogenic defects (glycogen storage disease), fatty acid oxidation defects, and galactosemia.[50]

Other Etiologies for Neonatal Encephalopathy

Bilirubin toxicity represents a rare but preventable cause of encephalopathy; some hereditary causes of hyperbilirubinemia are so difficult to control that toxicity may be unavoidable. Similar to encephalopathy in general, the diagnosis of bilirubin encephalopathy is easier to establish in the late preterm and term infant compared to the preterm infant given multiple morbidities of prematurity. Neurological features of bilirubin toxicity are protean and include poor suck and feeding, lethargy, high-pitched cry, abnormal tone, opisthotonic posturing, seizures, and thermal instability. Key to establishing a diagnosis of kernicterus is the onset of neurological abnormalities in a neonate with a high bilirubin concentration who previously was neurologically appropriate.[51,52]

Structural abnormalities of the brain may be associated with an altered neurological state and encephalopathy. There are many abnormalities of brain development that are associated with clinically abnormal neurological features. Examples include holoprosencephaly, absence of the corpus callosum, Dandy-Walker malformation, neuronal proliferative disorders, and neuronal migrational disorders.[6] Many of these malformations will be suspected based on abnormalities of head size or associated dysmorphic features or abnormalities in non-CNS structures. Abnormalities of tone, seizures, decreased responsiveness, limited movement, and poor feeding are hallmarks of many of these conditions.

SUMMARY

Although estimates of the incidence of encephalopathy attributable to hypoxia-ischemia are variable among population-based studies, it is not a common diagnosis. Clinicians are further challenged in dealing with this diagnosis because the clinical manifestations are nonspecific, and it may be difficult to distinguish other nonencephalopathic diagnoses. The interval immediately following birth can be particularly difficult to establish a diagnosis because of transitional physiology, effects of maternal medications and anesthesia, and other potential neonatal morbidities manifesting at birth. Nevertheless, neonatal encephalopathy is an important diagnosis for clinicians to be aware of because some etiologies have interventions that can modify outcome.

REFERENCES

1. Kurinczuk JJ, White-Koning M, Badawi N. Epidemiology of neonatal encephalopathy and hypoxic-ischaemic encephalopathy. *Early Hum Dev.* 2010;86(6):329–338.
2. Badawi N, Kurinczuk JJ, Keogh JM, et al. Antepartum risk factors for newborn encephalopathy: the Western Australian case-control study. *BMJ.* 1998;317(7172):1549–1553.
3. Evans K, Rigby AS, Hamilton P, Titchiner N, Hall DM. The relationships between neonatal encephalopathy and cerebral palsy: a cohort study. *J Obstet Gynaecol.* 2001;21(2):114–120.
4. Pierrat V, Haouari N, Liska A, Thomas D, Subtil D, Truffert P. Prevalence, causes, and outcome at 2 years of age of newborn encephalopathy: population based study. *Arch Dis Child Fetal Neonatal Ed.* 2005;90(3):F257–F261.
5. Dubowitz LMS, Dubowitz V, Mercuri E. The neurological profile of normal preterm and term infants. In: *The Neurological Assessment of the Preterm and Full Term Newborn Infant.* 2nd ed. London, UK: Mac Keith Press; 1999:68–84.
6. Volpe JJ. *Neurology of the Newborn.* 5th ed. Philadelphia, PA: Saunders Elsevier; 2008.
7. Logitharajah P, Rutherford MA, Cowan FM. Hypoxic-ischemic encephalopathy in preterm infants: antecedent factors, brain imaging, and outcome. *Pediatr Res.* 2009;66(2):222–229.
8. Badawi N, Kurinczuk JJ, Keogh JM, et al. Intrapartum risk factors for newborn encephalopathy: the Western Australian case-control study. *BMJ.* 1998;317(7172):1554–1558.
9. Dixon G, Badawi N, Kurinczuk JJ, et al. Early developmental outcomes after newborn encephalopathy. *Pediatrics.* 2002;109(1):26–33.
10. Sarnat HB, Sarnat MS. Neonatal encephalopathy following fetal distress. A clinical and electroencephalographic study. *Arch Neurol.* 1976;33(10):696–705.
11. Dammann O, Ferriero D, Gressens P. Neonatal encephalopathy or hypoxic-ischemic encephalopathy? Appropriate terminology matters. *Pediatr Res.* 2011;70(1):1–2.
12. Edwards AD, Brocklehurst P, Gunn AJ, et al. Neurological outcomes at 18 months of age after moderate hypothermia for perinatal hypoxic ischaemic encephalopathy: synthesis and meta-analysis of trial data. *BMJ* 2010;340:c363.
13. Busto R, Dietrich WD, Globus MY, Valdes I, Scheinberg P, Ginsberg MD. Small differences in intraischemic brain temperature critically determine the extent of ischemic neuronal injury. *J Cereb Blood Flow Metab.* 1987;7(6):729–738.
14. Gunn AJ, Gunn TR, Gunning MI, Williams CE, Gluckman PD. Neuroprotection with prolonged head cooling started before postischemic seizures in fetal sheep. *Pediatrics.* 1998;102(5):1098–1106.
15. Laptook AR, Corbett RJ, Sterett R, Burns DK, Garcia D, Tollefsbol G. Modest hypothermia provides partial neuroprotection when used for immediate resuscitation after brain ischemia. *Pediatr Res.* 1997;42(1):17–23.
16. Thoresen M, Bagenholm R, Loberg EM, Apricena F, Kjellmer I. Posthypoxic cooling of neonatal rats provides protection against brain injury. *Arch Dis Child Fetal Neonatal Ed.* 1996;74(1):F3–F9.
17. Shah PS. Hypothermia: a systematic review and meta-analysis of clinical trials. *Semin Fetal Neonatal Med.* 2010;15(5):238–246.
18. Corbett RJ, Sterett R, Laptook AR. Evaluation of potential effectors of agonal glycolytic rate in developing brain measured in vivo by 31P and 1H nuclear magnetic resonance spectroscopy. *J Neurochem.* 1995;64(1):322–331.
19. Vannucci RC, Towfighi J, Heitjan DF, Brucklacher RM. Carbon dioxide protects the perinatal brain from hypoxic-ischemic damage: an experimental study in the immature rat. *Pediatrics.* 1995;95(6):868–874.
20. Thompson CM, Puterman AS, Linley LL, et al. The value of a scoring system for hypoxic ischaemic encephalopathy in predicting neurodevelopmental outcome. *Acta Paediatr.* 1997;86(7):757–761.
21. Gluckman PD, Wyatt JS, Azzopardi D, et al. Selective head cooling with mild systemic hypothermia after neonatal encephalopathy: multicentre randomised trial. *Lancet.* 2005;365(9460):663–670.
22. Shankaran S, Laptook AR, Ehrenkranz RA, et al. Whole-body hypothermia for neonates with hypoxic-ischemic encephalopathy. *N Engl J Med.* 2005;353(15):1574–1584.
23. Azzopardi DV, Strohm B, Edwards AD, et al. Moderate hypothermia to treat perinatal asphyxial encephalopathy. *N Engl J Med.* 2009;361(14):1349–1358.
24. Simbruner G, Mittal RA, Rohlmann F, Muche R. Systemic hypothermia after neonatal encephalopathy: outcomes of neo.nEURO.network RCT. *Pediatrics.* 2010;126(4):e771–e778.
25. Zhou WH, Cheng GQ, Shao XM, et al. Selective head cooling with mild systemic hypothermia after neonatal hypoxic-ischemic encephalopathy: a multicenter randomized controlled trial in China. *J Pediatr.* 2010;157(3):367–372. 372.e1–3.
26. Jacobs SE, Morley CJ, Inder TE, et al. Whole-body hypothermia for term and near-term newborns with hypoxic-ischemic encephalopathy: a randomized controlled trial. *Arch Pediatr Adolesc Med.* 2011;165(8):692–700.
27. Blair E. A research definition for 'birth asphyxia'? *Dev Med Child Neurol.* 1993;35(5):449–452.
28. Raju TN, Nelson KB, Ferriero D, Lynch JK. Ischemic perinatal stroke: summary of a workshop sponsored by the National Institute of Child Health and Human Development and the National Institute of Neurological Disorders and Stroke. *Pediatrics.* 2007;120(3):609–616.

29. Chabrier S, Husson B, Dinomais M, Landrieu P, Nguyen The Tich S. New insights (and new interrogations) in perinatal arterial ischemic stroke. *Thromb Res.* 2011;127(1):13–22.

30. Lee J, Croen LA, Backstrand KH, et al. Maternal and infant characteristics associated with perinatal arterial stroke in the infant. *JAMA.* 2005;293(6):723–729.

31. Chabrier S, Saliba E, Nguyen The Tich S, et al. Obstetrical and neonatal characteristics vary with birthweight in a cohort of 100 term newborns with symptomatic arterial ischemic stroke. *Eur J Paediatr Neurol.* 2010;14(3):206–213.

32. Ramaswamy V, Miller SP, Barkovich AJ, Partridge JC, Ferriero DM. Perinatal stroke in term infants with neonatal encephalopathy. *Neurology.* 2004;62(11):2088–2091.

33. Sehgal A. Perinatal stroke: a case-based review. *Eur J Pediatr.* 2012;171(2):225–234. Epub 2011 June 25.

34. Rutherford MA, Ramenghi LA, Cowan FM. Neonatal stroke. *Arch Dis Child Fetal Neonatal Ed.* 2012;97(5):F377–F384. Epub 2011 Aug 17.

35. Barkovich AJ, Hajnal BL, Vigneron D, et al. Prediction of neuromotor outcome in perinatal asphyxia: evaluation of MR scoring systems. *AJNR Am J Neuroradiol.* 1998;19(1):143–149.

36. Stoll BJ, Hansen NI, Sanchez PJ, et al. Early onset neonatal sepsis: the burden of group B streptococcal and *E. coli* disease continues. *Pediatrics.* 2011;127(5):817–826.

37. Stoll BJ, Hansen N, Fanaroff AA, et al. Late-onset sepsis in very low birth weight neonates: the experience of the NICHD Neonatal Research Network. *Pediatrics.* 2002;110(2 Pt 1):285–291.

38. American College of Chest Physicians/Society of Critical Care Medicine Consensus Conference: definitions for sepsis and organ failure and guidelines for the use of innovative therapies in sepsis. *Crit Care Med.* 1992;20(6):864–874.

39. Gotsch F, Romero R, Kusanovic JP, et al. The fetal inflammatory response syndrome. *Clin Obstet Gynecol.* 2007;50(3):652–683.

40. Wynn JL, Wong HR. Pathophysiology and treatment of septic shock in neonates. *Clin Perinatol.* 2010;37(2):439–479.

41. Siami S, Annane D, Sharshar T. The encephalopathy in sepsis. *Crit Care Clin.* 2008;24(1):67–82. viii.

42. Stoll BJ, Hansen NI, Bell EF, et al. Neonatal outcomes of extremely preterm infants from the NICHD Neonatal Research Network. *Pediatrics.* 2010;126(3):443–456.

43. Limperopoulos C, Benson CB, Bassan H, et al. Cerebellar hemorrhage in the preterm infant: ultrasonographic findings and risk factors. *Pediatrics.* 2005;116(3):717–724.

44. Gupta SN, Kechli AM, Kanamalla US. Intracranial hemorrhage in term newborns: management and outcomes. *Pediatr Neurol.* 2009;40(1):1–12.

45. Rutherford M, Ramenghi LA, Edwards AD, et al. Assessment of brain tissue injury after moderate hypothermia in neonates with hypoxic-ischaemic encephalopathy: a nested substudy of a randomised controlled trial. *Lancet Neurol.* 2010;9(1):39–45.

46. Norenberg MD, Jayakumar AR, Rama Rao KV, Panickar KS. New concepts in the mechanism of ammonia-induced astrocyte swelling. *Metab Brain Dis.* 2007;22(3–4):219–234.

47. Albrecht J, Norenberg MD. Glutamine: a Trojan horse in ammonia neurotoxicity. *Hepatology.* 2006;44(4):788–794.

48. Msall M, Batshaw ML, Suss R, Brusilow SW, Mellits ED. Neurologic outcome in children with inborn errors of urea synthesis. Outcome of urea-cycle enzymopathies. *N Engl J Med.* 1984;310(23):1500–1505.

49. Tan ES. Inborn errors of metabolism presenting as neonatal encephalopathy: practical tips for clinicians. *Ann Acad Med Singapore.* 2008;37(12 Suppl):94–93.

50. Cook P, Walker V. Investigation of the child with an acute metabolic disorder. *J Clin Pathol.* 2011;64(3):181–191.

51. AlOtaibi SF, Blaser S, MacGregor DL. Neurological complications of kernicterus. *Can J Neurol Sci.* 2005;32(3):311–315.

52. Connolly AM, Volpe JJ. Clinical features of bilirubin encephalopathy. *Clin Perinatol.* 1990;17(2):371–379.

Intracranial Hemorrhage

Lu-Ann Papile

INTRODUCTION

Periventricular/intraventricular hemorrhage (P/IVH) is the most common intracranial hemorrhage in premature infants. In the United States, approximately 14,000 very low birth weight (VLBW) infants are diagnosed with P/IVH each year; of these, approximately 7% will develop posthemorrhagic hydrocephalus (PHH). Numerous risk factors for developing P/IVH have been described, most of which are associated with premature birth. Because the majority of babies with P/IVH do not manifest clinical signs, the diagnosis relies on screening with noninvasive cranial imaging. There are no effective neonatal therapies to prevent P/IVH; however, antenatal steroids (ANSs) given to women who are anticipated to deliver preterm reduces the frequency and severity of P/IVH among their offspring. Infants with extensive P/IVH have an increased risk of later neurodevelopmental impairment, whereas those with less-extensive P/IVH may not.

EPIDEMIOLOGY

Since the 1990s, the overall incidence of P/IVH has dramatically decreased from 50% to 20%–25%; however, since the mid-1990s there has been little, if any, progress in reducing the overall incidence further.[1,2] This, in part, may be explained by an increase in the birth and survival rates of extremely low birth weight (ELBW) infants (birth weight ≤ 1000 g), the cohort at highest risk for developing not only P/IVH but also the complications associated with PI/VH.[3]

Distribution and Frequency

The site of origin of P/IVH typically is the microcirculation of the subependymal germinal matrix (see the discussion of pathogenesis). The hemorrhage may be isolated or may be accompanied by hemorrhage into the lateral ventricles that may spread throughout the ventricular system, through the foramina of Magendie and Luscka and into the basilar cisterns in the posterior fossa. The particulate matter in the intraventricular blood may obstruct the outflow tracks of the third and fourth ventricles or incite an obliterative arachnoiditis in the posterior fossa with obstruction of cerebrospinal fluid (CSF) flow, resulting in PHH. The reported overall incidence of P/IVH is approximately 20% for infants with a birth weight less than 2000 g and approximately 25% for those who weigh less than 1500 g.

The most frequently used description of P/IVH was developed in 1978 and demarcated P/IVH into 4 grades: grade I, isolated subependymal hemorrhage (Figure 13-1); grade II, intraventricular hemorrhage (IVH); grade III, IVH with cerebral ventricular dilation (Figure 13-2); and grade IV, parenchymal hemorrhage (Figure 13-3).[4] Although the description was intended to characterize findings on computed tomographic brain scans, it continues to be used to describe lesions visualized on cranial ultrasonography (CUS). Isolated subependymal hemorrhage (grade I) is the most common lesion detected (approximately 40% of lesions), while parenchymal hemorrhage (grade IV) is the least frequent (approximately 10% of lesions)[2] (Figure 13-4). Since the mid-2000s, the frequency of grade II P/IVH has markedly decreased. The most likely explanation relates to the increasing survival of

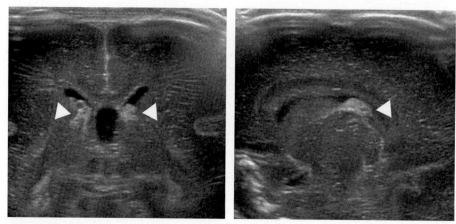

FIGURE 13-1 Subependymal germinal matrix hemorrhage (grade I periventricular/intraventricular hemorrhage) shown in the coronal and parasagittal planes (arrowheads). A homogeneously echogenic mass consistent with acute hemorrhage is noted in the caudothalamic groove. (Used with permission of Benjamin Brann IV, MD.)

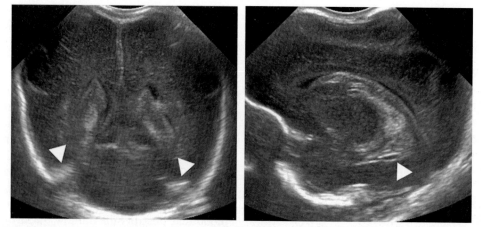

FIGURE 13-2 Intraventricular hemorrhage with ventricular dilation (grade III periventricular/intraventricular hemorrhage) is shown in the coronal and parasagittal planes (arrowheads). (Used with permission of Benjamin Brann IV, MD.)

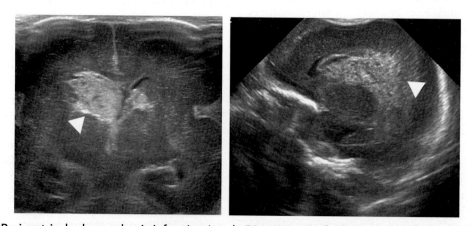

FIGURE 13-3 Periventricular hemorrhagic infarction (grade IV periventricular/intraventricular hemorrhage) is shown in the coronal and sagittal planes. A hemorrhagic infarction is noted adjacent to the left lateral ventricle that is filled with blood. The right lateral ventricle also contains a hemorrhagic clot. (Used with permission of Benjamin Brann IV, MD.)

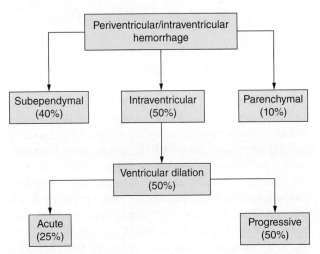

FIGURE 13-4 Distribution of periventricular/intraventricular hemorrhage (P/IVH) and subsequent development of ventricular dilation and posthemorrhagic hydrocephalus. (Used with permission of Lu-Ann Papile, University of Mexico. Unpublished personal data.)

extremely premature infants whose lateral ventricles are prominent to accommodate the choroid plexus.

The frequency of P/IVH is influenced by gestational age and birth weight. There is an inverse relationship of gestational age and P/IVH, with the most immature infants having the highest frequency and severity of P/IVH (Figures 13-5 and 13-6). Infants who weigh less than 751 g at birth have a 2-fold greater risk of having P/IVH than those whose birth weight is 1001–1500 g; the risk for infants who weigh 750–100 g is 1.5-fold greater.[2]

Although the overall reported frequency of P/IVH ranges from 20% to 25%, there is marked variability across centers. Centers participating in the National Institute of Child Health and Human Development Neonatal Research Network (NICHD NRN) reported frequencies of 7%–23% (grade I), 1%–11% (grade II), 3%–11% (grade III), and 3%–8% (grade IV).[2] Some of the difference can be attributed to interpretation

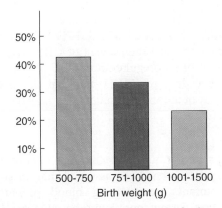

FIGURE 13-5 Frequency of periventricular/intraventricular hemorrhage (P/IVH) as a function of birth weight. (Adapted from Fanaroff et al.[2])

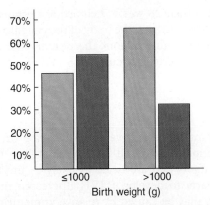

FIGURE 13-6 Frequency of grades I/II periventricular/intraventricular hemorrhage (P/IVH) (light) and grades III/IV P/IVH (dark) for infants 1000 g or less and greater than 1000 g birth weight. (Adapted from Fanaroff et al.[2])

of the head ultrasound (HUS) findings. When local interpretation of CUS was compared to that of central readers, the overall discrepancy in interpretation ranged from 21% to 28%, with the greatest disagreement occurring for grades I and II P/IVH (67% and 71%, respectively).[5] Other factors that might influence the frequency of P/IVH include population characteristics, neonatal practices, and obstetric management.

Risk Factors

Studies addressing the etiology of P/IVH have identified numerous environmental and medical risk factors including prematurity, male sex, respiratory failure and its attendant complication, and lack of exposure to ANS therapy.

Prematurity

The vast majority of P/IVH occurs in infants who are less than 32 weeks of gestational age. This relates to the prominence of the germinal matrix, a highly cellular and richly vascularized collection of neuronal-glial precursor cells in the developing brain where the majority of P/IVH originates. It is a source of neuronal precursors between 10 and 20 weeks of gestation, and during the third trimester provides glial elements that become oligodendroglia and astrocytes. The germinal matrix is most prominent between 20 and 25 weeks of gestation and involutes with increasing gestation as cells leave the region.[6] At 20–25 weeks of gestation, the germinal matrix surrounds the ventricular system and gradually involutes to reside over the body of the caudate nucleus between 25 and 28 weeks of gestation, the head of the caudate nucleus in the thalamus-striate groove between 28 and 34 weeks and usually dissipates at 36 weeks of gestation. The site of hemorrhage within the germinal matrix tends to shift with increasing gestational age. In infants less than 28 weeks, hemorrhage occurs mainly in the matrix overlying the body of the caudate nucleus, but in more mature infants, the primary site is at the head of the caudate nucleus at the level of the foramen of Munro.

Male Sex

Male infants have an overall higher rate of medical complications associated with prematurity than do female infants and are twice as likely as their female counterparts to develop P/IVH. Increased male vulnerability may be caused by relative immaturity of the male infant, increased genetic endowment related to redundancy in certain X-chromosome genes, genetic and environmental factors, or a combination of these.

PATHOGENESIS

The mechanism of P/IVH is multifactorial and most likely involves multiple environmental and genetic factors that affect the risk of P/IVH independently or interactively. They include immaturity of the cerebral vasculature, cerebral blood flow (CBF) dynamics, cardiovascular instability, and inflammatory and genetic factors.

Immaturity of the Cerebral Vasculature

Germinal Matrix Vasculature

Throughout gestation, the density and cross-sectional area of blood vessels in the human brain are largest in the germinal matrix.[7] This highly vascular network within the germinal matrix consists of high-caliber, irregular, thin-wall vessels that lack basement membrane deposition and glial end-foot ensheathing, both of which provide structural integrity to blood vessels.[8,9] The rich vascularity of the germinal matrix is essential to meeting the high metabolic demand of proliferating and maturing neuronal and glial precursor cells within the germinal matrix. However, the combination of a rich vascular network and the lack of structural integrity of these vessels enhances the propensity to hemorrhage.

Cerebral Venous System

The immature cerebral venous system may also contribute to the genesis of P/IVH. At 24 to 28 weeks of gestation, most of the cerebral venous blood flow is through the deep galenic system, which also drains the germinal matrix and most of the white matter. The major veins of the deep system pass directly through the germinal matrix, and any hemorrhage within the germinal matrix may result in venous congestion and stasis.

Alterations in Cerebral Blood Flow

Cerebral Pressure Autoregulation

The inability of preterm infants to maintain a relatively constant CBF despite fluctuations in arterial blood pressures (ie, cerebral pressure autoregulation) was first implicated in the genesis of P/IVH in the 1970s. Clinical studies using the xenon 133 clearance technique to measure CBF demonstrated a statistically significant correlation between CBF and arterial blood pressure in preterm infants, suggesting that cerebral pressure autoregulation in the preterm infant was impaired.[10] It was postulated that such impairment renders the preterm infant susceptible to both hypoperfusion with resultant ischemia and hyperfusion, which potentially could lead to rupture of germinal matrix vasculature.[11] The causal relationship of pressure passive CBF with P/IVH was reinforced by a subsequent study in which the effects of acute changes in blood pressure and partial pressure of carbon dioxide (Pco_2) on CBF were measured in preterm infants on mechanical ventilation using the xenon 133 clearance technique. P/IVH was noted only in infants who had pressure passive CBF and reduced CO_2 vasoreactivity.[12]

Near-infrared spectroscopy (NIRS) and spatially resolved spectroscopy (SRS) have been employed to continuously measure CBF. Used in conjunction with arterial blood pressure monitoring, NIRS measurements have been helpful in elucidating the role of cerebral pressure passivity in the genesis of P/IVH. An observational study using NIRS noted a high prevalence of cerebral pressure passivity among sick VLBW infants that waxed and waned over relatively short periods, being present 20% of the time and increasing in frequency with lower gestational age.[13] The investigators did not observe a relationship of CBF pressure passivity or systemic hypotension and P/IVH. In another observational study using SRS, impaired autoregulation of CBF was associated with mortality but not P/IVH.[14] Recent studies focusing on the magnitude of pressure passivity have shown that the magnitude is associated with P/IVH.[15] Thus, studies utilizing continuous monitoring of CBF suggest that impairment of autoregulation of CBF per se may not be an antecedent to P/IVH, but that the degree of impairment of autoregulation of CBF may be a factor.

Hemodynamic Factors

In the absence of bedside techniques to continuously measure CBF, it has been assumed that, in sick very preterm infants, maintaining blood pressure values between certain population-based normal limits would ensure adequate CBF and minimize the risk for cerebral injury. However, in clinical studies, neither mean blood pressure nor the duration of low blood pressure has been associated with P/IVH.[13,16] In 1 clinical study, CBF was significantly lower during the first 24 hours after birth in infants who incurred P/IVH compared to those who did not; however, mean arterial blood pressure was consistently higher.[17] Several investigators have suggested that cardiac function may be a more accurate measure of cerebral perfusion than blood pressure. Kluckow et al, using functional echocardiography to measure cardiac output and superior vena cava (SVC) blood flow demonstrated that low SVC flow is common in the first 24 hours after birth in extremely premature infants and is associated independently with subsequent P/IVH.[18] Additional studies for the same group indicated that systemic blood pressure measurements did not correlate with low-flow states in the SVC and were a poor predictor of P/IVH.[19,20] In subsequent follow-up studies, low SVC flow also was associated with poor neurodevelopmental outcome.[21,22] Kusaka and colleagues have measured CBF and left ventricular output simultaneously using multichannel NIRS and pulse dye densitometry with indocyanine green to show that there is a significant positive relationship between cardiac output and CBF, but not cardiac output and blood pressure.[23]

Both blood pressure fluctuations and a decrease in blood pressure variability have been implicated in the pathogenesis of P/IVH.[24] However, more recent studies using NIRS technology suggested that blood pressure variability is not a significant independent predictor for P/IVH.[13]

Biochemical Factors

Carbon dioxide is a potent and important mediator of CBF independent of autoregulation. Both hypocapnia and hypercapnia induce substantial alterations in CBF in newborn animal models. The vascular response to CO_2 is thought to be secondary to changes in intravascular pH. Hypercarbia as a risk factor for P/IVH was first proposed in the 1970s. Clinical studies using xenon 133 to measure CBF indicated that hypercarbia is associated with impaired cerebral autoregulation in ventilated VLBW infants and increased the risk of P/IVH.[25] It was postulated that infants who were hypercarbic were vulnerable to perturbations in blood pressure due to impaired autoregulation and at risk for P/IVH due to transmittance of arterial pressure to the capillaries in the germinal matrix. Any increase in blood pressure would cause CBF to increase in a passive manner due to ineffective vasoconstriction. Conversely, with hypotension, additional vasodilation might not be possible, resulting in pressure passive decreases in CBF. It was suggested that a possible intervention for the prevention of P/IVH would be to limit hypercapnia. However, there is extensive retrospective evidence that hypocapnia in preterm infants is associated with an increased risk of periventricular leukomalacia (PVL) and cerebral palsy,[26-28] possibly due to cerebral vasoconstriction, decreased CBF, and decreased cerebral oxygen delivery.

A more recent clinical study utilizing transcranial Doppler ultrasound suggested that autoregulation of CBF in ventilated preterm infants was intact at Pa_{CO_2} (partial pressure of carbon dioxide, arterial) values of 30 to 44 mm Hg, but there was a progressive loss of autoregulation between 45 and 60 mm Hg.[29] Because the study was cross sectional in design, data regarding brain injury are lacking. In a multicenter clinical trial of permissive hypercapnea ($Pa_{CO_2} > 52$ mm Hg) compared to routine ventilation ($Pa_{CO_2} < 48$ mm Hg), there was a small, but not significant, difference in the incidence of P/IVH and no difference in survival without neurodevelopmental impairment.[30] A single-center retrospective review of clinical and blood gas data during the first 4 days after birth suggested that extreme values of Pa_{CO_2}, whether high or low, and the wide variations in Pa_{CO_2} values for an individual infant are associated with grades III and IV P/IVH; the association persisted after adjustment for major perinatal variables.[31]

Genetic Factors

Since the mid-2000s, there has been an increasing interest in the potential role of genetic factors in the genesis of P/IVH. Twin studies suggested that shared environmental and genetic risk factors explain 41% of risk for developing P/IVH.[32] Observational studies of genetic association with P/IVH have focused primarily on genes related to inflammation or infection, mechanisms thought to be important in the pathophysiology of perinatal brain injury. Additional studies have focused on genes related to complement coagulation because of the possibility that increased fibrinolytic activity and decreased levels of clotting factors may contribute to the extent of the P/IVH lesion. *IL1β-511T*, *IL4-590T*, *IL6-174C*, and *TNF-α-308* have been associated with P/IVH.[33,34] The coagulation factor V Leiden mutation, a coagulation factor II, and prothrombin polymorphism have also been implicated.[35-39] Although factor V Leiden mutation is associated with an increased risk of P/IVH, several studies suggested that the P/IVH is limited to grades I and II.[35,38,39] However, many of the associations have not been evaluated in large cohorts of VLBW infants and have not been replicated across studies.

DIFFERENTIAL DIAGNOSIS

Germinal matrix hemorrhage and IVH are distinct entities that are readily detected with CUS. However, distinguishing parenchymal hemorrhage secondary to venous congestion (grade IV IVH) from hemorrhagic PVL may be challenging, and in some instances both lesions may be present.[40]

The typical HUS appearance of early parenchymal hemorrhage is that of a large, asymmetric, triangular, fan-shaped lesion that is located in the periventricular area just dorsal and lateral to the external angle of the lateral ventricle (Figure 13-2). Subependymal or IVH is almost always present on the same side as a parenchymal hemorrhage and is considered to be the underlying cause of venous compromise by compression of terminal veins underlying the germinal matrix. The lesion is usually unilateral and involves 2 or more lobar territories, typically the frontal and parietal regions. Bilateral lesions, although rare, are characterized by a grossly asymmetric appearance.[41] Approximately 50% of lesions are associated with a midline shift of cerebral structures. Eventually, the parenchymal hemorrhage evolves into multiple coalescent cysts or a large cyst that may or may not communicate with the lateral ventricle. In some cases, the lesion may resolve, resulting in ex vacuo dilation of the ipsilateral ventricle.

On CUS, hemorrhagic PVL typically appears as symmetrical bilateral lesions that are located in the regions adjacent to the trigone of the lateral ventricle or adjacent to the ventricles at the level of the foramina of Monro. The characteristic evolution of hemorrhagic PVL is the formation of multiple small cysts. The clinical usefulness of HUS criteria to distinguish grade IV P/IVH from hemorrhagic PVL has been evaluated. In a retrospective HUS study, 77% of lesions could be differentiated as either grade IV P/IVH or hemorrhagic PVL, with coexisting features noted in 11%. An additional 12% with persistent periventricular echo densities without cystic changes could not be classified.[40] In contrast, the results of a subsequent retrospective study indicated that only 53% of infants with white matter lesions on HUS could be allocated to periventricular hemorrhagic infarction or PVL. It was postulated that periventricular hemorrhagic infarction contributes to the risk of PVL.[42]

DIAGNOSTIC TESTS

Because most infants who develop P/IVH do not manifest clinical signs attributable to P/IVH, the diagnosis relies on screening with noninvasive cranial imaging. Some infants may exhibit subtle abnormalities in the level of consciousness, movement, tone, respirations, and eye movement; rarely, P/IVH will be accompanied by a catastrophic deterioration consisting of stupor, coma, decerebrate posturing, and generalized seizures. The majority of P/IVH is initiated within the first 24 hours after birth, and hemorrhages can progress over 48 hours or more. By the end of the first postnatal

week, 98% of P/IVH has occurred. The time frame in which P/IVH occurs is independent of gestational age, although extremely preterm infants tend to hemorrhage earlier than more mature infants. In 1 series, 62% of P/IVH in infants between 500 and 700 g birth weight occurred in the first 18 hours after birth.[43]

Cranial Sonography

In 2002, the American Academy of Neurology and the Child Neurology Society published a joint practice parameter for neuroimaging of the neonate.[44] In this report, screening with CUS was recommended for all preterm infants less than 30 weeks of gestational age at 2 time points. The first screening ultrasound was to be done at 7–14 days of age to detect P/IVH and the second ultrasound at 36–40 weeks' postmenstrual age to assess for cerebral ventriculomegaly and PVL. Because of its ease of use, CUS remains the imaging modality of choice to screen for P/IVH shortly after birth. Older studies have shown that the correlation of lesions noted on screening CUS and those detected at necropsy are excellent for both the frequency and extent of P/IVH.

Magnetic Resonance Imaging

Since the publication of the practice parameter in 2002, improvements in scanning procedures, the technique of bundling infants to minimize the use of sedative and anesthetic agents during a procedure, and the development of incubators compatible with magnetic resonance imaging (MRI) have enhanced the safety of MRI studies and, as a result, have led to its widespread use in ill neonates. Several observational studies have suggested that MRI is superior to CUS in the detection of brain lesions, especially in the extremely preterm infant, and should replace HUS as a screening tool for the detection of brain injury.[45,46] However, HUS data used for comparison in these reports were obtained early (2 to 6 weeks of age), precluding the inclusion of late CUS findings, such as diffuse gray and white matter loss and impaired brain growth, whereas the MRI data were obtained weeks later at term gestation. When comparing MRI and CUS evaluations done at term gestation and on the same day, cerebral lesions were detected equally well with both modalities.[47] A major drawback of using MRI routinely to diagnose neonatal brain injury is the lack of radiologists even in tertiary care centers with sufficient expertise in both neonatal neuroimaging and the interpretation of the MRI images. Based on available data, HUS remains the preferred modality for P/IVH screening shortly after birth. Whether CUS or MRI is used for the evaluation at 36 to 40 weeks' corrected age will depend on available equipment and expertise at a given center (see Figure 13-6).

MANAGEMENT

Management of P/IVH can be considered in terms of prevention of P/IVH and the treatment of PHH.

Prevention of P/IVH

The most effective strategy to prevent P/IVH would be to prevent preterm birth. Despite concerted efforts directed toward this end, there has been little change in the rate of premature birth, especially for infants who are less than 28 weeks of gestational age.[48] Strategies for the prevention of P/IVH have focused primarily on pharmacological interventions administered shortly before birth to women who are threatening premature birth or to premature infants shortly after birth (Table 13-1).

Antenatal Pharmacological Intervention

Because factors related to labor and delivery or the immediate postnatal period potentially may play a role in the pathogenesis of P/IVH, several investigators have explored the efficacy of interventions that could be instituted when premature delivery was imminent. Antenatal therapies that have been studied include glucocorticosteroids, phenobarbital, magnesium sulfate, and vitamin K.

Antenatal administration of glucocorticoids is the most effective antenatal strategy to prevent P/IVH. Interestingly, the initial report regarding the beneficial effect of corticosteroids for the prevention of P/IVH was based on meta-analysis of data from studies in which antenatal glucocorticoids were used to promote fetal lung maturation.[49] Numerous retrospective observational studies since the initial report have shown that ANSs reduce not only the overall incidence but also the severity of P/IVH. Multivariate analyses indicated that the beneficial effect of ANS on the incidence of P/IVH is independent of its beneficial effect of reducing respiratory disease. The mechanism of beneficial effect is not known, but it is thought to be related to maturation of brain structures and improved cardiovascular stability. The effectiveness of an ANS is greatest when a complete course is given; however, a partial course is also

Table 13-1 Effective Pharmacological Intervention for the Prevention of Periventricular/Intraventricular Hemorrhage

Antenatal therapy
Antenatal steroids (betamethasone and dexamethasone)
Postnatal therapy
Pancuronium bromide
Indomethacin

associated with a decrease in the frequency and severity of P/IVH. In addition, there does not appear to be any benefit accrued from repeated courses of ANS.[50] Retrospective analyses in which the outcome of infants exposed to antenatal betamethasone was compared to those exposed to dexamethasone suggested that betamethasone is associated with a reduced risk of death and less respiratory distress and chronic lung disease; however, there was no statistical difference in the frequency and severity of P/IVH.[51,52] Thus, it would appear that both pharmacological agents are equally effective in the prevention of P/IVH.

Coagulation disorders have been described in infants with P/IVH, and it is known that the function of vitamin K–dependent clotting factors in preterm infants is 30% to 60% of the function in adults. There have been 8 published trials of vitamin K given as an injection to women immediately before a very preterm birth. Comprehensive meta-analyses of these published trials showed no significant difference in the risk of having any grade of P/IVH between babies exposed to prenatal vitamin K and control babies.[53] The apparent lack of effect of vitamin K is most likely explained by poor placental transfer of vitamin K and therefore poor effect on fetal coagulation factors.

The beneficial effect of antenatal magnesium sulfate in the prevention of P/IVH is unproven. In several large randomized, placebo-controlled trials, antenatal magnesium sulfate did not reduce the incidence of P/IVH or PVL.[54,55] Despite this, there was a significant reduction in the risk of cerebral palsy among children who survived early preterm birth. The mechanism of neuroprotection is unknown.

Postnatal Pharmacological Intervention

Because a good proportion of P/IVH occurs within the first postnatal 12 hours after birth, postnatal strategies to prevent P/IVH need to be given at or shortly after birth to be effective. Pharmacological interventions that have been evaluated include phenobarbital, pavulon, vitamin E, ethamsylate, indomethacin, and ibuprofen. Of these, only pancuronium bromide and indomethacin therapy have proved effective in multiple clinical trials.

Before the availability of synchronous ventilation, it was noted that ventilated infants who "fought the ventilator" had a fluctuating pattern of CBF velocity that was associated with a high risk of developing P/IVH. Several small clinical trials were conducted after it was observed that abolishing this fluctuating pattern with muscle paralysis using pancuronium bromide markedly reduced the risk of developing P/IVH. A 2004 comprehensive review of published clinical trials using pancuronium bromide for short-term muscle paralysis of ventilated infants concluded that this intervention leads to a reduction in the incidence, but not the severity, of P/IVH.[55] However, since the studies were completed the use of synchronous and assist control ventilation has been widely implemented in the United States, making this strategy somewhat dated.

Initial trials of prophylactic indomethacin therapy to prevent P/IVH noted a significant decrease in the frequency and severity of P/IVH. The potentially beneficial effects of indomethacin include accelerated maturation of microvessels within the germinal matrix, alterations in CBF, and inhibition of the formation of free radicals. A recent detailed meta-analysis of published data of prophylactic indomethacin found no evidence of an effect on the overall incidence of P/IVH but did confirm a beneficial effect on the incidence of severe P/IVH.[56] However, despite the fact that indomethacin reduces the frequency of severe P/IVH, it does not improve the rate of survival without neurosensory impairment. Both mortality and neurosensory impairment in early childhood did not differ between children treated with prophylactic indomethacin and those who were not. It has been suggested that the beneficial effects of indomethacin prophylaxis may be restricted to male infants since secondary analyses of several studies have shown a differential effect of indomethacin by sex on the frequency of P/IVH.[57,58]

Posthemorrhagic Hydrocephalus

Prevention

Efforts to prevent the development of PHH have included repeated lumbar punctures at the time of diagnosis of IVH and the use of intraventricular fibrinolytic therapy in infants developing posthemorrhagic ventricular dilation. When repeated lumbar punctures were compared to conservative treatment, there was no difference in the relative risks for shunt placement, death, or disability.[59] Likewise, when intraventricular instillation of streptokinase was compared to conservative management of posthemorrhagic ventricular dilation, the numbers of deaths and infants who required the placement of a permanent shunt were similar.[60]

Management

Ventricular dilation occurs in approximately 50% of infants who develop an IVH (Figure 13-4). Approximately half of affected infants will undergo spontaneous arrest or resolution of the dilation; the other half will develop progressive ventricular dilation (ie, PHH) (see Figure 13-4). PHH may be communicating or noncommunicating. Noncommunicating PHH occurs when a large intraventricular clot or ependymal scarring impedes the flow of CSF through the outflow tracts of the lateral, third, and fourth ventricles.

Communicating PHH is thought to be secondary to an impairment of CSF absorption caused by an obliterative arachnoiditis at the posterior fossa or a chemical arachnoiditis caused by blood within the CSF.

Since progressive ventricular dilation typically occurs before there is clinical evidence of hydrocephalus (eg, increased rate of head growth and the presence of a full anterior fontanelle), early diagnosis is dependent on serial CUS evaluations (Figure 13-7). The main therapeutic dilemma in the management of ventricular dilation is identifying early which infants will develop PHH and will need intervention to minimize additional brain injury that may be caused by increasing distortion of the ventricles. However, because there are no universally accepted criteria for deciding when intervention is needed, the decision for treatment varies by center and surgeon and is generally dictated by local experience.

Despite many treatment options, there is no consensus on the management of PHH in VLBW infants. The large amount of blood and protein in the CSF, combined with the infant's small size, are deterrents to early ventriculoperitoneal shunt placement because of the high risk of blockage and infection. The most common initial approach to the management of PHH is the placement of a temporary CSF diversion device, usually either a ventriculosubgaleal (VSG) shunt, in which CSF is shunted into the subgaleal space of the scalp and absorbed into the bloodstream, or a ventricular reservoir that is intermittently tapped. In a large multicenter retrospective observational study, the use of VSG shunts was associated with a greater need for permanent CSF diversion compared to the use of intermittent tapping of ventricular reservoirs.[61] The rates of infection during temporization and for the initial 6 months after conversion to a ventriculoperitoneal (VP) shunt system were comparable for both groups.

OUTCOME

Prognosis can be considered in terms of short-term outcome, especially mortality, and the somewhat longer outcome of neurodevelopmental impairment in early childhood. The short-term outcome relates to the extent of the P/IVH and the degree of prematurity. The reported mortality rates for VLBW infants with isolated germinal matrix hemorrhages (grade I) are comparable to those of infants of the same gestational age without P/IVH. With both IVHs and normal ventricular size (grade II P/IVH) and IVHs with ventricular dilation (grade III P/IVH), the reported mortality rates are higher only for infants of extremely low gestational age. For those infants with P/IVH and parenchymal hemorrhage (grade IV P/IVH), the reported mortality rate is approximately 40%, a rate that is much higher than that for comparable infants without P/IVH.[62]

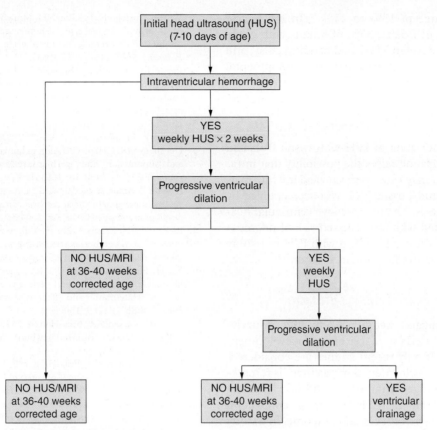

FIGURE 13-7 Management of periventricular/intraventricular hemorrhage. MRI, magnetic resonance imaging.

Although the spectrum and attendant complications of P/IVH have been well documented with non-invasive cranial imaging techniques, data regarding the impact of P/IVH on neurological and developmental outcome of affected infants are sparse. In addition, the heterogeneity between published studies makes interpretation of the data difficult. Two factors, the extent of hemorrhage and ventricular dilation, appear to be critical determinants of neurodevelopmental outcome.

Extent of Hemorrhage

In the majority of published studies, the incidence of neurodevelopmental impairment for infants who develop grades I or II P/IVH is essentially the same as that for infants with no evidence of P/IVH on CUS.[63–65] However, there are several reports that suggested the occurrence of these lesions is associated with a 2- to 5-fold higher odds of cerebral palsy and intellectual disability.[66–68]

Short-term outcome studies of preterm children who sustained a neonatal grade IV IVH (periventricular hemorrhagic infarction) have reported a high rate of cerebral palsy, ranging from 40% to 90%; however, there has been no consensus regarding cognitive outcome, with normal cognition noted in 20% to 79%.[69–72] Although available data on long-term outcome are sparse, published studies suggested that despite a high rate of cerebral palsy, the majority of affected children have limited functional impairment and attend regular education classes.[69,73] The discrepancy between outcome in early childhood and later childhood most likely relates to the shortcomings of infant neurodevelopmental testing. Because the successful completion of many test items relies heavily on intact motor function, the scores achieved by infants with motor impairment, such as cerebral palsy, underestimate their true ability and may lead to an unduly pessimistic view regarding their ultimate outcome. An additional finding that has not been emphasized is the risk for a visual field defect due to injury to the optic radiation. In 1 study, the frequency of a visual field defect was 25%.[74]

Acute Ventricular Dilation

Ventricular dilation can occur acutely, as seen with grade III P/IVH, or it may not be evident for weeks or months after birth. Later ventricular dilation may be progressive or nonprogressive. Nonprogressive ventriculomegaly is presumed to be a surrogate for white matter injury.

When the data from multiple published studies are combined, the pooled probability of an abnormal motor outcome when IVH is accompanied by acute ventricular dilation (grade III P/IVH) is approximately

26%, with a range of 13% to 45%.[75] In the largest published series of P/IVH, 35% of infants with grade III who did not develop PHH had cerebral palsy, and 55% were determined to have a neurodevelopmental impairment in early childhood.[72]

Nonprogressive Ventricular Dilation

The frequent association of IVH with cystic PVL and late ventricular dilation raises the possibility that intraventricular blood may cause periventricular white matter injury. In 1 study, cystic PVL was accompanied by IVH in 67% of cases.[76] Nonprogressive ventricular dilation was associated with an increased risk of neurodevelopmental impairment in infants with IVH in 1 study and impaired cognitive function in another.[77,78]

Progressive Ventricular Dilation

Historical data suggest that only 5% to 30% of surviving children with PHH were free of neurodevelopmental impairment. If only recent studies are considered, the rate of neurodevelopmental impairment is remarkably lower and ranges from 40% to 64%.[72,79] Among infants with PHH, there is a strong connection between the severity of P/IVH and outcome. In a study that included 128 infants with P/IVH who underwent surgical placement of a shunt, 60% of infants with grade III P/IVH and hydrocephalus were neurodevelopmentally impaired compared to 92% of infants with grade IV P/IVH and hydrocephalus.[72] A smaller study of 5- to 8-year-old children who required neurosurgical intervention for posthemorrhagic hydrocephalus as infants noted that none of the children with grade III P/IVH and 53% of those with grade IV P/IVH developed cerebral palsy.[79] The mean IQ of the cohort was 93.4, and 29% of the children had an IQ less than 85.

Comparison of children with and without PHH suggests that PHH per se may pose an additional risk for poor neurodevelopmental outcome beyond that associated with P/IVH. The rate of neurodevelopmental impairment for infants with uncomplicated grade III P/IVH was 55% compared to 78% for infants who had a shunt placed for PHH; the rates for infants with grade IV P/IVH were 63% and 92%, respectively.[72]

REFERENCES

1. Horbar JD, Badger GJ, Carpenter JH, et al; members of the Vermont Oxford Network. Trends in mortality and morbidity for very low birth weight infants, 1991–1999. *Pediatrics.* 2002;110(1 Pt 1):143–151.
2. Fanaroff AA, Stoll BJ, Wright LL, Carlo WA, et al. Trends in neonatal morbidity and mortality for very low birthweight infants; NICHD Neonatal Research Network. *Am J Obstet Gynecol.* 2007;196(2):147.el-8.
3. Wilson-Costello D, Friedman H, Minich N, Fanaroff AA, Hack M. Improved survival rates with increased neurodevelopmental disability for extremely low birth weight infants in the 1990's. *Pediatrics.* 2005;115(4):997–1003.
4. Papile LA, Burstein J, Burstein R, Koffler H. Incidence and evolution of subependymal and intraventricular hemorrhage: a study of infants with birthweights less than 1500 grams. *J Pediatr.* 1978;92(4):529–534.
5. Hintz SR, Slovis T, Bulas D, et al. NICHD Neonatal Research Network. *J Pediatr.* 2007;150(6):592–596.
6. Del Bigio MR. Cell proliferation in human ganglionic eminence and suppression after prematurity-associated haemorrhage. *Brain.* 2011;134(Pt 5):1344–1361.
7. Ballabh P, Braun A, Nedergaard M. Anatomic analysis of blood vessels in germinal matrix, cerebral cortex, and white matter in developing infants. *Pediatr Res.* 2004;56(1):117–124.
8. El-Khoury N, Braun A, Hu F, et al. Astrocyte end-feet in germinal matrix, cerebral cortex, and white matter in developing infants. *Pediatr Res.* 2006;59(5):673–679.
9. Xu H, Hu F, Sado Y, et al. Maturational changes in lamina, fibronectin, collagen IV, and perlecan in germinal matrix, cortex, and white matter and effect of bethamethasone. *J Neurosci Res.* 2008;86(7):1482–1500.
10. Lou HC, Lassen NA, Friis-Hansen B. Low cerebral blood flow in the hypotensive distressed newborn. *Acta Neurol Scand Suppl.* 1977;64:428–429.
11. Lou HC, Lassen NA, Friis-Hansen B. Is arterial hypertension crucial for the development of cerebral haemorrhage in premature infants? *Lancet.* 1979;1(8128):1215–1217.
12. Pryds O, Greisen G, Lou H. Friis-Hansen B. Heterogeneity of cerebral vasoreactivity in preterm infants supported by mechanical ventilation. *J Pediatr.* 1989;115(4):638–645.
13. Soul JS, Hammer PE, Tsuji M, et al. Fluctuating pressure-passivity is common in the cerebral circulation of sick preterm infants. *Pediatr Res.* 2007;61(4):467–473.
14. Wong FY, Leung TS, Austin T, et al. Impaired autoregulation in preterm infants identified by using spatially resolved spectroscopy. *Pediatrics.* 2008;121(3):e604–e611. Epub 2008 Feb 4.
15. O'Leary H, Gregas MC, Limperopolous C, et al. Elevated cerebral pressure passivity is associated with prematurity-related intracranial hemorrhage. *Pediatrics.* 2009;124(1):302–309.
16. Limperopoulos C, Bassan H, Kalish LA, et al. Current definitions of hypotension do not predict abnormal cranial ultrasound findings in preterm infants. *Pediatrics.* 2007;120(5):966–977.
17. Meek JH, Tyszczuk L, Elwell CE, Wyatt JS. Low cerebral blood flow is a risk factor for severe intraventricular haemorrhage. *Arch Dis Child Fetal Neonatal Ed.* 1999;81(1):F15–F18.
18. Kluckow M, Evans N. Relationship between blood pressure and cardiac output in preterm infants requiring mechanical ventilation. *J Pediatr.* 1996;129(4):506–512.
19. Kluckow M, Evans N. Low superior vena cava flow and intraventricular haemorrhage in preterm infants. *Arch Dis Child Fetal Neonatal Ed.* 2000;82(3):F188–F194.
20. Osborn DA, Evans N, Kluckow M. Hemodynamic and antecedent risk factors for severe intraventricular hemorrhage in premature infants. *Pediatrics.* 2003;112 (1 Pt 1):33–39.
21. Osborn DA, Evans N, Kluckow M, Bowen JR, Rieger I. Low superior vena cava flow and effect of inotropes on neurodevelopment to 3 years in preterm infants. *Pediatrics.* 2007;120(2):372–380.
22. Hunt RW, Evans N, Rieger I, Kluckow M. Low superior vena cava flow and neurodevelopment at 3 years in very preterm infants. *J Pediatr* 2004;145(5):588–592.
23. Kusaka T, Okubo K, Nagano K. Cerebral distribution of cardiac output in newborn infants. *Arch Dis Child Fetal Neonatal Ed.* 2005;90(1): F77–F78.
24. D'Souza SW, Janakova H, Minors D, et al. Blood pressure, heart rate, and skin temperature in preterm infants: associations

with periventricular haemorrhage. *Arch Dis Child Fetal Neonatal Ed.* 1995;72(3):F162–F167.

25. Lou HC, Lassen NA, Friis-Hansen B. Impaired autoregulation of cerebral blood flow in the distressed newborn infant. *J Pediatr.* 1979;94(1):118–121.

26. Greisin G, Trojaborg W. Cerebral blood flow, $PaCO_2$ changes, and visually evoked potentials in mechanically ventilated, preterm infants. *Acta Pediatr Scand.* 1987,76(3):394–400.

27. Okumura A, Hayakawa F, Kato T, et al. Hypocarbia in preterm infants with periventricular leukomalacia: the relation between hypocarbia and mechanical ventilation. *Pediatrics.* 2001;107(3):469–475.

28. Collins MP, Lorenz JM, Jetton JR, Paneth N. Hypocapnia and other ventilation-related risk factors for cerebral palsy in low birth weight infants. *Pediatr Res.* 2001;50(6):712–719.

29. Kaiser JR, Gauss CH, Williams DK. The effects of hypercapnia on cerebral autoregulation in ventilated very low birth weight infants. *Pediatr Res.* 2005;58(5):931–935.

30. Carlo WA, Stark AR, Wright LL, et al. Minimal ventilation to prevent bronchopulmonary dysplasia in extremely-low-birth-weight infants. *J Pediatr.* 2002;141(3):370–374.

31. McKee LA, Fabres J, Howard G, Peralta-Carcelen M, Carlo WA, Ambalavanan N. $PaCO_2$ and neurodevelopment in extremely low birth weight infants. *J Pediatr.* 2009;155(2):217–221.e1. Epub 2009 May 17.

32. Bhandari V, Bizzarro MJ, Shetty A, et al. Familial and genetic susceptibility to major neonatal morbidities in preterm twins. *Pediatrics.* 2006;117(6):1901–1906.

33. Baier RJ. Genetics of perinatal brain injury in the preterm infant. *Front Biosci.* 2006;11:1371–1387.

34. Harding DR, Dhamrait S, Whitelaw A, Humphries SE, Marlow N, Montgomery HE. Does interleukin-6 genotype influence cerebral injury or developmental progress after preterm birth? *Pediatrics.* 2004;114(4):941–947.

35. Göpel W, Kattner E, Seidenberg J, Kohlmann T, Segerer H, Möller J; Genetic Factors in Neonatology Study Group. The effect of the Val34Leu polymorphism in the factor XIII gene in infants with a birth weight below 1500 g. *J Pediatr.* 2002;140(6):688–692.

36. Komlósi K, Havasi V, Bene J, et al. Increased prevalence of factor V Leiden mutation in premature but not in full-term infants with grade I intracranial haemorrhage. *Biol Neonate.* 2005;87(1):56–59. Epub 2004 Sep 30.

37. Aronis S, Bouza H, Pergantou H, Kapsimalis Z, Platokouki H, Xanthou M. Prothrombotic factors in neonates with cerebral thrombosis and intraventricular hemorrhage. *Acta Paediatr Suppl.* 2002;91(438):87–91.

38. Göpel W, Gortner L, Kohlmann T, Schultz C, Möller J. Low prevalence of large intraventricular haemorrhage in very low birthweight infants carrying the factor V Leiden or prothrombin G20210A mutation. *Acta Paediatr.* 2001;90(9):1021–1024.

39. Ryckman KK, Dagle JM, Kelsey K, Momany AM, Murray JC. Replication of genetic associations in the inflammation, complement, and coagulation pathways with intraventricular hemorrhage in LBW preterm neonates. *Pediatr Res.* 2011;70(1):90–95.

40. Bass WT, Jones MA, White LE, Montgomery TR, Aiello F 3rd, Karlowicz MG. Ultrasonographic differential diagnosis and neurodevelopmental outcome of cerebral white matter lesions in premature infants. *J Perinatol.* 1999;19(5):330–336.

41. Bassan H, Benson CB, Limperopolous C, et al. Ultrasonographic features and severity scoring of periventricular hemorrhagic infarction in relation to risk factors and outcome. *Pediatrics.* 2006;117(6):2111–2118.

42. Kuban KC, Allred EN, Dammann O, et al. Topography of cerebral white-matter disease of prematurity studied prospectively in 1607 very-low-birthweight infants. *J Child Neurol.* 2001;16(6):401–408.

43. Perlman JM, Volpe JJ. Intraventricular hemorrhage in extremely preterm infants. *Am J Dis Child.* 1986;140(11):1122–1126.

44. Ment LR, Bada HS, Barnes P, et al. Practice parameter: neuroimaging of the neonate: report of the Quality Standards Subcommittee of the American Academy of Neurology and the Practice Committee of the Child Neurology Society. *Neurology.* 2002;58:1726–1738.

45. Woodward LJ, Anderson PJ, Austin NC, et al. Neonatal MRI to predict neurodevelopmental outcomes in preterm infants. *N Engl J Med.* 2006;355(7):685–694.

46. Mirmiran M, Barnes PD, Keller, et al. Neonatal brain magnetic resonance imaging before discharge is better than cranial ultrasound in predicting cerebral palsy in very low birth weight preterm infants. *Pediatrics.* 2004;114(4):992–998.

47. Horsch S, Skiold B, Hallberg B, et al. Cranial ultrasound and MRI at term age in extremely preterm infants. *Arch Dis Child Fetal Neonatal Ed.* 2010;95(5):F310–F314. Epub 2009 Oct 19.

48. Martin JA, Hamilton BE, Ventura SJ, et al. Births: final data for 2009. *Natl Vital Stat Rep.* 2011;60(1):1–70.

49. Crowley P, Chalmers I, Keirse I. The effects of corticosteroid administration before preterm delivery: an overview of the evidence from controlled trials. *Br J Obstet Gynecol.* 1990;97(1):11–25.

50. McKinlay CJ, Crowther CA, Middleton P, Harding JE. Repeat antenatal glucocorticoids for women at risk of preterm birth: a Cochrane Systematic Review. *Am J Obstet Gynecol.* 2012;206(3):187–194. Epub 2011 Jul 30.

51. Lee BH, Stoll BJ, McDonald SA, et al. Adverse neonatal outcomes associated with antenatal dexamethasone versus antenatal betamethasone. *Pediatrics.* 2006;117(5):1503–1510.

52. Feldman DM, Carbone J, Belden L, et al. Betamethasone vs. dexamethasone for the prevention of morbidity in very low-birth-weight neonates. *Am J Obstet Gynecol.* 2007;197(3):284.e1-4.

53. Crowther CA, Crosby DD, Henderson-Smart DJ. Vitamin K prior to preterm birth for preventing neonatal periventricular haemorrhage. *Cochrane Database Syst Rev.* 2010;(1):CD000229.

54. Doyle LW, Crowther CA, Middleton P, Marret S, Rouse D. Magnesium sulphate for women at risk of preterm birth for neuroprotection of the fetus. *Cochrane Database Syst Rev.* 2009;(1):CD004661.

55. Cools F, Offringa M. Neuromuscular paralysis for newborn infants receiving mechanical ventilation. *Cochrane Database Syst Rev.* 2005;(2):CD002773.

56. Fowlie PW, Davis PG, McGuire W. Prophylactic intravenous indomethacin for preventing mortality and morbidity in preterm infants. *Cochrane Database Syst Rev.* 2010;(7):CD000174.

57. Ment LR, Vohr BR, Makuch RW, et al. Prevention of intraventricular hemorrhage by indomethacin in male preterm infants. *J Pediatr.* 2004;145(6):832–834.

58. Ohlsson A, Roberts RS, Schmidt B, Davis P, et al. Male/female differences in indomethacin effects in preterm infants. *J Pediatr.* 2005;147(6):860–862.

59. Whitelaw A. Repeated lumbar or ventricular punctures in newborns with intraventricular hemorrhage. *Cochrane Database Syst Rev.* 2001;(1):CD000216.

60. Whitelaw A, Odd DE. Intraventricular streptokinase after intraventricular hemorrhage in newborn infants. *Cochrane Database Syst Rev.* 2007;(4):CD000496.

61. Wellons JC, Shannon CN, Kulkarni AV, et al. A multicenter retrospective comparison of conversion from temporary to permanent cerebrospinal fluid diversion in very low birth weight infants with posthemorrhagic hydrocephalus. *J Neurosurg Pediatr.* 2009;4(1):50–55.

62. Bassan H, Feldman HA, Limperopoulos C, et al. Periventricular hemorrhagic infarction: risk factors and neonatal outcome. *Pediatr Neurol.* 2006;35(2):85–92.

63. Kuban KC, Allred EN, O'Shea TM, et al. Cranial ultrasound lesions in the NICU predicts cerebral palsy at age 2 years in

children born at extremely low gestational age. *J Child Neurol.* 2009;24(1):63–72.

64. Laptook AR, O'Shea TM, Shankaran S, et al. Adverse neurodevelopmental outcomes among extremely low birth weight infants with a normal head ultrasound: prevalence and antecedents. *Pediatrics.* 2005;115(3):673–680.

65. O'Shea TM, Allred EN, Kiban KC, et al. Intraventricular hemorrhage and developmental outcome at 24 months of age in extremely preterm infants. *J Child Neurol.* 2012;27(1):22–29.

66. Pinto-Martin JA, Riolo S, Cnaan A, Holzman C, Susser MW, Paneth N. Cranial ultrasound prediction of disabling and nondisabling cerebral palsy at age two in a low birth weight population. *Pediatrics.* 1995;95(2):249–254.

67. Whitaker AH, Feldman JF, Van Rossem R, et al. Neonatal cranial ultrasound abnormalities in low birth weight infants: relation to cognitive outcomes at six years of age. *Pediatrics.* 1996;98(4):719–729.

68. Patra K, Wilson-Costello D, Taylor HG, Mercuri-Minich N, Hack M. grades I–II intraventricular hemorrhage in extremely low birth weight infants: effects on neurodevelopment. *J Pediatr.* 2006;149(2):169–173.

69. Hausler M, Merz U, Tuil C, Ramaekers VT. Long-term outcome after neonatal parenchymous brain lesions. *Klin Pediatr.* 2004;216(4):244–251.

70. Broitman E, Ambalavanam N, Higgins RD, et al. Clinical data predict neurodevelopmental outcome better than head ultrasound in extremely low birth weight infants. *J Pediatr.* 2007;151(5):500–505.

71. Brouwer A, Groenendaal F, van Haastert I-L, Rademaker K, Hanlo P, deVries L. Neurodevelopmental outcome of preterm infants with severe intraventricular hemorrhage and therapy for post-hemorrhagic hydrocephalus. *J Pediatr.* 2008;152(5):648–654.

72. Adams-Chapman I, Hansen NI, Stoll BJ, Higgins R, for the NICHD Neonatal Research Network. Neurodevelopmental outcome of extremely low birth weight infants with posthemorrhagic hydrocephalus requiring shunt insertion. *Pediatrics.* 2008;121(5):e1167–e1177.

73. Roze ER, Van Braeckel KN, van der Veere CN, Maatius CG, tijn A, Bos AF. Functional outcome at school age of preterm infants with periventricular hemorrhagic infarction. *Pediatrics.* 2009;123(6):1493–1500.

74. Bassan H, Limperopolous C, Visconti K, et al. Neurodevelopmental outcome in survivors of periventricular hemorrhagic infarction. *Pediatrics* 2007;120(4):785–792.

75. Nongena P, Ederies A, Azzopardi DV, Edwards AD. Confidence in the prediction of neurodevelopmental outcome by cranial ultrasound and MRI in preterm infants. *Arch Dis Child Fetal Neonatal Ed.* 2010;95(6):F388–F390. Epub 2010 Sep 24.

76. Hamrick SE, Miller SP, Leonard C, Glidden DV, et al. Trends in severe brain injury and neurodevelopmental outcome in premature newborn infants: the role of cystic periventricular leukomalacia. *J Pediatr.* 2004;145(5):593–599.

77. Miller SP, Ferriero DM, Leonard C, et al. Early brain injury in premature newborn detected with magnetic resonance imaging is associated with adverse neurodevelopmental outcome. *J Pediatr.* 2005;147(5):609–616.

78. Vollmer B, Roth S, Riley K, Sellwood MW. Neurodevelopmental outcome of preterm infants with ventricular dilatation with and without associated hemorrhage. *Dev Med Child Neurol.* 2006;48(5):348–352.

79. Brouwer AJ, van Stam C, Uniken VM, Koopman C, Groenendaal F, de Vries LS. Cognitive and neurological outcome at age of 5–8 years of preterm infants with post-hemorrhagic ventricular dilatation requiring neurosurgical intervention. *Neonatology.* 2011;101(3):210–216.

14 Perinatal Stroke

Alexa Craig and Donna M. Ferriero

INTRODUCTION

Neonatal stroke is estimated to occur in 1 per 2300 to 5000 live births.[1] This estimate may be an under-representation of the true incidence of neonatal stroke because of the inherent challenges in diagnosing this condition. In the adult, stroke is defined as "rapidly developed signs of focal (or global) disturbance of cerebral function lasting greater than 24 hours (unless interrupted by surgery or death), with no apparent nonvascular cause."[2] In this definition, there is heavy reliance on the clinical signs of neurological dysfunction. These signs are not usually apparent in the neonate because motor dysfunction is not easily appreciated, and sophisticated repertoires of behaviors such as language or the ability to follow commands have not yet developed. In the newborn, symptoms are vague, including encephalopathy, seizures, hypotonia, poor feeding, and apnea. This list of symptoms may be present in many of the diseases treated in the neonatal intensive care unit; therefore, trying to ascertain which are caused by stroke can be immensely challenging. The correct identification of stroke, however, is paramount for many reasons, ranging from identifying potentially modifiable risk factors to acute therapeutic intervention (particularly for sinus venous thrombosis). Managing long-term outcomes, which tend to be poor, is difficult but may improve with aggressive early intervention and emerging therapies such as transcranial magnetic stimulation and constraint-induced therapy.

In neonates, a proposed definition of stroke is as follows: "A group of heterogeneous conditions in which there is a focal disruption of cerebral blood flow secondary to arterial or venous thrombosis or embolization, between 20 weeks of fetal life through the 28th post-natal day, and confirmed by neuroimaging or neuropathological studies."[3] In this definition, there is a conspicuous absence of any clinical sign or physical exam finding suggesting neurologic dysfunction caused by stroke. As in adults, stroke in neonates can be subcategorized based on the affected vascular distribution (arterial vs venous), by whether the primary mechanism is ischemic or hemorrhagic, and by the presumed timing of the event (prenatal or post-natal). In this chapter, arterial ischemic stroke is discussed first, followed by venous stroke (better known as cerebral venous sinus thrombosis, CVST), and then hemorrhagic stroke. Prenatal and perinatal ischemic events defined by the term *presumed perinatal ischemic stroke* (PPIS) are also discussed.

PERINATAL ARTERIAL ISCHEMIC STROKE

Definitions

Arterial ischemic stroke occurs when an arterial vessel is occluded by a thrombus or an embolus, resulting in ischemic injury to the brain tissue distal to the occlusion. A thrombus is defined as a clot that is adherent to the wall of a vessel, whereas an embolus is a nonadherent thrombus. The embolus may be moving within arterial vessels or venous vessels or may become paradoxical by crossing from venous to arterial circulation. Paradoxical emboli may be more likely to occur in the neonate as right-to-left shunts are a necessary part of cardiovascular physiology during the transition from fetal to neonatal circulation.

Epidemiology

Perinatal arterial ischemic stroke (PAIS) is often a single lesion (70%) and is frequently located in the anterior circulation (71%).[4] A large international cohort revealed that there is a predominance of left-sided strokes affecting the middle cerebral artery (MCA) when only 1 hemisphere is involved (51% for isolated left vs 25% for isolated right) and that bilateral strokes occur in approximately 24% of patients. The left-sided predominance often leads to language deficits and right hemiparesis.[4] Seizures are a common presenting symptom and are often focal in manifestation.[5] Mortality was estimated in 1 study as 18 of 134 or 13.4% (8 died of hemorrhagic stroke, 9 died from arterial ischemic stroke, and 1 died from asphyxia and sinus thrombosis).[6]

Pathophysiology

Perinatal arterial ischemic stroke is dominated by necrosis. After 24 hours, activated microglia invade the lesion. They become foamy macrophages in 36–48 hours,

and astrocytic hypertrophy develops over 3–5 days. Over the longer term, the lesion becomes gliotic as glial fibrillary processes are laid down. There may be mineralization or cavity formation over the next weeks to months. After 4 to 6 weeks, cystic evolution occurs, leading frequently to ex vacuo dilation of the ipsilateral ventricle. The ischemic penumbra is the area surrounding the focal ischemic area destined for necrosis. In the penumbra, cellular metabolism is deranged because of decreased cerebral blood flow.

Risk factors for PAIS (see Figure 14-1) can be grouped according to maternal, fetal, or placental origin; naturally, there is great overlap among the 3 categories. Pregnancy itself is a hypercoagulable state because of innate protective thrombophilic factors that come into play to protect the mother from postpartum hemorrhage. In fact, this is true to such an extent that the maternal risk of stroke in the 3 days postpartum is elevated 34-fold when compared to the nonpregnant state.[1] In a normal pregnancy, there is a marked increase in the procoagulant activity in the maternal blood, characterized by elevation of factors V, VII, VIII, IX, X, and XII and fibrinogen (increases 2-fold) and von Willebrand factor, which is maximal around term.[7] In addition, there is a decrease in protein S activity and an acquired activated protein C resistance, leading to

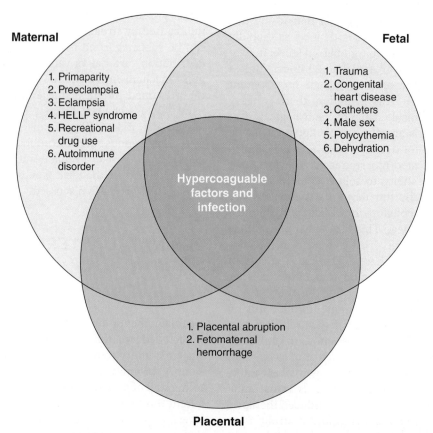

Maternal

1. Primaparity
2. Preeclampsia
3. Eclampsia
4. HELLP syndrome
5. Recreational drug use
6. Autoimmune disorder

Fetal

1. Trauma
2. Congenital heart disease
3. Catheters
4. Male sex
5. Polycythemia
6. Dehydration

Hypercoaguable factors and infection

1. Placental abruption
2. Fetomaternal hemorrhage

Placental

FIGURE 14-1 Risk factors associated with perinatal stroke. Hypercoagulable states and infection affect maternal, fetal, and placental categories. HELLP, hemolysis, elevated liver enzyme levels, and low platelets.

less-effective thrombolysis.[7] Other maternal factors increasing stroke risk include preeclampsia[3]; eclampsia; hemolysis, elevated liver enzyme levels, and low platelets (HELLP syndrome); elevated homocysteine and 677 C → T mutation in MTHFR gene; factor V Leiden mutation; chorioamnionitis; drug exposure (cocaine or amphetamine with associated vasospasm and poor perfusion of placenta); primiparity with a prolonged second stage of labor[8]; and autoimmune diseases such as lupus with associated autoantibodies. Fetal risk factors include birth-related trauma, which may result in stretch injury of carotid or vertebral arteries, leading to dissection, thrombus formation, and subsequent stroke. Congenital cardiac disease may lead to embolic stroke from thrombus that may occur in the heart because of diminished flow or the presence of right to left shunts. Cardiac surgery,[9] atrial septostomy,[10] and the presence of catheters[11] have been shown to increase the risk of stroke. Infection, such as meningitis, increases the risk of stroke. Interestingly, there is a male predominance among children with stroke, and in neonates in the International Pediatric Stroke Study (IPSS) registry, there were 249 with PAIS, 149 (57%) of whom were boys.[12]

The placenta is a low-flow system, which makes it more susceptible to clotting because of stasis effects. Thrombotic lesions are often found in the placenta of those neonates diagnosed with stroke. In a paper dedicated to the role of placental pathology in neonatal stroke, Elbers described abnormal placental pathology in 10 of 12 patients with neonatal stroke (7 with arterial ischemic stroke and 5 with CVST). In these patients, 50% demonstrated thromboinflammatory processes. A further 42% demonstrated acute catastrophic events, and 25% demonstrated decreased placental reserve.

Two patients had evidence of chorioamnionitis,[13] suggesting that infection also plays an important role.

Clinical Presentation

Seizures are the most common sign of PAIS. Seizures commonly occur in the first hours or days of life and are focal and clonic[5] (see Figure 14-2). A focal seizure in a neonate who is not encephalopathic is highly suggestive of PAIS. Stroke, however, can also be the etiology for severe encephalopathy to the extent that it is no longer uncommon to provide therapeutic hypothermia to an encephalopathic infant and later discover evidence of stroke on imaging rather than global injury caused by hypoxic ischemic encephalopathy. In a prospective cohort of 124 encephalopathic neonates, 6 (5%) were found to have focal stroke on imaging.[14]

Recognition of seizures can be challenging because of the variable clinical presentation of seizures, the complete lack of clinical correlate with many neonatal seizures, the dissociation between electrographic events and clinical events that occurs frequently after seizures are treated, and the frequent use of paralytic or sedating agents, especially during therapeutic hypothermia. A subclinical seizure is defined as one that occurs in the absence of any overt clinical repetitive or rhythmic movement that would be readily identified as seizure. In a study of 41 neonates, there were a total of 293 electrographic seizures (seizure apparent on electroencephalogram [EEG] only), 84 of which had a clinical correlate,[15] thus illustrating the fact that many neonatal seizures have no clinically visible features. In another study, 51 neonates at high risk for seizure were monitored with EEG, and 12 had a total of 526 seizures. Of these 526 electrographic seizures, only 179 or 34%

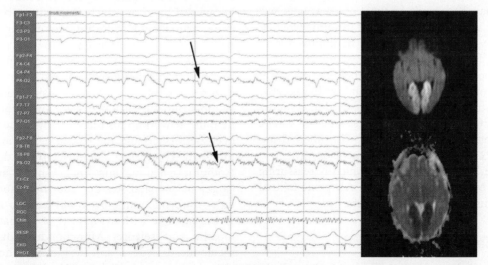

FIGURE 14-2 Conventional electroencephalogram (EEG) demonstrating a typical focal seizure. This is a 2-Hz occipital seizure on the right (P4-O2 and P8-O2 leads; see arrows) that was associated with a posterior cerebral artery infarct (see magnetic resonance image).

had clinically recognizable symptoms when the video and EEG were reviewed simultaneously. Of the 179 seizures with clinical correlate, only 48 were recognized as seizures by care providers. Conversely, there were 129 clinical seizure-like events documented by providers that had no EEG correlate. In other words, 73% of the time, seizure-like events were incorrectly identified at the bedside as seizures.[16] This study clearly illustrates the need to monitor with EEG not only to correctly identify true seizures but also to limit the incorrect identification of seizure-like events and inappropriate administration of anticonvulsant drugs.

Another challenge to the recognition of seizures is that treatment with anticonvulsants can cause "electro-clinical dissociation." This condition exists after administration of a drug such as phenobarbital, which may lead to the cessation of clinical seizures while electrographic seizures continue. Last, there is the unanswered question regarding whether aggressive treatment of subclinical seizures has any positive impact on developmental outcome or whether overtreatment of movements incorrectly perceived as seizures has potential adverse effect on neurodevelopmental outcome.

Because of the challenges of correctly identifying seizures, EEG monitoring should be used to identify seizures, monitor for electroclinical dissociation, and monitor the effectiveness of treatment. Conventional EEG (cEEG) is preferred because full coverage of the head using the 10- to 20-electrode placement system yields more accurate identification of the area of brain from which the seizure originates. However, cEEG is of limited utility at the bedside for non-neurology-based personnel because of the difficulty of interpreting the complex waveforms. Limited channel-monitoring devices, such as amplitude-integrated EEG (aEEG), are being used as an adjunct or in place of cEEG to improve bedside seizure detection. Although short seizures, those lasting less than 30 seconds, or those of low voltage will be missed by aEEG,[17] it is unclear at this time whether treating these seizures is imperative or improves outcome. aEEG is capable of detecting status epilepticus, and there is no ambiguity about whether prolonged status is deleterious to the newborn brain.[18] aEEG is easily employed by trained personnel, and if used in conjunction with cEEG, artifacts that appear seizure-like can be readily evaluated with great accuracy. The other advantage to aEEG is the ability to comment on prognosis based on the background activity, which is reassuring when there is evidence of state change in hypoxic-injured term newborns in the first 24–48 hours.[19]

Differential Diagnosis

The differential diagnosis (see Table 14-1) for PAIS and CVST is essentially the same as for neonatal encephalopathy, a broad term used to describe a

Table 14-1 Differential Diagnosis of Stroke

- Neonatal encephalopathy (hypoxic ischemic encephalopathy)
- Intracranial hemorrhage
  - Intraventricular, subarachnoid, subdural, or intraparenchymal hemorrhage
- Cerebral venous sinus thrombosis
- Central nervous system infection
  - Meningitis (bacterial or viral)
  - Encephalitis
- Electrolyte derangement
  - Hyponatremia
  - Hypocalcemia
  - Hypomagnesemia
- Hypoglycemia
- Metabolic diseases
  - Mitochondrial disease
  - Inborn errors of metabolism
  - Kernicterus
- Tumors
- Trauma

heterogeneous syndrome characterized by neurological dysfunction in the neonate. Hypoxic ischemic encephalopathy should be considered foremost for this differential diagnosis, and because of the significant overlap of symptoms, it is not uncommon for neonates with PAIS or CVST to be treated with therapeutic hypothermia. Any form of intracranial hemorrhage, including intraventricular (IVH), subarachnoid (SAH), subdural (SDH), or intraparenchymal hemorrhage (IPH), may have symptoms similar to PAIS or CVST (especially seizures and depressed mental status). Bedside cranial ultrasound can be used to quickly assess for the presence of blood. Trauma (incidental because of birth or inflicted) must not be overlooked as a potential etiology for intracranial hemorrhage and stroke.[20] Central nervous system infection, whether bacterial or viral (encephalitis or meningitis), may also present similarly with altered mental status and seizures and should prompt consideration of stroke. Lumbar puncture is a necessary and frequent component of the workup for these infants once imaging has been performed and the risk of herniation is deemed minimal. Hypoglycemia and electrolyte derangements (sodium, calcium, and magnesium) are treatable causes of neonatal seizures and thus should be ruled out. More uncommonly, brain tumors may present in the neonate with symptoms of neonatal encephalopathy and seizure. Mitochondrial disease, other metabolic disorders, and kernicterus should also be considered as part of the wider differential diagnosis when there is persistence of seizures and progressive alterations in mental status.

Diagnostic Tests

Imaging

Cranial ultrasound has a low likelihood of diagnosing PAIS.[21] Computed tomography (CT) is another option, but there is higher risk to the neonate because of the significant dose of ionizing radiation,[22] and CT may not be sensitive for infarcts that are less than 24 hours old.[21] The advantages of CT, however, are the relative speed of image acquisition (several minutes) as opposed to upward of 30 minutes for magnetic resonance imaging (MRI) and could be of utility in the unstable neonate for whom redirection of care is a consideration. CT is particularly sensitive at detecting intracranial blood, but this can be achieved equally well with MRI or even with ultrasound.

The gold standard for diagnosing PAIS is MRI. This provides the highest-resolution detail regarding the extent and timing of injury. It is essential to have a basic comprehension of diffusion sequences and conventional T1 and T2 sequences when evaluating stroke. In the first 1–14 days of life (maximal in the normothermic patient by day of life 4),[23] diffusion-weighted images (DWIs) depict areas of "diffusion restriction" as bright with "high signal intensity" compared to the surrounding noninjured brain tissue (see Figure 14-3, images A and E). Areas with restricted diffusion are areas where there has been injury resulting in energy depletion and failure of molecular pump machinery with subsequent decreased movement or "diffusion" of water molecules in the extracellular compartment. DWIs are compared to an apparent diffusion coefficient (ADC) map, where the areas of injury on the DWIs have areas of corresponding darkness (see Figure 14-3, images B and F). After approximately 10 to 14 days, these diffusion changes normalize, and the injury is no longer apparent on these sequences. Care must be taken with interpretation of diffusion images as the extent of injury may appear greater than what is ultimately seen on the conventional images. Pseudonormalization occurs 7 to 8 days after the injury; therefore, caution must be used in the interpretation of diffusion imaging as the absence of high signal intensity could represent the absence of injury or equally that the study was performed after day 7 or 8 when the diffusion changes are no longer apparent.[24]

The conventional T1- and T2-weighted images are useful to clarify the injury because these abnormalities should be visible on these sequences by day 7 or 8. On T1 images in the neonate, the white matter appears gray, the gray matter appears white, and the cerebral spinal fluid (CSF) is dark. Both injured cortex and injured white matter appear relatively hypointense or have "low signal intensity" (see Figure 14-3, images C and G) compared to normal tissue and, most important, lose the distinct boundary delineating gray vs white matter (blurring of the cortical ribbon). This change is evident from day 2 onward until the injured area undergoes

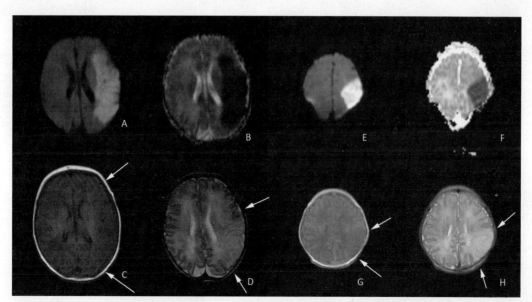

FIGURE 14-3 Diffusion-weighted and conventional magnetic resonance imaging (MRI) images of entire middle cerebral artery (MCA) distribution stroke on the left and partial MCA stroke on the right. A, hyperintensity in the left MCA distribution indicates acute MCA stroke confirmed by corresponding darkness on the apparent diffusion coefficient (ADC) map in image B. The T1 sequence shown on C reveals subtle changes in the affected area that are more prominent in the T2 sequence shown on image D (loss of cortical ribbon; see arrows). Images E (diffusion weighted) and F (ADC map) demonstrate a partial MCA territory stroke with corresponding T1 and T2 images again demonstrating subtle loss of the cortical ribbon on T1 and more apparent loss on T2 (see arrows).

cystic degeneration, at which point it appears dark like CSF. On T2-weighted images in the neonate, the white matter appears white, the gray matter appears gray, and the CSF is bright. Injured areas, including both cortex and white matter, appear relatively hyperintense or have "high signal intensity" compared to uninjured tissue, and the loss of the cortical ribbon is more evident than on T1 (see Figure 14-3, images D and H). This change can be appreciated from day 2 onward and is eventually replaced with bright CSF signal as the injured area undergoes cystic degeneration.

Magnetic resonance angiography (MRA) permits the evaluation of the intracranial and neck arterial vasculature. This technique is sensitive to motion artifact but may be useful to reveal underlying vessel pathology, such as dissection from birth trauma or arterial malformation. MRI and MRA are often performed with anesthesia to improve image quality by sedating the neonate so there is no movement. Wrapping techniques have been developed that employ vacuum devices to immobilize the unsedated neonate (see Figure 14-4),[25] thus eliminating risk of sedation with minimal to no sacrifice of image quality.

Management

Currently, the acute management of neonatal stroke is predominantly supportive. In adult stroke, normothermia, euglycemia, and permissive hypertension are accepted principles. Hyperthermia in animal models is known to increase metabolic demands if there is diminished capacity to deliver both oxygen and nutrients, leading to additional neuronal injury. In adults with stroke, hyperthermia is associated with a poorer prognosis, and in children with traumatic brain injury, hyperthermia is associated with longer hospitalization and lower Glasgow Coma Scale score.[26] Hyperthermia has not been specifically studied in children or neonates with stroke, but based on the known adverse outcomes in adults, normothermia is a reasonable goal in the management of neonatal stroke. In the subset of encephalopathic neonates who receive therapeutic hypothermia and are subsequently found to have PAIS, one study has shown a decrease in the frequency of seizures (0/5 cooled neonates had seizures vs 7/10 with seizures who were not cooled)[27] and thus suggests at least a need for future investigation into hypothermia

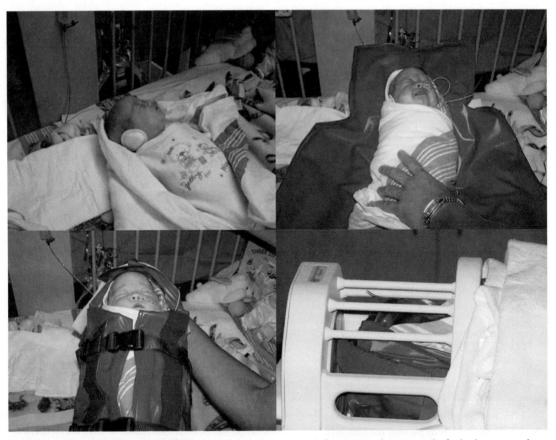

FIGURE 14-4 Transporting the unsedated neonate. In the upper left corner, the recently fed, sleepy, and unsedated neonate has ear protection applied and then is wrapped snugly in a blanket. The blue vacuum device is then wrapped around the neonate and secured with straps. A wall suction device is then used to remove the air from the vacuum device and the neonate is immobilized. The final image shows the neonate in the appropriate size head coil ready for magnetic resonance imaging (MRI). (From Mathur et al.[22])

as an intentional treatment for PAIS. Likewise, this study also suggests that treating seizures may decrease secondary neuronal injury. There is currently no evidenced-based approach to guide seizure treatment in the neonate; however, consensus seems to exist that status epilepticus (either clinical or subclinical) merits aggressive intervention[18] and, depending on the institution, will often result in escalating doses of phenobarbital, followed by fosphenytoin. There is less clarity regarding the treatment of subclinical seizures, and ongoing research efforts are under way to assess this.

In terms of euglycemia, neonates do not tend to have the same elevations in serum glucose as adults because of the absence of comorbid diabetes and hyperglycemia; therefore, this tends to be less of an issue. It is important, however, to avoid hypoglycemia as symptomatic hypoglycemia in term newborns has been shown on early MRI to have an association with white matter, cortex, basal ganglia, posterior limb of the internal capsule, and thalamic injury.[28] It is justified, then, to make a theoretical leap and assume that hypoglycemia can conceivably worsen an existing injury caused by PAIS and should therefore be avoided.

Adjunctive treatments currently investigated for hypoxic ischemic encephalopathy include xenon gas, erythropoeitin, and prophylactic use of anticonvulsant drugs, including phenobarbital, levetiracetam, and topiramate, but these are not yet being studied clinically for PAIS. Neonates are not usually treated with aspirin or antiplatelet drugs. On a case-by-case basis, particular disorders of hypercoagulability or cardiac diseases with large clot burden have been treated with either low molecular weight heparin (LMWH) or heparin drip. In one report, 3 neonates were discovered to have aortic arch thrombosis and were successfully treated with LMWH.[29]

With respect to the workup of neonatal stroke, it is essential to obtain MRI of the brain and vasculature and is reasonable to consider echocardiogram in the context of congenital heart disease and to perform Doppler ultrasound to evaluate flow. The hypercoagulable workup may be deferred from the acute setting, in which values are often reflective of the pregnancy state rather than intrinsic abnormalities of the neonate. The mother, especially in a first pregnancy, should have a hypercoagulable workup that includes examination of antiphospholipid antibodies and anticardiolipin antibodies. The neonate as part of outpatient follow-up can receive routine testing, including for antithrombin III, protein C, protein S, activated protein C resistance, factor V Leiden mutation, prothrombin gene mutation (*G20210A*), and antiphospholipid antibodies.

Outcome and Follow-up

Cerebral palsy (CP) is defined as a static, predominantly motor, deficit that results in spasticity in the extremities because of upper motor neuron injury of the cortical spinal tract. Of 36 infants with arterial stroke, 58% had CP,[30] and other estimates of motor deficit after stroke range from 30% to 40%.[31] Injury to the internal capsule (motor fibers), Broca's area/Wernicke's area (language centers), or basal ganglia or a large stroke (greater than two-thirds the area of a major vessel) are correlated with an increased risk of CP.[30] Types of CP include spastic (about 80%), ataxic (about 10% caused by damage of the cerebellum), and athetoid/dystonic (10% to 20% with a mixed picture of hyper- and hypotonia because of injury of basal ganglia and corticospinal tracts). MRI is a useful tool for prognosis, and in 37 neonates with stroke, 7 (19.4%) developed unilateral spastic CP (hemiplegia) and had pre-Wallerian degeneration changes evident on MRI that were predictive of this outcome.[32] In those who did not develop CP, 27 of 29 patients had no measurable change in the internal capsule or cerebral peduncle, which are components of the descending corticospinal tract.[32] In another study of 14 neonates with PAIS, diffusion-weighted MRI signal was abnormal in the descending corticospinal tract of 10, and this correlated well with motor outcomes.[31]

With respect to cognitive function, a recent study examined cognitive performance in 18 neonates at 12 and 24 months following stroke. At 12 months, children scored significantly below the normative sample on the Bayley Psychomotor Development Index and at 24 months significantly below the normative sample on both the Bayley Mental Development Index and the Psychomotor Development Index.[33] There were no differences found in this small sample based on stroke type (PAIS vs CVST) or based on which hemisphere was affected. A study of 26 older children also with unilateral stroke found that when tested at age 3.5 years and then again at almost 6 years, there was little difference among preschool-aged children when compared to normal controls. However, school-aged children (particularly males) had impaired performance on Full Scale IQ Working Memory and Processing Speed but not on Verbal IQ or Performance IQ. This suggests a trend toward later emergence of deficits reflective of dysfunction in higher levels of cognition and the potential need for ongoing educational support and assessment.[34]

CEREBRAL VENOUS SINUS THROMBOSIS

Definition

Cerebral venous sinus thrombosis occurs when a venous sinus, deep vein, or cortical vein is completely or partially obstructed by thrombus. This may occur without measurable parenchymal injury when there is incomplete occlusion of the vessel or good collateralization (blood flows out of the affected area through alternate routes) or may be associated with venous infarct. The term *bland infarct* is used to denote an infarct that does not have secondary hemorrhage. Typically, venous infarcts accompany 40% to 60% of CVSTs, and in one study, 29 of 69 neonates (42%) had infarct associated with CVST.[35] In this same study, secondary hemorrhagic conversion of the venous infarct was a frequent finding seen in 24 of 69 neonates (35%), whereas in another study of 109 neonates, 38% of infarcts remained bland and 62% became hemorrhagic.[36] Blood is not limited to the confines of the infarct as there is also frequent intraventricular and extraparenchymal hemorrhage (28% and 26%, respectively, in the Moharir study).[36]

The anatomical distribution of infarct is different in CVST compared to PAIS. In PAIS, the injured area is attributable to a lack of blood flow in a known arterial territory. In CVST, the findings of injury do not correspond to arterial territories, but predictable patterns are seen based on the areas drained by the affected sinus. For instance, with a straight sinus thrombosis, there may be evidence of injury to unilateral or bilateral basal ganglia and thalami, whereas with sagittal sinus thrombosis, there may be evidence of injury in a parasagittal watershed distribution.[37] Hemorrhagic lesions have been reported with the following associations: thalamo-ventricular hemorrhage with internal cerebral vein occlusion, bilateral thalamo-ventricular hemorrhage with vein of Galen occlusion, striato-hippocampal hemorrhage with basal vein thrombosis, temporal lobe or cerebellar hemorrhage with transverse sinus thrombosis, or temporal lobe hemorrhage alone with vein of Labbe thrombosis.[38]

Epidemiology

The incidence of venous ischemic stroke is estimated at 0.41 to 0.67 per 1000 live births,[39] with most recent estimates ranging from 2.6 to 12 per 100,000.[36] CVST is being diagnosed with increasing frequency because of greater clinical awareness of the disease and imaging techniques that are more sensitive. Mortality estimates range from 6% for CVST[36] to perhaps as high as 19%,[40] depending on the study and in which country it was done.

Pathophysiology

Venous infarcts occur because of the obstruction of cerebral veins by thrombus, which results in localized edema with pathologic evidence of swollen vessels and neurons with ischemic damage. Petechial hemorrhages occur that may coalesce into larger areas of hemorrhage. There may also be external mechanical factors, such as compression of the sagittal sinus from skull

bones caused by molding or positioning,[41] that confer a higher risk of venous thrombus formation because of interference with one or more of the components of Virchow's triad and result in hemodynamic flow changes, such as stasis, endothelial injury, and liberation of hypercoagulable factors.

The superior sagittal sinus is affected most frequently (62%), followed by the lateral sinuses (39%), then the straight sinus (30%), then the internal cerebral vein (10%), vein of Galen (8%), cortical veins (3%), and finally the jugular vein (1%).[35] In Moharir's study, 80% of neonates had multiple-sinus involvement.[36] Risk factors for CVST are multiple and like PAIS can be divided on the basis of maternal, fetal, or placental origin with natural overlap between these categories (see Figure 14-1).

Maternal risk factors are known to include premature rupture of membranes, chorioamnionitis, gestational diabetes, and preeclampsia with associated endothelial dysfunction. Fetal risk factors include acute systemic illness, polycythemia, and dehydration. A difficult delivery with or without trauma to the skull and injury to superior sagittal sinus has also been associated with increased risk of CVST; hypoxic ischemic encephalopathy is present in as many as 20% of cases later found to have CVST.[36] Male neonates have an increased frequency of CVST, but the underlying reason for this is unknown. Referring to the IPSS registry, of 92 neonates identified with CVST, 68 were male (74%).[35] In the Berfelo study, 75% of those with proven CVST were male.[40] In a 2004 paper, Golomb hypothesized that the size of the male infant (which at term is slightly larger than the female) may contribute to the increased risk.[42]

Given that the inciting factor in this mechanism of stroke occurs because of the presence of clot, it is essential to evaluate the neonate (and mother) for the presence of a hypercoagulable state. In children, prothrombotic disorders are present in one-to two-thirds of patients with CVST.[43] In neonates, however, the frequency of prothrombotic states seems lower, with one study showing 3 of 15 (20%) neonates with abnormalities, including 2 with (*MTHFR*) mutations and 1 with factor V Leiden mutation.[44] Assessment of antithrombin III, protein C, protein S, factor V Leiden, and prothrombin 20210A gene mutation is standard. *MTHFR*, homocysteine level, and lipoprotein (a) should also be evaluated. In a larger study of 52 neonates with CVST, 29 of the 52 were tested for antithrombin III, and all tests were normal.[40] In this same study, 32 of 52 were tested for both protein C and S levels, and all tests were normal. Forty-one of 52 were tested for G1691A factor V Leiden mutation, and a mutation was present in 2. The G20210A prothrombin gene mutation was tested in 18 of 52 and was present in 2. *MTHFR* C677T and A1298C mutations were tested in 23 and present in 13, but interestingly, all 23 had normal homocysteine levels.[40] Anticardiolipin antibody, lupus anticoagulant, prothrombin time (PT), partial thromboplastin time (PTT), and fibrinogen should not be overlooked. It is also critical to ensure that the results obtained are compared to age-adjusted normal controls. At this time, there is no consensus regarding the optimal timing of these studies and whether results from the acute period vs several months later are more reflective of the true state of coagulation.

Clinical Presentation

In CVST, seizures are often the presenting sign. In a study of 52 neonates, 29 or 55.8% presented with seizures that developed at a median time of 1.5 days.[40] In the Moharir study,[36] seizures occurred in 69% and encephalopathy in 53%. A term infant with intraventricular blood, thalamic hemorrhage, and seizures has a common triad suggestive of venous sinus thrombosis.[44] Other presentations include lethargy, a full fontanelle, and prominent scalp veins. As in PAIS, the next most common findings are apnea, temperature instability, hypotonia, poor feeding, and encephalopathy. Encephalopathy can be further defined as inappropriate level of consciousness, lack of spontaneous activity, low tone, absence of primitive reflexes, and autonomic dysfunction, including tachycardia or apnea.

Differential Diagnosis

For information on differential diagnosis, see the section on PAIS and Table 14-1.

Diagnostic Tests

Ultrasound findings in the term neonate with intraventricular and thalamic hemorrhage, especially if the patient has had clinical seizures, should be considered highly suspicious for CVST.[44] In the hands of experienced technicians and radiologists with color Doppler ultrasound, it is possible to view the sinuses clearly and diagnose absent flow, which is consistent with CVST.[37]

Computed tomography without contrast may show linear hyperintensities in places consistent with venous structures, suggesting the presence of thrombosis. On a CT scan with contrast, the term *empty delta sign* is used in the context of suspected CVST. This term refers to the pattern of thrombus evolution within the triangular-shaped sagittal sinus (the delta sign) that may appear to have a central hypointensity (the empty part of the delta). If imaging occurs within the first several days or after 2 months, this sign is not likely to be present. It also only applies to the sagittal sinus and can easily be missed if the thrombus does not extend into the posterior third of the sinus. This sign is not reliable in neonates because of the tendency for physiologic polycythemia in conjunction with the normal hypomyelinated neonatal brain to mimic the empty delta sign.[45]

Magnetic resonance imaging with magnetic resonance venogram (MRV) is the preferred method for diagnosing CVST because of the lack of exposure to harmful radiation and the sensitivity of the technique. On MRI, in the subacute stages, the thrombus will appear hyperintense on T1-weighted images (see Figure 14-5, image D). MRV should be obtained simultaneously because, in the acute phase, the thrombus is likely to appear isointense on T1 and hypointense on T2; this could be easy to misinterpret as normal flow. MRV is a study with images dedicated to evaluation of the venous structures and is the most effective at delineating areas where flow is absent (see Figure 14-6, image C). If there is an associated infarct, diffusion imaging techniques will reveal this. Infarcts that are *not* confined to known vascular territories or those that are bilateral and involve deep gray nuclei should prompt suspicion for CVST and acquisition of MRV sequences. Hemorrhage is frequently associated with CVST (see Figure 14-5, images A and B) and can be seen on MRI with susceptibility-weighted images (blood appears black with blooming artifact; see Figure 14-6, images E and F). In one study of 67 neonates who had full imaging data,[46] an infarct or hemorrhage was present in 66%. Serial imaging is required if a clot is present in order to evaluate for extension or propagation, in which case treatment is recommended[43,47] (see section on management). EEG monitoring for seizures and a hypercoagulable workup as described for PAIS should be undertaken in the case of CVST.

Management

Appropriate supportive care, such as correcting dehydration and treating infection and seizures if present, is undisputed in the literature on CVST. Unlike many conditions affecting the neonatal central nervous system, CVST is unique in that there is the potential for treatment with anticoagulation. Previous studies have shown that untreated CVST results in greater than 50% of patients having adverse outcomes with cognitive and motor impairments and epilepsy in 46% to 79%.[39] If associated infarct and seizure exist, outcome tends to be even worse,[35] thus heightening the urge to treat. In this context of urgency, however, current clinical guidelines do not align with respect to whom to treat. Recommendations in 2008 from the American Heart Association suggest considering anticoagulation in selected neonates with severe thrombophilic disorders, multiple cerebral or systemic emboli, or clinical

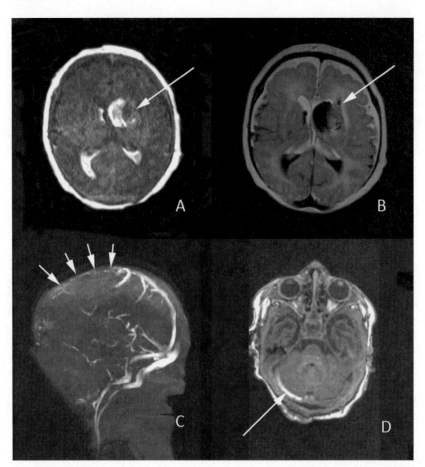

FIGURE 14-5 Cerebral venous sinus thrombosis. Image A is a T1 sequence showing hyperintense blood within both lateral ventricles as well as extension into the parenchyma at the left frontal pole of the lateral ventricle. The T2 sequence in image B displays more clearly the intraparenchymal extension of hemorrhage (see arrows). This hemorrhage is the sequelae of a cerebral venous sinus thrombosis (CVST). C, Magnetic resonance venogram (MRV) with occlusion of the anterior portion of the superior sagittal sinus indicated by absent flow (no hyperintense signal seen near arrows). D, T1 image with right transverse sinus thrombosis. Careful interpretation of this finding must be made as thrombus can easily be confused with subdural blood in this location.

or radiological evidence of propagating clot.[43] The recommendations from the American College of Chest Physicians (also in 2008) are more inclusive and recommend treating CVST when there is no extensive intracranial hemorrhage and to consider treating when clot is propagating even in the presence of extensive hemorrhage.[47]

In one retrospective study, 43 of 81 neonates with CVST were treated.[46] Fourteen received unfractionated heparin (UH), 34 received LMWH, 2 were treated with aspirin, and 1 received warfarin. There were no treatment-related adverse outcomes, and in the treated infants, clot propagation occurred in only 1 after LMWH was discontinued at 49 days. In a prospective study, Moharir enrolled 104 neonates with CVST, 53 of whom received anticoagulation therapy as either UH or LMWH.[36] Anticoagulation was initiated at diagnosis in 41 (39%) neonates and after thrombus propagation was discovered on serial MRI

in 12. In the treated group, there were no anticoagulant-related deaths or extensive systemic hemorrhage during the period of anticoagulation. There were 14 neonates with significant pretreatment hemorrhage who were anticoagulated, and none experienced worsening hemorrhage. One of 41 (2%) treated neonates experienced thrombus propagation, whereas 14 of 47 (30%) of untreated neonates experienced thrombus propagation. Clinically, propagation was silent in all but 1 neonate, who presented with worsening seizures, but new venous infarction was documented in 6 of 15 with clot propagation (40%). Outcomes for those with clot propagation were unfavorable (death or any neurologic deficit at last follow-up) in 10 of 15 neonates.

Repeat MRI and MRV are often obtained 5 to 7 days after the first studies to evaluate whether clot propagation is occurring. Serial Doppler ultrasound studies may detect a propagating thrombus. Full recanalization

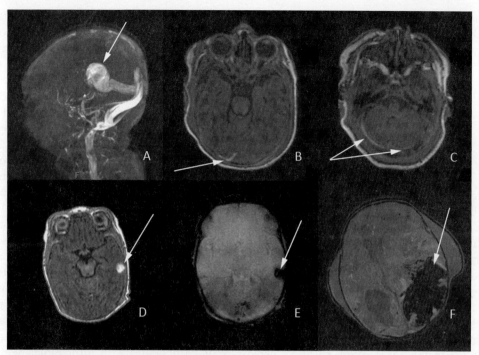

FIGURE 14-6 Intracranial hemorrhage: A, Magnetic resonance venogram (MRV) of a vein of Galen malformation with widely dilated venous system. B, T1 image with subdural hemorrhage (SDH) shown in the right occipital lobe (see arrow). C, SDH in the posterior fossa (see arrows). Note the similarity to image D in Figure 14-7. Image D reveals a small left-sided intraparenchymal hemorrhage (IPH) caused by a presumed cortical vein thrombosis that is characteristically hyperintense on T1. Image E shows this same hemorrhage with blooming artifact on a susceptibility-weighted image (SWI). Finally, image F shows a massive left-sided IPH (blood is dark on SWI) with midline shift, leading ultimately to herniation in this unfortunate neonate.

was demonstrated in 89% by 3 months.[36] Among other variables, intracranial hemorrhage, propagation of thrombus, and anticoagulant use did not predict the severity of neurodevelopmental outcome.

Outcome and Follow-up

With respect to developmental outcomes in the Moharir study, the mean follow-up was 2.5 years, and of those 85 neonates who survived, 35 were normal, 12 had mild deficits, and 38 had moderate-to-severe deficits.[36] Deficits ranged from sensorimotor deficits, to receptive and expressive language problems, to cognitive and behavioral concerns. Seizures were present in 69% at the time of diagnosis, and epilepsy was documented in only 18% of survivors.

In another study, DeVeber found that 77% of neonates followed to 1.6 years were "normal,"[35] but this finding applied to the group of children and neonates as a whole and was not analyzed by treatment. Long-term outcome in 1 study with only 9-month follow-up was notable for 45% being "uncomplicated" and a severely abnormal outcome in 19% of survivors.[40] It is clear that more studies are needed to better delineate outcomes, with particular emphasis on studying outcome as affected by treatment with anticoagulation.

HEMORRHAGIC STROKE

Definitions

There are 5 major, clinically relevant types of intracranial hemorrhage in the neonate: SAH, SDH, IPH, cerebellar hemorrhage, and IVH.[48] Intra-axial blood is defined as blood within the brain or within the ventricle; hence, this category includes IPH, cerebellar hemorrhage, and IVH. Extra-axial hemorrhage is by definition blood outside the brain parenchyma and is named according to the location of blood compared to the surrounding meninges. This category includes SAH and SDH. IVH in the term newborn is pathologically distinct from IVH in the preterm newborn, which is discussed elsewhere in this text. IPH, SDH, and SAH commonly occur in term newborns, whereas IVH and cerebellar hemorrhage tend to occur in prematurely born infants.

With more frequent use of MRI, cerebellar hemorrhage is increasingly diagnosed in preterm infants. This is important as the incidence is highest in those born weighing less than 750 g, for whom there is a 17% incidence of cerebellar hemorrhage according to the largest reported series.[49] In one small study of 15 preterm infants (median gestational age 25 weeks and 2 days and median birth weight 730 g), 13 experienced "notable, otherwise unexplained motor agitation in the days preceding the diagnosis" of cerebellar hemorrhage.[50] Cerebellar hemorrhage is associated with adverse developmental outcomes, including neuromotor disability, expressive and receptive language deficits, as well as socialization and behavioral abnormalities.

Epidemiology

The true incidence of intracranial hemorrhage in the full-term newborn is likely underestimated. When 101 asymptomatic term newborns were examined with MRI within the first 72 hours of life, 46 of them (46%) had SDHs and 20 of these (43%) also had hemorrhage in the posterior fossa.[51] In a study of 53 full-term symptomatic neonates with intracranial hemorrhage, all had both intra-axial and extra-axial hemorrhage. SDH was present in 50/53 (94%), whereas SAH was only present in 8/53 (15%). Associated IVH was seen in 12/53 (23%).[52] In this same study, 13 of 53 neonates died or had care withdrawn based on the severity of the hemorrhage and poor prognosis indicated by EEG, yielding a mortality rate of 24.5%.

Pathophysiology

Infrequently, neonatal intracranial hemorrhage is the result of a vascular defect. The 2 most common defects are aneurysms and arteriovenous malformations.[48] Intracranial hemorrhage related to aneurysm rupture is often characterized by rapid neurologic deterioration and SAH that may be later identified by MRI and cerebral angiography as secondary to aneurysm. Arteriovenous malformation is most commonly encountered in the context of a vein of Galen malformation (which is more likely to present with high-output congestive heart failure) (see Figure 14-6, image A). With this malformation, the hemorrhage is likely to be intraparenchymal or intraventricular.

Intracranial hemorrhage is more often associated with risk factors related to the delivery rather than vascular defects. SDH and IPH are more often the result of prolonged or precipitous delivery, vaginal breech delivery, instrumental delivery (forceps or vacuum assist), primaparity, or extreme multiparity.[52] According to a large retrospective study of greater than 500,000 deliveries, the risk of intracranial hemorrhage (including SDH, IPH, IVH, or SAH) with vacuum assist is estimated to be 1 in 860 compared to 1 in 1900 of those neonates who were delivered vaginally without use of the vacuum device. With forceps delivery, the ratio is increased to 1 in 664 for intracranial hemorrhage. If both forceps and vacuum assist are employed, the ratio further increases to 1

in 256. For cesarean section, the ratio is 1 in 907 for cesarean delivery performed after trial of labor. With failed attempt at "operative delivery," which is either vacuum assist or forceps, the rate for cesarean section increases to 1 in 334. In summary, there is an incremental increase in the frequency of intracranial hemorrhage if more than one surgical technique is employed.[53] The mechanism of injury caused by birth-related factors is likely because of mechanical stress from elongation of the head and subsequent stretching of the falx and tearing of the tentorium. The venous sinuses are exposed to these same mechanical forces and can also be ruptured.[48]

Risk factors other than the mode of delivery include thrombocytopenia, vitamin K status, and deficiency of coagulation factors. Intracranial hemorrhage is a rare complication of each of these diseases. Thrombocytopenia was present in 11 of the 50 neonates in the Brouwer study, and low platelet levels (less than 150×10^9 L^{-1}) were more commonly seen in those who died.[52] In another retrospective study, 2 of 23 neonates with intracranial hemorrhage were found to have thrombocytopenia.[54] Neonatal isoimmune thrombocytopenia occurs in 0.2 per 1000 live births, and cranial imaging should be part of the management of these infants so that this rare complication is diagnosed.

Vitamin K administration at the time of birth is now considered standard of care, but vitamin K status must not be overlooked as a possible etiology for intracranial hemorrhage. Treatment of mothers with phenobarbital, coumadin, aspirin, or antituberculosis drugs may indirectly cause vitamin K deficiency in the newborn, subsequently increasing the risk of intracranial hemorrhage. In one case report, a mother treated with 100 mg of phenobarbital daily for seizures gave birth to a term infant via vaginal delivery with vacuum assist; the infant subsequently developed a large left hemispheric SDH.[55]

Clinical Presentation

Hemorrhage occurs because of rupture of veins, and blood accumulates in the various spaces described previously. If this occurs in the posterior fossa around the cerebellum, increased intracranial pressure may result because of blockage of the cerebral aqueduct as well as mass effect from the blood itself. Clinical symptoms can include a tense or bulging anterior fontanelle, increasing head circumference, lethargy, apnea, and bradycardia. Urgent imaging and consideration of neurosurgical intervention are required. Later complications of intracranial hemorrhage can include hydrocephalus caused by CSF outflow obstruction or difficulty with resorption of CSF at the level of the arachnoid granulations (communicating hydrocephalus). Shunting may be required if this occurs.

As in the case of PAIS or CVST, intracranial hemorrhage presents with seizures the majority of the time (72%).[52] In one study, with temporal lobe hemorrhage particularly, there was an association with apneic seizures and a further 10 infants (19%) presented in this manner, thus bringing the total with seizure as the presenting sign to 91%. The other 5 infants in the study were admitted because of perinatal asphyxia, respiratory distress, and development of posthemorrhagic ventricular dilation. Seizures in the context of intracranial hemorrhage can be challenging to treat, as evidenced by the fact that 12 of 53 infants in this study needed 2 anticonvulsant drugs and another group of 18 required 3 anticonvulsant drugs.[52]

Differential Diagnosis

For information regarding a differential diagnosis, see the section on PAIS and Table 14-1.

Diagnostic Tests

Cranial ultrasound can be readily used at the bedside to identify IPH, which appears as a homogeneous area of increased echogenicity. CT scan without contrast is extremely sensitive to the presence of blood products, but the adverse effects of ionizing radiation are undesirable. MRI of the brain is the gold standard for evaluating intracranial pathology in the neonate both from a safety perspective and for obtaining the most accurate information. If blood is present, on the conventional images it will appear hyperintense on T1-weighted images (see Figure 14-6, images B and D) and hypointense or black on T2-weighted images. The appearance of blood can be easily remembered by the fact that blood signal is the opposite of the corresponding CSF signal in that sequence. Susceptibility images or gradient echo (GRE) sequences can be used to demonstrate the presence of blood products (see Figure 14-7, images E and F) and is as sensitive as CT scan.[56]

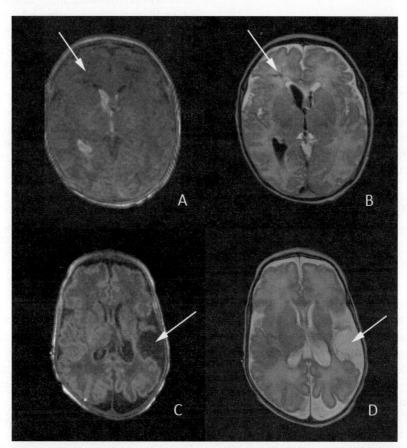

FIGURE 14-7 Presumed perinatal ischemic stroke: A, T1 image demonstrating hyperintense intraventricular hemorrhage in both ventricles (right greater than left). There is a subtle hint of pathology in the right frontal white matter that is clearly seen on the accompanying T2 image (image B; see arrows), with dark-appearing linear structures that may correspond to clotted vessels. This injury is presumed caused by compression of the medullary veins in this right frontal area and is termed a PVI or periventricular venous infarction. C and D, T1 and T2 images, respectively, of arterial presumed perinatal ischemic stroke (APPIS); these demonstrate the typical findings of chronicity of injury with encephalomalacia (see arrows) as the only evidence remaining of this in utero event.

Management

Much of the management of intracranial hemorrhage is supportive. Serial imaging and sequential neurological examination in the asymptomatic newborn is an appropriate approach. If, however, a large lesion is present or if there are signs of increased intracranial pressure or brainstem compromise, then neurosurgical evaluation is acutely necessary. In the Brouwer study, 3 of 21 infants with significant midline shift needed craniotomy for evacuation of hematoma.[52] In another study, 5 of 24 infants with intracranial hemorrhage required surgical intervention.[54]

Thrombocytopenia should be corrected if present. If vitamin K is deficient, this also should be addressed as well as any other coagulopathy. In both the acute and chronic phases of the illness, daily head circumference should be measured to monitor for posthemorrhagic hydrocephalus. In the Brouwer study, 16 infants developed hydrocephalus, 6 of whom needed subcutaneous reservoirs and 3 of those 6 went on to convert from reservoir to ventriculoperitoneal shunt.[52]

Outcome and Follow-up

Of the 40 surviving infants in the Brouwer study, 37 were seen in follow-up at a mean age of 20 months.[52] The mean developmental quotient (DQ) was 97, and there was no difference among groups based on neurosurgical intervention. Only 1 infant developed epilepsy and 3 developed CP.[52] There are few long-term studies evaluating outcome; therefore, although one can be cautiously optimistic, data are not available.

PRESUMED PERINATAL ISCHEMIC STROKE

Definitions and Mechanism

Much research has focused on acute, symptomatic stroke in the neonate that commonly presents with seizures. There is, however, increasing interest and research in stroke that is asymptomatic in the newborn period and later diagnosed by asymmetric early motor development or early hand preference.[57] Presumed perinatal ischemic stroke (PPIS) is defined as occurring in a neonate over the age of 28 days with a normal perinatal neurologic history who develops neurologic deficits attributable to a remote focal infarction confirmed on neuroimaging performed later in infancy.[3] PPIS, like acute stroke in the term neonate, can be subdivided based on the vascular territory affected: arterial vs venous. The vast majority of PPISs (80%) seems to affect arterial territories, and most are in the MCA distribution.[57] This type of stroke is referred to as APPIS to emphasize the arterial distribution. As with PAIS,

the implied mechanism is thrombotic or embolic, but interestingly, unlike PAIS, for which congenital cardiac disease plays a more prominent role, of 15 children with PPIS who were evaluated by echocardiogram, none was found to have clinically significant structural or functional abnormalities.[58] In contrast, when venous structures are affected, the term *periventricular venous infarction* (PVI) is used. The mechanism is suspected to be related to fetal germinal matrix hemorrhage, with the mass effect of this hemorrhage on the nearby medullary veins causing subsequent infarction.[59]

Hemorrhagic stroke can also occur prior to birth and has been described in families with early handedness and a history of porencephaly (a fluid-filled cavity in the brain communicating with the ventricles).[60] This disease is termed *familial porencephaly* and has been linked to a mutation in the *COL4A1* gene, which encodes the $\alpha1$ chain of type IV collagen.[61] The $\alpha1$ chain binds with 2 $\alpha2$ chains, and this heterotrimer becomes a crucial component of the basement membrane of blood vessels forming a "sheet-like network beneath the endothelium and surrounding smooth muscle cells."[61] Because of early research in a mouse model, it was thought that there was an interaction between this autosomal-dominant genetic predisposition and the environment, as mouse pups born via surgical delivery did not have the same intracranial hemorrhage burden as those born vaginally.[61] In humans, there seems to be a wide phenotypic spectrum, ranging from preterm infants born with resolving hemorrhage[60] to adults who have migraine headache, nephropathy, and tortuosity of the retinal vasculature,[61] thus making it challenging to define a relationship between genetics and the environment. Consideration should be given to genetic testing for the *COL4A1* mutation in the following circumstances: preterm infants who develop atypical IPH and all infants who are born with porencephalic cysts.[60]

Epidemiology

In a retrospective analysis of 59 children with PPIS, 63% were male.[57] Typically, PPIS has been described in infants who were born at term; however, there is also emerging data on PPIS in the preterm infant, with as many as 15% of those known to have PPIS having been born before 37 weeks' gestation.[3]

Clinical Presentation

Early hand preference, particularly in the first 12 months of life, is likely pathologic and should prompt neuroimaging with MRI of the brain. Of the 59 children studied by Kirton et al, 44 presented with early hand preference.[57] Seizure is the next most frequently occurring symptom, with 10 of 59 or 17% presenting this way.[57] When the APPIS group was compared to the PVI group, a pattern emerged, with the majority of PVI patients (92%) presenting with motor asymmetries, whereas the APPIS group had a much higher likelihood of presenting with a seizure (25% for APPIS vs 0% for PVI). The explanation for this may relate to the fact that the cortex, the epileptogenic component of brain tissue, is injured with APPIS but not with PVI. The median age in Kirton's study for parental concern of motor asymmetry was 5 months. Physician concern was raised by a median of 7 months and diagnosis made eventually by a median age of 12 months.[57]

Diagnostic Tests

The emphasis in the diagnosis of PPIS is on the remoteness of the injury; hence, there cannot be evidence of acute injury, and diffusion-weighted MRI images are therefore of no utility. On conventional images from MRI, there should be evidence that indicates chronicity of the injury, with features such as encephalomalacia, gliosis, and atrophy (see Figure 14-7, images C and D). MRI must have the following features to diagnose PVI: unilateral periventricular white matter infarction in a medullary vein territory (see Figure 14-7, image B) with 4 or more of focal periventricular encephalomalacia, T2 prolongation in the posterior limb of the internal capsule, cortical sparing, hemosiderin within the lesion, germinal matrix or ventricle, and relative sparing of the basal ganglia.[57]

Outcome and Follow-up

In a retrospective study of 22 children diagnosed with PPIS at a mean age of 6 months, 21 of the 22 (95%) had clinically significant hemiparesis.[58] Twelve of the 22 (55%) had speech, cognitive, or behavioral deficits.[58] Five of 22 developed persistent seizures, 1 with infantile spasms.[58] In a larger study of 59 children, which included the 22 children just discussed, 87% were described as having a poor outcome, with 82% having motor disability and 42% having epilepsy.[59]

Management

There is no acute management involved in the diagnosis of PPIS, but nonetheless it is important to identify stroke as the etiology so that early intervention with supportive services such as physical therapy, occupational therapy, and speech therapy can be employed.

SUMMARY

Stroke in the neonate is common, and with better detection through clinical awareness and the use of appropriate imaging modalities, better long-term outcomes in this group of infants can be achieved.

REFERENCES

1. Nelson KB. Perinatal ischemic stroke. *Stroke.* 2007;38(2 Suppl):742–745.
2. Thorvaldsen P, Asplund K, Kuulasmaa K, Rajakangas AM, Schroll M. Stroke incidence, case fatality, and mortality in the WHO MONICA project. World Health Organization Monitoring Trends and Determinants in Cardiovascular Disease. *Stroke.* 1995;26(3):361–367.
3. Raju TN, Nelson KB, Ferriero D, Lynch JK. Ischemic perinatal stroke: summary of a workshop sponsored by the National Institute of Child Health and Human Development and the National Institute of Neurological Disorders and Stroke. *Pediatrics.* 2007;120(3):609–616.
4. Kirton A, Armstrong-Wells J, Chang T, et al. Symptomatic neonatal arterial ischemic stroke: the International Pediatric Stroke Study. *Pediatrics.* 2011;128(6):e1402–e1410.
5. Barnette AR, Inder TE. Evaluation and management of stroke in the neonate. *Clin Perinatol.* 2009;36(1):125–136.
6. Govaert P, Ramenghi L, Taal R, Dudink J, Lequin M. Diagnosis of perinatal stroke II: mechanisms and clinical phenotypes. *Acta Paediatr.* 2009;98(11):1720–1726.
7. Brenner B. Haemostatic changes in pregnancy. *Thromb Res.* 2004;114(5–6):409–414.
8. Cheong JL, Cowan FM. Neonatal arterial ischaemic stroke: obstetric issues. *Semin Fetal Neonatal Med.* 2009;14(5):267–271.
9. Chen J, Zimmerman RA, Jarvik GP, et al. Perioperative stroke in infants undergoing open heart operations for congenital heart disease. *Ann Thorac Surg.* 2009;88(3):823–829.
10. Mukherjee D, Lindsay M, Zhang Y, et al. Analysis of 8681 neonates with transposition of the great arteries: outcomes with and without Rashkind balloon atrial septostomy. *Cardiol Young.* 2010;20(4):373–380.
11. Schmidt B, Andrew M. Neonatal thrombosis: report of a prospective Canadian and international registry. *Pediatrics.* 1995;96(5 Pt 1):939–943.
12. Golomb MR, Fullerton HJ, Nowak-Gottl U, Deveber G. Male predominance in childhood ischemic stroke: findings from the International Pediatric Stroke Study. *Stroke.* 2009;40(1):52–57.
13. Elbers J, Viero S, MacGregor D, DeVeber G, Moore AM. Placental pathology in neonatal stroke. *Pediatrics.* 2011;127(3):e722–e729.
14. Ramaswamy V, Miller SP, Barkovich AJ, Partridge JC, Ferriero DM. Perinatal stroke in term infants with neonatal encephalopathy. *Neurology.* 2004;62(11):2088–2091.
15. Clancy RR, Legido A, Lewis D. Occult neonatal seizures. *Epilepsia.* 1988;29(3):256–261.
16. Murray DM, Boylan GB, Ali I, Ryan CA, Murphy BP, Connolly S. Defining the gap between electrographic seizure burden, clinical expression and staff recognition of neonatal seizures. *Arch Dis Child Fetal Neonatal Ed.* 2008;93(3):F187–F191.
17. Hellström-Westas L, De Vries LS, Rosén I. *Atlas of Amplitude-Integrated EEGs in the Newborn.* 2nd ed. London, UK: Informa Healthcare; 2008.
18. Lawrence R, Inder T. Neonatal status epilepticus. *Semin Pediatr Neurol.* 2010;17(3):163–168.
19. Thoresen M, Hellstrom-Westas L, Liu X, de Vries LS. Effect of hypothermia on amplitude-integrated electroencephalogram in infants with asphyxia. *Pediatrics.* 2010;126(1):e131–e139.
20. Riel-Romero RM. Neonatal stroke. *Neurol Res.* 2008;30(8):839–844.
21. Golomb MR, Dick PT, MacGregor DL, Armstrong DC, DeVeber GA. Cranial ultrasonography has a low sensitivity for detecting arterial ischemic stroke in term neonates. *J Child Neurol.* 2003;18(2):98–103.

22. King MA, Kanal KM, Relyea-Chew A, Bittles M, Vavilala MS, Hollingworth W. Radiation exposure from pediatric head CT: a bi-institutional study. *Pediatr Radiol.* 2009;39(10):1059–1065.

23. Dudink J, Mercuri E, Al-Nakib L, et al. Evolution of unilateral perinatal arterial ischemic stroke on conventional and diffusion-weighted MR imaging. *AJNR Am J Neuroradiol.* 2009;30(5):998–1004.

24. McKinstry RC, Miller JH, Snyder AZ, et al. A prospective, longitudinal diffusion tensor imaging study of brain injury in newborns. *Neurology.* 2002;59(6):824–833.

25. Mathur AM, Neil JJ, McKinstry RC, Inder TE. Transport, monitoring, and successful brain MR imaging in unsedated neonates. *Pediatr Radiol.* 2008;38(3):260–264.

26. Bernard TJ, Goldenberg NA, Armstrong-Wells J, Amlie-Lefond C, Fullerton HJ. Treatment of childhood arterial ischemic stroke. *Ann Neurol.* 2008;63(6):679–696.

27. Harbert MJ, Tam EW, Glass HC, et al. Hypothermia is correlated with seizure absence in perinatal stroke. *J Child Neurol.* 2011;26(9):1126–1130.

28. Burns CM, Rutherford MA, Boardman JP, Cowan FM. Patterns of cerebral injury and neurodevelopmental outcomes after symptomatic neonatal hypoglycemia. *Pediatrics.* 2008;122(1):65–74.

29. Sharathkumar AA, Lamear N, Pipe S, et al. Management of neonatal aortic thrombosis with low-molecular weight heparin: a case series. *J Pediatr Hematol Oncol.* 2009;31(7):516–521.

30. Lee J, Croen LA, Lindan C, et al. Predictors of outcome in perinatal arterial stroke: a population-based study. *Ann Neurol.* 2005;58(2):303–308.

31. Kirton A, Shroff M, Visvanathan T, deVeber G. Quantified corticospinal tract diffusion restriction predicts neonatal stroke outcome. *Stroke.* 2007;38(3):974–980.

32. de Vries LS, van Haastert IC, Benders MJ, Groenendaal F. Myth: cerebral palsy cannot be predicted by neonatal brain imaging. *Semin Fetal Neonatal Med.* 2011;16(5):279–287.

33. McLinden A, Baird AD, Westmacott R, Anderson PE, deVeber G. Early cognitive outcome after neonatal stroke. *J Child Neurol.* 2007;22(9):1111–1116.

34. Westmacott R, MacGregor D, Askalan R, deVeber G. Late emergence of cognitive deficits after unilateral neonatal stroke. *Stroke.* 2009;40(6):2012–2019.

35. deVeber G, Andrew M, Adams C, et al. Cerebral sinovenous thrombosis in children. *N Engl J Med.* 2001;345(6):417–423.

36. Moharir MD, Shroff M, Pontigon AM, et al. A prospective outcome study of neonatal cerebral sinovenous thrombosis. *J Child Neurol.* 2011;26(9):1137–1144.

37. Govaert P. Sonographic stroke templates. *Semin Fetal Neonatal Med.* 2009;14(5):284–298.

38. Govaert P, Ramenghi L, Taal R, de Vries L, Deveber G. Diagnosis of perinatal stroke I: definitions, differential diagnosis and registration. *Acta Paediatr.* 2009;98(10):1556–1567.

39. Kersbergen KJ, de Vries LS, van Straaten HL, Benders MJ, Nievelstein RA, Groenendaal F. Anticoagulation therapy and imaging in neonates with a unilateral thalamic hemorrhage due to cerebral sinovenous thrombosis. *Stroke.* 2009;40(8):2754–2760.

40. Berfelo FJ, Kersbergen KJ, van Ommen CH, et al. Neonatal cerebral sinovenous thrombosis from symptom to outcome. *Stroke.* 2010;41(7):1382–1388.

41. Tan M, Deveber G, Shroff M, et al. Sagittal sinus compression is associated with neonatal cerebral sinovenous thrombosis. *Pediatrics.* 2011;128(2):e429–e435.

42. Golomb MR, Dick PT, MacGregor DL, Curtis R, Sofronas M, deVeber GA. Neonatal arterial ischemic stroke and cerebral sinovenous thrombosis are more commonly diagnosed in boys. *J Child Neurol.* 2004;19(7):493–497.

43. Roach ES, Golomb MR, Adams R, et al. Management of stroke in infants and children: a scientific statement from a Special Writing Group of the American Heart Association Stroke Council and the Council on Cardiovascular Disease in the Young. *Stroke.* 2008;39(9):2644–2691.

44. Wu YW, Hamrick SE, Miller SP, et al. Intraventricular hemorrhage in term neonates caused by sinovenous thrombosis. *Ann Neurol.* 2003;54(1):123–126.

45. Lee EJ. The empty delta sign. *Radiology.* 2002;224(3):788–789.

46. Jordan LC, Rafay MF, Smith SE, et al. Antithrombotic treatment in neonatal cerebral sinovenous thrombosis: results of the International Pediatric Stroke Study. *J Pediatr.* 2010;156(5):704–710. 710.e1–710.e2.

47. Monagle P, Chalmers E, Chan A, et al. Antithrombotic therapy in neonates and children: American College of Chest Physicians Evidence-Based Clinical Practice Guidelines (8th edition). *Chest.* 2008;133(6 Suppl):887S–968S.

48. Volpe JJ. *Neurology of the newborn.* 5th ed. Philadelphia, Pa.: Saunders; 2008.

49. Volpe JJ. Cerebellum of the premature infant: rapidly developing, vulnerable, clinically important. *J Child Neurol.* 2009;24(9):1085–1104.

50. Ecury-Goossen GM, Dudink J, Lequin M, Feijen-Roon M, Horsch S, Govaert P. The clinical presentation of preterm cerebellar haemorrhage. *Eur J Pediatr.* 2010;169(10):1249–1253.

51. Rooks VJ, Eaton JP, Ruess L, Petermann GW, Keck-Wherley J, Pedersen RC. Prevalence and evolution of intracranial hemorrhage in asymptomatic term infants. *AJNR Am J Neuroradiol.* 2008;29(6):1082–1089.

52. Brouwer AJ, Groenendaal F, Koopman C, Nievelstein RJ, Han SK, de Vries LS. Intracranial hemorrhage in full-term newborns: a hospital-based cohort study. *Neuroradiology.* 2010;52(6):567–576.

53. Towner D, Castro MA, Eby-Wilkens E, Gilbert WM. Effect of mode of delivery in nulliparous women on neonatal intracranial injury. *N Engl J Med.* 1999;341(23):1709–1714.

54. Ou-Yang MC, Huang CB, Huang HC, et al. Clinical manifestations of symptomatic intracranial hemorrhage in term neonates: 18 years of experience in a medical center. *Pediatr Neonatol.* 2010;51(4):208–213.

55. Renzulli P, Tuchschmid P, Eich G, Fanconi S, Schwobel MG. Early vitamin K deficiency bleeding after maternal phenobarbital intake: management of massive intracranial haemorrhage by minimal surgical intervention. *Eur J Pediatr.* 1998;157(8):663–665.

56. Tong KA, Ashwal S, Obenaus A, Nickerson JP, Kido D, Haacke EM. Susceptibility-weighted MR imaging: a review of clinical applications in children. *AJNR Am J Neuroradiol.* 2008;29(1):9–17.

57. Kirton A, Shroff M, Pontigon AM, deVeber G. Risk factors and presentations of periventricular venous infarction vs arterial presumed perinatal ischemic stroke. *Arch Neurol.* 2010;67(7):842–848.

58. Golomb MR, MacGregor DL, Domi T, et al. Presumed pre- or perinatal arterial ischemic stroke: risk factors and outcomes. *Ann Neurol.* 2001;50(2):163–168.

59. Kirton A, Deveber G, Pontigon AM, Macgregor D, Shroff M. Presumed perinatal ischemic stroke: vascular classification predicts outcomes. *Ann Neurol.* 2008;63(4):436–443.

60. de Vries LS, Koopman C, Groenendaal F, et al. *COL4A1* mutation in two preterm siblings with antenatal onset of parenchymal hemorrhage. *Ann Neurol.* 2009;65(1):12–18.

61. Vahedi K, Alamowitch S. Clinical spectrum of type IV collagen (*COL4A1*) mutations: a novel genetic multisystem disease. *Curr Opin Neurol.* 2011;24(1):63–68.

Neonatal Seizures

Donald M. Olson

INTRODUCTION

A seizure may be the first sign of neurological dysfunction and serious systemic disease. The potential etiologies are diverse and range from very serious brain injury to benign, age-limited genetic conditions. Because the underlying cause of the seizures may be an acute, potentially harmful, and treatable metabolic derangement (eg, hypoglycemia) or infection, early recognition, evaluation, and treatment are important.

EPIDEMIOLOGY

Seizures occur more often during the first week of life than at any other time.[1] The reported incidence ranges from 1 to 5 per 1000 newborns in developed countries.[2-4] The incidence is much higher in developing countries.[5] Premature and low birth weight infants also have a higher incidence of seizures than term and normal weight newborns.[4,6,7]

Etiology of Seizures in the Neonate

The most common etiology of seizures in the neonate is a hypoxic-ischemic insult as a result of conditions such as perinatal asphyxia, cardiac disease, and respiratory distress. Other common causes include infections, cerebral dysgenesis, and stroke. Less-common etiologies are the benign epilepsy syndromes that present in the neonatal period. A large variety of rare genetic and metabolic conditions are associated with severe seizures and a poor long-term prognosis,

although some are treatable. The most severe seizure disorders in neonates are caused by early infantile epileptic encephalopathy (EIEE; Otahara syndrome) and early myoclonic epilepsy (EME).[8,9]

Hypoxic-Ischemic Encephalopathy

Hypoxic-ischemic encephalopathy is the most common etiology of neonatal seizures. Approximately two-thirds of all neonatal seizures are a result of this cause.[10] Both animal studies and human case studies showed that the frequency and severity of neonatal seizures in the setting of hypoxic-ischemic encephalopathy usually parallel that of the encephalopathy.[11,12]

Seizures caused by hypoxic encephalopathy usually manifest in the first 2 days of life.[13] They are often persistent and difficult to control acutely. When they do come under control from a clinical perspective, they frequently persist on electroencephalogram (EEG). Seizures caused by an acute hypoxic insult are often transient, so seizure medication may only be needed in the short term. However, there is an independent long-term risk of epilepsy later in life. Approximately one-third of these infants will develop epilepsy.[14]

Infections

Meningitis

The organisms most commonly responsible for neonatal seizures during the first few days of life are β-hemolytic group B streptococci (GBS), *Escherichia coli*, and other gram-negative organisms reflecting maternal flora. Later-onset meningitis may be the result of community exposure as well.[15] Seizures are among the common presenting signs of meningitis in the neonate, along with irritability, lethargy, poor feeding, poor tone, and apnea.[16] Furthermore, seizures in the setting of neonatal meningitis are a concerning prognostic sign indicating a higher risk of an abnormal neurological outcome.[17]

Encephalitis

Central nervous system infection with herpes simplex virus (HSV) commonly presents with lethargy, poor temperature regulation, and seizures. The neonatal form is most often caused by type 2 HSV. Seizures are a poor prognostic sign. But, treatment with a full course of acyclovir does correlate with a better outcome. Still, over 50% of children with neonatal herpes will develop epilepsy.[18–21]

Congenital cytomegalovirus (CMV) infection is a relatively common infection, affecting as many as 1% of newborns worldwide. Seizures may be caused by either the active infection or, in most cases, brain injury and malformation caused by intrauterine infection.[22]

Intracranial Hemorrhage and Stroke

Hemorrhage

Subarachnoid, intraventricular, and intraparenchymal hemorrhages may cause seizures in term and preterm infants. Subdural and subarachnoid hemorrhages may cause seizures in infants even when a vaginal delivery does not appear to have been traumatic.[23] Focal clonic seizures, presumably caused by irritation of primary motor cortex, are a common manifestation. Typically, these seizures are easier to control than those caused by more diffuse insults, such as hypoxia-ischemia. Exclusion of systemic metabolic and infectious disease is important to have confidence that the hemorrhage is the etiology and not merely incidental. Computed tomography (CT) and magnetic resonance imaging (MRI) of the brain will show subarachnoid blood over the convexities of the hemispheres and along the tentorium. The seizures are usually self-limited, and the prognosis is favorable.[24]

In the premature infant, intraventricular hemorrhages occur as a result of bleeding in the subependymal germinal matrix. Large hemorrhages can be associated with parenchymal injury and may present with seizures. Intraventricular hemorrhage accounts for a large proportion of seizures presenting in premature infants.[25]

Parenchymal hemorrhage, including hemorrhage with subdural and subarachnoid extension, may result from venous sinus thrombosis. Perinatal risk factors such as complicated delivery and preeclampsia are frequently present and are more common than prothrombotic factors.[26] Seizures occur in about half of cases.[27] Symptoms are commonly present in the first

2 days after birth. Babies with intraparenchymal hemorrhage caused by sinovenous thrombosis are at significant risk for an abnormal neurological outcome.[28] Acute treatment with anticoagulation is controversial because of the perceived risk of additional hemorrhage and the high rate of spontaneous recanalization.

Stroke

Arterial occlusion may occur acutely because of complicated delivery, but stroke, particularly involving the middle cerebral artery distribution, may occur in utero. Thromboembolism caused by congenital heart disease may also lead to ischemic stroke. An acute stroke in a neonate will usually be associated with encephalopathy. But, a baby with a remote intrauterine stroke may look entirely normal at birth and have good bilateral motor function. Seizures, particularly focal clonic seizures, are a frequent first symptom of an ischemic stroke in the neonate. Infants frequently develop spastic hemiparesis as a long-term sequela of stroke, but fewer than half of such infants will develop epilepsy.[29]

Cerebral Malformations

Malformations of cortical development are a common cause of epilepsy in children. The majority present before 16 years of age. A sizable proportion present at less than a month of age.[30] The type of lesions range from diffuse malformations with dismal prognoses, such as lissencephaly, to subtle focal cortical dysplasia that may not be apparent with initial neuroimaging.[31]

Tuberous sclerosis (TS) is a particular genetic disorder associated with multifocal cortical malformations ("tubers"). The seizures commonly associated with TS may present in the neonate in conjunction with cutaneous hypopigmented macules, cardiac rhabdomyomas, and renal angiomyolipomas.[32,33] TS may present in the neonatal period with a variety of seizure types, ranging from infantile spasms to more subtle partial seizures.[34] When TS presents with seizures in the neonatal period, the prognosis for normal neurological development is poor. Epilepsy and mental retardation are common.[33]

Transient Metabolic Disorders

Hypoglycemia

When hypoglycemia is a cause of seizures in the neonate, the condition must be recognized quickly so appropriate therapy can be instituted and brain injury averted. Hypoglycemic seizures will be seen most commonly in infants born to mothers with gestational diabetes. Other conditions associated with hypoglycemia include hypoxic-ischemic encephalopathy, sepsis, intrauterine growth retardation, genetic disorders of glycogen metabolism, and hyperinsulinism.

Hypocalcemia/Hypomagnesemia

Although most newborns with hypocalcemia are asymptomatic, seizures can be a sign of low calcium. Focal clonic seizures are most common. There are both early and late causes of hypocalcemia. Early causes include prematurity, birth asphyxia, and intrauterine growth retardation. Later presentation after 2 or 3 days of age may be because of genetic disorders such as DiGeorge syndrome (22q11 deletion), maternal hyperparathyroidism, or deficient calcium intake. As with hypoglycemia, early recognition and correction of the underlying electrolyte abnormality will be more efficacious than simply administering antiseizure medication. Hypomagnesemia most often occurs in conjunction with hypocalcemia, although isolated cases are reported.

Hyponatremia

Hyponatremia is described less often than hypoglycemia and hypocalcemia as a cause of neonatal seizures. There are case reports of maternal water intoxication leading to neonatal seizures. Other reported causes include congenital adrenal hypoplasia, congenital hypothyroidism, and oxytocin administration.[35]

Persistent Metabolic Disorders

Inborn Errors of Metabolism

There are numerous inborn errors of metabolism associated with seizures during the newborn period. Most of these disorders present with seizures and progressive encephalopathy after a few days of age, once the baby has begun feeding and is dependent on his or her own metabolism instead of the mother's. Among the more common of these rare disorders are urea cycle defects, organic acidurias, and aminoacidopathies. Some of these are amenable to treatment with cofactor administration (eg, biotinidase deficiency) or avoidance of "toxic" nutrients via feeding with a specially formulated diet (eg, maple syrup urine disease). Measurement of ammonia, urine organic acids, and serum amino acids will usually reveal diagnostic abnormalities.

Nonketotic hyperglycinemia (glycine encephalopathy) is caused by a defect in cleavage of the excitatory amino acid glycine. This disorder often causes seizures characterized by frequent myoclonic seizures. Nearly all patients with nonketotic hyperglycinemia have severe neurologic sequelae, although a rare, transient form does exist and carries a more favorable prognosis. Measurement of glycine concentration in the cerebrospinal fluid (CSF) will suggest the diagnosis.

Pyridoxine dependency is caused by an inborn abnormality in the synthesis of γ-aminobutyric acid (GABA). This is a rare autosomal recessive disorder. Neonates without obvious seizure risk factors present with frequent, medically refractory seizures or status epilepticus in the newborn period or early infancy. Seizures may be present from the time of birth, an exception to the general rule that seizures caused by inborn errors of metabolism present after feeding has begun. EEGs are typically dramatically abnormal with burst suppression or hypsarrhythmia. Treatment with B6 (pyridoxine) may lead to a rapid resolution of the seizures and the EEG abnormalities, but the absence of an immediate EEG improvement does not preclude the diagnosis. Serum and CSF analysis show elevated α-aminoadipic semialdehyde and pipecolic acid.[36,37]

Folinic acid-responsive seizures are the result of another rare, cofactor-responsive inborn error of metabolism. As with pyridoxine dependency, the seizures are distressingly refractory to routine seizure medications. The seizures respond promptly to administration of folinic acid. CSF analysis shows elevated α-aminoadipic semialdehyde and pipecolic acid as in pyridoxine dependency, and the 2 disorders may be allelic.[38,39]

Familial or Idiopathic Epilepsies

There are 2 benign idiopathic epilepsy syndromes routinely considered in the neonate. One is benign familial neonatal seizures (BFNSs), and the other is benign idiopathic (nonfamilial) neonatal seizures (BINSs). Two other neonatal epilepsy syndromes are considered "catastrophic" seizure disorders: EME and EIEE.

The BFNS was the first idiopathic epilepsy proven to have a genetic etiology. The syndrome was recognized as an autosomal dominant condition with high penetrance (85%). It was first linked to chromosome 20 and soon afterward was attributed to mutations in genes encoding for voltage-gated potassium channels (KCNQ2 and KCNQ3). It is estimated to occur in 14 per 100,000 births. The seizures typically present in the first week of life as focal (or multifocal) clonic seizures or as tonic seizures. The babies respond well to treatment with traditional antiseizure medications. The interictal EEG is usually normal or only mildly abnormal. The seizures typically remit spontaneously at less than a year of life.[40,41]

The BINSs are distinguished from BFNSs by the absence of a family history. The etiology is therefore less clear. There still may be a genetic etiology with seizures arising because of de novo mutations. Most children affected by BINSs have seizure onset between 4 and 6 days of life (fifth-day fits). Most of the time, the seizures present as focal clonic seizures. Remarkably, the seizures typically remit within a few days, and there may not be a need to treat with seizure medication beyond a few days. BINSs are diagnosed by exclusion of other seizure-producing conditions and by the characteristic benign clinical course.

Early myoclonic epilepsy is characterized by erratic, fragmentary myoclonic jerks that begin in the first month of life. The myoclonus is eventually replaced by partial seizures, massive erratic myoclonus, and tonic seizures. The EEG reveals a burst-suppression pattern. There are a variety of possible etiologies, particularly inborn errors of metabolism (eg, nonketotic hyperglycinemia, pyridoxine dependency, urea cycle defects) and certain congenital structural abnormalities, such as Aicardi syndrome. The prognosis is, unfortunately, poor. Affected infants are developmentally delayed and have a variety of other symptoms, such as abnormal muscle tone and microcephaly.[42]

Early infantile epileptic encephalopathy presents with frequent tonic spasms in the neonatal period or early infancy. The EEG is characterized by an interictal burst-suppression pattern and diffuse attenuation during the spasms. The underlying cause is most frequently a structural abnormality, such as lissencephaly, porencephaly, hemimegalencephaly, and Aicardi syndrome. Congenital metabolic disorders are less frequently found than with EME. Infants with EIEE are severely developmentally delayed and have medically refractory seizures.

SEIZURE CLASSIFICATION

There are numerous neonatal seizure classification schemes that have been used over the years. The most recent classification proposed by the Commission on Classification and Terminology of the International League Against Epilepsy does not classify neonatal seizures separately from seizures in older individuals.[43] Nevertheless, there are common differences in the way seizures appear in neonates compared with older children and adults.

The most widely used scheme divides neonatal seizures into the following descriptive types (Table 15-1)[44]:

Focal clonic seizures: These seizures consist of rhythmic jerking of the hand, arm, leg, face, or trunk. The rhythmic clonic movements of focal clonic seizures in the neonate are usually slow (0.5–2 Hz) compared to the clonic movements in an older child or adult. Focal clonic seizures most commonly have a distinct ictal EEG pattern that correlates with the rhythmic clonic movements (Figure 15-1). Focal clonic seizures may be multifocal and sometimes have a generalized appearance, although EEG will typically show that there are bilateral, independent seizures occurring (Figure 15-2).

Focal tonic seizures: These consist of sustained posturing of one or more limbs, sometimes with more complex features, such as head and eye deviation. The seizures are transient, usually lasting seconds. They can be differentiated from nonepileptic movements by their repeated, stereotyped appearance and their persistence after repositioning or restraining the affected limb. Focal tonic seizures most often have a corresponding ictal EEG pattern.

Generalized tonic seizures: These seizures consist of bilateral tonic stiffening of the limbs and trunk. These seizures last for seconds and may evolve slowly or rapidly (spasms). They are often triggered by stimulation or a state change. These seizures, along with the "subtle seizures" described further in this list, may be thought of as a reflex phenomenon secondary to a depressed cortex that is not inhibiting the brainstem and other subcortical structures. The EEG will usually not show a characteristic evolving, rhythmic ictal pattern. There may be nonspecific paroxysmal changes on the EEG (eg, an electrodecrement) that reflects a sudden state change, but this pattern is not generally

Table 15-1 Seizure Types in Neonates

Seizure Type	Description	EEG Correlate
Focal clonic (multifocal clonic)	Rhythmic jerking of a limb (or limbs); usually slow, 0.5–2 Hz	Close correlation with a rhythmic, ictal pattern over the contralateral hemisphere
Focal tonic	Stiffening or posturing of a limb, sometimes with head and eye deviation	Usually correlates with an ictal pattern over the contralateral hemisphere
Generalized tonic	Bilateral tonic stiffening involving limbs and trunk	Nonspecific EEG changes; often a generalized electrodecrement
Myoclonic	Brief jerks of limbs or trunk; no sustained stiffening component	Often absent; single, time-locked burst of spikes in some
Subtle	Motor: chewing, blinking, eye deviation, bicycling, swimming movements. Autonomic: apnea, tachycardia, changes in blood pressure	Variable; often absent

Abbreviation: EEG, electroencephalogram.

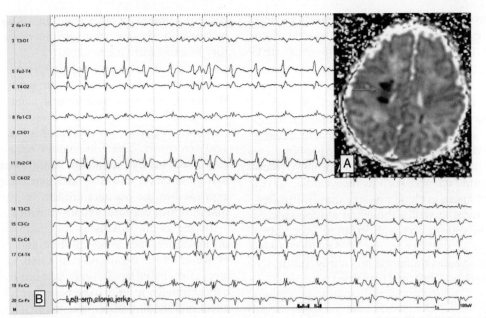

FIGURE 15-1 A, Magnetic resonance imaging (apparent diffusion coefficient map) showing focal abnormality (stroke; arrow) in the right posterior frontal lobe in a 2-day-old term baby with venous infarction caused by polycythemia. B, Electroencephalogram with rhythmic ictal discharge over the right central-temporal region; correlates with focal left arm clonic jerking.

regarded as "epileptic" in the same way as an evolving rhythmic discharge is.

Myoclonic seizures: Myoclonic seizures are sudden jerks of a limb, the face, or the trunk. They may be focal or generalized. The jerks are sudden and do not have sustained stiffening. This distinguishes them from brief focal or generalized tonic seizures. Sometimes, they are localized to the same body region; at other times, they may be multifocal. Myoclonic seizures may be generated by cortical or subcortical structures. When they have a cortical origin, there is often a clear ictal EEG correlate simultaneous with the clinical myoclonus.

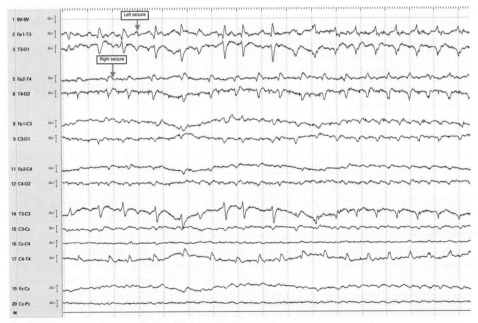

FIGURE 15-2 Independent bilateral ictal electroencephalographic rhythms (arrows) in a 1-day-old term baby with severe neonatal encephalopathy after decreased fetal movement, Apgar scores of 0 at 1 and 5 minutes, and 14 minutes of resuscitation. No ictal movements noted.

When the myoclonus is caused by an insult to deep gray nuclei (eg, acute hypoxic-ischemic insults), there will usually be no consistent, simultaneous EEG correlate.

Subtle seizures: These behaviors present the greatest diagnostic and treatment challenge among the various seizure types. Subtle seizures may be complex motor phenomena, such as rhythmic chewing and sucking movements, rhythmic tongue thrusting, blinking, eye deviation, or movements resembling swimming or bicycling. Autonomic changes such as tachycardia, apnea, and sudden changes in blood pressure may be manifestations of seizures as well, although in a nonparalyzed patient, apnea seldom occurs in isolation from subtle or overt motor seizure phenomena.[44,45] As with the generalized tonic seizures described previously, subtle seizures often have no EEG ictal correlate.

PATHOPHYSIOLOGY

An "epileptic seizure" is a transient behavior caused by abnormal excessive or synchronous neuronal activity in the brain.[46] Seizures are usually generated by abnormal excitatory activity in the cerebral cortex. Other types of stereotyped, paroxysmal behavior may be designated "seizures" as well. These may be generated from subcortical brain structures and have been characterized as a type of primitive reflex. The term *brainstem release phenomenon* was originally used by Mizrahi and Kellaway to describe these behaviors that have a seizure-like appearance because of the abnormal paroxysmal stereotyped nature of the behavior but do not have a consistent ictal EEG.[44]

Another important concept is that of "electroencephalographic seizures." Sometimes referred to as "subclinical seizures," these are apparent on EEG as paroxysmal, evolving, rhythmic, ictal discharges. However, the EEG seizures are not correlated with clinically apparent seizure behavior.[47]

Neonatal seizures are usually not generalized. The immature brain does not sustain truly generalized tonic clonic seizures (GTCs). There is immaturity of myelination that leads to multifocal and minimal seizure expression.[48] In addition, synaptic and dendritic density and the overall balance of excitatory and inhibitory neuronal activity contribute to a milieu in which seizures are expressed differently from those in a more mature brain.[49] When a neonate has what looks like a GTC, there are usually bilateral independent seizures evident on EEG (Figure 15-2).

It has long been recognized that the neonatal brain is particularly vulnerable to seizures. Although this no doubt reflects the number and severity of seizure-provoking insults to which the neonate is prone, there are also significant maturational differences between the neonate's brain and older children's. This also provides insight into why neonatal seizures are so often refractory to antiseizure medication.

Glutamate is the major excitatory neurotransmitter. Glutamate mediates changes in neuronal excitation through its action on sodium and calcium channels via binding to NMDA (N-methyl-d-aspartate) and AMPA (α-amino-3-hydroxy-5-methyl-4-isoxazole propionic acid) receptors. These excitatory receptors are overexpressed in the neonatal brain relative to more mature animals, and the particular receptor subtypes expressed in the neonate are less responsive to drugs that diminish excitatory neurotransmission.[49]

In the brain, GABA is the main inhibitory neurotransmitter, mediating chloride and potassium flux. However, in the neonatal brain, GABA has a net excitatory effect based largely on greater intracellular chloride concentrations in immature neurons.[50] This excitatory effect rapidly diminishes over the first months of life.[51] Because two major antiseizure medication classes typically used in the neonate, barbiturates and benzodiazepines, have predominantly GABAergic mechanisms of action, this provides some rationale for the often-incomplete effect of these. Furthermore, there is a well-described caudal-to-rostral maturation of the inhibitory GABA system.[52] This provides a plausible explanation for the frequently observed occurrence of EEG seizures in the absence of clinical manifestations. GABAergic drugs such as phenobarbital and benzodiazepines may suppress neurotransmission at a brainstem and diencephalic level, mitigating the clinical manifestations, while seizures persist at a cortical level apparent on EEG. Also of interest is the fact that neurons in certain types of brain malformations from older patients exhibit "epileptogenic" properties that resemble those of the immature neurons of neonates.[53]

DIFFERENTIAL DIAGNOSIS

There are numerous normal behaviors that may be mistaken for seizures, such as stretching, hiccupping, startle movements, chewing movements, and various limb twitching typical during the baby's active sleep state. Most of these nonepileptic behaviors are not truly stereotypical in appearance. When focal or multifocal limb movements are suspected of being seizures, a useful bedside intervention is to try to stimulate the baby in a way that will interrupt the behavior. Moving and repositioning a limb will usually stop simple clonus or cause a change in jittery behavior. Epileptic seizures most often occur spontaneously, and they do not stop with physical stimulation.

Apnea, bradycardia, and tachycardia, along with variations in blood pressure, are nonspecific and have many different underlying causes. Apnea is frequently

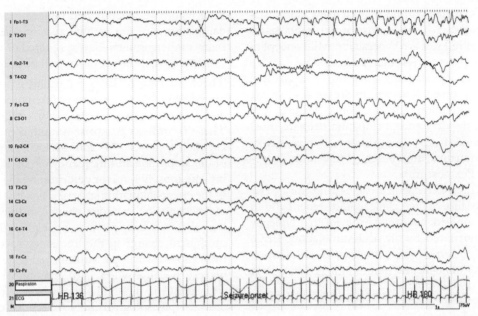

FIGURE 15-3 Subtle seizure manifested only by tachycardia. Heart rate just before seizure onset was 136 beats per minute. Immediately after left temporal seizure activity begins in the left temporal region (arrow), the heart rate increased to 180 beats per minute. Infant was 1 day old with choanal atresia and perinatal asphyxia.

suspected of being a sign of seizures, particularly in neonates who are encephalopathic because of a systemic insult or necessary interventions such as sedation and pharmacologic neuromuscular blockade. Apneic seizures are often accompanied by other subtle, stereotyped seizure manifestations, such as eye deviation or limb posturing. Tachycardia more frequently accompanies seizures than does bradycardia (Figure 15-3).

However, apnea and bradycardia may be postictal phenomena (Figure 15-4). Continuous EEG monitoring is the primary diagnostic test for differentiating seizures from other causes of apnea and bradycardia.

Neonates with a mild degree of encephalopathy often have varying levels of consciousness in which periods of lethargy alternate with periods of irritability and "hyperalertness." They often manifest jitteriness or

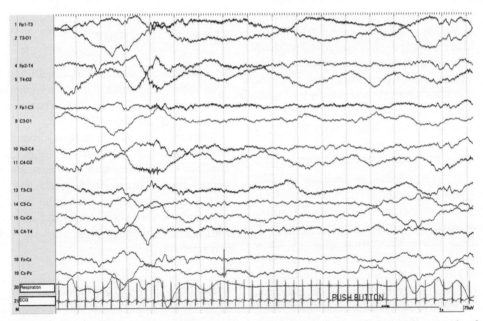

FIGURE 15-4 Postictal 7-second apnea recorded in respiratory monitor channel (arrow) 30 seconds after the seizure shown in Figure 15-3 ended. Annotation "Push Button" indicates when nurse pressed the event marker button because of oxygen desaturation alarm.

tremulousness, which can be mistaken for clonic seizures or myoclonus. Muscle tone is normal or increased, and the tendon reflexes are hyperactive. Mild encephalopathy usually lasts for less than 24 hours.[54]

Moderate encephalopathy presents a depressed level of consciousness (lethargy or stupor with some reactivity to stimulation) and hypotonia. Seizures that occur in a moderately encephalopathic neonate must be differentiated from other abnormal movements, such as spontaneous myoclonus, clonic limb movements, and reflex posturing.

It is important to recognize babies who are at risk for seizures because of their clinical predicament and to watch for stereotyped, abnormal behavior that typically cannot be interrupted by physical stimulation. EEG, particularly long-term studies, can prove useful when the epileptic vs nonepileptic nature of a behavior is in question.

DIAGNOSTIC TESTS

Depending on the type of presentation, testing for various metabolic, infectious, and structural abnormalities is appropriate (Table 15-2). EEG is the most helpful diagnostic test for determining whether frequent stereotyped behaviors in babies are epileptic seizures. There are 3 basic EEG approaches:

The first is routine bedside EEG done using a conventional neonatal array of electrodes. Physiologic monitoring channels (electrocardiogram [ECG], respiration, chin electromyography [EMG], and eye movement) are often included. Besides the obvious advantage of seeing changes in heart rate and respiration simultaneous with seizure activity on an EEG, the physiological channels allow discrimination between active and quiet sleep states and assist in determining if EEG activity is appropriate to the infant's postconception age. The recordings are run for a relatively brief amount of time, usually 45 to 60 minutes in a neonate. The duration of a routine neonatal EEG is longer than the 20 to 30 minutes typical of routine EEGs in older children and adults to record both active and quiet sleep states.

The second is long-term EEG monitoring (LTM). LTM can last from hours to days. The recordings usually include physiological channels to record respiration, eye movements, and muscle activity along with time-synchronized video. The usual goal of these longer recordings is to record suspicious, seizure-like behavior on the EEG and thereby determine the epileptic vs nonepileptic nature of the spells in question. LTM may reveal electrographic seizures without clinical signs and symptoms. It remains uncertain what this means in terms of necessity for aggressive treatment. It is increasingly recognized that infants who are very

ill or who have recently had major procedures such as cardiac surgery are at high risk of seizures. Because many of these infants may be sedated or pharmacologically paralyzed, seizures may well be masked.[55,56]

The third type of EEG recording is amplitude-integrated EEG (aEEG). It is most often used as a screening and monitoring tool in the newborn intensive care unit. These recordings comprise a limited number of EEG channels (often 2 or 4) and display a graphic depiction of the amplitude and frequency of EEG. These recordings are most helpful for determining the overall degree of the encephalopathic state of a sick infant and providing evidence of a sudden change in the baby's neurological status. Seizures may appear on the aEEG as a prominent change in the frequency spectrum distinct from those associated with normal state changes. The biggest challenge with regard to monitoring for seizures with aEEG is differentiating seizures from the other changes (physiological and artifact) that can cause sudden changes in the graphic display. For that reason, systems that provide a means of checking the actual EEG trace at the time in question are important.[57]

The EEGs performed on newborns use a more limited electrode array than is typical for older children and adults because (1) the newborn baby has a smaller head size, and (2) neonates manifest generally slower frequencies. Neonatal EEG is usually displayed with longer periods of time on screen to better show the overall background pattern of continuous vs discontinuous activity. The slower seizure patterns often characteristic of neonatal seizures may also be more apparent with longer periods of time displayed.

MANAGEMENT

This discussion of seizure treatment assumes there has been appropriate initial attention to maintaining a patent airway and adequate oxygenation while monitoring heart rate and blood pressure.

Seizures may be the primary manifestation of an underlying acute metabolic derangement or an infection. The earlier these remediable causes of seizures are treated, the less the risk of further brain injury. In addition, if there is an acute metabolic disorder (eg, hypocalcemia), it will likely be harder to control seizures with antiseizure medication until the derangement is corrected.

Electrolyte Disturbances

Hypoglycemia

Hypoglycemia is important to recognize as early as possible. There is no complete agreement on the definition

Table 15-2 Etiologies of Neonatal Seizures

Category	Etiology	Evaluation
Acute metabolic derangements	Hypoglycemia, hypocalcemia, hypomagnesemia, hyponatremia	Serum concentration of glucose, calcium, magnesium, sodium
Infectious	Bacterial meningitis, viral encephalitis, intrauterine infection (TORCH)	Lumbar puncture, herpes PCR, TORCH titers Neuroimaging may suggest TORCH infection
Benign neonatal seizures	BINS, BFNS	Exclusion of other etiologies BFNS: Characteristic family history in the absence of encephalopathy and acute seizure precipitants BINS: Normal-appearing baby without acute or chronic seizure precipitants; early resolution of seizures
Epileptic encephalopathies	EME, EIEE	EME: Multifocal myoclonic jerks; often associated with a metabolic derangement (see text) EIEE: Tonic and clonic seizures; imaging studies commonly show brain malformation
Hypoxic-ischemic	Perinatal asphyxia, circulatory arrest	Umbilical cord venous and arterial blood gases, neonatal blood gas, liver and renal function, electrolytes (especially calcium, serum lactate)
Hemorrhagic and stroke	Subdural, subarachnoid, venous thrombosis Arterial occlusion, trauma, malformation	Neuroimaging: CT, MRI, MR venography, MR angiography Head ultrasound LP may reveal hemorrhage
Malformations of cortical development	Generalized/multifocal: eg, hydranencephaly, lissencephaly, diffuse polymicrogyria, tuberous sclerosis Focal: eg, focal cortical dysplasia, heterotopia, agenesis of corpus callosum, holoprosencephaly	Neuroimaging: MRI most useful
Inborn errors of metabolism	Numerous Amino acidopathies Organic acidopathies Carbohydrate disorders Purine and pyrimidine disorders Sulfite oxidase deficiency CSF neurotransmitter disorders Biotinidase deficiency Pyridoxine dependency Folinic acid responsiveness Fatty acid oxidation disorders Carnitine transporter deficiency	Serum amino acids, ammonia, lactate, pyruvate, glucose, electrolytes Urine organic acids, purine and pyrimidine metabolites, sulfites, nitrites, ketones CSF glucose, neurotransmitters, lactate, glycine Biotinidase serum concentration Empirical administration of pyridoxine, folinic acid during EEG monitoring (Additional targeted testing depending on presentation and findings on screening labs)

BFNS, benign familial neonatal seizure; BINS, benign idiopathic (nonfamilial) neonatal seizure; CSF, cerebrospinal fluid; CT, computed tomography; EIEE, early infantile epileptic encephalopathy; EME, early myoclonic epilepsy; LP, lumbar puncture; MR, magnetic resonance; MRI, magnetic resonance imaging; PCR, polymerase chain reaction.

of hypoglycemia in the newborn,[58] but for a baby with seizures and a blood sugar below 45 mg/dL, there should be an assumption that the low glucose is the primary cause. Correction with 10% glucose solution administered parenterally is a reasonable first step. It is important to evaluate for the many possible causes of hypoglycemia in the newborn.

Hypocalcemia

Seizures are a possible manifestation of hypocalcemia. Babies with hypocalcemia may be jittery and have myoclonus. The treatment is administration of calcium gluconate. The baby must be closely monitored during calcium infusion because of risks that include bradycardia and tissue necrosis. As with hypoglycemia, there are many possible causes of hypocalcaemia, and further investigation for the etiology is necessary.

Hypomagnesemia

Hypomagnesemia often occurs in conjunction with hypocalcemia. When evaluating the etiology of acute neonatal seizures, both calcium and magnesium concentrations should be measured. Treatment of hypomagnesemia consists of infusion or injection of magnesium sulfate.

Hyponatremia

Hyponatremia may occur because of hypothyroidism, congenital adrenal hypoplasia, and maternal water intoxication. Iatrogenic causes include oxytocin administration and infusion of intravenous fluid without adequate sodium content. Correction must be gradual to avoid osmotic demyelination syndrome (central pontine myelinolysis), a complication of overly rapid correction of serum sodium.

Infectious Etiologies

Seizures may be the initial symptom of meningitis or encephalitis. The occurrence of seizures should prompt a careful evaluation for possible intracranial infection and appropriate treatment with antibiotics. Common bacterial causes of meningitis in the newborn include group B β-strep and *E. coli*. CMV and herpes simplex are relatively common viral causes of encephalitis.

Antiseizure Medications

There are few data from controlled trials of antiseizure medication in neonates and almost no head-to-head data comparing efficacy between seizure medications. An exception is a 1999 study that randomly assigned neonates to receive either phenobarbital or phenytoin for initial treatment of EEG-confirmed seizures. The medications were equally efficacious, but only about half of the babies responded initially to either drug.[59]

The most common treatment strategy is to initiate drug treatment and titrate the initial medication (usually phenobarbital or phenytoin/fosphenytoin) to the point at which clinically apparent seizures are controlled or high therapeutic serum concentrations are attained. If seizures are not controlled with the initial agent, it is reasonable to introduce a second antiseizure medication with a different mechanism of action. For example, both barbiturates and benzodiazepines have GABAergic mechanisms of action. If high serum concentrations of phenobarbital fail to achieve seizure control, a rational approach is to add a drug such as phenytoin/fosphenytoin because it has a different mechanism of action: blockade of sodium channels.

When clinical seizures remit, EEG seizures may persist. In many cases, these EEG seizures will prove resistant to further medication administration despite introduction of more medications and the exposure of the infant to greater risk of adverse effects. Often, EEG-only seizures will be targeted for additional treatment if the seizures are continuous or frequent. Determining the long-term benefit of aggressively treating EEG-only seizures remains difficult. As discussed further in the chapter, the outcome of neonates with seizures is more dependent on etiology than the seizures themselves.

When antiseizure medication is started, it is ideal to give a drug that can be administered parenterally. This will achieve reasonable serum concentrations quickly and avoid the uncertainties of enteral absorption in a sick neonate. Ideally, the seizure medication will be one that can later be given via the enteral route, assuming a baby needs to remain on chronic antiseizure therapy.

Phenobarbital

Phenobarbital is a barbiturate. Its primary mechanism of action is via increasing neuronal inhibition through increased chloride channel conductance. It undergoes hepatic metabolism and has a longer half-life in premature infants than in more mature babies. However, as a baby matures, these serum concentrations often fall as liver metabolism improves and the drug induces its own metabolism. It will also have a longer half-life in babies who have sustained an asphyxial insult with resulting hepatic dysfunction. They will likely need lower and less-frequent maintenance doses initially. Therapeutic hypothermia also results in a longer half-life.[60]

Phenytoin and Fosphenytoin

Phenytoin has long been the second drug of choice for intractable neonatal seizures and is sometimes used as the initial antiseizure medication, particularly when there is a concern that a loading dose of phenobarbital may be too sedating.

Phenytoin is highly insoluble in aqueous solutions, so it is formulated with various buffers to maintain the parenteral solution at a pH of 12. It must be administered slowly (<1 mg/kg/min) to avoid bradycardia and hypotension. Extravasation into the soft tissues can cause local injury. Fosphenytoin is substituted for phenytoin in many hospitals because patients tolerate a faster rate of administration (up to 3 mg/kg/min), and there is better compatibility with dextrose-containing intravenous fluid. Fosphenytoin is rapidly metabolized to phenytoin in the blood via hydrolysis.

It is typically difficult to sustain consistent therapeutic serum concentrations of phenytoin with oral (enteral) phenytoin in infants. There are differences in bioavailability with various formulations, and there is substantial interindividual variability in metabolism.[61] Phenytoin is highly protein bound and may displace other medications, leading to unexpected pharmacologic interactions. An ability to measure unbound ("free") phenytoin levels is useful.

Benzodiazepines

Benzodiazepines such as lorazepam, midazolam, and diazepam are often used when initial therapies fail to adequately control neonatal seizures. These are all relatively short-acting medications. Lorazepam has the longest duration of action, midazolam the shortest. For refractory status epilepticus, they will usually have to be given frequently or by continuous infusion. Respiratory depression and hypotension may complicate benzodiazepine administration, particularly in infants already medicated with phenobarbital.

Other Seizure Medications

There are small case series reporting the neonatal use of many of the antiseizure medications commonly administered to older children. Series reporting the use of carbamazepine, topiramate, zonisamide, and valproic acid have been published. For the most part, use of these medications will be limited to babies with refractory seizures and in whom more routinely used antiseizure medications have failed.[62–64]

Levetiracetam is an antiseizure medication increasingly being used in neonates. There are no controlled studies of levetiracetam in neonates, although there are numerous small case series reporting efficacy and safety.[65–67] Levetiracetam has many favorable pharmacologic properties. It is not metabolized in the liver, so it is not subject to the rapid changes in hepatic function seen in normal and sick neonates. It is excreted unchanged through the kidneys, so babies with renal dysfunction may need lower doses and less-frequent dosing. There are no drug-drug interactions. It is not protein bound. The drug has a higher volume of distribution and a longer half-life in the neonate.[68] It can be administered parenterally, and there is also an oral solution.

Lidocaine infusion is another potentially effective medication for management of neonatal seizures. It is more commonly used in Europe than in the United States. There are concerns about inducing a cardiac arrhythmia, although the concern may be excessive.[69]

Pyridoxine and Folinic Acid

When seizures are unresponsive to routinely administered antiseizure medications, and particularly when there is a very abnormal EEG in a baby without major seizure risk factors, consideration of pyridoxine- or folinic-acid-responsive seizures is warranted. Pyridoxine is usually given empirically as a 50- or 100-mg dose. Ideally, it is administered while the EEG is being monitored because there are reports of rapid EEG improvement shortly after B6 injection.[37,70]

If seizures do not respond to pyridoxine, a trial of folinic acid may be effective.[38]

OUTCOME

Neonates with seizures are at increased risk of cerebral palsy, epilepsy, behavior problems, and an abnormal cognitive outcome. Estimates of morbidity indicate some 35% to 60% of neonates with seizures will have an abnormal outcome. Three prognostic factors are most important: the etiology of the seizures, the timing of the insult, and the adverse effect of the seizures (and their treatment?) on the baby.

Seizure etiology is the primary determinant of outcome. Perinatal asphyxia is a well-recognized cause of long-term morbidity, and the presence of seizures in the setting of asphyxia confers a greater risk of an abnormal outcome.[14] Similarly, seizures in the setting of group B streptococcal meningitis,[17] sinovenous thrombosis,[27] and brain malformations are associated with a greater degree of abnormal outcome. Seizures caused by these conditions are typically regarded as markers of the extent of the injury.[71]

Seizures in extremely low birth weight infants are associated with a worse outcome than seizures in more mature neonates. Cerebral palsy, cognitive impairment, and epilepsy are more common following seizures in these immature, smaller babies. Their risk of abnormal outcome appears to be independent of factors such as intraventricular hemorrhage, sepsis, and meningitis.[24,72]

The unique contribution of the seizure burden (the percentage of time an EEG reveals seizure activity) to the child's outcome remains difficult to distinguish from the etiology of the seizures because injuries that have greater impact on cerebral cortex will more commonly manifest with seizures than will lesions not affecting cortex.[71] There is good evidence from animal studies that seizures in the immature brain do have an adverse effect on the development of neural networks, subpopulations of ion channels, and neurotransmitter receptors.[73,74] Seizures can potentially add to brain injury by increasing metabolic demands and disrupting neuronal repair mechanisms.[75] Increasingly, studies showing similar degrees of severity of underlying insult find worse neurodevelopmental outcomes in babies who also manifest seizures.[76] Still, there is little consensus on whether aggressive treatment of brief, self-limited EEG-only seizures results in a better outcome.

REFERENCES

1. Annegers JF, Hauser WA, Lee JR, et al. Incidence of acute symptomatic seizures in Rochester, Minnesota, 1935–1984. *Epilepsia.* 1995;36(4):327–333.
2. Glass HC, Pham TN, Danielsen B, et al. Antenatal and intrapartum risk factors for seizures in term newborns: a population-based study, California 1998–2002. *J Pediatr.* 2009;154(1): 24–28.e1.
3. Lanska MJ, Lanska DJ, Baumann RJ, et al. A population-based study of neonatal seizures in Fayette County, Kentucky. *Neurology.* 1995;45(4):724–732.
4. Ronen GM, Penney S, Andrews W. The epidemiology of clinical neonatal seizures in Newfoundland: a population-based study. *J Pediatr.* 1999;134(1):71–75.
5. Mwaniki M, Mathenge A, Gwer S, et al. Neonatal seizures in a rural Kenyan District hospital: aetiology, incidence and outcome of hospitalization. *BMC Med.* 2010;8:16.
6. Saliba RM, Annegers FJ, Waller DK, et al. Risk factors for neonatal seizures: a population-based study, Harris County, Texas, 1992–1994. *Am J Epidemiol.* 2001;154(1):14–20.
7. Sheth RD, Hobbs GR, Mullett M. Neonatal seizures: incidence, onset, and etiology by gestational age. *J Perinatol.* 1999;19(1):40–43.
8. Guerrini R, Aicardi J. Epileptic encephalopathies with myoclonic seizures in infants and children (severe myoclonic epilepsy and myoclonic-astatic epilepsy). *J Clin Neurophysiol.* 2003; 20(6):449–461.
9. Ohtahara S, Yamatogi Y. Epileptic encephalopathies in early infancy with suppression-burst. *J Clin Neurophysiol.* 2003; 20(6):398–407.
10. Tekgul H, Gauvreau K, Soul J, et al. The current etiologic profile and neurodevelopmental outcome of seizures in term newborn infants. *Pediatrics.* 2006;117(4):1270–1280.
11. Bjorkman ST, Miller SM, Rose SE, et al. Seizures are associated with brain injury severity in a neonatal model of hypoxia-ischemia. *Neuroscience.* 2010;166(1):157–167.
12. Scher MS, Steppe DA, Beggarly M. Timing of neonatal seizures and intrapartum obstetrical factors. *J Child Neurol.* 2008;23(6):640–643.
13. Wusthoff CJ, Dlugos DJ, Gutierrez-Colina A, et al. Electrographic seizures during therapeutic hypothermia for neonatal hypoxic-ischemic encephalopathy. *J Child Neurol.* 2011;26(6):724–728.
14. Garfinkle J, Shevell MI. Predictors of outcome in term infants with neonatal seizures subsequent to intrapartum asphyxia. *J Child Neurol.* 2011;26(4):453–459.
15. Stoll BJ, Hansen NI, Sanchez PJ, et al. Early onset neonatal sepsis: the burden of group B Streptococcal and E. coli disease continues. *Pediatrics.* 2011;127(5):817–826.
16. Gaschignard J, Levy C, Romain O, et al. Neonatal bacterial meningitis: 444 cases in 7 years. *Pediatr Infect Dis J.* 2011; 30(3):212–217.
17. Levent F, Baker CJ, Rench MA, et al. Early outcomes of group B streptococcal meningitis in the 21st century. *Pediatr Infect Dis J.* 2010;29(11):1009–1012.
18. Kimberlin DW. Herpes simplex virus infections of the newborn. *Semin Perinatol.* 2007;31(1):19–25.

19. Toth C, Harder S, Yager J. Neonatal herpes encephalitis: a case series and review of clinical presentation. *Can J Neurol Sci.* 2003;30(1):36–40.
20. Kimberlin DW, Lin CY, Jacobs RF, et al. Safety and efficacy of high-dose intravenous acyclovir in the management of neonatal herpes simplex virus infections. *Pediatrics.* 2001;108(2):230–238.
21. Whitley R, Arvin A, Prober C, et al. Predictors of morbidity and mortality in neonates with herpes simplex virus infections. The National Institute of Allergy and Infectious Diseases Collaborative Antiviral Study Group. *N Engl J Med.* 1991;324(7):450–454.
22. Lombardi G, Garofoli F, and Stronati M. Congenital cytomegalovirus infection: treatment, sequelae and follow-up. *J Matern. Fetal Neonatal Med.* 2010;23(Suppl 3):45–48.
23. Huang AH, Robertson RL. Spontaneous superficial parenchymal and leptomeningeal hemorrhage in term neonates. *AJNR. Am J Neuroradiol.* 2004;25(3):469–475.
24. Ronen GM, Buckley D, Penney S, et al. Long-term prognosis in children with neonatal seizures: a population-based study. *Neurology.* 2007;69(19):1816–1822.
25. Scher MS, Aso K, Beggarly ME, et al. Electrographic seizures in preterm and full-term neonates: clinical correlates, associated brain lesions, and risk for neurologic sequelae. *Pediatrics.* 1993;91(1):128–134.
26. Yang JY, Chan AK, Callen DJ, et al. Neonatal cerebral sinovenous thrombosis: sifting the evidence for a diagnostic plan and treatment strategy. *Pediatrics.* 2010;126(3):e693–e700.
27. Berfelo FJ, Kersbergen KJ, van Ommen CH, et al. Neonatal cerebral sinovenous thrombosis from symptom to outcome. *Stroke.* 2010;41(7):1382–1388.
28. Fitzgerald KC, Williams LS, Garg BP, et al. Cerebral sinovenous thrombosis in the neonate. *Arch Neurol.* 2006;63(3):405–409.
29. Wusthoff CJ, Kessler SK, Vossough A, et al. Risk of later seizure after perinatal arterial ischemic stroke: a prospective cohort study. *Pediatrics.* 2011;127(6):e1550–e1557.
30. Lortie A, Plouin P, Chiron C, et al. Characteristics of epilepsy in focal cortical dysplasia in infancy. *Epilepsy Res.* 2002;51(1–2):133–145.
31. Yoshida F, Morioka T, Hashiguchi K, et al. Appearance of focal cortical dysplasia on serial MRI after maturation of myelination. *Child's Nerv Syst.* 2008;24(2):269–273.
32. Miller SP, Tasch T, Sylvain M, et al. Tuberous sclerosis complex and neonatal seizures. *J Child Neurol.* 1998;13(12):619–623.
33. Isaacs H. Perinatal (fetal and neonatal) tuberous sclerosis: a review. *Am J Perinatol.* 2009;26(10):755–760.
34. Chu-Shore CJ, Major P, Camposano S, et al. The natural history of epilepsy in tuberous sclerosis complex. *Epilepsia.* 2010;51(7):1236–1241.
35. West CR, Harding JE. Maternal water intoxication as a cause of neonatal seizures. *J Paediatr Child Health.* 2004;40(12):709–710.
36. Koul R. Pyridoxine-dependent seizures: 10-year follow-up of eight cases. *Neurol India.* 2009;57(4):460–463.
37. Gospe SM. Pyridoxine-dependent seizures. In: Pagon RA, et al., eds. *GeneReviews.* Seattle, Wash.: University of Washington; 1993.
38. Torres OA, Miller VS, Buist NM, et al. Folinic acid-responsive neonatal seizures. *J Child Neurol.* 1999;14(8):529–532.
39. Gallagher RC, Van Hove JL, Scharer G, et al. Folinic acid-responsive seizures are identical to pyridoxine-dependent epilepsy. *Ann Neurol.* 2009;65(5):550–556.
40. Leppert M, Anderson VE, Quattlebaum T, et al. Benign familial neonatal convulsions linked to genetic markers on chromosome 20. *Nature.* 1989;337(6208):647–648.
41. Bellini G, Miceli F, Soldovieri MV, et al. Benign familial neonatal seizures. In: Pagon RA, et al., eds. *GeneReviews.* Seattle, Wash.: University of Washington; 1993.

42. Rossi S, Daniele I, Bastrenta P, et al. Early myoclonic encephalopathy and nonketotic hyperglycinemia. *Pediatr Neurol*. 2009;41(5):371–374.

43. Berg AT, Berkovic SF, Brodie MJ, et al. Revised terminology and concepts for organization of seizures and epilepsies: report of the ILAE Commission on Classification and Terminology, 2005–2009. *Epilepsia*. 2010;51(4):676–685.

44. Mizrahi EM, Kellaway P. Characterization and classification of neonatal seizures. *Neurology*. 1987;37(12):1837–1844.

45. Sirsi D, Nadiminti L, Packard MA, et al. Apneic seizures: a sign of temporal lobe hemorrhage in full-term neonates. *Pediatr Neurol*. 2007;37(5):366–370.

46. Fisher RS, van Emde Boas W, Blume W, et al. Epileptic seizures and epilepsy: definitions proposed by the International League Against Epilepsy (ILAE) and the International Bureau for Epilepsy (IBE). *Epilepsia*. 2005;46(4):470–472.

47. Weiner SP, Painter MJ, Geva D, et al. Neonatal seizures: electroclinical dissociation. *Pediatr Neurol*. 1991;7(5):363–368.

48. Haynes RL, Borenstein NS, Desilva TM, et al. Axonal development in the cerebral white matter of the human fetus and infant. *J Comp Neurol*. 2005;484(2):156–167.

49. Jensen FE. Neonatal seizures: an update on mechanisms and management. *Clin Perinatol*. 2009;36(4):881–900. vii.

50. Kirmse K, Witte OW, Holthoff K. GABAergic depolarization during early cortical development and implications for anticonvulsive therapy in neonates. *Epilepsia*. 2011;52(9):1532–1543.

51. Dzhala VI, Talos DM, Sdrulla DA, et al. NKCC1 transporter facilitates seizures in the developing brain. *Nat Med*. 2005;11(11):1205–1213.

52. Glykys J, Dzhala VI, Kuchibhotla KV, et al. Differences in cortical versus subcortical GABAergic signaling: a candidate mechanism of electroclinical uncoupling of neonatal seizures. *Neuron*. 2009;63(5):657–672.

53. Andre VM, Cepeda C, Vinters HV, et al. Interneurons, GABAA currents, and subunit composition of the GABAA receptor in type I and type II cortical dysplasia. *Epilepsia*. 2010;51(Suppl 3):166–170.

54. Sarnat HB, Sarnat MS. Neonatal encephalopathy following fetal distress. A clinical and electroencephalographic study. *Arch Neurol*. 1976;33(10):696–705.

55. Andropoulos DB, Mizrahi EM, Hrachovy RA, et al. Electroencephalographic seizures after neonatal cardiac surgery with high-flow cardiopulmonary bypass. *Anesth Analg*. 2010;110(6):1680–1685.

56. Clancy RR, Sharif U, Ichord R, et al. Electrographic neonatal seizures after infant heart surgery. *Epilepsia*. 2005;46(1):84–90.

57. Shah DK, Boylan GB, Rennie JM. Monitoring of seizures in the newborn. *Arch Dis Child Fetal Neonatal Ed*. 2012;97(1):F65–F69.

58. Adamkin DH. Postnatal glucose homeostasis in late-preterm and term infants. *Pediatrics*. 2011;127(3):575–579.

59. Painter MJ, Scher MS, Stein AD, et al. Phenobarbital compared with phenytoin for the treatment of neonatal seizures. *N Engl J Med*. 1999;341(7):485–489.

60. Filippi L, la Marca G, Cavallaro G, et al. Phenobarbital for neonatal seizures in hypoxic ischemic encephalopathy: a pharmacokinetic study during whole body hypothermia. *Epilepsia*. 2011;52(4):794–801.

61. Bourgeois BF, Dodson WE. Phenytoin elimination in newborns. *Neurology*. 1983;33(2):173–178.

62. Steinberg A, Shalev RS, Amir N. Valproic acid in neonatal status convulsivus. *Brain Dev*. 1986;8(3):278–279.

63. Glass HC, Poulin C, Shevell MI. Topiramate for the treatment of neonatal seizures. *Pediatr Neurol*. 2011;44(6):439–442.

64. Hoppen T, Elger CE, Bartmann P. Carbamazepine in phenobarbital-nonresponders: experience with ten preterm infants. *Eur J Pediatr*. 2001;160(7):444–447.

65. Abend NS, Gutierrez-Colina AM, Monk HM, et al. Levetiracetam for treatment of neonatal seizures. *J Child Neurol*. 2011;26(4):465–470.

66. Christensen KV, Leffers H, Watson WP, et al. Levetiracetam attenuates hippocampal expression of synaptic plasticity-related immediate early and late response genes in amygdala-kindled rats. *BMC Neurosci*. 2010;11:9.

67. Khan O, Chang E, Cipriani C, et al. Use of intravenous levetiracetam for management of acute seizures in neonates. *Pediatr Neurol*. 2011;44(4):265–269.

68. Merhar SL, Schibler KR, Sherwin CM, et al. Pharmacokinetics of levetiracetam in neonates with seizures. *J Pediatr*. 2011;159(1):152–154. e3.

69. Malingre MM, Van Rooij LG, Rademaker CM, et al. Development of an optimal lidocaine infusion strategy for neonatal seizures. *Eur J Pediatr*. 2006;165(9):598–604.

70. Gospe SM Jr. Pyridoxine-dependent seizures: new genetic and biochemical clues to help with diagnosis and treatment. *Curr Opin Neurol*. 2006;19(2):148–153.

71. Kwon JM, Guillet R, Shankaran S, et al. Clinical seizures in neonatal hypoxic-ischemic encephalopathy have no independent impact on neurodevelopmental outcome: secondary analyses of data from the neonatal research network hypothermia trial. *J Child Neurol*. 2011;26(3):322–328.

72. Davis AS, Hintz SR, Van Meurs KP, et al. Seizures in extremely low birth weight infants are associated with adverse outcome. *J Pediatr*. 2010;157(5):720–725. e1–e2.

73. Holmes GL. The long-term effects of neonatal seizures. *Clin Perinatol*. 2009;36(4):901–914. vii–viii.

74. Isaeva E, Isaev D, Savrasova A, et al. Recurrent neonatal seizures result in long-term increases in neuronal network excitability in the rat neocortex. *Eur J Neurosci*. 2010;31(8):1446–1455.

75. Silverstein FS. Do seizures contribute to neonatal hypoxic-ischemic brain injury? *J Pediatr*. 2009;155(3):305–306.

76. Glass HC, Glidden D, Jeremy RJ, et al. Clinical neonatal seizures are independently associated with outcome in infants at risk for hypoxic-ischemic brain injury. *J Pediatr*. 2009;155(3):318–323.

16 Neonatal Bacterial Meningitis

Alistair G. S. Philip

EPIDEMIOLOGY

Prior to the introduction of sulfonamides (late 1930s) and antibiotics (mid-1940s), a diagnosis of neonatal meningitis was almost always a death sentence. For the few who survived, severe neurologic sequelae were likely to occur. Subsequent to the introduction of antimicrobials, deaths were still common.

During the last 25 years, there has been an apparent decrease in both the incidence and the case fatality of neonatal bacterial meningitis in developed countries. The probable reason for this is a more aggressive approach to eradication of maternal colonization by those bacteria most commonly associated with early-onset (EO) meningitis. One of the most common organisms causing EO meningitis in the latter part of the 20th century was the group B streptococcus (GBS; also called *Streptococcus agalactiae*). However, in the 1990s, an aggressive approach to the elimination of GBS in both mother and infant was adopted to prevent neonatal sepsis and meningitis. Nevertheless, GBS and *Escherichia coli* (*E. coli*) remain the predominant organisms causing EO neonatal sepsis and meningitis. Recent figures from the USA (using the National Institute for Child Health and Human Development [NICHD] network) indicate that 43% of EO sepsis and meningitis were caused by GBS and 29% by *E. coli*. GBS occurred mostly in term infants (73%), whereas *E. coli* occurred predominantly in preterm infants (81%).[1]

It may be difficult to distinguish between sepsis and meningitis in the neonate, and they are often reported together. EO sepsis and meningitis are sometimes considered to be that which occurs within the first 3 days after birth (which may be considered as perinatal, with infection transmitted by the mother) and sometimes as that which occurs within the first week after birth (which might also include some cases of nosocomial infection, ie, hospital-acquired). There seems to be greater unanimity about the definition of late-onset (LO) meningitis, which is generally regarded as that which occurs more than 7 days after birth. At present, most cases of GBS meningitis are LO.

Although it may be difficult to distinguish clinically between sepsis and meningitis in the neonate, a diagnosis of bacterial meningitis usually requires a culture of cerebrospinal fluid (CSF) that is positive for pathogenic bacteria. However, if CSF cannot be obtained before administration of antibiotics, a diagnosis of meningitis *may* be supported by CSF pleocytosis and decreased CSF glucose (and increased CSF protein).

In addition to GBS, the other major organism associated with neonatal meningitis is *E. coli*, but *Klebsiella* species have also been implicated frequently in some countries, and *Listeria monocytogenes* accounts for a substantial number of LO cases in other countries. GBS and *E. coli* remain the predominant organisms causing both EO and LO meningitis in France. The distribution of organisms at different gestational ages, as well as different ages of onset, can be seen in Figure 16-1.[2] Although only a handful of bacteria are commonly associated with neonatal meningitis, an enormous number of bacteria have been implicated during the past 50 years. Details can be found elsewhere.[3] Especially in the very preterm infant, both *Staphylococcus aureus* and coagulase-negative staphylococci (mostly *Staphylococcus epidermidis*)

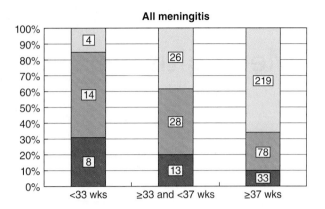

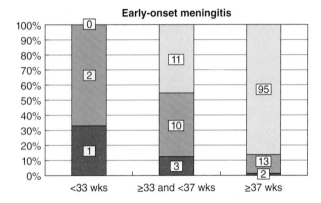

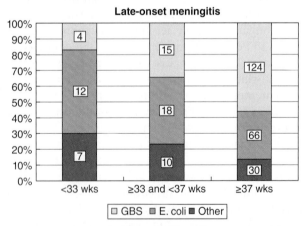

FIGURE 16-1 Distribution of all, early-onset, and late-onset neonatal meningitis according to gestational age at birth and causative organism. GBS, group B streptococci. (From Gaschinard et al.,[2] Figure 2.)

have been implicated,[4,5] and *Citrobacter koseri* (formerly *Citrobacter diversus*) deserves special mention because of the frequent association with brain abscesses.[6]

Incidence

Because neonatal bacterial meningitis is comparatively infrequent, especially since the start of the new millennium, it is difficult to derive useful data from single centers. There have been a number of national studies

over the years, which have provided useful information and allow incidence and case fatality rates (CFRs) to be derived.

Among developed countries, the lowest incidence of neonatal bacterial meningitis has been reported from Australia. In the 1990s, the incidence of neonatal meningitis in Australia was 0.15–0.17 per 1000 live births (LB), and a report from 2006, which also included New Zealand, documented an incidence of 0.10/1000 LB.[7] Reports from England and Wales in the mid-1980s and mid-1990s revealed little change, with incidence figures of 0.32 and 0.31/1000 LB, respectively.[8] In the Netherlands, the incidence was 0.23/1000 LB in the period 1976–1982.[9]

The introduction of widespread intrapartum chemoprophylaxis to prevent neonatal GBS sepsis and meningitis has resulted in a marked decrease in the incidence of GBS meningitis in some countries, whereas there was little change in the incidence of *E. coli* meningitis. A report from Australasia (Australia and New Zealand) in 2005 showed that EO GBS meningitis in 2002 fell from 0.24/1000 LB in 1993 to 0.03/1000 LB[10] (see Figure 16-2). On the other hand, gram-negative bacilli did not obviously decrease (see Figure 16-3). In contrast, a report from the Netherlands in 2007 documented a reduction in EO GBS sepsis from 0.54/1000 LB in 1997–1998 to 0.36/1000 LB in 1999–2001, but a slight increase in GBS meningitis from 0.14 to 0.17/1000 LB for the 2 time periods, respectively.[11] It is much more likely that GBS sepsis will be accompanied by meningitis after the first week of age. In the Netherlands study, babies investigated within 12 hours

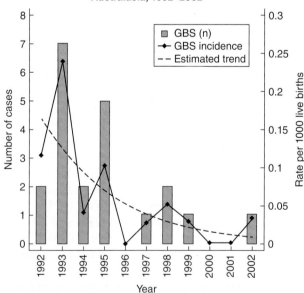

FIGURE 16-2 Decreasing incidence of early-onset group B streptococcal meningitis in Australasia, 1992–2002.

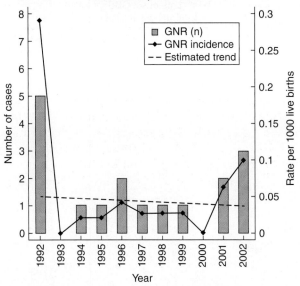

Early onset Gram negative bacillary (GNR) meningitis, Australasia, 1992–2002

FIGURE 16-3 Minimal change in incidence of early-onset gram-negative bacillary meningitis in Australasia, 1992–2002.

of birth who had GBS sepsis, had meningitis in only 6% of cases, whereas when investigated at greater than 7 days of age, 53% had accompanying meningitis.[11]

Incidence in the 21st Century

Further reductions in the incidence of bacterial meningitis have probably occurred in the last decade because there have been few reports dealing exclusively with neonatal meningitis, from single centers, during these years. The incidence of GBS sepsis has fallen substantially in the United States, with EO sepsis at 1.7/1000 LB in 1990 and 0.4/1000 LB in 2005, with a presumed reduction in EO meningitis[12] (see Figure 16-4). However, LO GBS sepsis has remained constant at about 0.4/1000 LB, which suggests that LO GBS meningitis has also stayed about the same.[12] In northern Italy, the incidence of EO GBS sepsis was 0.27/1000 LB, with only 2 cases of GBS meningitis in the years 2003–2005, whereas LO GBS sepsis was 0.23/1000 LB with 12/26 cases of sepsis accompanied by meningitis in the same time period.[13]

Using the Active Bacterial Core (ABC) surveillance system, a recent US national report documented rates of meningitis at less than 2 months of age as 0.65/1000 LB in 1998–2001 and 0.63/1000 LB in 2002–2007 and indicated that most cases were of LO.[14]

As with most forms of neonatal infection, the incidence of sepsis and meningitis is higher in low birth weight (<2500 g) infants and especially among very low birth weight (VLBW; <1500 g) infants.[1]

Most studies also reported higher incidence in males than females.

Case Fatality

In an earlier era, the CFRs for neonatal meningitis were high, but they seem to have decreased in recent years. Although it is comforting to think that this is the result of improved care, it could (in part) be because of the decreased virulence of the infecting bacteria. In England and Wales, among 450 cases seen in 1985–1987, the CFR was 29%; the CFR was 32% with gram-negative infections. In the years 1996–1997, a similar study of neonatal meningitis from England and Wales reported only a 10% CFR.[8] In southern Taiwan, the CFR was 17% in 1986–1993 but decreased[15] to 8% in 1994–2001. In less-well-developed countries,[16] CFRs of 30% to 40% were still being reported in the late 1990s.

The CFR in Toronto, Canada,[17] for the years 1979–1998 was 13%, and in a report from Greece in the year 2000, a remarkable 70 of 72 term infants with gram-negative bacterial meningitis survived to discharge with few sequelae.[18] Recent information from the United States suggests a CFR of 11% in meningitis occurring in infants under the age of 2 months (mostly because of GBS), with a somewhat higher rate (18%) with *L. monocytogenes*.[14] Rather similar data come from a national study in France, which reported on 444 cases seen between 2001 and 2007. In term infants (*n* = 330), the CFR was 10%, but in preterm infants, it was 26%. Also of interest is the fact that growth-restricted babies had a rate that was double (25%) that for appropriately grown infants (12%).[2]

Susceptibility

As mentioned, male infants appear to be more susceptible to neonatal infection than female infants. The reason for this is not clearly understood, but some protection seems to be conferred by the presence of the extra X chromosome in females. Increased susceptibility to infection in VLBW infants is caused (in part) by minimal transfer of protective antibodies from the mother until after 32 weeks' gestation. Although twins have been reported to be at increased risk for GBS infection, this is probably related to a greater likelihood of twins being born preterm.

A specific susceptibility may occur in infants with galactosemia, who are at particular risk of developing infection with *E. coli*. During a 12-year period, in an era when GBS was predominant, 35 infants with galactosemia were detected on routine neonatal metabolic screening. Of this group, 10 developed systemic infection with *E. coli*. All 9 with bacteremia died, despite antibiotic therapy.[19]

CHAPTER 16

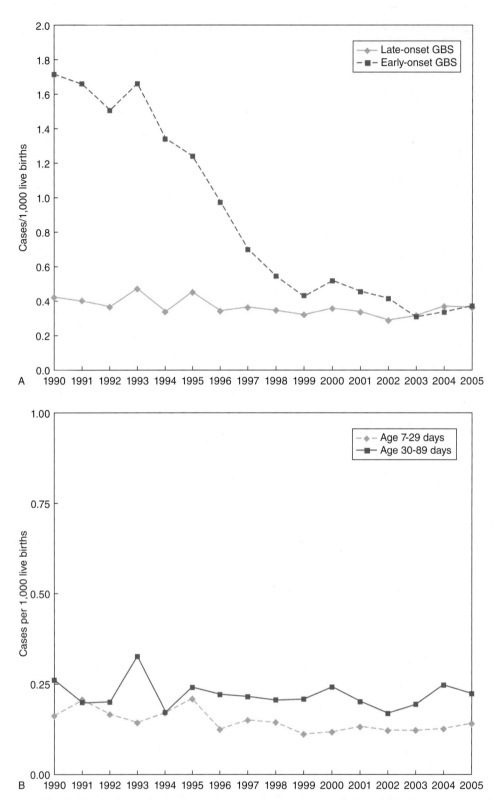

FIGURE 16-4 Marked decrease in incidence of early-onset group B streptococcal (GBS) disease in the United States, 1990–2005 (upper portion of panel A), with little change in the incidence of late-onset GBS disease (lower portion of panel A). Rates may have decreased slightly for late-onset meningitis in infants aged 7 to 29 days compared to those aged 30–89 days (panel B).

PATHOPHYSIOLOGY

Meningitis refers to inflammation of the leptomeninges covering the surface of the brain. With bacterial infection, this usually results in a purulent exudate. In the neonate, there may be difficulty localizing infection and inflammation, with the result that the brain (cerebral hemispheres and cerebellum) may be involved in a process of meningoencephalitis.

One of the factors limiting the spread of infection in older infants and children is the blood-brain barrier. This barrier seems to be less effective in the neonate. An additional concern for the preterm infant is that considerable brain growth occurs during the third trimester of pregnancy, and meningoencephalitis in the preterm infant can interfere with the normal processes of brain growth, with resultant developmental deficits.

Acquisition of Bacteria

As might be surmised from the fact that neonatal septicemia (sepsis) and meningitis are difficult to separate clinically, bloodstream infection is probably the most important route of transmission of bacteria to the meninges. Nevertheless, other routes are possible.[20] The most common route probably involves bacteria traversing placental blood vessels of the mother to infect the fetus. Nasopharyngeal colonization may occur, and access could possibly be gained by traversing the cribriform plate. Perhaps more important is intestinal colonization, with subsequent uptake into the bloodstream. This could result from contamination of the amniotic fluid, which the fetus is swallowing. Yet another portal of entry is a congenital dermal sinus, which needs to be looked for in the midline of the back; whenever an infant has a CSF shunt in place (eg, for posthemorrhagic hydrocephalus), there is a possibility for infection of the spinal fluid. It has also been reported that, later in the neonatal period, meningitis may frequently be preceded by a urinary tract infection.

In most cases of EO infection, it is difficult to know if bacteria are transmitted transplacentally or if infection is "ascending" secondary to infection of the amniotic fluid or colonization of the maternal genital tract with pathogenic organisms. In LO infection, acquisition of pathogenic bacteria may come from direct contact with colonized caregivers, the equipment surrounding or inserted into the infant (incubators, endotracheal tubes, ventilators, and intravenous catheters), as well as community-acquired sources.

Transfer of Maternal Antibody

There is a strong correlation between colonization of the mother and colonization of the infant. Although few infants who are colonized with pathogenic bacteria become infected, the more frequently mothers are colonized, the more likely is it that neonates will become infected. One of the key factors allowing neonates to become infected is the lack of specific antibody to a specific organism. Neonates born to mothers who have developed an antibody to certain bacteria are unlikely to become infected if they are born at term. This is less true in the preterm infant because the majority of maternal antibody transfer to the fetus occurs after 32 weeks' gestation, although *some* protection may be provided by the small amounts that manage to be transferred prior to 32 weeks.

As mentioned, susceptibility to infection is related to absence of antibody to common bacteria. With regard to GBS infection, this was strikingly demonstrated some time ago by Vogel et al.[21] They documented the lack of serospecifc antibody in neonates who acquired GBS infection. Only immunoglobulin G (IgG) usually traverses the placenta, by an active process, largely after 32 weeks' gestation. Because immunoglobulin M (IgM) does not cross the placenta, this may explain to some extent why *E. coli* is prominent in neonatal infection because antibody to *E. coli* and other gram-negative bacteria is found predominantly in the IgM fraction. Nevertheless, a small amount of antibody is in the IgG fraction and can provide some protection even in very preterm infants.[22]

Bacterial Characteristics

The characteristics of certain bacteria seem to increase the likelihood that they will cause neonatal meningitis. Organisms that have the propensity to cause neonatal meningitis are usually protected from the neonate's defense mechanisms (such as complement-mediated lysis and phagocytosis) by a polysaccharide capsule. One feature associated with this propensity is the presence of sialic acid in high concentrations in the capsule of some bacteria. Such is the case for the capsular polysaccharide of GBS serotype III, *E. coli* K1, and *L. monocytogenes* serotype IVb, the bacteria most commonly associated with neonatal meningitis. Another feature is the ability of bacteria to interact with neutrophils and affect their virulence. It has been shown that virulent clones of *E. coli* have impaired interaction with neutrophils, which makes them more likely to produce invasive infection.[23]

Although it has been known for many years[24] that certain strains of GBS are more likely to produce meningitis, particularly serotype III (but also IA and V), more recently the biotype has received increasing attention when it is related to loss of catabolic function.[25] Invasion of the central nervous system (CNS) of the neonate was 13 times more likely with biotypes B1 to B6 than with biotypes B7 to B15. Biotypes B1 to B6 were identified in 86% of 42 GBS strains associated with neonatal meningitis.[25]

Additional highly virulent clones of GBS have been noted in France, with ST-17 sequence type being important.[26] Using polymerase chain reaction (PCR) techniques, 156 strains of GBS were evaluated, and 40 were positive for ST-17. Among neonates with LO GBS disease (with a high incidence of meningitis), 78% of strains were ST-17.

With *E. coli* meningitis, the predominant strains are those carrying the K1 capsular antigen. K1 strains have been demonstrated in approximately 75% of cases of neonatal meningitis caused by *E. coli* and in 1 report accounted for 88% of cases.[9]

Recently, the "hypervirulence" of the ST-17 strain of GBS has been attributed to a specific surface-anchored protein called hypervirulent GBS adhesion (HvgA) protein.[26] The authors suggested that GBS that express HvgA adhere more efficiently to intestinal epithelial cells, choroid plexus epithelial cells, and microvascular epithelial cells, which constitute the blood-brain barrier. They also suggested that entry of bacteria may be from colonization of the intestine, followed by translocation across the intestinal barrier, as well as the blood-brain barrier, resulting in meningitis. In this study, evaluation of LO GBS meningitis revealed 88% of cases caused by serotype III and 83% had ST-17.[27]

There is also recent evidence concerning meningitis caused by *E. coli*. It is suggested that extracellular loops of *E. coli* (RS218) contained on the outer membrane protein A are important in bacterial survival in serum, as well as in entry into brain microvascular endothelial cells. Cellular invasion requires activation of host cytosolic phospholipase A2.[28] Apparently, the K1 capsule does not play a specific role in the invasion of the blood-brain barrier but seems to be important in maintaining bacterial viability during the invasion.[28]

The ability of certain bacteria, such as *E. coli* K1, *L. monocytogenes*, and GBS type III, to breech the blood-brain barrier seems to be because of an increased capacity to penetrate the cerebrovascular endothelium while increasing blood-brain barrier permeability. There are receptors on various elements of the neurovascular unit that allow endotoxins and proinflammatory cytokines to bind to them.[29]

Basic Mechanisms in Pathophysiology

It may be useful to consider that the pathophysiology of neonatal meningitis consists of 3 main phases[23]: (1) infection (colonization and invasion), (2) bacterial multiplication and CNS inflammation, and (3) brain damage. The mechanisms are complex and beyond the scope of this discussion, but include initial stages of immune recognition, activating brain cells to produce cytokines (such as tumor necrosis factor α and interleukin [IL] 6) and chemokines, matrix metalloproteinases, and reactive oxygen species. These may all contribute to an increase in the number of cells in the CSF (pleocytosis), which is usually a characteristic feature of meningitis. However, as discussed in the section on diagnosis, the CSF cell count can be remarkably normal in the early stages of neonatal bacterial meningitis, although CSF culture may be positive for bacteria.

CLINICAL MANIFESTATIONS AND DIFFERENTIAL DIAGNOSIS

Although some clinical features of bacterial meningitis may be more or less pathognomonic, these are all findings that are seen late in the course of the infection. To make an early diagnosis, clinicians need to be aware of findings that may point toward systemic infection (sepsis or meningitis). Early diagnosis and treatment are likely to result in a good outcome, whereas delay in diagnosis is more likely to produce a bad outcome. Clearly, late findings are more likely to be associated with a poor prognosis.

There are 2 specific "clusters" of disorders that should be kept in mind in the differential diagnosis. These are inborn errors of metabolism[30] and the more recently described autoinflammatory diseases in the neonate.[31]

The list of clinical features that should raise the suspicion of sepsis and meningitis is long. On the other hand, investigation of the neonate, soon after delivery, solely on the basis of maternal risk factors (such as prolonged rupture of the membranes or maternal fever) is unlikely to reveal meningitis. Beyond the first few hours (approximately 12 hours) after birth, investigation for sepsis will almost always be because of a number of clinical manifestations that are detailed in the following material. These findings include those presented in *Table 16-1*.

Table 16-1 Clinical Features of Meningitis

Early Signs	Late Signs
Lethargy	Pallor
Poor feeding	Poor perfusion
Temperature instability	Shock (systemic hypotension)
Abdominal distension	Sclerema
Apnea	Convulsions (seizures)
Cyanotic episodes	Bulging anterior fontanelle
Dyspnea (respiratory distress)	Nuchal rigidity

Early Signs

Lethargy

It is difficult to objectively define lethargy, but it is reasonable to think of a "lethargic" baby as one who is difficult to arouse at times when one would expect to be able to arouse him or her. For instance, a term baby who has recently been fed would not be considered lethargic, despite the difficulties one might encounter in arousing the baby from sleep. Similarly, the infant born following prolonged magnesium sulfate administration or following prolapse of the umbilical cord might be difficult to arouse because of hypermagnesemia or asphyxia, but a diagnosis of sepsis would not be entertained immediately. On the other hand, one of the earliest manifestations of sepsis/meningitis might be a "depressed" (poorly responsive) baby with low Apgar scores. Maternal administration of general anesthesia or analgesia, or fetal asphyxia, would need to be considered.

Poor Feeding

Similar difficulty to that of defining lethargy is encountered when trying to define poor feeding. The implication is that a baby who was formerly feeding (breast or bottle) quite vigorously now does so reluctantly, or not at all. Thus, an infant of less than 32 weeks' gestation would not usually fit into this category because adequate coordination of sucking and swallowing does not occur until after 32 weeks' gestation. However, "difficulty with feeding" could apply to preterm infants (or others) who are fed by intragastric tube (gavage), as increasing gastric residuals, or poor gastric emptying, may suggest an underlying infectious problem.

Temperature Instability

In contrast to older infants and children, fever in the neonate is comparatively uncommon in response to bacterial infection. Particularly in preterm infants, a low body temperature (hypothermia) is a more typical finding. In one study of 67 babies with hypothermia (defined as body temperature < 35°C) beyond 72 hours, but less than 28 days of age, 44 were found to have infection, with 12 cases of sepsis and 7 with meningitis.[32] However, it is probably more typical to have neither fever nor hypothermia. Fluctuating body temperature may require investigation, and concern about infection should be stimulated when difficulty in maintaining body temperature is encountered in infants attached to servo-control temperature devices.

Soon after delivery (approximately the first 4 hours), it may be difficult to evaluate abnormal temperatures. Fever in the neonate may occur because of maternal fever, because of infection such as chorioamnionitis, or secondary to prolonged epidural anesthesia of the mother.[33] Hypothermia may be the result of cooling in the delivery room, especially in smaller babies, unless care is taken to pay attention to maintenance of body temperature. Although rarely seen currently, environmental hypothermia (neonatal cold injury) can occur in babies who have been discharged to poorly heated housing. This itself can predispose to neonatal infection, although it is more likely to result in pneumonia than meningitis.

Another temperature-related phenomenon in neonatal sepsis was described many years ago but is now frequently neglected. This is the observation that babies who have fever on the basis of increased environmental temperature (eg, an overheated incubator) feel warm all over. On the other hand, babies who have an elevated core temperature on the basis of sepsis have an elevated core temperature (trunk feels warm), but have cooling of the extremities. This "tummy-toe" differential was first described[34] in 1965 and later more accurately documented with a skin thermistor that detected abdomen-leg temperature differences.[35] The conclusion of the latter study was that differences greater than 3°F (especially > 5°F) were indicative of bacterial infection (sepsis and meningitis).

Abdominal Distension

Because the abdominal circumference can be measured sequentially, it is a little easier to provide objective evidence to document abdominal distension. Nevertheless, a vigorous infant, who cries a lot and swallows a lot of air, may have an increased abdominal circumference because of air-filled loops of bowel. Under such circumstances, the abdomen is usually soft. An abdomen that appears tense (particularly if it is shiny) would be more indicative of sepsis, and there could be associated peritonitis. In the baby with birth weight less than 1500 g, the presence of abdominal distension could be caused by necrotizing enterocolitis (NEC), but many cases of NEC also have associated sepsis (and occasionally meningitis).

It should be remembered that abdominal distension occurring within the first 2 or 3 days after delivery is more likely to be the result of mid- or lower-intestinal obstruction.

Apnea

One of the more common reasons to evaluate an infant for sepsis and meningitis is apnea. However, of the clinical features suggesting systemic infection, apnea probably has the largest number of differential diagnoses. Among other possible disorders producing apnea are a large number of disorders of the lung; acidosis; metabolic disorders (eg, hypoglycemia, inborn errors, and hypocalcemia); intracranial hemorrhage; any disorder likely to produce seizures (apnea can be a "seizure equivalent"); and most commonly "apnea of prematurity."

Despite the large number of differential diagnoses, apnea frequently is the clinical feature that triggers an investigation for systemic infection. Most clinicians would hesitate to make a diagnosis of apnea of prematurity without first trying to rule out sepsis. In the absence of lung disease, apnea occurring after the first week of extrauterine life would definitely raise the possibility of meningitis.

Cyanotic Episodes and Dyspnea

As with apnea, cyanotic episodes (or "dusky spells" or prolonged oxygen desaturation) can be caused by a multitude of disorders other than infection. Among the most common disorders to be considered are "potentially cyanotic" congenital heart disease; hyperviscosity syndrome (most likely caused by high hematocrit); and a variety of lung disorders.

Although apnea and cyanotic episodes could certainly be considered as forms of respiratory distress, the more usual implication of respiratory distress is labored breathing or dyspnea. This is more commonly associated with pneumonia, which needs to be distinguished from respiratory distress syndrome (RDS) in the preterm infant. Pneumonia is often accompanied by sepsis and occasionally by meningitis.

Irritability

Just as it is difficult to define lethargy, it is not easy to define irritability. It is usually considered present when an infant seems more restless than usual. This may manifest as tremulousness (jitteriness) or increased activity with even minor stimuli or intermittent crying for no apparent reason. Disorders of the CNS (such as hypoxic-ischemic encephalopathy and intracranial hemorrhage) need to be considered seriously, but so does meningitis. Irritability in the first 2 to 3 days after birth is most likely caused by CNS disorders, but after 3 days (especially if this is the first time that irritability has been observed) meningitis becomes the most important consideration. After 7 days of age, infants *must* be investigated for possible meningitis.

Metabolic disorders, such as hypoglycemia, hypocalcemia, and inborn errors of metabolism, also need to be considered and can usually be eliminated quickly with a few laboratory tests.

Late Signs

Pallor and Poor Perfusion

The most likely cause of pallor in the neonate is peripheral vasoconstriction, which can result from metabolic acidosis, although causes of anemia should

also be considered. In the absence of obvious blood loss, the finding of metabolic acidosis should always raise the possibility of sepsis (and meningitis, after the first 24 hours). Both pallor and peripheral vasoconstriction can be the response to release of endotoxin or "endotoxin-like substances" released from pathogenic bacteria. When this sign is seen, evaluation for infection and initiation of treatment are urgent.

Because of increased vigilance, these findings are now seen less frequently. However, some years ago, in a retrospective study of 83 infants with septicemia (sepsis), it was reported that abnormal skin color, impaired capillary filling time, and metabolic acidosis were seen in 75%, 46%, and 24%, respectively, at the onset of the illness and in 95%, 95%, and 66%, respectively, at the peak of the disease.[36]

Shock

Markedly compromised peripheral perfusion is usually an indication of systemic hypotension. This can be corroborated by blood pressure measurements. Shock is one stage worse than pallor and may be accompanied by mottling or blotchiness of the skin (alternating areas of pallor and erythema), which is a late sign of sepsis.

Sclerema

Firmness of the subcutaneous tissues similar to hard wax (a tallow-like feel) is termed *sclerema* and is an ominous sign. Almost certainly, this is another manifestation of decreased peripheral perfusion, which results in cooling of the periphery, particularly the arms and legs (see section on temperature instability). This may produce a physical alteration in subcutaneous fat. When this sign is present, extreme measures (such as exchange transfusion) may be needed.[37]

Convulsions (Seizures)

As mentioned, irritability may suggest neonatal infection. A more extreme form of irritability would be convulsions or seizures. Seizures are relatively uncommon in the early stages of meningitis, so their presence is an ominous sign. Neonatal seizures have a broad differential diagnosis, with hypoxic-ischemic encephalopathy, metabolic disorders, intracranial hemorrhage, and drug withdrawal needing to be considered in addition to meningitis. Particularly after the first 2 to 3 days, when seizures occur in a neonate, meningitis needs to be considered, and a lumbar puncture (LP; spinal tap) becomes mandatory.

Bulging Fontanelle and Nuchal Rigidity

Palpation of the anterior fontanelle whenever a neonate is examined is a good practice to adopt as one becomes familiar with the normal size and tension. It is unlikely that a bulging fontanelle would be seen in an infant who has not been discharged from the hospital, as other signs would almost always be seen earlier. However, it might be seen in an infant who has been at home for several days or weeks, in whom the diagnosis of meningitis has been delayed. Other reasons for increased tension in the anterior fontanelle would be intracranial hemorrhage or cerebral edema.

Nuchal rigidity, which is common in older children, is rarely seen in the neonate. To some extent, this is explained by the fact that the neonatal skull is compliant. Particularly in the preterm infant, spreading of the sutures can accommodate some increase in pressure.

DIAGNOSTIC TESTS

Cerebrospinal Fluid Culture

A definitive diagnosis of bacterial meningitis requires a positive culture of CSF. To obtain CSF, an LP (spinal tap) is needed. Although the procedure is generally without incident, it can be destabilizing in the preterm infant, particularly those of VLBW (<1500 g). The question frequently arises regarding whether an LP should be performed in every case for which an evaluation for sepsis is initiated. There is considerable evidence to suggest that LP is not needed when sepsis evaluation is initiated for maternal risk factors alone.[38] However, LP should always be attempted in the term infant in the presence of clinical signs pointing to systemic infection. This also applies to most preterm infants, but if positioning of the baby compromises an already-unstable infant (producing blood oxygen desaturation), it may be wise to defer the procedure and evaluate adjunctive tests that may point to meningitis. In addition, a very low platelet count may also be considered as a possible contraindication to performing an LP because of the risk of bleeding.

In a recent study from Israel, a selective approach to performing LP was adopted (requiring evaluation by a senior neonatologist), with only 49% of extremely low birth weight (ELBW; < 1000 g) infants including LP in the sepsis evaluation, whereas LP was performed in 80% of sepsis evaluations in infants with birth weight greater than 1000 g. LO meningitis was found in only 1.4% of infants evaluated.[39]

Cerebrospinal Fluid Analysis

Interpretation of CSF findings can present difficulties. Early in the course of meningitis, the cellular changes indicative of meningitis may be absent. The upper limit of normal for the number of white blood cells (WBCs) in CSF also seems to be higher than in older infants and children. A number of studies over several years suggested that the upper limit of normal in the first week after delivery might be as high as 32/μL, although the number of 21/μL is often used. Presence of more cells than in older infants could be related to head compression during the birth process. A recent study in an emergency department evaluated a large number of infants less than 56 days of age for infection. They were able to exclude a variety of conditions that might have affected the CSF WBC count. In 142 infants aged less than 28 days, the median number of WBCs in CSF was 3/μL, with the 95th percentile being 19/μL (a number close to the number of 21 mentioned previously). Values in the older infants (29–56 days) were somewhat lower.[40]

Obtaining CSF that is uncontaminated by blood can also prove challenging, particularly in the small preterm infant. This can further complicate the interpretation of cellular findings. Although formulae for making corrections have been proposed, they do not always provide reliable estimates.

Cerebrospinal fluid glucose and protein have also been used as markers of meningitis, with CSF glucose to blood glucose ratio less than 50% in bacterial meningitis. An increase in CSF protein can be useful if it is extremely elevated.

Having said this, it should be noted that a comparatively recent analysis of CSF findings in a very large number of infants who underwent LP for suspected meningitis concluded that no single CSF value can reliably exclude the presence of meningitis in neonates.[41] Of 9111 infants greater than 33 weeks' gestation evaluated in 150 neonatal intensive care units (NICUs) between 1997 and 2004, culture-positive meningitis existed in 95 (1%). Using *any* WBC in CSF as the test, sensitivity for culture-positive meningitis was 97%, but the specificity was only 11%. Using a cutoff of 21 WBC/mm^3 (frequently considered the upper limit of normal), sensitivity decreased to 79%, while specificity increased to 81%. CSF glucose and protein did not diagnose meningitis accurately. Median WBC in CSF with negative CSF culture was 6/mm^3, compared to 477/mm^3 in those with a positive culture, but there was a huge range for each group. They were able to confirm previous reports, documenting that 10% with proven meningitis had fewer than 4 WBC/mm^3 CSF.[41]

Polymerase Chain Reaction

Although not yet available for routine use in most centers, it seems probable that in the future detection of systemic bacterial infection will become much more rapid using PCR techniques, which can detect specific bacterial genomes. To date, PCR has been used more for detection of viral infections (eg, enteroviruses and herpes simplex virus). In some centers, PCR has been able to detect sepsis more frequently than cultures. As might be expected, most studies have looked primarily at blood (serum) to detect bacterial organisms, but some have also included CSF and urine. In contrast to culture, which may take 48 hours for a positive result, PCR can be performed in as little as 2 hours.

In a study from France,[26] the highly virulent ST-17 clone of GBS was detected in 78% of neonates with LO GBS disease (the number with meningitis was not stated, but as mentioned previously, LO GBS infection frequently includes meningitis). Another study involving GBS compared standard culture with rapid fluorescent real-time PCR in 94 infants with suspected sepsis. Blood culture was positive in 17%, whereas PCR was positive in 54%.[42] Although some have suggested that PCR might be *too* sensitive, it should be remembered that blood culture may not be positive if the sample size is too small.

Further information concerning the value of PCR comes from a study of 200 women in labor in Geneva, Switzerland. Rectovaginal culture for GBS was positive in 16%, whereas PCR was positive in 27%. Vaginal culture for *E. coli* K1 was positive in 3.5%, whereas PCR was positive in 10%. Compared to culture, PCR sensitivity for GBS was 97%, with a specificity of 86%, but the possibility of false negatives for blood culture was mentioned. PCR sensitivity for *E. coli* K1 was only 71%, with specificity 92%. Nevertheless, although not entirely satisfactory for *E. coli* K1, this could allow earlier detection, with concomitant introduction of earlier antibiotic therapy.[43]

Nonspecific Tests

Leukocytes Counts in Blood

One of the most widely used indicators of neonatal infection is the WBC (leukocyte) count and differential count. Although leukocyte counts (total and differential) may suggest infection, they certainly do not indicate specifically that meningitis is present. In the large study mentioned, there was a wide range of leukocyte counts.[41] Of the 95 infants with proven meningitis, 85 had a peripheral WBC count close to the time of LP. Counts were less than 3000/µL in 17; 3–10,000/µL in 36; 10–15,000/µL in 13 and more than 15,000 to less than 30,000/µL in 9. In addition, although the immature to total neutrophil ratio (I:T ratio) may be markedly increased and a useful indicator of infection, it does not confirm meningitis.

C-Reactive Protein

C-reactive protein (CRP) is an acute-phase protein that can provide considerable help in establishing a diagnosis of neonatal sepsis and tends to be markedly increased in cases of meningitis. It should be emphasized that CRP may not be increased early in the course of infection. Its production in the liver seems to be stimulated by IL-6 (and possibly IL-8), but this process may take 6 to 8 hours to occur. Therefore, in cases of suspected sepsis and meningitis, sequential determinations need to be performed. The value of CRP has been described previously,[16] and it is noteworthy that the initial report of its value appeared in 1974, with increased levels noted particularly in cases of *E. coli* meningitis. Peak levels of CRP are almost always above 7 mg/dL, frequently above 10 mg/dL, and sometimes above 20 mg/dL in neonatal meningitis. Higher levels (those above 20 mg/dL) may be associated with brain destruction and are a somewhat ominous finding.

Other Nonspecific Biomarkers

A huge number of tests have been proposed as valuable in assessing neonatal infection in addition to CRP.[44] The most consistent findings have been seen with IL-6, IL-8, procalcitonin, and certain cell-surface markers. However, none can be relied on to make a definitive diagnosis of neonatal meningitis. On the other hand, levels of certain cytokines in CSF may have a role in predicting outcome.[45]

Imaging Studies

Data concerning imaging studies in neonatal meningitis remain comparatively sparse. Ultrasonography remains the most practical imaging technique because the evaluation can be performed at the bedside. Ultrasound evaluation may reveal ventriculitis, as well as echogenic sulci, ventriculomegaly, or infarction, all of which may be indicative of, or associated with, meningitis.[46] In addition, brain abscesses (seen with *C. koseri*) can be detected.[47]

Magnetic resonance imaging (MRI) has not been used extensively in neonatal meningitis but could also provide useful prognostic information. Indeed, in a report from Australia, 6 neonates with *E. coli* meningitis were evaluated by MRI. Five had the K1 strain, but all 6 displayed significant white matter injury.[48] Similarly, in a report from Chile, 8 neonates with GBS meningitis had evidence of "stroke patterns" with focal infarction, both deep and superficial.[49]

MANAGEMENT

Antibiotic Therapy

The most important aspect of management is antibiotic therapy. As was mentioned in the introduction, prior to the antimicrobial era, mortality from meningitis was high, and those who survived usually had severe neurological deficits. Antibiotics alone have not been the sole influence on mortality and morbidity, but outcome has depended in large measure on initiation of antibiotic therapy whenever meningitis is suspected. Whenever possible, obtaining CSF prior to starting antibiotics is desirable so that CSF culture can be performed. In the future, the use of PCR may make the time that CSF is obtained less important.

The decision about which antibiotics to use depends to a considerable extent on the age at which sepsis or meningitis is suspected. This is because the organism most likely to be causative changes according to postnatal age and gestational age. In the first few days after delivery, the most likely bacteria associated with meningitis in developing countries will be GBS and *E. coli*, so that coverage for these organisms is essential.[50] For infants who remain hospitalized after the first week (usually preterm infants in the NICU), *S. aureus* and coagulase-negative staphylococci become increasingly more likely, although gram-negative organisms such as *Klebsiella* and *Enterobacter* are common if ventilators or venous catheters are in use.[51]

One of the most important questions that should be asked before entering into antibiotic decisions is, What is the local experience regarding neonatal infection? If there has been a recent cluster of infections caused by an unusual organism, the appropriate antibiotic might be different from the one(s) normally selected for empirical therapy. Similarly, although GBS and *E. coli* would be the most likely organisms in North America, Australasia, Europe, and Scandinavia, this might not be true in other parts of the world. Consequently, the choice of antibiotic would be determined according to local experience, knowing the antibiotic sensitivities for the bacteria most likely to be encountered. Once an organism has been identified, specific sensitivities can be determined and antibiotics changed accordingly.

For the most part, and somewhat remarkably, using a combination of a penicillin and an aminoglycoside has proved successful in treating most cases of suspected neonatal meningitis. It is remarkable because it would have been anticipated that the commonly encountered bacteria would have developed resistance after so many years (decades) of using this strategy. This fear is certainly justified based on the experience with *S. aureus* in the 1950s and 1960s, with resistance to penicillin and then more recently methicillin. More recently, the development of resistance to vancomycin emphasizes the need to use antibiotics judiciously: using them when indicated, but using them for as short a time as possible.[52]

Group B streptococci remain sensitive to both penicillin and ampicillin, but *E. coli* is frequently resistant to the penicillins and is still sensitive (usually) to the aminoglycosides. Nevertheless, there does not seem to have been an increase in the incidence of ampicillin-resistant bacteria causing EO sepsis since the mid-1990s.[53] Consequently, the most common combination of antibiotics for EO infection in North America is ampicillin and gentamicin.[50] In areas where resistance to gentamicin occurs, it may be preferable to add a third-generation cephalosporin, such as cefotaxime (which has superior penetration into CSF),[50] to ampicillin. Some prefer this combination anyway, so that concern about gentamicin levels is mitigated, but there has recently been some concern about a possible increase in mortality with this combination.[50] With recent guidelines for gentamicin administration, it is unlikely that potentially toxic levels of gentamicin will be reached in term infants.[54] Ceftriaxone is often used in older infants but is not recommended for EO sepsis and meningitis because it may displace bilirubin from albumin.[50]

In older preterm infants, for whom staphylococcal infection is more likely, initial therapy might begin with oxacillin or nafcillin, possibly combined with vancomycin.[51] Although it was suggested that aminoglycosides and vancomycin penetrate poorly into CSF, there are older data to support their effectiveness in the presence of inflamed meninges.

Dosages of commonly used antibiotics are outlined in *Table 16-2*.

Table 16-2 Dosage of Commonly Used Antibiotics in Neonatal Bacterial Meningitis[a]

	<1 Week	>1 Week	Frequency
Penicillin G	100,000 units	200,000 units	Twice daily/four times daily
Ampicillin	200 mg	300 mg	Twice daily/four times daily
Gentamicin[b]	4 mg load, then 3 mg		Daily
Cefotaxime	100 mg	150 mg	Twice daily/three times daily
Vancomycin[b]	30 mg	45 mg	Twice daily/three times daily
Nafcillin	50 mg	100 mg	Twice daily/three times daily

[a]All are per kilogram per day.
[b]Serum levels may need to be monitored and administration less frequent in very preterm infants.

Adjunctive Therapy

In addition to constant vigilance, which should result in antibiotics being started whenever meningitis is first suspected, improvements in case fatality and morbidity are the result of improvements in the general management of neonates. Among the more important forms of adjunctive therapy are (1) monitoring of, and treatment for, hypotension and poor perfusion (to minimize the production of metabolic acidosis); (2) control of seizures; and (3) supporting defense mechanisms with agents such as serospecific IgG or anticytokine agents.

An additional therapy might be assisted ventilation, if respiratory failure occurs, and mild hyperventilation may minimize cerebral edema. Minimizing renal consequences by careful fluid administration and diuretics may also be beneficial.

Prevention

There are two major forms of prevention: chemoprophylaxis and immunoprophylaxis. Both of these can be further subdivided into maternal and neonatal forms.

Since the mid-2000s or so, as mentioned in the section on epidemiology, huge strides in reducing the incidence of GBS infection have been made by using maternal chemoprophylaxis in the form of intrapartum antibiotics. Previously, there had been considerable enthusiasm in some centers for the use of neonatal chemoprophylaxis in attempting to eliminate GBS, with all neonates receiving penicillin or ampicillin soon after delivery.[55] Because of the success of maternal prophylaxis, this approach is now promoted less enthusiastically. With either approach, there are concerns that resistant organisms or an increasing number of gram-negative organisms may emerge,[56] although this does not seem to have been a major problem so far.[50]

Neonatal immunoprophylaxis has been largely concerned with the use of prophylactic IgG. Earlier reports were contradictory, probably because of variability in the amount of specific antibody to common pathogens available in the preparations of IgG used. More reliable results might be obtained if preparations with species-specific antibody could be administered. The most recent report, in a large randomized controlled trial (approximately 3500 neonates) of immune globulin, showed no benefit in preventing infection.[57]

Maternal immunoprophylaxis still offers the best hope for reducing LO meningitis caused by GBS, although difficulties in producing immunogenic vaccines have hindered production of effective vaccines. It now appears that polyvalent vaccines to prevent GBS infection caused by serotypes III, IA, and V should soon be available and might be most beneficial when administered to adolescents.[12,58] Difficulties continue to prevent production of effective vaccines for other organisms, especially *E. coli*, because of the very large number of serotypes that can cause infection.

OUTCOME AND FOLLOW-UP

Case Fatality Rates

As mentioned, the CFRs for neonatal bacterial meningitis have decreased substantially since the 1990s or so. However, the outlook for survivors continues to be guarded. Many will have no discernible deficit, but a substantial percentage will demonstrate moderate-to-severe neurodevelopmental deficits.

In the Netherlands, CFR fell from 62% in 1977–1981 to 13% in 1997–2001 for EO GBS sepsis and from 80% in 1977–1981 to 10% in 1997–2001 for LO GBS sepsis.[11] In the same study, although EO GBS sepsis decreased significantly from 0.54/1000 LB in 1997–1998 to 0.36/1000 LB in 1999–2001, LO sepsis did not change. EO GBS meningitis was 0.14/1000 LB and 0.17/1000 LB in the same time periods.

With regard to EO GBS infection, which includes a sizable percentage with meningitis, CFR is affected by gestational age. Infants with greater than 37 weeks' gestation had a CFR of 2%, whereas those less than 33 weeks' gestation had a CFR of 30% in infants born in the 1990s.[59]

In a study of infants born between 2003 and 2005 in northern Italy, there were 30 cases of EO GBS infection, 2 of whom had meningitis and both died. Of 26 LO GBS infections, 12 had meningitis, with death occurring in 4 of 26 (number with meningitis who died was not stated).[13]

A recent report on bacterial meningitis in the United States, using the ABC surveillance system (which excludes *E. coli* and *S. aureus*) showed that 86% of cases under the age of 2 months were caused by GBS with a CFR of 11%. For cases caused by *L. monocytogenes*, the CFR was 18%.[14] As mentioned, figures from France, for the years 2001 to 2007, documented an overall CFR of 13%, but the CFR in term infants was 10%, whereas in preterm infants it was 26%. There was a similar discrepancy when appropriate-for-gestational age infants (CFR 12%) were compared to small-for-gestational age infants (CFR 25%).[2] Interestingly, in that study, there were no cases of EO GBS meningitis at less than 33 weeks' gestation.

Neurodevelopmental Disability

In two national studies conducted in England and Wales a decade apart, there was a dramatic fall in the acute-phase mortality in neonatal bacterial meningitis from 22% in 1985–1987 to 6.6% in 1996–1997. However, there was a minimal decrease in serious

Table 16-3 Outcome of Group B β-Hemolytic Streptococci (GBS) Meningitis

Study	Case Fatality (%)	Survivors	Major Neuro Sequelae
Edwards et al[60] 1985 (1974–1979)[a]	38	38	11 (29%)
Klinger et al[17] 2000 (1978–1998)[a]	13[b]	50	15 (30%)
De Louvois et al[8] 2005 (1996–1997)[a]	6.6[b]	41	14 (34%)
Levent et al[61] 2010 (1998–2006)[a]	5.7	50	11 (22%)

[a]Year study published, with years included in the study in parentheses.
[b]Based on all cases, not just GBS.

neurodevelopmental disability from 25.5% for the 1985–1987 cohort to 23.5% for the 1996–1997 cohort.[8] Looking only at GBS meningitis, the results were little different for major neurological sequelae than those seen 20 years earlier from the United States[60] (see *Table 16-3*).

A recent study from Texas Children's Hospital, looking at the outcome of GBS meningitis in neonates from 1998 to 2006 suggests that the outlook remains equally uncertain. While only 3 of the 53 cases died (5.7%), 11 of 53 were neurologically impaired (20.8%, or 22% of survivors).[61]

Some years ago, Unhanand et al reported on an experience with gram-negative enteric bacillary meningitis seen in Texas and documented hydrocephalus, seizure disorder, cerebral palsy, developmental delay, and hearing loss in 28%, 28%, 19%, 25%, and 16%, respectively, in 32 term infants and somewhat higher percentages for each category in 11 preterm infants who survived.[62]

More recently, a high survival rate and low incidence of sequelae were reported from Greece in term infants with gram-negative meningitis. Persisting seizures, spastic paralysis, developmental delay, and hearing deficit were found in 4%, 3%, 4%, and 6%, respectively. The authors suggested that delay in achieving sterile CSF may be correlated with an increased frequency of sequelae.[18]

Although the numbers of ELBW (<1000 g) infants with bacterial meningitis in any one institution is small, large numbers have been reported from the hospitals of the NICHD network. ELBW infants born between 1993 and 2001 were followed up at 18–22 months of age. The outcome for those with sepsis alone was little different from those with meningitis (with or without sepsis) but was substantially worse than the uninfected. Table 16-4 illustrates this.[63]

Factors Associated with Poor Outcome

From a review of the literature, there are a number of factors that have proved to be predictive of a poor outcome in cases of neonatal bacterial meningitis.[17,60,64]

Table 16-4 Neurodevelopmental Outcome in ELBW Infants Born in the NICHD Network, 1993 to 2001, with Follow-up at 18 to 22 Months of Age

Outcome (n)	Uninfected (%) (2161)	Sepsis Alone (%) (1922)	Meningitis ± Sepsis (%) (193)
MDI < 70	22	37	38
PDI < 70	13	27	27
CP	8	17	19
Impaired vision	5	15	16
Impaired hearing	1	3	2
Impaired neurodevelopment	29	48	48

CP, cerebral palsy; ELBW, extremely low birth weight; MDI, Mental Development Index; NICHD, National Institute of Child Health and Human Development; PDI, Physical Development Index.
Source: Modified from Stoll BJ et al.[63]

The factors that have been associated are as follows:

Very low birth weight

Coma (or semicoma)

Decreased perfusion

Need for inotropes to maintain blood pressure

Seizures (>12-h duration)

Peripheral white blood cell count <5,000/mm^3 (5.0 × 10^9/L)

Absolute neutrophil count less than 1000/mm^3 (1.0 × 10^9/L)

CSF protein greater than 300 mg/dL (3 g/L)

Delay in achieving sterile CSF

Abnormal electroencephalography reading (more than mild)

Although this list may be helpful in counseling parents, there are many babies who have a good outcome despite these findings, and parents should not be misinformed that a bad outcome will inevitably follow from any of these factors.

REFERENCES

1. Stoll BJ, Hansen NI, Sanchez PJ, et al. Early-onset neonatal sepsis: the burden of group streptococcal and *E. coli* disease continues. *Pediatrics.* 2011;127:817–826.
2. Gaschinard J, Levy C, Romain O, et al. Neonatal bacterial meningitis: 444 cases in 7 years. *Pediatr Infect Dis J.* 2011;30:212–217.
3. Davies PA, Rudd PT. Neonatal meningitis. In: *Clinics in Developmental Medicine.* Number 132. Cambridge, UK: Cambridge University Press; 1994:22–23.
4. Carey AJ, Saiman L, Polin RA. Hospital-acquired infections in the NICU, epidemiology for the new millennium. *Clin Perinatol.* 2008;35:223–249.
5. Carey AJ, Long SS. *Staphylococcus aureus*: a continuously evolving and formidable pathogen in the neonatal intensive care unit. *Clin Perinatol.* 2010;37:5535–5546.
6. Agarwal D, Mahapatra AK. Vertically acquired neonatal citrobacter brain abscess—case report and review of the literature. *J Clin Neurosci.* 2005;12:188–190.
7. Gordon A, Isaacs D. Late-onset neonatal gram-negative bacillary infection in Australia and New Zealand, 1992–2002. *Pediatr Infect Dis J.* 2006;25:25–29.
8. De Louvois J, Halket S, Harvey D. Neonatal meningitis in England and Wales: sequelae at 5 years of age. *Eur J Pediatr.* 2005;164:730–734.
9. Mulder CJ, Zanen HC. A study of 280 cases of neonatal meningitis in the Netherlands. *J Infect.* 1984;9:177–184.
10. May M, Daley AJ, Donath S, Isaacs D. Early-onset meningitis in Australia and New Zealand, 1992–2002. *Arch Dis Child Fetal Neonatal Ed.* 2005;99:F324–F327.
11. Trijbels-Smeulders M, de Jonge GA, Pasker-de Jonge PC et al. Epidemiology of neonatal group B streptococcal disease in the Netherlands before and after introduction of guidelines for prevention. *Arch Dis Child Fetal Neonatal Ed.* 2007;92:F271–F27.
12. Jordan HT, Farley MM, Craig A, et al. Revisiting the need for vaccine prevention of late-onset neonatal GBS disease: a multi-state, population-based analysis. *Pediatr Infect Dis J.* 2008;27:1057–1064.
13. Berardi A, Lugli L, Baronciani D, et al. Group B streptococcal infections in a northern region of Italy. *Pediatrics* 2007;120:e487–e493.
14. Thigpen MC, Whitney CG, Messonnier NE, et al. Bacterial meningitis in the United States 1998–2007. *N Engl J Med.* 2011;364:2016–2025.
15. Chang CJ, Chang WN, Huang LT, et al. Neonatal bacterial meningitis in southern Taiwan. *Pediatr Neurol* 2003;29:288–294.
16. Philip AGS. Neonatal meningitis in the new millennium. *NeoReviews.* 2003;4:e73–e80.
17. Klinger G, Chin CN, Beyene J, et al. Predicting the outcome of neonatal bacterial meningitis. *Pediatrics.* 2000;106:477–482.
18. Dellagrammaticas HD, Christodoulou C, Megaloyanni E, et al. Treatment of gram-negative neonatal meningitis in term neonates with third generation cephalosporins plus amikacin. *Biol Neonate.* 2000;77:139–146.
19. Levy HL, Sepe SJ, Shih VE, Vawter GF, Klein JO. Sepsis due to *Escherichia coli* in neonates with galactosemia. *N Engl J Med.* 1977;297:823–825.
20. Polin RA, Harris MC. Neonatal bacterial meningitis. *Semin Neonatol.* 2001;6:157–172.
21. Vogel LC, Boyer KM, Gadzala CA, Gotoff SP. Prevalence of type-specific group B streptococcal antibody in pregnant women. *J Pediatr.* 1980;96:1047–1051.
22. Sennhauser FH, Balloch A, MacDonald RA, Shelton MJ, Robertson DM. Maternofetal transfer of IgG anti-*Escherichia coli* antibodies with enhanced avidity and opsonic activity in very premature neonates. *Pediatr Res.* 1990;27:365–371.
23. Grandgirard D, Leib SL. Meningitis in neonates: bench to bedside. *Clin Perinatol.* 2010;37:655–676.
24. Baker CJ. Group B streptococcal infections in neonates. *Pediatr Rev.* 1979;1:5–15.
25. Domelier AS, van der Mee-Marquet N, Grandet A, Mereghetti L, Rosenau A, Quentin R. Loss of catabolic function in *Streptococcus agalactiae* strains and its association with neonatal meningitis. *J Clin Microbiol.* 2006;44(9):3245–3250.
26. Lamy MC, Dramsi S, Billoet A, et al. Rapid detection of the "highly virulent" group B streptococcus ST-17 clone. *Microbe Infect.* 2006;8:1714–1722.
27. Tazi A, Disson O, Bellais S, et al. The surface protein HvgA mediates group B streptococcus hypervirulence and meningeal tropism in neonates. *J Exp Med.* 2010;207:2313–2322.
28. Maruvada R, Kim KS. Extracellular loops of the *Escherichia coli* outer membrane protein A contribute to the pathogenesis of meningitis. *J Infect Dis.* 2011;203:131–140.
29. Malaeb SN, Cohen S, Stonestreet BS. Development of the blood-brain barrier: relationship to perinatal medicine. *NeoReviews.* 2012;13(4):e231–e250.
30. Enns GM. Diagnosing inborn errors of metabolism in the newborn: clinical features. *NeoReviews.* 2001;2:e183–e191.
31. Lionetti G, Lapidus S, Goldbach-Mansky R, Frankovich J. Auto-inflammatory disorders in the neonate: mimickers of neonatal infection. *NeoReviews.* 2010;11:e566–e577.
32. El-Radhi AS, Jawad M, Mansor N, Jamil I, Ibrahim M. Sepsis and hypothermia in the newborn infant: value of gastric aspirate examination. *J Pediatr.* 1983;103:300–302.
33. Riley LE, Celi AC, Onderdonk AB, et al. Association of epidural related fever and non-infectious inflammation in term labor. *Obstet Gynecol.* 2011;117:588–595.
34. Oliver TK, Jr. Temperature regulation and heat production in the newborn. *Pediatr Clin North Am.* 1965;12:765–778.
35. Pomerance JJ, Brand RJ, Meredith JL. Differentiating environmental from disease-related fevers in the term newborn. *Pediatrics.* 1981;67:485–488.

36. Tollner U. Early diagnosis of septicemia in the newborn: clinical studies and sepsis score. *Eur J Pediatr.* 1982;138:331–337.

37. Xanthou M, Xypolyta A, Anagnostakis D, Economou-Mavrou C, Matsaniotis N. Exchange transfusion in severe neonatal infection with sclerema. *Arch Dis Child.* 1975;50:901–902.

38. Ray B, Mangalore J, Harikumar C, Tuladhar A. Is lumbar puncture necessary for evaluation of early neonatal sepsis? *Arch Dis Child.* 2006;91:1033–1035.

39. Flidel-Ramon O, Leibovitz E, Eventov-Friedman S, Juster-Reicher A, Shinwell ES. Is lumbar puncture (LP) required in every workup for suspected late-onset sepsis in neonates. *Acta Paediatr.* 2011;100:303–304.

40. Kestenbaum LA, Ebberson J, Zorc JJ, Hodinka RL, Shah SS. Defining cerebrospinal fluid white blood cell count reference values in neonates and young infants. *Pediatrics.* 2010;125:257–264.

41. Garges HP, Moody MA, Cotton CM, et al. Neonatal meningitis: what is the correlation among cerebrospinal fluid culture, blood culture and cerebrospinal fluid parameters? *Pediatrics.* 2006;117:1094–1100.

42. Natarajan G, Johnson YR, Zhang F, Chen KM, Worsham MJ. Real-time polymerase chain reaction for the rapid detection of group B streptococcal colonization in neonates. *Pediatrics.* 2006;118:14–22.

43. Martinez de Tejada B, Stan CM, Boulvain M, et al. Development of a rapid PCR assay for screening of maternal colonization by group B streptococcus and neonatal invasive *Escherichia coli* during labor. *Gynecol Obstet Invest.* 2010;70:250–255.

44. Ng PC, Lam HS. Biomarkers for late-onset neonatal sepsis: cytokines and beyond. *Clin Perinatol.* 2010;37:599–610.

45. Damman O, O'Shea TM. Cytokines and perinatal brain damage. *Clin Perinatol.* 2008;35:643–663.

46. Raju VSN, Rao MN, Rao VSRM. Cranial sonography in pyogenic meningitis in meonates and infants. *J Trop Pediatr.* 1995;41:68–73.

47. Wilson DA, Nguyen DL, Marshall K. Sonography of brain abscesses complicating *Citrobacter* neonatal meningitis. *Am J Perinatol.* 1988;5:37–39.

48. Shah DK, Daley AJ, Hunt RW, Volpe JJ, Inder TE. Cerebral white matter injury in the newborn following *Escherichia coli* meningitis. *Eur J Paediatr Neurol.* 2005;9:13–17.

49. Hernandez MI, Sandoval CC, Tapia JL, et al. Stroke patterns in neonatal group B streptococcal meningitis. *Pediatr Neurol.* 2011;44:282–288.

50. Falciglia G, Hageman JR, Schreiber M, Alexander K. Antibiotic therapy and early-onset sepsis. *NeoReviews.* 2012;13(2):e86–e93.

51. Chu A, Hageman JR, Schreiber M, Alexander K. Antimicrobial therapy and late-onset sepsis. *NeoReviews.* 2012;13(2):e94–e102.

52. Isaacs D. Unnatural selection: reducing antibiotic resistance in neonatal units. *Arch Dis Child Fetal Neonatal Ed.* 2006;91:F72–F74.

53. Puopolo KM, Eichenwald EC. No change in incidence of ampicillin-resistant, neonatal early-onset sepsis over 18 years. *Pediatrics.* 2010;125:e1031–e1038.

54. Serane TV, Zengeya S, Penford G, Cooke J, Khanna G, McGregor-Colman E. Once daily dose gentamicin in neonates - is our dosing correct? *Acta Paediatr.* 2009;98:1100–1105.

55. Siegel JD, McCracken GH, Threlkeld N, et al. Single dose penicillin prophylaxis of neonatal group B streptococcal disease: conclusion of a 41 month controlled trial. *Lancet.* 1982;i:1426–1430.

56. Glasgow TS, Young PC, Wallin J, et al. Association of intrapartum antibiotic exposure and late-onset serious bacterial infections in infants. *Pediatrics.* 2005;116:696–702.

57. The INIS Collaborative Group. Treatment of neonatal sepsis with intravenous immune globulin. *N Engl J Med.* 2011;365:2101–1211.

58. Verani JR, Schrag SJ. Group B streptococcal disease in infants: progress in prevention and continued challenges. *Clin Perinatol.* 2010;37:375–392.

59. Schrag SJ, Zywicki S, Farley MM, et al. Group B streptococcal disease in the era of intrapartum prophylaxis. *N Engl J Med.* 2000;342:15–20.

60. Edwards MS, Rench MA, Beyene J, et al. Long-term sequelae of group B streptococcal meningitis in infants. *J Pediatr.* 1985;106:717–722.

61. Levent F, Baker CJ, Rench MA, Edwards MS. Early outcomes of group B streptococcal meningitis in the 21st century. *Pediatr Infect Dis J.* 2010;29:1009–1112.

62. Unhanand M, Mustafa MM, McCracken GH Jr, Nelson JD. Gram-negative enteric bacillary meningitis: a twenty-one-year experience. *J Pediatr.* 1993;122:15–21.

63. Stoll BJ, Hansen NI, Adams-Chapman I, et al. Neurodevelopmental and growth impairment among extremely low-birth-weight infants with neonatal infection. *JAMA.* 2004;292:2357–2365.

64. Klinger G, Chin CN, Otsobu H, et al. Prognostic value of EEG in neonatal bacterial meningitis. *Pediatr Neurol.* 2001;24:28–31.

17 Neonatal Hypotonia

Jean-Baptiste Le Pichon and Steven M. Shapiro

HISTORICAL PERSPECTIVE

It is difficult to find any reference to neonatal hypotonia before the beginning of the 20th century. This may be in part related to the very high infant mortality rate and the fact that for most of history children were not considered of much value until they had reached the age of 7 or so, when they had survived the vicissitudes of childhood and could start working.[1] With the advent of the Industrial Revolution and the fundamental changes in medicine that accompanied it, the first reports of infantile hypotonia were published (for an excellent summary of this history, refer to Victor Dubowitz's seminal work on the floppy infant[2]). Since the 1970s, and likely as a result of the exponential improvements in diagnostic tools, the scientific publications dedicated to hypotonia have steadily accumulated (Figure 17-1).

The earliest reports[2] of congenital hypotonia are probably those by Werdnig in 1891 and Hoffman in 1893. They independently described infants, apparently healthy at birth, who subsequently developed hypotonia and respiratory failure. Both of these authors described the pathology associated with spinal muscular atrophy (SMA). In 1900, Oppenheim described a series of infants born hypotonic and hyporeflexic who subsequently appeared to improve with no obvious residual pathology. He suggested the term *myatonia congenita*, later renamed *amyotonia congenita*. In 1957, Walton suggested the term *benign congenital hypotonia* to refer to cases in which the prognosis was "mild and may be overcome in time."[3] His major point was to distinguish patients with a grim prognosis, as is the

case in SMA, from those who faired better. Although the choice of the term *benign* was an unfortunate one that has led to considerable confusion, the diagnostic challenge that he was facing is still the dilemma that faces today's clinician. That is, what is the pathology behind the apparent hypotonia, and perhaps more importantly, what is the prognosis? The object of this chapter is to offer a rational approach to the diagnostic workup of the hypotonic infant.

DEFINITION: HYPOTONIA VS WEAKNESS

The first and perhaps most important step in evaluating a hypotonic infant is to ask the question: Is the infant truly hypotonic, or does the perceived hypotonia reflect weakness? The difference can be subtle but is of the essence since this difference is the first step in elucidating the etiology of the observed phenotype. Tone is generally defined as resistance to passive movement.[4] Tone can be further divided into postural or truncal tone (proximal muscle groups) and phasic or peripheral tone (extremities). In contrast, weakness refers to lack of muscle strength.[5] Therefore, in its simplest terms, strength can be thought of as the ability to generate movement and tone the ability to generate posture. It follows that weakness is the inability to maintain movement while hypotonia is the inability to generate posture. Thus, a 1-year-old child with a history of hypoxic ischemic encephalopathy (HIE) will likely demonstrate truncal hypotonia, peripheral spastic hypertonia, and diffuse weakness. This introduces

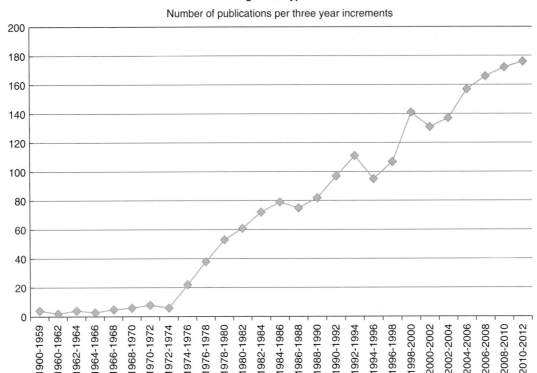

FIGURE 17-1 Scientific publications dedicated to congenital hypotonia have steadily increased since 1972–1974.

one last concept that needs to be defined: spasticity. Spasticity is generally defined as velocity-dependent increase in tone. In other words, tone increases with increased speed of movement about a joint.

EPIDEMIOLOGY

There are no studies that have looked at the incidence or prevalence of neonatal hypotonia. This likely reflects the broad range of etiologies associated with congenital hypotonia as well as the challenges associated with objectively defining hypotonia. However, by gleaning information from papers reporting the incidence of specific etiologies of neonatal hypotonia, one can estimate the overall incidence. There seems to be a consensus that HIE and intracranial hemorrhage account for approximately one-third of all cases of hypotonia in term infants.[6,7] In a retrospective chart review, Takenouchi et al reported the incidence and etiology of perinatal brain injury in term infants admitted to the New York Presbyterian Hospital neonatal intensive care unit (NICU).[8] In their study, the reported incidence of HIE in term infants was 0.27 per 1000 births. Assuming that these numbers are representative of the larger population, one can then extrapolate the incidence of congenital hypotonia in term infants to be on the order of

0.8/1000 births. However, the incidence of "neonatal encephalopathy," a global nonspecific term encompassing any congenital injury to the brain, is reported as 1 to 6 per 1000 live births. Since the most frequent presentation of neonatal encephalopathy is hypotonia,[9] it is probable that the incidence of neonatal hypotonia is much higher than was extrapolated from the study mentioned above.

The etiology of neonatal hypotonia has been addressed in several retrospective studies.[6,7,10,11] Most of these studies gave a similar distribution with regard to etiology (Figure 17-2). Typically, 66% to 88% of the hypotonia is classified as central, referring to causes in the central nervous system (CNS), while 9% to 34% is classified as peripheral, referring to causes in the peripheral nervous system, the neuromuscular junction, or the muscle itself. Of the central causes, HIE and intracerebral hemorrhage account for 28% to 42% of cases, chromosomal abnormalities and syndromic disorders (presumably chromosomal) account for 26% to 34% of cases, while the rest of the etiologies are spread among a wide variety of causes, ranging from migrational to metabolic disorders, each accounting for less than 10% of cases.

One retrospective study is unique in that it focused exclusively on causes of peripheral hypotonia.[12] The purpose of this study was to evaluate whether

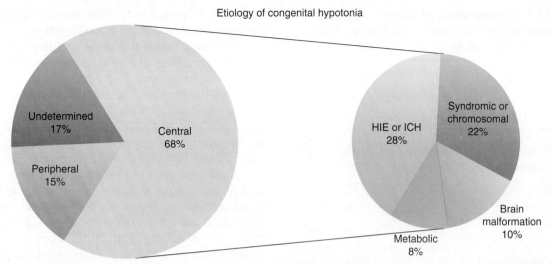

FIGURE 17-2 Etiology of congenital hypotonia among 144 infants. On the left is the percentage of congenital hypotonia due to central, peripheral, and undetermined causes. On the right is a further breakdown of the causes of central congenital hypotonia. HIE, hypoxic ischemic encephalopathy; ICH, intracranial hemorrhage. (Data from Laugel et al.[11])

classification of hypotonia as peripheral using standard physical examination parameters was an effective diagnostic approach to these infants. In this study, approximately 80% of the hypotonic infants had an identifiable disorder, and of those, 47% had a neuromuscular disorder. Interestingly, of the remaining 53% of infants, 10% had a genetic disorder, 10% a metabolic disorder, and 5% a CNS injury. Therefore, even after a careful clinical examination, more than a quarter of the infants were found to have evidence of CNS involvement (combining the genetic disorders, the metabolic disorders, and CNS injury). This illustrates well the conundrum clinicians face when evaluating the hypotonic infant: Even after a careful examination, hypotonia may appear peripheral in nature, yet the etiology will turn out to be central in many of the cases.

A SYSTEMATIC APPROACH TO CONGENITAL HYPOTONIA

So, how does one approach the hypotonic infant? Many different diagnostic approaches to the hypotonic infant have been proposed, starting with Walton in 1957, who classified the hypotonia into infantile muscular atrophy and related disorders, symptomatic hypotonia, and benign congenital hypotonia.[13] In 1964, Rabe proposed a classification based on neuroanatomical location: CNS, spinal cord, spinal roots and peripheral nerves, myoneural junction, and muscle.[14] Dubowitz, in his classic monograph on the floppy infant, argued for a classification of hypotonic infants in 2 groups: paralytic and nonparalytic.[2] Dubowitz's approach has

the advantage of simplifying the initial evaluation of the hypotonic infant. In this system, the child is classified on the basis of his or her ability to generate any movement against gravity and to maintain posture. If either of these findings is present, the infant can be classified as belonging to the nonparalytic group, the vast majority of whom will have a CNS etiology for the hypotonia. A similar approach was advocated by Bodensteiner,[4] who divided the hypotonic infants into (1) supraspinal conditions or central hypotonia and (2) segmental conditions or motor unit hypotonia. Both of these approaches have the merit of simplifying the initial evaluation of the hypotonic infant. However, additional clues that can help further delineate the etiology of the hypotonia can often be gleaned from the history and examination. In this chapter, we adopt a nomenclature similar to that proposed by Bodensteiner,[4] dividing the hypotonia into central vs peripheral.

It is worth noting that the terminology has its limitations. For example, the spinal cord is part of the CNS. Yet, we (and many others) choose to group SMA (a disorder of the motor neurons as it originates in the ventral horn of the spinal cord) in the peripheral hypotonia group. This makes sense since it is the motor neuron, the first component of the neuromuscular unit, that is affected. One might argue that the "segmental" nomenclature suggested by Bodensteiner is more accurate. However, the terms *central* and *peripheral* are widely used and generally well accepted. Therefore, we keep this nomenclature.

The following discussion reviews clues that can be uncovered from a careful history and physical examination. The importance of a good history and physical examination cannot be overstated. In a retrospective

Table 17-1 Contribution of Various Aspects of evaluation to Diagnosis in Neonates With Congenital Hypotonia

Workup	Percentage	Cumulative Percentage
History and physical examination	50	50
Neuroimaging	13	63
Genetic databases	9	72
Karyotype, FISH	7	79
Biochemical tests	6	85
Muscle/nerve investigations	6	91
Follow-up tests	7	97
Unclassified	3	100

Abbreviation: Fish, fluorescence in situ hybridization.
[a]Data from Paro-Panjan and Neubauer.[7]

study of 138 hypotonic infants, Paro-Panjan and Neubauer[7] found that 50% were properly classified on the basis of the history and physical examination alone, another 13% by neuroimaging, and the rest by other ancillary tests. None of the additional ancillary tests contributed to the classification of more than 10% of the study group[7] (Table 17–1).

Yet, the clues gleaned from the history and physical examination are often neither sensitive nor specific and should be framed within the larger clinical context, including ancillary tests. We believe that the best approach to the hypotonic infant is a staged approach. The initial classification into central vs peripheral hypotonia advocated by Dubowitz and many others is useful in establishing the initial diagnostic approach to the child. However, as further information becomes available, the differential diagnosis will evolve. The next section is written with this in mind. It reviews findings from the history, examination, and initial ancillary tests and how these might help narrow the wide spectrum of etiologies for congenital hypotonia.

History and Physical

It is essential to obtain a good history, as it will often uncover important clues regarding the diagnosis. The history should start with a careful history of the pregnancy. Was there poor prenatal care? Was there a history of alcohol or drug abuse? Was there a history of maternal illness during the pregnancy? A positive answer to any one of these questions markedly increases the risk for central hypotonia. This is in contrast to eliciting a

history of decreased fetal movements, which is more frequently observed in peripheral hypotonia.[11]

A thorough family history is also important. In a retrospective review of 83 infants with hypotonia consistent with motor unit disorders, 50% of the infants who were the product of a consanguineous union had a metabolic disorder, while 20% of infants with a diagnosed condition had a positive family history of a similar condition.[12]

A detailed birth history is also essential. In a retrospective cohort study of 144 hypotonic infants, Laugel et al found that polyhydramnios was much more frequent in peripheral hypotonia, while delivery via cesarean section or a history of perinatal asphyxia was more frequently associated with central hypotonia.[11] The contributions of the history and physical examination in distinguishing central from peripheral hypotonia are summarized in Table 17-2.

Anatomical Localization

Cerebral Hypotonia

Central hypotonia can be divided in disorders caused by cerebral hypotonia and those caused by spinal cord dysfunction. Cerebral hypotonia, meaning hypotonia

Table 17-2 Distinguishing Central From Peripheral Hypotonia by History and Physical Examination in Neonates Presenting With Congenital Hypotonia

	Central Hypotonia	Peripheral Hypotonia
History of the pregnancy	Poor prenatal care Alcohol or drug abuse Maternal illness	Decreased fetal movements
Family history	Positive: Metabolic disorders	Positive: Motor unit or myopathic disorder
Birth history	Perinatal asphyxia Cesarean	Polyhydramnios
Exam	**Early:** ↓Tone and ↓deep tendon reflexes, little or no weakness **Late:** ↑ Tone, ↑ deep tendon reflexes and spasticity Dysmorphic features	↓↓ Tone, ↓↓ or absent deep tendon reflexes, ↓↓ strength (little to no antigravity movement) Persists with time Poor suck and swallow

caused by abnormalities in the brain, has many etiologies, and it is unlikely that one can differentiate the causes of cerebral hypotonia based on examination alone. Nevertheless, some concepts may be useful when examining these infants. First and foremost, central hypotonia is usually not accompanied by weakness or hyporeflexia. If anything, in time the infant will display increased tone and reflexes, although initially, cerebral hypotonia may be easily confused as peripheral hypotonia, especially during the early phase of the illness, when there may be transient weakness and hyporeflexia.

When evaluating central hypotonia, it is useful to keep in mind the following broad categories of etiologies: systemic illness, genetic disorders, cortical dysgenesis and other malformations, deep-brain nuclei injury, brainstem and cerebellar dysfunction, and finally, spinal cord disruption. We return to each of these later in the chapter. The purpose of this section is to highlight common threads that may help with localization.

Systemic Illnesses

Systemic illnesses will often cause profound hypotonia from what can be thought of as an energy crisis imposed on the brain by the demands of the concurrent illnesses. These processes include sepsis and other infectious processes, congenital cardiac malformations, necrotizing enterocolitis, gastroschisis, and so on. Congenital metabolic disorders figure prominently in this group as well. Infants with such disorders will often appear normal at birth but will rapidly decompensate within the first 72 hours of life.

Genetic Disorders

Perhaps the most useful finding in identifying genetic disorders as a cause of cerebral hypotonia is the presence of dysmorphic features. Evidence for holoprosencephaly can be obvious (cyclopia) or much less obvious (single central incisor). If such abnormalities are found, it is important to look for other midline abnormalities, such as cleft lip or palate and congenital heart malformations. The presence of up- or down-slanting palpebral fissures, hypertelorism, or prominent bilateral epicanthal folds are often good indicators of a genetic disorder.

Cortical Dysgenesis and Other Malformations

Further clues may help sort the anatomical location of the central hypotonia. The presence of seizures is highly consistent with cortical abnormalities of both acquired and developmental etiologies.

Deep-Brain Nuclei Injury

With injury to deep-brain nuclei, as is seen in severe hypoxia (putamen) or severe hyperbilirubinemia (globus pallidus [GP] and subthalamic nucleus), one often observes hypotonia rapidly followed by increased tone, often within a few days to a few weeks of the injury.[9]

Brainstem and Cerebellar Dysfunction

Severe hypoxia, as can be seen with catastrophic peripartum events, can cause brainstem injury. This will often be clinically evident by cranial nerve dysfunction and feeding difficulties and is associated with high neonatal mortality.[9] Cerebellar and brainstem malformations are often associated with profound hypotonia. For example, infants with Joubert syndrome[15] (vermian and midbrain atrophy with the "molar tooth sign" on magnetic resonance imaging [MRI] or pontocerebellar hypoplasia[16] [cerebellar hemisphere and pontine hypoplasia]) almost always present with congenital hypotonia.

Spinal Cord Disruption

Spinal cord disruption may occur as a result of trauma at the time of delivery or, more commonly, of spinal cord dysraphism. Spinal cord injury as a result of trauma during delivery remains a relatively rare event. The prevalence was reported as 1 per 29,000 live births in 1 study.[17] The injuries are felt to be the result of both traction and compression injuries, with most of the injuries occurring in the cervical spine. The infants present with flaccid tetraplegia or paraplegia depending on the level of the injury and in time develop spasticity. Due to the mechanics of the injury, cervical and high-level thoracic spine injuries are much more common than lower-level injuries. It is important to keep in mind that the withdrawal reflex is a spinal reflex; thus, the withdrawal reflex will be present in spinal cord injury. Spinal dysraphisms resulting in spinal cord disruption sufficiently severe to cause congenital hypotonia will generally be evident in that almost all of these will be open malformations, with the 2 most common being myelomeningocele and myelocele.[18] As opposed to traumatic birth injury, spinal dysraphisms tend to be more common at the lower thoracic and lumbar levels.

Peripheral Hypotonia

In contrast to cerebral hypotonia, peripheral hypotonia usually presents with profound weakness and an inability to maintain posture. This is often evident on examination by the classic "frog posture" or, as described by Dubowitz, the rag doll appearance of the infant.[2] When lying prone on the examination table, these infants appear splayed out: the legs externally rotated, the arms inert parallel to the trunk, the shoulders falling backward. On horizontal suspension, the child will wrap around the hand of the examiner, while on vertical suspension the child will tend to slip due to the lack of tone in the shoulder girdle muscles. On traction of the upper extremities, the head will have a significant lag, and these infants often have a scarf sign, whereas on pulling 1 upper extremity across the chest the elbow will reach well beyond the midline. One consideration when examining the infant is the gestational age. As infants are delivered more and more prematurely, they have decreased tone that may be interpreted as pathogenic. In a longitudinal landmark study of 69 premature infants, Allen and Caputo documented the average gestational age at which tone and reflexes develop[19] (Figure 17-3). For example, all premature infants initially had a positive scarf sign and slip through on vertical suspension. It was not until 35 to 38 weeks' gestational age that these signs remitted.

It is useful to divide peripheral hypotonia into its 3 functional units: the motor nerve unit, the neuromuscular junction, and the muscle itself. Some general comments can be made with regard to the clinical presentation of a dysfunction for each functional unit.

Motor Nerve Unit Dysfunction

The prototypic motor neuron unit disorder is SMA.[20] In the neonatal form of this disorder, the α-motor neurons' ability to survive is affected, resulting in a clinical picture consisting of profound hypotonia and absent deep-tendon reflexes. Although the neck muscles are weak, bulbar function is usually preserved, and the CNS is unaffected, resulting in infants with a normal level of alertness that often contrasts markedly to the observed profound hypotonia and weakness.

Neuromuscular Junction Dysfunction

While SMA presents with profound hypotonia but usually preserved bulbar function, congenital myasthenic syndromes, in addition to hypotonia, usually present with cranial nerve dysfunction, including ophthalmoparesis.[21] Congenital myasthenias are frequently accompanied by

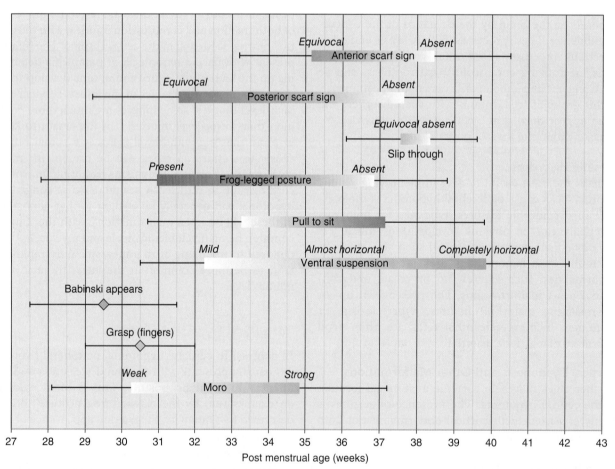

FIGURE 17-3 Neurological signs during development. The mean postmenstrual age of appearance of neurological signs relevant to muscle tone and strength are shown. The range of mean appearance or presence of each sign is shown as a thick, colored bar or a diamond, with the thin error bars before and after representing 1 standard deviation. (Data from Allen and Caputo.[19])

fatigue, although this feature can be difficult to elicit in infants.

Muscle Dysfunction

Congenital muscle diseases include 2 broad categories based on their pathological appearance: the congenital myopathies[22] and the congenital muscular dystrophies.[23] These 2 categories encompass many disorders with phenotypes ranging the gamut from mild to severe. As a general rule, the muscular dystrophies present with markedly elevated serum creatine kinase (CK), while the congenital myopathies have normal-to-slightly-elevated CK levels. Most of these disorders, when present at birth, involve the bulbar muscles. Muscular dystrophies tend to affect more proximal muscles first.

ETIOLOGY OF HYPOTONIA BASED ON ANATOMICAL LOCALIZATION

In this section, we examine in more detail the most common etiologies of congenital hypotonia. Whereas the previous section described typical presentations by anatomical location, this section focuses on clinical presentations by etiology. It is important to keep in mind that we do not intend this section as a systematic review of each condition or intend to cover every possible etiology of congenital hypotonia. Either proposition is well beyond the scope of this chapter. Nevertheless, we offer a tool we hope can be used as a reference in the evaluation of the hypotonic infant, a tool that will cover the most common causes of hypotonia and will offer a good start in the evaluation of the more unusual disorders.

As described previously, a careful history and physical examination should allow the clinician to classify the hypotonia as central vs peripheral and it is hoped further localize the pathology. Based on this information, the clinician can now proceed to further refine the differential diagnosis. This section is designed to help in this second step. It is divided in etiologies by localization: systemic, cerebral, spinal cord, motor nerve unit, and finally muscle.

Systemic Hypotonia

Systemic hypotonia defines a group of disorders in which a systemic disorder, either directly or indirectly, has an impact on cerebral function with a resultant clinical hypotonia. Systemic hypotonias can be subdivided in 3 groups: acquired or congenital systemic illnesses indirectly causing a cerebral energy crisis, congenital metabolic syndromes, and acquired metabolic illnesses.

Acute Congenital or Acquired Illnesses Resulting in a Cerebral Energy Crisis

It is well established that hypotonia is a common presentation of systemic illnesses in the newborn. Although the pathophysiology of the hypotonia is not well defined, it is useful to think of it in the context of a cerebral energy crisis. In other words, the metabolic demand on the rest of the body is such that the brain enters a deficient state with resultant encephalopathy and hypotonia. Two good examples of systemic acquired and congenital illnesses with hypotonia as one of the prominent features are septicemia and congenital heart defects. In a retrospective study of 83 newborn infants with septicemia,[24] only 6% of the infants had evidence of hypotonia before the onset of the infection, while the numbers rose to 54% at onset and 91% at the peak of the illness. In fact, it was one of the most consistent findings in septic infants (along with skin color and microcirculation). A similar result was reported in a study of infants with congenital heart defects.[25] In this study, 28 of 50 patients examined demonstrated abnormalities on neurological examination, and 20 of these 28 presented with diffuse hypotonia and 5 with weakness in the upper extremities. Most of the time, these illnesses will be evident from the clinical context. However, occasionally hypotonia will be the first clinical clue that the child is ill and the etiology should be investigated aggressively.

Congenital Metabolic Syndromes

As a group, congenital metabolic syndromes are daunting to the clinician. They are relatively rare, they often have complicated metabolic pathways, and their clinical presentations vary widely even within a single disorder due to variable residual activity of the enzymes affected. Saudubray et al presented a useful approach to inherited metabolic disorders.[26] They suggested classifying the disorders in 3 groups: disorders that give rise to intoxication, disorders of energy metabolism, and disorders involving complex molecules (Table 17-3). This classification has the merit of grouping the metabolic disorders in 3 groups with roughly distinguishable clinical presentations and with very different clinical managements. While the disorders that give rise to intoxication are mostly amenable to intervention, often urgently, the disorders in the other 2 groups are, as a general rule, poorly or not at all responsive to treatment.

Disorders that give rise to intoxication: This group of disorders includes the aminoacidemias, organic acidurias, abnormalities of galactose and fructose metabolism, and congenital urea cycle defects. Infants with these disorders typically present with progressive deterioration over the first week of life, often with onset of symptoms following the first feeding. Many of these disorders are treatable and require early intervention.

Disorders of energy metabolism: These disorders include the glycogen storage diseases (glucose deficiency), fatty acid oxidation disorders (carnitine metabolism defects; small-, medium-, and long-chain acyl-coenzyme A deficiency) and congenital lactic acidemias (pyruvate metabolism disorders, Krebs cycle and mitochondrial disorders). This group of disorders typically presents with severe hypoglycemia, hyperlactic acidemia, hypotonia, organomegaly, and myopathy. While the congenital lactic acidemias are not amenable to treatment, the rest of these disorders respond at least partially to clinical intervention. Mitochondrial myopathies presenting in the neonatal period are rare and are briefly discussed in a separate section.

Disorders involving complex molecules: This group of disorders includes all of the lysosomal storage disorders, peroxisomal disorders, congenital disorders of glycosylation, and inborn errors of cholesterol synthesis (see Table 17-3). With few exceptions, none of these disorders are treatable.

Acquired Metabolic Illnesses

A number of entities can be classified in this group of acquired metabolic illnesses. They all present with neonatal hypotonia as a prominent feature. By definition, they are transient and acquired and caused by toxicity transmitted to the infant by the mother. Examples of such illnesses include lithium toxicity,[27] magnesium toxicity,[28] and transient neonatal myasthenia.[29]

Lithium toxicity: Prenatal exposure to lithium used to treat maternal bipolar illness may pose an increased risk of teratogenesis. Infants without malformations may have transiently depressed neurological function, including hypotonia, respiratory distress syndrome, cyanosis, lethargy, weak suck and Moro, apnea, and bradycardia.[27] Lithium crosses the placenta freely, but the half-life in the fetus is increased. Most of these symptoms resolve as lithium is excreted, which may take up to 14 days. Transient nephrogenic diabetes insipidus, cardiac disorders, and thyroid goiters have been reported as well as cardiac anomalies, especially the Ebstein anomaly.

Magnesium toxicity: Magnesium sulfate is the most commonly used tocolytic and is now used for prevention of cerebral palsy.[30] In a recent retrospective cohort analysis, 6% of infants born to 6654 women with preeclampsia treated with intravenous magnesium sulfate were diagnosed with hypotonia.[28] Other clinical findings included significantly lower 1-minute Apgar scores and Apgar scores of 3 or less at 1 and 5 minutes. The probability of hypotonia increased with increasing magnesium concentration (13% when maternal magnesium levels were 7 mEq/L or greater).

Transient neonatal myasthenia: Transient neonatal myasthenia is a rare complication occurring in infants of mothers with acquired myasthenia gravis.[29] The pathophysiology is felt to be secondary to passive transfer of maternal acetylcholine receptor (AChR) antibodies across the placental blood barrier. However, this mechanism is clearly not sufficient since all infants born to mothers with positive AChR antibody myasthenia are found to have elevated AChR titer, yet only a small proportion develop symptoms. In a retrospective cohort study of 127 births to mothers with acquired myasthenia, 5 (4%) infants were diagnosed with neonatal myasthenia.[31] This is lower than the 10% to 20% previously reported and may relate to underreporting in this retrospective study or overreporting in the previous study (hypotonia secondary to causes other than neonatal myasthenia). The onset of symptoms in these infants occurs within the first day of life and usually presents with hypotonia, poor sucking, weak cry, facial paresis, difficulty swallowing, and in severe cases, respiratory failure. These children respond well to anticholinesterase treatment and typically make a complete recovery within 2 to 4 months.

Cerebral Hypotonia

Cerebral hypotonia encompasses a group of disorders in which cerebral dysfunction is the primary cause of the hypotonia. As mentioned, these infants typically present with hypotonia but with little or no weakness and with normal or increased deep-tendon reflexes. Additional clues to a cerebral etiology include seizures, developmental delays, and dysmorphic features. In time, almost all these infants develop spasticity. Cerebral hypotonia disorders can be roughly grouped in 4 categories: disorders resulting from a toxic insult to the brain, as in HIE or kernicterus; disorders resulting from cerebral dysgenesis; disorders resulting from white matter dysfunction; and disorders secondary to genetic syndromes.

Hypoxic Ischemic Encephalopathy

Hypoxic ischemic encephalopathy is the most common cause of cerebral hypotonia,[9] and in mild HIE, hypotonia may be the most prominent feature. In an 11-year retrospective cohort study of 50 neonates with hypotonia, with two-thirds central and one-third peripheral hypotonia, HIE was the most frequent diagnosis, accounting for 26% overall and 39% of the central hypotonias.[6] Decreased or absent reflexes were observed more frequently in the peripheral hypotonia group (88%) vs the central group (36%); similarly, decreased antigravity movement was more in the peripheral (88%) vs the central group (39%). Intubation for more than 5 days was found in 100% of peripheral and only 36% of the central group. Finally,

Table 17-3 Metabolic Disorders Presenting With Congenital Hypotonia

	Presents With	Disease	Initial Diagnostic Workup
Group 1: Intoxication disorders	Neurologic deterioration (often following first feeds), acidosis, ketosis	Maple syrup urine disease Methylmalonic aciduria Proprionic acidemia Isovaleric acidemia Urea cycle defects	**Serum:** gas chromatography, mass spectrometry, plasma amino acids
	Seizures	B₆ (pyridoxine) Folinic acid Biotin[a] Nonketotic hyperglycinemia	**Electroencephalogram (EEG) Cerebral Spinal Fluid (CSF):** neurotransmitters and amino acids
	Jaundice, liver failure	Galactosemia[a] Tyrosinemia Congenital disorder of glycosilation type Ib	**Serum:** plasma amino acids, specific enzyme testing, serum transferrin isoform analysis[b]
Group 2: Disorders of energy metabolism	Persistent hypoglycemia	Hyperinsulinism Glycogenosis Gluconeogenesis FAO disorders	**Serum:** acylcarnitine profile analysis, insulin, creatine kinase, β-hydroxybutyrate, lactate, free fatty acids **Urine:** oligosaccharides, organic acids
	Cardiac failure	Fatty acid oxidation disorders	**Serum:** acylcarnitine profile analysis
	Persistent lactic acidemia	Pyruvate carboxylase Pyruvate dehydrogenase Krebs cycle Mitochondrial respiratory chain disorders	**Serum:** lactate, spectrometry, plasma amino acids **CSF:** lactate, pyruvate (consider CSF amino acids)
Group 3: Disorders involving complex molecules		Lysosomal disorders Peroxisomal disorders Congenital disorders of glycosylation Cholesterol metabolism	**Serum:** very long chain fatty acids, serum transferrin isoform analysis,[b] cholesterol, and 7-dehydrocholesterol.

Abbreviation: FAO, Fatty acid oxidation.

[a] Biotinidase deficiency and galactosemia are now a part of the newborn screen in every state in the United States.

[b] Serum transferrin isoform analysis (for congenital disorders of glycosylation) is often inconclusive or misleading in infants younger than 3 weeks.

HIE was a frequent cause of neonatal hypotonia without other overt manifestations.

Most term infants with severe HIE have marked and diffuse hypotonia with minimal spontaneous or provoked movements in the first 12 hours after injury. Other signs of HIE in the CNS (eg, stupor, coma, seizures, and dysfunction in other organ systems) help establish the diagnosis. Less-severely involved infants may have normal tone, and those with prominent basal ganglia involvement may even have hypertonia initially. With time, the examination changes, and weakness in a proximal upper- more than lower-extremity distribution may be seen in term infants with ischemic parasagittal infarcts in a watershed distribution between the middle and anterior cerebral arteries. In premature infants, the distribution of hypotonia and weakness may favor the lower extremities. At 72 hours after injury, generalized hypotonia may persist, with evidence of hypertonia on moving the extremities; with time, the hypertonia may become more prominent.

Bilirubin Encephalopathy (Also Known as Kernicterus)

Kernicterus (bilirubin encephalopathy) results from bilirubin neurotoxicity, in which excessive amounts of free bilirubin enter the CNS and selectively damage specific neurons and areas of the CNS, including the GP and subthalamic nucleus of the basal ganglia, specific brainstem nuclei, cerebellar Purkinjee cells, and the CA2 area of the hippocampus.[32-34] Acutely, these infants present with central hypotonia and lethargy and, with worsening severity of the toxicity, variable hypo- and hypertonia, retrocollis, opisthotonus, high-pitched cry, and setting sun sign; fever and seizures may occur. In subsequent days, infants may become strikingly hypotonic, which over time (weeks to month) may progress to hypertonia, dystonia, and athetosis (slow, writhing movements) and in some cases a mixture of variable hypotonia and hypertonia. Reflexes may be hard to obtain but should be present. MRI shows bilateral symmetrical hyperintensity of the GP and, on high-quality scans, the subthalamic nuclei (STN). Initially, in the first days to weeks after the bilirubin neurotoxicity, the hyperintensity is seen in the GP and STN on T1-weighted and fluid-attenuated inversion recovery (FLAIR) MRI sequences, whereas months to years later, the hyperintensity is seen in T2-weighted and FLAIR images.[34]

Cerebral Dysgenesis: Migrational Disorders and Lissencephalies

Neuronal migrational disorders result in various cerebral malformations and are almost always associated with variable severity in developmental delays and epilepsy (Table 17-4). Structurally, they can be divided in 3 categories: disorders affecting the layering of the cerebral cortex (lissencephaly, polymicrogyria, pachygyria, subcortical heterotopias, and band heterotopia); disorders interfering with the normal development of the brain (holoprosencephaly, schizencephaly); and disorders affecting the brainstem (Joubert syndrome, pontocerebellar hypoplasia).[35] Although this is an oversimplification because many of these disorders overlap, it is a useful one, as it allows judicious genetic testing. For example, a lissencephaly that is more severe anteriorly is most consistent with a *DCX* mutation, while the reverse, a lissencephaly more severe in the occipital areas, is more consistent with *LIS1*. Prominent involvement of the infratentorial cortex is more consistent with cobblestone lissencephalies. Evidence of molar tooth sign in the midbrain is pathognomic for Joubert syndrome (vermis hypoplasia, deep interpeduncular fossa, and elongated superior cerebral peduncles), while cerebellar hemisphere atrophy and a thin pons are suggestive of pontocerebellar hypoplasia.

Disorders Resulting From Demyelination or Hypomyelination

Leukoencephalopathies encompass a broad group of disorders affecting the white matter. These can be categorized into demyelinating or hypomyelinating disorders[36] (Table 17-5). Infants with leukoencephalopathies typically present with axial hypotonia and often seizures.[37] Other clues can help in the differential diagnosis, for example, the presence of congenital cataracts in hypomyelination with congenital cataracts syndrome or macrocephaly in Alexander or Canavan disease. The pattern of myelin abnormality on MRI is also essential in developing a differential diagnosis. Hypomyelinating syndromes have mild or no T1 changes and mild T2 hyperintense white matter changes; in contrast, demyelination syndromes show much more intense changes (both in T1 hypointensity and T2 hyperintensity). Furthermore, the distribution of myelination change can give a clue as to the disorder. For example, Alexander disease will show a pattern of white matter change with frontal predominance, while Krabbe disease shows posterior predominance and vanishing white matter and Canavan disease will show diffuse involvement. The most common leukoencephalopathies presenting in infancy along with clinical characteristics and genetic testing when available are summarized in Table 17-5.

Genetic Syndromes

Hypotonia secondary to genetic disorders is often revealed by a careful physical examination, evidenced by dysmorphic features. The observed abnormalities

Table 17-4 Migrational Disorders and Lissencephalies

Classification	Disorder	Inheritance	Gene	Magnetic Resonance Imaging Findings	Distinguishing Clinical Features
Disorders affecting layering of the cortex[a] Lissencephalies	Lissencephaly with abnormal genitalia	XL	ARX	Three layer cortex	Usually lethal in males, in females intractable epilepsy, severe cognitive impairment, ambiguous enitalia
	Double-cortex syndrome	XL	DCX	Subcortical band heterotopia	Females with mild-to-moderate intellectual disability
	Isolated lissencephaly	XL	DCX	Four-layer cortex with anterior predominance	Males with severe intellectual disability and epilepsy
	Classic lissencephaly	LIS1 haploinsufficiency	LIS1	Four-layer cortex with posterior predominance	Mild dysmorphic features, severe intellectual disability, and epilepsy
	Miller-Dieker syndrome	Microdeletion	YWHAE	Four-layer cortex with posterior predominance	Dysmorphic features, severe intellectual disability and epilepsy
	Lissencephaly with cerebellar hypoplasia	AR	RELN	Severe cerebellar and hippocampal involvement	Dysmorphic features, severe intellectual disability, and epilepsy
Dystroglycanopathies	Fukuyama	AR	FKTN	Varies from mild to severe with cerebellar hypoplasia	Moderate-to-severe disability, cardiac malformations, microcephaly
	Walker-Warburg	AR	POMT1, POMT2, LARGE, FKRP	Cobblestone lissencephaly, hypoplastic vermis, and brainstem	Severe hypotonia, epilepsy, and eye abnormalities
	Muscle-eye-brain	AR	POMGNT1	Frontoparietal pachygyria with hypoplastic vermis and brainstem	Macrocephaly and epilepsy

(Continued)

Table 17-4 Migrational Disorders and Lissencephalies (Continued)

Classification	Disorder	Inheritance	Gene	Magnetic Resonance Imaging Findings	Distinguishing Clinical Features
Disorders affecting global structural anatomy	Holoprosencephaly[b]	Varies	To date 12 different genes identified including *SHH*	Varies in severity from mild, lobar, to severe, alobar holoprosencephaly	Severe (cyclopia) to mild (midface hypoplasia and single maxillary central incisor)
	Schizencephaly	Varies, may be acquired during gestation	Undefined in most cases	Open or closed lip gray matter cleft extending from the surface to the lateral ventricle	Frequent cause of epilepsy, often seen as part of a syndromic condition
Disorders affecting the brainstem	Joubert syndrome[c]	AR or XL	18 different genes to date with no known gene in 50% of the cases	Molar tooth sign: Vermian hypoplasia, deep interpeduncular fossa, thick and long superior cerebellar peduncles	Cognitive impairment hypotonia, and often tachypnea and abnormal eye movements
	Pontocerebellar hypoplasia[d]	AR	*TSEN54* and others	Cerebellar hypoplasia, pons with loss of ventral nuclei and transverse fibers	Hypotonia, may present with arthrogryposis, hypoventilation acquired microcephaly

Abbreviations: AR, autosonal recessive; XL, X linked.
Note: There is considerable overlap between clinical lissencephalies; therefore, the genes identified in this table are not meant to be exclusive of other disorders.
[a]Liu, 2011.[65]
[b]Jissendi-Tchofodo et al,[35].
[c]Brancati et al,[15]
[d]Namavar et al.[16]

Table 17-5 Leukodystrophies That Frequently Present in the Neonatal Period or Early Infancy[a]

Disease	Type of Leukodystrophy	Distribution of Demyelination on MRI	Key Clinical Findings in Infancy	Inheritance	Gene	Diagnostic Test
Alexander	Demyelinating	Frontal predominant with brainstem and cerebellar involvement	Hypotonia, macrocephaly, missing milestones	AD de novo	GFAP	Molecular
Canavan	Demyelinating	Subcortical and diffuse involvement	Hypotonia, irritability macrocephaly	AR	ASPA	Elevated urine and MRSNAA
Krabbe	Demyelinating	Parieto-occipital and periventricular predominant with cerebellar involvement	Irritability and excessive startle	AR	GALC	GALC enzyme testing
Megalencephalic leukoencephalopathy with subcortical cysts	Demyelinating	Diffuse with frontal or temporal cysts and cerebellar involvement	Macrocephaly, developmental delay and seizures	AR or AD	MLC1 HEPACAM	Molecular
Vanishing white matter disease	Demyelinating	Diffuse	Episodic decompensation associated with illnesses	AR	ARSA	Molecular
Pelizaeus-Merzbacher	Hypomyelinating	Diffuse, more prominent in periatrial regions with cerebellar involvement	Nystagmus, hypotonia and developmental delay	XL	PLP1	Molecular

Abbreviations: AD, autosomal dominant; AR, autosomal recessive: MRI, magnetic resonance imaging; NAA, N-acetyl aspartate; MRS, Magnetic resonance spectroscopy; XL, X-linked (table modified from Osterman et al, 2012 and Schiffmann and van der Knaap, 2009).
[a]Data from Osterman B et al., 2012[66] and Schiffmann R et al., 2009.[67]

can be at the level of the chromosome (trisomy 21, 18, or 13), large deletions or duplications (Alfi syndrome, 9p deletion; cri-du-chat syndrome, 5p deletion), or more subtle, as in microdeletion or duplication syndromes (Williams syndrome, 7q21.23 microdeletion; 1p36 deletion syndrome).

Prader-Willi syndrome and Angelman syndrome are most often caused by microdeletions in the 15q11q13 region, resulting in loss of function of the *UBE3A* gene. (It is worth mentioning that a small number of cases are caused by point mutations in the *UBE3A* gene. Therefore, if there is a strong suspicion of either syndrome in the presence of a normal methylation pattern, gene sequencing should be pursued.) These disorders are of special interest to this topic for 2 reasons. They both frequently present with congenital hypotonia, and they are inherited through genomic imprinting mechanisms.[38] Deletion of the paternal gene (or maternal monosomy) causes Prader-Willi syndrome; deletion of the maternal gene (or paternal monosomy) is responsible for Angelman syndrome.

With the advent of chromosomal microarrays, increasing numbers of microdeletion and microduplication syndromes are being described. Most of these occur in regions of the genome fragilized by repetitive DNA sequences highly subject to chromosomal rearrangements, so-called breakpoints, with resultant deletions, duplications, and translocations.[39] Two such regions are 15q11q13 and 22q11. Interestingly, many of the newly described disorders on 15q11q13 sit just outside the imprinting region and have been reported as causing varying degrees of congenital hypotonia, seizures, and intellectual disabilities, ranging from mild to severe.[40,41] Rearrangements in 22q11 give rise to multiple syndromes (DiGeorge, velocardiofacial, and cat eye syndrome, to name a few), all of which can present with hypotonia.

Fragile X syndrome is another example of a disorder caused by abnormalities of a gene highly susceptible to rearrangements via a slightly different mechanism.[42] Fragile X syndrome, the most common cause of inherited intellectual disability and a leading cause of autism spectrum disorder, is caused by an expansion of CGG triplet repeats in the *FMR1* gene. The resulting expansion results in hypermethylation and silencing of the *FMR1* gene.

Point mutations, resulting in missense (substitution of one amino acid for another) or nonsense (insertion of a stop codon, resulting in protein truncation) mutations account for a multitude of syndromes. Mutations in the *MECP2* and *CDKL5* genes deserve special notice here. While most of these mutations result in Rett syndrome, an X-linked disorder typically manifesting in girls during the toddler years with regression in cognitive skills and stereotypical hand-wringing movements, a subset of mutations in these genes can manifest in boys (MECP2 duplications) and girls (CDKL5 mutations) with congenital hypotonia, seizures, and developmental delay.[43]

Spinal Cord Hypotonia

Traumatic: Spinal Shock

Spinal cord injuries as a result of birth trauma are rare; in fact, most of the literature regarding these injuries dates back 20 years or more. The rarity of these injuries is felt to be due in part to the high resilience of the neck's soft tissues, bones, and ligaments and to the underdevelopment of the neck musculature.[44] These injuries most often involve the cervical spinal cord and less frequently the thoracic cord. The injuries tend to be more frequent with forceps deliveries or deliveries involving entrapment of the fetal head.[17] They are frequently severe, typically resulting in quadriplegia or diplegia, depending on the level of the injury. In work dating to the 1960s, spinal cord injuries were found to be present in 10% to 33% of newborn deaths and frequently were associated with brainstem injury.[45] Therefore, although rare, spinal cord injury should be suspected in hypotonic infants, especially in the context of a traumatic delivery. It is important to emphasize that standard radiographic studies will often miss spinal cord injuries in the newborn[44]; thus, it is important to obtain an MRI if such an injury is suspected.

Spinal Dysraphism

Most of the spinal dysraphisms presenting at birth with hypotonia consist of open neural tube defects; closed neural tube defects more often than not are asymptomatic at birth.[18] Myelomeningocele and myelocele are the 2 most common forms of open neural tube defects. The incidence of neural tube defects has dramatically decreased in developed countries over the last 30 years, likely as a result of folate supplementation, prenatal screening (α-fetoprotein and imaging), and termination of at-risk pregnancies.[46] For example, the incidence of myelomeningocele decreased 10-fold from 1981 to 2001. The causes of spinal dysraphisms are both genetic and environmental. For example, mutations in the 5,10-methyltetrahydrofolate reductase (*MTHFR*) gene are a known risk factor for the development of neural tube defects. MTHFR is a rate-limiting enzyme in the metabolism of folate. Its dysfunction results in accumulation of homocysteine and low levels of methionine. Environmental factors also play an important role. Dietary folic acid deficiency and maternal diabetes are 2 well-documented risk factors for neural tube defects.

Motor Unit Hypotonia

Motor unit hypotonia usually presents clinically with profound hypotonia and hyporeflexia. This group of disorders encompasses the prototypic clinical presentation of peripheral hypotonia. The pathology in these disorders (Figure 17-4) can occur at the level of the cell body of the motor neuron in the ventral horn of the spinal cord (as is the case in SMA), the myelin sheath of the axon (as in the hereditary motor and sensory neuropathies), or the synaptic terminal of the motor unit (as in the congenital myasthenic syndromes). This section is divided following this anatomical distribution.

Spinal Muscular Atrophy

Spinal muscular atrophy is an autosomal recessive disease and is the second-most-common genetic cause of death in infants (second only to cystic fibrosis).[20] SMA is caused by failure of the survival motor neuron 1 (*SMN1*) gene and results in degeneration of the α motor neurons in the spinal cord (Figure 17-4). The *SMN* genes localize to chromosome 5q13 and are unusual in that 2 variants of the gene (*SMN1* and *SMN2*) are present as part of 2 inverted, almost-identical DNA fragments. While there is only 1 copy of the *SMN1* gene, there are usually multiple copies of the *SMN2* gene. The only difference between *SMN1* and *SMN2* is a single base-pair change that results in alternative slicing of the gene. The resultant SMN2 gene product is a truncated and unstable protein. While the disease is caused by loss of *SMN1* gene function, the phenotype of the disease depends on the number of copies of the *SMN2* gene. Infants presenting with the classic form of the disease (Werdnig-Hoffmann disease or SMA type 1) usually have 1 or 2 copies of the *SMN2* gene.

SMA is classified according to its severity and time of onset. SMA type 1 is the classic infantile form of the disease. It presents with profound hypotonia, areflexia, and weakness with no antigravity movements. Because the facial muscles are usually spared, the children have a paradoxical appearance, appearing alert when awake but profoundly weak. They often show tongue fasciculations as a result of hypoglossal motor neuron degeneration. The weakness is more severe proximally, and a paradoxical breathing pattern is usually present due to impairment of the intercostal muscles but preservation of the diaphragm. In contrast to the hereditary sensory neuropathies (discussed separately), sensation is preserved in SMA. Children with SMA type 1 rarely live beyond the age of 1 year. A severe form of SMA is occasionally referred to as SMA type 0. In this form of the disease, the mother often describes diminished fetal movements, and the infants are born with arthrogryposis multiplex congenita.

The diagnosis of SMA is now largely based on molecular testing. The initial test looks for the absence of *SMN1* exon 7. It has a rapid turnaround, is relatively cheap, and will provide a diagnosis in 95% to 98% of the cases of type 1 SMA.[47] Compound heterozygotes account for the rest of the cases, and diagnosis requires sequencing of the *SMN1* gene. Prior to sending for *SMN1* sequencing, there should be a fairly convincing clinical picture as this is a rather expensive proposition. In this case, a nerve conduction study may be necessary to confirm the typical neurogenic picture seen in SMA.

Hereditary Motor and Sensory Neuropathies

Hereditary motor and sensory neuropathies form a heterogeneous group of disorders with complicated genetics. They are all disorders of peripheral myelination. Fortunately, only a few of these present in the neonatal period or early infancy with hypotonia.[48] Historically, 2 forms of congenital hereditary motor and sensory neuropathies were recognized: congenital hypomyelinating neuropathy and Dejerine-Sottas neuropathy. It is important to emphasize that the distinction between these 2 entities is largely artificial. These diseases exist along a continuum of Schwann cell dysfunction, ranging from complete absence of myelin to a demyelination-remyelination pattern resulting in the classic "onion bulb" formation seen on nerve biopsy. Clinically, these infants present with a distal greater than proximal weakness, sensory impairment, and respiratory compromise. The palpable nerve hypertrophy that is classically associated with Dejerine-Sottas disease is typically not present in newborns. Severe cases can present with arthrogryposis multiplex congenita.

In a cohort study of 77 patients who presented in the first year of life with hereditary motor and sensory neuropathy, more than half of the patients (55%) had no known gene diagnosis; 38% were found to have mutations in 11 different genes, and the remaining 7% had duplications in the 17p11.2–12 region.[49] The most frequent mutations in patients who presented with neonatal onset were de novo point mutations in the *PMP22*, *EGR2*, and *MPZ* genes. Given the genetic complexity of this group of disorders, the diagnostic workup should start with electromyographic (EMG) and nerve conduction studies. If these studies confirm hereditary motor and sensory neuropathy, then sequencing of the *PMP22*, *EGR2*, and *MPZ* genes is indicated. Duplication and deletion analysis of *PMP22* may be considered, although it should be remembered that, in contrast to presentation at an older age, the majority of hereditary motor and sensory neuropathies secondary to *PMP22* gene changes will be point mutations rather than duplications. As a general rule, nerve biopsy is not necessary to establish a diagnosis, although it may have a role to help sort particularly difficult cases.

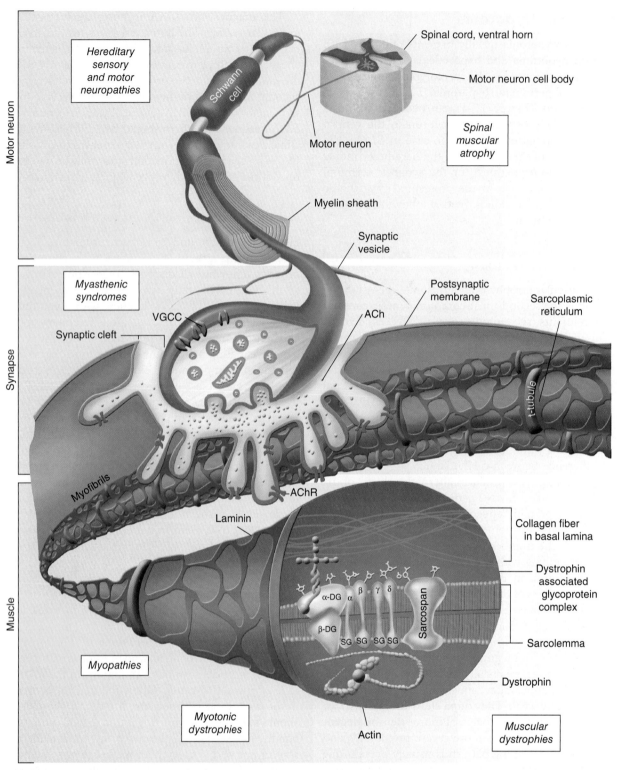

FIGURE 17-4 Peripheral neuroanatomy of congenital hypotonia. The lower motor neuron arising from the ventral horn of the spinal cord (actually, part of the central nervous system), the neuromuscular synapse, and the muscle. The peripheral hypotonias arising from each of these areas are highlighted in the panels. Abbreviations: VGCC, voltage-gated calcium channel; ACh, acetylcholine; AChR, acetylcholine receptor; α-DG, α-dystroglycan; β-DG, β-dystroglycan; α-SG, α-sarcoglycan; β-SG, β-sarcoglycan; γ-SG, γ-sarcoglycan; δ-SG, δ-sarcoglycan. (Used with permission of Marie E. Le Pichon.)

Congenital Myasthenic Syndromes

Congenital myasthenic syndromes are caused by a dysfunction of the neuromuscular junction.[21,50] The disorder can be the result of a presynaptic, synaptic, or postsynaptic defect (Figure 17-4). While in older children and adults fatigability is a hallmark of the disease, it may not be as obvious in infants. In a 15-year retrospective study of 46 patients with a confirmed diagnosis of congenital myasthenic syndromes, 63% of the patients presented in the neonatal period, 26% presented in the first 2 years of life, and 11% presented later in life.[51] Of those presenting in the neonatal period, 100% had feeding problems, 72% were hypotonic, 66% were weak, 66% developed ptosis, and 38% developed respiratory insufficiency. In this study, 60% of the children were initially misdiagnosed as having congenital myopathies or muscular dystrophies. The diagnostic challenge presented by these patients is illustrated by the fact that no study is definitive. In the study cited, electromyograms were interpreted as normal in 50% of the cases (importantly, repetitive stimulation testing is notoriously unreliable); muscle biopsies showed nonspecific changes, such as myopathic changes, variations in fiber size, and fiber-type predominance; and a definitive genetic diagnosis was only established in two-thirds of the patients. Ultimately, the diagnosis of a congenital myasthenic syndrome is based on a combination of clinical suspicion, supportive ancillary studies, and when possible, genetic confirmation. One additional useful tool is a pyridostigmine therapeutic trial. However, care should be used in patients suspected of having *COLQ, DOK7,* or slow-channel syndrome because pyridostigmine can worsen the symptoms in these children. It follows that such a therapeutic trial should only be done in the hospital setting.

While the vast majority (75%–80%) of congenital myasthenic syndromes are postsynaptic,[21] a few of the presynaptic and synaptic syndromes bear brief mention as they have characteristic clinical presentations.

Presynaptic: **Congenital myasthenic syndrome with episodic apnea** classically presents with bulbar weakness and intermittent and acute respiratory distress, often associated with an intercurrent illness. The disease is caused by a defect in the enzyme choline acetyltransferase, resulting in acetylcholine synaptic vesicle packaging defects. It responds to treatment with pyridostigmine.

Synaptic: **End-plate acetylcholinesterase deficiency** is typically reported in toddlers. However, it is important to keep this syndrome in mind as it is one of the congenital myasthenic syndromes that does not respond, and can potentially worsen, with pyridostigmine or other cholinesterase inhibitors. It is caused by a mutation in the *COLQ* gene that codes for the collagen tail subunit of acetylcholinesterase. Acetylcholinesterase hydrolyses the acetylcholine released in the synaptic terminal, thus terminating postsynaptic potentiation. Prolonged exposure to acetylcholine results in a desensitized AChR. Desensitized receptors are a possible mechanism implicated in the pathology of this syndrome. There is no effective treatment of this form of congenital myasthenic syndrome, although ephedrine or albuterol have been reported to alleviate the symptoms.

Postsynaptic: The postsynaptic AChR complex involves several proteins, any one of which can cause dysfunction of the end-plate terminal. Only the defects known to present in the neonatal period are presented here:

Slow- and fast-channel syndrome: These syndromes are caused by mutations in the AChR subunits, resulting in altered channel kinetics. In the slow-channel syndrome, the ion pore fails to close properly, resulting in excessive cation influx and subsequent excessive depolarization. By contrast, the fast-channel syndrome results in excessively rapid closure of the channel, in essence resulting in a failure to open. Both of these syndromes can present in the neonatal period and infancy.[50,52] They typically involve the bulbar, neck, and upper limb muscles. The management of each of these disorders follows its kinetic dysfunction. The slow-channel syndrome is a "gain-of-function" mutation and thus will become worse with cholinesterase inhibitors. This group of disorders is treated with AChR channel blockers such as quinidine sulfate. Conversely, the fast-channel syndromes respond nicely to cholinesterase inhibitors.

Acetylcholine aggregation complex defects: Proper distribution of the AChRs at the neuromuscular junction depends on a complex of proteins acting in concert; these include Dok-7, Rapsyn, and MuSK.[50,51] The phenotypic expression of mutations in these proteins is highly variable, resulting in onset of symptoms from infancy to later in life. Rapsyn and Dok-7 mutations can present with arthrogryposis, while MuSK, when it manifests in infancy, presents with respiratory compromise. Interestingly, while Rapsyn and MuSK myasthenic syndromes respond to cholinesterase inhibitors, Dok-7 can be paradoxically worsened by the same therapeutic intervention.

Muscle Disorders

The nomenclature of congenital muscle disorders can be rather confusing. It is based on clinical presentation and pathological and functional changes. It is worth having a clear understanding of this classification before further discussion. Congenital muscle disorders can be grouped into 3 broad categories: congenital myopathies, congenital muscular dystrophies, and congenital myotonic dystrophies (Table 17-6).

Table 17-6 Congenital Muscular Dystrophies and Myotonic Myopathies[a]

Classification	Disorder	Clinical Presentation	Creatine Kinase	Pathology	Genes	Inheritance
Congenital myopathies	Nemaline rod myopathy	Hypotonia and generalized weakness; respiratory compromise out of proportion to clinical presentation	Normal to mildly elevated	Rod-like inclusions in the sarcoplasm	ACTA1 NEB TPM2 TPM3 TNNT1 CFL2 KBTBD13	AD or AR AR AD AR or AD AR AR
	Central core myopathy	Hypotonia and proximal muscle weakness, respiratory compromise, poor suck	Normal to mildly elevated	Long, thin well-demarcated rods running an extended length of the type 1 fibers	RYRI	AD or AR
	Multiminicore myopathy	Axial hypotonia, spinal rigidity, respiratory compromise, often with cardiac involvement	Normal to mildly elevated	Small, poorly organized cores present in both type 1 and type 2 fibers	SEPN1	AR
	Centronuclear myopathy	Proximal weakness with bulbar muscle involvement (notably ophthalmoplegia), high arched palate and lower limb deformities	Normal to mildly elevated	Numerous centrally placed nuclei often surrounded by an area of pallor	DNM2 BIN1 RYR1 MTM1	AD AR AD XL
Congenital muscular dystrophies (all of these disorders show dystrophic changes on muscle biopsy)	Merosin-deficient myopathy	Profound hypotonia and weakness, weak cry, often with contractures, progressive respiratory failure	Moderately elevated	Absence of laminin α2 staining on muscle biopsy	LAMA2	AR

				Gene	Inheritance
	Ullrich disease	Profound hypotonia and weakness, often with contractures joint hyperlaxicity; eventually develop spine rigidity and scoliosis	Normal to mildly elevated	Collagen type VI staining reduced or absent	COL6A1 COL6A2 COL6A3	AR[b] AR[b] AR[b]
	Fukuyama	Profound hypotonia, generalized muscle weakness, migrational disorder[c]	Elevated (10 to 60x)	α-Dystroglycan staining absent or reduced	FKTN	AR
	Walker-Warburg	Severe hypotonia and weakness, eye abnormalities, hydrocephalus, epilepsy, Cobblestone lissencephaly[c]	Typically high to very high (>1000x)	α-Dystroglycan staining absent or reduced	POMT1 POMT2 LARGE FKRP	AR AR AR AR
	Muscle-eye-brain	Hypotonia (milder than WWS), dysmorphic facial traits, macrocephaly, congenital eye abnormalities, neuronal migrational disorder[c]	Mildly elevated	Decreased α-dystroglycan and merosin staining, laminin-β2 increased	POMGnT1	AR
Myotonic dystrophies	Congenital myotonic dystrophy	Hypotonia, often with contractures, facial weakness, tented upper lip, high arched palate, respiratory distress, NO MYOTONIA	Normal	Immature muscle pattern, central nucleus, peripheral sarcoplasmic halos	DMPK	Trinucleotide repeat expansion (>1000)

Abbreviations: AR, autosomal recessive; AD, autosomal dominant; XL, X-linked.
[a]Washington University Neuromuscular Disease Center (neuromuscular.wustl.edu); GeneReviews (ncbi.nlm.nih.gov jsitesjGeneTestjreview); Campbell[59]; Wallgreen-Pettersson et al,[55]; Nance et al,[22]; Sewry, 2008.[68]
[b]Ullrich's congenital muscular dystrophy is typically related in an autosomal recessive pattern. However, the related disorder, Bethlem myopathy, caused by partial absence of collagen type VI, is usually inherited in an autosomal recessive pattern.
[c]Refer to Table 17-4 for further details of magnetic resonance imaging findings.

To understand this classification, it is useful to start by comparing and contrasting *congenital myopathies* and *muscular dystrophies*[53]:

1. The pathological dystrophic changes observed in the muscular dystrophies consist of degenerative patterns with necrosis, regeneration, and extensive fibrosis. This is in contrast to the myopathies that show neither necrosis nor fibrosis. Therefore, dystrophinopathies can be thought of as disorders with a degenerative tissue process and myopathies as disorders resulting from muscle fiber structural changes in the absence of necrosis.

2. The second distinguishing feature is a direct consequence of the first. Whereas dystrophinopathies usually present with markedly elevated creatine phosphokinase (CK), it is normal to slightly elevated in congenital myopathies.

3. The third distinguishing feature is a clinical one. Congenital muscular dystrophies often involve the CNS, while congenital myopathies do not.

The third category, congenital myotonic dystrophies, encompasses a group of diseases with a common functional change, myotonia. Myotonia refers to the inability of the muscle fiber to relax following a contraction. The only myotonic dystrophy that typically presents at birth is congenital myotonic dystrophy. Myotonia congenita and paramyotonia congenita are channelopathies that typically present later in infancy or childhood and are not discussed here.

Finally, mitochondrial myopathies are discussed last. This group of disorders is generally classified as congenital myopathies whose unifying feature is mitochondrial dysfunction. Most of the mitochondrial myopathies are systemic disorders and were briefly mentioned in the section on systemic illnesses (see also Table 17-3). However, they are revisited in this section to discuss in more detail the myopathic aspect of these diseases.

Congenital Myopathies

Congenital myopathies consist of a group of disorders with characteristic and unique pathological changes in the absence of degenerative muscle fiber changes, normal to mildly elevated CK levels, and as a rule, no CNS involvement.[22] Typically, their clinical course is more indolent than the congenital muscular dystrophies. They can be grouped in 3 categories based on their pathology: nemaline rod myopathies, core myopathies, and centronuclear myopathies.

An important point needs to be made here about congenital myopathies. Several of the congenital myopathies are caused by mutations in a skeletal isoform of the ryanodine receptor *RYR1*. Mutations in the same gene can also cause malignant hyperthermia,

most notably when certain anesthetics are used.[54] Therefore, any person with a congenital myopathy caused by an *RYR1* mutation or with a genetically undetermined myopathy should be cautioned that they are at risk for developing malignant hyperthermia during surgical interventions.

Nemaline Rod Myopathies

Nemaline rod myopathies are a group of disorders that share common features, including abnormal myofibrils with rod-like structures (thus the name *nemaline* from the Greek "nema" for thread) and serum CK levels that are either normal or slightly elevated.[55] The clinical presentation varies widely, from severe with arthrogryposis and respiratory failure to a mild presentation with adult onset. However, the classic presentation is onset in the neonatal period with hypotonia and weakness that is more severe proximally and involves the bulbar muscles. In its classic form, nemaline myopathy is a slowly progressive disease. All of the cases are caused by autosomal mutations, although they can be recessive or dominant. Seven genes have been identified to date, yet many patients do not have a genetic diagnosis. There are good reasons for this: For many of the congenital myopathies, a gene has not yet been identified. For those that have a known gene disorder, identification relies on sequencing the entire gene. This can be done sequentially or in parallel; either way, it is an expensive proposition. It is probable that with the introduction of disease panels based on next-generation sequencing (allowing parallel and rapid sequencing of multiple genes at minimal cost), this will soon no longer be an issue. In the meantime, for this group of disorders, muscle biopsy remains the diagnostic investigation of choice.

Core Myopathies

Core myopathies[56] are characterized by a typical appearance on muscle biopsy consisting of a more or less circular area of pallor extending along the length of the myofibrils (it is important to keep in mind that the cores develop over time, and a muscle biopsy obtained early may not be diagnostic). The pallor is the result of the loss of mitochondria, itself likely secondary to excessive intracellular calcium concentration or loss of normal oxidative cellular protection. Depending on the shape and length of the rods, these myopathies are classified as *central core myopathies* (long and thinner rods running the length of the myofibril) or *multiminicore myopathies* (thicker, shorter rods, typically with a greater width than length). All of the core myopathies are autosomal, although they can be either dominant or recessive.

Central core myopathies are most often secondary to mutations in the *RYR1* gene. They present in the neonatal period with proximal and axial hypotonia. Bulbar and respiratory functions are rarely compromised. The prognosis is usually that of a static or slowly progressive disease. This is in contrast to the *multiminicore myopathies,* which often present with a prominent axial myopathy, spinal rigidity, and progressively worsening respiratory compromise. The course is that of a progressive disease, and the respiratory compromise will worsen over years. Mutations in the *SEPN1* gene cause the classic multiminicore disease, although many cases are caused by mutations in the ryanodine receptor, while others remain of unknown genetic etiology. Muscle biopsy remains the diagnostic modality of choice.

Centronuclear Myopathies

The myopathology of centronuclear myopathies is characterized by numerous centrally placed nuclei.[57] These can be surrounded by an area of pallor consistent with a defect in oxidative enzyme activity reminiscent of the pallor seen in the core myopathies. The centronuclear myopathies can be X-linked recessive, autosomal dominant, or autosomal recessive. The X-linked recessive form, caused by myotubularin gene (*MTM1*) mutations, is the best characterized. Both the X-linked and the autosomal recessive forms typically present in infancy. An important clue to the X-linked form is a family history of neonatal demise of male infants and decreased fetal movements. The male infants with myotubularin mutations are often macrosomic and profoundly hypotonic. The prognosis of the X-linked recessive form is poor, with demise often occurring within the first few months of life. The autosomal recessive forms usually present with proximal weakness, bulbar muscle involvement (notably ophthalmoplegia), high arched palate, and lower-limb deformities. The genetics of centronuclear myopathies are rather complex, with many cases still without a known gene defect. The most important diagnostic tool remains a muscle biopsy.

Congenital Muscular Dystrophies

The spectrum of congenital muscular dystrophies is extensive, and much of it is not covered in this section since many of these diseases present later in infancy or childhood. The congenital muscular dystrophies that present in the neonatal period with hypotonia can be grouped in 2 categories: congenital muscular dystrophies secondary to mutations in genes affecting structural proteins (including merosin and Ullrich congenital muscular dystrophies) and those affecting glycosylation of α-dystroglycan (as a group, these are referred to as dystroglycanopathies and include disorders such as Fukuyama congenital muscular dystrophy, muscle-eye-brain disease, and Walker-Warburg syndrome).[23]

Congenital Muscular Dystrophies Affecting Structural Proteins

The 2 most common congenital muscular dystrophies affecting structural proteins are merosin myopathy and Ullrich congenital muscular dystrophy.

Merosin myopathy: Merosin myopathy (properly referred to as congenital muscular dystrophy type 1A, MDC1A) is caused by a mutation in the laminin-α2 subunit (*LAMA2*).[58] Laminin is an important component of the basement membrane of myofibers and provides structural support to the dystroglycan/integrin complex. It is now recognized that there are wide phenotypic variations in the severity of merosin myopathies. While complete absence of the protein leads to a severe phenotype, point mutations cause variable severity of illnesses. MDC1A accounts for 20% to 40% of all cases of congenital muscular dystrophy.[23,58] The classic presentation is that of a profoundly hypotonic and weak infant, often accompanied by the presence of contractures. The CK levels are moderately elevated. The prognosis is grim, although with supportive care these children may achieve independent sitting and may live into their first decade, occasionally longer. As laminin-α2 is also expressed in the CNS and heart tissue, the children will typically develop white matter changes beyond the age of 1 year old and may have decreased ventricular function. Diagnosis is based on muscle biopsy but should be confirmed by sequencing of the *LAMA2* gene.

Ullrich's disease: *Ullrich's disease* is caused by a deficiency in collagen VI.[23] This muscular dystrophy is rather unusual in that the CK levels are usually normal to mildly elevated. It is caused by mutations in any of 3 genes encoding for 1 of the 3 chains of collagen VI: *COL6A1, COL6A2,* and *COL6A3.* Diagnosis is based on muscle biopsy and should be confirmed by genetic analysis. Clinically, these infants usually present with profound hypotonia and weakness and often contractures. One useful clinical characteristic is joint hyperlaxity. All patients eventually develop spine rigidity and scoliosis. Most patients are no longer ambulatory by the time they reach the second decade, and respiratory compromise or failure is a frequent complication.

Congenital Disorders of Glycosylation Affecting Glycosylation of α-Dystroglycan (Dystroglycanopathies)

The 3 most common dystroglycanopathies are Fukuyama congenital muscular dystrophy, muscle-eye-brain disease, and Walker-Warburg syndrome.[23] The common features of all of these disorders are elevated CK levels, CNS involvement, and a weakness with proximal predominance. Diagnosis is based on the detection of hypoglycosylated α-dystroglycan by immunolabeling or Western blot of tissue obtained from a muscle biopsy. It is important to emphasize that only half of the dystroglycanopathies have known gene disorders. There is also wide phenotypic variability, and a milder presentation later in life is common. MRI of the brain can provide important clues regarding the type of dystroglycanopathy and help in judicious choice for gene testing.[35]

Congenital Myotonic Dystrophy

Congenital myotonic dystrophy is an autosomal dominant disease caused by a CTG triplet-repeat expansion in the *DM1* gene.[59] (It is worth noting that congenital myotonic dystrophy can be caused by a repeat in the *DM2* gene. However, this form of the disease usually does not present in the neonatal period.) The *DM1* gene codes for the myotonic dystrophy protein kinase, a protein present in skeletal muscle and smooth muscle. The normal gene contains less than 35 CTG repeats. When the repeats exceed 1000, the disorder can present in the neonatal period or infancy, and with repeats greater than 1500, all cases present congenitally. The pattern of inheritance is autosomal dominant with the classic phenomenon of genetic anticipation seen in triplet-repeat diseases (meaning that onset of disease is earlier with successive generations).

In its congenital form, the disease presents with profound hypotonia and weakness. The weakness and hypotonia extend to the facial muscles and result in a typical appearance with an elongated face and tenting of the upper lip. Interestingly, the myotonia is generally not present in infants. These infants are at high risk for respiratory compromise and should be managed aggressively. With support, these children can become ventilator independent and live into the mid-30s. Multiple other organ systems can be affected, including slow gastrointestinal motility, arrhythmias and other cardiac malformations, obstructive hydrocephalus, seizures, endocrine disorders, and mild global cognitive impairment.

Diagnosis is primarily by genetic testing. Contrary to other muscular dystrophies, there are usually no dystrophic changes observed on biopsies, and serum CK levels are only mildly elevated. Targeted mutation analysis for the trinucleotide repeats will detect 100% of the cases and is the test of choice.[60]

Mitochondrial Myopathies

Mitochondrial myopathies encompass a large group of diseases, the vast majority of which are caused by nuclear mitochondrial DNA mutations.[61] The common theme for most of these diseases is profound hypotonia associated with a mixed central and peripheral clinical presentation and most often metabolic acidosis and lactic acidosis. These disorders are rare and can usually be diagnosed by muscle biopsy if appropriate special stains are included (cytochrome c oxidase and succinate dehydrogenase). It is important to keep in mind that these disorders are exceedingly rare (most mitochondrial diseases present later in infancy and childhood). Therefore, unless the clinical picture is highly suggestive of a mitochondrial disorder, other avenues should be investigated before engaging in mitochondrial testing. If a muscle biopsy is obtained and shows cytochrome oxidase or succinate dehydrogenase stain abnormalities, it is reasonable to send for respiratory enzyme chain function. However, this test has its own limitations and should be interpreted with caution. Mitochondrial DNA can be sent for sequencing, but with a couple of notable exceptions (infantile reversible cytochrome c oxidase deficiency and infantile Leigh syndrome), the vast majority of mitochondrial myopathies presenting in the neonatal period are caused by nuclear DNA mutations (diseases with mutations of mitochondrial DNA genes typically present later in life). With the advent of next-generation sequencing, there are panels available that will test multiple mitochondrial genes in a single test, greatly simplifying the approach to these diseases.

GENETIC ANALYSIS: A RAPIDLY CHANGING FIELD

Further in this book, there is an entire chapter devoted to laboratory studies, imaging, and ancillary testing in neonatal hypotonia. Therefore, it is not our purpose to revisit this topic. However, a few comments on the subject are appropriate in closing this chapter. With the advent of next-generation sequencing, it is probable that our entire approach to the hypotonic neonate, indeed to any condition of likely genetic etiology, will fundamentally change over the next decade. A good understanding of these new techniques and their limitations is becoming increasingly important to the practice of medicine. In this section, we briefly describe these techniques, review some of their potential uses, and discuss their inherent limitations.

Before broaching the topic, it is worth mentioning one last time that the history and physical examination will remain the most important elements of the evaluation of neonatal hypotonia. Indeed, as central hypotonia is the most common cause of neonatal hypotonia and as HIE is the most common cause of central hypotonia, no amount of genetic testing will ever replace a good history and physical examination (and may in fact be futile as the case may be). A good history and physical examination may direct the clinician to obtain an MRI before any gene testing is done. This study may obviate the need for gene testing (as in HIE) or markedly reduce the number of genes to be tested (eg, lissencephaly with a clear gradient favoring the occipital region would favor an *LIS1* gene mutation).

These points being made, let us review next-generation sequencing. Next-generation sequencing, or massive parallel sequencing, is based on new sequencing technologies that allow rapid sequencing of multiple target DNA fragments at once. One way to think about the difference between classic Sanger sequencing and next-generation sequencing is to describe the first as a sequential method of sequencing by which a single strand of DNA is analyzed at any one time, and the second as a parallel method of sequencing by which millions of stands of DNA are analyzed at once. It is a bit of an oversimplification, but it illustrates the point. The advantage of next-generation sequencing is that it can be performed rapidly for massive amounts of DNA at a fraction of the cost of Sanger sequencing. For example, the human genome, completed in 2003, took 10 years to complete at a total cost of approximately $3 billion. By comparison, using massive parallel sequencing methods, Saunders et al recently described a method that allowed them to sequence the complete genome of 4 infants in a NICU in roughly 50 hours for less $8000 per genome.[62]

The technique has its limitations. First and foremost, next-generation sequencing is not yet as reliable as Sanger sequencing. It is highly dependent on "depth" of sequencing. This means that each DNA sample is sequenced repeatedly, allowing for the elimination of sequencing errors (presumably the same sequence error will be not be present in multiple sequences of the same DNA sample). The depth of sequencing varies from 30 to 100 (meaning each DNA strand is sequenced 30 to 100 times). Greater depth increases reliability, but it also comes at a price in terms of complexity of the analysis, time, and cost. Furthermore, certain DNA sequences are notoriously difficult to sequence through (eg, GC-rich regions) and are underrepresented in next-generation sequencing.

Another major analytical barrier is that the average genome has on average 4 million variants. In the study cited, approximately half of those variants were gene associated. This wealth of data causes obvious issues. Cooper and Shendure recently characterized the problem as looking for "needles in stacks of needles."[63] Mardis, in an opinion piece published in *Genome Medicine* in 2010, framed the problem differently: "The $1,000 genome, the $100,000 analysis?"[64]

There are several ways to simplify the problem. One method is to limit the sequencing analysis to the roughly 22,000 genes (representing less than 2% of our genome). In this approach, whole-exome sequencing, the analysis is limited to material with the most potential for identifying pathogenic mutations. With this method, the average individual will be found to have about 20,000 variants. When combined with analysis of unaffected parents or siblings, this method lends itself particularly well to the identification of homozygous recessive diseases. Another approach is to design panels capable of sequencing multiple candidate genes in a single run. Such panels are already available commercially for multiple conditions, including, for example, epileptic encephalopathies of infancy.

As sequencing technologies continue to improve, it is probable that most causes of neonatal hypotonia will eventually be sorted out. The diagnosis of benign congenital hypotonia is likely to become a thing of the past, to be replaced by subtle but characterizable disorders based on the identification of the causative genes. As genetic information continues to accumulate, a clear-and-concise approach to the hypotonic infant will, more than ever, be crucial. We believe that Dubowitz elegantly outlined such a method in his monogram on floppy infants first published in 1984, and it is proper to end this chapter by referring the interested reader to this seminal work.

REFERENCES

1. Tuchman BW. *A Distant Mirror: The Calamitous 14th Century*. 1st trade ed. New York: Knopf; 1978.
2. Dubowitz V. *The floppy infant*. 2nd ed. London: Spastics International Medical Publications in association with Heinemann; Lippincott; 1980.
3. Walton JN. The limp child. *J Neurol Neurosurg Psychiatry*. 1957;20(2):144–154.
4. Bodensteiner JB. The evaluation of the hypotonic infant. *Semin Pediatr Neurol*. 2008;15(1):10–20.
5. Crawford TO. Clinical evaluation of the floppy infant. *Pediatr Ann*. 1992;21(6):348–354.
6. Richer LP, Shevell MI, Miller SP. Diagnostic profile of neonatal hypotonia: an 11-year study. *Pediatr Neurol*. 2001;25(1):32–37.
7. Paro-Panjan D, Neubauer D. Congenital hypotonia: is there an algorithm? *J Child Neurol*. 2004;19(6):439–442.
8. Takenouchi T, Kasdorf E, Engel M, Grunebaum A, Perlman JM. Changing pattern of perinatal brain injury in term infants in recent years. *Pediatr Neurol*. 2012;46(2):106–110.
9. Volpe JJ. Neonatal encephalopathy: an inadequate term for hypoxic-ischemic encephalopathy. *Ann Neurol*. 2012;72(2):156–166.
10. Birdi K, Prasad AN, Prasad C, Chodirker B, Chudley AE. The floppy infant: retrospective analysis of clinical experience (1990–2000) in a tertiary care facility. *J Child Neurol*. 2005;20(10):803–808.
11. Laugel V, Cossee M, Matis J, et al. Diagnostic approach to neonatal hypotonia: retrospective study on 144 neonates. *Eur J Pediatr*. 2008;167(5):517–523.
12. Vasta I, Kinali M, Messina S, et al. Can clinical signs identify newborns with neuromuscular disorders? *J Pediatr*. 2005;146(1):73–79.
13. Walton JN. The amyotonia congenita syndrome. *Proc R Soc Med*. 1957;50(5):301–308.
14. Rabe EF. The hypotonic infant. A review. *J Pediatr*. 1964;64:422–440.
15. Brancati F, Dallapiccola B, Valente EM. Joubert syndrome and related disorders. *Orphanet J Rare Dis*. 2010;5:20.

16. Namavar Y, Barth PG, Poll-The BT, Baas F. Classification, diagnosis and potential mechanisms in pontocerebellar hypoplasia. *Orphanet J Rare Dis.* 2011;6:50.

17. Vialle R, Pietin-Vialle C, Ilharreborde B, Dauger S, Vinchon M, Glorion C. Spinal cord injuries at birth: a multicenter review of nine cases. *J Matern Fetal Neonatal Med.* 2007;20(6):435–440.

18. Amarante MA, Shrensel JA, Tomei KL, Carmel PW, Gandhi CD. Management of urological dysfunction in pediatric patients with spinal dysraphism: review of the literature. *Neurosurg Focus.* 2012;33(4):E4.

19. Allen MC, Capute AJ. Tone and reflex development before term. *Pediatrics.* 1990;85(3 Pt 2):393–399.

20. D'Amico A, Mercuri E, Tiziano FD, Bertini E. Spinal muscular atrophy. *Orphanet J Rare Dis.* 2011;6:71.

21. Lorenzoni PJ, Scola RH, Kay CS, Werneck LC. Congenital myasthenic syndrome: a brief review. *Pediatr Neurol.* 2012;46(3):141–148.

22. Nance JR, Dowling JJ, Gibbs EM, Bonnemann CG. Congenital myopathies: an update. *Curr Neurol Neurosci Rep.* 2012;12(2):165–174.

23. Mercuri E, Muntoni F. The ever-expanding spectrum of congenital muscular dystrophies. *Ann Neurol.* 2012;72(1):9–17.

24. Tollner U. Early diagnosis of septicemia in the newborn. Clinical studies and sepsis score. *Eur J Pediatr.* 1982;138(4):331–337.

25. Limperopoulos C, Majnemer A, Shevell MI, Rosenblatt B, Rohlicek C, Tchervenkov C. Neurologic status of newborns with congenital heart defects before open heart surgery. *Pediatrics.* 1999;103(2):402–408.

26. Saudubray JM, Nassogne MC, de Lonlay P, Touati G. Clinical approach to inherited metabolic disorders in neonates: an overview. *Semin Neonatol.* 2002;7(1):3–15.

27. Kozma C. Neonatal toxicity and transient neurodevelopmental deficits following prenatal exposure to lithium: another clinical report and a review of the literature. *Am J Med Genet A.* 2005;132(4):441–444.

28. Abbassi-Ghanavati M, Alexander JM, McIntire DD, Savani RC, Leveno KJ. Neonatal effects of magnesium sulfate given to the mother. *Am J Perinatol.* 2012;29(10):795–800.

29. Papazian O. Transient neonatal myasthenia gravis. *J Child Neurol.* 1992;7(2):135–141.

30. Rouse DJ, Hirtz DG, Thom E, et al. A randomized, controlled trial of magnesium sulfate for the prevention of cerebral palsy. *N Engl J Med.* 2008;359(9):895–905.

31. Hoff JM, Daltveit AK, Gilhus NE. Myasthenia gravis: consequences for pregnancy, delivery, and the newborn. *Neurology.* 2003;61(10):1362–1366.

32. Wennberg RP, Ahlfors CE, Bhutani VK, Johnson LH, Shapiro SM. Toward understanding kernicterus: a challenge to improve the management of jaundiced newborns. *Pediatrics.* 2006;117(2):474–485.

33. Malamud N. Pathogenesis of kernicterus in the light of its sequelae. In: Swinyard CA, ed. *Kernicterus and Its Importance in Cerebral Palsy.* Springfield, IL: Thomas; 1961:230–246.

34. Shapiro SM. Chronic bilirubin encephalopathy: diagnosis and outcome. *Semin Fetal Neonatal Med.* 2010;15(3):157–163.

35. Jissendi-Tchofo P, Kara S, Barkovich AJ. Midbrain-hindbrain involvement in lissencephalies. *Neurology.* 2009;72(5):410–418.

36. Schiffmann R, van der Knaap MS. Invited article: an MRI-based approach to the diagnosis of white matter disorders. *Neurology.* 2009;72(8):750–759.

37. Phelan JA, Lowe LH, Glasier CM. Pediatric neurodegenerative white matter processes: leukodystrophies and beyond. *Pediatr Radiol.* 2008;38(7):729–749.

38. Buiting K. Prader-Willi syndrome and Angelman syndrome. *Am J Medical Genet C Semin Med Genet.* 2010;154C(3):365–376.

39. Kato T, Kurahashi H, Emanuel BS. Chromosomal translocations and palindromic AT-rich repeats. *Curr Opin Genet Dev.* 2012;22(3):221–228.

40. Lepichon JB, Bittel DC, Graf WD, Yu S. A 15q13.3 homozygous microdeletion associated with a severe neurodevelopmental disorder suggests putative functions of the TRPM1, CHRNA7, and other homozygously deleted genes. *Am J Med Genet A.* 2010;152A(5):1300–1304.

41. Abdelmoity AT, LePichon JB, Nyp SS, Soden SE, Daniel CA, Yu S. 15q11.2 proximal imbalances associated with a diverse array of neuropsychiatric disorders and mild dysmorphic features. *J Dev Behav Pediatr.* 2012;33(7):570–576.

42. Wang T, Bray SM, Warren ST. New perspectives on the biology of fragile X syndrome. *Curr Opin Genet Dev.* 2012;22(3):256–263.

43. Lisi EC, Cohn RD. Genetic evaluation of the pediatric patient with hypotonia: perspective from a hypotonia specialty clinic and review of the literature. *Dev Med Child Neurol.* 2011;53(7):586–599.

44. d'Amato C. Pediatric spinal trauma: injuries in very young children. *Clin Orthop Relat Res.* 2005(432):34–40.

45. Towbin A. Central nervous system damage in the human fetus and newborn infant. Mechanical and hypoxic injury incurred in the fetal-neonatal period. *Am J Dis Child.* 1970;119(6):529–542.

46. Kondo A, Kamihira O, Ozawa H. Neural tube defects: prevalence, etiology and prevention. *Int J Urol.* 2009;16(1):49–57.

47. Prior TW, Nagan N, Sugarman EA, Batish SD, Braastad C. Technical standards and guidelines for spinal muscular atrophy testing. *Genet Med.* 2011;13(7):686–694.

48. Plante-Bordeneuve V, Said G. Dejerine-Sottas disease and hereditary demyelinating polyneuropathy of infancy. *Muscle Nerve.* 2002;26(5):608–621.

49. Baets J, Deconinck T, De Vriendt E, et al. Genetic spectrum of hereditary neuropathies with onset in the first year of life. *Brain.* 2011;134(Pt 9):2664–2676.

50. Barisic N, Chaouch A, Muller JS, Lochmuller H. Genetic heterogeneity and pathophysiological mechanisms in congenital myasthenic syndromes. *Eur J Paediatr Neurol.* 2011;15(3):189–196.

51. Kinali M, Beeson D, Pitt MC, et al. Congenital myasthenic syndromes in childhood: diagnostic and management challenges. *J Neuroimmunol.* 2008;201–202:6–12.

52. Chaouch A, Muller JS, Guergueltcheva V, et al. A retrospective clinical study of the treatment of slow-channel congenital myasthenic syndrome. *J Neurol.* 2012;259(3):474–481.

53. Tubridy N, Fontaine B, Eymard B. Congenital myopathies and congenital muscular dystrophies. *Curr Opin Neurol.* 2001;14(5):575–582.

54. Taylor A, Lachlan K, Manners RM, Lotery AJ. A study of a family with the skeletal muscle RYR1 mutation (c.7354C>T) associated with central core myopathy and malignant hyperthermia susceptibility. *J Clin Neurosci.* 2012;19(1):65–70.

55. Wallgren-Pettersson C, Sewry CA, Nowak KJ, Laing NG. Nemaline myopathies. *Semin Pediatr Neurol.* 2011;18(4):230–238.

56. Jungbluth H, Sewry CA, Muntoni F. Core myopathies. *Semin Pediatr Neurol.* 2011;18(4):239–249.

57. Jungbluth H, Wallgren-Pettersson C, Laporte J. Centronuclear (myotubular) myopathy. *Orphanet J Rare Dis.* 2008;3:26.

58. Gawlik KI, Durbeej M. Skeletal muscle laminin and MDC1A: pathogenesis and treatment strategies. *Skelet Muscle.* 2011;1(1):9.

59. Campbell C. Congenital myotonic dystrophy. *J Neurol Neurophysiol.* 2012(S7):1-8.

60. Prior TW, American College of Medical Genetics Laboratory Quality Assurance Committee. Technical standards and

guidelines for myotonic dystrophy type 1 testing. *Genet Med.* 2009;11(7):552–555.

61. Tulinius M, Oldfors A. Neonatal muscular manifestations in mitochondrial disorders. *Semin Fetal Neonatal Med.* 2011;16(4):229–235.

62. Saunders CJ, Miller NA, Soden SE, et al. Rapid whole-genome sequencing for genetic disease diagnosis in neonatal intensive care units. *Sci Transl Med.* 2012;4(154):154ra135.

63. Cooper GM, Shendure J. Needles in stacks of needles: finding disease-causal variants in a wealth of genomic data. *Nat Rev Genet.* 2011;12(9):628–640.

64. Mardis ER. The $1,000 genome, the $100,000 analysis? *Genome Med.* 2010;2(11):84.

65. Liu JS. Molecular genetics of neuronal migration disorders. *Curr Neurol Neurosci Rep.* 2011;11(2):171–178.

66. Osterman B, Piana RL, Bernard G. Advances in the diagnosis of leukodystrophies. *Future Neurol.* 2012;7(5):595–612.

67. Schiffmann R, and van der Knaap MS. Invited article: an MRI-based approach to the diagnosis of white matter disorders. *Neurology.* 2009;72(8):750–759.

68. Sewr CA. Pathological defects in congenital myopathies. *J Muscle Res Cell Motil.* 2008;29:231–238.

Part B: Heart

Cyanotic Congenital Heart Defects

V. Mohan Reddy and Katsuhide Maeda

INTRODUCTION

Cyanotic congenital heart defects are the most important group of defects necessitating surgical intervention in the neonatal period. In general, this group of defects is characterized by ductal dependency of pulmonary blood flow (or effective pulmonary blood flow) but with notable exceptions of truncus arteriosus (TrA) and obstructed total anomalous pulmonary venous return or connection (TAPVR).

Cyanotic heart defects should be considered and ruled out or confirmed in any newborn presenting with cyanosis (see Chapter 80 for differential diagnosis of cyanosis in the neonate), although in a cyanotic neonate the response to oxygen, heart murmurs, chest roentgenogram, and electrocardiogram (ECG) can offer clues to cardiac defects and prompt further evaluation. The echocardiogram is the mainstay of diagnosis to delineate the morphology of the heart defect and plan intervention.

In the current era, fetal obstetric ultrasound and fetal echocardiography have enabled us to accurately diagnose congenital heart defects in the majority of neonates before they are born.

This modality has changed the presentation and management of this group of neonates. Because the diagnosis is often established before birth, the emphasis has shifted more on planning the management immediately after birth rather than establishing the diagnosis as in the past. However, a neonatologist still is faced with undiagnosed cyanotic newborns for which all clinical skills can be tested.

Once the diagnosis is confirmed, adequacy of pulmonary blood flow and systemic blood flow should be assessed and pulmonary venous obstruction should be ruled out. Physiology-specific therapeutic medical management should be instituted, and surgical treatment should be planned. In patients with low birth weight or in premature neonates, the approach to "wait and grow the patient" has not been promising. Waiting prior to surgical palliation increases preoperative complications without gaining any benefits.[1] Even in this group of patients, an early correction is indicated, and in patients with functional single ventricles, appropriate early surgical palliation is indicated.

TOTAL ANOMALOUS PULMONARY VENOUS RETURN

Introduction

Total anomalous pulmonary venous return (TAPVR) or connection is a cardiac malformation in which there is no direct connection between any pulmonary vein and the left atrium; rather, all the pulmonary veins connect to the right atrium or one of its tributaries. A patent foramen ovale (PFO) or atrial septal defect (ASD) is present and is necessary for survival after birth in all newborns with TAPVR.[2]

TAPVR is a rare congenital cardiac anomaly occurring in about 1.5% of children born with congenital heart defects. In addition, it can occur as an associated defect with many other congenital cardiac defects, especially in newborns with heterotaxy syndromes with single functional ventricles. Nevertheless, it is one of the few lesions necessitating urgent or emergent cardiac surgery in the neonatal period.

Morphology

TAPVR morphology (Figure 18-1A) can be categorized into 4 broad anatomic types:

1. The supracardiac type is the most common (45%); here, the pulmonary veins drain via either the ascending vertical vein to the innominate vein or directly to the superior vena cava (SVC) and rarely to the azygos vein. About two-thirds of these have pulmonary venous obstruction, often at the junction of the vertical vein to the systemic vein.

2. In the cardiac type (20%), drainage is directly into the right atrium or into the coronary sinus (CS). Pulmonary venous obstruction is rare but may be seen in up to 20% at the CS ostia or orifices of individual veins or their confluence.

3. In the infracardiac type (25%), drainage occurs via the descending vertical vein into the portal vein or rarely into the inferior vena cava. These are by definition always obstructed to some extent because the pulmonary venous return has to pass through the hepatic capillary system. In addition, they have a high incidence (80% to 90%) of obstruction, often at the junction of the vertical vein to the systemic vein.

4. The mixed type (the least common at 5%–10%) consists of a combination of one or more of the 3 other types described. It can be technically most challenging to repair.

In patients with isolated TAPVR, atrial septal communication, which is essential for survival, and a patent ductus arteriosus (PDA) are the only associated defects. The cardiac chambers and valves are almost always normally formed.

Even the youngest infants dying with the malformation often have structural changes in the lungs. Increased pulmonary arterial (PA) muscularity is seen in all infants dying with TAPVR, as evidenced by arterial wall thickness and vein wall thickness. There is also extension of muscle into smaller and more peripheral arteries than normal.

Clinical Presentation, Pathophysiology, and Diagnosis

Neonates usually present with tachypnea and respiratory distress.[3] Cyanosis is prominent when there is pulmonary venous obstruction. In the absence of obstruction, cyanosis is often overshadowed by tachypnea. Right-to-left shunting at the level of the PDA also adds to the cyanosis.

The neonate with obstructed TAPVR often is in critical condition, requiring tracheal intubation and ventilator support. It is not uncommon to see these patients mistakenly diagnosed as having pulmonary pathology such as respiratory distress syndrome, meconium aspiration, bronchiolitis, and so on. TAPVR should always be considered in the differential diagnosis of any neonate presenting with cyanosis or tachypnea.

In TAPVR, the right atrium is the common mixing chamber, which often is reflected in the frequent

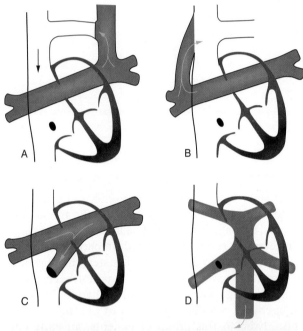

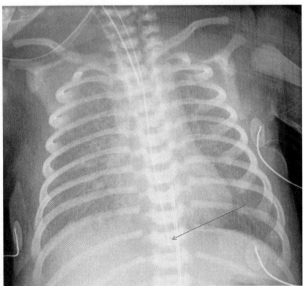

FIGURE 18-1 A, Types of total anomalous pulmonary venous return (TAPVR): a and b, supracardiac; c, cardiac; d, infracardiac. (From Stark et al.[58]) **B,** Chest x-ay of 1-day-old with obstructed infracardiac total anomalous Pulmonary venous connection, showing a ground-glass appearance in bilateral lung fields with a small cardiac shadow.

finding of the close similarity of oxygen content and saturations from the right atrium, left atrium, PA, and systemic artery. However, because of streaming of systemic venous return in the right atrium, directing inferior vena caval blood through the foramen ovale to the mitral valve and SVC blood through the tricuspid valve (TV), there can be considerable variation in different patients. This can be affected further by the size of the atrial communication. The hemodynamics of the nonobstructive types of TAPVR is similar to that of a large ASD. These neonates may present later in the neonatal period as the right ventricular (RV) compliance increases and the pulmonary vascular resistance (PVR) falls, and the ASD may become relatively inadequate in size.

A chest x-ray (Figure 18-1B) of neonates with TAPVR and pulmonary venous obstruction shows diffuse haziness or, in severe forms, a ground-glass appearance. In the supracardiac type, the appearance often is described as a "snowman sign." These signs are less marked when the pulmonary circuit can decompress via a PDA.

In the current era, even with fetal screening, TAPVR is often undiagnosed unless a fetal cardiac echocardiogram is part of prenatal evaluation. Postnatally, cardiac echo (Figure 18-2) is the definitive means of diagnosis. In some, a cardiac catheterization and angiography or a high-resolution computed tomographic (CT) scan may be needed to define the pulmonary venous anatomy.

Neonates born with TAPVR in general have an unfavorable prognosis. Mortality during the first few weeks or months of life is common in most neonates in whom tachypnea, cyanosis, and clinical evidence of low cardiac output develop, with only about 50% surviving beyond 3 months of life. Such neonates usually have pulmonary venous obstruction, long pulmonary venous pathways, and a small interatrial communication. Only about half the neonates surviving to age 3 months survive to 1 year.

Management

Regarding management,[4-6] surgery should be undertaken emergently, often immediately after diagnosis, in neonates and infants who are critically ill. These are usually neonates with obstructed TAPVR. A brief period of preoperative preparation and stabilization while the diagnosis is being confirmed is all that should be expected. This involves correcting metabolic acidosis and optimizing the ventilation. Prostaglandin E (PGE) is not indicated unless suprasystemic RV pressure is documented by echo. In such instances, right-to-left ductal shunting may improve systemic cardiac output. Rarely, the neonate is so critically ill with significant pulmonary injury that extracorporeal membrane oxygenation (ECMO) may be indicated for a few days prior to surgery. However, in stable neonates, typically without pulmonary venous obstruction, the operation can be scheduled electively.

Surgery is performed on cardiopulmonary bypass with or without circulatory arrest. This commonly involves anastomosing the common pulmonary venous chamber to the back of the left atrium (Figure 18-3). In TAPVR to the CS, the CS is flayed open into the left atrium. If the pulmonary veins are stenotic, each individual vein is flayed open; currently, a suture-less

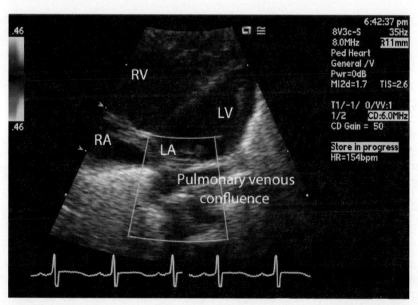

FIGURE 18-2 Echocardiography. Pulmonary venous confluence below the small left atrium pulmonary veins does not connect to the left atrium. Because of the pulmonary hypertension, the right ventricle is enlarged and the left ventricle is relatively small because of underfilling.

CHAPTER 18

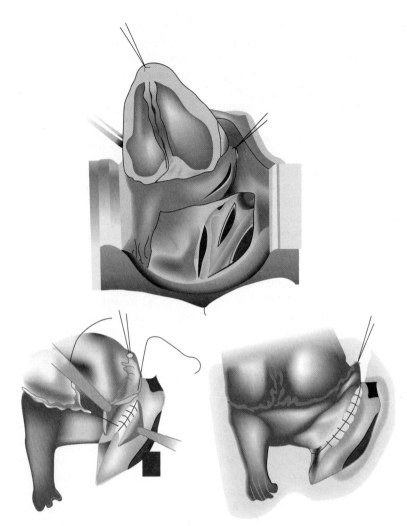

FIGURE 18-3 Repair of infracardiac-type total anomalous pulmonary venous drainage. Pulmonary venous chamber is opened and anastomosed into the back of the left atrium. (From Khonsari et al.[59])

technique is favored in this group. This involves suturing the margins of the cut-open back wall of the left atrium to the pericardium beyond the pulmonary venous openings.

Postoperative management can be challenging in these neonates. They often have high PVR, which will require aggressive treatment of acidosis, hyperventilation, and inhaled nitric oxide. The left ventricle (LV) is also often noncompliant and is sensitive to preload. Monitoring right atrial, left atrial, and PA pressure with indwelling catheters placed during surgery is helpful.

Outcomes

Surgical outcome[7–9] in neonates has steadily improved in the decades since 1970. Data from the database of the Society of Thoracic Surgeons show overall early mortality was 12.0% between 2002 and 2004. For infants falling within the normal weight range, mortality was 9.9%; it was 29.2% for infants less than 2.5 kg body weight.

Recurrent pulmonary venous obstruction is seen in 5% to 10% of neonates and often occurs within a few weeks to months after surgery. While anastomotic stenosis is uncommon and can easily be corrected by reoperation, true pulmonary vein obstruction is often not amenable to surgical or any other form of intervention.

TRANSPOSITION OF GREAT ARTERIES

Introduction

Complete transposition of the great arteries (TGA) is probably the most common cyanotic congenital heart defect in neonates. It accounts for approximately 5% of all congenital heart defects with male preponderance. If untreated (without PGE or balloon septostomy), mortality is high: 30% at 1 week, 50% at 1 month, and 90% at 1 year.

Morphology

Morphologically,[10,11] in TGA, as the name implies, the aorta is transposed to the RV and the PA to the LV. The aorta is anterior and commonly to the right of the PA; therefore, the prefix *d* is used for dextroposition, which is the most common type of complete transposition (d-TGA). The atria and ventricles are in normal relationship. Although the coronary arteries arise from the aorta, in at least a third the coronary artery origins and course are abnormal. All patients with TGA have an interatrial septal communication (PFO or ASD) and a PDA at birth. In about 70% of patients with d-TGA, the ventricular septum is intact (d-TGA/IVS), and the remaining 30% have a ventricular septal defect (d-TGA/VSD). Pulmonary stenosis, coarctation of the aorta (COA), and aortic arch obstruction are seen in about 25% to 35% of patients with d-TGA/VSD but they are rare in patients with d-TGA/IVS.

Coronary arteries originate from the sinuses of Valsalva facing the PA and are normal in two-thirds of the patients, with the left coronary artery originating from the leftward anterior-facing sinus and the right coronary artery (RCA) from the rightward posterior-facing sinus. In the rest, the pattern of origin and course is abnormal. The most common is the origin of the circumflex coronary artery from the RCA. A single origin of all coronary arteries and an intramural course of the coronary artery within the aortic wall are not infrequent and can pose technical challenges for the surgeon.

Pathophysiology

In d-TGA, the systemic venous blood returning to the RV is ejected back into the systemic bed through the aorta without passing through the lungs, and the pulmonary venous blood returning to the LV is ejected back into the lungs through the PA. This arrangement of 2 parallel circulations does not affect fetal survival because the placenta is the source of oxygenated blood but is incompatible with life in the postnatal period. Hence, after birth survival depends on adequate communication between the 2 parallel circuits at the level of PDA, ASD, and VSD (if present). The extent of mixing is determined by vascular resistance in each of the circulations, size of the communications between the 2 circuits, compliance of the ventricles, and volume of blood flow. Inadequate mixing results in hypoxia, hypercapnia, metabolic acidosis, and eventually death if untreated. Immediate postnatal interventions are primarily designed to maximize mixing of oxygenated and deoxygenated blood.

Clinical Presentation and Diagnosis

Cyanosis is the dominant clinical feature of these neonates, and it is often unresponsive to inhaled oxygen.

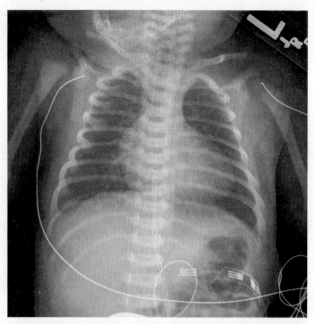

FIGURE 18-4 Chest x-ray. The heart is enlarged with a narrow pedicle, showing an "egg-on-a-string" sign.

Cyanosis may be less apparent in neonates with large ASDs and large PDAs, except occasionally because of streaming there is inadequate mixing of oxygenated and deoxygenated blood resulting in intractable cyanosis. In neonates with d-TGA/VSD, cyanosis is less apparent.

At presentation, these neonates often have unstable hemodynamics and a varying degree of acidosis. Physical examination may reveal a mildly hyperactive precordium with prominent single second heart sound and soft systolic murmurs. Peripheral arterial pulses may be prominent if the PDA is large. This may also result in symptoms of congested lungs. Chest x-ray often shows a mildly enlarged heart with a typical appearance (Figure 18-4).

Depending on the institution and country, in the current era prenatal diagnosis of TGA varies from 20% to 75%, and in such instances planned management almost always results in a stable neonate. Echocardiography is the mainstay of diagnosis and most often the only modality of imaging needed (Figure 18-5). Echocardiography can give all the necessary information, including the coronary anatomy needed for surgical planning. Rarely, a CT angiogram or a cardiac catheterization is needed.

Cardiac catheterization is usually a palliative tool in TGA to perform balloon septostomy.

Management

The preoperative management of a neonate with TGA/IVS is directed to increase mixing of oxygenated and deoxygenated blood between the 2 parallel circulations with the goal of increasing systemic oxygen delivery. PGE_2 infusion is started, and if necessary, a balloon

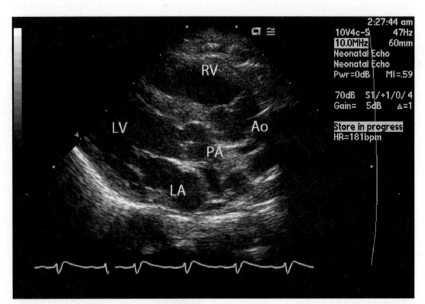

FIGURE 18-5 Echocardiography of the transposition of the great arteries. The aorta (Ao) arises from the right ventricle (RV) anteriorly, whereas the pulmonary trunk arises from the left ventricle (LV) posteriorly. LA, left atrium; PA, pulmonary artery.

atrial septostomy is performed either at the bedside in the neonatal intensive care unit (NICU) under echo guidance or in the cardiac catheterization lab. Most neonates do not require mechanical ventilation.

Some patients may not have adequate mixing of the oxygenated and deoxygenated blood despite these interventions; in such patients, inotropic support to increase the cardiac output and paralyzing the neonate and providing mechanical ventilation to decrease the metabolic needs may be necessary. Rarely, emergent surgery may be needed. In addition to these measures, correcting the metabolic abnormalities may be necessary.

On the other hand, neonates with TGA/VSD generally do not require PGE_2 or balloon septostomy if the VSD is large.

Surgical treatment is undertaken within the first few days of life, and it is not advisable to delay beyond 2 weeks of birth.[12] If there is a large VSD, some surgeons elect to wait for 2 to 4 weeks. The current procedure of choice is the arterial switch operation (ASO; Figure 18-6), which has replaced the atrial switch procedures, such as the Senning and Mustard operations.

The ASO is performed with cardiopulmonary bypass under cardiac arrest with cardioplegia with or without hypothermia. The procedure consists of transferring the aorta and coronary arteries to the LV and the PA with its branches to the RV.

In this procedure, the native pulmonary valve becomes the neoaortic valve and the native aortic valve becomes the neopulmonary valve. In addition, the PAs are translocated anterior to the aorta (Lecompte maneuver). Transferring the coronary arteries, the neoaorta[13] is the critical step in ASO. The PDA is ligated and divided. The ASD and VSD, if present, are closed.

Associated defects like COA or aortic arch obstruction are also repaired. In patients with LV outflow tract obstruction (LVOTO), an assessment is made whether it is dynamic or if it can be resected. In some patients with TGA/VSD/LVOTO, the pulmonary annulus is hypoplastic, the subpulmonary LV outflow tract (LVOT) is hypoplastic, or both. In such instances, a palliative procedure such as a systemic-to-PA shunt is undertaken; a primary repair is preferred by some surgeons. The operations for this subset of patients are known as the Rastelli procedure, REV procedure, or Bex-Nikkaidoh procedure. In the Rastelli or REV procedures, the LV is baffled to the aorta through the VSD; in the Bex-Nikkaidoh procedure, the aorta along with the valve and coronaries are translocated to the LV.

Outcomes

The early results[12,14–17] for the ASO have significantly improved since the late 1980s. The current survival rate for the ASO in those with TGA with or without VSD is less than 5%. If one excludes the high-risk patients, then the mortality is about 1% or less in most major centers. The risk factors for early death are also variable with experience. However, prematurity, low birth weight, single intramural coronary artery, aortic arch obstruction, multiple VSDs, hypoplasia of the RV, and older neonate/infant with TGA/IVS are some important risk factors. Many of these are neutralized in experienced hands. Preoperative physiologic state is also an important contributor to early death.

Late supravalvar PA stenosis and coronary artery obstruction are uncommon but important complications that require continued follow-up in these infants.

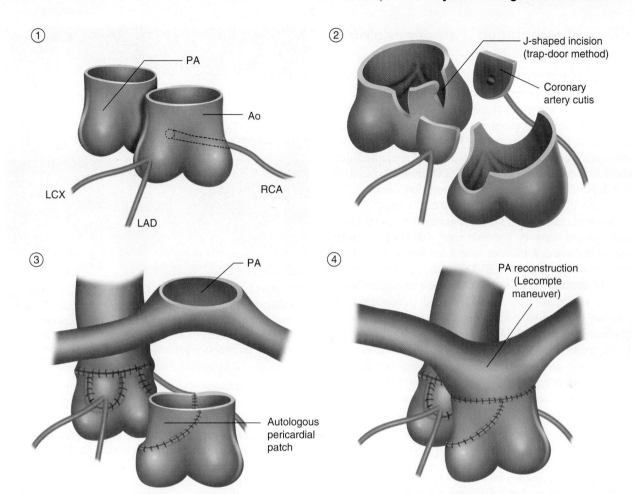

FIGURE 18-6 Surgical repair of arterial switch operation. Two coronary arteries are harvested and transferred into neo-aorta. The pulmonary artery is usually moved anterior to the aorta (Lecompte maneuver to prevent obstruction). LCx, left circumflex branch; LAD, left anterior descending branch; RCA, right coronary artery. (From Yasui et al.[60])

Another rarer complication, neoaortic valve regurgitation, may require even longer follow-up to determine its extent and significance.

TETRALOGY OF FALLOT

Introduction

Tetralogy of Fallot (TOF) is a common cyanotic congenital heart defect and accounts for 10% of all congenital heart defects. In 1888, Fallot described 4 related cardiac abnormalities, which together are known as TOF: VSD; PA stenosis; dextrorotation of the aorta (rightward), which overrides the VSD; and RV hypertrophy. Untreated, about 30% do not survive beyond 3 months, and 10% survive to the age of 21.

Morphology

Morphologically,[18,19] most likely the anterocephalad deviation of the outlet septum and an abnormal relationship of this outlet septum to the rest of the interventricular septum result in all 4 morphologic features. The VSD in TOF is typically conoventricular or perimembranous, but it can also be subarterial with an absent outlet septum. In about 5% of patients, an additional VSD may be present. The crowding of the RV outflow tract (RVOT) causes RV outflow tract obstruction (RVOTO). This results in varying degrees of pulmonary valve abnormality (stenosis, hypoplasia, or atresia) and sometimes supravalvar PA narrowing. The subvalvar infundibulum is narrow and muscle bound in a majority of patients. In a small number of patients, the PAs can be hypoplastic. In the subgroup of patients with pulmonary valve atresia, the PAs are typically duct dependent. In about 25% of these patients, the pulmonary blood flow is derived from aortopulmonary collaterals.

In about 5% of patients with TOF, the coronary artery abnormalities are the most common and are the origin of the left anterior descending (LAD) branch from the RCA.

Clinical Presentation, Pathophysiology, and Diagnosis

Because of RVOTO, the venous blood from the RV is ejected into the aorta through the VSD; this is facilitated to some extent by the overriding of the aorta into the RV. Cyanosis becomes more pronounced as the severity of RVOTO increases. In patients with pulmonary valve atresia, all the venous blood is ejected into the aorta. As the severity of RVOTO increases, so does the dependency of pulmonary blood flow on the presence of a PDA or aortopulmonary collaterals.

Most neonates with TOF are asymptomatic at birth, and cyanosis may be the only sign; this is often undetected if there is a PDA or in milder forms of TOF. In neonates with significant RVOTO, the cyanosis is obvious. In those with severe RVOTO or pulmonary valve atresia, the pulmonary blood flow is dependent on the patency of the ductus arteriosus. The neonates quickly become hypoxic as the PDA starts to close and require PGE$_2$ infusion to maintain systemic oxygenation.

Cyanotic spells are episodes of severe hypoxia and can be seen in newborns with moderate-to-severe RVOTO. The exact mechanism of these spells is unclear but may be multifactorial; the decrease in systemic vascular resistance and infundibular muscular hyperactivity are thought to be important.

Most neonates with TOF who have well-balanced systemic-to-pulmonary blood flow and systemic arterial oxygen saturation above 85% are discharged and have elective surgery between 2 and 6 months of age. The neonates who are on PGE$_2$ and who have cyanotic spells require surgical intervention in the neonatal period.

Clinical examination often reveals a systolic ejection murmur and a soft second heart sound. A continuous murmur of a PDA may be present. Chest x-ray (Figure 18-7) and ECG are often not diagnostic in neonates. Echocardiography (Figures 18-8 and 18-9) is the mainstay of diagnosis. With this modality, the diagnosis can be accurately established and all other morphologic features clearly defined except the details of pulmonary blood supply in patients with hypoplastic PAs or those with pulmonary atresia. In these neonates, cardiac catheterization and angiography or CT angiography is indicated.

Management

Most neonates with TOF do not require any intervention other than a period of observation until the PDA closes to ensure that they have adequate antegrade pulmonary blood flow to maintain systemic arterial oxygen saturation (preferably above 85% on room air).

If the neonate has cyanotic spells, aggressive medical management is immediately indicated. These spells are often amenable to maneuvers to increase systemic

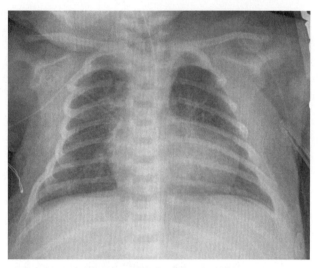

FIGURE 18-7 Chest x-ray of 1-month-old with tetralogy of Fallot (TOF) with severe pulmonary stenosis. Because of the diminutive pulmonary artery, a characteristic pattern, called the *couer en Sabot* "boot-shaped heart" is seen. The pulmonary vascular bed is hypoperfused.

vascular resistance (knee-to-chest position), volume administration, sedation, and sometimes β-blockers. Any cyanotic spell would indicate early surgery. If the cyanotic spells are frequent or difficult to manage, then emergency surgery may be indicated. However, in neonates, often PGE$_2$ infusion can reopen the closed PDA and stabilize the patient. In neonates who are PDA dependent from birth, surgery is indicated within a few days after birth. The small subset of patients with major aortopulmonary collaterals and multiple sources of pulmonary blood flow most often do not require surgery in the neonatal period unless they have pulmonary overcirculation or significant hypoxia.

Surgery

Initial surgical management of TOF can be either palliative or reparative. Alfred Blalock, at the persuasion of Helen Tausig, performed the first palliative systemic-to-PA shunt, widely known as the Blalock-Tausig shunt (BT shunt) to increase the pulmonary blood flow to improve the hypoxia. In this operation, the subclavian artery was transected distally, turned down, and anastomosed to the right or left PA. This historic surgery marked the emergence of cardiac surgery for congenital heart defects. Alternative shunts, such as Potts and Waterston shunts, also were advocated but fell out of favor because of complications. The modified BT shunt with the use of an expanded polytetrafluoroethylene (ePTFE) tube graft or a central aorta-to-pulmonary shunt with an ePTFE tube graft is widely practiced for palliation of not only TOF but also many other forms of congenital heart defects with decreased pulmonary blood flow.

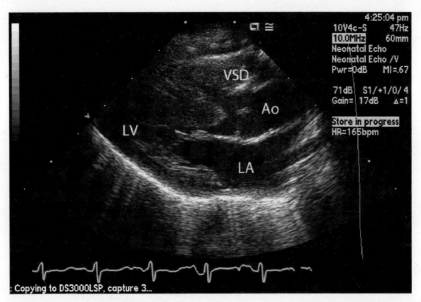

FIGURE 18-8 Echocardiography. Aorta (Ao) is overriding significantly to the right ventricle (RV). Because of pulmonary artery stenosis, the shunt through the ventricular septal defect (VSD) is right to left. LA, left atrium; LV, left ventricle.

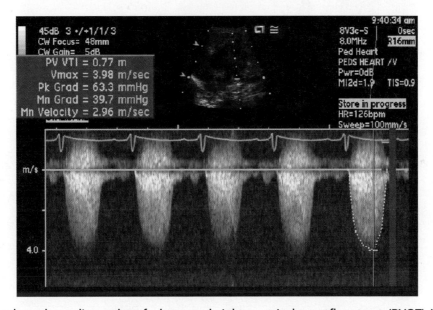

FIGURE 18-9 Doppler echocardiography of obstructed right ventricular outflow tract (RVOT) in a neonate with tetralogy of Fallot (TOF). The flow across the RVOT is accelerated significantly (V_{max} 3.98 m/s).

In the current era, repair not palliation even in neonates is preferred by many large centers. Palliation with shunts carries a higher mortality than repair and has the potential for PA distortion and shunt occlusion or thrombosis, resulting in interstage morbidity or mortality.

Surgical repair consists of patch closure of VSD with an RVOT procedure. The RVOT procedure varies depending on the size of the pulmonary annulus (Figure 18-10). If the pulmonary valve annulus is better than a z score of −2 to 2.5, then pulmonary valve commisurotomy and main PA enlargement along with infundibular muscle resection are performed. This results in little or no pulmonary insufficiency and no or mild pulmonary stenosis.

On the other hand, if the pulmonary valve is hypoplastic, a transannular patch RVOT augmentation is performed. This by definition means cutting across the pulmonary valve annulus, which results in pulmonary insufficiency. To avoid pulmonary insufficiency, some surgeons create a monocusp pulmonary valve from autologous pericardium or prosthetic material. The longevity of such monocusps is unreliable.

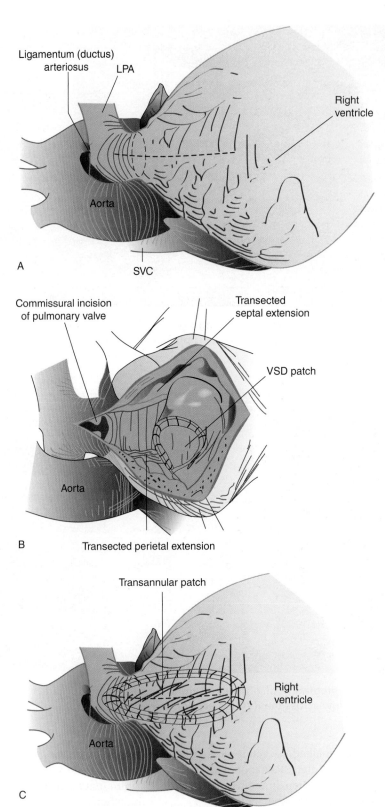

FIGURE 18-10 Repair of tetralogy of Fallot. In neonates, a transannular right ventricular–pulmonary artery incision is made. Hypertrophied muscle in the right ventricular outflow tract is resected, and the ventricular septal defect (VSD) is closed through a ventriculotomy. The transannular incision is then augmented with a patch. LPA, left pulmonary artery; SVC, superior vena cava. (From Kouchoukos et al.[61])

In patients with TOF with pulmonary atresia, a conduit (mostly a valved homograft conduit) is used to create continuity between the RV and PAs.

Outcomes

The surgical results of repair of TOF in the neonatal period have improved consistently since the 1990s.[20–26] In large centers, the mortality is less than 1% to 2% for repair in the neonatal period, thereby avoiding palliation. In comparable neonates, the mortality and morbidity of a palliation are equal to or worse than repair, hence the shift toward repair rather than palliation. However, in asymptomatic neonates, whether neonatal repair is really a good choice is controversial. Our approach is to perform an elective repair around 2 months of age in the asymptomatic group. Over the long run, many of these patients will require a pulmonary valve replacement or a conduit replacement if one has been used in the neonatal repair.

TRUNCUS ARTERIOSUS

In persistent truncus arteriosus (TrA), a single arterial blood vessel arises from the heart. A large VSD is almost always present in this condition with very rare exception. The PAs arise from this main arterial trunk, which then continues as the ascending aorta.

Morphology

Morphologically,[27–29] the TrA is classified[27] simply as type I when the main PA arises from the left lateral aspect of the truncus and divides into right and left PAs, type II when the right and left PAs arise as separate orifices but are close to each other from the left posterolateral aspect of the truncus, and type III when the right and left PAs arise separately from the right and left lateral sides of the truncus, respectively. This classification has no bearing on the outcomes but has implications in surgical reconstruction of the PAs.

Truncal valve morphology is variable. Most often, the valve is tricuspid but can also be bicuspid or quadricuspid. More important than the morphology of the valve is its function. Truncal valve regurgitation is seen in nearly a third to half of the patients and is moderate to severe in about 15% to 20%. True truncal valve stenosis is uncommon; more often, it is flow related.

Ventricular septal defect is almost always a subtruncal conoventricular defect and is unrestrictive. Occasionally, it is perimembranous, and additional muscular defects may be present. Coronary artery anomalies are common and seen in up to 60% of patients. In about 5% of patients, the aortic arch is interrupted; this is the only subgroup of patients who have a PDA. Rarely, the aortic arch is right sided, and in these patients tracheobronchial compression may be present.

Clinical Presentation, Pathophysiology, and Diagnosis

The most common presenting feature in the neonate is cyanosis. In neonates who present, late signs of congestive heart failure (CHF) are predominant, and the cyanosis may be minimal.

There is almost complete mixing of systemic and pulmonary venous blood, and pressures in both ventricles are identical. The level of oxygen saturation in the systemic circulation is proportional to the magnitude of pulmonary blood flow (PBF), which is dependent primarily on PVR and the size of the PAs. When the PBF is large, the patient is minimally cyanotic but may develop CHF because of excessive volume overload placed on the ventricle. When the PVR is high in the early neonatal period, the patient is cyanotic and does not develop CHF. In general, the neonate will start to develop pulmonary overcirculation within a few days after birth as the PVR continues to drop. As the PVR drops, patients develop CHF because of increasing PBF, and for a while the cyanosis abates until such time that pulmonary interstitial edema results in pulmonary venous desaturation.

Physical examination reveals varying degrees of cyanosis, depending on the magnitude of PBF. A heart murmur of the VSD is rarely audible because it is often large, and there is no pressure gradient between the 2 ventricles. If truncal valve regurgitation is significant, an early diastolic murmur may be heard. The ECG usually shows combined ventricular hypertrophy. The QRS complexes in all precordial leads are similar (poor R/S progression).

Chest x-ray (Figure 18-11) findings are consistent with the magnitude of PBF. In the early neonatal period, it may be relatively normal. Within a few days with increasing PBF, the chest x-ray shows signs of pulmonary congestion. Rarely, if the neonate has persistent pulmonary hypertension, the lung fields may look normal or hypoperfused.

The echocardiogram (Figure 18-12) is the gold standard for diagnosis of TrA. Often, it is the only diagnostic modality needed before surgery. Occasionally, it may be necessary to do a CT angiogram or cardiac catheterization to delineate the coronary anatomy or obtain hemodynamic data.

Management

In the neonatal period, these patients do not need any active management other than avoiding inhaled oxygen. As the PVR drops and CHF begins, anticongestant therapy may be needed. But, in the current era, surgical repair is undertaken within the first week of life.

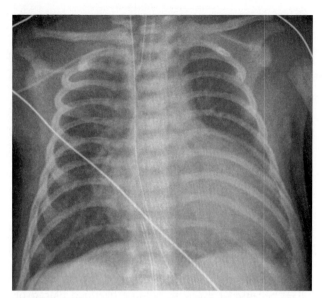

FIGURE 18-11 Chest x-ray. Because of the excessive pulmonary blood flow, the lungs are congested bilaterally and the heart is enlarged.

Palliative surgical treatment of bilateral pulmonary banding is no longer practiced; instead, a complete repair is the surgical treatment of choice.

The surgical procedure (Figure 18-13) consists of closure of the VSD, detaching the PAs from the truncal vessel, and placement of the RV-to-PA conduit. The conduit can be valved or nonvalved[30] and either a homograft or a bioprosthetic. The truncal vessel from where the PAs are detached is reconstructed with a patch.

In patients with associated interrupted aortic arch, the arch reconstruction is performed with a direct anastomosis of the descending aorta to the ascending aorta with or without a patch to augment the reconstruction.

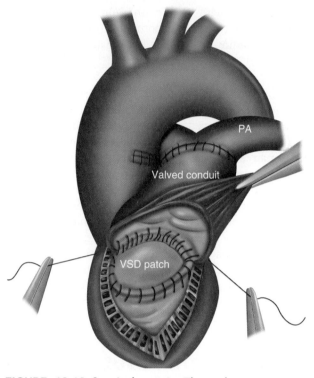

FIGURE 18-13 Surgical repair. The pulmonary artery (PA) is detached from the truncal artery, and the resulting defect is direct closed. The associated ventricular septal defect (VSD) is closed through a right ventriculotomy. A homograft is placed from the right ventricle to the pulmonary artery in the end. (From Khonsari et al.[59])

If the truncal valve regurgitation is more than mild, often an attempt is made to repair the valve; fairly good success is achieved. The need for neonatal truncal valve replacement is uncommon.

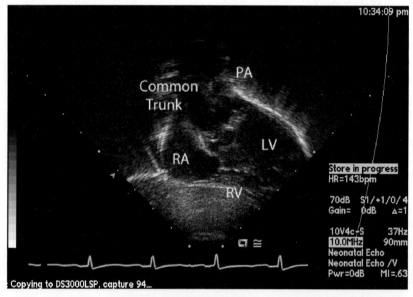

FIGURE 18-12 Pulmonary artery (PA) arises from the back of the large common trunk. LV, left ventricle; RA, right atrium; RV, right ventricle.

The surgery is performed on cardiopulmonary bypass with or without deep hypothermia and with or without circulatory arrest based on the surgeon's preference.

Results

The results of repair of TrA have improved over the last few decades; currently, the early mortality is below 5% in most centers.[31,32] The major risk factor for mortality is severe truncal valve regurgitation. Early reoperation for progressive truncal valve regurgitation is not uncommon and may be needed in 5% to 15% of patients within the first year after surgery.[31–35]

HYPOPLASTIC LEFT HEART SYNDROME

Introduction

Hypoplastic left heart syndrome (HLHS) is a spectrum of lesions, which are characterized by hypoplasia or underdevelopment of left heart structures: LV, aortic valve, mitral valve, ascending aorta, and aortic arch. At one end of the spectrum is an isolated hypoplastic aortic arch, and at the other end of the spectrum is severe hypoplasia of the LV, atresia of the aortic and mitral valves, and very hypoplastic ascending aorta. However, in practice, the term HLHS more commonly is used to describe a constellation of these morphologic features that together necessitate a Norwood operation.

Morphology

Broadly, HLHS[36,37] can be divided into 4 categories, all of which have the common feature of hypoplastic LV (which by definition is unsuitable to function as an independent ventricle) and varying degrees of hypoplasia of the ascending aorta. The 4 subcategories are (1) aortic stenosis and mitral stenosis; (2) aortic atresia and mitral atresia; (3) aortic stenosis and mitral atresia; and (4) aortic atresia and mitral stenosis. Although there is no significant difference in outcomes, the subset of aortic atresia and mitral stenosis is considered higher risk because of the presence of a hypertensive LV and sometimes significant communication between the LV and coronary arteries and rarely LV-dependent coronary arteries. On the other hand, the subset of patients with aortic and mitral stenosis with a small but functioning ventricle are at the good end of the spectrum. These patients often have some antegrade blood flow through the aortic valve. Hypoplasia of the ascending aorta is more severe in patients with aortic atresia, and it is often less than 2 mm in diameter.

The more important factors that make HLHS high risk are RV function, the presence of moderate or severe TV regurgitation, and intact or severely restrictive atrial septum, resulting in pulmonary venous obstruction. Patients in this group are critically ill after birth and require immediate postnatal catheter or surgical intervention. In addition, the presence of any significant noncardiac abnormalities are unfavorable for survival of these neonates.

Clinical Presentation, Pathophysiology, and Diagnosis

Neonates who are undiagnosed prenatally may be overlooked in the period immediately after birth. As the PDA starts closing, cyanosis becomes more apparent, and symptoms of low cardiac output begin. If unrecognized, the patients soon go into circulatory shock because of low cardiac output. Closure of the ductus arteriosus to any significant degree is incompatible with life unless PGE_2 is started immediately.

Patients with aortic and mitral stenosis with some antegrade blood flow in the ascending aorta are more fortunate in this regard.

In HLHS, there is complete mixing of oxygenated and deoxygenated blood at the atrial and ventricular levels. The mixed blood is ejected through the pulmonary valve (some through the LV to the aorta in the subset of patients with aortic and mitral stenosis), and the systemic circulation is dependent on the patency of the ductus arteriosus (Figure 18-15A). In most patients, even the coronary and cerebral blood flow is retrograde from the PDA. The PVR of the pulmonary blood flow increases at the expense of systemic blood flow. If unrecognized tachypnea, CHF, and low cardiac output follow, they result in metabolic acidosis, multiorgan failure, and eventually death.

If untreated, most patients with HLHS die within the first week, and 90% of them do not survive beyond the first 2 weeks of life.

Diagnosis is established or confirmed by echocardiography, which is the mainstay of diagnosis. Cardiac catheterization is indicated if there is suspicion of LV coronary sinusoids or to define coronary anatomy. Rarely, other modalities such as CT angiogram or magnetic resonance imaging (MRI) are needed to define other associated defects, such as venous anomalies or tracheal or diaphragmatic abnormalities.

Management

Immediate medical attention is essential for establishing stable hemodynamics and ensuring survival. Once the diagnosis is made, the neonate is started on PGE infusion. If necessary, mechanical ventilation is also instituted. Often, this is planned because of prenatal diagnosis.

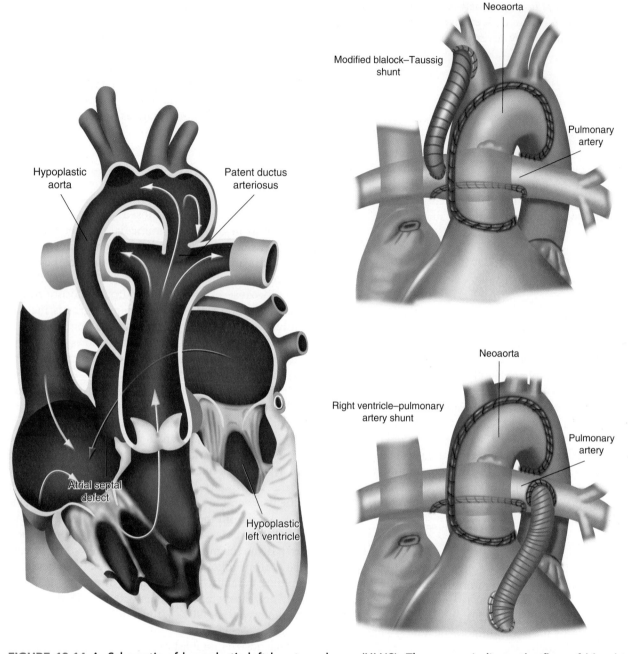

FIGURE 18-14 A, Schematic of hypoplastic left heart syndrome (HLHS). The arrows indicate the flow of blood in HLHS. B, top: Norwood procedure with a modified Blalock-Taussig shunt; bottom: modified Norwood procedure with a shunt from right ventricle to the pulmonary artery. (From Ohye et al.[42])

In patients with intact or a severely restrictive atrial septum, the neonate is immediately taken to the cardiac catheterization lab, and ASD creation or enlargement with a stent is performed.

All associated metabolic defects are corrected, and blood transfusion to raise the hematocrit may be needed. It is necessary to correct any pulmonary overcirculation. The neonate should be on room air, and if ventilated, maintaining the $PaCO_2$ in the range of 50 to 55 mm Hg is helpful. Despite these measures, if the neonate is still overcircualting, especially if there

is clinical evidence of systemic hypoperfusion, early surgery is indicated.

The surgical management for a long time has been a Norwood procedure[38] (Figure 18-14B), which involves creating a neoaorta using the native pulmonary outflow tract, providing controlled pulmonary blood flow through a systemic-to-pulmonary shunt (often a modified BT shunt), and atrial septectomy. A modification of the Norwood procedure was introduced by Japanese surgeons and is often referred to as the "Sano or Kishimoto shunt"; it is an RV-to-PA shunt instead of

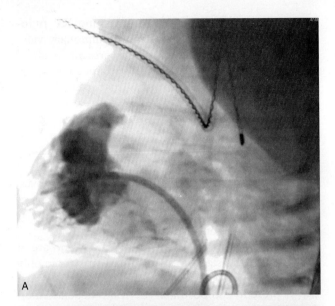

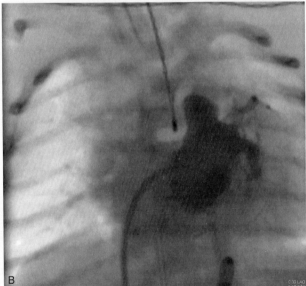

FIGURE 18-15 A and B, Angiography of pulmonary atresia with intact ventricular septum. There is no forward flow into the pulmonary artery. The right ventricle is hypertrophied with a small cavity. The coronary artery is opacified through sinusoidal communication.

a BT shunt.[39] Because this is systolic-only shunting of blood in the PAs, it is believed to be more beneficial, especially in the early postoperative period, because there is no diastolic runoff into the shunt and coronary perfusion is better preserved. Currently, most surgeons and institutions prefer this approach.

More recently, another approach to neonatal management of HLHS called the hybrid approach has been introduced.[40] This approach involves avoiding a Norwood procedure in the newborn period. Instead, the neonate undergoes bilateral branch PA banding and at the same time (in hybrid catheter lab/operating room suites) or immediately thereafter stenting of the PDA and, if needed, the atrial septum. In essence,

it is a way of replacing PGE therapy and controlling pulmonary blood flow. In Japan, oral PGE is used instead of a PDA stent, which probably is a better approach because it avoids all stent-related problems. This approach is not widely accepted yet but has its place, especially in neonates at high risk for whom avoiding cardiopulmonary bypass in the neonatal period is deemed beneficial: neonates with depressed ventricular function, associated significant noncardiac abnormalities, intact atrial septum, cerebral bleeding, and so on.

Outcomes

Surgical outcome of neonates with HLHS has steadily improved over the last few decades.[41–44] More recent reports with a standard Norwood procedure or with an RV-to-PA shunt suggest a survival rate of over 90%.[41,42] A recent report in the *New England Journal of Medicine* from a randomized multicenter study comparing the Norwood procedure with the BT shunt versus the Norwood procedure with an RV-to-PA shunt appeared to favor the latter approach. The results of hybrid approach have been variable but have a high incidence of multiple interventions before the second stage. Overall, about 70% to 85% of hospital survivors of the Norwood procedure make it to the subsequent stage of cavopulmonary shunt. Home monitoring programs between stage I and stage II have also improved the survival interval.[44]

PULMONARY VALVE ATRESIA WITH INTACT VENTRICULAR SEPTUM

Introduction

With rare exceptions, pulmonary valve atresia with IVS occurs with situs solitus and normal atrioventricular and ventriculoarterial connections. Pulmonary valve atresia with IVS is characterized by (1) complete obstruction of the pulmonary valve, (2) 2 distinct ventricles, (3) intact ventricular septum, and (4) a patent tricuspid orifice. Pulmonary valve atresia with IVS is a rare lesion, accounting for about 1%–1.5% of all congenital heart defects. The exact cause of this lesion is not known. The presence of abnormalities in the pulmonary valve without abnormalities in the aortic valve suggests that the etiology occurs after the valve cusps have formed. The majority of the cases have well-developed, fused pulmonary cusps with the typical triradiate appearance. The PA diameter is almost always normal in size in pulmonary valve atresia with IVS, and the ductus arteriosus is invariably present and is normal.

Morphology

Although the pulmonary valve lesion is presumably the primary event, much of the morbidity and mortality of this condition results from the severe secondary morphologic changes.[45–47] Marked morphologic heterogeneity is the hallmark of this lesion. All the secondary morphologic abnormalities in pulmonary valve atresia with IVS occur proximal to the right ventriculoarterial junction, in contrast to pulmonary atresia with a VSD, for which the major abnormalities occur distal to this junction.

The **pulmonary valve** is often well formed with definable but fused commissures. Bicuspid and quadricuspid valves are rare. However, not uncommonly the ventriculoarterial junction may be fibrous, which is presumed to be a remnant or pulmonary valvular tissue or imperforate fibrous tissue overlying muscular infundibular atresia.

An **interatrial communication** is virtually always present, most commonly a stretched foramen ovale (PFO). A true secundum ASD is present in about 20% of cases,[29] and in about 5%–10% of cases, the interatrial communication is restrictive, with the septum primum bulging into the left atrium.[26] The **right atrium** is often dilated, with the degree of dilation often proportional to the severity of tricuspid regurgitation.

Typically, the **TV** is smaller than normal, but it may range from the Ebstein anomaly with an enlarged dilated annulus on the one hand to an extremely stenotic valve on the other. In the Congenital Heart Surgeons Society (CHSS) study,[28] the median z value of the tricuspid annulus was −2.2 (the z value represents the normalized tricuspid annulus diameter, with 0 being normal[30] and the values above and below it representing the number of standard deviations from the normal). The size of the TV correlates well with the RV cavity size and is important in the prognosis of pulmonary valve atresia with IVS; it is discussed further in this chapter. Varying degrees of TV dysplasia are seen. In about 5%–10% of cases, the Ebstein deformity of the TV is present. Functionally, the TV may be regurgitant, stenotic, or both. Some degree of tricuspid regurgitation is present in most cases, with severe tricuspid regurgitation present in about 25% of cases.[28]

The **RV** is hypertrophied with a reduced cavity in 90% of cases, severely so in about 60% of cases. In about 5%–10% of cases, an enlarged and dilated RV is found in association with more severe degrees of tricuspid regurgitation and with an Ebstein anomaly. Even the smallest RVs are thought to have all 3 components; however, the massive hypertrophy may obliterate the trabecular or outlet parts. Associated diffuse fibrosis of the hypertrophied ventricular muscle may be present, and in severe cases, varying degrees of endocardial fibroelastosis are seen.

Coronary artery abnormalities and **RV myocardial sinusoids** are common in pulmonary valve atresia with IVS. RV sinusoids are present in about 50% of cases. These fistulous communications seem to be most prominent with small hypertensive RVs, occurring in 8% to 55% of reported cases. These fistulas from the coronary artery to the RV are present in the majority of cases in which sinusoids are present, and the prevalence of these lesions correlates inversely with TV diameter, RV cavity size, and the degree of tricuspid incompetence. In about 20% of these cases, the coronary circulation or some important part of it is solely derived from the RV. This is described as RV-dependent coronary circulation.

The **PAs** nearly always branch normally and are of normal size, with significant hypoplasia present in only about 6% of cases. The **ductus arteriosus** is almost always present, and postnatal survival is dependent on ductal patency.

Clinical Presentation, Pathophysiology, and Diagnosis

The infant born with pulmonary valve atresia with IVS is compromised physiologically almost immediately. The atretic pulmonary valve causes an obligatory dependence on patency of the ductus arteriosus for pulmonary blood flow. An ASD allows for complete mixing of deoxygenated and oxygenated blood. Pulmonary blood, and hence systemic oxygen delivery, depends on the patency of the ductus arteriosus.

Systemic arterial blood pressure usually shows a somewhat widened pulse pressure, secondary to runoff through the ductus arteriosus into the pulmonary circuit. RV pressure tends to correlate inversely with the degree of tricuspid insufficiency. RV pressure is typically systemic or suprasystemic in the small hypoplastic RV but may be lower in a completely decompensated dilated RV with profound tricuspid regurgitation.

In infants with pulmonary valve atresia with IVS, the extremely high pressure in the RV reduces coronary flow, which results in chronic ischemic changes, especially in the subendothelial layers, and may account for the subendocardial fibrosis of the RV seen in many of these patients.

In cases of RV-dependent coronary blood supply (Figure 18-15A, 18-15B), the myocardium is supplied partly or completely by desaturated blood at systemic-to-suprasystemic systolic pressures and relatively low diastolic pressures. The extremely marginal coronary reserve in these patients can be easily compromised if RV systolic pressure is reduced by any means.

Most infants born with pulmonary valve atresia with IVS are at term gestational age. Signs of cyanosis and hypoxia occur variably from a few hours to several days after birth and depend on ductal flow. However, the

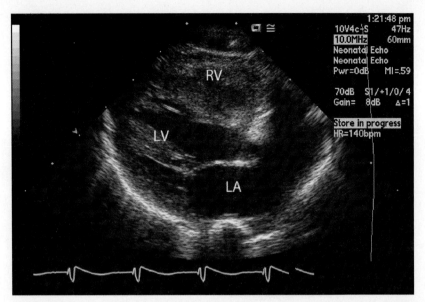

FIGURE 18-16 Echocardiography of pulmonary valve atresia with intact ventricular septum (IVS). The right ventricle (RV) is severely hypertrophied and does not have a normal cavity. LA, left atrium; LV, left ventricle.

majority (over 90%) of patients with pulmonary valve atresia with IVS present in the first 3 days of life as the ductus arteriosus begins to close. Currently, most often a fetal diagnosis is made, and PGE is instituted immediately after birth.

Chest roentgenograms in pulmonary valve atresia with IVS vary with anatomic type. In cases with a tiny RV and little or no tricuspid insufficiency, the heart is normal in size. The vascularity is reduced, normal, or occasionally increased, depending on the patency and size of the ductus arteriosus and the PVR. If the RV is normal or large with tricuspid insufficiency, the overall heart size is increased, and the enlarged right atrium gives considerable convexity to the right heart border.

Echocardiography allows a definitive and detailed diagnosis (Figure 18-16). Morphologic details of the RVOT, RV cavity, TV, atrial septum, and ductus arteriosus patency can be evaluated thoroughly and accurately. RV dependency on coronary blood flow cannot be reliably assessed by echocardiography, and cardiac catheterization and angiocardiography are necessary.

If untreated, pulmonary atresia with an intact septum carries a dismal prognosis. Within 2 weeks of birth, 50% of patients die, and by 6 months of age, 85% succumb. Death commonly results from severe metabolic acidosis caused by hypoxia following ductal narrowing or closure.

Management

As soon as the diagnosis is made, an infusion of PGE_1 (0.05 to 0.1 mg/kg/min) is started to maintain patency of the ductus arteriosus. Mechanical ventilation and inotropic support may be required in about one-third of patients.

If the diagnosis is delayed, profound cyanosis secondary to ductal constriction may be the mode of patient presentation. In this case, aggressive resuscitation with PGE_1, sodium bicarbonate, inotropic support, and mechanical ventilation may be necessary. Patients should be adequately stabilized whenever possible and thoroughly evaluated before performing the initial surgical procedure.

Catheter Intervention

During cardiac catheterization, a balloon atrial septostomy should be performed if deemed necessary to allow unrestricted right-to-left shunt. In selected cases of membranous pulmonary valve atresia with well-formed cusps, balloon valvotomy has been accomplished with acceptable initial results. Prostaglandins are generally weaned gradually over hours to days. This approach is an exception rather than a standard approach, and further follow-up is necessary to determine its success. More recently, radio-frequency and laser-guided pulmonary valve perforation and dilation have been undertaken successfully in a select group of patients.

Surgical Management

The ideal outcome for a patient with pulmonary atresia with IVS is completely separated in series 2-ventricle circulation. The central issue in achieving this is whether the RV can function as the sole provider of pulmonary blood flow at normal filling pressures. The primary goal of neonatal surgical management is to minimize mortality. The secondary goal should be to promote growth of the RV, thereby optimizing the chances of 2-ventricle circulation.

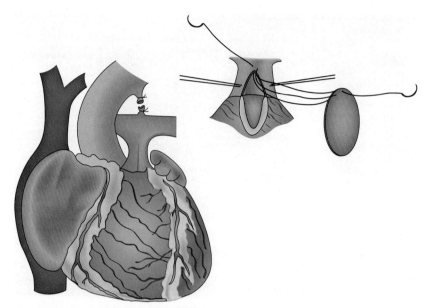

FIGURE 18-17 Surgical repair of pulmonary atresia with intact ventricular septum. Right ventricular outflow tract is enlarged with a patch. (From Yasui et al.[60])

The following morphology-specific treatment guidelines seem to give the best chances of fulfilling the goals mentioned, with these guidelines based on the data from the CHSS study[48]:

In a small subset of patients for which the TV diameter ($z = 0$ to -2) and RV cavity approach normal size, it may be ideal to perform an RVOT procedure (balloon or surgical pulmonary valvotomy or transannular patch) alone (Figure 18-17). With any of these procedures, profound postoperative cyanosis indicates the need for a shunt. This is likely to be necessary in slightly less than half of patients by 1 month of life.

For the patient with mild-to-moderate TV annular hypoplasia ($z = -2$ to -3), the goal of 2-ventricle circulation is achievable. However, the likelihood of this outcome decreases as the TV annular size decreases. The RVOT procedure with concomitant shunt is favored.

For the subset of patients with severe TV annular hypoplasia ($z = -3$ or less), the preferred procedure is a shunt alone because an ultimate 2-ventricle repair is unlikely in this subset. In the CHSS study, no patient with a TV annulus size less than 3 standard deviations below normal ($z = \leq 3$) has achieved a 2-ventricle repair.

In any patient with RV-dependent coronary circulation, RV decompression is contraindicated and shunt alone is the procedure of choice.

The subsequent surgical management of pulmonary valve atresia with IVS is also complex. It is generally accepted that 2-ventricle circulation with completely separated pulmonary and systemic circuits is ideal. But, it is also realized that some patients can never achieve this. Close follow-up is indicated in all patients irrespective of the initial procedure.

Results

The recent data from the CHSS study appear to be representative of general experience with this lesion.[47-52] In this study, the overall survival was 81% at 1 month and 64% at 4 years. This study also showed that a TV with a small diameter and marked RV coronary artery dependency were important morphologic risk factors for death. In addition, 55% of the survivors required subsequent procedures, mainly to address the inadequacy of the original procedure. Although Fontan repairs and "one-and-a-half-ventricle repairs" have been successfully achieved in patients with pulmonary valve atresia with IVS, follow-up data are needed to identify the predictors of successful long-term outcome.

TRICUSPID ATRESIA AND OTHER FORMS OF FUNCTIONALLY SINGLE VENTRICLES

Introduction

Tricuspid atresia[53] is the lack of a direct connection between the right atrium and RV because of complete atresia of the TV. This atresia is most often muscular but can be membranous.

Morphology

In tricuspid atresia, the TV is usually completely absent or can be vestigial or Ebstenoid, but in all cases, there is no opening in the TV.[54] The right atrium is usually enlarged to some degree, and there is an unrestricted ASD.

In patients without a VSD, the RV is severely hypoplastic, and the pulmonary valve is atretic or rudimentary. If there is a VSD, the RV and pulmonary valve are hypoplastic to varying degrees. The great arteries are normally related in the majority and transposed in about 20% to 30% of patients. In patients with TGA, there is a subgroup that has systemic subaortic obstruction without hypoplasia of the aortic valve and ascending aorta.

Other Miscellaneous Defects

Various forms of functionally single ventricles can cause cyanosis, although they are relatively rare. Embryologically, these single ventricles occur because of poor alignment of the common atrioventricular valve with the ventricles or incomplete septation of the ventricle chambers. These abnormalities in the fetal period of life end in double-inlet ventricles (usually, a double-inlet LV, the most common form of single ventricle), tricuspid atresia, mitral atresia, unbalanced atrioventricular canal defect, and a functional single ventricle with heterotaxy syndromes (asplenia, polysplenia, or atrial isomerism).

Pathophysiology, Clinical Features, and Diagnosis

The common unifying feature of these lesions is complete mixing of deoxygenated and oxygenated blood in the single functional ventricle. Patients may or may not be dependent on the patency of the ductus arteriosus. Patients with severe pulmonary stenosis or atresia are PDA dependent. In the absence of significant pulmonary stenosis, there is often pulmonary overcirculation, and the cyanosis is mild. On the other side of the spectrum, there is obstruction to systemic blood flow, and these patients have physiology similar to those with HLHS.

The lung fields on chest x-ray reflect the pulmonary blood flow status. Also, the atrial and visceral situs can be discerned. Echocardiography (Figure 18-18) is the mainstay of diagnosis and often is enough to plan surgical management. These neonates often have abnormal systemic and pulmonary venous connections that have to be delineated accurately. A CT angiogram can accurately define the venous anatomy in addition to pulmonary situs and visceral situs. Cardiac catheterization may be necessary in some patients, especially if there is potential for therapeutic palliative intervention such as balloon dilation of pulmonary stenosis or ductal stenting, which some institutions prefer.

Management

For a neonatologist, once the diagnosis is made, the next step is to assess the patient and determine the pathway of clinical management. Despite the complexity of morphology in terms of various atrial, ventricular, and venous abnormalities, the most important thing to consider is assessment of pulmonary blood flow: rule out any systemic outflow obstruction and pulmonary venous obstruction (including at the level of the atrial septum).

Assessment of pulmonary blood flow: Occasionally, a patient has just the appropriate amount of pulmonary blood flow because of natural stenosis in various levels of pulmonary stenosis. However, many

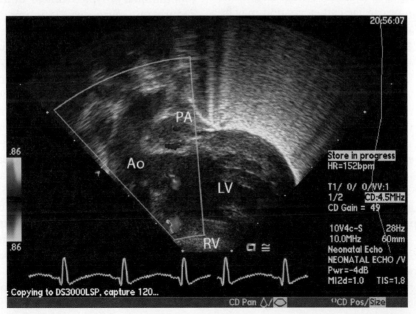

FIGURE 18-18 The right ventricle (RV) is hypoplastic, and a small ventricular septal defect is seen. The pulmonary blood flow is mainly supplied by a patent ductus arteriosus. Ao, aorta; LV, left ventricle; RV, right ventricle.

of them present with either high or low oxygen saturation, depending on the balance between the systemic and PVR. The low arterial oxygen saturation level can hinder normal growth and impair organ function. The high arterial saturation level results in pulmonary hypertension and impaired ventricular function. Generally, an arterial oxygen saturation level between 75% and 85% indicates a reasonable amount of pulmonary blood flow in terms of protection of the pulmonary vascular bed and ventricular function.

In addition to arterial oxygen saturation level, the plain chest x-ray helps assess pulmonary blood flow. A congested lung field and an enlarged heart imply pulmonary overflow and an oligemic lung field, and a small heart implies diminished pulmonary flow, with the exception of pulmonary venous pathway obstruction, which shows a congested lung field with diminished blood flow. Echocardiography is essential to determine the segmental classification of the patient's cardiac anatomy. Echocardiography should carefully examine any levels of obstruction in systemic and pulmonary circulation.

Assessment of systemic outflow obstruction: Clinically, the cyanosis is variable and depends on the amount of pulmonary blood flow. More important, the neonate should be assessed for signs of systemic hypoperfusion, which necessitates institution of PGE_1. Systemic outflow obstruction can be accurately assessed by echocardiography and cardiac catheterization is usually not necessary.

Assessment of pulmonary venous obstruction: Pulmonary venous obstruction, if severe, can be catastrophic and should be ruled out. A cyanotic patient in respiratory distress should prompt immediate attention. Chest x-ray shows signs of pulmonary venous congestion, and echocardiography is almost always diagnostic, but a CT angiogram or cardiac catheterization may be necessary to delineate the pulmonary venous anatomy. Occasionally, if the pulmonary venous obstruction is at the level of the atrial septum, a balloon septostomy is urgently indicated.

Palliative Surgical Intervention in the Neonatal Period and Outcome

The goal of intervention for all forms of single-ventricle physiology has 2 prongs: (1) achievement of an adequate balance between systemic and pulmonary blood flow; and (2) relief of obstructed systemic cardiac output.

Inadequate Pulmonary Blood Flow

In neonates with low saturation, it is critical to assess the cause of pulmonary blood flow obstruction. It can be one of the following or a combination of them: (1) pulmonary outflow obstruction, (2) pulmonary venous obstruction, and (3) poor mixing at the atrial level.

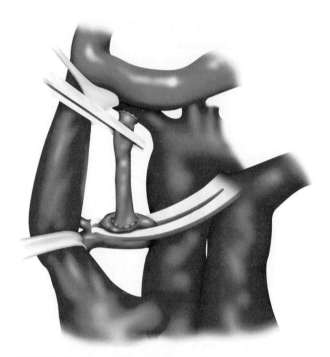

FIGURE 18-19 Modified Blalock-Taussig shunt. After proximal anastomosis of a Goretex tubing graft on the base of the innominate artery, the side-biting clamp has been placed on the superior edge of the right pulmonary artery to complete the distal anastomosis. (From Khonsari et al.[59])

The most common cause of inadequate flow is pulmonary outflow obstruction at various levels. To increase the pulmonary blood flow, a systemic-to-pulmonary shunt, either a modified Blalock-Tausig shunt (Figure 18-19) or a central shunt is employed. Usually, we can perform this procedure without cardiopulmonary bypass unless other intracardiac procedures are necessary. It is important to select the appropriate size shunt to achieve an arterial oxygen saturation of 80%–85%. An oversize shunt can create pulmonary overcirculation, which results not only in systemic hypoperfusion but also in volume overloading of the ventricle. It impairs myocardial contractility subsequently and causes long-term cardiac dysfunction. The shunt is also known to result in scarring and distortion of the PAs. Even though the Blalock-Tausig shunt was introduced almost 70 years ago, the mortality remains relatively high in a patient with a single ventricle (hospital mortality is 15% in those with a single ventricle vs 3% in a biventricular patient).

Particularly in the case of patients with heterotaxy syndrome, it is known that they may present with a severe degree of cyanosis because of an obstructed TAPVR. To prevent the damage in the pulmonary parenchyma and optimize development of the PA, it is important to repair the TAPVR soon after the diagnosis is made. This anomaly significantly complicates the care of a patient, and although early survival in these patient has improved, intermediate survival is still approximately only 50%.[3]

In patients with stenosis or atresia of the left atrioventricular valve, it is obligatory to have an unobstructed left-to-right flow at the atrial septal level. If the ASD is not adequate, it can cause pulmonary venous hypertension, resulting in cyanosis. For these patients, atrial septectomy is indicated. This can be performed with relatively low mortality either as an isolated procedure or combined with a systemic-to-pulmonary shunt or PA banding.

Excessive Pulmonary Blood Flow

Neonates with single-ventricular physiology without any PA or venous obstruction will develop pulmonary overcirculation as the PVR declines in the first couple of weeks of life. Excessive pulmonary flow can result in persistent pulmonary hypertension or impaired ventricular function, which make subsequent right heart bypass procedures, such as a Glenn or Fontan operation, difficult. Usually, to control the excessive pulmonary flow, creation of stenosis in the pulmonary trunk by banding is indicated (Figure 18-20). It is crucial to assess the status of the LVOT before proceeding to PA banding. As stated, in a single ventricle, pulmonary circulation and systemic circulation are parallel. Excessive pulmonary blood flow can be caused by either low PVR or high systemic vascular resistance. The PA banding can be performed without cardiopulmonary bypass in a safe manner. The degree of the banding is usually decided based on intraoperative echocardiography, pressure measurement, and oxygen saturation. The target oxygen saturation is usually 80%–85% under room air. According to a recent study of patients with single-ventricle physiology who underwent PA banding, the actual overall survival was 84% at 1 year and 76% at 5 and 15 years.[4]

In case of LV outflow obstruction, the patient instead should have systemic outflow augmentation procedures such as a Norwood or Damus-Kaye-Stansel procedure.

Systemic Outflow Obstruction

Systemic outflow obstruction can cause 2 problems: development of ventricular hypertrophy and pulmonary overcirculation. Ventricular hypertrophy results in ventricular dysfunction and late arrhythmia. It is important to address this problem early in life; otherwise, it will have a significant impact on patient mortality and morbidity. In the case of subaortic obstruction, the Damus-Kaye-Stansel procedure (the creation of an anastomosis between the proximal pulmonary trunk and the ascending aorta) has been employed. For LVOTO associated with a hypoplastic arch, a Norwood-type operation that requires major reconstruction of the arch in addition to the pulmonary trunk and ascending aorta anastomosis has been used. In either of these surgeries, pulmonary blood circulation is ensured by placing a graft between systemic and PA (or ventricle) circulation.

Results

The results of surgery are in general best for patients with tricuspid atresia who require pulmonary banding (over 95% survival) and worst with obstructed pulmonary

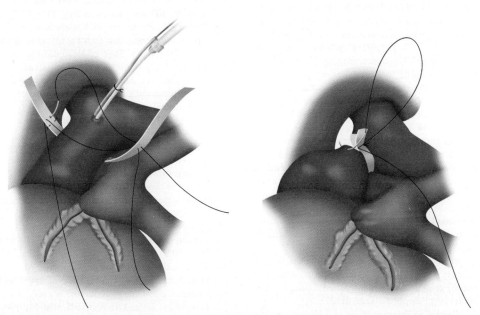

FIGURE 18-20 Pulmonary artery banding. The band is placed around the pulmonary trunk and tightened, monitoring the distal pulmonary artery pressure. To prevent the migration of the band, the band is anchored to the pulmonary trunk. (From Yasui et al.[60])

venous drainage (up to 50% to 75% early mortality).[55-57] The subsequent management of these patients requires a cavopulmonary shunt at 4 to 6 months of age and a Fontan procedure between 18 months and 4 years.

REFERENCES

1. Reddy VM, McElhinney DB, Sagrado T, et al. Results of 102 cases of complete repair of congenital heart defects in patients weighing 700 to 2500 grams. *J Thorac Cardiovasc Surg.* 1999;117:324–331.

2. Delisle G, Ando M, Calder AL, et al. Total anomalous pulmonary venous connection: report of 93 autopsied cases with emphasis on diagnostic and surgical considerations. *Am Heart J.* 1976;91:99–122.

3. Gathman GE, Nadas AS. Total anomalous pulmonary venous connection: Clinical and physiologic observations of 75 pediatric patients. *Circulation.* 1970;42:143–154.

4. Bando K, Turrentine MW, Ensing GJ, et al. Surgical management of total anomalous pulmonary venous connection: thirty-year trends. *Circulation.* 1996; 94(9 Suppl):II12–II16.

5. Boger AJ, Baak R, Lee PC, et al. Early results and long-term follow-up after corrective surgery for total anomalous pulmonary venous return. *Eur J Cardio-Thorac Surg.* 1999;16:296–299.

6. Hancock Friesen CL, Zurakowski D, Thiagarajan RR, et al. Total anomalous pulmonary venous connection: an analysis of current management strategies in a single institution. *Ann Thorac Surg.* 2005;79:596–606.

7. Karamlou T, Gurofsky R, Al Sukhni E, et al. Factors associated with mortality and reoperation in 377 children with total anomalous pulmonary venous connection. *Circulation.* 2007; 115:1591–1598.

8. Yun TJ, Coles JG, Konstantinov IE, et al. Conventional and sutureless techniques for management of the pulmonary veins: evolution of indications from postrepair pulmonary vein stenosis to primary pulmonary vein anomalies. *J Thorac Cardiovasc Surg.* 2005;129:167–174.

9. Alton GY, Robertson CMT, Sauve R, et al. Early childhood health, growth, and neurodevelopmental outcomes after complete repair of total anomalous pulmonary venous connection at 6 weeks or younger. *J Thorac Cardiovasc Surg.* 2007;133:905–911.e903.

10. Anderson RH, Weinberg PM. The clinical anatomy of transposition. *Cardiol Young.* 2005;15(Suppl 1):76–87.

11. Carvalho JS, Ho SY, Shinebourne EA. Sequential segmental analysis in complex fetal cardiac abnormalities: a logical approach to diagnosis. *Ultrasound Obstet Gynecol.* 2005;26:105–111.

12. Castaneda AR, Norwood WI, Jonas RA, et al. Transposition of the great arteries and intact ventricular septum: anatomical repair in the neonate. *Ann Thorac Surg.* 1984;38:438–443.

13. Lacour-Gayet F, Anderson RH. A uniform surgical technique for transfer of both simple and complex patterns of the coronary arteries during the arterial switch procedure. *Cardiol Young.* 2005;15(Suppl 1):93–101.

14. Soongswang J, Adatia I, Newman C, et al. Mortality in potential arterial switch candidates with transposition of the great arteries. *J Am Coll Cardiol.* 1998;32:753–757.

15. Kang N, de Leval MR, Elliott M, et al. Extending the boundaries of the primary arterial switch operation in patients with transposition of the great arteries and intact ventricular septum. *Circulation.* 2004;110(11 Suppl 1):II123–II127.

16. Qamar ZA, Goldberg CS, Devaney EJ, et al. Current risk factors and outcomes for the arterial switch operation. *Ann Thorac Surg.* 2007;84:871–878.

17. Losay J, Touchot A, Serraf A, et al. Late outcome after arterial switch operation for transposition of the great arteries. *Circulation.* 2001;104 (Suppl I):I-121–I-126.

18. Lev M, Eckner FAO. The pathologic anatomy of tetralogy of Fallot and its variants. *Dis Chest.* 1961;45:251–261.

19. Anderson RH, Weinberg PM. The clinical anatomy of tetralogy of Fallot. *Cardiol Young.* 2005;15(Suppl 1):38–47.

20. Kirklin JW, Blackstone EH, Pacifico AD, et al. Risk factors of early and late failure after repair of tetralogy of Fallot, and their neutralization. *Thorac Cardiovasc Surg.* 1984;32:208–214.

21. Reddy VM, Liddicoat JR, McElhinney DB, Brook MM, Stanger P, Hanley FL. Routine primary repair of tetralogy of Fallot in neonates and infants less than 3 months of age. *Ann Thorac Surg.* 1995;60:S592–S596.

22. Murphy JG, Gersh BJ, Mair DD, et al. Long-term outcome in patients undergoing surgical repair of tetralogy of Fallot. *N Engl J Med.* 1993;329:593–599.

23. Gatzoulis MA, Balaji S, Webber SA, et al. Risk factors for arrhythmia and sudden death late after repair of tetralogy of Fallot: a multicentre study. *Lancet.* 2000:356:975–981.

24. Therrien J, Siu SC, McLaughlin PR, et al. Pulmonary valve replacement in adults late after repair of tetralogy of Fallot: are we operating too late? *J Am Coll Cardiol.* 2000;36:1670–1675.

25. Del Nido PJ. Surgical management of right ventricular dysfunction late after repair of tetralogy of Fallot: right ventricular remodeling surgery. *Semin Thorac Cardiovasc Surg Pediatr Card Surg Annu.* 2006:29–34.

26. Therrien J, Marx GR, Gatzoulis MA. Late problems in tetralogy of Fallot: recognition, management, and prevention. *Cardiol Clin.* 2002;20:395–404.

27. Collett RW, Edwards JE. Persistent truncus arteriosus: a classification according to anatomic types. *Surg Clin North Am.* 1949;29:1245–1269.

28. Crupi G, Macartney FJ, Anderson RH. Persistent truncus arteriosus: a study of 66 autopsy cases with special reference to definition and morphogenesis. *Am J Cardiol.* 1977;40:569–578.

29. Calder L, Van Praagh R, Van Praagh S, et al. Truncus arteriosus communis: clinical, angiocardiographic, and pathologic findings in 100 patients. *Am Heart J.* 1976;92:23–38.

30. Barbero-Marcial M, Riso A, Atik E, Jatene A. A technique for correction of truncus arteriosus types I and II without extracardiac conduits. *J Thorac Cardiovasc Surg.* 1990;99:364–369.

31. Brown JW, Ruzmetov M, Okada Y, et al. Truncus arteriosus repair: outcomes, risk factors, reoperation and management. *Eur J Cardiothorac Surg.* 2001;20:221–227.

32. Thompson LD, McElhinney DB, Reddy VM, Petrossian E, Silverman NH, Hanley FL. Neonatal repair of truncus arteriosus: continuing improvement in outcomes. *Ann Thorac Surg.* 2001;72:391–395.

33. Danton MH, Barron DJ, Stumper O, et al. Repair of truncus arteriosus: a considered approach to right ventricular outflow tract reconstruction. *Eur J Cardiothorac Surg.* 2001;20:95–103; discussion 103–104.

34. Konstantinov IE, Karamlou T, Blackstone EH, et al. Truncus arteriosus associated with interrupted aortic arch in 50 neonates: a Congenital Heart Surgeons Society study. *Ann Thorac Surg.* 2006;81:214–222.

35. Hanley FL, Heinemann MK, Jonas RA, et al. Repair of truncus arteriosus in the neonate. *J Thorac Cardiovasc Surg.* 1993;105:1047–1056.

36. Tchervenkov CI, Jacobs JP, Weinberg PM, et al. The nomenclature, definition and classification of hypoplastic left heart syndrome. *Cardiol Young.* 2006;16:339–368.

37. Ilbawi AM, Spicer DE, Bharati S, et al. Morphologic study of the ascending aorta and aortic arch in hypoplastic left hearts: surgical implications. *J Thorac Cardiovasc Surg.* 2007;134:99–105.

38. Norwood WI, Lang P, Hansen DD. Physiologic repair of aortic atresia–hypoplastic left heart syndrome. *N Engl J Med.* 1983;308:23–26.

39. Sano S, Ishino K, Kawada M, et al. Right ventricle–pulmonary artery shunt in first-stage palliation of hypoplastic left heart syndrome. *J Thorac Cardiovasc Surg.* 2003;126:504–509.

40. Akintuerk H, Michel-Behnke I, Valeske K, et al. Stenting of the arterial duct and banding of the pulmonary arteries: basis for combined Norwood stage I and II repair in hypoplastic left heart. *Circulation.* 2002;105:1099–1103.

41. Reinhart O, Reddy VM, Petrossian E, et al. Homograft valved right ventricle to pulmonary artery conduit as a modification of the Norwood procedure. *Circulation.* 2006;114(1 Suppl): I594–I599.

42. Ohye RG, Sleeper LA, Mahony L, et al. Comparison of shunt types in the Norwood procedure for single ventricle lesions. *N Engl J Med.* 2010;362:1980–1992.

43. Wernovsky G, Chrisant MR. Long-term follow-up after staged reconstruction or transplantation for patients with functionally univentricular heart. *Cardiol Young.* 2004;14(Suppl 1):115–126.

44. Ghanayem NS, Hoffman GM, Mussatto KA, et al. Home surveillance program prevents interstage mortality after the Norwood procedure. *J Thorac Cardiovasc Surg.* 2003;126:1367–1377.

45. Freedom RM, ed. *Pulmonary Atresia with Intact Ventricular Septum.* Mount Kisco, NY: Futura; 1989.

46. Freedom RM, Anderson RH, Perrin D. The significance of ventriculo-coronary arterial connections in the setting of pulmonary atresia with an intact ventricular septum. *Cardiol Young.* 2005;15:447–468.

47. Daubeney PE, Delany DJ, Anderson RH, et al. Pulmonary atresia with intact ventricular septum: range of morphology in a population-based study. *J Am Coll Cardiol.* 2002;39:1670–1679.

48. Hanley FL, Sade RM, Blackstone EH, et al. Outcomes in neonatal pulmonary atresia with intact ventricular septum. *J Thorac Cardiovasc Surg.* 1993;105:406–427.

49. Powell AJ, Mayer JE, Lang P, Lock JE. Outcome in infants with pulmonary atresia, intact ventricular septum, and right ventricle-dependent coronary circulation. *Am J Cardiol.* 2000;86: 1272–1274.

50. Ashburn MD, Blackstone EH, Wells WJ, et al. Determinants of mortality and type of repair in neonates with pulmonary atresia and intact ventricular septum. *J Thorac Cardiovasc Surg.* 2004;127:1000–1008.

51. Daubeney PEF, Wang D, Delany DJ, et al. Pulmonary atresia with intact ventricular septum: predictors of early and medium-term outcome in a population-based study. *J Thorac Cardiovasc Surg.* 2005;130:1071.

52. Dyamenahalli U, McCrindle BW, McDonald C, et al. Pulmonary atresia with intact ventricular septum: management of, and outcomes for, a cohort of 210 consecutive patients. *Cardiol Young.* 2004;14:299–308.

53. Jacobs ML, Anderson RH. Nomenclature of the functionally univentricular heart. *Cardiol Young.* 2006;16(Suppl 1):3–8.

54. Kiraly L, Hubay M, Cook AC, et al. Morphologic features of the uniatrial but biventricular atrioventricular connection. *J Thorac Cardiovasc Surg.* 2007;133:229–234.

55. Karamlou T, Ashnurn DA, Caldarone CA, et al, Members of the Congenital Heart Surgeons Society. Matching procedure to morphology improves outcomes in neonates with tricuspid atresia. *J Thorac Cardiovasc Surg.* 2005;130:1503–1510.

56. Wald RM, Tham EB, McCrindle BW, et al. Outcome after prenatal diagnosis of tricuspid atresia: amulticenter experience. *Am Heart J.* 2007; 153:772–778.

57. Scheurer MA, Hill EG, Vasuki N, et al. Survival after bidirectional cavopulmonary anastomosis: analysis of preoperative risk factors. *J Thorac Cardiovasc Surg.* 2007; 134:82–89.

58. Stark J, de Leval M, Tsang. Surgery for Congenital Heart Defects. 3rd ed. London, UK: Wiley; 2006.

59. Khonsari S, Sintek CS, Ardehali A. *Cardiac Surgery: Safeguards and Pitfalls in Operative Technique.* 4th ed. Philadelphia, PA: Lippincott Williams and Wilkins; 2008.

60. Yasui H, Kado H, Masuda M. *Cardiovascular Surgery for Congenital Heart Disease.* New York, NY: Springer; 2009.

61. Kouchoukos N, Blackstone EH, Hanley FL, et al. *Kirklin/Barratt-Boyes Cardiac Surgery.* 4th ed. New York, NY: Elsevier Saunders; 2013.

SUGGESTED READING

Allen HD, Driscoll D, Shaddy RE, Feltes TF, eds. *Moss & Adams' Heart Disease in Infants, Children, and Adolescents: Including the Fetus and Young Adult.* 8th ed. Philadelphia, PA: Lippincott; 2012.

Kouchoukos N, Blackstone E, Hanley FL, Kirklin J, eds. *Kirklin/Barratt-Boyes Cardiac Surgery.* New York: Elsevier; 2012.

CHAPTER 18

Noncyanotic Congenital Heart Disease

Rajesh Punn

INTRODUCTION

This chapter focuses on noncyanotic congenital heart disease with a basic description of the epidemiology, embryology, clinical manifestation, diagnostic testing, management, treatment, and prognosis of each lesion. The intent is to provide a framework for the major types of noncyanotic congenital heart disease, ranging from septal defects, left ventricular outflow tract (LVOT) obstruction disease, and right ventricular outflow tract obstruction disease. The chapter forms a guide for managing neonates with these common heart conditions.

SEPTAL DEFECTS

Atrial Septal Defect

The atrial septal defect (ASD) is one of the first forms of congenital heart disease that was corrected surgically. It represents a communication between the left and right atria and does not usually manifest in the neonatal period unless there is associated congenital heart disease, which usually makes it difficult to diagnose. There are 3 major types: secundum ASD, primum ASD, and sinus venosus ASD. The primum ASD is discussed as a part of the atrioventricular canal (AVC) defect (Figure 19-1).

Epidemiology

The ASD represents the second-most-common form of congenital heart disease behind the ventricular septal defect (VSD). The occurrence is between 3% and 4.1% of 1000 live births[1,2] and 7% and 15% of all

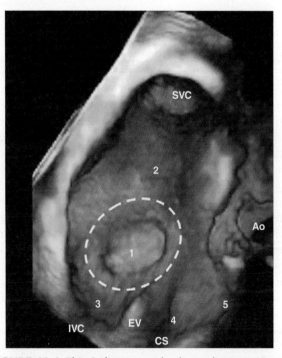

FIGURE 19-1 This 3-dimensional echocardiogram image depicts the interatrial septum from the perspective of the right atrial side. The superior vena cava (SVC) drains superiorly into the right atrium, while the inferior vena cava (IVC) drains from below. The fossa ovalis is central, and a secundum atrial septal defect (ASD) would lie in region 1. A superior or inferior sinus venosus ASD is located in regions 2 or 3, respectively. The primum ASD is located anteroinferiorly at region 5. The rare coronary sinus (CS) ASD, not discussed in this chapter, is located near the CS. The aorta (Ao), which is anteriorly located, is diagrammed as a point of reference. EV, Eustachian valve. (Reproduced with permission from Faletra et al.[160])

Table 19-1 Common Forms of Atrial Septal Defect (ASD) (%)

Type of ASD	Craig and Selzer,[9] 1968	Tandon and Edwards,[162] 1974	Helgason and Jonsdottir,[23] 1999
Secundum	85	93	92.5
Sinus venosus	8	6	4
Primum	6	Excluded	3.5
Single atrium	<1	1	0

congenital heart disease cases.[3,4] For defects that are larger and measure over 5 mm in diameter, there tends to be a female predominance.[5,6] The secundum ASD is by far the most common type (Table 19-1). Nearly 1 of every neonates will have an atrial communication that is difficult to distinguish from a patent foramen ovale.[7] Approximately 15% of trisomy 21 patients will have a secundum ASD, and 1% of ASD patients will have Holt-Oram syndrome.[8] Of note, patients with Holt-Oram tend to have very large ASDs and can have a common atrium with no wall separating the atria.

Pathophysiology

Patients with ASDs that are hemodynamically significant tend to have problems later in life and do not present in the neonatal period. Specifically, there is a chronic left-to-right atrial shunt that enlarges the right atrium and right ventricle. This shunt increases blood flow to the pulmonary arteries, which chronically can change the pulmonary vascular bed, leading to pulmonary hypertension. Approximately 22% of ASD patients will develop pulmonary hypertension in adulthood if the ASD is left unrepaired, and 15% will have elevated pulmonary vascular resistance.[9] Eisenmenger syndrome develops if a chronic left-to-right shunt lesion causes severe pulmonary vascular changes such that there is significant elevation in the pulmonary vascular resistance and a reversal of the shunt. Thus, blood would flow from the right atrium to the left atrium, resulting in arterial hypoxemia. Eisenmenger syndrome occurs 14% of the time in patients with an ASD.[9] Again, if left untreated another complication is right heart failure from the chronic volume overload as well as atrial arrhythmias from right atrial distension.[9] Fewer than 1% of infants with an isolated secundum ASD will develop significant symptoms that may lead to death.[10]

Infants can develop early right heart failure, which is presumably from a rapid drop in the pulmonary vascular resistance.[11] The degree of shunting is related to the relative compliance of the left ventricle in comparison to the right ventricle. As the resistance in the pulmonary bed drops, the right ventricular "stiffness" decreases, leading to the left-to-right shunt. Thus, ASD should be considered in the differential diagnosis of any infant with congestive heart failure or failure to thrive.[12]

The secundum ASD represents a defect in the flap of the foramen ovale where it is incompetent, leading to left-right shunting. The sinus venosus ASD, however, is quite separate and high, where the right pulmonary veins and superior vena cava drain; frequently, there is no associated shunting across the foramen ovale. Thus, anomalous drainage of the right pulmonary veins into the superior vena cava is associated with the sinus venosus ASD.

Regardless of the type of ASD, most patients are asymptomatic in early childhood; however, congestive heart failure symptoms begin before the age of 6 years in 84% of patients and, as mentioned, symptoms can develop during infancy if there is a rapid drop in the pulmonary vascular resistance.[9,11,13] The symptoms in the infant would include failure to thrive, tachypnea, feeding difficulties, and diaphoresis with feeds. Cyanosis would be unlikely because this defect does not produce Eisenmenger syndrome until adulthood. In the older patient, easy fatigability, syncope, and hemoptysis may also be present along with frequent pulmonary infections from the chronic left-to-right shunt. Unfortunately, 30% of children have only 1 or no typical physical sign from an ASD, which makes the diagnosis in the young child difficult.[14]

As a result of the extra volume of blood traversing the pulmonary valve, there is a relative pulmonary valve stenosis murmur. The systolic ejection-type murmur is present in 87% to 100% of the time.[14,15] In addition, extra volume across the tricuspid valve may lead to diastolic murmur from relative tricuspid stenosis in some cases. As a result of this volume-loaded right ventricle, the pulmonary valve closes later than the aortic valve throughout the cardiac cycle, resulting in the "fixed" split in S2, which is present 57% of the time.[14] Again, the neonate presents a challenge because in most patients the right ventricle is not volume loaded since the pulmonary vascular resistance remains relatively high and the right ventricle is "stiff." Thus, the physical examination findings may not be present during infancy.[12]

A few etiologies have been discovered for the ASD. The only reported maternal exposure associated with ASD is maternal alcohol consumption, which appears to double the risk of ASD.[16] Mutations in the fetus NKX2.5 gene have been identified in patients with many forms of congenital heart malformations, and ASD is common among them.[17,18]

Differential Diagnosis

Because the child with an ASD can have signs of congestive heart failure, other disease processes that cause congestive heart failure should be included in the differential diagnosis. Specifically, congenital heart disease that leads to a chronic left-to-right shunt should be considered, such as a VSD, patent ductus arteriosus, or an AVC defect. Infants with cardiomyopathy may also have the same symptoms noted for ASD. Finally, other noncardiac conditions that can cause congestive heart failure should also be considered, such as sepsis, severe anemia, or pulmonary infection.

Diagnostic Tests

Prior to the advent of echocardiography, the cardiac catheterization was used in patients with a clinical suspicion of ASD for diagnostic purposes, and repair was considered if the relative pulmonary blood was 50% greater than the flow across the aorta.[3] The electrocardiogram (ECG) in the neonate and infant may not demonstrate the classic RSR′ pattern because this is a marker for volume load, and right ventricular hypertrophy is a common finding in normal neonates (Figure 19-2). Also, ECG findings are often missing in children with ASD.[14]

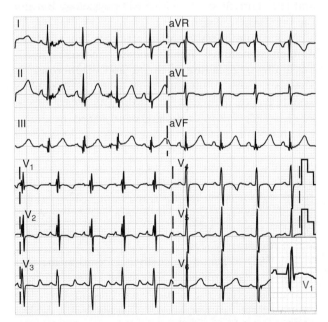

FIGURE 19-2 This electrocardiogram shows the classic RSR′ pattern in lead V1, which represents a volume load on the right ventricle. Note that the R′ is larger than the R in the bottom right inset.

Currently, the echocardiogram remains the gold standard for the diagnosis of all types of ASD. In addition to identifying the type of ASD, this technique is used to guide transcatheter closure and evaluate the surgical repair of an ASD.

Management

The decision to close a secundum ASD depends on the size of the defect, the degree of shunting, and the evidence of right ventricular enlargement. Traditionally, if the relative flow across the pulmonary artery is 50% more than the flow across the aorta because of the ASD, then an intervention is recommended.[3] Surgical closure or modern-day device closure with interventional cardiology of secundum ASDs is generally low risk and curative. The sinus venosus ASD is surgically repaired because there is no intervention available for this defect at this time.

In general, the closure of an ASD should be done in early childhood; however, as mentioned, there are cases where an infant would have evidence of congestive heart failure and secondary failure to thrive, which would warrant an earlier intervention.[19] Infants can also safely undergo ASD device closure in the catheterization laboratory, which would avoid a sternotomy and cardiopulmonary bypass.[20]

Spontaneous closure occurs in 26% of patients before the age of 2 years, and in general an ASD is unlikely to close after this age, which supports the idea of repair in early childhood.[21] Ninety-eight percent of ASDs less than 3 mm in diameter in neonates close by 18 months of age, and defects greater than 3 mm take longer to close.[6,22] Thus, size of the defect at initial presentation has an impact on the spontaneous closure rate. The ASDs in premature infants take longer to close; however, an associated patent ductus arteriosus tends to close the ASD sooner, presumably because of elevated left atrial pressure, which causes the septum primum flap to abut against the septum, resulting in closure of the defect.[6]

Outcome and Follow-up

Death is rare in patients with unrepaired ASD; however, atrial arrhythmias in adult patients with chronic atrial distension from the left-to-right shunt is much more common.[3] Cerebrovascular accidents are even rarer than mortality but still may occur.[3] Most patients are not symptomatic until the third decade of life; however, intervention is recommended in early childhood.[3,9]

With the advent of echocardiography and color Doppler, ASDs are recognized more readily at an earlier age. Over 70% to 80% of all secundum ASDs close spontaneously by 18 months of age.[1,5] A defect less than 3 mm in diameter has a nearly 100% spontaneous closure rate, while a defect greater than 8 mm is unlikely to close,[8,23] confirmed by later studies.[24-26]

Ventricular Septal Defect

The VSD represents a communication between the right and left ventricles and varies significantly in presentation. For the most part, the neonate may not have symptoms from a VSD even when it is large because flow across it relies on a drop in the pulmonary vascular resistance. The defect is classified by its location within the ventricular wall, the size, and the number of defects. Essentially, there are 3 major types: perimembranous, doubly committed subarterial (supracristal), inlet, and muscular (Figure 19-3). The perimembranous VSD lies superior and anterior within the region of the membranous septum, which is bordered by the tricuspid valve and aortic valve. The supracristal VSD is also anterior but represents a defect below the pulmonary and aortic valves. Both of these defects are outlet VSDs. The inlet VSD is a defect that is near the atrioventricular valves and located quite posteriorly. This defect is most commonly discovered with a complete atrioventricular canal (CAVC) defect, which is discussed further in this chapter. The muscular VSD represents a defect in the trabecular end of the ventricular septum and is bordered completely by muscle. Any combination of these defects may coexist; thus, the clinician should always be suspicious of multiple defects.

Epidemiology

The VSDs occur approximately in 0.95 of 1000 live births and represent the most common form of congenital heart disease other than bicuspid aortic valve.

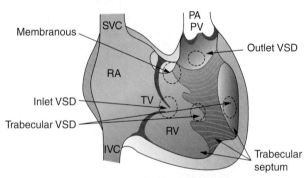

FIGURE 19-3 This diagram of the right ventricular aspect of the interventricular septum demonstrates the different types of ventricular septal defects (VSDs). Note that the inlet VSD is near the atrioventricular valves, and the outlet VSD tends to be near the outflow tract. IVC, inferior vena cava; PA, pulmonary artery; PV, pulmonary vein; RA, right atrium; RV, right ventricle; SVC, superior vena cava; TV, tricuspid valve. (Reproduced with permission from Axt-Fliedner et al.[40])

The majority of defects are perimembranous, ranging between 62% and 83%, followed by muscular defects, which vary between 9% and 12%.[27-30] Supracristal defects are much less common and occur between 2% and 3% of the time.[27,29] Muscular defects are less likely to be associated with a syndrome or a karyotype anomaly.[1]

Pathophysiology

The primary issue with the VSD is related to the degree of shunting from the left to the right ventricle. Multiple variables influence the degree of shunting and resultant symptoms from this type of defect. Specifically, the size and location of the defect are important in that small defects tend to protect against congestive heart failure. However, multiple small defects, known as a "Swiss cheese" VSD, may cause significant heart failure because of the collective size of all of the defects. Swiss cheese–type defects account for 0.5% of VSDs.[28] The other variable of importance is the relative resistance of the systemic and pulmonary vascular bed. In the neonatal period, the pulmonary vascular resistance is high; therefore, there is minimal shunting. As the pulmonary vascular resistance falls dramatically in the first few weeks of life, more left-to-right systolic shunting occurs across the defect. Because the relative pressures in diastole are similar between the ventricles, there is minimal diastolic shunting. Blood that shunts in systole enters directly into the main pulmonary artery; therefore, there is no nidus for right ventricular enlargement. The main pulmonary artery, left atrium, and left ventricle dilate with VSD physiology but not the right heart structures.

As the pulmonary vascular resistance drops, infants develop symptoms, which include tachypnea, feeding intolerance, failure to thrive, and diaphoresis.[27,31] However, 50% of infants may have no symptoms despite having a large defect. If the pulmonary vascular resistance fails to drop significantly, then the shunting and congestive heart failure symptoms would be minimal. Of note, premature infants tend to go into congestive heart failure much quicker than term infants; however, the proportion of patients in either group with these symptoms is the same.[31] The pulmonary vascular resistance drops with age, as expected in the setting of a VSD, but the resistance is generally higher for larger VSDs.[31]

The VSD murmur is usually not heard in the first few days of life unless it is a small defect. In fact, the murmur typically occurs within the first week to month of life in most cases.[31] Classically, the VSD's murmur is holosystolic in that it blends with the first heart sound, which generally cannot be auscultated. In addition, there may be excessive flow across the pulmonary and mitral valves, which would lead to a relative stenosis murmur in systole and diastole, respectively. In the case of a large VSD, the murmur may be difficult to hear.

Spontaneous closure of the VSD has been noted for the perimembranous and muscular VSD through various mechanisms. Tricuspid valve tissue may adhere to the perimembranous defect, resulting in occlusion of the defect over time.[32,33] The aortic valve sinus of Valsalva may also occlude the defect over time; however, this may be associated with herniation or rupture of the sinus into the right ventricle or aortic insufficiency. The margins of the muscular defect become relatively small as the child grows and the interventricular septum thickens, which is believed to be the mechanism of spontaneous closure.

Many associations have been noted with the outlet VSDs. Specifically, there can be a subaortic membrane or ridge associated with the defect that causes stenosis.[28,34] As noted, aortic insufficiency is associated with perimembranous defects but is also associated with supracristal defects because of the lack of tissue supporting the subvalvar apparatus.[28,35] However, subacute bacterial endocarditis associated with having a high-velocity jet and endothelial damage has also been noted to occur in 6% of all VSDs and can lead to aortic insufficiency secondary to direct damage; this will only exaggerate the congestive heart failure symptoms.[36] Subacute bacterial endocarditis and aortic insufficiency tend to be manifestations of a VSD later in life; congestive heart failure begins in infancy. An additional association is double-chamber right ventricle, for which a callous formation develops on the opposing wall of the right ventricle, which causes subpulmonary valve obstruction. Any outlet VSD can have an association with a coarctation of the aorta, which is discussed further in this chapter. VSD has an association with other forms of more complex cyanotic congenital heart disease; discussion of this is beyond the scope of this chapter.

The associated noncardiac conditions include trisomy 21, the VACTERL (vertebral defects, anal atresia, cardiac defects, tracheoesophageal fistula, renal anomalies, and limb abnormalities) association of congenital defects, cleft palate, bronchopulmonary dysplasia, chondrodysplasia, Klippel-Feil syndrome plus omphalocele, and polysplenia syndrome.[37]

Differential Diagnosis

Given that the VSD presents with signs of congestive heart failure in the infant after decreases in pulmonary vascular resistance, any other disease process that causes congestive heart failure must be ruled out. As with the ASD differential diagnosis, the left-to-right shunt lesions must be considered, such as AVC, patent ductus arteriosus, and aortopulmonary window.

Also, as the pulmonary vascular resistance drops, infants with anomalous origin of the coronary artery from the pulmonary artery would present as well because of coronary ischemia and steal. These patients would present with heart failure symptoms as well. In addition, lesions that cause high-output failure can mimic symptoms of a VSD. These include and are not limited to sepsis, severe anemia, and hepatic and cerebral arteriovenous malformations.

Diagnostic Tests

Ascultatory findings may not be evident on large defects because a VSD murmur may not be present. The ECG will demonstrate left atrial enlargement and left ventricular hypertrophy in the setting of large defects; chest x-ray will show evidence of cardiomegaly with increased pulmonary vascular markings. These findings, however, are nonspecific, and the diagnosis is usually made by echocardiography.[38] In fact, detection and closure of a VSD can be determined by fetal echocardiography as well.[39,40] In the past, these defects were confirmed by cardiac catheterization, which is no longer necessary.

Management

Large VSDs need to be repaired during infancy, and the elevated pulmonary vascular resistance as a result of the chronic shunt should improve postoperatively.[27] There is no difference in outcome for large VSD closure in children less than 4 kg vs greater than 4 kg; thus, it is recommended to intervene early to prevent recurrent respiratory infection, failure to thrive, and feeding difficulties.[37]

In the past, a pulmonary artery band (PAB) was positioned to limit pulmonary blood flow, and the VSD was closed as a separate procedure to minimize morbidity and mortality; however, VSDs are now closed in 1 step with primary closure regardless of the type. The indications for surgery include left heart failure, failure to thrive, feeding problems, and elevated pulmonary artery pressure. VSDs are usually closed through the right atrium[41,42] as opposed to a ventriculotomy, which can create a scar on the myocardium. For defects closer to the semilunar valves, repair can also occur through the pulmonary valve.[43] Multiple muscular VSDs can be closed primarily instead of with a PAB; however, if the septum is Swiss cheese, a PAB may be necessary because a patch across all of the defects may be difficult and may result in ventricular dysfunction.[44] After PAB placement, the defects may close spontaneously. Perventricular device closure of muscular VSDs in the cardiac catheterization lab may be an option in some select patients[45,46]; however, closure of perimembranous VSDs was not available when this chapter was written. This option is attractive to avoid a sternotomy, PAB, or cardiopulmonary bypass.

Outcome and Follow-up

The natural history of a VSD is for spontaneous closure, reduction in size, or development of pulmonary vascular disease. Death in infancy is most probably related to congestive heart failure.[47] The overall mortality is approximately 3% in all patients.[36] In general, muscular defects tend to have less congestive heart failure, higher closure rate, and less need for operative intervention compared to outlet defects.[48]

The natural closure rate for all VSDs is 22% to 36%.[31,33,49] The vast majority of defects that close do so before the eighth year of life and tend to be less than 6 mm in diameter.[49] Approximately 15% to 29% of perimembranous defects close compared to 57% to 65% of muscular defects.[1,28,50] Muscular defects tend to close during the first 6 to 12 months of life.[51] The most common complications after cardiac surgery include a residual VSD, right bundle branch block, complete heart block, death, persistent pulmonary hypertension, cerebrovascular accident, or tricuspid valve regurgitation, which may be related to perimembranous patch closure. However, in a recent article, the surgical results for isolated VSD were noted to be good, with 0% reoperation for residual defect, 0.5% mortality, 99.5% of patients asymptomatic, and none had more than mild new-onset tricuspid valve regurgitation.[30]

Atrioventricular Septal Defect

An atrioventricular septal, or canal, defect represents a malformation of the AVC whereby the crux of the heart does not develop, which potentially renders a primum ASD and inlet VSD. Thus, there is a spectrum of disease ranging from an isolated primum ASD with a cleft mitral valve to a CAVC defect with a large inlet VSD and primum ASD (Figure 19-4). As a result of these communications, patients can develop a chronic left-to-right shunt and atrioventricular valve regurgitation. As with other ASDs, a patient with an isolated primum ASD and cleft mitral valve does not usually present with heart failure in infancy; however, a CAVC can cause significant congestive heart failure in the first few months of life.

Epidemiology

The diagnosis of AVC defect often occurs with trisomy 21. In fact, about 50% of patients with trisomy 21 and congenital heart disease have this defect. Specifically, 36% of patients with trisomy 21 have AVC defects.[52]

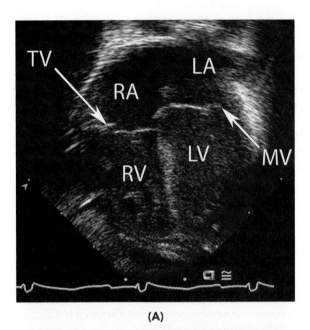

(A)

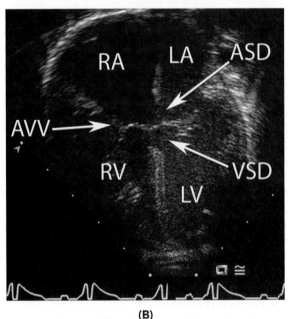

(B)

FIGURE 19-4 A, A normal 4-chamber view in diastole obtained by echocardiography. Note the atrial wall separating the right (RA) and left atrium (LA). The tricuspid valve (TV) is slightly lower and closer to the apex compared to the mitral valve (MV). LV, left ventricle; RV, right ventricle. B, This image shows a patient with a complete atrioventricular canal defect. There is a common atrioventricular valve that is not offset like the normal heart. A large atrial septal defect (ASD) and inlet ventricular septal defect (VSD) are also noted.

The AVC defect represents the most common form of heart disease in trisomy 21,[53] followed by VSD, ASD, and then tetralogy of Fallot. Importantly, about 40% to 50% of patients with Down syndrome have congenital heart disease in general.[52,54] For trisomy 21, a CAVC defect is more common than an isolated primum ASD with cleft mitral valve, which only occurs in 3% to 25% of patients with isolated primum ASD and cleft mitral valve series.[13,52,55] A CAVC defect can also occur in the setting of tetralogy of Fallot, which is associated with a genetic abnormality about 88% of the time, 67.2% of which is trisomy 21.[56]

Pathophysiology

As with the VSD and ASD, the shunt for a CAVC or isolated primum ASD is related to a drop in pulmonary vascular resistance. Thus, neonates may not have symptoms unless there are associated abnormalities. As the pulmonary vascular resistance falls, the infant can have symptoms of tachypnea, diaphoresis, and feeding difficulties, which can lead to failure to thrive. Of course, the VSD physiology of the AVC has a higher likelihood of causing symptoms than an isolated primum ASD with mitral valve cleft because the pulmonary arterial bed is under a pressure load and not just a volume load.

In addition to the left-to-right shunt, patients may have significant left atrioventricular, mitral valve, regurgitation, which elevates the left atrial pressure and can lead to worsening pulmonary venous congestion and respiratory symptoms. As with any of the left-to-right shunts, patients are at risk of recurrent respiratory infections if left untreated. Given that a large portion of patients with AVC have trisomy 21, it is important to note that children with trisomy 21 can have persistently elevated pulmonary vascular resistance in the first year of life compared to the normal patient population, which would make them potentially asymptomatic with no significant shunt.[57] However, children with trisomy 21 have a higher risk of fixed pulmonary vascular disease compared to children without trisomy 21, making the need for repair even greater.[57]

Several important associated anomalies must be accounted for when treating neonates with AVC. If the canal is unbalanced, the atrioventricular valve favors 1 ventricle over the other, making the other somewhat hypoplastic. In some cases, the ventricles are so unbalanced that the hypoplastic chamber is inadequate to serve the needs of the systemic or pulmonary circulation. Most of the time, this is an unbalanced left ventricular AVC, which renders hypoplastic left heart syndrome. Coarctation of the aorta, atrioventricular valve regurgitation, LVOT obstruction, and tetralogy of Fallot (discussed previously) are other conditions associated with AVC defects. Rarer anomalies would include heterotaxy with either right or left atrial isomerism, double-orifice mitral valve,[58–61] and cor triatriatum, a membrane that obstructs flow into the left ventricle.[62,63]

Differential Diagnosis

The AVC defect usually presents with symptoms of a chronic left-to-right shunt just like the ASD or VSD; however, the patients may present sooner given the multiple levels of shunting and the association with other congenital heart disease noted previously. Thus, these patients can present with congestive heart failure, and other diseases that present in this manner must be excluded. Namely, noncardiac conditions would include sepsis, severe anemia, and hepatic and cerebral arteriovenous malformations, and an additional cardiac condition would be a patent ductus arteriosus or aortopulmonary window.

Diagnostic Tests

The ECG in patients with AVC defect have an unusual counterclockwise direction of the frontal electrical conduction vector, resulting in the classic northwestern QRS axis[52] (Figure 19-5). Thus, a patient with this classic ECG finding along with the stigmata of trisomy 21 has an AVC defect until proven otherwise. Nonetheless, the echocardiogram can help determine the diagnosis more specifically. In addition, the associated lesions, such as balancing of the ventricles, valve regurgitation, left or ventricular outflow tract obstruction, and coarctation of the aorta, can be entertained. The typical appearance of the AVC is readily recognized from the 4-chamber view (Figure 19-4). The cardiac catheterization is reserved for those cases where the pulmonary vascular resistance is called into question if a child does not receive a repair early in infancy.

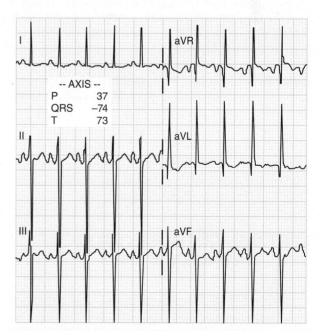

FIGURE 19-5 Classic electrocardiogram for a patient with complete atrioventricular canal. Notice that the QRS axis derived from these limb leads is −78°.

Management

Initial management in the past was PAB placement in infancy because of the poor results in infancy from CAVC defect repair.[64] Now, with improved techniques, surgery occurs predominantly in infancy without the need for a PAB. In the setting of a CAVC defect, there is no reason to wait beyond the 3-month age group to repair if there is a large VSD, which will only cause pulmonary vascular disease, especially in the large subgroup of trisomy 21 patients with pulmonary resistance issues from the start.[57] A primum ASD with a cleft mitral valve can be corrected later in life, and the timing of surgery is dependent on the institution's practice. At the time of repair, the primum ASD and inlet VSD are repaired along with an associated lesion, with patching of the defects and repair of a cleft in the mitral valve. In the past, the CAVC defect was repaired late in infancy; however, improved morbidity and mortality associated with earlier repair supports the idea of not delaying surgical intervention.[65]

Outcome and Follow-up

Without surgery, the survival for CAVC defect is 54% at 6 months of age and 35% at 12 months of age, 15% reach 24 months, and 4% reach 5 years of age[66]; thus, surgery is recommended for the children at risk for florid heart failure as the pulmonary vascular resistance decreases and there are multiple shunts. Heart failure in combination and severe respiratory infections are the modes of death among patients with trisomy 21.[52] However, there is no difference in outcomes comparing the patients with trisomy 21 with the nonsyndromic patients for AVC defect, ASD, or VSD lesions, which eventually lead to more children with trisomy 21 having congenital heart disease surgery.[53,67] The operative mortality has decreased significantly,[68–70] from 25% before 1976 to less than 4% after 1987. Complications after repair include death, 1.6%; postpericardiotomy syndrome, 13%; atrial arrhythmia, 3%; transient heart block, 1.6% to 3.5%; sternal wound infection, 0.5%; and left hemiparesis, 0.5%.[55,70] The 10-year survival is 98% in patients with AVC repair.[55] Some patients will require reintervention for mitral valve regurgitation (4%–7%)[70,71] or LVOT obstruction.

LEFT VENTRICULAR OUTFLOW TRACT ABNORMALITIES

Aortic Stenosis

The aortic valve in patients with aortic stenosis can have a variable morphology, appearing dysplastic, thickened, bicuspid, or hypoplastic. As a result of this aortic valve disease, neonates tend to present with variable degrees of obstruction; however, it is rare for infants to have significant aortic insufficiency without intervention. The presentation of aortic stenosis can be variable and depends on the degree of obstruction. In the most severe examples, the neonate is ductal dependent for systemic blood flow because of inadequate output from the left ventricle, and there is retrograde flow from the ductus arteriosus and aortic arch that feeds the brachiocephalic vessels and descending aorta. This clinical presentation is an example of critical aortic stenosis; however, much milder forms of aortic stenosis render the neonate asymptomatic.

Epidemiology

Aortic stenosis represents approximately 6% of all congenital heart disease and occurs in 6 of 10,000 live births.[72] Twenty-five percent of cases will also have a fibrous or muscular subaortic stenosis associated with the aortic stenosis. Rarely, this condition can be associated with pulmonary stenosis, especially in the setting of congenital rubella syndrome.[73] Genetic syndromes are also known to be associated with aortic stenosis and include Turner, Goltz, Costello, and Williams syndrome. If these genetic syndromes are suspected, an evaluation for aortic stenosis and other congenital heart disease should be initiated.

Pathophysiology

As discussed, the presentation of aortic stenosis will vary depending on the degree of obstruction, which can be mild to severe. The aortic valve leaflets typically are bicuspid and thickened with a decrease in cross-sectional area and can have associated supravalvar or subvalvar narrowing. Because of the obstruction to the aortic valve, the left ventricle can be hypertrophied in accordance with the degree of stenosis. In some cases with severe obstruction, the left ventricle begins to fail, resulting in a dilated ventricle with diminished systolic function. As a result of the high afterload, there can be endocardial fibroelastosis, which can impair both systolic and diastolic function of the left ventricle. With impaired diastolic function, the left ventricle fails to relax, resulting in high end-diastolic pressure and thus high left atrial and pulmonary arterial pressure from the back pressure.

The other common associated lesions include patent ductus arteriosus, coarctation of the aorta, VSD, ASD, mitral stenosis, and Shone's complex.[73,74] Shone's complex is a heart condition with multiple left heart obstruction lesions that traditionally include parachute mitral valve (single papillary muscle), supravalvar mitral ring, congenital mitral stenosis, subaortic stenosis (and valvar aortic stenosis), and coarctation of the aorta. Eight percent of patients with aortic stenosis have Shone's complex.[75] Often with Shone's complex, the left ventricle is deemed inadequate to handle the work of the systemic circulation, and the neonate must undergo a Norwood procedure for hypoplastic left heart syndrome.

Approximately 63% of the time, however, there is no associated pathology. As a result of the high left atrial pressure from decreased relaxation, there can be associated pulmonary hypertension 7% of the time.[75]

Neonates with aortic stenosis will present with the symptoms of congestive heart failure only if there is a significant amount of obstruction across the valve, and they can have tachypnea, diaphoresis, feeding difficulties, and failure to thrive. On physical examination, there should be a systolic ejection murmur that radiates to the neck with or without an associated thrill. A click should accompany the murmur because there is valvar involvement while the apical impulse will be increased.[73,76] Patients with even mild aortic stenosis should have the murmur findings but would probably be asymptomatic; however, patients with significant obstruction may also have a narrow pulse pressure.[73]

Differential Diagnosis

Neonates with critical aortic stenosis tend to be very ill and present in shock unless the ductus arteriosus is open and there is retrograde flow from the descending aorta to the ascending aorta. Thus, any lesion in the neonate that can cause symptoms of shock should be present in the differential diagnosis, such as sepsis, severe anemia, or hypovolemic shock from blood loss. In addition, any cardiac condition that is ductal dependent for systemic blood flow can present similarly, such as coarctation of the aorta, hypoplastic left heart syndrome, or aortic arch interruption.

The neonate with aortic stenosis who is not ductal dependent for systemic blood flow may still have severe aortic stenosis and would present with a heart murmur. The location of the heart murmur should be at the right upper sternal border with radiation to the neck; however, this distinction may be difficult in the neonate with faster heart rates and smaller chests. Thus, pulmonary stenosis may be confused with the diagnosis of aortic stenosis. Also, valvar aortic stenosis would present with the same type of murmur as supravalvar aortic stenosis or subvalvar aortic stenosis given the location of turbulent blood flow. However, valvar aortic stenosis is accompanied by a click, which should be absent in the last 2.

Diagnostic Tests

On ECG, the neonate may have ECG features of left ventricular hypertrophy with a strain pattern. This feature on the ECG would be unusual because most neonates have right-dominant forces. A chest x-ray in a patient with severe aortic stenosis would have a cardiothoracic ratio greater than 50% and would not necessarily have poststenotic dilation of the ascending

aorta.[72,73] Again, both of these tests would be nonspecific, and the echocardiogram would provide more definitive information, such as aortic valve thickening, bicuspid aortic valve, patent ductus arteriosus, aortic arch issues, or coarctation (Figure 19-6). Some features of the aortic valve, mitral valve, endocardial fibrosis, and left ventricle size help determine if the neonate has merely severe aortic stenosis or features of hypoplastic left heart syndrome.[77,78] In addition,

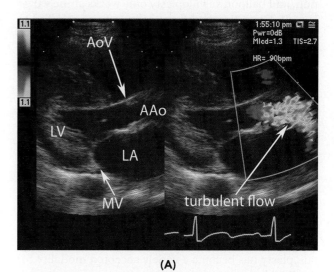

(A)

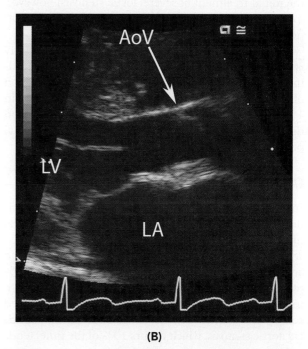

(B)

FIGURE 19-6 A, Parasternal echocardiogram for a patient with aortic stenosis. Note the turbulent flow entering the ascending aorta (AAo) with a mosaic color Doppler pattern after the aortic valve (AoV). The left ventricle (LV) has hypertrophy from the aortic stenosis. **B,** Close-up of the AoV shows thickened and doming leaflets in the same patient. LA, left atrium; MV, mitral valve, which is closed.

Doppler techniques define the aortic valve gradient, which aids in the management of this lesion.

Management

The mainstay of treatment of either critical or severe aortic stenosis with a normal-size left ventricle and no significant mitral valve disease is balloon aortic valvuloplasty as opposed to surgical valvotomy. Aortic valve stenosis is the most common type of LVOT obstruction, and balloon valvuloplasty only works at the valvar level.[79] The efficacy and mortality rate are similar to surgical techniques without the need of cardiopulmonary bypass and sternotomy.[80] The aortic valve gradient improves to acceptable levels without severe aortic insufficiency in most cases. Critical aortic stenosis is defined as enough left ventricular outflow obstruction such that the neonate is ductal dependent for systemic blood flow, an indication for balloon valvuloplasty. Severe aortic stenosis presentation and management strategies, however, vary. Nonetheless, the guidelines for valvuloplasty in severe aortic stenosis are a peak systolic gradient by echocardiographic Doppler techniques of 75 mm Hg, presence of strain on ECG, syncope, angina pectoris, fatigue with exercise, or severe left ventricular dysfunction.[81] Thus, balloon aortic valvuloplasty has become a widely accepted modality for the initial treatment of severe aortic stenosis; however, more complicated cases may require direct visualization with surgery.[82-87]

A major complication from balloon valvuloplasty is aortic wall injury, specifically creation of an intimal flap, which is an underrecognized complication of neonatal balloon aortic valvuloplasty, occurring in 15% of cases even in the recent era.[88] Repeat balloon dilation may be necessary, especially in the neonatal period with the risk of increasing aortic regurgitation.

Outcome and Follow-up

In cases of aortic stenosis for which there is heart failure in patients under the age of 18 months, the natural history is that 72% of these patients die.[73] Untreated severe aortic stenosis also has a poor prognosis.[76] Mild aortic stenosis still needs follow-up because only 20% of patients with mild aortic valve stenosis remain with mild symptoms into adulthood and may likely need some form of intervention.[89] In general, neonatal critical aortic stenosis, which occurs 10% of the time, tends to have a worse prognosis.[90]

Other factors also influence prognosis and increase mortality in severe aortic stenosis and include small aortic annulus, depressed systolic function, low aortic valve gradient, and endocardial fibroelastosis.[86] In addition, the size of the aortic valve and mitral valve calls into question the possibility of whether the left ventricle is suitable as a systemic pump given the relatively smaller size. Thus, some studies have investigated the use of certain morphologic characteristics of the left heart structures to determine if a single ventricle or biventricular physiology is superior.[77,91]

In those patients who are deemed to be amenable to an aortic balloon valvuloplasty, the prognosis is good, with about two-thirds of the patients needing no further surgical intervention 10 years after intervention.[81] Mortality is predominantly limited to the neonatal period around the time of aortic valve intervention. Beyond this period, mortality is nearly absent; however, many may require reintervention at some point for either recurrent aortic stenosis or aortic insufficiency from the balloon valvuloplasty.[92] The rate of progression of the aortic valve gradient tends to be slow over time.[92] Sudden death after balloon aortic valvuloplasty is extremely low, at 18 of 100,000 patient-years in children over 4 years of age.[93]

Coarctation of the Aorta

The coarctation of the aorta represents a narrowing in the aortic arch, typically beyond the left subclavian artery near the ductus arteriosus. Usually, there is a localized, narrow, constrictive lesion that appears as an infolding of the aortic media into the lumen.[94] As a result of this obstruction, neonates can present with shock from the lack of blood flow into the descending aorta to just a murmur with some systemic hypertension. Diminished lower-extremity pulses are the hallmark of this lesion and are the best, most reliable method of detecting it. Given that patients with aortic coarctation can present in shock, the clinician managing neonates should always attempt to detect this lesion.

Epidemiology

Coarctation is 1 of the 4 most common cardiac malformations, representing 14.8% of cardiac lesions.[95] As a frame of reference, VSD occurs 18% and transposition occurs 16% of the time in the same series.[95] Approximately 50% of deaths from neonatal coarctation occur after 7 days of life, and it is rare the first 2 days of life.[95] Noncardiac anomalies associated coarctation which include urinary tract malformations and tracheoesophageal fistula. The natural history of aortic coarctation is that 60% will die during infancy, with only 1 additional cardiac lesion, while 76% die if there are multiple cardiac defects.[94]

Simple coarctation occurs 61% of the time if there is no associated lesion. Complex coarctation with a VSD occurs 33% of the time; the remaining 6% of coarctation lesions are more complicated lesions.[96] One of the more common genetic syndromes associated with aortic coarctation is Turner syndrome.[97]

Pathophysiology

The primary issue in neonates with critical coarctation of the aorta is the ventricular dysfunction and shock that accompany the lack of cardiac output distal to the obstruction, leading to metabolic acidosis. Neonates do not present with symptoms usually until after 48 hours of life because the ductus arteriosus is protective and allows for distal perfusion.[95] The ductus arteriosus, with the blood flow from the right ventricle, usually supplies the descending aorta distal to the obstruction, and when the ductus arteriosus closes, the obstruction to the aortic arch is unmasked. Another mechanism of obstruction is where the aortic arch has an associated sling of ductal tissue that forms a ring around the aorta.[98] When the ductus arteriosus closes, the aortic arch becomes obstructed.

In 1 series, all infants with coarctation develop signs of congestive heart failure by 6 months of age; however, there are other series in which patients do not present until later with systemic hypertension.[94] Usually, in addition to the aortic isthmus obstruction, there is tubular hypoplasia of the distal transverse arch in a majority of neonatal coarctation.[94,98] Rarer forms of coarctation can occur between the left common carotid and left subclavian artery as well as the abdominal aorta.[99] The former will give rise to discrepant arm blood pressures, while an abdominal aorta coarctation will appear similar to the standard isthmus coarctation on physical examination.

Complex coarctation can occur with a VSD, ASD, or aortic stenosis.[94] Often, the aortic valve will be malformed, with a dysplastic or bicuspid aortic valve.[99] The VSD with aortic coarctation is often a posterior malalignment type, which can lead to subaortic obstruction and a somewhat smaller aortic valve. Coarctation can also occur with AVC defects, as previously described in this chapter.[99] Other reported associations include double-outlet right ventricle and complete transposition.[100]

Bicuspid aortic valve with fusion of the left and right coronary cusps is associated with coarctation, while those with right noncoronary fusion are associated with severe aortic stenosis and valve dysfunction.[101] Both forms of bicuspid aortic valve are associated with aortic root dilation, but this is more common in the latter form.[101] Bicuspid aortic valve with coarctation tends to have less aortic root dilation over time compared to isolated bicuspid aortic valve.[102]

Neonates who present with coarctation of the aorta tend to have symptoms of tachypnea, respiratory distress, and feeding intolerance.[103–105] As mentioned, coarctation of the aorta symptoms develop usually after the ductus arteriosus begins to close. With the development of symptoms, the pulses will be diminished or absent on physical examination. There will be radial-to-femoral delay in pulses. In critical coarctation of the aorta, the lower-extremity pulses will have lower oxygen saturations compared to upper-extremity pulses because the less-oxygenated blood of the right ventricle supplies the descending aorta. However, this may not be appreciable in the setting of a VSD because there can be left-to-right shunting that increases the ductal oxygen saturations. Upper- and lower-extremity blood pressure should be obtained whenever coarctation of the aorta is suspected to confirm a decrease in the lower-extremity blood pressure.

For neonates with coarctation that is not severe or critical, the presenting sign may be merely diminished pulses and upper-extremity hypertension. Upper- and lower-extremity blood pressure would also be discrepant in milder forms of coarctation.

Differential Diagnosis

Because shock and metabolic acidosis may be the presenting symptoms of coarctation, any disease process that can give those types of symptoms ought to be ruled out, such as sepsis, severe anemia, hypovolemic shock from blood loss, or other metabolic processes. Again, neonates with hypoplastic left heart syndrome and critical coarctation will also present in shock as a result of ductal closure and should be included in the differential diagnosis as well.

Diagnostic Tests

The physical examination is the single most important diagnostic test for coarctation with the presentation of absent or weak pulses. An ECG may demonstrate right axis deviation with right ventricular hypertrophy in 63% to 73% of cases[94]; however, this test is nonspecific. Echocardiography accurately detects coarctation of the aorta using suprasternal notch imaging[99]; however, the presence of a bicuspid aortic valve or VSD should provide some clues for coarctation as well. Computed tomographic (CT) angiography can provide excellent visualization of the aortic arch and coarctation when ultrasound imaging is deficient or the arch anatomy is complicated (Figure 19-7). With modern fetal echocardiography, the prenatal diagnosis of coarctation is feasible; however, the normal presence of the ductus arteriosus makes the diagnosis difficult.[96]

Management

The initial management strategy in the most severe forms of coarctation is to reverse the congestive heart failure and reverse metabolic acidosis, especially when neonates present in shock. Mechanical ventilation aids with removing the work of breathing. Most important, prostaglandin E_1 (PGE_1) should be used to dilate

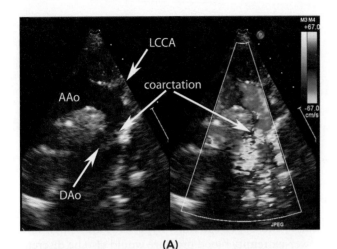

FIGURE 19-7 A, Suprasternal notch imaging of a coarctation is demonstrated by echocardiography. Notice the color flow disturbance and narrowing at the coarctation site after the ascending aorta (AAo) and before the descending aorta (Dao). **B,** Computed tomographic angiogram in the sagittal plane for a different patient demonstrates a discrete coarctation of the aorta after the take-off of the head and neck vessels. BCA, brachiocephalic artery; LCCA, left common carotid artery.

the ductus arteriosus, improve systemic output, and increase renal blood flow and urine output. Thus, as the ductus arteriosus opens, the ductal sling around the aorta opens, and the right ventricle can help with supplying descending aorta flow with right-to-left

ductal shunting. Surgery is used in the neonatal period to avoid systemic hypertension even with milder forms of coarctation. Unrepaired, there can also be left ventricular failure, myocardial fibrosis, or death. If the ductus arteriosus does not open in critical coarctation despite high-dose PGE_1 therapy, urgent surgery will become necessary because there is a failure in medical management. In neonates who present with shock and the ductus opens, time should be provided to allow for end-organ recovery from the shock.

The surgical treatment of coarctation has evolved from the subclavian flap to the end-to-end anastomosis and synthetic graft to fix coarctation.[106,107] Most centers elect to perform an extended end-end or an end-to-side anastomosis.[108,109] With modern techniques, the recoarctation rate is much less at less than 6% (Figure 19-8).[108-110]

Balloon angioplasty of native coarctation is not a great option because of the residual coarctation, greater than 20 mm Hg in 38% of patients.[111] In addition, this technique does not address distal hypoplasia of the arch, and there can be an intimal tear in 2.5%, resulting in aneurysm formation.[111-113] After surgical repair, echocardiogram Doppler techniques along with 4-limb blood pressure measurements can be used to assess the surgical repair.

Outcome and Follow-up

Medical management alone is inadequate, and there is no survival for critical coarctation with additional defects.[94] However, even with critically ill patients treated with PGE_1, mechanical ventilation, and catecholamines, at least 84% survive to at least 24 months.[114]

After surgical repair, many complications may arise and include spinal cord injury, left hemidiaphragm paralysis, left vocal cord paralysis, weak left radial pulse (subclavian flap-type repair), scoliosis about 3 years after surgery,[115] and residual systemic hypertension.[103,116,117] Persistent residual systemic hypertension is highly unlikely for neonates.[103,116] The mortality rate is low even when the neonate presents with shock and severe metabolic acidosis and is typically less than 5% in more recent series.[109,118,119]

Aortic Arch Interruption

The aortic arch interruption lesion, like the double-outlet right ventricle, tetralogy of Fallot, or transposition of the great vessels, is thought of as a conotruncal abnormality. The aortic arch can be completely interrupted in 3 primary locations between the left subclavian artery and the descending aorta (type A), the left common carotid artery and the left subclavian artery (type B), and the right innominate artery and the left common carotid artery (Figure 19-9). Type A

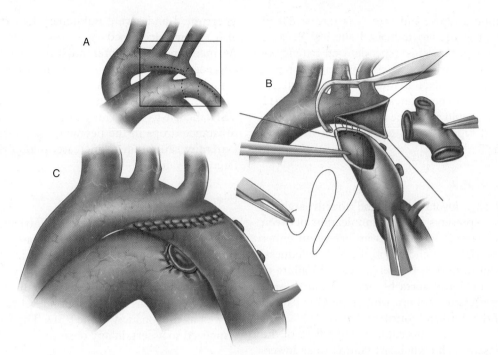

FIGURE 19-8 Diagram of a typical coarctation of the aorta repair before surgery (A), during resection of the narrowing (B), and the final extended end-to-end anastomosis (C). (Reproduced with permission from Dodge-Khatami et al.[161])

interruption could represent the most severe form of aortic coarctation given its location. In coarctation, there is some prograde flow across the narrowing, and in interruption, there is no communication between the vessels. Because there is no communication between the proximal and distal arch, a patent ductus arteriosus must be present to supply the distal perfusion. If the ductus arteriosus were to close in neonates with aortic arch interruption, profound shock and metabolic acidosis would ensue. The lower-extremity

oxygen saturation tends to be decreased when compared to the right upper extremity because deoxygenated blood arises from the right ventricle, which pumps to the ductus arteriosus and feeds the distal arch.

Epidemiology

Type B aortic arch interruption between the left common carotid and left subclavian artery is the most common form of arch interruption at 67%.[120] Type A

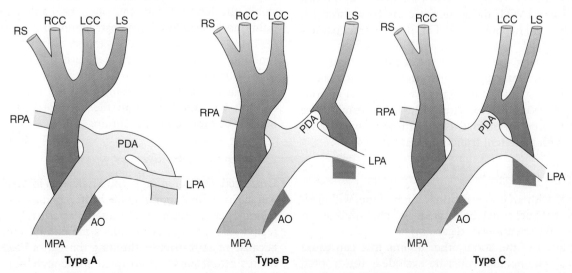

FIGURE 19-9 Types of aortic arch interruption. AO, aorta; LCC, left common carotid; LPA, left pulmonary artery; MPA, main pulmonary artery; PDA, patent ductus arteriosus; RCC, right common carotid; RPA, right pulmonary artery. (Reproduced with permission from Kinsley et al.[136])

is less common at 25%, and type C is rare at 8%.[120] The advent of PGE$_1$ has increased survival because lower-extremity perfusion is dependent on patency of the ductus arteriosus[121]; otherwise, surgery to repair the arch must take place before the ductus arteriosus closes. Like all conotruncal abnormalities, 22q11 microdeletion should always be considered and is present in 82% of type B but is less common in type A interruption.[122,123]

Pathophysiology

Embryologically, involution of the fourth arch in utero, which represents the communication between the common carotid and subclavian artery on either the left or the right depending on the arch sidedness, is the mechanism of type B interruption.[124] Failure of the left or right dorsal aorta beyond the fourth arch creates a type A interruption, while type C is caused by failure of the third and fourth arches.

Neonates with arch interruption, regardless of the type, will present with early heart failure, weak lower-extremity pulses, strong carotid pulses, and differential cyanosis from the desaturated blood exiting the right ventricle and supplying the lower extremities via a ductus arteriosus. Often with arch interruption, the right subclavian artery can arise anomalously and also be the ductus arteriosus, resulting in lower oxygen saturation in all limbs compared to the cerebral saturation.

There is almost always a ductus arteriosus to supply the lower-extremity perfusion; however, there are case reports of collateral flow from the vertebral arteries and thyrocervical trunk.[125] In 94% of cases, there is a large, posterior malalignment-type VSD[126]; there are also case reports of direct connections between the aorta and pulmonary artery, also known as an aortopulmonary window, and no VSD.[127–129] Most important, as a result of a narrow LVOT, the aortic valve can be malformed, bicuspid, and hypoplastic.[130] This outflow tract pathology may lead to severe subaortic or aortic stenosis, which can alter the management of these patients significantly. An interrupted aortic arch is also associated with mitral stenosis/atresia, persistent truncus arteriosus, or double-outlet right ventricle. The mortality rate for arch interruption increases significantly when associated with persistent truncus arteriosus.[131]

Differential Diagnosis

Patients with arch interruption, if left alone, will present with shock, metabolic acidosis, and diminished pulses. As mentioned regarding aortic stenosis or coarctation of the aorta, other lesions that can cause shock in the neonate must be excluded. Interrupted aortic arch has an interesting diagnostic feature of differential cyanosis as well; however, this is not necessarily unique because severe coarctation that is nearly interrupted and severe pulmonary hypertension may also show decreased lower-extremity saturation. As mentioned, the differential cyanosis may not be appreciable if the right subclavian artery also arises below the interruption and all extremities are fed by the ductus arteriosus. In addition, because there is a VSD, the left-to-right shunt as the pulmonary vascular resistance drops in the neonate may cause the lower-extremity saturation to increase, minimizing any differential cyanosis.

Diagnostic Tests

An ECG may show left or right ventricular hypertrophy; the chest x-ray may demonstrate cardiomegaly with increased pulmonary vascular markings. Both findings would be nonspecific and not diagnostic. Echocardiography is the mainstay of diagnosis even in fetal life.[132] The arch interruption level can be defined as well as the location of the VSD. The LVOT can be visualized to ascertain any obstruction or hypoplasia.

Management

Once the diagnosis of aortic arch obstruction has been identified, PGE$_1$ can be initiated to ensure adequate systemic perfusion. PGE$_1$ therapy can be accompanied by fever, irritability, hypotension, or apnea. Thus, the clinician should search for these side effects. Given the presence of a VSD and runoff diastolic flow into the branch pulmonary arteries from the ductus arteriosus, neonates can quickly develop pulmonary edema. Therefore, surgical intervention should not be delayed too long because of this complication.

The surgical procedure involves an aortic arch reconstruction and repairing any VSD or subaortic obstruction.[133,134] If the LVOT is deemed to be too small, the left ventricle can often be baffled to the pulmonary valve to relieve obstruction, and a conduit from the right ventricle to pulmonary arteries would function as the right ventricular outflow. This procedure with the arch reconstruction is not as ideal as repairing the arch and closing the VSD because the conduit will not grow with the neonate and would need to be replaced in the future.

Outcome and Follow-up

Untreated, 80% of infants with aortic arch interruption will die in the first month of life.[135] If a child survives the infancy period because of a ductus arteriosus, uncorrected Eisenmenger syndrome is the natural outcome because of unrestrictive shunting through a VSD and ductus arteriosus.[136] Interrupted aortic arch with subaortic obstruction is a more complicated lesion because of residual subaortic obstruction or the complex baffling the left ventricular flow to the pulmonary valve.

In fact, this combination of defects is met with 13% mortality and risk for need of reoperation.[134,137] However, with modern techniques and the advent of PGE_1, the operative mortality of all aortic arch interruption has decreased dramatically from 65% to less than 5%.[138–140] Most heart centers now advocate for a single-stage repair approach.[140,141]

RIGHT VENTRICULAR OUTFLOW TRACT ABNORMALITY

Pulmonary Stenosis

As with aortic stenosis, pulmonary stenosis is a result of a malformed, dysplastic, thickened, or bicuspid pulmonary valve. The clinical manifestations vary significantly from just a heart murmur to critical pulmonary stenosis by which the neonate is dependent on a patent ductus arteriosus for pulmonary blood flow. Management strategies will depend mostly on the degree of obstruction across the right ventricular outflow tract.

Epidemiology

The frequency of pulmonary stenosis is similar to that of aortic stenosis, occurring in 6 of 10,000 live births and 6 of 100 live births with congenital heart disease.[72] In the past, there was a high association with congenital rubella syndrome, for which there can be multiple levels of obstruction at the pulmonary valve, main pulmonary artery, or the branches.[142] Genetic syndromes are also heavily implicated with pulmonary stenosis, especially Williams and Noonan syndromes.[143] The valve is highly dysplastic when there is an associated genetic condition.

Pathophysiology

When there is severe obstruction as a result of pulmonary stenosis, the majority of neonates will have some degree of cyanosis, and some will have right ventricular failure as a result of the high afterload on the myocardium.[144] Because of severely elevated right ventricular end-diastolic pressure from the pulmonary stenosis and sometimes somewhat hypoplastic tricuspid valves, neonates will frequently shunt right to left across a patent foramen ovale, which (although it causes cyanosis) also allows the left ventricle to fill. Some neonates will have a true secundum ASD in association with pulmonary valve stenosis. As a result of pulmonary stenosis, older children may have dilation of the main pulmonary artery; however, this is unlikely in a neonate or infant.[144]

The pulmonary valve is supposed to have 3 thin mobile leaflets with excellent excursion; however, with pulmonary stenosis, the leaflets may dome in systole with fusion of the cusps or have a pinhole orifice,

resulting in right ventricular hypertrophy and near obliteration of the cavity.[145] As a result of the pulmonary stenosis, the infundibulum will also hypertrophy, which can lead to subpulmonary valve obstruction as well. In fact, the most severe form of pulmonary stenosis would be atresia of the pulmonary valve with an intact ventricular septum. This particular lesion can have a similar presentation to critical pulmonary stenosis with a pinhole orifice. Despite all of the pathology associated with the pulmonary valve, it is rare to have significant pulmonary insufficiency in the neonatal period.[72]

Neonates will present quickly with dyspnea, feeding difficulties, hepatomegaly, and a harsh systolic ejection-type murmur with a thrill if there is severe pulmonary stenosis.[145] In fact, the right ventricular pressure can be above systemic levels as a result of pulmonary stenosis. Despite the high afterload on the right ventricle, rarely do newborns or infants present with edema.[145] Neonates with mild-to-moderate pulmonary stenosis will in all likelihood be relatively asymptomatic.[72]

Differential Diagnosis

The murmur of aortic stenosis may sound similar to that of pulmonary stenosis; however, in the latter there is radiation of the murmur to the back. If there is significant obstruction, the clinician must differentiate this lesion from cyanotic congenital heart disease, which is discussed in another chapter. If there is significant obstruction, the tricuspid valve regurgitation may also be audible and would be holosystolic. Given that there can be a paucity of pulmonary vascular markings and an increase in right ventricular forces in neonates with severe pulmonary stenosis, this lesion must be differentiated from pulmonary hypertension.

Diagnostic Tests

The classic ECG findings in neonates with severe pulmonary stenosis would include right atrial enlargement and right ventricular hypertrophy with voltages exceeding 20 mm; however, the ECG can be normal in milder forms of the disease.[144,145] As discussed previously, the chest x-ray can demonstrate cardiomegaly with decreased pulmonary vascular markings; however, the enlargement of the main pulmonary artery from poststenotic dilation may not be apparent until after infancy.[144]

The echocardiogram is the mainstay for the diagnosis, can provide accurate Doppler-derived pulmonary stenosis gradients, and can provide an anatomic view of the pulmonary valve.[146] The gradient by echo correlates well with the cardiac catheterization-derived pressure gradient[146] ($r = 0.98$). Of note, careful attention should be placed on the pulmonary and tricuspid valve annulus size to see if surgical or cardiac catheterization interventions would be successful.

Management

Even in the early surgical era, the mortality rate for pulmonary valve repair was low at 4%.[144] Management has been altered, however, with the advent of advanced interventional cardiac techniques (Figure 19-10). Pulmonary valvuloplasty has become the standard of care for patients with critical pulmonary stenosis, with great short- and long-term results. Surgery should be reserved for those patients with a hypoplastic tricuspid valve and right ventricle.[147–153] In these cases with hypoplastic right ventricle associated with severe pulmonary stenosis, an aortopulmonary shunt may be necessary with a single- or "1.5-ventricle" repair strategy in the future.[154]

The advantage of balloon intervention is that there is no need for cardiopulmonary bypass, blood products, and sternotomy. Results are variable when the pulmonary valve is very dysplastic and thickened, however.[148,149] The mechanism by which balloon valvuloplasty works is by splitting the commissural fusion of the pulmonary valve and thereby relieving the stenosis.[149]

Outcome and Follow-up

Survival has improved with the advent of PGE_1 as a part of therapy to augment pulmonary blood flow in cases of critical pulmonary stenosis. Patients with critical pulmonary stenosis have not done well in the past prior to the use of PGE_1 therapy.[155] Severe pulmonary stenosis is a grave condition, leading to death if no intervention is conducted early in life.[144,145]

In 1 large series of 68 patients with pulmonary stenosis but no congestive heart failure or cyanosis, pulmonary stenosis was unlikely to progress, and the patient generally had a good prognosis.[156] If pulmonary stenosis remains mild after 1 year of life, it is unlikely to progress, while moderate-to-severe pulmonary stenosis can worsen in severity.[156–158] At older ages, it is unlikely for mild pulmonary stenosis to progress. In fact, there are cases of a natural cure for mild pulmonary stenosis by which the gradient across the valve goes away.[159]

After pulmonary valvuloplasty, there might still be right-to-left shunting across an atrial communication despite adequate relief of the pulmonary outflow obstruction because the right ventricular end-diastolic pressure might be high from impaired right ventricular compliance.[155] However, as the obstruction is most often relieved with adequate balloon dilation, the right ventricle relaxes over time, and the cyanosis improves.

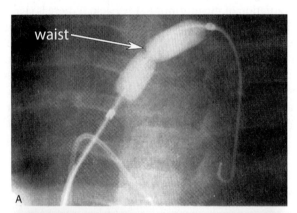

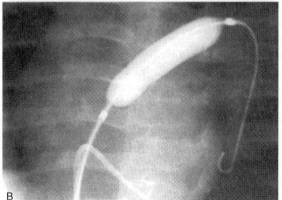

FIGURE 19-10 Balloon angioplasty of the pulmonary valve using cardiac catheterization. The waist represents the narrowing within the pulmonary valve (A), which disappears (B). (Reproduced with permission from Kan et al.[148])

REFERENCES

1. Garne E. Atrial and ventricular septal defects—epidemiology and spontaneous closure. *J Matern Fetal Neonatal Med.* 2006;19:271–276.
2. Marelli AJ, Mackie AS, Ionescu-Ittu R, Rahme E, Pilote L. Congenital heart disease in the general population: changing prevalence and age distribution. *Circulation.* 2007;115:163–172.
3. Reed WA, Dunn MI. Long-term results of repair of atrial septal defects. *Am J Surg.* 1971;121:724–727.
4. Hoffman JI, Christianson R. Congenital heart disease in a cohort of 19,502 births with long-term follow-up. *Am J Cardiol.* 1978;42:641–647.
5. Radzik D, Davignon A, van Doesburg N, Fournier A, Marchand T, Ducharme G. Predictive factors for spontaneous closure of atrial septal defects diagnosed in the first 3 months of life. *J Am Coll Cardiol.* 1993;22:851–853.
6. Riggs T, Sharp SE, Batton D, Hussey ME, Weinhouse E. Spontaneous closure of atrial septal defects in premature vs. full-term neonates. *Pediatr Cardiol.* 2000;21:129–134.
7. Takami T, Kawashima H, Kamikawa A, Takei Y, Miyajima T, Hoshika A. Characteristics of 11 neonates with atrial septal defects detected by heart murmurs. *Am J Perinatol.* 2003;20:195–199.
8. Azhari N, Shihata MS, Al-Fatani A. Spontaneous closure of atrial septal defects within the oval fossa. *Cardiol Young.* 2004;14:148–155.
9. Craig RJ, Selzer A. Natural history and prognosis of atrial septal defect. *Circulation.* 1968;37:805–815.
10. Spangler JG, Feldt RH, Danielson GK. Secundum atrial septal defect encountered in infancy. *J Thorac Cardiovasc Surg.* 1976;71:398–401.

11. Wyler F, Rutishauser M. Symptomatic atrial septal defect in the neonate and infant. *Helv Paediat Acta.* 1976;30:399–408.

12. Bull C, Deanfield J, de Leval M, Stark J, Taylor JF, Macartney FJ. Correction of isolated secundum atrial septal defect in infancy. *Arch Dis Child.* 1981;56:784–786.

13. Weyn AS, Bartle SH, Nolan TB, Dammann JF Jr. Atrial septal defect—primum type. *Circulation.* 1965;32:III13–III23.

14. Christensen DD, Vincent RN, Campbell RM. Presentation of atrial septal defect in the pediatric population. *Pediatr Cardiol.* 2005;26:812–814.

15. Zaver AG, Nadas AS. Atrial septal defect—secundum type. *Circulation.* 1965;32:III24–III32.

16. Tikkanen J, Heinonen OP. Risk factors for atrial septal defect. *Eur J Epidemiol.* 1992;8:509–515.

17. Reamon-Buettner SM, Borlak J. NKX2-5: an update on this hypermutable homeodomain protein and its role in human congenital heart disease (CHD). *Hum Mutat.* 2010;31:1185–1194.

18. Stallmeyer B, Fenge H, Nowak-Gottl U, Schulze-Bahr E. Mutational spectrum in the cardiac transcription factor gene NKX2.5 (CSX) associated with congenital heart disease. *Clin Genet.* 2010;78:533–540.

19. Phillips SJ, Okies JE, Henken D, Sunderland CO, Starr A. Complex of secundum atrial septal defect and congestive heart failure in infants. *J Thorac Cardiovasc Surg.* 1975;70:696–700.

20. Diab KA, Cao QL, Bacha EA, Hijazi ZM. Device closure of atrial septal defects with the Amplatzer septal occluder: safety and outcome in infants. *J Thorac Cardiovasc Surg.* 2007;134:960–966.

21. Cockerham JT, Martin TC, Gutierrez FR, Hartmann AF Jr, Goldring D, Strauss AW. Spontaneous closure of secundum atrial septal defect in infants and young children. *Am J Cardiol.* 1983;52:1267–1271.

22. Senocak F, Karademir S, Cabuk F, Onat N, Koc S, Duman A. Spontaneous closure of interatrial septal openings in infants: an echocardiographic study. *Int J Cardiol.* 1996;53:221–226.

23. Helgason H, Jonsdottir G. Spontaneous closure of atrial septal defects. *Pediatr Cardiol* 1999;20:195–199.

24. Saxena A, Divekar A, Soni NR. Natural history of secundum atrial septal defect revisited in the era of transcatheter closure. *Indian Heart J.* 2005;57:35–38.

25. Hanslik A, Pospisil U, Salzer-Muhar U, Greber-Platzer S, Male C. Predictors of spontaneous closure of isolated secundum atrial septal defect in children: a longitudinal study. *Pediatrics.* 2006;118:1560–1565.

26. Bostan OM, Cil E, Ercan I. The prospective follow-up of the natural course of interatrial communications diagnosed in 847 newborns. *Eur Heart J.* 2007;28:2001–2005.

27. Richardson JV, Schieken RM, Lauer RM, Stewart P, Doty DB. Repair of large ventricular septal defects in infants and small children. *Ann Surg.* 1982;195:318–322.

28. Eroglu AG, Oztunc F, Saltik L, Bakari S, Dedeoglu S, Ahunbay G. Evolution of ventricular septal defect with special reference to spontaneous closure rate, subaortic ridge and aortic valve prolapse. *Pediatr Cardiol.* 2003;24:31–35.

29. Kazmi U, Sadiq M, Hyder SN. Pattern of ventricular septal defects and associated complications. *J Coll Physicians Surg Pak* 2009;19:342–345.

30. Scully BB, Morales DL, Zafar F, McKenzie ED, Fraser CD Jr, Heinle JS. Current expectations for surgical repair of isolated ventricular septal defects. *Ann Thorac Surg.* 2010;89:544–549. discussion 550–551.

31. Hoffman JI, Rudolph AM. The natural history of ventricular septal defects in infancy. *Am J Cardiol.* 1965;16:634–653.

32. Varghese PJ, Rowe RD. Spontaneous closure of ventricular septal defects by aneurysmal formation of the membranous septum. *J Pediatr.* 1969;75:700–703.

33. Moe DG, Guntheroth WG. Spontaneous closure of uncomplicated ventricular septal defect. *Am J Cardiol.* 1987;60:674–678.

34. Fisher DJ, Snider AR, Silverman NH, Stanger P. Ventricular septal defect with silent discrete subaortic stenosis. *Pediatr Cardiol.* 1982;2:265–269.

35. Menahem S, Johns JA, del Torso S, Goh TH, Venables AW. Evaluation of aortic valve prolapse in ventricular septal defect. *Br Heart J.* 1986;56:242–249.

36. Corone P, Doyon F, Gaudeau S, et al. Natural history of ventricular septal defect. A study involving 790 cases. *Circulation.* 1977;55:908–915.

37. Hardin JT, Muskett AD, Canter CE, Martin TC, Spray TL. Primary surgical closure of large ventricular septal defects in small infants. *Ann Thorac Surg.* 1992;53:397–401.

38. Nygren A, Sunnegardh J, Berggren H. Preoperative evaluation and surgery in isolated ventricular septal defects: a 21 year perspective. *Heart.* 2000;83:198–204.

39. Paladini D, Palmieri S, Lamberti A, Teodoro A, Martinelli P, Nappi C. Characterization and natural history of ventricular septal defects in the fetus. *Ultrasound Obstet Gynecol.* 2000; 16:118–122.

40. Axt-Fliedner R, Schwarze A, Smrcek J, Germer U, Krapp M, Gembruch U. Isolated ventricular septal defects detected by color Doppler imaging: evolution during fetal and first year of postnatal life. *Ultrasound Obstet Gynecol.* 2006;27:266–273.

41. Henze A, Koul BL, Wallgren G, Settergren G, Bjork VO. Repair of ventricular septal defect in the first year of life. *Scand J Thorac Cardiovasc Surg.* 1984;18:151–154.

42. Doty DB, Lamberth WC. Repair of ventricular septal defects. *World J Surg.* 1985;9:516–521.

43. Monro JL, Keenan DJ, Keeton BR. Closure of ventricular septal defect through the pulmonary artery. *Pediatr Cardiol.* 1986;7:195–198.

44. Seddio F, Reddy VM, McElhinney DB, Tworetzky W, Silverman NH, Hanley FL. Multiple ventricular septal defects: how and when should they be repaired? *J Thorac Cardiovasc Surg.* 1999;117:134–139. discussion 139–140.

45. Bacha EA, Cao QL, Starr JP, Waight D, Ebeid MR, Hijazi ZM. Periventricular device closure of muscular ventricular septal defects on the beating heart: technique and results. *J Thorac Cardiovasc Surg.* 2003;126:1718–1723.

46. Michel-Behnke I, Ewert P, Koch A, Bertram H, Emmel M, Fischer G, et al. Device closure of ventricular septal defects by hybrid procedures: a multicenter retrospective study. *Catheter Cardiovasc Interv.* 2011;77:242–251.

47. Weidman WH, Blount SG Jr, DuShane JW, Gersony WM, Hayes CJ, Nadas AS. Clinical course in ventricular septal defect. *Circulation.* 1977;56:I56–I69.

48. Mehta AV, Chidambaram B. Ventricular septal defect in the first year of life. *Am J Cardiol.* 1992;70:364–366.

49. Collins G, Disenhouse R, Keith JD. Spontaneous closure of ventricular septal defect. *Can Med Assoc J.* 1969;100: 737–743.

50. Turner SW, Hunter S, Wyllie JP. The natural history of ventricular septal defects. *Arch Dis Child.* 1999;81:413–416.

51. Hiraishi S, Agata Y, Nowatari M, et al. Incidence and natural course of trabecular ventricular septal defect: two-dimensional echocardiography and color Doppler flow imaging study. *J Pediatr.* 1992;120:409–415.

52. Rowe RD, Uchida IA. Cardiac malformation in mongolism: a prospective study of 184 mongoloid children. *Am J Med.* 1961;31:726–735.

53. Baciewicz FA Jr, Melvin WS, Basilius D, Davis JT. Congenital heart disease in Down's syndrome patients: a decade of surgical experience. *Thorac Cardiovasc Surg.* 1989;37:369–371.

54. Vida VL, Barnoya J, Larrazabal LA, Gaitan G, de Maria Garcia F, Castaneda AR. Congenital cardiac disease in children with Down's syndrome in Guatemala. *Cardiol Young.* 2005; 15:286–290.

CHAPTER 19

55. Najm HK, Williams WG, Chuaratanaphong S, Watzka SB, Coles JG, Freedom RM. Primum atrial septal defect in children: early results, risk factors, and freedom from reoperation. *Ann Thorac Surg.* 1998;66:829–835.

56. Vergara P, Digilio MC, De Zorzi A, et al. Genetic heterogeneity and phenotypic anomalies in children with atrioventricular canal defect and tetralogy of Fallot. *Clin Dysmorphol.* 2006;15:65–70.

57. Clapp S, Perry BL, Farooki ZQ, et al. Down's syndrome, complete atrioventricular canal, and pulmonary vascular obstructive disease. *J Thorac Cardiovasc Surg.* 1990;100:115–121.

58. Lee CN, Danielson GK, Schaff HV, Puga FJ, Mair DD. Surgical treatment of double-orifice mitral valve in atrioventricular canal defects. Experience in 25 patients. *J Thorac Cardiovasc. Surg* 1985;90:700–705.

59. Anzai N, Yamada M, Tsuchida K, Yoshioka Y, Iida Y, Wakabayashi Y. Double orifice mitral valve associated with endocardial cushion defect. *Jpn Circ J.* 1986;50:455–458.

60. Prendergast B, Tometzki A, Mankad PS. Double-orifice right atrioventricular valve associated with partial atrioventricular septal defect. *Ann Thorac Surg.* 1996;62:893–895.

61. Ohta N, Sakamoto K, Kado M, et al. Surgical repair of double-orifice of the mitral valve in cases with an atrioventricular canal defects. *Jpn J Thorac Cardiovasc Surg.* 2001;49:656–659.

62. Reddy TD, Valderrama E, Bierman FZ. Images in cardiology. Atrioventricular septal defect with cor triatriatum. Heart. 2002;87:215.

63. Varma PK, Warrier G, Ramachandran P, et al. Partial atrioventricular canal defect with cor triatriatum sinister: report of three cases. *J Thorac Cardiovasc Surg.* 2004;127:572–573.

64. Silverman N, Levitsky S, Fisher E, DuBrow I, Hastreiter A, Scagliotti D. Efficacy of pulmonary artery banding in infants with complete atrioventricular canal. *Circulation.* 1983;68:II148–II153.

65. Frontera-Izquierdo P, Cabezuelo-Huerta G. Natural and modified history of complete atrioventricular septal defect—a 17 year study. *Arch Dis Child.* 1990;65:964–966. discussion 966–967.

66. Berger TJ, Blackstone EH, Kirklin JW, Bargeron LM Jr, Hazelrig JB, Turner ME Jr. Survival and probability of cure without and with operation in complete atrioventricular canal. *Ann Thorac Surg.* 1979;27:104–111.

67. Rizzoli G, Mazzucco A, Maizza F, et al. Does Down syndrome affect prognosis of surgically managed atrioventricular canal defects? *J Thorac Cardiovasc Surg.* 1992;104:945–953.

68. Bando K, Turrentine MW, Sun K, et al. Surgical management of complete atrioventricular septal defects. A twenty-year experience. *J Thorac Cardiovasc Surg.* 1995;110:1543–1552. discussion 1552–1554.

69. Tweddell JS, Litwin SB, Berger S, et al. Twenty-year experience with repair of complete atrioventricular septal defects. *Ann Thorac Surg.* 1996;62:419–424.

70. Hanley FL, Fenton KN, Jonas RA, et al. Surgical repair of complete atrioventricular canal defects in infancy. Twenty-year trends. *J Thorac Cardiovasc Surg.* 1993;106:387–394. discussion 394–397.

71. Backer CL, Mavroudis C, Alboliras ET, Zales VR. Repair of complete atrioventricular canal defects: results with the two-patch technique. *Ann Thorac Surg.* 1995;60:530–537.

72. Hoffman JI. The natural history of congenital isolated pulmonic and aortic stenosis. *Annu Rev Med.* 1969;20:15–28.

73. Peckham GB, Keith JD, Evans JR. Congenital aortic stenosis: some observations on the natural history and clinical assessment. *Can Med Assoc J.* 1964;91:639–643.

74. Shone JD, Sellers RD, Anderson RC, Adams P Jr, Lillehei CW, Edwards JE. The developmental complex of "parachute mitral valve," supravalvular ring of left atrium, subaortic stenosis, and coarctation of aorta. *Am J Cardiol.* 1963;11:714–725.

75. Brown DW, Dipilato AE, Chong EC, et al. Sudden unexpected death after balloon valvuloplasty for congenital aortic stenosis. *J Am Coll Cardiol.* 2010;56:1939–1946.

76. Lakier JB, Lewis AB, Heymann MA, Stanger P, Hoffman JI, Rudolph AM. Isolated aortic stenosis in the neonate. Natural history and hemodynamic considerations. *Circulation.* 1974;50:801–808.

77. Rhodes LA, Colan SD, Perry SB, Jonas RA, Sanders SP. Predictors of survival in neonates with critical aortic stenosis. *Circulation.* 1991;84:2325–2335.

78. Lofland GK, McCrindle BW, Williams WG, et al. Critical aortic stenosis in the neonate: a multi-institutional study of management, outcomes, and risk factors. Congenital Heart Surgeons Society. *J Thorac Cardiovasc Surg.* 2001;121:10–27.

79. Kitchiner D, Jackson M, Malaiya N, Walsh K, Peart I, Arnold R. Incidence and prognosis of obstruction of the left ventricular outflow tract in Liverpool (1960–91): a study of 313 patients. *Br Heart J.* 1994;71:588–595.

80. Zeevi B, Keane JF, Castaneda AR, Perry SB, Lock JE. Neonatal critical valvar aortic stenosis. A comparison of surgical and balloon dilation therapy. *Circulation.* 1989;80:831–839.

81. Fratz S, Gildein HP, Balling G, et al. Aortic valvuloplasty in pediatric patients substantially postpones the need for aortic valve surgery: a single-center experience of 188 patients after up to 17.5 years of follow-up. *Circulation.* 2008;117:1201–1206.

82. Moore P, Egito E, Mowrey H, Perry SB, Lock JE, Keane JF. Midterm results of balloon dilation of congenital aortic stenosis: predictors of success. *J Am Coll Cardiol.* 1996;27:1257–1263.

83. Egito ES, Moore P, O'Sullivan J, et al. Transvascular balloon dilation for neonatal critical aortic stenosis: early and midterm results. *J Am Coll Cardiol.* 1997;29:442–447.

84. O'Connor BK, Beekman RH, Rocchini AP, Rosenthal A. Intermediate-term effectiveness of balloon valvuloplasty for congenital aortic stenosis. A prospective follow-up study. *Circulation.* 1991;84:732–738.

85. Sholler GF, Keane JF, Perry SB, Sanders SP, Lock JE. Balloon dilation of congenital aortic valve stenosis. Results and influence of technical and morphological features on outcome. *Circulation.* 1988;78:351–360.

86. Agnoletti G, Raisky O, Boudjemline Y, et al. Neonatal surgical aortic commissurotomy: predictors of outcome and long-term results. *Ann Thorac Surg.* 2006;82:1585–1592.

87. Miyamoto T, Sinzobahamvya N, Wetter J, Kallenberg R, Brecher AM, Asfour B, et al. Twenty years experience of surgical aortic valvotomy for critical aortic stenosis in early infancy. *Eur J Cardiothorac Surg.* 2006;30:35–40.

88. Brown DW, Chong EC, Gauvreau K, Keane JF, Lock JE, Marshall AC. Aortic wall injury as a complication of neonatal aortic valvuloplasty: incidence and risk factors. *Circ Cardiovasc Interv.* 2008;1:53–59.

89. Kitchiner D, Jackson M, Walsh K, Peart I, Arnold R. The progression of mild congenital aortic valve stenosis from childhood into adult life. *Int J Cardiol.* 1993;42:217–223.

90. Brown JW, Ruzmetov M, Vijay P, Rodefeld MD, Turrentine MW. Surgery for aortic stenosis in children: a 40-year experience. *Ann Thorac Surg.* 2003;76:1398–1411.

91. Kovalchin JP, Brook MM, Rosenthal GL, Suda K, Hoffman JI, Silverman NH. Echocardiographic hemodynamic and morphometric predictors of survival after two-ventricle repair in infants with critical aortic stenosis. *J Am Coll Cardiol.* 1998;32:237–244.

92. Ten Harkel AD, Van Osch-Gevers M, Helbing WA. Real-time transthoracic three dimensional echocardiography: normal reference data for left ventricular dyssynchrony in adolescents. *J Am Soc Echocardiogr.* 2009;22:933–938.

93. Brown DW, Dipilato AE, Chong EC, Lock JE, McElhinney DB. Aortic valve reinterventions after balloon aortic

valvuloplasty for congenital aortic stenosis intermediate and late follow-up. *J Am Coll Cardiol.* 2010;56:1740–1749.

94. Sinha SN, Kardatzke ML, Cole RB, Muster AJ, Wessel HU, Paul MH. Coarctation of the aorta in infancy. *Circulation.* 1969;40:385–398.

95. Mehrizi A, Hirsch MS, Taussig HB. Congenital heart disease in the neonatal period: autopsy study of 170 cases. *J Pediatr.* 1964;65:721–726.

96. Carrico A, Moura C, Monterroso J, et al. Patients with aortic coarctation operated during the first year of life, different surgical techniques and prognostic factors—21 years of experience. *Rev Port Cardiol.* 2003;22:1185–1193.

97. Ravelo HR, Stephenson LW, Friedman S, et al. Coarctation resection in children with Turner's syndrome: a note of caution. *J Thorac Cardiovasc Surg.* 1980;80:427–430.

98. Ho SY, Anderson RH. Coarctation, tubular hypoplasia, and the ductus arteriosus. Histological study of 35 specimens. *Br Heart J.* 1979;41:268–274.

99. Smallhorn JF, Huhta JC, Adams PA, Anderson RH, Wilkinson JL, Macartney FJ. Cross-sectional echocardiographic assessment of coarctation in the sick neonate and infant. *Br Heart J.* 1983;50:349–361.

100. Kobayashi M, Ando M, Wada N, Takahashi Y. Outcomes following surgical repair of aortic arch obstructions with associated cardiac anomalies. *Eur J Cardiothorac Surg.* 2009;35:565–568.

101. Ciotti GR, Vlahos AP, Silverman NH. Morphology and function of the bicuspid aortic valve with and without coarctation of the aorta in the young. *Am J Cardiol.* 2006;98:1096–1102.

102. Beaton AZ, Nguyen T, Lai WW, et al. Relation of coarctation of the aorta to the occurrence of ascending aortic dilation in children and young adults with bicuspid aortic valves. *Am J Cardiol.* 2009;103:266–270.

103. Zehr KJ, Gillinov AM, Redmond JM, et al. Repair of coarctation of the aorta in neonates and infants: a thirty-year experience. *Ann Thorac Surg.* 1995;59:33–41.

104. Cobanoglu A, Thyagarajan GK, Dobbs JL. Surgery for coarctation of the aorta in infants younger than 3 months: end-to-end repair versus subclavian flap angioplasty: is either operation better? *Eur J Cardiothorac Surg.* 1998;14:19–25. discussion 25–26.

105. McElhinney DB, Yang SG, Hogarty AN, et al. Recurrent arch obstruction after repair of isolated coarctation of the aorta in neonates and young infants: is low weight a risk factor? *J Thorac Cardiovasc Surg.* 2001;122:883–890.

106. Beekman RH, Rocchini AP, Behrendt DM, et al. Long-term outcome after repair of coarctation in infancy: subclavian angioplasty does not reduce the need for reoperation. *J Am Coll Cardiol.* 1986;8:1406–1411.

107. Kino K, Sano S, Sugawara E, Kohmoto T, Kamada M. Late aneurysm after subclavian flap aortoplasty for coarctation of the aorta. *Ann Thorac Surg.* 1996;61:1262–1264.

108. Rajasinghe HA, Reddy VM, van Son JA, et al. Coarctation repair using end-to-side anastomosis of descending aorta to proximal aortic arch. *Ann Thorac Surg.* 1996;61:840–844.

109. Younoszai AK, Reddy VM, Hanley FL, Brook MM. Intermediate term follow-up of the end-to-side aortic anastomosis for coarctation of the aorta. *Ann Thorac Surg.* 2002;74:1631–1634.

110. Wright GE, Nowak CA, Goldberg CS, Ohye RG, Bove EL, Rocchini AP. Extended resection and end-to-end anastomosis for aortic coarctation in infants: results of a tailored surgical approach. *Ann Thorac Surg.* 2005;80:1453–1459.

111. Galal MO, Schmaltz AA, Joufan M, Benson L, Samatou L, Halees Z. Balloon dilation of native aortic coarctation in infancy. *Z Kardiol.* 2003;92:735–741.

112. Fiore AC, Fischer LK, Schwartz T, et al. Comparison of angioplasty and surgery for neonatal aortic coarctation. *Ann Thorac Surg.* 2005;80:1659–1664. discussion 1664–1665.

113. McGuinness JG, Elhassan Y, Lee SY, et al. Do high-risk infants have a poorer outcome from primary repair of coarctation? Analysis of 192 infants over 20 years. *Ann Thorac Surg.* 2010;90:2023–2027.

114. Quaegebeur JM, Jonas RA, Weinberg AD, Blackstone EH, Kirklin JW. Outcomes in seriously ill neonates with coarctation of the aorta. A multiinstitutional study. *J Thorac Cardiovasc Surg.* 1994;108:841–851. discussion 852–854.

115. Van Biezen FC, Bakx PA, De Villeneuve VH, Hop WC. Scoliosis in children after thoracotomy for aortic coarctation. *J Bone Joint Surg Am.* 1993;75:514–518.

116. Abdulla S, Malmgren N, Bjorkhem G, Lundstrom NR. A postoperative follow-up study of infantile coarctation of the aorta. *Acta Paediatr Suppl.* 1995;410:69–73.

117. Hjortdal VE, Khambadkone S, de Leval MR, Tsang VT. Implications of anomalous right subclavian artery in the repair of neonatal aortic coarctation. *Ann Thorac Surg.* 2003;76:572–575.

118. Hager A, Schreiber C, Nutzl S, Hess J. Mortality and restenosis rate of surgical coarctation repair in infancy: a study of 191 patients. *Cardiology.* 2009;112:36–41.

119. Fesseha AK, Eidem BW, Dibardino DJ, et al. Neonates with aortic coarctation and cardiogenic shock: presentation and outcomes. *Ann Thorac Surg.* 2005;79:1650–1655.

120. Schumacher G, Schreiber R, Meisner H, Lorenz HP, Sebening F, Buhlmeyer K. Interrupted aortic arch: natural history and operative results. *Pediatr Cardiol.* 1986;7:89–93.

121. Radford DJ, Bloom KR, Coceani F, Fariello R, Olley PM. Letter: Prostaglandin E1 for interrupted aortic arch in the neonate. *Lancet.* 1976;2:95.

122. Rauch A, Hofbeck M, Leipold G, et al. Incidence and significance of 22q11.2 hemizygosity in patients with interrupted aortic arch. *Am J Med Genet.* 1998;78:322–331.

123. Cuturilo G, Drakulic D, Stevanovic M, et al. A rare association of interrupted aortic arch type C and microdeletion 22q11.2. *Eur J Pediatr.* 2008;167:1195–1198.

124. Foley BV. Congenital interruption of the aortic arch. *Arch Dis Child.* 1958;33:131–133.

125. Morgan JR, Forker AD, Fosburg RG, Neugebauer MK, Rogers AK, Bemiller CR. Interruption of the aortic arch without a patent ductus arteriosus. *Circulation.* 1970;42:961–965.

126. Tawes RL Jr, Panagopoulos P, Aberdeen E, Waterston DJ, Bonham-Carter RE. Aortic arch atresia and interruption of the aortic arch. Experience in 11 cases of operation. *J Thorac Cardiovasc Surg.* 1969;58:492–501.

127. Chiemmongkoltip P, Moulder PV, Cassels DE. Interruption of the aortic arch with aortico-pulmonary septal defect and intact ventricular septum in a teenage girl. *Chest.* 1971;60:324–327.

128. Judez VM, Maitre MJ, De Artaza M, De Miguel JM, Valles F, Marquez J. Interruption of aortic arch without associated cardiac abnormalities. *Br Heart J.* 1974;36:313–317.

129. Ingram MT, Ott DA. Concomitant repair of aortopulmonary window and interrupted aortic arch. *Ann Thorac Surg.* 1992;53:909–911.

130. Ilbawi MN, Idriss FS, DeLeon SY, Muster AJ, Benson DW Jr, Paul MH. Surgical management of patients with interrupted aortic arch and severe subaortic stenosis. *Ann Thorac Surg.* 1988;45:174–180.

131. Konstantinov IE, Karamlou T, Blackstone EH, et al. Truncus arteriosus associated with interrupted aortic arch in 50 neonates: a Congenital Heart Surgeons Society study. *Ann Thorac Surg.* 2006;81:214–222.

132. Vogel M, Vernon MM, McElhinney DB, Brown DW, Colan SD, Tworetzky W. Fetal diagnosis of interrupted aortic arch. *Am J Cardiol.* 2010;105:727–734.

133. Suzuki Y, Kuga T, Minakawa M, Itaya H, Fukui K, Fukuda I. Surgical management of tunnel-like subaortic stenosis via ventricular septal defect in a patient with the interrupted aortic arch. *Jpn J Thorac Cardiovasc Surg.* 2004;52:480–483.

134. Suzuki T, Ohye RG, Devaney EJ, et al. Selective management of the left ventricular outflow tract for repair of interrupted aortic arch with ventricular septal defect: management of left ventricular outflow tract obstruction. *J Thorac Cardiovasc Surg.* 2006;131:779–784.

135. Roberts WC, Morrow AG, Braunwald E. Complete interruption of the aortic arch. *Circulation.* 1962;26:39–59.

136. Kinsley RH, Utian HL, Fuller DN, Marchand PE. Interruption of the aortic arch. *Thorax.* 1972;27:93–99.

137. Hirata Y, Quaegebeur JM, Mosca RS, Takayama H, Chen JM. Impact of aortic annular size on rate of reoperation for left ventricular outflow tract obstruction after repair of interrupted aortic arch and ventricular septal defect. *Ann Thorac Surg.* 2010;90:588–592.

138. Menahem S, Rahayoe AU, Brawn WJ, Mee RB. Interrupted aortic arch in infancy: a 10-year experience. *Pediatr Cardiol.* 1992;13:214–221.

139. Brown JW, Ruzmetov M, Okada Y, Vijay P, Rodefeld MD, Turrentine MW. Outcomes in patients with interrupted aortic arch and associated anomalies: a 20-year experience. *Eur J Cardiothorac Surg.* 2006;29:666–673. discussion 673–674.

140. Flint JD, Gentles TL, MacCormick J, Spinetto H, Finucane AK. Outcomes using predominantly single-stage approach to interrupted aortic arch and associated defects. *Ann Thorac Surg.* 2010;89:564–569.

141. Hussein A, Iyengar AJ, Jones B, et al. Twenty-three years of single-stage end-to-side anastomosis repair of interrupted aortic arches. *J Thorac Cardiovasc Surg.* 2010;139:942–947, 949; discussion 948.

142. Ellis JG, Kuzman WJ. Pulmonary artery stenosis, a frequent part of the congenital rubella syndrome. *Calif Med.* 1966;105:435–439.

143. Roberts N, Moes CA. Supravalvular pulmonary stenosis. *J Pediatr.* 1973;82:838–844.

144. Mustard WT, Jain SC, Trusler GA. Pulmonary stenosis in the first year of life. *Br Heart J.* 1968;30:255–257.

145. Anderson IM, Nouri-Moghaddam S. Severe pulmonary stenosis in infancy and early childhood. *Thorax.* 1969;24:312–326.

146. Lima CO, Sahn DJ, Valdes-Cruz LM, et al. Noninvasive prediction of transvalvular pressure gradient in patients with pulmonary stenosis by quantitative two-dimensional echocardiographic Doppler studies. *Circulation.* 1983;67:866–871.

147. Tynan M, Jones O, Joseph MC, Deverall PB, Yates AK. Relief of pulmonary valve stenosis in first week of life by percutaneous balloon valvuloplasty. *Lancet.* 1984;1:273.

148. Kan JS, White RI Jr, Mitchell SE, Anderson JH, Gardner TJ. Percutaneous transluminal balloon valvuloplasty for pulmonary valve stenosis. *Circulation.* 1984;69:554–560.

149. Rao PS. Balloon dilatation in infants and children with dysplastic pulmonary valves: short-term and intermediate-term results. *Am Heart J.* 1988;116:1168–1173.

150. Ballerini L, Mullins CE, Cifarelli A, et al. Percutaneous balloon valvuloplasty of pulmonary valve stenosis, dysplasia, and residual stenosis after surgical valvotomy for pulmonary atresia with intact ventricular septum: long-term results. *Cathet Cardiovasc Diagn.* 1990;19:165–169.

151. Melgares R, Prieto JA, Azpitarte J. Success determining factors in percutaneous transluminal balloon valvuloplasty of pulmonary valve stenosis. *Eur Heart J.* 1991;12:15–23.

152. Masura J, Burch M, Deanfield JE, Sullivan ID. Five-year follow-up after balloon pulmonary valvuloplasty. *J Am Coll Cardiol.* 1993;21:132–136.

153. Tabatabaei H, Boutin C, Nykanen DG, Freedom RM, Benson LN. Morphologic and hemodynamic consequences after percutaneous balloon valvotomy for neonatal pulmonary stenosis: medium-term follow-up. *J Am Coll Cardiol.* 1996;27:473–478.

154. Trowitzsch E, Colan SD, Sanders SP. Two-dimensional echocardiographic evaluation of right ventricular size and function in newborns with severe right ventricular outflow tract obstruction. *J Am Coll Cardiol.* 1985;6:388–393.

155. Coles JG, Freedom RM, Olley PM, Coceani F, Williams WG, Trusler GA. Surgical management of critical pulmonary stenosis in the neonate. *Ann Thorac Surg.* 1984;38:458–465.

156. Mody MR. The natural history of uncomplicated valvular pulmonic stenosis. *Am Heart J.* 1975;90:317–321.

157. Lange PE, Onnasch DG, Heintzen PH. Valvular pulmonary stenosis. Natural history and right ventricular function in infants and children. *Eur Heart J.* 1985;6:706–709.

158. Rowland DG, Hammill WW, Allen HD, Gutgesell HP. Natural course of isolated pulmonary valve stenosis in infants and children utilizing Doppler echocardiography. *Am J Cardiol.* 1997;79:344–349.

159. Atik E. [Mild pulmonary valve stenosis: the possible spontaneous cure in the natural history of the defect]. *Arq Bras Cardiol.* 2006;86:378–381.

160. Faletra FF, Nucifora G, Ho SY. Imaging the atrial septum using real-time three-dimensional transesophageal echocardiography: technical tips, normal anatomy, and its role in transseptal puncture. *J Am Soc Echocardiogr.* 2011;24:593–599.

161. Dodge-Khatami A, Backer CL, Mavroudis C. Risk factors for recoarctation and results of reoperation: a 40-year review. *J Card Surg.* 2000;15:369–377.

162. Tandon R, Edwards JE. Clinicopathologic correlations. Atrial septal defect in infancy: common association with other anomalies. *Circulation.* 1974;49:1005–1010.

20 | Hypotension

Shahab Noori and Istvan Seri

EPIDEMIOLOGY

Incidence and Definitions

Hypotension is a common problem in the neonatal intensive care unit (NICU).[1] More than half of neonates admitted to the NICU also carry the diagnosis of hypotension. Although the incidence is higher with lower gestational age at birth, the exact incidence is not known. This is primarily because of the lack of consensus on what constitutes hypotension.[2] Indeed, there are many ways to define neonatal hypotension, and the differences among the definitions obviously affect the reported incidence of hypotension and the decision to treat the condition.[3,4] As the ultimate goal is to ensure that oxygen delivery matches tissue oxygen demand in all organs, hypotension best can be defined based on *physiologic principles*, that is, by assessing the effects of decreased perfusion pressure on organ blood flow and oxygen delivery. However, because in the first, "compensated" phase of shock, vital organ (brain, myocardium, adrenal glands) blood flow and blood pressure (BP) are maintained by the neuroendocrine mechanism-driven redistribution of blood flow from nonvital organs, hypotension only presents when shock enters its second, "uncompensated" phase and vital organ blood flow also declines. Therefore, hypotension can be best defined as the BP below which vital organ (eg, brain) blood flow autoregulation is lost and cerebral blood flow (CBF) starts decreasing in proportion to the decrease in BP (the so-called autoregulatory threshold of hypotension; Figure 20-1).[5] On further decrease in BP and oxygen delivery, cellular function cannot be appropriately maintained, but structural integrity is not yet significantly affected (the so-called functional threshold of hypotension; Figure 20-1).[5] Finally, on further decline in BP and oxygen delivery, structural integrity of tissues becomes affected, resulting in permanent organ damage (the so-called ischemic threshold of hypotension; Figure 20-1).[5] Unfortunately, there are few data on the cutoff values, and because the capacity of the cardiovascular and neuroendocrine systems to appropriately compensate is affected by gestational and postnatal age as well as the underlying pathophysiology, these values likely vary in the individual patient and even for the same patient at different times.

On the other hand, the clinical definition of hypotension is straightforward because it is absolutely arbitrary. In clinical practice, hypotension in very low birth weight (VLBW) infants has been defined as a mean BP below the gestational age in numerical value[5] as this number is close to the 5th (or 10th) percentile of the population-based mean normative BP values for gestational age for the given patient population.[6] A number of researchers and clinicians also define hypotension in VLBW neonates during the first postnatal days as a mean BP below 28 to 30 mm Hg.[7–9] The last definition of hypotension is based on findings suggesting that the lower elbow of the CBF autoregulatory curve is around these values in VLBW neonates (Figure 20-1).[9–11]

More recently, likely because of the lack of a clinically relevant (ie, mortality and long-term outcome-based) definition of hypotension, the idea of "permissive hypotension" has been introduced in the literature.[12]

281

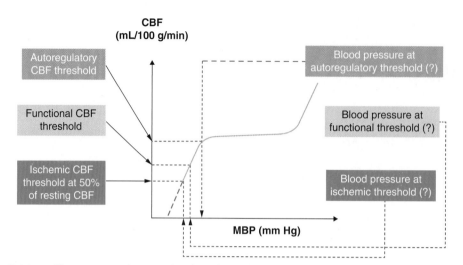

FIGURE 20-1 Definition of hypotension by 3 pathophysiologic phenomena[5] of increasing severity: autoregulatory, functional, and ischemic thresholds of hypotension. The mean blood pressure (MBP) associated with the loss of cerebral blood flow (CBF) autoregulation is the generally accepted definition of hypotension (*autoregulatory blood pressure threshold*). Preliminary data suggest that the autoregulatory blood pressure threshold might be around 28 to 30 mm Hg in the very low birth weight (VLBW) neonate during the first postnatal days.[5] However, at present it remains unclear what to do with this information in clinical practice. If blood pressure continues to fall, it reaches a value at which cerebral function becomes compromised (*functional blood pressure threshold*). Available preliminary data suggest that the functional blood pressure threshold might be around 22 to 24 mm Hg in the VLBW neonate during the first postnatal days.[5] Finally, if blood pressure decreases even further, it reaches a value at which structural integrity becomes compromised (*ischemic blood pressure threshold*). Findings in immature animals suggest that the ischemic CBF threshold is around 50% of the resting CBF. However, the gestational and postnatal age-dependent ischemic blood pressure is not known for the preterm or term neonate. Finally, it is of note that the forebrain in general and certain forebrain structures in particular are more vulnerable than the structures of the hindbrain. **See text for details.** (Modified from McLean et al.[5])

The permissive hypotension strategy calls for disregard of BP in the clinical assessment of the patient's cardiovascular status. Instead, the strategy calls for focusing *only* on assessment of adequacy of organ perfusion by evaluating clinical and laboratory indicators of tissue perfusion. Although BP is the dependent variable among the factors defining macrohemodynamics (see the section on pathophysiology), appropriate perfusion pressure is absolutely necessary to drive blood flow through the entire circulatory system (macro- and microcirculations). Therefore, the idea to discard BP as one of the hemodynamic factors in the assessment of the cardiovascular status essentially disregards the basic principles of cardiovascular physiology.

In addition, the clinical and laboratory indicators of adequacy of perfusion are either unreliable or delayed in presentation, rendering them less useful.[13] However, as none of the definitions of hypotension in itself has been shown to be associated with improved outcomes when "hypotension" is treated, the BP values are indeed arbitrarily used to trigger initiation of treatment. Finally, to make matters worse (ie, even more complex), having a BP above the cutoff value also does not ensure adequacy of perfusion in part because patients first enter the compensated phase of shock where BP remains within the "normal range" (see also the BP and blood flow interaction discussion that follows).

Figure 20-2 shows an example of statistically defined normal BP.[14] The lines represent the lower limit of the 80% confidence interval of BP for each gestational age group during the first 3 days of postnatal life. Therefore, 90% of neonates will have a mean BP value at or above this lower limit. Although adequacy

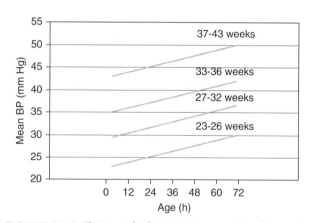

FIGURE 20-2 This graph depicts an example of statistically defined normal blood pressure (BP) values. The lines represent the lower limit of the 80% confidence interval of mean BP in neonates during the first 3 postnatal days. Ninety percent of neonates will have a mean BP value at or above this lower-limit confidence interval. (Modified from Nuntnarumit et al.[14] See the text for details.)

of organ perfusion cannot be deduced from these data or similar, statistically derived normative values, the graph clearly demonstrates that BP is directly related to both gestational and postnatal age and therefore can be used as a guideline in the initial assessment of neonates with suspected hemodynamic instability.[15]

Risk Factors

Certain neonatal patient populations are more likely to develop hypotension and circulatory failure and suffer from the complications associated with inadequate tissue perfusion. Prematurity, lack of exposure to antenatal steroids, chorioamnionitis, perinatal infection, perinatal depression, pre- and postnatal exposure to certain medications, respiratory distress syndrome, and persistent pulmonary hypertension are among the risk factors for developing hypotension. There are many reasons that the neonate, especially the preterm neonate, is vulnerable to the hemodynamic effects of hypotension. The immaturity of organ systems in general and the brain in particular predisposes the preterm infant to organ damage. The narrow BP range of CBF autoregulation[10] and its attenuation or complete loss in situations that are all

but too common (eg, hypercarbia and hypotension) in the preterm neonate can adversely affect CBF and contribute to the development of brain injury.

Recently, we have proposed that vital organ assignment might be developmentally regulated, and that in extremely preterm infants the forebrain is a nonvital organ during the first 24 to 48 hours following delivery.[16] Indirect evidence in preterm neonates and studies in developing animals support this hypothesis and demonstrate that, unlike in the hindbrain, vessels in the forebrain constrict in response to hypoxia or hypoperfusion.[17,18]

PATHOPHYSIOLOGY

Careful attention to the principles of cardiovascular physiology and the interaction between BP and systemic and organ blood flow are important in understanding the pathophysiology of hypotension and shock (Figure 20-3).[19,20] According to Poiseuille's law, flow is directly related to the pressure gradient and diameter of the vessel and inversely related to the length of the vessel and the viscosity of the fluid. Thus, pressure is the driving force behind moving blood through

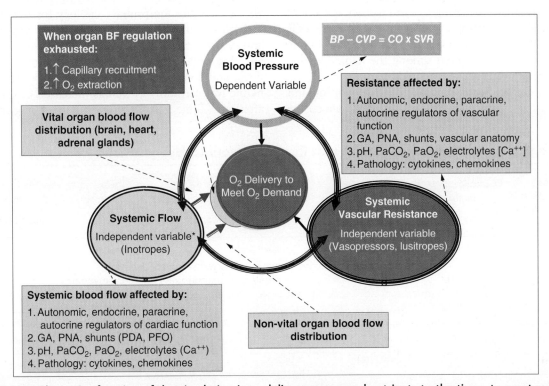

FIGURE 20-3 The major function of the circulation is to deliver oxygen and nutrients to the tissue to meet metabolic demand. The interaction between 2 factors, systemic flow and systemic resistance, ensures adequate oxygen delivery. These 2 relatively independent factors are regulated and controlled by autonomic, endocrine, and paracrine factors and affected by a host of other physiologic and pathologic mechanisms. The interaction between systemic flow and resistance ultimately determines blood pressure. Finally, if organ blood flow is insufficient, capillary recruitment and increase in oxygen extraction will keep the demand in check to maintain adequate oxygen delivery. BF, blood flow; [Ca++], calcium concentration; CO, cardiac output; CVP, central venous pressure; GA, gestational age; PaCO2, partial pressure of arterial carbon dioxide; PaO2, partial pressure of arterial oxygen; PDA, patent ductus arteriosus; PFO, patent foramen ovale; PNA, postnatal age; SVR, systemic vascular resistance. (Modified with permission from Soleymani S, Borzage M, Seri I. Hemodynamic monitoring in neonates: advances and challenges. J Perinatol. 2010;30 Suppl:S38–S45.)

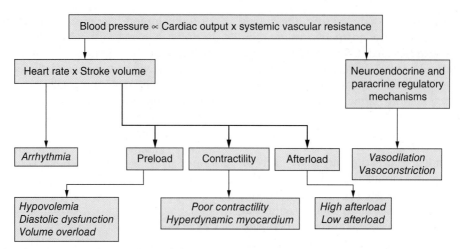

FIGURE 20-4 Blood pressure is the product of the interaction between cardiac output and systemic vascular resistance. Assessment of each component of this interaction is important and useful in identifying the underlying cause of cardiovascular compromise. (See the text for details.)

the vasculature. In clinical practice, Ohm's law is used to describe the interaction between BP, blood flow (cardiac output, CO), and systemic vascular resistance (SVR): $BP \propto SVR \times CO$. Accordingly, physiologic and pathologic changes in the 2 relatively independent parameters (CO and SVR) determine the dependent parameter, BP. Considering this interaction, BP would not change if, for example, CO drops by 50% and SVR doubles. This also illustrates the fact that BP is one of the principle parameters among the hemodynamic indicators of perfusion that should be monitored.

In defining the pathophysiology of hypotension and cardiovascular compromise, it is useful to evaluate the components of SVR and CO, the two so-called independent variables (Figure 20-4). Disturbances in regulation of or pathologic alterations in vascular tone, heart rate, preload, contractility, or afterload can all lead to hypotension and cardiovascular compromise. Therefore, based on the underlying pathophysiology, we can identify the primary etiology for hypotension, including disturbances of vascular tone (vasodilation and vasoconstriction); arrhythmia; conditions primarily affecting preload (hypovolemia and diastolic dysfunction); and contractility (myocardial injury or hyperdynamic myocardium) as well as increased or decreased afterload (Table 20-1). Among the underlying causes of

Table 20-1 Cardiovascular Mechanisms that Result in Neonatal Hypotension

Hypovolemia	Diastolic Dysfunction	Poor Contractility	Vasodilation	Shunt	High Afterload	Arrhythmia
Acute blood loss	Tension pneumothorax	Cardiovascular maladaptation after birth	Septic shock	Patent ductus arteriosus	CVS maladaptation after birth	Supraventricular tachycardia
Umbilical cord avulsion	Cardiac tamponade	Asphyxia	Systemic inflammatory response	Arteriovenous malformation	Dilated cardiomyopathy	Hyperkalemia
Subgaleal hemorrhage	Hypertrophic cardiomyopathy	Prenatal depression	Adrenal insufficiency			
Excessive insensible water loss	Inotrope overdose	Septic shock (late stage)	Pressor-resistant hypotension			
Polyuria		Dilated cardiomyopathy				
		Left ventricular noncompaction				

The table summarizes the most important cardiovascular mechanisms resulting in the development of hypotension in neonates and shows the leading clinical causes associated with each mechanism. See text for details.

hypotension and shock, vasodilation and poor contractility are the most common etiological factors in neonates, especially in preterm infants.

Disturbances of Vascular Tone

Regulation of vascular smooth muscle tone is complex and involves a delicate balance between vasodilator and vasoconstrictor signals controlled by the autonomic nervous system as well as endocrine mechanisms and paracrine and local vasoactive factors. The most important endocrine, paracrine, and local regulators of vascular tone include nitric oxide, eicosanoids, vasopressin, catecholamines, renin-angiotensin system, and endothelin. Some of the factors, such as locally generated nitric oxide and vasodilatory eicosanoids, are increased in septic shock and generalized inflammatory diseases and are considered the main cause of the associated poor vascular tone and vasodilatory shock in these conditions. Given the high incidence of clinical conditions with elevated inflammatory mediators such as chorioamnionitis, respiratory distress syndrome, necrotizing enterocolitis, inappropriate oxygen exposure, and immaturity of the autonomic nervous system, especially in the very preterm neonate, it is not surprising that vasodilation plays a significant role in the pathogenesis of circulatory failure in these patients.

Disturbances in Heart Rate and Rhythm

Although transient sinus bradycardia and tachycardia are common in neonates, it is the more sustained problems with cardiac rhythm that can lead to hypotension and circulatory failure. Among arrhythmias potentially leading to circulatory compromise, supraventricular tachycardia and hyperkalemia-related tachyarrhythmia are the most frequently occurring clinical presentations.

Disturbances of Preload

In general, conditions that decrease preload by resulting in absolute hypovolemia, such as acute blood loss, are rare. Moreover, the lack of evidence of a well-defined relationship between blood volume and BP in preterm neonates further supports the generally accepted notion that absolute hypovolemia is not a common cause of hypotension in the neonatal period.[21-23] However, it must be noted that these studies[21-23] were performed on more mature preterm neonates. Moreover, the recent findings of improved hemodynamics associated with delayed cord clamping suggest that some degree of decreased circulating blood volume is indeed not uncommon, especially in the very preterm neonate, and that having a higher absolute circulatory volume

at birth might be beneficial.[24,25] Of course, there may be additional mechanisms in play contributing to the improved hemodynamics seen following delayed cord clamping. For example, a more gradual increase in afterload when cord clamping is delayed rather than the abrupt afterload increase associated with the immediate clamping of the cord might allow for improved adaptation of the immature myocardium of the very preterm neonate.

On the other hand, reduced preload, despite the absence of significant absolute hypovolemia, is not uncommon. High intrathoracic pressure due to an inappropriately high mean airway pressure or a tension pneumothorax as well as the presence of a pericardial effusion can significantly decrease CO by decreasing venous return. Furthermore, although its role in the pathogenesis of hypotension has not been adequately studied, the decreased compliance of the immature myocardium could also limit the filling of the heart. Finally, significant diastolic dysfunction can contribute to decreased filling and thus decreased preload in patients with hypertrophic cardiomyopathy or in patients treated with inappropriately high doses of inotropes, especially dobutamine. Patients with hypertrophic cardiomyopathy are usually born to mothers with diabetes, and the small ventricular cavity and hyperdynamic myocardium result in significant reductions in preload.

Disturbances of Myocardial Contractility

Because of both structural and functional immaturity, the myocardium of the neonate is more prone to decreased contractility (Figure 20-5).[26] Myocardial dysfunction has been documented in about one-third to a half of very preterm infants presenting with hypotension or poor perfusion.[27,28] It has been postulated that the higher sensitivity of the immature myocardium to afterload compared to infants, children, and adults results in poor contractility in preterm, especially very preterm, neonates. Accordingly, the abrupt increase in left ventricular afterload following the sudden removal of the low-resistance placental vascular bed at the time of cord clamping is thought to be one of the primary causes of myocardial dysfunction in very preterm neonates in the immediate postnatal period.

Another major cause of myocardial dysfunction is hypoxic-ischemic injury associated with perinatal depression.[29-31] In this setting, the compensatory vasoconstriction may mask the impending circulatory failure by maintaining BP in the perceived normal range. Therefore, assessment of myocardial function by echocardiography has been recommended in all patients with low Apgar scores or evidence of perinatal depression.[32]

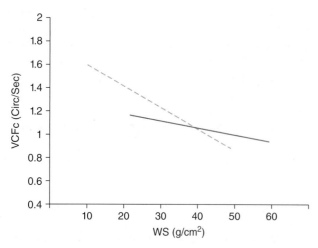

FIGURE 20-5 The solid line represents the normal inverse relationship between myocardial contractility (VCFc) and the afterload (WS) in children. The dotted line depicts this regression line in neonates. Because the slope of the regression line is steeper in neonates compared to older children, with an increase in afterload, the contractility of the immature myocardium of neonates decreases more rapidly than that of the mature heart of older children. (Modified from Rowland and Gutgesell.[26] See the text for details.)

Disturbances of Afterload

Afterload and SVR are often used interchangeably. However, although related, they do not represent the same hemodynamic entity. SVR is a calculated value based on the pressure gradient (the pressure difference between systemic mean arterial BP and central venous pressure) and CO. Conversely, afterload is the pressure or force that the myocardium has to overcome during the isovolumetric contraction time to eject blood out of the left ventricle into the aorta during the ejection time. The Laplace law describes afterload as the ventricular muscle tension being directly related to the pressure and the diameter of the left ventricle and inversely related to muscle thickness. Because the intraventricular pressure needed to open the aortic valve depends on the BP in the aorta and because SVR, through its interaction with CO, determines the BP, SVR is directly related to afterload. However, changes in left ventricular diameter or myocardial wall thickness will also alter the afterload without changes in the SVR. In summary, afterload and SVR are not the same and should not be used interchangeably.

As mentioned, high afterload has been implicated in the pathogenesis of circulatory failure in very preterm infants in the immediate postnatal period. Increased afterload also contributes to worsening hypotension and impaired tissue perfusion in settings of a dilated ventricle, such as dilated cardiomyopathy or failing left ventricle, more frequently seen

in neonates with asphyxia. Thus, only judicious use of volume expanders is recommended in these settings as the volume administration-associated increases in ventricular size lead to further increases in afterload and worsen the existing myocardial dysfunction.

In certain clinical situations, in addition to low SVR, low afterload can contribute to the development of circulatory failure. For example, in cases with hypertrophic cardiomyopathy, the low afterload caused by the small ventricular cavity and thick myocardium can lead to hyperdynamic myocardial function and therefore worsen the dynamic left ventricular tract obstruction associated with the hypertrophic cardiomyopathy.

Others

Circulatory compromise can also develop when an arterial shunt is present between the systemic and pulmonary circulations, such as seen with a hemodynamically significant patent ductus arteriosus (PDA) or an aortopulmonary collateral. Similarly, arteriovenous connections seen in patients with a large arteriovenous malformation can lead to circulatory compromise. PDA is discussed in another chapter of this book. Suffice it to say that, because of systolic or diastolic "steal" or myocardial dysfunction secondary to left ventricular volume overload with or without reduced coronary blood flow, a persistent hemodynamically significant PDA can result in the development of systemic hypotension and hypoperfusion.[33,34] Although aortopulmonary collaterals are not uncommon in preterm infants with chronic lung disease, they usually are not large enough to cause circulatory failure. Finally, in patients with a large arteriovenous malformation, the left ventricular volume overload can result in heart failure and circulatory compromise.

DIFFERENTIAL DIAGNOSIS

"True" systemic hypotension should be differentiated from factitious ones. Accordingly, when making the diagnosis of hypotension, potential problems with the measurement of BP itself and the uncertainty about the definition of *true hypotension* both need to be considered.

Blood pressure can be measured noninvasively (most commonly by using the oscillometric technique) or invasively via an umbilical or peripheral artery catheter connected to a pressure transducer. If using the noninvasive oscillometric technique, one must use the correct BP cuff with a ratio of cuff width to arm circumference between 0.45 and 0.7.[13,35] If the cuff size is too small or too large for the given patient, erroneously high or low BP readings, respectively, will be obtained.[13,35] However, with an appropriate-size cuff, accurate estimations of BP are generally obtained, with most studies finding good agreement between oscillometric and invasive techniques.[36] On the other hand, in very preterm infants (the population with the highest risk for the development of hypotension), the noninvasive technique might overestimate the BP.[37] When invasive BP monitoring via arterial catheters is used, improper setup of the BP monitoring system can result in significant errors. The presence of air bubbles or blood clots in the system can result in dampened waveforms and yield an erroneously low systolic and high diastolic BP, usually resulting in an underestimated mean BP.[36,38] In addition, if the pressure transducer is placed above or below the level of a patient's heart, an erroneously low or high BP, respectively, is recorded. However, these technical issues can be readily addressed once identified.

On the other hand, the problem of appropriately defining true hypotension, which will then merit treatment, is much more difficult to solve (see the section on the definition of hypotension). At present, the available bedside monitoring tools and clinical and laboratory indicators used in the assessment of the status of the cardiovascular system are unreliable and not evidence based. However, by using the appropriately obtained BP value in combination with the concurrently monitored additional cardiovascular parameters, such as heart rate, arterial oxygen saturation, and perhaps regional tissue oxygen saturation obtained via near-infrared spectroscopy, as well as by taking the findings of the physical examination and laboratory studies (capillary refill time [CRT], urine output, and serum lactate levels) into consideration, one may be able to more appropriately assess the status of the cardiovascular system and make a reasonable decision about the need for treatment. Once it has been decided that the given BP represents true hypotension, the next step is to identify the underlying etiology (Table 20-1) because the treatment must be tailored to the etiology and pathophysiology of the cardiovascular compromise. Finally, it must be emphasized again that, although we have evidence on short-term hemodynamic effects of the medications most frequently used in the treatment of neonatal hypotension, such as dopamine, dobutamine, epinephrine, and perhaps milrinone, we do not have evidence-based mortality and long-term outcome data and thus clinically relevant evidence on the safety and appropriateness of the presently used treatment of neonatal hypotension.[3–5,19]

DIAGNOSTIC TESTS

In the assessment of the adequacy of tissue perfusion in neonates with the clinical diagnosis of hypotension, a number of clinical and laboratory tests have been used.

Although these tests, especially when used in combination, enhance our ability to detect circulatory compromise, they also carry significant limitations. Newer bedside tools such as near-infrared and visible light spectroscopy, laser tissue Doppler, amplitude-integrated electroencephalography, electrical impedance cardiometry, and functional echocardiography provide more objective data on the status of the cardiovascular system and are promising.[20]

Among the clinical tests, CRT is commonly used and can provide information on the peripheral circulation. CRT is assessed by pressing the skin for 3 to 5 seconds to cause blanching by emptying the capillary bed; then, the time it takes for the capillary bed to refill and return to the baseline color is measured. Forehead and sternum are most likely the best places to measure CRT.[39,40] A CRT greater than 3 seconds is considered abnormal.[39,40] However, the predictive value of CRT for systemic hypoperfusion is poor. Although some improvements can be achieved by combining prolonged CRT with hypotension or other markers of hypoperfusion (eg, serum lactate levels), the sensitivity remains too low for CRT to be clinically useful.[39–42]

Another parameter that usually changes during circulatory compromise is the heart rate, and an elevated heart rate compared to the baseline may indicate low CO. However, as tachycardia can occur with many conditions (eg, fever, sepsis, pain, agitation, and as a side effect of certain medications), its value in the diagnosis of shock is limited. On the other hand, changes in heart rate pattern can be used to predict impending sepsis and thus, potentially, septic shock.[43]

Urine output can be used as an indirect method of assessment of adequacy of renal blood flow. Because, from a hemodynamic standpoint, the kidneys are considered nonvital organs, renal perfusion is among the first to change. Therefore, a decrease in urine output could be a sign of impending cardiovascular failure. In general, a urine output greater than 1–2 mL/kg/min suggests adequate renal perfusion during the first postnatal days. However, monitoring urine output to determine the adequacy of BP in a timely manner can be problematic as detection of low urine output usually takes hours after renal perfusion has decreased. In addition, low urine output may also be the result of causes unrelated to BP.

Serum lactate level is another indirect marker of tissue perfusion. In the absence of an inborn error of metabolism, elevated serum lactate levels suggest anaerobic metabolism as a consequence of poor tissue perfusion. However, similar to low urine output, high serum lactate only tells us about the lack of adequate tissue perfusion hours earlier and therefore may not be useful in determining the adequacy of BP and tissue perfusion in real time. Furthermore, as serum lactate is increased with epinephrine infusion independently of the status of tissue perfusion, a high serum lactate level may not be reflective of a perfusion problem in the epinephrine-exposed neonate.[44] However, repeated follow-up of serum lactate over time can be useful for the assessment of longer-term hemodynamic response to treatment.

Assessment of tissue perfusion using near-infrared and visible light spectroscopy might also be useful in the overall assessment of circulatory function.[46–49] However, routine application of these new techniques requires further evaluation. [46,48,49] Functional echocardiography allows for identifying the underlying pathophysiology of hypotension and should be considered in all patients with hemodynamic instability.[32,50] Assessment of myocardial contractility and the presence of pericardial effusion or a large PDA with a left-to-right shunt is relatively straightforward and important in determining the cause of hypotension. More detailed interrogation of cardiovascular function may include estimation of left and right ventricular output and superior vena cava flow as well as assessment of the load-dependent and load-independent measures of myocardial contractility (shortening fraction and stress-velocity index, respectively), diastolic function, pulmonary artery pressure, the hemodynamic significance of a PDA, and selective organ blood flows.

Although functional echocardiography can be helpful in the diagnosis and management of neonatal hypotension and shock, it has a number of shortcomings as well. Functional echocardiography requires the availability of expensive equipment and expert operators with the skill needed to perform and interpret the studies in the NICU 24/7, and it only provides a non-continuous assessment of the dynamically changing cardiovascular system.[32,50]

Recent findings suggest that noninvasive, continuous, beat-to-beat CO monitoring using thoracic bioimpedance technology (electrical impedance cardiometry) has an accuracy and precision in neonates comparable to those of echocardiography.[51,52] However, further studies are needed to validate the utility of electrical cardiometry in the clinical setting. It must also be noted that, if appropriately validated, electrical impedance cardiometry will be used in conjunction with and not instead of echocardiography.

MANAGEMENT

As stated previously, when discussing the management of neonates presenting with hypotension and systemic hypoperfusion, we must acknowledge the lack of information from randomized placebo-controlled clinical trials on the safety and clinically relevant, long-term benefits of correcting systemic hypotension, especially in the very preterm neonate in the immediate postnatal period. However, designing such a trial is challenging. Uncertainty about the gestational and chronological age-specific definition of hypotension, the type of treatment (volume, vasopressor-inotropes, inotropes, or lusitropes) appropriate for the underlying pathophysiology of the cardiovascular compromise in each patient (individualized treatment strategy); and the ability to adequately monitor in real time the comprehensive hemodynamic response elicited (BP, CO, SVR, and organ blood flow together) rather than only heart rate, oxygen saturation, and BP are among the main challenges of designing such a clinical trial. Furthermore, timely enrollment of the subjects and willingness of the participating clinician to randomize the hypotensive patients to the placebo arm are other issues to be resolved before such a trial may become feasible.[53]

In summary, the use of comprehensive hemodynamic monitoring allowing for the timely diagnosis and recognition of the underlying pathophysiology of the cardiovascular compromise and for appropriate selection and monitoring of the hemodynamic response of treatment as well as the selection of the most appropriate short-term hemodynamic and long-term, clinically relevant outcome measures are the most important challenges the designers of these trials face. In addition, patient populations with different gestational and postnatal ages will have to be stratified and studied separately. It is no wonder we do not have evidence yet on the safety and clinically relevant long-term effects of treatment of neonatal hypotension in preterm or term neonates.

While awaiting the findings of such well-designed placebo-controlled and appropriately executed studies, attention to the principles of developmental cardiovascular physiology, pathophysiology, and pharmacology[54] will likely aid in increasing the likelihood of recovery and decreasing the rate of adverse effects of hypotension and its treatment. Accordingly, taking into consideration the following points might help the clinician in the decision making process: (1) using one of the most relevant current definitions of hypotension as one of the available screening tools; (2) using clinical and laboratory indicators of adequacy of perfusion as adjuncts to BP; (3) identifying the underlying pathophysiology using the history, physical examination, and appropriate hemodynamic monitoring, including functional echocardiography; (4) addressing the underlying pathophysiology with an appropriate treatment strategy by choosing the most appropriate medication based on the hemodynamic derangement and the pharmacokinetics and pharmacodynamics of the given drug; (5) appropriately titrating the medication to the desired effect; (6) considering downregulation of adrenergic receptors to adjust the dose or use additional treatment, such as hydrocortisone,[55] to upregulate the receptors and intracellular enzyme systems involved in eliciting the hemodynamic response in the heart and vasculature; and (7) avoiding, or at least minimizing, significant fluctuations in BP and systemic and organ blood flow in response to treatment.

OUTCOME AND FOLLOW-UP

The impact of hypotension and its treatment on clinically relevant long-term outcome measures is unclear. There are many obstacles in evaluating the true effects of hypotension on neurodevelopmental outcome. The main challenge is the lack of any data from prospective studies or randomized controlled trials on the effects of untreated hypotension on short- and long-term outcome measures. The lack of appropriate data stems from the notion that, via its adverse effect on CBF and oxygen delivery, hypotension leads to brain injury. The association between hypotension and brain injury described in the literature has strengthened this notion.[6,56–59] Therefore, clinicians have been reluctant to enroll hypotensive patients in placebo-controlled randomized clinical trials designed to define hypotension based on the known effects on organ injury of true hypotension. Indeed, a recent clinical study found that a randomized clinical trial of treatment vs placebo in the very preterm population was not feasible.[53] While obtaining parental consent was the main obstacle in this trial, the clinicians' bias also played a major role as 22% of the eligible patients were not considered for enrollment by the treating neonatologists and 85% of the eligible patients who were not enrolled received treatment for hypotension.

Another challenge in elucidating the potential role of hypotension in extremely preterm infants with impaired long-term neurodevelopmental outcome is the presence of confounding factors. As hypotension most commonly occurs during the first few days after birth, other coexisting hemodynamic factors during the transitional period, such as myocardial dysfunction, PDA, upregulated inflammatory mediators, oxygen toxicity, and acid-base imbalance, are frequently present, and these factors by themselves have been associated with poor outcome.[16] In addition, the intended (eg, permissive hypercarbia) and unintended (high mean airway pressure) consequences of the respiratory management also affect CBF independent of the presence or absence of hypotension.[60–64] Finally, the lack of a gestational and postnatal age-dependent definition of hypotension based on physiology, pathophysiology, and clinically relevant outcome measures makes it difficult and, at present, likely not even feasible to appropriately define the patient population that truly has hypotension and thus could benefit from treatment.[16,19]

Among the hemodynamic factors that may determine whether a hypotensive preterm infant would have a poor outcome, the duration of hypotension,[56,64,65] response to treatment,[66] presence of metabolic acidosis,[57] and problems with perfusion[12,65] have been identified as potentially important factors. Of course, many other factors unrelated to hypotension or hemodynamic instability, including but not restricted to the degree of immaturity, presence of brain injury, infection, oxygen toxicity, maternal socioeconomic status, and other things, play a major role in long-term outcome.

Although some studies suggest otherwise,[67,68] the current literature is fairly consistent in that patients who have BP in the perceived normal range have better outcomes in general than those who become hypotensive.[7,8,12,55,56,62–66,69–71] However, it is unclear whether hypotension itself, its treatment, both, neither, or a combination of some or all of these factors are responsible for the poor outcomes. Most of the earlier studies have attributed the associated poor outcome to hypotension, while some of the more recent studies blamed the treatment for the complications. However, the fact is that the relationship between hypotension or its treatment with poor outcomes is one of association, and causality cannot be determined from the available data. Therefore, depending on our bias, we will continue to attribute the poor outcome to hypotension or its treatment until appropriately designed and executed clinical trials finally address this long-lasting controversy.

REFERENCES

1. Al-Aweel I, Pursley DM, Rubin LP, Shah B, Weisberger S, Richardson DK. Variations in prevalence of hypotension, hypertension, and vasopressor use in NICUs. *J Perinatol.* 2001;21(5):272–278.
2. Short BL, Van Meurs K, Evans JR. Summary proceedings from the cardiology group on cardiovascular instability in preterm infants. *Pediatrics.* 2006;117:S34–S39.
3. Limperopoulos C, Bassan H, Kalish LA, et al. Current definitions of hypotension do not predict abnormal cranial ultrasound findings in preterm infants. *Pediatrics.* 2007;120:966–977.
4. Laughon M, Bose C, Allred E, et al; ELGAN Study Investigators. Factors associated with treatment for hypotension in extremely low gestational age newborns during the first postnatal week. *Pediatrics.* 2007;119:273–280.
5. McLean CW, Noori S, Cayabyab R, Seri I. Cerebral circulation and hypotension in the premature infant—diagnosis and treatment. In: Perlman JM, ed. *Questions and Controversies in Neonatology—Neurology.* 2nd ed.
6. Development of audit measures and guidelines for good practice in the management of neonatal respiratory distress syndrome. Report of a Joint Working Group of the British Association of Perinatal Medicine and the Research Unit of the Royal College of Physicians. *Arch Dis Child.* 1992;67:1221–1227.
7. Watkins AM, West CR, Cooke RW. Blood pressure and cerebral haemorrhage and ischaemia in very low birthweight infants. *Early Hum Dev.* 1989;19:103–110.
8. Martens SE, Rijken M, Stoelhorst GM, et al. Is hypotension a major risk factor for neurological morbidity at term age in very preterm infants? *Early Hum Dev.* 2003;75(1–2):79–89.

9. Munro MJ, Walker AM, Barfield CP. Hypotensive extremely low birth weight infants have reduced cerebral blood flow. *Pediatrics*. 2004;114:1591–1596.

10. Greisen G. Autoregulation of cerebral blood flow in newborn babies. *Early Hum Dev*. 2005;81:423–428.

11. Børch K, Lou HC, Greisen G. Cerebral white matter blood flow and arterial blood pressure in preterm infants. *Acta Paediatr*. 2010;99:1489–1492.

12. Dempsey EM, Al Hazzani F, Barrington KJ. Permissive hypotension in the extremely low birthweight infant with signs of good perfusion. *Arch Dis Child. Fetal Neonatal Ed*. 2009;94:F241–F244.

13. de Boode W-P Clinical monitoring of systemic hemodynamics in critically ill newborns. *Early Hum Dev*. 2010;86:137–141.

14. Nuntnarumit P, Yang W, Bada-Ellzey HS. Blood pressure measurements in the newborn. *Clin Perinatol*. 1999;26:981–996. x.

15. Zubrow AB, Hulman S, Kushner H, Falkner B. Determinants of blood pressure in infants admitted to neonatal intensive care units: a prospective multicenter study. Philadelphia Neonatal Blood Pressure Study Group. *J Perinatol*. 1995;15:470–479.

16. Noori S, Stavroudis TA, Seri I. Systemic and cerebral hemodynamics during the transitional period after premature birth. *Clin Perinatol*. 2009;36:723–736. v.

17. Hernandez M, Hawkins R, Brennan R. Sympathetic control of regional cerebral blood flow in the asphyxiated newborn dog. In: Heistad DD, Marcus ML, eds. *Cerebral Blood Flow, Effects of Nerves and Neurotransmitters*. New York, NY: Elsevier; 1982:359–366.

18. Ashwal S, Dale PS, Longo LD. Regional cerebral blood flow: studies in the fetal lamb during hypoxia, hypercapnia, acidosis, and hypotension. *Pediatr Res*. 1984;18:1309–1316.

19. Noori S, Stavroudis TA, Seri I. Principles of developmental cardiovascular physiology and pathophysiology. In: Kleinman CS, Seri I, eds. *Questions and Controversies in Neonatology—Hemodynamics and Cardiology*. 2nd ed. New York, NY: Saunders/Elsevier; 2012:3–27.

20. Soleymani S, Borzage M, Noori S, Seri I. Hemodynamic monitoring in neonates: advances and challenges. *Expert Rev Med Devices*. 2012;9(5):00–00.

21. Barr PA, Bailey PE, Sumners J, Cassady G. Relation between arterial blood pressure and blood volume and effect of infused albumin in sick preterm infants. *Pediatrics*. 1977;60:282–289.

22. Bauer K, Linderkamp O, Versmold HT. Systolic blood pressure and blood volume in preterm infants. *Arch Dis Child*. 1993;69:521–522.

23. Wright IM, Goodall SR. Blood pressure and blood volume in preterm infants. *Arch Dis Child Fetal Neonatal Ed*. 1994;70:F230–F231.

24. Rabe H, Reynolds G, Diaz-Rossello J. A systematic review and meta-analysis of a brief delay in clamping the umbilical cord of preterm infants. *Neonatology*. 2008;93:138–144.

25. Sommers R, Stonestreet BS, Oh W, et al. Hemodynamic effects of delayed cord clamping in premature infants. *Pediatrics*. 2012;129(3):e667–e672.

26. Rowland DG, Gutgesell HP. Noninvasive assessment of myocardial contractility, preload, and afterload in healthy newborn infants. *Am J Cardiol*. 1995;75:818–821.

27. Gill AB, Weindling AM. Echocardiographic assessment of cardiac function in shocked very low birthweight infants. *Arch Dis Child*. 1993;68:17–21.

28. Osborn DA, Evans N, Kluckow M. Left ventricular contractility in extremely premature infants in the first day and response to inotropes. *Pediatr Res*. 2007;61:335–340.

29. Barberi I, Calabro MP, Cordero S, et al. Myocardial ischaemia in neonates with perinatal asphyxia. Electrocardiographic, echocardiographic and enzymatic correlations. *Eur J Pediatr*. 1999;158(9):742–747.

30. Wei Y, Xu J, Xu T, Fan J, Tao S. Left ventricular systolic function of newborns with asphyxia evaluated by tissue Doppler imaging. *Pediatr Cardiol*. 2009;30:741–746.

31. Nestaas E, Støylen A, Brunvand L, Fugelseth D. Longitudinal strain and strain rate by tissue Doppler are more sensitive indices than fractional shortening for assessing the reduced myocardial function in asphyxiated neonates. *Cardiol Young*. 2011;21:1–7.

32. Mertens L, Seri I, Barker P, et al. Targeted neonatal echocardiography in the neonatal intensive care unit: practice guidelines and recommendations for training. Writing Group of the American Society of Echocardiography (ASE) in collaboration with the European Association of Echocardiography (EAE) and the Association for European Pediatric Cardiologists (AEPC). *J Am Soc Echocardiogr*. 2011;24:1057–1078.

33. Clyman TA, Noori S. Principles of developmental cardiovascular physiology and pathophysiology. In: Kleinman CS, Seri I, eds. *Questions and Controversies in Neonatology—Hemodynamics and Cardiology*. 2nd ed. New York, NY: Saunders/Elsevier; 2012:267–289.

34. Sehgal A, McNamara PJ. Coronary artery perfusion and myocardial performance after patent ductus arteriosus ligation. *J Thorac Cardiovasc Surg*. 2012;143:1271–1278.

35. Kimble KJ, Darnall RA Jr, Yelderman M, Ariagno RL, Ream AK. An automated oscillometric technique for estimating mean arterial pressure in critically ill newborns. *Anesthesiology*. 1981;54:423–425.

36. Engle W. Definition of normal blood pressure range. The elusive target. In: Kleinman CS, Seri I, eds. *Questions and Controversies in Neonatology—Hemodynamics and Cardiology*. 2nd ed. New York, NY: Saunders/Elsevier; 2012:49–77.

37. Dannevig I, Dale HC, Liestøl K, Lindemann R. Blood pressure in the neonate: three non-invasive oscillometric pressure monitors compared with invasively measured blood pressure. *Acta Paediatr*. 2005;94:191–196.

38. Cunningham S, Symon AG, McIntosh N. Changes in mean blood pressure caused by damping of the arterial pressure waveform. *Early Hum Dev*. 1994;36:27–30.

39. Strozik KS, Pieper CH, Cools F. Capillary refilling time in newborns—optimal pressing time, sites of testing and normal values. *Acta Paediatr*. 1998;87:310–312.

40. Weindling M, Paize F. Peripheral haemodynamics in newborns: best practice guidelines. *Early Hum Dev*. 2010;86:159–165.

41. Osborn DA, Evans N, Kluckow M. Clinical detection of low upper body blood flow in very premature infants using blood pressure, capillary refill time, and central-peripheral temperature difference. *Arch Dis Child Fetal Neonatal Ed*. 2004;89:F168–F173.

42. Miletin J, Pichova K, Dempsey EM. Bedside detection of low systemic flow in the very low birth weight infant on day 1 of life. *Eur J Pediatr*. 2009;168:809–813.

43. Fairchild KD, O'Shea TM. Heart rate characteristics: physiomarkers for detection of late-onset neonatal sepsis. *Clin Perinatol*. 2010;37:581–598.

44. Valverde E, Pellicer A, Madero R, Elorza D, Quero J, Cabañas F. Dopamine versus epinephrine for cardiovascular support in low birth weight infants: analysis of systemic effects and neonatal clinical outcomes. *Pediatrics*. 2006;117:e1213–e1222.

45. Weindling AM. Peripheral oxygenation and management in the perinatal period. *Semin Fetal Neonatal Med*. 2010;15:208–215.

46. Wolfberg AJ, du Plessis AJ. Near-infrared spectroscopy in the fetus and neonate. *Clin Perinatol*. 2006;33:707–728. viii.

47. Benaron DA, Parachikov IH, Friedland S, et al. Continuous, noninvasive, and localized microvascular tissue oximetry using visible light spectroscopy. *Anesthesiology*. 2004;100:1469–1475.

48. Noori S, Drabu B, McCoy M, Sekar K. Non-invasive measurement of local tissue perfusion and its correlation with hemodynamic indices during the early postnatal period in term neonates. *J Perinatol*. 2011;31:785–788.

49. Lemmers P, Naulaers G, Van Bell F. Clinical applications of near-infrared spectroscopy in neonates. In: Kleinman CS, Seri I, eds. *Questions and Controversies in Neonatology—Hemodynamics and Cardiology.* 2nd ed. New York, NY: Saunders/Elsevier; 2012:Chap. 8.

50. Kluckow M, Seri I, Evans N. Functional echocardiography: an emerging clinical tool for the neonatologist. *J. Pediatr.* 2007;150:125–130.

51. Noori S, Drabu B, Soleymani S, Seri I. Continuous non-invasive cardiac output measurements in the neonate by electrical velocimetry: a comparison with echocardiography. *Arch Dis Child Fetal Neonatal Ed.* 2012;97(5):F340–F343. doi:10.1136/archdischild-2011-301090.

52. Weisz DE, Jain A, McNamara PJ, El-Khuffash A. Non-invasive cardiac output monitoring in neonates using bioreactance: a comparison with echocardiography. *Neonatology.* 2012;102:61–67.

53. Batton BJ, Li L, Newman NS, et al. Feasibility study of early blood pressure management in extremely preterm infants. *J Pediatr.* 2012;161(1):65–69.e1.

54. Noori S, Seri I. Neonatal blood pressure support: the use of inotropes, lusitropes, and other vasopressor agents. *Clin Perinatol.* 2012;39:221–238.

55. Noori S, Friedlich P, Wong P, Ebrahimi M, Siassi B, Seri I. Hemodynamic changes following low-dose hydrocortisone administration in vasopressor-treated neonates. *Pediatrics.* 2006;118:1456–1466.

56. Bada HS, Korones SB, Perry EH, et al. Mean arterial blood pressure changes in premature infants and those at risk for intraventricular hemorrhage. *J Pediatr.* 1990;117(4):607–614.

57. Goldstein RF, Thompson RJ Jr, Oehler JM, Brazy JE. Influence of acidosis, hypoxemia, and hypotension on neurodevelopmental outcome in very low birth weight infants. *Pediatrics.* 1995;95:238–243.

58. Miall-Allen VM, de Vries LS, Whitelaw AG. Mean arterial blood pressure and neonatal cerebral lesions. *Arch Dis Child.* 1987;62:1068–1069.

59. Seri I. Circulatory support of the sick preterm infant. *Semin Neonatol.* 2001;6:85–95.

60. Kaiser JR, Gauss CH, Williams DK. The effects of hypercapnia on cerebral autoregulation in ventilated very low birth weight infants. *Pediatr Res.* 2005;58:931–935.

61. Kaiser JR, Gauss CH, Pont MM, Williams DK. Hypercapnia during the first 3 days of life is associated with severe intraventricular hemorrhage in very low birth weight infants. *J Perinatol.* 2006;26:279–285.

62. Fabres J, Carlo WA, Phillips V, Howard G, Ambalavanan N. Both extremes of arterial carbon dioxide pressure and the magnitude of fluctuations in arterial carbon dioxide pressure are associated with severe intraventricular hemorrhage in preterm infants. *Pediatrics.* 2007;119:299–305.

63. McKee LA, Fabres J, Howard G, Peralta-Carcelen M, Carlo WA, Ambalavanan N. $PaCO_2$ and neurodevelopment in extremely low birth weight infants. *J Pediatr.* 2009;155(5):217–221.e1.

64. Low JA, Froese AB, Galbraith RS, Smith JT, Sauerbrei EE, Derrick EJ. The association between preterm newborn hypotension and hypoxemia and outcome during the first year. *Acta Paediatr.* 1993;82(5):433–437.

65. Hunt RW, Evans N, Rieger I, Kluckow M. Low superior vena cava flow and neurodevelopment at 3 years in very preterm infants. *J Pediatr.* 2004;145:588–592.

66. Pellicer A, Bravo MC, Madero R, Salas S, Quero J, Cabañas F. Early systemic hypotension and vasopressor support in low birth weight infants: impact on neurodevelopment. *Pediatrics.* 2009;123(5):1369–1376.

67. Logan JW, O'Shea TM, Allred EM, et al. Early postnatal hypotension and developmental delay at 24 months of age among extremely low gestational age newborns. *Arch Dis Child Fetal Neonatal Ed.* 2011;96(5):F321–F328.

68. Logan JW, O'Shea TM, Allred EM, et al. Early postnatal hypotension is not associated with indicators of white matter damage or cerebral palsy in extremely low gestational age newborns. *J Perinatol.* 2011;31(8):524–534.

69. Fanaroff JM, Wilson-Costello DE, Newman NS, Montpetite MM, Fanaroff AA. Treated hypotension is associated with neonatal morbidity and hearing loss in extremely low birth weight infants. *Pediatrics.* 2006;117:1131–1135.

70. Batton B, Batton D, Riggs T. Blood pressure during the first 7 days in premature infants born at postmenstrual age 23 to 25 weeks. *Am J Perinatol.* 2007;24:107–115.

71. Kuint J, Barak M, Morag I, Maayan-Metzger A. Early treated hypotension and outcome in very low birth weight infants. *Neonatology.* 2009;95:311–316.

Neonatal Arrhythmias

Elizabeth A. Greene and George Van Hare

DEFINITION

Arrhythmias, alterations in the heartbeat rhythm, are a common problem in the newborn period. Many are now diagnosed in utero. We consider the tachycardias (rapid heart rhythms) first, then the bradycardias (slowed heart rhythms).

TACHYCARDIAS

The most commonly diagnosed fetal arrhythmias are premature atrial contractions (PACs), which often resolve soon after birth. The other tachycardias frequently seen in the fetus and the newborn period are atrial tachycardia, atrial flutter, and the more usual reentrant-type supraventricular tachycardia (SVT).[1-3]

Differential Diagnosis

It is often necessary to distinguish sinus tachycardia from a true tachyarrhythmia. The normal resting heart rate for infants varies with gestational age, with term infants at 130–150 beats per minute (bpm). Preterm infants have slightly faster rates, with an average resting heart rate of 160 bpm at 32 weeks. The average heart rate[4] of a newborn is 145 with a range of 110–150 bpm.

It can be difficult to tell the difference between sinus tachycardia and an atrial tachycardia that originates close to the sinoatrial (SA) node based on the electrocardiographic appearance. If the clinical evidence is consistent with sepsis, dehydration, or blood loss, then it is likely that the rhythm is a reactive sinus tachycardia. Another helpful clue to sinus rhythm is the morphology of the P waves. With normal sinus rhythm, P waves are upright in leads I and aVF. In addition, one should see a biphasic P wave in V1. This is caused by the normal electrical depolarization of the atria that begins in the right atrium, spreads to the left atrium, then proceeds to the AV node.

If the baby is being monitored on telemetry, there may be a clear change in P-wave morphology or axis that will suggest PACs or an ectopic atrial rhythm. The PR interval may also prolong.[5] Figure 21-1 shows a comparison of sinus tachycardia and atrial tachycardia.

The PACs look similar to sinus beats with a P wave preceding each QRS complex, but these occur earlier than expected. The P wave may be buried in the preceding T wave if the heart rate is increased. If they occur in a pattern of every other beat with sinus beats, they are called atrial bigeminy. Both of these rhythms are usually benign and self-limited but can occur if there is a central line within the right atrium or electrolyte disturbances.

If the PAC is conducted aberrantly, there is often a question regarding whether it is a premature ventricular contraction (PVC) or PAC. It is helpful to invoke the 2 R-R rule to differentiate the origin of the premature beat. If the 2 R-R interval just prior to the premature beat is longer than the 2 R-R interval that contains the premature beat, that suggests a PAC. If the 2 R-R interval containing the premature beat is identical to the previous one, this is consistent with a PVC. This is because, typically, the atrium as unaffected by the early beat, continues its own timing, sends out the next P wave on time, and is then conducted normally.

A: Sinus tachycardia

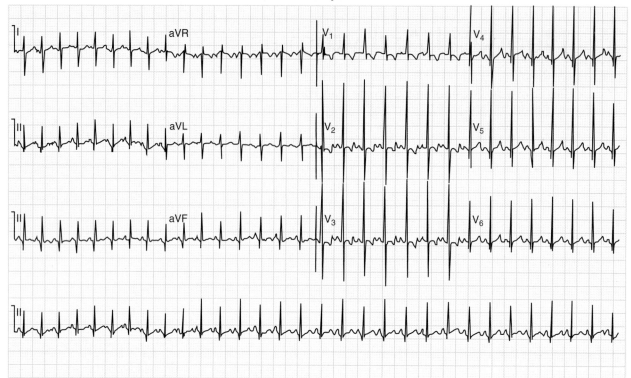

B: Ectopic atrial tachycardia, at least 2 P wave morphologies are seen

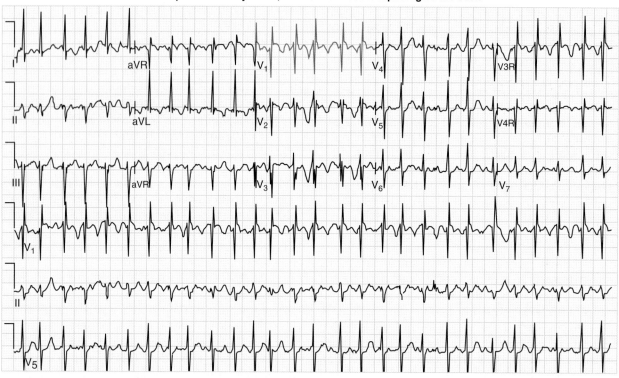

FIGURE 21-1 A, Sinus tachycardia vs B, ectopic atrial tachycardia (EAT). In sinus tachycardia, there is 1 P-wave morphology; in EAT there are at least 2 different P-wave morphologies.

PVC with 2 R-R interval to differentiate PAC from PVC

The premature beat causes the 2 R-R interval to shorten suggesting PAC
There is also a short run of atrial tachycardia to confirm the diagnosis

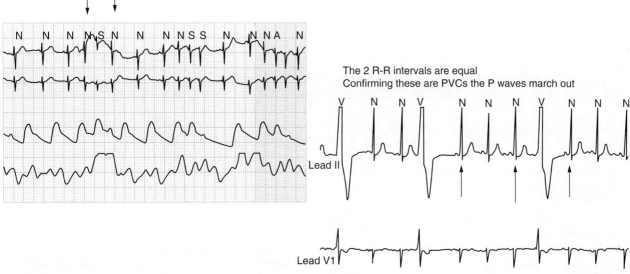

The 2 R-R intervals are equal
Confirming these are PVCs the P waves march out

Lead II

Lead V1

FIGURE 21-2 Premature atrial contraction (PAC) vs premature ventricular contraction (PVC). On left, PACs with normal conduction will be narrow. On right, simultaneous tracing in leads II and V1. PVCs will have a wide complex. PVCs do not affect the next atrial beat and therefore cause a compensatory pause in the ventricular beat. PACs do affect the next atrial beat, making it come earlier (or advancing it); therefore, no compensatory pause is seen.

The atrium does not change its timing, and this creates what is called the "compensatory pause" for the QRS or ventricular complex. On the other hand, if the premature beat came from the atrium, it will penetrate the sinus node and reset the pacemaker, and the 2 R-R interval that includes the premature beat will be shorter than the preceding one (Figure 21-2).

The pathophysiology of each tachycardia is different. Table 21-1 provides the differential diagnosis of SVT and response to adenosine. Ectopic atrial tachycardia comes from an area of atrial tissue that depolarizes and activates the atrium at a rate more rapid than the sinus node. The ectopic focus may be sensitive to catecholamines and inotropic medications.

The more usual form of reentrant SVT is caused by an accessory pathway. In Wolff-Parkinson-White (WPW) syndrome, the pathway conducts in sinus rhythm and is therefore evident on the electrocardiogram (ECG). By depolarizing an area of ventricular myocardium earlier than would happen if conduction were only via the AV node, the accessory pathway causes the QRS complex to widen on the ECG in the pattern we refer to as preexcitation or a delta wave. Many patients do not have WPW syndrome or a delta wave, but do have SVT, which is caused by a concealed accessory pathway or one that does not conduct in sinus rhythm or show itself on an ECG. The most common ECG appearance of SVT will be a narrow complex at a rate of 240–300 bpm (Figure 21-3).

If the infant is in SVT, it is not possible to tell if there is WPW syndrome. Once in sinus rhythm, delta waves may become apparent (Figure 21-4).

Staying within the atrium, another common tachyarrhythmia in neonates is atrial flutter. This rhythm is a reentrant circuit, contained within the atrium in a stereotypic pattern. The circuit ascends the atrial septum, crosses over the superior portion of the atrium, and then descends along the lateral atrial wall, where it then traverses the isthmus between the inferior vena cava (IVC) and the tricuspid valve and then turns back up the atrial septum. This creates the classic "sawtooth" flutter waves seen best in V1. The rate of the atrial flutter is usually 240 to 300 bpm in older children and adults, but it is substantially faster in newborns (400–600 bpm). The flutter rate is determined by the physics of the atrium and the distance covered in each lap. This is also a common arrhythmia in fetal life.[6] If the rhythm does not convert spontaneously at birth, it is easily treated with cardioversion and usually does not recur.

Fast Rhythms that Involve the Atrium, the AV Node, and the Ventricle

Fast rhythms that involve the atrium, AV node, and ventricle are otherwise known as typical reentrant SVTs. Many of these patients will have WPW syndrome, but not all; SVT and WPW syndrome are not synonymous. This is confounded by the phenomenon

Table 21-1 Differential Diagnosis of Supraventricular Tachycardia

Rhythm	Usual Rate in Term Infant	ECG Diagnostics	Response to Vagal	Response to Adenosine
Ectopic atrial tachycardia; fairly common	190–220	May gradually warm; change in P-wave axis and morphology; can be multifocal; may cause cardiomyopathy	May slow; may create block and reveal underlying atrial rhythm	May slow; may create block and reveal underlying atrial rhythm
Atrial flutter; fairly common	200–300	May be regular or irregular depending on the degree of block; P waves large and sawtooth, especially in V1	May see higher-grade block and unmask underlying rhythm	May see higher-grade block and unmask underlying rhythm
Atrial fibrillation (multiple foci usually in the left atrium); very rare but could be seen in WPW syndrome	200–340	Very irregular; P waves are tiny	Would not expect effect	Can cause atrial fibrillation; do not give
Reentrant SVT AVRT (due to an accessory pathway such as but not limited to WPW syndrome); common AVNRT; very rare in infants, utilizes dual AV node physiology	220–340	Sudden onset; very regular; may see retrograde P waves, which follow the QRS and will be very close to the QRS in AVNRT and close to halfway between R waves in AVRT	Often able to terminate the rhythm	Often able to convert the rhythm
Junctional ectopic tachycardia; rare	180–200	Often incessant; may cause cardiomyopathy; look for dissociation on ECG with more QRS complexes than P waves; may need long rhythm strips	May slow	May slow

Abbreviations: AVNRT, atrioventricular node reentry tachycardia; AVRT, atrioventricular reciprocating tachycardia; ECG, electrocardiogram; SVT, supraventricular tachycardia; WPW, Wolff-Parkinson-White.

of a delay in the appearance of preexcitation or delta waves for several days after birth or conversion to sinus rhythm. ECGs done in tachycardia will usually show narrow-complex tachycardia in the range of 270–320 bpm. At that rate, P waves are almost impossible to see but may be appreciated on the upstroke of the T wave. If that is seen, it helps to envision the mechanism of tachycardia in these patients; the SVT circuit in these patients is usually down the AV node and then back up the accessory pathway. The circuit involves both atrium and ventricle, and conduction time from ventricle to atrium via the pathway is shorter than conduction time from atrium to ventricle over the AV node.

Figure 21-5 shows atrial flutter with variable block and transesophageal pacing used to convert reentrant SVT.[7,8] This type of pacing may also be used for conversion of atrial flutter.

Atrial fibrillation would be an unusual rhythm to see in a neonate with normal cardiac anatomy and function but might be seen in the setting of an inflammatory process such as myocarditis. It is recognizable by its irregularity and small, sometimes almost invisible, P waves. More often in infants, one may see chaotic atrial tachycardia, characterized by irregular discrete P waves of varying morphology.

Table 21-2 indicates the treatment of SVT.[9–12]

Moving lower in the heart and its conduction system, we come to the AV node or junction. This part of the heart is capable of becoming the auxiliary pacemaker if the sinus node fails; it may become inflamed and become an origin for ectopic tachycardia or cause too slow or blocked conduction if traumatized by surgery, inflammation, or intrauterine exposure to antibodies against itself. The ECG pattern in junctional tachycardia will characteristically show a narrow-complex rhythm and may or may not show P waves. If P waves are seen, they will typically be in a pattern of AV dissociation, with a slower atrial rate than ventricular rate

Newborn SVT with easily seen retrograde P waves

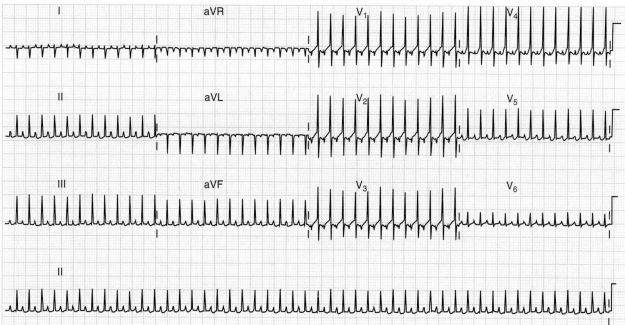

FIGURE 21-3 Narrow-complex supraventricular tachycardia (SVT). The mechanism for this rhythm is a reentrant circuit that uses the atrioventricular (AV) node as the antegrade limb and an accessory pathway as the retrograde limb. The P wave is almost equidistant between the R waves, which suggests the retrograde conduction time along the accessory pathway.

and occasional sinus capture beats that advance the tachycardia.[13] If there is, instead, 1:1 retrograde conduction from the focus to the atrium, P waves will be superimposed on the QRS complex and therefore not visible. Occasionally, they can be appreciated immediately after the QRS complex. In this case, one may appreciate the axis of the P waves as negative in II, III,

and aVF as well, which suggests that the origin is from an area inferior to the sinus node.

Negative P waves seen before the QRS complex do not have the same significance; there may be an inferior atrial origin of the rhythm, but it is not junctional. Another feature of junctional rhythm, whether fast of slow, is that it is not driven by the atrial rate. If you are

Baby with WPW

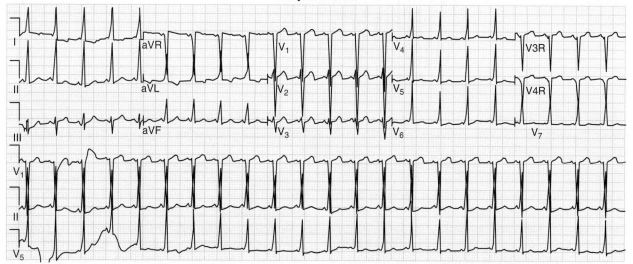

FIGURE 21-4 Electrocardiogram (ECG) in sinus rhythm shows Wolff-Parkinson-White (WPW) syndrome. There is a pattern of preexcitation with delta waves.

Neonatal flutter with variable block in 35 week Preemie

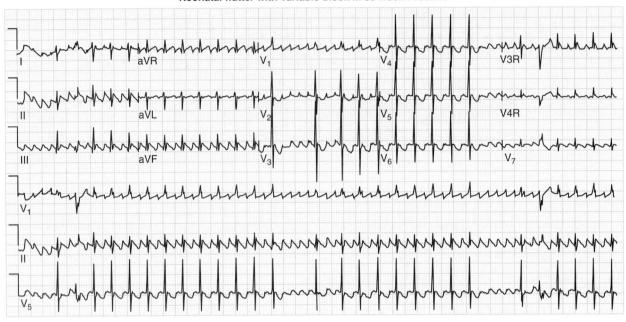

Transesophageal pacing used to convert SVT in newborn, also useful in Flutter

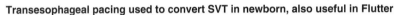

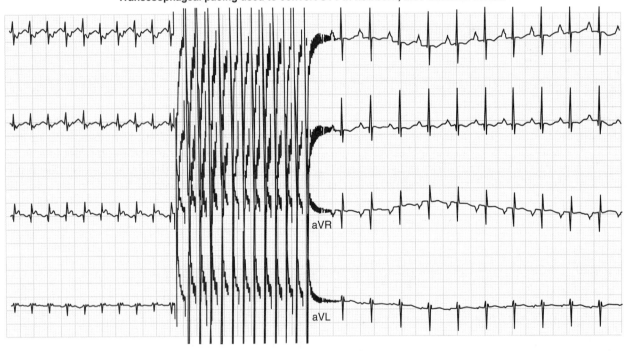

FIGURE 21-5 A, Atrial flutter: a macroreentrant rhythm confined to the atrium that produces large, sawtooth P waves. There is also variable atrioventricular (AV) block. **B,** Transesophageal pacing may be used to convert supraventricular tachycardia (SVT) as in this case or for atrial flutter.

able to document dissociation, in that there are different atrial and junctional rates, with the junctional rate faster than the atrial and a regular rate for both, you have good evidence of junctional rhythm (Figure 21-6).

A rare rhythm that is confused with junctional rhythm is persistent (permanent form of) junctional reciprocating tachycardia (PJRT). This rhythm has

inverted P waves, but they occur just prior to the QRS complex and are due to retrograde conduction along a slow-conducting accessory pathway. The negative P waves are seen in the inferior leads because the pathway comes near the posterior inferior portion of the right atrium near the coronary sinus os and the AV node. Because the tachycardia utilizes such a

Table 21-2 Treatment of Supraventricular Tachycardia

Treatment Recommendations for Supraventricular Tachycardias	Cardioversion Transesophageal Pacing	Recommended Medications
Ectopic atrial tachycardia (EAT)	Pacing may accelerate; cardioversion will not convert	Digoxin, β-blocker, flecainide, procaineamide, amiodarone
Atrial flutter	Pacing may convert; cardioversion usually curative	If cardioverted, digoxin for 3 months; sotalol second-line treatment (especially if congenital heart disease)
Atrial Fibrillation	Pacing will not help; cardioversion often needed to achieve sinus rhythm	If cardioverted, will need medication to prevent recurrence; avoid digoxin in WPW syndrome; β-blocker, flecainide, and amiodarone reasonable choices
Reentrant SVT from accessory pathway (including WPW syndrome)	Pacing may convert; cardioversion if unstable	Avoid digoxin if WPW syndrome; inderol first-line treatment; second-line treatment with flecainide, amiodarone if difficult to control
Junctional ectopic tachycardia	Pacing will not convert; cardioversion will not convert	Inderol first-line treatment; may require amiodarone

Abbreviations: SVT, supraventricular tachycardia; WPW, Wolff-Parkinson-White. Cardioversion dose is 0.5 to 2 joules per kilogram, synchronized.

slow-conducting pathway, the patients tolerate it for much longer than the usual reentrant SVT. Eventually, it can cause a decrease in function and cardiomyopathy (Figure 21-7).

Fast Rhythms that Originate in the Ventricle

The epidemiology of ventricular tachycardia (VT) includes systemic problems, such as viral myocarditis, metabolic disease, electrolyte abnormalities, and genetic channelopathies, including long QT syndrome (LQTS). This rhythm, possibly more than any other, taxes clinicians in terms of the immediate response. The dilemma is to make the diagnosis and then to decide whether the patient is stable.

The differential diagnosis of wide-complex tachycardia includes benign ventricular accelerated rhythm of the newborn, sinus rhythm with a bundle branch block, SVT with aberrancy, SVT with antegrade conduction along the accessory pathway, and VT.

Benign ventricular rhythm of the newborn occurs when the ventricular pacemaker is slightly faster than the sinus pacemaker at a rate that is usually 140 to 170 bpm. It may require a long rhythm strip to demonstrate dissociation. It resolves spontaneously but can also be suppressed with beta blockers (Figure 21-8).

Pathophysiology

Rhythms coming from 1 of the ventricles will have a widened QRS duration for age. For a neonate, the normal QRS duration is 40 ms or 1 small box on the ECG paper at the usual recording speed of 25 mm/s. If the QRS duration is 80 ms, it is considered wide. This occurs because of the ventricle being activated gradually as the electrical depolarization makes its way across the myocardium without the aid of the usual conducting tissue. VT from the left ventricle will make the ECG look like there is a right bundle branch block. VT from the right ventricle will make the ECG look like there is a left bundle branch block. Just as with a junctional rhythm, there will be dissociation with 2 separate rhythms in progress, the atrial and the ventricular, without 1 affecting the other consistently. The AV node is capable of both antegrade (the usual pattern of conduction from the atrium to the ventricle) and retrograde (from the ventricle to the atrium) conduction, especially in the young. If that phenomenon is occurring, one may see retrograde (after the QRS) P waves in VT similar to that seen in junctional rhythm. Unlike junctional rhythm, in VT the QRS complex should be wide for age (Figure 21-9).

Treatment

If there is sinus tachycardia, the baby needs to be treated for the underlying cause, such as dehydration. Medications or treatments to address a primary tachycardia in this setting may make the infant more ill. For example, if the baby has a heart rate above normal (210 bpm for an infant at 36 weeks' gestation) and is hypotensive secondary to sepsis, drugs such as β-blockers can make the hemodynamic situation worse.

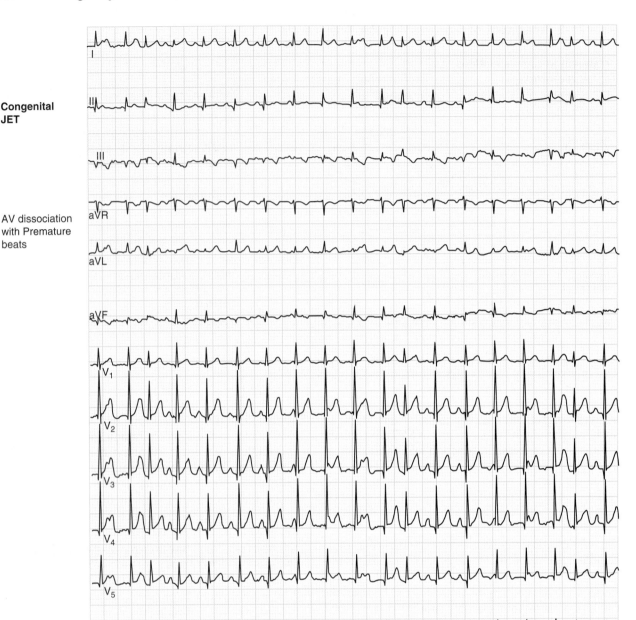

Congenital JET

AV dissociation with Premature beats

FIGURE 21-6 Junctional ectopic tachycardia (JET; after repair of tetralogy of Fallot) with atrioventricular (AV) dissociation. There are also premature atrial contractions (PACs), which conduct with a slightly wider QRS complex. This helps differentiate JET from ventricular tachycardia (VT), for which the QRS duration in the tachycardia would normally be wider or longer than the sinus capture beats.

Treatment options for tachyarrhythmias above the ventricle depend on the exact rhythm. Table 21-3 presents a selected formulary.

Once a diagnosis of hemodynamically significant VT is made, then therapy is either electrical or medication. If the baby is in VT and is stable, then initial treatment with lidocaine can be considered while preparations are made to perform elective cardioversion. If the baby is unstable, then cardioversion may need to be emergent.

If the baby has sinus bradycardia or heart block in addition to VT, that is highly suggestive of LQTS. VT in LQTS is usually polymorphic, with a pattern known as torsades de pointes. For monomorphic VT, treatment with lidocaine and cardioversion or defibrillation if there is no pulse will be needed emergently. Amiodarone would not be advised if LQTS is known as it will prolong the QT interval further. Magnesium may be given for torsades de pointes (Figure 21-10).

PJRT with negative P waves in the inferior leads but not consistent with junctional rhythm

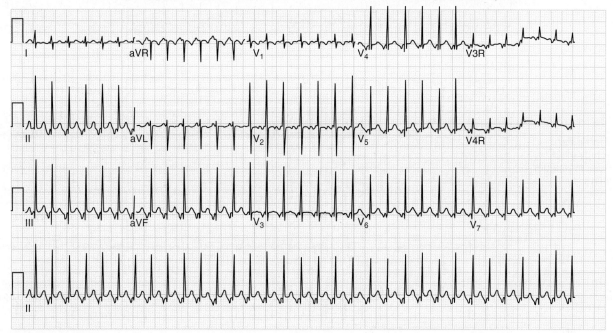

FIGURE 21-7 Persistent (permanent form of) junctional reciprocating tachycardia (PJRT) caused by a slow-conducting accessory pathway, which may cause incessant tachycardia. In this form of supraventricular tachycardia (SVT), the time taken to conduct retrograde from the ventricle to the atrium is reflected by the long V-to-A time (or R to P). The resultant P waves are also negative in the inferior leads, consistent with a right-sided posterior and inferior accessory pathway.

Idioventricular rhythm of the newborn, atrial rate approx 160, ventricular rate 170

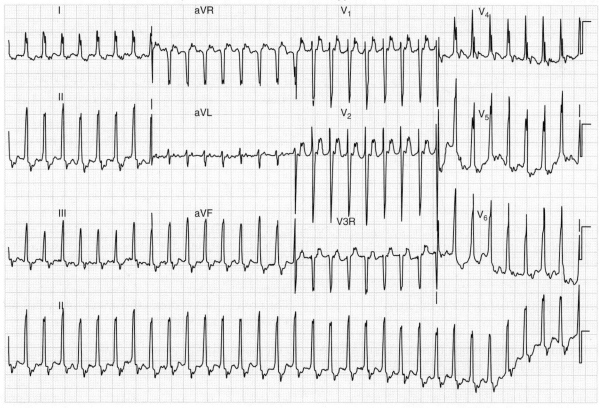

FIGURE 21-8 Idioventricular rhythm of the newborn. The ventricular rate is slightly faster than the atrial rate.

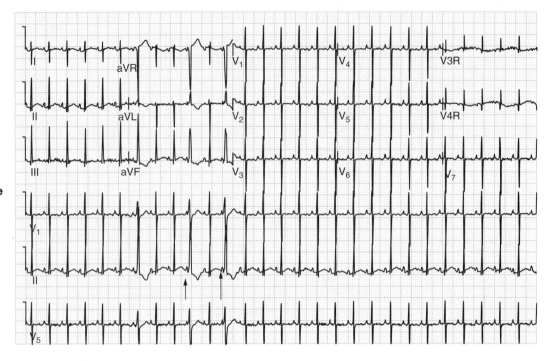

Ventricular ectopy ex 25 week premature infant

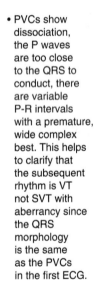

- PVCs show dissociation, the P waves are too close to the QRS to conduct, there are variable P-R intervals with a premature, wide complex best. This helps to clarify that the subsequent rhythm is VT not SVT with aberrancy since the QRS morphology is the same as the PVCs in the first ECG.

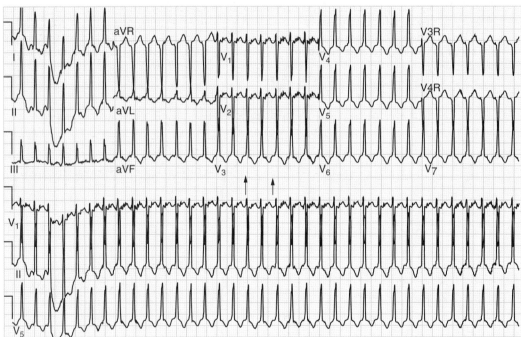

FIGURE 21-9 A, Premature ventricular contractions (PVCs) and B, ventricular tachycardia in an ex 25-week preemie. The PVCs show dissociation and widened QRS complex. This helps to clarify that the subsequent rhythm is ventricular tachycardia (VT) and not supraventricular tachycardia (SVT) with aberrancy. ECG, electrocardiogram.

Troubleshooting or Diagnostic Redirections

If a rhythm is initially thought to be SVT and adenosine is given to a patient in VT, realize the following:

Diagnostic use of the ECG obtained at that time.

Danger of doing that maneuver

The need to always be ready to cardiovert when using adenosine in any situation.

If the rhythm is initially thought to be VT and lidocaine is given to a patient in SVT:

A lack of response does not make the diagnosis of SVT but is suggestive.

Table 21-3 Drug Doses: Selected Formulary

Adenosine
Indication: Convert reentrant SVT that utilized the AV node as part of the circuit. Diagnostically, it can be helpful in unmasking atrial flutter or tachycardia.
Dose recommendations: 100 μg/kg, fast intravenous push; increase to 200 μg/kg for second dose; may increase to 400 μg/kg if unsuccessful.
Caution: May cause prolonged heart block if infant is acidotic. The usual half-life is 10–15 s.
Esmolol (β-blocker for patients who can have nothing by mouth or are more ill)
Indication: SVT that has been recurrent after adenosine. May help subsequent dosing of adenosine to be successful and may convert SVT as well. Can use this to suppress ectopic focus of EAT or VT. Can be used to lower the rate of more incessant tachycardias such as PJRT or junctional ectopic tachycardia.
Dose recommendations: Bolus of up to 200 μg/kg over 1 minute. Starting dose for infusion of 50 μg/kg/min; often need to increase dosing to 100 μg/kg/min but may need dosing up to 200 μg/kg/min.
Caution: May cause hypotension, especially in patients with poor function. β-Blocker effects such as bradycardia and hypoglycemia must be monitored. Half-life is approximately 10 minutes.
Propranolol (oral β-blocker)
Indication: SVT, EAT, VT for maintenance therapy. May be used in combination for rhythms more difficult to control, such as PJRT.
Dosing: 1–2 mg/kg/d divided every 6 hours. This can be changed to every 8 hours when the infants are a few months old if there is good control.
Caution: Same as for esmolol but less pronounced. Usually recommend checking blood sugar an hour after dosing for the first 3 doses. Maintain usual infant feeding of at least every 3–4 hours as newborn. If the infant can have nothing by mouth except for medication, another source of glucose must be provided to prevent hypoglycemia.
Sotalol (combination of oral β-blocker and potassium channel blocker)
Indication: Control of atrial tachycardia, atrial flutter, and VT.
Dosing: 2–8 mg/kg/d divided twice a day.
Caution: Can cause bradycardia and heart block. Because it is almost entirely a potassium channel blocker at higher doses (as opposed to amiodarone, which has many other effects as well), there is more risk of torsades. Follow ECG daily; if QTc is 500 ms, may need to consider different medication or dose reduction.
Procaineamide (intravenous sodium channel blocker)
Indication: Difficult-to-control atrial tachycardia, junctional tachycardia, and SVT.
Dosing: Bolus dosing of 5 to 15 mg/kg but given in 5-mg/kg increments over 20 minutes each, then continuous drip at 20 to 100 μg/kg/min.
Caution: Half-life is 13 hours in neonates; can cause conduction defects and bradycardia; monitor QRS duration and if greater than 25%, no further dose increase; if the QTc is greater than 500 ms, stop drug. Check drug interactions. Follow procaineamide and NAPA (N-acetylprocainamide) levels for toxicity.
Lidocaine (intravenous sodium channel blocker)
Indication: Ventricular tachycardia.
Dosing: 1 mg/kg IV bolus or IV push if necessary. Continuous infusion at 20–50 μg/kg/min.
Caution: Half-life is 3.2 hours in neonates. Monitor for neurologic symptoms, including seizures. Decrease rate by 50% after 24 hours. Follow lidocaine levels.
Flecainide (oral sodium channel blocker)
Indication: Often added to β-blocker for control of recurrent SVT. Also used for atrial tachycardia.
Dosing: Can be dosed by body surface area or by weight. Starting dose of 1–3 mg/kg/d. Usually will need to be in the 3–6 mg/kg/d range. Dosing interval in infants is every 8 hours.
Caution: Narrow therapeutic window. Follow levels. Serum level is dependent on milk-based feedings as Ca^{2+} blocks absorption. If feeding regimen is changed or the infant can have nothing by mouth except for medication, the dose will need to be reduced by 50%. For all patients, follow QRS duration when medication is started and acquire serum levels as needed. There are multiple drug interactions.
Amiodarone (has effects of each type of antiarrhythmic drug class)
Indication: Recurrent and persistent EAT, atrial flutter, SVT, PJRT, JET, VT. Amiodarone helps to suppress both ectopic and reentrant tachycardias in the atrium and the ventricle by increasing the refractory period of every tissue in the heart. This helps to prevent any arrhythmia from recurring by making the tissues less excitable.
Dosing: There is both intravenous and oral dosing. Most likely a neonate requiring this medication would receive it intravenously. Recommended intravenous bolus dose would be 2.5 mg/kg over 30 minutes. During this time, the infant must be monitored for bradycardia and hypotension. If the rhythm is controlled with this dose, then a continuous infusion of 10 mg/kg/d is started. If necessary, subsequent boluses can be given; usually, a total of 10 mg/kg is sufficient to control most tachycardias. It takes approximately 10 days to load with amiodarone whether it is given intravenously or orally. Initial maintenance dosing is 50% of the loading dose or 5 mg/kg/d. Half-life is very long, maybe weeks.

(Continued)

Table 21-3 Drug Doses: Selected Formulary (*Continued*)

Caution: Amiodarone is 35% iodine. Because of its multiple effects, there are multiple cautions and multiple drug interactions. There are thyroid, pulmonary, cutaneous, and hepatic effects to monitor. Daily ECGs are needed to evaluate the QTc. Bradycardia and conduction defects can occur. If QTc is greater than 500 ms, dosing must be reassessed and likely decreased. Multiple drug interactions in particular will increase digoxin and flecainide levels and potentiate the effects of all other antiarrhythmics.

Digoxin (the aspirin of electrophysiology; oldest antiarrhythmic agent)

Indication: Control of SVT in patients without WPW syndrome. May also be used to prevent recurrence of atrial flutter or atrial tachycardia after sinus rhythm is restored.

Dosing: Depending on the circumstance, may give loading dose first or begin maintenance.
  Intravenous dosing is 75% of oral dosing.
  Dosing is by gestational age.
  Loading doses given over 24 hours.
  Premature infant: 20 μg/kg.
  Term infant: 30 μg/kg.
  Maintenance: 25% of the loading dose daily, divided twice a day.

Caution: Digoxin may cause preferential block in the AV node and allow the accessory pathway to conduct more rapidly if patients also develop atrial fibrillation and have a rapidly conducting pathway. May cause heart block and ventricular arrhythmia if toxic. Half-life is 2–3 days in neonates.

Abbreviations: AV, atrioventricular; EAT, ectopic atrial tachycardia; ECG, electrocardiogram; JET, junctional ectopic tachycardia; PJRT, persistent (permanent form of) junctional reciprocating tachycardia; SVT, supraventricular tachycardia; VT, ventricular tachycardia.

The danger of giving lidocaine is predominantly that of neurologic sequelae.

You must always be ready to cardiovert if using lidocaine for VT.

If the rhythm is thought to be SVT and adenosine is given to a patient in atrial flutter:

The ECG may be diagnostic and unmask flutter.

The danger of giving adenosine is that it may cause atrial fibrillation or prolonged AV block in an acidotic premature infant.

You must always be ready to cardiovert when using adenosine.

If rhythm is thought to be SVT and adenosine is given to a patient with sinus tachycardia:

The ECG may be diagnostic in that there will be slowing but no conversion.

The danger would be of prolonged AV block or atrial fibrillation in a patient who is stressed by an underlying issue.

You must always be ready to cardiovert and to treat acidosis, hypovolemia, and blood loss.

If the rhythm is thought to be SVT and adenosine is given to a patient in atrial tachycardia:

The ECG may be diagnostic. It not only may slow the rhythm but also may cause a block to reveal an underlying atrial tachycardia.

The danger is atrial fibrillation and heart block.

You must always be ready to cardiovert and treat acidosis.

BRADYCARDIAS

Slow Rhythms in the Atrium

In the delivery room, a heart rate under 60 is a criterion for resuscitation. The list of causes for sinus bradycardia after birth is long but commonly includes sedation, vagal stimulation such as seen with gastroesophageal reflux, hypoxemia, sepsis, hypothermia, or other metabolic causes. As in any patient with a rhythm concern, a 12- or 15-lead ECG is needed. In the case of sinus bradycardia, the ECG is needed not only to confirm the rhythm but also to look for LQTS. The QTc is not reliable until day 3 of life as the stress of delivery can cause the QTc to prolong. Despite that, a QTc of over 500 ms, especially if there is also sinus bradycardia, would prompt a detailed family history for sudden death, syncope, seizures, or deafness and consideration for genetic testing if the finding persists.[14]

Slow Rhythms at the AV Node

A slow junctional rhythm in a patient with no structural heart disease would most likely be an escape rhythm secondary to complete heart block. A common reason for heart block in neonates is maternal systemic lupus erythematosus (SLE).[15] This may be diagnosed in utero by fetal echo.[16]

CHB and LQTS in newborn

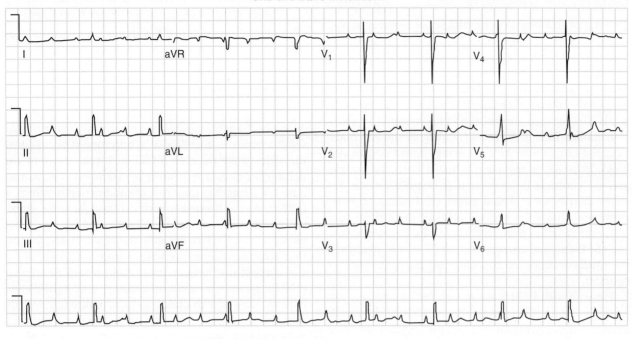

Torsades De Pointe Which may occur in LQTS

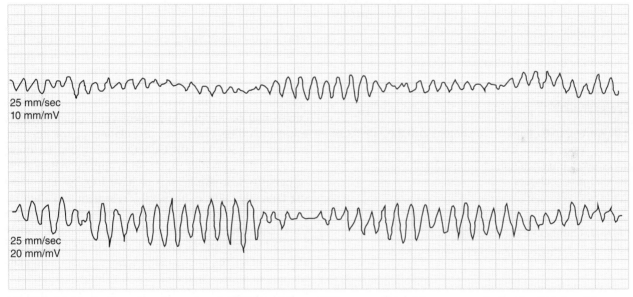

FIGURE 21-10 **A,** Complete heart block (CHB) and long QT in a newborn. The escape rhythm is slightly wide, suggesting an origin below the atrioventricular (AV) node. The QTc is prolonged with T waves, which are best seen in V5 and V6. **B,** Torsades de pointe, which may occur in long QT syndrome (LQTS), especially if there is bradycardia.

Dissociation is the key to diagnosing complete heart block. In this case, the junctional or AV nodal rhythm is regular, the atrial or sinus rhythm is also regular, and they are different.

Other, less-complete forms of heart block occur when some of the input from the atrium gets through and some does not. First-degree AV block has a prolonged PR interval, which designates a longer transit time through the AV node, but all signals get through.

Second-degree AV block implies that some but not all atrial signals make it through the AV node. With Mobitz type 1 (Wenckebach conduction), there is progressive PR prolongation, leading to a blocked beat, followed by normalization of the PR in a repetitive pattern. With Mobitz type II, one does not see this progressive prolongation of conduction time. Higher grades of AV block are also seen (2:1, 3:1, 4:1, and so on) and are more ominous.

Differential Diagnosis

The important point of the difference between first-, second-, and third-degree AV block is that third-degree block implies no association between the atrial and ventricular outputs. One would expect first-degree block to have a regular heart rate. Second-degree block will have an irregular ventricular rate, especially if it is Wenckebach conduction. This irregularity actually implies that there is still ability of the AV node to conduct and can be reassuring. Third-degree AV block is usually a regular rhythm in both the atrium and the ventricle because neither one is affecting the other. It may take several pages of rhythm strips to document dissociation if the rates of the atrium and the junction are similar. Eventually, the P waves, if you can see them, will emerge onto the T waves, overlying the QRS, or show up too close to the next QRS to conduct.

Patients with LQTS are at risk for heart block for several reasons. There may also be a defect in the K currents in the neonatal conducting tissue, which can cause conduction delay and true heart block, either second or third degree. If the QTc is very prolonged, it reflects the length of time it takes for the ventricles to repolarize. If a P wave arrives when the ventricle is still refractory or unexcitable, then it will not conduct. There may be a 2:1 pattern in this case.[17]

Treatment

The American College of Cardiology and the American Heart Association have determined guidelines for pacemaker implantation.[18] These 2002 guidelines are divided into 3 classes:

Class I: Evidence/agreement of usefulness

Class II: Conflict of evidence/opinion

Class III: Not useful; may be harmful

It was also noted that there was a difference in indications for pacing in children because of difference in heart rate needed for age as well as other factors. Class I indications would be met in a patient with complete heart block and LQTS especially if the QRS duration were wide for age, as in the example.

Class I: Evidence/agreement of usefulness

- Sinus node dysfunction with symptomatic bradycardia
- Advanced second- or third-degree AV block with symptomatic bradycardia, ventricular dysfunction, or low cardiac output , wide QRS, complex ventricular ectopy, *heart rate 50 bpm or less or 70 bpm or less with congenital heart disease in infants*
- Postoperative second- or third-degree AV block not expected to resolve or longer than 7days
- Pause-dependent VT with proven pacing efficacy

LONG-TERM OUTCOME AND FOLLOW-UP

Many of the tachycardias will resolve by 1 year of age. Of the patients with WPW syndrome, 50% will lose the delta wave on their ECG at 1 year. Loss of the delta wave does not mean that patients will no longer have SVT but that their risk of sudden death (which is 0.2% per year if symptomatic) is thought to be eliminated. Medications are usually weaned by a year for patients with SVT to evaluate the clinical need for further treatment. Patients who continue to have SVT, especially if they remain preexcited, would be considered for an invasive electrophysiology study (EPS) and pathway ablation in childhood and will likely remain on medication. Of patients with atrial tachycardia, 50% will have spontaneous resolution by 1 year of age as well, and medications are usually weaned at this time to determine clinical need.[19–22]

The long-term prognosis for VT depends a great deal on the underlying etiology.[23] If the patient had a history of myocarditis and persistently decreased function, ongoing treatment of ventricular arrhythmias will need to be based on Holter monitoring and clinical status. If the baby has LQTS, lifelong medication will be needed to prevent ventricular arrhythmias, including ventricular fibrillation or torsades de pointes (Figure 21-10). Genetic testing can be done to reveal the causative mutation in approximately 80% of patients who are known to have LQTS. This testing typically takes 6–8 weeks. Treatment can then be planned more specifically geared to the predicted risk for malignant ventricular arrhythmias. Types I and II LQTS, which are K-channel defects and catecholamine sensitive, are usually treated with β-blocker therapy in infancy and childhood, as long as there is no associated heart block. If there is heart block, a pacemaker will also be needed. Type III LQTS, which is a sodium channel defect, most likely is not protected by β-blocker therapy, and most will require implantation of a cardioverter-defibrillator. In the future, some may be treated with a combination approach, including a sodium channel blocker.

Overall long-term prognosis for patients with bradycardia and heart block due to maternal lupus is good, with an average of 86% survival at 10 years of age for live birth. Not all patients require a pacemaker at birth if the heart rate and function are adequate and the heart is structurally normal as per the guidelines discussed. Often, patients will be able to wait until childhood before that is needed.

REFERENCES

1. Zaidi AN, Ro PS. Treatment of fetal and neonatal arrhythmias. *US Cardiology.* 2006;3:1–4.

2. Killen SAS, Fish FA. Fetal and neonatal arrhythmias. *NeoReviews.* 2008;9(6);e242–e252.

3. Singh GK. Management of fetal tachyarrhythmias. *Curr Treat Options Cardiovasc Med.* 2004;6:399–406.

4. Park M. *Pediatric Cardiology Handbook.* Maryland Heights, MO: Mosby; 2010:34.

5. Kothari DS, Skinner JR. Neonatal tachycardias: an update. *Arch Dis child Fetal Neonatal Ed.* 2006;91:F136–F144.

6. Wu Th, Huang LC, Ho M. Fetal atrial flutter: a case report and experience of sotalol treatment. *Taiwan J Obstet Gynecol.* 2006;45(1):79–82.

7. Benson DW, Dunnigan A, Benditt DG. Follow up evaluation of infant paroxysmal atrial tachycardia: transesophageal study. *Circulation.* 1987;75(3):542–549.

8. Tester KM, Kertesz NJ, Friedman RA. Atrial flutter in infants. *Pediatr Cardiol.* 2006;48(5):1040–1046.

9. Saul JP1, Scott WA, Brown S, Marantz P, Acevedo V, Etheridge SP, Perry JC, Triedman JK, Burriss SW, Cargo P, Graepel J, Koskelo EK, Wang R. Intravenous amiodarone pediatric investigators. Intravenous amiodarone for incessant tachyarrhythmias in children: a randomized, double-blind, antiarrhythmic drug trial. *Circulation.* 2005;112(22):3470–3477.

10. Bink-Boelkens MT. Pharmacologic management of arrhythmias. *Pediatr Cardiol.* 2000;21:508–515.

11. Price JF, Kertesz NJ, Snyder CS, et al. Flecainide and sotalol: a new combination therapy for refractory supraventricular tachycardia in children less than 1 year of age. *J Am Coll Cardiol.* 2002;39(3):517–520.

12. Laer S, Elshoff JP, Meibohm B. Development of a safe and effective pediatric dosing regimen for sotalol based on population pharmacokinetics and pharmacodynamics in children with supraventricular tachycardia. *J Am Coll Cardiol.* 2005;46(7):1322–1330.

13. Sarubbi B, Vergara P, D'Alto M, Calabrò R. Congenital junctional ectopic tachycardia: presentation and outcome. *Indian Pacing Electrophysiol J.* 2003;3(3):143.

14. Ackerman MJ, Prioi SG, Willems S, et al. HRS/EHRA expert consensus statement on the state of genetic testing for the channelopathies and cardiomyopathies. *Heart Rhythm.* 2011; 8(8):1308–1339.

15. Donofrio MT, Guillquist SD, Mehta ID, et al. Congenital complete heart block: fetal management protocol, review of the literature, and report of the smallest successful pacemaker implantation. *J Perinatol.* 2004;24(2):112–117.

16. Buyon JP, Clancy RM, Freidman DM. Cardiac manifestations of neonatal lupus erythematosus: guidelines to management, integrating clues from the bench and bedside. *Nat Clin Pract Rheumatol.* 2009;5(3):139–148.

17. Van Hare G, Franz MR, Roge C, Sheinman MM. Persistent functional atrioventricular block in two patients with prolonged QT intervals: elucidation of the mechanism of block. *Pace Clin Electrophy.* 1990;13(5):608–618.

18. Gregoratos F, Abrams J, Epstein AE, et al. ACC/AHA/NASPE 2002 guideline update for implantation of cardiac pacemakers and antiarrhythmic devices. Executive summary. *Circulation.* 2002;106(16):2145–2161.

19. Lundberg A. Paroxysmal atrial tachycardia in infancy: long-term follow-up of 49 subjects. *Pediatrics.* 1982;70(4):638–642.

20. Salerno JC, Kertesz NJ, Friednman RA. Clinical course of atrial ectopic tachycardia is age dependent: results and treat in children less than 3 or greater than 3 years of age. *J Am Coll Cardiol.* 2004;43(3):438–444.

21. Gilljam T, Jaeggi E, Gow RM. Neonatal supraventricular tachycardia: outcomes over a 27-year period at a single institution. *Acta Paediatr.* 2008;97(8):1035–1039. Epub 2008 May 16.

22. Munger TM, Packer DL, Hammill SC, et al. A population study of the natural history of WPW syndrome in Olmsted County, Minnesota, 1953–1989. *Circulation.* 1993; 87(3):866–873.

23. Iwamoto M. Idiopathic ventricular tachycardia in children. *Circulation J.* 2011;75:544–545.

CHAPTER 21

22 Patent Ductus Arteriosus

Jeff Reese and Robert B. Cotton

INTRODUCTION

The ductus arteriosus is a central vascular shunt that interconnects the pulmonary artery and aorta during fetal life. A ductus or similar structure is present in mammals and most other vertebrates and is embryologically derived from the distal portion of the left sixth branchial arch.[1,2] As a result of the relatively large size of the ductus and the high resistance of the pulmonary vascular circuit in utero, approximately 90% of right ventricular output flows though the ductus and into the systemic circulation, thus bypassing the unaerated fetal lung.

Constriction of the ductus arteriosus is a critical step in postnatal circulatory transition. The normal physiological shift from a placental to a pulmonary respiration pattern is marked by a rapid sequence of events, including loss of umbilical flow and a subsequent fall in right atrial pressures, along with separation from the low-resistance vascular bed of the placenta and an accompanying increase in systemic vascular resistance (SVR)[3] (Figure 22-1). The abrupt decrease in pulmonary vascular resistance (PVR) that occurs with the onset of respiration leads to an 8- to 10-fold increase in pulmonary blood flow. As a result, left atrial pressure increases, facilitating closure of the foramen ovale. The combined increase in SVR and arterial blood pressure and decrease in PVR redirects blood flow through the ductus arteriosus in a left-to-right pattern until closure takes place via smooth muscle constriction and obstruction of the lumen. Luminal obstruction is a result of subendothelial thickening, the formation of intimal mounds that protrude into the vessel lumen,

and endothelial cell proliferation and crowding with ongoing muscular constriction. The formation of cell-cell adhesions and recruitment of circulating leukocytes or platelets might also contribute to ductus closure.[4–7]

Normal closure of the ductus arteriosus involves well-characterized anatomic changes that result in the remodeling of this structure to become the *ligamentum arteriosum*. Full-term infants with persistent patency of the ductus arteriosus do not undergo this remodeling. The result is a structural defect that occurs in full-term infants and often is associated with other cardiovascular anomalies.

In contrast to the timely closure of the ductus in full-term infants, premature infants, particularly those with lung disease, do not always undergo ductus closure shortly after birth. Unlike the full-term infant, in whom the patent ductus arteriosus (PDA) is a congenital structural defect, the ductus of a premature infant with symptomatic PDA would have closed normally but for the misfortune of the infant being delivered prematurely.

EPIDEMIOLOGY

A large proportion of premature infants will undergo spontaneous closure of the ductus arteriosus sometime during the neonatal period. Other premature infants will not experience ductus closure for weeks or more after birth. Hemodynamic symptoms of PDA are present in 55% to 70% of infants less than 1000 g birth weight or prior to 28 weeks of gestation.[8]

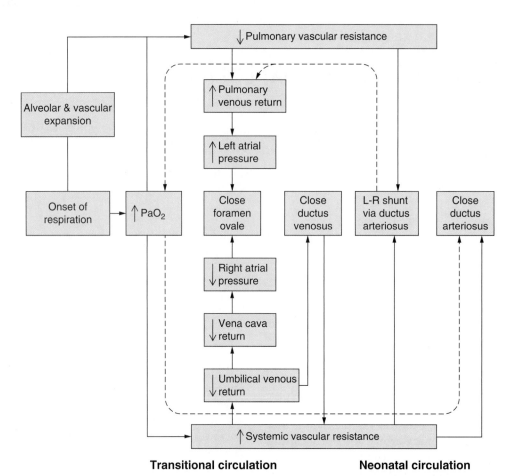

FIGURE 22-1 Cardiopulmonary transition at birth. The normal physiological shift from a placental to a pulmonary respiration pattern is marked by a rapid sequence of events illustrated by this block diagram of the transitional circulation. (Adapted from Smith and Nelson.[3])

To avoid ambiguities and inconsistencies, at least within this chapter, the following definitions are used:

- *Patent ductus arteriosus* (PDA) refers to the anatomic state of the ductus arteriosus.
  - Normal in fetal life
  - Abnormal when present after birth (sometimes referred to as persistent PDA)
  - When present after birth implies some degree of left-to-right shunt
- *Hemodynamically significant PDA* (hsPDA) is an echocardiographic definition referring to left-to-right ductus shunting with
  - diastolic flow reversal in the descending aorta, OR
  - evidence of LV failure (eg, LA or LV enlargement)
- *Symptomatic PDA* involves left-to-right shunting through a persistent PDA associated with clinical evidence of related pulmonary or cardiovascular compromise; some, but not all, infants with persistent PDA will also have symptomatic PDA. All infants with symptomatic PDA also have persistent PDA.

PDA in the Preterm Infant

Efforts to reevaluate the necessity to close a symptomatic PDA have led to renewed interest in the natural history of this disorder and suggest that current predictions of anticipated ductus closure in extremely low birth weight (ELBW) infants may need to be reevaluated. Spontaneous ductus closure may occur in 30% to 35% of immature infants less than 28 weeks' gestational age[9,10]; however, interpretation of these rates is difficult because they are based only on infants (by definition) who did not undergo intervention to close the ductus. Spontaneous closure rates are higher in more mature infants and lower when the clinical course is complicated by significant lung disease. In general, there is a significant negative correlation between length of time before spontaneous ductus closure occurs and gestational age, underscoring the strong developmental influence on when the ductus will close if left alone. Most infants with persistent ductus shunting will eventually undergo spontaneous closure. Reports from centers where medical management is emphasized as an alternative to pharmacologic or surgical intervention indicate that final spontaneous closure may not occur for weeks or longer, and that some infants may be discharged home with a persistent PDA and not experience final spontaneous closure until 60–76 weeks postmenstrual age.[9–11]

The strong influence of gestational immaturity on persistent ductus patency most likely reflects biological immaturity of the developing ductus smooth muscle, the presence of ongoing vasodilatory stimuli,[12] or incomplete acquisition of multiple-signaling systems that contribute to ductus closure.[13,14] Other factors associated with ductus patency are shown in Table 22-1.

There is growing evidence in preterm as well as full-term infants that hereditary and genetic factors play a role in susceptibility to persistent ductus patency after birth. In 1 study, comparison of monozygotic and dizygotic twin pairs indicated a significant genetic contribution to persistent PDA requiring indomethacin treatment, an effect that remained significant after taking environmental factors into consideration.[15] In another study of preterm twin pairs,[16] environmental factors rather than genetic factors accounted for a significant hereditary susceptibility to persistent PDA, indicating the inherent complexity of these kinds of studies.[17] In a population study designed to determine if genetic risk factors play a role in persistent PDA in preterm infants, 377 single-nucleotide polymorphisms from 130 genes of interest were evaluated in DNA samples collected from 204 infants with a gestational age of less than 32 weeks. The results of this study support a role for genetic variations in transcription factor AP-2β, tumor necrosis factor receptor–associated factor 1, and prostacyclin synthase in the persistent patency of the ductus arteriosus in preterm infants.[18] Although it would be premature to assume that these genetic variations reveal a biological etiology, it is reasonable to regard these findings as genetic risk factors for persistent PDA that can be added to the list of established clinical risk factors such as birth weight, gestational age, acute perinatal stress, and hyaline membrane disease. In the absence of genetic risk factors for persistent PDA, the 28-week preterm infant might not have persistent PDA even though the infant had the same clinical risk factors as the 28-week preterm infant who is positive for the genetic risk factors and who develops persistent PDA.[19]

Table 22-1 Factors Associated with Patent Ductus Arteriosus (PDA)[a,b]

Established Risk Factors for PDA	Other Factors Associated with PDA	
Early gestational age[19,127,170,385,425,426]	IUGR[19,427]	Maternal drugs:
Low birth weight[385,426,438]	Delay in indocin treatment[425]	Antihistamine[428]
RDS[19,127,426,438]	Furosemide treatment[166,439]	Magnesium[429,430]
Persistence of DA flow[394]	Use of HFOV[348,440]	ACE inhibitors[431,432]
Sepsis[389,393]	Race:	Anticonvulsants[433]
Excess fluid administration[170,172]	Caucasian (PT)[127,170,428]	Ca channel blockers[434]
Antenatal NSAID exposure[390,392]	African American (T)[441]	Cocaine[435]
Initial hypotension[428,438]		Maternal PKU (T)[436,437]
Need for intubation/CPAP[19,428]	Gender:	
Lack of antenatal betamethasone[127]	Male (PT)[428,442] Female (T)[443,444]	
Maternal diabetes (T)[442,446]	Prolonged ROM[426]	Genetic Conditions (T)[445]
Birth at high altitude (T)[447,448]	Twins[442,449,450]	Trisomy 21, 18, 13; Char, Holt-Oram, DiGeorge, Noonan, Cantu, CHARGE, TAAD/PDA
Congenital rubella (T)[451]	Perinatal stress[19]	Genetic susceptibility[16,18]
Hypothyroidism (T, PT)[452,453]	Antenatal hemorrhage[170,442]	Familial PDA[445]
	Breech[428]	
	Phototherapy[454]	

Abbreviations: ACE, angiotensin-converting enzyme; CPAP, continuous positive airway pressure; DA, ductus arteriosus; HFOV, high-frequency oscillatory ventilation; IUGR, intrauterine growth retardation; NSAID, nonsteroidal anti-inflammatory drug; PKU, phenylketonuria; PT, preterm; RDS, respiratory distress syndrome; ROM, rupture of membranes; T, term; TAAD, thoracic aortic aneurysms and dissection.
[a]Adapted from Reese et al.[12]
[b]Risk factors for PDA were considered to be well established if they were identified by studies that sought causative factors for PDA, remained significant after multivariate analysis, or were consistently found in multiple controlled trials in different patient populations. Other factors that have been shown to have an association with PDA were drawn from single studies, epidemiologic surveys, birth defect registry reports, case reports, or small studies that did not control for confounding variables. Conflicting studies that did not detect an association of PDA with these factors are not presented. Genetic conditions were considered separately. Only a subset of representative citations are shown for risk factors that were consistently identified in numerous studies.

Persistent PDA in the Term Infant

Persistent PDA in full-term infants is the result of different pathological processes than in preterm infants. Anatomic studies have shown that the ductus in term infants with persistent PDA is abnormally formed.[20] The full-term infant with persistent PDA maintains an intact internal elastic lamina rather than undergoing fragmentation to facilitate the migration of underlying smooth muscle cells into the subendothelial space, with a corresponding reduction in the formation of intimal cushions for occlusion of the ductus lumen. The ductus in full-term infants with persistent PDA also has altered formation of elastic lamina, reduced subendothelial swelling and matrix deposition, reduced proliferation of the muscular media, and reduced smooth muscle layers.[4,20,21]

Prematurity does not protect against the pathophysiology underlying persistent PDA in the full-term infant. If a premature infant happens to have a "full-term-like" persistent PDA, it would probably be thought (mistakenly) to have a preterm persistent PDA that did not close spontaneously, unless it was associated with other anomalies.

The ductus usually closes by 48 hours of age in nearly all term gestation newborns. The prevalence of persistent PDA in term infants is approximately 2 to 8 per 10,000 live births.[22] A 2:1 to 3:1 preponderance of PDA cases in female infants is historically based on surveys that include other congenital cardiac anomalies or those that require ductus ligation.[23,24] More recent studies showed mixed results for female predominance at term.[25-28] Infants who are born at high altitude or experience sustained hypoxia have an increased incidence of PDA. Genetic syndromes and congenital rubella have also been associated with a large proportion of the full-term variety of PDA. Other factors that contribute to PDA in the term infant are given in Table 22-1.

PATHOPHYSIOLOGY

Effects of a Symptomatic PDA on the Cardiopulmonary System

The normal postnatal fall in PVR leads to reversal of blood flow across the ductus in the first few hours after birth.[29,30] The adverse effects of a persistent PDA depend on the size of the left-to-right shunt and the capacity for left ventricular compensation. Blood flow across the ductus is primarily influenced by PVR but is also the product of many interacting factors, including the balance between SVR and PVR, myocardial function and systemic blood pressure, the relative size and flow-restrictive characteristics of the PDA, viscosity of the blood, and other factors that regulate the flow of fluids. In the face of falling PVR after birth, freshly oxygenated blood from the aorta is redirected back into the pulmonary bed via the ductus, diverting blood from the systemic circulation and sending excessive blood flow through the lungs into the left atrium and ventricle. Left-to-right shunting through the PDA results in increased blood volume (preload) and excess work for the left heart. In most neonates, maintenance of cardiac output in the face of an increasing left-to-right shunt through the ductus is accomplished by changes in stroke volume rather than heart rate.[30-32] The corresponding increase in left ventricular stroke volume is proportional to the size of the shunt. A small PDA may not cause significant hemodynamic effects, and infants with significant or long-standing left-to-right shunt through a large PDA may experience left-sided chamber enlargement that can progress to failure. Right heart or biventricular failure is eventually possible in the presence of pulmonary hypertension due to increased PVR.

The premature heart is more vulnerable to excess volume load from significant left-to-right flow through a PDA, although shunts of up to 4:1 or greater have been documented,[33,34] and some studies show no adverse effects on contractility.[35] Compared to the adult heart, the fetal or immature myocardium has several features that contribute to enhanced sensitivity to volume overload. Fetal myocardial cells are less compliant than adult cells and have decreased ability to generate active tension. Immature myocardial cells are more dependent on extracellular calcium and the function of L-type calcium channels and have less available calcium via the sacroplasmic reticulum than adult cells. Immature myocytes are disorganized, and their myofibrils are less oriented than adult cells. The shape and dimensions of immature myocytes also contribute to their diminished contractile force and speed. The immature myocardium also has increased water content and an increased mass of noncontractile components (nuclei, mitochondria, cell membranes) compared to adults, which reduce their biomechanical advantage. The immature ventricle is thus less distensible with less-contractile force-generating ability, although individual myofilaments within fetal and adult myocardial cells have similar contractile potential when normalized for these differences.[36,37]

Increased flow through the preterm PDA distends the pulmonary arteries, with enlargement of the pulmonary veins, left atrium, and left ventricle due to volume overload and the less-favorable characteristics of the immature myocardium. Left heart failure and associated pulmonary edema may ensue. The immature lung is more susceptible to transmural fluid shifts caused by low plasma oncotic pressures in premature infants and increased microvascular pressures from an hsPDA. Increased capillary permeability may be present because of structural impairments and hormonal influences in the immature lung, combined with adverse effects on endothelial integrity in the presence of respiratory distress syndrome (RDS), mechanical ventilation, and inflammatory mediators in the local and systemic circulations. Fluid displacement or leak of plasma proteins into the interstitial and alveolar spaces can interfere with respiratory function and inhibit surfactant function. Lymphatic function in the preterm lung can temporarily compensate for the presence of increased interstitial fluid and protein. Pulmonary edema may be a presenting sign of symptomatic PDA and is common in infants with longer exposure to left-to-right ductus shunting. Improvements in pulmonary function occur following pharmacologic or surgical closure of the PDA. Pulmonary hemorrhage is another possible consequence of pulmonary microvascular fragility, reduced myocardial compliance, and increased back pressure in the presence of an hsPDA. The relationship between surfactant administration and pulmonary hemorrhage is partially explained by the presence of an increasing left-to-right ductus shunt consequent to improved alveolar PaO_2 and decreasing PVR, resulting in increasing pulmonary microvascular pressure. The pulmonary response to left-to-right shunting varies according to the degree of shunt and the host response but may be reflected by an increased oxygen requirement, diminished ventilation, and worsening pulmonary compliance, leading to an increased need for respiratory support. Closure of the ductus under these conditions improves pulmonary mechanical properties and reduces the risks for pulmonary hemorrhage, chronic lung disease, and the need for ventilatory support.[14,38–42]

Effects of Left-to-Right Ductus Shunting on Other Organs

Redistribution of blood flow away from the systemic circulation by a left-to-right ductus shunt also affects the perfusion of other organ systems. Hypotension is a common early manifestation of excess flow through a symptomatic PDA. Diastolic runoff and the compensatory increase in stroke volume are typically able to maintain systolic blood pressure while diastolic pressures decrease, leading to widened pulse pressure.

Preservation of cerebral perfusion and oxygenation in the presence of lower blood pressures are of paramount importance in the perinatal period. PDA has been associated with intraventricular hemorrhage (IVH) and adverse neurodevelopment.[43–45] Indomethacin given as prophylaxis (see the section discussing this specifically) decreases the incidence and severity of IVH and as well as any left-to-right ductus shunt that may be present. However, long-term outcomes are not necessarily improved.[46–48] Most

studies indicated that the presence of an hsPDA has some form of deleterious effect on cerebral blood flow, perfusion, or oxygenation.[49–53]

The effects of a large PDA on systemic blood flow may be greater for the renal, mesenteric, and other postductal vascular beds than for preductal cerebral perfusion, consistent with a ductal steal phenomenon.[54–56] Reversal of blood flow during diastole in the descending aorta is a distinguishing characteristic of an hsPDA, with corresponding hypoperfusion of distal tissues.[51,54,57,58] Decreased blood flow or tissue perfusion because of significant left-to-right shunt from an hsPDA is associated with abnormalities of the gut, including feeding intolerance and necrotizing enterocolitis (NEC).[55,57,59–65] Spontaneous intestinal perforation (SIP) is distinct from NEC.[66–69] The presence of a PDA may be a risk factor for SIP,[70–73] but this observation requires further study. Efforts to close or significantly constrict the hsPDA are generally beneficial for the gut.

Reversal of diastolic blood flow in the renal vasculature is a common feature of an hsPDA.[54,55,74,75] Oliguria is considered a reflection of hypoperfusion and prerenal insufficiency in association with left-to-right ductus shunting. Treatment with indomethacin poses an additional risk to the underperfused kidney unless systemic flow is restored by closing the ductus. Attempts to negate the renal side effects of indomethacin with furosemide, dopamine, and other agents have been advocated[76,77] but with limited success.[78–83]

Mechanisms Responsible for Normal Postnatal Ductus Closure

Constriction and permanent closure of the ductus arteriosus is a complex process involving alterations in ductus blood flow, endothelial–smooth muscle interactions, cell trafficking, apoptosis and cell turnover, and unique responses to changes in oxygen and other endocrine and paracrine molecular signals.[13,14] Preparation for postnatal ductus constriction begins several weeks prior to birth. Localized areas of subintimal thickening eventually form large mounds, or intimal cushions, that protrude into the ductus lumen[4,84–86] (Figure 22-2). Delivery at premature gestation or disruption of this process in large-animal models can result in PDA.[87,88]

After birth, the abrupt increase in oxygen tension with the onset of respiration triggers initial constriction of the postnatal ductus arteriosus (Figure 22-1). Although closure of the ductus is a continuous event that begins with precocious maturation in utero, the postnatal steps that contribute to closure are considered to occur in 2 phases: (1) a functional closure that occurs within hours of birth and is the product of muscular constriction and luminal obstruction and (2) a

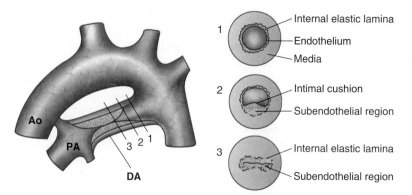

FIGURE 22-2 Schematic structure of the closing ductus arteriosus (DA). In a canine model of DA closure, the following occur: (1) The aortic end of the DA (near the aortic isthmus) still lacks intimal thickening. (2) Intimal thickening starts at the "bottom" of the DA; later stages of this process can be observed toward the pulmonary end. (3) Luminal closure is observed from approximately the middle of the DA to the pulmonary end. Ao, aorta; PA, pulmonary artery. (Adapted from de Reeder et al.[84])

permanent anatomic occlusion that involves fibromuscular transformation of the ductus into a persisting vascular remnant, the *ligamentum arteriosum*.[14]

The initial functional phase is characterized by potent vasoconstriction in response to oxygen. The mechanisms for oxygen-induced ductus constriction are still under investigation but may include the actions of cytochrome P450 (CYP) enzymes and endothelin-1 (ET-1), which acts as a downstream effector of ductus constriction.[89–91] A second mechanism involves the presence of oxygen-sensitive, voltage-gated potassium channels.[92–94] Here, oxygen exposure triggers a redox cascade in the mitochondria of sensitive cells[95] with the production of peroxide or other diffusible mediators, leading to inhibition of Kv channels and disruption of the normal resting potential of the cell membrane. Stimulation of membrane depolarization by alterations in resting membrane potential triggers entry of calcium from the sarcoplasmic reticulum and extracellular sources.[96] Calcium influx into ductus smooth muscle cells is primarily mediated through voltage-dependent L-type calcium channels, resulting in vessel constriction,[92,97–99] although other calcium channels contribute.[100–104]

Functional closure also results from prompt withdrawal of the vasodilatory effects of prostaglandins. Although prostaglandins are locally synthesized by both cyclooxygenase 1 (COX-1) and cyclooxygenase 2 (COX-2) isoforms in the ductus wall,[105–107] the acute decrease in circulating prostaglandin E_2 (PGE_2) is primarily due to loss of the placenta as a source and increased PGE catabolism by upregulation of prostaglandin dehydrogenase (PGDH) in the lung and peripheral tissues. A postnatal decrease in ductus PGE receptors may also contribute to reduced prostaglandin sensitivity after birth.[108–110]

In the second phase, permanent anatomic closure of the ductus takes place over a period of several weeks.

At term gestation, initial ductus constriction is accompanied by impairment of vasa vasorum perfusion of the thick muscular media, producing circumferential watershed-like regions of hypoxic and ischemic injury in the vessel wall.[111,112] Decreased local production of vasodilatory prostaglandins and nitric oxide (NO) permit ongoing contractile forces to maintain ductus closure. Hypoxic signals stimulate local production of growth factors such as vascular endothelial growth factor (VEGF) and transforming growth factor β (TGF-β)[113–115] that contribute to a fibrous transformation of the vessel into a ligamentous cord. Permanent remodeling involves localized hypoglycemia and depletion of adenosine triphosphate (ATP) and other nutrients with corresponding energy failure and cell death.[116,117] Apoptosis is a prerequisite for permanent ductus remodeling[118] and is accompanied by changes in hyaluronic acid, chondroitin sulfate, fibronectin, and other extracellular matrix constituents.[85] The presence of a persistent PDA in preterm infants may be due to failure of initial ductus closure or reopening of a previously constricted ductus and failure of vessel remodeling. If the preterm ductus is able to close, the normal process of involution and cell turnover can proceed. However, the preterm ductus with incomplete luminal constriction fails to undergo ATP depletion, nutrient restriction, and energy failure, preventing the necessary cell death and turnover that is required for fibrous transformation.[119] Permanent closure of the ductus also involves the recruitment of circulating leukocytes that invade the ductus wall to promote intimal cushion formation.[5,7] A role for platelet adhesion in permanent ductus constriction has been proposed, although this observation has not been confirmed in other patient populations.[6,120–123]

Pharmacologic agents that promote maturation of the ductus also contribute to its postnatal closure. Antenatal steroids are consistently identified as contributing to successful ductus closure.[124–127] Postnatal glucocorticoid treatment of BPD is also associated with reduction in the incidence of PDA.[128–130] Routine use of postnatal glucocorticoids to promote sensitivity of the ductus to contractile stimuli is not yet supported by clinical trials, although improved use of antenatal steroids should be encouraged. Retinoids have important roles in cardiovascular development and are linked to ductus arteriosus formation and maturation.[131–133] However, despite the large number of infants exposed to vitamin A in clinical trials,[134] evidence has not emerged linking vitamin A status or treatment with PDA.[135,136] Maturation of the ductus may also be enhanced by intrauterine stress and exposure to thyroid hormones or progesterone,[137–140] but there are no current therapies to exploit these advantages. Avoidance of drugs and other pharmacologic compounds that contribute to ductus relaxation should also be considered as a conservative measure to prevent symptomatic PDA.[12]

CLINICAL PRESENTATION AND DIFFERENTIAL DIAGNOSIS

Clinical Presentation of Symptomatic PDA

A persistent PDA becomes symptomatic when left-to-right shunting through the ductus arteriosus becomes of sufficient magnitude to compromise pulmonary or cardiovascular function. For the most part, this occurs in premature infants, not full-term infants. The "symptoms" of a symptomatic PDA relate to pulmonary, cardiac, or systemic findings. *Pulmonary symptoms* include increasing oxygen requirement, episodes of apnea and bradycardia, ventilator dependence, and pulmonary edema. The pulmonary edema may be severe, resulting in a "white-out" on chest x-ray and requiring substantial increases in ventilatory support. *Cardiac symptoms* include congestive heart failure; tachycardia, sometimes with a gallop rhythm; increasing heart size; and deterioration of cardiac function. *Systemic symptoms* reflect inadequate systemic circulatory perfusion due to the diversion of left ventricular output away from the systemic circulation and include feeding intolerance with abdominal distention or NEC, compromised caloric intake, metabolic acidosis, renal insufficiency and even central nervous system depression.[141]

Infants with symptomatic PDA have heterogeneous findings on physical examination.[141] The presenting signs are proportional to the size of the left-to-right shunt (see the section on pathophysiology). Typical features evolve over the first few days of life. The physical findings of symptomatic PDA include a hyperactive precordium, increased pulses and pulse pressure (usually > 30 or 40 mm Hg), a low diastolic pressure (usually lower than 30 mm Hg), loud heart sounds, murmur, decreased perfusion of skin with a capillary refill time longer than 3 s, rales, and diminished air entry into the lungs, causing diminished breath sounds.

The classic "machinery" murmur described in 1898 by Gibson[142] occurs due to turbulent flow across the ductus throughout the cardiac cycle. The continuous murmur of a persistent PDA is not always present. A holosystolic murmur is frequently described, although the murmur of a persistent PDA can take many forms.[142–144] A "silent" ductus in the presence of a widely patent ductus has been recognized for over 50 years.[145–148] Burnard (1958) first recognized that the association between a systolic murmur and cardiomegaly on the chest radiograph of newborn premature infants represented a persistent PDA that sometimes evolved into an overt symptomatic PDA.[143]

While echocardiography is immensely useful in documenting cardiovascular structure and function, it has not made the physical examination obsolete. Findings such as rales and diminished breath sounds, poor capillary perfusion, decreased level of consciousness, and abdominal distention may help provide clinical evidence that a premature infant with persistent PDA has become symptomatic, requiring consideration of different treatment options.

DIFFERENTIAL DIAGNOSIS

The physical findings of a persistent PDA may be similar to other cardiovascular lesions with a continuous murmur or features of pulmonary congestion and diastolic runoff related to left-to-right shunt. These defects include aortico-pulmonary window; arteriovenous fistulae in coronary, pulmonary, or systemic systems; systemic-to-pulmonary collaterals; absent pulmonary valve syndrome; truncus arteriosus; hemitruncus; ruptured sinus of Valsalva aneurysm; and ventricular septal defect with aortic regurgitation. An innocent venous hum or peripheral pulmonary artery stenosis may have auscultory findings similar to a persistent PDA. Differentiation of these conditions from persistent PDA must be made by Doppler echocardiography.

DIAGNOSTIC TESTS

Radiographic findings include cardiomegaly, presenting as an increase or relative increase in cardiothoracic ratio over time. Pulmonary overcirculation is reflected by increased vascular markings or fullness of the outflow tract on anterior-posterior (A-P) views.

CHAPTER 22

Pulmonary infiltrates may obscure these findings. The overall diagnostic accuracy of radiographic findings is poor.[149]

The electrocardiogram is usually normal. Long-standing persistent PDAs or those with large shunts may show signs of left-sided strain, left ventricular hypertrophy, or left atrial enlargement, but these findings are nondiagnostic. Tachycardia may be present but is not specific for left-to-right ductus shunting.

Echocardiography is the definitive method for diagnosis of persistent PDA. Combined with color Doppler, information can be obtained on the size of the ductus, magnitude and direction of shunt, and assessment of diastolic blood flow disturbance. Effects on cardiac chamber size and flow in other regions can be measured. Two-dimensional echocardiography permits detection of associated abnormalities, including aneurysm of the ductus, coarctation, or right-sided aortic arch. In the presence of high PVR, detection of ductus flow by color Doppler may be more difficult.

Consensus criteria for the echocardiographic diagnosis of an hsPDA are lacking.[29,150,151] The functional significance of a persistent PDA is indirectly assessed by values that reflect the degree of left-to-right shunt. Retrograde flow in the descending aorta during diastole represents a large-volume shunt.[29,56] However, the use of echocardiography to determine whether a persistent PDA is hemodynamically significant requires more than 1 echocardiographic measurement of a single parameter.[29,150,152] Commonly used schemes include combinations of the following criteria to define a moderate-to-large ductus: ductus diameter 1.5 mm or greater, left atrial-to-aortic root (LA/Ao) ratio 1.5 or greater, the presence of reversed diastolic flow in the descending aorta, or left pulmonary artery end-diastolic flow 2.0 m/s or greater.[29,153] Cutoff values may be indexed for birth weight (eg, ductus diameter ≥ 1.4 mm/kg).[153] Echocardiographic criteria should be used in combination with clinical signs of persistent PDA and interpreted with respect to each individual's clinical condition, postnatal age, and potential for spontaneous closure. The development of uniform staging criteria that incorporate both clinical and echocardiographic parameters will be beneficial.[154]

Additional criteria have been developed to assess the physiological impact of a persistent PDA. Serum levels of atrial natriuretic peptide (ANP), brain-type natriuretic peptide (BNP), troponin, endothelin, or combinations of these measurements reflect the degree of cardiac distension or myocardial injury in the presence of an hsPDA.[155-161] However, changes in BNP levels are poorly predictive of changes in ductus shunt or response to treatment,[162,163] while other serological measurements remain incompletely characterized.

MANAGEMENT

Medical Management (Conservative Approach)

All premature infants who develop a symptomatic PDA should have certain anticongestive measures implemented to control pulmonary edema and to maintain adequate systemic perfusion. These measures can be regarded as intervention to "hold the fort" while waiting for the ductus to close, whether spontaneously (weeks or longer), pharmacologically (hours), or with surgery (until tomorrow). Some refer to this regimen as medical management of symptomatic PDA, and others regard it as less-aggressive or conservative management. These approaches may reduce the risk that a persistent PDA will become symptomatic.

Medical management of symptomatic PDA is based on an understanding of the pathophysiology of this condition (see the section on this topic). Management of a symptomatic PDA is a balancing act that attempts to promote adequate systemic flow without causing excessive pulmonary blood flow. Measures to limit pulmonary blood flow and control pulmonary edema may result in inadequate systemic perfusion. On the other hand, measures to achieve adequate systemic perfusion may result in increased pulmonary blood flow and pulmonary edema.

Pulmonary edema can be controlled by regulating fluid balance, which can be achieved by fluid restriction (as low as 60 mL/kg/d and no more than 130 mL/kg/d) and the judicious use of a diuretic. The effects of diuretic therapy need to be assessed by monitoring body weight, serum sodium, urine output, and physical findings such as rales and peripheral edema. When diuretic therapy is used, it should be given on a "one-time" basis to adjust for prior excessive fluid intake rather than being given as a scheduled dose. Choice of diuretic should take into consideration the potentially beneficial extrarenal effects of furosemide[164,165] as well as the possibility that loop diuretics may increase the risks for PDA.[166,167]

Exposure to excess fluid administration, either through early treatment with volume expanders or by increased daily fluid intake, is associated with development of PDA.[168-170] An increased risk for PDA exists for fluid intake of more than 170 mL/kg/d, even after controlling for gestational age and illness severity. For small preterm infants, every 10 mL/kg increase in fluid administration rate on the second or third day of life adds additional risk.[171] In nurseries where PDA is an ongoing problem, a restrictive fluid management strategy is likely to result in lower risks for PDA.[172]

The quickest way to control pulmonary edema is to increase distending airway pressure. This can be done with nasal continuous positive airway pressure (CPAP) or with mechanical ventilation. A periodic "sigh" may also help reclaim lung volume previously lost to pulmonary edema. The efficacy of these efforts to control pulmonary edema will result in improved blood gases and the physical findings of improved air entry and decreased rales. Positive end-expiratory pressure (PEEP) and other forms of distending airway pressure decrease pulmonary edema by increasing intraluminal hydrostatic pressure in the terminal airways. In addition, the use of PEEP decreases the degree of left-to-right shunting through the ductus and improves systemic blood flow.[173,174] Improved ventilation and reduced work of breathing help improve tissue perfusion and systemic oxygen delivery and relieve increased demands on left ventricular output that is already burdened by much of the left ventricular output being shunted through the pulmonary circulation.

Adequate oxygenation is important to stimulate and maintain postnatal ductus constriction. Recommendations to lower the oxygen saturation target range in small preterm infants have successfully reduced the frequency and severity of retinopathy of prematurity (ROP) but may adversely affect ductus constriction. Noori et al found a 1.7-fold increased risk for hsPDA after chronic exposure to reduced saturation ranges. The need for ligation of the ductus was unchanged, however, suggesting that pharmacological therapy or spontaneous ductus closure was still possible despite lower levels of oxygenation.[175] Increased incidence of symptomatic PDA has not been reported in other studies that target lower saturation limits.[176] It is also unclear whether resuscitation of preterm infants with room air or reduced oxygen concentrations will have an impact on ductus closure rates. Any protocol to target the risks of oxygen injury will need to be balanced against the risks for symptomatic PDA and other neonatal morbidities.

Systemic perfusion must be supported in patients with symptomatic PDA. An increase in the capacity of the left heart and pulmonary vascular bed that occurs in symptomatic PDA may require blood transfusions with packed red cells to maintain an adequate blood volume and an adequate hematocrit for oxygen transport to the systemic circulation. Increasing the hematocrit increases PVR more than SVR and as a result reduces left-to-right shunt[177] and provides improved forward systemic flow and oxygen-carrying capacity to peripheral tissues. The left ventricle must supply an adequate output to perfuse the systemic circulation in the face of the additional left ventricular output diverted back across the ductus and into the pulmonary circulation. For this reason, care should be taken to reduce other demands on the left ventricle. Under these circumstances, it may become necessary to support myocardial performance with inotropes such as dobutamine. Drugs such as dopamine, which increase SVR, may shift cardiac output from the systemic

circulation and into the lungs, thereby aggravating pulmonary edema.

Less-Aggressive Intervention (to Close or Not to Close)

Measures that optimize fluid and respiratory management, hemodynamic status, and hematologic parameters may minimize the complications of symptomatic PDA, but they do not necessarily obviate the need for closure of the ductus. Recommendations to pursue ductus closure aggressively have been traditionally based on evidence that prolonged exposure to the complications of a symptomatic PDA leads to substantial morbidity, if not mortality.[38,39,178–180] The comorbidities associated with a symptomatic PDA include an increased need for prolonged respiratory support related to ventilatory failure and BPD, as well as complications such as recurrent sepsis, NEC, feeding intolerance requiring prolonged use of total parenteral nutrition (TPN), metabolic bone disease, and others.

On the other hand, recent studies questioned whether the association between these complications and prolonged ductus shunting is an independent effect that can be decreased by ductus closure. For example, a systematic review of randomized trials[181,182] cautioned that infants undergoing ductus closure were no better off than their declared controls with regard to survival, BPD, NEC, or ROP. In addition, outcomes have been no better in infants undergoing ductus closure prior to development of symptomatic PDA.[182–184] However, these kinds of studies must be carefully interpreted because some of the "control" infants also underwent backup intervention (surgical ligation or nonsteroidal anti-inflammatory drug [NSAID] treatment) to close the ductus.

Routine closure of the symptomatic PDA has been challenged as the standard of care[184,185] for several reasons. First, it is becoming more widely accepted that the vast majority of infants with symptomatic PDA will eventually experience spontaneous closure of the ductus, even when there has been a recurrence of symptomatic PDA following unsuccessful treatment with NSAIDs. Second, the complications related to either surgical ligation or treatment with NSAIDs may outweigh any beneficial effect of attaining ductus closure soon after the PDA of an infant becomes symptomatic. These reasons are the basis of an increased interest in managing infants with symptomatic PDA medically while waiting for spontaneous closure of the ductus, a paradigm that is already practiced in some nurseries, as reflected by the content of surveys and large registries of premature infants.[186–192] It has even been suggested that active interventions to close the ductus should be limited to clinical trials.[185,193–195] In fact, the lack of information comparing the outcome of this practice of withholding intervention to close the ductus underscores the need for a properly controlled randomized trial to address this question.[196]

There is accumulating evidence that a patent ductus will eventually close spontaneously even in very immature infants. In a retrospective assessment of medical management without intervention to close the ductus, Herrman et al observed spontaneous ductus closure in the majority of very low birth weight (VLBW) infants who had left-to-right ductus shunting at the time of discharge. Spontaneous closure of small, persistent PDA occurred as late as 60–76 weeks post-menstrual age (PMA).[11] Other investigators also have noted spontaneous ductus closure in small preterm infants.[9,10,185,187]

Until comparisons of long-term outcomes have been made between medical management with and without intervention to close the ductus, it will be difficult, if not impossible, to identify the group of infants who are most likely to benefit from active intervention to close the ductus without incurring unacceptable complications, short or long term. In the meantime, withholding intervention to close a symptomatic PDA should be limited to patients whose systemic circulation is adequately perfused and whose ductus is predicted to close spontaneously sooner rather than later, keeping in mind that even these patients may benefit from ductus closure.

Prophylactic (Preemptive) Indomethacin

Prophylactic indomethacin has consistently been shown to reduce the incidence of symptomatic PDA and the need for ductus ligation, along with a reduction in severe IVH (grades 3 and 4) and pulmonary hemorrhage.[42,46,197,198] A prophylactic approach (<24 hours of age) to preempt symptomatic PDA with the administration of indomethacin within the first 24 hours after birth[199–201] came into consideration at the time when indomethacin was found to be an effective approach for prevention of IVH.[202–208] The beneficial effects of indomethacin for IVH prevention do not appear to be related to ductus closure.[203,204] However, the observation that prophylactic indomethacin treatment reduced the incidence of severe IVH legitimized its widespread adoption as a management strategy of symptomatic PDA as well as a means to prevent severe IVH.[46,209]

Even though prophylactic indomethacin has been shown to prevent symptomatic PDA, reduce the need for ductus ligation, and prevent severe IVH, it is disappointing that its use does not reduce the incidence of BPD or improve survival without neurosensory impairment at 18 months of age or improve other long-term outcomes of interest for preterm infants.[46,181,182,198,210] On the other hand, common complications of extreme prematurity such as NEC or gastrointestinal perforation, ROP, chronic lung disease, or cerebral white matter injury were not observed. In addition, it was estimated

that only 20 infants would need to be treated with prophylactic indomethacin to avert the need to ligate the ductus of 1 high-risk infant. Given the favorable benefit-to-risk ratio of prophylactic indomethacin, its use would be appropriate in patient populations that experience higher-than-expected rates of severe IVH, pulmonary hemorrhage, or need for surgical ligation.[42,197,211] Another beneficial feature of prophylactic indomethacin is that, given the prolonged clearance in the first few days of life, it is possible that a single 0.2-mg/kg dose of indomethacin in the first 24 hours of life can be used as an effective prophylaxis strategy with limited exposure to indomethacin toxicities.[201]

Ibuprofen has potential benefits for closure of a persistent PDA and prevention of ligation[212] but is no longer considered an alternative for prophylaxis of a symptomatic PDA due to unforeseen risks of treatment.[213–217] A meta-analysis of 7 trials (931 infants) concluded that prophylactic ibuprofen effectively reduced the incidence of symptomatic PDA, the need for rescue treatment with NSAIDs, and the need for surgical ligation, but exposed many infants to a drug with concerning renal and gastrointestinal side effects without conferring important short-term benefits.[218]

Pharmacologic Ductus Closure with NSAIDs

Current pharmacological approaches to stimulate ductus closure are based on inhibition of vasodilatory forces (PGE_2) rather than triggers for vascular smooth muscle contraction because vasoconstrictive agents (other than oxygen) that specifically target the ductus are not yet available. An important role for prostaglandins in ductus relaxation was suspected when fetal ductus constriction occurred in pregnant women who were treated with salicylates or indomethacin.[219,220] Prostaglandins or their inhibitors were concurrently found to have potent effects on ductus tone in various animal models.[221–224] In 1975, prolongation of human ductus patency by PGE infusion was noted.[225] In 1976, two clinical trials established the effectiveness of indomethacin for ductus closure in premature infants.[226,227] Ibuprofen was found to have similar effects on ductus closure soon thereafter,[228,229] but until 1995, clinical trials in preterm infants were not reported.[230–232]

Indomethacin and ibuprofen, the most commonly used NSAIDs for pharmacologic constriction of the ductus, inhibit the prostaglandin synthase (or cyclooxygenase) enzymes, COX-1 and COX-2. NSAIDs exert their effects by binding inside the cyclooxygenase channel to prevent arachidonic acid catabolism and formation of prostaglandins.[233] Indomethacin inhibits both COX isoforms in a competitive, time-dependent, slowly reversible manner. The COX-1 and COX-2 enzymes are both present in the human ductus,[107] although inhibition of prostaglandin synthesis in peripheral tissues might also be important for ductus closure.[234-236] Indomethacin and ibuprofen inhibit COX-1-derived prostaglandins, which are essential for homeostatic functions in the gut, kidney, brain, and elsewhere, leading to the potential toxicities of these drugs and other nonselective NSAIDs.

There are several recommendations for the timing of initial indomethacin treatment. Optimal dosing remains the subject of ongoing debate.[237,238,239-241] Clinical trials designed to answer questions about the timing of pharmacologic treatment all suffer from lack of true controls because these trials have used crossover designs and provision for backup treatment.[242] A meta-analysis showed that early treatment of a symptomatic PDA (1–3 days of age) compared to treatment at a later stage (7–10 days of age) was effective for ductus closure and reduced the need for ligation, along with less pulmonary morbidity and reduced association with NEC.[197] A subsequent prospective trial of early (day 3) vs late (day 7) indomethacin treatment in ventilator-dependent infants also found improved ductus closure rates but did not confirm the pulmonary benefits while raising concerns for renal compromise and more severe adverse outcomes.[243] A delay in treatment to close the ductus is a reasonable choice because early treatment of a symptomatic PDA might unnecessarily expose infants to NSAIDs who would otherwise undergo spontaneous ductus closure without the drug. On the other hand, the beneficial effects realized with prophylactic ductus closure may be a justification for early treatment of symptomatic PDA. Moreover, NSAIDs lose their effectiveness with advancing postnatal age.[244-248] Taking all of these factors into consideration, the benefit/risk ratio of early treatment appears to justify beginning a pharmacologic agent to close the ductus as soon as the diagnosis of *symptomatic* PDA is made. Medical management measures discussed previously in this chapter should also be considered as soon as the diagnosis of left-to-right ductus shunting is established.

The FDA-approved package insert for indomethacin calls for the intravenous administration of 3 doses at 12- to 24-hour intervals with an initial dose of 0.2 mg/kg and second and third doses of 0.1, 0.2, or 0.25 mg/kg, depending on the postnatal age (<48 hours, 2–7 days, or > 7days) that the first dose is administered. Administration over a minimum of 20 to 30 minutes is recommended. Another commonly used regimen is to administer 0.2 mg/kg as the initial dose; then, for infants younger than 28 weeks, 0.1-mg/kg doses are given at 12 and 36 hours after the first dose; for infants older than 28 weeks, 0.2 mg/kg is given for each dose.[8]

Plasma clearance is dependent on postnatal age, resulting in a long half-life on the first day after birth but more rapid elimination by the end of the first

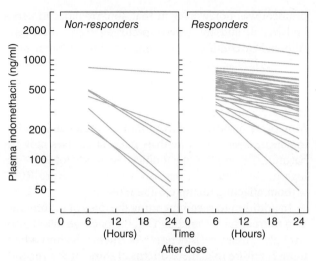

FIGURE 22-3 Concentration-dependent response of the patent ductus arteriosus (PDA) to indomethacin. Plasma indomethacin levels between 6 and 24 hours after the administration of 0.2 mg/kg of the drug intravenously to premature infants with symptomatic PDA. Each line is derived from the regression analysis of drug levels from 6 hours to as long as 5 days after administration. In 6 of 7 studies not associated with a major constrictive effect (panel on left), the plasma level of indomethacin at 24 hours was less than 250 ng/mL. The corresponding level was greater than 250 ng/mL in 28 of 32 studies that were accompanied by a major constrictive effect. (From Cotton RB. Patency of the ductus arteriosus—its etiologic and pathogenetic relationship in the respiratory distress syndrome. In: Stern L, ed. *Respiratory Distress Syndrome*. New York, NY: Grune & Stratton; 1984.)

week.[249-253] Pharmacokinetic studies have shown that efficacy of indomethacin to close the ductus requires a threshold plasma level of 200 ng/mL at 24 hours after infusion[251] (Figure 22-3). Although achievement of threshold indomethacin concentrations has been emphasized,[248,253-255] a sufficiently quick turnaround time for assays is generally not available on a routine basis to adjust dosing based on plasma levels.

Reopening of the ductus after successful closure with indomethacin may occur and is partially related to immaturity and incomplete luminal constriction.[256,257] For this reason, additional doses of the drug may be given based on mid- or posttreatment echocardiographic Doppler examination because ongoing flow through the ductus lumen is associated with treatment failure.[8,257-260]

A variety of dosing protocols have been studied in an effort to reduce treatment failure and late recurrence of symptomatic PDA. Improved efficacy has been reported with prolonged low-dose administration,[259,261-263] repeated short (3-day) courses,[264] stepwise advancement up to a 1-mg/kg dose,[265] and continuous infusion over 36 hours.[266,267] These studies showed no excess adverse effects over standard dosing. The continuous infusion protocol was noteworthy in that abnormalities in cerebral, renal, and mesenteric perfusion were alleviated. Although a continuous infusion of indomethacin over 36 hours is an appealing protocol in view of the amelioration of peripheral vascular effects, additional studies and long-term follow-up are required before this approach can be recommended for routine clinical practice.[237,268,269] Moreover, protocols incorporating prolonged indomethacin dosing or more than 2 repeat courses may be harmful.[238,264,270,271] One multicenter study of low- vs high-dosage strategies was associated with severe ROP without affecting ductus closure rates.[272]

In addition to recommending the dose of indomethacin to treat symptomatic PDA, the package insert also strongly advises consideration of ductus ligation when there is failure to achieve ductus closure after a second course of the drug. This is reasonable advice in view of the increasing risk of adverse effects, such as renal failure and continued feeding intolerance, that will only be prolonged by the likely failure of subsequent courses to result in ductus closure. In this scenario, the most vexing side effect of indomethacin in the treatment of symptomatic PDA is postponement of a decision regarding ductus ligation.

Ibuprofen is another effective NSAID to constrict a persistent PDA.[230–232,273] Ibuprofen is a competitive, rapidly reversible inhibitor that nonselectively blocks both COX-1 and COX-2. Ibuprofen-lysine is preferable to formulations containing tromethamine (THAM).[274] Standard ibuprofen dosing is 10 mg/kg on day 1, followed by 5-mg/kg doses 24 and 48 hours later.[231,232] Doses up to 20, 10, and 10 mg/kg on the same schedule have been given with similar success.[275] Taking maturation into account, pharmacology studies suggested that drug dosing can be increased with advancing postnatal age (10-5-5 mg/kg at less than 70 hours; 14-7-7 mg/kg from 70 to 108 hours; and 18-9-9 mg/kg from 108 to 180 hours of age).[276] Similar to indomethacin,[277] successful ductus closure is less likely when a subsequent course of ibuprofen is required.[278–280] Two separate meta-analyses came to different conclusions on whether the risks and benefits significantly favored ibuprofen over indomethacin.[281,282] A more recent systematic review that evaluated 20 randomized controlled trials ($n = 1092$ infants) comparing ibuprofen to indomethacin found that both drugs were equally efficacious for ductus closure. There were no statistically significant differences in mortality, reopening of the ductus arteriosus, surgical ligation, duration of ventilator support, IVH, cerebral white matter injury, time to full enteral feeds, gastrointestinal bleeding, ROP, sepsis, or duration of hospital stay. Ibuprofen was associated with a lower incidence of NEC and had fewer adverse effects on renal function (urine output, creatinine levels).[283] The modest, at best, therapeutic advantage of ibuprofen is tempered by rare reports of pulmonary hypertensive crises that were

originally attributed to ibuprofen-THAM but have also occurred with the lysine formulation.[217] Because ibuprofen is 95% to 99% protein bound, concerns also exist regarding bilirubin displacement and the potential for kernicterus.[284,285] Retrospective studies showed an association of ibuprofen with higher serum levels or longer need for phototherapy,[286,287] but most clinical studies showed that these risks are limited.[274,288–290]

Other NSAIDs used for constriction of a persistent PDA in preterm infants are limited by their side effects or efficacy. Mefenamic acid is a member of the fenamate class of NSAIDs. There is limited information from randomized clinical trials on the use of mefenamic acid in preterm infants. Several small observational and pharmacokinetic studies indicated its potential usefulness for ductus closure.[32,260,291,292] Side effect concerns have prevented widespread use of this NSAID. Acetaminophen inhibits prostaglandin synthesis and has analgesic and antipyretic properties like other NSAIDs but has limited anti-inflammatory effects. The mechanisms for COX inhibition by acetaminophen are more complex than other NSAIDs. Acetaminophen crosses the placenta and is known to constrict the ductus arteriosus in utero,[293–295] but clinical studies of the ductus of newborns are lacking. Recently, Hammerman and colleagues demonstrated the efficacy of acetaminophen for ductus closure in a small series of cases.[296] Although there may be fewer vasoconstrictive concerns with acetaminophen, hepatic toxicity might be a greater concern than other NSAID complications.

Medical Treatment: Adverse Effects

The adverse effects of indomethacin and ibuprofen are primarily related to constrictive effects in other vascular beds. Indomethacin treatment causes significant reductions in mesenteric blood flow.[32,57,267,297–300] Exposure to indomethacin has been associated with NEC, SIP, gastrointestinal hemorrhage, and feeding intolerance.[61,62,64,70,72,200,238,270,271,301–306] Despite these concerns, there is no clear evidence that the incidence or severity of NEC is related to treatment with indomethacin or that a causative relationship exists.[185,193,242] Combined administration of indomethacin and glucocorticoids, on the other hand, significantly increases the risk for NEC or viscus perforation[307–310] and should be avoided. A postprandial intestinal hyperemic response is present in preterm infants[300,311,312] that may protect gut integrity. As such, there is an increasing willingness to provide feedings in the presence of a symptomatic PDA or during indomethacin treatment,[64,313–315] albeit with more hesitant adoption in US nurseries.[190,315,316]

Indomethacin is also associated with reduced renal perfusion and function.[300,317–319] Fluid intake should be adjusted accordingly, but dehydration should be avoided to prevent additional renal compromise.

Indomethacin-induced prostaglandin suppression occurs for 6 to 7 days before circulating levels return to pretreatment values,[320] coinciding with the transient nature of indomethacin-associated renal impairment.

Indomethacin causes significant reductions in cerebral blood flow.[321-330] Cerebral oxygenation is also compromised by indomethacin treatment[53,328,330-332] or by the presence of an hsPDA.[53,333] Regional oxygen saturation levels eventually normalize after effective PDA closure.[52,53] Given these concerns, it is reassuring that neurodevelopmental outcomes are unchanged[46,334-336] or possibly improved[48,337-339] in indomethacin-treated infants. Indomethacin can also inhibit platelet COX-1 and cause decreased platelet function that might lead to PDA or coagulation abnormalities.

Many of the vascular effects of indomethacin are associated with a bolus infusion of the drug. These effects are ameliorated when the drug is given over a period of 30 minutes or longer. By 24 hours after completion of the infusion, these effects are not detectable. The return of these measurements to baseline well before indomethacin levels have decreased below those that are clinically effective in COX-1 and COX-2 inhibition suggests that these vascular effects are related more to the nonspecific vasoconstrictive properties of indomethacin than to COX-1/COX-2 suppression.[340-343]

Ibuprofen appears to have fewer side effects than indomethacin[231,274,344,345] and is less selective for COX-1 even though both are considered nonselective COX inhibitors.[346] Ibuprofen has limited effects on mesenteric blood flow compared to indomethacin[300,340] and is less associated with NEC in combined analyses,[283] although SIP and other events are increasingly reported.[347] Renal perfusion and urine output are less impaired with ibuprofen than indomethacin.[218,282,300,329,345,348-350] Despite the overall reduction in risk, ibuprofen has been associated with transient or prolonged renal dysfunction[214,273,278,279,348,351,352] and causes intense vasoconstriction in animal models.[353] In addition, reports of acute renal failure[354-358] indicate that ibuprofen treatment still poses nephrotoxic risks for preterm infants. Ibuprofen has limited effects on cerebral blood flow[329,330,359,360] and improves autoregulation.[359,361,362] These features confer a potential advantage for ibuprofen treatment of symptomatic PDA. However, the improvements in cerebral blood flow and autoregulation are insufficient for prevention of IVH in preterm infants.[213,214,216,344] An increased risk of chronic lung disease after ibuprofen treatment was observed in some meta-analyses[282,363] but not others.[283]

Surgical Treatment

Ligation or division of the ductus is an effective measure to eliminate the symptomatic PDA. However, the merits of surgical closure relative to its risks are an area of controversy.[364,365] A single study on prophylactic ligation of the ductus found a reduction in NEC but was also associated with increased risks for chronic lung disease[366,367] and is not currently recommended.[368] Compared to pharmacologic closure, early surgical closure (<1 week of age) of an open ductus in ventilator-dependent preterm infants reduced the duration of mechanical ventilation, improved hemodynamics and lung compliance, and allowed earlier enteral nutrition.[39] Similar benefits were observed in infants who required earlier ligation (<2-3 weeks of age) compared to later ligation (>2-3 weeks) due to NSAID treatment failure or contraindications.[369,370] However, early ligation and cessation of feedings may not be preferable to a more conservative approach by which ductus ligation is restricted to infants with cardiopulmonary compromise and enteral feedings are encouraged in the meantime. A brief delay in the decision to ligate may also reduce other comorbidities.[191] Surgical ligation has been favored over indomethacin treatment,[371-373] and in some neonatal intensive care units (NICUs), surgery is the preferred first-line treatment of an hsPDA in small preterm infants.[179,188,192,374-378] However, surgical closure in the neonatal period is usually reserved for infants who fail to respond to pharmacologic agents or when contraindications to these agents are present. Enthusiasm for surgical ligation is also limited by growing concerns for adverse outcomes among infants who require ligation (see next section).

OUTCOME AND FOLLOW-UP

Medical Management Without Intervention to Close the Ductus

The occurrence of spontaneous closure, particularly in infants over 1000 g at birth or 29 weeks' gestation,[9,10] suggests that medical management of a symptomatic PDA and careful observation may be a reasonable option. Adoption of conservative measures that optimize conditions for ductus closure (see the section on management) and attention to risk factors that are associated with PDA (Table 22-1) are the mainstay of this approach. Medications that contribute to ductus relaxation should be avoided.[12] Episodes of sepsis, hypotension, acidosis, or overhydration may prevent ductus closure or provoke its reopening. Timely follow-up, including periodic echocardiography as required by individual patient characteristics, is important for predischarge management.

The prognosis for infants who are discharged home with persistent PDA has not been systematically evaluated. Historical concerns for bacterial endocarditis have been largely resolved, although not eradicated, and antibiotic prophylaxis is only used infrequently.[379-382] Information from various studies suggests that a small or clinically insignificant persistent PDA at the time of discharge may be well tolerated and undergo later spontaneous closure[9–11,144,185,383–385] much like a small muscular ventricular septal defect. However, untoward outcomes may also become more apparent as this approach is embraced.[196] Outpatient follow-up is therefore critical for infants who are discharged home with a persistent PDA. Interventional management may be required in infants with persistent PDA after 6 months of age, although the criteria to reach the threshold for treatment and the optimal timing and approach for closure have not been resolved.[379,386,387]

Outcome Following Pharmacologic Treatment

The outcome of NSAID treatment is well defined, although the long-term benefits are debated. Indomethacin and ibuprofen are effective measures for infants who require pharmacological treatment of a symptomatic PDA. Early studies showed that treatment efficacy for ductus closure ranged from 18% to 85%, based on variations in enteral vs intravenous preparations, timing of administration, definitions of symptomatic PDA, and pathophysiologic condition of the infant.[249] Current studies suggested that NSAIDs have an overall success rate of 60% to 92%.[248,257,264,278,282,348,349] Rates of reopening after successful initial closure range from 21% to 45%,[10,179,257,258,260,318,349,375,388] prompting consideration of additional NSAID courses. Various factors contribute to treatment failure, including immaturity, residual blood flow through the ductus lumen, delayed initiation of NSAID treatment, sepsis, absence of antenatal steroids, or exposure to antenatal indomethacin.[8,127,257–260,389–393] A second NSAID course will achieve additional ductus closures, but treatment failures still occur.[259,264,277,278,388,394] Ligation should be considered if a symptomatic PDA persists after 2 courses of NSAIDs.[264,280,388,394]

Surgical Outcome

Unlike NSAID treatment, surgical ligation results in definitive closure of the ductus in virtually every case. Operative mortality is usually low, and systemic hypoperfusion and pulmonary overcirculation are promptly relieved. Depending on the approach used, there is an approximately 1% to 3% risk of residual flow or recurrent patency because of recanalization.[386] In this case, a second procedure is rarely required but may be needed if hemodynamic compromise recurs or in cases of aneurysmal dilation or inadvertent ligation of adjacent vessels.

The beneficial outcome of ligation in preterm neonates may not outweigh the associated risks. Immediate complications related to the surgical procedure include pneumothorax, pulmonary interstitial emphysema, chylothorax, hemorrhage, infection, or renal impairment.[395,396] Postoperative hypotension occurs in approximately one-third of VLBW infants, and a postligation syndrome has been described.[397–401] Myocardial dysfunction after ligation is the result of recovery from cardiac distension and altered loading conditions,[398,400] frequently necessitating the use of inotropic support. Early postoperative echocardiography may be able to identify infants who require early intervention for myocardial dysfunction.[402] Phrenic nerve injury is uncommon, but damage to the left recurrent laryngeal nerve remains an ongoing concern. Paralysis of the left vocal cord is reported in up to 40% to 67% of ELBW infants after ligation, occurs more commonly in the most immature infants, and may not be recognized until adulthood.[403–406] Vocal cord paralysis in ELBW infants is associated with long-term respiratory and feeding difficulties.[403,404] Preoperative examination is recommended to document vocal cord mobility. Scoliosis and chest wall deformities after lateral thoracotomy are increasingly recognized long-term complications of ductus ligation.[407–409]

More recent studies have raised concerns for the long-term pulmonary and neurodevelopmental consequences of ductus ligation. Although there are initial improvements in lung compliance and gas exchange, ligation has been identified as an independent risk factor for the development of chronic lung disease.[364,367,410–412] The cause for this is unclear. Animal studies suggested that the beneficial effects of pharmacological closure of the ductus on alveolar growth are not present after ductus ligation, and an unfavorable gene expression profile for lung development may exist.[413,414] Ligation also appears to pose a risk for cognitive and developmental delay. Retrospective analysis of subsets of infants who underwent ductus ligation revealed cognitive delays or neurosensory impairment at 18 months of age.[411,412] Among preterm infants who manifest developmental disabilities, ductus ligation was also found to be an independently associated risk factor.[415–417] However, it should be kept in mind that infants undergoing ligation are usually the most severely affected, an effect that might account for these late complications. Although these findings are not consistently observed,[410,418] they do warrant attention when considering treatment options.

Development of Future Management Strategies

The optimal management strategy for a symptomatic PDA remains elusive. Improved definition of an hsPDA[151] or development of combined diagnostic criteria[19,154,160] will allow comparisons that are more uniform across clinical trials and reduce unnecessary treatment. It is hoped that pharmacological advances will identify therapies beyond the currently used NSAIDs that stimulate ductus constriction with less toxicity or greater efficacy.[13,91,296,419] The use of targeted echocardiography to tailor NSAID regimens reduces overall drug exposure and can be used to guide therapy for those infants who qualify for treatment.[280,420-422] Future studies of the genetic susceptibility to persistent ductus patency will support pharmacogenomic approaches that optimize treatment of individual patients[18,423,424] and lay the foundations for personalized medicine in the NICU.

REFERENCES

1. Bergwerff M, DeRuiter MC, Gittenberger-de Groot AC. Comparative anatomy and ontogeny of the ductus arteriosus, a vascular outsider. *Anat Embryol (Berl)*. 1999;200(6):559–571.
2. Dzialowski EM, Sirsat T, van der Sterren S, Villamor E. Prenatal cardiovascular shunts in amniotic vertebrates. *Respir Physiol Neurobiol*. 2011;178(1):66–74.
3. Smith CA, Nelson NM. *The Physiology of the Newborn Infant*. 4th ed. Springfield, IL: Charles C. Thomas; 1976.
4. Slomp J, van Munsteren JC, Poelmann RE, de Reeder EG, Bogers AJ, Gittenberger-de Groot AC. Formation of intimal cushions in the ductus arteriosus as a model for vascular intimal thickening. An immunohistochemical study of changes in extracellular matrix components. *Atherosclerosis*. 1992;93(1–2):25–39.
5. Waleh N, Seidner S, McCurnin D, et al. The role of monocyte-derived cells and inflammation in baboon ductus arteriosus remodeling. *Pediatr Res*. 2005;57(2):254–262.
6. Echtler K, Stark K, Lorenz M, et al. Platelets contribute to postnatal occlusion of the ductus arteriosus. *Nat Med*. 2010;16(1):75–82.
7. Waleh N, Seidner S, McCurnin D, et al. Anatomic closure of the premature patent ductus arteriosus: The role of CD14+/CD163+ mononuclear cells and VEGF in neointimal mound formation. *Pediatr Res*. 2011;70(4):332–338.
8. Hermes-DeSantis ER, Clyman RI. Patent ductus arteriosus: pathophysiology and management. *J Perinatol*. 2006;26 (Suppl 1):S14–S18. discussion S22–S13.
9. Koch J, Hensley G, Roy L, Brown S, Ramaciotti C, Rosenfeld CR. Prevalence of spontaneous closure of the ductus arteriosus in neonates at a birth weight of 1000 grams or less. *Pediatrics*. 2006;117(4):1113–1121.
10. Nemerofsky SL, Parravicini E, Bateman D, Kleinman C, Polin RA, Lorenz JM. The ductus arteriosus rarely requires treatment in infants > 1000 grams. *Am J Perinatol*. 2008;25(10):661–666.
11. Herrman K, Bose C, Lewis K, Laughon M. Spontaneous closure of the patent ductus arteriosus in very low birth weight infants following discharge from the neonatal unit. *Arch Dis Child Fetal Neonatal Ed*. 2009;94(1):F48–F50.
12. Reese J, Veldman A, Shah L, Vucovich M, Cotton RB. Inadvertent relaxation of the ductus arteriosus by pharmacologic agents that are commonly used in the neonatal period. *Semin Perinatol*. 2010;34(3):222–230.
13. Smith GC. The pharmacology of the ductus arteriosus. *Pharmacol Rev*. 1998;50(1):35–58.
14. Clyman RI. Mechanisms regulating the ductus arteriosus. *Biol Neonate*. 2006;89(4):330–335.
15. Lavoie PM, Pham C, Jang KL. Heritability of bronchopulmonary dysplasia, defined according to the consensus statement of the National Institutes of Health. *Pediatrics*. 2008;122(3):479–485.
16. Bhandari V, Zhou G, Bizzarro MJ, et al. Genetic contribution to patent ductus arteriosus in the premature newborn. *Pediatrics*. 2009;123(2):669–673.
17. Hallman M, Marttila R, Pertile R, Ojaniemi M, Haataja R. Genes and environment in common neonatal lung disease. *Neonatology*. 2007;91(4):298–302.
18. Dagle JM, Lepp NT, Cooper ME, et al. Determination of genetic predisposition to patent ductus arteriosus in preterm infants. *Pediatrics*. 2009;123(4):1116–1123.
19. Cotton RB, Lindstrom DP, Stahlman MT. Early prediction of symptomatic patent ductus arteriosus from perinatal risk factors: a discriminant analysis model. *Acta Paediatr Scand*. 1981;70(5):723–727.
20. Gittenberger-de Groot AC. Persistent ductus arteriosus: most probably a primary congenital malformation. *Br Heart J*. 1977;39(6):610–618.
21. Ho SY, Anderson RH. Anatomical closure of the ductus arteriosus: a study in 35 specimens. *J Anat*. 1979;128(Pt 4):829–836.
22. Hajj H, Dagle J. Genetics of patent ductus arteriosus susceptibility and treatment. *Semin Perinatol*. 2012;36(2):98–104.
23. Krovetz LJ, Lester RG, Warden HE. The diagnosis of patent ductus arteriosus in infancy. *Dis Chest*. 1962;42:241–250.
24. Zetterquist P. *A Clinical and Genetic Study of Congenital Heart Defects*. Uppsala, Sweden: Institute for Medical Genetics, University of Uppsala; 1972:1–80.
25. Jan SL, Hwang B, Fu YC, Chi CS. Prediction of ductus arteriosus closure by neonatal screening echocardiography. *Int J Cardiovasc Imaging*. 2004;20(5):349–356.
26. Takami T, Yoda H, Kawakami T, et al. Usefulness of indomethacin for patent ductus arteriosus in full-term infants. *Pediatr Cardiol*. 2007;28(1):46–50.
27. Amoozgar H, Ghodstehrani M, Pishva N. Oral ibuprofen and ductus arteriosus closure in full-term neonates: a prospective case-control study. *Pediatr Cardiol*. 2010;31(1):40–43.
28. Lin YC, Huang HR, Lien R, et al. Management of patent ductus arteriosus in term or near-term neonates with respiratory distress. *Pediatr Neonatol*. 2010;51(3):160–165.
29. Skinner J. Diagnosis of patent ductus arteriosus. *Semin Neonatol*. 2001;6(1):49–61.
30. Noori S, Seri I. The very low birth weight neonate with a hemodynamically significant ductus arteriosus during the first postnatal week. In: Kleinman C, Seri I, eds. *Neonatology Questions and Controversies: Hemodynamics and Cardiology*. Philadelphia, PA: Saunders/Elsevier Co.; 2008:178–194.
31. Clyman RI, Mauray F, Heymann MA, Roman C. Cardiovascular effects of patent ductus arteriosus in preterm lambs with respiratory distress. *J Pediatr*. 1987;111(4):579–587.
32. Shimada S, Kasai T, Konishi M, Fujiwara T. Effects of patent ductus arteriosus on left ventricular output and organ blood flows in preterm infants with respiratory distress syndrome treated with surfactant. *J Pediatr*. 1994;125(2):270–277.
33. Rudolph AM, Drorbaugh JE, Auld PA, et al. Studies on the circulation in the neonatal period. The circulation in the respiratory distress syndrome. *Pediatrics*. 1961;27:551–566.
34. Stahlman M. Treatment of cardiovascular disorders of the newborn. *Pediatr Clin North Am*. 1964;11(2):363–400.
35. Barlow AJ, Ward C, Webber SA, Sinclair BG, Potts JE, Sandor GG. Myocardial contractility in premature neonates with and without patent ductus arteriosus. *Pediatr Cardiol*. 2004;25(2):102–107.
36. Friedman WF. The intrinsic physiologic properties of the developing heart. *Prog Cardiovasc Dis*. 1972;15(1):87–111.

37. Anderson PA. The heart and development. *Semin Perinatol.* 1996;20(6):482–509.

38. Cotton RB, Stahlman MT, Kovar I, Catterton WZ. Medical management of small preterm infants with symptomatic patent ductus arteriosus. *J Pediatr.* 1978;92(3):467–473.

39. Cotton RB, Stahlman MT, Bender HW, Graham TP, Catterton WZ, Kovar I. Randomized trial of early closure of symptomatic patent ductus arteriosus in small preterm infants. *J Pediatr.* 1978;93(4):647–651.

40. Kluckow M, Evans N. Ductal shunting, high pulmonary blood flow, and pulmonary hemorrhage. *J Pediatr.* 2000;137(1):68–72.

41. Bancalari E, Claure N, Gonzalez A. Patent ductus arteriosus and respiratory outcome in premature infants. *Biol Neonate.* 2005;88(3):192–201.

42. Alfaleh K, Smyth JA, Roberts RS, Solimano A, Asztalos EV, Schmidt B. Prevention and 18-month outcomes of serious pulmonary hemorrhage in extremely low birth weight infants: results from the trial of indomethacin prophylaxis in preterms. *Pediatrics.* 2008;121(2):e233–e238.

43. Evans N, Kluckow M. Early ductal shunting and intraventricular haemorrhage in ventilated preterm infants. *Arch Dis Child Fetal Neonatal Ed.* 1996;75(3):F183–F186.

44. Jim WT, Chiu NC, Chen MR, et al. Cerebral hemodynamic change and intraventricular hemorrhage in very low birth weight infants with patent ductus arteriosus. *Ultrasound Med Biol.* 2005;31(2):197–202.

45. Drougia A, Giapros V, Krallis N, et al. Incidence and risk factors for cerebral palsy in infants with perinatal problems: a 15-year review. *Early Hum Dev.* 2007;83(8):541–547.

46. Schmidt B, Davis P, Moddemann D, et al. Long-term effects of indomethacin prophylaxis in extremely-low-birth-weight infants. *N Engl J Med.* 2001;344(26):1966–1972.

47. Fowlie PW, Davis PG. Prophylactic indomethacin for preterm infants: a systematic review and meta-analysis. *Arch Dis Child Fetal Neonatal Ed.* 2003;88(6):F464–F466.

48. Ment LR, Vohr BR, Makuch RW, et al. Prevention of intraventricular hemorrhage by indomethacin in male preterm infants. *J Pediatr.* 2004;145(6):832–834.

49. Perlman JM, Hill A, Volpe JJ. The effect of patent ductus arteriosus on flow velocity in the anterior cerebral arteries: ductal steal in the premature newborn infant. *J Pediatr.* 1981;99(5):767–771.

50. Lipman B, Serwer GA, Brazy JE. Abnormal cerebral hemodynamics in preterm infants with patent ductus arteriosus. *Pediatrics.* 1982;69(6):778–781.

51. Martin CG, Snider AR, Katz SM, Peabody JL, Brady JP. Abnormal cerebral blood flow patterns in preterm infants with a large patent ductus arteriosus. *J Pediatr.* 1982;101(4):587–593.

52. Zaramella P, Freato F, Quaresima V, et al. Surgical closure of patent ductus arteriosus reduces the cerebral tissue oxygenation index in preterm infants: a near-infrared spectroscopy and Doppler study. *Pediatr Int.* 2006;48(3):305–312.

53. Lemmers PM, Toet MC, van Bel F. Impact of patent ductus arteriosus and subsequent therapy with indomethacin on cerebral oxygenation in preterm infants. *Pediatrics.* 2008;121(1):142–147.

54. Wong SN, Lo RN, Hui PW. Abnormal renal and splanchnic arterial Doppler pattern in premature babies with symptomatic patent ductus arteriosus. *J Ultrasound Med.* 1990;9(3):125–130.

55. Shimada S, Kasai T, Hoshi A, Murata A, Chida S. Cardiocirculatory effects of patent ductus arteriosus in extremely low-birth-weight infants with respiratory distress syndrome. *Pediatr Int.* 2003;45(3):255–262.

56. Groves AM, Kuschel CA, Knight DB, Skinner JR. Does retrograde diastolic flow in the descending aorta signify impaired systemic perfusion in preterm infants? *Pediatr Res.* 2008;63(1):89–94.

57. Coombs RC, Morgan ME, Durbin GM, Booth IW, McNeish AS. Gut blood flow velocities in the newborn: effects of patent ductus arteriosus and parenteral indomethacin. *Arch Dis Child.* 1990;65 (10 Spec No):1067–1071.

58. Petrova A, Bhatt M, Mehta R. Regional tissue oxygenation in preterm born infants in association with echocardiographically significant patent ductus arteriosus. *J Perinatol.* 2011;31(7):460–464.

59. Milner ME, de la Monte SM, Moore GW, Hutchins GM. Risk factors for developing and dying from necrotizing enterocolitis. *J Pediatr Gastroenterol Nutr.* 1986;5(3):359–364.

60. Meyers RL, Alpan G, Lin E, Clyman RI. Patent ductus arteriosus, indomethacin, and intestinal distension: effects on intestinal blood flow and oxygen consumption. *Pediatr Res.* 1991;29(6):569–574.

61. Sankaran K, Puckett B, Lee DS, et al. Variations in incidence of necrotizing enterocolitis in Canadian neonatal intensive care units. *J Pediatr Gastroenterol Nutr.* 2004;39(4):366–372.

62. Dollberg S, Lusky A, Reichman B. Patent ductus arteriosus, indomethacin and necrotizing enterocolitis in very low birth weight infants: a population-based study. *J Pediatr Gastroenterol Nutr.* 2005;40(2):184–188.

63. Luig M, Lui K. Epidemiology of necrotizing enterocolitis—Part II: Risks and susceptibility of premature infants during the surfactant era: a regional study. *J Paediatr Child Health.* 2005;41(4):174–179.

64. Patole SK, Kumaran V, Travadi JN, Brooks JM, Doherty DA. Does patent ductus arteriosus affect feed tolerance in preterm neonates? *Arch Dis Child Fetal Neonatal Ed.* 2007;92(1):F53–F55.

65. Bertino E, Giuliani F, Prandi G, Coscia A, Martano C, Fabris C. Necrotizing enterocolitis: risk factor analysis and role of gastric residuals in very low birth weight infants. *J Pediatr Gastroenterol Nutr.* 2009;48(4):437–442.

66. Meyer CL, Payne NR, Roback SA. Spontaneous, isolated intestinal perforations in neonates with birth weight less than 1000 g not associated with necrotizing enterocolitis. *J Pediatr Surg.* 1991;26(6):714–717.

67. Pumberger W, Mayr M, Kohlhauser C, Weninger M. Spontaneous localized intestinal perforation in very-low-birth-weight infants: a distinct clinical entity different from necrotizing enterocolitis. *J Am Coll Surg.* 2002;195(6):796–803.

68. Gordon PV. Understanding intestinal vulnerability to perforation in the extremely low birth weight infant. *Pediatr Res.* 2009;65(2):138–144.

69. Messina M, Molinaro F, Ferrara F, Messina G, Di Maggio G. Idiopathic spontaneous intestinal perforation: a distinct pathological entity in the preterm infant. *Minerva Pediatr.* 2009;61(4):355–360.

70. Aschner JL, Deluga KS, Metlay LA, Emmens RW, Hendricks-Munoz KD. Spontaneous focal gastrointestinal perforation in very low birth weight infants. *J Pediatr.* 1988;113(2):364–367.

71. Raghuveer G, Speidel B, Marlow N, Porter H. Focal intestinal perforation in preterm infants is an emerging disease. *Acta Paediatr.* 1996;85(2):237–239.

72. Attridge JT, Clark R, Walker MW, Gordon PV. New insights into spontaneous intestinal perforation using a national data set: (1) SIP is associated with early indomethacin exposure. *J Perinatol.* 2006;26(2):93–99.

73. Bloom BT. Attridge et al. present an analysis of a complex data set, which offers important confirmation of the differences between the clinical presentation of spontaneous intestinal perforations (SIP) and surgical necrotizing enterocolitis (NEC). *J Perinatol.* 2006;26(6):384; author reply 384–386.

74. Bomelburg T, Jorch G. Abnormal blood flow patterns in renal arteries of small preterm infants with patent ductus arteriosus detected by Doppler ultrasonography. *Eur J Pediatr.* 1989;148(7):660–664.

75. Visser MO, Leighton JO, van de Bor M, Walther FJ. Renal blood flow in neonates: quantification with color flow and pulsed Doppler US. *Radiology.* 1992;183(2):441–444.

76. Yeh TF, Wilks A, Singh J, Betkerur M, Lilien L, Pildes RS. Furosemide prevents the renal side effects of indomethacin therapy in premature infants with patent ductus arteriosus. *J Pediatr.* 1982;101(3):433–437.

77. Seri I, Abbasi S, Wood DC, Gerdes JS. Regional hemodynamic effects of dopamine in the indomethacin-treated preterm infant. *J Perinatol.* 2002;22(4):300–305.

78. Romagnoli C, Zecca E, Papacci P, et al. Furosemide does not prevent indomethacin-induced renal side effects in preterm infants. *Clin Pharmacol Ther.* 1997;62(2):181–186.

79. Baenziger O, Waldvogel K, Ghelfi D, Arbenz U, Fanconi S. Can dopamine prevent the renal side effects of indomethacin? A prospective randomized clinical study. *Klin Padiatr.* 1999;211(6):438–441.

80. Brion LP, Campbell DE. Furosemide for symptomatic patent ductus arteriosus in indomethacin-treated infants. *Cochrane Database Syst Rev.* 2001;(3):CD001148.

81. Barrington K, Brion LP. Dopamine versus no treatment to prevent renal dysfunction in indomethacin-treated preterm newborn infants. *Cochrane Database Syst Rev.* 2002;(3):CD003213.

82. Andriessen P, Struis NC, Niemarkt H, Oetomo SB, Tanke RB, Van Overmeire B. Furosemide in preterm infants treated with indomethacin for patent ductus arteriosus. *Acta Paediatr.* 2009;98(5):797–803.

83. Lee BS, Byun SY, Chung ML, et al. Effect of furosemide on ductal closure and renal function in indomethacin-treated preterm infants during the early neonatal period. *Neonatology.* 2010;98(2):191–199.

84. de Reeder EG, Gittenberger-de Groot AC, van Munsteren JC, Poelmann RE, Patterson DF, Keirse MJ. Distribution of prostacyclin synthase, 6-keto-prostaglandin F1 alpha, and 15-hydroxyprostaglandin dehydrogenase in the normal and persistent ductus arteriosus of the dog. *Am J Pathol.* 1989;135(5):881–887.

85. Rabinovitch M. Cell-extracellular matrix interactions in the ductus arteriosus and perinatal pulmonary circulation. *Semin Perinatol.* 1996;20(6):531–541.

86. Tada T, Wakabayashi T, Nakao Y, et al. Human ductus arteriosus. A histological study on the relation between ductal maturation and gestational age. *Acta Pathol Jpn.* 1985;35(1):23–34.

87. Bokenkamp R, DeRuiter MC, van Munsteren C, Gittenberger-de Groot AC. Insights into the pathogenesis and genetic background of patency of the ductus arteriosus. *Neonatology.* 2010;98(1):6–17.

88. Mason CA, Bigras JL, O'Blenes SB, et al. Gene transfer in utero biologically engineers a patent ductus arteriosus in lambs by arresting fibronectin-dependent neointimal formation. *Nat Med.* 1999;5(2):176–182.

89. Coceani F. Cytochrome P450 in the contractile tone of the ductus arteriosus: regulatory and effector mechanisms. In: Weir EK, Archer SL, Reeves JT, eds. *The Fetal and Neonatal Pulmonary Circulations.* Armonk, NY: Futura Publishing Company, Inc.; 1999:331–341.

90. Baragatti B, Ciofini E, Scebba F, et al. Cytochrome P-450 3A13 and endothelin jointly mediate ductus arteriosus constriction to oxygen in mice. *Am J Physiol Heart Circ Physiol.* 2011;300(3):H892–H901.

91. Baragatti B, Coceani F. Arachidonic acid epoxygenase and 12(S)-lipoxygenase: evidence of their concerted involvement in ductus arteriosus constriction to oxygen. *Can J Physiol Pharmacol.* 2011;89(5):329–334.

92. Michelakis E, Rebeyka I, Bateson J, Olley P, Puttagunta L, Archer S. Voltage-gated potassium channels in human ductus arteriosus. *Lancet.* 2000;356(9224):134–137.

93. Thebaud B, Michelakis ED, Wu XC, et al. Oxygen-sensitive Kv channel gene transfer confers oxygen responsiveness to preterm rabbit and remodeled human ductus arteriosus: implications for infants with patent ductus arteriosus. *Circulation.* 2004;110(11):1372–1379.

94. Thebaud B, Wu XC, Kajimoto H, et al. Developmental absence of the O_2 sensitivity of L-type calcium channels in preterm ductus arteriosus smooth muscle cells impairs O_2 constriction contributing to patent ductus arteriosus. *Pediatr Res.* 2008;63(2):176–181.

95. Reeve HL, Tolarova S, Nelson DP, Archer S, Weir EK. Redox control of oxygen sensing in the rabbit ductus arteriosus. *J Physiol.* 2001;533(Pt 1):253–261.

96. Weir EK, Archer SL. The role of redox changes in oxygen sensing. *Respir Physiol Neurobiol.* 2010;174(3):182–191.

97. Tristani-Firouzi M, Reeve HL, Tolarova S, Weir EK, Archer SL. Oxygen-induced constriction of rabbit ductus arteriosus occurs via inhibition of a 4-aminopyridine-, voltage-sensitive potassium channel. *J Clin Invest.* 1996;98(9):1959–1965.

98. Michelakis ED, Rebeyka I, Wu X, et al. O_2 sensing in the human ductus arteriosus: regulation of voltage-gated K$^+$ channels in smooth muscle cells by a mitochondrial redox sensor. *Circ Res.* 2002;91(6):478–486.

99. Archer SL, Wu XC, Thebaud B, Moudgil R, Hashimoto K, Michelakis ED. O_2 sensing in the human ductus arteriosus: redox-sensitive K$^+$ channels are regulated by mitochondria-derived hydrogen peroxide. *Biol Chem.* 2004;385(3–4):205–216.

100. Keck M, Resnik E, Linden B, et al. Oxygen increases ductus arteriosus smooth muscle cytosolic calcium via release of calcium from inositol triphosphate-sensitive stores. *Am J Physiol Lung Cell Mol Physiol.* 2005;288(5):L917–L923.

101. Yokoyama U, Minamisawa S, Adachi-Akahane S, et al. Multiple transcripts of Ca^{2+} channel alpha1-subunits and a novel spliced variant of the alpha1C-subunit in rat ductus arteriosus. *Am J Physiol Heart Circ Physiol.* 2006;290(4):H1660–H1670.

102. Clyman RI, Waleh N, Kajino H, Roman C, Mauray F. Calcium-dependent and calcium-sensitizing pathways in the mature and immature ductus arteriosus. *Am J Physiol Regul Integr Comp Physiol.* 2007;293(4):R1650–R1656.

103. Akaike T, Jin MH, Yokoyama U, et al. T-type Ca^{2+} channels promote oxygenation-induced closure of the rat ductus arteriosus not only by vasoconstriction but also by neointima formation. *J Biol Chem.* 2009;284(36):24025–24034.

104. Waleh N, Reese J, Kajino H, et al. Oxygen-induced tension in the sheep ductus arteriosus: effects of gestation on potassium and calcium channel regulation. *Pediatr Res.* 2009;65(3):285–290.

105. Guerguerian AM, Hardy P, Bhattacharya M, et al. Expression of cyclooxygenases in ductus arteriosus of fetal and newborn pigs. *Am J Obstet Gynecol.* 1998;179(6 Pt 1):1618–1626.

106. Takahashi Y, Roman C, Chemtob S, et al. Cyclooxygenase-2 inhibitors constrict the fetal lamb ductus arteriosus both in vitro and in vivo. *Am J Physiol Regul Integr Comp Physiol.* 2000;278(6):R1496–R1505.

107. Rheinlaender C, Weber SC, Sarioglu N, Strauss E, Obladen M, Koehne P. Changing expression of cyclooxygenases and prostaglandin receptor EP4 during development of the human ductus arteriosus. *Pediatr Res.* 2006;60(3):270–275.

108. Bhattacharya M, Asselin P, Hardy P, et al. Developmental changes in prostaglandin E(2) receptor subtypes in porcine ductus arteriosus. Possible contribution in altered responsiveness to prostaglandin E(2). *Circulation.* 1999;100(16):1751–1756.

CHAPTER 22

109. Bouayad A, Bernier SG, Asselin P, et al. Characterization of PGE$_2$ receptors in fetal and newborn ductus arteriosus in the pig. *Semin Perinatol.* 2001;25(2):70–75.

110. Bouayad A, Kajino H, Waleh N, et al. Characterization of PGE$_2$ receptors in fetal and newborn lamb ductus arteriosus. *Am J Physiol Heart Circ Physiol.* 2001;280(5):H2342–H2349.

111. Clyman RI, Chan CY, Mauray F, et al. Permanent anatomic closure of the ductus arteriosus in newborn baboons: the roles of postnatal constriction, hypoxia, and gestation. *Pediatr Res.* 1999;45(1):19–29.

112. Kajino H, Goldbarg S, Roman C, et al. Vasa vasorum hypoperfusion is responsible for medial hypoxia and anatomic remodeling in the newborn lamb ductus arteriosus. *Pediatr Res.* 2002;51(2):228–235.

113. Clyman RI, Seidner SR, Kajino H, et al. VEGF regulates remodeling during permanent anatomic closure of the ductus arteriosus. *Am J Physiol Regul Integr Comp Physiol.* 2002;282(1):R199–R206.

114. Boudreau N, Clausell N, Boyle J, Rabinovitch M. Transforming growth factor-beta regulates increased ductus arteriosus endothelial glycosaminoglycan synthesis and a post-transcriptional mechanism controls increased smooth muscle fibronectin, features associated with intimal proliferation. *Lab Invest.* 1992;67(3):350–359.

115. Tannenbaum JE, Waleh NS, Mauray F, Gold L, Perkett EA, Clyman RI. Transforming growth factor-beta protein and messenger RNA expression is increased in the closing ductus arteriosus. *Pediatr Res.* 1996;39(3):427–434.

116. Goldbarg S, Quinn T, Waleh N, et al. Effects of hypoxia, hypoglycemia, and muscle shortening on cell death in the sheep ductus arteriosus. *Pediatr Res.* 2003;54(2):204–211.

117. Levin M, Goldbarg S, Lindqvist A, et al. ATP depletion and cell death in the neonatal lamb ductus arteriosus. *Pediatr Res.* 2005;57(6):801–805.

118. Reese J. Death, dying, and exhaustion in the ductus arteriosus: prerequisites for permanent closure. *Am J Physiol Regul Integr Comp Physiol.* 2006;290(2):R357–R358.

119. Levin M, McCurnin D, Seidner SR, et al. Postnatal constriction, ATP depletion, and cell death in the mature and immature ductus arteriosus. *Am J Physiol Regul Integr Comp Physiol.* 2006;290(2):359–364.

120. Fujioka K, Morioka I, Miwa A, et al. Does thrombocytopenia contribute to patent ductus arteriosus? *Nat Med.* 2011;17(1):29–30. author reply 30–21.

121. Shah NA, Hills NK, Waleh N, et al. Relationship between circulating platelet counts and ductus arteriosus patency after indomethacin treatment. *J Pediatr.* 2011;158(6):919–923. e911–e912.

122. Boo NY, Mohd-Amin I, Bilkis AA, Yong-Junina F. Predictors of failed closure of patent ductus arteriosus with indomethacin. *Singapore Med J.* 2006;47(9):763–768.

123. Sallmon H, Weber SC, von Gise A, Koehne P, Hansmann G. Ductal closure in neonates: a developmental perspective on platelet-endothelial interactions. *Blood Coagul Fibrinolysis.* 2011;22(3):242–244.

124. Clyman RI, Mauray F, Roman C, et al. Effects of antenatal glucocorticoid administration on ductus arteriosus of preterm lambs. *Am J Physiol.* 1981;241(3):H415–H420.

125. Tsai MY, Brown DM. Effect of dexamethasone on fetal lung 15-hydroxy-prostaglandin dehydrogenase: possible mechanism for the prevention of patent ductus arteriosus by maternal dexamethasone therapy. *Prostaglandins Leukot Med.* 1987;27(2–3):237–245.

126. Eronen M, Kari A, Pesonen E, Hallman M. The effect of antenatal dexamethasone administration on the fetal and neonatal ductus arteriosus. A randomized double-blind study. *Am J Dis Child.* 1993;147(2):187–192.

127. Chorne N, Jegatheesan P, Lin E, Shi R, Clyman RI. Risk factors for persistent ductus arteriosus patency during indomethacin treatment. *J Pediatr.* 2007;151(6):629–634.

128. Heyman E, Ohlsson A, Shennan AT, Heilbut M, Coceani F. Closure of patent ductus arteriosus after treatment with dexamethasone. *Acta Paediatr Scand.* 1990;79(6–7):698–700.

129. Halliday HL, Ehrenkranz RA, Doyle LW. Early postnatal (<96 hours) corticosteroids for preventing chronic lung disease in preterm infants. *Cochrane Database Syst Rev.* 2003;(1): CD001146.

130. Doyle LW, Ehrenkranz RA, Halliday HL. Dexamethasone treatment in the first week of life for preventing bronchopulmonary dysplasia in preterm infants: a systematic review. *Neonatology.* 2010;98(3):217–224.

131. Colbert MC, Kirby ML, Robbins J. Endogenous retinoic acid signaling colocalizes with advanced expression of the adult smooth muscle myosin heavy chain isoform during development of the ductus arteriosus. *Circ Res.* 1996;78(5): 790–798.

132. Momma K, Toyono M, Miyagawa-Tomita S. Accelerated maturation of fetal ductus arteriosus by maternally administered vitamin A in rats. *Pediatr Res.* 1998;43(5):629–632.

133. Yokoyama U, Sato Y, Akaike T, et al. Maternal vitamin A alters gene profiles and structural maturation of the rat ductus arteriosus. *Physiol Genomics.* 2007;31(1):139–157.

134. Darlow BA, Graham PJ. Vitamin A supplementation to prevent mortality and short- and long-term morbidity in very low birthweight infants. *Cochrane Database Syst Rev.* 2011;(10):CD000501.

135. Wardle SP, Hughes A, Chen S, Shaw NJ. Randomised controlled trial of oral vitamin A supplementation in preterm infants to prevent chronic lung disease. *Arch Dis Child Fetal Neonatal Ed.* 2001;84(1):F9–F13.

136. Ravishankar C, Nafday S, Green RS, et al. A trial of vitamin A therapy to facilitate ductal closure in premature infants. *J Pediatr.* 2003;143(5):644–648.

137. King DT, Emmanouilides GC, Andrews JC, Hirose FM. Morphologic evidence of accelerated closure of the ductus arteriosus in preterm infants. *Pediatrics.* 1980;65(5):872–880.

138. Ibara S, Tokunaga M, Ikenoue T, et al. Histologic observation of the ductus arteriosus in premature infants with intrauterine growth retardation. *J Perinatol.* 1994;14(5):411–416.

139. van Wassenaer AG, Kok JH. Trials with thyroid hormone in preterm infants: clinical and neurodevelopmental effects. *Semin Perinatol.* 2008;32(6):423–430.

140. Pulkkinen MO, Momma K, Pulkkinen J. Constriction of the fetal ductus arteriosus by progesterone. *Biol Neonate.* 1986;50(5):270–273.

141. Cotton RB. The relationship of symptomatic patent ductus arteriosus to respiratory distress in premature newborn infants. *Clin Perinatol.* 1987;14(3):621–633.

142. Marquis RM. The continuous murmur of persistence of the ductus arteriosus—an historical review. *Eur Heart J.* 1980;1(6):465–478.

143. Burnard ED. A murmur from the ductus arteriosus in the newborn baby. *Br Med J.* 1958;1(5074):806–810.

144. Hallidie-Smith KA. Murmur of persistent ductus arteriosus in premature infants. *Arch Dis Child.* 1972;47(255):725–730.

145. Rudolph AM, Mayer FE, Nadas AS, Gross RE. A clinical and hemodynamic study of 23 patients in the first year of life. *Pediatrics.* 1958;22(5):892–904.

146. Rowe RD, Lowe JB. Auscultation in the diagnosis of persistent ductus arteriosus in infancy. A study of 50 patients. *N Z Med J.* 1964;63:195–199.

147. McGrath RL, McGuinness GA, Way GL, Wolfe RR, Nora JJ, Simmons MA. The silent ductus arteriosus. *J Pediatr.* 1978;93(1):110–113.

148. Zanardo V, Trevisanuto D, Dani C, et al. "Silent" patent ductus arteriosus and bronchopulmonary dysplasia in low birth weight infants. *J Perinat Med.* 1995;23(6):493–499.

149. Davis P, Turner-Gomes S, Cunningham K, Way C, Roberts R, Schmidt B. Precision and accuracy of clinical and radiological signs in premature infants at risk of patent ductus arteriosus. *Arch Pediatr Adolesc Med.* 1995;149(10):1136–1141.

150. Sehgal A, McNamara PJ. Does echocardiography facilitate determination of hemodynamic significance attributable to the ductus arteriosus? *Eur J Pediatr.* 2009;168(8):907–914.

151. Zonnenberg I, de Waal K. The definition of a haemodynamic significant duct in randomized controlled trials: a systematic literature review. *Acta Paediatr.* 2012;101(3):247–251.

152. Evans N. Diagnosis of patent ductus arteriosus in the preterm newborn. *Arch Dis Child.* 1993;68 (1 Spec No):58–61.

153. El Hajjar M, Vaksmann G, Rakza T, Kongolo G, Storme L. Severity of the ductal shunt: a comparison of different markers. *Arch Dis Child Fetal Neonatal Ed.* 2005;90(5):F419–F422.

154. McNamara PJ, Sehgal A. Towards rational management of the patent ductus arteriosus: the need for disease staging. *Arch Dis Child Fetal Neonatal Ed.* 2007;92(6):F424–F427.

155. Andersson S, Tikkanen I, Pesonen E, Meretoja O, Hynynen M, Fyhrquist F. Atrial natriuretic peptide in patent ductus arteriosus. *Pediatr Res.* 1987;21(4):396–398.

156. Rascher W, Bald M, Kreis J, Tulassay T, Heinrich U, Scharer K. Atrial natriuretic peptide in infants and children. *Horm Res.* 1987;28(1):58–63.

157. Holmstrom H, Hall C, Thaulow E. Plasma levels of natriuretic peptides and hemodynamic assessment of patent ductus arteriosus in preterm infants. *Acta Paediatr.* 2001;90(2):184–191.

158. El-Khuffash AF, Barry D, Walsh K, Davis PG, Molloy EJ. Biochemical markers may identify preterm infants with a patent ductus arteriosus at high risk of death of severe intraventricular haemorrhage. *Arch Dis Child Fetal Neonatal Ed.* 2008;93(6):F407–F412.

159. Zanardo V, Vedovato S, Chiozza L, Faggian D, Favaro F, Trevisanuto D. Pharmacological closure of patent ductus arteriosus: effects on pulse pressure and on endothelin-1 and vasopressin excretion. *Am J Perinatol.* 2008;25(6):353–358.

160. Cambonie G, Dupuy AM, Combes C, Vincenti M, Mesnage R, Cristol JP. Can a clinical decision rule help ductus arteriosus management in preterm neonates? *Acta Paediatr.* 2012;101(5): e213–e218.

161. Letzner J, Berger F, Schwabe S, et al. Plasma C-terminal pro-endothelin-1 and the natriuretic pro-peptides NT-proBNP and MR-proANP in very preterm infants with patent ductus arteriosus. *Neonatology.* 2011;101(2):116–124.

162. Chen S, Tacy T, Clyman R. How useful are B-type natriuretic peptide measurements for monitoring changes in patent ductus arteriosus shunt magnitude? *J Perinatol.* 2010;30(12): 780–785.

163. Hammerman C, Shchors I, Schimmel MS, Bromiker R, Kaplan M, Nir A. N-Terminal-pro-B-type natriuretic peptide in premature patent ductus arteriosus: a physiologic biomarker, but is it a clinical tool? *Pediatr Cardiol.* 2010;31(1):62–65.

164. Dikshit K, Vyden JK, Forrester JS, Chatterjee K, Prakash R, Swan HJ. Renal and extrarenal hemodynamic effects of furosemide in congestive heart failure after acute myocardial infarction. *N Engl J Med.* 1973;288(21):1087–1090.

165. Johnston GD, Nicholls DP, Leahey WJ. The dose-response characteristics of the acute non-diuretic peripheral vascular effects of frusemide in normal subjects. *Br J Clin Pharmacol.* 1984;18(1):75–81.

166. Green TP, Thompson TR, Johnson DE, Lock JE. Furosemide promotes patent ductus arteriosus in premature infants with the respiratory-distress syndrome. *N Engl J Med.* 1983;308(13): 743–748.

167. Toyoshima K, Momma K, Nakanishi T. In vivo dilatation of the ductus arteriosus induced by furosemide in the rat. *Pediatr Res.* 2010;67(2):173–176.

168. Stevenson JG. Fluid administration in the association of patent ductus arteriosus complicating respiratory distress syndrome. *J Pediatr.* 1977;90(2):257–261.

169. Bell EF, Warburton D, Stonestreet BS, Oh W. Effect of fluid administration on the development of symptomatic patent ductus arteriosus and congestive heart failure in premature infants. *N Engl J Med.* 1980;302(11):598–604.

170. Furzan JA, Reisch J, Tyson JE, Laird P, Rosenfeld CR. Incidence and risk factors for symptomatic patent ductus arteriosus among inborn very-low-birth-weight infants. *Early Hum Dev.* 1985;12(1):39–48.

171. Stephens BE, Gargus RA, Walden RV, et al. Fluid regimens in the first week of life increase risk of patent ductus arteriosus in extremely low birth weight infants. *J Perinatol.* 2008;28(2):123–128.

172. Bell EF, Acarregui MJ. Restricted versus liberal water intake for preventing morbidity and mortality in preterm infants. *Cochrane Database Syst Rev.* 2008;(1):CD000503.

173. Roberton NR. Prolonged continuous positive airways pressure for pulmonary oedema due to persistent ductus arteriosus in the newborn. *Arch Dis Child.* 1974;49(7):585–587.

174. Cotton RB, Lindstrom DP, Kanarek KS, Sundell H, Stahlman MT. Effect of positive-end-expiratory-pressure on right ventricular output in lambs with hyaline membrane disease. *Acta Paediatr Scand.* 1980;69(5):603–606.

175. Noori S, Patel D, Friedlich P, Siassi B, Seri I, Ramanathan R. Effects of low oxygen saturation limits on the ductus arteriosus in extremely low birth weight infants. *J Perinatol.* 2009;29(8):553–557.

176. Carlo WA, Finer NN, Walsh MC, et al. Target ranges of oxygen saturation in extremely preterm infants. *N Engl J Med.* 2010;362(21):1959–1969.

177. Lister G, Hellenbrand WE, Kleinman CS, Talner NS. Physiologic effects of increasing hemoglobin concentration in left-to-right shunting in infants with ventricular septal defects. *N Engl J Med.* 1982;306(9):502–506.

178. Brooks JM, Travadi JN, Patole SK, Doherty DA, Simmer K. Is surgical ligation of patent ductus arteriosus necessary? The Western Australian experience of conservative management. *Arch Dis Child Fetal Neonatal Ed.* 2005;90(3):F235–F239.

179. Alexander F, Chiu L, Kroh M, Hammel J, Moore J. Analysis of outcome in 298 extremely low-birth-weight infants with patent ductus arteriosus. *J Pediatr Surg.* 2009;44(1):112–117. discussion 117.

180. Noori S, McCoy M, Friedlich P, et al. Failure of ductus arteriosus closure is associated with increased mortality in preterm infants. *Pediatrics.* 2009;123(1):e138–e144.

181. Knight DB. Patent ductus arteriosus: how important to which babies? *Early Hum Dev.* 1992;29(1–3):287–292.

182. Knight DB. The treatment of patent ductus arteriosus in preterm infants. A review and overview of randomized trials. *Semin Neonatol.* 2001;6(1):63–73.

183. Cooke L, Steer P, Woodgate P. Indomethacin for asymptomatic patent ductus arteriosus in preterm infants. *Cochrane Database Syst Rev.* 2003;(2):CD003745.

184. Laughon MM, Simmons MA, Bose CL. Patency of the ductus arteriosus in the premature infant: is it pathologic? Should it be treated? *Curr Opin Pediatr.* 2004;16(2):146–151.

185. Benitz WE. Treatment of persistent patent ductus arteriosus in preterm infants: time to accept the null hypothesis? *J Perinatol.* 2010;30(4):241–252.

186. Laughon M, Bose C, Clark R. Treatment strategies to prevent or close a patent ductus arteriosus in preterm infants and outcomes. *J Perinatol.* 2007;27(3):164–170.

187. Vanhaesebrouck S, Zonnenberg I, Vandervoort P, Bruneel E, Van Hoestenberghe MR, Theyskens C. Conservative treatment for patent ductus arteriosus in the preterm. *Arch Dis Child Fetal Neonatal Ed.* 2007;92(4):F244–F247.

188. Guimaraes H, Rocha G, Tome T, Anatolitou F, Sarafidis K, Fanos V. Non-steroid anti-inflammatory drugs in the treatment of patent ductus arteriosus in European newborns. *J Matern Fetal Neonatal Med.* 2009;22(Suppl 3):77–80.

189. Hoellering AB, Cooke L. The management of patent ductus arteriosus in Australia and New Zealand. *J Paediatr Child Health.* 2009;45(4):204–209.

190. Kiefer AS, Wickremasinghe AC, Johnson JN, et al. Medical management of extremely low-birth-weight infants in the first week of life: a survey of practices in the United States. *Am J Perinatol.* 2009;26(6):407–418.

191. Jhaveri N, Moon-Grady A, Clyman RI. Early surgical ligation versus a conservative approach for management of patent ductus arteriosus that fails to close after indomethacin treatment. *J Pediatr.* 2010;157(3):381–387. 387.e381.

192. Brissaud O, Guichoux J. Patent ductus arteriosus in the preterm infant: a survey of clinical practices in French neonatal intensive care units. *Pediatr Cardiol.* 2011;32(5):607–614.

193. Bose CL, Laughon MM. Patent ductus arteriosus: lack of evidence for common treatments. *Arch Dis Child Fetal Neonatal Ed.* 2007;92(6):F498–F502.

194. Benitz WE. Learning to live with patency of the ductus arteriosus in preterm infants. *J Perinatol.* 2011;31(Suppl 1):S42–S48.

195. Benitz WE. Patent ductus arteriosus: to treat or not to treat? *Arch Dis Child Fetal Neonatal Ed.* 2012;97(2):F80–F82.

196. Kaempf JW, Wu YX, Kaempf AJ, Kaempf AM, Wang L, Grunkemeier G. What happens when the patent ductus arteriosus is treated less aggressively in very low birth weight infants? *J Perinatol.* 2012;32(5):344–348.

197. Clyman RI. Recommendations for the postnatal use of indomethacin: an analysis of four separate treatment strategies. *J Pediatr.* 1996;128(5 Pt 1):601–607.

198. Fowlie PW, Davis PG, McGuire W. Prophylactic intravenous indomethacin for preventing mortality and morbidity in preterm infants. *Cochrane Database Syst Rev.* 2010;(7):CD000174.

199. Mahony L, Caldwell RL, Girod DA, et al. Indomethacin therapy on the first day of life in infants with very low birth weight. *J Pediatr.* 1985;106(5):801–805.

200. Rennie JM, Doyle J, Cooke RW. Early administration of indomethacin to preterm infants. *Arch Dis Child.* 1986;61(3):233–238.

201. Krueger E, Mellander M, Bratton D, Cotton R. Prevention of symptomatic patent ductus arteriosus with a single dose of indomethacin. *J Pediatr.* 1987;111(5):749–754.

202. Ment LR, Stewart WB, Scott DT, Duncan CC. Beagle puppy model of intraventricular hemorrhage: randomized indomethacin prevention trial. *Neurology.* 1983;33(2):179–184.

203. Ment LR, Duncan CC, Ehrenkranz RA, et al. Randomized indomethacin trial for prevention of intraventricular hemorrhage in very low birth weight infants. *J Pediatr.* 1985;107(6):937–943.

204. Ment LR, Duncan CC, Ehrenkranz RA, et al. Randomized low-dose indomethacin trial for prevention of intraventricular hemorrhage in very low birth weight neonates. *J Pediatr.* 1988;112(6):948–955.

205. Bandstra ES, Montalvo BM, Goldberg RN, et al. Prophylactic indomethacin for prevention of intraventricular hemorrhage in premature infants. *Pediatrics.* 1988;82(4):533–542.

206. Hanigan WC, Kennedy G, Roemisch F, Anderson R, Cusack T, Powers W. Administration of indomethacin for the prevention of periventricular-intraventricular hemorrhage in high-risk neonates. *J Pediatr.* 1988;112(6):941–947.

207. Bada HS, Green RS, Pourcyrous M, et al. Indomethacin reduces the risks of severe intraventricular hemorrhage. *J Pediatr.* 1989;115(4):631–637.

208. Ment LR, Oh W, Ehrenkranz RA, et al. Low-dose indomethacin and prevention of intraventricular hemorrhage: a multicenter randomized trial. *Pediatrics.* 1994;93(4):543–550.

209. Clyman RI, Saha S, Jobe A, Oh W. Indomethacin prophylaxis for preterm infants: the impact of 2 multicentered randomized controlled trials on clinical practice. *J Pediatr.* 2007;150(1):46–50.e42.

210. Hammerman C, Strates E, Komar K, Bui K. Failure of prophylactic indomethacin to improve the outcome of the very low birth weight infant. *Dev Pharmacol Ther.* 1987;10(6):393–404.

211. Yanowitz TD, Baker RW, Sobchak Brozanski B. Prophylactic indomethacin reduces grades III and IV intraventricular hemorrhages when compared to early indomethacin treatment of a patent ductus arteriosus. *J Perinatol.* 2003;23(4):317–322.

212. Tefft RG. The impact of an early Ibuprofen treatment protocol on the incidence of surgical ligation of the ductus arteriosus. *Am J Perinatol.* 2010;27(1):83–90.

213. Dani C, Bertini G, Pezzati M, et al. Prophylactic ibuprofen for the prevention of intraventricular hemorrhage among preterm infants: a multicenter, randomized study. *Pediatrics.* 2005;115(6):1529–1535.

214. Gournay V, Roze JC, Kuster A, et al. Prophylactic ibuprofen versus placebo in very premature infants: a randomised, double-blind, placebo-controlled trial. *Lancet.* 2004;364(9449):1939–1944.

215. Hammerman C, Kaplan M. Primum non nocere: prophylactic versus curative ibuprofen. *Lancet.* 2004;364(9449):1920–1922.

216. Van Overmeire B, Allegaert K, Casaer A, et al. Prophylactic ibuprofen in premature infants: a multicentre, randomised, double-blind, placebo-controlled trial. *Lancet.* 2004;364(9449):1945–1949.

217. Bellini C, Campone F, Serra G. Pulmonary hypertension following L-lysine ibuprofen therapy in a preterm infant with patent ductus arteriosus. *CMAJ.* 2006;174(13):1843–1844.

218. Ohlsson A, Shah SS. Ibuprofen for the prevention of patent ductus arteriosus in preterm and/or low birth weight infants. *Cochrane Database Syst Rev.* 2011;(7):CD004213.

219. Arcilla RA, Thilenius OG, Ranniger K. Congestive heart failure from suspected ductal closure in utero. *J Pediatr.* 1969;75(1):74–78.

220. Zuckerman H, Reiss U, Rubinstein I. Inhibition of human premature labor by indomethacin. *Obstet Gynecol.* 1974;44(6):787–792.

221. Coceani F, Olley PM. The response of the ductus arteriosus to prostaglandins. *Can J Physiol Pharmacol.* 1973;51(3):220–225.

222. Coceani F, Olley PM, Bodach E. Lamb ductus arteriosus: effect of prostaglandin synthesis inhibitors on the muscle tone and the response to prostaglandin E_2. *Prostaglandins.* 1975;9(2):299–308.

223. Sharpe GL, Thalme B, Larsson KS. Studies on closure of the ductus arteriosus. XI. Ductal closure in utero by a prostaglandin synthetase inhibitor. *Prostaglandins.* 1974;8(5):363–368.

224. Starling MB, Elliott RB. The effects of prostaglandins, prostaglandin inhibitors, and oxygen on the closure of the ductus arteriosus, pulmonary arteries and umbilical vessels in vitro. *Prostaglandins.* 1974;8(3):187–203.

225. Elliott RB, Starling MB, Neutze JM. Medical manipulation of the ductus arteriosus. *Lancet.* 1975;1(7899):140–142.

226. Friedman WF, Hirschklau MJ, Printz MP, Pitlick PT, Kirkpatrick SE. Pharmacologic closure of patent ductus arteriosus in the premature infant. *N Engl J Med.* 1976;295(10):526–529.

227. Heymann MA, Rudolph AM, Silverman NH. Closure of the ductus arteriosus in premature infants by inhibition of prostaglandin synthesis. *N Engl J Med.* 1976;295(10):530–533.

228. Coceani F, Olley PM, Bishai I, et al. Prostaglandins and the control of muscle tone in the ductus arteriosus. *Adv Exp Med Biol.* 1977;78:135–142.

229. Coceani F, White E, Bodach E, Olley PM. Age-dependent changes in the response of the lamb ductus arteriosus to oxygen and ibuprofen. *Can J Physiol Pharmacol.* 1979;57(8):825–831.

230. Patel J, Marks KA, Roberts I, Azzopardi D, Edwards AD. Ibuprofen treatment of patent ductus arteriosus. *Lancet.* 1995; 346(8969):255.

231. Van Overmeire B, Follens I, Hartmann S, Creten WL, Van Acker KJ. Treatment of patent ductus arteriosus with ibuprofen. *Arch Dis Child Fetal Neonatal Ed.* 1997;76(3):F179–F184.

232. Varvarigou A, Bardin CL, Beharry K, Chemtob S, Papageorgiou A, Aranda JV. Early ibuprofen administration to prevent patent ductus arteriosus in premature newborn infants. *JAMA.* 1996;275(7):539–544.

233. Smith WL, DeWitt DL, Garavito RM. Cyclooxygenases: structural, cellular, and molecular biology. *Annu Rev Biochem.* 2000;69:145–182.

234. Clyman RI. Ductus arteriosus: current theories of prenatal and postnatal regulation. *Semin Perinatol.* 1987;11(1):64–71.

235. Reese J, O'Mara PW, Poole SD, et al. Regulation of the fetal mouse ductus arteriosus is dependent on interaction of nitric oxide and COX enzymes in the ductal wall. *Prostaglandins Other Lipid Mediat.* 2009;88(3–4):89–96.

236. Reese J, Waleh N, Poole SD, Brown N, Roman C, Clyman RI. Chronic in utero cyclooxygenase inhibition alters PGE_2-regulated ductus arteriosus contractile pathways and prevents postnatal closure. *Pediatr Res.* 2009;66(2):155–161.

237. Gork AS, Ehrenkranz RA, Bracken MB. Continuous infusion versus intermittent bolus doses of indomethacin for patent ductus arteriosus closure in symptomatic preterm infants. *Cochrane Database Syst Rev.* 2008;(1):CD006071.

238. Herrera C, Holberton J, Davis P. Prolonged versus short course of indomethacin for the treatment of patent ductus arteriosus in preterm infants. *Cochrane Database Syst Rev.* 2007;(2):CD003480.

239. Clyman R. Patent ductus arteriosus: are current neonatal treatment options better or worse than no treatment at all? *Semin Perinatol.* 2012;36(2):123–129.

240. Hammerman C, Bin-Nun A, Kaplan M. Managing the PDA in the premature neonate: a new look at what we thought we knew. *Semin Perinatol.* 2012;36(2):130–138.

241. Johnston PG, Gillam-Krakauer M, Fuller MP, Reese J. Evidence-based use of indomethacin and ibuprofen in the neonatal intensive care unit. *Clin Perinatol.* 2012;39(1):111–136.

242. Clyman RI, Chorne N. Patent ductus arteriosus: evidence for and against treatment. *J Pediatr.* 2007;150(3):216–219.

243. Van Overmeire B, Van de Broek H, Van Laer P, Weyler J, Vanhaesebrouck P. Early versus late indomethacin treatment for patent ductus arteriosus in premature infants with respiratory distress syndrome. *J Pediatr.* 2001;138(2):205–211.

244. McCarthy JS, Zies LG, Gelband H. Age-dependent closure of the patent ductus arteriosus by indomethacin. *Pediatrics.* 1978;62(5):706–712.

245. Achanti B, Yeh TF, Pildes RS. Indomethacin therapy in infants with advanced postnatal age and patent ductus arteriosus. *Clin Invest Med.* 1986;9(4):250–253.

246. Kresch MJ, Moya FR, Ascuitto RJ, Ross-Ascuitto NT, Heusser F. Late closure of the ductus arteriosus using indomethacin in the preterm infant. *Clin Pediatr (Phila).* 1988;27(3):140–143.

247. Sterniste W, Gabriel C, Sacher M. Successful closure of the patent ductus arteriosus by indomethacin in an extremely low birth weight infant of very advanced postnatal age. *Pediatr Cardiol.* 1998;19(3):256–258.

248. Shaffer CL, Gal P, Ransom JL, et al. Effect of age and birth weight on indomethacin pharmacodynamics in

249. Vert P, Bianchetti G, Marchal F, Monin P, Morselli PL. Effectiveness and pharmacokinetics of indomethacin in premature newborns with patent ductus arteriosus. *Eur J Clin Pharmacol.* 1980;18(1):83–88.

250. Yaffe SJ, Friedman WF, Rogers D, Lang P, Ragni M, Saccar C. The disposition of indomethacin in preterm babies. *J Pediatr.* 1980;97(6):1001–1006.

251. Brash AR, Hickey DE, Graham TP, Stahlman MT, Oates JA, Cotton RB. Pharmacokinetics of indomethacin in the neonate. Relation of plasma indomethacin levels to response of the ductus arteriosus. *N Engl J Med.* 1981;305(2):67–72.

252. Yeh TF, Achanti B, Patel H, Pildes RS. Indomethacin therapy in premature infants with patent ductus arteriosus–determination of therapeutic plasma levels. *Dev Pharmacol Ther.* 1989;12(4):169–178.

253. Smyth JM, Collier PS, Darwish M, et al. Intravenous indomethacin in preterm infants with symptomatic patent ductus arteriosus. A population pharmacokinetic study. *Br J Clin Pharmacol.* 2004;58(3):249–258.

254. Friedman CA, Parks BR, Rawson JE, Serwer GA, Anderson PA. Indomethacin and the preterm infant with a patent ductus arteriosus: relationship between plasma concentration and ductus closure. *Dev Pharmacol Ther.* 1982;4(1–2):37–46.

255. Seyberth HW, Knapp G, Wolf D, Ulmer HE. Introduction of plasma indomethacin level monitoring and evaluation of an effective threshold level in very low birth weight infants with symptomatic patent ductus arteriosus. *Eur J Pediatr.* 1983;141(2):71–76.

256. Cotton RB, Haywood JL, FitzGerald GA. Symptomatic patent ductus arteriosus following prophylactic indomethacin. A clinical and biochemical appraisal. *Biol Neonate.* 1991; 60(5):273–282.

257. Narayanan M, Cooper B, Weiss H, Clyman RI. Prophylactic indomethacin: factors determining permanent ductus arteriosus closure. *J Pediatr.* 2000;136(3):330–337.

258. Weiss H, Cooper B, Brook M, Schlueter M, Clyman R. Factors determining reopening of the ductus arteriosus after successful clinical closure with indomethacin. *J Pediatr.* 1995;127(3): 466–471.

259. Quinn D, Cooper B, Clyman RI. Factors associated with permanent closure of the ductus arteriosus: a role for prolonged indomethacin therapy. *Pediatrics.* 2002;110(1 Pt 1):e10.

260. Uchiyama A, Nagasawa H, Yamamoto Y, et al. Clinical aspects of very-low-birthweight infants showing reopening of ductus arteriosus. *Pediatr Int.* 2011;53(3):322–327.

261. Hammerman C, Aramburo MJ. Prolonged indomethacin therapy for the prevention of recurrences of patent ductus arteriosus. *J Pediatr.* 1990;117(5):771–776.

262. Rennie JM, Cooke RW. Prolonged low dose indomethacin for persistent ductus arteriosus of prematurity. *Arch Dis Child.* 1991;66 (1 Spec No):55–58.

263. Rhodes PG, Ferguson MG, Reddy NS, Joransen JA, Gibson J. Effects of prolonged versus acute indomethacin therapy in very low birth-weight infants with patent ductus arteriosus. *Eur J Pediatr.* 1988;147(5):481–484.

264. Sangem M, Asthana S, Amin S. Multiple courses of indomethacin and neonatal outcomes in premature infants. *Pediatr Cardiol.* 2008;29(5):878–884.

265. Sperandio M, Beedgen B, Feneberg R, et al. Effectiveness and side effects of an escalating, stepwise approach to indomethacin treatment for symptomatic patent ductus arteriosus in premature infants below 33 weeks of gestation. *Pediatrics.* 2005;116(6):1361–1366.

266. Hammerman C. Patent ductus arteriosus. Clinical relevance of prostaglandins and prostaglandin inhibitors in PDA pathophysiology and treatment. *Clin Perinatol.* 1995;22(2):457–479.

neonates treated for patent ductus arteriosus. *Crit Care Med.* 2002;30(2):343–348.

CHAPTER 22

267. Christmann V, Liem KD, Semmekrot BA, van de Bor M. Changes in cerebral, renal and mesenteric blood flow velocity during continuous and bolus infusion of indomethacin. *Acta Paediatr.* 2002;91(4):440–446.

268. Cotton RB. Indomethacin: continuous versus bolus administration. *Acta Paediatr.* 2002;91(4):369–370.

269. de Vries NK, Jagroep FK, Jaarsma AS, Elzenga NJ, Bos AF. Continuous indomethacin infusion may be less effective than bolus infusions for ductal closure in very low birth weight infants. *Am J Perinatol.* 2005;22(2):71–75.

270. Tammela O, Ojala R, Iivainen T, et al. Short versus prolonged indomethacin therapy for patent ductus arteriosus in preterm infants. *J Pediatr.* 1999;134(5):552–557.

271. Lee J, Rajadurai VS, Tan KW, Wong KY, Wong EH, Leong JY. Randomized trial of prolonged low-dose versus conventional-dose indomethacin for treating patent ductus arteriosus in very low birth weight infants. *Pediatrics.* 2003;112(2):345–350.

272. Jegatheesan P, Ianus V, Buchh B, et al. Increased indomethacin dosing for persistent patent ductus arteriosus in preterm infants: a multicenter, randomized, controlled trial. *J Pediatr.* 2008;153(2):183–189.

273. Aranda JV, Clyman R, Cox B, et al. A randomized, double-blind, placebo-controlled trial on intravenous ibuprofen L-lysine for the early closure of nonsymptomatic patent ductus arteriosus within 72 hours of birth in extremely low-birth-weight infants. *Am J Perinatol.* 2009;26(3):235–245.

274. Aranda JV, Thomas R. Systematic review: intravenous Ibuprofen in preterm newborns. *Semin Perinatol.* 2006;30(3):114–120.

275. Desfrere L, Zohar S, Morville P, et al. Dose-finding study of ibuprofen in patent ductus arteriosus using the continual reassessment method. *J Clin Pharm Ther.* 2005;30(2):121–132.

276. Hirt D, Van Overmeire B, Treluyer JM, et al. An optimized ibuprofen dosing scheme for preterm neonates with patent ductus arteriosus, based on a population pharmacokinetic and pharmacodynamic study. *Br J Clin Pharmacol.* 2008;65(5):629–636.

277. Madan J, Fiascone J, Balasubramanian V, Griffith J, Hagadorn JI. Predictors of ductal closure and intestinal complications in very low birth weight infants treated with indomethacin. *Neonatology.* 2008;94(1):45–51.

278. Richards J, Johnson A, Fox G, Campbell M. A second course of ibuprofen is effective in the closure of a clinically significant PDA in ELBW infants. *Pediatrics.* 2009;124(2):e287–e293.

279. Kushnir A, Pinheiro JM. Comparison of renal effects of ibuprofen versus indomethacin during treatment of patent ductus arteriosus in contiguous historical cohorts. *BMC Clin Pharmacol.* 2011;11:8.

280. Pees C, Walch E, Obladen M, Koehne P. Echocardiography predicts closure of patent ductus arteriosus in response to ibuprofen in infants less than 28 week gestational age. *Early Hum Dev.* 2010;86(8):503–508.

281. Ohlsson A, Walia R, Shah S. Ibuprofen for the treatment of patent ductus arteriosus in preterm and/or low birth weight infants. *Cochrane Database Syst Rev.* 2005;(4):CD003481.

282. Thomas RL, Parker GC, Van Overmeire B, Aranda JV. A meta-analysis of ibuprofen versus indomethacin for closure of patent ductus arteriosus. *Eur J Pediatr.* 2005;164(3):135–140.

283. Ohlsson A, Walia R, Shah SS. Ibuprofen for the treatment of patent ductus arteriosus in preterm and/or low birth weight infants. *Cochrane Database Syst Rev.* 2010;(4):CD003481.

284. Cooper-Peel C, Brodersen R, Robertson A. Does ibuprofen affect bilirubin-albumin binding in newborn infant serum? *Pharmacol Toxicol.* 1996;79(6):297–299.

285. Ahlfors CE. Effect of ibuprofen on bilirubin-albumin binding. *J Pediatr.* 2004;144(3):386–388.

286. Rheinlaender C, Helfenstein D, Walch E, Berns M, Obladen M, Koehne P. Total serum bilirubin levels during cyclooxygenase inhibitor treatment for patent ductus arteriosus in preterm infants. *Acta Paediatr.* 2009;98(1):36–42.

287. Zecca E, Romagnoli C, De Carolis MP, Costa S, Marra R, De Luca D. Does ibuprofen increase neonatal hyperbilirubinemia? *Pediatrics.* 2009;124(2):480–484.

288. Linder N, Bello R, Hernandez A, et al. Treatment of patent ductus arteriosus: indomethacin or ibuprofen? *Am J Perinatol.* 2010;27(5):399–404.

289. Amin SB, Miravalle N. Effect of ibuprofen on bilirubin-albumin binding affinity in premature infants. *J Perinat Med.* 2011;39(1):55–58.

290. Desfrere L, Thibaut C, Kibleur Y, Barbier A, Bordarier C, Moriette G. Unbound bilirubin does not increase during ibuprofen treatment of patent ductus arteriosus in preterm infants. *J Pediatr.* 2012;160(2):258–264.

291. Sakhalkar VS, Merchant RH. Therapy of symptomatic patent ductus arteriosus in preterms using mefenemic acid and indomethacin. *Indian Pediatr.* 1992;29(3):313–318.

292. Ito K, Niida Y, Sato J, Owada E, Ito K, Umetsu M. Pharmacokinetics of mefenamic acid in preterm infants with patent ductus arteriosus. *Acta Paediatr Jpn.* 1994;36(4):387–391.

293. Peterson RG. Consequences associated with nonnarcotic analgesics in the fetus and newborn. *Fed Proc.* 1985;44(7):2309–2313.

294. Momma K, Takao A. Transplacental cardiovascular effects of four popular analgesics in rats. *Am J Obstet Gynecol.* 1990;162(5):1304–1310.

295. Simbi KA, Secchieri S, Rinaldo M, Demi M, Zanardo V. In utero ductal closure following near-term maternal self-medication with nimesulide and acetaminophen. *J Obstet Gynaecol.* 2002;22(4):440–441.

296. Hammerman C, Bin-Nun A, Markovitch E, Schimmel MS, Kaplan M, Fink D. Ductal closure with paracetamol: a surprising new approach to patent ductus arteriosus treatment. *Pediatrics.* 2011;128(6):e1618–e1621.

297. Grosfeld JL, Kamman K, Gross K, et al. Comparative effects of indomethacin, prostaglandin E1, and ibuprofen on bowel ischemia. *J Pediatr Surg.* 1983;18(6):738–742.

298. Van Bel F, Van Zoeren D, Schipper J, Guit GL, Baan J. Effect of indomethacin on superior mesenteric artery blood flow velocity in preterm infants. *J Pediatr.* 1990;116(6):965–970.

299. Yanowitz TD, Yao AC, Werner JC, Pettigrew KD, Oh W, Stonestreet BS. Effects of prophylactic low-dose indomethacin on hemodynamics in very low birth weight infants. *J Pediatr.* 1998;132(1):28–34.

300. Pezzati M, Vangi V, Biagiotti R, Bertini G, Cianciulli D, Rubaltelli FF. Effects of indomethacin and ibuprofen on mesenteric and renal blood flow in preterm infants with patent ductus arteriosus. *J Pediatr.* 1999;135(6):733–738.

301. Ryder RW, Shelton JD, Guinan ME. Necrotizing enterocolitis: a prospective multicenter investigation. *Am J Epidemiol.* 1980;112(1):113–123.

302. Alpan G, Eyal F, Vinograd I, et al. Localized intestinal perforations after enteral administration of indomethacin in premature infants. *J Pediatr.* 1985;106(2):277–281.

303. Rajadurai VS, Yu VY. Intravenous indomethacin therapy in preterm neonates with patent ductus arteriosus. *J Paediatr Child Health.* 1991;27(6):370–375.

304. Grosfeld JL, Chaet M, Molinari F, et al. Increased risk of necrotizing enterocolitis in premature infants with patent ductus arteriosus treated with indomethacin. *Ann Surg.* 1996;224(3):350–355. discussion 355–357.

305. Shorter NA, Liu JY, Mooney DP, Harmon BJ. Indomethacin-associated bowel perforations: a study of possible risk factors. *J Pediatr Surg.* 1999;34(3):442–444.

306. Fujii AM, Brown E, Mirochnick M, O'Brien S, Kaufman G. Neonatal necrotizing enterocolitis with intestinal perforation

in extremely premature infants receiving early indomethacin treatment for patent ductus arteriosus. *J Perinatol.* 2002;22(7):535–540.

307. Stark AR, Carlo WA, Tyson JE, et al. Adverse effects of early dexamethasone in extremely-low-birth-weight infants. National Institute of Child Health and Human Development Neonatal Research Network. *N Engl J Med.* 2001;344(2):95–101.

308. Watterberg KL, Gerdes JS, Cole CH, et al. Prophylaxis of early adrenal insufficiency to prevent bronchopulmonary dysplasia: a multicenter trial. *Pediatrics.* 2004;114(6):1649–1657.

309. Peltoniemi O, Kari MA, Heinonen K, et al. Pretreatment cortisol values may predict responses to hydrocortisone administration for the prevention of bronchopulmonary dysplasia in high-risk infants. *J Pediatr.* 2005;146(5):632–637.

310. Paquette L, Friedlich P, Ramanathan R, Seri I. Concurrent use of indomethacin and dexamethasone increases the risk of spontaneous intestinal perforation in very low birth weight neonates. *J Perinatol.* 2006;26(8):486–492.

311. Leidig E. Doppler analysis of superior mesenteric artery blood flow in preterm infants. *Arch Dis Child.* 1989;64 (4 Spec No): 476–480.

312. Martinussen M, Brubakk AM, Linker DT, Vik T, Yao AC. Mesenteric blood flow velocity and its relation to circulatory adaptation during the first week of life in healthy term infants. *Pediatr Res.* 1994;36(3):334–339.

313. Bellander M, Ley D, Polberger S, Hellstrom-Westas L. Tolerance to early human milk feeding is not compromised by indomethacin in preterm infants with persistent ductus arteriosus. *Acta Paediatr.* 2003;92(9):1074–1078.

314. Berseth CL. Feeding strategies and necrotizing enterocolitis. *Curr Opin Pediatr.* 2005;17(2):170–173.

315. Jhaveri N, Soll RF, Clyman RI. Feeding practices and patent ductus arteriosus ligation preferences-are they related? *Am J Perinatol.* 2010;27(8):667–674.

316. Hans DM, Pylipow M, Long JD, Thureen PJ, Georgieff MK. Nutritional practices in the neonatal intensive care unit: analysis of a 2006 neonatal nutrition survey. *Pediatrics.* 2009;123(1):51–57.

317. Betkerur MV, Yeh TF, Miller K, Glasser RJ, Pildes RS. Indomethacin and its effect on renal function and urinary kallikrein excretion in premature infants with patent ductus arteriosus. *Pediatrics.* 1981;68(1):99–102.

318. Gersony WM, Peckham GJ, Ellison RC, Miettinen OS, Nadas AS. Effects of indomethacin in premature infants with patent ductus arteriosus: results of a national collaborative study. *J Pediatr.* 1983;102(6):895–906.

319. van Bel F, Guit GL, Schipper J, van de Bor M, Baan J. Indomethacin-induced changes in renal blood flow velocity waveform in premature infants investigated with color Doppler imaging. *J Pediatr.* 1991;118(4 Pt 1):621–626.

320. Seyberth HW, Muller H, Wille L, Pluckthun H, Wolf D, Ulmer HE. Recovery of prostaglandin production associated with reopening of the ductus arteriosus after indomethacin treatment in preterm infants with respiratory distress syndrome. *Pediatr Pharmacol (New York).* 1982;2(2):127–141.

321. Laudignon N, Chemtob S, Bard H, Aranda JV. Effect of indomethacin on cerebral blood flow velocity of premature newborns. *Biol Neonate.* 1988;54(5):254–262.

322. Pryds O, Greisen G, Johansen KH. Indomethacin and cerebral blood flow in premature infants treated for patent ductus arteriosus. *Eur J Pediatr.* 1988;147(3):315–316.

323. Van Bel F, Van de Bor M, Stijnen T, Baan J, Ruys JH. Cerebral blood flow velocity changes in preterm infants after a single dose of indomethacin: duration of its effect. *Pediatrics.* 1989;84(5):802–807.

324. Edwards AD, Wyatt JS, Richardson C, et al. Effects of indomethacin on cerebral haemodynamics in very preterm infants. *Lancet.* 1990;335(8704):1491–1495.

325. Austin NC, Pairaudeau PW, Hames TK, Hall MA. Regional cerebral blood flow velocity changes after indomethacin infusion in preterm infants. *Arch Dis Child.* 1992;67 (7 Spec No): 851–854.

326. Ohlsson A, Bottu J, Govan J, Ryan ML, Fong K, Myhr T. Effect of indomethacin on cerebral blood flow velocities in very low birth weight neonates with a patent ductus arteriosus. *Dev Pharmacol Ther.* 1993;20(1–2):100–106.

327. Simko A, Mardoum R, Merritt TA, Bejar R. Effects on cerebral blood flow velocities of slow and rapid infusion of indomethacin. *J Perinatol.* 1994;14(1):29–35.

328. Benders MJ, Dorrepaal CA, van de Bor M, van Bel F. Acute effects of indomethacin on cerebral hemodynamics and oxygenation. *Biol Neonate.* 1995;68(2):91–99.

329. Mosca F, Bray M, Lattanzio M, Fumagalli M, Tosetto C. Comparative evaluation of the effects of indomethacin and ibuprofen on cerebral perfusion and oxygenation in preterm infants with patent ductus arteriosus. *J Pediatr.* 1997;131(4):549–554.

330. Patel J, Roberts I, Azzopardi D, Hamilton P, Edwards AD. Randomized double-blind controlled trial comparing the effects of ibuprofen with indomethacin on cerebral hemodynamics in preterm infants with patent ductus arteriosus. *Pediatr Res.* 2000;47(1):36–42.

331. McCormick DC, Edwards AD, Brown GC, et al. Effect of indomethacin on cerebral oxidized cytochrome oxidase in preterm infants. *Pediatr Res.* 1993;33(6):603–608.

332. Liem KD, Hopman JC, Kollee LA, Oeseburg B. Effects of repeated indomethacin administration on cerebral oxygenation and haemodynamics in preterm infants: combined near infrared spectrophotometry and Doppler ultrasound study. *Eur J Pediatr.* 1994;153(7):504–509.

333. Chock VY, Ramamoorthy C, Van Meurs KP. Cerebral oxygenation during different treatment strategies for a patent ductus arteriosus. *Neonatology.* 2011;100(3):233–240.

334. Couser RJ, Hoekstra RE, Ferrara TB, Wright GB, Cabalka AK, Connett JE. Neurodevelopmental follow-up at 36 months' corrected age of preterm infants treated with prophylactic indomethacin. *Arch Pediatr Adolesc Med.* 2000;154(6): 598–602.

335. Luu TM, Ment LR, Schneider KC, Katz KH, Allan WC, Vohr BR. Lasting effects of preterm birth and neonatal brain hemorrhage at 12 years of age. *Pediatrics.* 2009;123(3): 1037–1044.

336. Rheinlaender C, Helfenstein D, Pees C, et al. Neurodevelopmental outcome after COX inhibitor treatment for patent ductus arteriosus. *Early Hum Dev.* 2010;86(2):87–92.

337. Ment LR, Vohr B, Allan W, et al. Outcome of children in the indomethacin intraventricular hemorrhage prevention trial. *Pediatrics.* 2000;105(3 Pt 1):485–491.

338. Vohr BR, Allan WC, Westerveld M, et al. School-age outcomes of very low birth weight infants in the indomethacin intraventricular hemorrhage prevention trial. *Pediatrics.* 2003;111(4 Pt 1): e340–e346.

339. Miller SP, Mayer EE, Clyman RI, Glidden DV, Hamrick SE, Barkovich AJ. Prolonged indomethacin exposure is associated with decreased white matter injury detected with magnetic resonance imaging in premature newborns at 24 to 28 weeks' gestation at birth. *Pediatrics.* 2006;117(5):1626–1631.

340. Malcolm DD, Segar JL, Robillard JE, Chemtob S. Indomethacin compromises hemodynamics during positive-pressure ventilation, independently of prostanoids. *J Appl Physiol.* 1993;74(4):1672–1678.

341. Lehmann T, Day RO, Brooks PM. Toxicity of antirheumatic drugs. *Med J Aust.* 1997;166(7):378–383.

342. Tegeder I, Pfeilschifter J, Geisslinger G. Cyclooxygenase-independent actions of cyclooxygenase inhibitors. *FASEB J.* 2001;15(12):2057–2072.

CHAPTER 22

343. Sagi SA, Weggen S, Eriksen J, Golde TE, Koo EH. The non-cyclooxygenase targets of non-steroidal anti-inflammatory drugs, lipoxygenases, peroxisome proliferator-activated receptor, inhibitor of kappa B kinase, and NF kappa B, do not reduce amyloid beta 42 production. *J Biol Chem.* 2003;278(34):31825–31830.

344. Shah SS, Ohlsson A. Ibuprofen for the prevention of patent ductus arteriosus in preterm and/or low birth weight infants. *Cochrane Database Syst Rev.* 2003;(2):CD004213.

345. Fanos V, Benini D, Verlato G, Errico G, Cuzzolin L. Efficacy and renal tolerability of ibuprofen vs indomethacin in preterm infants with patent ductus arteriosus. *Fundam Clin Pharmacol.* 2005;19(2):187–193.

346. Warner TD, Mitchell JA. Cyclooxygenases: new forms, new inhibitors, and lessons from the clinic. *FASEB J.* 2004;18(7):790–804.

347. Rao R, Bryowsky K, Mao J, Bunton D, McPherson C, Mathur A. Gastrointestinal complications associated with ibuprofen therapy for patent ductus arteriosus. *J Perinatol.* 2011;31(7):465–470.

348. Van Overmeire B, Smets K, Lecoutere D, et al. A comparison of ibuprofen and indomethacin for closure of patent ductus arteriosus. *N Engl J Med.* 2000;343(10):674–681.

349. Lago P, Bettiol T, Salvadori S, et al. Safety and efficacy of ibuprofen versus indomethacin in preterm infants treated for patent ductus arteriosus: a randomised controlled trial. *Eur J Pediatr.* 2002;161(4):202–207.

350. Giniger RP, Buffat C, Millet V, Simeoni U. Renal effects of ibuprofen for the treatment of patent ductus arteriosus in premature infants. *J Matern Fetal Neonatal Med.* 2007;20(4):275–283.

351. Su BH, Lin HC, Chiu HY, Hsieh HY, Chen HH, Tsai YC. Comparison of ibuprofen and indomethacin for early-targeted treatment of patent ductus arteriosus in extremely premature infants: a randomised controlled trial. *Arch Dis Child Fetal Neonatal Ed.* 2008;93(2):F94–F99.

352. Vieux R, Desandes R, Boubred F, et al. Ibuprofen in very preterm infants impairs renal function for the first month of life. *Pediatr Nephrol.* 2010;25(2):267–274.

353. Guignard JP. The adverse renal effects of prostaglandin-synthesis inhibitors in the newborn rabbit. *Semin Perinatol.* 2002;26(6):398–405.

354. Cataldi L, Leone R, Moretti U, et al. Potential risk factors for the development of acute renal failure in preterm newborn infants: a case-control study. *Arch Dis Child Fetal Neonatal Ed.* 2005;90(6):F514–F519.

355. Cuzzolin L, Fanos V, Pinna B, et al. Postnatal renal function in preterm newborns: a role of diseases, drugs and therapeutic interventions. *Pediatr Nephrol.* 2006;21(7):931–938.

356. Tiker F, Yildirim SV. Acute renal impairment after oral ibuprofen for medical closure of patent ductus arteriosus. *Indian Pediatr.* 2007;44(1):54–55.

357. Erdeve O, Sarici SU, Sari E, Gok F. Oral-ibuprofen-induced acute renal failure in a preterm infant. *Pediatr Nephrol.* 2008;23(9):1565–1567.

358. Fanos V, Antonucci R, Zaffanello M. Ibuprofen and acute kidney injury in the newborn. *Turk J Pediatr.* 2010;52(3):231–238.

359. Chemtob S, Beharry K, Rex J, Varma DR, Aranda JV. Prostanoids determine the range of cerebral blood flow autoregulation of newborn piglets. *Stroke.* 1990;21(5):777–784.

360. Romagnoli C, De Carolis MP, Papacci P, et al. Effects of prophylactic ibuprofen on cerebral and renal hemodynamics in very preterm neonates. *Clin Pharmacol Ther.* 2000;67(6):676–683.

361. Li DY, Hardy P, Abran D, et al. Key role for cyclooxygenase-2 in PGE_2 and PGF_{2alpha} receptor regulation and cerebral blood flow of the newborn. *Am J Physiol.* 1997;273(4 Pt 2):R1283–R1290.

362. Mosca F, Bray M, Colnaghi MR, Fumagalli M, Compagnoni G. Cerebral vasoreactivity to arterial carbon dioxide tension in preterm infants: the effect of ibuprofen. *J Pediatr.* 1999;135(5):644–646.

363. Jones LJ, Craven PD, Attia J, Thakkinstian A, Wright I. Network meta-analysis of indomethacin versus ibuprofen versus placebo for PDA in preterm infants. *Arch Dis Child Fetal Neonatal Ed.* 2011;96(1):F45–F52.

364. Raval MV, Laughon MM, Bose CL, Phillips JD. Patent ductus arteriosus ligation in premature infants: who really benefits, and at what cost? *J Pediatr Surg.* 2007;42(1):69–75. discussion 75.

365. Noori S. Pros and cons of PDA ligation: Hemodynamic changes and other morbidities after PDA ligation. *Semin Perinatol.* 2012;36(2):139–145.

366. Cassady G, Crouse DT, Kirklin JW, et al. A randomized, controlled trial of very early prophylactic ligation of the ductus arteriosus in babies who weighed 1000 g or less at birth. *N Engl J Med.* 1989;320(23):1511–1516.

367. Clyman R, Cassady G, Kirklin JK, Collins M, Philips JB 3rd. The role of patent ductus arteriosus ligation in bronchopulmonary dysplasia: reexamining a randomized controlled trial. *J Pediatr.* 2009;154(6):873–876.

368. Mosalli R, Alfaleh K, Paes B. Role of prophylactic surgical ligation of patent ductus arteriosus in extremely low birth weight infants: systematic review and implications for clinical practice. *Ann Pediatr Cardiol.* 2009;2(2):120–126.

369. Jaillard S, Larrue B, Rakza T, Magnenant E, Warembourg H, Storme L. Consequences of delayed surgical closure of patent ductus arteriosus in very premature infants. *Ann Thorac Surg.* 2006;81(1):231–234.

370. Hsiao CC, Wung JT, Tsao LY, Chang WC. Early or late surgical ligation of medical refractory patent ductus arteriosus in premature infants. *J Formos Med Assoc.* 2009;108(1):72–77.

371. Edmunds LH Jr. Operation or indomethacin for the premature ductus. *Ann Thorac Surg.* 1978;26(6):586–589.

372. Ivey HH, Kattwinkel J, Park TS, Krovetz LJ. Failure of indomethacin to close persistent ductus arteriosus in infants weighing under 1000 grams. *Br Heart J.* 1979;41(3):304–307.

373. Little DC, Pratt TC, Blalock SE, Krauss DR, Cooney DR, Custer MD. Patent ductus arteriosus in micropreemies and full-term infants: the relative merits of surgical ligation versus indomethacin treatment. *J Pediatr Surg.* 2003;38(3):492–496.

374. Palder SB, Schwartz MZ, Tyson KR, Marr CC. Management of patent ductus arteriosus: a comparison of operative v pharmacologic treatment. *J Pediatr Surg.* 1987;22(12):1171–1174.

375. Trus T, Winthrop AL, Pipe S, Shah J, Langer JC, Lau GY. Optimal management of patent ductus arteriosus in the neonate weighing less than 800 g. *J Pediatr Surg.* 1993;28(9):1137–1139.

376. Perez CA, Bustorff-Silva JM, Villasenor E, Fonkalsrud EW, Atkinson JB. Surgical ligation of patent ductus arteriosus in very low birth weight infants: is it safe? *Am Surg.* 1998;64(10):1007–1009.

377. Lee SK, McMillan DD, Ohlsson A, et al. Variations in practice and outcomes in the Canadian NICU network: 1996–1997. *Pediatrics.* 2000;106(5):1070–1079.

378. Niinikoski H, Alanen M, Parvinen T, Aantaa R, Ekblad H, Kero P. Surgical closure of patent ductus arteriosus in very-low-birth-weight infants. *Pediatr Surg Int.* 2001;17(5–6):338–341.

379. Fortescue EB, Lock JE, Galvin T, McElhinney DB. To close or not to close: the very small patent ductus arteriosus. *Congenit Heart Dis.* 2010;5(4):354–365.

380. Onji K, Matsuura W. Pulmonary endarteritis and subsequent pulmonary embolism associated with clinically silent patent ductus arteriosus. *Intern Med.* 2007;46(19):1663–1667.

381. Pharis CS, Conway J, Warren AE, Bullock A, Mackie AS. The impact of 2007 infective endocarditis prophylaxis guidelines on the practice of congenital heart disease specialists. *Am Heart J.* 2011;161(1):123–129.

382. Schneider DJ, Moore JW. Patent ductus arteriosus. *Circulation.* 2006;114(17):1873–1882.

383. Danilowicz D, Rudolph AM, Hoffman JI. Delayed closure of the ductus arteriosus in premature infants. *Pediatrics.* 1966;37(1):74–78.

384. Powell ML. Patent ductus arteriosus in premature infants. *Med J Aust.* 1963;2:58–60.

385. Siassi B, Blanco C, Cabal LA, Coran AG. Incidence and clinical features of patent ductus arteriosus in low-birthweight infants: a prospective analysis of 150 consecutively born infants. *Pediatrics.* 1976;57(3):347–351.

386. Peirone AR, Benson LN. The patent arterial duct. In: Freedom RM, Yoo S-J, Midailian H, Williams WG, eds. *The Natural and Modified History of Congenital Heart Disease.* Elmsford, NY: Blackwell Publishing Ltd.; 2004:72–82.

387. Schneider DJ. The patent ductus arteriosus in term infants, children, and adults. *Semin Perinatol.* 2012;36(2):146–153.

388. Vida VL, Lago P, Salvatori S, et al. Is there an optimal timing for surgical ligation of patent ductus arteriosus in preterm infants? *Ann Thorac Surg.* 2009;87(5):1509–1515. discussion 1515–1506.

389. Gonzalez A, Sosenko IR, Chandar J, Hummler H, Claure N, Bancalari E. Influence of infection on patent ductus arteriosus and chronic lung disease in premature infants weighing 1000 grams or less. *J Pediatr.* 1996;128(4):470–478.

390. Hammerman C, Glaser J, Kaplan M, Schimmel MS, Ferber B, Eidelman AI. Indomethacin tocolysis increases postnatal patent ductus arteriosus severity. *Pediatrics.* 1998;102(5):E56.

391. Kim ES, Kim EK, Choi CW, et al. Intrauterine inflammation as a risk factor for persistent ductus arteriosus patency after cyclooxygenase inhibition in extremely low birth weight infants. *J Pediatr.* 2010;157(5):745–750. e741.

392. Norton ME, Merrill J, Cooper BA, Kuller JA, Clyman RI. Neonatal complications after the administration of indomethacin for preterm labor. *N Engl J Med.* 1993;329(22):1602–1607.

393. Rojas MA, Gonzalez A, Bancalari E, Claure N, Poole C, Silva-Neto G. Changing trends in the epidemiology and pathogenesis of neonatal chronic lung disease. *J Pediatr.* 1995;126(4):605–610.

394. Keller RL, Clyman RI. Persistent Doppler flow predicts lack of response to multiple courses of indomethacin in premature infants with recurrent patent ductus arteriosus. *Pediatrics.* 2003;112(3 Pt 1):583–587.

395. Koehne PS, Bein G, Alexi-Meskhishvili V, Weng Y, Buhrer C, Obladen M. Patent ductus arteriosus in very low birthweight infants: complications of pharmacological and surgical treatment. *J Perinat Med.* 2001;29(4):327–334.

396. Mandhan P, Brown S, Kukkady A, Samarakkody U. Surgical closure of patent ductus arteriosus in preterm low birth weight infants. *Congenit Heart Dis.* 2009;4(1):34–37.

397. Harting MT, Blakely ML, Cox CS Jr, Lantin-Hermoso R, Andrassy RJ, Lally KP. Acute hemodynamic decompensation following patent ductus arteriosus ligation in premature infants. *J Invest Surg.* 2008;21(3):133–138.

398. McNamara PJ, Stewart L, Shivananda SP, Stephens D, Sehgal A. Patent ductus arteriosus ligation is associated with impaired left ventricular systolic performance in premature infants weighing less than 1000 g. *J Thorac Cardiovasc Surg.* 2010;140(1):150–157.

399. Moin F, Kennedy KA, Moya FR. Risk factors predicting vasopressor use after patent ductus arteriosus ligation. *Am J Perinatol.* 2003;20(6):313–320.

400. Noori S, Friedlich P, Seri I, Wong P. Changes in myocardial function and hemodynamics after ligation of the ductus arteriosus in preterm infants. *J Pediatr.* 2007;150(6):597–602.

401. Teixeira LS, Shivananda SP, Stephens D, Van Arsdell G, McNamara PJ. Postoperative cardiorespiratory instability following ligation of the preterm ductus arteriosus is related to early need for intervention. *J Perinatol.* 2008;28(12):803–810.

402. Jain A, Sahni M, El-Khuffash A, Khadawardi E, Sehgal A, McNamara PJ. Use of targeted neonatal echocardiography to prevent postoperative cardiorespiratory instability after patent ductus arteriosus ligation. *J Pediatr.* 2012;160(4):584–589.e1.

403. Benjamin JR, Smith PB, Cotten CM, Jaggers J, Goldstein RF, Malcolm WF. Long-term morbidities associated with vocal cord paralysis after surgical closure of a patent ductus arteriosus in extremely low birth weight infants. *J Perinatol.* 2010;30(6):408–413.

404. Clement WA, El-Hakim H, Phillipos EZ, Cote JJ. Unilateral vocal cord paralysis following patent ductus arteriosus ligation in extremely low-birth-weight infants. *Arch Otolaryngol Head Neck Surg.* 2008;134(1):28–33.

405. Roksund OD, Clemm H, Heimdal JH, et al. Left vocal cord paralysis after extreme preterm birth, a new clinical scenario in adults. *Pediatrics.* 2010;126(6):e1569–e1577.

406. Spanos WC, Brookes JT, Smith MC, Burkhart HM, Bell EF, Smith RJ. Unilateral vocal fold paralysis in premature infants after ligation of patent ductus arteriosus: vascular clip versus suture ligature. *Ann Otol Rhinol Laryngol.* 2009;118(10):750–753.

407. Roclawski M, Sabiniewicz R, Potaz P, et al. Scoliosis in patients with aortic coarctation and patent ductus arteriosus: does standard posterolateral thoracotomy play a role in the development of the lateral curve of the spine? *Pediatr Cardiol.* 2009;30(7):941–945.

408. Seghaye MC, Grabitz R, Alzen G, et al. Thoracic sequelae after surgical closure of the patent ductus arteriosus in premature infants. *Acta Paediatr.* 1997;86(2):213–216.

409. Shelton JE, Julian R, Walburgh E, Schneider E. Functional scoliosis as a long-term complication of surgical ligation for patent ductus arteriosus in premature infants. *J Pediatr Surg.* 1986;21(10):855–857.

410. Chorne N, Leonard C, Piecuch R, Clyman RI. Patent ductus arteriosus and its treatment as risk factors for neonatal and neurodevelopmental morbidity. *Pediatrics.* 2007;119(6):1165–1174.

411. Kabra NS, Schmidt B, Roberts RS, Doyle LW, Papile L, Fanaroff A. Neurosensory impairment after surgical closure of patent ductus arteriosus in extremely low birth weight infants: results from the Trial of Indomethacin Prophylaxis in Preterms. *J Pediatr.* 2007;150(3):229–234. 234.e221.

412. Madan JC, Kendrick D, Hagadorn JI, Frantz ID 3rd. Patent ductus arteriosus therapy: impact on neonatal and 18-month outcome. *Pediatrics.* 2009;123(2):674–681.

413. Chang LY, McCurnin D, Yoder B, Shaul PW, Clyman RI. Ductus arteriosus ligation and alveolar growth in preterm baboons with a patent ductus arteriosus. *Pediatr Res.* 2008;63(3):299–302.

414. Waleh N, McCurnin DC, Yoder BA, Shaul PW, Clyman RI. Patent ductus arteriosus ligation alters pulmonary gene expression in preterm baboons. *Pediatr Res.* 2011;69(2):212–216.

415. Kobaly K, Schluchter M, Minich N, et al. Outcomes of extremely low birth weight (<1 kg) and extremely low gestational age (<28 weeks) infants with bronchopulmonary dysplasia: effects of practice changes in 2000 to 2003. *Pediatrics.* 2008;121(1):73–81.

416. Lee GY, Sohn YB, Kim MJ, et al. Outcome following surgical closure of patent ductus arteriosus in very low birth weight infants in neonatal intensive care unit. *Yonsei Med J.* 2008;49(2):265–271.

417. Tran U, Gray PH, O'Callaghan MJ. Neonatal antecedents for cerebral palsy in extremely preterm babies and interaction with maternal factors. *Early Hum Dev.* 2005;81(6):555–561.

418. Merritt TA, White CL, Coen RW, Friedman WF, Gluck L, Rosenberg M. Preschool assessment of infants with a patent ductus arteriosus: comparison of ligation and indomethacin therapy. *Am J Dis Child.* 1982;136(6):507–512.

419. Momma K, Toyoshima K, Takeuchi D, Imamura S, Nakanishi T. In vivo constriction of the fetal and neonatal ductus arteriosus by a prostanoid EP4-receptor antagonist in rats. *Pediatr Res.* 2005;58(5):971–975.

420. Carmo KB, Evans N, Paradisis M. Duration of indomethacin treatment of the preterm patent ductus arteriosus as directed by echocardiography. *J Pediatr.* 2009;155(6):819–822.e811.

421. Desandes R, Jellimann JM, Rouabah M, et al. Echocardiography as a guide for patent ductus arteriosus ibuprofen treatment and efficacy prediction. *Pediatr Crit Care Med.* 2012;13(3):324–327.

422. Su BH, Peng CT, Tsai CH. Echocardiographic flow pattern of patent ductus arteriosus: a guide to indomethacin treatment in premature infants. *Arch Dis Child Fetal Neonatal Ed.* 1999;81(3):F197–F200.

423. Chen YW, Zhao W, Zhang ZF, et al. Familial nonsyndromic patent ductus arteriosus caused by mutations in TFAP2B. *Pediatr Cardiol.* 2011;32(7):958–965.

424. Waleh N, Hodnick R, Jhaveri N, et al. Patterns of gene expression in the ductus arteriosus are related to environmental and genetic risk factors for persistent ductus patency. *Pediatr Res.* 2010;68(4):292–297.

425. Itabashi K, Ohno T, Nishida H. Indomethacin responsiveness of patent ductus arteriosus and renal abnormalities in preterm infants treated with indomethacin. *J Pediatr.* 2003;143(2):203–207.

426. van de Bor M, Verloove-Vanhorick SP, Brand R, Ruys JH. Patent ductus arteriosus in a cohort of 1338 preterm infants: a collaborative study. *Paediatr Perinat Epidemiol.* 1988;2(4):328–336.

427. Robel-Tillig E, Knupfer M, Vogtmann C. Cardiac adaptation in small for gestational age neonates after prenatal hemodynamic disturbances. *Early Hum Dev.* 2003;72(2):123–129.

428. Cunningham MD, Ellison RC, Zierler S, Kanto WP Jr, Miettinen OS, Nadas AS. Perinatal risk assessment for patent ductus arteriosus in premature infants. *Obstet Gynecol.* 1986;68(1):41–45.

429. del moral T, Gonzalez-Quintero VH, Claure N, Vanbuskirk S, Bancalari E. Antenatal exposure to magnesium sulfate and the incidence of patent ductus arteriosus in extremely low birth weight infants. *J Perinatol.* 2007;27(3):154–157.

430. Stigson L, Kjellmer I. Serum levels of magnesium at birth related to complications of immaturity. *Acta Paediatr.* 1997;86(9):991–994.

431. Kreft-Jais C, Plouin PF, Tchobroutsky C, Boutroy MJ. Angiotensin-converting enzyme inhibitors during pregnancy: a survey of 22 patients given captopril and nine given enalapril. *Br J Obstet Gynaecol.* 1988;95(4):420–422.

432. Shotan A, Widerhorn J, Hurst A, Elkayam U. Risks of angiotensin-converting enzyme inhibition during pregnancy: experimental and clinical evidence, potential mechanisms, and recommendations for use. *Am J Med.* 1994;96(5):451–456.

433. Thomas SV, Ajayku B, Sindhu K, et al. Cardiac malformations are increased in infants of mothers with epilepsy. *Pediatr Cardiol.* 2008;29(3):604–608.

434. McGuirl J, Arzuaga B, Lee B. Increased risk for patent ductus arteriosus with antenatal calcium channel blocker exposure in extremely low birth weight infants. *Annual Meeting of the Pediatric Academic Societies, 2009.* 2009;E-PAS2009: 461 (abstr).

435. Dusick AM, Covert RF, Schreiber MD, et al. Risk of intracranial hemorrhage and other adverse outcomes after cocaine exposure in a cohort of 323 very low birth weight infants. *J Pediatr.* 1993;122(3):438–445.

436. Levy HL, Guldberg P, Guttler F, et al. Congenital heart disease in maternal phenylketonuria: report from the Maternal PKU Collaborative Study. *Pediatr Res.* 2001;49(5):636–642.

437. Rouse B, Matalon R, Koch R, et al. Maternal phenylketonuria syndrome: congenital heart defects, microcephaly, and developmental outcomes. *J Pediatr.* 2000;136(1):57–61.

438. Treszl A, Szabo M, Dunai G, et al. Angiotensin II type 1 receptor A1166C polymorphism and prophylactic indomethacin treatment induced ductus arteriosus closure in very low birth weight neonates. *Pediatr Res.* 2003;54(5):753–755.

439. Friedman Z, Demers LM, Marks KH, Uhrmann S, Maisels MJ. Urinary excretion of prostaglandin E following the administration of furosemide and indomethacin to sick low-birth-weight infants. *J Pediatr.* 1978;93(3):512–515.

440. Cambonie G, Guillaumont S, Luc F, Vergnes C, Milesi C, Voisin M. Haemodynamic features during high-frequency oscillatory ventilation in preterms. *Acta Paediatr.* 2003;92(9):1068–1073.

441. Botto LD, Correa A, Erickson JD. Racial and temporal variations in the prevalence of heart defects. *Pediatrics.* 2001;107(3):E32.

442. Hammoud MS, Elsori HA, Hanafi EA, Shalabi AA, Fouda IA, Devara LV. Incidence and risk factors associated with the patency of ductus arteriosus in preterm infants with respiratory distress syndrome in Kuwait. *Saudi Med J.* 2003;24(9):982–985.

443. Rothman KJ, Fyler DC. Sex, birth order, and maternal age characteristics of infants with congenital heart defects. *Am J Epidemiol.* 1976;104(5):527–534.

444. Samanek M, Voriskova M. Congenital heart disease among 815,569 children born between 1980 and 1990 and their 15-year survival: a prospective Bohemia survival study. *Pediatr Cardiol.* 1999;20(6):411–417.

445. Forsey JT, Elmasry OA, Martin RP. Patent arterial duct. *Orphanet J Rare Dis.* 2009;4:17.

446. Seppanen MP, Ojanpera OS, Kaapa PO, Kero PO. Delayed postnatal adaptation of pulmonary hemodynamics in infants of diabetic mothers. *J Pediatr.* 1997;131(4):545–548.

447. Alzamora-Castro V, Battilana G, Abugattas R, Sialer S. Patent ductus arteriosus and high altitude. *Am J Cardiol.* 1960;5:761–763.

448. Miao CY, Zuberbuhler JS, Zuberbuhler JR. Prevalence of congenital cardiac anomalies at high altitude. *J Am Coll Cardiol.* 1988;12(1):224–228.

449. Doyle PE, Beral V, Botting B, Wale CJ. Congenital malformations in twins in England and Wales. *J Epidemiol Community Health.* 1991;45(1):43–48.

450. Layde PM, Erickson JD, Falek A, McCarthy BJ. Congenital malformation in twins. *Am J Hum Genet.* 1980;32(1):69–78.

451. Gibson S, Lewis KC. Congenital heart disease following maternal rubella during pregnancy. *AMA Am J Dis Child.* 1952;83(3):317–319.

452. Nakagawa T. Delayed closure of ductus arteriosus in premature infants with transient hypothyroidism. *Lancet.* 1993;341(8848):839.

453. Williams FL, Ogston SA, van Toor H, Visser TJ, Hume R. Serum thyroid hormones in preterm infants: associations with postnatal illnesses and drug usage. *J Clin Endocrinol Metab.* 2005;90(11):5954–5963.

454. Barefield ES, Dwyer MD, Cassady G. Association of patent ductus arteriosus and phototherapy in infants weighing less than 1000 grams. *J Perinatol.* 1993;13(5):376–380.

Part C: Lungs

Respiratory Distress Syndrome

Alan Jobe

EPIDEMIOLOGY

The disease that has defined the history of neonatology is what we now call respiratory distress syndrome (RDS). The enigmatic hyaline membrane disease was uniformly fatal for preterm infants before neonatal care was available.[1] The atelectasis, epithelial injury, and accumulation of eosinophilic proteinaceous material in the airspaces were attributed primarily to aspiration or infection. The recognition that the early respiratory failure of some preterm infants could be treated with oxygen in the 1950s contributed to the development of early newborn care centers that have morphed into modern neonatal intensive care units. However, excessive oxygen use resulted in an epidemic of retrolental fibroplasia (now called retinopathy of prematurity).[2]

The seminal 1959 observation of Avery and Mead[3] that the lungs of preterm infants who died of hyaline membrane disease had decreased amounts of surfactant finally identified the primary abnormality that caused the respiratory failure. However, little progress in treatment other than oxygen occurred until the invention of continuous positive airway pressure (CPAP) by Gregory et al[4] in 1971 and the concurrent development of mechanical ventilators with positive end-expiratory pressure (PEEP) for infants. Maternal treatment with corticosteroids was described by Liggins and Howie[5] in 1972 and to date is the only therapy to prevent RDS. In 1971, Gluck et al[6] reported that the L/S (lecithin/sphingomyelin) ratio, a test to measure surfactant components in amniotic fluid, could predict infants at risk of RDS prior to birth. These advances, together with improvements in the general care for preterm infants (better temperature control, fluid therapy, nutrition, physiological monitoring) resulted in high survival rates for the larger and more mature preterm infants, but with the appearance of a new lung disease— bronchopulmonary dysplasia (BPD), caused primarily by oxygen and mechanical ventilation.[7] With increased survival, the name of the disease changed from the signature pathologic finding—the hyaline membrane to the physiologic descriptor—respiratory distress.

Experimental studies with premature animals demonstrated that surfactant given via the trachea could improve lung function,[8,9] and the first report of successful surfactant treatment of RDS was published in 1980 by Fujiwara et al.[10] Surfactants were licensed for general clinical use in 1999–2000 by the Food and Drug Administration (FDA). Subsequent technological improvements in infant ventilators, in the general care of very preterm infants, and in physician skills for the treatment of RDS have resulted in remarkable survival rates with minimal complications for infants with RDS who are greater than 28 weeks' gestational age at birth.[11] Thus, the epidemiology of RDS has changed as the recognition and treatment of the disease has evolved.

In the current era, about 500,000 preterm infants are born in the United States each year, representing about 13% of all live births. Most of these infants are late-preterm infants born between 35 and 37 weeks' gestational age who have an increased incidence of transient tachypnea of the newborn (TTN) but about a 1% low risk of RDS.[12] More immature infants with birth gestations of 32 to 35 weeks have about a 10% RDS incidence.[11] The frequency of RDS increases

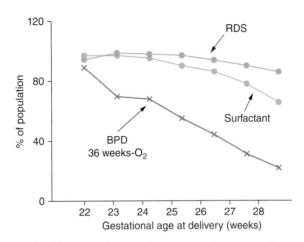

FIGURE 23-1 Respiratory distress syndrome (RDS), surfactant treatments, and bronchopulmonary dysplasia (BPD) relative to gestational age. Data for 9575 infants born at 22–28 weeks' gestational age from 2003 to 2007 reported by the National Institute of Child Health and Human Development (NICHD) Neonatal Research Network. (Data from Reference 14.)

strikingly below gestational ages of 32 weeks to about 50% at 30 weeks' gestation,[13] and the diagnosis of RDS approaches 100% for infants born at less than 28 weeks' gestation[14] (Figure 23-1). The occurrence of RDS is decreased with obstetric interventions to maintain preterm pregnancies at risk of delivery and with antenatal treatments with corticosteroids. As developed in the discussion of differential diagnoses, the epidemiology of RDS does not accurately reflect the true incidence of the disease.

PATHOPHYSIOLOGY

Surfactant

Respiratory distress syndrome is a disease caused by lung immaturity. The developmental/biochemical problem is surfactant deficiency. The clinical result is respiratory distress caused by inadequate gas exchange from atelectasis, nonuniform aeration of distal lung units that progresses to epithelial injury, proteinaceous pulmonary edema, and ultimately respiratory failure. The central factor is the complex function and metabolism of surfactant in the preterm lung.

Surfactant is a mixture of phospholipids and specific surfactant proteins (SPs) that are produced by type II cells in the alveoli epithelium of air-breathing mammals (Figure 23-2). Surfactant is synthesized in type II cells, packaged into intracellular organelles called lamellar bodies for storage and secretion to the gas exchange surface.[15] The composition of surfactant is about 50% phosphatidylcholine with 2 saturated fatty acids, generally palmitic acid, esterified to the glycerol backbone of the molecule.

This "saturated" phosphatidylcholine is extremely surface active as its hydrophilic choline head group solubilizes into water, while the palmitic acids repel water. Surfactant will form a surface film that decreases the equilibrium surface tension of water from about 72 nM/m^2 to about 20 nM/m^2. With compression of saturated phosphatidylcholine at an air-liquid interface, surface tensions fall to very low values. However, saturated phosphatidylcholine is a solid at 37°C and requires other components to allow it to spread.

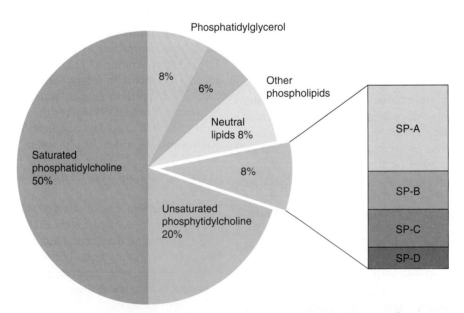

FIGURE 23-2 Composition of surfactant. The major class of surface-active lipids in surfactant are saturated phosphatidylcholines. Surfactant also contains the innate host defense surfactant proteins (SPs) SP-A and SP-D and the lipoproteins SP-B and SP-C.

Major contributors to the in vivo behavior of surfactant are phosphatidylglycerol, unsaturated phosphatidylcholines, and in surfactant from immature mammals, phosphatidylinositol. These lipids and other minor lipid components interact with 2 small lipophilic SPs, SP-B and SP-C, which are highly conserved across mammalian species.[15] The mature form of SP-B is an 8-kDa protein that is required for the intracellular packaging and secretion of the surfactant lipids. The SP-B intercalates in the lipids, facilitating surface adsorption. SP-C is a 4-kDa lipophilic protein that also intercalates with the surfactant lipids to enhance function. A genetic deficiency of SP-C does not cause acute respiratory failure at birth because surfactant lipids with SP-B have good function, although abnormal SP-C can result in interstitial lung disease in later life.[16] In contrast, a rare form of lethal RDS primarily in term infants is a genetic deficiency of SP-B because an absence of SP-B disrupts lamellar body formation and the secretion of other surfactant components. The other surfactant-associated proteins, SP-A and SP-D, are collectin family proteins that primarily function as innate host defense proteins. SP-D also regulates surfactant pool sizes, and SP-A makes surfactant more resistant to inactivation by inhibitors (see below).

Early Lung Maturation

Infants have RDS because the synthetic machinery for surfactant is immature, resulting in surfactant deficiency. The lungs of infants are predictably mature when the L/S ratio in amniotic fluid is greater than 2 or when phosphatidylglycerol is detected, which is at about 34–36 weeks for normal pregnancies[17] (Figure 23-3). Although measurements of the L/S ratio are primarily of historical interest because easier-to-perform (although less-accurate) tests are in current use, the L/S ratios for normal pregnancies at different gestational ages contrast sharply with the frequency of RDS in clinical practice at these gestational ages. The differences between the timing of normal lung maturation and clinical experience result from the early maturational potential of the fetal lung. As a general perspective, all preterm deliveries should be considered to be abnormal because of the stresses associated with prematurity. There are 2 main pathways to prematurity: (1) vascular developmental abnormalities associated with maternal/fetal diagnoses such as pregnancy-associated hypertension (preeclampsia) and intrauterine growth restriction and (2) intrauterine infection, which can be chronic and clinically silent prior to preterm labor.[18] These 2 pathways contribute to most of the very preterm deliveries and contribute to lung maturation earlier in gestation than would occur normally.

There are 2 clinically relevant factors that cause early maturation of the fetal lung: corticosteroids and intrauterine exposure to inflammation. Maternal corticosteroid treatments decrease the incidence of RDS for infants born at 28–34 weeks' gestation by about 50% and are standard of care for women at risk of preterm delivery.[19] This simple and inexpensive treatment not only matures the fetal lungs but also has pleotropic and beneficial effects to increase blood pressure, improve postdelivery bilirubin metabolism, decrease intraventricular hemorrhage, and decrease death.

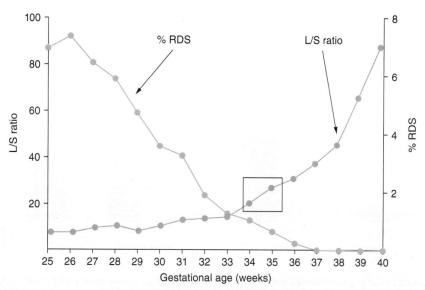

FIGURE 23-3 Incidence of respiratory distress syndrome (RDS) in preterm infants relative to L/S (lecithin/sphingomyelin) ratios for normal pregnancies not delivering preterm. The L/S ratio for normal pregnancies does not indicate maturity with a value greater than 2 until about 35 weeks' gestational age, as indicated by the box. In contrast, RDS occurs frequently in more preterm infants. (Data from References 6 and 13.)

The effects on preterm fetal lungs include increased surfactant lipid and surfactant-specific protein synthesis and changes in lung structure to decrease interstitial tissue and increase the potential gas volume.[20] Other effects include more rapid clearance of fetal lung fluid after birth and decreased epithelial permeability to protein with ventilation.

The second clinical association with less RDS is fetal exposure to histologic chorioamnionitis. In animal models, fetal exposure to intra-amniotic lipopolysaccharide (a toll-like receptor 4 agonist) or live *Ureaplasma parvum* (the organism most associated with preterm delivery) results in more induced lung maturation than does maternal corticosteroid treatment (Figure 23-4).[21] Curiously, the proinflammation and anti-inflammatory maternal corticosteroids have similar net effects on the fetal lung in that both increase surfactant lipids and proteins and change lung structure to improve gas exchange. In clinical practice, more than 50% of infants born at less than 28 weeks' gestation have been exposed to histologic chorioamnionitis, and 80% of these pregnancies will be treated with antenatal corticosteroids.[22] In both animal models and clinical practice, the 2 exposures decrease RDS and improve outcomes.[23] In animal models, the combined fetal exposures to corticosteroids and chorioamnionitis have additive or synergistic effects to increase lung maturation, which should translate clinically to less RDS.[24,25] Clinically maternal corticosteroid treatments also decrease RDS in pregnancies with histologic chorioamnionitis.[23] Given the available information, the explanations for the frequent birth of infants prior to 34–36 weeks who do not have RDS are fetal stresses that increase fetal cortisol levels, maternal corticosteroid treatments, or fetal exposures to inflammation that mature the fetal lungs.

Surfactant Pool Sizes and Metabolism

As the fetus matures, the distal epithelium of the lung differentiates into immature type II cells and type I cells beginning at about 20 weeks' gestational age.[26] The lamellar body storage granules for surfactant begin to appear after about 22–24 weeks, and an immature surfactant begins to be stored and secreted. This immature surfactant contains less saturated phosphatidylcholine to total phosphatidylcholine, low amounts of the SPs and phosphatidylinositol, and no phosphatidylglycerol. With advancing gestation, more surfactant is stored and secreted and that surfactant is more "mature"—more saturated phosphatidylcholine, more of all of the SPs, and less phosphatidylinositol, and phosphatidylglycerol appears. Surfactant that is secreted is carried into the oral pharynx by the continuously produced fetal lung fluid and fetal breathing. Some of this fluid is swallowed, and some mixes with amniotic fluid, where the increasing amounts of surfactant components can be sampled by amniocentesis for lung maturational testing.

The fetal lung at term contains large amounts of stored surfactant that is secreted just prior to and at delivery in response to redundant stimuli from lung stretch, increases in catecholamines, and purinoreceptor agonists to increase the concentration of surfactant in the fetal lung fluid. This high surfactant concentration facilitates the lowering of surface tensions on menisci of fluid in the airways and facilitates the recruitment of an initial functional residual capacity. The amount of surfactant in the airspaces of term mammals after birth is about 100 mg/kg body weight. In contrast, the adult human lung has about 5 mg/kg surfactant in the airspaces.[27] The large amounts in the airspaces at term are presumably a

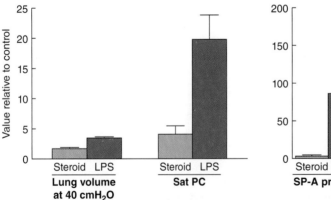
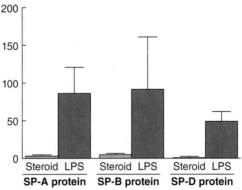

FIGURE 23-4 Increases in lung gas volumes measured at 40 cm H_2O pressure and surfactant components measured 7 days after fetal exposure to intra-amniotic lipopolysaccharide (LPS) or betamethasone (steroid) in preterm sheep. The LPS exposure increased lung gas volumes and the surfactant components in surfactant recovered by bronchoalveolar lavage more than did the steroid exposure. All values are expressed relative to a control value of 1. PC, phosphatidylcholine; SP, surfactant protein. (Data from references 20 and 21.)

developmental adaptation to ensure the successful transition to air breathing.

Preterm infants destined to develop RDS have greatly decreased stores of surfactant. At birth, the available stores are secreted, and the initial severity of respiratory failure is determined by the pool size of surfactant. Some very preterm infants have almost no surfactant and cannot achieve initial aeration of the lungs without positive pressure recruitment and ventilation. Other, often more mature, infants have a "honeymoon period" during which initial respiratory distress and oxygen needs are minimal, but the RDS progresses over hours. The pool sizes of surfactant estimated by lavages of lungs of infants who died of RDS prior to the era of mechanical ventilation ranged from 0 to 10 mg/kg.[28] Preterm lambs or rabbits have minimal RDS if surfactant pool sizes are greater than about 4 mg/kg.[29] Measurements in ventilated preterm infants with RDS using stable isotopes supported these values for the amount of surfactant associated with RDS.[30]

Infants with RDS had progressive respiratory failure in the hours after birth that peaked at about 2–3 days in the presurfactant treatment era. The metabolic behavior of surfactant contributes to this progressive respiratory failure. Over weeks, the fetal lung has accumulated the surfactant pool to be secreted at birth. Once that surfactant is secreted, the accumulation of more surfactant is a slow process that includes new synthesis and recycling of surfactant components from the airspaces back through type II cells for reprocessing and secretion. Measurements of bulk surfactant metabolism in both large animal models and preterm infants with RDS demonstrated that surfactant pool sizes in airspaces take days to increase substantially.

Labeled precursors of saturated phosphatidylcholine appear in the airway surfactant slowly, with a time to maximal labeling (maximal accumulation of newly synthesized surfactant) of about 3 days.[31] Once surfactant is in the airspaces, the half-life for clearance is also about 3 days.[32] Simultaneously, surfactant components are being recycled efficiently in the preterm lung. The overview is that surfactant components are being slowly, but dynamically, synthesized and recycled because surfactant function depends on newly synthesized surfactant as surfactant is "used" with breathing. Variables known to change surfactant metabolism are lung injury and antenatal corticosteroids, but type of mechanical ventilation (conventional relative to high-frequency oscillation) is a less-important variable.[33]

Surfactant Inhibition

Another factor contributing to the progression of the symptoms of RDS over several days is the function of the surfactant. The preterm lung at birth that has only surfactant deficiency is immature, but not injured.

Fetal lung fluid has very low protein levels, but this fluid must be cleared via ion pumps that are immature. Thus, the surfactant-deficient preterm lung with low surfactant pools has high surface tensions in the small airways. The movement of air-fluid interfaces across epithelial surfaces can disrupt those epithelial barriers, causing the bronchiolar epithelial lesions noted with ventilation of the surfactant-deficient and fluid-filled lung.[34] Epithelial disruptions and cell injury increase the permeability of the epithelial barrier to interstitial and intravascular components, resulting in protein-aceous fluid accumulation in the airspace.[9] Surfactant function—its ability to adsorb to an air-fluid interface, to spread, and to decrease surface tension—is strikingly inhibited by the proteins in interstitial and intravascular fluid, by inflammatory products, and by fibrin degradation products.[26] Surfactant lipids can function as a thromboplastin to promote clotting in the airspaces, which forms the hyaline membranes that then can trap the surfactant and deplete the functional pool.

The potent effects of inhibition of surfactant can be demonstrated with tracheal aspirates from infants with RDS requiring intubation for respiratory failure (Figure 23-5).[35] The material recovered by tracheal aspirate had high surface tension, but good surfactant was recovered by centrifugation, demonstrating that surfactant function was inhibited. In a surfactant treatment model using a very preterm lung injured with mechanical ventilation, surfactant treatment quickly increased oxygenation and decreased surface tension.[36] However, the effect on oxygenation was lost as surface tensions increased because of inhibition.

The net sequence is that spontaneous or assisted ventilation of the surfactant-deficient lung will injure the epithelium and cause stretch injury. The combination of soluble proteins and inflammatory products in airspaces can inhibit surfactant function. The inhibitory activities are more potent when surfactant concentrations are low and when surfactant contains less of the SPs, particularly SP-A and SP-D.[37]

The explanation for the honeymoon period for some infants with RDS is that the initial release of surfactant at birth is sufficient for the initial recruitment of functional residual capacity (FRC) and for breathing. Because of the slow replacement of surfactant, inactivation of surfactant by progressive injury/edema formation degrades the function of the small surfactant pool. New synthesis and recycling are inadequate to replace functional surfactant, resulting in progressive respiratory failure. In model systems, clinically relevant variables can decrease the inhibition of surfactant. Ventilation strategies such as the use of PEEP or CPAP to recruit and sustain FRC can decrease injury and preserve surfactant function.[29] Antenatal corticosteroid treatments can mature the airspace epithelium such that the lung is less easily injured and thus less proteinaceous pulmonary

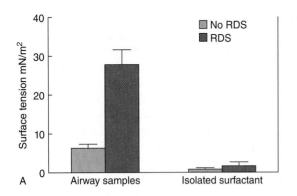

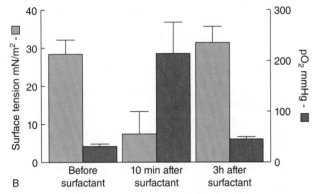

FIGURE 23-5 Surface tensions and oxygenation. A, Airway samples from infants with respiratory distress syndrome (RDS) at the time of intubation had high minimum surface tensions relative to samples from infants without RDS. The airway samples from the infants with RDS contained good surfactant that could be isolated by centrifugation to remove soluble proteins. (Data redrawn from Reference 35.) **B,** Surface tensions in airway samples and arterial pO_2 values for ventilated preterm lambs before surfactant treatment, 10 minutes after surfactant treatment, and 3 hours after surfactant treatment. The low pO_2 values and high surface tensions at 3 hours resulted from inhibition of surfactant function. (Data from Reference 36.)

edema develops.[38] Antenatal corticosteroids and more advanced gestational age mature the surfactant by increasing the relative amounts of saturated phosphatidylcholine and SPs, which decrease the sensitivity of the surfactant to inhibition.[39] Finally, a surfactant treatment before much injury has occurred has 2 benefits: The surfactant pool is greatly increased, making surfactant inactivation less of a problem, and the extra surfactant will decrease further injury.

DIFFERENTIAL DIAGNOSES/ DIAGNOSTIC TESTS

The diagnosis of RDS is not straightforward because there are no laboratory tests or radiologic findings that uniquely demonstrate surfactant deficiency. An immature L/S ratio or other test of amniotic fluid can identify fetuses at risk for RDS.[17] With an increasing interval from amniotic fluid sampling to delivery and with maternal exposure to antenatal corticosteroids, the probability of RDS decreases. The more premature the infant is, the more likely is the diagnosis of RDS. However, there are no measures of surfactant adequacy after birth other than lung performance, which can be abnormal for multiple reasons other than RDS. Assessments of surfactant using tracheal aspirates from intubated infants or gastric aspirates collected at birth can help identify infants with surfactant deficiency, but these tests are not generally used in clinical practice.

The traditional diagnosis used clinically for RDS was respiratory distress in a preterm infant requiring supplemental oxygen at or soon after delivery that persists and is accompanied by a compatible chest roentgenogram showing low-to-normal lung expansion with diffuse, usually uniformly, hazy lung fields with air bronchograms. Those diagnostic criteria are inherently subjective and can be altered by treatment interventions. For example, early surfactant treatment can clear the hazy and granular chest roentgenogram and prevent disease progression. Early introduction of mechanical ventilation with PEEP also can decrease oxygen need and clear the chest film. Fetal pneumonias caused by organisms such as group B streptococcal sepsis/pneumonia can perfectly mimic the roentgenographic findings in RDS.

As described further here, surfactant treatment responses that cause rapid and large improvements in oxygenation and lung function may be the clinical indicators that best test the surfactant deficiency state of the infant. Infants born with surfactant deficiency and treated with surfactant soon after birth may develop no respiratory distress and thus will not have a diagnosis of RDS. Similarly, the practice of initiating CPAP in the delivery room to stabilize the lung of the preterm is a care strategy that can mask the features of mild RDS.[40] Many very preterm infants do not have RDS based on the need for surfactant therapy if treated with CPAP[41-43] (Table 23-1). Infants generally will be given the diagnosis of RDS if they were intubated and ventilated from birth.

For epidemiologic purposes, the National Institute of Child Health and Human Development (NICHD) Neonatal Research Network diagnosis of RDS is presentation in an infant of grunting, flaring, retractions, paradoxical breathing (the respiratory distress), and cyanosis or the need for oxygen within the first 24 hours of life. There is no radiologic component to the diagnosis, and most infants with transient tachypnea or pneumonia would fit this diagnosis. The diagnostic criteria used by the Vermont Oxford Network are a PaO_2 less than 50 mm Hg in room air,

Table 23-1 Incidence of Respiratory Distress Syndrome Based on Need for Surfactant Treatments[a]

Study	Infants	Treated with Surfactant (%)
Danish Experience	27 ± 2 weeks	30
Vermont Oxford, 2008	<1250 g	64
COIN Trial	950 g average	38 (CPAP arm)
NICHD, Support Trial	24–27 weeks	67 (CPAP arm)

Abbreviations: CPAP, continuous positive airway pressure; NICHD, National Institute of Child Health and Human Development.
[a]Data from References 41–43.

a requirement for supplemental oxygen to maintain a PaO_2 above 50 mm Hg or supplemental oxygen to keep the oxygen saturation greater than 85% as measured by pulse oximetry, and a chest radiograph consistent with RDS within the first 24 hours of age. This definition of RDS is more specific but does not specifically identify surfactant deficiency. In practice, the diagnosis of a preterm infant on CPAP, on room air with a relatively clear chest radiograph is unclear—the infant is on ventilatory support with CPAP and is perhaps tachypneic. The diagnosis of RDS is not supported by an oxygen requirement or the radiographic findings. However, if the infant is taken off CPAP, the infant is likely to have more radiographic findings and an oxygen requirement and achieve the criteria for a diagnosis of RDS. For coding and reimbursement purposes, most infants with birth weights less than 1 kg will have a diagnosis of RDS, although they may not have strict criteria for a diagnosis of RDS.

The diagnosis of RDS in more mature infants also is not straightforward. Infants with gestational ages greater than about 32 weeks who deliver after spontaneous labor seldom have much respiratory distress and will only occasionally have RDS. However, with increased early inductions of labor and cesarean sections to manage pregnancies complicated by preeclampsia or multiple births, for example, these more mature infants often have problems with respiratory adaptation.[44] Other infants delivered by elective cesarean section without labor at term will also have an increased incidence of respiratory adaptation difficulties, especially if the delivery was prior to 39 weeks' gestation. Although the incidence is low, the cesarean section rate in the United States is about 30%, such that many infants are at risk. Some of these infants will have TTN, a disease thought to result from delayed clearance of fetal lung fluid, and a few will have moderate-to-severe RDS. In fact, mild RDS and TTN are probably a continuum of lung immaturity with the

surfactant deficiency being more prominent in RDS and with delayed fluid clearance identified for infants with TTN, although infants with TTN also may have low amounts of surfactant, as indicated by low lamellar body counts.[45]

A question without a clear answer is if antenatal corticosteroids should be given to those with pregnancies delivering after 32–34 weeks' gestation or for women scheduled for elective surgical deliveries. Two trials have provided conflicting results,[12,46] and other trials are ongoing.

MANAGEMENT OF RDS

Lung Injury

From a historical perspective, the management of RDS before the availability of surfactant was with oxygen to treat the hypoxia. If oxygen therapy alone was insufficient, the infant was supported with CPAP or intubated and ventilated with a mechanical ventilator. The sequence of interventions was guided by the severity of the RDS, the respiratory drive of the infant, and other problems of prematurity the infant might have.[1] After the availability of surfactant, the therapies have evolved to try to minimize lung injury and prevent BPD, the major adverse lung outcome of RDS. Surfactant therapy is a specific treatment to reverse much of the pathophysiology of RDS.

The physiologic basis for the difficulties with ventilation of the preterm lung result from the small lung volumes for a preterm infant with RDS relative to an adult lung (Figure 23-6). The adult lung inflates from collapse at lower pressures to a maximal lung volume V_T of about 90 mL/kg; the preterm lung with RDS requires higher pressures to achieve a lower V_T of perhaps 30 mL/kg. The preterm lung will optimally function with an FRC of perhaps 20 mL/kg, and the adult lung has a higher optimal FRC of about 30 mL/kg. However, the FRC to V_T fraction is 0.33 for the adult; that fraction for the preterm infant is 0.66.

Lung injury from mechanical ventilation occurs when the FRC is low or when tidal volumes plus FRC approach V_T.[47] Thus, strategies to ventilate preterm lungs, especially lungs with RDS, are constrained by the low lung volumes of the preterm. Ventilation of infants without the use of PEEP resulted in high mortality and BPD in the 1960s. Conventional ventilation with PEEP greatly improved outcomes for larger infants, but the incidence of BPD was high in very small infants in the 1970s and 1980s. The factors that have improved mechanical ventilation for preterm infants have not been carefully evaluated in trials. However, the use of high-frequency ventilators demonstrated the benefits of higher mean airway pressures and small tidal

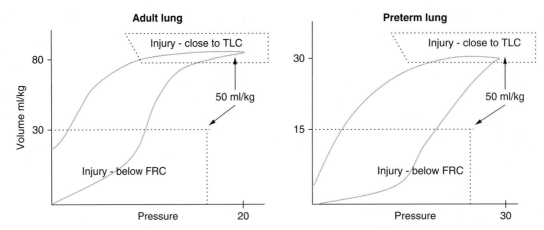

FIGURE 23-6 Idealized pressure-volume curves for the preterm lung with respiratory distress syndrome (RDS) and a normal adult lung. The preterm lung has a lower total lung capacity (TLC), a lower functional residual capacity (FRC), and less lung gas volume between the zones of injury for ventilation of the lungs, indicated by dashed boxes.

volumes in animal studies and some clinical studies.[48] Clinicians adapted their use of conventional ventilators to lower tidal volume strategies with careful avoidance of hyperventilation and selective use of higher PCO_2 targets to decrease injury. The net effect is that trials that are more recent demonstrated minimal differences in BPD between conventional ventilation using patient synchronization and high-frequency oscillation. The monitoring of V_T and more aggressive extubation policies have also decreased ventilator-mediated injury for infants with RDS.

Surfactant Treatment Response

With availability of surfactant treatments, mortality and morbidity from RDS decreased. The responses of the surfactant-deficient lung to surfactant are quite striking, as illustrated by the changes in the static pressure-volume curve (Figure 23-7). This example gives idealized curves for the effects of a surfactant treatment at birth on lung gas volumes of preterm rabbits.[49] The lungs not given surfactant did not inflate until the distending pressure was greater than 20 cm H_2O, and maximal lung volume was only about 25 mL/kg. The lungs completely collapsed at low transpulmonary pressures. The surfactant treatment decreased the pressure required to initially open the lungs, increased maximal lung gas volume to over 80 mL/kg, and caused the lung to retain about 30 mL/kg on deflation.

These striking changes in the static pressure-volume curve with surfactant treatment have clear clinical correlates. For infants that fail CPAP, intubation and

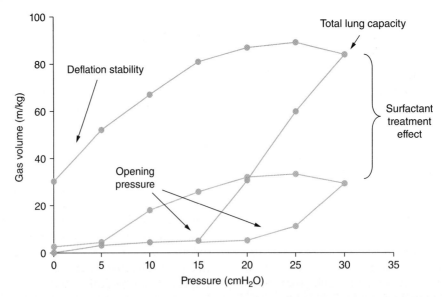

FIGURE 23-7 Idealized pressure-volume curves from measurements with preterm rabbit lungs (○) and surfactant-treated lungs (●). Surfactant decreased the opening pressure, increased the total lung capacity, and increased deflation stability on deflation. (Data from Reference 49.)

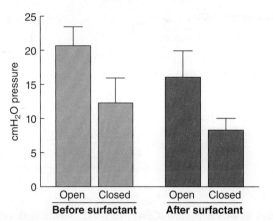

FIGURE 23-8 Mean air pressures required to decrease oxygen to 25% or less for infants with respiratory distress syndrome (RDS) ventilated with high-frequency oscillators. Following intubation for respiratory failure, mean airway pressures were increased to about 21 cm H_2O to improve oxygenation until the oxygen requirement was 25% or less, indicating that the lungs were "open." The mean airway pressures were then progressively decreased until the oxygenation decreased, indicating that the lungs were "closed." Surfactant treatment decreased the pressures. (Data from reference 50.)

ventilation with high-frequency ventilators demonstrate the high pressures needed to "open" the lungs to optimize oxygenation of infants with RDS.[50] In the example in Figure 23-8, the mean airway pressure was increased repetitively by 2 cm H_2O until the oxygen could be decreased to less than 25%, which occurred when the mean airway pressure averaged about 21 cm H_2O for a group of over 100 infants. The investigators then decreased mean airway pressure until the oxygen needs increased, indicating lung closure—moving the lungs down the deflation limb of the P-V curve—and that occurred at about 14 cmH$_2$O pressure. A surfactant treatment resulted in lower pressures to open the lung and a lung closing pressure of only 8 cm H_2O. In clinical practice, surfactant treatments result in rapid increases in PO$_2$, decreases in compliance if overinflation is avoided, lower ventilation support settings, and a large decrease in the risk of pneumothorax.

Surfactant was approved for treatments soon after birth to prevent RDS in high-risk infants—generally infants less than 28 weeks' gestational age—or to treat infants in the first hours of life with RDS. Although the trials demonstrated clear benefit to the very early treatments, such treatments give surfactant needlessly to many infants who may not have RDS. The current practice is to treat infants when RDS is first diagnosed, and such a strategy results in similar outcomes to early treatments.[51]

Infants with a clinical diagnosis of RDS who receive surfactant should respond with improved lung function. Term infants with pneumonia will improve with surfactant treatments, but the clinical responses are more modest than for preterm infants with RDS.[52] Similarly, very preterm infants with RDS and with a fetal inflammatory response syndrome and a history of exposure to chorioamnionitis may have decreased responses to surfactant.[53] The probable explanation is lung inflammation that inhibits the function of the surfactant used for treatment. Infants exposed to antenatal corticosteroids will have a lower incidence of RDS, and those with RDS will have good clinical responses to surfactant treatments.[19,54] Not all infants with a clinical diagnosis of RDS have striking treatment responses. This variability has multiple explanations that include coexisting inflammation, lung injury prior to treatment, structurally more immature lungs, and delayed fluid clearance. If an infant with a clinical diagnosis of RDS does not respond to treatment, multiple re-treatments are unlikely to be of benefit. The infant should be reevaluated for other conditions, such as congenital heart disease.

The major interventions to treat and manage severe RDS have been surfactant treatments and mechanical ventilation. However, the use of CPAP soon after birth may help recruit FRC, facilitate breathing, and perhaps preserve marginal surfactant pools in preterm infants.[41] Recent trials have evaluated the relative benefits of the very early use of CPAP relative to intubation and surfactant treatment.[42,43] Some trials have included the strategy to intubate, surfactant treat, and then extubate soon after birth.[55] The individual trials have similar primary outcomes for BPD or death, with a tendency to favor the CPAP strategies. This early use of CPAP coupled with efforts to minimize ventilator-mediated injury and promote early extubation is thought to decrease the severity, if not the incidence, of BPD. The flow diagram in Figure 23-9 illustrates options for clinicians to use CPAP for the treatment of RDS.

OUTCOME AND FOLLOW-UP

In the recent past, RDS was a major cause of death of preterm infants. Now, few infants die of RDS alone. Infants who are greater than 28 weeks' gestational age have almost no mortality from RDS unless there are other complications of development or prematurity. For example, some degree of pulmonary hypoplasia is probably more frequent than recognized and can be difficult to distinguish from RDS. Pulmonary hypoplasia can result in a poor lung outcome or death. Intrauterine growth restriction is a strong predictor of BPD, and these infants often will have RDS.[56] The growth restriction is thought to cause abnormal lung development. Very preterm infants of less than 25 weeks' gestational age may have RDS listed as the

Opportunities for CPAP for infants with RDS

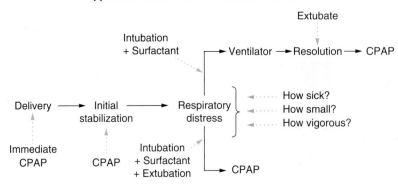

FIGURE 23-9 Outline of opportunities to use continuous positive airway pressure (CPAP) to treat infants with respiratory distress syndrome (RDS).

proximal cause of death, but severe immaturity of multiple organ systems often contribute to the death.

With the availability of surfactant treatments and the use of gentler approaches to ventilation, pneumothorax is much less frequent than in previous eras. There is about a 7% incidence of pneumothorax in infants less than 29 weeks' gestation.[14] The incidence of pulmonary interstitial emphysema is also low if gentle approaches to ventilation are used. However, occasional infants have unmanageable problems with pulmonary interstitial emphysema and pneumothorax, probably resulting from immature lung structure on a developmental basis.

The major adverse outcome from RDS is BPD. The occurrence of BPD can be predicted in very preterm infants based on gestational age, birth weight, race, sex, and respiratory support.[57] The respiratory support variable becomes more predictive as the infant ages. Table 23-2 demonstrates that the risk for BPD is low for those infants on low oxygen through 14 days of age (presumably they had minimal RDS, although 78% received surfactant).[58] About 40% of the infants had persistently high oxygen requirements despite surfactant treatments, demonstrating that surfactant does not prevent severe lung disease in many infants with a diagnosis of RDS. The risks of RDS and BPD at early gestational ages are shown in Figure 23-1. In a population of almost 10,000 infants who had a diagnosis of RDS, BPD was most highly associated with decreasing gestational age.[14]

Long-term outcomes for infants diagnosed with RDS relative to infants born at equivalent gestational ages have not been carefully documented. Longer-term pulmonary outcomes for infants with RDS depend in part on the progression to BPD. However, there is good information on the pulmonary outcomes for populations of very preterm infants, most of whom would have had RDS. Infants with birth gestations less than 26 weeks in the United Kingdom in 1995 had decreased lung function primarily from airway narrowing when tested at 6 years of life, and BPD predicted more abnormalities.[59] The airway disease is often treated as asthma in childhood, as demonstrated by the use of asthma medications that increases as gestational age decreases.[60] The deficits in lung function of preterm infants with RDS and not BPD probably are similar to those of infants of comparable gestational ages who did not have RDS. These abnormalities result from poorly understood lung structural consequences of very preterm birth and not RDS per se.

Table 23-2 Oxygen Use, Surfactant Treatment, and Diagnosis of Bronchopulmonary Dysplasia (BPD) in a Population of 1309 Infants with Gestational Ages Less than 28 Weeks[a]

Oxygen Use (%)			Population Percentage	
1 d	7 d	14 d	Surfactant Treatment	BPD
37	42	49	97	67
28	27	41	89	51
24	22	21	78	17

[a]Data from Laughon et al.[58]

REFERENCES

1. Kamath BD, Macguire ER, McClure EM, Goldenberg RL, Jobe AH. Neonatal mortality from respiratory distress syndrome: lessons for low-resource countries. *Pediatrics* 2011;127:1139–1146.
2. Silverman, WA. *Retrolental Fibroplasia. A Modern Parable.* New York, NY: Grune Stratton; 1980.
3. Avery ME, Mead J. Surface properties in relation to atelectasis and hyaline membrane disease. *Am J Dis. Child.* 1959; 97:517–523.
4. Gregory GA, Kitterman JA, Phibbs RH, Tooley WA, Hamilton WK. Treatment of the ideopathic respiratory distress system with continuous positive airway pressure. *N Engl J Med.* 1971;284:1333–1340.

5. Liggins GC, Howie RN. A controlled trial of antepartium glucocorticoid treatment for prevention of RDS in premature infants. *Pediatric.* 1972;50:515–525.

6. Gluck L, Kulovich M, Borer RC, et al. Diagnosis of the respiratory distress syndrome by amniocentesis. *Am J Obstet Gynecol.* 1971;109:440–445.

7. Northway WH Jr, Rosan RC, Porter DY. Pulmonary disease following respirator therapy of hyaline-membrane disease. Bronchopulmonary dysplasia. *N Engl J Med.* 1967;276:357–368.

8. Enhörning G, Robertson B. Lung expansion in the premature rabbit fetus after tracheal deposition of surfactant. *Pediatrics.* 1972;50:58–66.

9. Robertson D. Pathology and pathophysiology of neonatal surfactant deficiency. In: Robertson B, Van Golde L, Batenburg JJ, eds. *Pulmonary Surfactant.* Amsterdam, the Netherlands: Elsevier Science Publishers; 1984:383–418.

10. Fujiwara T, Chida S, Watabe Y, et al. Artificial surfactant therapy in hyaline-membrane disease. *Lancet.* 1980;1:55–59.

11. Altman M, Vanpee M, Cnattingius S, Norman M. Neonatal morbidity in moderately preterm infants: a Swedish national population-based study. *J Pediatr.* 2011;158:239–244.e231.

12. Porto AM, Coutinho IC, Correia JB, Amorim MM. Effectiveness of antenatal corticosteroids in reducing respiratory disorders in late preterm infants: randomised clinical trial. *BMJ.* 2011;342:d1696.

13. Chang EY, Menard MK, Vermillion ST, Hulsey T, Ebeling M. The association between hyaline membrane disease and preeclampsia. *Am J Obstet Gynecol.* 2004;191:1414–1417.

14. Stoll BJ, Hansen NI, Bell EF, et al. Neonatal outcomes of extremely preterm infants from the NICHD Neonatal Research Network. *Pediatrics.* 2010;126:443–456.

15. Perez-Gil J, Weaver TE. Pulmonary surfactant pathophysiology: current models and open questions. *Physiology (Bethesda).* 2010;25:132–141.

16. Whitsett JA, Wert SE, Weaver TE. Alveolar surfactant homeostasis and the pathogenesis of pulmonary disease. *Annu Rev Med.* 2010;61:105–119.

17. Hallman M, Kulovich M, Kirkpatrick E, Sugarman RG, Gluck L. Phosphatidylinositol and phosphatidylglycerol in amniotic fluid: indices of lung maturity. *Am J Obstet Gynecol.* 1976;125:613–617.

18. McElrath TF, Hecht JL, Dammann O, et al. Pregnancy disorders that lead to delivery before the 28th week of gestation: an epidemiologic approach to classification. *Am J Epidemiol.* 2008;168:980–989.

19. Roberts D, Dalziel S. Antenatal corticosteroids for accelerating fetal lung maturation for women at risk of preterm birth. *Cochrane Database Syst Rev.* 2006;3:CD004454.

20. Jobe AH. Prenatal corticosteroids: a neonatologist's perspective. *NeoReviews.* 2006;7:e259–e267.

21. Kramer BW, Kallapur S, Newnham J, Jobe AH. Prenatal inflammation and lung development. *Semin Fetal Neonatal Med.* 2009;14:2–7.

22. Goldenberg RL, Culhane JF, Iams JD, Romero R. Epidemiology and causes of preterm birth. *Lancet.* 2008;371:75–84.

23. Goldenberg RL, Andrews WW, Faye-Petersen OM, et al. The Alabama preterm birth study: corticosteroids and neonatal outcomes in 23- to 32-week newborns with various markers of intrauterine infection. *Am J Obstet Gynecol.* 2006;195:1020–1024.

24. Newnham JP, Moss TJ, Padbury JF, et al. The interactive effects of endotoxin with prenatal glucocorticoids on short-term lung function in sheep. *Am J Obstet Gynecol.* 2001;185:190–197.

25. Moss TJM, Nitsos I, Knox CL, et al. Ureaplasma colonization of amniotic fluid and efficacy of antenatal corticosteroids for preterm lung maturation in sheep. *Am J Obstet Gynecol.* 2009;200:96. e91–e96.

26. Jobe AH. Why surfactant works for respiratory distress syndrome. *NeoReviews.* 2006;7:e95–e105.

27. Rebello CM, Job, AH, Eisele JW, Ikegami M. Alveolar and tissue surfactant pool sizes in humans. *Am J Respir Crit Care Med.* 1996;154:625–628.

28. Adams FH, Fujiwara T, Emmanouilides GC, Raiha N. Lung phospholipid of the human fetus and infants with and without hyaline membrane disease. *J Pediatr.* 1970;77:833.

29. Mulrooney N, Champion Z, Moss TJ, et al. Surfactant and physiological responses of preterm lambs to continuous positive airway pressure. *Am J Respir Crit Care Med.* 2005;171:1–6.

30. Carnielli VP, Zimmermann LJ, Hamvas A, Cogo PE. Pulmonary surfactant kinetics of the newborn infant: novel insights from studies with stable isotopes. *J Perinatol.* 2009;29(Suppl 2): S29–S37.

31. Bunt JE, Carnielli VP, Darcos Wattimena JL, et al. The effect in premature infants of prenatal corticosteroids on endogenous surfactant synthesis as measured with stable isotopes. *Am J Respir Crit Care Med.* 2000;162:844–849.

32. Torresin M, Zimmermann LJ, Cogo PE, et al. Exogenous surfactant kinetics in infant respiratory distress syndrome: a novel method with stable isotopes. *Am J Respir Crit Care Med.* 2000;161:1584–1589.

33. Merchak A, Janssen DJ, Bohlin K, et al. Endogenous pulmonary surfactant metabolism is not affected by mode of ventilation in premature infants with respiratory distress syndrome. *J Pediatr.* 2002;140:693–698.

34. Hillman NH, Moss TJ, Kallapur SG, et al. Brief, large tidal volume ventilation initiates lung injury and a systemic response in fetal sheep. *Am J Respir Crit Care Med.* 2007;176:575–581.

35. Ikegami M, Jacobs H, Jobe AH. Surfactant function in the respiratory distress syndrome. *J Pediatr.* 1983;102:443–447.

36. Ikegami M, Jobe A, Glatz T. Surface activity following natural surfactant treatment in premature lambs. *Am J Physiol Lung Cell Mol Physiol.* 1981;51:L306–L312.

37. Sato A, Whitsett JA, Scheule RK, Ikegami M. Surfactant protein-D inhibits lung inflammation caused by ventilation in premature newborn lambs. *Am J Respir Crit Care Med.* 2010;181:1098–1105.

38. Ikegami M, Berry D, Elkady T, et al. Corticosteroids and surfactant change lung function and protein leaks in the lungs of ventilated premature rabbits. *J Clin Invest.* 1987;79:1371–1378.

39. Ueda T, Ikegami M, Polk D, Mizuno K, Jobe A. Effects of fetal corticosteroid treatments on postnatal surfactant function in preterm lambs. *J Appl Physiol.* 1995;79:846–851.

40. Soll RF, Morley C. Prophylactic versus selective use of surfactant for preventing morbidity and mortality in preterm infants. *Cochrane Database Syst Rev.* 2001;(2):CD000510.

41. Verder H, Albertsen P, Ebbesen F, et al. Nasal continuous positive airway pressure and early surfactant therapy for respiratory distress syndrome in newborns of less than 30 weeks' gestation. *Pediatrics.* 1999;103:E24.

42. Morley CJ, Davis PG, Doyle LW, et al. Nasal CPAP or intubation at birth for very preterm infants. *N Engl J Med.* 2008;358:700–708.

43. Finer NN, Carlo WA, Walsh MC, et al. Early CPAP versus surfactant in extremely preterm infants. *N Engl J Med.* 2010;362:1970–1979.

44. Shapiro-Mendoza CK, Tomashek KM, Kotelchuck M, et al. Effect of late-preterm birth and maternal medical conditions on newborn morbidity risk. *Pediatrics.* 2008;121:e223–e232.

45. Machado LU, Fiori HH, Baldisserotto M, et al. Surfactant deficiency in transient tachypnea of the newborn. *J Pediatr.* 2011;159:750–754.

46. Stutchfield P, Whitaker R, Russell, I. Antenatal betamethasone and incidence of neonatal respiratory distress after elective caesarean section: pragmatic randomised trial. *BMJ.* 2005;331:662.

47. Dreyfuss D, Saumon G. Ventilator-induced lung injury. *Am J Respir Crit Care Med.* 1998;157:294–323.

48. Bollen CW, Uiterwaal CS, van Vught AJ. Cumulative meta-analysis of high-frequency versus conventional ventilation in premature neonates. *Am J Respir Crit Care Med.* 2003;168:1150–1155.

49. Rider ED, Ikegami M, Whitsett JA, et al. Treatment responses to surfactants containing natural surfactant proteins in preterm rabbits. *Am Rev Respir Dis.* 1993;147:669–676.

50. de Jaegere A, van Veenendaal MB, Michiels A, van Kaam AH. Lung recruitment using oxygenation during open lung high-frequency ventilation in preterm infants. *Am J Respir Crit Care Med.* 2006;174:639–645.

51. Horbar JD, Carpenter JH, Buzas J, et al. Collaborative quality improvement to promote evidence based surfactant for preterm infants: a cluster randomised trial. *BMJ.* 2004;329:1004–1010.

52. Herting E, Gefeller O, Land M, et al. Surfactant treatment of neonates with respiratory failure and group B streptococcal infection. *Pediatrics.* 2000;106:957–964.

53. Been JV, Rours IG, Kornelisse RF, et al. Chorioamnionitis alters the response to surfactant in preterm infants. *J Pediatr.* 2010;156:10–15.e11.

54. Jobe AH, Mitchell BR, Gunkel JH. Beneficial effects of the combined use of prenatal corticosteroids and postnatal surfactant on preterm infants. *Am J Obstet Gynecol.* 1993;168:508–513.

55. Sandri F, Plavka R, Ancora G, et al. Prophylactic or early selective surfactant combined with nCPAP in very preterm infants. *Pediatrics.* 2010;125:e1402–e1409.

56. Zeitlin J, El Ayoubi M, Jarreau PH, et al. Impact of fetal growth restriction on mortality and morbidity in a very preterm birth cohort. *J Pediatr.* 2010;157:733–739.e731.

57. Laughon MM, Langer JC, Bose CL, et al. Prediction of bronchopulmonary dysplasia by postnatal age in extremely premature infants. *Am J Respir Critical Care Med.* 2011;183:1715–1722.

58. Laughon M, Allred EN, Bose C, et al. Patterns of respiratory disease during the first 2 postnatal weeks in extremely premature infants. *Pediatrics.* 2009;123:1124–1131.

59. Fawke J, Lum S, Kirkby J, et al. Lung function and respiratory symptoms at 11 years in children born extremely preterm: the EPICure study. *Am J Respir Crit Care Med.* 2010;182:237–245.

60. Vogt H, Lindstrom K, Braback L, Hjern A. Preterm birth and inhaled corticosteroid use in 6- to 19-year-olds: a Swedish national cohort study. *Pediatrics.* 2011;127:1052–1059.

Transient Tachypnea of the Newborn

Sarah Keene and Lucky Jain

INTRODUCTION

Transient tachypnea of the newborn (TTN) was the name given by Mary Ellen Avery in 1966 to describe a similar clinical presentation in a group of 8 neonates with: marked tachypnea on the first day of life (80–140 breaths/minute), mild cyanosis, mild work of breathing, no evidence of infection, similar chest x-ray findings, and resolution by 2 to 5 days.[1] It was also known as type II respiratory distress in the early years in an effort to differentiate it from the better-known respiratory distress syndrome (RDS). It is the most common cause of respiratory distress in the term infant and a frequent reason for admission to the neonatal intensive care unit (NICU).[2,3] TTN results from a failure of the normal transition from placental gas exchange in utero to pulmonary gas exchange and breathing. The primary mechanism causing TTN is delayed resorption of fetal lung fluid, a complex process that is now understood to begin several days before spontaneous delivery.[4,5] Although our understanding of the processes involved in the clearance of fetal lung fluid has increased, the clinical picture has remained much the same as described in 1966 (Table 24-1).

EPIDEMIOLOGY

Incidence

Transient tachypnea of the newborn is the most common cause of respiratory distress in the full-term neonate (37–41 weeks) and is responsible for almost half (42.7%–50.3%) of NICU admissions for respiratory distress at term, with an overall incidence of 4.3 to 5.7/1000 live births.[6,7] The majority of affected infants are admitted to NICUs for 48 to 72 hours and receive therapies that include respiratory support, intravenous fluids, and antibiotics, resulting in a substantial health care burden. Incidence in premature infants and those with risk factors is substantially higher but often underreported because of overlap with other respiratory disorders associated with prematurity.

Multiple studies have shown that the risk of all types of respiratory distress, and of TTN specifically, increases with each week less than 39 weeks' gestation.[6,8,9] The Consortium on Safe Labor evaluated respiratory outcomes at delivery in 233,844 infants with gestational age greater than 34 weeks, with a special focus on late-preterm infants (34 to 36 and 6/7 weeks) and found the incidence of TTN was highest at 34 weeks (64/1000 births) and 35 weeks (46/1000 births) and decreased with advancing gestational age. The gestational age effect is augmented when delivery is by elective cesarean section, so that even infants delivered at 39 weeks (39 and 0/7 to 39 and 6/7 weeks) have almost double the risk of TTN than their vaginally delivered counterparts.[9] TTN in more premature infants, those under 34 weeks, is likely significantly underdiagnosed, as the clinical picture is often complicated by surfactant deficiency and RDS. However, retained fetal lung fluid may contribute significantly to respiratory illness in these infants.

Risk Factors

A number of maternal and perinatal factors have repeatedly been associated with an increased risk of the development of TTN (Table 24-2).[10–12] The majority

347

Table 24-1 Key Diagnostic Features of Transient Tachypnea of the Newborn

Tachypnea with respiratory rate > 60 breaths/minute, often > 100 breaths/minute
Typical chest x-ray findings (hyperinflation, increased perihilar markings, diffuse mild opacities, residual pleural fluid in the interlobar fissures)
Hypoxemia and increased work of breathing (usually mild)
No evidence of systemic illness or infection
Onset in the first few hours of life and lasting more than 6 hours
Complete resolution usually by 72 hours, always by 7 days

of risk factors are related, directly or indirectly, to relative fetal immaturity and lack of preparedness for labor. Modifiable risk factors, such as mode of delivery, glycemic control in a diabetic mother, and in some cases, prematurity, deserve special attention.

Cesarean Section

Elective cesarean section performed before 39 weeks is one of the clearly modifiable risk factors in the development of TTN; for this reason, the current American Congress of Obstetricians and Gynecologists (ACOG) guidelines specify such deliveries should occur after 39 completed weeks.[13] However, the relationship between cesarean delivery of all types and TTN is complex. It is clear that cesarean delivery increases the risk of respiratory distress at birth, which is especially pronounced at lower gestational ages.[9,14] Multiple works have shown an increased rate of TTN among infants delivered by cesarean as well as an increased rate of RDS.[15] Late-preterm infants (34–36 and 6/7 weeks) and early term infants (37–38 and 6/7 weeks) are at increased risk of TTN regardless of delivery type, but especially

Table 24-2 Risk Factors for Transient Tachypnea of the Newborn

Prematurity
Maternal diabetes
Maternal asthma
Macrosomia
Polyhydramnios
Cesarean delivery
Male gender
Low Apgar score

after elective repeat cesarean.[8,16] However, it is unclear whether onset of labor prior to cesarean delivery is protective against developing TTN, with some work showing a difference between studied infants but others finding no difference.[7,14,15,17]

Genetics

Epidemiologic studies provide evidence for a genetic contribution to the risk of developing TTN.[18] Familial clustering is seen of cases of TTN without known risk factors,[19] and infants born to mothers with a history of asthma have a higher rate of development of TTN.[12] Perhaps unsurprisingly, some work showed affected infants are also at a higher risk of developing asthma in childhood.[20] Polymorphisms have been studied in a number of genes that produce substances known to have a role in neonatal transition, including surfactant, epithelial sodium channels (ENaCs), and catecholamine.[21,22]

The majority of studies failed to find an association between polymorphisms of selected introns and TTN. An association was seen for the β-adrenergic receptor (ADRB)[21]: Infants diagnosed with TTN were significantly more likely to carry loss-of-function polymorphisms for this gene. The role of genetics in TTN, much like the role of genetics in asthma, is complex and multifactorial, with many areas of active research.

PATHOPHYSIOLOGY

The fetal lung is a secretory organ during fetal life, a process essential to normal development of the pulmonary system.[23] This must change, and fluid must be cleared rapidly during labor and then delivery for the normal transition to air breathing to occur. Events that interfere with or delay this process cause respiratory distress, especially tachypnea.

Fluid in the Fetal Lung

Fetal lung fluid is actively secreted from alveolar type I and II cells at a rate of up to 20 mL/kg/d.[24,25] This fluid is chloride rich and low in protein, the product of chloride secretion into the nascent airspaces after the creation of an electrochemical gradient by basolateral channels in epithelial cells.[24,26] In the fetus, sodium follows chloride, and water follows the newly developed osmotic gradient to result in a net secretion of fluid by the fetal lung. Underlying mechanisms that allow the volume of fluid to be sensed and adjusted are still unknown, as is the identity of the primary chloride channel involved. What is clear is that this fluid is essential to normal lung growth and provides a distending volume similar to functional residual capacity (FRC). Processes that interfere with normal production and volume of fetal lung fluid, such as oligohydramnios and pulmonary artery ligation, result in pulmonary hypoplasia and respiratory distress.[23,27]

Newborn Transition

At the time of delivery after spontaneous labor, the transition from fluid-filled lungs to air-filled lungs has already begun. Animal studies have shown a decrease in the production of fetal lung fluid and net volume of fluid in the lungs occurs in the days prior to delivery.[25,28,29] The initial stimulus for this process is still unknown, much as many factors in the onset of labor itself are still a mystery. Hormonal changes that accompany labor, including production of steroid hormones, catecholamines, thyroid hormone, and vasopressin, have all been shown to decrease the production of fluid by the fetal lung.[25,28–30] With the addition of exposure to oxygen and mechanical stretch that follow delivery, the lung epithelium ultimately becomes a highly effective absorptive surface, with the majority of fetal lung fluid taken up into the pulmonary blood vessels and lymphatic system instead of out the mouth

and trachea as the vaginal squeeze theory previously postulated.[5]

Studies performed on lung explants and fetal lambs revealed that sodium flux from the lung lumen to the plasma occurs, resulting in net lung fluid absorption.[31,32] Sodium transport, and thus lung fluid resorption, is inhibited by administration of the diuretic amiloride,[32] and administration to fetal rabbits resulted in heavier lungs, respiratory distress, and hypoxia at birth.[33] The identification of ENaC, which is specifically sensitive to amiloride, helped to clarify further the essential role that secondary active sodium transport plays in the process.[34] As shown in Figure 24-1, the basolateral Na^+/K^+ adenosine triphosphatase (ATPase) creates an electrochemical gradient that draws sodium into the cell through sodium channels that are newly present in the apical membrane. Anions and water follow, causing net fluid absorption. ENaC is responsible for 40% to 70% of the sodium resorption in the newborn period and has been extensively studied. Steroid hormones and catecholamines, shown to decrease the production of fetal lung fluid, have also been demonstrated to enhance ENaC activity and production,[35–39] and serum cortisol levels were shown to correlate with α-ENaC levels in neonates.[40]

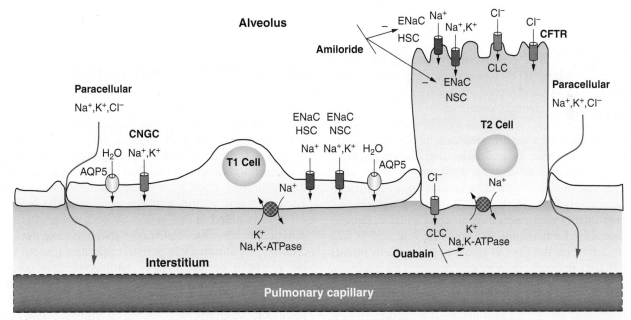

FIGURE 24-1 Epithelial sodium absorption in the fetal lung near birth. Near birth, Na^+/K^+ adenosine triphosphatase (ATPase) activity on the basolateral aspect of the cell membrane increases, which drives out 3 Na ions in exchange for 2 K ions, increasing the electrochemical gradient at the apical membrane. This process can be blocked by the cardiac glycoside ouabain. Na^+ enters the cell through the apical surface of both alveolar type 1 (ATI) and type 2 (ATII) cells via amiloride-sensitive epithelial Na channels (ENaCs), both highly selective channels (HSCs) and nonselective channels (NSCs), and cyclic nucleotide gated channels (CNGC) (seen only in ATI cells). Electroneutrality is conserved with chloride movement through cystic fibrosis transmembrane conductance regulator (CFTR) or through chloride channels (CLCs) in ATI and ATII cells or paracellularly through tight junctions. Net ion movement is from the apical surface to the interstitium, creating an osmotic gradient, which in turn directs water transport in the same direction, either through aquaporins (Aquaporin-5, AQP5) or by diffusion.

There are 4 identified subunits of the ENaC channel: α, β, γ, and δ, with the role of δ-ENaC the least well known as it was only recently identified in respiratory epithelium.[41] The α subunit has been the most studied, and its deficiency has been shown to cause respiratory failure that is neonatally lethal in mice; deficiency in the β and γ subunits does lead to an increase in lung water content but caused death of the mice from electrolyte abnormalities.[36,42] The relative importance of the subunits is not clearly defined in humans, but all are necessary for normal function.[39]

Abnormalities in Transition

Nasal potential difference studies, which are performed on nasal epithelium as a surrogate for respiratory epithelium, indicated levels of sodium transport and thus ENaC activity. Support for the role of ENaC in the pathogenesis of TTN was demonstrated by Gowen et al in 1988; they showed that infants with TTN had a significantly higher nasal potential difference than healthy controls and did not show the typical decrease in response to amiloride, both indicative of low levels of ENaC.[43] This was mirrored in infants delivered by cesarean section prior to the onset of labor, although they were often asymptomatic. Elevated respiratory rate and elevated nasal potential difference were correlated, and both decreased together over time and were equal to those of healthy controls at 72 hours of life.

It is clear that prematurely born infants are at increased risk for TTN. This is in part explained by evidence in animal and human studies that ENaC expression is developmentally regulated.[31,35] Nasal potential difference studies in preterm infants with respiratory distress showed a smaller decrease in potential difference in response to amiloride than preterm infants without respiratory distress, indicating a lower level of ENaC activity.[44] Further studies have confirmed quantatively lower levels of α-, β-, and γ-ENaC in preterm infants with respiratory distress when compared to healthy term infants.[45,46] Trending levels of ENaC subunits over the first 30 hours of life in term infants delivered vaginally, term infants delivered via cesarean, and preterm infants have shown term infants have a decrease in ENaC levels as lung fluid is cleared, but this decrease is slower in those delivered by cesarean, as it is in premature infants.[45] Thus, lower levels of epithelial sodium transport due to low levels of ENaC production, whether due to gestational immaturity, lack of spontaneous labor, or both, contribute to the development of TTN.

How retention of fetal lung fluid leads to such predictable tachypnea, in spite of usually normal or even low arterial CO_2 levels, is a puzzling biological phenomenon. Early studies by Paintal et al[47] suggested a role for pulmonary C fibers (J receptors) in initiating reflex activity leading to tachypnea and bronchoconstriction among other effects. Paintal postulated that C fibers respond to excess fluid in the interstitial space as interstitial stretch receptors triggering rapid shallow breathing, which may occur even in the presence of hypocapnia. A similar role has since been described for bronchial C fibers as well.[48,49]

CLINICAL PICTURE

The hallmark of TTN, as the name implies, is tachypnea appearing shortly after birth with respiratory rates greater than 60 breaths per minute (Table 24-1). Tachypnea may be accompanied by grunting, flaring, retractions, and cyanosis but is distinctly disproportionate to other signs of respiratory distress. Infants may have an increased oxygen requirement, but there is generally no hypercapnia. There is no clear consensus for the minimum duration of tachypnea needed to justify the label of TTN. Many experts recommend more than 6 hours of respiratory symptoms to differentiate the condition from the more transient delayed neonatal transition. Resolution of symptoms by 72 hours is seen in a majority of the infants. However, secondary complications such as pulmonary hypertension, acidosis, and air leak syndrome can alter the course and lead to severe hypoxic respiratory failure.[50,51]

DIFFERENTIAL DIAGNOSIS

Neonatal tachypnea can be caused by a wide variety of factors that encompass the full spectrum of illness in the neonate. These can be grouped into 3 categories as seen in Table 24-3, with a good amount of expected overlap. The first group includes acquired illnesses of the respiratory tract, such as infection, processes not associated with an inherent abnormality of the lungs. TTN is included in this group. Second, congenital or genetic abnormalities that cause aberrant lung development or pulmonary hypoplasia may also present in the newborn period. Finally, pathophysiologic processes involving other organ systems, or the body as a whole, may present with tachypnea as an initial, predominant symptom.

It is worth remembering that, on initial presentation, TTN can be clinically indistinguishable from neonatal pneumonia or a host of other etiologies of tachypnea that can be life threatening.[52] TTN is a classic diagnosis of exclusion. The extent of the workup for other causes should be determined on a case-by-case basis in response to the clinical presentation and degree of illness. An infant can be definitively diagnosed with TTN only once other etiologies have been

Table 24-3 Differential Diagnosis of Neonatal Tachypnea

Acquired lung disease	Neonatal pneumonia Aspiration syndromes Respiratory distress syndrome Pulmonary hemorrhage Pneumothorax Transient tachypnea of the newborn
Congenital abnormality of the lung	Primary pulmonary hypertension Congenital diaphragmatic hernia Cystic lung disease Congenital chylothorax Chest wall deformity Genetic abnormalities in lung development
Systemic illness involving the respiratory system	Sepsis Congenital heart disease/heart failure Cerebral hyperventilation Metabolic acidosis Polycythemia

excluded and the clinical course has been shown to be characteristic, relatively short, and self-limited.

Lung Disease

Acquired Lung Disease

The category of acquired lung disease includes processes that occur before, during, and after birth, such as infection, aspiration, and fluid retention. RDS is also included. Neonatal pneumonia deserves special consideration, as the initial presentation is often similar to that of TTN and chest x-ray findings may not be diagnostic. Infants with pneumonia are more likely to have known risk factors for infection, such as maternal fever, chorioamnionitis, malodorous amniotic fluid, prolonged rupture of membranes, and fetal tachycardia.[53] However, multiple studies have shown the majority of infants ultimately diagnosed with pneumonia have no identified risk factors.[52,54] Ultimately, hospital course, severity of illness, and if possible, identification of a pathogen make the diagnosis clear. Common pathogens include bacteria that typically colonize the vaginal tract (group B streptococci, *Escherichia coli*); viruses (herpes simplex virus, enterovirus); and atypical bacteria (*Listeria*) and overlap with those that commonly cause neonatal sepsis.[53] Neonatal sepsis and severe pneumonia often occur together.

Meconium aspiration syndrome is estimated to occur in 5% of infants born into meconium-stained fluid and is a common cause of respiratory distress

requiring intubation in term infants.[55] The clinical picture can vary from mild tachypnea to fulminant respiratory failure and pulmonary hypertension. Clinical history should be suggestive of this etiology, although it may not be clearly stated. Meconium in the respiratory tract creates an anatomic obstruction and causes irritation, resulting in a pneumonitis that can be severe. Although less common, blood aspiration can produce a similar clinical picture, as can pulmonary hemorrhage (discussed in Chapter 25).

Respiratory distress syndrome or hyaline membrane disease is a disorder of lung immaturity caused in large part by surfactant deficiency. It is discussed extensively in Chapter 23, but it is worth noting that there can be substantial overlap with TTN. Because of the developmental nature of the mechanisms for clearance of fetal lung fluid, preterm infants are at increased risk for TTN, which can occur separately or exacerbate RDS. Full-term infants, especially those born in the early term period of 37–38 weeks' gestation, are still at risk for lung immaturity and surfactant deficiency.[9,56,57] Typical chest x-ray findings include atelectasis and a ground-glass appearance but may not be characteristic enough to allow for differentiation. RDS should be considered, especially in infants with suggestive history and a high oxygen requirement.

Pneumothorax can develop in the neonate and does more frequently in those with RDS; it is uncommon but can occur in infants with TTN. Spontaneous, symptomatic pneumothorax is rare, but pneumothorax and pneumomediastinum occurring after resuscitation with positive pressure ventilation or in conjunction with meconium aspiration syndrome or RDS are more common.[58]

Congenital Lung Disease

Congenital lung disease encompasses a lengthy list of disorders that are developmental, genetic, or both. Many, including congenital diaphragmatic hernia and the cystic lung lesions, are readily seen on chest x-ray and are fairly easily distinguished from TTN. These disorders are discussed extensively elsewhere in this book. As with abnormalities of the thorax or muscular system causing restrictive lung disease, the common final pathway is pulmonary hypoplasia. Other, much less common, congenital disorders in lung structure and function may be less evident at patient presentation. This list is extensive and includes disorders such as alveolar capillary dysplasia and surfactant protein deficiency in which clinical presentation can initially be similar to TTN in mild cases, with tachypnea as a prevailing symptom. However, these patients worsen with time rather than improve, becoming severely ill and staying so. Genetic evaluation is necessary only in rare cases.

Systemic Illness Involving the Respiratory System

Tachypnea may be the presenting symptom for many serious and not uncommon neonatal disorders that do not affect the respiratory system primarily. Chief among these are neonatal sepsis and congenital heart disease, both discussed elsewhere in this book. The inability to clinically distinguish neonatal sepsis/pneumonia from TTN in the first few hours is the reason many infants are treated initially with antibiotics until the picture becomes clear. Septic infants may rapidly progress from simple tachypnea to fulminant respiratory failure.

The clinical picture of tachypnea, significant cyanosis, but only mildly increased work of breathing is classic for the early stages of cyanotic heart disease before the infant becomes significantly ill.[59] Acyanotic heart disease may also present initially with tachypnea as the infant attempts to compensate for a progressive acidosis.

Additional systemic causes of neonatal tachypnea include cerebral hyperventilation in response to a central nervous system insult, such as a stroke or hypoxic ischemic encephalopathy. Tachypnea may be the presenting symptom for intracranial hemorrhage, although apnea is more common.[60] Such patients will often have alkalosis as the degree of tachypnea is excessive for demand. Conversely, infants with acidosis from any cause, including not only sepsis but also inherited metabolic disorders, are often tachypneic. These infants usually present at days to weeks old rather than a few hours, but an excessive, unexplained acidosis should be investigated. Hypoglycemia, hypocalcemia, and polycythemia are all fairly common in the neonate and can cause tachypnea, which should resolve rapidly with treatment of the underlying disorder.[61]

DIAGNOSIS

Patient Evaluation

An infant with mild tachypnea (60–80 breaths/minute) and no hypoxia who are systemically well appearing may be observed initially without specific therapy or evaluation. Respiratory rate, heart rate, and pulse oximetry levels should be monitored until tachypnea resolves. Tachypnea that is accompanied by additional signs of respiratory distress or hypoxia, persists longer than 6 hours, or is accompanied by other systemic symptoms merits laboratory and radiologic studies.

A complete blood cell count (CBC) with differential and blood culture should be performed to evaluate for an infectious etiology of tachypnea. Inflammatory markers, such as C-reactive protein (CRP) and erythrocyte sedimentation rate (ESR) are nonspecific, and mild elevations may occur due to delivery, but trending values can be useful in infants with a prolonged course.[62,63] Patients with TTN will typically have a normal CBC for age without increased white blood cell count or a high percentage of immature cells.

Hypoxia; signs of more severe respiratory distress (retractions, persistent grunting); or severe (>100 breaths/minute) tachypnea are indications for arterial blood gas analysis to assess oxygenation and ventilation and evaluate for acidosis. Significant respiratory failure with derangements in oxygenation and ventilation is unusual in TTN but can occur. Blood gas results and examination will guide the need for increased respiratory support or intubation.

For infants requiring admission to the NICU or with risk factors (maternal diabetes, large for gestational age, small for gestational age), glucose screening should be performed. A serum calcium level may also be helpful. Infants remaining on intravenous fluids for more than 24 hours because of persistent tachypnea should have a full serum chemistry and bilirubin level performed.

Diagnostic Tests and Imaging

Chest x-ray should be performed on any infant admitted to the NICU with respiratory symptoms. This may make clear a diagnosis of aspiration or congenital anomaly or support the diagnosis of TTN. A typical chest x-ray is seen in Figure 24-2. Findings consistent with TTN include hyperinflation with flattened diaphragms; signs of vascular congestion, including increased perihilar markings and fluid in the interlobar fissures; and mild streaky opacity that is uniform across lung fields.[1,10] A slightly increased cardiac silhouette may also be noted. These chest x-ray findings may also be seen in asymptomatic infants just after birth, so symptomatology is key in making a diagnosis.[64] Findings of atelectasis, significant opacification, or air bronchograms are not typically seen in TTN and are more compatible with RDS. A single anterioposterior film may be sufficient, although a lateral view will be helpful in identifying pneumomediastinum or pneumothorax, which can occur in TTN. Follow-up studies have shown chest x-ray findings will normalize in most patients as symptoms resolve, usually by 72 hours.[65] However, repeat x-rays are unnecessary in the infant who is improving and should be reserved for those with tachypnea lasting longer than 3 days or of worsening severity.

Cardiac imaging, via echocardiography, is necessary in the small percentage of infants initially thought to have TTN who have either severe hypoxia or prolonged symptomatology. Infants with oxygen requirements persistently in excess of 60% or saturations unresponsive to oxygen administration should have an

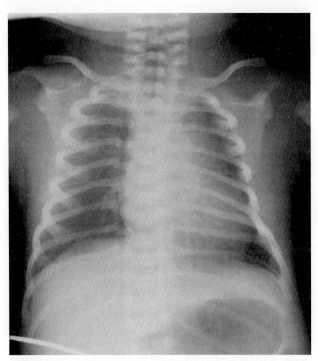

FIGURE 24-2 Chest x-ray findings in transient tachypnea of the newborn. This chest x-ray exhibits many of the typical findings: increased perihilar markings, mild streaky opacification, hyperinflation with flat diaphragms, and residual pleural fluid in the lobar fissures (seen at right).

evaluation performed for congenital heart disease and pulmonary hypertension, which can occur in TTN.[50] Those with tachypnea lasting longer than 5 days, even without hypoxia, may merit an echocardiogram to evaluate function and anatomy.

There is no specific testing that confirms the diagnosis of TTN. Rather, a compatible medical history, lack of systemic illness, normal laboratory evaluation, typical chest x-ray findings, and ultimately a characteristic clinical course with recovery usually by 72 hours will confirm the diagnosis.

TREATMENT

Supportive Care

The mainstay of treatment of TTN is supportive care. Because this disorder is usually benign and self-limited, no treatment may be required, and any treatment should be used with careful consideration of the risks and benefits. Infants whose primary symptom is tachypnea, without hypoxia or signs of increased work of breathing such as grunting or retractions, may be observed without specific respiratory treatment. They are at risk for hypoglycemia, so supplemental glucose may be necessary in the form of intravenous dextrose

or nasogastric feeds. For term infants, a total fluid rate of 60–80 mL/kg/d is adequate. Until the diagnosis of TTN has become clear, caregivers should consider treating infants with antibiotics given the possibility of neonatal sepsis or pneumonia, although in specific cases this may not be necessary.[66] Ampicillin, which covers group B streptocci and *Listeria*, is usually appropriate in combination with a gram-negative agent, such as gentamicin. Local resistance patterns and any antibiotic treatment of the mother during pregnancy should be taken into account. If infection markers and cultures are negative and the clinical picture fits TTN, then antibiotics should be stopped.

The degree of respiratory support should be guided by the degree of illness. Close observation, pulse oximetry, and monitoring for apnea should be undertaken in all infants until symptoms have improved. As stated, isolated tachypnea may not require specific treatment. Hypoxia should be treated with supplemental oxygen to keep saturations above 90%. If the oxygen requirement is persistently greater than 40% or there is clearly increased work of breathing, an arterial blood gas value should be obtained to evaluate for hypoxemia and hypercarbia, which may herald worsening respiratory failure. High levels of supplemental oxygen, such as is sometimes provided by 100% oxyhood, should be used with caution unless clearly necessary to maintain saturations. This treatment has historically been used for moderate-size pneumothoraces but has not been well studied and is controversial. There is increasing information about the morbidities of exposure to even brief periods (30 minutes) of 100% oxygen in both term and preterm infants,[67,68] including concerns about free radical production and worsened atelectasis. Large or symptomatic air leaks should be treated with syringe decompression or chest tube placement. A small subgroup of infants with TTN may have a more severe clinical picture, evidenced by high oxygen requirement and respiratory failure, and require continuous positive airway pressure (CPAP) or mechanical ventilation.[50,57] These infants should be evaluated carefully for other causes of illness and, if oxygen requirement is substantial, for pulmonary hypertension.

Targeted Therapy

No specific targeted therapies are considered standard of care in the treatment of TTN. Small trials have been done with the diuretic furosemide, administered both orally and intravenously, with increased postnatal weight loss but without effect on the duration of symptoms or need for respiratory support.[69,70] In a recent study, Stroustrup et al[66] evaluated mild fluid restriction (40 mL/kg/d in full-term infants) in neonates with TTN and found a benefit of decreased duration of respiratory support in a subgroup of 26 infants with severe TTN, but no overall effect. No ill effects of fluid restriction were found.

Inhalational supplementation of catecholamines, which are essential in the normal process of fetal lung fluid clearance, has been trialed in 2 pilot studies. Epinephrine treatment did not change outcomes, but inhaled salbutamol, a β-2 agonist, decreased maximum oxygen requirements and length of stay in a group of 54 neonates.[71,72]

Because the duration of illness is often brief, some focus has shifted to prevention of TTN prior to birth. Chief among this is ensuring adherence to the recommendation that elective cesarean delivery not occur until at least 39 weeks' gestation. The role of prenatal betamethasone, known to improve morbidity due to RDS in premature infants less than 34 weeks, has been evaluated as a potential preventive strategy for TTN. Basic science studies suggested that antenatal steroids should enhance lung fluid clearance and thus facilitate transition, particularly if the normal endogenous steroid surge that accompanies labor has not occurred.[5,73]

One randomized trial has been conducted in the term population.[74] Betamethasone prior to elective cesarean delivery was shown to decrease the risk of NICU admission for respiratory distress but not the overall rate of NICU admission. In the late-preterm population (34 to 36 and 6/7 weeks), prenatal steroid administration has not been shown to decrease the rate of RDS, but the study was underpowered to detect a difference in rates of TTN.[75] A large study sponsored by the National Institutes of Health to evaluate the role of antenatal betamethasone in late-preterm gestation infants is under way.

OUTCOMES

The prognosis for TTN is generally excellent, with full recovery expected in two-thirds to three-quarters of infants by 72 hours.[10,76] Hospital stays are usually fairly short, but a day or 2 longer than that for a healthy term infant. Long-term sequelae are generally uncommon. In rare cases, tachypnea can be prolonged or severe, requiring a lengthier hospital stay or mechanical respiratory support. Infants with symptoms lasting more than 5 to 7 days should prompt evaluation for other causes of respiratory distress. There are few outcome data available in the modern era, but this is estimated to occur in around 10% of infants with TTN.[76] Those requiring prolonged respiratory support and nasogastric feedings often have poor oromotor skills, although this is temporary and usually recoverable.

Finally, a small subset of infants with TTN will have severe hypoxic respiratory failure, often accompanied by pulmonary hypertension. Several case series described neonates with clinical pictures and chest x-ray findings classic for TTN who went on to have severe pulmonary hypertension and even require extracorporeal membrane oxygenation (ECMO) therapy.[50,51] This is a rare outcome with unknown exact incidence, but it is clear that infants delivered by elective cesarean section are overrepresented in the ECMO population. The consequences of severe illness and multiple medical therapies put this subgroup of patients at substantial risk for residual lung disease throughout childhood.

REFERENCES

1. Avery ME, Gatewood OB, Brumley G. Transient tachypnea of newborn. Possible delayed resorption of fluid at birth. *Am J Dis Child.* 1966;111(4):380–385.
2. Horowitz K, Feldman D, Stuart B, Borgida A, Ming Victor Fang Y, Herson V. Full-term neonatal intensive care unit admission in an urban community hospital: the role of respiratory morbidity. *J Matern Fetal Neonatal Med.* 2011;24(11):1407–1410.
3. Kumar A, Bhat BV. Epidemiology of respiratory distress of newborns. *Indian J Pediatr.* 1996;63(1):93–98.
4. Helve O, Pitkanen O, Janer C, Andersson S. Pulmonary fluid balance in the human newborn infant. *Neonatology.* 2009; 95(4):347–352.
5. Jain L, Eaton DC. Physiology of fetal lung fluid clearance and the effect of labor. *Semin Perinatol.* 2006;30(1):34–43.
6. Hibbard JU, Wilkins I, Sun L, et al. Respiratory morbidity in late preterm births. *JAMA.* 2010;304(4):419–425.
7. Morrison JJ, Rennie JM, Milton PJ. Neonatal respiratory morbidity and mode of delivery at term: influence of timing of elective caesarean section. *Br J Obstet Gynaecol.* 1995;102(2):101–106.
8. Tita AT, Landon MB, Spong CY, et al. Timing of elective repeat cesarean delivery at term and neonatal outcomes. *N Engl J Med.* 2009;360(2):111–120.
9. Hansen AK, Wisborg K, Uldbjerg N, Henriksen TB. Risk of respiratory morbidity in term infants delivered by elective cesarean section: cohort study. *BMJ.* 2008;336(7635):85–87.
10. Guglani L, Lakshminrusimha S, Ryan RM. Transient tachypnea of the newborn. *Pediatr Rev.* 2008;29(11):e59–e65.
11. Perez Molina JJ, Romero DM, Ramirez Valdivia JM, Corona MQ. [Transient tachypnea of the newborn, obstetric and neonatal risk factors.] *Ginecol Obstet Mex.* 2006;74(2):95–103.
12. Demissie K, Marcella SW, Breckenridge MB, Rhoads GG. Maternal asthma and transient tachypnea of the newborn. *Pediatrics.* 1998;102(1 Pt 1):84–90.
13. ACOG Committee Opinion No. 394, December 2007. Cesarean delivery on maternal request. *Obstet Gynecol.* 2007;110(6):1501.
14. Tutdibi E, Gries K, Bucheler M, Misselwitz B, Schlosser RL, Gortner L. Impact of labor on outcomes in transient tachypnea of the newborn: population-based study. *Pediatrics.* 2010; 125(3):e577–e583.
15. Silasi M, Coonrod DV, Kim M, Drachman D. Transient tachypnea of the newborn: is labor prior to cesarean delivery protective? *Am J Perinatol.* 2010;27(10):797–802.
16. Derbent A, Tatli MM, Duran M, et al. Transient tachypnea of the newborn: effects of labor and delivery type in term and preterm pregnancies. *Arch Gynecol Obstet.* 2011;283(5):947–951.
17. Hales KA, Morgan MA, Thurnau GR. Influence of labor and route of delivery on the frequency of respiratory morbidity in term neonates. *Int J Gynaecol Obstet.* 1993;43(1):35–40.
18. Yurdakok M. Transient tachypnea of the newborn: what is new? *J Matern Fetal Neonatal Med.* 2010;23(Suppl 3):24–26.

19. Guala A, Carrera P, Pastore G, et al. Familial clustering of unexplained transient respiratory distress in 12 newborns from three unrelated families suggests an autosomal-recessive inheritance. *Sci World J*. 2007;7:1611–1616.

20. Birnkrant DJ, Picone C, Markowitz W, El Khwad M, Shen WH, Tafari N. Association of transient tachypnea of the newborn and childhood asthma. *Pediatr Pulmonol*. 2006;41(10):978–984.

21. Aslan E, Tutdibi E, Martens S, Han Y, Monz D, Gortner L. Transient tachypnea of the newborn (TTN): a role for polymorphisms in the beta-adrenergic receptor (ADRB) encoding genes? *Acta Paediatr*. 2008;97(10):1346–1350.

22. Tutdibi E, Hospes B, Landmann E, et al. Transient tachypnea of the newborn (TTN): a role for polymorphisms of surfactant protein B (SP-B) encoding gene? *Klin Padiatr*. 2003;215(5):248–252.

23. Moessinger AC, Singh M, Donnelly DF, Haddad GG, Collins MH, James LS. The effect of prolonged oligohydramnios on fetal lung development, maturation and ventilatory patterns in the newborn guinea pig. *J Dev Physiol*. 1987;9(5):419–427.

24. Cassin S, Gause G, Perks AM. The effects of bumetanide and furosemide on lung liquid secretion in fetal sheep. *Proc Soc Exp Biol Med*. 1986;181(3):427–431.

25. Bland RD, Hansen TN, Haberkern CM, et al. Lung fluid balance in lambs before and after birth. *J Appl Physiol*. 1982;53(4):992–1004.

26. Wilson SM, Olver RE, Walters DV. Developmental regulation of lumenal lung fluid and electrolyte transport. *Respir Physiol Neurobiol*. 2007;159(3):247–255.

27. Wallen LD, Perry SF, Alston JT, Maloney JE. Fetal lung growth. Influence of pulmonary arterial flow and surgery in sheep. *Am J Respir Crit Care Med*. 1994;149(4 Pt 1):1005–1011.

28. Brown MJ, Olver RE, Ramsden CA, Strang LB, Walters DV. Effects of adrenaline and of spontaneous labour on the secretion and absorption of lung liquid in the fetal lamb. *J Physiol*. 1983;344:137–152.

29. Kitterman JA, Ballard PL, Clements JA, Mescher EJ, Tooley WH. Tracheal fluid in fetal lambs: spontaneous decrease prior to birth. *J Appl Physiol*. 1979;47(5):985–989.

30. Gandhi SG, Law C, Duan W, Otulakowski G, O'Brodovich H. Pulmonary neuroendocrine cell-secreted factors may alter fetal lung liquid clearance. *Pediatr Res*. 2009;65(3):274–278.

31. O'Brodovich H, Yang P, Gandhi S, Otulakowski G. Amiloride-insensitive Na$^+$ and fluid absorption in the mammalian distal lung. *Am J Physiol Lung Cell Mol Physiol*. 2008;294(3):L401–L408.

32. Olver RE, Ramsden CA, Strang LB, Walters DV. The role of amiloride-blockable sodium transport in adrenaline-induced lung liquid reabsorption in the fetal lamb. *J Physiol*. 1986;376:321–340.

33. Song GW, Sun B, Curstedt T, Grossmann G, Robertson B. Effect of amiloride and surfactant on lung liquid clearance in newborn rabbits. *Respir Physiol*. 1992;88(1–2):233–246.

34. Canessa CM, Merillat AM, Rossier BC. Membrane topology of the epithelial sodium channel in intact cells. *Am J Physiol*. 1994;267(6 Pt 1):C1682–C1690.

35. Jesse NM, McCartney J, Feng X, Richards EM, Wood CE, Keller-Wood M. Expression of ENaC subunits, chloride channels, and aquaporins in ovine fetal lung: ontogeny of expression and effects of altered fetal cortisol concentrations. *Am J Physiol Regul Integr Comp Physiol*. 2009;297(2):R453–R461.

36. Hummler E, Barker P, Gatzy J, et al. Early death due to defective neonatal lung liquid clearance in alpha-ENaC-deficient mice. *Nat Genet*. 1996;12(3):325–328.

37. Helms MN, Chen XJ, Ramosevac S, Eaton DC, Jain L. Dopamine regulation of amiloride-sensitive sodium channels in lung cells. *Am J Physiol Lung Cell Mol Physiol*. 2006;290(4):L710–L722.

38. Jain L, Chen XJ, Ramosevac S, Brown LA, Eaton DC. Expression of highly selective sodium channels in alveolar type II cells is determined by culture conditions. *Am J Physiol Lung Cell Mol Physiol*. 2001;280(4):L646–L658.

39. Elias N, Rafii B, Rahman M, Otulakowski G, Cutz E, O'Brodovich H. The role of alpha-, beta-, and gamma-ENaC subunits in distal lung epithelial fluid absorption induced by pulmonary edema fluid. *Am J Physiol Lung Cell Mol Physiol*. 2007;293(3):L537–L545.

40. Janer C, Pitkanen OM, Helve O, Andersson S. Airway expression of the epithelial sodium channel alpha-subunit correlates with cortisol in term newborns. *Pediatrics*. 2011;128(2):e414–e421.

41. Bangel-Ruland N, Sobczak K, Christmann T, et al. Characterization of the epithelial sodium channel delta-subunit in human nasal epithelium. *Am J Respir Cell Mol Biol*. 2010;42(4):498–505.

42. Hummler E, Planes C. Importance of ENaC-mediated sodium transport in alveolar fluid clearance using genetically-engineered mice. *Cell Physiol Biochem*. 2010;25(1):63–70.

43. Gowen CW Jr, Lawson EE, Gingras J, Boucher RC, Gatzy JT, Knowles MR. Electrical potential difference and ion transport across nasal epithelium of term neonates: correlation with mode of delivery, transient tachypnea of the newborn, and respiratory rate. *J Pediatr*. 1988;113(1 Pt 1):121–127.

44. Barker PM, Gowen CW, Lawson EE, Knowles MR. Decreased sodium ion absorption across nasal epithelium of very premature infants with respiratory distress syndrome. *J Pediatr*. 1997;130(3):373–377.

45. Helve O, Janer C, Pitkanen O, Andersson S. Expression of the epithelial sodium channel in airway epithelium of newborn infants depends on gestational age. *Pediatrics*. 2007;120(6):1311–1316.

46. Helve O, Pitkanen OM, Andersson S, O'Brodovich H, Kirjavainen T, Otulakowski G. Low expression of human epithelial sodium channel in airway epithelium of preterm infants with respiratory distress. *Pediatrics*. 2004;113(5):1267–1272.

47. Paintal AS. Mechanism of stimulation of type J pulmonary receptors. *J Physiol*. 1969;203(3):511–532.

48. Roberts AM, Bhattacharya J, Schultz HD, Coleridge HM, Coleridge JC. Stimulation of pulmonary vagal afferent C-fibers by lung edema in dogs. *Circ Res*. 1986;58(4):512–522.

49. Widdicombe J. Reflexes from the lungs and airways: historical perspective. *J Appl Physiol*. 2006;101(2):628–634.

50. Keszler M, Carbone MT, Cox C, Schumacher RE. Severe respiratory failure after elective repeat cesarean delivery: a potentially preventable condition leading to extracorporeal membrane oxygenation. *Pediatrics*. 1992;89(4 Pt 1):670–672.

51. Ramachandrappa A, Rosenberg ES, Wagoner S, Jain L. Morbidity and mortality in late preterm infants with severe hypoxic respiratory failure on extra-corporeal membrane oxygenation. *J Pediatr*. 2011;159(2):192–198.e193.

52. Costa S, Rocha G, Leitao A, Guimaraes H. Transient tachypnea of the newborn and congenital pneumonia: a comparative study. *J Matern Fetal Neonatal Med*. 2012;25(7):992–994.

53. Nissen MD. Congenital and neonatal pneumonia. *Paediatr Respir Rev*. 2007;8(3):195–203.

54. Mathur NB, Garg K, Kumar S. Respiratory distress in neonates with special reference to pneumonia. *Indian Pediatr*. 2002;39(6):529–537.

55. Ramadan G, Paul N, Morton M, Peacock JL, Greenough A. Outcome of ventilated infants born at term without major congenital abnormalities. *Eur J Pediatr*. 2012;171(2):331–336.

56. Ayachi A, Rigourd V, Kieffer F, Dommergues MA, Voyer M, Magny JF. [Hyaline membrane disease in full-term neonates.] *Arch Pediatr*. 2005;12(2):156–159.

57. Liu J, Shi Y, Dong JY, et al. Clinical characteristics, diagnosis and management of respiratory distress syndrome in full-term neonates. *Chin Med J (Engl)*. 2010;123(19):2640–2644.

CHAPTER 24

58. Kim SK, Kim WH. Tension pneumothorax in a newborn after Cesarean-section delivery—a case report. *Korean J Anesthesiol.* 2010;59(6):420–424.

59. Hunt EA, Brunetti M, Nelson KL, Shilkofski NA, Peddy SB. Recognition and initial management of cardiac emergencies in children. *Minerva Pediatr.* 2009;61(2):141–162.

60. Brouwer AJ, Groenendaal F, Koopman C, Nievelstein RJ, Han SK, de Vries LS. Intracranial hemorrhage in full-term newborns: a hospital-based cohort study. *Neuroradiology.* 2010;52(6):567–576.

61. Sarkar S, Rosenkrantz TS. Neonatal polycythemia and hyperviscosity. *Semin Fetal Neonatal Med.* 2008;13(4):248–255.

62. Kordek A, Torbe A, Podraza W, Loniewska B, Jursa-Kulesza J, Rudnicki J. Does prenatal antibiotic therapy compromise the diagnosis of early-onset infection and management of the neonate? *J Perinat Med.* 2011;39(3):337–342.

63. Zuppa AA, Calabrese V, D'Andrea V, et al. [Evaluation of C reactive protein and others immunologic markers in the diagnosis of neonatal sepsis.] *Minerva Pediatr.* 2007;59(3):267–274.

64. Steele RW, Copeland GA. Delayed resorption of pulmonary alveolar fluid in the neonate. *Radiology.* 1972;103(3):637–639.

65. Wesenberg RL, Graven SN, McCabe EB. Radiological findings in wet-lung disease. *Radiology.* 1971;98(1):69–74.

66. Stroustrup A, Trasande L, Holzman IR. Randomized controlled trial of restrictive fluid management in transient tachypnea of the newborn. *J Pediatr.* 2012;160(1):38–43.

67. Wiswell TE. Resuscitation in the delivery room: lung protection from the first breath. *Respir Care.* 2011;56(9):1360–1367. discussion 1367–1368.

68. Vento M, Sastre J, Asensi MA, Vina J. Room-air resuscitation causes less damage to heart and kidney than 100% oxygen. *Am J Respir Crit Care Med.* 2005;172(11):1393–1398.

69. Lewis V, Whitelaw A. Furosemide for transient tachypnea of the newborn. *Cochrane Database Syst Rev.* 2002;(1):CD003064.

70. Wiswell TE, Rawlings JS, Smith FR, Goo ED. Effect of furosemide on the clinical course of transient tachypnea of the newborn. *Pediatrics.* 1985;75(5):908–910.

71. Armangil D, Yurdakok M, Korkmaz A, Yigit S, Tekinalp G. Inhaled beta-2 agonist salbutamol for the treatment of transient tachypnea of the newborn. *J Pediatr.* 2011;159(3):398–403.e391.

72. Kao B, Stewart de Ramirez SA, Belfort MB, Hansen A. Inhaled epinephrine for the treatment of transient tachypnea of the newborn. *J Perinatol.* 2008;28(3):205–210.

73. Venkatesh VC, Katzberg HD. Glucocorticoid regulation of epithelial sodium channel genes in human fetal lung. *Am J Physiol.* 1997;273(1 Pt 1):L227–L233.

74. Stutchfield P, Whitaker R, Russell I. Antenatal betamethasone and incidence of neonatal respiratory distress after elective caesarean section: pragmatic randomised trial. *BMJ.* 2005; 331(7518):662.

75. Porto AM, Coutinho IC, Correia JB, Amorim MM. Effectiveness of antenatal corticosteroids in reducing respiratory disorders in late preterm infants: randomised clinical trial. *BMJ.* 2011;342:d1696.

76. Kasap B, Duman N, Ozer E, Tatli M, Kumral A, Ozkan H. Transient tachypnea of the newborn: predictive factor for prolonged tachypnea. *Pediatr Int.* 2008;50(1):81–84.

25 Pulmonary Hemorrhage

Elaine Barefield St. John and Waldemar A. Carlo

DEFINITION, HISTORY, AND EPIDEMIOLOGY

Pulmonary hemorrhage (PH) is the appearance of bright red blood from the trachea in association with acute pulmonary compromise and radiographic changes. Prior to the advent of exogenous surfactant, PH was described as a disorder primarily in term infants, in addition to the occasional very ill preterm infant, with sepsis, asphyxia, hypothermia, Rh disease, intrauterine growth retardation (IUGR), heart failure, or coagulopathy. The incidence was estimated at 1.3/1000 births[1] and 18/1000 in very low birth weight (VLBW) infants.[2] In recent decades, PH is more often a complication of extreme prematurity and is becoming more common as smaller, more immature infants are provided intensive care. PH is most often seen in extremely immature infants after surfactant administration,[3,4] particularly when the ductus arteriosus is still patent.[5-7] The incidence of PH in VLBW infants in the immediate postsurfactant era was estimated between 3% (according to Braun et al[2]) and 5.7% (according to Tomaszewska et al[3]) and has progressively increased since 1998 (Figure 25-1).[8] Although once viewed as almost uniformly fatal, the mortality now is closer to 50% in VLBW infants.[3] PH accounted for 18% of all deaths in a large series of infants at 23 weeks' gestation.[9]

Data from the Trial of Indomethacin Prophylaxis in Preterms (TIPP) study conducted from 1996 to 1998 in 1202 infants who weighed 500–999 g was reanalyzed in 2007 with respect to the effect of indomethacin prophylaxis on PH.[7] The information from this analysis yields a wealth of information on the likely etiopathology of this much-feared complication. The original analysis of TIPP data included pink-tinged endotracheal secretions without accompanying ventilatory worsening or x-ray changes under the definition of PH. Infants receiving indomethacin prophylaxis had no significant reduction on PH compared to control infants.[10] This is likely evidence that transient minor bleeding could be due to trauma such as suctioning.[11] Infants in TIPP with serious PH were less mature, more likely male and products of multiple gestation, and to have received surfactant on the first day after birth.

These risk factors along with a protective trend with antenatal steroids have been observed in a number of other studies as well.[12-14] Prophylactic indomethacin reduced the incidence of symptomatic patent ductus arteriosus (PDA) by 50% and serious PH in the first week by 35% (Figure 25-2). After adjustment for other risk factors and accounting for timing of left-to-right ductal shunt, promotion of PDA closure accounted for 80% of the protective effect of indomethacin prophylaxis on PH. This effect became less prominent after the first week, such that the 23% lower risk of PH in the indomethacin prophylaxis group was not significantly different by the end of the hospital stay.[7] This fits with the well-recognized phenomenon of ductal reopening after prophylactic use of indomethacin.

PATHOPHYSIOLOGY

The frequent occurrence of PH after surfactant administration in the presence of a patent ductus has given rise to the theory that relative pulmonary

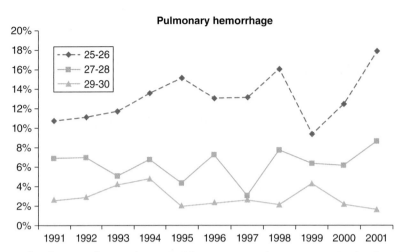

FIGURE 25-1 Incidence of pulmonary hemorrhage (PH) by gestational age groups in the first 10 years after routine use of surfactant. (From St. John and Carlo.[8])

overperfusion occurs with improvement in compliance and lower pulmonary vascular resistance (PVR) after surfactant. "Overtransfusion" was thought as early as 1973 to be related to left ventricular (LV) failure and PH.[1] In a study of sequential echocardiography in 126 babies at 23 to 29 weeks' gestation, PH was associated with greater left-to-right ductal shunting and higher pulmonary blood flow.[6] This hyperperfusion is thought to be the culprit in PH. Indeed, pulmonary congestion with certain types of congenital heart defects and the LV failure sometimes observed in asphyxia fit with this hydrostatic theory of PH,[15] although coagulopathy that occurs after acidemia and hypoxia could certainly contribute. Coagulopathy from any cause is a

risk factor for PH; and in this circumstance, PH may accompany bleeding at other sites.

Increased risk of PH in growth-restricted infants and IUGR infants with elevated nucleated red blood cell (NRBC) counts[16] implicates chronic hypoxemia in the etiology.

Pulmonary hemorrhage in term infants is most likely to occur with asphyxia, meconium aspiration syndrome (MAS), and sepsis.[12,13] The timing of PH in very preterm infants vs near-term and term infants also reflects the differing etiologies. PH in very preterm infants occurred at a mean age of 2–4 days, whereas in late-preterm and term infants, PH occurred at a mean of 6–18 hours.[12,13]

Environmental exposure to mycotoxins has been reported to cause spontaneous PH in otherwise-healthy term infants.[17–19] Exposure to mold in ventilator circuits or humid incubators or fungal infections have not been reported in relation to PH in preterm infants.

CLINICAL PRESENTATION

Diagnosis of PH is made with recognition of blood in the trachea or its secretions, often at the time of endotracheal tube suctioning. This last observation may lead to the conclusion that trauma caused the bleeding. Although trauma may play a role in transient minor bleeding, large hemorrhages are likely related to pathophysiologic causes[7] and can occur without antecedent or recent suctioning. A prodromal period with frothy pink edema prior to serious hemorrhage has been observed.[3] This phenomenon is likely responsible for the coining of the term *hemorrhagic pulmonary edema* (PE),[1] in which the hematocrit of blood from the endotracheal tube was found to be lower than that

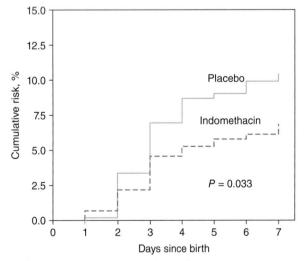

FIGURE 25-2 Kaplan-Meier estimates of the cumulative risk for serious pulmonary hemorrhage in prophylactic indomethacin and placebo groups in the Trial of Indomethacin Prophylaxis in Preterms (TIPP). (From Alfaleh et al.[7])

of arterial blood but in some instances increased over time. Epidemiologic studies have used a definition of PH as bright red blood from the endotracheal tube in conjunction with increased ventilatory support and new infiltrates on chest radiograph.

Oxygenation is first to be impaired with this alveolar-filling process. Impaired ventilation can be seen with more severe hemorrhages. When x-ray changes are seen, they are generally multilobar infiltrates.[2] Massive hemorrhage can cause bilateral complete opacification of the chest film.

PREVENTION AND TREATMENT

Prevention is geared toward avoiding pulmonary over-perfusion, as can be seen with PDA with left-to-right shunt. Refraining from injudicious use of surfactant in infants with minimal oxygen or ventilator requirements may decrease the incidence of PH. Yoshimoto et al reported elimination of PH in fifteen 23- to 24-week infants treated with a 12-hour, 0.01-mg/kg/h dose of indomethacin within 6 hours of life compared to 7% occurrence in untreated case-controls.[20]

Once PH has occurred, elimination of causes of overcirculation should be undertaken to reduce continued bleeding. Transfusion and volume expansion should be done slowly if they cannot be avoided completely. Correction of coagulopathy should be undertaken only if there is laboratory evidence of dysfunction or bleeding at other sites. Empiric platelet or plasma transfusion may worsen the pulmonary congestion. Pressure stops bleeding. A temporary increase in positive end-expiratory pressure may stanch the bleeding and improve oxygenation.[12] Use of high-frequency ventilation or avoidance of tidal ventilation are reported[5,21] but have not been rigorously evaluated in the prevention or treatment of PH. There are anecdotal reports of coagulants such as hemocoagulase (batroxobin) and recombinant activated factor VII used for prevention[22] and treatment[22–24] of PH. Use of vasoconstrictors, such as epinephrine and cocaine, has been reported as well.[12] Moderate and severe hemorrhages are likely to cause a secondary surfactant dysfunction and may improve with surfactant treatment.[25,26]

OUTCOME

The long-term outcome of VLBW infants is dramatically altered by the occurrence of a serious PH. A doubling of mortality, cerebral palsy, and cognitive delay was associated with PH in VLBW infants in the TIPP examination.[7] Trends toward increased risk of blindness or deafness did not reach statistical significance.

Increased rates of periventricular leukomalacia and seizures have been reported after PH.[3]

REFERENCES

1. Cole VA, Normand IC, Reynolds WQ, Rivers RP. Pathogenesis of hemorrhagic pulmonary edema and massive pulmonary hemorrhage in the newborn. *Pediatrics.* 1973;51(2):175–187.
2. Braun KR, Davidson KNM, Henry M, Nielsen HC. Severe pulmonary hemorrhage in the premature newborn infant: analysis of presurfactant and surfactant eras. *Biol Neonate.* 1999;75(1):18–30.
3. Tomaszewska M, Stork E, Minich NM, Friedman H, Berlin S, Hack M. Pulmonary hemorrhage: clinical course and outcomes among very low-birth-weight infants. *Arch Pediatr Adolesc Med.* 1999;153(7):715–721.
4. Soll R, Ozek E. Prophylactic protein free synthetic surfactant for preventing morbidity and mortality in preterm infants. *Cochrane Database Syst Rev.* 2000;(2):CD001079. Review. Update in: *Cochrane Database Syst Rev.* 2010;(1):CD001079.
5. Ko SY, Chang YS, Park WS. Massive pulmonary hemorrhage in newborn infants successfully treated with high frequency oscillatory ventilation. *J Korean Med Sci.* 1998;13(5):495–499.
6. Kluckow M, Evans N. Ductal shunting, high pulmonary blood flow, and pulmonary hemorrhage. *J Pediatr.* 2000;137(1):68–72.
7. Alfaleh K, Smyth JA, Roberts RS, Solimano A, Asztalos EV, Schmidt B. Trial of Indomethacin Prophylaxis in Preterms Investigators. Prevention and 18-month outcomes of serious pulmonary hemorrhage in extremely low birth weight infants: results from the trial of indomethacin prophylaxis in preterms. *Pediatrics.* 2008;121(2):e233–e238.
8. St John EB, Carlo WA. Respiratory distress syndrome in VLBW infants: changes in management and outcomes observed by the NICHD Neonatal Research Network. *Semin Perinatol.* 2003;27(4):288–292.
9. Batton DG, DeWitte DB, Pryce CJ. One hundred consecutive infants born at 23 weeks and resuscitated. *Am J Perinatol.* 2011;28(4):299–304. Epub 2010 Nov 29.
10. Schmidt B, Davis P, Moddemann D, et al. Trial of indomethacin prophylaxis in preterms investigators. long-term effects of indomethacin prophylaxis in extremely-low-birth-weight infants. *N Engl J Med.* 2001;344(26):1966–1972.
11. Turner BS, Loan LA. Tracheobronchial trauma associated with airway management in neonates. *AACN Clin Issues.* 2000;11(2):283–299.
12. Bhandari V, Gagnon C, Rosenkrantz T, Hussain N. Pulmonary hemorrhage in neonates of early and late gestation. *J Perinat. Med* 1999;27(5):369–375.
13. Berger TM, Allred EN, Van Marter L. Antecedents of clinically significant pulmonary hemorrhage among newborn infants. *J Perinatol.* 2000;20(5):295–300.
14. Lin TW, Su BH, Lin HC, et al. Risk factors of pulmonary hemorrhage in very-low-birth-weight infants: a two-year retrospective study. *Acta Paediatr Taiwan.* 2000;42(5):255–258.
15. Goretsky MJ, Martinasek D, Warner BW. Pulmonary hemorrhage: a novel complication after extracorporeal life support. *J Pediatr Surg.* 1996;31(9):1276–1281.
16. Steurer MA, Berger TM. Massively elevated nucleated red blood cells and cerebral or pulmonary hemorrhage in severely growth-restricted infants—is there more than coincidence? *Neonatology.* 2008;94(4):314–319.
17. Etzel RA. *Stachybotrys. Curr Opin Pediatr.* 2003;15(1):103–106.
18. Weiss A, Chidekel AS. Acute pulmonary hemorrhage in a Delaware infant after exposure to *Stachybotrys atra. Del Med J.* 2002;74(9):363–368.

19. Vesper SJ, Dearborn DG, Yike I, Sorenson WG, Haugland RA. Hemolysis, toxicity, and randomly amplified polymorphic DNA analysis of *Stachybotrys chartarum* strains. *Appl Environ Microbiol.* 1999;65(7):3175–3181.

20. Yoshimoto S, Sakai H, Ueda M, Yoshikata M, Mizobuchi M, Nakao H. Prophylactic indomethacin in extremely premature infants between 23 and 24 weeks gestation. *Pediatr Int.* 2010;52(3):374–377.

21. AlKharfy TM. High-frequency ventilation in the management of very-low-birth-weight infants with pulmonary hemorrhage. *Am J Perinatol.* 2004;21(1):19–26.

22. Shi Y, Zhio J, Tang S, et al. Effect of hemocoagulase for prevention of pulmonary hemorrhage in critical newborns on mechanical ventilation: a randomized controlled trial. *Indian Pediatr.* 2008;45(3):199–202.

23. Cetin H, Yalaz M, Akisu M, Karapinar DY, Lavakli K, Kultursay N. The use of recombinant activated factor VII in the treatment of massive pulmonary hemorrhage in a preterm infant. *Blood Coagul Fibrinolysis.* 2006;17(3):213–216.

24. Olomu N, Kulkarni R, Manco-Johnson M. Treatment of severe pulmonary hemorrhage with activated recombinant factor VII (rFVlla) in very low birth weight infants. *J Perinatol.* 2022;22(8):672–674.

25. Bissinger R, Carlson C, Hulsey T, Eicher D. Secondary surfactant deficiency in neonates. *J Perinatol.* 2004;24(10):663–666.

26. Neumayr TM, Watson AM, Wylam ME, Ouellette Y. Surfactant treatment of an infant with acute idiopathic pulmonary hemorrhage. *Pediatr Crit Care Med.* 2008;9(1):e4–e6.

Refractory Hypoxemic Respiratory Failure

Robin H. Steinhorn

EPIDEMIOLOGY

Definitions and Incidence

Respiratory failure severe enough to require mechanical ventilation or other advanced respiratory support affects about 2% of all live births.[1] In adult critical care, the term *hypoxemic respiratory failure* (HRF) defines the patient with respiratory failure and an arterial oxygen tension (PaO_2) below 60 mm Hg. In neonatal intensive care, most babies with respiratory failure are preterm, while the term *hypoxemic respiratory failure* typically refers to the substantial subset of infants with respiratory failure that are term or near term. The term is often used interchangeably with persistent pulmonary hypertension of the newborn (PPHN), the clinical syndrome defined by the failure to achieve the normal neonatal drop in pulmonary vascular resistance (PVR) and increase in pulmonary blood flow and oxygenation. HRF or PPHN complicates a wide range of neonatal cardiopulmonary diseases and affects up to 10% of neonates who require neonatal intensive care unit (NICU) hospitalization. Timely recognition and therapy are important because of high associated rates of neonatal mortality as well as short- and long-term morbidities, including significant neurodevelopmental sequelae.

The incidence of PPHN is not well understood. An important study from the mid-1990s estimated its prevalence at 1.9/1000 live births,[2] but only included infants referred to Level III NICUs in the United States; the majority of these infants were mechanically ventilated and receiving an FiO_2 (fraction of inspired oxygen) greater than 0.9. More study is needed to

better understand the incidence of more moderate disease, as well as the incidence of pulmonary arterial hypertension in mildly symptomatic or even asymptomatic babies. New national initiatives to perform routine pulse oximetry screening for critical congenital heart disease may provide valuable data to address the latter.[3]

General Risk Factors

A recent case-control surveillance study sought to determine risk factors for PPHN by interviewing mothers of infants who met criteria for PPHN and matched control subjects after discharge from the hospital.[4] Maternal factors that were independently associated with an elevated risk for PPHN were black or Asian maternal race, elevated body mass index (BMI) (>27), diabetes, and asthma. Neonatal risk factors included male gender, delivery by cesarean section, infants large for gestational age, and delivery before 37 weeks' gestation or after 41 weeks.

Genetic Risk Factors

Unlike pulmonary hypertension, which affects adults and older children, PPHN is rarely familial, and few genetic causes have been identified. A recent single-center report described the results of rigorous genotype analysis of 88 neonates with documented PPHN.[5] No differences were noted in most candidate genes, including bone morphogenetic protein receptor type II (BMPR2) and nitric oxide synthase. However, a significant association was identified in the genes for corticotropin-releasing hormone receptor 1 (*CRHR1*) and CRH-binding protein. Significantly increased levels of 17-hydroxyprogesterone were also noted, adding weight to the hypothesis that genetic disorders of cortisol metabolism could contribute to PPHN. These data are supported by animal data indicating that antenatal and postnatal steroids reduce oxidant stress and normalize nitric oxide synthase and phosphodiesterase (PDE) function in experimental PPHN.[6,7]

Several studies have reported that children with Down syndrome (trisomy 21) have an elevated incidence of PPHN.[8,9] In a Dutch cohort with excellent early ascertainment of Down syndrome, PPHN was documented in 5.2% of the infants.[10] Infants with Down syndrome are also overrepresented in the registry maintained by the Extracorporeal Life Support Organization, and their survival to discharge is significantly decreased compared to the general population.[11]

Maternal Medications

The potential risk of maternal medications has also been examined for at least 2 commonly used agents. Maternal use of nonsteroidal anti-inflammatory drugs (NSAIDs) was identified as an independent risk factor in several studies.[4,12] Upregulation of cyclooxygenases (COXs; both COX-1 and COX-2) in late gestation allows for increased production of prostacyclin (PGI_2) at the time of birth,[13,14] and maternal use of salicylates was 1 of the earliest triggers identified for PPHN.[15,16] More recently, a single-center case-control study of 40 patients revealed a strong association between clinically significant PPHN and the presence of at least 1 NSAID (aspirin, ibuprofen, naproxen) in the meconium.[17] At least 2 studies have indicated that NSAID levels correlate with the absence of a patent ductus arteriosus (PDA), suggesting that antenatal ductal constriction was a contributing factor.[17,18]

Selective serotonin reuptake inhibitors (SSRIs) are commonly used to treat maternal depression during pregnancy. In this case, conflicting evidence exists whether maternal SSRI use during pregnancy increases the risk of PPHN. In animal studies, newborn rats exposed in utero to fluoxetine developed pulmonary vascular remodeling and had clinical findings of abnormal oxygenation and higher mortality when compared with vehicle-treated controls.[19] Brief infusions of sertraline and fluoxetine in fetal lambs directly increased PVR, and this elevation was sustained for at least 1 hour after the infusion was stopped.[20] To date, 6 retrospective population-based studies have presented a range of findings: Three of the studies reported a positive association with adjusted odd ratios of 2.1 to 6.1, although little information is provided on the severity of PPHN.[21–23] Three additional retrospective cohort studies did not find an association.[24–26]

In addition, other reviews have highlighted the challenges of distinguishing the impact of SSRI use from the impact of depression (including an increased risk of prematurity) on the risk for PPHN.[27] The Food and Drug Administration (FDA) concluded (December 14, 2011) that the evidence is currently insufficient to conclude that SSRI use in pregnancy causes PPHN (Selective Serotonin Reuptake Inhibitor [SSRI] Antidepressant Use During Pregnancy and Reports of a Rare Heart and Lung Condition in Newborn Babies, http://www.fda.gov/Drugs/DrugSafety/ucm283375.htm) and currently recommends that health care professionals treat depression during pregnancy as clinically appropriate.

PATHOPHYSIOLOGY

General Categories of HRF

Table 26-1 outlines a broad range of diseases that can be associated with HRF or PPHN. Severe HRF usually presents as 1 of 3 types: (1) *maladaptation*, with constricted but structurally normal pulmonary vasculature, commonly associated with lung parenchymal diseases such as meconium aspiration syndrome, respiratory distress syndrome (RDS), or pneumonia; (2) *excessive muscularization*, in which the lung has normal parenchyma but remodeled pulmonary vasculature characterized by increased smooth muscle cell thickness and distal extension of muscle to vessels that are usually nonmuscular; or (3) the *hypoplastic vasculature*, associated with underdevelopment of the pulmonary vasculature, as seen in congenital diaphragmatic hernia (CDH). However, these designations are imprecise, and many patients have respiratory failure due to changes that overlap among these categories. For example, neonates with meconium aspiration typically have clinical evidence of altered vasoreactivity, but excessive muscularization is often found at autopsy. Neonates with CDH are primarily classified as having vascular hypoplasia, yet lung histology of fatal cases typically shows marked muscularization of pulmonary arteries, and clinically, these patients frequently respond to vasodilator therapy.

Pulmonary Vascular Remodeling

The first reports of PPHN described term newborns with profound hypoxemic pulmonary hypertension who lacked radiographic evidence of parenchymal lung disease. Idiopathic PPHN is sometimes called "black lung PPHN" because of the predominant vascular disease with little or no underlying parenchymal lung disease (Figure 26-1). It can cause profound hypoxemia due to shunting of blood through

Table 26-1 Disorders Associated with Hypoxemic Respiratory Failure

Pulmonary
Idiopathic pulmonary hypertension
Meconium aspiration syndrome
Respiratory distress syndrome
Transient tachypnea of the newborn
Pneumonia/sepsis
Lung hypoplasia
Congenital diaphragmatic hernia
Associated abnormalities in lung development:
• Alveolar-capillary dysplasia
• Surfactant protein B deficiency
• ABCA3 deficiency
• Pulmonary lymphangiectasis
• Congenital lobar emphysema (rare association)
• Cystic adenomatoid malformation (rare association)

Cardiovascular
Myocardial dysfunction (asphyxia; infection; stress)
Structural cardiac diseases
• Mitral stenosis, cor triatriatum
• Endocardial fibroelastosis
• Pompe disease
• Aortic atresia, coarctation of the aorta, interrupted aortic arch
• Transposition of the great vessels
• Ebstein anomaly, tricuspid atresia
Pulmonary venous disease
• Pulmonary vein stenosis (isolated)
• Total anomalous pulmonary venous return
Pulmonary atresia
Hepatic arteriovenous malformations (AVMs)
Cerebral arteriovascular malformations

Associations with other diseases
Neuromuscular disease
Metabolic disease
Polycythemia
Thrombocytopenia
Maternal factors: nonsteroidal anti-inflammatory drug use, maternal diabetes or smoking

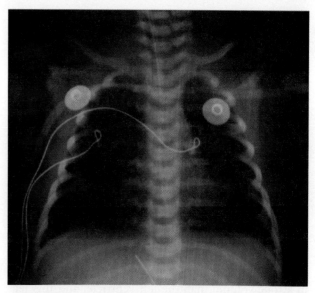

FIGURE 26-1 Typical chest radiograph of an infant with persistent pulmonary hypertension showing mild hyperexpansion and oligemic lung fields.

Idiopathic PPHN is perhaps the best-studied form of neonatal pulmonary hypertension in the laboratory setting, and many groups have developed models to explain the fetal and neonatal pathophysiology that underlies the abnormal remodeling and vascular dysfunction of the fetal and early neonatal pulmonary vasculature. For instance, a well-known cause of idiopathic PPHN is constriction of the fetal ductus arteriosus in utero from exposure to NSAIDs during the third trimester. Subsequent studies developed a fetal lamb model in which the ductus is surgically closed in

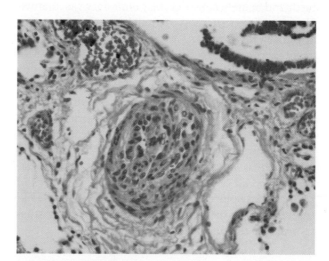

FIGURE 26-2 Histology of a pulmonary vessel from an infant who died of fatal hypoxemic respiratory failure (HRF); this illustrates the dramatic remodeling that can be associated with severe persistent pulmonary hypertension of the newborn.

the extrapulmonary channels of the foramen ovale and ductus arteriosus. Autopsy studies of fatal PPHN suggest that severe hypertensive structural remodeling with vessel wall thickening and smooth muscle hyperplasia develops in utero, likely as a result of chronic intrauterine stress (Figure 26-2). In addition, the vascular smooth muscle extends to the level of the intra-acinar arteries, which does not normally occur until much later in postnatal lung development. Pulmonary vascular remodeling and extrapulmonary shunting can also contribute to the severity of disease in babies with meconium aspiration syndrome and other parenchymal lung diseases.

utero, which induces rapid increases in fetal pulmonary artery pressure, pulmonary vascular remodeling, and a subsequent failure to transition to extrauterine life.

Right ventricular dysfunction is a critically important component of severe PPHN and is a major contributor to poor outcomes.[28] Although PVR is high during fetal life, the right ventricle pumps against the low-resistance placental circulation by directing most of its output through the ductus arteriosus. If transition occurs normally, the right ventricle continues to pump against a low-resistance circuit as PVR falls. On the other hand, if PPHN develops, the fetal right ventricle must rapidly adapt to a high-resistance circuit. Data from fetal lambs indicated that, when presented with elevated afterload,[29] the fetal and neonatal right ventricle responded with a more dramatic reduction in stroke volume than the left ventricle, and this feature helps explain why right ventricular dysfunction is such an important determinant of outcome for HRF (Figure 26-3).

Parenchymal Lung Disease

Meconium Aspiration Syndrome

Approximately 13% of all live births are associated with meconium-stained fluid, although only 5% of these infants will go on to develop meconium aspiration syndrome. Intrauterine hypoxia and other stressful stimuli trigger passage meconium in utero. Aspiration of meconium either before or during delivery will obstruct small airways, cause severe pneumonitis, and induce inflammatory changes in the lung; all of these abnormalities will impair oxygenation after birth and acutely constrict the pulmonary vasculature. Hypertensive structural remodeling of small intraacinar arteries is present in the most severe cases, most likely in response to chronic intrauterine hypoxia or lung injury.[30] In support of this idea, another study found depressed expression of endothelial nitric oxide synthase in umbilical venous endothelial cells in infants who had severe PPHN in association with meconium-stained amniotic fluid.[31] Meconium also induces postnatal release of pulmonary vasoconstrictors such as endothelin, thromboxane, and prostaglandin E_2, all of which promote the development of pulmonary hypertension and proliferation of vascular smooth muscle that will lead to antenatal and postnatal vascular remodeling.[32-34]

Surfactant Deficiency

Surfactant deficiency (RDS) or inactivation (eg, from meconium aspiration syndrome or pneumonia) is a relatively common cause of HRF. Even subtle

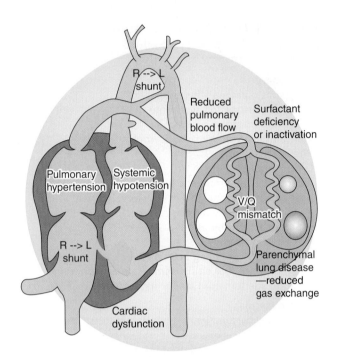

FIGURE 26-3 Hemodynamic changes in persistent pulmonary hypertension of the newborn/hypoxemic respiratory failure, demonstrating the interrelationship of cardiac, pulmonary, and vascular function. Surfactant deficiency (respiratory distress syndrome) or inactivation (meconium aspiration syndrome or pneumonia) produces parenchymal lung disease and ventilation-perfusion (V/Q) mismatch. Increased pulmonary vascular resistance results in reduced pulmonary blood flow and right-to-left shunt through the patent ductus arteriosus or patent foramen ovale. Pulmonary hypertension, often associated with systemic hypotension, results in septal deviation to the left. Left ventricular dysfunction secondary to asphyxia, sepsis, or congenital heart disease may contribute to pulmonary venous hypertension and complicate hypoxemic respiratory failure. (Used with permission of Satyan Lakshminrusimha.)

deficiencies of surfactant function or lung development may contribute to the development of HRF. Delivery prior to 39 weeks' gestation is now appreciated to worsen neonatal outcomes, in large part because of an elevated incidence of neonatal respiratory failure.[35,36] Furthermore, late-preterm and early-term infants are overrepresented in infants with the most severe respiratory distress who require extracorporeal membrane oxygenation (ECMO) support.[37] Respiratory failure and alveolar hypoxia can trigger PPHN, adding further evidence that supports the ongoing national initiatives to reduce delivery prior to 39 weeks. When HRF is severe or does not resolve within the first week of life, an inherited disorder of surfactant synthesis should be considered.

Pulmonary Hypoplasia

Congenital Diaphragmatic Hernia

Congenital diaphragmatic hernia affects approximately 1 in 2000 to 3000 births and is the most common cause of pulmonary hypoplasia in the neonate. The majority are left-sided Bochdalek defects. CDH is characterized by a variable degree of pulmonary hypoplasia that reduces the alveolar surface area for gas exchange and may alter surfactant production or function. These epithelial abnormalities are accompanied by a decrease in the cross-sectional area of the pulmonary vasculature, increased muscularization of the intra-acinar pulmonary arteries, and in the most severe cases, left ventricular hypoplasia. Pulmonary capillary blood flow is decreased because of the small cross-sectional area of the pulmonary vascular bed, and flow may be further decreased by abnormal pulmonary vasoconstriction. Chromosomal abnormalities have been reported in as many as 30% of infants with CDH. CDH is a recognized finding in Cornelia de Lange syndrome, and as a prominent feature of Fryns syndrome, an autosomal recessive disorder with variable features, including diaphragmatic hernia, cleft lip and palate, and distal digital hypoplasia. Pallister-Killian syndrome (tetrasomy 12p mosaicism) presents with findings that are similar to those of Fryns syndrome, including coarse facial features, aortic stenosis, cardiac septal defects, and abnormal genitalia. Chromosome deletions on chromosomes 1q, 8p, and 15q have been reported in association with CDH, and deletions of chromosomes 8p and 15q appear to be associated with heart malformations.

DIFFERENTIAL DIAGNOSIS

The initial evaluation could also reveal whether rare lung abnormalities such as a congenital cystic adenomatoid malformation are causing cyanosis or pulmonary hypertension. Because infants with PPHN often present with cyanosis that is poorly responsive to oxygen therapy or mechanical ventilation, an early echocardiogram is essential to rule out congenital heart disease as a cause of fixed hypoxemia. Careful examination is required to ensure that there are no abnormalities of the pulmonary veins, and this component of the examination can be challenging in the presence of extensive right-to-left shunting across the ductus arteriosus.

Another diagnostic dilemma occurs in infants with severe refractory HRF that does not reverse despite optimal management. In these cases, the clinician must consider congenital abnormalities of surfactant synthesis or developmental lung defects such as lymphangiectasis or alveolar capillary dysplasia (ACD). This is particularly important for children with HRF that does not respond to ECMO.

Genetic Abnormalities of Surfactant Function

Genetic abnormalities of surfactant function were initially recognized in infants with PPHN who were refractory to inhaled nitric oxide (iNO) and ECMO. Surfactant protein B (SP-B) deficiency was the first to be reported and is characterized by early presentation, radiographic findings of severe RDS, and progressive respiratory failure and early death. The most common mutation is in codon 121 of the SP-B gene. Deficiencies in SP-C also occur, but PPHN is not a known association. Mutations in the adenosine triphosphate (ATP) binding cassette (ABC) transporter 3 gene are now recognized to occur in neonates with severe neonatal lung disease and symptoms of surfactant deficiency,[38] are more common than SP-B deficiency, and have been reported to cause lethal PPHN.[39]

Alveolar Capillary Dysplasia

Alveolar capillary dysplasia with misalignment of the pulmonary veins is a rare form of interstitial lung disease that presents as severe pulmonary hypertension and hypoxemia early in life. It remains uniformly fatal despite treatment with all known modalities, including extracorporeal support.[40] The etiology of ACD is not well understood, but the prevailing opinion is that an early antenatal injury or a genetic defect leads to insufficient development of the pulmonary capillary bed, followed by remodeling and muscularization of the pulmonary arterioles and the development of congested "misaligned pulmonary veins" residing in the same adventitial sheath. Approximately 10% of reported ACD cases have a familial association, indicating a probable genetic component. Mutations or deletions in the FOXF1 transcription factor gene or deletions upstream to FOXF1 are identified in up to 40% of infants with ACD.[41]

DIAGNOSTIC TESTING

Chest X-ray

Early evaluation with a chest x-ray is mandatory. The chest x-ray in classic idiopathic PPHN is oligemic, normally or slightly hyperinflated, and without parenchymal infiltrates (Figure 26-1). The chest x-ray will also evaluate for parenchymal lung disease, such as pneumonia, RDS, and meconium aspiration syndrome, as well as lung abnormalities such as CDH or cystic adenomatoid malformation.

Electrocardiogram

An electrocardiogram is occasionally performed but is not usually much help because a predominance of right-sided forces and moderate right ventricular hypertrophy are common and relatively nonspecific findings in newborn infants.

Echocardiography

The echocardiogram plays an essential diagnostic role and can serve as an important tool for the ongoing management of newborns with severe HRF. The initial echocardiographic evaluation rules out structural heart disease causing hypoxemia or ductal shunting (eg, coarctation of the aorta or total anomalous pulmonary venous return), determines the predominant direction of shunting at the patent foramen ovale and PDA, and assesses ventricular function. The echocardiogram will also help determine whether an infant with HRF has hypoxemia due to pulmonary hypertension. Although elevated pulmonary artery pressure is commonly found in association with neonatal lung disease, the diagnosis of PPHN is only established when there is evidence of bidirectional or predominantly right-to-left shunting across the foramen ovale or ductus arteriosus. Echocardiographic signs such as increased right ventricular systolic time intervals and septal flattening are suggestive, but less definitive, in establishing a diagnosis of pulmonary hypertension.

In addition to examining for the physiologic features of PPHN, the echocardiogram is critical for evaluation of left ventricular function. Some infants may develop the worrisome finding of predominant right-to-left shunting at the ductus and left-to-right shunting at the foramen ovale, a combination of findings that indicates that left ventricular dysfunction is contributing to the underlying pathophysiology. When this occurs, left ventricular dysfunction increases left atrial and pulmonary venous pressure, which elevates pulmonary arterial pressure and causes right-to-left shunting with little vasoconstriction. In such cases, pulmonary vasodilators will not improve oxygenation and may cause or aggravate pulmonary edema, so they must be accompanied by therapies targeted to increase cardiac performance and decrease left ventricular afterload. Careful and sequential echocardiographic assessment provides invaluable information that will help guide the course of treatment.

Laboratory Findings

Common laboratory abnormalities may include hypoglycemia, hypocalcemia, polycythemia, or thrombocytopenia. At present, there is no single biochemical marker that has emerged with sufficient sensitivity and specificity for the diagnosis and management of PPHN. Serial lactate levels can be useful for monitoring the adequacy of systemic perfusion and tissue oxygenation and have been used to provide early predictive information about the outcome of neonates treated with ECMO.[42]

Brain-type natriuretic peptide (BNP), an endogenous peptide hormone secreted by the cardiac ventricles in response to increased wall stress, may help determine the contribution of vascular disease and right ventricular strain. Several reports indicated a positive correlation between BNP levels and echocardiographic findings of pulmonary hypertension in pediatric populations,[43–45] although it is not clear that BNP levels can be used to directly assess the severity of PPHN. One report suggested that high BNP levels (particularly those > 850 pg/mL) help differentiate infants with PPHN physiology from those with pulmonary causes of respiratory failure.[45] Because BNP levels are widely used for rapid assessment of cardiac failure in adults, they can be easily and rapidly measured in most hospitals. Currently, the test is most helpful when used in combination with other clinical and echocardiographic data.

MANAGEMENT

General management principles for all newborns with HRF include maintenance of normal temperature; electrolytes (particularly calcium, an ion critical for normal cardiac and vascular function); glucose; hemoglobin; and intravascular volume. Mechanical ventilation is almost always required to achieve normal lung volumes, and some newborns with parenchymal lung disease associated with PPHN physiology demonstrate marked improvements in oxygenation as well as decreased right-to-left extrapulmonary shunting following lung recruitment during high-frequency ventilation.[46] Particular care should be taken to avoid high lung volumes that will compress the capillary bed and elevate PVR. Maintaining normal tidal volumes will also prevent ventilator-induced lung injury, with its associated inflammatory changes, pulmonary edema, and decreased lung compliance.

Oxygen

Alveolar hypoxia increases PVR and can trigger or greatly exacerbate the pathophysiology of PPHN. The use of supplemental oxygen, often in combination with mechanical ventilation, is therefore a cornerstone of PPHN management. However, the optimal amount of supplemental oxygen or ideal PaO_2 in the management of PPHN remains a topic of intense investigation.

When PPHN occurs as a component of HRF, it is characterized by hypoxemia that is poorly responsive to supplemental oxygen, and this finding will frequently prompt use of oxygen concentrations up to 100%. However, exposure to such extreme hyperoxia will result in formation of oxygen free radicals and promote lung inflammation and injury. An approach of "gentle ventilation" with avoidance of hyperoxia and hyperventilation was proposed almost 20 years ago as an approach that could improve outcomes in a series of neonates with respiratory failure.[47] Furthermore, data from animal models indicate that although hypoxemia (<45–50 mm Hg) is a powerful vasoconstrictor,[48,49] the vasodilatory effects of supplemental oxygen reach a plateau at about 50% inspired oxygen or a PaO_2 of 60 mm Hg, and that higher FiO_2 or a PaO_2 of greater than 70 mm Hg does not significantly augment the decrease in PVR.[48–50] In addition, even brief exposure to 100% oxygen in neonatal lambs increases the contractility of the pulmonary arteries, promotes formation of oxygen radicals such as superoxide, and decreases cyclic guanosine monophosphate (cGMP) and relaxation responses to endogenous and exogenous nitric oxide (NO).[48,50–54] Maintaining preductal oxygen saturations in the 90% to 97% range has been proposed to optimize the drop in PVR in an animal model of PPHN (Figure 26-4).[55] Taken as a whole, the data suggest that avoiding hyperoxia is as important as avoiding hypoxia in the management of HRF.[55,56]

Forced Alkalosis

Acidosis acts as a pulmonary vasoconstrictor, potentiates the effects of hypoxia,[49] and should be avoided. Alkalosis induced by hyperventilation or infusion of sodium bicarbonate was frequently used to drop PVR prior to the approval of iNO.[2] Although forced alkalosis will often produce transient improvements in PaO_2, no studies have demonstrated long-term benefit in survival or other outcomes. In fact, prolonged alkalosis may paradoxically worsen pulmonary vascular reactivity and permeability edema[57] and may produce cerebral constriction, reduced cerebral blood flow, and worse neurodevelopmental outcomes.[58] It is now recommended to maintain pH and pCO_2 in the normal range.

Surfactant

Single-center trials have shown that administration of up to 3 doses of surfactant improves oxygenation, reduces air leak, and reduces need for ECMO in infants with meconium aspiration.[59] A large multicenter trial showed that surfactant reduced the need for ECMO in infants with parenchymal lung diseases such as meconium aspiration syndrome and sepsis, and surfactant is now commonly used to facilitate lung recruitment

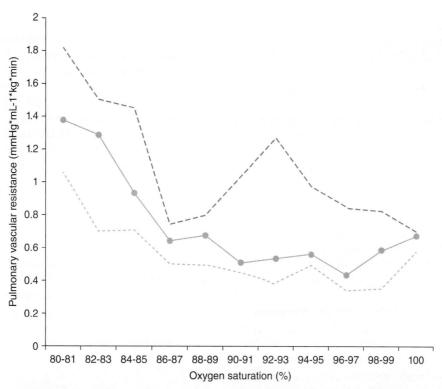

FIGURE 26-4 The relationship between oxygen saturation and pulmonary vascular resistance in lambs born after chronic intrauterine hypertension. Median (solid line) and 25th and 75th percentile lines (dashed lines) are shown in the figure. A saturation range of 90% to 97% is associated with the lowest pulmonary vascular resistance. (From Lakshminrusimha et al.[48])

in infants with severe HRF.[60] The benefit appears to be greatest for infants with lower disease severity (oxygenation index [OI] of 15–22), suggesting that earlier administration may prevent lung injury.[61] Importantly, this trial also failed to show a reduction in ECMO utilization in the subset of newborns with idiopathic PPHN, and carried a risk of acute airway obstruction. As such, surfactant should only be considered for infants with significant parenchymal lung disease.

Cardiac Support

Elevated PVR is a hallmark of HRF and PPHN, and high PVR in combination with hypoxia and other factors such as sepsis will often depress cardiac function and systemic blood pressure (Figure 26-3). Patients with HRF and PPHN typically have right-to-left shunting at the level of the ductus arteriosus and foramen ovale. Because extrapulmonary shunting may produce severe hypoxemia, it is often tempting to elevate systemic vascular resistance to reverse the ductal shunt and improve pulmonary blood flow and oxygenation. While this may be temporarily effective, the neonatal right ventricle is poorly adapted to handle an acute elevation in afterload[28,29] and may be at risk of failure if PVR does not also fall. It is also important to remember that an open ductus can also protect the right ventricle by providing a "pop-off" that relieves some of the right ventricular afterload.

Dopamine is a commonly used first-line agent that stimulates dopaminergic, α_1, α_2, and β_1 receptors and will reliably increase systemic blood pressure in neonates. However, the action of dopamine does not appear to be specific to the systemic vascular bed, and some animal studies showed that dopamine will elevate both systemic vascular resistance and PVR.[62] A recent study in newborn lambs indicated the effects of dopamine may depend on whether pulmonary vascular remodeling is present. In normal lambs, dopamine selectively increased systemic arterial pressure without significantly increasing pulmonary arterial pressure. In contrast, in PPHN lambs, the pulmonary circulation was highly sensitive to the vasoconstrictor effects of dopamine, particularly for doses greater than 10 µg/kg/min.[55] Therefore, high doses of dopamine may paradoxically worsen ventricular afterload or decrease oxygen delivery in PPHN.

The addition of dobutamine to dopamine in patients with impaired myocardial function is a commonly used but poorly studied approach in PPHN.[63] Dobutamine acts on both α and β receptors, but its β effects could theoretically drop systemic resistance and favor right-to-left shunt, and high doses may directly increase pulmonary artery pressure.[64] It has also been recently appreciated that higher doses of dobutamine may lead to tachycardia and decreased myocardial

compliance, both of which may diminish diastolic function and restrict ventricular filling in patients with myocardial hypertrophy.

Epinephrine stimulates α_1, α_2, β_1, and β_2 receptors. At lower dose ranges (<0.2 µg/kg/min), epinephrine will preferentially target β_2 receptors that promote vasodilation and improve cardiac contractility. Although low-dose epinephrine can be an excellent drug for infants with PPHN, it may interfere with interpretation of lactate levels because stimulation of β_2 receptors in the liver and skeletal muscle may increase lactate production even in the face of clinical improvement. Norepinephrine, which acts primarily through α receptors, would be expected to carry risks of increased afterload similar to dopamine and is not commonly used for infants with HRF, although 1 report suggested that norepinephrine improved cardiac performance and decreased the pulmonary/systemic pressure ratio in infants with PPHN.[65] The effects of arginine-vasopressin have not been well studied to date, but this drug may be well suited to the treatment of PPHN. For instance, terlipressin decreases pulmonary arterial pressure in animal models of hypoxic vasoconstriction, and recent case reports suggested the same may be true in infants with PPHN.[66]

Left ventricular dysfunction deserves special mention because it is an especially important problem for the infant with HRF. Increased left atrial pressures will produce pulmonary venous hypertension, and left ventricular dysfunction must be reversed prior to administration of pulmonary vasodilators, as they may aggravate pulmonary venous hypertension and cause severe pulmonary edema. An "inodilator" such as milrinone may improve left ventricular function and reduce pulmonary venous hypertension, both of which may improve pulmonary blood flow and oxygenation in infants with refractory HRF. Interestingly, milrinone also inhibits PDE3A activity in vascular smooth muscle, thus increasing cyclic adenosine monophosphate (cAMP) levels and promoting vascular relaxation. Recent studies in animal models and clinical series suggested that milrinone may be especially effective in promoting pulmonary vasodilation and improving oxygenation in PPHN that is poorly responsive to iNO.[67–71] Because of the complex interrelationships, serial echocardiography may be especially helpful if a patient with HRF is poorly responsive to inotropic support.

Pulmonary Vasodilators

Nitric Oxide

Inhaled nitric oxide is well suited for the treatment of PPHN: It is a rapid and potent vasodilator that can be delivered as inhalation therapy to the airspaces adjacent to the pulmonary vascular bed. Several multicenter trials have shown that iNO acutely improves oxygenation and decreases the need for ECMO support in newborns with PPHN and an OI greater than 25, and it remains the only FDA-approved pulmonary vasodilator for PPHN. iNO should be initiated at a dose of 20 ppm as higher doses do not tend to improve the clinical response but will promote increased methemoglobin and nitrogen dioxide levels. In all studies to date, nearly 30% to 40% of infants do not achieve a sustained improvement in oxygenation, and iNO has not been found to reduce mortality or length of hospitalization. Close attention to cardiac function and lung recruitment is essential for achieving the best clinical response. One important trial enrolled infants with respiratory failure that was in an earlier stage of evolution (OI of 15 to 25) and found that iNO did not decrease the incidence of ECMO or death or improve other outcomes, such as chronic lung disease or neurodevelopmental impairment.[72,73] On the other hand, 1 smaller single-center study suggested that delaying iNO initiation until respiratory failure is advanced (OI greater than 40) could increase the length of time on oxygen.[74]

Most infants will require treatment with iNO for less than 5 days. After oxygenation improves and stabilizes, iNO usually can be weaned to 5 ppm without difficulty over a 24-hour period and then gradually weaned to 1 ppm prior to discontinuation. Gradual weaning of inspired oxygen should occur at the same time, and FiO_2 levels of 0.4 to 0.6 generally indicate that discontinuation of iNO will be well tolerated. If NO is stopped abruptly, "rebound" pulmonary hypertension can develop. This interesting phenomenon may occur even if no improvement in oxygenation was observed, can be life-threatening, and has raised questions about whether vascular cells respond to NO by upregulating vasoconstrictor pathways.[43,75,76] Rebound pulmonary hypertension also indicates that care must be taken to ensure continuous delivery of the drug during suctioning, transport, and so on. Infants who remain hypoxemic with evidence of PPHN beyond 5 to 7 days of iNO therapy should be evaluated for an underlying developmental lung abnormality, such as ACD, pulmonary hypoplasia, defects in surfactant metabolism, or progressive lung injury.

Sildenafil

Phosphodiesterases regulate concentrations of cGMP, the critical second messenger that regulates contractility of vascular smooth muscle (Figure 26-5). PDE5 is the primary enzyme responsible for regulating cGMP in the lung and is 1 of the most important regulators of NO-mediated vascular relaxation in the neonatal pulmonary vasculature. PDE5 activity is elevated in fetal lambs with chronic intrauterine pulmonary hypertension,[52,77] and even more striking increases in activity

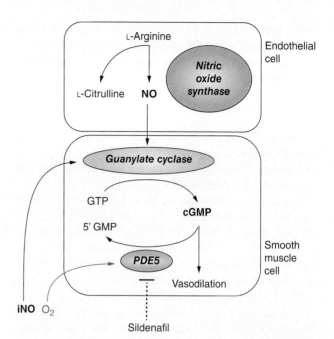

FIGURE 26-5 Nitric oxide (NO) signaling pathway. NO is synthesized by nitric oxide synthase (NOS) from the terminal nitrogen of L-arginine. NO from endogenous sources, or delivered as an inhaled gas, stimulates soluble guanylate cyclase (sGC) to increase intracellular cyclic guanosine monophosphate (cGMP), which produces smooth muscle relaxation. Specific phosphodiesterases (PDEs) such as phosphodiesterase 5 (PDE5) hydrolyze cGMP, thus regulating the intensity and duration of its vascular effects. Hyperoxia stimulates activity and expression of PDE5, thus reducing cGMP accumulation in response to endogenous or exogenous NO. Inhibition of cGMP phosphodiesterases with agents such as sildenafil may enhance pulmonary vasodilation. GMP, guanosine monophosphate; GTP, guanine triphosphate; iNO, inhaled nitric oxide.

occur following birth and initiation of mechanical ventilation and oxygen therapy.[52,78] Increased PDE5 activity would be expected to diminish responses to both endogenous and exogenous NO and could explain why iNO is not sufficient to reverse pulmonary hypertension in some patients.

The first clinical report of the use of the PDE5 inhibitor sildenafil in infants was to facilitate weaning from iNO following corrective surgery for congenital heart disease.[79] The use of enteral sildenafil has also been reported in infants with PPHN, including 1 small, randomized controlled trial that showed a dramatic improvement in oxygenation and survival.[80] An open-label pilot trial of intravenous sildenafil demonstrated improved oxygenation in infants with PPHN.[81] Most of these patients were refractory to iNO, but sildenafil also improved oxygenation in 7 patients who were NO naive. A loading dose (0.4 mg/kg) is generally required, but this should be delivered over a 3-hour interval to avoid hypotension.[82] These promising results indicate that sildenafil is a useful adjunctive therapy for PPHN, but more study is needed to determine whether sildenafil will improve outcomes.

Other Agents

Prostacyclin increases vascular concentrations of cAMP and is a common systemically administered pulmonary vasodilator in children and adults. On the other hand, intravenous PGI_2 is rarely used in neonates because of concerns about systemic hypotension or ventilation-perfusion mismatch.[83] In limited case series reports, inhaled PGI_2 (50–100 ng/kg/min) enhanced oxygenation in infants who were poorly responsive to iNO.[84,85] However, the alkaline solution needed to maintain drug stability could irritate the airway, and delivery of precise doses can be difficult because of loss of medication into the nebulization circuit.[83] Further investigations should focus on preparations specifically designed for inhalation, such as iloprost or treprostinil. These preparations are much more stable than PGI_2 and have longer half-lives that allow for intermittent dosing using ultrasonic nebulizers. Milrinone inhibits PDEs that regulate cAMP concentrations and thus potentiate the cAMP signaling pathway.[83] Interestingly, iNO has been shown to dramatically increase PDE3A levels in preclinical studies, which suggests that, in addition to its inotropic effects, milrinone may enhance the vasodilatory effects of iNO/cGMP signaling.[68]

Endothelin-1 is a potent vasoconstrictor, and its plasma levels are increased in infants with PPHN and appear to correlate with the severity of illness.[86,87] Endothelin blockade enhances pulmonary vasodilation in experimental PPHN,[88] and recent case reports suggested that the endothelin receptor antagonist bosentan improves oxygenation in neonates with PPHN.[89,90] A randomized controlled trial is currently under way to investigate the efficacy of bosentan in infants with severe PPHN.

Extracorporeal Support

Infants who fail to respond to medical management with sustained improvement in oxygenation and good hemodynamic function should receive prompt evaluation for ECMO treatment in a center that is equipped with appropriate equipment and personnel.[91] The OI [calculated as (mean airway pressure * FiO_2 * 100)/PaO_2] is a useful gauge for the severity of disease, with OI greater than 40 often used as an indication for evaluation for ECMO. There are fewer than 200 ECMO centers worldwide, meaning that most patients will need to be transferred to an ECMO center, and each local center should maintain open communication with the closest ECMO center to facilitate safe and

timely transfers. Although ECMO can be lifesaving, it is also costly, labor intensive, and associated with many potential adverse effects, such as intracranial hemorrhage and ligation of the right common carotid artery. ECMO programs should belong to the registry maintained by the Extracorporeal Life Support Organization to facilitate sharing of data and to support decision making for individual patients.

OUTCOME AND FOLLOW-UP

Mortality and Medical Outcomes

Prior to the introduction of ECMO in the late 1980s, the mortality rate for severe HRF was nearly 40%, and the prevalence of major neurologic disability in survivors was estimated at 25% to 60%. ECMO produced remarkable reductions in the mortality rate of PPHN, and based on the recent iNO clinical trials, contemporary mortality rates are approximately 7% to 9%. It is interesting to note that no further improvement in mortality was observed with iNO use, but this is probably because of the availability of ECMO in all the major trials. Furthermore, a trial that enrolled infants with moderate HRF (OI of 15–25) reported lower rates of ECMO, but mortality rates remained in the 7% to 9% range.

Postdischarge medical problems for the first year of life include a greater than 25% incidence of reactive airway disease and a 15% to 20% incidence of significant feeding difficulty or poor weight gain (less than fifth percentile for age).[92] The need for supplemental oxygen decreases substantially by 2 years of age, although the incidence of reactive airway disease and rehospitalization remains high through school age.[93] Adult pulmonary outcomes are not yet known.

Neurodevelopmental Sequelae

Approximately 25% of survivors of neonatal HRF will display significant neurodevelopmental impairment when tested at 12–24 months of age. Similar to the mortality findings discussed, neurodevelopmental disability rates are similar in infants with moderate vs severe HRF,[83] and iNO therapy does not improve developmental outcomes.[73,93] The lack of iNO effect was somewhat unexpected because of the decreased need for ECMO but may indicate that antenatal stress or commonly used therapies such as hyperventilation, hyperoxia, or drugs such as pancuronium play a significant role in adverse outcomes. Serial screening for late sensorineural hearing loss is mandatory, as its prevalence is 6% to 10%, and will persist through school age. Comprehensive follow-up of a large PPHN cohort through school age found a 9% incidence of severe intellectual disability (Full Scale Intelligence Quotient [FSIQ] < 70) and a 7% incidence of moderate intellectual disability (FSIQ of 70 to 84).[93] Worse outcomes were noted in the children with CDH, with a 33% rate of moderate or severe handicap. Comprehensive screening is recommended for all HRF survivors before they enter school to determine if any subtle deficits may predispose them to learning disabilities.

REFERENCES

1. Angus DC, Linde-Swirble WT, Clermont G, Griffin MF, Clark RH. Epidemiology of neonatal respiratory failure in the United States. *Am J Resp Crit Care Med.* 2001;164:1154–1160.

2. Walsh-Sukys MC, Tyson JE, Wright LL, et al. Persistent pulmonary hypertension of the newborn in the era before nitric oxide: practice variation and outcomes. *Pediatrics.* 2000;105:14–20.

3. Mahle WT, Martin GR, Beekman RH 3rd, Morrow WR. Endorsement of Health and Human Services recommendation for pulse oximetry screening for critical congenital heart disease. *Pediatrics.* 2012;129:190–192.

4. Hernandez-Diaz S, Van Marter LJ, Werler MM, Louik C, Mitchell AA. Risk factors for persistent pulmonary hypertension of the newborn. *Pediatrics.* 2007;120:e272–e282.

5. Byers HM, Dagle JM, Klein JM, et al. Variations in CRHR1 are associated with persistent pulmonary hypertension of the newborn. *Pediatr Res.* 2012;71:162–167.

6. Chandrasekar I, Eis A, Konduri GG. Betamethasone attenuates oxidant stress in endothelial cells from fetal lambs with persistent pulmonary hypertension. *Pediatr Res.* 2008;63:67–72.

7. Perez M, Lakshminrusimha S, Wedgwood S, et al. Hydrocortisone normalizes oxygenation and cGMP regulation in lambs with persistent pulmonary hypertension of the newborn. *Am J Physiol Lung Cell Mol Physiol.* 2012;302(6):L595–L603.

8. Shah PS, Hellmann J, Adatia I. Clinical characteristics and follow up of Down syndrome infants without congenital heart disease who presented with persistent pulmonary hypertension of newborn. *J Perinat Med.* 2004;32:168–170.

9. Cua CL, Blankenship A, North AL, Hayes J, Nelin LD. Increased incidence of idiopathic persistent pulmonary hypertension in Down syndrome neonates. *Pediatr Cardiol.* 2007;28:250–254.

10. Weijerman ME, van Furth AM, van der Mooren MD, et al. Prevalence of congenital heart defects and persistent pulmonary hypertension of the neonate with Down syndrome. *Eur J Pediatr.* 2010;169:1195–1199.

11. Southgate WM, Annibale DJ, Hulsey TC, Purohit DM. International experience with trisomy 21 infants placed on extracorporeal membrane oxygenation. *Pediatrics.* 2001;107:549–552.

12. Van Marter LJ, Leviton A, Allred EN. PPHN and smoking and aspirin and nonsteroidal antiinflammatory drug consumption during pregnancy. *Pediatrics.* 1996;97:658–663.

13. Brannon TS, North AJ, Wells LB, Shaul PW. Prostacyclin synthesis in ovine pulmonary artery is developmentally regulated by changes in cyclooxygenase-1 gene expression. *J Clin Invest.* 1994;93:2230–2235.

14. Leffler CW, Hessler JR, Green RS. Mechanism of stimulation of pulmonary prostacyclin synthesis at birth. *Prostaglandins.* 1984;28:877–887.

15. Levin DL, Mills LJ, Weinberg AG. Hemodynamic, pulmonary vascular, and myocardial abnormalities secondary to pharmacologic constriction of the fetal ductus arteriosus. A possible mechanism for persistent pulmonary hypertension and transient tricuspid insufficiency in the newborn infant. *Circulation.* 1979;60:360–364.

16. Levin DL, Fixler DE, Morriss FC, Tyson J. Morphologic analysis of the pulmonary vascular bed in infants exposed in utero to prostaglandin synthetase inhibitors. *J Pediatr.* 1978;92:478–483.

17. Alano MA, Ngougmna E, Ostrea EM Jr, Konduri GG. Analysis of nonsteroidal antiinflammatory drugs in meconium and its relation to persistent pulmonary hypertension of the newborn. *Pediatrics.* 2001;107:519–523.

18. Perkin RM, Levin DL, Clark R. Serum salicylate levels and right-to-left ductus shunts in newborn infants with persistent pulmonary hypertension. *J Pediatr.* 1980;96:721–726.

19. Fornaro E, Li D, Pan J, Belik J. Prenatal exposure to fluoxetine induces fetal pulmonary hypertension in the rat. *Am J Respir Crit Care Med.* 2007;176:1035–1040.

20. Delaney C, Gien J, Grover TR, Roe G, Abman SH. Pulmonary vascular effects of serotonin and selective serotonin reuptake inhibitors in the late-gestation ovine fetus. *Am J Physiol Lung Cell Mol Physiol.* 2011;301:L937–L944.

21. Chambers CD, Hernandez-Diaz S, Van Marter LJ, et al. Selective serotonin-reuptake inhibitors and risk of persistent pulmonary hypertension of the newborn. *N Engl J Med.* 2006;354:579–587.

22. Kallen B, Olausson PO. Maternal use of selective serotonin reuptake inhibitors and persistent pulmonary hypertension of the newborn. *Pharmacoepidemiol Drug Saf.* 2008;17:801–806.

23. Kieler H, Artama M, Engeland A, et al. Selective serotonin reuptake inhibitors during pregnancy and risk of persistent pulmonary hypertension in the newborn: population based cohort study from the five Nordic countries. *BMJ.* 2012;344:d8012.

24. Andrade SE, McPhillips H, Loren D, et al. Antidepressant medication use and risk of persistent pulmonary hypertension of the newborn. *Pharmacoepidemiol Drug Saf.* 2009;18:246–252.

25. Wichman CL, Moore KM, Lang TR, et al. Congenital heart disease associated with selective serotonin reuptake inhibitor use during pregnancy. *Mayo Clin Proc.* 2009;84:23–27.

26. Wilson KL, Zelig CM, Harvey JP, et al. Persistent pulmonary hypertension of the newborn is associated with mode of delivery and not with maternal use of selective serotonin reuptake inhibitors. *Am J Perinatol.* 2011;28:19–24.

27. Occhiogrosso M, Omran SS, Altemus M. Persistent pulmonary hypertension of the newborn and selective serotonin reuptake inhibitors: lessons from clinical and translational studies. *Am J Psychiatry.* 2012;169:134–140.

28. Lapointe A, Barrington KJ. Pulmonary hypertension and the asphyxiated newborn. *J Pediatr.* 2011;158:e19–e24.

29. Reller MD, Morton MJ, Reid DL, Thornburg KL. Fetal lamb ventricles respond differently to filling and arterial pressures and to in utero ventilation. *Pediatr Res.* 1987;22:621–626.

30. Murphy JD, Vawter GF, Reid LM. Pulmonary vascular disease in fatal meconium aspiration. *J Pediatr.* 1984;104:758–762.

31. Villanueva ME, Zaher FM, Svinarich DM, Konduri GG. Decreased gene expression of endothelial nitric oxide synthase in newborns with persistent pulmonary hypertension. *Pediatr Res.* 1998;44:338–343.

32. Zagariya A, Doherty J, Bhat R, et al. Elevated immunoreactive endothelin-1 levels in newborn rabbit lungs after meconium aspiration. *Pediatr Crit Care Med.* 2002;3:297–302.

33. Soukka H, Jalonen J, Kero P, Kaapa P. Endothelin-1, atrial natriuretic peptide and pathophysiology of pulmonary hypertension in porcine meconium aspiration. *Acta Paediatr.* 1998;87:424–428.

34. Soukka H, Viinikka L, Kaapa P. Involvement of thromboxane A2 and prostacyclin in the early pulmonary hypertension after porcine meconium aspiration. *Pediatr Res.* 1998;44:838–842.

35. Tita AT, Landon MB, Spong CY, et al. Timing of elective repeat cesarean delivery at term and neonatal outcomes. *N Engl J Med.* 2009;360:111–120.

CHAPTER 26

36. Tomashek KM, Shapiro-Mendoza CK, Davidoff MJ, Petrini JR. Differences in mortality between late-preterm and term singleton infants in the United States, 1995–2002. *J Pediatr.* 2007;151:450–456. 456.e451.

37. Ramachandrappa A, Rosenberg ES, Wagoner S, Jain L. Morbidity and mortality in late preterm infants with severe hypoxic respiratory failure on extra-corporeal membrane oxygenation. *J Pediatr.* 2011;159:192–198.e193.

38. Shulenin S, Nogee LM, Annilo T, et al. ABCA3 gene mutations in newborns with fatal surfactant deficiency. *N Engl J Med.* 2004;350:1296–1303.

39. Kunig AM, Parker TA, Nogee LM, Abman SH, Kinsella JP. ABCA3 deficiency presenting as persistent pulmonary hypertension of the newborn. *J Pediatr.* 2007;151:322–324.

40. Bishop NB, Stankiewicz P, Steinhorn RH. Alveolar capillary dysplasia. *Am J Respir Crit Care Med.* 2011;184:172–179.

41. Stankiewicz P, Sen P, Bhatt SS, et al. Genomic and genic deletions of the FOX gene cluster on 16q24.1 and inactivating mutations of FOXF1 cause alveolar capillary dysplasia and other malformations. *Am J Hum Genet.* 2009;84:780–791.

42. Cheung PY, Etches PC, Weardon M, et al. Use of plasma lactate to predict early mortality and adverse outcome after neonatal extracorporeal membrane oxygenation: a prospective cohort in early childhood. *Crit Care Med.* 2002;30:2135–2139.

43. Vijlbrief DC, Benders MJ, Kemperman H, van Bel F, de Vries WB. B-type natriuretic peptide and rebound during treatment for persistent pulmonary hypertension. *J Pediatr.* 2012;160:111–115.e111.

44. Vijlbrief DC, Benders MJ, Kemperman H, van Bel F, de Vries WB. Use of cardiac biomarkers in neonatology. *Pediatr Res.* 2012;72:337–343.

45. Reynolds EW, Ellington JG, Vranicar M, Bada HS. Brain-type natriuretic peptide in the diagnosis and management of persistent pulmonary hypertension of the newborn. *Pediatrics.* 2004;114:1297–1304.

46. Kinsella JP, Abman SH. Clinical approach to inhaled NO therapy in the newborn. *J Pediatr.* 2000;136:717–726.

47. Wung JT, James LS, Kilchevsky E, James E. Management of infants with severe respiratory failure and persistence of the fetal circulation, without hyperventilation. *Pediatrics.* 1985;76:488–494.

48. Lakshminrusimha S, Swartz DD, Gugino SF, et al. Oxygen concentration and pulmonary hemodynamics in newborn lambs with pulmonary hypertension. *Pediatr Res.* 2009;66:539–544.

49. Rudolph AM, Yuan S. Response of the pulmonary vasculature to hypoxia and H⁺ ion concentration changes. *J Clin Invest.* 1966;45:399–411.

50. Lakshminrusimha S, Russell JA, Steinhorn RH, et al. Pulmonary hemodynamics in neonatal lambs resuscitated with 21%, 50%, and 100% oxygen. *Pediatr Res.* 2007;62:313–318.

51. Farrow KN, Groh BS, Schumacker PT, et al. Hyperoxia increases phosphodiesterase 5 expression and activity in ovine fetal pulmonary artery smooth muscle cells. *Circ Res.* 2008;102:226–233.

52. Farrow KN, Wedgwood S, Lee KJ, et al. Mitochondrial oxidant stress increases PDE5 activity in persistent pulmonary hypertension of the newborn. *Respir Physiol Neurobiol.* 2010;174:272–281.

53. Lakshminrusimha S, Russell JA, Steinhorn RH, et al. Pulmonary arterial contractility in neonatal lambs increases with 100% oxygen resuscitation. *Pediatr Res.* 2006;59:137–141.

54. Lakshminrusimha S, Steinhorn RH, Wedgwood S, et al. Pulmonary hemodynamics and vascular reactivity in asphyxiated term lambs resuscitated with 21 and 100% oxygen. *J Appl Physiol.* 2011;111:1441–1447.

55. Lakshminrusimha S. The pulmonary circulation in neonatal respiratory failure. *Clin Perinatol.* 2012;39:655–683.

56. Saugstad OD. Resuscitation of newborn infants: from oxygen to room air. *Lancet.* 2010;376(9757):1970–1971.

57. Laffey JG, Engelberts D, Kavanaugh BP. Injurious effects of hypocapnic alkalosis in the isolated lung. *Am J Resp Crit Care Med.* 2000;162:399–405.

58. Ferrara B, Johsnon DE, Chang PN, Thompson TR. Efficacy and neurologic outcome of profound hypocapneic alkalosis for the treatment of persistent pulmonary hypertension in infancy. *J Pediatr.* 1984;105:457–461.

59. Findlay RD, Taeusch W, Walther FJ. Surfactant replacement therapy for meconium aspiration syndrome. *Pediatrics.* 1996;97:48–52.

60. Fliman PJ, deRegnier RA, Kinsella JP, et al. Neonatal extracorporeal life support: impact of new therapies on survival. *J Pediatr.* 2006;148:595–599.

61. Lotze A, Mitchell BR, Bulas DI, et al. Multicenter study of surfactant (beractant) use in the treatment of term infants with severe respiratory failure. Survanta in Term Infants Study Group. *J Pediatr.* 1998;132:40–47.

62. Cheung PY, Barrington KJ. The effects of dopamine and epinephrine on hemodynamics and oxygen metabolism in hypoxic anesthetized piglets. *Crit Care.* 2001;5:158–166.

63. Noori S, Seri I. Neonatal blood pressure support: the use of inotropes, lusitropes, and other vasopressor agents. *Clin Perinatol.* 2012;39:221–238.

64. Cheung PY, Barrington KJ, Bigam D. The hemodynamic effects of dobutamine infusion in the chronically instrumented newborn piglet. *Crit Care Med.* 1999;27:558–564.

65. Tourneux P, Rakza T, Bouissou A, Krim G, Storme L. Pulmonary circulatory effects of norepinephrine in newborn infants with persistent pulmonary hypertension. *J Pediatr.* 2008;153:345–349.

66. Stathopoulos L, Nicaise C, Michel F, et al. Terlipressin as rescue therapy for refractory pulmonary hypertension in a neonate with a congenital diaphragmatic hernia. *J Pediatr Surg.* 2011;46:e19–e21.

67. Chen B, Lakshminrusimha S, Czech L, et al. Regulation of phosphodiesterase 3 in the pulmonary arteries during the perinatal period in sheep. *Pediatr Res.* 2009;66:682–687.

68. Lakshminrusimha S, Porta NF, Farrow KN, et al. Milrinone enhances relaxation to prostacyclin and iloprost in pulmonary arteries isolated from lambs with persistent pulmonary hypertension of the newborn. *Pediatr Crit Care Med.* 2009;10:106–112.

69. McNamara PJ, Laique F, Muang-In S, Whyte HE. Milrinone improves oxygenation in neonates with severe persistent pulmonary hypertension of the newborn. *J Crit Care.* 2006;21:217–222.

70. McNamara PJ, Shivananda SP, Sahni M, Freeman D, Taddio A. Pharmacology of milrinone in neonates with persistent pulmonary hypertension of the newborn (PPHN) and suboptimal response to inhaled nitric oxide. *Pediatr Crit Care Med.* 2013;14(1):74–84.

71. Thelitz S, Oishi P, Sanchez LS, et al. Phosphodiesterase-3 inhibition prevents the increase in pulmonary vascular resistance following inhaled nitric oxide withdrawal in lambs. *Pediatr Crit Care Med.* 2004;5:234–239.

72. Konduri GG, Solimani A, Sokol GM, et al. A randomized trial of early versus standard inhaled nitric oxide therapy in term and near-term newborn infants with hypoxic respiratory failure. *Pediatrics.* 2004;113:559–564.

73. Konduri GG, Vohr B, Robertson C, et al. Early inhaled nitric oxide therapy for term and near-term newborn infants with hypoxic respiratory failure: neurodevelopmental follow-up. *J Pediatr.* 2007;150:235–240. 240.e231.

74. Gonzalez A, Fabres J, D'Apremont I, et al. Randomized controlled trial of early compared with delayed use of inhaled nitric oxide in newborns with a moderate respiratory failure and pulmonary hypertension. *J Perinatol.* 2010;30:420–424.

75. Atz AM, Adatia I, Wessel DL. Rebound pulmonary hypertension after inhalation of nitric oxide. *Ann Thorac Surg.* 1996;62:1759–1764.

76. Lavoie A, Hall JB, Olson DM, Wylam ME. Life-threatening effects of discontinuing inhaled nitric oxide in severe respiratory failure. *Am J Resp Crit Care Med.* 1996;153:1985–1987.

77. Hanson KA, Abman SH, Clarke WR. Elevation of pulmonary PDE5-specific activity in an experimental fetal ovine perinatal pulmonary hypertension model. *Pediatr Res.* 1996;39:334A.

78. Farrow KN, Lakshminrusimha S, Czech L, et al. Superoxide dismutase and inhaled nitric oxide normalize phosphodiesterase 5 expression and activity in neonatal lambs with persistent pulmonary hypertension. *Am J Physiol Lung Cell Mol Physiol.* 2010;299:L109–L116.

79. Atz AM, Wessel DL. Sildenafil ameliorates effects of inhaled nitric oxide withdrawal. *Anesthesiology.* 1999;91:307–310.

80. Baquero H, Soliz A, Neira F, Venegas ME, Sola A. Oral sildenafil in infants with persistent pulmonary hypertension of the newborn: a pilot randomized blinded study. *Pediatrics.* 2006;117:1077–1083.

81. Steinhorn RH, Kinsella JP, Pierce C, et al. Intravenous sildenafil in the treatment of neonates with persistent pulmonary hypertension. *J Pediatr.* 2009;155:841–847.

82. Mukherjee A, Dombi T, Wittke B, Lalonde R. Population pharmacokinetics of sildenafil in term neonates: Evidence of rapid maturation of metabolic clearance in the early postnatal period. *Clin Pharmacol Ther.* 2008;85:56–63.

83. Porta NF, Steinhorn RH. Pulmonary vasodilator therapy in the NICU: inhaled nitric oxide, sildenafil, and other pulmonary vasodilating agents. *Clin Perinatol.* 2012;39:149–164.

84. Kelly LK, Porta NF, Goodman DM, Carroll CL, Steinhorn RH. Inhaled prostacyclin for term infants with persistent pulmonary hypertension refractory to inhaled nitric oxide. *J Pediatr.* 2002;141:830–832.

85. Brown AT, Gillespie JV, Miquel-Verges F, et al. Inhaled epoprostenol therapy for pulmonary hypertension: Improves oxygenation index more consistently in neonates than in older children. *Pulm Circ.* 2012;2:61–66.

86. Keller RL, Tacy TA, Hendricks-Munoz K, et al. Congenital diaphragmatic hernia: endothelin-1, pulmonary hypertension, and disease severity. *Am J Respir Crit Care Med.* 2010;182:555–561.

87. Rosenberg AA, Kennaugh J, Koppenhafer SL, et al. Elevated immunoreactive endothelin-1 levels in newborn infants with persistent pulmonary hypertension. *J Pediatr.* 1993;123:109–114.

88. Abman SH. Role of endothelin receptor antagonists in the treatment of pulmonary arterial hypertension. *Annu Rev Med.* 2009;60:13–23.

89. Nakwan N, Choksuchat D, Saksawad R, Thammachote P. Successful treatment of persistent pulmonary hypertension of the newborn with bosentan. *Acta Paediatr.* 2009;98:1683–1685.

90. Goissen C, Ghyselen L, Tourneux P, et al. Persistent pulmonary hypertension of the newborn with transposition of the great arteries: successful treatment with bosentan. *Eur J Pediatr.* 2008;167:437–440.

91. UK Collaborative ECMO Trial Group. UK collaborative randomised trial of neonatal extracorporeal membrane oxygenation. *Lancet.* 1996;348:75–82.

92. Rosenberg AA, Kennaugh JM, Moreland SG, et al. Longitudinal follow-up of a cohort of newborn infants treated with inhaled nitric oxide for persistent pulmonary hypertension. *J Pediatr.* 1997;131:70–75.

93. Rosenberg AA, Lee NR, Vaver KN, et al. School-age outcomes of newborns treated for persistent pulmonary hypertension. *J Perinatol.* 2010;30:127–134.

CHAPTER 26

Congenital Diaphragmatic Hernia

Björn Frenckner and Krisa Van Meurs

INTRODUCTION

Congenital diaphragmatic hernia (CDH) is a developmental defect in the diaphragm associated with herniation of the abdominal viscera and ipsilateral pulmonary hypoplasia most pronounced on the ipsilateral side. In the current era, approximately 64% of cases in the United States will be diagnosed prenatally by midtrimester ultrasound, and the majority of the remaining newborns will present in the first few hours of life with varying degrees of respiratory distress. Herniation occurring later in gestation is associated with less-significant pulmonary hypoplasia and milder respiratory distress in the newborn period and is often not prenatally diagnosed. Prenatal diagnosis and advances in neonatal care have improved survival to 75% for isolated CDH. However, newborns with more severe CDH and those with other congenital anomalies or chromosomal defects continue to have a significant risk of death and morbidities, such as chronic lung disease, pulmonary hypertension, gastroesophageal reflux, failure to thrive, hernia recurrence, chest wall deformities, scoliosis, and adverse neurodevelopmental outcome.

A voluntary international registry for CDH infants was established in 1995 by Dr. Kevin Lally to collect data on infants with CDH with the goal of advancing the care and outcome for such infants.[1] The CDH Study Group Registry now includes data from over 6000 patients from 93 centers in 10 countries and has provided important information regarding the efficacy of various therapies and predictors of outcome.

EPIDEMIOLOGY

The birth prevalence of CDH in population-based studies ranges from 0.17 to 0.57 per 1000 live births.[2,3] CDH is more frequent in males, with a ratio of 1.4 to 1, and less frequent among African Americans.[3] Associated congenital anomalies occur in 25%, abnormal karyotype in 16%, and genetic syndromes in 5%. Cardiac malformations are the most frequent congenital anomalies seen in the CDH population, followed by anomalies of the ribs and sternum, brain, and spine. Chromosomal abnormalities seen include trisomy 18, 13, 21, 22, and 9 as well as other nontrisomy chromosomal anomalies.[3] Fryns syndrome is the most common autosomal recessive syndrome seen in the CDH population, occurring in 1% to 10%, and is associated with a high mortality rate and extremely poor quality of life.[4]

PATHOPHYSIOLOGY

The diaphragm is formed by fusion of the septum transversum and the pleuroperitoneal folds around the eighth week of gestation, thereby separating the pleural cavities from the peritoneal cavity. Failure of this closure will result in a diaphragmatic hernia, which most frequently appears in the posterior/lateral part, referred to as a Bochdalek hernia. Hernias in the anterior part of the diaphragm, known as Morgagni hernias, are less frequent. About 85% to 90% of diaphragmatic hernias occur on the left side and 10% to

15% on the right side. Bilateral hernias are uncommon (1%-2%). Most commonly, the defect is complete with a direct communication between the pleural and peritoneal cavities. In about 10% to 15%, however, the defect is covered by a thin membrane, or hernia sac, consisting of the pleural and peritoneal membranes.[5,6]

Failure of diaphragmatic closure occurs in the transition between the embryonic phase and the pseudoglandular phase of lung development. Subsequent lung development is characterized by a reduction in the number of airway generations, resulting in a decreased number of terminal bronchioles and alveoli. Alveolar septa are thickened, and the general histologic appearance is that of an immature lung. The number of arterial generations is also decreased, and the pulmonary arteries have a thicker muscle layer than normal. Furthermore, muscularized arterioles are seen more peripheral than in the normal lung. The weight, DNA, and protein content of the lungs are decreased. The pulmonary hypoplasia affects both lungs but is more severe on the ipsilateral side.[5,6]

During fetal life, the lungs are a liquid-producing organ and are the main producers of amniotic fluid. This occurs through an active transport of chloride ions across the alveoli. The ion transporter NKCC-1 (Na^+-K^+-$2Cl^-$ cotransporter) is localized in the basolateral membranes of the alveolar cells and is considered rate limiting for this process. Fetal lung liquid production is essential for lung growth.[7] Around birth, the lungs instead change to become a water-reabsorbing organ, which occurs through active sodium transport through the ion channel ENaC (epithelial sodium channel) in the alveolar cells. In recent experiments, the expression of ENaC in rat lungs with experimentally induced CDH was reduced,[7,8] and in newborns with CDH, ENaC was reduced in tracheal aspirates compared to controls.[9] This fits well with the clinical observation that newborn babies with CDH need more frequent airway suctioning than other newborns and indicates that, in addition to hypoplasticity, CDH lungs are immature.

The etiology of the diaphragmatic defect and the concomitant pulmonary hypoplasia seen with CDH is unknown. Classically, the primary defect was considered to be the failure of diaphragmatic closure, allowing the abdominal viscera to herniate into the thoracic cavity, thereby interfering with pulmonary development and causing pulmonary hypoplasia. Recent data, however, have supported a more complex mechanism mainly based on concomitant abnormalities in diaphragmatic and pulmonary development.[10–12] An interesting combination is the "dual-hit hypothesis"[13] explaining the pathogenesis of pulmonary development by 2 different insults. The first event, caused by unidentified genetic and environmental factors, occurs early in development before normal diaphragmatic closure, and the second insult is caused by interference from the herniated abdominal viscera.

In the fetus, the pulmonary vascular resistance is normally high, and blood is shunted from the pulmonary artery through the ductus arteriosus to the aorta. In healthy babies, the vascular resistance drops after birth, leading to a rapid fall in pulmonary artery pressure, change of direction in ductal shunt, and eventually closure of the ductus. Probably due to decreased cross-sectional area and increased musculature of the pulmonary vascular bed, the pulmonary vascular resistance remains high in patients with CDH and pulmonary hypoplasia, which in severe cases will lead to suprasystemic pressure in the pulmonary artery and to right-to-left shunting at the level of the ductus and foramen ovale. Decreased blood flow through the lungs results in hypoxemia, hypercarbia, and acidosis and initiates a vicious cycle, as hypoxia and acidosis are potent stimuli for the pulmonary artery smooth muscle cells to contract, which further increases pulmonary vascular resistance. Other important stimuli that cause increased pulmonary vascular resistance are hypothermia and stress.[5,14–16] Severe and progressive respiratory failure will ensue unless the vicious cycle is broken.

The majority of newborns with CDH will present within 24 hours after birth with respiratory distress. The more severe the pulmonary hypoplasia is, the earlier the symptoms will present. The most severe cases will need immediate ventilator support and intensive care directly after birth. By contrast, mild cases can occasionally present later with diffuse respiratory symptoms or be diagnosed by incidental chest radiograph. In rare instances, the bowel can be herniated through a small diaphragmatic defect later in life, leading to an incarcerated hernia with classical signs of intestinal obstruction.

DIFFERENTIAL DIAGNOSIS

Most CDH cases are diagnosed prenatally by ultrasound or postnatally by chest radiograph (Figure 27-1). The differential diagnosis includes diaphragmatic eventration, congenital cystic adenomatoid malformation (CCAM), bronchopulmonary sequestration, bronchogenic cysts, bronchial atresia, enteric cysts, and teratomas. Definitive prenatal sonographic diagnosis is made when abdominal organs are present in the fetal chest. Right-sided CDH is more frequently missed or misdiagnosed, as liver can have a similar echogenicity to lung.

DIAGNOSTIC TESTS

Prenatal ultrasonography (US) will identify most fetuses with CDH. Diagnosis has been described as early as the 11th week of gestation, and in many developed

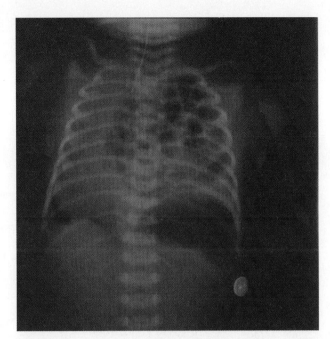

FIGURE 27-1 Postnatal chest radiograph demonstrating a newborn with a left congenital diaphragmatic hernia (CDH) with dilated loops of bowel in the left hemithorax and shift of the heart to the right.

countries, CDH is diagnosed during routine ultrasound screening during the first part of the second trimester. Mediastinal shift and abdominal organs within the thoracic cavity will be the hallmark. In left-sided hernias, the mediastinum is shifted to the right, and intestines, sometimes together with the stomach, and the left liver lobe are found in the thorax. In right-sided hernias, often the liver is herniated. In a strict 4-chamber view, the cross-sectional area of the contralateral lung can be calculated, and when this is divided by the head circumference measured at the standard biparietal view, the lung-to-head ratio (LHR) is obtained. In left-sided hernias, this ratio is felt to correlate with outcome. As the LHR normally varies during gestation, a better prognostic parameter is the observed LHR divided by the expected LHR at that time point of gestation. US can also identify the position of the liver in left-sided hernias, which influences prognosis.[17,18]

Prenatal magnetic resonance imaging (MRI) assessment is used more frequently in the current era. Besides confirming the diagnosis and position of the liver, it allows for a more accurate estimation of lung volume with subsequent correlation to outcome. In cases with equivocal US findings, MRI will also be of value.

Postnatally, classical signs at physical examination of a newborn with CDH are respiratory distress in conjunction with a scaphoid abdomen. In left-sided hernias, the heart sounds will be heard more clearly to the right. Breath sounds, on the other hand, are easily transmitted over the chest and can be fairly symmetrical despite unilateral lung hypoplasia.

The diagnosis of CDH is confirmed by a plain chest radiograph, which demonstrates a mediastinal shift to the contralateral side and bowel loops in the thorax. Air is frequently seen in the esophagus. Rarely, the radiograph can mimic that of a patient with CCAM involving the left lower lobe. However, with CCAM, both diaphragms can be visualized on the lateral view. In doubtful cases, contrast medium given in the gastric tube can be useful. Computed tomographic (CT) scan is rarely needed for diagnosis.

MANAGEMENT

Prenatal Evaluation, Counseling, and Planning for Delivery

Once CDH has been diagnosed in utero, it is important to determine if the defect is isolated or associated with other congenital or chromosomal anomalies known to affect outcome. Level 2 US to screen for other anatomic abnormalities should be performed, and an amniocentesis should be considered to identify chromosomal abnormalities. After this evaluation, the medical team is faced with presenting the various options to the parents. At most centers, the options include pregnancy termination or delivery at a tertiary-level center with multimodality support available. Pregnancy termination may or may not be an option depending on the gestational age at the time of diagnosis. Fetal surgery is now offered to selected prenatally diagnosed infants at a few centers.

Fetal Therapy

In a classical work performed by Harrison et al, a balloon was inserted into 1 pleural cavity in fetal lambs during the third trimester. If the balloon was left inflated, the lambs died soon after birth and had pulmonary hypoplasia much resembling what is seen in human CDH. In another group of sheep, the balloon was instead deflated after 20 days. The lungs were better developed in these lambs compared to the previous group.[19] These preliminary experiments were followed by others in which a diaphragmatic defect was surgically created in fetal lambs during the first trimester. Typical signs of CDH with pulmonary hypoplasia were seen after birth. If the defect was surgically repaired during the second trimester, the pulmonary hypoplasia was significantly less pronounced. Success in large-animal studies led to attempts in humans with prenatally diagnosed CDH.

However, the results from human open repair of CDH in utero were disappointing. Of 14 patients with isolated left-sided CDH, there were only 4 survivors. The major problem was technical, as it was not possible to reduce the herniated liver into the abdomen without kinking the umbilical vein. The investigators concluded that open fetal repair was not possible in the group of left-sided hernia patients with the worst prognosis (ie, those with herniated liver). Following this, a prospective study was conducted in which patients with nonherniated livers were randomized to open fetal repair or conventional therapy. The study failed to demonstrate any difference in outcome. Open fetal repair has since been abandoned.[20]

In contrast to patients with CDH, the lungs of fetuses with rare malformations leading to congenital high-airway obstruction syndrome are hyperplastic. During fetal life, the lungs produce fluid through active excretion of chloride ions, and the lung water escapes through the trachea to the amniotic fluid when the glottis periodically opens. High-airway obstruction prevents escape of fluid and causes an increased airway pressure in the fetus, leading to stimulated lung growth. This has been extensively studied in animal experiments. The hyperplastic lungs exhibit a normal histologic architecture and consist of a larger number of alveoli and capillaries. Experimentally performed tracheal obstruction (TO) in the fetal lamb model enhances lung growth, abdominal viscera are reduced to the abdominal cavity, and postnatal lung function is improved. However, type II pneumocytes producing surfactant are decreased after TO, but this effect may be reduced if TO is discontinued prior to birth.

Tracheal obstruction in human fetuses with CDH was first performed by Harrison et al in 1996[21] by maternal laparotomy, hysterotomy, and open fetal neck dissection. A special technique called the ex utero intrapartum treatment (EXIT) procedure was developed for delivery. The mother was anesthetized and the uterus relaxed. The fetal head and neck were mobilized through a hysterotomy, and the fetal airway was secured before the placental circulation was interrupted. Despite stimulated lung growth, the mortality after TO was initially high, which mainly was attributed to complications from preterm labor.

Improved techniques and the development of smaller laparoscopic instruments enabled the fetal endoscopic (FETENDO) surgical procedure, in which laparoscopic trocars are placed in the uterus under ultrasound guidance. Subsequently, intratracheal balloons were developed, making the technique less invasive and decreasing the risk for tracheal and recurrent laryngeal nerve damage. The results were encouraging in comparison to historical controls, but in a randomized controlled trial, the survival of fetuses with left-sided CDH, liver-up, and LHR less than 1.4 treated with FETENDO was 73%, which was equivalent to the control group.[22]

A technique for complete percutaneous TO has subsequently been developed by Deprest and coworkers[23] using a small fetoscope and intratracheal balloons.

With this method, which currently is practiced in some European centers, it is possible to remove the TO before birth so that the babies can be delivered normally. Again, significantly higher survival rates have been published compared to historical controls, but results from randomized controlled trials have not yet been published.

Postnatal Medical Management

The antenatal diagnosis of CDH allows the immediate neonatal care of infants with CDH to be optimized. Not only are parents able to be educated regarding the diagnosis and treatment, but also the delivery of medical and surgical care can be coordinated between perinatology, neonatology, and pediatric surgical services. Birth at a tertiary center with pediatric surgery, neonatology, and the availability of advanced therapies such as high-frequency ventilation, inhaled nitric oxide, and extracorporeal membrane oxygenation (ECMO) is desirable. Two studies performed by the Canadian Neonatal Network found a survival benefit for newborns with CDH who were delivered at high-volume tertiary centers.[24,25]

Prompt intubation, avoidance of bag-mask ventilation, placement of a nasogastric tube for decompression, and ongoing intensive care provided by medical personnel experienced in the management of CDH is now the norm. Hyperventilation and escalation of peak inspiratory pressure are avoided to decrease the risk of contralateral pneumothorax as well as lung injury secondary to barotrauma. Wung et al first described the use of "gentle ventilation" for infants with persistent pulmonary hypertension of the newborn (PPHN). Kays and colleagues reported improved survival with the use of a lung protective strategy with maximum peak inspiratory pressure (PIP) of 20–24 and a modified strategy for critically ill infants who do not meet the ideal goals.[26] Using this approach involves targeting preductal saturations greater than 85% and PaO_2 (partial pressure of oxygen in arterial blood) greater than 30 as long as the perfusion is adequate as measured by pH and lactate. ECMO was used only if these goals were not attainable. Improved survival, when compared to historical results, has been described by a number of groups using a lung protective strategy with consistent, standardized treatment guidelines, often developed jointly by neonatology, pediatric surgery, ECMO, and respiratory therapy groups.

The use of adjunctive therapies varies. Using the CDH Study Group Registry, surfactant use was found to have no beneficial effect on the need for ECMO, CLD rates, or mortality and anecdotally is associated with acute decompensation in infants with CDH.[27] A randomized controlled trial of inhaled nitric oxide in

53 infants with CDH found no benefit of oxygenation, ECMO use, and mortality.[28] High-frequency ventilation is often used with success as either a primary or a rescue strategy; however, there is no evidence directly supporting its use in the CDH population.

A useful adjunct in the care of the newborn with CDH and is now the most common indication for neonatal ECMO use reported to the Extracorporeal Life Support Organization. Authors vary in their conclusion regarding whether ECMO improves survival.[29-31] The difficulty lies in comparing statistics across differing time periods in patient cohorts with discrepant severity of illness. The CDH Study Group demonstrated a significant survival benefit for newborns with a mortality risk greater than 80% when compared to those who were not treated with ECMO.[31] Timing of CDH repair relative to ECMO also remains controversial. The CDH Study Group found that CDH repair following ECMO was associated with an improved survival when compared to repair on ECMO despite controlling for factors known to influence survival (77% vs 48%, $p = .03$, HR 1.41, 95% CH 1.03–1.92).[32]

Surgical Repair

The surgical repair of the diaphragmatic defect aims to separate the pleural and the 2 cavities and thereby provide space for the thoracic organs and restore prerequisites for normal mechanical breathing. Although this is a fairly simple and uncomplicated surgical procedure, there are still some controversies, such as when the patient should be operated on, when a patch repair is necessary, if and when patients should be operated on during an ECMO course, and if minimally invasive surgery (MIS) is preferable to open surgery.

Historically, it was believed that surgical repair of CDH was an emergent procedure to reduce intrathoracic pressure by reduction of abdominal viscera. However, since the early 1990s, there has been a major paradigm shift, and it is now widely accepted that surgery should not be undertaken until the patient is in a stable condition. There have been no prospective randomized trials supporting this, but numerous case series with delayed surgery and preoperative stabilization have shown improved results compared to earlier strategies. Specific criteria in terms of ventilator settings, requirement for inotropic support, blood pressure, and blood gases to define what constitutes a "stable condition" are lacking, however, and there is wide heterogeneity in practice between centers. Another unresolved issue concerns the few patients who neither meet ECMO criteria nor are stable enough to be operated on. Of almost 4000 patients reported to the CDH Study Group Registry, the majority (67%) were operated at an age greater than 48 hours, and only 5% received surgery within 24 hours.[6] In addition, 18% were never received an operation.

The standard approach for an open repair is a subcostal abdominal incision, although a thoracic approach is also possible. The abdominal viscera are reduced from the thoracic cavity. If there is a hernia sac, this should be removed, and the diaphragm is repaired. A small defect is closed by a primary suture, but a larger defect needs to be closed by a patch. A thoracic drain is rarely necessary. The abdominal cavity is smaller than normal, and abdominal closure can occasionally be troublesome. An abdominal wall patch or silo was needed in 10% of the patients in the CDH Study Group Registry.

Patch repair of the diaphragmatic defect is needed in about half of the cases. The mortality and morbidity are significantly higher if a patch is needed, which mainly reflects the severity of the defect. Several types of material have been used for patches, such as completely synthetic (eg, Gore-Tex®, Marlex®) or biosynthetic biodegradable products (eg, Surgisis®, Permacol®). Autologous muscle flaps have also been used for both primary and secondary repair. A tissue-engineered diaphragm substitute has been proposed as a future possibility.[33] A cone or dome shape of the patch has been suggested to decrease the risk for recurrence as synthetic patches do not grow.[6,16] This shape also increases the volume of the abdominal cavity and may facilitate abdominal closure.

Surgical repair while the patient is on ECMO is a special challenge as these patients are prone to bleeding complications caused by the requirement for systemic heparinization and damage to platelets and coagulation factors by the ECMO circuit. There is no universal agreement on when in the ECMO course the patients should be operated on or if attempts to come off ECMO should be done before surgical repair. These patients will almost invariably need a patch repair because of the strong correlation between the defect size and the severity of the disease. Use of antifibrinolytic agents and fibrin sealants has been suggested, and meticulous surgical hemostasis is of utmost importance to minimize postoperative bleeding. In contrast to other patients, a thoracic drain may be beneficial in patients operated on while on ECMO.

Minimally invasive surgery for CDH can either be from the thorax (thoracoscopic approach) or from the abdomen (laparoscopic approach). The theoretical advantages of MIS are cosmesis, reduced postoperative pain, decreased risk for incisional hernias, and possibly decreased risk for chest wall deformities and adhesive intestinal obstruction. Concerns for using MIS techniques have focused mainly on the risk for hypercarbia and acidosis as well as consequences of elevated abdominal and thoracic cavity pressures during surgery. MIS can be used for both primary repair and patch repair, and case series have shown that it is even feasible in infants who have required preoperative stabilization on ECMO. However, as the technique is comparatively new, long-term experience is limited. The results available today indicate a higher recurrence rate with the MIS approach, and the future role of MIS is yet to be determined.[34,35]

OUTCOME AND FOLLOW-UP

Survival

Historically, the survival rate to discharge from the hospital in infants born with isolated CDH has been around 50%. With improvement in neonatal intensive care as outlined previously, the outcome has improved substantially, and many centers today report survival rates between 80% and 90%.[5,36] The CDH Study Group reports a survival of 75% for isolated CDH for the 1712 patients born after January 1, 2007. The survival for all patients with CDH was 71% (Table 27-1).

The severity of the malformation mainly depends on pulmonary development, and by fetal US and MRI, the size of the fetal lung can be estimated. The LHR is measured by US. The product of the orthogonal diameters of the contralateral lung in a 4-chamber view is divided by the head circumference (all measurements in millimeters). A LHR at 24 to 26 weeks' gestation below 1.0 defines a very poor prognosis, whereas a ratio above 1.4 defines a good prognosis.[17] This measurement is dependent on gestational age, and a more accurate predictor is the observed LHR divided by the expected LHR at the specific gestational age.[18] Other US markers associated with a poor prognosis are early diagnosis (before 25 weeks' gestation), intrathoracic stomach, polyhydramnios, and hydrops. Liver herniation in left-sided hernias also defines a more unfavorable outcome.[37] Three-dimensional US and MRI permit calculation of the combined lung volumes, and when this is related to the expected lung volumes, it can predict outcome in terms of both survival and need for ECMO.

Several postnatal factors have been found to correlate with outcome. Age at clinical presentation reflects the severity of the pulmonary hypoplasia, and early presenters (within hours after birth) have a worse prognosis compared to late presenters. Low birth weight, lower gestational age, low Apgar score at 5 minutes, presence of cardiac or chromosomal anomaly, and large size of the defect all correlate with poor outcome. Patients with right-sided hernia seem to have a slightly worse prognosis compared to patients with left-sided hernia. Newborns with bilateral diaphragmatic hernia have a uniformly poor prognosis. The size of the defect seems to be the major single factor influencing

outcome and is likely a surrogate marker for the degree of pulmonary hypoplasia.[38] Patients whose defect size permits a primary repair have a 95% chance of survival according to the CDH Study Group Registry.

However, the improvements in survival seen during the last decades have not come without a price. Modern neonatal intensive care permits infants with malformations that are more severe to survive, and as a consequence, today there is a significant long-term morbidity in some survivors as well as late mortality.

Chronic Lung Disease

The CDH Study Group Registry reported that approximately 60% of CDH survivors are in room air at 30 days; however, significant respiratory illness persists, including recurrent wheezing and reactive airway disease seen frequently in CDH survivors requiring ECMO. In a Canadian Pediatric Surgery Network study by Safavi and colleagues, only 11% of CDH survivors at 24 months of age and beyond had respiratory complications, and Davis reported that 48% of CDH survivors treated with ECMO had long-term respiratory morbidity with recurrent asthma or wheezing requiring medications, oxygen use following discharge, or need for rehospitalization for respiratory infections.[39,40] Respiratory complications in CDH survivors appear to correspond to the severity of the underlying pulmonary hypoplasia.

Pulmonary Hypertension

Pulmonary hypertension related to the decreased cross-sectional area of the pulmonary vascular bed and reactive pulmonary vasoconstriction is a significant problem in the immediate newborn period for many infants with CDH, but typically improves with or without specific therapy. In a small number of infants, symptomatic or asymptomatic pulmonary hypertension is evident on echocardiography at discharge and beyond, resulting in late morbidity and mortality. Keller et al. found that the severity of pulmonary hypertension and outcome can be predicted from endothelin-1 levels at 1 and 2 weeks of age. They concluded that critical changes in the pulmonary parenchyma and vascular bed during this period result in irrecoverable arrest of growth and development, reflecting biochemical and structural differences.[41] Kinsella found that 20% of infants with CDH had suprasystemic pulmonary pressures prior to extubation while on inhaled nitric oxide and treated them with nasal cannula nitric oxide.[42] Often, the severity of the pulmonary hypertension was disproportionate to the respiratory status at the time of extubation, with marked elevations in pulmonary arterial pressure despite low FiO_2 and adequate oxygenation.

Table 27-1 Characteristics of Patients Reported to the CDH Study Group Registry over Three Time Periods

	1995–1999 (n = 1780)	2000–2004 (n = 1854)	2005–2011 (n = 2900)	All (n = 6534)
Inborn, n (%)	615 (34.8)	722 (38.9)	1265 (43.7)	2602 (39.9)
Male, n (%)	1056 (59.7)	1069 (57.8)	1784 (61.6)	3909 (60.0)
Race, n (%)				
White	1293 (72.6)	1265 (68.2)	1745 (60.2)	4303 (65.9)
Black	149 (8.4)	134 (7.3)	206 (7.1)	489 (7.5)
Hispanic	175 (9.8)	204 (11.0)	321 (11.1)	700 (10.7)
Asian	22 (1.2)	131 (7.1)	196 (6.8)	349 (5.3)
Native American	9 (0.5)	18 (0.9)	22 (0.7)	49 (0.7)
Other/unknown	132 (7.4)	102 (5.5)	410 (14.1)	644 (9.9)
Birth weight, g (± SD)	3000 ± 645	2952 ± 652	2952 ± 642	2965 ± 645
GA weeks (± SD)	37.9 ± 2.5	37.6 ± 2.5	37.6 ± 2.4	37.7 ± 2.5
Prenatal diagnosis, n (%)	826 (46.7)	1042 (56.4)	1885 (65.2)	3753 (57.7)
Side, n (%)				
Left	1403 (79.6)	1485 (80.6)	2406 (83.3)	5294 (81.5)
Right	345 (19.5)	331 (17.9)	462 (16.0)	1138 (17.5)
Bilateral	15 (0.9)	27 (1.5)	20 (0.7)	62 (1.0)
Isolated, n (%)	1605 (90.2)	1636 (88.2)	2558 (88.2)	5799 (88.8)
Repaired, n (%)	1473 (82.8)	1528 (82.4)	2391 (82.3)	5392 (82.5)
ECMO, n (%)	99 (15.4)	34 (6.1)	53 (6.6)	186 (9.3)
Repair prior to ECMO	298 (46.4)	248 (44.3)	396 (49.2)	942 (47.0)
Repair on ECMO	156 (24.3)	189 (33.8)	201 (25.0)	546 (27.2)
Repair after ECMO	89 (13.9)	89 (15.8)	154 (19.2)	332 (16.6)
ECMO but no repair				
Survival, n (%)				
All	1204 (67.6)	1265 (68.2)	2030 (70.0)	4499 (68.9)
Isolated CDH	1149 (71.6)	1183 (72.3)	1905 (74.5)	4237 (73.1)
ECMO	338 (52.6)	281 (50.2)	383 (47.6)	1002 (50.0)

Abbreviations: CDH, congenital diaphragmatic hernia; ECMO, extracorporeal membrane oxygenation; GA, gestational age.

Growth and Gastroesophageal Reflux

Although rarely recognized before 1990, a significant number of CDH survivors show evidence of failure to thrive with growth retardation.[43,44] Several factors might contribute to this finding. Chronic lung disease and pulmonary hypoplasia lead to increased breathing effort with increased caloric demand. Gastroesophageal reflux disease (GERD) and oral aversion result in inadequate nutrition, and even if adequate caloric intake is secured by tube or gastrostomy feeding, growth retardation remains a problem. ECMO and need for oxygen at discharge are predictive for failure to thrive. Half of ECMO-treated CDH survivors had a weight below the fifth percentile at 2 years of age.[45] The management of these patients is difficult, and there is no general consensus regarding the best strategy.

The incidence of GERD depends on the diagnostic methods used and has been reported to be from 20% to 72%. Several reasons for GERD have been proposed. Increased intra-abdominal pressure in combination with reduced intrathoracic pressure increase the abdominothoracic pressure gradient and could predispose for GERD. The malformation involves an underdeveloped diaphragmatic crus, and the surgical repair may cause tension and further distortion of the anatomy, adversely affecting the angle of His. Furthermore, in many newborns with CDH, the esophagus is dilated and ectactic, which may be caused by a primary disturbance of its motility. GERD seems to be more common in patients who require ECMO and patch repair (ie, in patients with the most severe initial malformations).[46] There is no consensus in the literature regarding indications for surgical treatment of GERD in patients with CDH, and long-term results are lacking.

Other Gastrointestinal Problems

Intestinal malrotation occurs in most patients with CDH and should be considered part of the malformation because the intrathoracic location of the intestines prevents the normal fixation of the bowel during fetal life. Intestinal obstruction is a common problem and has been reported to occur in 10% to 20% of the patients.[46] This is far more common than after other neonatal abdominal procedures and is in a similar range as patients operated for gastroschisis. The cause of bowel obstruction is mostly midgut volvulus or bowel adhesions. The latter may be enhanced by prolonged intestinal paralysis in the critical neonatal period and by increased intra-abdominal pressure causing bowel ischemia after the initial diaphragmatic repair.[47]

Recurrent Hernia

The reported incidence of recurrence of the diaphragmatic hernia varies from 3% to 50%.[48,49] It seems to be most common in patients requiring patch repair and in ECMO-treated patients.[50] The recurrence can present from months to years after the initial repair. The most common presentation is gastrointestinal complaints with vomiting and signs of partial intestinal obstruction followed by pulmonary problems. A significant number of patients with recurrence are asymptomatic and are discovered by routine follow-up chest radiograph.[50]

Chest Asymmetry and Scoliosis

Chest wall asymmetry, usually in the form of a pectus excavatum, is commonly described in the follow-up of patients with CDH. However, surgical intervention for this is rarely necessary. The true incidence cannot be reliably assessed before cessation of growth,[43] but varies from 16% to 48%.[46] It has been suggested that the pectus excavatum is caused by the fact that the lung volume, and thereby also the thoracic cavity, is smaller than normal. The increased work of breathing in combination with the compliant cartilaginous anterior wall of the chest may also contribute.

Scoliosis has been reported in 5% to 27% of CDH survivors at follow-up.[43,44] The risk of scoliosis is greater in patients with large defects and patch repair.[47,51] Tension of the diaphragmatic repair is felt to be the cause. In general, however, the spinal defect is mild and rarely requires surgical intervention.

Neurodevelopmental Outcome

Poor neurodevelopmental outcome is one of the most common significant morbidities seen in CDH survivors. Unfortunately, there are relatively few studies that reported long-term or longitudinal neurodevelopmental and functional outcomes of population-based cohorts and allow a comprehensive view of the full range of outcomes of CDH survivors. In addition, the majority of studies have been performed on CDH infants less than 36 months of age; testing at this age is not predictive of long-term outcome and functioning. Although the rates of central nervous system sequelae such as seizures, cerebral palsy, and stroke are low, there is a significant incidence of fine and gross motor skill abnormalities, behavioral problems, executive functioning issues, learning disabilities, and cognitive impairment. In general, neurocognitive outcomes were normal in approximately 50% of CDH survivors, suspect in 25%, and abnormal in 25%; neuromotor scores were typically lower, often due to persistent hypotonia.[39,40,45,52,53] Few later school aged and longitudinal studies are published, and the rate of abnormal outcome is similar to studies at earlier ages.

Hearing loss—specifically, delayed-onset, high-frequency sensorineural hearing loss—is seen commonly in CDH survivors despite normal hearing screens in the newborn period. The cause remains unknown, and its occurrence has been associated with high pH, longer duration of mechanical ventilation and hyperoxia, and the use of drugs such as aminoglycosides, vancomycin, loop diuretics, and muscle relaxants. Given the important impact of hearing impairment on neurodevelopmental outcome, frequent audiologic evaluation is critical in this patient population starting at 6 months of age.

Recommended Clinical Follow-Up

The morbidity of CDH survivors varies a great deal. Mild cases have an excellent chance of being perfectly healthy after initial discharge from hospital, whereas patients with a severe malformation can exhibit a significant morbidity throughout childhood and require multiple interventions. Early recognition of problems is of great importance to ameliorate their consequences. All patients with CDH should therefore be followed in the clinic at intervals depending on the severity of the malformation. General health, respiratory function, cardiac function, gastrointestinal function, nutritional status, hearing, neurological status, and musculoskeletal function should be evaluated. Ideally, the patients should be seen in a multidisciplinary clinic with availability of all required specialists.[43,47,54] The American Academy of Pediatrics has recommended a detailed schedule (Table 27-2) for clinical follow-up.[49]

Table 27-2 Suggested Postdischarge Follow-Up for Congenital Diaphragmatic Hernia (CDH) Survivors [a]

	Before Discharge	1–3 months	4–6 months	9–12 months	15–18 months	Annual
Weight, length, head circumference	×	×	×	×	×	×
Chest radiograph	×	If patched	If patched	If patched	If patched	If patched
Pulmonary function testing			If indicated		If indicated	If indicated
Childhood immunizations	As indicated throughout childhood	×	×	×	×	×
RSV prophylaxis	RVS season during first 2 years	×	×	×	×	×
Echocardiogram and cardiology follow-up	×	If previously abnormal or on oxygen	If previously abnormal or on oxygen	If previously abnormal or on oxygen	If previously abnormal or on oxygen	If previously abnormal or on oxygen
Head CT or MRI	If (1) abnormal finding on head ultrasound; (2) seizures/abnormal neurologic findings: or (3) ECMO or patch repair	As indicated	As indicated	As indicated	As indicated	As indicated
Audiology	Auditory brainstem evoked response or otoacoustic emissions screen	×	×	×	×	Every 6 months to age 3 years, then annually to age 5 years
Developmental screening evaluation	×		×	×		Annually to age 5 years
Neurodevelopmental evaluation	×			×		Annually to age 5 years
Assessment oral feeding problems	×	×	If oral feeding problems	If oral feeding problems	If oral feeding problems	If oral feeding problems
Upper GI, pH probe, gastric scintiscan	Consider all patients	If symptoms	If symptoms	Consider all patients	If symptoms	If symptoms
Esophagoscopy		If symptoms	If symptoms	If symptoms	If symptoms	If symptoms
Scoliosis and chest wall deformity screening (physical examination, chest radiograph and/or CT)				×		×

[a]Reproduced with permission from American Academy of Pediatrics Section on Surgery; American Academy of Pediatrics Committee on Fetus and Newborn, Lally KP, Engle W: Postdischarge follow-up of infants with congenital diaphragmatic hernia. Pediatrics. 2008;121(3):627–632.

REFERENCES

1. Tsai K, Lally KP. The congenital diaphragmatic hernia study group: a voluntary international registry. *Sem Ped Surg.* 2008;17:90–97.

2. Skari H, Bjornland K, Haugen G, Egeland T, Emblem R. Congenital diaphragmatic hernia: a meta-analysis of mortality factors. *J Pediatr Surg.* 2000;35:1187–1197.

3. Yang W, Carmichael SL, Harris JA, et al. Epidemiologic characteristics of congenital diaphragmatic hernia among 2.5 million California births, 1989–1997. *Birth Defects Rese.* 2006;76:170–174.

4. The Congenital Diaphragmatic Hernia Study Group. Frynns syndrome and congenital diaphragmatic hernia. *J Pediatr Surg.* 2002;37;1685–1687.

5. Muratore CS, Wilson JM. Congenital diaphragmatic hernia: where are we and where do we go from here? *Semin Perinatol.* 2000;24:418–428.

6. Kotecha S, Barbato A, Bush A, et al. European Respiratory Society Task Force on Congenital Diaphragmatic Hernia. *Eur Respir J.* 2012;39:820–829.

7. Ringman A, Zelenina M, Eklof AC, et al. NKCC-1 and ENaC are down-regulated in nitrofen-induced hypoplastic lungs with congenital diaphragmatic hernia. *Pediatr Surg Int.* 2008;24:993–1000.

8. Folkesson HG, Chapin CJ, Beard LL, et al. Congenital diaphragmatic hernia prevents absorption of distal air space fluid in late-gestation rat fetuses. *Am J Physiol Lung Cell Mol Physiol.* 2006;290:L478–L484.

9. Ringman Uggla A, von Schewelov K, Zelenina M, et al. Low pulmonary expression of epithelial Na(+) channel and Na(+), K(+)-ATPase in newborn infants with congenital diaphragmatic hernia. *Neonatology.* 2011;99:14–22.

10. Rottier R, Tibboel D. Fetal lung and diaphragm development in congenital diaphragmatic hernia. *Semin Perinatol.* 2005;29:86–93.

11. Ackerman KG, Greer JJ. Development of the diaphragm and genetic mouse models of diaphragmatic defects. *Am J Med Genet C Semin Med Genet.* 2007;145C:109–116.

12. Clugston RD, Greer JJ. Diaphragm development and congenital diaphragmatic hernia. *Semin Pediatr Surg.* 2007;16:94–100.

13. Keijzer R, Liu J, Deimling J, et al. Dual-hit hypothesis explains pulmonary hypoplasia in the nitrofen model of congenital diaphragmatic hernia. *Am J Pathol.* 2000;156:1299–1306.

14. Bosenberg AT, Brown RA. Management of congenital diaphragmatic hernia. *Curr Opin Anaesthesiol.* 2008;21:323–331.

15. Hartnett KS. Congenital diaphragmatic hernia: advanced physiology and care concepts. *Adv Neonatal Care.* 2008;8:107–115.

16. Waag KL, Loff S, Zahn K, et al. Congenital diaphragmatic hernia: a modern day approach. *Semin Pediatr Surg.* 2008;17:244–254.

17. Graham G, Devine PC. Antenatal diagnosis of congenital diaphragmatic hernia. *Semin Perinatol.* 2005;29:69–76.

18. Claus F, Sandaite I, DeKoninck P, et al. Prenatal anatomical imaging in fetuses with congenital diaphragmatic hernia. *Fetal Diagn Ther.* 2011;29:88–100.

19. Harrison MR, Bressack MA, Churg AM, et al. Correction of congenital diaphragmatic hernia in utero. II. Simulated correction permits fetal lung growth with survival at birth. *Surgery.* 1980;88:260–268.

20. Jelin E, Lee H. Tracheal occlusion for fetal congenital diaphragmatic hernia: the US experience. *Clin Perinatol.* 2009;36: 349–361. ix.

21. Harrison MR, Adzick NS, Flake AW, et al. Correction of congenital diaphragmatic hernia in utero VIII: response of the hypoplastic lung to tracheal occlusion. *J Pediatr Surg.* 1996;31:1339–1348.

22. Harrison MR, Keller RL, Hawgood SB, et al. A randomized trial of fetal endoscopic tracheal occlusion for severe fetal congenital diaphragmatic hernia. *N Engl J Med.* 2003;349:1916–1924.

23. Deprest J, Gratacos E, Nicolaides KH. Fetoscopic tracheal occlusion (FETO) for severe congenital diaphragmatic hernia: evolution of a technique and preliminary results. *Ultrasound Obstet Gynecol.* 2004;24:121–126.

24. Javid PJ, Jaksic T, Skarsgard ED, et al. Survival rate in congenital diaphragmatic hernia: the experience of the Canadian Neonatal Network. *J Pediatr Surg.* 2004;39:657–660.

25. Nasr A, Langer JC. Influence of location of delivery on outcome in neonates with congenital diaphragmatic hernia. *J Pediatr Surg.* 2011;46:814–816.

26. Kays DW, Langham MR, Ledbetter DJ, Talbert JL. Detrimental effects of standard medical therapy in congenital diaphragmatic hernia. *Ann Surg.* 1999;230:340–351.

27. Van Meurs K and the Congenital Diaphragmatic Hernia Study Group. Is surfactant therapy beneficial in the treatment of the term newborn infant with congenital diaphragmatic hernia? *J Pediatr.* 2004;145:312–316.

28. The Neonatal Inhaled Nitric Oxide Study Group (NINOS). Inhaled nitric oxide and hypoxic respiratory failure in infants with congenital diaphragmatic hernia. *Pediatrics.* 1997;99:838–845.

29. Van Meurs KP, Newman KD, Anderson KD, Short BL. Effect of extracorporeal membrane oxygenation on survival of infants with congenital diaphragmatic hernia. *J Pediatr.* 1990: 117:954–960.

30. Wung JT, Sahni R, Moffitt ST, Lipsitz E, Stolar CJ. Congenital diaphragmatic hernia: survival treated with very delayed surgery, spontaneous respiration, and no chest tube. *J Pediatr Surg.* 1995;30(3):406–409.

31. The Congenital Diaphragmatic Hernia Study Group. Does extracorporeal membrane oxygenation improve survival in neonates with congenital diaphragmatic hernia? *J Pediatr Surg.* 1999;34:720–725.

32. The Congenital Diaphragmatic Hernia Study Group. Congenital diaphragmatic hernia requiring extracorporeal membrane oxygenation: does timing of repair matter? *J Pediatr Surg.* 2009;44:1165–1172.

33. Tsao K, Lally KP. Surgical management of the newborn with congenital diaphragmatic hernia. *Fetal Diagn Ther.* 2011;29:46–54.

34. Lansdale N, Alam S, Losty PD, et al. Neonatal endosurgical congenital diaphragmatic hernia repair: a systematic review and meta-analysis. *Ann Surg.* 2010;252:20–26.

35. Gander JW, Fisher JC, Gross ER, et al. Early recurrence of congenital diaphragmatic hernia is higher after thoracoscopic than open repair: a single institutional study. *J Pediatr Surg.* 2011;46:1303–1308.

36. Logan JW, Rice HE, Goldberg RN, et al. Congenital diaphragmatic hernia: a systematic review and summary of best-evidence practice strategies. *J Perinatol.* 2007;27:535–549.

37. Mullassery D, Ba'ath ME, Jesudason EC, et al. Value of liver herniation in prediction of outcome in fetal congenital diaphragmatic hernia: a systematic review and meta-analysis. *Ultrasound Obstet Gynecol.* 2010;35:609–614.

38. Lally KP, Lally PA, Lasky RE, et al. Defect size determines survival in infants with congenital diaphragmatic hernia. *Pediatrics.* 2007;120:e651–e657.

39. Safavi A, Synnes AR, O'Brien K, et al. Multi-institutional follow-up of patients with congenital diaphragmatic hernia reveals severe disability and variations in practice. *J Pediatr Surg.* 2012;47:836–841.

40. Davis PJ, Firmin RK, Manktelow B, et al. Long-term outcome following extracorporeal membrane oxygenation for congenital diaphragmatic hernia: the UK experience. *J Pediatr.* 2004;144:309–315.

41. Keller RL, Tacy TA, Hendricks-Munoz K, et al. Congenital diaphragmatic hernia: Endothelin-1, pulmonary hypertension, and disease severity. *Am J Respir Crit Care Med.* 2010;182:555–561.

42. Kinsella JP, Parker TA, Ivy DD, Abman SH. Noninvasive delivery of inhaled nitric oxide therapy for late pulmonary hypertension in newborn infants with congenital diaphragmatic hernia. *J Pediatr.* 2003;142:397–401.

43. West SD, Wilson JM. Follow up of infants with congenital diaphragmatic hernia. *Semin Perinatol.* 2005;29:129–133.

44. Jaillard SM, Pierrat V, Dubois A, et al. Outcome at 2 years of infants with congenital diaphragmatic hernia: a population-based study. *Ann Thorac Surg.* 2003;75:250–256.

45. Van Meurs KP, Robbins ST, Reed VL, et al. Congenital diaphragmatic hernia: long-term outcome in neonates treated with extracorporeal membrane oxygenation. *J Pediatr.* 1993;122:893–899.

46. Peetsold MG, Heij HA, Kneepkens CM, et al. The long-term follow-up of patients with a congenital diaphragmatic hernia: a broad spectrum of morbidity. *Pediatr Surg Int.* 2009;25:1-17.

47. Bagolan P, Morini F. Long-term follow up of infants with congenital diaphragmatic hernia. *Semin Pediatr Surg.* 2007;16:134–144.

48. Rowe DH, Stolar CJ. Recurrent diaphragmatic hernia. *Semin Pediatr Surg.* 2003;12:107-109.

49. Lally KP, Engle W. Post-discharge follow-up of infants with congenital diaphragmatic hernia. *Pediatrics.* 2008;121:627–632.

50. Moss RL, Chen CM, Harrison MR. Prosthetic patch durability in congenital diaphragmatic hernia: a long-term follow-up study. *J Pediatr Surg.* 2001;36:152–154.

51. Jancelewicz T, Vu LT, Keller RL, et al. Long-term surgical outcomes in congenital diaphragmatic hernia: observations from a single institution. *J Pediatr Surg.* 2010;45:155–160.

52. Danzer E, Hedrick HL. Neurodevelopmental and neurofunctional outcomes in children with congenital diaphragmatic hernia. *Early Hum Dev.* 2011;87:625–632.

53. Frisk V, Jakobson LS, Unger S, Trachsel D, O'Brien K. Long-term neurodevelopmental outcomes of congenital diaphragmatic hernia survivors not treated with extracorporeal membrane oxygenation. *J Pediatr Surg.* 2011;46:1309–1318.

54. Chiu P, Hedrick HL. Postnatal management and long-term outcome for survivors with congenital diaphragmatic hernia. *Prenat Diagn.* 2008;28:592–603.

28 Cystic Lung Lesions

Erik D. Skarsgard

INTRODUCTION

Congenital cystic lung disease covers a spectrum of lung malformations that include congenital cystic adenomatoid malformation (CCAM; which is also defined by the term *congenital pulmonary airway malformation* or CPAM), bronchopulmonary sequestration (BPS), congenital lobar emphysema (CLE), and bronchogenic cysts. The intricate process of lung development begins at about 4 weeks' gestation and consists of 6 discrete phases: (1) the embryonic stage (4–7 weeks' gestation); (2) the pseudoglandular stage (5–17 weeks' gestation); (3) the canalicular stage (16- to 26-weeks' gestation); (4) the saccular stage (24- to 38-weeks' gestation); (5) the alveolar stage (36-weeks' gestation to 2 years of age); and (6) microvascular maturation (birth to 2–3 years of age).[1]

A key stage in the development of congenital cystic lung disease appears to be the pseudoglandular stage, when branching morphogenesis occurs. Branching morphogenesis results in the formation of the conductive airway system, which is an essential prerequisite to alveolization. Lung development is influenced at all stages by the spatial and temporal distribution of a variety of signaling molecules and their receptors and by the positive and negative control of signaling by paracrine, autocrine, and endocrine mechanisms. It is likely that a developmental arrest or maturation disorder in the pseudoglandular stage is responsible for the vast majority of developmental lung anomalies, and although many of the responsible genes and gene products have been identified, the precise mechanisms involved are unknown.[2-5] Analysis of resected fetal lung lesions have shown an imbalance between cellular proliferation and apoptosis, suggesting a loss of growth regulation.[6]

Although there is a tendency to compartmentalize congenital cystic lung disease into discrete pathological conditions, there is considerable overlap between conditions. An example is the shared features of CCAM and BPS within so-called hybrid lesions, which exhibit the histological features of CCAM combined with the anomalous vascular anatomy of BPS.

Epidemiology of Neonatal Cystic Lung Lesions

There are few data on the epidemiology of cystic lung lesions. One frequently quoted study using population-based data estimated the incidence of CCAM to be 1 per 25,000 to 35,000 pregnancies.[7] Most cystic lung lesions occur with equal frequency in the right and left lungs and have a slight preponderance for males.[8]

Differential Diagnosis

The differential diagnosis of cystic lung lesions in an infant include CPAM, BPS, CLE, bronchogenic cysts, as well as congenital diaphragmatic hernia (CDH) and a variety of congenital and acquired cystic lesions of the lung and mediastinum. Some of the acquired cystic lung conditions include pulmonary interstitial emphysema, postinfectious pulmonary cysts, lung abscesses, and rare tumors, including bronchioloalveolar carcinoma (BAC) and pleuropulmonary blastoma (PPB).

CONGENITAL CYSTIC ADENOMATOID MALFORMATION AND CONGENITAL PULMONARY AIRWAY MALFORMATION

The CCAM and CPAM cystic lung hamartomas are associated with a proliferative increase in terminal bronchioles relative to alveoli. The result is an intrapulmonary mass that is usually confined to 1 lobe of the lung. The nomenclature and descriptive classification of these lesions has changed significantly since the original description in 1949 of a "congenital adenomatoid lesion" of the lung.[9] In 1977, Stocker et al proposed a classification scheme (types I, II, and III) based on the clinicopathologic attributes of CCAMs.[10] The most common type (type I) accounts for over 50% of cases and is characterized by single or multiple cysts larger than 2 cm. Based on the increased frequency of prenatal diagnosis and the realization that the natural history of a fetal lung lesion could be predicted by its sonographic appearance, Adzick et al proposed a classification system that defined CCAMs as either microcystic (appearing solid or "echogenic" on ultrasound and more often associated with fetal hydrops) or macrocystic, with definitive cysts larger than 5 mm in diameter.[11] More recently, the term *congenital pulmonary airway malformation* has been coined that provides a unifying classification of lung malformations into CPAM 0, 1, 2, 3, and 4 based on the site of suspected malformation development along the tracheobronchial/acinar structural unit pathway.[12] In this classification system, the vast majority of malformations are CPAM 1 (Figure 28-1), implying that these are developmentally derived from the bronchial or bronchiolar units. The relationship between these 2 nomenclature systems is summarized in Table 28-1.

CPAM 1 accounts for 60% to 65% of postnatal cases.[12] It arises from a single lobe (Figure 28-2) and consists of single or multiple large, intercommunicating cysts that are surrounded by smaller cysts and atelectatic normal lung. The cyst walls are thin and lined by an epithelium that varies from low cuboidal to ciliated pseudostratified columnar epithelium. The walls contain fibromuscular connective tissue that in some areas forms a muscular wall resembling bronchi. Cartilage islands may be present within the walls along with arteries and veins, which are classically derived from the pulmonary circulation. There are rare case reports of adenocarcinoma developing in association with a CPAM 1, suggesting the possibility of a preinvasive lesion that becomes cancerous over time.[13]

CPAM 2 lesions, which account for about 20% of postnatally diagnosed cases, contain numerous smaller cysts (less than 2 cm), which appear as "back-to-back" bronchiole-like structures lined by a simple cuboidal to columnar epithelium. A key feature of CPAM 2 lesions is their association in 50% of cases with other malformations, including CDH, cardiovascular abnormalities, and rarely lethal malformations such as bilateral renal agenesis or dysplasia.[14,15]

CPAM 3 represents the microcystic variant, which is now recognized antenatally as being at greatest risk for the development of hydrops.[16] The microscopic appearance is that of irregular bronchiole-like structures lined by cuboidal epithelium.

CPAM 4 accounts for about 10% of cases and results when disordered acinar development produces a hamartomatous cyst of variable size in the lung periphery. The cysts are lined by types 1 and 2 alveolar cells.[12] The clinical presentation may be variable (asymptomatic, pneumonia, spontaneous pneumothorax).

An area of controversy has been an understanding of the relationship between CPAM and PPB. The clinical, radiologic, and even histologic overlap between cystic PPB and CPAM 4 is well recognized, and for a time it was thought that PPB resulted from "malignant transformation" of a CPAM. However, that view has been discounted by thorough histological characterization and subtyping of PPB,[17] and it is now accepted that CPAM and PPB represent pathologically discrete entities.[18]

Fetal Diagnosis and Outcome

With advances in ultrasound technology and widespread screening, the detection of fetal lung lesions has become increasingly common. The combination of high-resolution ultrasound, vascular Doppler, and magnetic resonance imaging (MRI) usually results in an accurate fetal lung anomaly diagnosis. A suspected fetal lung anomaly should prompt additional diagnostic testing, including echocardiography and amniocentesis for karyotyping, to exclude significant associated cardiovascular or chromosomal malformations.

Once a fetal lung malformation has been identified, it should be closely monitored because its behavior may be difficult to predict. It has been reported that approximately 40% of CCAMs will grow rapidly between 18 and 26 weeks, leading to mediastinal compression and the development of fetal hydrops.[19] Conversely, the phenomenon of spontaneous regression, regardless of cyst morphology (ie, macro vs microcystic), is well documented.[7,20–24] Whether CCAMs can permanently spontaneously resolve is debatable. Most apparently vanishing fetal CCAMs are detectable on postnatal computed tomographic (CT) scans[25,26]; however, the phenomenon of postnatal disappearance documented by CT scan has been reported.[27]

Fetal hydrops occurs when the rapidly growing lung mass causes vena caval compression and cardiac failure. Polyhydramnios, pleural effusions and ascites,

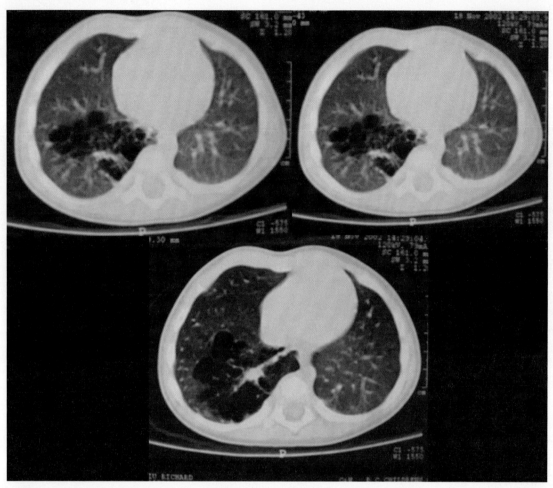

FIGURE 28-1 Computed tomographic scan showing macrocystic, multilocular congenital pulmonary airway malformation type 1.

and subcutaneous edema are all signs of fetal hydrops. The development of hydrops portends a poor prognosis for the fetus and may be an indication for fetal intervention, including catheter drainage for macrocystic disease or fetal thoracotomy and lung resection for microcystic disease. The latter requires multidisciplinary expertise in fetomaternal care and therefore should only be undertaken in specialized fetal treatment centers. A small proportion of CCAMs associated with fetal hydrops may also manifest the maternal mirror syndrome.[28] In this scenario, the mother's condition begins to mirror that of her fetus, as she develops progressive symptoms of preeclampsia. The pathophysiology of this condition is poorly understood; however, fetectomy and removal of the placenta is lifesaving for the mother.

The ability to predict which fetuses may develop hydrops has been enabled by the development of an ultrasound prediction tool called the CCAM volume-to-head-circumference ratio (CVR).[19] Using an elliptical volume approximation of the CCAM that is gestationally adjusted by dividing by the head circumference, the CVR allows estimation of the risk of hydrops development prior to 28 weeks' gestation (after which the risk of developing hydrops is significantly reduced). If the calculated CVR is greater than 1.6 and there is no dominant cyst, the risk that a fetus will develop hydrops is approximately 80%. Such fetuses should be closely monitored (twice-weekly ultrasound) for developing signs of hydrops.

Fetal Intervention

With an evolved understanding of the natural history of fetal CCAMs, the potential lifesaving benefit of fetal intervention for the development of hydrops has been realized. The options for intervention are maternal steroid administration, and fetal thoracotomy and lung resection for microcystic CCAM and ultrasound-guided thoracoamniotic shunting for macrocystic CCAM. The largest reported experience to date with maternal steroid treatment of fetal CCAM is 13 patients, all with a CVR greater than 1.6, of whom 9 had developed hydrops. Following a single dose of

Table 28-1 Comparisons of Features of CPAM and CCAM Subtypes[a]

CPAM Type	Type 0	Type I	Type 2	Type 3	Type 4
CCAM Type		Type I	Type II	Type III	
Developmental origin	Tracheal/bronchial	Bronchial/Bronchiolar	Bronchiolar	Bronchiolar/alveolar	Acinar
Proportion of CPAM	<2%	60%–65%	15%–20%	5%–10%	10%
Timing of presentation	Birth	Prenatal (especially if large cysts)	Postnatally	Prenatal (if large)	Postnatal
Clinical presentation	Lethal pulmonary hypoplasia, absence or lack of alveoli	Asymptomatic, or immediate or delayed respiratory distress or infection	Respiratory presentation often less significant than associated anomalies	Prenatal (development of hydrops) Postnatal (depending on size) respiratory distress	Incidental finding, pneumonia or pneumothorax
Cyst size	None	0.5–10 cm	0.5–2 cm	Microcystic (solid)	Large multilocular
Lung involvement	All lobes involved (incompatible with life)	Lobar	Lobar	Lobar or entire lung	Lobar
Associated anomalies	CV anomalies, renal hypoplasia		50% associated anomalies (CV, CDH, BPS, renal dysplasia agenesis)	None	Pleuropulmonary blastoma
Malignancy risk	None	Bronchoalveolar carcinoma (rare)	None	None	Pleuropulmonary blastoma

Abbreviations: BPS, bronchopulmonary sequestration; CCAM, congenital cystic adenomatoid malformation; CDH, congenital diaphragmatic hernia; CPAM, congenital pulmonary airway malformation.
Data from References 12–18.

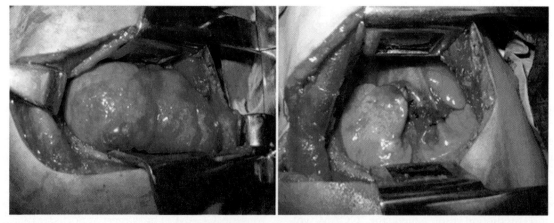

FIGURE 28-2 Operative photograph demonstrating large type congenital pulmonary airway malformation arising from right upper lobe, pre- (left panel) and postresection (right panel).

steroids, the CVR decreased in 8 (62%), and hydrops resolved in 7 (78%). All fetuses survived to delivery, and 11/13 (85%) survived to hospital discharge.[29]

For fetuses with a large CCAM and a dominant cyst, there may be a role for fetal thoracentesis and cyst aspiration or placement of a thoracoamniotic shunt. It is important to remember that fetuses with large CCAMs are also at risk of having significant pulmonary hypoplasia, so despite an apparently favorable response to maternal steroids or catheter drainage, there is the potential for marked respiratory insufficiency at birth, which may require significant ventilatory support or even extracorporeal membrane oxygenation (ECMO). In rare instances if the risk of severe pulmonary hypoplasia at birth is high, there may be a role for an ex utero intrapartum treatment (EXIT) to lung resection approach. In this highly specialized procedure, the baby is delivered by cesarean section and maintained on the placental circulation while thoracotomy and lung resection are undertaken. This approach has been used successfully in 9 high-risk cases of fetal CCAM. In this series, 8 of 9 patients survived, although 4 did require ECMO following lung resection, attesting to the severity of associated pulmonary hypoplasia.[30]

Postnatal Diagnosis and Management

If a prenatal diagnosis of a CCAM has been made, a decision needs to be made regarding location of delivery. Because of the unpredictability of respiratory distress at birth due to underlying pulmonary hypoplasia or worsening mediastinal shift and adjacent lung collapse caused by air or fluid trapping, any fetus with a history of a large CCAM should be delivered in a center with access to urgent pediatric surgical care. Fetuses with "disappearing" or small, peripheral cystic lesions can be safely delivered outside a specialty perinatal center as long as the baby can be expeditiously transferred to a specialty center if needed.

The assessment of a baby with a history of fetal CCAM or a baby without a prenatal diagnosis who has respiratory symptoms begins with a chest radiograph. The differential diagnosis of a postnatally diagnosed CCAM includes CDH, especially when the left side is involved. However, the 2 conditions can usually be distinguished based on the identification of a nasogastric tube in an intrathoracic stomach or by instilling contrast and obtaining a limited study of the gastrointestinal tract. If a CCAM diagnosed antenatally is not seen on postnatal chest radiograph, a follow-up CT scan should be done, although certainly this is not required in the immediate postnatal period.

Infants with CCAMs who are symptomatic in the newborn period should undergo urgent surgical treatment, consisting of thoracotomy and either lobectomy or occasionally segmental resection if the lesion is amenable to this. The management of CCAMs that are asymptomatic at birth remains somewhat controversial, with some authors recommending observation and others advocating planned, elective excision. The most common complication of CCAMs that are asymptomatic at birth are the development of symptoms from air or fluid trapping and the development of infection in the cyst, which presents as acute-onset respiratory distress or pneumonia and is estimated to occur in at least 10% of patients who are initially asymptomatic.[31]

The other important consideration in the management of asymptomatic cystic lung lesions is the risk of malignancy. Malignant processes have historically been described in association with CPAM types 1 and 4: PPB in CPAM types 1 and 4 and much more rarely BAC in CPAM type 1. It should be restated that cystic PPB is not a preexisting CPAM that has undergone malignant transformation; rather, cystic PPB is a discrete low-grade tumor that evolves over 2–4 years to a high-grade, solid, overtly sarcomatous disease. Patients with PPB may have associated tumors, most commonly cystic nephroma.[18] Over 90% of patients with PPB present before age 6, and the youngest patient to be diagnosed with PPB was only 2 months old.[32]

On the basis of the risks of infection and malignancy, the very low morbidity of infant thoracotomy, and the potential for compensatory lung growth up to approximately age 7, most pediatric surgeons favor elective resection of CCAMs after approximately 3 months of age.

BRONCHOPULMONARY SEQUESTRATION

Bronchopulmonary sequestrations are bronchopulmonary foregut malformations consisting of lung tissue that lacks connection to the tracheobronchial tree and account for 20% to 40% of congenital lung anomalies.[33] Sequestrations may be invested by their own visceral pleura (extralobar) or are located within normal lung (intralobar), with the 2 forms occurring with approximately equal incidence. Extralobar sequestrations can be found above, below, and even within the diaphragm (Figure 28-3). Another characteristic feature of sequestrations is a systemic arterial supply, which typically arises from the descending thoracic aorta and occasionally the infradiaphragmatic aorta. Venous drainage may be either systemic (extralobar) or through the appropriate pulmonary vein (intralobar).

Given their origin from foregut, there may occasionally be a connection between the sequestration

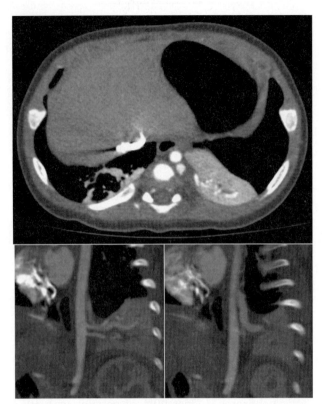

FIGURE 28-3 Computed tomographic scan demonstrating extralobar bronchopulmonary sequestration (BPS) located between left lower lobe and diaphragm. A, Axial view through BPS; B and C, left parasagittal views demonstrating two systemic arteries arising from the descending aorta (B) and systemic venous drainage into the hemiazygous vein (C).

and the proximal gastrointestinal tract, hence the term bronchopulmonary foregut malformation. In these instances, the sequestration (which may be intralobar or extralobar) communicates via a bronchus-like structure with the esophagus (67%) or stomach (15%). A classification scheme for these rare malformations has been proposed: Group I (16%) is associated with esophageal atresia; for group II (33%), the entire lung takes origin from the distal esophagus; in group III (46%), an isolated lobe or lung segment is connected to the distal esophagus or stomach; and in group IV (5%), a portion of the normal bronchial tree communicates with the esophagus.[34]

Prenatal diagnosis of sequestrations by ultrasound occurs frequently. These lesions appear solid, and the documentation of a systemic blood supply by Doppler ultrasound usually confirms the diagnosis. However, the phenomenon of hybrid CPAMs/BPSs, which are typically cystic with a systemic arterial supply, is well described.[35,36] Another significant prenatal consideration is the association of extralobar BPS with other malformations, including CDH, congenital heart disease, and chest wall and vertebral anomalies, and these

should be specifically sought. The natural history of a fetal diagnosis of BPS has the same potential for the development of hydrops by 1 of 2 mechanisms: (1) mediastinal shift and heart or inferior vena caval (IVC) compression leading to impaired cardiac output and (2) high-output cardiac failure resulting from shunting between the anomalous arterial inflow and venous drainage. If either condition results in hydrops, there is a risk of fetal demise, so, as for CPAM, there may be a role for fetal surgery if hydrops develops by either mechanism.

Extralobar BPS has features that distinguish it from intralobar BPS (Table 28-2). Extralobar BPS occurs 3 times as frequently in males compared to females and has a higher likelihood of associated anomalies. The diagnosis is either suspected at birth based on findings on antenatal ultrasound or, in about 25% of babies with extralobar BPS, respiratory distress or feeding difficulties may become evident in the first few months of life. Slightly older children can present with respiratory distress from congestive cardiac failure.[37-40] Approximately two-thirds of extralobar BPSs are left sided, with the majority located between the lower lobe and diaphragm. Intralobar BPSs affect the genders with equal incidence and have a lower rate of associated anomalies compared to extralobar BPSs.[41,42] Unless a prenatal diagnosis has been made, intralobar BPS usually presents after age 2, usually with chronic or recurrent pneumonia and less often with high-output congestive heart failure or hemoptysis.[43,44] More than 95% of intralobar BPSs occur in the lower lobes (typically the posterior medial and basal segments), with the left lung (60%) more commonly involved than the right.[42,45] Arterial supply is most commonly from the thoracic aorta (75%), followed by the abdominal aorta in 20% of cases.[42]

Diagnosis of BPS

If a diagnosis of BPS has been made antenatally, a postnatal chest CT scan usually confirms the diagnosis and demonstrates the anomalous arterial supply and venous drainage. If the BPS appears to have diminished or disappeared prior to birth, a CT scan will invariably demonstrate persistence of the sequestration.[46,47] MRI has also been used to image these lesions and their blood supply.[48] Infants and children with respiratory symptoms caused by a BPS will typically show a triangular-shaped infiltrate in the lower lobes. The presence of an air fluid level suggests communication with the gastrointestinal tract, and contrast studies should be undertaken.

Symptomatic infants require expeditious surgical excision. Knowledge of the anomalous vascularity (especially if the arterial supply is from the subdiaphragmatic aorta) is the key to a safe resection and will be facilitated

Table 28-2 Comparison of Extralobar and Intralobar Sequestration

	Extralobar Sequestration	Intralobar Sequestration
Thoracic location	Above, in, below diaphragm (separate from lung mass, with own pleural investment)	Within lung
Laterality % (L:R)	65:35	60:40
Site	Between lower lobe, diaphragm (65%) Anterior mediastinum (10%) Posterior mediastinum (5%) Intra-abdominal (10%–15%)	>95% in lower lobe
Associated anomalies	60% (congenital heart disease, congenital diaphragmatic hernia, vertebral, chest wall)	10%
Gender prevalence (M:F)	3:1	1:1
Arterial (A) supply/venous (V) drainage	A: Thoracic/abdominal aorta (90%) V: Systemic venous: azygos, hemiazygos (80%); pulmonary venous (20%)	A: Thoracic/abdominal aorta (95%) V: Systemic venous (5%); pulmonary venous (95%)

Data from References 41–45.

by a preoperative CT scan if time permits. If a high-flow sequestration has resulted in cardiac decompensation, coil embolization of the aberrant artery may be performed as definitive therapy or in combination with surgical resection.[49,50] Transumbilical embolization has been described as definitive therapy for asymptomatic intralobar sequestration in antenatally diagnosed newborns, with some evidence of regression.[51]

Intra-abdominal BPS may present antenatally as a left-sided suprarenal mass and may therefore be misdiagnosed as a congenital neuroblastoma.[52,53] Negative postnatal neuroblastoma screening combined with a CT scan that demonstrates a feeding artery from the infradiaphragmatic aorta will confirm the diagnosis of BPS.

CONGENITAL LOBAR EMPHYSEMA

Congenital lobar emphysema or overdistension is a rare lung anomaly that usually presents in the neonatal period with respiratory distress and radiographic evidence of progressive air trapping in 1 or more pulmonary lobes (Figure 28-4). Like the other congenital lung anomalies, it may be diagnosed antenatally by ultrasound and fetal MRI, with its echogenic, homogeneous appearance similar to that of a microcystic CPAM or sequestration, which are the 2 conditions more commonly considered in the differential diagnosis. The absence of a systemic arterial supply should exclude BPS from the differential diagnosis. Like other congenital lung lesions, antenatally diagnosed CLE may progressively increase in size, resulting in

progressive mediastinal shift and compression of adjacent unaffected lobes and the contralateral lung, raising concerns over the possibility of the development of hydrops and longer-term concerns of pulmonary hypoplasia in the unaffected lung. However, CLE can also regress spontaneously and appear indistinguishable from adjacent lung by ultrasound.[54,55] Complete atresia of a mainstem bronchus leads to massive fetal lung enlargement, mediastinal shift and cardiac compression, hydrops, and fetal death. MRI demonstrates involvement of the entire lung and dilated bronchi distal to the mainstem atresia.[56]

There are several pathophysiological mechanisms by which fluid trapping (prenatally) or air trapping (postnatally) may occur: (1) the presence of dysplastic bronchial cartilages that produce "ball-valve" endobronchial obstruction[57]; (2) luminal mucus inspissation[58] or mucosal proliferation and infolding[59]; (3) extrinsic compression from a bronchogenic cyst[60] or aberrant cardiopulmonary vasculature or enlarged cardiac chambers[61]; (4) diffuse bronchial abnormalities that may be due in part to infection[62,63]; and (5) polyalveolosis or the polyalveolar lobe, in which total alveolar numbers are disproportionately increased relative to bronchial structure numbers, which are normal for age.[64]

Approximately 50% of cases of CLE will have a mechanistic explanation identified by a combination of preoperative bronchoscopy or histopathologic evaluation of resected lung; in the remainder, the cause is unknown. The most common sites of involvement are left upper lobe (45%), followed by the right middle lobe (35%), right upper lobe (20%), and the

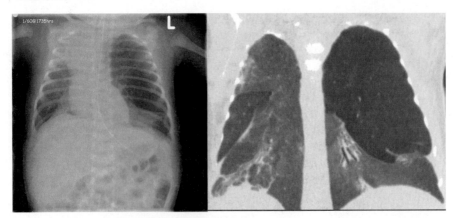

FIGURE 28-4 Chest radiograph (left panel) and coronal view from computed tomographic scan demonstrating bilobar (left upper lobe, right middle lobe) congenital lobar emphysema. The patient underwent left upper lobectomy for respiratory distress and remains asymptomatic and under observation for the remaining involved lobe.

lower lobes in less than 1%. Multiple-lobe involvement has been reported in 10% to 15% of patients.[65] Approximately 20% of patients have associated congenital cardiac anomalies, which should be sought in the evaluation of a symptomatic infant with CLE.[66]

Approximately 50% of infants who will require surgery for symptomatic CLE present within the first month of life; presentation after 6 months is rare. When a newborn with CLE develops respiratory distress, a chest radiograph and CT scan will usually confirm the diagnosis. The hyperlucency of the overinflated lung may lead to an errant diagnosis of pneumothorax and unnecessary chest tube placement prior to surgical referral.[67]

Surgical resection is required for symptomatic CLE, and the anesthetic management of patients is critical to avoid profound cardiopulmonary collapse caused by precipitous severe air trapping due to positive pressure ventilation. Therefore, it is important for the surgeon to be present during anesthetic induction in case urgent thoracotomy is required. Selective bronchial intubation,[68] flexible bronchoscopic decompression,[69] and high-frequency jet ventilation[70] have all been described as useful adjuncts to the perioperative management of patients with CLE and respiratory distress. Some infants with CLE have no or mild respiratory symptoms and may be followed clinically and radiographically, with the expectation that some mildly symptomatic patients may improve spontaneously.[71]

BRONCHOGENIC CYSTS

Developmental cysts arising from the tracheobronchial tree are called bronchogenic cysts and may be located in the mediastinum (trachea) (Figure 28-5), lung hilum (hilar bronchi), or lung parenchyma (intraparenchymal bronchi). Approximately two-thirds of bronchogenic cysts are located within the lung itself[72]; bronchogenic cysts have also been reported in a variety

of ectopic sites, including the neck, tongue, chest wall, paraesophageal, subcarinal, and pericardial locations. The proportion of reported bronchogenic cysts among clinical cohorts of congenital cystic bronchopulmonary foregut malformations ranges from 22% to 50%.[73,74] Bronchogenic cysts are unilocular and are lined by ciliated cuboidal, columnar, or squamous epithelium with mucous glands. The cysts can be quite variable in size, ranging from subcentimeter to several centimeters, and typically do not communicate with the functional tracheobronchial tree.

It is difficult to identify bronchogenic cysts as a single diagnostic entity as they may share features with a heterogeneous group of cystic lesions that occur in the mediastinum and are beyond the scope of discussion in this chapter. These entities include cystic hygroma, thymic cysts, esophageal duplication cysts, neurenteric cysts, and cystic tumors, including neuroblastoma and

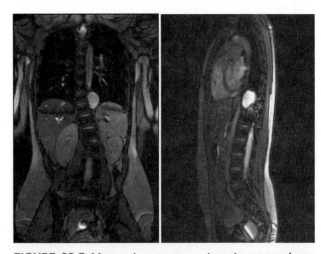

FIGURE 28-5 Magnetic resonance imaging scan showing coronal (right panel) and left parasagittal (left panel) views of a bronchogenic cyst located in the left posterior mediastinum.

teratoma. These disparate cystic lesions may share attributes of origin of symptoms depending on their location, whether they compress adjacent viscera, and because of the development of secondary infection. The classification of the mediastinum into anatomic subdivisions (superior, anterior, middle, and posterior) and a knowledge of the regional predilection of the different cyst types can aid in differential diagnosis. For example, bronchogenic cysts will tend to localize to the anterior or middle mediastinum, thymic cysts to the anterior or superior mediastinum, teratomas to the anterior mediastinum, and esophageal duplication cysts, neurenteric cysts, and cystic neuroblastoma to the posterior mediastinum.

Newborns with large cysts adjacent to the trachea or proximal airways can present with respiratory distress from tracheal obstruction or air trapping from lobar overdistension, as noted in the section on CLE.[60] Nonobstructive lesions may be asymptomatic but detected coincidentally as a mediastinal mass on anteroposterior and lateral chest radiographs. The choices for cross-sectional imaging include contrast-enhanced CT scan or MRI. Each has its own advantages.[75] CT demonstrates calcification, which may be a feature of teratomas; MRI is more useful for vascular lesions or those that may be associated with spinal abnormalities, such as neurenteric cysts. For cystic lesions in the middle mediastinum that enlarge the cardiac silhouette, an echocardiogram may be useful for defining the location of the cyst as intra- or extra-pericardial.[76] In addition to imaging, the considered differential diagnosis of tumors should invoke a urine screen for neuroblastoma and serum screening for germ cell tumors (α-fetoprotein and β-human chorionic gonadotropin).

The preferred treatment of these cystic tumors is surgical resection at diagnosis, with exceptions being small, asymptomatic cystic masses provided they can be followed clinically and radiographically.

ACQUIRED CYSTIC LUNG DISEASE

A final category of cystic lung disease in newborns is acquired cystic disease arising from ventilator-induced lung injury in premature infants with respiratory distress syndrome (RDS). Pneumatoceles represent 1 category of acquired cystic lung disease in ex-premature infants that has seen a reduction in incidence with the routine use of surfactant.[77] Another category of ventilation-induced lung injury is interstitial pulmonary emphysema (IPE), which results when alveolar rupture allows air tracking into the interlobular septum, which can dissect centrally or peripherally, resulting in pneumothorax and occasionally pneumopericardium.[12]

For both of these acquired conditions, reduction of ventilatory mean airway pressure will usually result in cyst resolution; however, the development of pneumothorax and a chronic air leak is associated with higher rates of mortality. The third category of acquired cystic lung disease in infancy is postinfectious cysts, which represent either necrotized tissue cavities or lung abscesses.[78,79]

Regardless of etiology, the majority of acquired cystic lung disease can be managed conservatively. An important determinant of success of conservative management is resolution of the underlying lung disease and its cause, especially the need for high-pressure mechanical ventilation or infection. Some infants develop large-volume pneumatoceles that result in symptoms from compression of adjacent lung or mediastinal shift. Some of these may require pigtail catheter decompression or occasionally surgical resection. Infant lung resection for symptomatic acquired cystic lung disease is infrequently necessary, but when it is, ventilatory adjuncts such as selective lung ventilation may be helpful.[80]

REFERENCES

1. Correia-Pinto J, Gonzaga S, Huang Y, Rottier R. Congenital lung lesions—underlying molecular mechanisms. *Semin Pediatr Surg*. 2010;19:171–179.
2. Miura T. Modeling lung branching morphogenesis. *Curr Top Dev Biol*. 2008;81:291–310.
3. Maeda Y, Dave V, Whitsett JA. Transcriptional control of lung morphogenesis. *Physiol Rev*. 2007;87:219–244.
4. Cardoso WV, Lu J. Regulation of early lung morphogenesis: questions, facts and controversies. *Development*. 2006;133:1611–1624.
5. Roth-Kleiner M, Post M. Similarities and dissimilarities of branching and septation during lung development. *Pediatr Pulmonol*. 2005;40:113–134.
6. Cass DL, Quinn TM, Yang EY, et al. Increased cell proliferation and decreased apoptosis characterize congenital cystic adenomatoid malformation of the lung. *J Pediatr Surg*. 1998;33:1043–1046. discussion 1047.
7. Laberge JM, Flageole H, Pugash D, et al. Outcome of the prenatally diagnosed congenital cystic adenomatoid lung malformation: a Canadian experience. *Fetal Diagn Ther*. 2001;16:178–186.
8. Hernanz-Schulman M. Cysts and cystlike lesions of the lung. *Radiol Clin North Am*. 1993;31:631–649.
9. Ch'in KY, Tang MY. Congenital adenomatoid malformation of one lobe of a lung with general anasarca. *Arch Path*. 1949;48:221–225.
10. Stocker JT, Madewell JE, Drake RM. Congenital cystic adenomatoid malformation of the lung. classification and morphologic spectrum. *Hum Pathol*. 1977;8:155–171.
11. Adzick NS, Harrison MR, Glick PL, et al. Fetal cystic adenomatoid malformation: prenatal diagnosis and natural history. *J Pediatr Surg*. 1985;20:483–488.
12. Stocker JT. Cystic lung disease in infants and children. *Fetal Pediatr Pathol*. 2009;28:155–184.
13. Summers RJ, Shehata BM, Bleacher JC, Stockwell C, Rapkin L. Mucinous adenocarcinoma of the lung in association with congenital pulmonary airway malformation. *J Pediatr Surg*. 2010;45:2256–2259.

14. Carles D, Dallay D, Serville F, et al. Cystic adenomatoid malformation of the lung, bilateral renal agenesis and left heart hypoplasia. an unusual association in potter's syndrome. *Ann Pathol.* 1992;12:367–370.

15. Pham TT, Benirschke K, Masliah E, Stocker JT, Yi ES. Congenital pulmonary airway malformation (congenital cystic adenomatoid malformation) with multiple extrapulmonary anomalies: autopsy report of a fetus at 19 weeks of gestation. *Pediatr Dev Pathol.* 2004;7:661–666.

16. Harrison MR, Adzick NS, Jennings RW, et al. Antenatal intervention for congenital cystic adenomatoid malformation. *Lancet.* 1990;336:965–967.

17. Priest JR, McDermott MB, Bhatia S, Watterson J, Manivel JC, Dehner LP. Pleuropulmonary blastoma: a clinicopathologic study of 50 cases. *Cancer.* 1997;80:147–161.

18. Priest JR, Williams GM, Hill DA, Dehner LP, Jaffe A. Pulmonary cysts in early childhood and the risk of malignancy. *Pediatr Pulmonol.* 2009;44:14–30.

19. Crombleholme TM, Coleman B, Hedrick H, et al. Cystic adenomatoid malformation volume ratio predicts outcome in prenatally diagnosed cystic adenomatoid malformation of the lung. *J Pediatr Surg.* 2002;37:331–338.

20. Revillon Y, Jan D, Plattner V, et al. Congenital cystic adenomatoid malformation of the lung: prenatal management and prognosis. *J Pediatr Surg.* 1993;28:1009–1011.

21. MacGillivray TE, Harrison MR, Goldstein RB, Adzick NS. Disappearing fetal lung lesions. *J Pediatr Surg.* 1993;28:1321–1324. discussion 1324–1325.

22. McCullagh M, MacConnachie I, Garvie D, Dykes E. Accuracy of prenatal diagnosis of congenital cystic adenomatoid malformation. *Arch Dis Child.* 1994;71:F111–F113.

23. Taguchi T, Suita S, Yamanouchi T, et al. Antenatal diagnosis and surgical management of congenital cystic adenomatoid malformation of the lung. *Fetal Diagn Ther.* 1995;10:400–407.

24. Davenport M, Warne SA, Cacciaguerra S, Patel S, Greenough A, Nicolaides K. Current outcome of antenatally diagnosed cystic lung disease. *J Pediatr Surg.* 2004;39:549–556.

25. Winters WD, Effmann EL, Nghiem HV, Nyberg DA. Disappearing fetal lung masses: importance of postnatal imaging studies. *Pediatr Radiol.* 1997;27:535–539.

26. Sauvat F, Michel JL, Benachi A, Emond S, Revillon Y. Management of asymptomatic neonatal cystic adenomatoid malformations. *J Pediatr Surg.* 2003;38:548–552.

27. Butterworth SA, Blair GK. Postnatal spontaneous resolution of congenital cystic adenomatoid malformations. *J Pediatr Surg.* 2005;40:832–834.

28. Adzick NS. Management of fetal lung lesions. *Clin Perinatol.* 2003;30:481–492.

29. Curran PF, Jelin EB, Rand L, et al. Prenatal steroids for microcystic congenital cystic adenomatoid malformations. *J Pediatr Surg.* 2010;45:145–150.

30. Hedrick HL, Flake AW, Crombleholme TM, et al. The ex utero intrapartum therapy procedure for high-risk fetal lung lesions. *J Pediatr Surg.* 2005;40:1038–1043. discussion 1044.

31. Aziz D, Langer JC, Tuuha SE, Ryan G, Ein SH, Kim PC. Perinatally diagnosed asymptomatic congenital cystic adenomatoid malformation: to resect or not? *J Pediatr Surg.* 2004;39:329–334. discussion 329–334.

32. Indolfi P, Casale F, Carli M, et al. Pleuropulmonary blastoma: management and prognosis of 11 cases. *Cancer.* 2000;89:1396–1401.

33. Pinkerton HJ, Oldham KT. Lung. In: Oldham KT, Colombani PM, Foglia RP, Skinner MA, eds. *Principles and Practice of Pediatric Surgery.* Philadelphia, PA: Lippincott, Williams and Wilkins; 2005:951–982.

34. Srikanth MS, Ford EG, Stanley P, Mahour GH. Communicating bronchopulmonary foregut malformations: classification and embryogenesis. *J Pediatr Surg.* 1992;27:732–736.

35. Cass DL, Crombleholme TM, Howell LJ, Stafford PW, Ruchelli ED, Adzick NS. Cystic lung lesions with systemic arterial blood supply: a hybrid of congenital cystic adenomatoid malformation and bronchopulmonary sequestration. *J Pediatr Surg.* 1997;32:986–990.

36. Hirose R, Suita S, Taguchi T, Koyanagi T, Nakano H. Extralobar pulmonary sequestration mimicking cystic adenomatoid malformation in prenatal sonographic appearance and histological findings. *J Pediatr Surg.* 1995;30:1390–1393.

37. Thilenius OG, Ruschhaupt DG, Replogle RL, Bharati S, Herman T, Arcilla RA. Spectrum of pulmonary sequestration: association with anomalous pulmonary venous drainage in infants. *Pediatr Cardiol.* 1983;4:97–103.

38. White JJ, Donahoo JS, Ostrow PT, Murphy J, Haller JA Jr. Cardiovascular and respiratory manifestations of pulmonary sequestration in childhood. *Ann Thorac Surg.* 1974;18:286–294.

39. Choplin RH, Siegel MJ. Pulmonary sequestration: six unusual presentations. *AJR Am J Roentgenol.* 1980;134:695–700.

40. Corbett HJ, Humphrey GM. Pulmonary sequestration. *Paediatr Respir Rev.* 2004;5:59–68.

41. Arcomano JP, Azzoni AA. Intralobar pulmonary sequestration and intralobar enteric sequestration associated with vertebral anomalies. *J Thorac Cardiovasc Surg.* 1967;53:470–476.

42. Savic B, Birtel FJ, Tholen W, Funke HD, Knoche R. Lung sequestration: report of 7 cases and review of 540 published cases. *Thorax.* 1979;34:96–101.

43. Sade RM, Clouse M, Ellis FH Jr. The spectrum of pulmonary sequestration. *Ann Thorac Surg.* 1974;18:644–658.

44. Laurin S, Aronson S, Schuller H, Henrikson H. Spontaneous hemothorax from bronchopulmonary sequestration: unusual angiographic and pathologic-anatomic findings. *Pediatr Radiol.* 1980;10:54–56.

45. DeParedes CG, Pierce WS, Johnson DG, Waldhausen JA. Pulmonary sequestration in infants and children: a 20-year experience and review of the literature. *J Pediatr Surg.* 1970;5:136–147.

46. Adzick NS, Harrison MR, Crombleholme TM, Flake AW, Howell LJ. Fetal lung lesions: management and outcome. *Am J Obstet Gynecol.* 1998;179:884–889.

47. Bromley B, Parad R, Estroff JA, Benacerraf BR. Fetal lung masses: prenatal course and outcome. *J Ultrasound Med.* 1995;14:927–936. quiz p1378.

48. Shanmugam G, MacArthur K, Pollock JC. Congenital lung malformations—antenatal and postnatal evaluation and management. *Eur J Cardiothorac Surg.* 2005;27:45–52.

49. Curros F, Chigot V, Emond S, et al. Role of embolisation in the treatment of bronchopulmonary sequestration. *Pediatr Radiol.* 2000;30:769–773.

50. Chien KJ, Huang TC, Lin CC, Lee CL, Hsieh KS, Weng KP. Early and late outcomes of coil embolization of pulmonary sequestration in children. *Circ J.* 2009;73:938–942.

51. Lee BS, Kim JT, Kim EA, et al. Neonatal pulmonary sequestration: clinical experience with transumbilical arterial embolization. *Pediatr Pulmonol.* 2008;43:404–413.

52. Gross E, Chen MK, Lobe TE, Nuchtern JG, Rao BN. Infradiaphragmatic extralobar pulmonary sequestration masquerading as an intraabdominal, suprarenal mass. *Pediatr Surg Int.* 1997;12:529–531.

53. Agayev A, Yilmaz S, Cekrezi B, Yekeler E. Extralobar pulmonary sequestration mimicking neuroblastoma. *J Pediatr Surg.* 2007;42:1627–1629.

54. Olutoye OO, Coleman BG, Hubbard AM, Adzick NS. Prenatal diagnosis and management of congenital lobar emphysema. *J Pediatr Surg.* 2000;35:792–795.

55. Richards DS, Langham MR Jr, Dolson LH. Antenatal presentation of a child with congenital lobar emphysema. *J Ultrasound Med.* 1992;11:165–168.

56. Keswani SG, Crombleholme TM, Pawel BR, et al. Prenatal diagnosis and management of mainstem bronchial atresia. *Fetal Diagn Ther.* 2005;20:74–78.

57. Doull IJ, Connett GJ, Warner JO. Bronchoscopic appearances of congenital lobar emphysema. *Pediatr Pulmonol.* 1996;21:195–197.

58. Thompson J, Forfar JO. Regional obstructive emphysema in infancy. *Arch Dis Child.* 1958;33:97–101.

59. Hendren WH, McKee DM. Lobar emphysema in infancy. *J Pediatr Surg.* 1966;1:24–32.

60. Khemiri M, Ouederni M, Ben Mansour F, Barsaoui S. Bronchogenic cyst: an uncommon cause of congenital lobar emphysema. *Respir Med.* 2008;102:1663–1666.

61. Gordon I, Dempsey JE. Infantile lobar emphysema in association with congenital heart disease. *Clin Radiol.* 1990;41:48–52.

62. Leape LL, Longino LA. Infantile lobar emphysema. *Pediatrics.* 1964;34:246–255.

63. Bolande RB, Schneider AF, Boggs JD. Infantile lobar emphysema; an etiological concept. *AMA Arch Pathol.* 1956;61:289–294.

64. Hislop A, Reid L. New pathological findings in emphysema of childhood. 1. Polyalveolar lobe with emphysema. *Thorax.* 1970;25:682–690.

65. Ozcelik U, Gocmen A, Kiper N, Dogru D, Dilber E, Yalcin EG. Congenital lobar emphysema: evaluation and long-term follow-up of thirty cases at a single center. *Pediatr Pulmonol.* 2003;35:384–391.

66. Roguin N, Peleg H, Lemer J, Naveh Y, Riss E. The value of cardiac catheterization and cineangiography in infantile lobar emphysema. *Pediatr Radiol.* 1980;10:71–74.

67. Choudhury SR, Chadha R, Mishra A, Kumar V, Singh V, Dubey NK. Lung resections in children for congenital and acquired lesions. *Pediatr Surg Int.* 2007;23:851–859.

68. Glenski JA, Thibeault DW, Hall FK, Hall RT, Germann DR. Selective bronchial intubation in infants with lobar emphysema: indications, complications, and long-term outcome. *Am J Perinatol.* 1986;3:199–204.

69. Phillipos EZ, Libsekal K. Flexible bronchoscopy in the management of congenital lobar emphysema in the neonate. *Can Respir J.* 1998;5:219–221.

70. Goto H, Boozalis ST, Benson KT, Arakawa K. High-frequency jet ventilation for resection of congenital lobar emphysema. *Anesth Analg.* 1987;66:684–686.

71. Mei-Zahav M, Konen O, Manson D, Langer JC. Is congenital lobar emphysema a surgical disease? *J Pediatr Surg.* 2006;41:1058–1061.

72. deLorimier AA. Respiratory problems related to the airway and lung. In: O'Neill JA, Rowe MI, Grosfeld JL, Fonkalsrud EW, Coran AG, eds. *Pediatric Surgery.* 5th ed. St Louis, MO: Mosby; 1998:891.

73. Buntain WL, Isaacs H Jr, Payne VC Jr, Lindesmith GG, Rosenkrantz JG. Lobar emphysema, cystic adenomaloid malformation, pulmonary sequestration, and bronchogenic cyst in infancy and childhood: a clinical group. *J Pediatr Surg.* 1974;9:85–93.

74. Takeda S, Miyoshi S, Inoue M, et al. Clinical spectrum of congenital cystic disease of the lung in children. *Eur J Cardiothorac Surg.* 1999;15:11–17.

75. Merten DF. Diagnostic imaging of mediastinal masses in children. *AJR Am J Roentgenol.* 1992;158:825–832.

76. Kumar S, Jain P, Sen R, Rattan K, Agarwal R, Garg S. Giant pericardial cyst in a 5-year-old child: a rare anomaly. *Ann Pediatr Cardiol.* 2011;4:68–70.

77. Hussain N, Noce T, Sharma P, et al. Pneumatoceles in preterm infants-incidence and outcome in the post-surfactant era. *J Perinatol.* 2010;30:330–336.

78. Hoffer FA, Bloom DA, Colin AA, Fishman SJ. Lung abscess versus necrotizing pneumonia: implications for interventional therapy. *Pediatr Radiol.* 1999;29:87–91.

79. Kunyoshi V, Cataneo DC, Cataneo AJ. Complicated pneumonias with empyema and/or pneumatocele in children. *Pediatr Surg Int.* 2006;22:186–190.

80. Liu CM, Huang CH, Lau HP, Yeh HM. Anesthetic management for two infants undergoing surgery for tension pneumatoceles. *Paediatr Anaesth.* 2007;17:189–190.

CHAPTER 28

Bronchopulmonary Dysplasia

Anne Hilgendorff

EPIDEMIOLOGY

Chronic lung disease (CLD) of the newborn, also known as bronchopulmonary dysplasia (BPD), is the most common CLD in early infancy.[1] The incidence of BPD varies between newborn care centers, reflecting differences in patient population and infant management practices.[2–4] Recent publications reported a BPD incidence of 68% in very low birth weight (401- to 1500-g) infants born prior to 29 weeks' gestation or 77% in infants born at less than 32 weeks' gestation with a birth weight below 1 kg.[3,5,6] The latest studies in Europe reported a BPD rate of up to 25% in infants below 32 weeks' gestational age (GA).[2] The overall incidence in the United States is approximately 10–15,000 cases per year.[7] The incidence of BPD is inversely related to GA, varying from 80% or more among the most immature infants at 24 weeks' gestation to less than 5% among infants greater than 32 weeks' gestation.[2,3,8] Infants who are born very prematurely often require prolonged assisted ventilation to treat acute respiratory failure caused by primary surfactant deficiency (ie, respiratory distress syndrome, RDS), sustained or recurrent apnea, or infections. BPD also can develop in term infants who are treated with long-term mechanical ventilation for respiratory failure from meconium aspiration, bacterial or viral pneumonia, lung hypoplasia, or cardiopulmonary malformations.

Although the rate of severe BPD was found to decrease between 1994 and 2002, the overall incidence did not change.[7] The incidence of long-term sequelae remained unchanged or increased among the most immature infants,[9] presumably because of a significant reduction of mortality rates.

PATHOPHYSIOLOGY

Definitions

Bronchopulmonary dysplasia, as a pulmonary disease following mechanical ventilation of hyaline membrane disease, was first described 1967 by Northway et al.[10] In 1989, the Bureau of Maternal and Child Health and Resources Development proposed the following diagnostic criteria for BPD: (1) Requirement for positive pressure ventilation during the first 2 weeks of life, (2) minimum requirement of ventilation for 3 days, (3) clinical signs of respiratory compromise persisting beyond 28 days of age, (4) requirement for supplemental oxygen beyond 28 days of age to maintain a PaO_2 of greater than 50 torr, and (5) chest radiographs showing characteristic lung abnormalities (diffuse bilateral densities, often associated with areas of hyperinflation). More recently, the definition has been modified to specify a need for supplemental oxygen for greater than 28 days or beyond 36 weeks' postmenstrual age (PMA), accompanied by characteristic radiographic abnormalities.

This and subsequent modifications of the earlier definition were initiated by substantial changes in the BPD patient cohort, where application of different ventilation regimens and other significant changes in treatment procedures yielded not only an increased survival rate in the most immature infants but also a different appearance of lung injury, with the characteristic

Table 29-1 Degrees of Bronchopulmonary Dysplasia[a]

Gestational Age	<32 wk 36 wk PMA	≥32 wk > 28 d and < 56 d
	FiO$_2$ > 0.21 for 28 d plus	
Mild	FiO$_2$ 0.21 at 36 wk PMA	FiO$_2$ 0.21 at 56 d
Moderate	FiO$_2$ < 0.30 at 36 wk PMA	FiO$_2$ < 0.30 at 56 d
Severe	FiO$_2$ ≥ 0.30 and/or PPV/CPAP at 36 wk PMA	FiO$_2$ ≥ 0.30 and/or PPV/CPAP at 56 d

Abbreviations: CPAP, continuous positive airway pressure; PMA, postmenstrual age; PPV, positive pressure ventilation.
[a]Adapted with permission from Reference 1.

Table 29-2 Pathophysiologic Characteristics of "Old" and "New" Bronchopulmonary Dysplasia (BPD)

Old BPD	New BPD
Atelectasis and overinflation	Alveolar hypoplasia
	Dysmorphic capillaries, reduction of capillary number
Hyper- and metaplasia of epithelium	Variable degree of epithelial lesions
Hyperplasia of smooth muscle cells	Variable degree of smooth muscle cell hyperplasia
Fibroproliferation	Variable degree of fibroproliferation
Reduction of gas exchange by thickening of interstitial tissue	Reduction of gas exchange by reduction of alveolar and capillary surface area

arrest of lung development at a very early stage. This form of the disease was called "new BPD."

In 2000, a workshop on BPD sponsored by the National Institutes of Health (NIH) proposed an extensive definition that uses O$_2$ dependency at 36 weeks' postconceptual age (failure to maintain normal O$_2$ saturation when breathing room air) and defined mild, moderate, and severe disease (Table 29-1). This definition "corrects" for the degree of immaturity in the moderate and severe stages of the disease as the definition refers to 36 weeks' postconception.[1] A study investigating the predictive validity of the severity-based, consensus definition of BPD by identifying a spectrum of risk for adverse pulmonary and neurodevelopmental outcomes in early infancy supported the more refined definitions of BPD grades according to need for supplemental O$_2$ or positive pressure breathing at 36 weeks' PMA.[6]

Pathophysiologic Findings

A variety of experimental and clinical studies have shown that BPD is characterized by a decrease in alveolarization accompanied by a decrease in small-vessel development.[11] Structural and molecular abnormalities of the lung in BPD include increased smooth muscle in small pulmonary arteries and airways, decreased numbers of terminal respiratory units (alveoli and alveolar septa), and a corresponding increase in alveolar size. When compared to cases treated in the presurfactant era, the amount of interstitial fibrosis is substantially less and tends to be more diffuse in the new BPD, associated with a partial-to-complete arrest in alveolarization[12] (Table 29-2; Figures 29-1 and 29-2).

Different processes were found to have an impact on lung development through alteration of growth factor signaling, apoptosis, and profound changes to the extracellular matrix (ECM). Figure 29-3 gives an overview of the pathophysiologic processes that contribute to the development of BPD. Injury to the lungs of preterm infants who later present with BPD takes places in the canalicular to the saccular stages of lung development, long before the general presence of defined alveolar structures as seen in term infants (Figure 29-4).

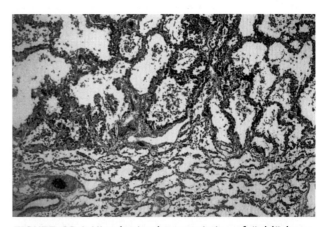

FIGURE 29-1 Histologic characteristics of "old" bronchopulmonary dysplasia. Infants not treated with surfactant display the "classic" features of long-standing healed bronchopulmonary dysplasia (LSHBPD), acini with severe alveolar septal fibrosis (top) adjacent to those with little or no septal fibrosis (bottom) (hematoxy and eosin; original magnification ×20). (Reproduced with permission from Husain AN, Siddiqui NH, Stocker JT. Pathology of arrested acinar development in postsurfactant bronchopulmonary dysplasia. *Hum Pathol.* 1998;29(7):710–717.)

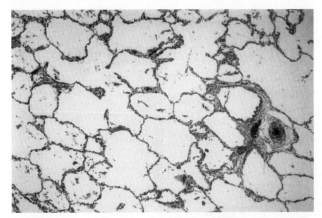

FIGURE 29-2 Histologic characteristics of "new" bronchopulmonary dysplasia (BPD). In the latest histological manifestation of BPD, surfactant-treated infants develop little or no alveolar septal fibrosis. The acini, however, display expanded, simplified alveolar ducts, saccules, and alveoli (hematoxy and eosin; original magnification ×25). (Reproduced with permission from Husain AN, Siddiqui NH, Stocker JT. Pathology of arrested acinar development in postsurfactant bronchopulmonary dysplasia. *Hum Pathol.* 1998;29(7):710–717.)

Inflammatory processes are considered crucial events for the initiation of BPD. The condition may be associated with chorioamnionitis before birth, systemic infection after birth, or pulmonary accumulation of activated neutrophils, which has been described in RDS, aspiration syndromes, pneumonia, and prolonged application of positive pressure ventilation.[13] The characteristic influx of neutrophils into the lung is accompanied by increased numbers of macrophages in the course of the disease.[14–16] Deficiency of antioxidant enzymes and inhibitors of proteolytic enzymes render the very immature infant's lungs especially vulnerable to the effects of toxic oxygen metabolites and proteases released by activated neutrophils and macrophages.[17–20] Pulmonary inflammation and the associated increase in protease activity then leads to the degradation of lung elastin in infants with BPD, manifested as increased urinary excretion of desmosine, a breakdown product of the mature elastic fiber.[21–23]

Following increased remodeling of the ECM, lungs of infants with BPD exhibit increased abundance and abnormal distribution of elastin in the pulmonary parenchyma and circulation, with increased pulmonary

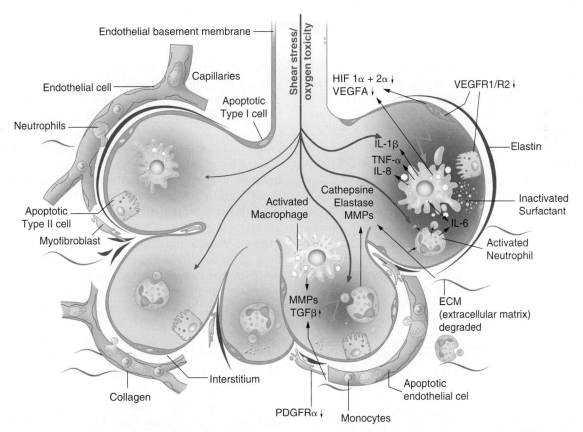

FIGURE 29-3 Bronchopulmonary dysplasia (BPD) pathophysiology. Pathological processes in the development of BPD as identified by clinical and experimental studies. HIF, hypoxia inducible factor; IL, interleukin; MMP, matrix metalloproteinase; PDGFR, platelet-derived growth factor receptor; TGF, transforming growth factor; TNF, tumor necrosis factor; VEGFA, vascular endothelial growth factor A; VEGFR, vascular endothelial growth factor receptor.

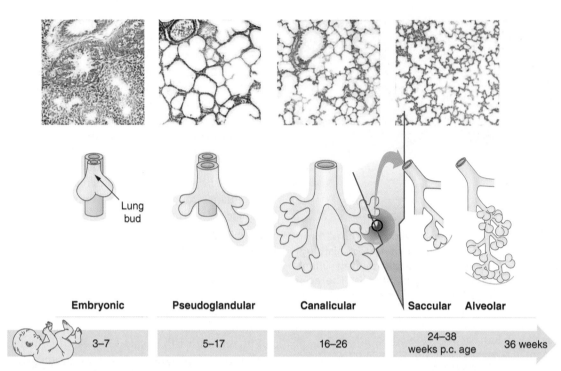

FIGURE 29-4 Stages of lung development. Progress from canalicular to alveolar stage in lung development. Upper row: Histological findings in preterm infants. Middle row: Schematic of lung budding to the formation of alveoli. Lower row: Corresponding age of fetus (p.c. postcongestional). The red arrow indicates the time of injury for the preterm lung in infants later developing BPD. (Adapted with permission from Whitsett JA, Wert SE, Trapnell BC. Genetic disorders influencing lung formation and function at birth. *Hum Mol Genet.* 2004;13.)

expression of tropoelastin (Figure 29-5)[24,25]. Changes to the structural integrity of the ECM potentially affect its function as a scaffold for the formation of new alveoli and capillaries. The release of various cytokines, activation of transcription factors (eg, nuclear factor kappa B [NF-kB]), and signaling of growth factors such as transforming growth factor (TGF) β lead to a characteristic increase in apoptosis.[26] The process of deficient alveolarization is characteristically associated with the presence of dysmorphic capillaries and an altered pattern of angiogenic growth factors (eg, a reduced pulmonary expression of vascular endothelial growth factor [VEGF] and VEGF receptors).[27–29] These changes are accompanied by diminished endothelial nitric oxide synthase (eNOS) and soluble guanylate cyclase (sGC) in lung blood vessels and airways,[30,31] contributing to the development of pulmonary hypertension and affecting lung lymphatic drainage.[32,33] Relevant factors in vascular abnormalities are depicted in Figure 29-6.

The Clinical Picture

Clinically, BPD is characterized by persistent oxygen requirement accompanied by varying signs of respiratory distress, including tachypnea, nasal flaring, and use of accessory muscles with intercostal and substernal retractions, grunting, and cyanosis. Impaired respiratory gas exchange (ie, hypoxemia with need for supplemental O_2 and alveolar hypoventilation with resultant hypercapnia) leads to a mismatch of ventilation and perfusion.[34] The increased lung vascular resistance, typically associated with impaired responsiveness to inhaled nitric oxide (iNO) and other vasodilators, can progress to reversible or sustained pulmonary hypertension and right heart failure.[32,33] Lung function at term shows increased respiratory tract resistance and hyperreactive airways,[35] which can manifest as episodic bronchoconstriction and cyanosis. Diminished lung compliance, tachypnea, and increased minute ventilation and work of breathing are accompanied by increased lung microvascular filtration pressure that may lead to interstitial pulmonary edema.

Risk Factors

Risk factors for the development of BPD as identified by clinical and experimental studies bear their impact on the structure and function of the immature lung beyond the background of genetic susceptibility (Figure 29-7). Factors directly related to preterm birth, such as the presence of a patent ductus arteriosus (PDA) or the immaturity of the immune system, rank next to independent pre- and postnatal risk factors

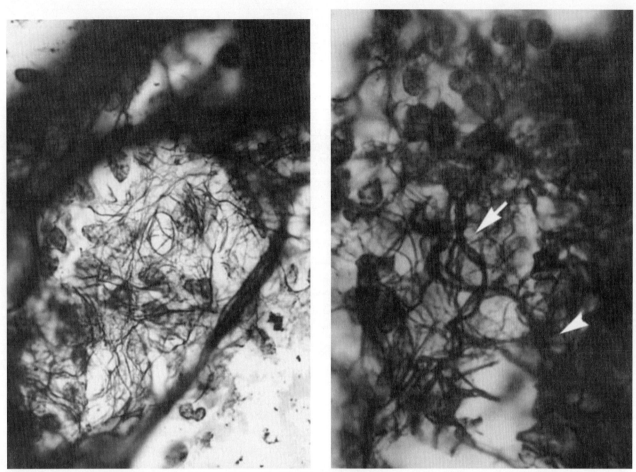

FIGURE 29-5 Extracellular matrix remodeling in bronchopulmonary dysplasia. Left: En face section through the lung septal wall of a 28-week postconceptional age (PCA) infant on mechanical ventilation at 31 days of life. The fibers appear generally coarser, but the pattern is disorganized, with spiraling fibers. Right: En face section through the septal wall of a 24.4-weeks' gestational age infant who died at a PCA of 28.8 weeks. The secondary collagen fibers are disorganized, tortuous, and thickened (arrow) (section 40 μm thick; Gomori reticulum stain; ×100 oil). (Reproduced with permission from Thibeault DW, Mabry SM, Ekekezie II. Collagen scaffolding during development and its deformation with chronic lung disease. *Pediatrics.* 2003;111(4 Pt 1):766–776.)

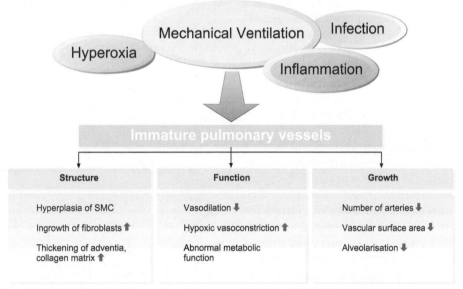

FIGURE 29-6 Vascular abnormalities in bronchopulmonary dysplasia (BPD). Characteristic factors indicating impaired vessel development in BPD.

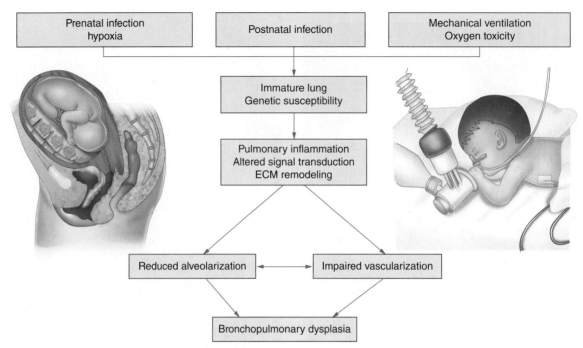

FIGURE 29-7 Risk factors for the development of bronchopulmonary dysplasia (BPD). ECM, extracellular matrix.

such as gender or growth retardation. Studies in twins and preterm infants with similar environmental risk factors suggested that genetic susceptibility may play a role in the pathogenesis of the disease.[36–38] After controlling for covariates, genetic factors accounted for 53% of the variance in liability for BPD in one study investigating twin preterm infants.[39] Furthermore, male preterm infants are at a higher risk for the development of long-term impairment, including BPD,[40] and hormonal regulation has been discussed as an underlying cause.[41] With respect to prenatal determination of pulmonary outcome, intrauterine growth retardation increases the risk of BPD 3- to 4-fold,[15,42–44] most likely through alteration of growth factor signaling and impaired alveolar and vascular growth.[45] In addition, the fetal inflammatory response syndrome as well as the full picture of amnion infection with histologic signs of chorioamnionitis are known to increase the risk of BPD.[13,46–48]

After birth, the presence of congenital and nosocomial systemic or pulmonary infections is an important risk factor for the development of the disease.[49,50] Prolonged mechanical ventilation using large tidal volumes and high inflation pressures together with oxygen toxicity related to the magnitude and duration of exposure to supplemental oxygen are major risk factors for the development of BPD.[51,52] The development of pulmonary complications (eg, air leaks, interstitial emphysema, and pneumothoraces) further increases the risk.[51]

Clinical conditions (eg, gastroesophageal reflux) leading to aspiration of gastric contents and associated aspiration pneumonitis, incorrect placement of the endotracheal tube or improper delivery of surfactant, airway obstruction from mucous plugs, and prolonged airway sucking need to be monitored closely as they may add to the overall risk by inducing acute lung injury and nonuniform lung expansion. Furthermore, excessive fluid and salt intake, the presence of a PDA as well as myocardial dysfunction increase the risk for BPD through induction of lung edema.[53–57] Poor nutritional support, vitamin A deficiency, and insufficient adrenal and thyroid hormone release in the very premature infant contribute to the development of the disease.[58–60] Table 29-3 gives an overview of relevant risk factors for the development of BPD.

Table 29-3 Risk Factors for the Development of Bronchopulmonary Dysplasia (Increase in Relative Risk, RR)[a]

	RR	95% Confidence Interval
Birth weight < 10th percentile	3.8	2.1–6.8
Gestational age (weeks)	0.7	0.6–0.8
Gender (female)	0.6	0.4–0.9
RDS and MV > 3 d	15.2	2.0–117.2
Sepsis	1.6	1.02.4
Surfactant therapy	1.6	1.0–2.4

Abbreviations: MV, mechanical ventilation; RDS, respiratory distress syndrome.
[a]Data from Reference 43.

DIFFERENTIAL DIAGNOSIS

The differential diagnosis for BPD mainly comprises interstitial lung diseases (ILDs) in children, which have been categorized in a new classification system.[61] Figure 29-8 is an overview of the diseases that have to be considered. Neonatal CLD accounts for many cases in the group of pulmonary growth abnormalities that reflect deficient alveolarization. Chromosomal disorders leading to defective lung growth, as well as pulmonary hypoplasia associated with birth defects such as diaphragmatic hernia, have to be included in the differential diagnosis. In the group of surfactant dysfunction disorders, lung diseases, caused by mutations in the surfactant protein C and the adenosine triphosphate (ATP) binding cassette transporter A3 (ABCA3) genes, both necessary for surfactant metabolism, have been shown to cause the picture of alveolar proteinosis and desquamative interstitial pneumonia (DIP).[62–64] Besides these, neuroendocrine cell hyperplasia of infancy and pulmonary interstitial glycogenosis, although of undefined etiology, need to be included in diagnostic considerations.[61] When recurrent infections occur, special diagnoses concerning the immunocompromised host, including most common opportunistic infections, need to be taken into account. Furthermore, several disorders that masquerade as ILD, such as congenital heart diseases, arterial hypertensive vasculopathy, or congenital lymphatic disorders, need to be considered.

The lack of the typical history, including extreme prematurity followed by mechanical ventilation, the presence of a suspect family history of (undiagnosed) pulmonary diseases, or signs for additional malformations, should lead to consideration of other differential diagnoses.

DIAGNOSTIC TESTS

The diagnosis of BPD is based on pulmonary function at term combined with the characteristic history or preterm birth and ventilator support. Oxygen requirement to maintain oxygen saturation above 85% is accompanied by an increase in pCO_2 (partial pressure of carbon dioxide) and bicarbonate in blood gas analyses.[65] Besides clinical signs, these measures of gas exchange are the main follow-up parameters. Lung function testing is used in some clinical studies but has not been introduced into the clinical routine yet. Chest radiographic appearance includes the presence of fibrosis/interstitial shadows, cystic elements, and hyperinflation at 7 days of age and was shown to facilitate prediction of outcome of infants born very prematurely.[66] In this study, infants who died before discharge differed significantly from the rest with respect to significantly higher

scores for cysts. Compared to radiologic findings in the presurfactant era, infants with new BPD show more subtle radiographic abnormalities.[67]

Findings in high-resolution computed tomography (HRCT) include linear and reticular opacities, areas of architectural distortion, and gas trapping/hyperaeration (Figure 29-9). Depending on the respective BPD definition applied, lung function abnormalities seem to be reflected by changes in chest radiographs or HRCT, showing fibrotic changes/interstitial shadowing to a varying degree, in some studies accompanied by (local) hyperinflation.[68–73]

Use of current magnetic resonance imaging (MRI) techniques, as applied in infants with chronic diaphragmatic hernia to estimate lung volume, would allow reducing exposure to radiation but is not part of clinical routine yet.[74] Advances in computed tomographic (CT) scanning or the application of newer techniques such as hyperpolarized gas MRI may increase the clinical role for imaging technologies in the diagnostic regimen for BPD.

Right heart function is assessed by echocardiography, and pulmonary pressure can be estimated when tricuspidal insufficiency is present. In severe cases, right heart catheter procedures might be indicated. The degree and reversibility of lung vascular resistance can be estimated by testing the responsiveness to iNO and other vasodilators such as oxygen.[32,33]

Regarding potential differential diagnoses, the workup needs to include genetic consultation, probable lung biopsy or lavage under critical consideration of the clinical picture, the patient history, and findings from imaging technologies.

MANAGEMENT

The best approach for preventing or reducing the severity of BPD is to adopt strategies that minimize or avoid conditions that likely contribute to lung injury.

Prenatal Management

Pre- or perinatal management critically affects not only the rate of preterm delivery but also the development of severe long-term sequelae, including BPD.[47] Antenatal glucocorticoid treatment is a major stimulant of lung maturation. Preterm infants whose mothers received a complete and timely course of antenatal steroids (ie, 2 doses of betamethasone more than 24 hours prior to birth, with the last dose given no earlier than 7 days before birth) had a significantly reduced risk of developing BPD.[75] A benefit of this treatment was also shown for incomplete courses of glucocorticoids, and stratification by gender and birth weight at 1 kg showed a benefit

CHAPTER 29

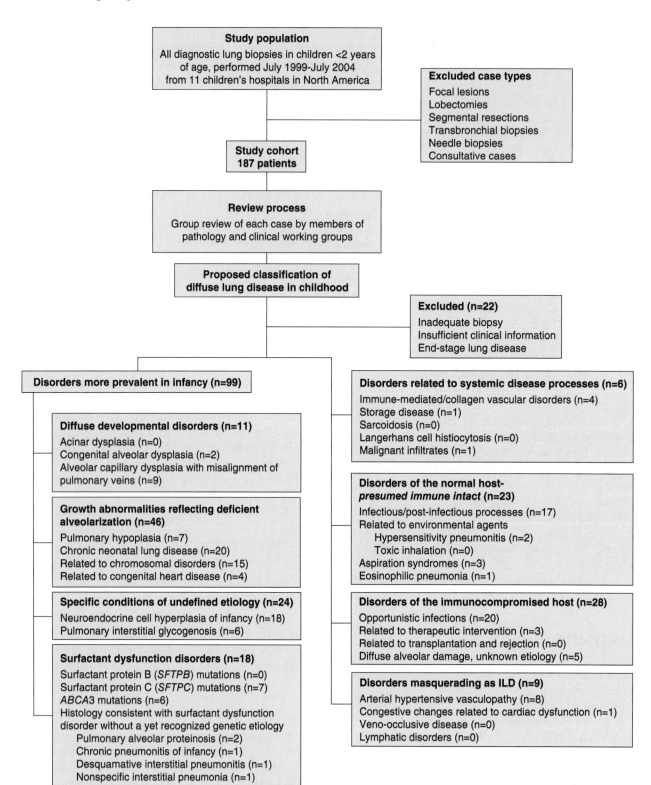

FIGURE 29-8 Classification system of diffuse lung disease in children. The study cohort was composed of patients under the age of 2 years who had a diagnostic lung biopsy during the designated 5-year interval; exclusion criteria are listed. The clinical–pathologic classification scheme is detailed with numbers of cases and specific entities identified within each category. Some unusual entities not seen are also listed, but there are clearly other entities associated with diffuse lung disease not seen in this cohort that have not been listed. (Reproduced with permission from Deutsch GH, Young LR, Deterding RR, et al. Diffuse lung disease in young children: application of a novel classification scheme. *Am J Respir Crit Care Med.* 2007;176(11):1120–1128.)

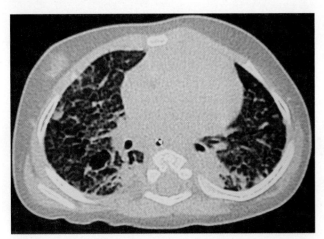

FIGURE 29-9 High-resolution computed tomography: findings in bronchopulmonary dysplasia (BPD). Structural changes in the lung of BPD patients. (Used with permission of Prof. Dr. Irwin Reiss, Intensive Care and Department of Pediatric Surgery, ErasmusMC–Sophia Children's Hospital, Rotterdam, the Netherlands.)

of therapy in all strata except that of extremely low birth weight male infants.[75] A meta-analysis in 2000 did not find enough evidence for the prevention of BPD.[76] With respect to repetitive doses of antenatal steroids, a meta-analysis recommended considering another course of treatment in women at risk of preterm birth 7 or more days after an initial course, in view of the neonatal benefits.[77,78] Although these neonatal benefits were associated with a small reduction in size at birth, up to current evidence no significant harm—or benefit—of the treatment regimen was observed in early childhood.

Prenatal infection/inflammation significantly contributes to the development of BPD, indicating careful consideration of either prolongation of pregnancy under maternal antibiotic and tocolytic treatment or the decision for preterm delivery.[79,80] As experimental studies and clinical findings suggested, strategies such as stimulation of lung growth through infectious agents such as lipopolysaccharides, tolerance of "low-grade" infections, or prevention of severe amnion infection syndrome need to be weighed against each other.[81] As markers to determine a "dose" and timeline in management of prenatal infections are missing, careful individual prenatal case management is needed.

Surfactant Replacement and Ventilation Regimen

The introduction of surfactant replacement into the care of preterm infants reduced mortality in very immature infants and considerably changed the picture of BPD. A meta-analysis showed that postnatal treatment with animal-derived surfactant extracts reduced the risk for BPD or death at 28 days of age.[82] This

can be considered to be the an effect of a reduction in the severity of acute lung disease after premature birth and the resultant need for long-term mechanical ventilation with high peak inflation pressure (PIP). In line with this, early surfactant replacement therapy with extubation to nasal continuous positive airway pressure (NCPAP) was found to be associated with a lower incidence of BPD, less need for mechanical ventilation, and fewer air leak syndromes compared with later selective surfactant replacement and continued mechanical ventilation.[83] Furthermore, lower treatment thresholds (forced inspiratory oxygen [FIO_2] > 0.45) conferred greater advantage in reducing the incidences of air leaks and BPD.[83]

To minimize ventilator-induced changes to the developing lung, assisted ventilation with low PIP, relatively short inspiratory times, and sufficient positive end-expiratory pressures (PEEPs) leading to high-frequency and low tidal volumes have been shown to be beneficial for the preterm lung.[84,85] A recent meta-analysis of 9 studies investigating the effect of pressure-limited and volume-targeted ventilation showed that volume-targeted ventilation reduced death/BPD, duration of ventilation, pneumothoraces, hypocarbia, and periventricular leukomalacia/severe intraventricular hemorrhage (IVH).[51] Adequate heating and humidification of the inspired gas and caution with endotracheal tube suctioning that provokes lung collapse are important steps in the prevention of airway injury.[86] Although application of NCPAP directly after birth reduced the incidence of the need for oxygen at 28 days as well as the number of days of ventilation in infants born at 25 to 28 weeks' gestation,[87] this approach did not significantly reduce the rate of death or BPD when compared to primary intubation. However, extubation to nasal intermittent positive pressure ventilation (NIPPV) or NCPAP in the first postnatal week was found to be associated with decreased probability of BPD/death.[88]

Treatment with a respiratory stimulant, specifically caffeine, reduces the risk of apnea and recently was shown to reduce the incidence of BPD.[89] Inspired O_2 concentrations need to be targeted not only to prevent hyperoxia (ie, O_2 saturation above 96% or PaO_2 above 80 mm Hg) but also to avoid hypoxemia (O_2 saturation < 80% or PaO_2 < 50 mm Hg), which causes pulmonary hypertension; increased fluid filtration (lung edema, potentially through lung epithelial sodium transport); increased airway resistance; and inhibition of alveolar and pulmonary vascular growth. A recent meta-analysis and systematic review of all published randomized studies concluded that a low compared with a high saturation reduced the relative risk of BPD in preterm babies by about 4% to 10%.[52,90] However, as 2 important trials reported slightly increased mortality rates for the group with low oxygen saturation,

O_2 saturation between 85% and 89% cannot currently be recommended in immature babies.[91] The optimal O_2 saturation is presently not known; current practice is to keep the O_2 saturation between 85% and 95% and PaO_2 between 50 and 80 mm Hg.

Despite a good rationale for the application of permissive hypercapnia ($PaCO_2$ 55 or 60 cm H_2O, with a pH of 7.25 or greater) to reduce lung injury in preterm infants during mechanical ventilation in the first week of life, a recent report showed an increased rate of BPD in infants with hypercarbia during that period of time.[92] Other studies showed no apparent benefit of this approach for infants between 23 and 28 weeks' gestation.[93,94]

To reduce oxygen free radical injury, administration of superoxide dismutase was evaluated in infants at risk to develop BPD, but the study failed to detect any benefit of this therapy.[95]

Fluid Management

Restricting fluid and salt intake and allowing for diuresis and a progressive loss of about 10% body weight in the first week of life has been shown to reduce the risk of BPD.[53,54] Excessive fluid and heat losses in the very immature infant should be minimized during the first days after birth by keeping the infant in a warm, humidified chamber.[96–98] Overall fluid balance can be monitored effectively by keeping the infant on a bed scale or by measuring body weight at frequent intervals, by keeping accurate records of fluid intake and urine output, and by considering invisible loss through evaporation through skin and airways. In a suitably humidified environment, appropriate initial rates of intravenous fluid intake for the premature infant are 80–90 mL/kg during the first day of life and 160–180 mL/kg on the sixth day of life, with a stepwise increase of 10 to 20 mL/kg per day.[99,100]

Frequent measurements of serum electrolytes are important in helping to guide fluid therapy. Sodium should be withheld from intravenous fluids for at least the first 24 hours, until adequate diuresis (>2 mL/kg/h) is obtained and the weight is at least 5% below birth weight.[101–103]

Diuretics must be used with caution because of their potential complications—electrolyte deficiencies (notably of sodium, potassium, and chloride), bone demineralization from urinary calcium loss, nephrocalcinosis, and hearing impairment—without benefits for long-term pulmonary outcome.[104] Furosemide is a potent diuretic that reduces pulmonary blood flow and lung vascular filtration pressure and thereby decreases interstitial pulmonary edema.[105] Early use of furosemide is associated with an increased incidence of PDA in preterm infants, as it stimulates the production of prostaglandin E_2 from the kidneys. Hydrochlorthiazide and spironolactone may have less-adverse effects on

urinary calcium or hearing loss. Prolonged use of diuretics can cause contraction alkalosis with associated potassium and chloride depletion, usually heralded by rising serum bicarbonate concentration and low serum chloride concentration.

Other studies have shown that dopamine, when delivered intravenously at low doses to support systemic blood pressure, can enhance lung epithelial Na^+ transport and thereby facilitate clearance of liquid from the airspaces and resolution of pulmonary edema.

Patent Ductus Arteriosus

Closure of the ductus arteriosus by pharmacologic intervention improves lung function in patients with RDS[56] but does not appear to reduce the risk of BPD.[54,106] Although the therapeutic efficiency of cyclo-oxygenase inhibitors, such as indomethacin and ibuprofen, is well documented, prophylactic administration is currently not justified. Short-term benefits of the prophylactic treatment approach for preterm infants, including a reduction in the incidence of symptomatic PDA, PDA surgical ligation, and severe IVH, did not lead to a reduction in either mortality or impaired neurodevelopment.[107] Prophylactic ligation significantly increased the incidence of BPD, defined as supplemental oxygen requirement at 36 weeks' PMA and/or the need for ventilatory support at 36 weeks.[15,108,109]

Management of Postnatal Infections

As nosocomial infections have been shown to increase the risk for BPD, careful and frequent evaluations to detect early signs of infection, meticulous monitoring of aseptic technique in infant handling as well as in the management of ventilatory circuits and airway care, and early initiation of appropriate antimicrobial treatment of infection are considered critical issues to help reduce the incidence and severity of BPD.[49] The pre- or postnatal exposure to *Ureaplasma* or *Chlamydia* species is associated with BPD and IVH in preterm infants even after adjustment for multiple risk factors.[110,111] Nonetheless, the use of erythromycin or azithromycin therapy has not been shown to reduce BPD and thus cannot be recommended.[112]

The use of α_1-proteinase as a way to counter the inflammatory changes to the lung showed a trend toward a reduction in the BPD rate, but without reaching statistical significance.[113]

Nutrition

Nutritional needs of the infant with BPD depend on environmental conditions. The goal should be a neutral thermal environment and the adaption of nutritional intake to work of breathing and general metabolism. Early delivery of parenteral nutrition, including protein and lipid, through an umbilical catheter or a peripherally placed central venous line is helpful in establishing early positive nitrogen balance and facilitating growth and lung repair. A retrospective analysis revealed that aggressive early parenteral nutrition and receipt of calorie-dense milk improved growth for early low birth weight infants with BPD.[114] Actual recommendations state a protein intake of a minimum of 3 g/kg body weight from the second day of life.[115] In orally fed infants, caloric, protein, and mineral needs can usually be met with fortification of mother's breast milk or with premature infant formula. Nonetheless, it has to be considered that there are no clear-cut recommendations to date with respect to increased energy intake for infants with BPD.[116] Nonetheless, latest studies demonstrated that the influence of critical illness on the risk of adverse outcomes was mediated by total daily energy intake during the first week of life.[117]

Furthermore, premature infants with BPD require nutritional supplements of calcium and phosphorus, in addition to adequate vitamins, and if they are receiving diuretics, their overall electrolyte balance needs to be monitored closely.[118] For the decision on early nutrition, long-term metabolic consequences have to be considered.[119]

Retinol (vitamin A) has been shown to decrease the incidence and severity of BPD in extremely premature infants, who are typically deficient in vitamin A. From a meta-analysis of 9 trials, vitamin A appears to be beneficial in reducing death or oxygen requirement at 1 month of age and oxygen requirement at 36 weeks' PMA, although neurodevelopmental outcome showed no differences between the groups at 18 to 22 months.[120,121] For intramuscular treatment in the smallest infants on ventilatory support, retinol was given at a dose of 5000 IU, 3 times/week, for a total of 12 injections.[122] The specific mechanism by which retinol treatment helps to prevent BPD is unclear; a recent report stated that retinol treatment of mechanically ventilated premature baboons yielded no apparent benefit in terms of either lung physiology or alveolar structure[123] but could be shown to increase capillary surface density as well as expression of VEGF.[124]

Glucocorticoids

Because immature infants often have low plasma cortisol levels and do not always respond appropriately to corticotropin (ACTH), hydrocortisone treatment has been considered beneficial. Nonetheless, prophylaxis of early adrenal insufficiency with hydrocortisone, 1 mg/kg per day for 12 days, then 0.5 mg/kg per day for 3 days, did not improve survival without BPD.[125] However, a subanalysis

in chorioamnionitis-exposed infants showed a significant decrease in mortality and improved survival without BPD in this study population, without suppressing adrenal function or compromising short-term growth.[125] The combination of indomethacin and hydrocortisone should be avoided as patients receiving both treatments showed increased spontaneous gastrointestinal perforation. Low cortisol concentrations were not predictive of adverse long-term outcomes, and high cortisol concentrations, although predictive of short-term adverse outcomes such as IVH and periventricular leukomalacia, did not predict adverse outcome of BPD.[126]

High doses of a much more potent anti-inflammatory steroid, dexamethasone, have been used to facilitate weaning from mechanical ventilation. This approach is contraindicated during the first week of life because of its serious side effects[127]: an increased incidence of cerebral palsy and poor neurologic outcome, perhaps related to impaired brain growth and periventricular leukomalacia discovered in infants who have received such therapy over a period of several days to weeks.[128] Low-dose dexamethasone treatment after the first week of life facilitated weaning from the respirator for chronically ventilator-dependent infants.[129–131] This approach should be limited to a short treatment period initiated after the first week of life, with close monitoring for complications such as hyperglycemia and hypertension. So far, no association has been identified between this treatment regimen and long-term morbidity at 2 years' corrected age.[132]

Inhaled steroids have not been shown to be beneficial in reducing the incidence or severity of BPD.[133]

Bronchodilator Therapy

Because infants with BPD have increased respiratory tract resistance and airway hyperreactivity, there is a good rationale for the use of bronchodilators, either by inhalation (β_2-adrenergic agonists) or by intravenous or oral (methylxanthine) delivery. The β_2-adrenergic agonists may be beneficial in BPD by relaxing smooth muscle constriction and by inducing sodium-potassium adenosine triphosphatase (ATPase) activity in the lung epithelium, which may improve pulmonary edema. In unusual circumstances, aerosolized bronchodilators, such as albuterol or atrovent, may induce hypoxemia resulting from vasodilation and mismatching of ventilation and perfusion. This may occur if the underlying problem is not bronchoconstriction but rather atelectasis or mucous plugging; hence, close observation of the response to the bronchodilator treatment to determine its effectiveness is important. Different studies reported controversial results on the benefit of either salbutamol or ipatropium bromide inhalation.[35,134–139] So far, one double-blind randomized control trial using inhaled salbutamol to prevent BPD found no evidence that this therapy reduced mortality, oxygen dependency at 28 days, duration of ventilation, or duration of oxygen supplementation in preterm infants.[140]

Methylxanthines, although helpful in relieving bronchospasm in selected infants with BPD, have significant side effects that may aggravate BPD, including tachycardia, seizures, and gastroesophageal reflux. If these drugs are used, plasma levels must be monitored to help establish therapeutic efficacy and prevent toxicity. As there is insufficient evidence to date with meaningful clinical outcomes following β-receptor agonist therapy, its routine use in prevention or treatment of BPD cannot be justified.

Inhaled Nitric Oxide

There is considerable experimental evidence that iNO can improve respiratory gas exchange, reduce lung inflammation, improve alveolarization and surfactant function, and reverse pulmonary hypertension and bronchoconstriction in newborn animals with acute and chronic lung injury.[141,142] Reports from clinical studies suggested that low-dose iNO may improve oxygenation in infants with BPD. Two multicenter, randomized, placebo-controlled trials showed that iNO treatment reduced the incidence of BPD in preterm infants who required mechanical ventilation.[143,144] In contrast, a recently published study performed in Europe did not confirm these beneficial effects.[145]

A recent meta-analysis showed a 7% reduction in the risk of the composite outcome of death or BPD at 36 weeks, but no reduction in death alone or BPD, for infants treated with iNO compared with controls and concluded that there is currently no evidence to support the use of iNO in preterm infants with respiratory failure outside the context of rigorously conducted randomized clinical trials.[146] This recommendation was supported by the NIH consensus conference in 2011[147,148] and holds true for iNO as a rescue therapy in preterm infants with respect to prevention of BPD.[149]

Potential toxicities of iNO therapy include oxidant lung injury and loss of surfactant function from the production of peroxynitrite, interference with normal platelet function that could affect the incidence of intracranial or pulmonary hemorrhage, and long-term neurodevelopmental disability.

Measures to Treat Gastroesophageal Reflux and Aspiration of Gastric Contents

If suspected, an esophageal pH study should be done to test for the presence of reflux and possible apnea to establish the severity and frequency of the problem. If significant reflux is documented, drugs that might contribute to the problem should be discontinued, and antireflux medications should be considered. To date, comprehensive studies that investigate the direct impact of these complications on the development of BPD are missing.

Assessment for Vocal Cord Injury

Stridor or persistent respiratory distress may be a sign of vocal cord injury, which sometimes occurs through neural injury during cardiovascular surgery, including PDA ligation, or as a direct injury to the vocal cords after prolonged tracheal intubation.[150] Injury of the vocal cords can contribute to respiratory symptoms associated with BPD and prolong weaning from assisted ventilation.

OUTCOME AND FOLLOW-UP

Preterm infants with BPD show acute and long-term pulmonary impairment. This outcome is complicated through the increased risk of neurologic complications associated with the disease. Affected infants can remain oxygen dependent for many months—or even years—although only a few remain oxygen dependant beyond 2 years of age.[151,152] Oxygen dependency therefore indicates the most severe lung disease, as these infants require twice as much hospital readmission compared to infants who are not home oxygen dependent.

Even after outgrowing oxygen dependency, this patient cohort still has more outpatient attendance, episodes of wheezing, and need for an inhaler. Overall, infants suffering from BPD have a high readmission rate, with up to 70% requiring a hospital stay and about 30% requiring 3 readmissions in the first 2 years of life,[153] with lower respiratory tract infections of respiratory syncytial virus a major cause for readmission among preterm infants regardless of BPD status.[154] Hospitalization rate then declines after the second year of life.[155] Regarding respiratory symptoms, BPD was found to be a significant risk factor for wheezing and medication requirement (odds ratios 2.7 and 2.4, respectively), with about 20% to 30% of infants with BPD having those symptoms at 6 and 12 months of age.[156] Respiratory symptoms remain common at preschool and school age,[151,157] with the most severely affected children remaining symptomatic into adulthood.[69] As adults, the effect of gender seems to be different compared to the neonatal period, when male preterm infants are at a higher risk of developing BPD. Later, female BPD patients are more severely affected.[158]

Long-term pulmonary function in patients with BPD has been characterized by different studies. Important data were generated by the EPICure study,[159] showing significantly lower peak oxygen consumption, forced expiratory volume at 1 second (FEV1) and gas transfer in preterm infants at school age, compared to age-matched controls. Preterm infants achieved significantly lower peak workload and employed greater breathing frequencies in combination with lower tidal volumes during peak exercise, whereas their residual capacity was increased. These changes may reflect the effect of hyperinflation due to airway obstruction or altered pulmonary chemoreceptor function and suggest persistent airflow limitation and reduced alveolar surface area. The study showed no gender differences.

Lower lung volumes and gas-mixing efficiency in patients with BPD during infancy have been confirmed by various studies, reflecting defective lung growth.[160,161] Up to 80% of preterm infants, particularly those who presented with wheezing, showed airway obstruction in early childhood and adolescence, with the majority symptomatic.[162–164] Some studies showed more rapid deterioration of lung function in adolescence in patients with a history of BPD.[165] Here, again, findings of lung function abnormalities must be viewed in the context of the underlying era in which the disease was diagnosed (ie, pre- or post-surfactant era).

Studies of long-term sequelae in extremely low birth weight infants showed BPD to be associated with poor neurologic outcome (cerebral palsy, cognitive delay, severe hearing loss, or bilateral blindness at 18 months of age) in about 40% of the infants.[166] Children with severe BPD exhibited lower IQ scores and language delay at 3 years of age as well as lower performance IQ and perceptual organization at 8 years of age compared to children diagnosed with mild or moderate BPD. Children with severe BPD also received more special education services than did children with mild BPD.[167] In very low birth weight infants, BPD predicts poorer motor outcome at 3 years, after controlling for other risks. Cohorts of infants with BPD also had higher rates of mental retardation, associated with greater neurologic and social risk.[168] A recent study showed no group differences in neuropsychological outcome based on categorical ranking of BPD severity. However, continuous measures of BPD severity accounted for a unique portion of the variance in fine motor performance.[169]

The severity of the disease affects long-term neurologic outcome as combined treatment with both mechanical ventilation and supplemental oxygen at 36 weeks' PMA strongly predicts the more common bilateral cerebral palsy phenotypes, whereas BPD without mechanical ventilation at 36 weeks' PMA was not significantly associated with any form of cerebral palsy.[170] Latest studies showed severe retinopathy of prematurity and brain injury but not BPD to correlate independently with poor outcome at 11 years of age.[171]

Adequate follow-up findings for somatic growth in infants with BPD are still missing. It is known that children born at the limit of viability attain poor growth in early childhood, followed by catchup growth to age 11 years, but remain smaller than their term-born peers.[172] Few studies specifically looked at the effect of BPD on growth in puberty or adulthood. Studies in younger infants, however, showed that despite an improvement in weight compared to infants with BPD from the last decade, poor growth attainment at birth, 40 weeks', and 20 months' corrected age remains a major problem among infants with BPD.[173]

ACKNOWLEDGMENT

Acknowledgment is given to Dr. Antje Brand and Dr. Harald Ehrhardt.

REFERENCES

1. Jobe AH, Bancalari E. Bronchopulmonary dysplasia. *Am J Respir Crit Care Med.* 2001;163(7):1723–1729.
2. Gortner L, Misselwitz B, Milligan D, et al. Rates of bronchopulmonary dysplasia in very preterm neonates in Europe: results from the MOSAIC cohort. *Neonatology.* 2010;99(2):112–117.
3. Stoll BJ, Hansen NI, Bell EF, et al. Neonatal outcomes of extremely preterm infants from the NICHD Neonatal Research Network. *Pediatrics.* 2010;126(3):443–456.
4. Van Marter LJ, Pagano M, Allred EN, et al. Rate of bronchopulmonary dysplasia as a function of neonatal intensive care practices. *J Pediatr.* 1992;120(6):938–946.
5. Johnson AH, Peacock JL, Greenough A, et al. High-frequency oscillatory ventilation for the prevention of chronic lung disease of prematurity. *N Engl J Med.* 2002;347(9):633–642.
6. Ehrenkranz RA, Walsh MC, Vohr BR, et al. Validation of the National Institutes of Health consensus definition of bronchopulmonary dysplasia. *Pediatrics.* 2005;116(6):1353–1360.
7. Smith VC, Zupancic JA, McCormick MC, et al. Trends in severe bronchopulmonary dysplasia rates between 1994 and 2002. *J Pediatr.* 2005;146(4):469–473.
8. Laughon MM, Langer JC, Bose CL, et al. Prediction of bronchopulmonary dysplasia by postnatal age in extremely premature infants. *Am J Respir Crit Care Med.* 183(12):1715–1722.
9. Doyle LW. Evaluation of neonatal intensive care for extremely-low-birth-weight infants. *Semin Fetal Neonatal Med.* 2006;11(2):139–145.
10. Northway WH Jr, Rosan RC, Porter DY. Pulmonary disease following respirator therapy of hyaline-membrane disease. Bronchopulmonary dysplasia. *N Engl J Med.* 1967;276(7):357–368.
11. Jobe AJ. The new BPD: an arrest of lung development. *Pediatr Res.* 1999;46(6):641–643.
12. Husain AN, Siddiqui NH, Stocker JT. Pathology of arrested acinar development in postsurfactant bronchopulmonary dysplasia. *Hum Pathol.* 1998;29(7):710–717.
13. Watterberg KL, Demers LM, Scott SM, et al. Chorioamnionitis and early lung inflammation in infants in whom bronchopulmonary dysplasia develops. *Pediatrics.* 1996;97(2):210–215.
14. Speer CP. Inflammation and bronchopulmonary dysplasia: a continuing story. *Semin Fetal Neonatal Med.* 2006;11(5):354–362. Epub 2006 May 15.

15. Walsh MC, Yao Q, Horbar JD, et al. Changes in the use of postnatal steroids for bronchopulmonary dysplasia in 3 large neonatal networks. *Pediatrics.* 2006;118(5):e1328–e1335.

16. Todd DA, Earl M, Lloyd J, et al. Cytological changes in endotracheal aspirates associated with chronic lung disease. *Early Hum Dev.* 1998;51(1):13–22.

17. Rose MJ, Stenger MR, Joshi MS, et al. Inhaled nitric oxide decreases leukocyte trafficking in the neonatal mouse lung during exposure to > 95% oxygen. *Pediatr Res.* 67(3):244–249.

18. Bose CL, Dammann CE, Laughon MM. Bronchopulmonary dysplasia and inflammatory biomarkers in the premature neonate. *Arch Dis Child Fetal Neonatal Ed.* 2008;93(6):F455–F461.

19. Vento G, Tirone C, Lulli P, et al. Bronchoalveolar lavage fluid peptidomics suggests a possible matrix metalloproteinase-3 role in bronchopulmonary dysplasia. *Intensive Care Med.* 2009;35(12):2115–2124.

20. Watterberg KL, Carmichael DF, Gerdes JS, et al. Secretory leukocyte protease inhibitor and lung inflammation in developing bronchopulmonary dysplasia. *J Pediatr.* 1994;125(2):264–269.

21. Bruce MC, Schuyler M, Martin RJ, et al. Risk factors for the degradation of lung elastic fibers in the ventilated neonate. Implications for impaired lung development in bronchopulmonary dysplasia. *Am Rev Respir Dis.* 1992;146(1):204–212.

22. Bruce MC, Wedig KE, Jentoft N, et al. Altered urinary excretion of elastin cross-links in premature infants who develop bronchopulmonary dysplasia. *Am Rev Respir Dis.* 1985;131(4):568–572.

23. Merritt TA, Cochrane CG, Holcomb K, et al. Elastase and alpha 1-proteinase inhibitor activity in tracheal aspirates during respiratory distress syndrome. Role of inflammation in the pathogenesis of bronchopulmonary dysplasia. *J Clin Invest.* 1983;72(2):656–666.

24. Thibeault DW, Mabry SM, Ekekezie II, et al. Lung elastic tissue maturation and perturbations during the evolution of chronic lung disease. *Pediatrics.* 2000;106(6):1452–1459.

25. Pierce RA, Albertine KH, Starcher BC, et al. Chronic lung injury in preterm lambs: disordered pulmonary elastin deposition. *Am J Physiol.* 1997;272(3 Pt 1):L452–L460.

26. Kunzmann S, Speer CP, Jobe AH, et al. Antenatal inflammation induced TGF-beta1 but suppressed CTGF in preterm lungs. *Am J Physiol Lung Cell Mol Physiol.* 2007;292(1):L223–231. Epub 2006 Aug 25.

27. Thebaud B. Angiogenesis in lung development, injury and repair: implications for chronic lung disease of prematurity. *Neonatology.* 2007;91(4):291–297.

28. De Paepe ME, Greco D, Mao Q. Angiogenesis-related gene expression profiling in ventilated preterm human lungs. *Exp Lung Res.* 36(7):399–410.

29. De Paepe ME, Mao Q, Powell J, et al. Growth of pulmonary microvasculature in ventilated preterm infants. *Am J Respir Crit Care Med.* 2006;173(2):204–211.

30. Bland RD, Ling CY, Albertine KH, et al. Pulmonary vascular dysfunction in preterm lambs with chronic lung disease. *Am J Physiol Lung Cell Mol Physiol.* 2003;285(1):L76–L85. Epub 2003 Mar 7.

31. Vyas-Read S, Shaul PW, Yuhanna IS, et al. Nitric oxide attenuates epithelial-mesenchymal transition in alveolar epithelial cells. *Am J Physiol Lung Cell Mol Physiol.* 2007;293(1):L212–L221. Epub 2007 May 11.

32. Kinsella JP, Greenough A, Abman SH. Bronchopulmonary dysplasia. *Lancet.* 2006;367(9520):1421–1431.

33. Steinhorn RH. Neonatal pulmonary hypertension. *Pediatr Crit Care Med.* 11(2 Suppl):S79–S84.

34. Lopez E, Mathlouthi J, Lescure S, et al. Capnography in spontaneously breathing preterm infants with bronchopulmonary dysplasia. *Pediatr Pulmonol.* 46(9):896–902.

35. Hilgendorff A, Reiss I, Gortner L, et al. Impact of airway obstruction on lung function in very preterm infants at term. *Pediatr Crit Care Med.* 2008;9(6):629–635.

36. Hallman M, Haataja R. Genetic influences and neonatal lung disease. *Semin Neonatol.* 2003;8(1):19–27.

37. Parker RA, Lindstrom DP, Cotton RB. Evidence from twin study implies possible genetic susceptibility to bronchopulmonary dysplasia. *Semin Perinatol.* 1996;20(3):206–209.

38. Bhandari V, Gruen JR. The genetics of bronchopulmonary dysplasia. *Semin Perinatol.* 2006;30(4):185–191.

39. Bhandari V, Bizzarro MJ, Shetty A, et al. Familial and genetic susceptibility to major neonatal morbidities in preterm twins. *Pediatrics.* 2006;117(6):1901–1906.

40. Binet ME, Bujold E, Lefebvre F, et al. Role of gender in morbidity and mortality of extremely premature neonates. *Am J Perinatol.* 2012;29(3):159–169.

41. Trotter A, Maier L, Kron M, et al. Effect of oestradiol and progesterone replacement on bronchopulmonary dysplasia in extremely preterm infants. *Arch Dis Child Fetal Neonatal Ed.* 2007;92(2):F94–F98.

42. Regev RH, Lusky A, Dolfin T, et al. Excess mortality and morbidity among small-for-gestational-age premature infants: a population-based study. *J Pediatr.* 2003;143(2):186–191.

43. Reiss I, Landmann E, Heckmann M, et al. Increased risk of bronchopulmonary dysplasia and increased mortality in very preterm infants being small for gestational age. *Arch Gynecol Obstet.* 2003;269(1):40–44.

44. Rieger-Fackeldey E, Schulze A, Pohlandt F, et al. Short-term outcome in infants with a birthweight less than 501 grams. *Acta Paediatr.* 2005;94(2):211–216.

45. Rozance PJ, Seedorf GJ, Brown A, et al. Intrauterine growth restriction decreases pulmonary alveolar and vessel growth and causes pulmonary artery endothelial cell dysfunction in vitro in fetal sheep. *Am J Physiol Lung Cell Mol Physiol.* 2011;301(6):L860–L871.

46. Yoon BH, Romero R, Jun JK, et al. Amniotic fluid cytokines (interleukin-6, tumor necrosis factor-alpha, interleukin-1 beta, and interleukin-8) and the risk for the development of bronchopulmonary dysplasia. *Am J Obstet Gynecol.* 1997;177(4):825–830.

47. Kramer BW. Antenatal inflammation and lung injury: prenatal origin of neonatal disease. *J Perinatol.* 2008;28(Suppl 1):S21–S27.

48. Stoll BJ, Gordon T, Korones SB, et al. Early-onset sepsis in very low birth weight neonates: a report from the National Institute of Child Health and Human Development Neonatal Research Network. *J Pediatr.* 1996;129(1):72–80.

49. Stoll BJ, Hansen N, Fanaroff AA, et al. Late-onset sepsis in very low birth weight neonates: the experience of the NICHD Neonatal Research Network. *Pediatrics.* 2002;110(2 Pt 1):285–291.

50. Van Marter LJ, Dammann O, Allred EN, et al. Chorioamnionitis, mechanical ventilation, and postnatal sepsis as modulators of chronic lung disease in preterm infants. *J Pediatr.* 2002;140(2):171–176.

51. Wheeler KI, Klingenberg C, Morley CJ, et al. Volume-targeted versus pressure-limited ventilation for preterm infants: a systematic review and meta-analysis. *Neonatology.* 2011;100(3):219–227.

52. Saugstad OD, Aune D. In search of the optimal oxygen saturation for extremely low birth weight infants: a systematic review and meta-analysis. *Neonatology.* 2011;100(1):1–8.

53. Van Marter LJ, Leviton A, Allred EN, et al. Hydration during the first days of life and the risk of bronchopulmonary dysplasia in low birth weight infants. *J Pediatr.* 1990;116(6):942–949.

54. Schmidt B, Roberts RS, Fanaroff A, et al. Indomethacin prophylaxis, patent ductus arteriosus, and the risk of

bronchopulmonary dysplasia: further analyses from the Trial of Indomethacin Prophylaxis in Preterms (TIPP). *J Pediatr.* 2006;148(6):730–734.

55. Marshall DD, Kotelchuck M, Young TE, et al. Risk factors for chronic lung disease in the surfactant era: a North Carolina population-based study of very low birth weight infants. North Carolina Neonatologists Association. *Pediatrics.* 1999;104(6):1345–1350.

56. Stefano JL, Abbasi S, Pearlman SA, et al. Closure of the ductus arteriosus with indomethacin in ventilated neonates with respiratory distress syndrome. Effects of pulmonary compliance and ventilation. *Am Rev Respir Dis.* 1991;143(2):236–239.

57. Laughon MM, Smith PB, Bose C. Prevention of bronchopulmonary dysplasia. *Semin Fetal Neonatal Med.* 2009;14(6):374–382.

58. Biniwale MA, Ehrenkranz RA. The role of nutrition in the prevention and management of bronchopulmonary dysplasia. *Semin Perinatol.* 2006;30(4):200–208.

59. Shenai JP, Chytil F, Stahlman MT. Vitamin A status of neonates with bronchopulmonary dysplasia. *Pediatr Res.* 1985;19(2):185–188.

60. Watterberg KL, Scott SM. Evidence of early adrenal insufficiency in babies who develop bronchopulmonary dysplasia. *Pediatrics.* 1995;95(1):120–125.

61. Deutsch GH, Young LR, Deterding RR, et al. Diffuse lung disease in young children: application of a novel classification scheme. *Am J Respir Crit Care Med.* 2007;176(11):1120–1128.

62. Bullard JE, Wert SE, Whitsett JA, et al. ABCA3 mutations associated with pediatric interstitial lung disease. *Am J Respir Crit Care Med.* 2005;172(8):1026–1031.

63. Nogee LM, Dunbar AE 3rd, Wert SE, et al. A mutation in the surfactant protein C gene associated with familial interstitial lung disease. *N Engl J Med.* 2001;344(8):573–579.

64. Shulenin S, Nogee LM, Annilo T, et al. ABCA3 gene mutations in newborns with fatal surfactant deficiency. *N Engl J Med.* 2004;350(13):1296–1303.

65. Kaempf JW, Campbell B, Brown A, et al. PCO_2 and room air saturation values in premature infants at risk for bronchopulmonary dysplasia. *J Perinatol.* 2008;28(1):48–54.

66. Greenough A, Thomas M, Dimitriou G, et al. Prediction of outcome from the chest radiograph appearance on day 7 of very prematurely born infants. *Eur J Pediatr.* 2004;163(1):14–18.

67. Agrons GA, Courtney SE, Stocker JT, et al. From the archives of the AFIP: Lung disease in premature neonates: radiologic-pathologic correlation. *Radiographics.* 2005;25(4):1047–1073.

68. Andreasson B, Lindroth M, Mortensson W, et al. Lung function eight years after neonatal ventilation. *Arch Dis Child.* 1989;64(1):108–113.

69. Northway WH Jr, Moss RB, Carlisle KB, et al. Late pulmonary sequelae of bronchopulmonary dysplasia. *N Engl J Med.* 1990;323(26):1793–1799.

70. Hakulinen AL, Heinonen K, Lansimies E, et al. Pulmonary function and respiratory morbidity in school-age children born prematurely and ventilated for neonatal respiratory insufficiency. *Pediatr Pulmonol.* 1990;8(4):226–232.

71. Oppenheim C, Mamou-Mani T, Sayegh N, et al. Bronchopulmonary dysplasia: value of CT in identifying pulmonary sequelae. *AJR Am J Roentgenol.* 1994;163(1):169–172.

72. Aquino SL, Schechter MS, Chiles C, et al. High-resolution inspiratory and expiratory CT in older children and adults with bronchopulmonary dysplasia. *AJR Am J Roentgenol.* 1999;173(4):963–967.

73. Howling SJ, Northway WH Jr, Hansell DM, et al. Pulmonary sequelae of bronchopulmonary dysplasia survivors: high-resolution CT findings. *AJR Am J Roentgenol.* 2000;174(5):1323–1326.

74. Mayer S, Klaritsch P, Petersen S, et al. The correlation between lung volume and liver herniation measurements by fetal MRI in isolated congenital diaphragmatic hernia: a systematic review and meta-analysis of observational studies. *Prenat Diagn.* 2011;31(11):1086–1096.

75. Van Marter LJ, Leviton A, Kuban KC, et al. Maternal glucocorticoid therapy and reduced risk of bronchopulmonary dysplasia. *Pediatrics.* 1990;86(3):331–336.

76. Crowley P. Prophylactic corticosteroids for preterm birth. *Cochrane Database Syst Rev.* 2000;(2):CD000065.

77. Crowther CA, McKinlay CJ, Middleton P, et al. Repeat doses of prenatal corticosteroids for women at risk of preterm birth for improving neonatal health outcomes. *Cochrane Database Syst Rev.* (6):CD003935.

78. McKinlay CJ, Crowther CA, Middleton P, et al. Repeat antenatal glucocorticoids for women at risk of preterm birth: a Cochrane Systematic Review. *Am J Obstet Gynecol.* 2012;206(3):187–194.

79. Mittendorf R, Covert R, Montag AG, et al. Special relationships between fetal inflammatory response syndrome and bronchopulmonary dysplasia in neonates. *J Perinat Med.* 2005;33(5):428–434.

80. Ikegami M, Jobe AH. Postnatal lung inflammation increased by ventilation of preterm lambs exposed antenatally to *Escherichia coli* endotoxin. *Pediatr Res.* 2002;52(3):356–362.

81. Jobe AH, Ikegami M. Antenatal infection/inflammation and postnatal lung maturation and injury. *Respir Res.* 2001;2:27–32.

82. Seger N, Soll R. Animal derived surfactant extract for treatment of respiratory distress syndrome. *Cochrane Database Syst Rev.* 2009(2):CD007836.

83. Stevens TP, Harrington EW, Blennow M, et al. Early surfactant administration with brief ventilation vs. selective surfactant and continued mechanical ventilation for preterm infants with or at risk for respiratory distress syndrome. *Cochrane Database Syst Rev.* 2007(4):CD003063.

84. Naik AS, Kallapur SG, Bachurski CJ, et al. Effects of ventilation with different positive end-expiratory pressures on cytokine expression in the preterm lamb lung. *Am J Respir Crit Care Med.* 2001;164(3):494–498.

85. Wada K, Jobe AH, Ikegami M. Tidal volume effects on surfactant treatment responses with the initiation of ventilation in preterm lambs. *J Appl Physiol.* 1997;83(4):1054–1061.

86. Schulze A. Respiratory gas conditioning and humidification. *Clin Perinatol.* 2007;34(1):19–33. v.

87. Morley CJ, Davis PG, Doyle LW, et al. Nasal CPAP or intubation at birth for very preterm infants. *N Engl J Med.* 2008;358(7):700–708.

88. Dumpa V, Northrup V, Bhandari V. Type and timing of ventilation in the first postnatal week is associated with bronchopulmonary dysplasia/death. *Am J Perinatol.* 28(4):321–330.

89. Schmidt B, Roberts RS, Davis P, et al. Caffeine therapy for apnea of prematurity. *N Engl J Med.* 2006;354(20):2112–2121.

90. Carlo WA, Finer NN, Walsh MC, et al. Target ranges of oxygen saturation in extremely preterm infants. *N Engl J Med.* 2010;362(21):1959–1969.

91. Saugstad OD, Speer CP, Halliday HL. Oxygen saturation in immature babies: revisited with updated recommendations. *Neonatology.* 2011;100(3):217–218.

92. Subramanian S, El-Mohandes A, Dhanireddy R, et al. Association of bronchopulmonary dysplasia and hypercarbia in ventilated infants with birth weights of 500–1,499 g. *Matern Child Health J.* 2011;15(Suppl 1):S17–S26.

93. Hardy P, Clemens F. Stopping a randomized trial early: from protocol to publication. Commentary to Thome at al: outcome of extremely preterm infants randomized at birth to different $PaCO_2$ targets during the first seven days of life (Biol Neonate 2006;90:218–225). *Biol Neonate.* 2006;90(4):226–228.

94. Thome UH, Carroll W, Wu TJ, et al. Outcome of extremely preterm infants randomized at birth to different $PaCO_2$

targets during the first seven days of life. *Biol Neonate.* 2006;90(4):218–225.

95. Stiskal JA, Dunn MS, Shennan AT, et al. alpha1-Proteinase inhibitor therapy for the prevention of chronic lung disease of prematurity: a randomized, controlled trial. *Pediatrics.* 1998;101(1 Pt 1):89–94.

96. Hammarlund K, Sedin G, Stromberg B. Transepidermal water loss in newborn infants. VII. Relation to post-natal age in very pre-term and full-term appropriate for gestational age infants. *Acta Paediatr Scand.* 1982;71(3):369–374.

97. Hammarlund K, Sedin G, Stromberg B. Transepidermal water loss in newborn infants. VIII. Relation to gestational age and post-natal age in appropriate and small for gestational age infants. *Acta Paediatr Scand.* 1983;72(5):721–728.

98. Baumgart S. Reduction of oxygen consumption, insensible water loss, and radiant heat demand with use of a plastic blanket for low-birth-weight infants under radiant warmers. *Pediatrics.* 1984;74(6):1022–1028.

99. Koletzko B, Goulet O, Hunt J, et al. 1. Guidelines on paediatric parenteral nutrition of the European Society of Paediatric Gastroenterology, Hepatology and Nutrition (ESPGHAN) and the European Society for Clinical Nutrition and Metabolism (ESPEN), supported by the European Society of Paediatric Research (ESPR). *J Pediatr Gastroenterol Nutr.* 2005;41(Suppl 2):S33–S38.

100. Oh W, Poindexter BB, Perritt R, et al. Association between fluid intake and weight loss during the first ten days of life and risk of bronchopulmonary dysplasia in extremely low birth weight infants. *J Pediatr.* 2005;147(6):786–790.

101. Costarino AT, Jr., Gruskay JA, Corcoran L, et al. Sodium restriction versus daily maintenance replacement in very low birth weight premature neonates: a randomized, blind therapeutic trial. *J Pediatr.* 1992;120(1):99–106.

102. Hartnoll G, Betremieux P, Modi N. Randomised controlled trial of postnatal sodium supplementation on oxygen dependency and body weight in 25–30 week gestational age infants. *Arch Dis Child Fetal Neonatal Ed.* 2000;82(1):F19–F23.

103. Sweet DG, Carnielli V, Greisen G, et al. European consensus guidelines on the management of neonatal respiratory distress syndrome in preterm infants—2010 update. *Neonatology.* 97(4):402–417.

104. Stewart A, Brion LP, Ambrosio-Perez I. Diuretics acting on the distal renal tubule for preterm infants with (or developing) chronic lung disease. *Cochrane Database Syst Rev.* 9:CD001817.

105. Thomas W, Speer CP. Management of infants with bronchopulmonary dysplasia in Germany. *Early Hum Dev.* 2005;81(2):155–163.

106. Schmidt B, Davis P, Moddemann D, et al. Long-term effects of indomethacin prophylaxis in extremely-low-birth-weight infants. *N Engl J Med.* 2001;344(26):1966–1972.

107. Fowlie PW, Davis PG, McGuire W. Prophylactic intravenous indomethacin for preventing mortality and morbidity in preterm infants. *Cochrane Database Syst Rev.* (7):CD000174.

108. Clyman R, Cassady G, Kirklin JK, et al. The role of patent ductus arteriosus ligation in bronchopulmonary dysplasia: reexamining a randomized controlled trial. *J Pediatr.* 2009;154(6):873–876.

109. Mosalli R, Alfaleh K, Paes B. Role of prophylactic surgical ligation of patent ductus arteriosus in extremely low birth weight infants: systematic review and implications for clinical practice. *Ann Pediatr Cardiol.* 2009;2(2):120–126.

110. Kasper DC, Mechtler TP, Bohm J, et al. In utero exposure to *Ureaplasma* spp. is associated with increased rate of bronchopulmonary dysplasia and intraventricular hemorrhage in preterm infants. *J Perinat Med.* 39(3):331–336.

111. Colaizy TT, Morris CD, Lapidus J, et al. Detection of *Ureaplasma* DNA in endotracheal samples is associated with

112. Ballard HO, Shook LA, Bernard P, et al. Use of azithromycin for the prevention of bronchopulmonary dysplasia in preterm infants: a randomized, double-blind, placebo controlled trial. *Pediatr Pulmonol.* 2011;46(2):111–118.

bronchopulmonary dysplasia after adjustment for multiple risk factors. *Pediatr Res.* 2007;61(5 Pt 1):578–583.

113. Suresh GK, Davis JM, Soll RF. Superoxide dismutase for preventing chronic lung disease in mechanically ventilated preterm infants. *Cochrane Database Syst Rev.* 2001(1):CD001968.

114. Theile AR, Radmacher PG, Anschutz TW, et al. Nutritional strategies and growth in extremely low birth weight infants with bronchopulmonary dysplasia over the past 10 years. *J Perinatol.* 2012;32(2):117–122.

115. Koletzko B, Goulet O, Hunt J, et al. 1. Guidelines on paediatric parenteral nutrition of the European Society of Paediatric Gastroenterology, Hepatology and Nutrition (ESPGHAN) and the European Society for Clinical Nutrition and Metabolism (ESPEN), supported by the European Society of Paediatric Research (ESPR). *J Pediatr Gastroenterol Nutr.* 2005;41(Suppl 2): S1–S87.

116. Lai NM, Rajadurai SV, Tan KH. Increased energy intake for preterm infants with (or developing) bronchopulmonary dysplasia/ chronic lung disease. *Cochrane Database Syst Rev.* 2006;(3):CD005093.

117. Ehrenkranz RA, Das A, Wrage LA, et al. Early nutrition mediates the influence of severity of illness on extremely LBW infants. *Pediatr Res.* 2011;69(6):522–529.

118. Pohlandt F. Prevention of postnatal bone demineralization in very low-birth-weight infants by individually monitored supplementation with calcium and phosphorus. *Pediatr Res.* 1994;35(1):125–129.

119. Singhal A, Cole TJ, Lucas A. Early nutrition in preterm infants and later blood pressure: two cohorts after randomised trials. *Lancet.* 2001;357(9254):413–419.

120. Darlow BA, Graham PJ. Vitamin A supplementation to prevent mortality and short and long-term morbidity in very low birth-weight infants. *Cochrane Database Syst Rev.* 2007;(4):CD000501.

121. Darlow BA, Graham PJ. Vitamin A supplementation to prevent mortality and short- and long-term morbidity in very low birth-weight infants. *Cochrane Database Syst Rev.* (10):CD000501.

122. Landman J, Sive A, Heese HD, et al. Comparison of enteral and intramuscular vitamin A supplementation in preterm infants. *Early Hum Dev.* 1992;30(2):163–170.

123. Pierce RA, Joyce B, Officer S, et al. Retinoids increase lung elastin expression but fail to alter morphology or angiogenesis genes in premature ventilated baboons. *Pediatr Res.* 2007;61(6):703–709.

124. Albertine KH, Jiancheng S, Dahl MJ, et al. Retinol treatment from birth increases expression of vascular endothelial growth factor (VEGF) and its receptor, fetal liver kinase (Flk-1), and is associated with greater lung capillary surface density in chronically ventilated preterm lambs. *Pediatr Res* 2002;51:A60.

125. Watterberg KL, Gerdes JS, Cole CH, et al. Prophylaxis of early adrenal insufficiency to prevent bronchopulmonary dysplasia: a multicenter trial. *Pediatrics.* 2004;114(6):1649–1657.

126. Aucott SW, Watterberg KL, Shaffer ML, et al. Early cortisol values and long-term outcomes in extremely low birth weight infants. *J Perinatol.* 2010;30(7):484–488.

127. Postnatal corticosteroids to treat or prevent chronic lung disease in preterm infants. *Pediatrics.* 2002;109(2):330–338.

128. Doyle LW, Ehrenkranz RA, Halliday HL. Dexamethasone treatment in the first week of life for preventing bronchopulmonary dysplasia in preterm infants: a systematic review. *Neonatology.* 2010;98(3):217–224.

129. Tanney K, Davis J, Halliday HL, et al. Extremely low-dose dexamethasone to facilitate extubation in mechanically ventilated preterm babies. *Neonatology.* 2011;100(3):285–289.

130. Doyle LW, Ehrenkranz RA, Halliday HL. Dexamethasone treatment after the first week of life for bronchopulmonary dysplasia in preterm infants: a systematic review. *Neonatology.* 98(4):289–296.

131. Doyle LW, Davis PG, Morley CJ, et al. Low-dose dexamethasone facilitates extubation among chronically ventilator-dependent infants: a multicenter, international, randomized, controlled trial. *Pediatrics.* 2006;117(1):75–83.

132. Doyle LW, Davis PG, Morley CJ, et al. Outcome at 2 years of age of infants from the DART study: a multicenter, international, randomized, controlled trial of low-dose dexamethasone. *Pediatrics.* 2007;119(4):716–721.

133. Jarreau PH, Fayon M, Baud O, et al. [The use of postnatal corticosteroid therapy in premature infants to prevent or treat bronchopulmonary dysplasia: current situation and recommendations.] *Arch Pediatr.*2010;17(10):1480–1487.

134. Brundage KL, Mohsini KG, Froese AB, et al. Bronchodilator response to ipratropium bromide in infants with bronchopulmonary dysplasia.*Am Rev Respir Dis.* 1990;142(5):1137–1142.

135. Wilkie RA, Bryan MH. Effect of bronchodilators on airway resistance in ventilator-dependent neonates with chronic lung disease. *J Pediatr.* 1987;111(2):278–282.

136. Yuksel B, Greenough A. Effect of nebulized salbutamol in preterm infants during the first year of life.*Eur Respir J.* 1991;4(9):1088–1092.

137. Yuksel B, Greenough A. Influence of lung function and postnatal age on the response to nebulized ipratropium bromide in children born prematurely. *Respir Med.* 1994;88(7):527–530.

138. Yuksel B, Greenough A. Ipratropium bromide for symptomatic preterm infants. *Eur J Pediatr.* 1991;150(12):854–857.

139. Yuksel B, Greenough A, Green S. Paradoxical response to nebulized ipratropium bromide in pre-term infants asymptomatic at follow-up. *Respir Med.* 1991;85(3):189–194.

140. Ng GY, da S, Ohlsson A. Bronchodilators for the prevention and treatment of chronic lung disease in preterm infants. *Cochrane Database Syst Rev.* 2001(3):CD003214.

141. Bland RD, Albertine KH, Carlton DP, et al. Inhaled nitric oxide effects on lung structure and function in chronically ventilated preterm lambs. *Am J Respir Crit Care Med.* 2005;172(7):899–906. Epub 2005 Jun 23.

142. Ballard PL, Gonzales LW, Godinez RI, et al. Surfactant composition and function in a primate model of infant chronic lung disease: effects of inhaled nitric oxide. *Pediatr Res.* 2006;59(1):157–162.

143. Ballard RA, Truog WE, Cnaan A, et al. Inhaled nitric oxide in preterm infants undergoing mechanical ventilation. *N Engl J Med.* 2006;355(4):343–353.

144. Kinsella JP, Cutter GR, Walsh WF, et al. Early inhaled nitric oxide therapy in premature newborns with respiratory failure. *N Engl J Med.* 2006;355(4):354–364.

145. Mercier JC, Hummler H, Durrmeyer X, et al. Inhaled nitric oxide for prevention of bronchopulmonary dysplasia in premature babies (EUNO): a randomised controlled trial. *Lancet.* 2010;376(9738):346–354.

146. Donohue PK, Gilmore MM, Cristofalo E, et al. Inhaled nitric oxide in preterm infants: a systematic review. *Pediatrics.*2011; 127(2):e414–422.

147. Cole FS, Alleyne C, Barks JD, et al. NIH Consensus Development Conference statement: inhaled nitric-oxide therapy for premature infants. *Pediatrics.*2011;127(2):363–369.

148. Cole FS, Alleyne C, Barks JD, et al. NIH Consensus Development Conference: inhaled nitric oxide therapy for premature infants. *NIH Consens State Sci Statements.* 2010;27(5):1–34.

149. Barrington KJ, Finer N. Inhaled nitric oxide for respiratory failure in preterm infants. *Cochrane Database Syst Rev.* (12):CD000509.

150. Zbar RI, Chen AH, Behrendt DM, et al. Incidence of vocal fold paralysis in infants undergoing ligation of patent ductus arteriosus. *Ann Thorac Surg.* 1996;61(3):814–816.

151. Greenough A, Alexander J, Burgess S, et al. Preschool healthcare utilisation related to home oxygen status. *Arch Dis Child Fetal Neonatal Ed.* 2006;91(5):F337–F341.

152. Greenough A, Alexander J, Burgess S, et al. Home oxygen status and rehospitalisation and primary care requirements of infants with chronic lung disease. *Arch Dis Child.* 2002;86(1):40–43.

153. Greenough A, Cox S, Alexander J, et al. Health care utilisation of infants with chronic lung disease, related to hospitalisation for RSV infection. *Arch Dis Child.* 2001;85(6):463–468.

154. Broughton S, Roberts A, Fox G, et al. Prospective study of healthcare utilisation and respiratory morbidity due to RSV infection in prematurely born infants. *Thorax.* 2005;60(12):1039–1044.

155. Doyle LW, Cheung MM, Ford GW, et al. Birth weight < 1501 g and respiratory health at age 14. *Arch Dis Child.* 2001;84(1):40–44.

156. Greenough A, Limb E, Marston L, et al. Risk factors for respiratory morbidity in infancy after very premature birth. *Arch Dis Child Fetal Neonatal Ed.* 2005;90(4):F320–F323.

157. Gross SJ, Iannuzzi DM, Kveselis DA, et al. Effect of preterm birth on pulmonary function at school age: a prospective controlled study. *J Pediatr.* 1998;133(2):188–192.

158. Vrijlandt EJ, Gerritsen J, Boezen HM, et al. Gender differences in respiratory symptoms in 19-year-old adults born preterm. *Respir Res* 2005;6:117.

159. Welsh L, Kirkby J, Lum S, et al. The EPICure study: maximal exercise and physical activity in school children born extremely preterm. *Thorax.* 65(2):165–172.

160. Greenough A, Dimitriou G, Bhat RY, et al. Lung volumes in infants who had mild to moderate bronchopulmonary dysplasia. *Eur J Pediatr.* 2005;164(9):583–586.

161. Hjalmarson O, Sandberg KL. Lung function at term reflects severity of bronchopulmonary dysplasia. *J Pediatr.* 2005;146(1):86–90.

162. Broughton S, Thomas MR, Marston L, et al. Very prematurely born infants wheezing at follow-up: lung function and risk factors. *Arch Dis Child.* 2007;92(9):776–780.

163. Yuksel B, Greenough A. Relationship of symptoms to lung function abnormalities in preterm infants at follow-up. *Pediatr Pulmonol.* 1991;11(3):202–206.

164. Pelkonen AS, Hakulinen AL, Turpeinen M. Bronchial lability and responsiveness in school children born very preterm. *Am J Respir Crit Care Med.* 1997;156(4 Pt 1):1178–1184.

165. Doyle LW, Faber B, Callanan C, et al. Bronchopulmonary dysplasia in very low birth weight subjects and lung function in late adolescence. *Pediatrics.* 2006;118(1):108–113.

166. Schmidt B, Asztalos EV, Roberts RS, et al. Impact of bronchopulmonary dysplasia, brain injury, and severe retinopathy on the outcome of extremely low-birth-weight infants at 18 months: results from the trial of indomethacin prophylaxis in preterms. *JAMA.* 2003;289(9):1124–1129.

167. Short EJ, Kirchner HL, Asaad GR, et al. Developmental sequelae in preterm infants having a diagnosis of bronchopulmonary dysplasia: analysis using a severity-based classification system. *Arch Pediatr Adolesc Med.* 2007;161(11):1082–1087.

168. Singer L, Yamashita T, Lilien L, et al. A longitudinal study of developmental outcome of infants with bronchopulmonary dysplasia and very low birth weight. *Pediatrics.* 1997;100(6):987–993.

169. Newman JB, Debastos AG, Batton D, et al. Neonatal respiratory dysfunction and neuropsychological performance at the preschool age: a study of very preterm infants with bronchopulmonary dysplasia. *Neuropsychology.*2011;25(5):666–678.

CHAPTER 29

170. Van Marter LJ, Kuban KC, Allred E, et al. Does broncho-pulmonary dysplasia contribute to the occurrence of cerebral palsy among infants born before 28 weeks of gestation? *Arch Dis Child Fetal Neonatal Ed.*2011;96(1):F20–F29.

171. Farooqi A, Hagglof B, Sedin G, et al. Impact at age 11 years of major neonatal morbidities in children born extremely pre-term. *Pediatrics.*2011;127(5):e1247–e1257.

172. Farooqi A, Hagglof B, Sedin G, et al. Growth in 10- to 12-year-old children born at 23 to 25 weeks' gestation in the 1990s: a Swedish national prospective follow-up study. *Pediatrics.* 2006;118(5):e1452–e1465.

173. Madden J, Kobaly K, Minich NM, et al. Improved weight attainment of extremely low-gestational-age infants with bronchopulmonary dysplasia. *J Perinatol.*2010;30(2):103–111.

30 Neonatal Jaundice and Hemolytic Disease of the Newborn

Michael Kaplan, Ruben Bromiker, and Cathy Hammerman

INTRODUCTION

Neonatal jaundice, implying a yellow color of the skin and mucous membranes due to bilirubin deposition, occurs in about 60% of infants and even more often in those exclusively breast feeding. In most cases, the jaundice will be mild or moderate, and the total serum bilirubin (TSB) will not endanger the newborn infant. Occasionally, the TSB may increase to potentially dangerous levels and require treatment with phototherapy or rarely exchange transfusion to offset any further increase. Rarely, the TSB may rise to hazardous levels, at which bilirubin may cross the blood-brain barrier and enter the brain cells. The result will be the complication of acute bilirubin encephalopathy (ABE), in many cases with the devastating chronic sequela of choreoathetotic cerebral palsy known as kernicterus, or death. Despite attempts to eliminate this condition, kernicterus, although a rare condition, is still with us and accompanies us into the third millennium. Many cases should be preventable. Because the implications for affected individuals are lifelong, the public health aspects are necessarily of major importance. Understanding of the metabolism of bilirubin and the pathophysiology of hyperbilirubinemia are crucial to the prevention of this condition, as discussed in this chapter.

EPIDEMIOLOGY

Was There a Disappearance and Resurgence of Kernicterus?

Some authors refer to a disappearance and then resurgence of reported cases of kernicterus in Westernized countries during the last decades.[1-4] Others opine that the condition never completely disappeared and is still being seen, both in countries with advanced medical systems and in developing countries.[5] There can be no doubt that widespread use of the 2 mainstays of treatment of hyperbilirubinemia, exchange transfusion and phototherapy, along with immune prophylaxis of Rh isoimmunization, have prevented many cases of extreme hyperbilirubinemia. If the condition did indeed disappear, however, there can be no explanation for the cases of kernicterus still occurring due to conditions including glucose-6-phosphate dehydrogenase (G-6-PD) deficiency and direct antiglobulin titer (DAT) positive ABO isoimmunization, conditions that, in themselves, did not disappear.[6,7]

In favor of the resurgence theory, following a period during which few cases of kernicterus were reported, several case reports were published from the United States,[8-10] followed by reports of the US-based Kernicterus Registry.[7,11] In Denmark, Ebbesen[12] did find cases of bilirubin encephalopathy between 1994 and 2001, whereas in a nationwide search, he uncovered no cases during the 20 years preceding 1994.

On the other hand, in the United States, Burke et al reported a 70% decrease in the number of hospitalizations between 1988 and 2005 of neonates diagnosed with kernicterus.[13] Brooks et al found a constant incidence of kernicterus in California occurring during 2 time epochs: 1988–1993 and 1994–1997.[14] On a national US basis, mortality data due to kernicterus from the Centers for Disease Control and Prevention databases revealed 31 kernicterus-related deaths between 1979 and 2006, the mortality during the first 14 years of the study period being similar to that of the second.[13]

The debate whether kernicterus did or did not disappear and then reappear is overshadowed by that fact that, well into the third millennium, cases of kernicterus are still being reported with major public health effects on neonatal and childhood morbidity and mortality.

How Frequent Is Kernicterus Currently?

National Statistics

Kernicterus is not a reportable disease, and the exact incidence may not be able to be accurately determined. From the data available, it appears that the incidence varies widely from country to country, as seen in Table 30-1.

Kernicterus in Westernized Countries

Series of affected neonates from Westernized countries have recently been published from the United States,[7] Canada,[15] the United Kingdom and Ireland,[16] and Denmark.[17] The US-based Kernicterus Registry has details of 125 infants who actually developed kernicterus. In addition to cases of kernicterus, the Canadian, UK and Ireland, and Danish studies also included infants with extreme hyperbilirubinemia but without evidence of ABE. The Canadian survey further included newborns who had undergone exchange transfusion. These reports shared several common epidemiologic and etiologic features, summarized in Table 30-2. It is of note that many of the infants had been discharged as healthy from birth hospitalization but were subsequently readmitted for extreme hyperbilirubinemia. Black ethnicity and minority groups were also overrepresented, relative to the home population, in the US and UK/Ireland groups.

In an Italian survey of 109 level III neonatal units, 16 cases of kernicterus (11 of these in term infants)

were reported[18] during the 10 years prior to 2010. A national surveillance system in Germany uncovered 11 cases of kernicterus in infants born between 2003 and 2005.[19] Late prematurity and readmission of previously healthy babies were commonly encountered in this series.

Kernicterus in the Non-Western World

Kernicterus continues to occur in countries to which G-6-PD deficiency is indigenous, as well as in developing countries with underdeveloped health services, or in war zones, at a high rate. Perhaps the most devastating example emanates from Baghdad, Iraq.[20] Of 162 hyperbilirubinemia-related neonatal admissions, 22% had advanced ABE, 12% died within 48 hours of admission, and 21% had posticteric sequelae. Other recent reports derive from Nigeria (115 babies with ABE, of whom 42 [36.5%] died)[21]; Oman (14 cases, of whom 4 [28.5%] died)[22]; and Turkey (10 G-6-PD-deficient neonates, of whom 5 [50%] developed kernicterus).[23] In Kuwait, newborns with kernicterus were reported following traditional henna applications to their skin.[24] Gamaleldin et al recently reported 249 newborns admitted during a 12-month period with a TSB level 25 to 76.4 mg/dL to Cairo University Children's Hospital.[25] Forty-four (18%) had evidence of ABE on admission; another 55 (22%) had subtle evidence of bilirubin-induced neurologic dysfunction (BIND). Twenty-six (10.4%) died, with the deaths attributable to bilirubin neurotoxicity. The most common cause for the hyperbilirubinemia was ABO incompatibility (24%), followed by Rh isoimmunization (8.8%) and G-6-PD deficiency (8.1% of 86 tested).

Surrogates for Assessing the Incidence of Kernicterus

As kernicterus is generally rare, it is difficult to assess the incidence in any specific population group with

Table 30-1 Incidence, per Live Births, of Acute Bilirubin Encephalopathy and Kernicterus in Westernized Countries[a]

Country/State	Years of Birth	Incidence	
		Acute Bilirubin Encephalopathy	**Kernicterus**
Denmark	1994–1998	1/53,000	1/64,000
Denmark	1994–2003	1/79,000	
United Kingdom	2003–2005	1/100,000	1/150,000
Canada	2007–2008	1/49,000	1/43,000
California	1988–1997	0.44/100,000	

[a]Adapted with permission from Maisels M. Neonatal hyperbilirubinemia and kernicterus—not gone but sometimes forgotten. *Early Hum Dev.* 2009;85(11):727–732. California data is compiled from Reference 14.

Table 30-2 Major Epidemiologic and Etiologic Factors for Severe Hyperbilirubinemia Common to Recent Series from Westernized Countries[a]

ABO heterospecificity
G-6-PD deficiency
Other isoimmunizations
Late prematurity
Breast feeding
Sepsis
Male gender
Discharge prior to 48 hours

[a]From References 7 and 15–17.

any precision. To assess the potential for developing ABE in any population groups, surrogates have been sought, including the incidence of extreme hyperbilirubinemia (serum total bilirubin [STB] > 25 mg/dL or 30 mg/dL) or the incidence of readmission for hyperbilirubinemia.[14,26] The reported range for readmission[27–37] for hyperbilirubinemia lies between 0.17% and 3.2%. The main reasons for readmission include lower gestational age, early discharge, unsuccessful breast feeding, and lack of predischarge assessment of the risk for subsequent hyperbilirubinemia. Punaro et al, in Brazil, recently emphasized an important effect of late prematurity on the rate of readmission for hyperbilirubinemia.[38]

Newman et al assessed the incidence of newborns developing extreme hyperbilirubinemia within a health care system. Despite the close surveillance and ready availability of treatment, 0.14% of newborns born at Kaiser Permanente centers in northern California developed an STB greater than 25 mg/dL; 0.01% had STB values ranging from 30.5 to 45.5 mg/dL.[39] Chou et al, after controlling for gestational age, sex, maternal race, feeding type, and maternal age, compared their data from the Henry Ford Health System, Detroit, Michigan, with those of Newman et al.[40] They found that the newborns under their care were less likely to have severe hyperbilirubinemia, defined as a TSB value greater than 20 mg/dL (0.6% vs 2%).[40] They attributed this difference to a rigorous bilirubin screening, follow-up, and treatment program. Under less-vigorous scrutiny, the incidence of extreme hyperbilirubinemia could be expected to be even higher.

DEFINING HYPEBILIRUBINEMIA

The Hour-Specific Bilirubin Nomogram

A major advance in our understanding of bilirubin dynamics during the first week of life has been the development of the hour-specific bilirubin nomogram.[41] As there are rapid changes in STB during the first postnatal days, it is inappropriate, for the purpose of bilirubin assessment, to regard units of time in days of life, but rather in hours. The higher the bilirubin value plots for postnatal hour, the higher becomes the chance of that infant developing subsequent hyperbilirubinemia. Examination of this graph will reveal an increase in STB during the first days of life, with a plateau at about 5 days. As a result, within the normal distribution of bilirubin values, no single bilirubin value can be designated to define hyperbilirubinemia. Whereas an STB value of 10 mg/dL at 12 hours of life lies above the 95th percentile, in the high-risk zone and predictive of severe hyperbilirubinemia, the same value at age 84 or 96 hours will be of little consequence. It is clear that all bilirubin values should be plotted on the nomogram to assess these values in relation to the baby's age.

Definition of Hyperbilirubinemia

The 95th percentile on the bilirubin nomogram has been used by some in recent years to define hyperbilirubinemia,[11] and several clinical research studies have incorporated this definition.[42–44] This definition may not be universally practical, as the American Academy of Pediatrics (AAP, 2004) guidelines indicate the need for phototherapy below that level in cases of premature neonates or those with risk factors.[45] Use of the 75th percentile for hour of life, to designate clinically significant jaundice,[46] or STB values approaching the AAP indications for phototherapy[47] may be viable alternatives.

PATHOPHYSIOLOGY

Bilirubin Formation and Metabolism

Bilirubin is formed from the metabolism of heme (Figure 30-1). The majority of the heme derives from the continual turnover of red blood cells (RBCs), releasing hemoglobin (Hb), although some other sources, such as myoglobin, also contribute to the heme pool. Heme is catabolized by heme oxygenase to biliverdin, by which process equimolar quantities of CO are released. Biliverdin is then reduced to bilirubin via bilirubin reductase. This form of bilirubin, also known as unconjugated or indirect bilirubin, complexes reversibly with serum albumin and in this form is transported to the liver. Intrahepatocytic uridine diphosphate (UDP)–glucuronosyltransferase 1A1 controls the conjugation of bilirubin to glucuronic acid, to form the mono- and diglucuronide forms of conjugated bilirubin. This water-soluble, polarized bilirubin

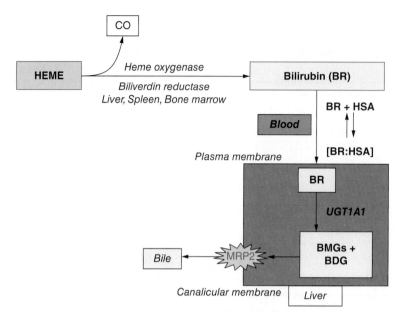

FIGURE 30-1 Main steps in the formation and elimination of bilirubin. BMG and BDG, bilirubin monoglucuronide and diglucuronide, respectively; BR, unconjugated bilirubin; HSA, human serum albumin; UGT1A1, uridine disphospho-glucuronosyl transferase 1A1. (Reproduced with permission from McDonagh AF. Controversies in bilirubin biochemistry and their clinical relevance. *Semin Fetal Neonatal Med.* 2010;15(3):141–147.)

form is now transported into the bile by the canalicular adenosine triphosphate (ATP)–dependent transport protein MRP2[49] and thence to the intestine from which most is excreted. Some bilirubin, however, may be reconverted to the unconjugated form by intestinal bacteria, thereby allowing its reabsorption and return to the bilirubin pool (enterohepatic circulation). This process is facilitated by the presence of the enteric mucosal enzyme β-glucuronidase in the newborn.

Several of the steps noted have important clinical implications.

Release of CO

Carbon monoxide released concomitant with heme breakdown combines with Hb to form carboxyhemoglobin (COHb). As the CO is released in equimolar quantities with the biliverdin, quantification of COHb or end-tidal CO, corrected for ambient CO, represents the endogenous production of CO, which can be used as an index of the rate of heme catabolism, or hemolysis.[50] Unfortunately, there is no bedside tool currently available for clinical use.

Heme Oxygenase

Heme oxygenase 1 (HO-1) controls the first step in heme catabolism and is the rate-limiting factor in the conversion of heme to bilirubin. Polymorphisms of the *HO-1* gene encoding HO-1 may have an effect on the bilirubin production rate. Although variations

in the gene promoter have been associated with higher TSB levels in adults,[51,52] no effect of *HO-1* polymorphisms has been reported in association with neonatal hyperbilirubinemia.[53] The enzyme may be important with regard to bilirubin pharmacotherapeutics. Synthetic heme analogues, metalloporphyrins, are competitive inhibitors of HO-1 and have been used clinically to inhibit the enzyme activity, thereby either preventing bilirubin formation or limiting further bilirubin production when treating established hyperbilirubinemia.[54] Some studies have documented successful use of metalloporphyrins, as reviewed,[54] but the Food and Drug Administration (FDA) has not yet approved the drug for routine clinical use.

Bilirubin Binding and Unbound Bilirubin

As long as the unconjugated bilirubin is bound to serum albumin, this complex is thought to be unable to cross the blood-brain barrier and enter the brain cells. Unbound bilirubin, on the other hand, is potentially neurotoxic and has the ability to cause neuronal damage. Indeed, the unbound bilirubin fraction concentration is a much better predictor of bilirubin neurotoxicity than the STB.[55,56] Unfortunately, there is currently no bedside tool to make unbound bilirubin measurement readily available or clinically useful, and the bilirubin-albumin ratio is sometimes used as a surrogate to determine the need for exchange transfusion.[45] Some factors that may facilitate the finding of increased serum unbound bilirubin and therefore precipitate the penetration of bilirubin into brain cells include hypoalbuminemia, asphyxia, hypothermia, metabolic acidosis, and sepsis.

Uptake Genes

Uptake of bilirubin into the liver is controlled by the solute carrier organic anion transporter protein 1B1, SLCO1B1, also known as OATP2.[57] This sinusoidal transporter facilitates the hepatic uptake of bilirubin as well as other substances, and varying expression of the gene may affect bilirubin kinetics and metabolism. SLCO1B1*1b variant is associated with neonatal hyperbilirubinemia in Tawainese newborns, especially when coupled with UGT1A1 (uridine disphospho-glucuronosyl transferase 1A1) variants.[58] In a US-based study, coexpression of SLCO1B1*1b with G-6-PD A- was associated with hyperbilirubinemia.[59] These studies and others[60] emphasized the importance of gene interactions and ethnic variation in the pathogenesis of hyperbilirubinemia.

Genetic Control of UGT1A1

The function of the UGT enzyme is to conjugate glucuronic acid to certain target substrates to facilitate their elimination from the body. Of major importance to the conjugation and elimination of bilirubin is the *UGT1A1* gene,[61] situated on chromosome 2q37. This gene encodes the UGT1A1 enzyme and is therefore of paramount importance in bilirubin conjugation. The gene consists of 4 common exons (exons 2, 3, 4, and 5) and 13 variable exons, but of the latter, only variable exon A1 is of importance regarding bilirubin conjugation (Figure 30-2). The variable exon A1 functions in conjunction with the common exons to regulate the synthesis of the individual enzyme isoform. Upstream of each variable exon is a regulatory noncoding promoter that contains a TATAA box sequence of nucleic acids. Mutations or polymorphisms of the variable exon A1,

its promoter, or the common exons 2–5, may interfere in the normal process of bilirubin conjugation. While polymorphisms of the noncoding promoter area may affect bilirubin conjugation by diminishing expression of a normally structured enzyme, mutations of the coding areas may alter the structure of the enzyme molecule, thereby interfering with or abolishing enzyme function.

Imbalance Between Bilirubin Production and Elimination

The STB concentration at any point reflects 2 major processes: bilirubin production and bilirubin elimination.[63] Most important is the concept of lack of equilibrium between bilirubin production and conjugation. As long as these processes remain in equilibrium, the STB should remain within normal limits. In the postnatal period, increased heme catabolism in combination with diminished UGT1A1 activity results in imbalance between these processes with increasing bilirubin levels. The enterohepatic circulation may add to the bilirubin load. Should this imbalance remain mild or moderate, STB concentrations should not exceed the 95th percentile on the hour-of-life-specific bilirubin nomogram.[41] However, should bilirubin production exceed its elimination, hyperbilirubinemia may occur. Some degree of increased heme catabolism, not necessarily severe, occurs in many cases of hyperbilirubinemia, even when no obvious hemolytic etiology is apparent.[42,46,64] Despite increased hemolysis and production of large amounts of bilirubin, some babies may not develop increased STB because their hepatic bilirubin-conjugating capacity is mature. On the other hand, minimally increased hemolysis in the face of immature bilirubin conjugation may well result in hyperbilirubinemia. This concept has been likened to a sink of water. Increased inflow relative to the drainage will result in a rise in the water level, whereas increased inflow along with an efficient drainage system will result in minimal rise of the water level.[63] Kaplan et al

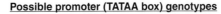

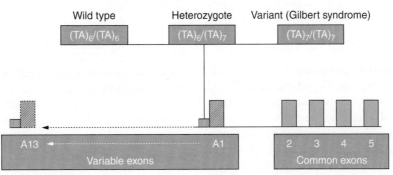

FIGURE 30-2 The uridine diphosphate (UDP)–glucuronosyltransferase gene. For explanation, see the text on the genetic control of UGT1A1. (From Ref. 62.)

demonstrated this concept mathematically.[65] Using blood carboxyhemoglobin corrected for ambient CO (COHbc) to index heme catabolism as the numerator of the equation and serum-conjugated bilirubin to reflect bilirubin conjugation as the denominator, they found that the combined effect of bilirubin production and conjugation correlated better with TSB levels than any of these processes individually.

Increased Danger Associated with Hemolysis

It is generally believed that neonates with hemolytic disease are at a higher risk of bilirubin neurotoxicity than those whose hyperbilirubinemia is not the result of hemolysis.[66,67] Indeed, many original reports of kernicterus emanated from infants with Rh isoimmunization.[68] Data from a few studies are supportive of this concept. In a Turkish study, a positive DAT (or direct Coombs test), due to Rh isoimmunization or ABO incompatibility, was used as a presumed marker of hemolysis.[69] In children with indirect hyperbilirubinemia, DAT positivity was associated with lower IQ scores and a higher incidence of neurologic abnormalities than controls without a positive test but with similar bilirubin concentrations. In DAT-positive Norwegian males who had TSB levels greater than 15 mg/dL for longer than 5 days, IQ scores were significantly lower than average for that population.[70] In the Jaundice and Infant Feeding Study, 5-year IQ values of infants with TSB greater than 25 mg/dL in combination with a positive DAT were significantly lower than hyperbilirubinemic counterparts but with a negative DAT (−17.8 IQ points, 95% confidence interval [CI] −26.8 to −8.8).[71] In a reanalysis of the data from the Collaborative Perinatal Project, Kuzniewicz and Newman found the presence of a positive DAT in those with a TSB of greater than 25 mg/dL was associated with a 6.7-point decrease in IQ scores.[72] An increase in the duration of exposure to high TSB levels was also associated with an increase in neurologic abnormalities. Hemolytic conditions were among the most common etiologies for hyperbilirubinemia in the previously mentioned neonates with ABE recently reported from Egypt: ABO incompatibility (24%), Rh isoimmunization (8.8%), and G-6-PD deficiency (8.1% of 86 who were tested).[25]

The reason for hemolysis increasing the risk for bilirubin neurotoxicity is not clear. Rapid rise in STB and earlier onset of the peak bilirubin value may contribute to this effect. Rapid saturation of the extravascular tissues with bilirubin may further increase the intravascular component. The AAP recommends institution of treatment of hyperbilirubinemia at lower levels of STB in newborns in whom hemolysis is recognized than in nonhemolyzing controls.[45]

THE DREADED COMPLICATION OF EXTREME HYPERBILIRUBINEMIA: ACUTE BILIRUBIN ENCEPHALOPATHY OR KERNICTERUS

Definitions

The term *kernicterus* is sometimes used interchangeably for acute encephalopathy and the chronic form of choreoathetotic cerebral palsy. The clinical picture of these conditions, however, is very different.[73] Bilirubin encephalopathy implies the central nervous system findings that result from bilirubin toxicity to the basal ganglia and other brainstem nuclei.[45] The Subcommittee on Hyperbilirubinemia of the AAP recommends using the term *acute bilirubin encephalopathy* to denote the acute manifestations of bilirubin toxicity seen in the first few weeks after the hyperbilirubinemic episode. The term *kernicterus*, in contrast, should be used in association with the chronic and permanent clinical sequelae of bilirubin toxicity.[45] The expression *bilirubin-induced neurologic dysfunction* (BIND) usually refers to a form of bilirubin neurotoxicity that is subtle, including neurodevelopmental and auditory disabilities that appear to be due to bilirubin toxicity but without the classic findings of kernicterus.[74,75]

Pathology of Bilirubin Toxicity

The pathologic hallmark of bilirubin neurologic damage is staining and necrosis of neurons in the basal ganglia, hippocampal cortex, subthalamic nuclei, and cerebellum followed by gliosis of these areas in survivors (Figure 30-3). The cerebral cortex is generally spared.

Clinical Picture of Kernicterus

Acute Bilirubin Encephalopathy

Early clinical features of ABE include with severe lethargy and poor feeding (phase 1). Although these signs are nonspecific, in the presence of severe hyperbilirubinemia, encephalopathy should be suspected to avoid delay in institution of therapy. During the middle of the first postnatal week (phase 2), muscle tone may fluctuate between hypo- and hypertonia, and a high-pitched cry develops. Spasm of the extensor muscles with back arching, opisthotonus, retrocollis, and impairment of upward gaze resulting in the "setting sun sign" ensue in phase 3, with fever, seizures, apnea, and death following[45,73,77] (Figure 30-4).

Chronic Kernicterus

The clinical picture of kernicterus in its chronic form has been well described.[73] Affected individuals may

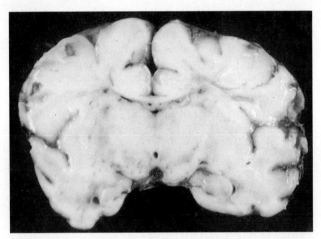

FIGURE 30-3 Bilirubin (yellow) staining of the basal ganglia of a newborn who died from acute bilirubin encephalopathy. (Reproduced with permission of Zangen S, Kidron D, Gelbart T, et al. Fatal kernicterus in a girl deficient in glucose-6-phosphate dehydrogenase: a paradigm of synergistic heterozygosity. *J Pediatr.* 2009;154(4): 616–619.)

display a dystonic or athetoid movement disorder, an auditory processing disturbance that may be associated with hearing loss, motor ocular impairment of upward gaze, enamel dysplasia of the teeth, and hypotonia and ataxia due to cerebellar involvement. Many are unable to walk, require a feeding tube, or have other feeding disabilities. Mental retardation is not uncommon, but some do not have evidence of mental impairment. Hearing and visual impairments occur frequently. Motor spasticity, ataxia, and dyskinesia or hypotonia may be seen.[14,45]

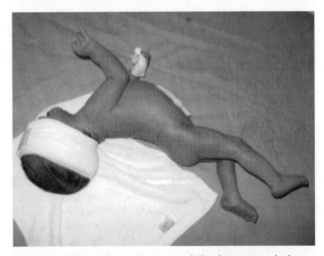

FIGURE 30-4 Baby with acute bilirubin encephalopathy. Note arching of extensor muscles of back and neck. (Reproduced with permission from Bhutani VK, Stevenson DK. The need for technologies to prevent bilirubin-induced neurologic dysfunction syndrome. *Semin Perinatol.* 2011;35(3):97–100.)

Subtle Bilirubin Encephalopathy and Auditory Neuropathy

Bilirubin encephalopathy may not always manifest as the classic, chronic picture of kernicterus. In some, bilirubin-induced neurological damage may result in subtle bilirubin encephalopathy, or BIND. These children have less-severe injury than those with classic kernicterus but may have cognitive disturbances, mild neurologic abnormalities, isolated hearing loss, or auditory neuropathy.[74,79] Auditory neuropathy associated with hyperbilirubinemia is not simply a sensorineural hearing loss, but rather is the result of dysfunction at the level of the auditory brainstem or nerve. Functionally, auditory neuropathy or dyssynchrony is characterized by absent or abnormal brainstem auditory evoked potentials, but with normal inner ear function. In these cases, hearing screening utilizing automated auditory brainstem responses will identify the condition. Evoked otoacoustic emission studies, reflecting inner ear function, may be normal, however, and if used alone, may result in the auditory neuropathy being missed. Awareness of bilirubin auditory neuropathy is of practical importance as cochlear implantation has been used successfully in children with this condition.[74] The mechanism by which hearing is improved is not clear, as the implant is actually proximal to the neural lesion.

DIFFERENTIAL DIAGNOSIS

A list of conditions associated with neonatal jaundice can be seen in Table 30-3. Some specific conditions, chosen because they are frequent, demonstrate a principle, or have public health implications, have been selected for further description in the following paragraphs.

Physiological Jaundice

About 60% of term newborns and even more breast-feeding infants will develop some degree of visible jaundice. During the first postnatal week, there is a natural increase in STB, reaching a mean peak of 5 to 6 mg/dL at about 5 days. Visible jaundice occurring during the first 24 hours should never be regarded as physiologic.[45] Any bilirubin concentration greater than the 95th percentile should not be regarded as physiologic. Following the fifth day, the STB values decrease gradually.

Physiologic jaundice occurs because of increased heme catabolism in combination with diminished bilirubin conjugation, even in the absence of known risk factors for jaundice. Newborn babies have a high rate of heme catabolism, the result of shorter RBC lifespan

Table 30-3 Common Conditions Associated with Neonatal Jaundice

General
Physiological jaundice
Breast milk jaundice
Hemolytic conditions
 Immune
  Rh
  ABO
  Other immunizations
Nonimmune
 G-6-PD deficiency
 Hereditary spherocytosis
 Pyruvate kinase deficiency
 Red cell membrane defects
 Unstable hemoglobinopathies
Conditions associated with diminished bilirubin
 conjugation or elimination
 Gilbert syndrome
 Crigler-Najjar syndromes types 1 and 2
 Hypothyroidism
 Breast milk jaundice
 Prematurity or late prematurity

and greater hematocrit and RBC volume than older counterparts. Also, UGT1A1 enzyme activity is immature in newborns, leading to bilirubin buildup in the immediate postnatal period.[80] This physiologic phenomenon can be exacerbated by breast feeding (below) or increased reabsorption of bilirubin from the bowel in newborns by way of the enterohepatic system, adding to the already-overloaded bilirubin pool and putting further strain on the limited conjugative system.

Jaundice in Breast-Feeding Infants

Healthy term and late-preterm infants who are breast-feeding have higher STB concentrations than formula-feeding counterparts. Some authorities recognize 2 specific entities with regard to jaundice in breast-fed infants, the first, related to inadequate feeding, leading to mild dehydration (breast feeding jaundice), and the second due to breast milk itself (breast milk jaundice).[81] Breast-feeding jaundice occurs during the first postnatal week. Many of these babies have excessive weight loss, the result of delayed initiation of breast feeding, insufficient frequency of feeding, and supplementation with water. These factors may result in increased bilirubin absorption via the enterohepatic circulation. Frequent and successful breast feeding not only will enhance the milk supply, thereby increasing caloric intake and providing sufficient fluid, but also will accelerate intestinal transit time and facilitate excretion of meconium, thereby reducing the enterohepatic bilirubin circulation. Phototherapy may be necessary. In contrast, breast milk jaundice appears

after the first week. The infants are healthy and vigorous and have been gaining weight appropriately. It is postulated that substances present in the breast milk may inhibit UGT1A1 activity. Suggested substances include the progesterone metabolite pregnane-3-alpha-20-beta-diol or beta-glucuronidase. It has been demonstrated that presence of the $(TA)_7$ *UGT1A1* promoter polymorphism (*UGT1A1*28*) may be responsible for prolonged jaundice in breast-feeding newborns.[82] Most infants with breast milk jaundice will respond to phototherapy, and in most cases, it is unnecessary to discontinue breast feeding during treatment.

Hemolytic Conditions

Neonatal hemolytic conditions may be divided into immune and nonimmune pathophysiologic subgroups (Table 30-4). Although Rh isoimmunization is today largely preventable, much of our knowledge regarding the pathophysiology of kernicterus derives from the study of babies affected with this hemolytic condition. ABO immune disease is now the most common immune condition encountered. Of the nonimmune causes, G-6-PD deficiency is the most important from a public health standpoint and is associated with the development of extreme hyperbilirubinemia and, in some cases, bilirubin encephalopathy.

Immune Hemolytic Conditions

The Direct Antiglobulin Test

The DAT, otherwise known as the direct Coombs test, is the hallmark of isoimmunization[83] and is indicative of maternally derived immunoglobulin (Ig) G directed against fetal/neonatal RBC antigenic sites. The antiglobulin reaches the fetus via the placenta. The DAT detects antibody but does not identify the specific

Table 30-4 Some Important and Commonly Encountered Risk Factors for Neonatal Hyperbilirubinemia[a]

Late prematurity
Breast feeding
Early discharge
Poorly established nursing, excessive weight loss
Hemolytic conditions
 Immune hemolytic disease (direct antiglobulin titer
 [DAT] positive)
 G-6-PD deficiency
Previous sibling with hyperbilirubinemia
Bruising, cephalhematoma
Infection

[a]A complete list of risk factors can be found in Reference 45.

antibody type; for this purpose, further tests are necessary. Agglutinated clumps of RBCs may be identified visually or microscopically. Although a positive DAT is potentially associated with increased hemolysis and hyperbilirubinemia, this may not be universally so. Herschel et al found that a newborn with a positive DAT had only a 59% chance of having a 12-hour corrected end-tidal CO (ETCOc) value greater than the 95th percentile, and only 14.8% of DAT-positive neonates developed a STB equal to or greater than the 75th percentile.[84] Ozolek et al found a similar relationship between DAT and hyperbilirubinemia/jaundice in ABO-heterospecific mother-infant pairs.[85]

Rh Isoimmune Hemolytic Disease

Rh disease in pregnancy may lead to intrauterine hemolysis, severe intrauterine anemia, hydrops fetalis, and intrauterine death. Following delivery, ongoing hemolysis may result in severe hemolytic disease of the newborn (HDN), anemia, and hyperbilirubinemia with the potential for bilirubin encephalopathy.

Background: The Immunization Process

Although the Rh group comprises the C, c, D, E, and e antigens, each of which may result in isoimmunization and hemolysis, RhD isommunization was formerly the most common, and when it does occur, is still the most severe. In white populations, 13% to 15% of individuals are Rh negative, but only about half that number are encountered in African Americans, and few Asian individuals are Rh negative. Because of paternal heterozygosity (D/d), an Rh-negative mother may have an Rh-negative fetus in about 50% of pregnancies. However, because of factors such as nonuniversal fetomaternal transmission of fetal blood and variable maternal immune responses, the overall incidence of Rh isoimmunization is infrequent and reported to be 6.8 cases per 1000 live births.[86]

Exposure of a D-negative woman to the D antigen, occurring either antepartum or intrapartum by fetomaternal passage of fetal RBCs containing the D antigen, sets the immunization process into action. Although first-pregnancy isoimmunization has been documented, in primigravidas the process usually begins too late to allow for sufficient maternal IgG antibody to be produced and transferred across the placenta.[87,88] Transfusion of Rh-positive RBCs may also occur during abortion, blood administration, amniocentesis, chorionic villus sampling, or fetal blood sampling, thereby sensitizing the mother. In response to the antigen, the mother's immune system produces anti-D IgG antibodies, which cross the placenta and adhere to the D-antigen sites of the fetal RBCs. The resulting antigen-antibody response culminates in hemolysis and anemia. During subsequent pregnancies, this response may become progressively more severe and rapid. The bone marrow now releases increased numbers of circulating immature RBCs (erythroblastosis), and hepatomegaly and splenomegaly may ensue due to extramedullary hematopoiesis. Fetal hydrops, including generalized tissue edema and pleural, pericardial, and peritoneal effusions, may result. Formation of this extravascular fluid results from hypoproteinemia, tissue hypoxia, and capillary leakage, along with congestive cardiac failure, itself the result of poor myocardial function and diminished cardiac output due to anemia and venous congestion.[89]

Management of the Pregnancy

Hydrops fetalis is associated with a high mortality rate. Should the fetus become anemic, the option to perform intrauterine transfusion must be weighed against delivery. This decision will depend primarily on the gestational age: With increasing maturity, the potential for inherent complications involved in preterm delivery will decrease relative to the dangers involved in performing intrauterine transfusion. Amniocentesis-based regimens for detecting fetal anemia[90] are being replaced by a combination of advancing ultrasonographic techniques and developing genetic technologies, as described further in this chapter. Furthermore, modern advances in DNA technologies allow for accurate determination of paternal RhD gene status; cell-free fetal DNA determination techniques may allow for minimally invasive determination of fetal Rh type in a maternal blood sample.[91-93] Administration of rhesus immune globulin during pregnancy to all nonimmunized, RhD-negative women, in combination with routine postpartum administration of the globulin to those delivering an Rh-positive newborn,[94] has reduced the incidence of antenatal immunization from 14% to 0.1%. The globulin should also be administered following spontaneous or elective abortion, amniocentesis, chorionic villus sampling, or fetal blood sampling. In developing countries where Rh immune prophylaxis is not yet routine, the incidence of Rh HDN in still common.[95]

Determination of the maternal anti-D titer to find the critical titer associated with a high risk of kernicterus is an important step in the monitoring of an RhD-sensitized woman. The critical titer[89] ranges from 1:8 to 1:32. Doppler assessment of the blood flow velocity in the middle cerebral artery of the fetus is replacing amniocentesis in the detection of fetal anemia, the fetal anemia resulting in increased blood flow velocity due to decreased blood viscosity and increased cardiac output.[96] Should the results suggest anemia, fetal blood is then sampled by cordocentesis. Intrauterine transfusion is an option when the hematocrit is less than 30% and the fetus less than 35 weeks' gestation. However, if the pregnancy has reached 35 weeks' gestation or more, delivery will be prudent. In experienced hands, the outcome of intrauterine transfusion should be good.[97]

Postnatal Management of the Newborn

Management of a hydropic, severely anemic neonate, especially if complicated by respiratory and other problems of prematurity, will require intubation and ventilation, sometimes with adjunctive use of surfactant, nitric oxide, and high-frequency ventilation, with emergency drainage of pleural and pericardial effusions.[53] Metabolic acidosis and hypoglycemia are common.[98,99]

Cord blood sample Hb values less than 10 g/dL and STB above 5 mg/dL suggest the presence of severe hemolysis. It may be preferable to correct the anemia isovolumetrically, titrating the hematocrit value until the desired concentration is obtained, using a partial exchange transfusion technique via umbilical venous or arterial catheter rather than by simple blood transfusion.

Following delivery, the placenta will no longer participate in bilirubin elimination. Extreme hyperbilirubinemia may develop, the result of continuing hemolysis and ongoing bilirubin elimination immaturity. Phototherapy and exchange transfusion, should the STB continue to rise despite intensive phototherapy, should be performed according to the 2004 AAP guidelines.[45]

Intravenous immune globulin (IVIG) may be effective in preventing or limiting the number of exchange transfusions in Rh disease.[100–104] Although the 2004 AAP guideline recommends the use of IVIG to prevent exchange transfusion in cases of failing phototherapy,[45] a Dutch study recently found no benefit from the prophylactic administration of IVIG to infants with Rh hemolytic disease.[105] A Cochrane report concluded that more information, based on well-designed studies, was needed before IVIG could be recommended for the treatment of isoimmune hemolytic disease.[106] Meanwhile, even if an exchange transfusion will ultimately be necessary, delay of this procedure by IVIG can be useful in gaining time for stabilization of the patient.

Hemolytic Disease of the Newborn Caused by ABO Heterospecificity

By the term *ABO setup*, we refer to a blood group A or B baby born to a group O mother, a combination seen in about 15% of pregnancies. About one-third of these pregnancies will have a positive DAT due to anti-A or -B antibodies attached to RBCs.[85] Because Rh hemolytic disease has been virtually eliminated in the Western world, ABO blood group heterospecificity has become the most frequent cause of immune hemolytic disease in the neonate. The hyperbilirubinemia may at times be severe and associated with bilirubin encephalopathy. For example, 31 (25%) of 125 babies reported in the US Kernicterus Registry were ABO incompatible.[7] A high incidence of ABO heterospecificity among infants with kernicterus or extreme hyperbilirubinemia was also reported from Canada, the United Kingdom and Ireland, Denmark, Nigeria, and Switzerland.[15–17,107,108]

In contrast to Rh isoimmunization, ABO disease does not follow an initial immunizing process during pregnancy. Some women with type O blood group have an inherently high titer of anti-A or anti-B antibodies even before their first pregnancy.[109] Furthermore, in group O individuals, anti-A or anti-B antibodies comprise IgG molecules that are able to cross the placenta. These IgG molecules may cross the placenta and attach to the corresponding A or B antigens on the fetal RBCs, thereby precipitating hemolysis in utero. Hemolysis of the IgG-coated RBCs is mediated by Fc-receptor-bearing cells within the reticuloendothelial system. The immune process is not usually sufficiently strong to result in severe hemolysis prior to delivery, but continuation of the hemolytic process following delivery can potentially result in severe hyperbilirubinemia.

It is important to realize that ABO heterospecificity, even if the DAT is positive, does not necessarily indicate the presence of ABO *hemolytic disease*, and many infants may not develop early jaundice or significant hyperbilirubinemia. The following criteria should be used to support the diagnosis of ABO hemolytic disease:

1. Mother blood group O, baby group A or B
2. Positive DAT
3. Indirect hyperbilirubinemia, especially during the first 24 hours of life
4. Microspherocytosis on peripheral blood smear
5. Increased reticulocyte count

Studies of Hemolysis Incorporating Endogenous Formation of Carbon Monoxide

Although not all ABO-heterospecific, DAT-positive neonates will necessarily develop hyperbilirubinemia, measurements of endogenous formation of CO, an index of heme catabolism, have demonstrated an increased rate of heme catabolism in these neonates compared with controls.[42,110–112] These studies confirmed the role of hemolysis in the pathogenesis of the hyperbilirubinemia and explained the high incidence of this condition in series of infants with bilirubin encephalopathy. However, not all hemolyzing babies will necessarily develop hyperbilirubinemia. In a multinational, multicenter study in which ETCOc was used to detect hemolysis, values were higher in 54 DAT-positive babies compared with the total.[42] However, only 18.5% of the DAT-positive newborns developed a TSB greater than the 95th percentile. Despite the increased hemolysis, many, by implication, had sufficiently mature conjugating mechanisms and were able to handle the increased bilirubin load. Kaplan et al found that ABO-heterospecific, DAT-positive neonates had higher COHbc values than previously published values for a DAT-negative reference group, and that those who developed hyperbilirubinemia (STB > 95th percentile) had even higher COHbc values.[44] The percentage of newborns who developed hyperbilirubinemia increased in tandem with COHbc, reaching 100% in those with COHbc values greater than the 90th percentile.

Incidence of Hyperbilirubinemia in ABO-Heterospecific Neonates

Not all affected neonates will develop severe or clinically significant hyperbilirubinemia. For example, Kanto et al found that only 11.3% of infants developed STB values greater than 12 mg/dL[113]; Ozolek et al reported that only 13.7% developed STB concentrations greater than 12.8 mg/dL.[85] On the other hand, Kaplan et al found that 51.8% DAT-positive, ABO-heterospecific neonates developed STB values greater than the 95th percentile, 67% of whom had their first TSB greater than the 95th percentile documented earlier than 24 hours.[44] As early jaundice has been recognized by the AAP (2004) as a risk factor for hyperbilirubinemia, any additional stress precipitated by further hemolysis or conjugating immaturity may upset the equilibrium between the bilirubin production and elimination processes with the potential for developing severe hyperbilirubinemia.[45,114]

ABO blood group incompatibility with a negative DAT, not usually predictive of hemolysis or hyperbilirubinemia, may occasionally cause early jaundice with progression to potentially dangerous bilirubin levels, reminiscent of DAT-positive hemolytic disease. Some of these infants may be displaying a manifestation of coexpression between ABO incompatibility and homozygosity for the (TA)$_7$ *UGT1A1* polymorphism (*UGT1A1*28*).[115] This concept is discussed in the section on the genetic interactions between hemolytic conditions and UGT1A1 polymorphisms.

Treatment of ABO Heterospecificity-Associated Neonatal Jaundice

A high degree of vigilance is necessary to detect developing jaundice in newborns born to blood group O mothers. STB or TcB should be measured if jaundice is seen in the first 12–24 hours. Phototherapy and exchange transfusions should be implemented according to the 2004 AAP guideline.[45] IVIG may be helpful in modifying the rate of rise of bilirubin and is indicated if the STB is approaching the exchange transfusion threshold despite a trial of intensive phototherapy. In an analysis of 4 randomized trials involving 226 babies affected with Rh and ABO immune disease, IVIG in combination with phototherapy significantly reduced the need for exchange transfusions compared with phototherapy alone (relative risk [RR], 0.28; 95% CI, 0.17–0.47).[104] In newborns who responded to IVIG administration with a decrease in STB, COHbc values decreased from baseline in tandem with diminishing STB concentrations, demonstrating the effect of IVIG on limiting heme catabolism.[116] The authors have found IVIG therapy useful in neonates who are approaching the indications for exchange transfusion despite phototherapy.

Tin mesoporphyrin (SnMP), a metalloporphyrin that inhibits HO, has been shown to reduce the need for and duration of phototherapy in DAT-positive, ABO-incompatible neonates,[117] but this drug has not yet been approved by the FDA.

Immunization Due to Antibodies Other than RhD and ABO

Because the number of pregnancies complicated by Rh isoimmunization has decreased, uncommon RBC antigens have now become relatively more clinically important. More than 50 RBC antigens may cause HDN.[118] Some clinically important antibodies with regard to intrauterine hemolysis include anti-c, -Kell, -Fy^a, -Jk^a, -C, -E, -C^w, -k, and -S. Anti-Kell isoimmunization warrants special mention as fetal anemia, rather than hyperbilirubinemia, often predominates the clinical picture.[119]

Fetal surveillance protocols and neonatal clinical strategies developed for RhD alloimmunization can be used for the monitoring of affected pregnancies and management of newborns affected by antibodies other than Rh.

Nonimmune Hemolytic Conditions

G-6-PD Deficiency

Deficiency of G-6-PD is a major etiologic factor in the pathogenesis of neonatal hyperbilirubinemia and a well-described cause of extreme hyperbilirubinemia and bilirubin toxicity, as reviewed in Reference 6. In the previously mentioned series of neonates with extreme hyperbilirubinemia or kernicterus from the United States, Canada, the United Kingdom, and Ireland, G-6-PD deficiency comprised a major proportion of affected infants and was overrepresented relative to the background frequency of this condition in these populations.[7,15,16] The condition therefore has major public health implications with regard to the newborn.

Deficiency of G-6-PD is estimated to affect hundreds of millions of individuals worldwide.[120–122] Immigration patterns and ease of travel have transformed G-6-PD deficiency into a condition that is now encountered in virtually every part of the globe and is no longer limited to its indigenous distribution, which included the Mediterranean basin, Africa, and the Middle and Far East.

Function of G-6-PD

G-6-PD[120–122] is a major stabilizing enzyme of the RBC membrane, protecting these cells from oxidative damage. By reducing NADP (nicotinomide adenine dinucleotide phosphate) to NADPH (reduced [hydrogenated] NADP) reduced glutathione can be regenerated from its oxidized form, a process that is essential to oxidative defenses. If there is a deficiency of G-6-PD, NADPH will not become available, regeneration of reduced glutathione will be compromised, and cells will be rendered susceptible to oxidation. The RBC is especially vulnerable because, in these cells, no alternative source of NADPH is available. Oxidative damage to the cell membrane may cause hemolysis.

As G-6-PD deficiency is an X-linked condition, males may be either normal hemizygotes or deficient hemizygotes, whereas females may be normal homozygotes, deficient homozygotes, or heterozygotes.[120–122] Although there should be no difficulty in differentiating between the 2 genotypes in males, in females, the heterozygotes may be difficult to classify because of the phenomenon of X chromosome inactivation. Varying ratios of active and inactivated mutated chromosomes within the cells result in differing degrees of enzyme activity. The most common G-6-PD mutations include G-6-PD A-, originally encountered in Africa; G-6-PD Mediterranean, indigenous to the Mediterranean basin and the Middle East; and G-6-PD Canton, indigenous to the Far East. Many other mutations have been described.[123]

G-6-PD Deficiency and Hemolysis

Deficiency of G-6-PD is notoriously associated with severe hemolytic episodes with resultant jaundice and anemia, which may occur in both children and adults, following exposure to a hemolytic trigger. Classically, these episodes occur following ingestion of or contact with the fava bean (*Vicia fava*). Other chemical triggers, such as antimalarials, sulfonamides, and naphthalene-containing mothballs, may be equally dangerous, as are infections.[120]

Extreme Neonatal Hyperbilirubinemia

The most extreme and dreaded form of hemolysis associated with G-6-PD deficiency occurs in neonates. Typically, there is acute, sudden, and unpredictable onset of jaundice. STB levels may rise exponentially, and bilirubin encephalopathy may ensue. Frequently,

no trigger can be identified. Extreme hyperbilirubinemia may develop, and exchange transfusion may be the only recourse.

Studies of endogenous CO formation have demonstrated the important role of increased hemolysis in association with the extreme hyperbilirubinemia associated with this condition.[124] Often, there is an absence of hematological evidence of hemolysis, leading some to conclude, erroneously, that these events are not the result of hemolysis.[125,126]

Moderate Neonatal Hyperbilirubinemia

Many G-6-PD-deficient neonates manifest a more moderate form of jaundice that usually responds to phototherapy, although exchange transfusion may sometimes be necessary.[43,127] Moderately increased COHbc concentrations do not correlate with the degree of hyperbilirubinemia, leading to the conclusion that this somewhat increased hemolysis cannot be implied as the primary icterogenic factor. Consequently, a predilection for diminished bilirubin conjugation has been demonstrated,[128,129] the result of an interaction between G-6-PD deficiency and the (TA)$_7$ *UGT1A1* promoter polymorphism[60] (Figure 30-5). These infants may be at high risk for subsequent development of severe hyperbilirubinemia as any further imbalance between bilirubin production and conjugation may result in severe hyperbilirubinemia.[130]

Testing for G-6-PD Deficiency

Qualitative or quantitative screening tests should accurately determine the hemizygous state in males

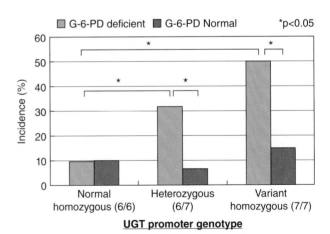

FIGURE 30-5 Interaction between G-6-PD (glucose-6-phosphate dehydrogenase) deficiency and the variant (TA)$_7$ UDP-glucuronosyltransferase 1A1 promoter polymorphism in the pathogenesis of neonatal hyperbilirubinemia (total serum bilirubin ≥15 mg/dL). UDP, uridine diphosphate; UGT, uridine disphosphoglucuronosyl transferase. (Reproduced with permission from Kaplan M, Renbaum P, Levy-Lahad E, et al. Gilbert syndrome and glucose-6-phosphate dehydrogenase deficiency: a dose-dependent genetic interaction crucial to neonatal hyperbilirubinemia. *Proc Natl Acad Sci USA*. 1997;94(22):1228–1232.)

or the homozygous state in females. Biochemical tests are based on the oxidation of glucose-6 phosphate by G-6-PD, which results in generation of NADPH, the NADPH production reflecting G-6-PD activity. NADPH fluoresces in ultraviolet light and is the basis of the fluorescent spot test.[131] Spectrophotometric measurement of absorbance at 340 nm reflects NADPH activity and is used in the quantitative measurement of G-6-PD activity. Neonatal G-6-PD enzyme values are frequently higher than adult values because neonates have many young RBCs with inherently high G-6-PD activity. Molecular screening methods will allow for heterozygote identification, but some newborns with mutations not included in any specific set of mutations tested for may be missed. The test time is substantially longer than biochemical screening tests. Neonatal G-6-PD screening programs, in combination with parental education regarding the development of jaundice and which foodstuffs or chemical substances to avoid, are in force in some countries and have been associated with a decrease in the number of cases of kernicterus, as reviewed elsewhere.[132,133]

The treatment of neonatal hyperbilirubinemia associated with G-6-PD deficiency should follow the guidelines of the AAP for neonates with hemolytic risk factors.[45]

Pyruvate Kinase Deficiency

Following on G-6-PD deficiency, pyruvate kinase (PK) deficiency is the second-most-common cause of nonspherocytic, Coombs-negative, hemolytic neonatal jaundice in the United States.[134] PK plays an important part in catalyzing the process resulting in formation of ATP from adenosine diphosphate in the Embden-Meyerhof pathway. It is therefore crucial to energy production. Four PK isoenzymes are encoded by 2 genes, for which 180 mutations have been identified. PK deficiency is inherited in an autosomal recessive manner.[135]

In the PK-deficiency state, ATP depletion and increased cell content of 2,3-disphosphoglycerate (2,3-DPG) result in stasis, acidosis, and hypoxia, contributing to entrapment and premature destruction of poorly deformable RBCs in the microcirculation of the reticuloendothelial system. Resultant hemolysis may lead to severe neonatal anemia and early hyperbilirubinemia.[136] In patients with homozygous null mutations, no functional enzyme is formed, and newborns may be born severely anemic or even die in utero.[137] Kernicterus has been reported in association with the enzyme deficiency.[138]

The condition should be suspected in cases of hemolysis and hyperbilirubinemia not associated with a positive direct Coombs test or spherocytosis. Enzyme-deficient patients have a 5% to 40% of normal enzyme activity. Molecular studies may confirm the diagnosis by identifying mutations in the coding area of the PK gene.[139] Treatment is supportive, consisting of exchange transfusion or blood transfusions when necessary. Iron overload is common, and chelation therapy may be required.

Hereditary Spherocytosis

Hereditary spherocytosis (HS) is an RBC membrane defect that can lead to acute hemolysis and hyperbilirubinemia in the newborn.[140-142] The condition is characterized by a deficiency in 1 or more RBC membrane proteins. Affected RBCs are abnormally shaped, have higher metabolic requirements, and are prematurely trapped and destroyed in the spleen.[143] The condition is usually inherited in an autosomal dominant fashion, but recessive or de novo mutations are also encountered. Protein deficiencies in the RBC membrane, including ankyrin, band 3, α-spectrin, β-spectrin, and protein 4.2, leave microscopic patches of the lipid bilayer inner surface bare of proteins. At these points, microvesicularization occurs, rendering the affected RBCs osmotically fragile. Affected RBCs become trapped in the spleen, the microvesicles are aspirated by macrophages, and the cell is destroyed. Hemolysis may result in jaundice, anemia, and splenomegaly. Clinically, in its most severe form, HS may result in hydrops fetalis with intrauterine death.[144] Hyperbilirubinemia may require exchange transfusion[145]; kernicterus has been described.[146] Frequently, there is a history of hyperbilirubinemia in a sibling or a parent.

The diagnosis of HS is based on the combination of a typical clinical picture with the presence of spherocytes on a peripheral blood smear, the setting of familial hemolytic anemia, and an abnormal osmotic fragility test.[143] Christensen and Henry recently demonstrated that a mean corpuscular Hb concentration of greater than 36.0 g/dL had an 82% sensitivity and 98% specificity for identifying HS.[147] Flow cytometric analysis techniques may be more specific diagnostically than osmotic fragility testing.[148]

The diagnosis of HS may be difficult in the neonatal period as splenomegaly is infrequent, and reticulocytosis may not be severe or universal. Many affected neonates may not have large numbers of spherocytes in their peripheral blood smears.[149,150] Also, the osmotic fragility test is less reliable for diagnosis of this disease in newborns than in adults. Postponement of testing until the infant is about 6 months of age may be prudent.[142,151]

Treatment of hyperbilirubinemia in the neonatal period should be guided by the 2004 AAP guideline.[45] Splenectomy may become necessary later during childhood to control the anemia resulting from ongoing hemolysis.

Hereditary Elliptocytosis, Hereditary Pyropoikilocytosis, Hereditary Ovalocytosis, and Hereditary Stomatocytosis

Hereditary elliptocytosis, hereditary pyropoikilocytosis, hereditary ovalocytosis, and hereditary stomatocytosis are rare conditions affecting the erythrocyte membrane. The diagnosis is usually made by microscopic examination of the peripheral blood smear. Hemolysis may occur in the neonatal period and result in anemia and hyperbilirubinemia.[141,152–155]

Unstable Hemoglobinopathies

Hemoglobinopathies are the result of mutations of the globin genes. These unstable hemoglobins[156,157] may decrease RBC survival time. Heinz body inclusions may be seen in the RBCs. The γ-globin mutations Hemoglobin Poole and Hemoglobin Hasharon have been reported to cause neonatal hemolysis with jaundice and anemia. Unstable hemoglobinopathies should be sought in cases of unexplained hemolytic anemias.

Conditions Associated with Diminished Bilirubin Uptake, Conjugation, or Elimination

Gilbert Syndrome

Gilbert syndrome is a benign disorder that produces mild unconjugated bilirubinemia in about 6% of adults. Both defective hepatic uptake of bilirubin and decreased hepatic UGT activity have been demonstrated. In individuals with Gilbert syndrome, the UGT1A1-conjugating enzyme is normally structured but not fully functional because of diminished gene expression. This is because the noncoding, rather than coding, area of the gene is affected. The genetic basis of the reduced gene expression lies in the presence of additional TA repeats [$(TA)_7$ or occasionally $(TA)_8$ instead of the wild-type $(TA)_6$] in the TATAA box in the promoter region of the *UGT1A1* gene[158,159] (Figure 30-2). In and of itself, the $(TA)_7$ promoter polymorphism has resulted in increased STB values compared with $(TA)_6$ controls, but not with hyperbilirubinemia. When in combination with additional icterogenic factors, however, the situation may be very different.

Kaplan et al described a dose-dependent genetic interaction between G-6-PD deficiency and $(TA)_7$ promoter polymorphism in which the incidence of any STB greater than 15 mg/dL increased dramatically when these 2 factors were in combination[60] (Figure 30-5). In Asian populations, interaction between G-6-PD deficiency and coding area *UGT1A1* mutations similarly exacerbate hyperbilirubinemia.[160] Iolascon et al described an interaction between $(TA)_7$ promoter

polymorphism and HS, also increasing the incidence of neonatal hyperbilirubinemia over and above that of HS, individually.[161]

Crigler-Najjar Syndrome Type I

Crigler-Najjar (CN) syndrome type I is a rare autosomal recessive disease characterized by an almost-complete absence of hepatic UGT activity. In contrast to Gilbert syndrome, the coding area of the UGT gene is mutated, so the enzyme itself is structurally abnormal with no or little bilirubin-conjugating ability. In homozygotes, severe unconjugated hyperbilirubinemia develops during the first days of life, and STB concentrations may reach 25 to 35 mg/dL. Kernicterus may occur. Stools are pale yellow, and bile bilirubin concentrations are low, with total absence of bilirubin glucuronide in bile. The diagnosis can now be obtained by sequencing the *UGT1A1* gene and identifying mutations.[162]

The management of these neonates involves containment of STB concentrations by phototherapy, sometimes in combination with exchange transfusion.[163] The advent of effective phototherapy systems has altered the course of this previously lethal disease, but patients remain at risk from bilirubin neurotoxicity throughout their lifetime.[163] Although liver transplant offers the only definitive treatment of the disease, in a multicenter report, 7 of 21 (33%) of transplanted children had already developed some form of brain damage by the time of their transplantation.[164] Hepatocyte transplantation and gene therapy may have promise for these children in the future.[165]

Crigler-Najjar Syndrome Type II

Crigler-Najjar syndrome type II is more common than type I disease and is typically benign. Unconjugated hyperbilirubinemia occurs in the first days of life and may be exacerbated by fasting, illness, and anesthesia. The occurrence of kernicterus is rare. Unconjugated hyperbilirubinemia may persist into adulthood. Less than 50% of the daily bilirubin production is excreted in bile, and the monoglucuronide is the predominant form due to inability to convert monoglucuronide to diglucuronide.[162]

Phenobarbital may be used as a simple clinical tool to differentiate between type II and type I diseases. Jaundiced neonates with type II disease respond to oral administration of phenobarbital with a sharp decline in TSB; individuals with type I disease do not respond in this way. Beyond the neonatal period, there should be no long-term risk of kernicterus.

Crigler-Najjar syndrome type II occurs as both an autosomal recessive and a dominant inheritance. The parents and other family members may appear icteric or have low-grade unconjugated hyperbilirubinemia. Testing of the neonate and the parents for the capacity to form glucuronides of bilirubin was used diagnostically in the past. Molecular diagnostic techniques with *UGT1A1* gene sequencing have replaced the older methods.[162]

Pyloric Stenosis

Pyloric stenosis may be associated with unconjugated hyperbilirubinemia. Hepatic UGT activity is diminished in jaundiced neonates, the result of the presence of the variant (TA)$_7$ *UGT1A1* gene promoter.[166]

Hypothyroidism

About 10% of congenitally hypothyroid neonates may develop prolonged jaundice due to diminished UGT activity, and testing for thyroid function should be performed in these cases. The mechanism of this association may be impairment of hepatic uptake and reduced hepatic ligandin concentrations. Absence of thyroid hormone may delay hepatic bilirubin enzyme and transport development.[167]

Jaundice Associated with Prematurity

Jaundice in premature infants is more common and severe than in full-term neonates. STB concentrations peak around the fifth day of life. The reason for the frequency of jaundice in premature infants is immaturity of the UGT1A1 bilirubin-conjugating enzyme, over and above the level of immaturity normally encountered in term infants.[80] In premature infants, bilirubin toxicity may occur at lower concentrations of bilirubin than in term infants. Any visible jaundice in a preterm infant should be closely monitored. Recommended STB values for commencing phototherapy or performing exchange transfusions are lower for premature infants than in term newborns.[168]

Jaundice Associated with Late Prematurity

Late-preterm gestation (newborns born who have completed between 34 weeks and 36 weeks 6 days) is becoming important as a risk factor for the development of neonatal hyperbilirubinemia. Kernicterus has been described in association with late prematurity. Immature bilirubin conjugative capacity may contribute to the greater prevalence and potential severity of jaundice in these infants. Coexpression of late prematurity with additional icterogenic factors such as G-6-PD deficiency may enhance the jaundice.[169] Management of late-preterm infants and discharge at 1 or 2 days, as if they were term infants, with lack of appropriate follow-up, is a major contributor to the bilirubin-related morbidity in these cases.

DIAGNOSTIC TESTS

Assessment of Level of Jaundice

Visual

Newborns should be assessed visually for the appearance of jaundice from birth and several times daily through the first days of life. Jaundice appears first on the head and progresses cephalocaudally. The point to which the jaundice has reached has been used to allow for visual assessment of the level of jaundice.[170] Assessment of the skin color may be facilitated by blanching the skin to reveal the skin and underlying tissue color. In dark-skinned newborns, inspection of the palms, soles, and mucous membranes may enhance the assessment. Visual assessment, however, is an inaccurate technique, and quantification of jaundice should be performed by obtaining a STB, especially in the presence of jaundice appearing during the first 24 hours. Transcutaneous bilirubinometry (TcB) technology should facilitate closer and more objective noninvasive evaluation than was available in the past (see the next sections).

Serum or Plasma Bilirubin Determinations

The STB is the mainstay of bilirubin determination for practical, clinical use. Although high-performance liquid chromatographic (HPLC) techniques are the "gold standard" of bilirubin determinations, this method of testing is expensive and labor intensive. There are still inaccuracies and variability in laboratory performance of bilirubin testing in the clinical laboratory, although efforts are being made to standardize systems and minimize inaccuracy.[171]

Transcutaneous Bilirubinometry

Transcutaneous bilirubinometry measurement techniques offer a rapid, noninvasive, point-of-care screen.[172] TcB does not measure the actual bilirubin but measures the intensity of the yellow color of the skin and translates that into a value estimating the STB. TcB is useful in that it eliminates the guesswork associated with visual assessment of jaundice and can give guidance regarding which babies require a serum or plasma test. TcB readings correlate well with actual STB determinations, although TcB tends to underestimate the actual TSB determination. It may be prudent to obtain a blood test to confirm TcB readings prior to institution of therapy or should the reading be greater than the 75th percentile on the bilirubin nomogram or greater than the 95th percentile on a TcB nomogram.[173]

Interpretation of the TcB or STB Value: Assessment of Risk

It is imperative to interpret the TcB or STB value by plotting the value on the hour-specific nomogram and determining the percentile for age.[41] There are rapid changes in STB during the first days of life, and the identical bilirubin value may have different implications when occurring at different ages during the first week. In general, the higher the percentile is, the greater the risk of subsequently developing significant hyperbilirubinemia will be. Newborns with readings less than the 40th percentile (low-risk zone) have a low, but not negligible, risk of subsequent hyperbilirubinemia. Risk factor assessment should be incorporated in the assessment of the STB value. The presence of factors such as late prematurity, DAT positivity, or G-6-PD deficiency may have an effect on exacerbating the risk of subsequent hyperbilirubinemia.

Blood Groups and DAT

Blood grouping and DAT determinations do not need to be performed routinely, except in infants born to Rh-negative mothers to determine the need for maternal anti-D administration. Blood groups and DAT should be determined in infants of group O mothers who are developing jaundice or in cases of unexplained, severe jaundice to identify possible isoimmunization due to causes other than ABO heterospecificity.

Complete Blood Count

The CBC may sometimes be useful as a falling Hb or HCT value or increased reticulocyte count may be adjunctive in assessing whether hemolysis is present. However, the CBC is not an accurate index of hemolysis in newborns, and there may be overlap between normal and abnormal CBC values in hemolytic and nonhemolytic situations.[174]

Examination of the blood smear may be useful in the identification of RBC morphology.

G-6-PD and Pyruvate Kinase Testing

In cases of unexplained jaundice or an unidentified cause of hemolysis, especially in families with a strong family background for G-6-PD deficiency, the G-6-PD status can be assessed by either qualitative screening tests or quantitative enzyme assays. PK can be tested by enzyme assay.

Magnetic Resonance Imaging

In many cases, ABE and kernicterus are accompanied by characteristic magnetic resonance imaging (MRI) changes. Typically noted is a bilateral, symmetric, high-intensity signal in the globus pallidus and sometimes in the hippocampus and thalamus.[74] In the acute stages of the disease process, these changes may not be universally present: Coskun et al recently reported only 8 of 13 affected neonates with this finding.[175] Absence of typical MRI changes does not exclude the diagnosis.[74] Gkoltsiou et al were not able to demonstrate a constant relationship between early imaging abnormality and motor outcome. Classic globus pallidus changes on T2-weighted images, however, were seen in all infants with cerebral palsy attributable to bilirubin neurotoxicity.[176]

Brainstem Auditory Evoked Potentials

As auditory neural tissue is sensitive to the effects of bilirubin toxicity, the brainstem auditory evoked potential (BAEP) offers an early and sensitive measure of bilirubin-induced central nervous system dysfunction. Increased latency and decreased amplitude of waves III and V are early signs of bilirubin toxicity, followed by absence of these waveforms and finally complete absence of all waveforms. Automated ABR can be used at the bedside as a rapid test of auditory function in a neonate with severe hyperbilirubinemia. Absence of automated ABR, or change from "pass" to "refer," may be an indication of bilirubin neurotoxicity.[73]

MANAGEMENT

Successful ongoing evaluation to detect the development of jaundice, predischarge assessment of the risk for subsequent hyperbilirubinemia, and the timely management of hyperbilirubinemia when it does occur to prevent bilirubin encephalopathy are essential to ensure a safe first week of life. Several countries, including the United States, Canada, United Kingdom, Norway, Israel, and South Africa, have set up national guidelines to standardize the management of neonatal jaundice in an attempt to minimize the number of babies developing kernicterus.

Ongoing assessment during birth hospitalization includes regular assessment of babies for development of jaundice and assessment of risk factors that may exacerbate the risk of hyperbilirubinemia. Some important risk factors include exclusive breast feeding, late prematurity, a previous sibling with significant jaundice, G-6-PD deficiency, and DAT positivity. Although babies born at 37 weeks' gestation are classified as term, their bilirubin-conjugating system is not as efficient as that of an infant at 40 weeks' gestation. It is now recommended that each infant is assessed predischarge for the risk of hyperbilirubinemia by determining a bilirubin value, either by the STB or

TcB routes, in addition to assessment of risk factors.[173] Should the risk be determined high, that baby should have a bilirubin test within 1 or 2 days of discharge. Because the bilirubin value may increase even in the absence of risk factors or a bilirubin percentile in the high-risk zone, all newborns should be seen by a health authority within 2 or 3 days of discharge to assess the success of breast feeding and to evaluate the need for bilirubin testing.[45,173]

Treatment of Hyperbilirubinemia

The mainstays of treatment include phototherapy and exchange transfusion.[177] The AAP has published graphs indicating specific TSB values at which treatment should be instituted.[45] These graphs, akin to the bilirubin nomogram, vary according to hour of life and with the presence of risk factors or prematurity. The technical aspects of phototherapy and exchange transfusion are discussed in the Atlas section of this book.

Therapy with IVIG may be useful in cases of immune hemolysis in which the STB is reaching exchange transfusion indications. The AAP has published guidelines for its use.[45]

Drug therapy has included phenobarbital administration to enhance UGT activity and facilitate bilirubin excretion. Mesoporphyrins have been demonstrated to successfully lower the STB and may in the future play a major role in the management of hyperbilirubinemia but, as discussed, have not yet been released by the FDA for routine use.

Once the chronic features of kernicterus have become established, the treatment is primarily supportive and directed toward improving the neurodevelopmental and other sequelae. Physiotherapy, occupational therapy, and speech therapy may be helpful in alleviating some of the symptoms. Additional related problems can include feeding and nutritional difficulties, sleep disturbances, and muscle hypertonicity. Hearing deficits may be alleviated by conventional hearing aid amplification. Cochlear implantation has been reported to be successful in improving hearing, even though the lesion may be proximal to the implant.[74]

OUTCOME AND FOLLOW-UP

Extreme Hyperbilirubinemia

The STB is a poor predictor of bilirubin-related neurologic outcome as not all newborns with extreme hyperbilirubinemia go on to develop choreoathetotic cerebral palsy.[55] In a study of 140 newborns with STB values greater than 25 mg/dL who were treated with phototherapy or exchange transfusion, 5-year outcomes were not significantly different from those of randomly selected controls.[71] Reanalyzing data from the Collaborative Perinatal Project, Kuzniewicz and Newman found no relationship between maximum STB levels and IQ scores.[72] However, in both these studies, the presence of a positive DAT did result in poorer prognosis than the general population studied. Of 249 newborns admitted with STB values greater than 25 mg/dL to a children's hospital in Cairo, Egypt, Gamaleldin et al found little correlation between admission STB and ABE.[25] However, the presence of risk factors, including Rh incompatibility, ABO incompatibility, and sepsis, decreased the threshold TSB for identifying babies with bilirubin encephalopathy relative to those without risk factors.

Acute Bilirubin Encephalopathy

Sgro et al recently documented the clinical picture of 32 Canadian newborns whose STB ranged from 24.9 to 45.2 mg/dL and who had neurological findings compatible with ABE at the time of admission.[77] The dominant clinical features included hypotonia, poor suck, lethargy, and abnormal auditory evoked responses. Opisthotonus, retrocollis, apnea, seizures, irritability, and hypertonia were also found. Infants in the highest peak bilirubin level group (>32 mg/dL), who presented within the first 2 days of life, or who had undergone exchange transfusion were at higher risk for presenting with signs of bilirubin encephalopathy. The authors suggested that the rapid increase in serum bilirubin may have potentiated the risk of ABE.

Many babies with ABE go on to develop chronic choreoathetotic cerebral palsy.

Chronic Kernicterus

The clinical picture of kernicterus in its chronic form has been well described.[73] A recent report of 25 California cases of strictly defined kernicterus provided a dismal picture of these severely disadvantaged children.[14] Seventy-two percent were male. At a mean (SD) age of 7.8 (3.9) years, 60% did not walk at all, and only 16% were able to walk unaided. Only 52% could self-feed; a feeding tube was in place in 12%. Severe or profound mental retardation or severe disablement was found in 36%, while only 32% had no evidence of mental retardation. Epilepsy was found in 20%. Severe, profound, or untestable visual impairment was documented in one-quarter of cases. Severe, profound, or untestable hearing impairment affected 56%, with only 36% having normal hearing. Motor spasticity was seen in 32%, ataxia and dyskinesia in 12% each, and hypotonia in 8%.

Does Acute Bilirubin Encephalopathy Necessarily Predict Chronic Outcome?

Although ABE usually precedes the permanent neurological sequelae of kernicterus, some reports suggested that this may not necessarily be so. There are reports of severely hyperbilirubinemic infants with signs of ABE on admission who subsequently did not demonstrate signs of bilirubin neurotoxicity.[16,17,178,179] These results, although most likely representing the minority of outcomes, are nevertheless encouraging. Should a baby present with features of ABE, exchange should be done as soon as feasible because of the potential for reversal of the severe outcome.

CONCLUSIONS

Despite growing awareness of the condition and the formulation of international as well as local guidelines, kernicterus continues to occur well into the third millennium. Kernicterus has been declared a never event, but because of conditions causing sudden and unpredictable rises to extreme levels of STB, such as G-6-PD deficiency, it is unlikely that kernicterus will be completely eliminated. However, if general principles and published guidelines are meticulously followed, most babies should be unaffected. It is imperative to assess each baby prior to discharge for TcB or STB as well as for risk factors and to evaluate each baby within a few days of discharge in accordance with AAP recommendations.[45] Severely hyperbilirubinemic neonates should be followed up closely clinically with auditory and MRI evaluation to detect and institute supportive therapy as indicated.

REFERENCES

1. Hansen TW. Kernicterus in term and near-term infants—the specter walks again. *Acta Paediatr.* 2000;89:1155–1157.
2. Johnson L, Bhutani VK. Guidelines for management of the jaundiced term and near term infant. *Clin Perinatol.* 1998;25:555–574.
3. Davidson L, Thilo EH. How to make kernicterus a "never event." *NeoReviews.* 2003;4:308–314.
4. Bhutani VK, Johnson L. Kernicterus in the 21st century: frequently asked questions. *J Perinatol.* 2009;29(Suppl 1): S20–S24.
5. Maisels MJ. Neonatal hyperbilirubinemia and kernicterus—not gone but sometimes forgotten. *Early Hum Dev.* 2009;85:727–732.
6. Kaplan M, Hammerman C. Glucose-6-phosphate dehydrogenase deficiency and severe neonatal hyperbilirubinemia: a complexity of interactions between genes and environment. *Semin Fetal Neonatal Med.* 2010;15:1448–1456.
7. Johnson L, Bhutani VK, Karp K, Sivieri EM, Shapiro SM. Clinical report from the pilot USA Kernicterus Registry (1992 to 2004). *J Perinatol.* 2009;29(Suppl 1):S25–S45.
8. MacDonald MG. Hidden risks: early discharge and bilirubin toxicity due to glucose 6-phosphate dehydrogenase deficiency. *Pediatrics.* 1995;96:734–738.
9. Maisels MJ, Newman TB. Kernicterus in otherwise healthy, breast-fed term newborns. *Pediatrics.* 1995;96:730–733.
10. Penn AA, Enzmann DR, Hahn JS, Stevenson DK. Kernicterus in a full term infant. *Pediatrics.* 1994;93:1003–1006.
11. Bhutani VK, Johnson LH, Jeffrey Maisels M, et al. Kernicterus: epidemiological strategies for its prevention through systems-based approaches. *J Perinatol.* 2004;24:650–662.
12. Ebbesen F. Recurrence of kernicterus in term and near-term infants in Denmark. *Acta Paediatr.* 2000;89:1213–1217.
13. Burke BL, Robbins JM, Bird TM, Hobbs CA, Nesmith C, Tilford JM. Trends in hospitalizations for neonatal jaundice and kernicterus in the United States, 1988–2005. *Pediatrics.* 2009;123:524–532.
14. Brooks JC, Fisher-Owens SA, Wu YW, Strauss DJ, Newman TB. Evidence suggests there was not a "resurgence" of kernicterus in the 1990s. *Pediatrics.* 2011;127:672–679.
15. Sgro M, Campbell D, Shah V. Incidence and causes of severe neonatal hyperbilirubinemia in Canada. *CMAJ* 2006;175:587–590.
16. Manning D, Todd P, Maxwell M, Jane Platt M. Prospective surveillance study of severe hyperbilirubinaemia in the newborn in the UK and Ireland. *Arch Dis Child Fetal Neonatal Ed.* 2007;92:F342–F346.
17. Bjerre JV, Petersen JR, Ebbesen F. Surveillance of extreme hyperbilirubinaemia in Denmark. A method to identify the newborn infants. *Acta Paediatr.* 2008;97:1030–1034.
18. Dani C, Poggi C, Barp J, Romagnoli C, Buonocore G. Current Italian practices regarding the management of hyperbilirubinaemia in preterm infants. *Acta Paediatr.* 2011;100:666–669.
19. Bartmann P, Schaaff F. Kernicterus in Germany 2003–2005. *Pediatric Academic Societies.* E-PAS 2007:617936.24.
20. Hameed NN, Na'Ma AM, Vilms R, Bhutani VK. Severe neonatal hyperbilirubinemia and adverse short-term consequences in Baghdad, Iraq. *Neonatology.* 2011;100:57–63.
21. Owa JA, Ogunlesi, TA. Why we are still doing so many exchange blood transfusion for neonatal jaundice in Nigeria? *World J Pediatr.* 2009;5:51–55.
22. Nair PA, Al Khusaiby SM. Kernicterus and G6PD deficiency—a case series from Oman. *J Trop Pediatr.* 2003;49:74–77.
23. Katar S. Glucose-6-phosphate dehydrogenase deficiency and kernicterus of South-East anatolia. *J Pediatr Hematol Oncol.* 2007;29:284–286.
24. Raupp P, Hassan JA, Varughese M, Kristiansson B. Henna causes life threatening haemolysis in glucose-6-phosphate dehydrogenase deficiency. *Arch Dis Child.* 2001;85:411–412.
25. Gamaleldin R, Iskander I, Seoud I, et al. Risk factors for neurotoxicity in newborns with severe neonatal hyperbilirubinemia. *Pediatrics.* 2011;128(4):e925–e931.
26. Escobar GJ, Greene JD, Hulac P, et al. Rehospitalisation after birth hospitalisation: patterns among infants of all gestations. *Arch Dis Child.* 2005;90(2):125–131.
27. Oddie SJ, Hammal D, Richmond S, Parker L. Early discharge and readmission to hospital in the first month of life in the northern region of the UK during 1998: a case cohort study. *Arch Dis Child.* 2005;90:119–124.
28. Meara E, Kotagal UR, Atherton HD, Lieu TA. Impact of early newborn discharge legislation and early follow-up visits on infant outcomes in a state Medicaid population. *Pediatrics.* 2004;113:1619–1627.
29. Madden JM, Soumerai SB, Lieu TA, Mandl KD, Zhang F, Ross-Degnan D. Length-of-stay policies and ascertainment of postdischarge problems in newborns. *Pediatrics.* 2004;113:42–49.

30. Lock M, Ray JG. Higher neonatal morbidity after routine early hospital discharge: are we sending newborns home too early? *CMAJ* 1999;161:249–253.

31. Grupp-Phelan J, Taylor JA, Liu LL, Davis RL. Early newborn hospital discharge and readmission for mild and severe jaundice. *Arch Pediatr Adolesc Med.* 1999;153:1283–1288.

32. Seidman DS, Stevenson DK, Ergaz Z, Gale R. Hospital readmission due to neonatal hyperbilirubinemia. *Pediatrics.* 1995;96:727–729.

33. Danielsen B, Castles AG, Damberg CL, Gould JB. Newborn discharge timing and readmissions: California, 1992–1995. *Pediatrics.* 2000;106:31–39.

34. Geiger AM, Petitti DB, Yao JF. Rehospitalisation for neonatal jaundice: risk factors and outcomes. *Paediatr Perinat Epidemiol.* 2001;15:352–358.

35. Eggert LD, Wiedmeier SE, Wilson J, Christensen RD. The effect of instituting a prehospital-discharge newborn bilirubin screening program in an 18-hospital health system. *Pediatrics.* 2006;117:e855–e862.

36. Slaughter J, Annibale D, Suresh G. False-negative results of pre-discharge neonatal bilirubin screening to predict severe hyperbilirubinemia: a need for caution. *Eur J Pediatr.* 2009;168(12):1461–1466.

37. Maisels MJ, Deridder JM, Kring EA, Balasubramaniam M. Routine transcutaneous bilirubin measurements combined with clinical risk factors improve the prediction of subsequent hyperbilirubinemia. *J Perinatol.* 2009;29(9):612–617.

38. Punaro E, Mezzacappa MA, Facchini FP. Systematic follow-up of hyperbilirubinemia in neonates with a gestational age of 35 to 37 weeks. *J Pediatr (Rio J).* 2011;87(4):301–306.

39. Newman TB, Xiong B, Gonzales VM, Escobar GJ. Prediction and prevention of extreme neonatal hyperbilirubinemia in a mature health maintenance organization. *Arch Pediatr Adolesc Med.* 2000;154(11):1140–1147.

40. Chou SC, Palmer RH, Ezhuthachan S, et al. Management of hyperbilirubinemia in newborns: measuring performance by using a benchmarking model. *Pediatrics.* 2003;112(6 Pt 1): 1264–1273.

41. Bhutani VK, Johnson L, Sivieri EM. Predictive ability of a predischarge hour-specific serum bilirubin for subsequent significant hyperbilirubinemia in healthy term and near-term newborns. *Pediatrics.* 1999;103:6–14.

42. Stevenson DK, Fanaroff AA, Maisels MJ, et al. Prediction of hyperbilirubinemia in near-term and term infants. *Pediatrics.* 2001;108(1):31–39.

43. Kaplan M, Herschel M, Hammerman C, Hoyer JD, Stevenson DK. Hyperbilirubinemia among African American, glucose-6-phosphate dehydrogenase-deficient neonates. *Pediatrics.* 2004;114:e213–e219.

44. Kaplan M, Hammerman C, Vreman HJ, Wong RJ, Stevenson DK. Hemolysis and hyperbilirubinemia in antiglobulin positive, direct ABO blood group heterospecific neonates. *J Pediatr.* 2010;157:772–777.

45. American Academy of Pediatrics Subcommittee on Hyperbilirubinemia. Management of hyperbilirubinemia in the newborn infant 35 or more weeks of gestation. *Pediatrics.* 2004;114:297–316.

46. Maisels MJ, Kring E. The contribution of hemolysis to early jaundice in normal newborns. *Pediatrics.* 2006;118(1):276–279.

47. Keren R, Luan X, Friedman S, Saddlemire S, Cnaan A, Bhutani VK. A comparison of alternative risk-assessment strategies for predicting significant neonatal hyperbilirubinemia in term and near-term infants. *Pediatrics.* 2008;121(1):e170–e179.

48. McDonagh AF. Controversies in bilirubin biochemistry and their clinical relevance. *Semin Fetal Neonatal Med.* 2010;15(3):141–147.

49. Nies A, Keppler D. The apical conjugate efflux pump ABCC2 (MRP2). *Pflugers Arch.* 2007;453:643–569.

50. Stevenson DK, Vreman HJ, Wong RJ. Bilirubin production and the risk of bilirubin neurotoxicity. *Semin Perinatol.* 2011;35(3):121–126.

51. Lin R, Wang X, Wang Y, et al. Association of polymorphisms in four bilirubin metabolism genes with serum bilirubin in three Asian populations. *Hum Mutat.* 2009;30(4):609–615.

52. Exner M, Minar E, Wagner O, Schillinger M. The role of heme oxygenase-1 promoter polymorphisms in human disease. *Free Radic Biol Med.* 2004;37(8):1097–1104.

53. Kanai M, Akaba K, Sasaki A, et al. Neonatal hyperbilirubinemia in Japanese neonates: analysis of the heme oxygenase-1 gene and fetal hemoglobin composition in cord blood. *Pediatr Res.* 2003;54(2):165–171.

54. Stevenson DK, Wong RJ. Metalloporphyrins in the management of neonatal hyperbilirubinemia. *Semin Fetal Neonatal Med.* 2010;15(3):164–168.

55. Wennberg RP, Ahlfors CE, Bhutani VK, Johnson LH, Shapiro SM. Toward understanding kernicterus: a challenge to improve the management of jaundiced newborns. *Pediatrics.* 2006;117:474–485.

56. Ahlfors CE, Wennberg RP, Ostrow JD, Tiribelli C. Unbound (free) bilirubin: improving the paradigm for evaluating neonatal jaundice. *Clin Chem.* 2009;55:1288–1299.

57. Cui Y, König J, Leier I, Buchholz U, Keppler D. Hepatic uptake of bilirubin and its conjugates by the human organic anion transporter SLC21A6. *J Biol Chem.* 2001;276(13):9626–9630.

58. Huang MJ, Kua KE, Teng HC, Tang KS, Weng HW, Huang CS. Risk factors for severe hyperbilirubinemia in neonates. *Pediatr Res.* 2004;56(5):682–689.

59. Watchko JF, Lin Z, Clark RH, Kelleher AS, Walker MW, Spitzer AR. Complex multifactorial nature of significant hyperbilirubinemia in neonates. *Pediatrics.* 2009;124(5):e868–e877.

60. Kaplan M, Renbaum P, Levy-Lahad E, Hammerman C, Lahad A, Beutler E. Gilbert syndrome and glucose-6-phosphate dehydrogenase deficiency: a dose-dependent genetic interaction crucial to neonatal hyperbilirubinemia. *Proc Natl Acad Sci. USA.* 1997;94(22):12128–12132.

61. van Es HH, Bout A, Liu J, et al. Assignment of the human UDP glucuronosyltransferase gene (UGT1A1) to chromosome region 2q37. *Cytogenet Cell Genet.* 1993;63:114–116.

62. Kaplan M, Hammerman C. Bilirubin and the genome: the hereditary basis of unconjugated neonatal hyperbilirubinemia. *Curr Pharmacogenom.* 2005;3:21–42.

63. Stevenson DK, Dennery PA, Hintz SR. Understanding newborn jaundice. *J Perinatol.* 2001;21(Suppl 1):S21–S24.

64. Kaplan M, Herschel M, Hammerman C, Karrison T, Hoyer JD, Stevenson DK. Studies in hemolysis in glucose-6-phosphate dehydrogenase-deficient African American neonates. *Clin Chim Acta.* 2006;365(1–2):177–182.

65. Kaplan M, Muraca M, Hammerman C, et al. Imbalance between production and conjugation of bilirubin: a fundamental concept in the mechanism of neonatal jaundice. *Pediatrics.* 2002;110:e47.

66. Newman TB, Maisels MJ. Does hyperbilirubinemia damage the brain of healthy full-term infants? *Clin Perinatol.* 1990;17:331–358.

67. Watchko JF, Oski FA. Bilirubin 20 mg/dL = vigintiphobia. *Pediatrics.* 1983;71:660–663.

68. Hsia DY, Allen FH Jr, Gellis SS, Diamond LK. Erythroblastosis fetalis. VIII. Studies of serum bilirubin in relation to Kernicterus. *N Engl J Med* 1952;247:668–671.

69. Ozmert E, Erdem G, Topçu M, et al. Long-term follow-up of indirect hyperbilirubinemia in full-term Turkish infants. *Acta Paediatr.* 1996;85:1440–1444.

70. Nilsen ST, Finne PH, Bergsj P, Stamnes O. Males with neonatal hyperbilirubinemia examined at 18 years of age. *Acta Paediatr Scand.* 1984;73:176–180.

71. Newman TB, Liljestrand P, Jeremy RJ, et al; Jaundice and Infant Feeding Study Team. Outcomes among newborns with total serum bilirubin levels of 25 mg per deciliter or more. *N Engl J Med.* 2006;354:1889–1900.

72. Kuzniewicz MW, Escobar GJ, Newman TB. Impact of universal bilirubin screening on severe hyperbilirubinemia and phototherapy use. *Pediatrics.* 2009;124:1031–1039.

73. Shapiro SM. Hyperbilirubinemia and the risk for brain injury. In Perlman J, Polin RA, eds. *Neurology: Neonatology Questions and Controversies.* Philadelphia, PA: Saunders Elsevier; 2008:195–209.

74. Shapiro SM. Chronic bilirubin encephalopathy: diagnosis and outcome. *Semin Fetal Neonatal Med.* 2010;15(3):157–163.

75. Johnson L, Bhutani VK. The clinical syndrome of bilirubin-induced neurologic dysfunction. *Semin Perinatol.* 2011;35(3):101–113.

76. Zangen S, Kidron D, Gelbart T, Roy-Chowdhury N, Wang X, Kaplan M. Fatal kernicterus in a girl deficient in glucose-6-phosphate dehydrogenase: a paradigm of synergistic heterozygosity. *J Pediatr.* 2009;154(4):616–619.

77. Sgro M, Campbell D, Barozzino T, Shah V. Acute neurological findings in a national cohort of neonates with severe neonatal hyperbilirubinemia. *J Perinatol.* 2011;31:392–396.

78. Bhutani VK, Stevenson DK. The need for technologies to prevent bilirubin-induced neurologic dysfunction syndrome. *Semin Perinatol.* 2011;35(3):97–100.

79. Johnson L, Bhutani VK. The clinical syndrome of bilirubin-induced neurologic dysfunction. *Semin Perinatol.* 2011;35:101–113.

80. Kawade N, Onishi S. The prenatal and postnatal development of UDP-glucuronyltransferase activity towards bilirubin and the effect of premature birth on this activity in the human liver. *Biochem J.* 1981;196(1):257–260.

81. Gartner LM, Herschel M. Jaundice and breastfeeding. *Pediatr Clin North Am.* 2001;48(2):389–399.

82. Monaghan G, McLellan A, McGeehan A, et al. Gilbert's syndrome is a contributory factor in prolonged unconjugated hyperbilirubinemia of the newborn. *J Pediatr.* 1999;134(4):441–446.

83. Coombs RR, Mourant AE, Race RR. In-vivo isosensitisation of red cells in babies with haemolytic disease. *Lancet.* 1946;1:264–266.

84. Herschel M, Karrison T, Wen M, Caldarelli L, Baron B. Evaluation of the direct antiglobulin (Coombs') test for identifying newborns at risk for hemolysis as determined by end-tidal carbon monoxide concentration (ETCOc); and comparison of the Coombs' test with ETCOc for detecting significant jaundice. *J Perinatol.* 2002;22:341–347.

85. Ozolek JA, Watchko JF, Mimouni F. Prevalence and lack of clinical significance of blood group incompatibility in mothers with blood type A or B. *J Pediatr.* 1994;125:87–91.

86. Martin JA, Hamilton BE, Sutton PD, et al. Births: final data for 2003. *Natl Vital Stat Rep.* 2005;54:1–116.

87. Goplerud CP, White CA, Bradbury JT, Briggs TL. The first Rh-isoimmunized pregnancy. *Am J Obstet Gynecol.* 1973;115:632–638.

88. Bowman JM, Chown B, Lewis M, Pollock JM. Rh isoimmunization during pregnancy: antenatal prophylaxis. *Can Med Assoc J.* 1978;118:623–627.

89. Moise KJ Jr. Management of rhesus alloimmunization in pregnancy. *Obstet Gynecol.* 2008;112:164–176.

90. Queenan JT, Tomai TP, Ural SH, King JC. Deviation in amniotic fluid optical density at a wavelength of 450 nm in Rh-immunized pregnancies from 14 to 40 weeks' gestation:

91. Lo YM, Hjelm NM, Fidler C, et al. Prenatal diagnosis of fetal RhD status by molecular analysis of maternal plasma. *N Engl J Med.* 1998;339:1734–1738.

92. Kolialexi A, Tounta G, Mavrou A. Noninvasive fetal RhD genotyping from maternal blood. *Expert Rev Mol Diagn.* 2010;10:285–296.

93. Rouillac-Le Sciellour C, Puillandre P, Gillot R, et al. Large-scale pre-diagnosis study of fetal RHD genotyping by PCR on plasma DNA from RhD-negative pregnant women. *Mol Diagn.* 2004;8:23–31.

94. Bowman JM. The prevention of Rh immunization. *Transfus Med Rev.* 1988;2:129–150.

95. Zipursky A, Paul VK. The global burden of Rh disease. *Arch Dis Child Fetal Neonatal Ed.* 2011;96:F84–F85.

96. Mari G, Deter RL, Carpenter RL, et al. Noninvasive diagnosis by Doppler ultrasonography of fetal anemia due to maternal red-cell alloimmunization. Collaborative Group for Doppler Assessment of the Blood Velocity in Anemic Fetuses. *N Engl J Med.* 2000;342:9–14.

97. Van Kamp IL, Klumper FJ, Oepkes D, et al. Complications of intrauterine intravascular transfusion for fetal anemia due to maternal red-cell alloimmunization. *Am J Obstet Gynecol.* 2005;192:171–177.

98. Greenough A. Rhesus disease: postnatal management and outcome. *Eur J Pediatr.* 1999;158:689–693.

99. Smits-Wintjens VE, Walther FJ, Lopriore E. Rhesus haemolytic disease of the newborn: postnatal management, associated morbidity and long-term outcome. *Semin Fetal Neonatal Med.* 2008;13:265–271.

100. Rübo J, Albrecht K, Lasch P, et al. High-dose intravenous immune globulin therapy for hyperbilirubinemia caused by Rh hemolytic disease. *J Pediatr.* 1992;121:93–97.

101. Alpay F, Sarici SU, Okutan V, et al. High-dose intravenous immunoglobulin therapy in neonatal immune haemolytic jaundice. *Acta Paediatr.* 1999;88:216–219.

102. Dağoğlu T, Ovali F, Samanci N, Bengisu E. High-dose intravenous immunoglobulin therapy for rhesus haemolytic disease. *J Int Med Res.* 1995;23:264–271.

103. Voto LS, Sexer H, Ferreiro G, et al. Neonatal administration of high-dose intravenous immunoglobulin in rhesus hemolytic disease. *J Perinat Med.* 1995;23:443–451.

104. Gottstein R, Cooke RW. Systematic review of intravenous immunoglobulin in haemolytic disease of the newborn. *Arch Dis Child Fetal Neonatal Ed.* 2003;88:F6–F10.

105. Smits-Wintjens VE, Walther FJ, Rath ME, et al. Intravenous immunoglobulin in neonates with rhesus hemolytic disease: a randomized controlled trial. *Pediatrics.* 2011;127:680–686.

106. Alcock GS, Liley H. Immunoglobulin infusion for isoimmune haemolytic jaundice in neonates. *Cochrane Database Syst Rev.* 2002;(3):CD003313.

107. Zoubir S, Arlettaz Mieth R, Berrut S, Roth-Kleiner M; the Swiss Paediatric Surveillance Unit (SPSU). Incidence of severe hyperbilirubinaemia in Switzerland: a nationwide population-based prospective study. *Arch Dis Child Fetal Neonatal Ed.* 2011;96(4):F310–F31.

108. Ogunlesi TA, Dedeke IO, Adekanmbi AF, Fetuga MB, Ogunfowora OB. The incidence and outcome of bilirubin encephalopathy in Nigeria: a bi-centre study. *Niger J Med.* 2007;16:354–359.

109. Grundbacher FJ. The etiology of ABO hemolytic disease of the newborn. *Transfusion.* 1980;20:563–568.

110. Fällström SP, Bjure J. Endogenous formation of carbon monoxide in newborn infants. 3. ABO incompatibility. *Acta Paediatr Scand.* 1968;57:137–144.

111. Uetani Y, Nakamura H, Okamoto O, et al. Carboxyhemoglobin measurements in the diagnosis of ABO hemolytic disease. *Acta Paediatr Jpn.* 1989;31:171–176.

112. Herschel M, Karrison T, Wen M, Caldarelli L, Baron B. Isoimmunization is unlikely to be the cause of hemolysis in ABO-incompatible but direct antiglobulin test-negative neonates. *Pediatrics.* 2002;110(1 Pt 1):127–130.

113. Kanto WP Jr, Marino B, Godwin AS, Bunyapen C. ABO hemolytic disease: a comparative study of clinical severity and delayed anemia. *Pediatrics.* 1978;62:365–369.

114. Kaplan M, Vreman HJ, Hammerman C, et al. Contribution of haemolysis to jaundice in Sephardic Jewish glucose-6-phosphate dehydrogenase deficient neonates. *Br J Haematol.* 1996;93:822–827.

115. Kaplan M, Hammerman C, Renbaum P, Klein G, Levy-Lahad E. Gilbert's syndrome and hyperbilirubinaemia in ABO-incompatible neonates. *Lancet.* 2000;356:652–653.

116. Hammerman C, Vreman HJ, Kaplan M, Stevenson DK. Intravenous immune globulin in neonatal immune hemolytic disease: does it reduce hemolysis? *Acta Paediatr.* 1996;85:1351–1353.

117. Kappas A, Drummond GS, Manola T, Petmezaki S, Valaes T. Sn-protoporphyrin use in the management of hyperbilirubinemia in term newborns with direct Coombs-positive ABO incompatibility. *Pediatrics.* 1988;81:485–489.

118. Moise KJ. Red blood cell alloimmunization in pregnancy. *Semin Hematol.* 2005;42:169–178.

119. McKenna DS, Nagaraja HN, O'Shaughnessy R. Management of pregnancies complicated by anti-Kell isoimmunization. *Obstet Gynecol.* 1999;93:667–673.

120. Beutler E. G6PD deficiency. *Blood* 1994;84:3613–3636.

121. Cappellini MD, Fiorelli G. Glucose-6-phosphate dehydrogenase deficiency. *Lancet.* 2008;371:64–74.

122. WHO Working Group. Glucose-6-phosphate dehydrogenase deficiency. *Bull World Health Organ.* 1989;67:601–611.

123. Luzzatto L. Glucose 6-phosphate dehydrogenase deficiency: from genotype to phenotype. *Haematologica.* 2006;91:1303–1306.

124. Slusher TM, Vreman HJ, McLaren DW, et al. Glucose-6-phosphate dehydrogenase deficiency and carboxyhemoglobin concentrations associated with bilirubin-related morbidity and death in Nigerian infants. *J Pediatr.* 1995;126:102–108.

125. Meloni T, Cutillo S, Testa U, Luzzatto L. Neonatal jaundice and severity of glucose-6-phosphate dehydrogenase deficiency in Sardinian babies. *Early Hum Dev.* 1987;15:317–322.

126. Kaplan M, Hammerman C, Vreman HJ, Wong RJ, Stevenson DK. Severe hemolysis with normal blood count in a glucose-6-phosphate dehydrogenase deficient neonate. *J Perinatol.* 2008;28:306–309.

127. Kaplan M, Abramov A. Neonatal hyperbilirubinemia associated with glucose-6-phosphate dehydrogenase deficiency in Sephardic-Jewish neonates: incidence, severity, and the effect of phototherapy. *Pediatrics.* 1992;90(3):401–405.

128. Kaplan M, Rubaltelli FF, Hammerman C, et al. Conjugated bilirubin in neonates with glucose-6-phosphate dehydrogenase deficiency. *J Pediatr.* 1996;128:695–697.

129. Kaplan M, Muraca M, Hammerman C, et al. Bilirubin conjugation, reflected by conjugated bilirubin fractions, in glucose-6-phosphate dehydrogenase-deficient neonates: a determining factor in the pathogenesis of hyperbilirubinemia. *Pediatrics.* 1998;102:E37.

130. Kaplan M, Muraca M, Vreman HJ, et al. Neonatal bilirubin production-conjugation imbalance: effect of glucose-6-phosphate dehydrogenase deficiency and borderline prematurity. *Arch Dis Child Fetal Neonatal Ed.* 2005;90:F123–F127.

131. Beutler E. A series of new screening procedures for pyruvate kinase deficiency, glucose-6-phosphate dehydrogenase deficiency, and glutathione reductase deficiency. *Blood.* 1966;28:553–562.

132. Kaplan M, Hammerman C. The need for neonatal glucose-6-phosphate dehydrogenase screening: a global perspective. *J Perinatol.* 2009;29(Suppl 1):S46–S52.

133. Kaplan M, Hammerman C. Neonatal screening for glucose-6-phosphate dehydrogenase deficiency: biochemical versus genetic technologies. *Semin Perinatol.* 2011;35(3):155–161.

134. Beutler E, Gelbart T. Estimating the prevalence of pyruvate kinase deficiency from the gene frequency in the general white population. *Blood.* 2000;95:3585–3588.

135. Mentzer WC. Pyruvate kinase deficiency and disorders of glycolysis. In: Nathan DG, Orkin SH, eds. *Nathan and Oski's Hematology of Infancy and Childhood.* Philadelphia, PA: Saunders; 1998:665–703.

136. Christensen RD, Eggert LD, Baer VL, Smith KN. Pyruvate kinase deficiency as a cause of extreme hyperbilirubinemia in neonates from a polygamist community. *J Perinatol.* 2010;30:233–236.

137. Zanella A, Bianchi P, Fermo E. Pyruvate kinase deficiency. *Haematologica.* 2007;92:721–723.

138. Oski FA, Nathan DG, Sidel VW, Diamond LK. Extreme hemolysis and red-cell distortion in erythrocyte puryvate kinase deficiency. *N Engl J Med.* 1964;270:1023–1030.

139. Bianchi P, Zanella A. Hematologically important mutations: red cell pyruvate kinase. (Third Update.) *Blood Cells Mol Dis.* 2000;26:47–53.

140. Iolascon A, Miraglia del Giudice E, Perrotta S, et al. Hereditary spherocytosis: from clinical to molecular defects. *Haematologica.* 1998;83:240–257.

141. Steiner LA, Gallagher PG. Erythrocyte disorders in the perinatal period. *Semin Perinatol.* 2007;31:254–261.

142. Perrotta S, Gallagher PG, Mohandas N. Hereditary spherocytosis. *Lancet.* 2008;372:1411–1426.

143. Iolascon A, Avvisati RA, Piscopo C. Hereditary spherocytosis. *Transfus Clin Biol.* 2010;17:138–142.

144. Whitfield CF, Follweiler JB, Lopresti-Morrow L, Miller BA. Deficiency of alpha-spectrin synthesis in burst-forming units-erythroid in lethal hereditary spherocytosis. *Blood.* 1991;78:3043–3051.

145. Iolascon A, Perrotta S, Stewart GW. Red blood cell membrane defects. *Rev Clin Exp Hematol.* 2003;7:1–35.

146. Berardi A, Lugli L, Ferrari F, et al. Kernicterus associated with hereditary spherocytosis and UGT1A1 promoter polymorphism. *Biol Neonate.* 2006;90:243–246.

147. Christensen RD, Henry E. Hereditary spherocytosis in neonates with hyperbilirubinemia. *Pediatrics.* 2010;125:120–125.

148. King MJ, Behrens J, Rogers C, et al. Rapid flow cytometric test for the diagnosis of membrane cytoskeleton associated haemolytic anaemia. *Br J Haematol.* 2000;111:924–933.

149. Eber SW, Armbrust R, Schröter W. Variable clinical severity of hereditary spherocytosis: relation to erythrocytic spectrin concentration, osmotic fragility, and autohemolysis. *J Pediatr.* 1990;117:409–416.

150. Delhommeau F, Cynober T, Schischmanoff PO, et al. Natural history of hereditary spherocytosis during the first year of life. *Blood.* 2000;95:393–397.

151. Schroter W, Kahsnitz E. Diagnosis of hereditary spherocytosis in newborn infants. *J Pediatr.* 1983;103:460–463.

152. Gallagher PG, Weed SA, Tse WT, et al. Recurrent fatal hydrops fetalis associated with a nucleotide substitution in the erythrocyte beta-spectrin gene. *J Clin Invest.* 1995;95:1174–1178.

153. Gallagher PG, Petruzzi MJ, Weed SA, et al. Mutation of a highly conserved residue of beta spectrin associated with fatal and near-fatal neonatal hemolytic anemia. *J Clin Invest.* 1997;99:267–277.

154. Delaunay J, Stewart G, Iolascon A. Hereditary dehydrated and overhydrated stomatocytosis: recent advances. *Curr Opin Hematol.* 1999;6:110–114.

155. Grootenboer-Mignot S, Cretien A, Laurendeau I, et al. Sublethal hydrops as a manifestation of dehydrated hereditary stomatocytosis in two consecutive pregnancies. *Prenat Diagn.* 2003;23:380–384.

156. Kutlar F. Diagnostic approach to hemoglobinopathies. *Hemoglobin.* 2007;31:243–250.

157. Murray NA, Roberts IA. Haemolytic disease of the newborn. *Arch Dis Child Fetal Neonatal Ed.* 2007;92:F83–F88.

158. Bosma PJ, Chowdhury JR, Bakker C, et al. The genetic basis of the reduced expression of bilirubin UDP-glucuronosyltransferase 1 in Gilbert's syndrome. *N Engl J Med.* 1995;333:1171–1175.

159. Monaghan G, Ryan M, Seddon R, Hume R, Burchell B. Genetic variation in bilirubin UPD-glucuronosyltransferase gene promoter and Gilbert's syndrome. *Lancet.* 1996;347:578–581.

160. Huang CS, Chang PF, Huang MJ, Chen ES, Chen WC. Glucose-6-phosphate dehydrogenase deficiency, the UDP-glucuronosyl transferase 1A1 gene, and neonatal hyperbilirubinemia. *Gastroenterology.* 2002;123:127–133.

161. Iolascon A, Faienza MF, Moretti A, Perrotta S, Miraglia del Giudice E. UGT1 promoter polymorphism accounts for increased neonatal appearance of hereditary spherocytosis. *Blood.* 1998;91:1093.

162. Bosma PJ. Inherited disorders of bilirubin metabolism. *J Hepatol.* 2003;38(1):107–117.

163. Strauss KA, Robinson DL, Vreman HJ, Puffenberger EG, Hart G, Morton DH. Management of hyperbilirubinemia and prevention of kernicterus in 20 patients with Crigler-Najjar disease. *Eur J Pediatr.* 2006;165(5):306–319.

164. van der Veere CN, Sinaasappel M, McDonagh AF, et al. Current therapy for Crigler-Najjar syndrome type 1: report of a world registry. *Hepatology.* 1996;24(2):311–315.

165. Miranda PS, Bosma PJ. Towards liver-directed gene therapy for Crigler-Najjar syndrome. *Curr Gene Ther.* 2009;9(2):72–82.

166. Trioche P, Chalas J, Francoual J, et al. Jaundice with hypertrophic pyloric stenosis as an early manifestation of Gilbert syndrome. *Arch Dis Child.* 1999;81:301–303.

167. Goudonnet H, Magdalou J, Mounie J, et al. Differential action of thyroid hormones and chemically related compounds on the activity of UDP-glucuronosyltransferases and cytochrome P-450 isozymes in rat liver. *Biochim Biophys Acta.* 1990;1035:12–19.

168. Maisels MJ, Watchko JF. Treatment of jaundice in low birthweight infants. *Arch Dis Child Fetal Neonatal Ed.* 2003;88(6):F459–F463.

169. Kaplan M, Herschel M, Hammerman C, Hoyer JD, Heller GZ, Stevenson DK. Neonatal hyperbilirubinemia in African American males: the importance of glucose-6-phosphate dehydrogenase deficiency. *J Pediatr.* 2006;149(1):83–88.

170. Kramer LI. Advancement of dermal icterus in the jaundiced newborn. *Am J Dis Child.* 1969;118(3):454–458.

171. Lo SF, Doumas BT. The status of bilirubin measurements in US laboratories: why is accuracy elusive? *Semin Perinatol.* 2011;35(3):141–147.

172. Maisels MJ. Transcutaneous bilirubinometry. *NeoReviews.* 2006;7:e217–e215.

173. Maisels MJ, Bhutani VK, Bogen D, Newman TB, Stark AR, Watchko JF. Hyperbilirubinemia in the newborn infant > or = 35 weeks' gestation: an update with clarifications. *Pediatrics.* 2009;124(4):1193–1198.

174. Blanchette V, Dror Y, Chan A. Hematology. In: MacDonald MG, Mullet MD, Seshia MMK, eds. *Avery's Neonatology. Pathophysiology and Management of the Newborn.* Philadelphia, PA: Lippincott, Williams and Wilkins; 2005:1169–1234.

175. Coskun A, Yikilmaz A, Kumandas S, Karahan OI, Akcakus M, Manav A. Hyperintense globus pallidus on T1-weighted MR imaging in acute kernicterus: is it common or rare? *Eur Radiol.* 2005;15:1263–1267.

176. Gkoltsiou K, Tzoufi M, Counsell S, Rutherford M, Cowan F. Serial brain MRI and ultrasound findings: relation to gestational age, bilirubin level, neonatal neurologic status and neurodevelopmental outcome in infants at risk of kernicterus. *Early Hum Dev.* 2008;84(12):829–838.

177. Maisels MJ, McDonagh AF. Phototherapy for neonatal jaundice. *N Engl J Med.* 2008;358(9):920–928.

178. Harris MC, Bernbaum JC, Polin JR, Zimmerman R, Polin RA. Developmental follow-up of breastfed term and near-term infants with marked hyperbilirubinemia. *Pediatrics.* 2001;107:1075–1080.

179. Hansen TW, Nietsch L, Norman E, et al. Reversibility of acute intermediate phase bilirubin encephalopathy. *Acta Paediatr.* 2009;98:1689–1694.

Anemia in the Neonatal Period

Robin K. Ohls, Nader Bishara, Wendy Wong, and Bertil Glader

INTRODUCTION

The newborn period marks a time when red blood cell (RBC) indices change significantly. Anemia can occur at various times in the neonatal period, from the perinatal and immediate postnatal period through the first months of life. Hematocrits 2 or more standard deviations below the normal range for gestation are seen frequently and should be evaluated. Conversely, true anemia, the inability to adequately deliver oxygen to tissues, is less common. Anemia can be classified into the following 3 major processes: hemolysis, hemorrhage, or hypoproliferative disease. Anemia can also result from overlapping processes. For example, sepsis can result in hemolysis, disseminated intravascular coagulation (DIC), and subsequent hemorrhage. This chapter reviews fetal and neonatal erythropoiesis, discusses the etiology and diagnosis of anemia in the neonatal period, and offers management options for anemic term and preterm infants.

Fetal Erythropoiesis

The growth factors stimulating fetal erythropoiesis during gestation are produced solely by the fetus. Erythropoietin, or Epo, is the primary growth factor responsible for erythropoiesis after birth and appears to be the principal growth factor for fetal erythropoiesis as well. Primary production of Epo occurs in the liver during fetal development. The kidney becomes the primary source of Epo following delivery; however, the etiology for the liver-to-kidney switch continues to be studied. Anephric fetuses have normal serum Epo concentrations and normal hematocrits, proving that renal Epo production is not required for erythropoiesis during fetal development. Methylation patterns in the promoter and enhancer regions of the Epo gene isolated from fetal liver and kidney suggest increased methylation in the kidney as a possible explanation for decreased Epo gene expression during fetal development.

During gestation, the site of red cell production transitions from yolk sac to liver to marrow. Primitive erythroblasts are produced in the fetal yolk sac during the first 3–4 weeks of gestation. By 6 to 8 weeks' gestation, definitive erythropoiesis is established in the fetal liver. Although erythrocytes are noted in the fetal marrow as early as 8–9 weeks' gestation, the liver remains the primary site of erythropoiesis until well into the second trimester. By the third trimester, erythropoiesis occurs primarily in the fetal marrow, although production can continue in extramedullary sites in the face of increased need, during times of hemolysis, or in fetal infection caused by a variety of bacteria or viruses.

Variations in hematologic indices for preterm and term infants reflect the dynamic nature of the erythron in late fetal development. The production of hemoglobin transitions from embryonic (Gower 1 [$\zeta_2\varepsilon_2$], Gower 2 [$\alpha_2\varepsilon_2$], and Portland [$\zeta_2\gamma_2$]) to fetal hemoglobin ($\alpha_2\gamma_2$) and finally to adult hemoglobin ($\alpha_2\beta_2$), as shown in Figure 31-1.

In conjunction with changes in globin gene expression and the transition from embryonic to fetal hemoglobin production, hemoglobin concentrations gradually increase, from approximately 14.5 g/dL at

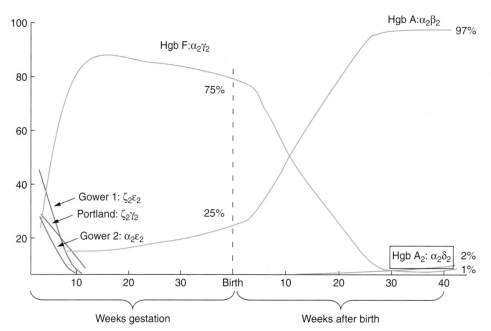

FIGURE 31-1 Changes in hemoglobin production from conception through 40 weeks postnatal age.

28 weeks' gestation to 15 g/dL at 34 weeks to 16.8 g/dL at 40 weeks.[1] The relationship between cord hemoglobin concentration and duration of pregnancy is linear for infants who are appropriate for gestational age (AGA). The mean corpuscular volume (MCV) is higher in preterm infants than in term infants and is inversely proportional to gestation, averaging 5–20 fL higher than the mean MCV of 108 fL in term infants.

Reticulocyte counts are elevated at birth, averaging 6% to 10%. Nucleated red blood cells (NRBCs) are not consistently elevated, but there does appear to be an inverse relationship between number of NRBCs and gestational age. Normoblasts are cleared rapidly from the circulation during the first postnatal days, although a few may still be observed in small preterm infants into the second week of life. Variations in red cell size and shape are somewhat greater than those observed in term infants.

Neonatal Erythropoiesis

The abrupt transition from the relatively hypoxic in utero environment to the oxygen-rich postnatal environment triggers erythropoietic responses that have a profound effect on the red cell mass. Over the first 2 to 6 months of life, the infant experiences both the highest and the lowest hemoglobin concentrations occurring at any time in development. Although variable, Epo levels at birth are above the normal adult range but decrease abruptly in the immediate postnatal period, with a half-life of no more than 4 hours (2.6 ± 0.5 hours in infants with polycythemia and 3.7 ± 0.9 hours in infants born to mothers with preeclampsia.)[2] By 24 hours, the Epo

value is nearly undetectable and remains so throughout the first month of life. The decrease in Epo is accompanied by a decrease in the number of erythroid progenitors and in the reticulocyte count.[3]

A combination of decreased red cell production, shortened cell survival, and growth-related expansion of the blood volume results in a progressive fall of the hemoglobin concentration to a mean of approximately 11 g/dL at 2–3 months of age.[1] The lower range of normal for infants of this age is approximately 9 g/dL. This nadir is called *physiologic anemia*, in that it is not associated with lack of oxygen delivery to tissues and is not abrogated by nutritional supplements. Stabilization of the hemoglobin concentration is heralded by an increase in reticulocytes in the second month of life. Thereafter, the hemoglobin concentration rises to an average of 12.5 g/dL, where it remains throughout infancy and early childhood.

ETIOLOGY

Hemolysis

Hemolysis is the premature destruction of erythrocytes and is generally categorized as *immune-mediated* or *non-immune-mediated* hemolysis (Table 31-1). Immune-mediated hemolysis occurs when immunoglobulin (Ig) G antibodies created by the maternal immune system cross the placenta and cause destruction of antigen-containing fetal red cells (isoimmunization). Hemolysis in the fetus can be severe enough to lead to *hydrops fetalis*. Non-immune-mediated hemolysis

Table 31-1 Differential Diagnosis of Hemolysis in the Fetal and Neonatal Period

Immune-Mediated Hemolysis	Non-Immune-Mediated Hemolysis	Nonspecified Hemolysis

Rh incompatibility (anti-D antibody)
ABO, c, C, e, E, G incompatibility
Minor blood group incompatibility:
  Fya (Duffy), Kell group, Jka, MNS, Vw
Drug induced (penicillin, alpha-methyl DOPA, Cephalothin)
Maternal autoimmune hemolytic anemia
	Congenital erythrocyte enzyme defects
	  Glucose-6-phosphate dehydrogenase deficiency
	  Pyruvate kinase (PK) deficiency
	  Hexokinase deficiency
	  Glucose phosphate isomerase deficiency
	  Pyrimidine 5′ nucleotidase deficiency
	Erythrocyte membrane disorders
	  Spherocytosis
	  Elliptocytosis
	  Stomatocytosis
	  Pyropoikylocytosis
	  Other membrane disorders
	Hemoglobin defects
	  α-Thalassemia syndromes
	  γ-Thalassemia syndromes
	  α- and γ-Chain structural anomalies
	Drug induced
	  Valproic acid
		Infection
		  Bacterial sepsis (*Escherichia coli*, group B streptococcus)
		  Parvovirus B-19 (can present with hydrops fetalis)
		  Congenital syphilis
		  Congenital malaria
		  Congenital TORCH infections (toxoplasmosis, cytomegalovirus, rubella, disseminated herpes)
		  Other congenital viral infections
		Disseminated intravascular coagulation
		Macro- and microangiopathic hemolysis
		  Cavernous hemangiomas
		  Arteriovenous malformations
		  Renal artery stenosis or thrombosis
		  Other large-vessel thrombi
		  Severe coartaction of the aorta
		  Severe vavular stenoses
		Associated with Systemic Disease
		  Galactosemia
		  Lysosomal storage diseases
		  Prolonged metabolic acidosis from metabolic disease (amino acid and organic acid disorders)
		  Transfusion reactions
		  TAR syndrome

occurs when intrinsic abnormalities in the fetal or neonatal red cell lead to premature destruction and a shortened red cell life span.

In older children and adults with congenital hemolytic anemia, there is usually clear evidence of hemolysis, as manifested by indirect hyperbilirubinemia, reticulocytosis, and low haptoglobin levels, all markers of increased red cell destruction. In neonates, however, the recognition of congenital hemolytic anemia utilizing these laboratory measurements is more challenging. Physiologic indirect hyperbilirubinemia is common in neonates because of the increased red cell mass at birth, decreased RBC survival, and reduced hepatic glucuronyl transferase activity. Also, the normal physiologic anemia of infancy can modulate reticulocytosis in the presence of mild hemolytic anemia. Finally, serum haptoglobin is not a reliable index of neonatal hemolysis because concentrations of this protein do not increase until after 6 months of age.

Neonates with congenital hemolytic anemia may have a normal-for-age hemoglobin or there may be mild-to-severe anemia. Indirect hyperbilirubinemia presenting earlier than expected and in excess of the usual physiologic levels is the most common and occasionally only sign of hemolytic anemia. Reticulocytosis and persistence of nucleated RBCs beyond the third day of life are other reasons to evaluate a neonate for hemolytic anemia. Acquired hemolytic anemia in neonates occurs with alloimmune hemolysis (chapter 34), hemolytic anemia secondary to maternal disease, and hemolysis secondary to infection or microangiopathic anemia.

Immune-Mediated Hemolysis

The most common cause for hemolysis in the neonatal period is immune-mediated hemolysis due to ABO incompatibility or Rh incompatibility. Following the advent of RhoGAM (RhD antibody), the incidence of hydrops fetalis due to RhD sensitization decreased significantly, from approximately 1 in 200 live births to now less than 1 in 1000 live births.[4] Immune-mediated hemolysis due to anti-A or anti-B antibodies crossing the placenta is now the most common etiology of immune-mediated hemolysis.

RhD Isoimmunization: RhD incompatibility occurs when a woman with RhD-negative blood type is exposed to Rh-positive blood cells, leading to the development of RhD antibodies (anti-D antibodies). Fifteen percent of the population lacks the D antigen (is Rh negative). RhD sensitization occurs in approximately 1 per 1000 births to women who are Rh negative.

RhD incompatibility occurs through 2 primary mechanisms. The most common route of exposure occurs when an Rh-negative pregnant mother is exposed to Rh-positive fetal RBCs secondary to fetomaternal hemorrhage (FMH), spontaneous abortion, or normal delivery. RhD incompatibility can also occur if an Rh-negative female accidentally receives Rh-positive blood. Maternal anti-D IgG antibodies freely cross the placenta into the fetal circulation, where they form antigen-antibody complexes with RhD-positive fetal RBCs. The red cells are eventually lysed, leading to isoimmune hemolytic anemia.[5] As a result, large amounts of bilirubin are produced from the breakdown of fetal hemoglobin and are transferred via the placenta to the mother, where they are conjugated and excreted.

Once the baby is born, low levels of glucuronyl transferase can lead to significant elevations of unconjugated hyperbilirubinemia. Erythroblastosis fetalis is a severe form of the disease characterized by severe hemolytic anemia and hydrops fetalis, involving placental and fetal edema, ascites, pericardial effusion, high-output cardiac failure, and extramedullary hematopoiesis. The risk and severity of sensitization increase with each subsequent pregnancy in which the fetus is Rh positive. The risk of sensitization depends on the volume of FMH, the extent of maternal immune response, and the concurrent presence of ABO incompatibility, which actually decreases the severity of hemolysis in Rh-positive fetuses.

Administration of RhoGAM decreases the production of maternal IgG antibodies by inhibiting immune memory. RhD immune globulin coats the surface of RhD-positive fetal RBCs. These antibody-antigen complexes inhibit the stimulation of maternal B cells to produce IgG antibodies. RhoGAM is administered once at 28–32 weeks' gestation. It has a short half-life of 23–28 days and is thus administered again within 72 hours after delivery. Rh-negative (nonsensitized) women presenting to the emergency room with antepartum bleeding or potential FMH should receive 300 μg of Rh IgG.[6] An additional 300 μg of Rh IgG should be administered for every 30 mL of fetal blood to which the Rh-negative mother is exposed. A lower 50-μg dose (MICRhoGAM) is available and recommended for Rh-negative women who have a termination of pregnancy in the first trimester when the volume of FMH is likely minimal.[7]

ABO Isoimmunization: Hemolysis of fetal red cells caused by ABO antibodies occurs almost exclusively in infants of blood group A or B who are born to group O mothers.[8] Anti-A and anti-B antibodies formed in group O individuals are mainly IgG antibodies and thus can cross the placenta, whereas anti-A and anti-B antibodies found in the serum of group A or group B individuals tend to be IgM antibodies. ABO incompatibility tends to be relatively mild in nature, mainly because fetal RBCs do not express adult levels of A and B antigens, resulting in few reactive sites. This allows the antibody-coated cells to remain in the circulation for a longer period of time compared to RhD disease. In addition, severity of ABO incompatibility is not dependent on birth order.[9]

The presence of microspherocytes on peripheral blood smear is a characteristic of ABO isoimmunization, with little or no increase in nucleated RBCs. In RhD isoimmunization, there are fewer spherocytes and a large number of nucleated RBCs.[10] ABO isoimmunization usually presents with hyperbilirubinemia and can be managed by phototherapy alone. Exchange transfusions are occasionally required. The direct antiglobulin test (DAT) is usually weakly positive but can be negative in some cases despite evidence of immune-mediated hemolysis.

Minor Blood Group Isoimmunization: Although RhD isoimmunization is the most common cause of severe hemolytic disease of the newborn, other antibodies belonging to Kell (K and k), Duffy (Fya), Lewis, Kidd (Jka and Jkb), and MNSs (M, N, S, and s) systems can cause severe hemolytic disease of the newborn.[11] Kell antigen is a minor blood group antigen that often results in isoimmunization. In addition, antibodies directed against Kell antigens can bind to erythroid progenitors in the fetal marrow and result in hypoproliferative anemia.[12] Minor Rhesus blood group antigens c and E can also cause severe hemolysis, requiring exchange transfusion.

Non-Immune-Mediated Hemolysis

Enzyme Disorders

Glucose is the major metabolic substrate for RBCs, and it is metabolized via the glycolytic pathway and hexose monophosphate (HMP) shunt. The glycolytic pathway generates adenosine triphosphate (ATP), NADH (reduced nicotinamide adenine dinucleotide), and 2,3-disphosphoglycerate (2,3-DPG), all important in maintaining RBC integrity. The HMP shunt pathway is critical for protecting RBCs against oxidative insult. Glucose-6-phosphate dehydrogenase (G-6-PD) is the initial step in the HMP pathway. Among hemolytic anemias due to hereditary enzyme deficiencies, G-6-PD deficiency is the most common. The remaining glycolytic pathway enzymopathies are relatively rare, with only a few thousand cases known and 90% due to pyruvate kinase deficiency.

Glucose-6-Phosphate Dehydrogenase Deficiency: Deficiency of G-6-PD is one of the most common genetic disorders in the world, affecting over 400 million people worldwide.[13] It is a sex-linked disorder affecting males, but females who are homozygous for G-6-PD deficiency or have skewed lyonization of the X chromosome can also have significant enzyme deficiency.

This enzymopathy is found most commonly in people from Africa, Asia, and the Mediterranean region. Three clinically important types of G-6-PD deficiency are classified by the World Health Organization (WHO). Class I G-6-PD deficiency is vanishingly rare, but it is the most severe form, characterized by lifelong mild-to-moderate chronic hemolytic anemia. Class II G-6-PD variants, commonly found in Mediterranean (G-6-PD^Mediterranean), Middle Eastern, and Asian people, have a marked enzyme deficiency that is associated with severe anemia after exposure to oxidant drugs and chemicals (eg, primaquine, ciprofloxacin, nitrofurans, sulfonamides, dapsone, naphthalene) or fava beans. Class III G-6-PD is the mildest deficiency, found in people of African (A-variant) and Asian background who experience moderate but self-limited hemolytic anemia with oxidant exposure. In patients with class II or III G-6-PD, there is no anemia or hemolysis in the steady state when there is no oxidant exposure.

G-6-PD deficiency in neonates is associated with high risk of severe jaundice and kernicterus.[14,15] It is much more common in neonates with class II variants than in infants with class III G-6-PD deficiency. The possibility of G-6-PD deficiency should be considered in infants with hyperbilirubinemia beyond expected physiologic levels. The neonatal jaundice associated with G-6-PD deficiency has a late peak at day 5–6 of life; it may be especially difficult to identify in preterm infants due to their later peak bilirubin levels. Of particular importance, hyperbilirubinemia often is the only abnormality, and there may be no other signs of hemolysis. This observation has suggested that hyperbilirubinemia might not be related solely to increased bilirubin production from red cell destruction but rather may be due to a defect in liver clearance of bilirubin.[16] Also, there are reports suggesting that marked hyperbilirubinemia in G-6-PD deficiency is associated with the simultaneous inheritance of the variant Gilbert polymorphism.[17] In the United States, severe hyperbilirubinemia due to G-6-PD deficiency is responsible for over 30% of kernicterus cases.[18] Neonates at risk for G-6-PD should have bilirubin levels measured prior to discharge. Close outpatient follow-up is particularly important given that many neonates are discharged early from the hospital. Neonatal discharge guidelines have been established by the American Academy of Pediatrics and the American College of Obstetricians and Gynecologists.[19]

Severe hyperbilirubinemia occurring in G-6-PD deficiency requires phototherapy and, occasionally, exchange transfusion. Packed RBC (PRBC) transfusion should be given for symptomatic anemia. Avoidance of oxidative medications and chemicals is important to prevent further hemolysis. Mothers who are breastfeeding should be counseled to avoid ingestion of fava beans and oxidant medications. Vitamin K injection is safe for neonates with class II and III variants and should be given to prevent hemorrhagic disease of the newborn.

Pyruvate Kinase Deficiency: Pyruvate kinase (PK) deficiency is the most common glycolytic pathway defect. Over 200 different mutations of the 2 different PK genes (*PKM2* and *PK-LR*) have been reported.[20] It is an autosomal disorder, with most patients compound heterozygous for 2 different mutations. The prevalence of PK deficiency among Caucasians in the United States has been estimated at 1 in 20,000. The disease is common among the Amish population in Pennsylvania and other inbred communities.[21]

Pyruvate kinase catalyzes the conversion of phosphoenolpyruvate to pyruvate, at the same time generating ATP, a critical source of energy for RBCs. Impaired ATP production occurs in PK-deficient cells, leading to loss of membrane plasticity and, ultimately, splenic destruction of red cells.

The clinical features of PK deficiency are highly variable, ranging from severe anemia and jaundice at birth to an incidental finding in adults. This is likely related to the many different known mutations and the often-compound heterozygosity for different mutations causing the deficiency.

Deficiency of PK should be part of the differential diagnosis of hydrops fetalis and neonatal jaundice. Jaundice can be pronounced, and kernicterus has been reported.[22] In contrast to G-6-PD deficiency, in addition to hyperbilirubinemia, there are usually obvious features of hemolysis, including anemia and reticulocytosis. PK deficiency should be suspected in a neonate with evidence of hemolytic anemia after immune-mediated hemolysis, hereditary spherocytosis (HS), and G-6-PD deficiency are ruled out.

Hyperbilirubinemia should be managed with phototherapy and exchange transfusion as needed. Severe anemia may require red cell transfusions to maintain hemoglobin or as needed to maintain normal neonatal growth and development. Many children with severe PK deficiency are transfusion dependent until they undergo splenectomy after 5 years of age.

Other RBC Enzymopathies Associated With Hemolysis: Abnormalities have been reported in all glycolytic enzymes. These conditions are rare, accounting for less than 1% of hemolytic anemia due to enzymopathies.[23] After PK deficiency, which accounts for 90% of glycolytic enzymopathies, glucose phosphate isomerase (GPI) deficiency is the next most common. All glycolytic enzymopathies are associated with chronic nonspherocytic hemolytic anemia. The degree of hemolytic anemia varies from mild to severe, and hydrops fetalis has been seen in those with the most severe hemolysis. Several glycolytic enzyme deficiencies are associated with myopathy or neurologic deficits. Most are inherited in an autosomal recessive (AR) pattern except phosphoglycerate kinase deficiency, which is X linked. This group of rare disorders should be considered when a neonate shows clear and persistent evidence of nonspherocytic hemolytic anemia and after other hemolytic causes such as immune-mediated hemolysis, membrane defects, and the more common enzymopathies discussed have been ruled out. Enzymopathies should also be considered in neonates with neurologic defects or myopathy in addition to hemolytic anemia. Specific assays of RBC enzyme activity are necessary for diagnosis of these rare conditions. In some cases, DNA-based molecular tests are available.

Membrane Disorders

Hemolytic anemias due to abnormalities of the erythrocyte membrane comprise an important group of inherited disorders. The most common disorder encountered is HS. Hemolysis due to hereditary elliptocytosis (HE), and the hereditary stomatocytosis (HSt) syndromes also occurs but is less common.

Hereditary Spherocytosis: Hereditary spherocytosis is the most common hereditary hemolytic anemia in people of northern European descent, occurring in up to 1 in 2500 individuals.[24] In the United States, it is estimated that 1 in 5000 people have HS. Most cases of HS are inherited in an autosomal dominant (AD) pattern. However, up to 25% of cases do not display this inheritance; some are new mutations, while others represent AR inheritance.

Hereditary spherocytosis is associated with deficiencies of membrane cytoskeleton proteins (spectrin, ankyrin, or band 3) that lead to destabilization of the RBC lipid bilayer, resulting in progressive membrane surface loss and microspherocyte formation.[25] Microspherocytes are vulnerable to entrapment by the spleen, which leads to further membrane loss and ultimately cell destruction by splenic macrophages. A characteristic feature of HS is the presence of spherocytes seen in the peripheral blood smear. However, even normal neonates can have a small population of spherocytes, and as noted previously, spherocytes also are found in neonates with hemolysis due to ABO incompatibility. Older children and adults with HS commonly have anemia, reticulocytosis, indirect hyperbilirubinemia, and splenomegaly.

In neonates, the most common presentation of HS is jaundice. Jaundice may present early, be more severe than usual, persist longer, and may require treatment with phototherapy. Infants with HS rarely require an exchange transfusion. Up to 50% of adults with HS have a history of jaundice during the first week of life.[26] Those who coinherit HS and the gene for Gilbert syndrome may develop marked jaundice requiring phototherapy.

The diagnosis of HS can be made in a neonate with a positive family history of HS who has evidence of hemolytic anemia, the presence of an increased number of spherocytes on peripheral smear, elevation of mean corpuscular hemoglobin concentration (MCHC), and a negative DAT. In these cases, further testing is not necessary. However, if the family history is in doubt or if there is coexistence of ABO incompatibility, further testing of the neonate or repeat testing of the affected family member might be necessary to confirm the diagnosis. The incubated RBC osmotic test is used to detect spherocytosis. However, it is important to recognize that this test does not differentiate the various causes of spherocytosis. If there is an ABO incompatibility setup, it is important to obtain a DAT. Occasionally, the establishment of the diagnosis of HS needs to be delayed until confounding factors (maternal antibodies, fetal RBC changes) are resolved. Since management and counseling of neonates with hemolytic anemia is not dependent on the exact cause, the complete laboratory workup can usually be deferred for 4 to 6 months.

Occasionally, severe symptomatic anemia can develop soon after birth and require a PRBC transfusion. More often, anemia develops after discharge from the nursery. It therefore is important to have close follow-up of these infants. While some neonates do not develop significant anemia at all, others may need PRBC transfusions during the first few months of life. Splenectomy is the definitive treatment of HS; however, even in the most severe cases, this surgery is often delayed until a child is at least 5 years old given the increased risk of life-threatening sepsis with encapsulated organisms in young children.

Hereditary Elliptocytosis: The HE syndromes are a heterogeneous group of disorders characterized by the presence of elliptical-shape RBCs in the peripheral blood smear.

Common HE is a dominantly inherited condition characterized by many elliptocytes in the peripheral blood smear. The clinical severity of common HE is extremely variable, ranging from an incidental asymptomatic condition, most commonly observed, to mild-to-moderate hemolytic anemia. The clinical expression of *hemolytic HE* ranges from a moderate hemolytic disorder to a severe, near-fatal or fatal hemolytic anemia. *Hereditary pyropoikilocytosis* (HPP) is a severe hemolytic anemia, with red cell fragments, poikilocytes, and microspherocytes seen on peripheral blood smear. From a clinical perspective, it is difficult to distinguish severe hemolytic HE from HPP. Once regarded as a separate condition, HPP is now recognized to be a variant of the HE disorders. *Spherocytic HE* is a rare condition in which both ovalocytes and spherocytes are present on the blood smear. *Southeast Asian ovalocytosis* (SAO), also known as stomatocytic elliptocytosis, is an HE variant prevalent in the malaria-infested belt of Southeast Asia and the South Pacific, and it is characterized by rigid spoon-shaped cells that have either a longitudinal slit or a transverse ridge. The varied clinical and hematologic manifestations of HE are an expression of the numerous molecular defects that give rise to an elliptocytic-shape erythrocyte. The most commonly encountered cases seen are nonhemolytic common HE, hemolytic HE, and HPP.

The incidence of HE is estimated at 1:2000–4000 in the United States.[27] It is found worldwide but is more common among people of African and Mediterranean decent. HE is inherited in an AD fashion. Heterozygous patients generally have asymptomatic elliptocytosis (common HE) that is often found incidentally. Overall, only 12%–15% of patients with HE are symptomatic at some time during their life.[27]

Similar to HS, this membrane disorder is due to qualitative and quantitative defects of RBC membrane cytoskeletal proteins. Alternation in the amount, function, and structure of these proteins leads to elliptocyte formation, instability of the RBC membrane, and in some cases hemolysis. In the last subset of HE patients, symptoms include anemia, splenomegaly, and intermittent jaundice.

Most neonates with HE are asymptomatic. However, infants with rare HE subtypes (common HE with infantile poikilocytosis and HPP) may present with severe hemolytic anemia. These neonates present with jaundice, moderate-to-severe anemia, and peripheral blood smear findings of marked poikilocytosis. In the neonatal period, common HE with infantile poikilocytosis and HPP are clinically indistinguishable. However, the poikilocytosis and severe hemolytic anemia are transient in patients with common HE. The distorted RBCs noted at birth morph into the typical HE elliptical shape by a few months of life, and there is complete resolution of the hemolytic anemia. At birth, it is difficult to predict if an infant has common HE or HPP. Hydrops fetalis has been described in association with unusually severe hemolytic HE.

Children with common HE have anywhere from a few up to all elliptocytic RBCs on their peripheral blood smear. However, these elliptocytes usually do not appear until 4–6 months of age, so infants who present to the neonatal units generally have severe hemolytic anemia with poikilocytosis. In all cases, however, infants with hemolytic HE need to be followed to see if their elliptocytosis persists or benign common HE evolves. In the hemolytic variants seen in infants, the peripheral smear may demonstrate red cell fragments, microspherocytes, and some elliptocytes. Osmotic fragility testing in these patients is abnormal, with increased fragility. In addition to typical features of hemolytic anemia, the MCV of those with HPP can be very low (25–75 fL) due to the presence of a large number of microspherocytes.

The management of neonates with hemolytic anemia due to HE is identical to any patient with hemolytic anemia. Most neonates require no treatment, but some may have significant hyperbilirubinemia and anemia requiring phototherapy, exchange transfusion, or PRBC transfusion. Splenectomy later in childhood is helpful in minimizing or resolving the chronic hemolytic anemia in those with severe hemolytic HE or HPP.

Hereditary Stomatocytoses (HSt): HSt syndromes are a group of inherited disorders characterized by erythrocytes with a mouth-shaped (stoma) area of central pallor on peripheral blood smear. HSt is associated with abnormalities in red cell cation permeability that lead to changes in red cell volume. MCV may be increased (hydrocytosis), decreased (xerocytosis), or in some cases, near normal.[28] Many patients present with hemolytic anemia in the neonatal period. Pallor, jaundice, hepatosplenomegaly, and signs of gallstone disease (in older patients) are the most common physical findings. Peripheral blood smears show an increased number of stomatocytes (up to 3% is normal). The reticulocyte count is elevated during hemolysis, and the stomatocytes are osmotically fragile in the overhydrated form of stomatocytosis and are resistant to osmotic lysis in the dehydrated form. Neonates with HSt may require phototherapy and occasionally exchange transfusions. Patients with HSt do not generally require splenectomy as the results vary. There is an increased risk of life-threatening thrombosis after splenectomy.[29] Cholecystectomy may be considered in patients with cholelithiasis.

Erythrocyte Hemoglobin Abnormalities

Hemoglobin is a tetrameric protein made up of 4 globin chains, each associated with a heme group. The production of globin chains is directed by the alpha (α) gene cluster on chromosome 16 and the beta (β) gene cluster on chromosome 11. The α-gene cluster contains the embryonic delta (ζ) gene and 2 adult α genes. The β-gene cluster contains the embryonic epsilon (ε) gene, the fetal gamma (γ) gene, and the adult β gene. During fetal development, embryonic globin production is switched to fetal or adult globin production at different times ($\zeta \rightarrow \alpha$, $\varepsilon \rightarrow \gamma$, and $\gamma \rightarrow \beta$). Various globin chains form different hemoglobin tetramers during embryonic, fetal, and postnatal life (Figure 31-1). Embryonic hemoglobins (Hb Gower 1, Hb Gower 2) are responsible for oxygen delivery during the first 8 weeks of gestation. By 10 weeks, embryonic chain production ceases, γ-chain synthesis ensues, and fetal hemoglobin (HbF: $\alpha_2\gamma_2$) becomes the dominant hemoglobin. HbF has a high oxygen affinity, allowing the fetus to extract oxygen across the placenta. At term, 60%–90% of hemoglobin in a newborn is HbF. Following birth, γ-chain production is replaced by β-chain synthesis. By 6 months of age, 95%

of hemoglobin will be adult hemoglobin (HbA), which is composed of 2 α and 2 β chains ($α_2β_2$). At birth, production of δ chains begins. The presence of HbA_2 ($α_2δ_2$), a minor hemoglobin, increases gradually to the adult level of 2%–3% during the first few months of life.

Congenital hemolytic anemias can be secondary to *deficient production of normal hemoglobin* (thalassemia syndromes) or *production of abnormal hemoglobins* (sickle cell disease). The α-globin chain disorders are manifest at birth, while β-globin chain abnormalities may not be clinically apparent until 4–6 months of age, after the switch from γ- to β-globin chain synthesis. Rare mutations affecting γ-globin chains also exist, and these can result in transient neonatal problems that resolve by 3 months of age.

Thalassemia Syndromes: Thalassemia disorders are due to decreased production of normal α- or β-globin chains, leading to a relative excess of the complementary unaffected globin chains. Thalassemias are one of the most common genetic disorders worldwide. Just like G-6-PD deficiency and sickle cell anemia, it is believed that thalassemia heterozygosity is protective against malaria. In the United States, the large influx of Southeast Asian people has led to a significant increase in the number of thalassemia syndromes seen in this country. Newborn screening programs for sickle cell disease also have led to discovery of nonsickling hemoglobinopathies, including thalassemia.

α-Thalassemia Disorders: These conditions are due to decreased or absent α-globin synthesis, a consequence of deletions or mutations of α-globin genes. More than 40 different deletions have been identified.[30] Most commonly, α thalassemia occurs in China and Southeast Asia and less frequently in India, Kuwait, the Middle East, Greece, Italy, and northern Europe. In African Americans, α-thalassemia trait is common, with up to 5% prevalence, but it rarely causes clinically significant problems. With increasing immigration to the United States from countries with high carrier rates of thalassemia, the prevalence of significant α thalassemia is rising. Data from the California newborn program, a state with a 13% Asian population, suggest that the prevalence rate of α-thalassemia disorder is 1/9000.[31]

Decreased α-globin chain production is associated with accumulation of the non-α-globin chains, leading to the formation of $γ_4$ tetramers (Hb Bart) and $β_4$ tetramers (HbH). The amount of Hb Bart or HbH will vary, depending on the number of α-globin genes deleted and the age of the patient.

The *silent carrier state* is due to deletion of one α-globin gene. There are no clinical symptoms, and the blood counts are normal.

The *α-thalassemia trait* is due to deletions of 2 α-globin genes. These individuals have no clinical symptoms but will have microcytosis, hypochromia,

and mild anemia with a normal hemoglobin electrophoresis. At birth, the MCV is less than 100 fL, and the Hb Bart level is 2%–10% (normal is 1%). Beyond infancy, Hb Bart disappears, and the only abnormality is mild microcytosis. This is a clinically benign condition; therefore, establishing the diagnoses is not necessary in the neonatal period. In people of African extraction, α-thalassemia trait is due to 2 deletions occurring in *trans* (2 different chromosomes) vs *cis* deletions (occurring on the same chromosome), which is what is observed in Asians. If an α-thalassemia syndrome is noted in any Asian child, the parents should be referred for α-thalassemia testing and genetic counseling to determine the risk of their future pregnancies being affected by a more severe type of α thalassemia (see further discussion this chapter). The risk of more serious α-thalassemia conditions is not an issue in people of African background unless the mating partner has α-thalassemia trait and is Asian.

Hemoglobin H disease is due to deletion of 3 α-globin genes (– –/– α). Also, a combination of 2 α-globin deletions and an α-globin gene mutation, most common constant spring (– –/αα^{cs}), results in HbH disease. The clinical features of HbH disease beyond infancy are characterized by mild-to-moderate chronic microcytic anemia with variable degrees of intermittent hemolysis. HbH is unstable and undergoes denaturation in the presence of oxidant stress, thereby forming intracellular inclusions that damage red cells, leading to early removal from circulation. Similar to G-6-PD deficiency, exposure to oxidants can lead to increased hemolysis and worsening anemia. In most cases, HbH disease does not cause clinical problems other than microcytic anemia in neonates. Diagnosis in the neonatal period generally results from newborn screening tests, which detect increased amounts of Hb Bart (usually greater than 20%). Beyond infancy, children with HbH disease have a mild-to-moderate microcytic anemia (Hb 9–10 g/dL), and there can be evidence of hemolysis, such as indirect hyperbilirubinemia and splenomegaly. These infants and children rarely require RBC transfusions.

Hb Barts hydrops fetalis is due to deletion of all 4 α-globin genes (– –/– –). There are no functional α-globin chains produced; non-α-globin chains accumulate, forming exclusively Hb Bart ($γ_4$) and HbH (β4). Embryos that lack 4 α-globin genes are well until 8 weeks of age, when production of embryonic hemoglobin ceases. Subsequently, due to lack of α-globin chains, Hb Bart becomes the predominant hemoglobin. Hb Bart has a very high oxygen affinity and is unable to efficiently deliver oxygen. Consequently, these fetuses develop anemia and have severe hypoxia, resulting in hydrops with heart failure, generalized edema, and severe growth failure. Most homozygous α-thalassemia fetuses die in utero, although some survive until term due to persistent expression of embryonic globin chains. These hydropic infants often have congenital anomalies and significant neurologic defects. There are case reports of infants with 4 α-globin gene deletions supported with intrauterine transfusions until delivery. Postdelivery, these infants received PRBC transfusions until bone marrow transplantation. This management strategy is controversial as there remain concerns regarding poor in utero neurodevelopment and long-term outcome.

Besides the fetal effects, there are serious maternal complications in pregnancies of homozygous α thalassemia. Up to 30% of women develop severe preeclampsia. Antepartum hemorrhage, hypertension, renal failure, congestive heart failure, and placental abruption are other known complications. Without proper medical care, up to a 50% mortality rate has been reported.[30] Hemoglobin Bart hydrops fetalis can be diagnosed prenatally by DNA-based testing of amniocytes from amniocentesis or chorionic villus sampling. It is important to establish this diagnosis early to avoid the serious maternal complications seen in these pregnancies.

β-Thalassemia Major: β-Thalassemia major, due to mutations in both β-globin genes, is not a neonatal disease. Anemia from β thalassemia is not notable until 3 months of age when γ-globin production decreases. There are 2 groups of β thalassemia. β[0] thalassemia is caused by complete absence of β-chain production; β[+] thalassemia has significantly decreased but some β-globin production. Hemoglobin electrophoresis during newborn screening of neonates with β[0] thalassemia reveals HbF only, consistent with absent HbA production, while β[+]-thalassemia patients will have HbF and very small traces of HbA. The diagnosis of β[+] thalassemia is therefore only possible after the neonatal period. Infants with β-thalassemia major will become anemic and transfusion dependent by 6–9 months of age. These patients require lifelong transfusions and treatment of iron overload. Bone marrow transplantation is the only curative option.

Hemoglobin E/β thalassemia is a result of coinheritance of HbE trait and β-thalassemia trait. HbE is a β-globin variant most commonly seen in individuals in India and Southeast Asia, including Thailand, Laos, and Cambodia. There is significant clinical heterogeneity among patients with HbE/β thalassemia, ranging from a mild hemolytic process to a severe chronic transfusion-dependent anemia, identical to that seen with β[0]-thalassemia major. HbE/β thalassemia is diagnosed by newborn screening hemoglobin electrophoresis, which will demonstrate an FE or FEA pattern. Just like β-thalassemia major, clinical symptoms do not arise until after 3 months of age. However, once the newborn screening tests reveal this hemoglobin disorder, the infant and family should be referred to a hematology treatment center for advice and guidance.

Sickle Cell Disease: Hemoglobin S is one of the most common β-globin mutations encountered worldwide. The most severe form of sickle cell disease results from inheritance of 2 β[s] mutations. This genetic pattern results in what is classically known as sickle cell anemia (HbSS disease). Inheritance of one β[s] mutation and one β-thalassemia trait mutation causes sickle β thalassemia (HbS-β thal), which is identical to sickle cell anemia phenotypically except there is also microcytosis. Coinheritance of β[s] mutations and β[c] mutations results in HbS-C disease, which is a milder form of sickle cell disease. All 50 US states have newborn screening programs for sickle cell disease. Hemoglobin patterns are reported in the order of decreasing hemoglobin concentration. The normal neonatal pattern is fetal/adult (FA). Infants with sickle cell anemia and HbS-β thal will have an FS pattern on their newborn screen, while HbS-C disease will provide an FSC pattern. FSA is seen in Hb S-β thal while FAS indicates sickle cell trait.

Neonates are protected from clinical symptoms of sickle cell disease due to the presence of fetal hemoglobin. However, as HbF concentration decreases after birth, and as HbS production increases, significant complications from cells sickling arise. Newborn screening for sickle cell disease was adopted to ensure early diagnosis to prevent life-threatening complications. Two major complications during infancy are sepsis from encapsulated organisms and splenic sequestration. All neonates with sickle cell anemia should be referred to a sickle cell treatment center for family education and care. Penicillin prophylaxis should begin by 2 months of age, and it is particularly important for sickle cell patients to receive all scheduled vaccines during their first year of life. Sickle cell center staff or primary physicians should provide appropriate education to parents to help them identify splenic sequestration and other sickle cell complications. Couples with a child with sickle cell disease or trait should be referred for further testing and genetic counseling.

Hypoproliferative Disorders

Hypoproliferative anemia refers to anemia caused by impaired erythrocyte production (Table 31-2) and is the least-common etiology of anemia in the neonatal period. Lack of specific growth factors stimulating erythropoiesis can lead to hypoproliferative anemia, such as the anemia of prematurity. Decreased erythrocyte progenitors, as seen in isoimmunization with Kell antibodies, can cause decreased red cell production. Abnormalities resulting in increased Epo resistance or abnormalities in Epo receptor expression can result in a decreased red cell mass. Finally, lack of specific

Table 31-2 Syndromes Associated With Hypoproliferative Anemia in the Neonatal Period

Syndrome	Features, Inheritance, and Mapping
Aase syndrome	Steroid-responsive hypoplastic anemia that improves with age Inheritance: autosomal recessive (AR), possible autosomal dominant (AD)
Congenital dyserythropoietic anemia (CDA)	Type I (rare): megaloblastoid erythroid hyperplasia and nuclear chromitin bridges between nuclei Type II (common): hereditary erythroblastic multinuclearity, positive acidified serum (HEMPAS) test, increased lysis to anti-i Type III: erythroblastic multinuclearity ("gigantoblasts"), macrocytosis Mapped to the following: type I: 15q15.1–q15.3; type II: 20q11.2; type III: 15q21
Diamond-Blackfan syndrome	Steroid-responsive hypoplastic anemia, often macrocytic After 5 months of age; inheritance: AR; sporadic mutations and AD inheritance described; mapped to 19q13.2, 8p23.3-p22
Dyskeratosis congenita	Hypoproliferative anemia usually presenting between 5 and 15 years of age; inheritance: X-linked recessive, locus on Xq28; some cases with AD inheritance
Fanconi pancytopenia	Androgen-responsive hypoplastic anemia, reticulocytopenia, some macrocytic red blood cells (RBCs), shortened RBC life span Cells are hypersensitive to DNA cross-linking agents Inheritance: AR, mapped to multiple genes: complementation group A: 16q24.3; B:; C: 9q22.3; D2: 3p25.3; E: 6p22-p21; F: 11p15; G: 9p13
Osteopetrosis	Hypoplastic anemia from marrow compression, extramedullary erythropoiesis; lethal form due to reduced osteoclasts AR form: mapped to 16p13, 11q13.4-q13.5 AD form: mapped to 1p21
Pearson syndrome	Hypoplastic sideroblastic anemia, marrow cell vacuolization caused by pleioplasmatic rearrangement of mitochondrial DNA; inheritance: X linked or AR
X-linked α-thalassemia/ mental retardation (ATR and ATR-16) syndromes	ATR-X: hypochromic, microcytic anemia; mild form of hemoglobin H disease ATR-16: more significant hemoglobin H disease/anemia present Inheritance: ATR-X: X-linked recessive, mapped to Xq13.3 ATR-16: mapped to 16p13.3, deletions of α-globin locus

substrates or their carriers (such as iron, folate, vitamin B_{12}, or transcobalamin II deficiency) can also lead to deficient production of red cells.

Congenital/Genetic Hypoproliferative Disorders: Congenital Hypoplastic Anemias

Congenital hypoplastic anemias refer to a rare group of inherited disorders with impaired RBC production. The most common congenital hypoplastic anemia is Diamond-Blackfan anemia (DBA). Other very rare causes include congenital dyserythropoietic anemia (CDA), and Pearson syndrome.

Diamond-Blackfan anemia is an AD disorder, estimated at 4–7 cases per million live births, occurring equally in males and females. With the discovery of multiple ribosomal gene mutations and deletions in patients with DBA, it is now firmly established that DBA is a ribosomopathy.[32] Mutations in 9 different ribosomal protein genes (*RPL 5, RPL 11, RPL 35A, RPS 7, RPS 10, RPS 17, RPS 19, RPS 24, and RPS 26*) have been confirmed to be associated with 50% of DBA patients. An additional 20% of patients

have deletions of these same ribosomal protein genes, while 30% of patients with DBA remain genetically unclassified.

In children 6 months of age to toddler years, the main differential diagnosis of RBC aplasia is DBA vs transient erythroblastopenia of childhood (TEC). However, TEC is rarely ever seen in newborns and is unusual in the first 6 months of life. Other causes of red cell aplasia include congenital parvovirus infection, maternal drug exposure, or a marrow infiltrative process such as congenital leukemia. Anemia with reticulocytopenia can also be seen in newborns who have received in utero PRBC transfusions.

Diamond-Blackfan anemia usually presents in infancy, with approximately 90% of patients diagnosed by 12 months of age. Over 25% of affected infants have severe anemia. Newborns with DBA are otherwise healthy (aside from associated congenital defects) but have severe anemia and reticulocytopenia. DBA is usually an isolated anemia, with other cell lines normal. The anemia is generally macrocytic, but the increased MCV is only appreciated beyond the neonatal period given the large RBC size during the first few months of life. If a bone marrow aspirate is done, it typically reveals normal overall cellularity with a marked decrease in erythroid precursors.

An important clinical feature of DBA is the presence of congenital anomalies in over 50% of patients. Craniofacial anomalies are most common, but upper limb, hand (particularly thumb), genitourinary, and cardiac anomalies are common. These features can be subtle and may be hard to recognize at birth. The constellation of congenital hypoplastic anemia associated with skeletal anomalies, cleft palate, growth failure, and triphalangial thumbs was previously coined Aase syndrome.[33] It is now recognized that this is one of the variants of DBA. Diagnosis of DBA is supported by detecting elevated erythrocyte adenosine deaminase (eADA) activity, found in over 80% of DBA patients.[34] Genetic testing for ribosomal protein mutations is available through some commercial gene diagnostic laboratories.

Packed RBC transfusions are recommended as initial treatment if needed until 1 year of age.[35] After this period, steroids are started if the child remains significantly anemic. About 80% of children will respond to steroids, with reticulocytosis noted within 1–2 weeks after initiation of therapy. The natural history of DBA is variable, ranging from a need for chronic red cell transfusions, to a need for continuous administration of small doses of steroids, to spontaneous remission after years of transfusion or steroids. Treatment for those who are steroid refractory or steroid intolerant includes regular PRBC transfusions and iron chelation therapy for preventing and treating iron overload. Hematopoietic stem cell transplantation is the only curative option for DBA, and outcome of matched sibling transplants has been encouraging, with overall survival of greater than 75%. Increasing amounts of data have arisen to support the observation that DBA is a cancer predisposition syndrome. Leukemia and solid tumors have both been reported.[36]

Congenital dyserythropoietic anemia is a rare disorder marked by ineffective erythropoiesis, macrocytic or normocytic anemia, and characteristic abnormalities of the nuclear membrane and cytoplasm seen on electron microscopy. Both AD and AR inheritance patterns have been reported. Three types of CDA have been described.[37] Type I CDA is characterized by AD inheritance, macrocytic anemia, nuclear chromatin bridges between marrow erythroblasts, and erythroid hyperplasia. Type I CDA has been linked to chromosome 15q15.1–15.3 in a large cohort, and the mutated gene is *CDAN1* (codanin-1). Type II, the most common form of CDA, is characterized by normocytic anemia, erythroblastic multinuclearity, and a positive acidified serum test result. A specific mutation in the *SEC23B* gene on chromosome 20p has been demonstrated in this condition. CDA II appears to result from enzymatic defects in the cellular glycosylation pathway that affects band 3 anion transport activity. Type III CDA is marked by erythroblastic multinuclearity and macrocytosis.

Congenital dyserythropoietic anemia can present in the newborn period with macrocytic anemia, early jaundice, hepatosplenomegaly, and intrauterine growth retardation. Infants with type I CDA may have bony abnormalities and syndactyly. Fetuses with CDA can present with hydrops fetalis. Although rare, this disorder should be included in the differential diagnosis of newborns with anemia, jaundice, and hepatosplenomegaly. Treatment of this disorder consists of supportive therapy and close observation for side effects of chronic transfusions. Splenectomy may be helpful in some older patients with severe anemia.

Pearson marrow pancreas syndrome is a disorder involving the hematopoietic system, exocrine pancreas, liver, and kidneys. It presents in infancy with macrocytic anemia, sometimes associated with neutropenia and thrombocytopenia. The bone marrow has normal cellularity but with erythrocyte abnormalities, including vacuolization of erythroid and myeloid precursors and ringed sideroblasts. The disorder is associated with deletions in mitochondrial DNA and appears to involve defects in oxidative phosphorylation. There is no specific therapy. The disorder is usually considered fatal. Some of the few children who survive the hematologic cytopenias later go on to have the clinical and laboratory features associated with Kearns-Sayre syndrome.

Fanconi anemia is an AR-inherited disorder characterized by marrow failure. In many patients, there are congenital anomalies, including abnormalities in skin pigmentation, gastrointestinal anomalies, renal defects, and upper limb anomalies. In addition, FA is associated with an increased risk of myeloid leukemia and squamous cell cancers, occurring at a relatively younger age than when these tumors usually appear. This disorder is due to a defect in DNA repair, and 13 different FA genes have been identified.[38] Peripheral blood lymphocytes are hypersensitive to DNA cross-linking agents such as diepoxybutane (DEB) and mitomycin C, representing a sensitive and specific diagnostic test for FA. The mean age of diagnosis is 6.5 years. The hematologic features of FA are rarely ever present in the newborn period. When FA is identified in neonates, it is because early recognition of congenital abnormalities initially led to specific testing for FA. Definitive treatment of FA necessitates stem cell transplantation, which can ameliorate the hematologic problems, although the increased risk of solid tumors remains.

Anemia of Prematurity

In utero, serum Epo concentrations gradually increase through the third trimester and are highest at term. Epo measurements made on neonatal cord blood of laboring and nonlaboring mothers can reflect hypoxic stress during labor and delivery. An increase in NRBCs can be seen with chronic in utero hypoxic stress; however, acute stress (less than 24 hours) may be associated with increased Epo concentrations alone. Serum Epo concentrations at birth normally range from 5 to 100 mU/mL, while Epo concentrations in anemic, nonuremic adults range from 300 to 400 mU/mL.

In preterm infants, adaptive mechanisms to the extrauterine environment are incomplete, and the transition to term organ function often follows gestational age, regardless of premature delivery. In anemic preterm infants, Epo concentrations are significantly lower than those found in adults, given the degree of their anemia. This normocytic, normochromic anemia is termed the anemia of prematurity. It commonly affects infants 32 weeks' gestation or less and is the most common anemia seen in the neonatal period.[39] The anemia of prematurity is minimally responsive to the addition of iron, folate, vitamin E, or other erythropoietic nutrients. Some infants may be asymptomatic despite hemoglobin concentrations below 8 g/dL, while others demonstrate signs of anemia that appear alleviated by transfusion. Signs associated with the anemia of prematurity include tachycardia, increased episodes of apnea and bradycardia, poor weight gain, tachypnea, an increased oxygen requirement, and elevated serum lactate concentrations that decrease following PRBC transfusion.

Multiple studies evaluating the use of recombinant Epo to prevent and treat the anemia of prematurity have been published to show that Epo is successful in preterm infants in stimulating erythropoiesis (described in the treatment section of this chapter).

Epo recipients will maintain hematocrits 4%–6% greater than placebo recipients (Figure 31-2), total transfusions are decreased, and the number of nontransfused infants are increased.

Fetal/Neonatal Anemia due to Congenital Infection

Infections before and after birth can lead to anemia through a hemorrhagic, hemolytic, or hypoproliferative process or a combination of processes. Neonatal sepsis due to *Escherichia coli*, group B streptococcus, and other perinatal organisms may result in hemolysis, DIC, and hemorrhage. Infants are often jaundiced and have hepatosplenomegaly, although the degree of hyperbilirubinemia does not always correlate with the degree of anemia. Infants may have an elevated direct bilirubin as well, possibly due to infectious involvement with the liver. Bacteria such as *E coli* will produce hemolytic endotoxins, which result in increased red cell destruction, often associated with a microangiopathic process.

Fetal and neonatal parvovirus B19 infection can cause severe anemia, hydrops, and fetal demise.[40] The infant generally presents with a hypoplastic anemia, but hemolysis can occur as well. The virus replicates in erythroid progenitor cells and shuts down erythropoiesis, resulting in aplastic anemia. In utero transfusions for hydropic fetuses have been investigated but are not successful in all patients. Treatment during aplastic crises with intravenous immunoglobulin (IVIG) leads to resolution of the anemia.

Both malaria and the human immunodeficiency virus (HIV) can be associated with neonatal anemia. Congenital malaria may occur in major urban

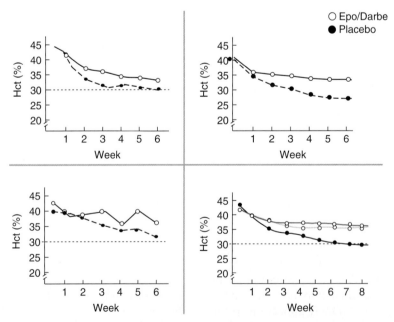

FIGURE 31-2 Hematocrit differences in erythropoietin (Epo) studies. Hct, hematocrit.[57,61–63]

areas, where imported cases of malaria are increasing. Congenital HIV infection can be asymptomatic in newborns. Infants born to mothers on zidovudine (AZT) may have hypoplastic anemia due to transplacental side effects of AZT.

Other Erythropoietin-Responsive Anemias in the Newborn Period

Late Anemia of Rh Disease. Early anemia in infants with Rh hemolytic disease is caused by ongoing antibody-mediated hemolysis, but a late (age 1 to 3 months) anemia resulting from diminished erythrocyte production can also occur. Late anemia appears to be more common in infants who receive intrauterine transfusions and is characterized by low serum concentrations of Epo but erythroid progenitors that remain highly responsive to recombinant Epo in vitro. Infants with this late anemia will often receive PRBC transfusions until the late anemia resolves, generally by the third or fourth month of life. Following the active hemolytic period when circulating anti-D antibody levels are elevated, the administration of Epo is effective at stimulating erythropoiesis and can serve as an alternative to erythrocyte transfusion.[41] Outpatient Epo administration may also diminish or eliminate the need for hospitalization in those centers in which infants are hospitalized for transfusions.

Kell isoimmunization is a unique hemolytic disorder that selectively impacts marrow erythroid precursors, resulting in both hemolytic and hypoproliferative anemia. Kell positive infants born to Kell-negative mothers can present with severe and protracted anemia.[37] Epo administration for neonatal anemia after active hemolysis is resolved can stimulate erythropoiesis.

Anemia of Bronchopulmonary Dysplasia. Anemia can develop in patients with bronchopulmonary dysplasia (BPD). The anemia of BPD is characterized as normocytic, normochromic, hypo-regenerative anemia, with marrow normoblast iron stains that are distinct from those observed in both the anemia of chronic disorders and the anemia of prematurity. Similar to the late anemia of Rh hemolytic disease, the anemia of BPD responds to Epo administration. The explanation for reduced Epo production in patients with BPD requires further study to determine if other factors that could create a relatively Epo-resistant environment are involved, such as interleukin (IL) 1, tumor necrosis factor, and interferon γ.

Anemia in Neonates Requiring Surgery. Neonates who are born with problems that require surgical repair, such as congenital diaphragmatic hernia, gastroschisis, omphalocele, meningomyelocele, and craniofacial abnormalities often undergo surgery during the period of physiologic anemia. These hospitalized infants undergo blood loss through phlebotomy, the surgery itself, and postoperative care. As a result, the physiologic anemia is exacerbated, and transfusions are often administered to increase hemoglobin concentrations, especially around the time of surgery. These infants respond to Epo administration by increasing erythropoiesis[42] and may also benefit from the non-hematopoietic, mitogenic effects of Epo, such as an increase in villous growth.

In addition to neonates who require surgery, other neonatal populations may benefit from Epo therapy. Epo has been used successfully to treat anemia in newborns with end-stage renal disease due to congenital nephrotic syndrome or polycystic kidney disease and in infants with congenital heart disease awaiting surgery. In addition, infants with hemolytic disease from ABO incompatibility and HS have been treated with Epo.[43] Further studies are required in these populations to determine whether treatment with Epo is beneficial and does not cause further harm through increased hemolysis and hyperbilirubinemia.

Hemorrhage

The process of blood loss from the intravascular space can be either acute or chronic and can occur at any time during the prenatal, perinatal, or postnatal periods (Table 31-3). Acute hemorrhage generally results in a change in hemoglobin and hematocrit only, while chronic hemorrhage can result in changes to other red cell indices, such as MCV, MCHC, reticulocyte count, and red cell distribution width (RDW).

Prenatal Hemorrhage

Twin-to-twin transfusion syndrome (TTS) is a complication of monochorionic twin gestations and occurs in 5% to 30% of these pregnancies. Depending on the timing and severity of presentation, the perinatal mortality rate can be as high as 70%–100%. In TTS, placental anastomoses allow transfer of blood from one twin to the other. Approximately 70% of monozygous twin pregnancies have monochorionic placentas. Although vascular anastomoses are present in almost all instances of monochorionic placentas, not all anastomoses result in TTS.

Acute TTS usually results in twins of similar size with hemoglobin concentrations that vary by more than 5 g/dL. Chronic TTS results in the donor twin becoming progressively anemic and growth retarded, while the recipient twin becomes polycythemic, macrosomic, and sometimes hypertensive. The donor twin can become hydropic from profound anemia, while the recipient twin can develop hydrops from congestive heart failure and hypervolemia. The donor twin exists in diminished amniotic fluid volumes, while the

Table 31-3 Etiology of Neonatal/Perinatal Hemorrhage

A. Prenatal:
- Chronic or acute twin-to-twin transfusion syndrome
- Chronic or acute fetal-maternal hemorrhage
- Hemorrhage into amniotic fluid following periumbilical blood sampling
- Traumatic amniocentesis
- Trauma following external cephalic version
- Maternal trauma

B. Perinatal:
- Placenta previa
- Vasa previa
- Placental abruption
- Trauma or incision of placenta during cesarean section
- Ruptured normal or abnormal (varices, aneurysms) umbilical cord
- Cord or placental hematoma
- Velamentous insertion of the cord
- Placental chorioangioma
- Nuchal cord

C. Postnatal:
- Subgaleal hemorrhage
- Cephalohematoma
- Intraventricular/intracranial hemorrhage (prematurity, trauma, isoimmune thrombocytopenia)
- Hemorrhage associated with disseminated intravascular coagulation/sepsis
- Organ trauma (liver, spleen, adrenal, renal)
- Pulmonary hemorrhage
- Iatrogenic blood loss (phlebotomy, umbilical or central line accidents, arterial line accidents)

recipient twin has increased amniotic fluid due to significant differences in blood volume, renal blood flow, and urine output.

Chronic TTS can be diagnosed by serial prenatal ultrasounds measuring cardiomegaly, discordant amniotic fluid volume, and fetal growth discrepancy of more than 20%. After birth, the donor twin may be anemic enough to require transfusions and can also experience hypoglycemia, neutropenia, hydrops from severe anemia, growth retardation, and congestive heart failure. The recipient is often the sicker twin, experiencing congestive heart failure associated with hypertrophic cardiomyopathy, hypocalcemia, hypoglycemia, polycythemia, hyperviscosity, and respiratory difficulties. Neurologic evaluation and imaging are important as the risk of antenatally acquired neurologic cerebral lesions is 20% to 30% in both twins. Morbidities include hypoperfusion syndromes from hypotension, multiple cerebral infarctions, and periventricular leukomalacia.[44] Long-term neurologic follow-up is necessary and important for all TTS survivors.

Treatment options vary but should include close monitoring and reduction amniocenteses if needed to decrease uterine stretch and prolong the pregnancy. The average survival rates with serial reduction amniocenteses range from 40% to 70%. Selective fetocide of the hydropic twin has also resulted in the survival of the healthier twin in some studies. Laser surgery to ablate bridging vessels has the best outcomes for TTS pregnancies, resulting in improved survival rates of up to around 50%, with approximately 70% of the pregnancies having at least one survivor. The survival rate without morbidity in the surviving twin is approximately 50%. Meta-analyses have found no differences in outcome between amnioreduction, fetoscopy, septostomy, or close observation for fetuses with TTS.[45]

Feto-Maternal Hemorrhage. Maternal and fetal circulating cells may cross the placental barrier at varying times during the pregnancy. The passage of fetal red cells into the maternal circulation is termed *feto-maternal hemorrhage* (FMH).

Approximately 50%–75% of pregnancies are associated with some degree of FMH, usually occurring after the first trimester. Commonly, the volume of fetal blood transferred into the maternal circulation is relatively small, usually on the order of 0.01 to 0.1 mL. About 1 pregnancy in 400 is associated with an FMH of 30 mL or greater, and about 1 pregnancy in 2000 is associated with an FMH of 100 mL or more.[46]

In an Rh-incompatible pregnancy, the overall risk of maternal blood group sensitization due to FMH is 16% if the fetus is Rh positive and ABO. The risk decreases to 1.5% if the fetus is Rh positive but ABO incompatible due to the destruction of incompatible cells early during placental transfer. Fetal transfer of cells to the mother occurs during abortions as well: there is a 2% incidence of such transfer with spontaneous abortion and a 4%–5% rate with therapeutic abortion.

The *Kleihauer-Betke stain* (KB stain) evaluates the acid elution of hemoglobin from red cells on a sample of maternal blood. Fetal hemoglobin resists acid elution to a greater degree than adult hemoglobin. Maternal cells (in which adult hemoglobin has been eluted from the cell) appear clear (termed *ghost cells*), while the contaminating fetal cells appear pink.

KB stains obtained from mothers with increased fetal hemoglobin synthesis, such as mothers with sickle cell disease, thalassemia, or hereditary persistence of fetal hemoglobin, are not reliable; in these cases, other methods should be used to detect FMH, such as flow cytometry using anti-HbF antibodies.[47] Diagnosis of a small-volume FMH may be difficult when the mother and infant are ABO incompatible as fetal cells are rapidly cleared from the maternal circulation.

One in 1000 deliveries is associated with severe (>200 mL) FMH. Severe FMH has been associated with decreased fetal movements and a fetal sinusoidal heart rate (SHR) pattern. Studies noted that decreased/absent fetal movements for a period ranging between 24 hours and 7 days were present for 10%–15% of cases evaluated.[48] In this group, two-thirds of the infants either died in utero or during the neonatal period. An SHR pattern was reported in 15% of cases and was associated with decreased fetal movement in 40% of the cases.

Infants need rapid evaluation and treatment if a significant hemorrhage is suspected. The infant with massive hemorrhage will present with pallor, tachypnea, and delayed capillary refill but may not have a significant oxygen requirement. Hemoglobin concentrations can be extremely low at birth, less than 6 g/dL. Significant metabolic acidosis is often present as a result of poor perfusion.

Other causes of pallor in the newborn period do exist and should be ruled out once the infant is stable. Infants with asphyxia and infants with chronic hemolytic anemia may also present with pallor (Table 31-4). These diagnoses can be distinguished from acute hemorrhage based on differences in clinical signs (Table 31-5). With chronic hemolytic anemia, clinical signs are mild or absent, and infants respond to conservative therapy with iron alone. Asphyxiated infants will be pale and floppy and may have poor peripheral circulation. The hemoglobin will be stable but may decrease if DIC and subsequent bleeding occur.

Other causes of prenatal hemorrhage include vaginal bleeding due to placenta previa or abruption, nonelective cesarean section, and deliveries associated with cord compression. Significant FMH has been described following trauma, and fetal hemorrhage into the placenta has been associated with placental chorioangioma.

Perinatal Hemorrhage

Obstetrical complications such as placenta previa, placental abruption, incision or tearing of the placenta during cesarean section, and cord evulsion of normal or abnormal umbilical cords can result in significant neonatal blood loss at the time of delivery. Placental anomalies such as a multilobed placenta and placental chorioangiomas may also be a source of hemorrhage during the perinatal period.

Placental abruption occurs when there is separation of the placenta from the uterus prior to delivery.

Table 31-4 Differential Diagnosis of the "Pale" Neonate

Etiology	Hematologic	Neurologic	Cardiovascular	Respiratory
Hypoxia/ischemia	Hematocrit/hemoglobin remains stable over time; may develop thrombocytopenia and DIC from hypoxic injury to marrow	Abnormal transition period, hypotonia, decreased arousal state; may have seizures in first 6–24 hours	Normal or bradycardia	Respiratory distress, O_2 requirement
Acute hemorrhage	Normal-to-low hematocrit; drop in hematocrit occurs within hours	Normal or hyperalert/hyperirritable ("catecholamine response")	Tachycardia, hypotension	Tachypnea, no O_2 requirement
Hemolytic anemia	Anemic from birth; hepatosplenomegaly; jaundice, positive Coombs test	Normal	May vary from normal to presence of congestive heart failure and hydrops, depending on degree of anemia	Normal
Congenital heart disease	Normal or elevated hematocrit	Normal	Normal or tachycardia; decreased perfusion/pulses when ductus closes with ductal-dependent lesion	Normal or respiratory distress depending on type of lesion
Septic shock	Hematocrit usually normal; may have moderate-to-severe neutropenia and thrombocytopenia, may develop DIC	Normal or decreased arousal state, depending on timing of infection	Tachycardia, hypotension	Respiratory distress or apnea

Abbreviation: DIC, disseminated intravascular coagulation.

Severe fetal growth restriction, prolonged rupture of membranes, chorioamnionitis, hypertension (chronic and pregnancy induced), cigarette smoking, advanced maternal age, and male gender are all risk factors for placental abruption.[49] Abruption occurs in approximately 1% of term deliveries, and the incidence of abruption increases with decreasing gestation. Mortality ranges 0.8 to 2 per 1000 births and can be as high as 15% to 20% of the deliveries in which significant abruption occurs. The risk of stillbirth increases significantly when abruption exceeds 50%.

Women with a history of a previous cesarean birth and increased parity are at increased risk of having a pregnancy complicated by placenta previa,[50] a condition in which part or all of the placenta overlies the cervical os. Cigarette smoking increases the risk of placenta previa 2.6- to 4.4-fold. Prenatal diagnosis of vasa previa (anomalous vessels overlying the internal os of the cervix) can be performed with transvaginal color Doppler and should be suspected in any case of antepartum or intrapartum hemorrhage. Although uncommon (1 in 3000 deliveries), the perinatal death rate is high, ranging from 33% to 100% when undetected before delivery.[51] Infants are often stillborn.

Infants born following placental abruption or placenta previa may be anemic and may also present with signs of hypoxia. In these infants, it is important to monitor changes in hematocrit and neurologic signs. The need for postnatal transfusions in the infants is generally associated with the volume of perinatal hemorrhage. The infant's hemoglobin should be measured at birth and again at 12 to 24 hours whenever there is evidence of placental abruption, placenta previa, or any significant vaginal bleeding. A KB stain can be performed on maternal blood to determine if FMH occurred. Monitoring mothers with a history of second- or third-trimester bleeding with Doppler flow ultrasound to detect placental abnormalities may decrease the incidence of fetal loss and anemia in newborns.

Cord rupture due to excess traction on a shortened or abnormal umbilical cord usually occurs closer to the fetus than the placenta. Cord aneurysms, varices, and cysts can all lead to a weakened cord. Cord infections, termed *funicitis*, can also weaken the cord and increase the risk of rupture. In addition, infants born precipitously may be at increased risk for a ruptured cord.

Hematomas of the cord occur infrequently (1 in 5000–6000 births) but can result in fetal blood loss and may be associated with significant perinatal mortality. Intrauterine fetal demise may occur due to compression of the umbilical vein and arteries by the hematoma. Cord hematomas can result from trauma due to percutaneous umbilical blood sampling (PUBS) and can also be associated with a high maternal α-fetoprotein. Cord hematomas can be accurately diagnosed in utero by ultrasound and differentiated from other lesions of the placenta and cord. The lesion can also result in poor fetal growth and FMH.

Velamentous insertion of the umbilical cord occurs when the umbilical cord enters the membranes distant from the placenta and is present in approximately 0.5% to 2% of pregnancies. Blood vessels left unprotected by Wharton's jelly are more vulnerable to tension on the cord, and rupture of anomalous vessels in the absence of traction or trauma can occur even if the cord itself attaches centrally or paracentrally. Fetal mortality is high with velementous insertion, often because detection by routine ultrasound is rare.[52]

Postnatal Hemorrhage

Blood loss into the placenta, termed *fetoplacental hemorrhage*, is one of the most common etiologies for a low hematocrit at birth. Of the 120 mL/kg of blood in the fetoplacental unit, approximately one-third remains in the placenta, and blood will continue to flow in the direction of gravity after birth. Fetoplacental hemorrhage occurs when the infant is held above the placenta after birth; for this reason, infants born by cesarean section have smaller blood volumes than those born vaginally.[53] In addition, infants can lose 10% to 20% of their total blood volume when born with a tight nuchal cord, which allows blood to be pumped through umbilical arteries toward the placenta while constricting flow through the umbilical vein.

Blood loss into the subgaleal space is referred to as a subgaleal hemorrhage and can occur during difficult deliveries requiring vacuum or forceps assistance, such as face presentation, occiput posterior presentation, and shoulder dystocia. It is a potentially life-threatening event and must be recognized as early as possible to prevent significant morbidity or mortality. Subgaleal hemorrhage occurs when emissary or "bridging" veins are torn, allowing blood to accumulate in the large potential space between the galea aponeurotica (the epicranial aponeurosis) and the periosteum of the skull (Figure 31-3). The subgaleal space extends from the orbital ridge to the base of the skull and can accommodate an infant's entire blood volume, or 80 to 90 mL/kg of blood.

A subgaleal hemorrhage may occur because of pre-existing risk factors, such as coagulopathy or asphyxia. The diagnosis should be considered in the presence of a ballotable fluid collection in dependent regions of the infant's head, coupled with signs of hypovolemia such as tachycardia and metabolic acidosis. A rule of thumb for estimating the volume of blood lost is that every centimeter increase in head circumference represents 38 mL of blood loss. Treatment requires restoration of blood volume and control of bleeding. Exsanguination due to subgaleal hemorrhage has been reported, and the mortality is high if the hemorrhage goes unrecognized.

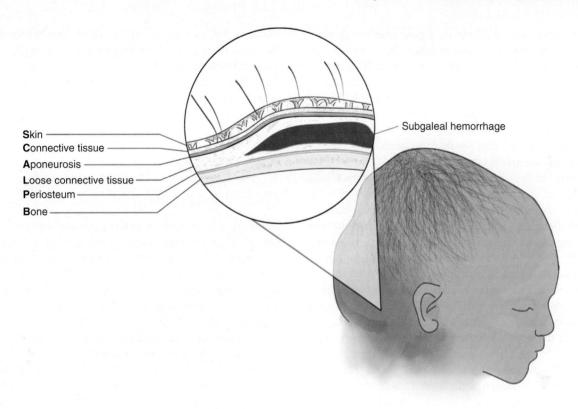

Skin
Connective tissue
Aponeurosis
Loose connective tissue
Periosteum
Bone

Subgaleal hemorrhage

FIGURE 31-3 Subgaleal hemorrhage: Perinatal and postnatal hemorrhage can occur into the subgaleal space. Sheering forces caused by traumatic delivery or vacuum extraction can cause tearing of veins within the loose connective tissue space (the *L* in the acronym SCALP), resulting in significant and sometimes lethal overwhelming hemorrhage as the space can expand to hold the entire neonatal blood volume.

Infants undergoing vacuum extraction have an increased risk for subgaleal hemorrhage.[54] The duration of vacuum application is thought to be the best predictor of scalp injury, followed by duration of second stage of labor and paramedian cup placement. Of those infants with reported subgaleal hemorrhages, 60%–90% had some history of vacuum or instrument-assisted delivery. A cesarean delivery does not preclude the use of vacuum or forceps, and subgaleal hemorrhage can still occur via this route of delivery. Limiting the frequency and duration of vacuum assistance in high-risk infants may decrease the risk.

Infants with neonatal alloimmune thrombocytopenia (NAIT) are at increased risk for pre- and postnatal intracranial hemorrhage. NAIT results from platelet-antigen incompatibility between the mother and fetus and occurs in 1 to 2 per 1000 live births. Antibodies to human platelet antigen (HPA) 1a antigen occur most commonly. Of newborns with platelet alloimmunization, 10%–20% will have an intracranial hemorrhage, of which half occur in utero.[55] The risk for intracranial hemorrhage is increased in newborns with an affected sibling who had an antenatal intracranial hemorrhage; similar to RhD isoimmunization, the subsequent affected newborns generally have more severe

disease than the first sibling. Treatment includes IVIG and platelet transfusions in severe cases.[56] Platelets obtained from the mother have a longer half-life because they lack the antigen causing consumption. Treatment of fetal thrombocytopenia includes maternal IVIG administration, maternal steroid administration, and fetal platelet transfusions.

Anemia appearing after the first 24 hours of life in an unjaundiced infant may result from postnatal hemorrhage. In addition to birth trauma causing visible hemorrhage such as a cephalohematoma, internal hemorrhage to liver, spleen, or other organs can occur. Breech deliveries may be associated with renal, adrenal, or splenic hemorrhage into the retroperitoneal space. Delivery of macrosomic infants, such as infants born to diabetic mothers, may also result in organ damage and hemorrhage.

The incidence of adrenal hemorrhage is not uncommon, occurring in 1.7 per 1000 births. In addition to causing anemia, adrenal hemorrhage may result in circulatory collapse due to the loss of organ function. Adrenal hemorrhage can also affect surrounding organs. Intestinal obstruction and kidney dysfunction have been reported in infants with adrenal hemorrhage. Diagnosis can be made using ultrasonography, which notes calcifications or cystic masses. Adrenal hemorrhage can be distinguished from renal vein thrombosis (RVT) by ultrasound, in that RVT generally results in a solid mass. Occasionally, both entities may coexist in the same patient. Infants with RVT may have gross or microscopic hematuria and may develop renal failure and hypertension.

Splenic rupture can result from birth trauma or as a result of distention caused by extramedullary hematopoiesis, such as that seen in erythroblastosis fetalis. Abdominal distension and discoloration, scrotal swelling, and pallor are clinical signs of splenic rupture.

The newborn liver is prone to iatrogenic rupture, resulting in high morbidity and mortality. Infants may appear asymptomatic until significant hemoperitoneum occurs. Hepatic rupture and hemorrhage occur in both term and preterm infants and have been associated with chest compressions during cardiopulmonary resuscitation. Surgical intervention involving vascular tamponade has been reported to save some infants; however, the mortality remains high.

Other rare causes of hemorrhage in the newborn include hemangiomas of the gastrointestinal tract, characteristic of Kassaback-Merrit syndrome; vascular malformations of the skin; and hemorrhage into soft tumors, such as giant sacrococcygeal teratomas, thoracic hamartomas, or cystic hygromas. Occult intra-abdominal hemorrhage can occur with fetal ovarian cysts, which are commonly benign and resolve spontaneously.

DIAGNOSIS

Clinical Assessment

The diagnosis of anemia in the perinatal and postnatal period often requires rapid investigation, laboratory evaluation, and treatment. An immediate assessment of the infant includes determining whether the infant is suffering from acute or chronic anemia, as treatments vary significantly (Table 31-5). Infants presenting in shock from their anemia have most likely suffered massive hemorrhage, and patient stabilization is of utmost importance to avoid organ damage and death. The "ABCs" of newborn resuscitation should be applied: stabilize the infant's airway, administer oxygen and intubate if necessary, and determine if the

Table 31-5 Symptoms of Acute vs Chronic Hemorrhage in the Neonate

	Acute Blood Loss	Chronic Blood Loss
Clinical symptoms		
Appearance	Hyperalert; may be pale; "stunned" gaze	Normal neurologic examination; pale
Hematologic:		
Indices	MCV 105–118 fL; reticulocytes 4%–10%	MCV < 100 fL, reticulocytes > 10%, RDW increased
Morphology	Macrocytic, normochromic (normal)	Microcytic, hypochromic
Hemoglobin	May be normal or decreased, continues to decrease over 24 hours	Decreased
Iron	Loss of iron in erythrocytes	Decreased
	Normal ferritin	
Cardiovascular	Tachycardic with weak pulses; low blood pressure	Normal or mildly tachycardic; rarely in congestive heart failure with hepatomegaly; blood pressure normal or even increased
Respiratory	Tachypneic, in mild-to-moderate distress, no or minimal oxygen requirement	Normal, rarely may be tachypneic; oxygen requirement if congestive heart failure is present
Course	Promptly treat hypovolemia, may need rapid volume expansion to prevent shock, DIC, and death	Usually uneventful hospital course, may need treatment of congestive heart failure and hydrops
Treatment	Volume expansion with isotonic fluid and PRBCs, FFP, and platelets Iron therapy later Epo therapy may be appropriate to enhance erythropoiesis	Initiate iron therapy PRBC transfusion rarely needed Epo therapy may be appropriate to enhance erythropoiesis

Abbreviations: DIC, disseminated intravascular coagulation; Epo, erythropoietin; FFP, fresh frozen plasma; MCV, mean corpuscular volume; PRBC, packed red blood cells; RDW, red cell distribution width.

infant's cardiovascular and intravascular volume status is adequate. Immediate volume expansion using normal saline should be performed when a significant acute hemorrhage is suspected. A transfusion of type O, Rh-negative blood ("trauma" blood) may be required in the first hour if massive hemorrhage has occurred. Repeat transfusions of cross-matched PRBCs may be necessary to treat lactic acidosis if oxygen delivery to the tissues is not improved with volume expansion.

It is helpful to identify the timing of presentation of anemia. Infants with significant acute blood loss before or during delivery may be anemic and hypovolemic at birth, while infants with TTS, chronic FMH, or chronic ongoing hemolysis from isoimmunization may not be immediately symptomatic. Infants with internal trauma and hemorrhage (hepatic, splenic, adrenal, or renal) may not initially be symptomatic but may rapidly decompensate as compensation for intravascular volume loss fails. Attention to details of the infant's transition period from fetal to postnatal life may be life-saving. As an example, an infant suffering from subgaleal hemorrhage will experience an increased heart and respiratory rate during stage 2 of transition (instead of the expected decrease in heart rate and respiratory rate) due to intravascular volume loss and worsening metabolic acidosis. Close observation during transition will allow rapid diagnosis and potentially life-saving treatment for the infant.

Maternal, Labor, and Delivery History

Once the infant is stable, information on maternal, labor, and delivery history can be gathered from both the mother's and infant's chart to help determine the cause of anemia. Any family history of anemia, bleeding, "low blood" counts, transfusions, jaundice, or unusual hematologic indices should be identified. Ethnicity of both parents is important to note, as some inherited disorders (eg, G-6-PD deficiency or thalassemia) are more prevalent in specific ethnic groups.

Obtaining a thorough labor and delivery history is important, including information on vaginal bleeding, trauma, infection or exposure to infected individuals, and any prescribed or nonprescribed drug use during the pregnancy. The use of cocaine prior to delivery may increase the potential for placental abruption, fetal infarction, and postinfarction hemorrhage. Important maternal laboratory information includes blood type and antibody screen, maternal hepatitis, and syphilis and rubella status.

Detailed information regarding labor and delivery can sometimes be difficult to obtain, especially if delivery was not anticipated, such as an emergent cesarean section for loss of fetal heart tones. Episodes of fetal tachycardia or decelerations or other evidence of fetal heart rate abnormalities such as loss of beat-to-beat variability should be noted. The length of labor, vaginal bleeding, evidence of placental abruption, knowledge of placenta previa or vasa previa, and route of delivery should be noted. Information regarding the placenta (cord hematoma, cord rupture, chorioangioma, velementous insertion of the cord) should be gathered and the placenta examined. The use of forceps, vacuum, or other manipulations is important to note. Finally, it is important to identify the presence of multiple gestations, especially those associated with discordant growth.

Laboratory Evaluation

Laboratory evaluation of the anemic infant includes a complete blood count including RBC indices and peripheral smear, a reticulocyte count, a direct Coombs test, and total and direct bilirubin. A KB stain of maternal blood can identify fetal cells in the maternal circulation if FMH is suspected. With a thorough history, physical examination, and minimal laboratory evaluation, most causes of anemia in the newborn period can be determined.

TREATMENT

PRBC Transfusion

Treatment of anemia in neonates should be guided by the timing and etiology of the anemia. The management of hemorrhage in the neonatal period depends in part on the etiology of the hemorrhage, its timing, and the extent of hemorrhage. Infants with chronic hemorrhage, such as those with chronic FMH or TTS, may have had time to compensate for a gradual decrease in hemoglobin and may therefore have an adequate intravascular volume despite a low circulating erythrocyte volume (Table 31-5). Those infants will require iron supplementation to replace iron stores depleted by the loss of red cells; however, they are unlikely to require an immediate PRBC transfusion or even volume expansion. Infants experiencing an acute hemorrhage will require volume expansion to improve circulation and organ perfusion.

Treatment of anemia due to hemolysis involves understanding the etiology of the hemolysis, the rate of red cell destruction, and the benefits of stimulating neonatal erythropoiesis vs administering an erythrocyte transfusion. Management of hemolytic anemia in neonates will first include managing hyperbilirubinemia. If hemolysis is significant enough and hyperbilirubinemia severe enough to require a double-volume exchange (generally with immune-mediated hemolysis), then correction of hematocrit can occur with the double-volume exchange transfusion. If a double-volume exchange transfusion is not required, acute anemia should be managed with PRBC transfusion. Epo is contraindicated when circulating antibodies directed against the infant's blood type are still significantly elevated, as stimulating neonatal erythropoiesis may result in increased hemolysis.

Treatment of anemia due to hypoproliferative disorders has expanded with the use of erythropoiesis-stimulating agents (ESAs). Most hypoproliferative disorders are associated to a varying degree with low Epo production; thus, treatment with ESAs to increase serum Epo concentrations is often effective.

The decision to administer an immediate transfusion of O-negative "trauma" PRBCs should be made carefully, and the emergency use of whole blood prior to type and cross match is generally discouraged. Type O-negative whole blood will contain antibodies directed against A and B blood groups and leukocytes. It should only be used in a hemorrhagic emergency or if the infant's blood type is known to be O negative.

Immediate transfusions will benefit those infants with significant metabolic acidosis and oxygen requirement, generally those with greater than 30%–40% acute blood loss. When considering a transfusion in a preterm infant with a low hematocrit (not associated with an acute drop in hematocrit), the clinician should first determine if the infant needs an immediate increase in oxygen to tissues. If the answer is yes, then treatment consists of a transfusion of PRBCs. If there is no evidence that an immediate increase in oxygen delivery is necessary, then treatment with red cell growth factors and appropriate substrates might be considered. An example of guidelines used to administer transfusions is shown in Table 31-6.

Treatment of anemic infants with modalities beyond volume expansion, PRBC transfusion, and vitamin and iron supplementation depends on the clinical care offered. The use of recombinant Epo to stimulate erythropoiesis has become more common in neonatal intensive care units; its role in the newborn nursery and in outpatient treatment continues to be refined.

Erythropoiesis-Stimulating Agents

The in vitro response of erythroid progenitors from preterm infants led investigators to begin evaluating Epo administration to preterm infants. Since the early 1990s, numerous studies evaluating the use of Epo to prevent and treat the anemia of prematurity have been performed.[39] The administration of Epo successfully stimulates erythropoiesis in preterm infants, and transfusion requirements are decreased. Success rates in preventing transfusions in preterm infants are dependent in part on transfusion criteria and the

Table 31-6 Transfusion Guidelines

1. A central hematocrit or hemoglobin should be obtained on admission. Further hematocrits should be specifically ordered.
2. Transfusions should be considered if acute blood loss of 10% or greater associated with symptoms of decreased oxygen delivery occurs or if significant hemorrhage of more than 20% total blood volume occurs.
3. For infants receiving erythropoietin, considerations of the previous guidelines should be made regarding the rate of decrease in hemoglobin or hematocrit, the infant's reticulocyte count, the postnatal day of age, the need for supplemental oxygen, and the overall stability of the infant.
4. Consider transfusions for the following conditions:

For infants **requiring moderate or significant mechanical ventilation** (MAP > 8 cm H_2O and FiO_2 > 0.40 on a conventional ventilator or MAP > 14 and FiO_2 > 0.40 on high-frequency ventilator), consider a transfusion if the **hematocrit is 30% or less (hemoglobin ≥ 10 g/dL)**.[a]

For infants **requiring minimal mechanical ventilation** (MAP ≤ 8 cm H_2O or FiO_2 ≤ 0.40 or MAP < 14 or FiO_2 < 0.40 on high-frequency ventilator), consider a transfusion if the **hematocrit is 25% or less (hemoglobin ≥ 8 g/dL)** or if the infant will undergo major surgery within 72 hours in which blood loss is likely.

For infants on supplemental oxygen who are **not requiring mechanical ventilation**, consider a transfusion if the **hematocrit is 21% or less (hemoglobin ≥ 7 g/dL)**, and one or more of the following is present:

- 24 hours or longer tachycardia (heart rate > 180) or tachypnea (respiratory rate > 60);
- doubling of the oxygen requirement from the previous 48 hours;
- lactate 2.5 mEq/L or greater or an acute metabolic acidosis (pH < 7.20);
- weight gain less than 10 g/kg/d over the previous 4 days while receiving 120 kcal/kg/day or more;
- if the infant will undergo major surgery within 72 hours in which blood loss is expected to be minimal.

For infants **without symptoms**, consider a transfusion if the **hematocrit is 18% or less (hemoglobin ≤ 6 g/dL)** associated with an absolute reticulocyte count less than 100,000 cells/μL (<2%)

Abbreviation: FiO2, forced inspiratory oxygen.
[a]Transfusion volume: 20 mL/kg PRBC unless the hematocrit is greater than 29% or if significant phlebotomy losses are anticipated in smaller infants with hematocrit greater than 29%.

volume of phlebotomy losses. Side effects of Epo in published randomized controlled trials (RCTs) have not differed from placebo, although meta-analyses have suggested an association between early Epo administration and retinopathy of prematurity (ROP). Because a single relevant study was mistakenly categorized in the early Epo analysis instead of the late analysis, this association was incorrectly determined to be statistically significant. This error will be corrected in the next analysis. The development of ROP in preterm infants is likely multifactorial. Moreover, there is evidence in some adult studies of protective effects of Epo in diabetic retinopathy.

Darbepoetin alfa (Darbe), a biologically modified version of Epo, was developed by Amgen in 1998. Darbe has a longer serum half-life than Epo in adults and preterm infants, so dosing can be spread over 1 to 2 weeks. Side effects are similar to Epo, and the production of anti-Epo antibodies has not been reported. Studies are under way to evaluate short- and long-term effects of extended courses of Darbe administered to preterm infants. Recent results showed decreased donor and transfusion exposure with weekly Darbe doses of 10 μg/kg.[57]

A minimal number of clinical studies evaluating Darbe administration to preterm infants have been published, and randomized trials are ongoing. In contrast, numerous RCTs evaluating Epo administration to preterm infants have consistently shown evidence of increased erythropoiesis and a decrease in transfusions.

A consistent finding in the largest RCTs has been an elevation in hematocrit in the Epo-treated infants compared to those treated with placebo/controls (Figure 31-2). For those neonatal practitioners electing to maintain the hematocrit at higher levels, the use of Epo generally results in an increase of 4%–6% hematocrit points and a decrease in the number of transfusions administered. The increased hematocrit may benefit the infant by increasing available oxygen to tissues and may also provide indirect benefit by avoiding transfusions, which have recently been associated with both necrotizing enterocolitis (NEC) and intraventricular hemorrhage (IVH).[58-60] Guidelines for Epo and vitamin/iron administration to preterm infants as part of clinical care are presented in Table 31-7.

Given the risks of transfusion, such as transmission of infectious agents like hepatitis, *Trypanosoma cruzi*, West Nile virus, and HIV[64]; the possible development of graft-vs-host disease; and possible associated risks, such as the development of NEC or the worsening of IVH, treatment of anemic neonates using recombinant Epo is an important alternative. Regardless of treatment strategy, a critical understanding of the physiologic influences affecting oxygen availability, delivery, and extraction at the tissue level will best serve clinicians in developing the best evidence-based approach to managing the red cell mass in term and preterm infants.

Table 31-7 Guidelines for Erythropoietin (Epo) and Supplement Administration

Epo Administration
Recommendations for infants receiving TPN:
200 units/kg/day, added to TPN
Begin dosing when infant is receiving protein
Intravenous administration (if not added to TPN) to run over at least 4 hours; use protein-containing solution to dilute
Recommendations for subcutaneous administration:
400 units/kg given 3 times a week
Begin dosing at 7 to 10 days of life or when intravenous access is gone
For preterm infants being discharged or for infants with late anemia due to Rh or ABO isoimmunization, a dose of 1000 U/kg SC once a week can be used to enhance erythropoiesis
Recommendations for length of treatment:
Continue dosing until 34–36 weeks corrected gestational age
Contraindications:
Epo is contraindicated in infants with thrombotic disease, hypertension, or seizures
Iron and Vitamin Administration
Iron:
Iron dextran, 3–5 mg/kg once a week added to TPN solution if available (1 mg/kg/d is acceptable; check ferritin after 2 weeks of dosing)
Ferrous sulfate 4–6 mg/kg/d depending on formula (4 mg/kg/d) or EBM (6 mg/kg/d)
Vitamin E: 25 IU/day PO
Folate: 50 μg/d PO
B_{12} (if available): 21 μg/week SC

Abbreviations: EBM, expressed breast milk; TPN, total parenteral nutrition.

ACKNOWLEDGMENTS

We wish to thank Erin Adair for figure production and Mary Merchant and Cyndie Suniga for their assistance editing the manuscript.

REFERENCES

1. Jopling J, et al. Reference ranges for hematocrit and blood hemoglobin concentration during the neonatal period: data from a multihospital health care system. *Pediatrics.* 2009;123(2):e333–e337.
2. Ruth V, et al. Postnatal changes in serum immunoreactive erythropoietin in relation to hypoxia before and after birth. *J Pediatr.* 1990;116(6):950–954.
3. Kling PJ, et al. Serum erythropoietin levels during infancy: associations with erythropoiesis. *J Pediatr.* 1996;128(6):791–796.
4. Chavez GF, Mulinare J, Edmonds LD. Epidemiology of Rh hemolytic disease of the newborn in the United States. *JAMA.* 1991;265(24):3270–3274.
5. Elalfy MS, Elbarbary NS, Abaza HW. Early intravenous immunoglobin (two-dose regimen) in the management of severe Rh hemolytic disease of newborn—a prospective randomized controlled trial. *Eur J Pediatr.* 2011;170(4):461–467.
6. Thorp JM. Utilization of anti-RhD in the emergency department after blunt trauma. *Obstet Gynecol Surv.* 2008;63(2):112–115.
7. Crowther C, Middleton P. Anti-D administration after childbirth for preventing Rhesus alloimmunisation. *Cochrane Database Syst Rev.* 2000(2):CD000021.
8. Wang M, et al. Hemolytic disease of the newborn caused by a high titer anti-group B IgG from a group A mother. *Pediatr Blood Cancer.* 2005;45(6):861–862.
9. Oski FA. The erythrocyte and its disorders. In: Orkin SH, Nathan DG, Ginsberg D, Look AT, Fisher DE, Lux SE, *Hematology of Infancy and Childhood.* Philadelphia, PA: Saunders; 2008:21–66.
10. Murray NA, Roberts IA. Haemolytic disease of the newborn. *Arch Dis Child Fetal Neonatal Ed.* 2007;92(2):F83–F88.
11. van der Schoot CE, et al. Prenatal typing of Rh and Kell blood group system antigens: the edge of a watershed. *Transfus Med Rev.* 2003;17(1):31–44.
12. Vaughan JI, et al. Inhibition of erythroid progenitor cells by anti-Kell antibodies in fetal alloimmune anemia. *N Engl J Med.* 1998;338(12):798–803.
13. Beutler E. G6PD deficiency. *Blood.* 1994;84(11):3613–3636.
14. Kaplan M, Hammerman C. Glucose-6-phosphate dehydrogenase deficiency: a hidden risk for kernicterus. *Semin Perinatol.* 2004;28(5):356–364.
15. Watchko JF. Identification of neonates at risk for hazardous hyperbilirubinemia: emerging clinical insights. *Pediatr Clin North Am.* 2009;56(3):671–687, table of contents.
16. Kaplan M, Hammerman C. Severe neonatal hyperbilirubinemia. A potential complication of glucose-6-phosphate dehydrogenase deficiency. *Clin Perinatol.* 1998;25(3):575–590, viii.
17. Kaplan M, et al. Gilbert syndrome and glucose-6-phosphate dehydrogenase deficiency: a dose-dependent genetic interaction crucial to neonatal hyperbilirubinemia. *Proc Natl Acad Sci U S A.* 1997;94(22):12128–12132.
18. Johnson L, et al. Clinical report from the pilot USA Kernicterus Registry (1992 to 2004). *J Perinatol.* 2009;29(Suppl 1):S25–S45.
19. Bhutani VK, Stark AR, Lazzeroni LC, et al. Predischarge screening for severe neonatal hyperbilirubinemia identifies infants who need phototherapy. *J Pediatr.* 2013;162(3):477–482.
20. Zanella A, et al. Red cell pyruvate kinase deficiency: molecular and clinical aspects. *Br J Haematol.* 2005;130(1):11–25.
21. Christensen RD, Eggert LD, Baer VL, Smith KN. Pyruvate kinase deficiency as a cause of extreme hyperbilirubinemia in neonates from a polygamist community. *J Perinatol.* 2010;30(3):233–236.
22. Zanella, A, et al. Pyruvate kinase deficiency: the genotype-phenotype association. *Blood Rev.* 2007;21(4):217–231.
23. Glader B Hereditary hemolytic anemias due to red blood cell enzyme disorders. In: Greer JP, et al, eds. *Wintrobe's Clinical Hematology.* Philadelphia, PA: Lippincott, Williams & Wilkins; 2009:933–955.
24. Steiner LA, Gallagher PG. Erythrocyte disorders in the perinatal period. *Semin Perinatol.* 2007;31(4):254–261.
25. Gallagher PG. Update on the clinical spectrum and genetics of red blood cell membrane disorders. *Curr Hematol Rep.* 2004;3(2):85–91.
26. Stamey CC, Diamond LK. Congenital hemolytic anemia in the newborn; relationship to kernicterus. *AMA J Dis Child.* 1957;94(6):616–622.
27. Gallagher PG. Hereditary elliptocytosis: spectrin and protein 4.1R. *Semin Hematol.* 2004;41(2):142–164.
28. Delaunay J, Stewart G, Iolascon A. Hereditary dehydrated and overhydrated stomatocytosis: recent advances. *Curr Opin Hematol.* 1999;6(2):110–114.
29. Stewart GW, et al. Thrombo-embolic disease after splenectomy for hereditary stomatocytosis. *Br J Haematol.* 1996;93(2):303–310.
30. Vichinsky EP. Alpha thalassemia major—new mutations, intrauterine management, and outcomes. *Hematology Am Soc Hematol Educ Program.* 2009:35–41.
31. Hoppe CC. Newborn screening for non-sickling hemoglobinopathies. *Hematology Am Soc Hematol Educ Program.* 2009:19–25.
32. Clinton C, Gazda HT. Diamond-Blackfan anemia. In: Pagon RA, et al, eds. *GeneReviews.* Seattle, WA; 1993.
33. Aase JM, Smith DW. Congenital anemia and triphalangeal thumbs: a new syndrome. *J Pediatr.* 1969;74(3):471–474.
34. Fargo JH, et al. Erythrocyte adenosine deaminase: diagnostic value for Diamond-Blackfan anaemia. *Br J Haematol.* 2013;160(4):547–554.
35. Vlachos A, et al. Diagnosing and treating Diamond Blackfan anaemia: results of an international clinical consensus conference. *Br J Haematol.* 2008;142(6):859–876.
36. Vlachos A, et al. Incidence of neoplasia in Diamond Blackfan anemia: a report from the Diamond Blackfan Anemia Registry. *Blood.* 2012;119(16):3815–3819.
37. Iolascon A, Russo R, Delaunay J. Congenital dyserythropoietic anemias. *Curr Opin Hematol.* 2011;18(3):146–151.
38. Shimamura A, Alter BP. Pathophysiology and management of inherited bone marrow failure syndromes. *Blood Rev.* 2010;24(3):101–122.
39. Bishara N, Ohls RK. Current controversies in the management of the anemia of prematurity. *Semin Perinatol.* 2009;33(1):29–34.
40. Chauvet A, et al. Ultrasound diagnosis, management and prognosis in a consecutive series of 27 cases of fetal hydrops following maternal parvovirus B19 infection. *Fetal Diagn Ther.* 2011;30(1):41–47.
41. Ohls RK, Wirkus PE, Christensen RD. Recombinant erythropoietin as treatment for the late hyporegenerative anemia of Rh hemolytic disease. *Pediatrics.* 1992;90(5):678–680.
42. Bierer R, et al. Erythropoietin increases reticulocyte counts and maintains hematocrit in neonates requiring surgery. *J Pediatr Surg.* 2009;44(8):1540–1545.
43. Hosono S, et al. Successful recombinant erythropoietin therapy for a developing anemic newborn with hereditary spherocytosis. *Pediatr Int.* 2006;48(2):178–180.

44. Lopriore E, Oepkes D, Walther FJ. Neonatal morbidity in twin-twin transfusion syndrome. *Early Hum Dev.* 2011;87(9):595–599.

45. Salomon LJ, et al. Long-term developmental follow-up of infants who participated in a randomized clinical trial of amniocentesis vs laser photocoagulation for the treatment of twin-to-twin transfusion syndrome. *Am J Obstet Gynecol.* 2010;203(5):444.e1–7.

46. Wylie BJ, D'Alton ME. Fetomaternal hemorrhage. *Obstet Gynecol.* 2010;115(5):1039–1051.

47. Chambers E, et al. Comparison of haemoglobin F detection by the acid elution test, flow cytometry and high-performance liquid chromatography in maternal blood samples analysed for fetomaternal haemorrhage. *Transfus Med.* 2012; 22(3):199–204.

48. Wilcock FM, Kadir RA. Fetomaternal haemorrhage—a cause for unexplained neonatal death, presenting with reduced fetal movements and non-reactive fetal heart trace. *J Obstet Gynaecol.* 2004;24(4):456–457.

49. Tikkanen M. Placental abruption: epidemiology, risk factors and consequences. *Acta Obstet Gynecol Scand.* 2011;90(2):140–149.

50. Fishman SG, Chasen ST, Maheshwari B. Risk factors for preterm delivery with placenta previa. *J Perinat Med.* 2011;40(1):39–42.

51. Rosenberg T, et al. Critical analysis of risk factors and outcome of placenta previa. *Arch Gynecol Obstet.* 2011;284(1):47–51.

52. Rao KP, et al. Abnormal placentation: evidence-based diagnosis and management of placenta previa, placenta accreta, and vasa previa. *Obstet Gynecol Surv.* 2012;67(8):503–519.

53. Garofalo M, Abenhaim HA. Early versus delayed cord clamping in term and preterm births: a review. *J Obstet Gynaecol Can.* 2012;34(6):525–531.

54. Chang HY, et al. Neonatal subgaleal hemorrhage: clinical presentation, treatment, and predictors of poor prognosis. *Pediatr Int.* 2007;49(6):903–907.

55. McQuilten ZK, et al. A review of pathophysiology and current treatment for neonatal alloimmune thrombocytopenia (NAIT) and introducing the Australian NAIT registry. *Aust N Z J Obstet Gynaecol.* 2011;51(3):191–198.

56. Symington A, Paes B. Fetal and neonatal alloimmune thrombocytopenia: harvesting the evidence to develop a clinical approach to management. *Am J Perinatol.* 2011;28(2):137–144.

57. Ohls RK, Christensen RD, Kamath-Rayne BD, et al. A randomized, masked, placebo-controlled study of darbepoetin alfa in preterm infants. *Pediatrics.* 2013;132:1–9.

58. Christensen RD. Association between red blood cell transfusions and necrotizing enterocolitis. *J Pediatr.* 2011;158(3):349–350.

59. Baer VL, et al. Red blood cell transfusion of preterm neonates with a grade 1 intraventricular hemorrhage is associated with extension to a grade 3 or 4 hemorrhage. *Transfusion.* 2011;51(9):1933–1939.

60. Christensen RD, et al. Postponing or eliminating red blood cell transfusions of very low birth weight neonates by obtaining all baseline laboratory blood tests from otherwise discarded fetal blood in the placenta. *Transfusion.* 2011;51(2):253–258.

61. Donato H, Vain N, Rendo P, et al. Effect of early versus late administration of human recombinant erythropoietin on transfusion requirements in premature infants: results of a randomized, placebo-controlled, multicenter trial. *Pediatrics.* 2000;105:1066–1072.

62. Ohls RK, Ehrenkranz RA, Wright LL, et al. Effects of early erythropoietin therapy on the transfusion requirements of preterm infants below 1250 grams birth weight: a multicenter, randomized, controlled trial. *Pediatrics.* 2001;108:934–942.

63. Haiden N, Schwindt J, Cardona F, et al. Effects of a combined therapy of erythropoietin, iron, folate, and vitamin B12 on the transfusion requirements of extremely low birth weight infants. *Pediatrics.* 2006;118:2004–2013.

64. Kleinman S, et al. The National Heart, Lung, and Blood Institute retrovirus epidemiology donor studies (Retrovirus Epidemiology Donor Study and Retrovirus Epidemiology Donor Study-II): twenty years of research to advance blood product safety and availability. *Transfus Med Rev.* 2012;26(4):281–304, 304.e1–2.

CHAPTER 31

Neonatal Thrombocytopenia

Clara Y. Lo, Bertil Glader and Wendy Wong

INTRODUCTION

Thrombocytopenia is a well-recognized phenomenon in the neonatal intensive care unit (NICU); it can lead to morbidity and mortality from severe and life-threatening bleeding. The epidemiology, pathophysiology, causes, management, and outcome of neonatal thrombocytopenia are reviewed in this chapter.

Thrombocytopenia is traditionally defined as a platelet count below 150,000/μL. This definition is based on several population studies, which have demonstrated that in mothers with normal platelet counts, over 98% of healthy term neonates have platelet counts greater than 150,000/μL at birth.[1–3] Thrombocytopenia is rare in healthy newborns; however, it affects up to one-third of patients in the NICU.[4,5] The increased incidence of thrombocytopenia in NICU patients is reflective of the inverse relationship of thrombocytopenia risk to birth weight and gestational age.[4,6] Christensen et al reported that up to 70% of infants with birth weight less than 1000 g are thrombocytopenic.[6] Preterm infants, particularly those at less than 24 weeks' gestation, have platelet counts as low as 100,000/μL in the first few days of life.[4,7]

Severe thrombocytopenia is defined as a platelet count of less than 50,000/μL. Severe thrombocytopenia occurs in less than 1% of healthy newborns[2,3], but affects 5%–10% of hospitalized neonates.[4,8,9]

CAUSES OF NEONATAL THROMBOCYTOPENIA

The causes of neonatal thrombocytopenia can be classified into 2 major pathophysiologic categories: increased destruction (including consumption) and decreased production. In some neonates, especially sick preterm infants, both processes can occur concomitantly. The time of thrombocytopenia onset has often been used to help with diagnosis. Early-onset thrombocytopenia occurs within 72 hours of birth, while late-onset thrombocytopenia occurs after 72 hours of life (Table 32-1). Diagnostic algorithms and general management of neonatal thrombocytopenia are highlighted in Chapter 92.

The diagnoses of thrombocytopenia based on underlying pathophysiologic classifications are summarized in Table 32-2. The most common causes include infection, necrotizing enterocolitis (NEC), neonatal alloimmune thrombocytopenia, maternal platelet autoantibodies, and chronic fetal hypoxia. The major causes of neonatal thrombocytopenia are reviewed next.

Congenital Infection

Congenital infections are a major cause of thrombocytopenia in the neonatal population. Cytomegalovirus and herpes simplex virus are the most likely of the congenital TORCH (toxoplasmosis, rubella, cytomegalovirus,

Table 32-1 Classification of Early-Onset (72 Hours Postbirth) Thrombocytopenias[a,b]

Early onset (<72 hours)	**Chronic fetal hypoxia** (eg, PIH, IUGR, gestational diabetes) **Perinatal asphyxia** **Perinatal infection** (eg, *E. coli*, GBS) **Congenital infection** (eg, CMV, rubella) **Sepsis/DIC** **Neonatal alloimmune thrombocytopenia** **Maternal platelet autoantibodies** Thrombosis Bone marrow replacement (eg, congenital leukemia) Kasabach-Merritt syndrome Metabolic disease (eg, proprionic academia) Inherited thrombocytopenias (eg, TAR, CAMT)
Late onset (>72 hours)	**Late-onset sepsis/DIC** **Necrotizing enterocolitis** **Congenital infection** (eg, CMV, rubella) **Maternal autoantibodies** Kasabach-Merritt syndrome Metabolic disease (eg, proprionic acidemia) Inherited thrombocytopenias (eg, TAR, CAMT)

Abbreviations: CAMT, congenital amegakaryocytic thrombocytopenia; CMV, cytomegalovirus; DIC, disseminated intravascular coagulation; *E. coli*, *Escherichia coli*; GBS, group B *Streptococcus*; IUGR, intrauterine growth restriction; PIH, pregnancy-induced hypertension; TAR, thrombocytopenia-absent radius syndrome.
[a]Adapted from Roberts, Stanworth, and Murray.[4]
[b]The more common conditions are in **bold**.

Table 32-2 Classification of Neonatal Thrombocytopenias by Underlying Pathophysiology: Increased Platelet Destruction and Decreased Platelet Production[a]

Increased destruction/ consumption	**Perinatal infection** (eg, *E. coli*, GBS) **Necrotizing enterocolitis** **Congenital infection** (eg, CMV, rubella) **Sepsis/DIC** **Neonatal alloimmune thrombocytopenia** **Maternal platelet autoantibodies** Thrombosis Kasabach-Merritt syndrome
Decreased production	**Chronic fetal hypoxia** (eg, PIH, IUGR, gestational diabetes) **Perinatal asphyxia** Bone marrow replacement (eg, congenital leukemia) Metabolic disease (eg, proprionic acidemia) Inherited thrombocytopenias (eg, TAR, CAMT)

Abbreviations: CAMT, congenital amegakaryocytic thrombocytopenia; CMV, cytomegalovirus; DIC, disseminated intravascular coagulation; *E. coli*, *Escherichia coli*; GBS, group B *Streptococcus*; IUGR, intrauterine growth restriction; PIH, pregnancy-induced hypertension; TAR, thrombocytopenia-absent radius syndrome.
[a]The more common conditions are in **bold**.

herpes simplex virus) infections to cause thrombocytopenia. Cytomegalovirus is the most common of the congenital infections, affecting 0.5%–1.5% of live births. Most of these neonates are asymptomatic, but up to 35% develop thrombocytopenia.[10] Other congenital infections that have been implicated include Coxsackievirus, syphilis, varicella zoster virus, human immunodeficiency virus (HIV), and parvovirus B19.

Mechanisms of thrombocytopenia with congenital infection include increased platelet aggregation, hypersplenism secondary to splenomegaly and platelet pooling, and platelet membrane damage secondary to viral neuraminidase cleavage of sialic acid. Infants with congenital infections are typically well appearing but can present with clinical manifestations such as a petechial rash, microcephaly, intracerebral calcifications, and hepatosplenomegaly. Thrombocytopenia is generally mild to moderate (>50,000/μL), and affected infants usually do not have bleeding apart from cutaneous manifestations. Positive results for a specific congenital infection typically confirm the diagnosis. Most patients do not require therapy for thrombocytopenia, and management generally is close observation. Platelet transfusions may be given for rare cases of severe thrombocytopenia or bleeding.

Bacterial and Fungal Infections

Perinatal bacterial infections particularly implicated in neonatal thrombocytopenia include group B *Streptococcus* (GBS) and *Escherichia coli* (*E. coli*). Other late-onset (>72 hours postdelivery) bacterial and fungal infections may also occur, particularly in vulnerable preterm infants. Mechanisms of thrombocytopenia include endothelial damage and increased platelet aggregation caused by adherence of bacterial products to platelet membranes. Neonates can present with vital sign instability, leukocytosis, and mild-to-severe thrombocytopenia. Sepsis and disseminated intravascular coagulation (DIC) may occur and are associated with rapid onset of severe thrombocytopenia, consumptive coagulopathy, and clinical bleeding or thrombosis. Management includes platelet transfusions for severe thrombocytopenia and bleeding, and most important, aggressive treatment of the underlying infection.

Necrotizing Enterocolitis

Necrotizing enterocolitis occurs in up to 10% of neonates, particularly in those with a birth weight less than 1500 g.[11] Platelets are destroyed at sites of gut ischemia, injury, and necrosis, resulting in thrombocytopenia. The degree of thrombocytopenia correlates with gut necrosis severity, particularly within the first 3 days of NEC onset.[12] The presence of severe thrombocytopenia may also be predictive of overall morbidity and mortality.[12] DIC can also complicate NEC, thereby increasing morbidity and mortality risk from significant bleeding or thrombosis. Platelet transfusions are given for severe thrombocytopenia and clinical bleeding. Thrombocytopenia typically improves with improvement and resolution of the NEC.

Immune-Mediated Thrombocytopenia

There are 2 major immune-mediated causes of neonatal thrombocytopenia: neonatal alloimmune thrombocytopenia (NAIT) and maternal platelet autoantibodies. Immune-mediated neonatal thrombocytopenia most commonly occurs in otherwise-well, term neonates without other reasons for thrombocytopenia. Patients typically have decreased platelet counts at birth (early-onset thrombocytopenia).

Neonatal Alloimmune Thrombocytopenia

Epidemiology

Neonatal alloimmune thrombocytopenia is estimated to occur in 1:1000 live births.[13] NAIT is the platelet equivalent of hemolytic disease of the newborn, or Rhesus (Rh) antigen incompatibility. It occurs in the first pregnancy in nearly half of cases, unlike Rh incompatibility, in which neonates are affected only after the index pregnancy.[13] Differences between Rh incompatibility and NAIT are outlined in Table 32-3. The majority of patients have severe thrombocytopenia, and often the thrombocytopenia is severe (platelets <20,000/μL).[14] Neonates are at high risk of major bleeding, including intracranial hemorrhage (ICH). Large retrospective studies have reported ICH in 10%–20% of untreated NAIT cases.[15,16] The bleeding may occur in utero, as thrombocytopenia develops after 20 weeks' gestation in untreated cases.[15,16]

Pathophysiology

Neonatal alloimmune thrombocytopenia results from transplacental passage of maternal alloantibodies against fetal platelets expressing paternal human platelet antigens (HPAs) that the mother lacks. Sixteen HPA antigens have been identified, and 3 of them cause 95% of NAIT in Caucasians[16,17]: HPA-1a, HPA-5b, and HPA-15b. HPA-4 has been implicated in NAIT

Table 32-3 Differences Between Rhesus Disease and Neonatal Alloimmune Thrombocytopenia[a]

	Rh Disease	NAIT
Incidence	1/100 (25% severe)	1/1000
First child affected	No	Yes
Routine screening in place	Yes	No
Testing readily available	Yes (any blood bank)	No (send out labs)
Prophylaxis available	Yes (anti-D immunoglobulin)	No
Severe clinical phenotype	Hydrops fetalis, kernicterus	ICH
Antenatal management of next pregnancy	In utero red cell transfusion	Maternal IVIG weekly

Abbreviations: ICH, intracranial hemorrhage; IVIG, intravenous immunoglobulin; NAIT, neonatal alloimmune thrombocytopenia; Rh, Rhesus disease.
[a]Adapted from Bussel.[14]

in Asians.[16,17] HPA-1a in particular causes nearly 75% of all NAIT cases.[16,17] HPA-1a incompatibility occurs in 1:350 pregnancies, but NAIT occurs in only 1:1500 cases.[16] The reason for this disparity is due to differences in human leukocyte antigen (HLA) alleles. Specifically, HLA DRB3*0101-positive women are up to 140 times more likely to form HPA-1a antibodies than are HLA DRB3*0101-negative women, thereby indicating a strong association of HLA with NAIT.[18,19]

Differential Diagnosis

The major and most important differential diagnoses are bacterial and congenital infections. Evaluation for bacteremia with blood counts and cultures is particularly important in the vulnerable neonatal population, and empiric broad-spectrum antibiotic therapy is warranted until bacteremia is excluded. Patients with congenital infections typically have other physical stigmata (see the section on congenital infections), which may aid in diagnosis.

Thrombocytopenia secondary to maternal autoantibodies (see the section on this topic) is an alternative diagnosis that can be excluded by the absence of maternal thrombocytopenia or maternal autoimmune disease (ie, systemic lupus erythmatosus). Thrombocytopenia secondary to hypoxia or acidosis may occur in neonates with complicated pregnancies or deliveries and thus can be excluded in cases of uncomplicated term pregnancies and deliveries. Inherited thrombocytopenia syndromes (see the section on this topic) may also present similarly but are much rarer. The diagnosis of inherited syndromes typically includes evaluation for specific physical examination or peripheral smear findings and genetic testing.

Diagnostic Tests

Thrombocytopenia is evident at birth. Generally, a diagnosis of NAIT requires both evidence of maternal-paternal platelet antigen incompatibility and maternal antiplatelet antibodies. Occasionally, maternal antibodies are found without evidence of platelet antigen incompatibility. In these cases, the reference laboratory should distinguish between "unimportant" antigens (ie, HLA) vs incompatibilities of a previously undefined platelet antigen.[14] Evidence of a platelet antigen incompatibility without maternal antibodies is insufficient for an NAIT diagnosis.

Management

Treatment involves platelet transfusions and intravenous immunoglobulin (IVIG; 1 g/kg administered over 1–2 days). Historically, recommendations were for transfusion of maternal platelet antigen-matched platelets or HPA-1a-negative platelets if maternal platelet antigen type was unavailable. However, recent studies showed no difference in outcome between antigen-specific and random donor platelets.[20,21] Therefore, given the often-lengthy delay in platelet typing or obtaining antigen-specific platelets, recommended initial therapy for NAIT is the administration of IVIG and random donor platelets. The duration of effect of a platelet transfusion needs to be closely monitored to evaluate the need for further transfusion. A head ultrasound should always be performed to evaluate for ICH.

Antenatal management of NAIT has been controversial. Previous recommendations were for fetal platelet monitoring and intrauterine transfusions. However, the invasiveness and complications associated with these procedures have since decreased their appeal. In cases of NAIT in index pregnancies, guidelines for subsequent pregnancies include maternal infusion of IVIG (1 g/kg) weekly, starting at 16 weeks if the previous sibling had ICH and at 32 weeks if not.[22] In some protocols, steroids also have been used antenatally in particularly difficult NAIT cases. Because of the intensity of antenatal management, it is important to be certain of NAIT diagnosis.

Outcome and Follow-up

The majority of neonates with thrombocytopenia do well, with the platelets resolving within 7 days after delivery, without relapses or long-term sequelae.[15,16] However, a small subset of infants has thrombocytopenia that lasts several weeks and may require additional platelet transfusions. Those neonates who develop ICH have poorer neurodevelopmental outcomes, including cerebral palsy and sensory impairment.[16]

Maternal Platelet Autoantibodies

Epidemiology

Neonatal thrombocytopenia can also occur in infants born to mothers with platelet autoantibodies. Immune thrombocytopenia (ITP) is the most common underlying disease in mothers, and 10%–15% of maternal ITP cases result in neonatal thrombocytopenia.[23] Platelet autoantibodies can also occur in mothers affected with systemic lupus erythematosis (SLE) and hyperthyroidism, among other less-common autoimmune disorders.

Fortunately, neonatal thrombocytopenia associated with maternal autoantibodies is much less of a clinical problem than NAIT. The thrombocytopenia is generally transient, though infants should be closely monitored in the first several days of life, as platelet counts can rapidly drop during this time. The majority of neonates have mild-to-moderate thrombocytopenia (50,000 to 100,000/μL), and most are clinically asymptomatic except for minimal bruising or petechiae.[24] However, up to 10% of affected neonates develop more severe thrombocytopenia. ICH is rare and has been reported in less than 1% of infants with severe thrombocytopenia. Predictive factors for clinical bleeding and severe neonatal thrombocytopenia include history of older sibling(s) with severe neonatal thrombocytopenia, maternal platelet count at delivery less than 100,000/μL, and maternal ITP refractory to splenectomy.[23]

Pathophysiology

Neonatal thrombocytopenia occurs secondary to maternal antiplatelet autoantibodies that cross the placenta to also affect the fetus and newborn. Autoantibodies are typically directed against platelet glycoprotein (Gp) IIbIIIa, although there are also cases of anti-Gp1b autoantibodies.

Differential Diagnosis

Maternal ITP should not be confused with gestational thrombocytopenia, a benign transient entity that occurs in women only during pregnancy and resolves spontaneously after delivery. Affected women are typically healthy, have no history of autoimmune disease, and have an uncomplicated pregnancy. Maternal platelet counts are mildly low in the majority of cases. Furthermore, neonatal thrombocytopenia rarely occurs. Both mothers and fetuses typically are asymptomatic and do not require any medical treatment.

Other major differential diagnoses include bacterial and congenital infections. Bacterial infections should be strongly considered and empirically treated until cultures are proven negative, particularly in high-risk neonates. NAIT may be excluded by the presence of maternal thrombocytopenia or maternal autoimmune disease.

Inherited thrombocytopenia syndromes are alternative diagnoses that are typically associated with distinct physical examination or peripheral smear findings and are often diagnosed with specific genetic testing.

Diagnostic Tests

There is no specific test for thrombocytopenia secondary to maternal autoantibodies. Tests for anti-GpI-IbIIIa or anti-Gp1b antibodies have low sensitivity. Instead, diagnosis is typically based on maternal and neonatal history and other laboratory findings. The greatest diagnostic clue is a maternal history of ITP or other autoimmune disorder. Affected mothers and neonates typically have isolated thrombocytopenia and variably large platelets on peripheral smear, typical of what is seen with ITP. Thrombocytopenia in the neonate is evident at birth. Mothers may also have a previous history of ITP treatment, including steroids, IVIG, and splenectomy. Previously splenectomized mothers actually may have a normal platelet count but still have circulating autoantibodies that can cross the placenta to destroy fetal platelets. Therefore, if maternal platelet counts are normal but maternal autoantibodies are suspected, it is important to query mothers regarding whether they previously had their spleen removed or if they have any other history of autoimmune disease.

Management

Treatment of thrombocytopenia is typically supportive. In the presence of severe thrombocytopenia or life-threatening bleeding, first-line therapy includes IVIG (1 g/kg administered over 1–2 days). Platelet transfusions also may be indicated, although since maternal antibodies are directed against common antigens, the transfusion may not be effective.

Previously, the antenatal management of known maternal ITP cases included removing the mother's spleen and fetal blood sampling to determine the safety of vaginal delivery. However, current recommendations are less invasive, with IVIG or steroids for the mother to delay splenectomy until at least after delivery. Fetal blood sampling is no longer done. Furthermore, cesarean sections now are recommended only for obstetric indications.

Outcome and Follow-up

Platelet counts typically nadir between day 2 and day 5 of life and recover 1 week after birth. There are a relatively small number of patients with persistent thrombocytopenia beyond 7 days, in which case anti-platelet antibodies persist.[25] With documented platelet normalization to greater than 150,000/μL, there is no risk of recurrent thrombocytopenia since the maternal autoantibodies will have been cleared from the neonate.

Chronic Fetal Hypoxia and Acidosis

Chronic fetal hypoxia typically occurs in neonates born to mothers with pregnancy-associated hypertension, intrauterine growth restriction (IUGR), and gestational diabetes mellitus. All result in placental insufficiency and therefore decreased fetal oxygenation. The underlying mechanism for the thrombocytopenia is thought to be related to decreased megakaryopoiesis.[5] Low platelet counts in these cases are evident at birth, are typically mild to moderate (eg, platelet counts of 50,000–100,000/μL), and commonly self-resolve within 1 to 2 weeks after birth. Most patients do not require treatment of their thrombocytopenia, but platelet transfusions can be given if indicated for bleeding or if there is risk of increased bleeding (eg, invasive procedures).

Kasabach-Merritt Syndrome

Kasabach-Merritt syndrome, associated with capillary hemangiomas, can present with neonatal thrombocytopenia, along with microangiopathic anemia and DIC. Affected neonates have one or more enlarging vascular lesions. Diagnosis is typically straightforward in cases of cutaneous lesions; however, approximately 20% of patients have visceral involvement (eg, of the liver) without cutaneous lesions.[26-28] Thrombocytopenia occurs secondary to sequestration of platelets within the vascular endothelium and is compounded in cases complicated by DIC. Supportive therapy entails replacement of platelets and clotting factors, along with definitive treatment of the vascular lesions. Definitive therapies used for Kasabach-Merritt syndrome include steroids, vincristine, interferon, and sirolimus.[26]

Inherited Thrombocytopenia Syndromes

Neonatal thrombocytopenia that persists more than 2 weeks after birth is unusual and warrants further investigation. As most other forms of thrombocytopenia resolve by this time, the likely cause of prolonged, otherwise-unexplained, thrombocytopenia is an inherited syndrome. Inherited thrombocytopenias can be classified into 3 major groups, based on platelet size: increased platelet size, normal platelet size, and decreased platelet size (Table 32-4).

Wiskott-Aldrich Syndrome and X-Linked Thrombocytopenia

Epidemiology

Wiskott-Aldrich syndrome (WAS) is a rare, X-linked recessive disorder, affecting 1–10:1 million live male births worldwide. Males with classic WAS present with microthrombocytopenia, eczema, and deficiencies in the

Table 32-4 Inherited Thrombocytopenia Syndromes

Thrombocytopenia with decreased platelet size	Wiskott-Aldrich syndrome X-linked thrombocytopenia
Thrombocytopenia with normal platelet size	Congenital amegakaryocytic thrombocytopenia Thrombocytopenia-absent radius syndrome Quebec platelet syndrome Trisomy 13, 18, 21 Turner syndrome

Thrombocytopenia with increased platelet size	Mediterranean macrothrombocytopenia
	DiGeorge/velocardiofacial syndrome
	Pseudo–von Willebrand disease
	Myosin heavy chain 9–related disorders
	  May-Hegglin anomaly
	  Fechtner syndrome
	  Sebastian syndrome
	  Epstein syndrome
	Jacobsen syndrome/Paris-Trousseau syndrome
	Gray platelet syndrome
	Bernard-Soulier syndrome

innate and adaptive immune system. These patients have problems with severe bleeding, recurrent and serious infections, and increased malignancy and autoimmune risks in later childhood. A less-severe variant of WAS is X-linked thrombocytopenia (XLT), in which affected males generally have isolated microthrombocytopenia.

Pathophysiology

Mutations for both WAS and XLT have been isolated to the WAS gene that encodes the protein (WASp). The WASp protein is important in cytoskeleton remodeling and cell signaling: Alterations in the protein impair cell, including T- and B-cell, function.[29,30] Several WAS gene mutational hot spots and genotype-phenotype correlations have been identified.[31] Furthermore, missense mutations, associated with abnormal but present WASp expression, seem to correlate with XLT and phenotypically milder WAS phenotype.[32] Alternatively, nonsense, deletion, and insertion mutations, associated with absent WASp expression, appear to correlate with severe microthrombocytopenia, gastrointestinal hemorrhage, ICH, severe eczema, and high infection and malignancy risk.[32]

Differential Diagnosis

Early-onset moderate-to-severe microthrombocytopenia is typically the earliest finding in WAS, as eczema and infections tend to develop in later infancy. Patients with XLT typically present with mild-to-moderate microthrombocytopenia at birth. Differentiation between WAS and XLT can be determined by phenotypic severity and genetic testing for the WAS gene mutation. There are several other alternate diagnoses for early-onset thrombocytopenia, but these are excluded by the presence of small platelets on a peripheral smear, a unique characteristic of WAS and XLT.

Diagnostic Tests

A peripheral smear reviewed by an expert hematologist or hematopathologist reveals uniformly small platelets (Figure 32–1). Further testing for WAS is done by flow cytometry using an anti-WASp antibody. Ultimately, the WAS mutation is identified through gene sequencing.

Management

Early management for WAS is primarily supportive. Platelet transfusions are indicated for severe thrombocytopenia with bleeding symptoms within the first few weeks of life, during which patients are at particularly high risk of ICH. Beyond this time, transfusions should be administered judiciously, as platelet refractoriness positively correlates with the number of platelet transfusions. Beyond the immediate newborn period, platelet replacement generally is reserved for cases of extremely severe thrombocytopenia (less than 20,000/μL), bleeding, and in preparation for surgical procedures.

Aminocaproic acid, an antifibrinolytic, is helpful in treatment or prevention of mucosal bleeding (eg, epistaxis, gingival bleeding). However, it is contraindicated in patients with hematuria as it may precipitate clots in the glomerular capillaries, renal pelvis, or ureters. IVIG has been given to patients with WAS who also have autoimmune hemolytic anemia; however, unlike NAIT and autoimmune thrombocytopenia,

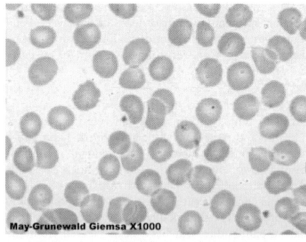

May-Grunewald Giemsa X1000

FIGURE 32-1 Wiskott-Aldrich: small platelet smear.

IVIG does not alleviate the thrombocytopenia in WAS as it is not an immune-mediated process. Splenectomy has been done in particularly severe cases in efforts to halt bleeding tendencies by increasing the circulating platelets. However, because patients with WAS are immunodeficient and already at high risk of sepsis, splenectomy is not routinely recommended. Prophylactic antimicrobial therapy is given to prevent serious bacterial, viral, fungal, and opportunistic infections. The ultimate curative treatment is hematopoietic stem cell transplantation (HSCT). Current data indicate that long-term outcomes are best for patients transplanted at younger than 2 years of age.[33]

Outcome and Follow-up
Untreated, patients with WAS uniformly have a decreased life span. The major cause of death is bleeding. Other reasons for premature death include autoimmune disease, sepsis, and malignancy. Lymphoma (primarily Epstein-Barr virus positive) and leukemia constitute the majority of malignancies associated with WAS, but this complication typically occurs later in childhood or adolescence. Fortunately, long-term outcome is dramatically improved after successful hematopoeitic stem cell transplant with reports of up to 90% overall survival for 5 years.[33] Alternatively, patients with XLT generally have a benign course, with minimal-to-absent bleeding and a normal life span.

If the WAS genetic mutation is known in a given family, antenatal diagnosis in future offspring of heterozygous carriers is possible. Prenatal diagnosis of a male fetus can be done by DNA analysis with chorionic villi sampling or cultured amniocytes.

Congenital Amegakaryocytic Thrombocytopenia

Epidemiology
Congenital amegakaryocytic thrombocytopenia (CAMT) is a bone marrow failure syndrome that typically presents with isolated, early-onset, severe thrombocytopenia. Nearly 70% of affected patients present at birth with a median platelet count of 16,000/μL.[34]

Pathophysiology
Congenital amegakaryocytic thrombocytopenia is inherited in an autosomal recessive pattern, with an increased proportion in offspring of consanguineous parents. The mutation has been isolated to the myeloproliferative leukemia (MPL) virus oncogene, the receptor of the hematopoietic growth factor thrombopoietin (Tpo). Together, MPL and Tpo are key regulators of megakaryocyte proliferation and platelet production. Males and females are equally affected by either homozygous or compound heterozygous mutations. The result is thrombocytopenia secondary to ineffective megakaryopoiesis.

Differential Diagnosis
Congenital amegakaryocytic thrombocytopenia is generally a diagnosis of exclusion. Early evaluation and empiric treatment of alternative diagnoses, particularly bacterial infections and NAIT, are important. CAMT should be considered in cases unresponsive to treatment of alternative diagnoses or in cases of prolonged thrombocytopenia.

Diagnostic Tests
Platelets, though decreased, appear normal in size on peripheral smear. Bone marrow examination demonstrates a reduced number of small, immature megakaryocytes. Definitive diagnosis involves genetic testing for an MPL mutation.

Management
Acute treatment involves platelet transfusion for severe thrombocytopenia or bleeding. Similar to WAS, judicious use of platelet transfusions is advised beyond the immediate newborn period given the increased risk of platelet refractoriness. HSCT is required for cure.

Outcome and Follow-up
The 2 major forms, CAMT1 and CAMT2, vary in clinical course: Patients with CAMT1 have persistently severe thrombocytopenia, whereas patients with CAMT2 can have thrombocytopenia of varying severity. Without HSCT, patients develop progressive aplastic anemia.

Thrombocytopenia-Absent Radius Syndrome

Epidemiology
Thrombocytopenia-absent radius (TAR) syndrome is an inherited disorder in which patients have limb anomalies and thrombocytopenia. It occurs with an approximate prevalence of 1–2:1 million live births.[35] Patients often present with early-onset thrombocytopenia. Approximately 50% of patients develop severe thrombocytopenia within the first week of life, and 90% of patients develop severe thrombocytopenia by 4 months of age.[36]

Pathophysiology
The exact mechanism of TAR is not fully known. Recently, Klopocki et al described a microdeletion of chromosome 1q21.1.[37] However, they also reported that mutations within this region were not found on the corresponding undeleted chromosome, implying that deletion of one allele with mutation of the other is not the mechanism of TAR. Furthermore, the deletion was inherited in the majority of cases, but all carrier parents were unaffected. Therefore, it is likely that additional genetic mutations, possibly at different loci, are necessary to result in the TAR phenotype.

Regardless of the genetic mutation, the result is decreased megakaryocyte size, maturity, and function, resulting in a hypomegakaryocytic thrombocytopenia as the primary hematologic manifestation. The megakaryocytes have decreased response to Tpo, despite normal MPL receptors.

Differential Diagnosis

Alternative diagnoses include other causes of early- and late-onset thrombocytopenia. TAR is generally easily distinguished from other etiologies by the presence of limb anomalies. However, there are several other inherited syndromes with limb anomalies that must be carefully excluded. These include Fanconi anemia, radioulnar synostosis with CAMT, and Holt-Oram syndrome (Table 32–5). TAR is distinguished from these other syndromes by the triad of an absent radius or radii, present thumbs, and isolated thrombocytopenia.

Diagnostic Tests

Generally, TAR diagnosis is based on clinical presentation. Patients have an absent radius or radii (Figure 32–2),

Table 32-5 Thrombocytopenia-Absent Radius (TAR) Syndrome Features and Differential Diagnosis[a]

	Upper Limb	Hematologic	Lower Limb	Molecular	Other
TAR syndrome	Absent radius, thumbs present	Thrombocytopenia, onset prenatal to first few months	Genu varum, small patellae	1q21.1 microdeletion plus other unknown genetic change	Relative macrocephaly, short stature, characteristic facial phenotype
FA	Hypoplasia of radius and thumb; thumb can also be duplicated or absent	Pancytopenia, onset first decade of life	None	Heterogeneous; several different genes can cause FA	Microcephaly, renal anomalies, short stature; can be mistaken for VACTERL association
Roberts syndrome	Radial defects with oligo- or syndactyly	None	Fibular defects with oligo- or syndactyly	Mutation in ESCO2	Multiple other anomalies can occur (eg, neural tube, renal, genitourinary, orofacial)
Holt-Oram syndrome	Thumb anomalies most common; reduction of upper limb rare	None	Usually none	Mutation in TBX5	Cardiac anomalies common, especially atrial septal defect
Rapadilino syndrome	Absent or hypoplastic radii and thumbs	None	Abnormal patellae, joint dislocations	Mutation in RECQL4	Characteristic facial phenotype, diarrhea
Radioulnar synostosis with congenital amegakaryocytic thrombocytopenia	Radioulnar synostosis	Congenital thrombocytopenia	None	Mutation in HOXA11	Clinodactyly
Ceballos-Quint TAR-like syndrome	Absent radius, hypoplastic thumbs	Thrombocytopenia	Hip anomalies	Unknown	Glaucoma, cataract, clavicular anomalies

Abbreviations: FA, Fanconi anemia; TAR, thrombocytopenia-absent radius; VACTERL, vertebral, anal, cardiac, tracheal, esophageal, renal, and limb.
[a]Adapted from Toriello.[35]

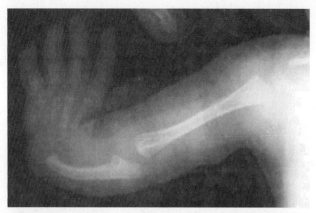

FIGURE 32-2 X-ray of newborn with thrombocytopenia-absent radius (TAR) syndrome.

present (though often hypoplastic) thumbs, and thrombocytopenia. In addition, patients can have other structural abnormalities, such as clinodactyly, hypoplasia of the ulna or humerus, cardiac and renal abnormalities, facial anomalies, and short stature.

Management

Management of thrombocytopenia in TAR syndrome is supportive, with platelet transfusions administered for severe thrombocytopenia and bleeding. Transfusions should be more liberally administered in the first several days of life to prevent ICH, with general platelet goals of greater than 20,000/µL for healthy term infants and greater than 50,000/µL for preterm or at-risk infants.

Outcome and Follow-up

Thrombocytopenia associated with TAR generally improves over time, with platelet counts approaching normal in older childhood. Management otherwise focuses on repair and management of the other structural abnormalities. Orthotics and prostheses may improve quality of life. Surgical correction may be warranted for facial, orthopedic, cardiac, and renal anomalies. Generally, it is prudent to delay surgery until improvement or resolution of thrombocytopenia to decrease bleeding risk. Long-term outcome for patients with TAR is good, with the majority having a normal life span once they have survived beyond the first year of life.

Myosin Heavy Chain 9–Related Disorders

Epidemiology

Myosin heavy chain 9–related disorders (MYH-RDs) are rare inherited platelet disorders, reported in 101 unrelated kindreds worldwide.[38] MYH9-RD is a unifying diagnosis for what was previously described as 4 distinct disorders: Fechtner, Sebastian, and Ebstein syndromes and the May-Hegglin anomaly.

Pathophysiology

MYH9 is the gene for the heavy chain of nonmuscle myosin heavy chain IIA, which is part of a family of motor proteins vital for several cellular processes. *MYH9* mutations are inherited in an autosomal dominant manner and result in congenital macrothrombocytopenia that is evident at birth. The thrombocytopenia is thought to be secondary to defects in megakaryocyte maturation and platelet formation.[39] Other abnormalities can evolve in later childhood and adulthood, including presenile cataracts, deafness, and nephropathy.

Differential Diagnosis

Neonates with MYH9-RD present with early-onset macrothrombocytopenia, which is usually mild to moderate in severity. Congenital macrothrombocytopenias often are confused with NAIT and maternal autoantibodies, in which platelets may also be large.

Diagnostic Tests

In contrast to immune-mediated thrombocytopenias, for which both normal and large platelets are seen, platelets are uniformly large in MYH9-RD. Platelets are often larger than red cells, ranging from 30 to 80 fL (normal platelet size 7–10 fL). These giant platelets are often mistaken for red cells on an automated cell counter. MYH-RD can be further distinguished from other congenital macrothrombocytopenias by the presence of leukocyte inclusions (Figure 32–3). These leukocyte inclusions, often referred to as Dohle bodies, are abnormal aggregates of the protein nonmuscle myosin

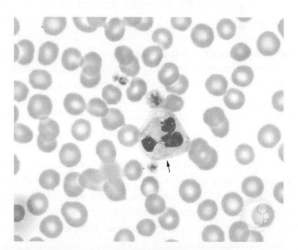

FIGURE 32-3 *MYH9*-related disorders. Hematoxylin and eosin stained peripheral smear of a patient with *myosin heavy chain 9–related disorder* (MYH-RD), showing a giant platelet (open arrow) and a neutrophil inclusion body (ie, Dohle body; closed arrow). NMMIIA, nonmuscle myosin IIA. (Reproduced with permission from American Society of Hematology. ASH Image Bank, by John Lazarchick, 2008 http://imagebank.hematology.org/AssetDetail.aspx?AssetID=3600&AssetType=Asset.)

IIA (NMMIIA). Ultimately, the presence of a specific *MYH9* mutation is detected by exon gene sequencing.

Management

Platelet transfusions are the mainstay of therapy for active bleeding and in preparation for surgical procedures. As with other causes of neonatal thrombocytopenia, platelet replacement should be given more liberally in the immediate neonatal period to prevent ICH. However, transfusions should be judiciously administered in older childhood, given the increased risk of platelet refractoriness and alloimmunization.

Outcome and Follow-up

The degree of thrombocytopenia is moderate, with platelets ranging from 30,000 to 100,000/μL. Bleeding generally is mild. However, patients may develop complications from nephropathy, sensorineural deafness, and cataracts in later childhood and adulthood. Progressive hearing loss is the most common of the extrahematologic complications, affecting up to 60% of patients.[39] The extrahematologic manifestations are dependent on the exact type and location of *MYH9* mutation.

Glycoprotein Ib-IX-V Deficiencies

Bernard-Soulier syndrome (BSS) is an exceedingly rare disorder characterized by macrothrombocytopenia. It is due to a deficiency in the glycoprotein Ib-IX-V platelet membrane complex essential for platelet adhesion. Patients are born with uniformly giant platelets and mild-to-moderate thrombocytopenia. It is inherited in an autosomal recessive pattern. BSS can be distinguished by the presence of abnormal platelet aggregation to ristocetin. Patients have lifelong stable macrothrombocytopenia and generally have mild-to-moderate bleeding symptoms. Platelet transfusions are utilized in the presence of clinical bleeding.

Mediterranean macrothrombocytopenia is common in individuals of southern European ancestry. Linkage analysis of affected kindreds isolates the mutation to an unknown locus on chromosome 17. Patients have mild-to-moderate macrothrombocytopenia, and flow cytometry demonstrates decreased expression glycoprotein Ib-IX-V. In comparison to BSS, individuals with Mediterranean macrothrombocytopenia have little, if any, bleeding symptoms and normal platelet function.[40]

Velocardiofacial syndrome (VCFS) is associated with a constellation of defects involving the skeletal, cardiac, endocrine, neurologic, and hematologic systems. It results from a mutation of 22q11. As the glycoprotein Ib-IX-V complex gene loci are all located in this region of chromosome 22, patients with VCFS present similarly to those with Mediterranean macrothrombocytopenia, with mild-to-moderate thrombocytopenia, decreased GpIb-IX-V expression, and little-to-no bleeding.

Thrombocytopenia With Storage Pool Defects

Jacobsen syndrome is a rare congenital disorder that results from a terminal deletion of 11q23. The mutation typically is spontaneous. Patients are born with mild-to-moderate thrombocytopenia, abnormal facies, and structural heart defects. Along with thrombocytopenia, platelets have functional defects secondary to storage pool deficiency.[41] Patients are particularly at high risk for bleeding and require lifelong platelet transfusion support.

Gray platelet syndrome results from mutations on 3p21. Patients are born with moderate macrothrombocytopenia and a marked decrease in platelet α granules. Platelets have a characteristic gray appearance under light microscopy due to decreased granules. Patients have stable lifelong mild-to-moderate bleeding tendencies.

Aneuploidy

Aneuploidy is another cause of neonatal thrombocytopenia. Trisomies 13, 18, and 21 are particularly associated with decreased platelet counts. Thrombocytopenia is typically mild to moderate, and patients have little-to-no bleeding symptoms.

Miscellaneous Causes

Other recognized causes of neonatal thrombocytopenia due to increased platelet destruction/consumption include hypersplenism, thrombosis, use of extracorporeal membrane oxygenation (ECMO), and exchange transfusions. Hypersplenism occurs in patients with splenomegaly; platelets are sequestered within the enlarged spleen, resulting in decreased platelet circulation. Thrombosis also can cause thrombocytopenia because platelets are consumed at the sites of clots. Thrombocytopenia associated with ECMO and exchange transfusion results from platelet adhesion to the oxygenator membrane or tubing.

Other rare causes of neonatal thrombocytopenia secondary to decreased production include storage disorders (eg, proprionic and methylmalonic acidemia) and bone marrow infiltrative malignancies (eg, congenital leukemia, neuroblastoma).

GENERAL MANAGEMENT

Timely recognition and diagnosis of neonatal thrombocytopenia is important in preventing morbidity and mortality. Diagnostic algorithms for neonatal thrombocytopenia in term and preterm infants are outlined in Figures 32–4 and 32–5.

In most affected infants, the degree of thrombocytopenia is mild to moderate and does not require treatment except for management of the underlying etiology.

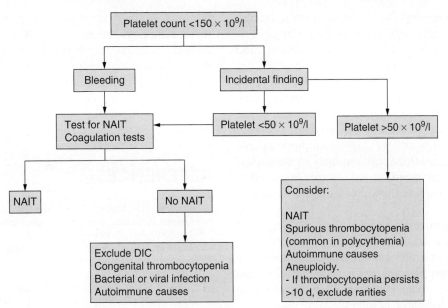

FIGURE 32-4 Diagnostic algorithm for neonatal thrombocytopenia in term neonates. DIC, disseminated intravascular coagulation; NAIT, neonatal alloimmune thrombocytopenia. (Reproduced with permission from Chakravorty and Roberts.[45])

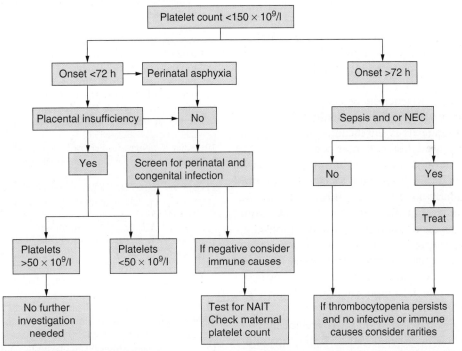

FIGURE 32-5 Diagnostic algorithm for neonatal thrombocytopenia in preterm neonates. NAIT, neonatal alloimmune thrombocytopenia; NEC, necrotizing enterocolitis. (Reproduced with permission from Chakravorty and Roberts.[45])

It is controversial whether the degree of thrombocytopenia confers increased bleeding risk. Stanworth et al performed a prospective observational study, using a bleeding assessment tool to objectively measure bleeding frequency in severely thrombocytopenic neonates.[9] In this study, the major determinant of severe bleeding (eg, intracranial, pulmonary) was gestational age less than 28 weeks rather than platelet count. A retrospective analysis of intraventricular hemorrhage (IVH) risk in thrombocytopenic neonates also reported no significant relationship between bleeding and the degree of thrombocytopenia.[42] Rather, it appears that IVH bleeding risk is multifactorial, involving other factors, such as gestational age, birth weight, and underlying illness. In preterm neonates, IVH has been particularly associated with blood vessel fragility, previously damaged blood vessels, and concomitant coagulopathies.[43] Furthermore, IVH has been discovered in one-third of thrombocytopenic neonates before the thrombocytopenia existed, which raises the question of whether IVH is the cause or the effect of thrombocytopenia.[8,9,43] In a recent prospective observational study of 169 thrombocytopenic neonates with a gestational age less than 34 weeks, the major independent bleeding risk factors were NEC and the onset of severe thrombocytopenia within 10 days of birth.[44]

Despite the controversies related to the degree of thrombocytopenia and bleeding risk, a general consensus among pediatric hematologists and neonatologists is to maintain platelets above 50,000/µL in term healthy infants and platelets above 30,000/µL for sick preterm infants and those at high bleeding risk.[8,9,44]

Platelet transfusions remain the mainstay of treatment. Recommendations are for 10–15 mL/kg aliquots of cytomegalovirus-negative and irradiated platelets. Directed donor (eg, maternal platelets) or antigen-specific (eg, HPA-1a negative) platelets may be indicated in certain cases of NAIT. A single platelet transfusion can increase counts by as much as 50,000–100,000/µL, particularly when thrombocytopenia is due to decreased platelet production. Increases can be substantially less or even negligible when there is ongoing platelet destruction or consumption. The life span of transfused platelets is usually 5 to 9 days, though platelet longevity is significantly diminished in disorders of increased destruction or consumption.

Given the often-unknown duration of a transfused platelet life span, it is important to closely monitor counts, particularly in a severely thrombocytopenic neonate or in an infant with a high bleeding risk. Until the pattern of transfused platelet survival is established, serial monitoring as frequent as every 4 to 6 hours may be warranted. Particular attention is necessary for neonates undergoing procedures or surgeries, as they may require increased platelet support to minimize intra- or postoperative bleeding.

Other therapies have been outlined previously and are specific to the underlying cause of the thrombocytopenia. These include treatments such as IVIG for maternal ITP and NAIT, antimicrobial treatment of infections, and steroids for Kasabach-Merritt syndrome.

SUMMARY

Neonatal thrombocytopenia is a common entity in the NICU population. Timely recognition and management are important to prevent clinical sequelae. Many cases are mild to moderate in severity, with minimal or no symptoms, and do not require treatment. However, patients with NAIT, sepsis, NEC, and certain inherited thrombocytopenic syndromes are at particularly high risk of severe and life-threatening bleeding and require close observation and medical management. Early recognition and intervention are particularly important in these cases to prevent poor clinical outcomes.

REFERENCES

1. Burrows RF, Kelton JG. Incidentally detected thrombocytopenia in healthy mothers and their infants. *N Engl J Med.* 1988;319(3):142–145.
2. Burrows RF, Kelton JG. Fetal thrombocytopenia and its relation to maternal thrombocytopenia. *N Engl J Med.* 1993;329(20):1463–1466.
3. Sainio S, et al. Thrombocytopenia in term infants: a population-based study. *Obstet Gynecol.* 2000;95(3):441–446.
4. Roberts I, Stanworth S, Murray NA. Thrombocytopenia in the neonate. *Blood Rev.* 2008;22(4):173–186.
5. Sola-Visner M, Saxonhouse MA, Brown RE. Neonatal thrombocytopenia: what we do and don't know. *Early Hum Dev.* 2008;84(8):499–506.
6. Christensen RD, et al. Thrombocytopenia among extremely low birth weight neonates: data from a multihospital healthcare system. *J Perinatol.* 2006;26(6):348–353.
7. Wiedmeier SE, et al. Platelet reference ranges for neonates, defined using data from over 47,000 patients in a multihospital healthcare system. *J Perinatol.* 2009;29(2):130–136.
8. Baer VL, et al. Severe thrombocytopenia in the NICU. *Pediatrics.* 2009;124(6):e1095–e1100.
9. Stanworth SJ, et al. Prospective, observational study of outcomes in neonates with severe thrombocytopenia. *Pediatrics.* 2009;124(5):e826–e834.
10. Adler SP, Nigro G, Pereira L. Recent advances in the prevention and treatment of congenital cytomegalovirus infections. *Semin Perinatol.* 2007;31(1):10–18.
11. Horbar JD, et al. Trends in mortality and morbidity for very low birth weight infants, 1991–1999. *Pediatrics.* 2002;110(1 Pt 1):143–151.
12. Kenton AB, et al. Severe thrombocytopenia predicts outcome in neonates with necrotizing enterocolitis. *J Perinatol.* 2005;25(1):14–20.
13. Pacheco LD, et al. Fetal and neonatal alloimmune thrombocytopenia: a management algorithm based on risk stratification. *Obstet Gynecol.* 2011;118(5):1157–1163.
14. Bussel J. Diagnosis and management of the fetus and neonate with alloimmune thrombocytopenia. *J Thromb Haemost.* 2009;7(Suppl 1):253–257.
15. Bussel JB, et al. Clinical and diagnostic comparison of neonatal alloimmune thrombocytopenia to non-immune cases of thrombocytopenia. *Pediatr Blood Cancer* 2005;45(2):176–183.
16. Ghevaert C, et al. Management and outcome of 200 cases of fetomaternal alloimmune thrombocytopenia. *Transfusion* 2007;47(5):901–910.
17. Bussel JB, Primiani A. Fetal and neonatal alloimmune thrombocytopenia: progress and ongoing debates. *Blood Rev.* 2008;22(1):33–52.
18. Stuge TB, et al. The cellular immunobiology associated with fetal and neonatal alloimmune thrombocytopenia. *Transfus Apher Sci.* 2011;45(1):53–59.
19. Loewenthal R, Rosenberg N, Kalt R, et al. Compound heterozygosity of HLA-DRB3*01:01 and HLA-DRB4*01:01 as a

potential predictor of fetal neonatal alloimmune thrombocytopenia. *Transfusion*. 2012;53(2):344–352.

20. Allen D, et al. Platelet transfusion in neonatal alloimmune thrombocytopenia. *Blood*. 2007;109(1):388–389.

21. Kiefel V, et al. Antigen-positive platelet transfusion in neonatal alloimmune thrombocytopenia (NAIT). *Blood*. 2006;107(9):3761–3763.

22. van den Akker ES, et al. Noninvasive antenatal management of fetal and neonatal alloimmune thrombocytopenia: safe and effective. *BJOG*. 2007;114(4):469–473.

23. Koyama S, et al. Reliable predictors of neonatal immune thrombocytopenia in pregnant women with idiopathic thrombocytopenic purpura. *Am J Hematol*. 2012;87(1):15–21.

24. Stavrou E, McCrae KR. Immune thrombocytopenia in pregnancy. *Hematol Oncol Clin North Am*. 2009;23(6):1299–1316.

25. Gill KK, Kelton JG. Management of idiopathic thrombocytopenic purpura in pregnancy. *Semin Hematol*. 2000;37(3):275–289.

26. Hall GW. Kasabach-Merritt syndrome: pathogenesis and management. *Br J Haematol*. 2001;112(4):851–862.

27. Enjolras O, et al. Residual lesions after Kasabach-Merritt phenomenon in 41 patients. *J Am Acad Dermatol*. 2000;42(2 Pt 1):225–235.

28. Kelly M. Kasabach-Merritt phenomenon. *Pediatr Clin North Am*. 2010;57(5):1085–1089.

29. Lafouresse F, et al. Wiskott-Aldrich syndrome protein controls antigen-presenting cell-driven CD4+ T-cell motility by regulating adhesion to intercellular adhesion molecule-1. *Immunology*. 2012;137(2):183–196.

30. Westerberg LS, et al. Wiskott-Aldrich syndrome protein (WASP) and N-WASP are critical for peripheral B-cell development and function. *Blood*. 2012;119(17):3966–3974.

31. Jin Y, et al. Mutations of the Wiskott-Aldrich Syndrome Protein (WASP): hotspots, effect on transcription, and translation and phenotype/genotype correlation. *Blood*. 2004;104(13):4010–4019.

32. Imai K, et al. Clinical course of patients with WASP gene mutations. *Blood*. 2004;103(2):456–464.

33. Shin CR, et al. Outcomes following hematopoietic cell transplantation for Wiskott-Aldrich syndrome. *Bone Marrow Transplant*. 2012;47(11):1428–1435.

34. Ballmaier M, Germeshausen M. Congenital amegakaryocytic thrombocytopenia: clinical presentation, diagnosis, and treatment. *Semin Thromb Hemost*. 2011;37(6):673–681.

35. Toriello HV. Thrombocytopenia-absent radius syndrome. *Semin Thromb Hemost*. 2011;37(6):707–712.

36. de Ybarrondo L, Barratt MS. Thrombocytopenia absent radius syndrome. *Pediatr Rev*. 2011;32(9):399–400; discussion 400.

37. Klopocki E, et al. Complex inheritance pattern resembling autosomal recessive inheritance involving a microdeletion in thrombocytopenia-absent radius syndrome. *Am J Hum Genet*. 2007; 80(2):232–240.

38. Althaus K, Greinacher A. MYH9-related platelet disorders. *Semin Thromb Hemost*. 2009;35(2):189–203.

39. Balduini CL, Pecci A, Savoia A. Recent advances in the understanding and management of MYH9-related inherited thrombocytopenias. *Br J Haematol*. 2011;154(2):161–174.

40. Savoia A, et al. Autosomal dominant macrothrombocytopenia in Italy is most frequently a type of heterozygous Bernard-Soulier syndrome. *Blood*. 2001;97(5):1330–1335.

41. White JG. Platelet storage pool deficiency in Jacobsen syndrome. *Platelets*. 2007;18(7):522–527.

42. von Lindern JS, et al. Thrombocytopenia in neonates and the risk of intraventricular hemorrhage: a retrospective cohort study. *BMC Pediatr*. 2011;11:16.

43. Stanworth SJ, Bennett C. How to tackle bleeding and thrombosis in the newborn. *Early Hum Dev*. 2008;84(8):507–513.

44. Muthukumar P, et al. Severe thrombocytopenia and patterns of bleeding in neonates: results from a prospective observational study and implications for use of platelet transfusions. *Transfus Med*. 2012;22(5):338–343.

45. Chakravorty S, Roberts I. How I manage neonatal thrombocytopenia. *Br J Haematol*. 2012;156(2):155–162.

Bleeding Disorders

Yaser A. Diab and Naomi L. C. Luban

INTRODUCTION

This chapter reviews common neonatal bleeding disorders. These disorders can present challenges in diagnosis and management. Most neonatal bleeding defects are acquired; however, some inherited hemorrhagic disorders can present in the neonatal period.

Understanding the normal hemostatic process and the developmental aspects of the neonatal hemostatic system is important when investigating a neonate with a suspected bleeding disorder. The physiology of hemostasis in newborn infants and the approach to evaluation of neonatal bleeding disorders are discussed in the following introductory sections.

Overview of Normal Hemostasis

The key elements of the hemostatic system include the vascular endothelium, platelets, and coagulation. The immediate response to vascular injury is transient arteriolar vasoconstriction due to reflex neurogenic mechanisms and local secretion of vasoactive factors. This is followed by activation of platelets and coagulation proteins. Finally, once bleeding is controlled, blood vessel patency is restored by the fibrinolytic system. Hence, the normal hemostatic response can be viewed to occur in the following three phases (Figure 33-1):

1. Initiation and formation of the platelet plug (primary hemostasis)
2. Propagation of the clotting process by the coagulation cascade followed by termination of clotting by antithrombotic control mechanisms (secondary hemostasis)
3. Removal of the clot by the fibrinolytic system (tertiary hemostasis)

Vitamin K Physiology in Neonates

Vitamin K is present in a variety of dietary sources and is produced by intestinal bacteria. Vitamin K is a cofactor for γ-glutamyl carboxylase, an enzyme that performs posttranslational carboxylation, converting glutamate residues in proteins to γ-carboxyglutamate residues (Figure 33-2). These residues facilitate membrane interactions mediated by calcium ions and are necessary for proper function of the coagulation factors II, VII, IX, and X and proteins C and S. The newborn infant has a particularly fragile vitamin K status because of (1) limited hepatic stores at birth; (2) limited placental transfer of vitamin K; (3) variable and limited content of vitamin K in breast milk; and (4) initially, a sterile gastrointestinal system.[1]

Developmental Hemostasis in the Neonate

Proteins required for hemostasis do not cross the placenta and are synthesized by the fetus. Distinctive, quantitative, and qualitative gestational-age-dependent differences involving various components of hemostasis have been well characterized in neonates[2,3] (Table 33-1). These differences are more pronounced

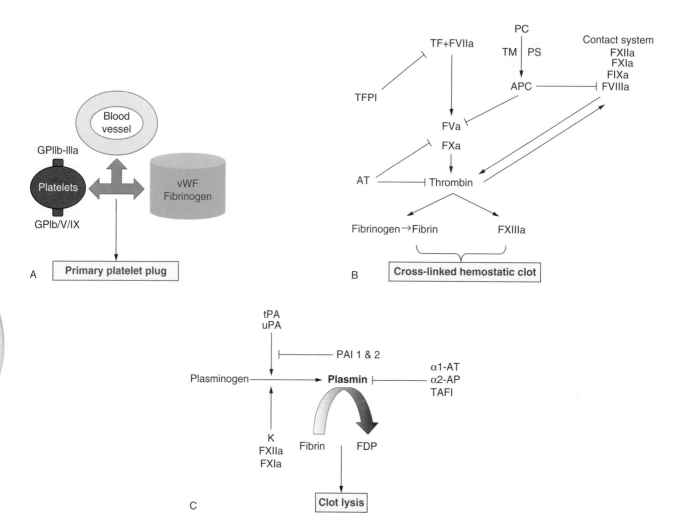

FIGURE 33-1 Overview of the three phases of hemostasis. A, Primary hemostasis is dependent on interactions between platelets, the vascular endothelium, and coagulation proteins (von Willebrand factor [vWF] and fibrinogen). vWF associated with collagen in the exposed subendothelial matrix interacts with platelet GpIb/V/IX complex to mediate "platelet adhesion," while vWF and fibrinogen bind platelet GpIIb-IIIa to mediate "platelet aggregation." B, Secondary hemostasis involves sequential activation of coagulation factors. Formation of factor VIIa-tissue factor (TF) complex is the major initiating event that results in the generation of small amounts of thrombin (initiation phase or intrinsic pathway). These amounts of thrombin activate platelets and additional coagulation factors (amplification phase or extrinsic pathway), which results in a burst of thrombin formation, so that a stable fibrin clot can be formed. This process is subsequently terminated by three types of natural anticoagulants: antithrombin (AT), which inhibits the activity of thrombin and factors IXa, Xa, XIa, and XIIa; protein C (PC), which is activated by thrombomodulin (TM), thrombin, and its cofactor protein S (PS), inhibits factors Va and VIIIa; and TF pathway inhibitor (TFPI), which inhibits factor Xa and TF/factor VIIa. C, Tertiary hemostasis (fibrinolysis) functions to remove formed clots after hemostasis is secured. α1-AT 1 and 2, α1-antitrypsin 1 and 2, respectively; F, factor; FDP, fibrin degradation products ; PAI 1 and 2, plasminogen activator inhibitor 1 and 2, respectively; tPA, tissue plasminogen activator; uPA, urokinase plasminogen activator.

in premature infants. Although neonatal platelets are hyporeactive, the concentration and function of von Willebrand factor (vWF) are increased in neonates due to the presence of ultralarge, more functionally potent vWF multimers.[4] Vitamin K–dependent factors II, VII, IX, and X and contact factors XI and XII are reduced to about 50% of normal adult values, while the levels of the factors V, VIII, and XIII are similar to adult ranges. Although fibrinogen concentration is within normal adult ranges, it exists in a "fetal" form in the

first 3 weeks of life. Fetal fibrinogen has a different composition compared to adult fibrinogen (increased sialic acid and phosphorous content) and shows a decreased rate of fibrin polymerization, which results in prolonged thrombin clotting time (TCT) in normal neonates.[5] Similarly, concentrations of antithrombin, protein C, and protein S are significantly lower at birth, and the overall fibrinolytic capacity is decreased in neonates. As a result of these counterbalanced differences, the neonatal hemostatic system remains physiologically

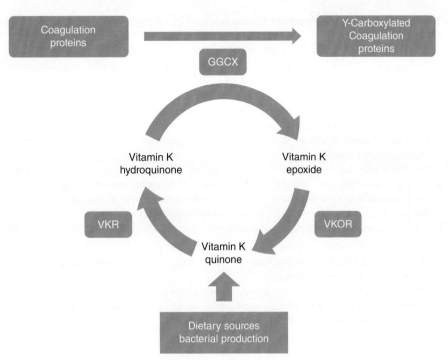

FIGURE 33-2 The vitamin K cycle. GGCX, vitamin K γ-glutamyl carboxylase; VKR, vitamin K reductase; VKOR, vitamin K epoxide reductase.

Table 33-1 Hemostatic Parameters in the Newborn[a]

Decreased Compared to Adult Reference Ranges	Within Normal Adult Reference Ranges	Increased Compared to Adult Reference Ranges
FII	Fibrinogen	FVIII (mildly)
FVII	FV	vWF[b]
FIX	FXIII	α2-macroglobulin
FX	α2-Antiplasmin	
FXI	tPA	
FXII	PAI-1	
Prekallikrin		
HMWK		
Antithrombin		
Heparin cofactor II		
Protein C		
Protein S		
TFPI		
Plasminogen		
Platelet count and mean platelet volume vary with gestational and postnatal ages with wider intervals than adult reference ranges; prothrombin time (PT) is minimally prolonged, and activated partial thromboplastin time (aPTT) is markedly prolonged. Thrombin clotting time (TCT) is also prolonged. Platelet function studies show shorter bleeding times, shorter closure times by the platelet function analyzer (PFA-100), and decreased platelet aggregation in response to thrombin, adenosine diphosphate (ADP), and epinephrine.		

Abbreviations: F, factor; HMWK, high molecular weight kininogen; PAI-1, plasminogen activator inhibitor 1; TFPI, tissue factor pathway inhibitor; tPA, tissue plasminogen activator; vFW, von Willebrand factor.
[a]Data from Andrew et al.[2,3]
[b]The vWF concentration and function are both increased and ultralarge molecular weight multimers are present in neonatal plasma.

Table 33-2 Pertinent History and Physical Examination Findings in Neonatal Bleeding Disorder

History	• Presentations suggestive of neonatal bleeding disorders include diffuse purpura/ecchymoses, oozing from the umbilical stump, excessive bleeding from peripheral puncture/heel stick sites, large cephalohematomas without significant birth trauma history, prolonged bleeding following circumcision, intracranial hemorrhage in a term or late preterm infant without history of birth trauma, and unexplained bleeding in a very low birth weight infant. • Bleeding in a well neonate is suggestive of an inherited coagulation disorder or an immune-mediated thrombocytopenia, whereas a sick preterm neonate is more likely to have acquired hemostatic disorder. • Vitamin K administration. • Maternal and obstetric history, including history of prior pregnancies and their outcomes, maternal medications (eg, anticonvulsants can cause neonatal vitamin K deficiency) and maternal immune thrombocytopenia, which can cause neonatal thrombocytopenia. • Family history, including parental ethnic background and consanguinity, and family history of bleeding.
Physical examination	• The findings of purpura, petechiae, ecchymoses, and mucosal bleeding in neonates are suggestive of a primary hemostatic defect. • The presence of dysmorphic features/congenital anomalies may suggest an underlying genetic defect since some genetic syndromes are associated with a congenital bleeding tendency, most commonly involving platelets.

intact but lacks adequate reserve under stress conditions. Therefore, the risk of bleeding is increased in sick neonates and is further increased in premature infants.

Approach to Neonatal Bleeding Disorders

Bleeding disorders in neonates can be congenital or inherited but are more often acquired. It is clinically useful to classify bleeding disorders into those affecting primary hemostasis (blood vessels, vWF, and platelets) and those affecting secondary hemostasis (coagulation proteins). Disorders involving tertiary hemostasis (fibrinolytic system) are exceedingly rare. Acquired bleeding disorders can affect multiple components in the hemostatic system, which can give rise to complex hemostatic abnormalities. The evaluation of bleeding disorders in neonates can be challenging due to subtle or nonspecific clinical presentations and difficulties in both obtaining adequate specimens for coagulation testing and interpreting the results of these tests in the context of developmental hemostasis. A systematic approach and involvement of a pediatric hematologist are vital to establish the diagnosis of and therapeutic approach to a bleeding disorder. A complete history and physical examination is an essential first step that can direct further laboratory workup (Table 33-2). The laboratory evaluation of neonates with suspected bleeding disorders is best carried out in a rational stepwise fashion (Figure 33-2) in which an initial hemostatic screen is performed, which is followed by additional testing if an abnormality is identified on the initial screen. Additional testing is also indicated if the clinical suspicion remains high despite

a normal hemostatic screen that cannot exclude several less-common or milder bleeding disorders (Figure 33-2). Moreover, several potential pitfalls should be kept in mind regarding laboratory evaluation of hemostasis in neonates[6] (Table 33-3). While many of these issues can be overcome, the major challenge in hemostatic testing in neonates remains the establishment of appropriate neonatal reference values that are analyzer and reagent specific and at the same time clinically relevant (ie, reference ranges that can accurately identify "disease").[6]

NEONATAL PLATELET DISORDERS

This group of disorders results when platelets are deficient in number (thrombocytopenia), functionally defective (thrombocytopathy), or both. Typical manifestations include petechiae (singly or in crops), bruising, and hemorrhage from mucosal surfaces. Bleeding from a heel stick puncture is often the first clinical indicator of an issue. Although generally rare, serious bleeding can complicate some of the more severe platelet defects. In this section, we review platelet disorders that present in neonates.

Neonatal Thrombocytopenia

Thrombocytopenia in a neonate of any viable gestational age is traditionally defined[7] as a platelet count of less than 150×10^9/L. However, recently gestational and postnatal age-specific reference intervals for platelet counts have been described that may need to be considered when defining thrombocytopenia in

Table 33-3 Special Considerations in Neonatal Hemostatic Laboratory Testing

Variable	Sources of Errors	Possible Solution(s)
Preanalytical	Insufficient sample volume and underfilling of collection tubes	Establishment of standard protocols, techniques for specimen collection and transport, and microtization of assays
	Heparin contamination (sample collected from indwelling catheters or into a preheparinized syringe)	
	Specimen activation	
	High hematocrit at birth (required citrate-to-blood ratio of 9:1 may not be achieved using standard collection tubes)	When the hematocrit exceeds 0.55 (55%), the reduced plasma volume requires a decrease in the volume of anticoagulant used to maintain the ratio of 9:1 using the following formula: $C\,(mL) = 1.85 \times 10^{-3} \times (100 - Hct\,(\%)) \times V\,(mL)$ C = milliliters of 3.2% sodium citrate anticoagulant; $Hct\,(\%)$ = hematocrit of the patient in percentage; and V = milliliters of whole blood in tube
Analytical	Elevated levels of bilirubin or lipids and hemolysis in neonates can interfere with optical density measurements used to determine end points of some coagulation tests	Additional centrifugation of the sample
Postanalytical	Defining appropriate reference ranges for neonates	Use of age-related reference ranges specific for analyzer-reagent combination used in the coagulation laboratory

premature neonates.[8] Thrombocytopenia is one of the most frequent hematological disorders encountered in the sick neonate.[9] This is evidenced by a fairly high incidence among neonates admitted to the neonatal intensive care unit (NICU) (22%–35%) compared to a relatively low overall incidence (0.7%–0.9%).[10] The incidence is inversely proportional to gestational age or birth weight.[11] Severe thrombocytopenia (platelet count $< 50 \times 10^9$/L) is less common, affecting 5%–10% of all neonates and 14% of extremely low birth weight (ELBW) infants.[7,12] The predisposition of neonates to develop thrombocytopenia in response to illness is likely due to limited ability of the neonatal megakaryopoietic axis to increase platelet production in response to platelet consumption.[13] While there are a large number of disease processes that have been associated with thrombocytopenia in neonates, impaired platelet production is the prevailing mechanism in most cases.[9] Consumption or sequestration underlie thrombocytopenia in 25%–35% of cases.[9] The differential diagnosis, and consequently diagnostic evaluation, of neonates with thrombocytopenia is usually based on onset (early onset ≤ 72 hours and late onset > 72 hours of life), overall presentation, and natural course (Table 33-4). While the most common identifiable causes are chronic fetal hypoxia in early-onset thrombocytopenia and sepsis and necrotizing

enterocolitis (NEC) in late-onset thrombocytopenia, no etiology is identified in a significant proportion of thrombocytopenic ELBW neonates.[11]

Neonatal Thrombocytopenic Disorders Requiring Special Attention

Immune-Mediated Thrombocytopenias

Fetal and Neonatal Alloimmune Thrombocytopenia (FNAIT): FNAIT is the most common cause of severe neonatal thrombocytopenia and of intracranial hemorrhage (ICH) in term neonates.[14] FNAIT occurs with an estimated incidence of 1/1000–2000 live births.[15] FNAIT results from transplacental passage of maternal antibodies to fetal platelets expressing paternal antigens that the mother lacks. Fetomaternal incompatibility involving certain human platelet antigens (HPAs) specifically expressed by platelets leads to the production of an immunoglobulin (Ig) G allo-antibody, which then crosses the placenta, often in early pregnancy, binding to fetal platelets and resulting in fetal and neonatal thrombocytopenia. Genetic incompatibility to platelet antigens is necessary, but not sufficient, for FNAIT, as the clinical syndrome is seen for less than what would be expected based on genetic frequency alone.[14] Thus, other

Table 33-4 Causes of Neonatal Thrombocytopenia[a]

Classification	Causes	Presentation
Early onset (≤72 hours)	Chronic fetal hypoxia/placental insufficiency (PIH, IUGR, diabetes)	Slowly evolving, mild-moderate thrombocytopenia, nadir at days 4–7, resolution by day 10
	Aneuploidy (trisomies 18, 13, 21; isochromosome 18q; triploidy; Turner syndrome)	Dysmorphism, congenital anomalies
	Perinatal asphyxia	Sick neonate with severe thrombocytopenia
	Early neonatal sepsis (*Escherichia coli*, group B *Streptococcus*, *Haemophilus influenzae*)	
	DIC	
	Immune-mediated thrombocytopenias (FNAIT, autoimmune thrombocytopenia from maternal ITP)	Well full-term neonate with severe thrombocytopenia
	Kasabach-Merritt syndrome	Severe thrombocytopenia, DIC, enlarging cutaneous or visceral vascular tumor
	Thrombosis (renal vein thrombosis, aortic thrombosis, portal vein thrombosis, CSVT)	Unexplained thrombocytopenia, clinical features of organ dysfunction (such as renal insufficiency in renal vein thrombosis, seizures in CSVT)
	Thrombotic microangiopathies (congenital TTP, familial atypical HUS)	Hemolysis, hyperbilirubinemia, multiorgan dysfunction
	Congenital infections (CMV, toxoplasma, others)	Stigmata of congenital infections
	Bone marrow failure/replacement (congenital leukemia, metastatic neuroblastoma, storage disorders, Fanconi anemia)	Pancytopenia, additional systemic manifestations
	Inborn errors of metabolism (organic acidemia)	Associated clinical features
	Inherited thrombocytopenias	Persistent unexplained thrombocytopenia, associated congenital anomalies
Late onset (>72 hours)	Late-onset sepsis (bacterial/fungal)	Rapid-onset severe thrombocytopenia with slow recovery
	NEC	
	Autoimmune thrombocytopenia from maternal ITP	History of maternal thrombocytopenia/SLE
	Congenital infection (CMV, toxoplasma, others)	Stigmata of congenital infections
	Kasabach-Merritt syndrome	
	Inborn errors of metabolism	
	Inherited thrombocytopenias	
	Drug-induced thrombocytopenia (β-lactams, vancomycin, indomethacin, ibuprofen, H$_2$-blockers, heparin)	Resolution on withdrawal of offending drug

Abbreviations: CMV, cytomegalovirus; CSVT, cerebral sinovenous thrombosis; DIC, disseminated intravascular coagulation; FNAIT, fetal and neonatal alloimmune thrombocytopenia; HUS, hemolytic uremic syndrome; ITP, immune thrombocytopenia; IUGR, intrauterine growth restriction; NEC, necrotizing enterocolitis; PIH, pregnancy-induced hypertension; SLE, systemic lupus erythematosus; TTP, thrombotic thrombocytopenic purpura.
[a]Data from Roberts et al.[7]

factors, including genetic immune response modifiers and HLA alleles, must be important in the pathophysiology.[16] The degree of significant bleeding in FNAIT is striking compared to other thrombocytopenic disorders, such as immune thrombocytopenia (ITP); alloantibody-mediated secondary effects may be responsible, including platelet dysfunction and megakaryocytic damage that causes prolonged thrombocytopenia and endothelial injury (eg, HPA-1a antigen is expressed by endothelial cells).[16] HPA frequencies vary among different ethnic groups, and the severity of FNAIT can correlate with the specific HPA incompatibility identified (Table 33-5).

Fetal and neonatal alloimmune thrombocytopenia should be strongly considered in one of two clinical scenarios: In the first scenario, an otherwise-healthy

Table 33-5 Platelet Antigens and FNAIT

Platelet Antigen	Clinical Implications
HPA-1a	• Implicated in 85% of serologically confirmed FNAIT • Accounts for the vast majority of FNAIT in the white population • Associated with severe FNAIT
HPA-5a, HPA-5b, HPA-15a, HPA-15b	• Anti-HPA-5b is the second-most-common cause of FNAIT and is a more important cause of FNAIT in African Americans than anti-HPA-1a. • Alloimmunization to these antigens accounts for most of the remaining cases and is generally associated with less-severe disease.
HPA-9b	• Despite being a relatively rare antigen, alloimmunization against HPA-9b has been recently found to be an important cause of FNAIT and is associated with particularly severe course.
HPA-2a, HPA-2b, HPA-3a, HPA-4a	• These account for a minority of FNAIT cases. • Alloimmunization to HPA-2b (like HPA-5b) is also a more important cause of FNAIT in African Americans. • Alloimmunization to HPA-3a is associated with severe FNAIT. • Anti-HPA-4a is the most important cause of FNAIT in Asian populations.
HPA-6b through HPA-14b (except 9b), and HPA-16b	• Private antigens are expressed in very few individuals in the general population; therefore, detection of FNAIT antibodies is more optimal using paternal platelets rather random donor platelets.
HPA-1b and HPA-3b	• Rarely associated with FNAIT

Abbreviations: FNAIT, fetal and neonatal alloimmune thrombocytopenia; HPA, human platelet antigen.

neonate, born after an uneventful pregnancy and delivery, exhibits petechiae or widespread purpura associated with severe thrombocytopenia (platelet count $< 50 \times 10^9$/L) within 24–48 hours of birth. For the second scenario, ICH, porencephaly, or ventriculomegaly is discovered during fetal life. About 10%–20% of clinically recognized cases will have ICH, which can be asymptomatic, discovered radiographically or symptomatically. Of ICH, 50%–75% occurs in utero and can be fatal (one-third of cases) or result in significant neurologic sequelae. To confirm a clinical diagnosis of FNAIT, two laboratory criteria need to be satisfied: platelet antigen incompatibility demonstrated by genotyping (polymerase chain reaction [PCR] techniques) and phenotyping (flow cytometry, various immunoassay methods) and evidence of maternal alloantibody directed against the identified alloantigen demonstrated by various immunoassays (eg, enzyme-linked immunosorbent assay [ELISA]) and using maternal serum tested against paternal platelets (preferably) or platelets from normal donors with known platelet alloantigen phenotypes.[14] In addition, neuroimaging of all neonates with suspected FNAIT is recommended because some will have asymptomatic central nervous system bleeding, requiring more aggressive treatment measures.

Autoimmune Thrombocytopenia in Infants Born to Mothers With ITP: Neonatal ITP due to transplacental passage of maternal IgG antiplatelet autoantibodies occurs in up to 25% of mothers who develop primary or secondary ITP (due to systemic lupus erythematosus)

during pregnancy.[7,17] The risk of severe thrombocytopenia and ICH in affected neonates is significantly lower compared to FNAIT (<15% and <2%, respectively). Importantly, maternal platelet counts during pregnancy cannot reliably predict the risk of neonatal thrombocytopenia; however, a maternal platelet count less than 50×10^9/L at delivery and a history of severe thrombocytopenia in a previous neonate may be useful indicators of the likelihood of significant neonatal thrombocytopenia complicating current pregnancy.[18,19] Typically, the nadir platelet count in affected neonates is observed between days 2 and 5 after birth, with resolution by day 7; however, some neonates may continue to have thrombocytopenia secondary to maternal ITP for months, necessitating long-term monitoring. Evaluation of affected neonates should include serial platelet counts and screening transcranial ultrasonography (US; if platelet count is $< 50 \times 10^9$).

Inherited Thrombocytopenias: The inherited thrombocytopenias (Table 33-6) belong to a rare group of heterogeneous disorders with highly variable bleeding tendency. Although far less common than acquired forms, inherited thrombocytopenias should be considered in neonates with (1) persistent unexplained thrombocytopenia since birth; (2) bleeding tendency disproportionate to the platelet counts; (3) family history of thrombocytopenia; (4) typical congenital anomalies/dysmorphism; and (5) suggestive blood smear abnormalities (consistently large or small platelets, abnormal platelet granules, or neutrophil inclusion "Döhle bodies"). Except for Wiskott-Aldrich

Table 33-6 Inherited Thrombocytopenic Syndromes That Can Present in the Neonatal Period

Syndrome	Genetics	Hemostatic Features	Additional Findings
Large/Giant Platelets, MPV Greater Than 11 fL			
MYH9-related thrombocytopenia (May-Hegglin anomaly and Fechtner, Epstein, and Sebastian syndromes)	AD (22q11)	Mild bleeding tendency Mild-moderate thrombocytopenia with mild platelet dysfunction	Neutrophil inclusions, ± sensorineural hearing loss, ± nephritis, ± cataracts
Bernard-Soulier syndrome	AR (17pter-p12; 22q11.2; 3q21)	Severe bleeding tendency Variable thrombocytopenia with defective platelet adhesion	None
X-linked thrombocytopenia with dyserythropoiesis	XL (Xp11.23)	Severe bleeding tendency Severe thrombocytopenia with defective platelet function	Microcytic anemia, dyserythropoiesis, thalassemia, splenomegaly
11q terminal deletion disorder (Paris-Trousseau thrombocytopenia/ Jacobsen syndrome)	AD (11q23)	Mild bleeding tendency Severe neonatal thrombocytopenia that resolves over time and persistent platelet dysfunction	Developmental delay, growth retardation, dysmorphism, and multiple congenital anomalies (Jacobsen syndrome)
Normal-Size Platelets, MPV 7–11 fL			
Congenital amegakaryocytic thrombocytopenia	AR (1p34)	Severe bleeding tendency Severe neonatal thrombocytopenia	Marrow failure during second decade
Thrombocytopenia and absent radii	AR (?)	Severe bleeding tendency Severe neonatal thrombocytopenia	Shortened/absent radii bilaterally Bleeding tendency and thrombocytopenia improve after infancy
Thrombocytopenia and radial synostosis	AD (7p15-p14.2)	Severe bleeding tendency Severe neonatal thrombocytopenia	Fused radius, incomplete range of motion, other skeletal problems and sensorineural hearing loss Thrombocytopenia usually does not improve with time
Small Platelets, MPV Less Than 7 fL			
Classic Wiskott-Aldrich syndrome	XL (Xp11.23-p11.22)	Severe bleeding tendency with significant risk of bleeding Severe neonatal thrombocytopenia	Immunodeficiency, autoimmunity, eczema, lymphoma
X-linked thrombocytopenia	XL (Xp11.23-p11.22)	Severe bleeding tendency with significant risk of bleeding Severe neonatal thrombocytopenia	Manifestations besides microthrombocytopenia uncommon

Abbreviations: AD, autosomal dominant; AR, autosomal recessive; MPV, mean platelet volume; XL, X linked.

Table 33-7 Causes of Platelet Function Defects

Acquired

Uremia

Liver disease

Extracorporeal membrane oxygenation and cardiopulmonary bypass

Disseminated intravascular coagulation

Medications (indomethacin, ibuprofen, nitric oxide, others)

Hypothermia

Inherited

Primary platelet function defects

Defective platelet adhesion (platelet-type vWD, Bernard-Soulier syndrome)

Defective platelet aggregation (Glanzmann thrombasthenia)

Defective receptor interactions and abnormal signal transduction

    Receptor defects (thromboxane A2 receptor defect, purinergic receptor defects for ADP and ATP, collagen receptor defects)

    Arachidonic acid pathway defects (cyclooxygenase-1 deficiency and thromboxane synthase deficiency)

    Signal transduction defects (defects in G-protein activation, defects in phosphatidylinositol metabolism, defects in calcium mobilization, and defects in protein phosphorylation)

Defective granule storage and secretion

    Deficiency of α granules (Gray platelet syndrome, Quebec platelet disorder, arthrogryposis–renal dysfunction–cholestasis syndrome)

    Deficiency of δ granules (idiopathic δ-storage pool disease, Chediak-Higashi syndrome, Hermansky-Pudlak syndrome)

    Deficiency of α and δ granules (11q terminal deletion disorder)

Defective procoagulant function (Scott syndrome)

Secondary platelet function defects

vWD

Congenital afibrinogenemia

Abbreviations: ADP, adenosine diphosphate; ATP, adenosine triphosphate; vWD, von Willebrand disease.

syndrome (WAS) and X-linked thrombocytopenia (XLT), in which increased consumption of platelets in addition to defective production are implicated, the thrombocytopenia in these disorders is generally thought to be the result of impaired production. In addition, associated platelet dysfunction can be identified in many inherited thrombocytopenias, which are often responsible for the significant bleeding tendency that is out of proportion to the measured platelet count—a characteristic feature of some of these disorders (eg, Bernard-Soulier syndrome [BSS]). The diagnostic evaluation of these disorders can be challenging and should be conducted by a clinician with expertise in this area and directed by clinical manifestations, physical examination findings, and results of complex laboratory tests, some of which are only available in research laboratories. Genetic or molecular studies are needed to confirm the diagnosis in some inherited platelet disorders (such as WAS/XLT).

Platelet Function Disorders

Platelet function disorders include a large number of disorders with either inherited or acquired mechanisms

(Table 33-7). These disorders pose diagnostic challenges because the tests needed to fully evaluate platelet function can be complex, requiring a great deal of expertise, and are often restricted to specialized coagulation or research laboratories (Figure 33-3). As a group, these disorders present as primary hemostatic defects of variable severity characterized by mucocutaneous bleeding (bruising, petechiae). Although most congenital platelet function defects rarely cause pathologic bleeding in the neonatal period, the severe platelet function disorders like Glanzmann thrombasthenia (GT) and Bernard-Soulier syndrome (BSS) can present in neonates (Table 33-8). Some of these congenital disorders are associated with thrombocytopenia, while others cause isolated platelet dysfunction with normal platelet counts. For more information about these disorders, excellent reviews are available.[20,21]

Management of Platelet Disorders in Neonates

Besides treating the underlying cause, platelet transfusions are the mainstay therapy for most neonates with platelet disorders. In neonatal thrombocytopenia,

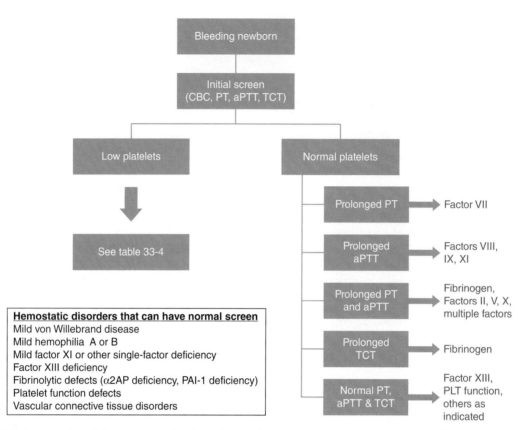

Hemostatic disorders that can have normal screen
Mild von Willebrand disease
Mild hemophilia A or B
Mild factor XI or other single-factor deficiency
Factor XIII deficiency
Fibrinolytic defects (α2AP deficiency, PAI-1 deficiency)
Platelet function defects
Vascular connective tissue disorders

FIGURE 33-3 Approach to laboratory evaluation of coagulation in neonates. aPTT, activated partial thromboplastin time; CBC, complete blood cell count; PAI, plasminogen activator inhibitor; PT, prothrombin time; TCT, thrombin clotting time.

platelet transfusions can be given for therapeutic indication in those with active bleeding or, in most cases, for prophylactic indication to prevent serious bleeding events, particularly ICH and intraventricular hemorrhage (IVH) in preterm infants. While the correlation between platelet count and the risk of a clinical hemorrhage is poor, the risk of bleeding is probably higher in neonates with FNAIT, sepsis, or NEC, particularly those with extreme prematurity.[22] Due to the paucity of controlled data to guide neonatal platelet transfusion decisions, considerable variability exists in practice as well as in published

Table 33-8 Glanzmann Thrombasthenia vs Bernard-Soulier Syndrome

	Glanzmann Thrombasthenia	Bernard-Soulier Syndrome
Epidemiology	International frequency data unknown; increased incidence in certain ethnic groups (South Indian Hindus, Iraqi Jews, French gypsies, and Jordanian nomadic tribes) and families with consanguinity	Estimated prevalence less than 1 in 1 million
Pathophysiology	Defective platelet aggregation due to quantitative or qualitative defect of platelet GpIIbIIIa (fibrinogen receptor)	Defective platelet adhesion due to quantitative or qualitative defects of platelet GpIb-IX-V receptor complex (von Willebrand factor receptor)
Inheritance	Autosomal recessive	Autosomal recessive
Thrombocytopenia	No	Yes (of variable severity)
Aggregation studies	Absent platelet aggregation in response to all agonists except ristocetin	Failure to aggregate with ristocetin, normal aggregation response to other agonists
Diagnosis	Flow cytometric studies of platelet surface glycoprotein expression, GpIIa/IIb	Flow cytometric studies of platelet surface glycoprotein expression, GpIb/IX

Table 33-9 Platelet Transfusion Thresholds in Neonates (Platelet Counts × 10⁹/L)[a]

Published Guidelines	Nonbleeding		Term	Bleeding	Prior to Invasive Procedure	ECMO
	Preterm					
	Stable	Unstable				
Most restrictive	<20	<30	<20	<50	<50	<100
Least restrictive	<50	<100	<30	<100	<100	

Abbreviations: ECMO, extracorporeal membrane oxygenation.
[a]Data from Blanchette et al[23] and Gibson et al.[24]

guidelines[23,24] (Table 33-9). Recent recommendations are, however, more restrictive, accepting lower platelet triggers for transfusions due to recognition that the clinical condition is an important determinant of the risk of bleeding and because of concerns regarding the risks of platelet transfusions (such as transfusion-related acute lung injury, bacterial contamination, and alloimmunization).

Treatment of infants with suspected FNAIT should be initiated promptly and without waiting for definitive test results. The mainstay therapy is platelet transfusions, which should be given in nonbleeding well neonates if the platelet count is less than 30×10^9/L and in neonates with ICH or other major bleeding events if the platelet count is less than $50–100 \times 10^9$/L.[14,24] HPA-1a/5b-negative platelets compatible in more than 90% of cases with FNAIT or washed, irradiated maternal platelets are the platelet products of choice because they result in higher and longer-lasting platelet count increments; if, however, matched platelets are not immediately available, random donor platelets should be given instead.[16] Intravenous immunoglobulin (IVIG) and corticosteroids can also be used as adjuvant therapies.[14] Antenatal management of pregnancies at risk for FNAIT is complex, requiring a multidisciplinary approach. Standard medical treatment consists of weekly IVIG in early pregnancy with or without systemic corticosteroids. Intrauterine platelet antigen-negative platelet transfusions are reserved for medical treatment failures and for prophylaxis of acute hemorrhage at the time of fetal blood sampling.[25] Early cesarean delivery has also been advocated to decrease the risk of ICH, although evidence is lacking.

Recommended management of neonatal ITP consists of close observation in those with platelet counts between 20 and 50×10^9/L at delivery and IVIG in neonates with clinical hemorrhage or platelet counts of less than 20×10^9/L.[26] In addition, cesarean section, unless otherwise indicated for obstetric reasons, and intrapartum fetal platelet count measurements are not recommended.[27]

Finally, in neonates with significant bleeding due to congenital platelet disorders or acquired platelet dysfunction, fibrinolytic inhibitor drugs (ε-aminocaproic acid and tranexamic acid) and recombinant activated factor VII can be used as adjuvants to, or, in some cases, in place of platelet transfusions in patients with BSS or GT who are at increased risk of isoimmunization or alloimmunization from platelet transfusion therapy, which can result in platelet transfusion refractoriness, rendering future platelet transfusions largely ineffective.[28] For certain inherited platelet disorders, such as congenital amegakaryocytic thrombocytopenia and WAS, hematopoietic stem cell transplantation from suitable donors can be curative.

NEONATAL COAGULATION DISORDERS

The neonatal coagulation group of disorders results in impairment of secondary hemostasis, resulting in bleeding that is typically delayed and in deep tissues. Like platelet disorders, inherited or, more commonly, acquired mechanisms are involved. In this section, we describe coagulation disorders that can present in neonates.

Inherited Coagulation Disorders

Inherited coagulation disorders usually present with abnormal bleeding in an otherwise-healthy neonate. Although a positive family history can confirm the diagnosis, an inherited bleeding disorder in the absence of family history is still possible in cases arising as a result new mutations or inherited in an autosomal recessive fashion.

Hemophilia

Hemophilia, the most common inherited bleeding disorder to present in the neonatal period, is due to deficiency of factor VIII (hemophilia A) or, less commonly, factor IX (hemophilia B). Hemophilia is classified according to severity on the basis of plasma procoagulant concentrations as follows:

- Mild hemophilia (<5% but < 40% normal factor [<0.05 to < 0.40 IU/mL])
- Moderately severe hemophilia (1%–5% normal factor [0.01–0.05 IU/mL])
- Severe hemophilia (<1% normal factor [<0.01 IU/mL])

The annual incidences of hemophilia A and B in the United States are 1 in 5000 and 1 in 30,000 male births, respectively; 60% and 44% of these new cases, respectively, have the severe phenotype. In both disorders, thrombin generation is markedly decreased, which leads to delayed formation and poor stability of the hemostatic clot. Both are X-linked recessive disorders caused by a variety of gene mutations (Table 33-10). Of the mutations in hemophilia A, 30%–50% are de novo mutations.

Hemophilia A and B are clinically indistinguishable, and clinical manifestations early in life are almost always confined to boys. Over 50% of hemophiliacs are diagnosed as neonates, of whom up to one-third have clinically significant bleeding.[29] The pattern of bleeding in newborns with hemophilia differs significantly from that in older children and adults. Iatrogenic bleeding is the most common hemorrhagic manifestation, typically presenting as significant oozing or hematoma formation following venous or arterial puncture, heel stick, intramuscular vitamin K injection, or circumcision. Extracranial hemorrhage (ECH), including subgaleal hemorrhage and cephalhematomas as well as ICH,

can also occur in neonates with hemophilia. There is a 1%–4% incidence of ICH in neonates with severe hemophilia.[30,31] ICH is more common than ECH, and the most frequent site of hemorrhage is subdural.[32] Risk factors for cranial bleeding include forceps/vacuum instrumentation during delivery, severe phenotype, and preterm delivery.

Intracranial hemorrhage can have dramatic (seizures, focal deficits) or subtle presentations or can be asymptomatic or "silent." ECH also demands attention as it can cause massive blood loss in neonates with hemophilia. Finally, umbilical, musculoskeletal, and gastrointestinal and other organ bleeding are infrequently encountered in hemophilic neonates.[33]

The diagnosis of hemophilia in neonates requires laboratory confirmation. Isolated prolongation of the activated partial thromboplastin time (aPTT) is usually found on routine coagulation testing. The definitive diagnosis of hemophilia requires measurement of factor levels in uncontaminated cord blood or neonatal venous blood samples. While it is usually possible to confirm a diagnosis of hemophilia A of any severity in the neonatal period irrespective of the gestational age, confirmation of mild hemophilia B is problematic because, unlike factor VIII, factor IX levels are reduced at birth and are further reduced in preterm infants. It is therefore possible to make a diagnosis of severe and moderate hemophilia B at birth, but for mildly affected neonates, confirmation requires repeat testing at 6 months of age or molecular analysis if the genetic defect is known.[33] Controversy exists regarding role, timing, and optimal technique for radiological assessment of ICH in neonates with hemophilia. Recently, the British Committee for Standards in Hematology published guidelines that recommend screening cranial US in all neonates with severe or moderate hemophilia prior to discharge and cranial magnetic resonance imaging (MRI) or computed tomographic (CT) scanning in symptomatic neonates even if the US is normal due to the low sensitivity of US for the detection of subdural bleeding.[34]

The management of neonatal hemophilia can be summarized as follows[34]:

- Management during delivery
  - The optimal mode of delivery remains unclear and may be best determined on an individual basis, taking into account obstetric and hemostatic factors.
  - Vacuum extraction, forceps, and invasive monitoring procedures, such as placement of fetal scalp electrodes and fetal scalp blood sampling, should all be avoided.
- Management in the postnatal period
  - Intramuscular vitamin K should be withheld until hemophilia is excluded. Oral vitamin K can be given instead if there is a delay in diagnosis or if hemophilia is confirmed.

Table 33-10 Genetic Defects in Hemophilia

Phenotype	Hemophilia A	Hemophilia B
Mild-moderate disease	• Missense mutations[a] • Splicing defects • Small deletions/insertions	• Missense mutations[a] • Small deletions/insertions
Severe disease	• Gross rearrangements (intron 22 inversion,[a] intron 1 inversion) • Missense mutations • Nonsense mutations • Splicing defects • Large deletions/insertions	• Missense mutations[a] • Nonsense mutations • Large deletions/insertions

[a]The most frequent causative gene defect responsible for the corresponding phenotype.

- Following confirmation of diagnosis, short-term prophylactic replacement therapy (with specific factor concentrates) may be given to neonates following traumatic, instrumented, or preterm delivery or a prolonged second stage of labor.
- Management of clinically significant bleeding in neonates
  - Prior to confirmation of diagnosis, fresh-frozen plasma (15–25 mL/kg) should be given.
  - After confirmation of diagnosis, recombinant factor VIII or IX concentrates should be given with close monitoring as neonates may require higher doses to achieve desired factor levels and may demonstrate a shortened factor half-life.

von Willebrand Disease

Despite being the most common inherited bleeding disorder overall, initial presentation/identification of most forms of von Willebrand disease (vWD) in neonates is rare owing to physiologically increased vWF concentration and function in neonates compared to adults. vWD is classified as type 1 disease, which is a partial quantitative deficiency in vWF; type 2 disease, which is characterized by various qualitative (functional) defects in vWF; and type 3 disease, which is caused by total quantitative deficiency of vWF. While most types of vWD are inherited in an autosomal dominant fashion, type 3 is recessively inherited. Laboratory tests in vWD usually include measurements of plasma vWF antigen (vWF:Ag), vWF function by vWF ristocetin cofactor assay (vWF:RCo), and factor VIII coagulant activity (FVIII:C) and assessment of the molecular weight profile of circulating plasma vWF (vWF multimers). Two types of vWD can present in neonates:

1. Type 2B vWD is characterized by increased affinity of vWF to platelets, leading to the formation of circulating platelet aggregates that are reversibly sequestered in the microcirculation. Neonates with this type can present with moderate thrombocytopenia and bleeding, and this rare type of vWD should be considered in the differential diagnosis of unexplained neonatal thrombocytopenia.

2. vWD type 3, the most severe form, represents 1% or less of all VWD cases but is the type most likely to present in neonates. Bleeding manifestations are variable; mucosal bleeding is more common than in hemophilia A, while ICH is almost unheard of in type 3 vWD, which may be attributed to low but residual factor VIII activity.[35] On coagulation testing, type 3 vWD is characterized by prolonged aPTT, undetectable vWF:Ag and vWF:Rco, very low FVIII:C (<1 IU/mL), and absent vWD multimers.

Due to clinical and laboratory overlap with severe hemophilia A, testing for type 3 vWD should be considered in neonates with suspected severe hemophilia A particularly when the clinical course or the laboratory data are not typical.

Management of bleeding in vWD requires factor replacement using plasma-derived vWF-containing factor VIII concentrate. Due to the risks of hyponatremia, desmopressin acetate (DDAVP, desamino-D-arginine vasopressin) should not be used in the treatment of neonatal vWD.[36]

Rare Inherited Coagulation Disorders

The group of rare inherited coagulopathies comprises less than 5% of all inherited deficiencies of coagulation. They are generally transmitted as autosomal recessive traits. Unlike hemophilia, causative mutations, identifiable in 80%–90% of patients, are private (ie, unique for each affected kindred).[37] Because of their rarity, data on clinical manifestations and management are relatively limited, but it is clear that a number of these disorders are associated with a severe bleeding tendency, which may manifest itself in neonates (Table 33-11).[39] Typical manifestations in neonates include soft tissue bleeding, umbilical stump bleeding, and postcircumcision bleeding. ICH is also a relatively common feature of these disorders.[39] These disorders should be suspected in neonates with bleeding tendency and prolonged clotting times. A prolonged prothrombin time (PT) with a normal aPTT is indicative of factor VII deficiency, whereas a prolonged aPTT with a normal PT is indicative of factor XI deficiency, provided that vWD and hemophilia have been ruled out. The prolongation of both tests should point to the possible deficiencies of factor X, factor V, prothrombin, or fibrinogen; dysfibrinogenemia; or combined factor deficiencies. Factor XIII deficiency is an exception in that both PT and aPTT are normal; factor XIII assays or urea clot stability assays are commonly used to screen for this factor deficiency. Confirmation of diagnosis is achieved by specific factor coagulant activity assays and rarely antigen assays. Although DNA mutation analysis is rarely performed, results can be useful for prenatal diagnosis.[37]

Acquired Coagulation Disorders

Acquired deficiency or impairment of coagulation is a frequently encountered complication of other disease processes in sick neonates. In this next section, we review three important acquired coagulopathies in neonates: vitamin K deficiency, disseminated intravascular coagulation (DIC), and coagulopathy of liver disease.

Vitamin K Deficiency

As previously discussed, vitamin K is a critical cofactor required for posttranslational modification of

Table 33-11 Rare Inherited Coagulation Disorders That Can Present in the Neonatal Period[a]

Disorder	Estimated Prevalence[b]	Treatment
Afibrinogenemia[c]	1	Cryoprecipitate and fibrinogen concentrates
Factor II deficiency	0.5	FFP and PCC
Factor V deficiency	1	FFP
Factor VII deficiency	2	FFP and recombinant factor VIIa
Factor X deficiency	1	FFP and PCC
Factor XI deficiency	1	FFP and factor XI concentrate
Factor XIII deficiency[d]	0.5	Cryoprecipitate, FFP, and factor XIII concentrate
Combined factor V and factor VIII deficiency	0.5	FFP
Combined vitamin K–dependent coagulation factor deficiency[e]	0.5	Vitamin K (oral or parentral), FFP

Abbreviations: FFP, fresh-frozen plasma; PCC, prothrombin complex concentrate.
[a]Data from Bolton-Maggs et al.[38]
[b]Per 1 million population.
[c]Inherited fibrinogen disorders can manifest as quantitative defects (afibrinogenemia and hypofibrinogenemia) or qualitative defects (dysfibrinogenemia). Neonatal presentation is usually seen in afibrinogenemia, which is characterized by the complete deficiency of plasma fibrinogen.
[d]In addition to bleeding tendency, affected neonates can have impaired wound healing
[e]Severely affected neonates may also exhibit features that resemble "warfarin embryopathy," including nasal hypoplasia, distal digital hypoplasia, epiphyseal stippling, and mild conductive hearing loss attributed to dysfunction of other vitamin K–dependent proteins (osteocalcin and matrix Gla proteins).

several coagulation proteins. In the absence of vitamin K, these proteins are dysfunctional and are released into the circulation in a decarboxylated form known as *proteins induced by vitamin K absence* (PIVKA). The presence of PIVKA without coagulation deficit indicates subclinical vitamin K deficiency.[1] The recommended daily dietary intake of vitamin K is 1 µg/kg body weight.[1] Vitamin K deficiency can be idiopathic or secondary. Secondary causes include the following:

1. Inadequate intake, which can occur in infants exclusively receiving unsupplemented breast feedings, on broad-spectrum antibiotics that eliminate intestinal vitamin K–producing bacteria, or are receiving total parenteral nutrition without vitamin K supplementation

2. Poor absorption or fat malabsorption state due to cholestatic liver disease, pancreatic insufficiency, or intestinal disorders (eg, short-bowel syndrome)

3. Poor utilization, as seen in significant liver disease

4. Vitamin K antagonism due to warfarin therapy

Vitamin K deficiency bleeding (VKDB) is a rare but potentially life-threatening bleeding disorder that presents in three different patterns (Table 33-12).

Isolated prolongation of the PT is the earliest laboratory evidence of vitamin K deficiency, followed

Table 33-12 Vitamin K Deficiency Bleeding Presentations in Neonates[a]

Presentation	Bleeding Sites	Etiologies
Early (first 24 hours)	Scalp, subperiosteal, skin, intracranial, intrathoracic, intra-abdominal	Maternal drugs (eg, warfarin, anticonvulsants)
Classical (days 1–7)	Gastrointestinal, umbilical, skin, nose, circumcision	Mainly idiopathic, breast feeding (low-milk intake)
Late (≥day 8; peak 3–8 weeks)	Intracranial, skin, gastrointestinal	Idiopathic or secondary, exclusive breast feeding in the absence of vitamin K administration, undiagnosed cholestasis often present; secondary cases from malabsorption due to underlying disease (eg, bilary atresia, α-1-antitrypsin, cystic fibrosis) or to chronic diarrhea; antibiotic therapy sometimes implicated

[a]Data from Van Winckel et al.[1]

by prolongation of the aPTT. The diagnosis is confirmed by correction of these parameters by vitamin K administration or by assays of the specific factors. Other confirmatory tests, such as measurement of decarboxyprothrombin (PIVKA-II) and measurement of vitamin K concentrations, are rarely available for routine laboratory use.[36]

Treatment of VKDB requires parenteral vitamin K administration by slow intravenous infusion or subcutaneously if venous access cannot be established. For neonates who are bleeding, fresh-frozen plasma should also be given. Prothrombin complex concentrates (PCCs) should be considered in the presence of life-threatening hemorrhage or ICH when it is necessary to rapidly normalize the levels of the depleted coagulation factors.[36] In the United States, prevention of VKDB by administration of a single intramuscular injection of vitamin K soon after birth is the current standard practice and has been almost universally effective.[40]

Disseminated Intravascular Coagulation

Disseminated intravascular coagulation (DIC) is a clinicopathological syndrome that is characterized by systemic activation of coagulation and fibrinolysis, consumption of platelets and coagulation factors, and generation of fibrin clots that can lead to ischemic organ damage or failure. DIC represents a continuum in severity, with definable phases characterized by initial localization and compensation (nonovert or compensated DIC) that progresses into widespread dysregulation of coagulation and fibrinolysis (overt or decompensated DIC).

Although the risk of developing DIC is believed to be highest in neonates, accurate data on the epidemiology of DIC in neonates are lacking due to difficulties in establishing the diagnosis and consequent underestimation of the true frequency of this disorder.[41] DIC in neonates can be triggered by a variety of pathological conditions (Table 33-13). The cardinal manifestations of overt DIC are due to excessive bleeding and microvascular thrombosis. Hemorrhagic symptoms include petechiae and bruising, oozing from venipuncture sites, bleeding from traumatic and surgical wounds, and in severe cases, bleeding involving internal organs; thrombosis typically manifests as biochemical or clinical evidence of end-organ dysfunction. Kasabach-Merritt syndrome (KMS) represents a localized form of DIC seen in association with cutaneous or occasionally visceral congenital vascular lesions. Although several cases of KMS complicating classic capillary hemangiomas of infancy have been published, kaposiform hemangioendothelioma and tufted angiomas are more frequently reported.[42] The pathophysiology of KMS is generally presumed to be that of platelet trapping by abnormally proliferating endothelium within the hemangioma.

This results in the activation of platelets with a secondary consumption of clotting factors. The diagnosis of DIC, particularly in the early stages, can be problematic because there is no single laboratory test that can establish or rule out DIC. Hence, the diagnosis is often made on the basis of an appropriate clinical suspicion supported by laboratory evidence of procoagulant and fibrinolytic system activation coupled with anticoagulant consumption. Laboratory abnormalities seen in DIC include thrombocytopenia, elevated fibrin degradation products (FDPs) or D-dimers, prolonged PT, prolonged aPTT, prolonged TCT, and low fibrinogen. In this regard, it is important to remember that serial testing may be necessary for diagnosis given the dynamic nature of DIC and that fibrinogen is an acute-phase reactant; therefore, plasma concentrations can remain well within the normal range despite ongoing consumption.

Successful treatment of DIC relies largely on reversal of the underlying condition and supporting adequate blood flow and oxygen delivery. Blood component transfusions (platelets, fresh-frozen plasma, and cryoprecipitate) are an important part of supportive treatment of DIC. In cases of DIC in which thrombosis predominates, such as arterial or venous thromboembolism or severe purpura fulminans (PF), therapeutic anticoagulation with unfractionated heparin may be considered. Except for the use of protein C concentrates in PF due to protein C deficiency, anticoagulant concentrates (protein C, antithrombin), recombinant factor VIIa, and recombinant tissue plasminogen activator are not generally indicated for the routine treatment of DIC.

Coagulopathy of Acute Liver Disease

Acute liver disease affects hemostasis in several different ways. Hemostatic abnormalities associated with acute liver failure include thrombocytopenia and thrombocytopathy, decreased production of coagulation factors, vitamin K deficiency, reduced vitamin K–dependent

Table 33-13 Common Causes of Disseminated Intravascular Coagulation in Neonates

- Sepsis
- Perinatal hypoxia-ischemia (perinatal asphyxia, placental abruption)
- Necrotizing enterocolitis
- Severe hepatic dysfunction
- Respiratory disorders (RDS, MAS)
- Metabolic disorders (galactosemia, others)
- Vascular anomalies (Kasabach-Merritt syndrome)
- Hematological disorders (purpura fulminans due to protein C/protein S deficiency, erythroblastosis fetalis)

Abbreviations: MAS, meconium aspiration syndrome; RDS, respiratory distress syndrome.

γ-carboxylase activity, acquired dysfibrinogenemia, decreased fibrinolytic activity, and DIC. The net result is a complex bleeding diathesis of variable severity. Although spontaneous bleeding is rare, serious bleeding after invasive procedures can occur.

Coagulation testing often shows prolonged PT and aPTT, thrombocytopenia, decreased fibrinogen level, and decreased concentrations of factors VII and V. A normal or elevated factor VIII concentration distinguishes primary liver disease from DIC.[43] Conventional coagulation assays, however, do not fully reflect the hemostatic status and do not predict risk of bleeding. Hence, there is no benefit to correcting coagulopathy in nonbleeding neonates. Treatment of active hemorrhage includes blood product transfusions (fresh-frozen plasma, cryoprecipitate, platelets) and vitamin K administration. Recombinant factor VIIa has also been used successfully to maintain hemostasis, although there is an increased risk of thrombosis in this setting.[43,44]

REFERENCES

1. Van Winckel M, De Bruyne R, Van De Velde S, Van Biervliet S. Vitamin K, an update for the paediatrician. *Eur J Pediatr.* 2009;168(2):127–134.
2. Andrew M, Paes B, Milner R, et al. Development of the human coagulation system in the healthy premature infant. *Blood.* 1988;72(5):1651–1657.
3. Andrew M, Paes B, Milner R, et al. Development of the human coagulation system in the full-term infant. *Blood.* 1987;70(1):165–172.
4. Israels SJ, Rand ML, Michelson AD. Neonatal platelet function. *Semin Thromb Hemost.* 2003;29(4):363–372.
5. Witt I, Muller H, Kunzer W. Evidence for the existence of foetal fibrinogen. *Thromb Diath Haemorrh.* 1969;22(1):101–109.
6. Monagle P, Ignjatovic V, Savoia H. Hemostasis in neonates and children: pitfalls and dilemmas. *Blood Rev.* 2010;24(2):63–68.
7. Roberts I, Stanworth S, Murray NA. Thrombocytopenia in the neonate. *Blood Rev.* 2008;22(4):173–186.
8. Wiedmeier SE, Henry E, Sola-Visner MC, Christensen RD. Platelet reference ranges for neonates, defined using data from over 47,000 patients in a multihospital healthcare system. *J Perinatol.* 2009;29(2):130–136.
9. Roberts I, Murray NA. Neonatal thrombocytopenia: causes and management. *Arch Dis Child Fetal Neonatal Ed.* 2003;88(5):F359–F364.
10. Sola-Visner M, Saxonhouse MA, Brown RE. Neonatal thrombocytopenia: what we do and don't know. *Early Hum Dev.* 2008;84(8):499–506.
11. Christensen RD, Henry E, Wiedmeier SE, et al. Thrombocytopenia among extremely low birth weight neonates: data from a multihospital healthcare system. *J Perinatol.* 2006;26(6):348–353.
12. Baer VL, Lambert DK, Henry E, Christensen RD. Severe thrombocytopenia in the NICU. *Pediatrics.* 2009;124(6):e1095–e1100.
13. Sola MC, Rimsza LM. Mechanisms underlying thrombocytopenia in the neonatal intensive care unit. *Acta Paediatr Suppl.* 2002;91(438):66–73.
14. Bussel J. Diagnosis and management of the fetus and neonate with alloimmune thrombocytopenia. *J Thromb Haemost.* 2009;7(Suppl 1):253–257.
15. Davoren A, Curtis BR, Aster RH, McFarland JG. Human platelet antigen-specific alloantibodies implicated in 1162 cases of neonatal alloimmune thrombocytopenia. *Transfusion.* 2004;44(8):1220–1225.
16. Arnold DM, Smith JW, Kelton JG. Diagnosis and management of neonatal alloimmune thrombocytopenia. *Transfus Med Rev.* 2008;22(4):255–267.
17. Webert KE, Mittal R, Sigouin C, Heddle NM, Kelton JG. A retrospective 11-year analysis of obstetric patients with idiopathic thrombocytopenic purpura. *Blood.* 2003;102(13):4306–4311.
18. Valat AS, Caulier MT, Devos P, et al. Relationships between severe neonatal thrombocytopenia and maternal characteristics in pregnancies associated with autoimmune thrombocytopenia. *Br J Haematol.* 1998;103(2):397–401.
19. Jensen JD, Wiedmeier SE, Henry E, Silver RM, Christensen RD. Linking maternal platelet counts with neonatal platelet counts and outcomes using the data repositories of a multihospital health care system. *Am J Perinatol.* 2011;28(8):597–604.
20. Bolton-Maggs PH, Chalmers EA, Collins PW, et al. A review of inherited platelet disorders with guidelines for their management on behalf of the UKHCDO. *Br J Haematol.* 2006;135(5):603–633.
21. Nurden P, Nurden AT. Congenital disorders associated with platelet dysfunctions. *Thromb Haemost.* 2008;99(2):253–263.
22. Christensen RD. Platelet transfusion in the neonatal intensive care unit: benefits, risks, alternatives. *Neonatology.* 2011;100(3):311–318.
23. Blanchette VS, Hume HA, Levy GJ, Luban NL, Strauss RG. Guidelines for auditing pediatric blood transfusion practices. *Am J Dis Child.* 1991;145(7):787–796.
24. Gibson BE, Todd A, Roberts I, et al. Transfusion guidelines for neonates and older children. *Br J Haematol.* 2004;124(4):433–453.
25. Bussel JB, Primiani A. Fetal and neonatal alloimmune thrombocytopenia: progress and ongoing debates. *Blood Rev.* 2008;22(1):33–52.
26. Provan D, Stasi R, Newland AC, et al. International consensus report on the investigation and management of primary immune thrombocytopenia. *Blood.* 2010;115(2):168–186.
27. Neunert C, Lim W, Crowther M, Cohen A, Solberg L Jr, Crowther MA. The American Society of Hematology 2011 evidence-based practice guideline for immune thrombocytopenia. *Blood.* 2011;117(16):4190–4207.
28. Simon D, Kunicki T, Nugent D. Platelet function defects. *Haemophilia.* 2008;14(6):1240–1249.
29. Conway JH, Hilgartner MW. Initial presentations of pediatric hemophiliacs. *Arch Pediatr Adolesc Med.* 1994;148(6):589–594.
30. Kulkarni R, Soucie JM, Lusher J, et al. Sites of initial bleeding episodes, mode of delivery and age of diagnosis in babies with haemophilia diagnosed before the age of 2 years: a report from the Centers for Disease Control and Prevention's (CDC) Universal Data Collection (UDC) project. *Haemophilia.* 2009;15(6):1281–1290.
31. Tarantino MD, Gupta SL, Brusky RM. The incidence and outcome of intracranial haemorrhage in newborns with haemophilia: analysis of the Nationwide Inpatient Sample database. *Haemophilia.* 2007;13(4):380–382.
32. Kulkarni R, Lusher JM. Intracranial and extracranial hemorrhages in newborns with hemophilia: a review of the literature. *J Pediatr Hematol Oncol.* 1999;21(4):289–295.
33. Chalmers EA. Haemophilia and the newborn. *Blood Rev.* 2004;18(2):85–92.

34. Chalmers E, Williams M, Brennand J, Liesner R, Collins P, Richards M. Guideline on the management of haemophilia in the fetus and neonate. *Br J Haematol.* 2011;154(2):208–215.

35. Wetzstein V, Budde U, Oyen F, et al. Intracranial hemorrhage in a term newborn with severe von Willebrand disease type 3 associated with sinus venous thrombosis. *Haematologica.* 2006;91(12 Suppl):ECR60.

36. Williams MD, Chalmers EA, Gibson BE. The investigation and management of neonatal haemostasis and thrombosis. *Br J Haematol.* 2002;119(2):295–309.

37. Mannucci PM, Duga S, Peyvandi F. Recessively inherited coagulation disorders. *Blood.* 2004;104(5):1243–1252.

38. Bolton-Maggs PH, Perry DJ, Chalmers EA, et al. The rare coagulation disorders—review with guidelines for management from the United Kingdom Haemophilia Centre Doctors' Organisation. *Haemophilia.* 2004;10(5):593–628.

39. Chalmers EA. Neonatal coagulation problems. *Arch Dis Child Fetal Neonatal Ed.* 2004;89(6):F475–F478.

40. American Academy of Pediatrics Vitamin K Ad Hoc Task Force. Controversies concerning vitamin K and the newborn. *Pediatrics.* 1993;91(5):1001–1003.

41. Veldman A, Fischer D, Nold MF, Wong FY. Disseminated intravascular coagulation in term and preterm neonates. *Semin Thromb Hemost.* 2010;36(4):419–428.

42. Hall GW. Kasabach-Merritt syndrome: pathogenesis and management. *Br J Haematol.* 2001;112(4):851–862.

43. Saxonhouse MA, Manco-Johnson MJ. The evaluation and management of neonatal coagulation disorders. *Semin Perinatol.* 2009;33(1):52–65.

44. Witmer CM, Huang YS, Lynch K, Raffini LJ, Shah SS. Off-label recombinant factor VIIa use and thrombosis in children: a multi-center cohort study. *J Pediatr.* 2011;158(5):820–825.e1.

Thrombophilic Disorders

Karen E. Effinger and Michael R. Jeng

INTRODUCTION

Thromboembolic events are rare in childhood; however, neonates are disproportionately affected by thrombosis. The propensity for neonates to clot may be due to several contributing factors. First, neonates have an immature hemostatic system, which generally gives them physiologic thrombophilia. In addition, they are at high risk for sepsis, which leads to thrombosis due to inflammation or disseminated intravascular coagulopathy (DIC). The high use of central catheters, both arterial and venous, in neonates also increases their risk of thrombosis. Although often considered in neonatal thrombosis, the contributing role of inherited thrombophilias in both arterial and venous thrombotic events in this age group remains poorly defined.

Clinicians caring for neonates should be especially aware of clinical thrombotic events common in the neonate, including portal vein thrombosis, renal vein thrombosis, purpura fulminans, and neonatal stroke. The portal vein is a commonly affected anatomic vein, which is attributed to the use of central catheters. Renal vein thromboses have long been recognized as occurring spontaneously in neonates. Neonatal purpura fulminans is a rare condition of dermal microvascular thrombosis associated with DIC and perivascular hemorrhage. This is often associated with inherited thrombophilias, specifically protein C deficiency. Neonatal central nervous system thrombotic events, including cerebral sinovenous thrombosis and neonatal ischemic stroke, are important thrombotic events. These are discussed in detail in another chapter. In addition to familiarity with these sites of thromboses, it is crucial for clinicians to be aware of the different treatments that may be considered for the best long-term outcomes.

VENOUS THROMBI

The majority of neonatal thrombi occur in the venous system, and most are associated with the placement of central venous catheters. Many of these cases are asymptomatic, though catheter-associated thrombi may present with catheter dysfunction. Symptomatic thrombi often present with swelling of the limbs and lower body in the case of inferior vena cava thrombosis versus swelling of the arm, head, and neck seen in superior vena cava thrombosis (otherwise known as SVC syndrome). Due to the frequent use of umbilical venous lines, neonates also may develop portal vein thrombosis, which can lead to hepatic lobar atrophy or portal hypertension. Intracardiac thrombosis may also develop. These thrombi are usually located in the right atrium and are often associated with central venous lines. The most frequent location for spontaneous venous thrombi in neonates is in the renal veins. Infants with renal vein thrombosis may present with macroscopic or microscopic hematuria, thrombocytopenia, or a palpable flank mass.

ARTERIAL THOMBI

Neonatal arterial thrombi outside the central nervous system are almost exclusively due to iatrogenic causes. Rarely, a spontaneous thrombus may develop in the aorta. Femoral artery catheters used for cardiac catheterization and umbilical artery or peripheral arterial catheters used for blood pressure and blood gas monitoring are the main risk factors for arterial thrombi. These cases may be asymptomatic or present with signs of ischemia or organ dysfunction. Involved extremities usually become cool and pale with poor perfusion. If the thrombus occludes the renal artery or mesenteric artery, the infant may develop hypertension with renal failure or necrotizing enterocolitis.

MATERNAL RISK FACTORS

The influence of maternal thrombophilia and prenatal risks on the development of neonatal thrombosis is not well defined. There have been reports of peri- and neonatal infarction associated with thrombosis and infarction of the placenta. Preeclampsia, gestational diabetes, chorioamnionitis, and maternal smoking or drug use have all been associated with increased risk of thrombosis (Table 34-1). Maternal antiphospholipid syndrome (APS) is another rare cause of neonatal thrombosis.

Table 34-1 Acquired Risk Factors for the Development of Neonatal Thrombosis[a]

Neonatal Risk Factors	Delivery Risk Factors	Maternal Risk Factors
Catheter placement Asphyxia Dehydration Sepsis Congenital heart disease Congenital nephrotic syndrome Polycythemia Total parenteral nutrition (TPN) use Surgery Extracorporeal membrane oxygenation (ECMO)	Bradycardia Cesarean section	Gestational diabetes Chorioamionitis Preeclampsia Antiphospholipid syndrome Smoking Polydrug use Oligohydramnios Maternal thrombosis

[a]From Revel-Vilk and Ergaz[1]; Saracco et al[2]; and Saxonhouse and Manco Johnson.[3]

INFANT RISK FACTORS

The majority of neonates who develop thrombi have associated risk factors. The most notable risk factor is the presence of a central venous catheter, which is present in approximately 90% of neonates with thrombosis.[4,5] In addition, neonatal thrombosis may be the initial presentation of an inherited thrombophilia. Other risk factors include sepsis, asphyxia, heart disease, surgery, dehydration, and nephrotic syndrome (Table 34-1).

Developmental Hemostasis

Prior to the 1980s, there was no concept of developmental hemostasis as it was presumed that children and adults had similar hemostatic systems. Dr. Maureen Andrew conducted 2 seminal studies to evaluate the human coagulation system in neonates. Her studies analyzed blood samples from 93 healthy, full-term infants and 137 healthy preterm infants born between 30 and 36 weeks estimated gestational age. At various time points throughout the first 6 months of life, she tested plasma concentration levels of coagulation and anticoagulation factors in the infants.

Her studies revealed that the neonatal hemostatic system evolves rapidly from birth through infancy. Plasma concentrations of coagulation and anticoagulation factors are drastically different from those found in adults. The results showed that levels of indigenous anticoagulants, such as antithrombin, protein C, and protein S, are less than 50% of the normal adult levels in the neonatal period, which is only somewhat balanced by an increase in serum concentrations of α2-macroglobulin (Tables 34-2 and 34-3). However, most of serum procoagulant concentrations are also decreased in newborns (see discussion in another chapter).

In addition, the fibrinolytic pathway is altered in newborns. Although newborns have increased tissue plasminogen activator (tPA), plasminogen levels are about 50% of adult levels, and neonatal plasminogen has a qualitative impairment, requiring more tPA for activation. Also, plasminogen activator inhibitor (PAI) is increased, making the fibrinolytic pathway in infants less active.[2]

These alterations in pro- and anticoagulant concentrations form an equilibrium in healthy infants that prevents significant hemorrhagic or thrombotic complications. However, due to these variations, neonates, especially preterm ones, are at an increased risk of shifting this equilibrium toward bleeding or thrombotic complications in the presence of illness, instrumentation, or other hemostatic challenges.

Table 34-2 Reference Values for the Inhibition of Coagulation in the Healthy Full-Term Infant During the First 6 Months of Life[a]

Inhibitors	Day 1 (n)	Day 5 (n)	Day 30 (n)	Day 90 (n)	Day 180 (n)	Adult (n)
Antithrombin	0.63 ± 0.12 (58)	0.67 ± 0.13 (74)	0.78 ± 0.15 (66)	0.97 ± 0.12 (60)[b]	1.04 ± 0.10 (56)[b]	1.05 ± 0.13 (28)
α_2-macroglobulin	1.39 ± 0.22 (54)	1.48 ± 0.25 (73)	1.50 ± 0.22 (61)	1.76 ± 0.25 (55)	1.91 ± 0.21 (55)	0.86 ± 0.17 (29)
α_2-antiplasmin	0.85 ± 0.15 (55)	100 ± 0.15 (75)[b]	1.00 ± 0.12 (62)[b]	1.08 ± 0.16 (55)[b]	1.11 ± 0.14 (53)[b]	1.02 ± 0.17 (29)
C1 esterase inhibitor	0.72 ± 0.18 (59)	0.90 ± 0.15 (76)[b]	0.89 ± 0.21 (63)	1.15 ± 0.22 (55)	1.41 ± 0.26 (55)	1.01 ± 0.15 (29)
α_1-antitrypsin	0.93 ± 0.22 (57)[b]	0.89 ± 0.20 (75)[b]	0.62 ± 0.13 (61)	0.72 ± 0.15 (56)	0.77 ± 0.15 (55)	0.93 ± 0.19 (29)
Heparin cofactor II	0.43 ± 0.25 (56)	0.48 ± 0.24 (72)	0.47 ± 0.20 (58)	0.72 ± 0.37 (58)	1.20 ± 0.35 (55)	0.96 ± 0.15 (29)
Protein C	0.35 ± 0.09 (41)	0.42 ± 0.11 (44)	0.43 ± 0.11 (43)	0.54 ± 0.13 (44)	0.59 ± 0.11 (52)	0.96 ± 0.16 (28)
Protein S	0.36 ± 0.12 (40)	0.50 ± 0.14 (48)	0.63 ± 0.15 (41)	0.86 ± 0.16 (46)[b]	0.87 ± 0.16 (49)[b]	0.92 ± 0.16 (29)

Note. All values are expressed in units per milliliter as the mean ± 1 SD.
[a]From Andrew et al.[6]
[b]Values that do not differ statistically from the adult values.

EPIDEMIOLOGY

The exact incidence of neonatal thrombosis is unknown. A German registry of symptomatic neonatal thrombosis over a 2-year period revealed an incidence of 0.51 per 10,000 births.[8] In a Canadian registry of cases submitted from neonatal intensive care units (NICUs) in North America, Europe, and Australia during a 3.5-year period, the incidence of clinically apparent thrombi, excluding stroke, in infants less than 1 month of age was 24 per 10,000 admissions.[4] Approximately two-thirds to three-fourths of the events were venous thrombi. A 2-year registry of venous thromboembolism from the Netherlands reported an annual incidence of 14.5 per 10,000 children aged 0–28 days.[5]

Renal Vein Thrombosis

Renal vein thrombosis is the most prevalent non-catheter-related thrombosis in neonates; however, its exact incidence is unknown due to the lack of large population-based studies. The estimated incidence in Germany from 1992 to 1994 was 2.2 per 100,000 births, and it accounted for 22%–44% of thrombi reported in 2 large neonatal registries.[4,8] Renal vein thrombosis is more prevalent in males, representing 67% of the cases. Although the cause of the gender difference is unknown, some hypothesize that it is due to differences in renal perfusion or the increased rate of congenital renal malformations in males.[9]

Renal vein thrombosis occurs in both preterm and full-term infants. The time of onset varies, with 67% of cases occurring within 3 days of birth. However, renal vein thrombosis presents antenatally in 7% of cases and in greater than 3 days after birth in 26% of patients.[10] In 70% of cases, renal vein thrombosis is unilateral, and the majority of these cases (64%) involve the left kidney.[10] These thrombi may extend into the inferior vena cava and are occasionally associated with adrenal hemorrhage. Although the classic triad of renal vein thrombosis includes macroscopic hematuria, palpable flank mass, and thrombocytopenia, all 3 are only seen in 13%–22% of cases.[9]

Perinatal risk factors have been found to be associated with renal vein thrombosis. Perinatal asphyxia has been associated in approximately 32% of cases.[10] Renal vein thrombosis is also associated with dehydration, sepsis, congenital heart disease, and maternal diabetes mellitus. These conditions allow for thrombus formation through endothelial injury from hypoxia or endotoxin in the setting of decreased vascular blood flow. In addition, neonates with renal vein thrombosis are more likely to have an inherited thrombophilia.

Neonatal Purpura Fulminans

Neonatal purpura fulminans is a rare, life-threatening disorder that presents with dermal microvascular thrombosis associated with DIC. Often, these

Table 34-3 Reference Values for Inhibitors of Coagulation in Healthy Premature Infants During First 6 Months of Life[a]

Tests	Day 1 M	Day 1 B	Day 5 M	Day 5 B	Day 30 M	Day 30 B	Day 90 M	Day 90 B	Day 180 M	Day 180 B	Adult M	Adult B
Antithrombin (U/mL)	0.38	(0.14–0.62)[b]	1.0.56	(0.30–0.82)[c]	0.59	(0.37–0.81)[d]	0.83	(0.45–1.21)[d]	0.90	(0.52–1.28)[d]	1.05	(0.79–1.31)
α_2 macroglobulin (U/mL)	1.10	(0.56–1.82)[b]	1.25	(0.71–1.77)[c]	1.38	(0.72–2.04)	1.80	(1.20–2.66)[b]	2.09	(1.10–3.21)[b]	0.86	(0.52–1.20)
α_2 antiplasmin (U/mL)	0.78	(0.40–1.16)	0.81	(0.49–1.13)[c]	0.89	(0.55–1.23)[d]	1.06	(0.64–1.48)[c]	1.15	(0.77–1.53)	1.02	(0.68–1.36)
C_1 esterase inhibitor (U/mL)	0.65	(0.31–0.99)	0.83	(0.45–1.21)	0.74	(0.40–1.24)[d]	1.14	(0.60–1.68)[c]	1.40	(0.98–2.04)[b]	1.01	(0.71–1.31)
α_1 antitrypsin (U/mL)	0.90	(0.36–1.44)[c]	0.94	(0.42–1.46)[d]	0.76	(0.38–1.12)[d]	0.81	(0.49–1.13)[c,d]	0.82	(0.48–1.16)[c]	0.93	(0.55–1.31)
Heparin cofactor II (U/mL)	0.32	(0.00–0.60)[d]	0.34	(0.00–0.69)[c]	0.43	(0.15–0.71)	0.61	(0.20–1.11)[b]	0.89	(0.45–1.40)[b–d]	0.96	(0.66–1.26)
Protein C (U/mL)	0.28	(0.12–0.44)[c,d]	0.31	(0.11–0.51)[c]	0.37	(10.15–0.59)[d]	0.45	(0.23–0.67)[d]	0.57	(0.31–0.83)	0.96	(0.64–1.28)
Protein S (U/mL)	0.26	(0.14–0.38)[d]	0.37	(0.13–0.61)[c]	0.56	(0.22–0.90)	0.76	(0.40–1.12)[d]	0.82	(0.44–1.20)	0.92	(0.60–1.24)

All values are expressed in U/mL, where pooled plasma contains 1.0 U/mL. All values are given as a mean (M) followed by lower and upper boundary encompassing 95% of the population (B). Between 40 and 75 samples were assayed for each value for the newborn.
[a]From Andrew et al.[7]
[b]Measurements are skewed owing to a disproportionate number of high values. Lower limit that excludes the lower 2.5% of the population is given (B).
[c]Values indistinguishable from those of adults.
[d]Values different from those of full-term infants.

neonates present 2–12 hours after birth with cutaneous purpura, frequently initiating at the site of previous trauma. The lesions progress from dark red to indurated, purple-black. If left untreated, the areas will become necrotic and gangrenous. In addition to the dermal findings, the neonates may have intracerebral thrombi, vitreous hemorrhage, retinal detachment, and large-vessel thrombosis.

The symptoms are caused by a deficiency of protein C or S. This deficiency may stem from inherited risk factors, such as homozygous protein C or S deficiency, compound heterozygosity, or coinheritance with another inherited thrombophilia. Acquired causes are primarily attributed to infection, with group B *Streptococcus* the most common. Severe hepatic dysfunction, galactosemia, and severe congenital heart disease have also been associated with neonatal purpura fulminans.[11]

PATHOPHYSIOLOGY

The activation of the coagulation cascade leads to thrombus formation. Natural anticoagulants and the fibrinolytic system help to keep the hemostatic system in equilibrium. In neonates, several factors may interfere with the hemostatic system, leading to thrombosis. Some of these factors may be inherited, while others are acquired. Inflammation, leading to damage of the endothelial surface, and foreign bodies, such as catheters, can activate the coagulation cascade. In addition, changes in blood flow that lead to increased stasis may increase an infant's propensity to clot. Often, multiple factors occur at the same time to tip the balance toward thrombosis. Since neonates have a more delicate hemostatic balance, they have a great propensity to develop thrombi with minimal disruptions.

Acquired Risk Factors

The majority of thrombi that develop in neonates occur due to acquired risk factors. Neonatal and maternal factors can lead to thrombosis (Table 34-1).

Catheter-Associated Thrombosis

The placement of central lines is almost ubiquitous in neonates admitted to the hospital. These lines are used for intravenous therapy, blood products, blood sampling and to measure arterial blood pressure. These catheters are typically placed in the umbilical vein, umbilical artery, or a peripheral vein. The thrombotic risks associated with these catheters are thought to be due to vessel injury, blocked blood flow due the large size of the catheter compared to the diameter of the vessel, and thrombogenic catheter materials.

Venous: Umbilical venous catheter (UVC) thrombosis has been documented in 22%–43% of neonates undergoing systemic ultrasound screening.[1] Many times, they are asymptomatic; however, UVC thrombus should be considered in dysfunctional lines, lines with persistent infections, and in infants with persistent thrombocytopenia of unknown etiology. The position of line placement is crucial. UVCs should be inserted to the inferior vena caval–right atrial junction. Of right atrial thrombi, 91% occur in the setting of a central venous line.[12] In addition, portal vein thrombosis is associated with a UVC approximately 75% of the time, and 50% of the time it is associated with aninappropriately placed UVC.[13] Current recommendations are to replace a UVC after 14 days.

Arterial: Arterial thrombi in the neonate are predominantly iatrogenic due to the presence of catheterization of the umbilical, femoral, and peripheral arteries. Studies using ultrasound and angiography evaluation reported an incidence of 14%–35% and 64%, respectively.[2] The majority of these thrombi occur several days after line removal. High-positioned catheters and end-hole catheters tend to have fewer clinical vascular complications. Spontaneous arterial thrombi occur in the aorta of the neonate occasionally, but this is exceedingly rare.

Other Infant Factors

Conditions that cause a hemostatic imbalance place neonates at risk for thrombosis due to alteration in blood flow. Congenital heart disease, asphyxia, dehydration, and polycythemia are all known risk factors. In addition, infection and sepsis increase the risk of thrombus formation by activating clotting factors through inflammation and DIC. Long-term administration of total parenteral nutrition (TPN) can increase endothelial damage and lead to thrombus formation at the catheter tip. Other events that damage the endothelium, such as surgery, can lead to increased risk in the neonate. Infants on extracorporeal membrane oxygenation (ECMO) are at increased risk of thrombosis due to alteration of blood flow as well as endothelial damage. Many of these factors occur in combination with the placement of an intravascular catheter, further increasing the risk to the neonate.

Antiphospholipid Syndrome (APS)

The mother and fetus share their circulatory systems through the placenta. There is an association between thrombosis and infarction of the placenta and thrombosis and infarction in the neonate that is thought to be due to embolization. APS, which is known to cause thrombosis in children and adults, is a rare cause of thrombosis in neonates and occurs in neonates of affected women. APS is defined as the presence of an antiphospholipid antibody and a disease manifestation, including thrombosis, recurrent miscarriages, or premature birth due to preeclampsia, eclampsia, or placental insufficiency. APS can be a primary disorder or associated with autoimmune disorders, such as systemic lupus erythematosus. The antibodies associated with APS include anticardiolipin antibody, lupus anticoagulant, and β2-glycoprotein-I antibody. APS in the mother may be diagnosed after the thrombotic complication in the neonate is observed.

The majority of neonatal thrombi associated with APS are arterial, and many involve the central nervous system. Anticardiolipin antibody, lupus anticoagulant, and β2-glycoprotein-I antibody have all been associated with APS in infants. These antibodies are usually tested in the mother, though they can be detected in the affected infant due to transplacental transfer of the immunoglobulin (Ig) G antibodies. Infants with APS often have additional neonatal risk factors for thrombosis, including catheters, asphyxia, or sepsis.[14]

Maternal Factors

Many maternal factors other than APS may lead to increased risk of neonatal thrombosis. Preeclampsia and gestational diabetes can lead to endothelial damage, which may predispose the placenta to thrombosis. Similarly, chorioamnionitis is associated with inflamed placental vessels and localized thrombosis. Maternal smoking and polydrug use can lead to a variety of placental changes, including vasospasm, endothelial activation, and thrombocytosis. Vascular changes to the placenta may disrupt the delicate hemostatic balance in the infant or lead to thrombosis due to placental embolism.[2]

Inherited Thrombophilias

Inherited thrombophilias are a well-known cause of thrombosis in children and adults. The role that they play in the formation of thrombi in neonates is not well defined. These conditions include protein deficiencies, such as antithrombin, protein C, and protein S. In addition, genetic mutations, including factor V Leiden, prothrombin gene mutation, and methylenetetrahydrofolate reductase (MTHFR) polymorphisms, play a role in thrombosis.

Antithrombin Deficiency

Antithrombin, formerly known as antithrombin III, is a vitamin K–independent protein primarily synthesized in the liver, which inhibits thrombin, factor Xa, and other coagulation serine proteases. A deficiency in this protein leads to a dysregulation of the serine proteases involved in the coagulation cascade, leading to a prothrombotic

Table 34-4 Thrombophilia Testing and Time Until Normalization

Condition	Test	Time of Normalization
Antithrombin deficiency	AT level	6 months of age and off heparin
Protein C deficiency	Protein C activity	6 months of age
Protein S deficiency	Protein S activity	Activity close to normal at birth, total antigen low until 6 months
Factor V Leiden gene mutation	G1691A gene testing	At birth
Prothrombin gene mutation	G20210A gene testing	At birth
MTHFR gene mutation	C677 T gene testing	At birth
Increased homocysteine	Level	At birth
Increased lipoprotein a	Level	1 year of age
Antiphospholipid syndrome	Anticardiolipin, lupus anticoagulant, and β2-glycoprotein-I	Maternal antibodies should be tested

state. The gene encoding antithrombin has been localized to chromosome 1. Mutations in this gene may lead to either a quantitative (type I) or qualitative (type II) deficiency. Familial antithrombin deficiency is inherited in an autosomal dominant fashion, with the homozygous state almost universally fatal in utero. Heterozygous deficiencies occur in 0.02%–0.2% of the general population.[15] In a recent meta-analysis of pediatric patients with deep vein thrombosis, there was an odds ratio of 9.4 for antithrombin deficiency.[16] It is important to note that neonates have a physiologically lower level of antithrombin, which may affect screening for the deficiency (Table 34-4).

Protein C Deficiency

Protein C is a vitamin K–dependent protein synthesized in the liver. It forms an activated complex in conjunction with a protein S cofactor called activated protein C (APC), which prevents excess coagulation through the inactivation of factors Va and VIIIa. Protein C deficiency is due to a mutation on chromosome 2, which may be a quantitative (type I) or qualitative (type II) deficiency. Asymptomatic protein C deficiency occurs in 0.2%–0.5% of the population; clinically significant mutations occur in 1/20,000 individuals.[17] The deficiency is inherited in an autosomal dominant fashion;

however, severe forms, including homozygotes and complex heterozygotes, are less frequent than predicted, presumably due to fetal demise. Protein C levels may be difficult to interpret in the neonate due to physiologically low levels (Table 34-4).

Protein S Deficiency

Protein S is an important vitamin K–dependent cofactor in the protein C complex that is also synthesized primarily in the liver. Deficiencies in this protein lead to a hypercoagulable state by decreasing the function of APC. Protein S deficiency is due to a mutation on chromosome 3 that is inherited in an autosomal dominant fashion. The quantitative type I and III deficiencies are much more common than the rare qualitative type II deficiency. Heterozygous protein S deficiency occurs in 1%–13% of all individuals with venous thrombosis.[18] Homozygous individuals are extremely rare as homozygosity is usually incompatible with life. Total protein S levels are markedly decreased in newborns, though functional levels may only be slightly reduced. Care should be taken in interpreting these values in newborns (Table 34-4).

Factor V Leiden Mutation

Factor Va Leiden, named for the town in which it was first discovered, is the most common cause of inherited thrombophilia. Factor Va Leiden mutation confers resistance of factor Va to inactivation by APC, leading to a hypercoagulable state. It is an autosomal dominant point mutation in the factor V gene on chromosome 1 that is characterized by a guanine-to-adenine substitution at position 1691 (G1691A). This mutation occurs in 0.5%–5% of the population, with Caucasians having the highest frequency. Homozygosity occurs in 1 in 5000 individuals and leads to a higher incidence of thrombosis at a younger age.[19]

Prothrombin G20210A Mutation

Prothrombin gene mutation, which leads to the substitution of an adenine for guanine at the 20210 position of the prothrombin (factor II) gene on chromosome 11, leads to increased levels of prothrombin. This increase in plasma prothrombin levels confers an increased thrombotic risk. Prothrombin G20210A mutation is autosomal dominant and occurs in approximately 2% of the US population. Like factor V Leiden, it is more prevalent in Caucasians. Approximately 1 in 10,000 individuals is a homozygote, which confers a higher rate of thrombosis.[19]

Homocysteine

Increased homocysteine levels have been associated with both venous and arterial thrombosis. A common genetic polymorphism that can affect homocysteine levels is mutation in the MTHFR gene. MTHFR is an enzyme that converts 5,10-methylenetetrahydrofolate to 5-methylenetetrahydrofolate. 5-Methylenetetrahydrofolate is a cofactor that is utilized in the conversion of homocysteine to methionine. A common polymorphism in the gene encoding for MTHFR, in which a cytosine is replaced with a thymine at position 677 (MTHFR C677T), is found in many populations. This polymorphism confers a decrease in activity of the MTHFR and thus lower availability of 5-methylenetetrahdrofolate and an increase in homocysteine levels. Therefore, testing for either MTHFR C677T mutations or, more directly, elevated homocysteine levels may be indicated in neonates with thrombosis. Both the heterozygous and homozygous states are commonly encountered, with the latter conferring a higher thrombophilic risk compared to the heterozygote state. However, MTHFR mutation does not confer risk without elevation in homocysteine.[19]

DIAGNOSTIC TESTING

Radiologic Testing

Thrombi are diagnosed using imaging. The gold standard for diagnosis of a thrombus is angiography; however, angiography requires contrast and radiation. Ultrasounds and echocardiograms are often used instead of angiography as they can be performed at bedside in the case of critically ill neonates. In studies, both ultrasound and echocardiography have been shown to have lower sensitivity when compared to venography.[1] Similarly, the incidence of arterial thrombosis was found to be 14%–35% using ultrasound and 64% with angiography.[2] This decrease in sensitivity may be attributed to the difficulty in interpreting whether the reduced compressibility of the vessel by the ultrasound probe is due to the catheter or a thrombus. In addition, the low pulse pressure of ill neonates may limit interpretation.

Renal Vein Thrombosis

Ultrasonography has replaced venography for the diagnosis of renal vein thrombosis as the sensitivity is high in evaluating the renal veins. The ultrasound findings vary depending on the time of onset and severity. Echogenic streaks are seen within the first few days and correlate to intralobular and interlobular thrombosis. In addition, the corticomedullary junction may be lost. Early changes, which typically occur in the first week, include renal enlargement with increased echogenicity of the renal parenchyma. During the second week, intermediate changes including prominent and diffuse renal enlargement and loss of corticomedullary differentiation are seen. At this time, there may be patchy hyperechoic and hypoechoic areas that represent hemorrhage and edema. After the first 2 weeks, the kidney may become normal in appearance or begin to atrophy. Thrombi may become calcified. Doppler images can detect high arterial resistance and reversal of flow. Currently, studies are trying to determine if ultrasound can be used to predict long-term prognosis in renal vein thrombosis.[9]

Thrombophilia Screening

The role of inherited thrombophilia in neonatal thrombosis is unclear. While some studies have found an increased association of inherited thrombophilia with catheter-related thrombosis, others have not.[2] Several inherited thrombophilias have been found in association with neonatal renal vein thrombosis.[9] In addition, neonatal purpura fulminans is often associated with protein C or S deficiency. Therefore, thrombophilia screening should be reserved for neonates with significant spontaneous thrombosis, recurrent thrombosis, or neonatal purpura fulminans.

Prior to undergoing thrombophilia screening, a detailed family history should be obtained, including the pregnancy history of the mother focused on miscarriages and premature births. Neonates with spontaneous thrombosis, recurrent thrombosis, or a strong family history of thrombosis should undergo the testing outline in Table 34-4. However, it must be noted that the levels of natural anticoagulants are decreased both during infancy and in the presence of a thrombus. Antithrombin, protein C, and protein S levels should be postponed to 6 months of age or repeated at that time if initial levels are low. In addition, lipoprotein a levels do not reach adult levels until approximately 1 year. If the level is low or normal, it should be repeated at 1 year of age.

In patients with neonatal purpura fulminans, protein C and S activity levels should be sent prior to treatment. If an individual is a homozygote, the level will be undetectable. As repeat testing in 3 to 6 months is not practical in these patients, testing the parents for heterozygous states is imperative and may require repeat analysis.

MANAGEMENT

The majority of neonatal thrombi are managed medically. Prior to initiating therapy, it is important to weigh the risks and benefits of antithrombotic therapy. Occasionally, surgical intervention may be considered in arterial and atrial thrombi; however, this is technically difficult due to the size of neonatal vessels. The choice of antithrombotic treatment is based on the location, size, and symptoms associated with the thrombus.

Medications

Currently, there are 2 common agents used for anticoagulation in neonates: unfractionated heparin and low molecular weight heparin, such as enoxaparin. Vitamin K antagonists, such as warfarin, are rarely used in infants due to the narrow therapeutic index and multiple dietary and medication interactions. In addition, there is concern for inconsistent dosing from crushing tablets as warfarin cannot be safely compounded. Newer anticoagulation agents, such as direct thrombin inhibitors and fondaparinux, are currently in development. The direct thrombin inhibitors, including bivalirudin and argatroban, have the advantage of being antithrombin independent; however, their study in neonates has been limited, and they require continuous administration. Fondaparinux is a synthetic antithrombin-dependent inhibitor of factor Xa that has a prolonged half-life, allowing for daily administration; however, dosing in neonates has not been established. In settings of life- or limb-threatening thrombosis, anticoagulation may not be enough. In these cases, thrombolytic agents, such as tPA, may be warranted if surgical thrombectomy is not possible.

Unfractionated Heparin

Unfractionated heparin works as an anticoagulant by potentiating the inhibitory effects of antithrombin on thrombin and factor Xa. Heparin is the treatment of choice for anticoagulation in the critically ill and is also used prophylactically to maintain catheter patency. It has a short half-life of 30 minutes and therefore must be administered continuously.

Due to high interpatient variability in dosing, it is essential to monitor for therapeutic activity levels. A heparin activity level, which is antifactor Xa, should be checked 6 and 12 hours after initiation of therapy and 6 hours after any adjustment to the dose. The heparin infusion should be adjusted to obtain a goal heparin activity level of 0.35–0.7. Once the level is therapeutic, it should continue to be monitored twice daily. Activated partial thromboplastin time (PTT) is not suggested for monitoring as levels may vary based on the age of the neonate and are not as reliable for evaluating the effects of heparin. Part of the variability in heparin activity is because infants are physiologically deficient in antithrombin. Antithrombin can be safely replaced to allow for better anticoagulation effects of heparin. Levels should be monitored to ensure they remain adequate (greater than 60%).

Heparin therapy is not without side effects. The main adverse effects associated with heparin therapy are associated with bleeding. Advantages of unfractionated heparin are that the half-life is short and the infusion can be stopped. In addition, protamine sulfate serves as a reversal agent by binding heparin. However, another major adverse effect is heparin-induced thrombocytopenia (HIT). HIT is initiated by the formation of antibodies to heparin that activates platelets, leading to further thrombus formation and thrombocytopenia. The incidence of HIT in neonates, particularly those with congenital heart disease, is approximately 1% and can lead to significant morbidity and mortality.[20]

Enoxaparin

Enoxaparin, or Lovenox®, is the most commonly used low molecular weight heparin. Like unfractionated heparin, enoxaparin works by potentiating the effects of antithrombin. However, it has a more profound effect on factor Xa than on thrombin. Enoxaparin is becoming more popular in the treatment of neonatal thrombosis due to the ease of dosing. It is administered via a subcutaneous injection and has a longer half-life than heparin, allowing twice-daily dosing. However, unlike heparin, enoxaparin does not have a reliable mechanism of reversal with protamine; therefore, it should not be used in infants requiring immediate invasive interventions or surgical procedures. In the case of a planned procedure, enoxaparin should be discontinued 24 hours prior to the event. In addition, enoxaparin is not recommended in premature infants who do not have sufficient subcutaneous tissue for administration.

In general, preterm neonates require higher doses of enoxaparin compared to term infants to reach the therapeutic goals. Similarly, infants require increased doses compared to older children and adults. These changes in pharmacodynamics may be due to the larger volume of distribution in infants and the developing hemostatic system. In addition, rapid weight gain in neonates contributes to the difficulty in maintaining therapeutic dosing once it is achieved. The current recommended starting dose of enoxaparin in neonates is 1.5 mg/kg every 12 hours; however, prospective and retrospective studies have suggested that doses of 1.7 mg/kg every 12 hours in term neonates and 2 mg/kg every 12 hours in preterm neonates allow for more rapid attainment of therapeutic levels without an increased number of bleeding events.[21] The increased dosage would not be suggested in infants with high risk of bleeding.

Enoxaparin requires antifactor Xa monitoring to ensure that levels remain in the therapeutic range of 0.5–1 U/mL. Levels should be checked 4 hours after the dose. Like heparin, enoxaparin works by activating antithrombin; therefore, it is important to ensure that the antithrombin level is adequate (greater than 60%) during therapy. While enoxaparin monitoring tends to require fewer venipunctures than heparin, obtaining therapeutic targets with enoxaparin poses a similar challenge to heparin therapy. Once levels are therapeutic, antifactor Xa monitoring should be performed at a minimum of weekly to ensure proper dosing.

Adverse events documented with the use of enoxaparin in infants primarily are bleeding events. Minor events, including bruising and oozing from the injection site, occurred in 0%–56% of patient cohorts. Major bleeding events occurred in 4% of neonates and included major bleeding at the injection site, compartment syndrome, bleeding from gastrointestinal ulcers, intracerebral hemorrhage, hemorrhagic infarction, and hemorrhagic pericardial effusion. All of these occurred while the enoxaparin level was therapeutic.[21] Enoxaparin can also affect bone metabolism, leading to osteopenia after prolonged periods of use, although there are no studies of this in infants. In addition, HIT can develop with the use of enoxaparin, though it occurs less with low molecular weight heparin compared with unfractionated heparin.

Thrombolytic Agents

Although anticoagulation is the mainstay of medical treatment in neonates with thrombosis, thrombolytic agents may be indicated in cases of thrombi obstructing blood flow to a limb or organ. These agents should be considered in thrombi causing tissue ischemia, superior vena cava syndrome due to thrombosis, massive pulmonary embolism, bilateral renal vein thrombosis, large atrial thrombi, congenital heart disease with shunt obstruction, and cerebral sinovenous thrombosis with progressive decline.[22] Thrombolytic drugs work by converting plasminogen to plasmin in order to promote fibrinolysis. They are most effective in thrombi that have been present for less than 2 weeks. tPA is the most common thrombolytic used in children and neonates; however, few clinical trials used these agents in neonates.

Thrombolytic agents can be used either systemically or locally. There are 2 distinct systemic dosing regimens that are commonly used for tPA. High-dose tPA consists of a 0.5–0.6 mg/kg/h infusion for 6 hours followed by an evaluation to determine if the course should be extended or repeated. This is commonly used for life- or limb-sparing thrombi. More recently, there is evidence that low-dose tPA may be as effective in treating peripheral venous and arterial thrombi. Low-dose tPA typically starts at 0.03 mg/kg/h with an hourly maximum of 2 mg and may be increased to 0.06 mg/kg/h. This infusion may be continued for 48 to 96 hours.[22] Catheter-directed thrombolysis is an alternative with decreased systemic effects by allowing delivery of the medication directly to the affected site. However, placement of a catheter in the affected area may be difficult in small neonates. There is no standard dosing range for catheter-directed therapy, though tPA doses of 0.015 to 0.2 mg/kg/h have been reported.[23]

The utility of thrombolytic therapy has been extrapolated in review articles that included multiple different types of thrombi and courses of treatment. In a review of 413 children of all ages who received thrombolytics, 64% of patients had complete clot resolution, 15% had partial resolution, and 21% had no resolution.[22] The most concerning factor limiting the use of these agents is the increased risk of bleeding, especially in neonates who are at a higher risk for intracranial hemorrhage. In the same cohort, 22% of the patients had a minor bleed, and 15% had a major bleed, defined as central nervous system hemorrhage or other hemorrhage requiring blood transfusion. Fatal bleeding occurred in 1.25% of these patients.[22] In a separate review of cases reported in the literature, intracranial hemorrhage was found in 14/929 children (1.5%) but was more common in preterm infants, with a prevalence of 25%.[22] To decrease the risk associated with thrombolytic therapy, a number of relative contraindications have been formulated (Table 34-5). The risk of bleeding due to one of these factors should be weighed against the risk of the thrombus.

Due to the increased risk of bleeding, patients should be monitored closely during thrombolytic administration. Neonates should have a baseline head ultrasound prior to initiation of treatment to evaluate for intracranial hemorrhage. In addition, procedures that include rectal temperatures, urinary catheterizations, and intramuscular injections should be avoided. Fibrinogen and platelet levels should be monitored closely to keep the fibrinogen level greater than 100 mg/dL and platelets greater than 100,000/μL.[23] In addition, hemoglobin levels should be followed to monitor for occult blood loss.

Table 34-5 Contraindications for Use of Thrombolytic Therapy[a]

Major surgery or hemorrhage within 10 days
Central nervous system (CNS) surgery, ischemia, trauma, or hemorrhage within 30 days
Invasive procedures within 3 days prior to initiation of therapy
Seizures within 48 hours
Prematurity: < 32 weeks gestation
Systemic septicemia
Active bleeding
Inability to maintain platelet count > 75,000/μL
Inability to maintain fibrinogen > 100mg/dL
Uncontrolled hypertension

[a]From Raffini[22] and Williams.[23]

Neonates, especially premature infants, have a reduced level of plasminogen when compared to older children and adults. These decreased levels lead to less plasmin formation and therefore less fibrinolysis. In the setting of low plasminogen, thrombolytic agents are not effective even with increasing dosages. Plasminogen should be replaced with daily infusion of fresh-frozen plasma (FFP; 10 mL/kg) prior to treatment with thrombolytic agents.

Unlike anticoagulants, thrombolytics do not inhibit clot formation. Low-dose unfractionated heparin (10 U/kg/h) has been used in conjunction with thrombolytic therapy, though the therapeutic effect has not been proven. Therapeutic anticoagulation should be initiated after thrombolytic therapy to prevent further thrombus formation.

Location Specific

The choice of treatment of neonatal thrombosis is largely based on the location and extent of the thrombus as well as the risk of bleeding in the patient.

Catheter-Associated

Most neonatal thrombi are associated with the presence of an intravenous line. The location of the catheter and the need for further intravenous treatment factor into the treatment recommendations for catheter-associated thrombi. The eighth edition of the American College of Chest Physicians Evidence-Based Clinical Practice Guidelines was published in 2008 and offers recommendations for treatment of catheter-associated thrombi in children and neonates. These recommendations were summarized by Revel-Vilk and Ergaz (Table 34-6)[1]. If a thrombus is associated with an arterial line, the line should be removed promptly and treatment with anticoagulation therapy consisting of unfractionated heparin or enoxaparin should be initiated for a minimum of 10 days. For venous-associated thrombi, the patient should be treated with 6 weeks to 3 months of anticoagulation therapy. If the line is no longer needed or is nonfunctioning, it should be removed after 3–5 days of anticoagulation therapy. If the line is required and functioning, it can be left in place. If it is still in place after the anticoagulation has ceased, prophylactic anticoagulation should be instituted until the line is removed.

If a thrombus is asymptomatic and detected radiographically, the recommendations are less distinct. Lines that are unnecessary should be removed. If the line is still required, there is no clear recommendation for anticoagulation. If the line was removed prior to the detection of the clot, for instance a thrombus located at the site of a previous umbilical catheter, the area should be followed closely with no initial therapy needed.[1]

Table 34-6 Recommended management of central-line-related thrombosis in neonates.[a]

Thrombotic event	Principles of management
Acute, symptomatic in arterial line	Prompt removal of the catheter. Anticoagulation therapy for at least 10 days.
Acute, symptomatic in venous line: the line is no longer required or is non-functioning	The line should be removed. Anticoagulation therapy 3-5 days prior to line removal. Anticoagulation therapy for between 6 weeks and 3 months. Option for radiologic monitoring after line removal without therapy: however, subsequent anticoagulation is needed if extension of the thrombosis occurs.
Acute, symptomatic in venous line: the line is required and functioning	The line may be left in place. Anticoagulation therapy for between 6 weeks and 3 months. If the line is still in place on completion of therapeutic anticoagulation, a prophylactic dose of LMWH should be given to prevent recurrent thrombosis until the line is removed.
Acute symptomatic, causing critical compromise of life, organs or limbs	Thrombolysis therapy with tPA. Supplement with plasminogen (fresh frozen plasma) prior to commencing therapy.
Radiographically detected, asymptomatic: the line is no longer required	The line should be removed. In venous lines, 3-5 days of anticoagulation prior to line removal is suggested.
Radiographically detected, asymptomatic: the line is required	No evidence-based data. Some suggest treatment with anticoagulation in the absence of contraindications. The need for full dose anticoagulation is not clear.
Radiographically detected, asymptomatic UAC- or UVC related thrombosis after the catheter has been removed	Close clinical follow-up and therapy only for symptomatic cases.

Abbreviations: LMWH, low molecular weight heparin; tPA, tissue plasminogen activator; UAC, umbilical artery catheter; UVC, umbilical vein catheter.
[a]From Revel-Vilk and Ergaz.[1]

Renal Vein Thrombosis

The treatment of renal vein thrombosis is based on the extent of the thrombosis as well as its effect on renal function. The current guidelines from the American College of Chest Physicians suggest treatment of bilateral renal vein thrombosis with or without renal impairment with thrombolysis using tPA followed by anticoagulation consisting of unfractionated heparin or enoxaparin. If the patient has unilateral renal vein thrombosis with extension into the inferior vena cava, the patient should be treated with anticoagulation alone consisting of unfractionated heparin or enoxaparin. For unilateral renal vein thrombosis without renal impairment, close follow-up with or without anticoagulation is recommended. There are no clear recommendations for unilateral renal vein thrombi that do not extend to the inferior vena cava but have renal impairment.[9] Whether infants with decreased levels of protein C, protein S, and antithrombin benefit from replacement is unknown.

Currently, the data on the long-term effects of treatment with antithrombotic therapy in renal vein thrombosis is sparse. One retrospective chart review of 23 neonates with renal vein thrombosis showed that 33% of patients treated with heparin had renal atrophy compared to 100% of those who did not receive anticoagulation. Those neonates who received anticoagulation also had less secondary hypertension. In contrast, 2 slightly larger reviews showed no significant difference in the renal outcome of those treated with anticoagulation, thrombolysis, or supportive care.[9]

Neonatal Purpura Fulminans

Neonatal purpura fulminans occurs in the presence of DIC. DIC should be managed with supportive blood products as needed. If the neonate has classical signs of neonatal purpura fulminans, blood samples should be drawn for protein C and S function and activity levels prior to any replacement therapy. Severe transient deficiencies of protein C or S are treated by aggressive therapy for the underlying cause. FFP or cryoprecipitate can be used as replacement therapy. If there is concern for congenital deficiencies, replacement should start promptly with FFP at 10–20 mL/kg every 6–12 hours. There is no protein S concentrate; however, protein C concentrate should be used as soon as it is available for those with congenital protein C deficiency. The goal trough of protein C activity is greater than 10 IU/dL while waiting for the concentrate and the plasma concentration is raised by 1 IU/dL for every 1 mL/kg of FFP. The most common side effects of treatment with FFP include fluid overload and exposure to multiple donors.[11]

There are currently 2 human plasma-derived, viral-inactivated protein C concentrates on the market: Ceprotin is licensed in the United States and Europe, and Protexel is licensed in Europe. The plasma protein C concentration is raised by 1 IU/dL for every 1 IU/kg of concentrate, and the half-life is 6–10 hours. Therefore, the initial dosage recommendation is 100 U/kg followed by 50 U/kg every 6 hours to maintain a trough protein C activity level of 50 IU/dL.[11] Treatment should continue until all lesions have resolved. Anticoagulation with unfractionated heparin or enoxaparin should also be initiated with administration of protein C replacement.

Individuals with congenital protein C deficiency will require maintenance therapy. Maintenance therapy consists of anticoagulation alone or protein C concentrate of 30–50 IU/kg every 1–3 days with anticoagulation. Currently, protein C concentrate is given intravenously, necessitating central line placement, which may lead to increased risk of thrombosis. Studies are currently ongoing to determine the pharmacokinetics of subcutaneous protein C concentrate. Many patients are placed on warfarin for long-term maintenance. Warfarin therapy initiation must occur after therapeutic levels of heparin have been attained due to the initial decrease in protein C levels. If protein C concentrate is not administered, the goal international normalized ratio (INR) for prophylaxis is 2.5–3.5. If protein C replacement is ongoing, the goal INR is 1.5–2.5. Prior to any surgery, individuals with protein C deficiency should receive 100 U/kg of protein C concentrate as a bolus, followed by 30–50 U/kg every 12–24 hours to reach a goal protein C activity level of 20–50 IU/dL.[11] Liver transplantation has been performed in individuals with congenital protein C deficiency when replacement therapy was not available.

OUTCOME AND FOLLOW-UP

While many small thrombi self-resolve, thrombosis may lead to significant morbidity depending on its location. Many catheter-associated thrombi are located in the extremities. Postthrombotic syndrome, including chronic limb edema, skin discoloration, poor wound healing, pain, and limitation of limb function, occurs in 12%–63% of children with deep vein thrombosis. Catheter-associated venous thrombi also may lead to pulmonary embolism or an embolic stroke, though the exact frequency in infants is unknown. Thrombi that develop in the portal vein lead to left lobe atrophy in 22.6% of infants and portal hypertension in 4.5% of infants.[24] In the Canadian registry, thrombi in the aorta, right atrium, and superior vena cava had a 33% mortality rate.[23] Idiopathic venous thromboembolism has a recurrence rate of approximately 3% in neonates.[16]

Renal vein thrombosis has the lowest mortality rate of thromboembolic events in neonates, with a rate of 5%. In addition, death in these cases was attributed to other medical conditions. Though the mortality rate is low, renal vein thrombi lead to significant morbidity. Acute events include adrenal hemorrhage, arterial ischemic stroke, central sinovenous thrombosis, and pulmonary embolism. Long-term complications include hypertension in 19%–22% of infants and chronic renal insufficiency from acute and chronic renal injury in 29% of patients. Progression to end-stage renal failure occurs in 3% of patients.[9] Due to these complications, children with a history of renal vein thrombosis should have their blood pressure monitored at every visit and their renal function monitored closely if it is abnormal. Depending on the renal dysfunction, renal ultrasounds should be performed at regular intervals, and urine microalbumin levels should be followed.

REFERENCES

1. Revel-Vilk S, Ergaz Z. Diagnosis and management of central-line-associated thrombosis in newborns and infants. *Semin Fetal Neonatal Med.* 2011;16(6):340–344. doi: 10.1016/j.siny.2011.07.003.
2. Saracco P, Parodi E, Fabris C, Cecinati V, Molinari AC, Giordano P. Management and investigation of neonatal thromboembolic events: genetic and acquired risk factors. *Thrombosis Res.* 2009;123(6):805–809.
3. Saxonhouse M, Manco Johnson M. The evaluation and management of neonatal coagulation disorders. *Semin Perinatol.* 2009;33(1):52–65.
4. Schmidt B, Andrew M. Neonatal thrombosis: report of a prospective Canadian and international registry. *Pediatrics.* 1995;96(5):939–943.
5. van Ommen CH, Heijboer H, Bller HR, Hirasing RA, Heijmans HS, Peters M. Venous thromboembolism in childhood: a prospective two-year registry in the Netherlands. *J Pediatr.* 2001;139(5):676–681.
6. Andrew M, Paes B, Milner R, et al. Development of the human coagulation system in the full-term infant. *Blood.* 1987;70(1):165–172.
7. Andrew M, Paes B, Milner R, et al. Development of the human coagulation system in the healthy premature infant. *Blood.* 1988;72(5):1651–1657.
8. Nowak-Göttl U, von Kries, R, Gobel, U. Neonatal symptomatic thromboembolism in Germany: two year survey. *Arch Dis Child Fetal Neonatal Ed.* 76(3), F163–F167.
9. Brando, L, Simpson, E, Lau, K. Neonatal renal vein thrombosis. *Seminars in fetal and neonatal medicine.*
10. Lau, K, Stoffman, J, Williams S, McCusker P, Brandao L, Patel S, Chan AKC. Neonatal renal vein thrombosis: review of the English-language literature between 1992 and 2006. *Pediatrics.* 2007;120(5):e1278–e1284.
11. Price VE, Ledingham DL, Krumpel A, Chan AK. Diagnosis and management of neonatal purpura fulminans. *Semin Fetal Neonatal Med.* 2011;16(6):318–322. doi: 10.1016/j.siny.2011.07.009.
12. Yang J, Williams S, Brando L, Chan A. Neonatal and childhood right atrial thrombosis: recognition and a risk-stratified treatment approach. *Blood Coagul Fibrinolysis.* 2010;21(4):301–307.
13. Morag I, Epelman M, Daneman A, et al. Portal vein thrombosis in the neonate: risk factors, course, and outcome. *J Pediatr.* 2006;148(6):735–739.

14. Boffa MC, Lachassinne E. Infant perinatal thrombosis and antiphospholipid antibodies: a review. *Lupus*. 2007;16(8):634–641.

15. Patnaik MM, Moll S. Inherited antithrombin deficiency: a review. *Haemophilia*. 2008;14(6):1229–1239.

16. Nowak-Göttl U, Kurnik K, Manner D, Kenet G. Thrombophilia testing in neonates and infants with thrombosis. *Semin Fetal Neonatal Med*. 2011;16(6):345–348.

17. Goldenberg NA, Manco Johnson MJ. Protein C deficiency. *Haemophilia*. 2008;14(6):1214–1221.

18. Marlar R, Gausman J. Protein S abnormalities: a diagnostic nightmare. *Am J Hematol*. 2011;86(5):418–421.

19. Varga E, Kujovich J. Management of inherited thrombophilia: guide for genetics professionals. *Clin Genet*. 2012;81(1):7–17.

20. Young G. Old and new antithrombotic drugs in neonates and infants. *Semin Fetal Neonatal Med*. 2011;16(6):349–354. doi: 10.1016/j.siny.2011.07.002.

21. Malowany J, Monagle P, Knoppert D, et al. Enoxaparin for neonatal thrombosis: a call for a higher dose for neonates. *Thromb Res*. 2008;122(6):826–830.

22. Raffini L. Thrombolysis for intravascular thrombosis in neonates and children. *Curr Opin Pediatr*. 2009;21(1):9–14.

23. Williams MD. Thrombolysis in children. *Br J Haematol*. 2010;148(1):26–36. doi: 10.1111/j.1365–2141.2009.07914.x.

24. Yang JYK, Chan AKC. Neonatal systemic venous thrombosis. *Thromb Res*. 2010;126(6):471–476.

Part E: Gastro-Intestinal

35   Gastroschisis and Omphalocele

Zachary Kastenberg and Sanjeev Dutta

INTRODUCTION

Gastroschisis and omphalocele (also referred to as exomphalos) are 2 of the most common abdominal wall defects requiring neonatal intensive care. Their similarities, most notably evisceration of abdominal structures through a defect at or near the umbilicus, misled generations of physicians and surgeons to inaccurately diagnose them as a single common disease. The pathologic differences between these 2 entities were formally realized when, in 1953, Thomas Moore and George Stokes defined gastroschisis as a large extraumbilical evisceration of intestines *without* a covering sac. They distinguished this from omphalocele, which was defined as the herniation of viscera into the base of the umbilical cord *with* a protective membranous sac.[1] The establishment of gastroschisis and omphalocele as 2 distinct pathologies with their own specific anatomic features and associated anomalies provides the basis for our management of these defects today.

EPIDEMIOLOGY

Historically, omphalocele was observed nearly twice as commonly as gastroschisis. More recent literature shows an increase in the incidence of gastroschisis,[2-4] suggesting that the actual relationship is approximately 1:1. This phenomenon remains unexplained but is probably related to a combination of improved diagnostic coding (prior to the incorporation of Moore and Stokes's definition, gastroschisis was commonly referred to as omphalocele) and the environmental factors noted in the discussion that follows. The approximate incidence is 1–3 per 10,000 live births for both gastroschisis and omphalocele.[4]

Population studies have found associations between a number of environmental factors and gastroschisis. Young maternal age (<20 years) reproducibly correlates with gastroschisis, while individual studies have found gastroschisis to be associated with low economic status, maternal use of over-the-counter vasoactive medications or salicylates, maternal smoking, alcohol consumption, and illicit substance use.[2,5-8] Omphalocele, on the other hand, is associated with advanced maternal age and karyotype abnormalities.[5,7,9]

GENETICS

The genetic basis for gastroschisis is poorly understood. Gastroschisis is most frequently sporadic, but there are rare familial cases documented in the literature, suggesting an underlying genetic component. Such case reports include concordance for gastroschisis in monozygotic twins,[10,11] dizygotic twins,[12] and distant relatives.[13]

Genotype analysis of patients with gastroschisis has led to the identification of associated single-nucleotide polymorphisms (SNPs) at the genes encoding endothelial nitric oxide synthase (NOS3/eNOS; odds ratio [OR] 1.9, 95% confidence interval [CI] 1.1–3.4); intracellular adhesion molecule 1 (ICAM1; OR 1.9, 95% CI 1.1–3.4); and atrial natriuretic peptide precursor α (NPPA; OR 1.9, 95% CI 1.0–3.4).[14] Both ICAM and NOS3/eNOS are intimately involved in the molecular cascades of angiogenesis.[15] Although inconclusive, these studies lend some weight to the vasculogenic theories of pathogenesis discussed in the following section. Interestingly, when these polymorphisms were analyzed in mothers who smoked during pregnancy, the odds ratio for developing gastroschisis increased substantially (NOS3/eNOS OR 5.2, 95% CI 2.4–11.4; ICAM1 OR 5.2, 95% CI 2.1–12.7; NPPA OR 6.4, CI 2.8–14.6), providing evidence for a gene-environment interaction.[14]

Omphalocele, in comparison, is associated with significant chromosomal abnormalities in approximately 30% of cases.[4] Trisomy 13, 18, and 21 are the most common karyotype abnormalities. Other genes have been implicated, including pituitary homeobox 2 (PITX2), a gene mutated frequently in Reiger syndrome[16]; insulin-like growth factor 2 (IGF2) and cyclin-dependent kinase inhibitor 1C (CDKN1C), both associated with Beckwith-Wiedemann syndrome[17]; and MTHFR, 677C-T, a polymorphism in the methylenetetrahydrofolate reductase gene.[18] Whether a causal relationship exists between these specific mutations and omphalocele remains to be defined.

EMBRYOLOGY

A sound understanding of the basic embryology of the ventral body wall is important for comprehending the pathology and management of abdominal wall defects. During the third week of gestation, the process of gastrulation leads to the formation of a trilaminar germ disk with an identifiable mesoderm sandwiched between the primitive ectoderm and endoderm (Figure 35-1). The subsequent rapid growth of the ectoderm and the mesoderm causes ventral folding of the embryo. The 4 body folds (cranial, caudal, and 2 lateral folds) approximate in the middle of the ventral surface to form the umbilicus (Figures 35-2 and 35-3).

During the sixth week of gestation, the rapid growth of the midgut leads to physiologic herniation at the base of the umbilicus. As the fetus grows, the intestine rotates 270° in the counterclockwise direction and returns to the peritoneal cavity spontaneously by the 10th week of gestation. Omphalocele is believed to arise from incomplete folding of the lateral body wall folds and failure of the intestines to return to the peritoneal cavity following this physiologic herniation.[19,20] As a result, intestinal nonrotation is almost always observed in infants with omphalocele. Importantly, the umbilical stalk persists as a broad-based protective sac and is composed of peritoneum and amnion with an intervening layer of Wharton's jelly.

Variants of omphalocele occur in the epigastrium and the infraumbilical region. The embryopathology of epigastric omphalocele is related to failure of the cranial body wall-folding process. This defect is often seen in combination with sternal cleft, ectopia cordis/cardiac defects, pericardial defects, and diaphragmatic hernia. When present concurrently, these defects are known as the pentalogy of Cantrell.[21] Infraumbilical omphalocele is thought to arise from a deficit in caudal body wall folding and is frequently associated with bladder or cloacal exstrophy.

Following successful ventral body wall folding, the early umbilical contents consist of the yolk stalk and its associated vitelline vessels, the umbilical vessels, and the allantois. The yolk sac maintains its connection to the embryonic intestine through the vitelline duct. It receives its blood supply from the vitelline arteries, which are a network of arteries originating from the dorsal aorta. As the yolk sac atrophies and the nutritional requirements of the fetus are supplied by the placenta and maternal circulation, the vitelline arteries regress. The proximal

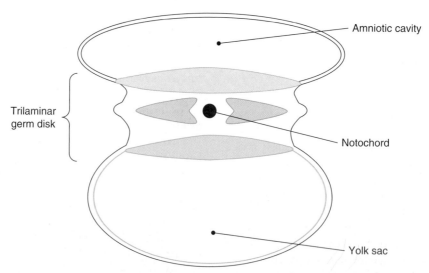

FIGURE 35-1 Formation of a trilaminar germ disk.

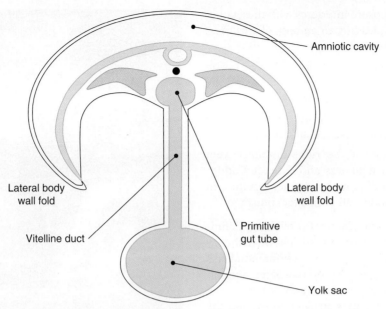

FIGURE 35-2 Beginning of umbilicus formation.

arterial segments persist as the celiac, superior mesenteric, and inferior mesenteric arteries, supplying the foregut, midgut, and hindgut, respectively.

The umbilical vessels supply the maternal-fetal circulation. The umbilical arteries are paired branches originating at the fetal iliac arteries and carry deoxygenated blood back to the maternal circulation through the umbilical cord. Postnatally, the umbilical arteries regress and become the medial umbilical ligaments, while the closely associated urachus (conduit from the fetal bladder to the allantois) fibroses to become the median umbilical ligament. The umbilical veins, on the other hand, carry oxygenated maternal blood to the fetus. The right umbilical vein regresses early in development; the left umbilical vein persists

as the conduit from the placenta to the fetal central venous system. Postnatally, the left umbilical vein atrophies to become the ligamentum teres, the intrahepatic portion of which is known as the ligamentum venosum.

While the exact embryologic etiology of gastroschisis remains much more controversial than that of omphalocele, a number of leading theories have emerged from the last half century, including the following:

1. Similar to omphalocele, failed reduction of the herniated bowel at the 10th week of gestation followed by rupture of the membrane at the base of the umbilical cord lead to the unprotected evisceration characteristic of gastroschisis.[22]

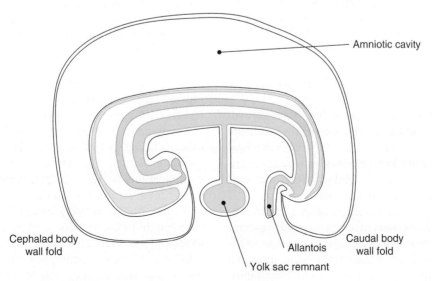

FIGURE 35-3 Approximation of the body folds to form the umbilicus.

2. Early teratogen exposure interferes with mesenchymal differentiation, leading to an area of weakness just lateral to the umbilicus.[23]

3. Incomplete body wall folding leads to failed fusion of the yolk sac with the umbilical stalk, leaving the yolk sac as a lead point for herniation.[24]

4. Untimely involution or disruption of the vitelline artery leads to body wall ischemia and necrosis.[25]

5. Abnormal involution of the right umbilical vein leads to an area of weakness and extended apoptosis in the surrounding mesenchyme, resulting in resorption of the body wall at this location.[26]

While these theories are thought provoking, definitive evidence is lacking in each case. The first theory does not explain the differences in environmental risk factors, maternal characteristics, or associated anomalies observed between gastroschisis and omphalocele. The second and third theories struggle to explain the right-sided predilection of the abdominal wall defect. In contradiction to the fourth theory is the fact that the abdominal wall receives the majority of its circulation from segmental perforating vessels originating at the aorta, not from the vitelline arteries. The umbilical vein theory, put forth by deVries in 1980, has been favored as it both explains the right-sided preponderance of the defect and fits with the genetic associations suggesting a vasculogenic etiology. This theory has also been supported by rare cases of left-sided gastroschisis found to have resorption of the left umbilical vein.[27]

PATHOPHYSIOLOGY

Gastroschisis

Gastroschisis is a congenital malformation resulting in a lateral abdominal wall defect almost always 1 to 2 cm to the right of the umbilicus (Figure 35-4). The eviscerated structures do not have a protective sac and are in direct contact with the amniotic fluid, leading to the characteristic edematous, foreshortened, fibrinous peel-covered small bowel. In the absence of significant gastrointestinal morbidity, the long-term outcomes are generally good.

Gastroschisis tends to occur as an isolated malformation. Comorbidities in the neonatal period are almost always directly related to the gastrointestinal tract and include intestinal atresia, stenosis, and nonrotation. Approximately 10% of infants born with gastroschisis will have a concurrent intestinal atresia.[28,29] The exact etiology of this phenomenon is unknown, but it is thought to be related to an in utero vascular accident, either volvulus or compression of the bowel at the abdominal wall defect. Like omphalocele, intestinal nonrotation is frequently encountered in affected individuals. In nonrotation, the small bowel occupies the

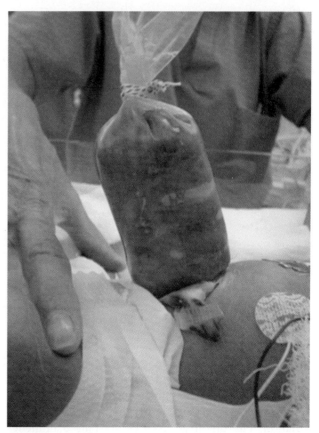

FIGURE 35-4 Gastroschisis is a congenital lateral abdominal wall defect.

right abdomen, the large bowel occupies the left abdomen, and there is a relatively wide mesentery; thus, the risk of volvulus is negligible. In fact, a Ladd procedure for rotational anomalies that is designed to prevent volvulus leaves the bowel in a nonrotated configuration.

Gastroschisis is almost ubiquitously associated with delayed initiation of enteral feeding and intestinal hypomotility. There is evidence to suggest that this is directly related to the damaging effects of in utero intestinal exposure to amniotic fluid and constriction of the intestines at the body wall.[30] Supporting this theory are animal studies in which removal of allantoic fluid (ie, urine) from the amniotic cavity[31] or complete amniotic fluid replacement[32] prevented the development of the characteristic edematous, fibrinous peel-covered intestine.

Prematurity is frequently associated with gastroschisis, with up to 28% of affected individuals delivered spontaneously at less than 37 weeks' gestation.[33] The complications frequent to prematurity and low birth weight are also observed in the setting of gastroschisis. Most notably, necrotizing enterocolitis (NEC) occurs in these individuals with a predilection for infants weighing less than 2500 kg at birth.[34] Furthermore, NEC can emerge as a complication following abdominal closure and the initiation of enteral feeds in these patients, regardless of gestational age.

Omphalocele

Omphalocele is a congenital malformation that results in a midline abdominal wall defect at the umbilicus (Figure 35-5). Less-common variants occur in the epigastrium or infraumbilical region. The eviscerated contents are contained within a protective sac and are not in contact with the amniotic fluid. The eviscerated structures almost always include small bowel and colon; solid organs, most frequently liver, are often involved. Omphalocele is associated with other anomalies approximately 50%–70% of the time, with 30%–50% of affected infants having significant congenital cardiac disease.[4] Long-term outcomes are dependent on the severity of the associated anomalies.

Significant gastrointestinal morbidity is less common in omphalocele than in gastroschisis. As mentioned, nonrotation of the intestine is common but does not predispose to volvulus, thus is left untouched. Prolonged ileus and delayed enteric feeding are less severe than in gastroschisis but can lead to prolonged hospitalizations for some individuals. Ruptured omphalocele presents a unique problem in which the gastrointestinal complications of gastroschisis are often present dependent on the length of time that the bowel was exposed to the amniotic fluid.

In addition to the sporadic cardiac defects and relatively rare gastrointestinal pathology, omphalocele is characterized by its frequent syndromic presentation. Patau syndrome (trisomy 13), Edward syndrome (trisomy 18), and Down syndrome (trisomy 21) are associated with omphalocele at rates greater than that seen in the general population. Gigantism, macroglossia, omphalocele, and hypoglycemia secondary to pancreatic hyperplasia cluster to form the Beckwith-Wiedemann syndrome, which is seen in roughly 10% of infants with omphalocele.[4,35] Other syndromes associated with omphalocele include pentalogy of Cantrell, as described in the preceding section, OEIS (omphalocele, exstrophy of the bladder, imperforate anus, and spinal defects) syndrome, CHARGE (coloboma, heart defects, choanal atresia, mental retardation, genitourinary and ear anomalies) syndrome, and in the well-documented VACTERL (vertebral, anal, cardiac, tracheoesophageal, renal, and limb) association.[5]

DIFFERENTIAL DIAGNOSIS

Umbilical Hernia

Umbilical hernias are a common occurrence caused by incomplete closure of the umbilical ring after separation of the umbilical cord remnant. They occur in roughly 80% of neonates with birth weights less than 1200 g and in 20% of neonates with birth weights less than 2500 g.[36] They are 10 times more common for unclear reasons in African Americans than in other races or ethnicities.[36] Nearly 90% of these hernias will spontaneously resolve by 3 to 4 years of age.[36] Because of this, umbilical hernias are rarely repaired electively before 5 years of age. Indications for urgent repair include incarceration, obstruction, or pain, all extremely infrequent occurrences. Umbilical hernias tend to be smaller than omphalocele without herniation of solid organs. They can be differentiated from gastroschisis and omphalocele by the presence of normal skin overlying the defect, with the exception of rare cases in which there is an omphalocoele sac that is partially epithelialized.

Prune-Belly Syndrome

Prune-belly (Eagle-Barrett) syndrome consists of deficiency or absence of abdominal wall musculature; a constellation of ureteral, bladder, and urethral anomalies; and bilateral cryptorchidism. The incidence is approximately 1 in 50,000 live births and almost always occurs in males.[37] The deficient abdominal wall musculature leads to the characteristic flaccidity and wrinkling of the abdominal skin. Prune-belly syndrome is distinguished from other abdominal wall defects by complete containment of the abdominal viscera within a continuous layer of skin with a normal umbilicus. There is no definitive treatment of the abdominal wall deficiency. In most cases, the lack of abdominal musculature does not cause significant functional impairment. It is important to note that omphalocele does occasionally occur in the setting of prune-belly syndrome. This represents the concurrent presentation of 2 distinct pathologies and should be treated as such. The long-term outcomes of prune-belly syndrome are directly related to the severity of the genitourinary anomalies and underlying renal function.

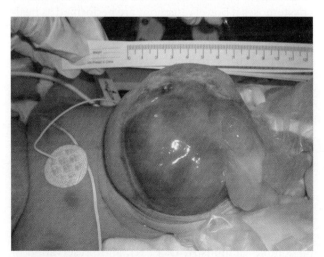

FIGURE 35-5 Omphalocele is a congenital midline abdominal wall defect at the umbilicus.

DIAGNOSTIC TESTS

Prenatal Imaging

Abdominal wall defects are most commonly identified on routine prenatal ultrasound. Conventional ultrasound identifies both gastroschisis and omphalocele with a specificity of greater than 95%. Unfortunately, the sensitivity is only 60%–75% due to the effects of the timing of the study and inherent operator dependence.[9,38] Once a fetus with an abdominal wall defect is identified, directed ultrasounds should be performed to look for associated anomalies and malformations. Serial ultrasounds will be needed to continually reassess fetal viability. The popularity and availability of fetal magnetic resonance imaging (MRI) has substantially increased in recent years. MRI offers superior image clarity and improved accuracy in the prenatal diagnosis of congenital neurologic, thoracic, abdominal (including abdominal wall defects), and urogenital malformations. At many facilities it is now used as a reflex imaging study if initial ultrasound is suspicious for gastroschisis or omphalocele.

Laboratory Tests

Assessment of maternal serum α-fetoprotein (AFP) is a common prenatal test used to screen for chromosomal abnormalities and neural tube defects but is also useful in identifying abdominal wall defects. Elevated maternal serum AFP correlates closely with both gastroschisis and omphalocele. Gastroschisis, perhaps due to the direct communication between the visceral structures and the amniotic cavity, usually presents with a dramatically elevated maternal serum AFP, while omphalocele tends to have a more modest elevation (7–9 multiples of the mean compared to 4 multiples of the mean, respectively).[39,40]

Positive ultrasound findings or a significant elevation of maternal serum AFP should lead to a discussion regarding possible amniocentesis or chorionic villus sampling. Early detection of significant karyotype abnormalities identifies high-risk pregnancies and allows for psychological preparation of the family, mobilization of the necessary health care resources, and if appropriate, may prompt a discussion on the possibility of pregnancy termination.

MANAGEMENT

Prenatal Management

Early diagnosis and referral to a specialized neonatal center is key to the management of congenital abdominal wall defects. Prenatal sonographic evidence of bowel dilation has been correlated with poorer outcomes and is considered a controversial indication for preterm delivery.[41–43] Others advocate for cesarean delivery for infants with omphalocele to avoid sac rupture.[44] The majority of the literature comparing various modes and timing of delivery in infants with abdominal wall defects, however, is equivocal.[45–49] There is currently no evidence to recommend early vs term delivery or elective cesarean sections vs vaginal delivery of neonates with abdominal wall defects.

Postnatal Management

Both gastroschisis and omphalocele present with varying degrees of severity; nonetheless, the presence of a neonatologist and pediatric surgeon should be considered mandatory in all cases whenever possible. After initial stabilization (ie, covering of exposed viscera with a plastic bag and warm saline, establishment of intravenous access, fluid resuscitation, and placement of an orogastric tube), the surgeon must assess the viability of the exposed structures. If bowel necrosis is present, the management is much more complicated, and the surgical strategy has to be tailored to each particular case. These surgeries include emergent resections, creation of stomas, tube diversions, and so on. In the absence of necrosis, the decisions hinge on the type and size of the defect (omphalocele vs gastroschisis) and the reducibility of the eviscerated structures.

Gastroschisis

Management begins with orogastric intubation for decompression, protection of the eviscerated structures with moist dressings and protective plastic bag, and adequate fluid resuscitation. The surgeon must then assess the bowel for viability. If there are segments of necrosis or perforation, emergent surgical resection is indicated. No attempt should be made at primary anastomoses if bowel resections are performed as healing of the inflamed bowel is severely compromised, and atretic segments are left untouched. Instead, blind segments can be reduced and the abdomen closed, with reexploration after 6 weeks to connect the intestinal segments after inflammation has cleared. The goal of any resection is to leave the infant with enough small bowel to avoid long-term total parenteral nutrition (TPN) dependence or short-bowel syndrome (SBS). The general rule is to preserve at least 40 cm of viable small bowel as well as the ileocecal valve whenever possible. The actual length of bowel necessary to prevent SBS is dependent on a number of factors, including gestational age, quality of remaining bowel, presence of viable ileum (for absorption of vitamin B_{12}, fat-soluble vitamins A, D, E, K), and preservation of the ileocecal valve for slowing the nutrient transit time.

In the absence of intestinal necrosis or perforation, the surgeon is faced with the question of primary vs delayed closure of the defect. This topic remains controversial, but there appears to be a consensus that primary closure is preferred when the eviscerated structures can be reduced without causing physiologic compromise (ie, increased peak inspiratory pressures, elevated bladder pressure, decreased urine output, or worsening acidosis). If delayed closure is planned, a spring-loaded silo is placed over the bowel and anchored with the circular spring around its base to the internal surface of the fascial defect. This can be done either at the bedside or in the operating room based on surgeon preference. The silo is then serially tied off starting at its apex until the eviscerated contents are entirely reduced back into the abdomen. This typically takes 5–7 days to complete.

Once reduction in the absence of physiologic compromise is possible (primary or delayed), the defect is closed using either the traditional sutured approach or a sutureless technique. The sutured technique involves closing the fascial defect with sutures and attempting a cosmetic reconstruction of the skin defect and umbilicus. The sutureless technique involves placement of a plastic-occlusive dressing over the defect to retain abdominal contents while the fascial defect closes by secondary healing and contraction. Closure can be achieved in as little as 5–7 days, with full epithelialization by 10–14 days. There is emerging evidence to suggest that the sutureless approach leads to outcomes comparable to the traditional sutured method.[50–52] Proponents of this technique describe improved cosmesis of the umbilicus when healing is allowed by secondary intention and reduction in post-operative ventilatory support. Long-term outcomes of the sutureless technique, however, remain to be established.

Omphalocele

Immediate measures for omphalocele include resuscitation, protection of the sac with saline-soaked dressings, and intubation with ventilatory support if necessary. In addition, postnatal karyotype analysis, echocardiography, renal ultrasound, and detailed physical examination to assess for musculoskeletal defects prior to operative intervention are performed.

The definitive management of omphalocele depends on the size of the omphalocele and whether the sac is intact or perforated. Giant omphaloceles with intact sacs undergo progressive epithelialization promoted by daily application of silver sulfadiazine to assist with escharization. Progressive compression using a body wrap technique is used to reduce the contents, with elective repair of the fascial defect at 6–24 months. If a giant omphalocele presents with a ruptured sac, a silastic silo is sutured to the fascial edges and serial

reduction is performed, similar to that with gastroschisis, with later closure of the fascial defect (which sometimes requires mesh closure).

Small omphaloceles may be closed primarily in the operating room or epithelialized with delayed closure. This decision is based on the surgeon's judgment of the feasibility of reduction of the eviscerated organs in addition to the presence or absence of associated anomalies requiring prioritized management. Interestingly, small omphaloceles are more frequently found to have karyotype abnormalities and associated anomalies when compared to giant omphaloceles, especially those containing liver.[53]

Postreduction Management

The management of both omphalocele and gastroschisis following reduction focuses on nutritional balance and early recognition of comorbidities. Most surgeons and neonatologists recommend 48 hours of antibiotics following reduction or establishment of silo protection. Parenteral nutrition is established early in all cases of gastroschisis given the near ubiquity of prolonged ileus and selectively in omphalocele if ileus is expected. Orogastric feeds are initiated as oral gastric tube (OGT) output decreases and bowel function returns, regardless of the status of the abdominal wall closure. Given the extent of the ileus in cases of gastroschisis, workup for stricture/atresia is not undertaken until approximately 6 weeks of life to allow for adequate time for resumption of gut function. If oral feeds are not tolerated at 6 weeks, a small-bowel contrast study is obtained, and delayed repair of any stricture or atresia is planned.

OUTCOMES AND FOLLOW-UP

The outcomes of gastroschisis are directly related to the presence or absence of gastrointestinal complications. Gastroschisis has an overall mortality rate of approximately 4%–7%.[54,55] The majority of these deaths are related to gastrointestinal catastrophes, including intestinal necrosis or multiple atresias resulting in SBS.[55] One recent series noted the most common nonlethal complications of gastroschisis were prolonged ileus (28%), catheter infections (25%), and sepsis (15%).[56]

In cases of omphalocele, the outcomes are directly related to the severity of the associated anomalies. The overall mortality rate for omphalocele is approximately 30%.[57] When associated anomalies are present, mortality approaches 60%, while isolated omphalocele has a mortality rate roughly equivalent to uncomplicated gastroschisis (~10%).[58,59] The most common complications related to the omphalocele itself include ileus (12%), wound infection (15%), and sepsis (12%).[56]

Advances in neonatal intensive care and surgical technique have led to excellent long-term outcomes for both uncomplicated gastroschisis and isolated omphalocele. These individuals advance to adulthood with relatively normal physical and cognitive development. In a questionnaire-based study, 88% of adults with a history of either gastroschisis or omphalocele considered themselves to be in good health.[60] The most frequent complaints in this group were displeasure with abdominal scar or lack of umbilicus (37%) and nondebilitating gastrointestinal symptoms (intermittent discomfort, 21%; symptoms of gastrointestinal reflux, 19%; or both 10%).[60] Importantly, while early childhood studies have found a higher frequency of learning disabilities in children with abdominal wall defects,[61] long-term follow-up revealed attainment of education and employment at rates commensurate with the normal population.[60]

REFERENCES

1. Moore TC, Stokes GE. Gastroschisis; report of two cases treated by a modification of the gross operation for omphalocele. *Surgery*. 1953;33(1):112–120.
2. Hwang PJ, Kousseff BG. Omphalocele and gastroschisis: an 18-year review study. *Genet Med*. 2004;6(4):232–236.
3. Brewer S, Williams T. Finally, a sense of closure? Animal models of human ventral body wall defects. *Bioessays*. 2004;26(12):1307–1321.
4. Ledbetter DJ. Gastroschisis and omphalocele. *Surg Clin North Am*. 2006;86(2):249–260, vii.
5. Frolov P, Alali J, Klein MD. Clinical risk factors for gastroschisis and omphalocele in humans: a review of the literature. *Pediatr Surg Int*. 2010;26(12):1135–1148.
6. Richardson S, Browne ML, Rasmussen SA, et al. Associations between periconceptional alcohol consumption and craniosynostosis, omphalocele, and gastroschisis. *Birth Defects Res A Clin Mol Teratol*. 2011;91(7):623–630.
7. Mac Bird T, Robbins JM, Druschel C, Cleves MA, Yang S, Hobbs CA. Demographic and environmental risk factors for gastroschisis and omphalocele in the National Birth Defects Prevention Study. *J Pediatr Surg*. 2009;44(8):1546–1551.
8. Tan KH, Kilby MD, Whittle MJ, Beattie BR, Booth IW, Botting BJ. Congenital anterior abdominal wall defects in England and Wales 1987–93: retrospective analysis of OPCS data. *BMJ*. 1996;313(7062):903–906.
9. Rankin J, Dillon E, Wright C. Congenital anterior abdominal wall defects in the north of England, 1986–1996: occurrence and outcome. *Prenat Diagn*. 1999;19(7):662–668.
10. Gorczyca DP, Lindfors KK, Giles KA, McGahan JP, Hanson FW, Tennant FP. Prenatally diagnosed gastroschisis in monozygotic twins. *J Clin Ultrasound*. 1989;17(3):216–218.
11. Hershey DW, Haesslein HC, Marr CC, Adkins JC. Familial abdominal wall defects. *Am J Med Genet*. 1989;34(2):174–176.
12. Sarda P, Bard H. Gastroschisis in a case of dizygotic twins: the possible role of maternal alcohol consumption. *Pediatrics*. 1984;74(1):94–96.
13. Torfs CP, Curry CJ. Familial cases of gastroschisis in a population-based registry. *Am J Med Genet*. 1993;45(4):465–467.
14. Torfs CP, Christianson RE, Iovannisci DM, Shaw GM, Lammer EJ. Selected gene polymorphisms and their interaction with maternal smoking, as risk factors for gastroschisis. *Birth Defects Res A Clin Mol Teratol*. 2006;76(10):723–730.
15. Lammer EJ, Iovannisci DM, Tom L, Schultz K, Shaw GM. Gastroschisis: a gene-environment model involving the VEGF-NOS3 pathway. *Am J Med Genet C Semin Med Genet*. 2008;148C(3):213–218.
16. Katz LA, Schultz RE, Semina EV, Torfs CP, Krahn KN, Murray JC. Mutations in PITX2 may contribute to cases of omphalocele and VATER-like syndromes. *Am J Med Genet A*. 2004;130A(3):277–283.
17. Lam WW, Hatada I, Ohishi S, et al. Analysis of germline CDKN1C (p57KIP2) mutations in familial and sporadic Beckwith-Wiedemann syndrome (BWS) provides a novel genotype-phenotype correlation. *J Med Genet*. 1999;36(7):518–523.
18. Mills JL, Druschel CM, Pangilinan F, et al. Folate-related genes and omphalocele. *Am J Med Genet A*. 2005;136(1):8–11.
19. Sadler TW. The embryologic origin of ventral body wall defects. *Semin Pediatr Surg*. 2010;19(3):209–214.
20. Sadler TW. *Langman's Medical Embryology*. 11th ed. Baltimore: Lippincott Williams & Wilkins; 2010.
21. Cantrell JR, Haller JA, Ravitch MM. A syndrome of congenital defects involving the abdominal wall, sternum, diaphragm, pericardium, and heart. *Surg Gynecol Obstet*. 1958;107(5):602–614.
22. Shaw A. The myth of gastroschisis. *J Pediatr Surg*. 1975;10(2):235–244.
23. Duhamel B. Embryology of exomphalos and allied malformations. *Arch Dis Child*. 1963;38(198):142–147.
24. Feldkamp ML, Carey JC, Sadler TW. Development of gastroschisis: review of hypotheses, a novel hypothesis, and implications for research. *Am J Med Genet A*. 2007;143(7):639–652.
25. Hoyme HE, Higginbottom MC, Jones KL. The vascular pathogenesis of gastroschisis: intrauterine interruption of the omphalomesenteric artery. *J Pediatr*. 1981;98(2):228–231.
26. deVries PA. The pathogenesis of gastroschisis and omphalocele. *J Pediatr Surg*. 1980;15(3):245–251.
27. Wang KS, Skarsgard ED. Left-sided gastroschisis associated with situs inversus. *J Pediatr Surg*. 2004;39(12):1883–1884.
28. Kronfli R, Bradnock TJ, Sabharwal A. Intestinal atresia in association with gastroschisis: a 26-year review. *Pediatr Surg Int*. 2010;26(9):891–894.
29. Snyder CL, Miller KA, Sharp RJ, et al. Management of intestinal atresia in patients with gastroschisis. *J Pediatr Surg*. 2001;36(10):1542–1545.
30. Langer JC. Abdominal wall defects. *World J Surg*. 2003;27(1):117–124.
31. Kluck P, Tibboel D, van der Kamp AW, Molenaar JC. The effect of fetal urine on the development of the bowel in gastroschisis. *J Pediatr Surg*. 1983;18(1):47–50.
32. Aktug T, Erdag G, Kargi A, Akgur FM, Tibboel D. Amnio-allantoic fluid exchange for the prevention of intestinal damage in gastroschisis: an experimental study on chick embryos. *J Pediatr Surg*. 1995;30(3):384–387.
33. Lausman AY, Langer JC, Tai M, et al. Gastroschisis: what is the average gestational age of spontaneous delivery? *J Pediatr Surg*. 2007;42(11):1816–1821.
34. Charlesworth P, Njere I, Allotey J, et al. Postnatal outcome in gastroschisis: effect of birth weight and gestational age. *J Pediatr Surg*. 2007;42(5):815–818.
35. Vachharajani AJ, Rao R, Keswani S, Mathur AM. Outcomes of exomphalos: an institutional experience. *Pediatr Surg Int*. 2009;25(2):139–144.
36. O'Donnell KA, Glick PL, Caty MG. Pediatric umbilical problems. *Pediatr Clin North Am*. 1998;45(4):791–799.
37. Sutherland RS, Mevorach RA, Kogan BA. The prune-belly syndrome: current insights. *Pediatr Nephrol*. 1995;9(6):770–778.

38. Walkinshaw SA, Renwick M, Hebisch G, Hey EN. How good is ultrasound in the detection and evaluation of anterior abdominal wall defects? *Br J Radiol*. 1992;65(772):298–301.

39. Palomaki GE, Hill LE, Knight GJ, Haddow JE, Carpenter M. Second-trimester maternal serum alpha-fetoprotein levels in pregnancies associated with gastroschisis and omphalocele. *Obstet Gynecol*. 1988;71(6 Pt 1):906–909.

40. Saller DN Jr, Canick JA, Palomaki GE, Knight GJ, Haddow JE. Second-trimester maternal serum alpha-fetoprotein, unconjugated estriol, and hCG levels in pregnancies with ventral wall defects. *Obstet Gynecol*. 1994;84(5):852–855.

41. Langer JC, Khanna J, Caco C, Dykes EH, Nicolaides KH. Prenatal diagnosis of gastroschisis: development of objective sonographic criteria for predicting outcome. *Obstet Gynecol*. 1993;81(1):53–56.

42. Adra AM, Landy HJ, Nahmias J, Gomez-Marin O. The fetus with gastroschisis: impact of route of delivery and prenatal ultrasonography. *Am J Obstet Gynecol*. 1996;174(2):540–546.

43. Hadidi A, Subotic U, Goeppl M, Waag KL. Early elective cesarean delivery before 36 weeks vs late spontaneous delivery in infants with gastroschisis. *J Pediatr Surg*. 2008;43(7):1342–1346.

44. Hasan S, Hermansen MC. The prenatal diagnosis of ventral abdominal wall defects. *Am J Obstet Gynecol*. 1986;155(4):842–845.

45. Davidson JM, Johnson TR Jr, Rigdon DT, Thompson BH. Gastroschisis and omphalocele: prenatal diagnosis and perinatal management. *Prenat Diagn*. 1984;4(5):355–363.

46. Calisti A, Manzoni C, Perrelli L. The fetus with an abdominal wall defect: management and outcome. *J Perinat Med*. 1987;15(1):105–111.

47. Lewis DF, Towers CV, Garite TJ, Jackson DN, Nageotte MP, Major CA. Fetal gastroschisis and omphalocele: is cesarean section the best mode of delivery? *Am J Obstet Gynecol*. 1990;163(3):773–775.

48. Moretti M, Khoury A, Rodriquez J, Lobe T, Shaver D, Sibai B. The effect of mode of delivery on the perinatal outcome in fetuses with abdominal wall defects. *Am J Obstet Gynecol*. 1990;163(3):833–838.

49. Soares H, Silva A, Rocha G, Pissarra S, Correia-Pinto J, Guimaraes H. Gastroschisis: preterm or term delivery? *Clinics (Sao Paulo)*. 2010;65(2):139–142.

50. Lansdale N, Hill R, Gull-Zamir S, et al. Staged reduction of gastroschisis using preformed silos: practicalities and problems. *J Pediatr Surg*. 2009;44(11):2126–2129.

51. Riboh J, Abrajano CT, Garber K, et al. Outcomes of sutureless gastroschisis closure. *J Pediatr Surg*. 2009;44(10):1947–1951.

52. Owen A, Marven S, Johnson P, et al. Gastroschisis: a national cohort study to describe contemporary surgical strategies and outcomes. *J Pediatr Surg*. 2010;45(9):1808–1816.

53. Nyberg DA, Fitzsimmons J, Mack LA, et al. Chromosomal abnormalities in fetuses with omphalocele. Significance of omphalocele contents. *J Ultrasound Med*. 1989;8(6):299–308.

54. Novotny DA, Klein RL, Boeckman CR. Gastroschisis: an 18-year review. *J Pediatr Surg*. 1993;28(5):650–652.

55. Baerg J, Kaban G, Tonita J, Pahwa P, Reid D. Gastroschisis: a sixteen-year review. *J Pediatr Surg*. 2003;38(5):771–774.

56. Henrich K, Huemmer HP, Reingruber B, Weber PG. Gastroschisis and omphalocele: treatments and long-term outcomes. *Pediatr Surg Int*. 2008;24(2):167–173.

57. Heider AL, Strauss RA, Kuller JA. Omphalocele: clinical outcomes in cases with normal karyotypes. *Am J Obstet Gynecol*. 2004;190(1):135–141.

58. Mabogunje OA, Mahour GH. Omphalocele and gastroschisis. Trends in survival across two decades. *Am J Surg*. 1984;148(5):679–686.

59. Hughes MD, Nyberg DA, Mack LA, Pretorius DH. Fetal omphalocele: prenatal US detection of concurrent anomalies and other predictors of outcome. *Radiology*. 1989;173(2):371–376.

60. Koivusalo A, Lindahl H, Rintala RJ. Morbidity and quality of life in adult patients with a congenital abdominal wall defect: a questionnaire survey. *J Pediatr Surg*. 2002;37(11):1594–1601.

61. Ginn-Pease ME, King DR, Tarnowski KJ, Green L, Young G, Linscheid TR. Psychosocial adjustment and physical growth in children with imperforate anus or abdominal wall defects. *J Pediatr Surg*. 1991;26(9):1129–1135.

Intestinal Obstruction

Gary E. Hartman

EPIDEMIOLOGY

Intestinal obstruction is a common condition in the neonatal period. Although precise data are not available, it is estimated to occur in approximately 1 in 2000 live births.[1] Esophageal obstruction generally presents with respiratory symptoms and is not discussed here. Intestinal obstruction is frequently complete, as in intestinal atresia, or incomplete, as in duodenal stenosis. While the majority of obstructions are mechanical, others are functional, such as Hirschprung disease or meconium ileus. The ileus associated with septic or metabolic conditions may mimic intestinal obstruction and must be distinguished from obstruction, as it does not require operative intervention.

Associated conditions include genetic abnormalities or associated malformations. Trisomy 21 and duodenal atresia are associated[2]; meconium ileus is associated with cystic fibrosis (CF) and familial forms of Hirschprung disease. Imperforate anus is associated with esophageal atresia and renal or musculoskeletal anomalies, as in the VACTERL (vertebral, anal, cardiac, tracheoesophageal, renal, and limb) association.

PATHOPHYSIOLOGY

The symptoms of intestinal obstruction may be catastrophic (eg, malrotation with midgut volvulus with ischemia or infarction) or relatively benign (eg, atresia of the duodenum or small intestine). The bowel proximal to the obstruction becomes dilated, presumably due to the effect of peristalsis against the obstruction, and the degree of dilation is considered to be related to the duration of the obstruction. The secretions of the intestine proximal to the obstruction accumulate in the dilated proximal bowel and result in vomiting or polyhydramnios. The vomitus is bilious in the majority of instances but will be nonbilious if the obstruction is proximal to the ampulla of Vater. If the vomiting is prolonged, the infant will become volume depleted and have electrolyte abnormalities.

Abdominal distension develops as the obstruction continues and is more prominent the more distal the obstruction is. Proximal obstructions (pyloric, duodenal, high jejunal) will have little or no distension. Distal obstructions, such as imperforate anus, Hirschprung disease, or distal ileal obstruction, will develop significant abdominal distension. Malrotation with volvulus will have no distension early in the process but once the bowel has become ischemic may have significant distension and abdominal tenderness. Abdominal tenderness and erythema are not associated with intestinal obstruction unless it is complicated by ischemia or perforation.

Failure to pass meconium or delayed passage may be associated with intestinal obstruction. Ninety-five percent of term infants will pass meconium during the first 24 hours of life.[3] Of infants with Hirschprung disease, 60% to 95% will pass meconium after 24 hours following birth.[4] Newborn boys with apparent imperforate anus are usually observed for up to 24 hours to identify passage of meconium through small openings on the perineum. The appearance of meconium or of white "pearls" on the perineum will identify a fistulous opening that can be probed to identify a low imperforate anus

Table 36-1 Other Causes of Neonatal Obstruction

Etiology	Location
Inguinal hernia	Small bowel, colon
Necrotizing enterocolitis stricture	Colon, small bowel
Intestinal duplication	Small bowel
Internal hernia	Small bowel
Mesenteric cyst	Small bowel

that is covered by an epithelial membrane as opposed to a high imperforate anus that will need either a colostomy or a primary pull-through procedure.

Other causes of obstruction are presented in Table 36-1.

DIFFERENTIAL DIAGNOSIS

The differential diagnosis of intestinal obstruction depends on the symptom of obstruction that is being evaluated: polyhydramnios, vomiting, abdominal distension, or delayed passage of meconium.

Polyhydramnios is an infrequent complication of pregnancy (1%) and is determined by qualitative or quantitative criteria. The majority (60%) of cases are classified as idiopathic. Other causes include fetal malformations and genetic conditions (8%–45%), maternal diabetes mellitus (5%–26%), multiple gestations (8%–10%), and fetal anemia (1%–11%).[5]

Vomiting is a common symptom in newborns and is classified as bilious vs nonbilious and projectile or effortless. The most common causes of vomiting in neonates are gastroesophageal (GE) reflux, overfeeding, and gastric dysfunction due to prematurity, gastritis, or metabolic conditions. The emesis in obstructions that are proximal to the ampulla of Vater will be nonbilious. The vomitus in newborns with gastritis is typically brown, "coffee grounds," or blood tinged. Infants with gastritis are also typically irritable due to the ongoing inflammation.

Abdominal distension (see Figures 36-1 and 36-2) is also common in newborns, particularly premature infants. Generalized abdominal distension may be due to ascites, gaseous or liquid accumulation in the gastrointestinal (GI) tract, or rarely, large masses in the liver, GI or genitourinary tract, or retroperitoneum. Gaseous distension of the entire GI tract is typical of the ileus due to sepsis, metabolic conditions such as congenital adrenal hyperplasia, or the dysmaturity of the GI tract in premature infants. This last condition, characterized by repeated episodes of abdominal distension and feeding intolerance, results in frequent

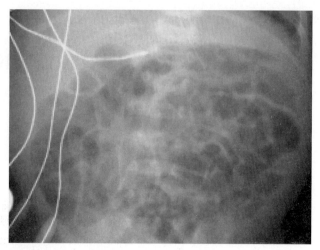

FIGURE 36-1 Abdominal x-ray of premature infant with normal gas pattern.

interruptions in enteral feeding and diagnostic investigations that may be unnecessary or associated with risk. These episodes are usually self-limited and eventually resolve as the infant approaches term.

Delayed passage of meconium is a characteristic symptom of Hirschprung disease, with reports of 95% of affected infants passing their first meconium after 24 hours of age. Paradoxically, infants with complete obstructions of the GI tract may pass meconium or mucous stools as they are evacuating material that accumulated before the obstruction became complete or are emptying distal intestinal secretions to the point of obstruction.

DIAGNOSTIC TESTS

The diagnosis of intestinal obstruction can be suspected or defined during the prenatal period with ultrasound or fetal magnetic resonance imaging (MRI). On ultrasound, obstruction is suggested by dilation of the bowel and vigorous peristalsis. Accuracy of ultrasound

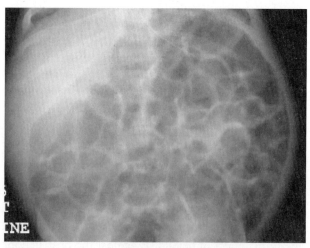

FIGURE 36-2 Same infant with diffuse distension.

in this setting is low (34%), with greater accuracy for proximal obstructions such as those of the duodenum (52%) and small intestine (40%). The sensitivity for anal atresia is low, %8–10%.[6,7] The sensitivity of ultrasound in detecting fetal obstruction is further compromised given that the routine timing for ultrasound anatomic survey is 20 weeks and that many of the obstructions may occur after this date.

Fetal bowel is well visualized by MRI, but the usefulness of MRI in diagnosing fetal obstructions appears limited as the majority of cases are identified by ultrasound; MRI has not been more accurate in the case of anal atresia.

After birth, most obstructions can be diagnosed accurately with the combination of history, physical examination, plain films of the abdomen, and contrast study of either the upper or lower GI tract. Ultrasound is useful in identifying ascites, abdominal mass, and malrotation. Ultrasound has also been used to evaluate malrotation.

MANAGEMENT

Stomach

Antral Web/Pyloric Atresia

Obstructions of the distal stomach and pylorus are rare, accounting for 1% or less of neonatal obstructions. Antral web was described in the 1970s as a mucosa-lined membrane near the pylorus that produces partial or high-grade obstruction. Recent reports have described more fibrous bands. The radiographic diagnosis consists of a thin band in the distal antrum. While operative resection of the web is the described treatment, there have been reports of responses to treatments directed at gastritis, such as acid blockers.

Pyloric atresia is extremely rare, with an incidence of 1:100,000 to 1:1 million live births. Approximately half of the cases are associated with epidermolysis bullosa,[8] which should be assumed until excluded with careful attention to wound care. Diagnosis is suspected by air contrast films and can be confirmed with contrast if needed. Operative correction has been described as pyloroplasty or gastroduodenostomy.

Pyloric Stenosis

Pyloric stenosis is a common cause of intestinal obstruction in infants and frequently occurs during the neonatal period. The vast majority of cases occur in term infants who have developed nonbilious vomiting at home after an initial asymptomatic period of days to weeks. The emesis is frequently described as forceful or projectile, and the infants are typically hungry and happy between feeds, in contrast to infants with gastritis, who are frequently irritable.

Ultrasound is the preferred method of diagnosis and has high reliability. Wall thickness greater than 3 mm and pyloric length greater than 12 mm are considered abnormal, especially if combined with failure to identify fluid passing through the pylorus during the examination.[9] The study must be performed systematically and with care to measure the wall thickness in a true perpendicular image. If the measurements are equivocal (2- to 3-mm wall thickness), a period of observation or repeat ultrasound is a reasonable strategy.

Once diagnosis is established, normalizing intravascular volume and electrolyte balance are the prime priority. Infants with pyloric stenosis may be 10%–15% dehydrated and suffer from hypochloremic alkalosis. This must be corrected before attempts at operative intervention to prevent arrhythmias associated with anesthesia. Fracture of the anterior wall of the pyloric muscle (pyloromyotomy) performed laparoscopically or by open approach has been the standard therapy for over 50 years. Recovery is rapid, with most centers allowing feedings beginning 4 to 6 hours following the operation and discharge at approximately 24 hours. In the days following operation, most infants continue to have emesis that is less severe and does not compromise hydration or electrolyte balance.

Gastric Volvulus

Rotation or twisting of the stomach along its long axis (organoaxial) or its short axis (mesenteroaxial) is a rare condition due to the normally extensive fixation of the stomach by its attachments to the diaphragm, spleen, and the anchoring effect of the immobile GE junction and the duodenum. Conditions such as malrotation, especially in the situation of asplenia or polysplenia, may predispose to gastric volvulus. This condition is marked by the sudden onset of severe vomiting or retching and rapid progression to cardiovascular collapse. Diagnosis is suspected from the unusual gastric bubble on plain films and confirmed by contrast studies that demonstrate obstruction at the GE junction or pylorus and elevation of the pylorus at times more cranial than the GE junction.

The treatment of gastric volvulus is operative anchoring of the stomach either by anterior gastropexy or gastrostomy. The procedure may be performed laparoscopically or open. Fixation of the stomach has been recommended at the time of correction of malrotation in the setting of poly- or asplenia and when the stomach is unusually mobile.

Duodenum

Atresia, Stenosis, Annular Pancreas, or Web

Atresia or stenosis of the duodenum occurs in 1:5000 to 1:10,000 live births, making it the most common intestinal atresia.[10,11] The duodenum is the only portion of the gastrointestinal tract that has a solid phase during development, and the etiology of atresia and stenosis in this area is postulated as a failure of the normal vacuolization of the solid phase that results in the formation of the duodenal lumen. Duodenal atresia and its associated conditions of stenosis, duodenal web, or annular pancreas are associated with trisomy 21, cardiac anomalies, and malrotation in approximately 30% of cases. Prematurity and infants small for gestational age are also common.

Polyhydramnios is present in up to 80% of cases, and ultrasound diagnosis can be apparent in the second or third trimester.[12] Fluid-filled distended stomach and proximal duodenum produce the "double bubble" that is characteristic of these anomalies. Exaggerated gastric peristalsis may also be appreciated. After birth, the fluid-filled double bubble is air filled and generally is diagnostic. Injection of 20–30 cc of air through a nasogastric (NG) or oral gastric (OG) tube can accentuate the radiographic findings in ambiguous cases. Upper gastrointestinal series (UGI) may be considered in cases of partial obstruction (stenosis, web) or to exclude malrotation with obstruction if operative repair will be deferred due to complications of prematurity or associated cardiac anomalies.

Treatment is by operative bypass of the obstruction (duodenoduodenostomy) or excision of the web, which may be performed laparoscopically or by an open approach. Attempts to "divide" the annular pancreas if present are ineffective as the obstruction in such cases is due to atresia or stenosis of the duodenum, not the failure of normal pancreatic rotation. Placement of a transanastomic feeding tube may be used to inspect the rest of the duodenum and small intestine for other atresias and may facilitate postoperative feeding.

Malrotation

Between the 5th and 12th weeks of gestation, the rapid elongation of the GI tract results in herniation of the bowel through the umbilical ring into the coelomic stalk. The bowel returns to the abdominal cavity and undergoes a process of rotation and finally fixation. Malrotation is the result of a disruption of the usual process of rotation and fixation. Symptomatic malrotation is estimated to occur in 1:6000 live births, while asymptomatic rotational abnormalities are estimated to affect up to 0.5% of the population.[13] Malrotational anomalies produce intestinal obstruction by duodenal compression from peritoneal attachments between the retroperitoneum and the cecum or by twisting of the midgut around the narrow pedicle formed by the adhesion of the duodenojejunal limb to the cecum. Symptomatic midgut volvulus progresses to intestinal ischemia and cardiovascular collapse within a matter of hours, generally believed to be less than 4 to 6 hours from the onset

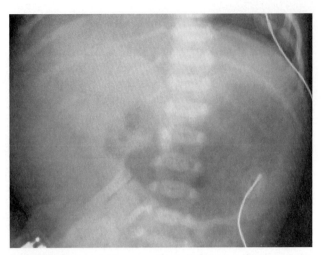

FIGURE 36-3 Newborn with malrotation. Film demonstrates dilated gas-filled stomach with paucity of other intestinal gas.

of the symptoms. Failure to reverse the ischemia results in loss of the entire midgut from the distal duodenum to the midtransverse colon, resulting in permanent intestinal insufficiency. The catastrophic consequences and the extremely short therapeutic window make identification of malrotation a high diagnostic priority.

Malrotation (Figure 36-3) is associated with other anomalies[14] in 30%–60% of cases, with cardiac, diaphragmatic, and GI anomalies most common. There are no diagnostic features of malrotation on plain film, which generally requires contrast study for confirmation (Figure 36-4). However, paucity of bowel gas in the appropriate clinical setting should suggest malrotation and prompt urgent confirmation. Ultrasound has been employed with reversal of position of the superior mesenteric artery and vein and Doppler blood flow findings of importance. The classical presentation of a reversible case of midgut volvulus would be a term infant less than a month of age who had been thriving but developed bilious emesis with a soft, nondistended abdomen and minimal bowel gas on plain film. The lack of worrisome physical findings or radiographic distension should not be reassuring. By the time the infant has developed abdominal distension, diffuse gas-filled loops on plain film with or without cardiovascular compromise, the ischemia is likely to be irreversible.

The treatment of symptomatic malrotation with volvulus is emergent operation with derotation, assessment of bowel viability, and either bowel resection or planned second-look operation if bowel viability is uncertain. If the bowel regains perfusion, the rest of the classical Ladd procedure (widening of the mesentery, appendectomy, and placement of small bowel to the right with colon to left) is completed. In asymptomatic cases, the procedure can be safely performed laparoscopically.

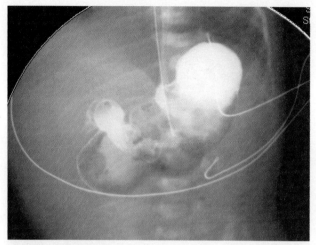

FIGURE 36-4 Contrast fails to pass second portion of displaced duodenum.

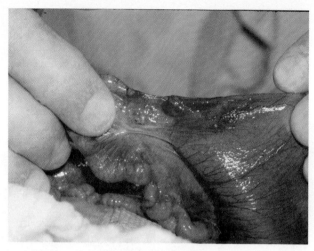

FIGURE 36-6 Jejunoileal atresia with small gap.

Jejunem/Ileum

Atresia

Atresia of the jejunem and ileum appear to be late-gestation events resulting from vascular insult to the developed bowel.[15] The amount of intestine involved depends on the magnitude of the vascular insult. The ischemic bowel is resorbed, producing a blind proximal and distal segment if the amount of bowel involved is significant (Figure 36-5). In cases of more limited vascular event, the bowel may remain in continuity with only a membrane between the proximal and distal segments (Figure 36-6). The proximal bowel becomes progressively dilated due to peristalsis against the obstruction (Figure 36-7). If the ischemic event occurs near delivery, the necrotic or resorbing bowel may still be present. Atresia of the jejunem (Figure 36-8) appears to be equal in frequency to that

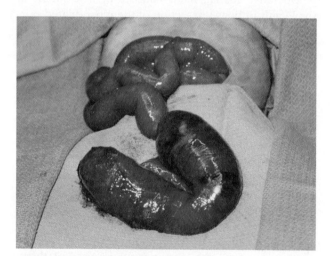

FIGURE 36-7 Jejunoileal atresia with large gap and volvulus of the dilated proximal limb.

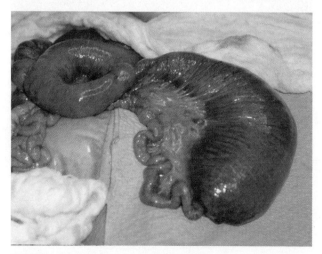

FIGURE 36-5 Jejunoileal atresia with no gap in mesentery. Note the dilated proximal bowel.

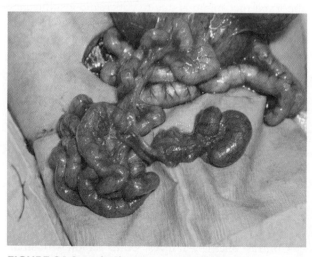

FIGURE 36-8 Multiple segmental atresias.

of the ileum, and together they affect approximately 1:5000 live births.[10]

The timing of symptoms and amount of distension depend on the level of the obstruction, with more distal atresias producing more distension over a period of many hours or days. Plain films reveal dilated loops of variable but sometimes-dramatic size. Contrast enema usually reveals a small-caliber colon ("microcolon") due to the lack of enteral contents entering the segment distal to the atresia. Contrast administered from above may show dilated loops of small bowel but is generally not helpful in defining the level of obstruction due to dilution of the contrast.

Management of jejunoileal atresias is operative after appropriate fluid resuscitation and evaluation for associated anomalies. Associated anomalies are infrequent (10%),[16] which is assumed to be due to the late-gestational timing of these anomalies.

Operative management consists of assessment of the length of bowel, resection of the most dilated portion of the proximal segment, and anastomosis. The disparity between proximal and distal segments may be challenging and occasionally requires tapering of the proximal segment or creation of stomas with delayed anastomosis after the proximal segment has decreased in size. Long-term outcome is primarily determined by the amount of viable bowel remaining. The limits of remaining bowel that will support enteral independence appear to be 25–30 cm with an intact ileocecal valve and 40–50 cm without it.

Meconium Ileus

Meconium ileus refers to a condition characterized by obstruction of the distal ileum due to inspissated, thickened meconium. It is reported to affect 1:3000 live births and is associated with CF in 95% of term infants with the condition. A similar syndrome occurs in very low birth weight infants without the association with CF. The abnormal meconium is due to pancreatic insufficiency and to the secretion of abnormal mucus from the intestinal glands in infants with CF. The obstruction begins in utero, resulting in established abdominal distension at birth, the only mechanical obstruction to present with distension at birth. In addition to the early distension, palpation of the abdomen may reveal a "doughy" texture with the persistence of an imprint if the examiner compresses the doughy material. Radiographic features of the plain films may also be suggestive of meconium ileus as the cause of the obstruction. The dilated loops are of a wide variety of calibers (Figures 36-9 to 36-12); there are few, if any, air-fluid levels, there is little difference between supine and upright films, and there may be a "soap bubble" appearance to many loops.

Contrast enema will reveal a microcolon with small beads of meconium in the lumen of the proximal colon

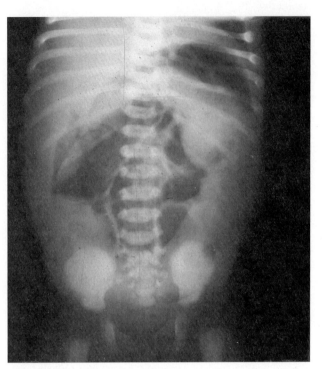

FIGURE 36-9 Plain film with dilated loops without air-fluid levels.

or distal ileum. The obstruction associated with meconium ileus may be uncomplicated or complicated by volvulus, ischemia, or perforation. In uncomplicated meconium ileus, treatment may be nonoperative. Contrast enema with a hyperosmolar contrast agent

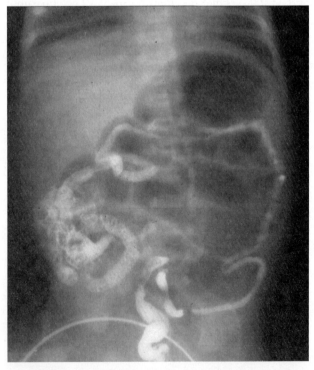

FIGURE 36-10 Contrast enema demonstrating microcolon and lucent beads of meconium in the distal ileum.

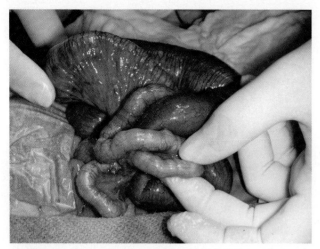

FIGURE 36-11 Operative photo demonstrating the firm beads of meconium inspissated in the distal ileum with proximal dilated loops of small bowel.

(Gastrografin) may successfully break up the luminal obstruction. The mechanism is uncertain but is thought to be due to the osmolar effect drawing fluid into the intestinal lumen as well as a direct "detergent" effect of disrupting disulfide bonds in the abnormal meconium. Undiluted Gastrografin is 1900 mosm and should not be used full strength or without secure intravenous access. The hyperosmolar enema may be repeated if not initially successful. Approximately 50% of uncomplicated cases will be successfully managed with contrast enema. If the radiographic attempts are not successful, the operative approach involves instillation of saline or Gastrografin into the lumen of the bowel proximal to the obstruction, followed by milking of the material into the colon.

Meconium ileus complicated by ischemia, perforation, or peritonitis should not be treated by contrast enema. Operative intervention may be associated with significant bleeding due to intense inflammatory

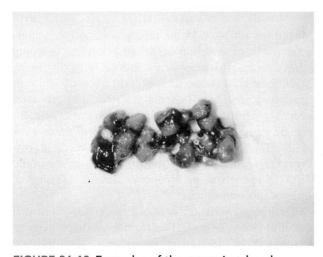

FIGURE 36-12 Examples of the meconium beads.

reaction and adhesions. Debridement of the necrotic tissue and extravasated meconium are accompanied by irrigation of any residual luminal obstruction and either intestinal anastomosis or enterostomy. Occasionally, prenatal perforation of meconium ileus will result in a large meconium "cyst" at birth that may be treated by initial drainage with definitive operative correction deferred until the inflammatory process has resolved. In addition, on occasion diffuse abdominal calcification will be observed in the absence of intestinal symptoms, presumably representing an in utero perforation that has resolved without resultant peritonitis or intestinal obstruction. Aggressive treatment of the accompanying CF should be instituted in the perioperative period.

Colon/Anus

Atresia

Atresia of the colon is the least-common atresia of the GI tract, with an estimated incidence of 1:20,000 live births.[17] While it is frequently an isolated anomaly, it may be associated with proximal jejunoileal atresia (10%–15%), gastroschisis (2%), or Hirschprung disease (1%–2%). Colonic atresia is also associated with several significant musculoskeletal anomalies.[18]

Like jejunoileal atresia, the mechanism of colonic atresia is assumed to be a vascular insult to the formed colon. The obstruction is rarely identified by prenatal ultrasound, and polyhydramnios is uncommon. The infants are usually born at term and develop progressive and severe abdominal distension with a significant risk of perforation. The abdominal distension may produce respiratory compromise that requires assisted ventilation.

Plain films of the abdomen reveal severely distended loops of bowel with multiple air-fluid levels consistent with a distal obstruction. Contrast enema will reveal microcolon distal to the blind-ending atresia. Following preoperative resuscitation and preparation, most authors recommended urgent operative correction due to the risk of perforation. Suction rectal biopsy is also frequently recommended due to the rare but consistent association with Hirschprung disease.

Operative treatment consists of resection of the atretic ends with primary anastomosis if feasible. Occasionally, colostomy will be required due to excessive size disparity or contamination from perforation.

Hirschprung Disease

Hirschprung disease is a cause of distal colonic and rectal functional obstruction due to absent innervation. The incidence is estimated at 1:5000 live births,[19] and there is a strong male (4:1) predominance except in the long-segment varieties.[20] The familial incidence is reported between 3.5% and 8% but is higher (13%–20%) in total colonic and total intestinal disease (50%). Approximately 12% of infants with Hirschprung disease have chromosomal abnormalities,[19] most commonly trisomy 21.

The abnormal innervation of the bowel is described as a continuous process extending proximally from the rectum. The "transition" zone from abnormal to normal innervation is in the rectosigmoid region in 75% of cases, with total colonic involvement in 5%–10%. Extension of the disease into the small intestine is unusual. Skip areas have been reported but also are considered rare.

The vast majority, up to 90%, of infants with Hirschprung disease will have their first passage of meconium delayed past 24 hours of life.[4] They develop progressive abdominal distension with vomiting, and the majority are diagnosed in the first month of life. While some authors believe that Hirschprung disease does not occur in premature infants, there are well-documented instances, although the frequency of prematurity in patients with Hirschprung disease appears decreased.

Plain films are consistent with a distal bowel obstruction, and contrast enema will show a small or normal-caliber rectum with funnel-shaped transition zone progressing to the dilated normally innervated bowel (Figures 36-13 and 36-14). Contrast enema may not be diagnostic in the early neonatal period or if excessive rectal dilations or irrigations have been instituted. The diagnosis is confirmed by rectal biopsy, which is usually performed by a suction biopsy device but may be done by open operative approach. The demonstration of the absence of ganglion cells may be challenging, particularly in premature infants. This fact has led many to recommend deferring biopsy until term or near term.

Treatment of Hirschprung disease is surgical removal of the aganglionic bowel with anastomosis of

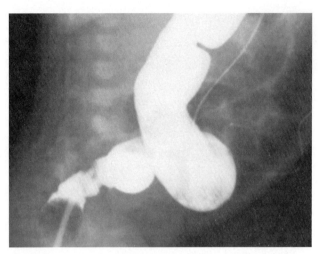

FIGURE 36-14 Contrast enema with normal-caliber rectum and funnel-shaped transition to dilated sigmoid.

normally innervated bowel to the anus just above the dentate line. In the past, this was accomplished in a two-stage procedure with initial colostomy proximal to the transition zone with subsequent pull-through procedure. Currently, most cases are managed with a one-stage pull-through procedure either in the first few days of life or after a period of stabilization with rectal irrigations substituted for the colostomy. Results of this current strategy appear equivalent to the two-stage procedure, although occasional infants will have persistent difficulties with constipation or rarely with continence.

Enterocolitis associated with Hirschprung disease is characterized by foul-smelling, liquid, green stool and may progress rapidly to cardiovascular collapse. It is treated with aggressive irrigations, volume resuscitation, antibiotics, and supportive care. Previously felt to be a risk only prior to surgical correction, it is well documented in postoperative patients.

Meconium Plug Syndrome

Meconium plug syndrome refers to a condition characterized by obstruction of the left colon due to a plug of meconium. It is relatively common, affecting up to 1:500 infants, who are usually term but may occur in premature infants. Maternal diabetes and neonatal hypothyroidism may be associated with this condition. Hirschprung disease has been reported in up to 15% of infants and argues for routine suction rectal biopsy. Previous reports linking meconium plug syndrome with CF are felt to be erroneous due to inclusion of cases of meconium ileus.[21]

Clinical presentation is of a distal obstruction with multiple dilated loops and air-fluid levels on plain films. Diagnosis and treatment are usually accomplished with water-soluble contrast enema or occasionally with

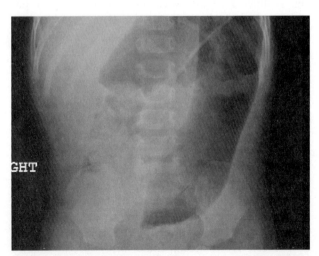

FIGURE 36-13 Plain film with dilated colon with air-fluid level in rectosigmoid area.

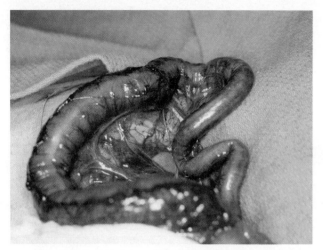

FIGURE 36-15 Operative photo of meconium plug syndrome with small-caliber left colon with meconium plug in place.

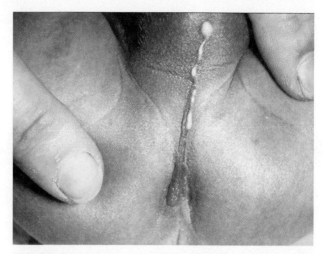

FIGURE 36-17 Perineum of infant with low imperforate anus revealing squamous pearls and small area of meconium visible.

spontaneous passage of the mucous plug (Figures 36-15 and 36-16). Symptoms generally resolve promptly following passage of the plug.

Imperforate Anus

Imperforate anus occurs in approximately 1:5000 live births and is usually obvious at birth, preventing progression to clinical obstruction. However, failure to recognize imperforate anus may occur in instances of a fistula to the perineum or high-grade anal stenosis. Low imperforate anus (Figure 36-17), characterized by a fistula to the perineum or meconium or squamous "beads" on the perineum, may be treated by an anoplasty in the neonatal period. High imperforate anus will generally require a colostomy before definitive repair, although many centers are performing primary pull-through procedures in selected cases.

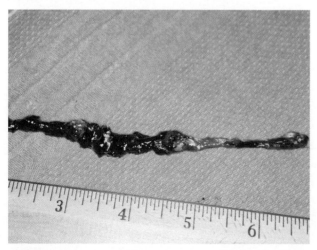

FIGURE 36-16 Meconium plug passes after contrast enema.

REFERENCES

1. Young JY, Kim DS, Muratore CS, et al. High incidence of postoperative bowel obstruction in newborns and infants. *J Pediatr Surg.* 2007;42(6):962–965.
2. Kimble RM, Harding J, Kolbe A. Additional congenital anomalies in babies with gut atresia or stenosis: when to investigate, and which investigation. *Pediatr Surg Int.* 1997;12(8):565–570.
3. Clark DA. Times of first void and first stool in 500 newborns. *Pediatrics.* 1977;60(4):457–459.
4. Singh SJ, Craoker GD, Manglick P, et al. Hirschprung's disease: the Australian Paediatric Surveillance Unit's experience. *Pediatr Surg Int.* 2003;19(4):247–250.
5. Hill LM, Breckle R, Thomas ML, Fries JK. Polyhydramnios: ultrasonically detected prevalence and neonatal outcome. *Obstet Gynecol.* 1987; 69:21.
6. Haeusler MC, Berghold A, Stoll C, et al. Prenatal ultrasonographic detection of gastrointestinal obstruction: results from 18 European congenital anomaly registries. *Prenat Diagn.* 2002;22:616.
7. Stoll C, Alembik Y, Dott B, Roth MP. Evaluation of prenatal diagnosis of congenital gastro-intestinal atresias. *Eur J Epidemiol.* 1996;12:611.
8. Nawaz A, Matta H, Jacobsz A, et al. Congenital pyloric atresia and junctional epidermolysis bullosa: a report of two cases. *Pediatr Surg Int.* 2000;16(3):206–208.
9. Lund Kofoed PE, Høst A, Elle B, Larsen C. Hypertrophic pyloric stenosis: determination of muscle dimensions by ultrasound. *Br J Radiol.* 1988; 61:19.
10. Dalla Vecchia LK, Grosfeld JL, West KW, et al. Intestinal atresia and stenosis: a 25 year experience with 277 cases. *Arch Surg.* 1998;133(5):490–497.
11. Kimura K, Mukohara N, Nishijima E, et al. Diamond shaped anastomosis for duodenal atresia: an experience with 44 patients over 15 years. *J Pediatr Surg.* 1990;25(9):977–979.
12. Bittencourt DG, Barini R, Marba S, et al. Congenital duodenal obstruction: does prenatal diagnosis improve the outcome? *Pediatr Surg Int.* 2004;20(8):582–585.
13. Kapfer SA, Rappold JF. Intestinal malrotation-not just the pediatric surgeon's problem. *J Am Coll Surg.* 2004;199(4):628–635.
14. Smith SD. Disorders of intestinal rotation and fixation. In: Grosfeld JL, Oneill JA, Fonkalsrud EW, et al, eds. *Pediatric Surgery.* 6th ed. Philadelphia, PA: Mosby Elsevier; 2006:1342–1357.

15. Louw JH, Barnard CN. Congenital intestinal atresia; observations on its origin. *Lancet.* 1955;269(6899):1065–1067.

16. Sweeney B, Surana R, Puri P. Jejunoileal atresia and associated malformations:correlation with the timing of in utero insult. *J Pediatr Surg.* 2001;36(5):774–776.

17. Powell RW, Raffensperger JG. Congenital colonic atresia. *J Pediatr Surg.* 1982;17(2):166–170.

18. Baglaj M, Carachi R, MacCormack B. Colonic atresia: a clinicopathological insight into its etiology. *Eur J Pediatr Surg.* 2010;20(2):102–105.

19. Amiel J, Sproat-Emison E, Garcia-Barcelo M, et al. Hirschprung disease, associated syndromes and genetics: a review. *J Med Genet.* 2008;45(1):1–14.

20. Badner JA, Sieber WK, Garver KL, et al. A genetic study of Hirschprung disease. *Am J Hum Genet.* 1990;46(3):568–580.

21. Keckler S, St Peter S, Spilde T, et al. Current significance of meconium plug syndrome. *J Pediatr Surg.* 2008;43(5):896–898.

CHAPTER 36

Necrotizing Enterocolitis and Spontaneous Intestinal Perforation

Jonathan L. Slaughter and R. Lawrence Moss

INTRODUCTION

Necrotizing enterocolitis (NEC) remains one of the most devastating diagnoses in the neonatal intensive care unit. Primarily affecting preterm infants, it is a leading cause of death and lifelong gastrointestinal and neurodevelopmental morbidities in the very low birth weight (VLBW) (birth weight < 1500 g) population. Despite decades of research, the specific etiology for NEC remains unknown. NEC appears to be precipitated by an insult that leads the immature neonatal immune system to mount an abnormal and deleterious inflammatory response. Since many neonates die or suffer unfavorable outcomes despite maximal medical and surgical therapy, a preventive strategy is greatly needed. This chapter reviews the epidemiology, pathophysiology, diagnostic criteria, and supportive treatment of NEC, as well as promising novel, preventive strategies currently under investigation.

EPIDEMIOLOGY

Necrotizing enterocolitis is estimated to occur in 1 per 1000 US live births each year.[1] Its annual rate in the highest-risk population, VLBW infants born prior to 29 weeks, is much higher (10%–15%). NEC frequency is inversely related to birth weight and gestational age in a nonlinear fashion, with a marked increase in NEC incidence as birth weight decreases below 1500 g.[2] In the United States, the incidence rate in the VLBW population has remained stable at 11% in recent years.[3] Despite this stability, the proportion of neonatal deaths secondary to NEC has actually increased over the past 2 decades, as preterm deaths from other causes have fallen due to advances in neonatal care.[4]

Although NEC is predominantly a disease of VLBW infants, it is occasionally seen in term infants following other illnesses. Concurrent diagnoses of congenital heart disease, bacterial sepsis, polycythemia, and hypotension are associated with NEC in term and late-preterm infants.[5]

Patient Demographics

Necrotizing enterocolitis is reported more frequently in male infants and non-Hispanic infants of African descent.[1] Timing of onset is inversely related to gestational age, with a median onset of nearly 4 postnatal weeks in infants born at less than 25 weeks' gestation, 2 weeks at 27–29 weeks' gestation, and within the first week in term infants.[6] Most NEC cases present sporadically, although temporal, nonseasonal clustering of NEC cases within neonatal intensive care units has been reported.[7]

Antenatal Risk Factors

The main antenatal risk factors for NEC are those associated with preterm birth, the leading risk factor for NEC.[8] Thus, at birth it is nearly impossible to predict which VLBW infants will be at higher risk for NEC. Recent investigations have reported an association between antenatal indomethacin administration for tocolysis and NEC.[9,10]

Postnatal Risk Factors

Prematurity is the leading postnatal risk factor for NEC, which only rarely occurs in term infants. The association between preterm birth and NEC has been consistently verified over time in numerous investigations.[1,3,4,8] Since NEC only affects a small fraction of preterm infants, clinical researchers continue to investigate other factors that may be associated with developing NEC.

Packed red blood cell (PRBC) transfusion in VLBW infants and empiric antibiotic use in infants with extremely low birth weight (ELBW) (<1000 g) have been associated with the development of NEC, although further research is needed before any causal relationship may be established.

In a retrospective cohort of VLBW infants, Paul et al found that those receiving PRBC transfusions had double the odds of NEC, even when transfusions after the diagnosis of NEC were excluded.[11] Other authors have found that patients with NEC have an increased likelihood of having been transfused with PRBC within 48 hours of NEC onset.[12,13] Infants who developed NEC after transfusion were older at presentation (mean age > 30 postnatal days) than those who were never transfused.[11,12]

In a retrospective cohort study of ELBW infants within the National Institute of Child Health and Human Development (NICHD) Neonatal Research Network (NRN) centers, Cotton et al found that empiric antibiotics started within the first 3 days of birth and continued for 5 days or greater with negative initial culture results were associated with an increased incidence of NEC.[14] A case-control study by Alexander et al determined an association between duration of antibiotic exposure in neonates without a prior bloodstream infection and risk of NEC.[15] A leading hypothesis for this association is that antibiotics disrupt normal bowel colonization and flora, thus predisposing the bowel to the inflammatory cascade associated with NEC. Normally, a commensal relationship exists between native microflora and the intestinal epithelium.[16] Normal epithelial cell development appears to be dependent on commensal bacteria, and the presence of a diverse microflora has been associated with both increased digestive tolerance and weight gain in preterm infants.[17]

Other postnatal risk factors associated with development of necrotizing enterocolitis are the need for resuscitation with chest compressions or resuscitative drugs immediately following birth and being born to a teenaged mother.[18] Recent case reporting led to a Food and Drug Administration (FDA) warning and voluntary recall of the use of a xanthan gum–based formula thickener (Simply Thick®) in preterm infants, and pending further investigation, the use of thickening agents in preterm infants should be avoided prior to 44 weeks' adjusted gestational age.[19,20]

Spontaneous Intestinal Perforation

Spontaneous intestinal perforation (SIP), also known as focal intestinal perforation, has been used to describe the occurrence of an isolated perforation of the ileum without other signs of NEC occurring in a premature infant.[21] SIP occurs in VLBW infants with a median gestational age of 25–26 weeks[22,23] and usually presents within the first 2 weeks of life. There is an association between indomethacin and corticosteroid administration within the first 3 days of life and SIP.[22] The diagnosis of SIP cannot be confirmed unless a laparotomy is performed and perforation in the absence of necrotic bowel is noted.

Debate exists regarding whether SIP is a mild variant of NEC or a unique illness. Proponents of classifying SIP as a distinct illness note that the pathology of SIP has been reported to differ from NEC. Instead of widespread inflammation and necrosis, histological examination reveals intact mucosal epithelium and absence of intestinal musculature limited to the focal area of perforation.[24] A diagnosis of SIP is associated with decreased mortality and better neurodevelopmental outcomes compared to NEC.[8,21]

Despite these conflicting viewpoints, the 2 entities present in a similar manner: a premature infant with free intraperitoneal air requiring operation. Data from the NICHD NRN and others suggest that the absence of pneumatosis does not rule out widespread NEC.[8] Necrosis is often found during laparotomy in infants with a preoperative diagnosis of SIP.[8] All infants with intestinal perforation require either peritoneal drain placement or laparotomy, regardless of the extent of additional disease.

PATHOPHYSIOLOGY

The pathophysiology of necrotizing enterocolitis results from a hyperactive intestinal inflammatory response. This is thought to be a maladaptive reaction of the immature neonatal intestine to a specific trigger(s), which remain(s) elusive and unknown. Bowel immaturity appears to be a key factor in NEC since the disease is only found in infancy.

Gross and Histological Bowel Pathology

On gross examination, necrosis is noted in the diseased bowel segments, which are distended with thin walls. These affected areas display dark red to black or gray-green discoloration, and the mucosa is often hemorrhagic, ulcerated, and friable. Both the small and large intestines may be involved, and the diseased area(s) may be either continuous or consist of discontinuous segments (Figures 37-1 and 37-2). Although any segment

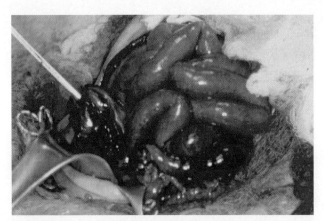

FIGURE 37-1 Intraoperative photograph showing segment of normal bowel (superiorly) and necrotized bowel (inferiorly).

of the intestine can be affected, the ileum and proximal colon are the most frequent sites. Pneumatosis intestinalis or gas within the wall of the intestine, when present, can be seen, and intestinal perforations may be noted.[25]

Histologically, ischemic (coagulation) necrosis and inflammatory changes are visible. These changes can be limited to the mucosa in mild disease but spread transmurally in severe cases. Acute inflammatory changes are noted, and neutrophil infiltrate is the dominant finding. Reparative tissue changes, including granulation and fibrosis, and bacterial overgrowth are often noted (Figures 37-3 and 37-4).[25]

Neonatal Gastrointestinal Immaturity

The preterm gastrointestinal tract is immature, which likely predisposes it to bacterial invasion and improper

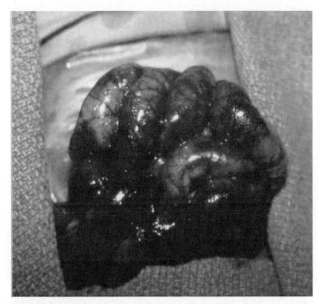

FIGURE 37-2 Photograph showing completely necrotic bowel (necrotizing enterocolitis totalis).

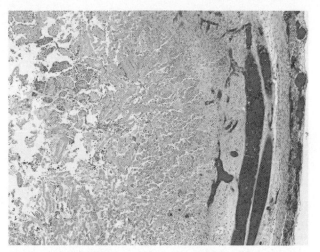

FIGURE 37-3 Histopathological bowel specimen showing necrotic changes.

immune responses. Relative deficiencies of growth factors involved in intestinal maturation, including epidermal growth factor (EGF)[26] and heparin-binding epidermal growth factor (HB-EGF)[27] may play a role in this immaturity. The epithelial cells normally provide a physical barrier between the intestine and the rest of body. With decreasing gestational age, the protective mucous layer overlying the epithelium is less mature, and the tight junctions between individual epithelial cells are more permeable to pathogenic invasion.[17] Motility is also decreased. In preterm infants, the gastrointestinal bacterial flora differ from that of healthy term infants, and their intestines are more likely to be colonized with pathogenic bacteria.[28]

Bacterial Role

Bacteria play an important role in NEC, and multiple bacterial species have been associated with the disease. The species of intestinal microflora and rate of colonization in extremely preterm infants differ from more mature infants.[17] Some have theorized that a change

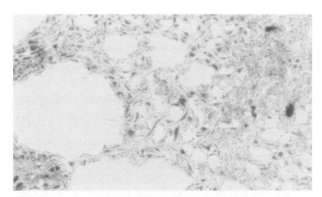

FIGURE 37-4 Histopathological bowel specimen showing pneumatosis intestinalis.

in normal gastrointestinal tract colonization precedes the onset of NEC. Since no particular bacterial strain appears causative, it is presumed that NEC is not an infectious disease but instead is related to opportunistic infection occurring during the disease process. It is unknown whether an inflammatory reaction responsible for increased permeability allows bacterial invasion to occur in early NEC or whether bacterial invasion occurs first and triggers the hyperactive immune response.[28]

Inflammation

Inflammation is responsible for the cellular destruction and necrosis that is central to NEC. Although the specific inflammatory pathways in NEC are not completely understood, certain cytokines and nitric oxide (NO) are thought to play key roles.[29,30]

Inflammatory mediators associated with NEC include platelet-activating factor (PAF), tumor necrosis factor α (TNF-α), and interleukins (ILs), including IL-1, IL-6, IL-8, IL-10, IL-12, and IL-18. The pattern recognition receptor, toll-Like receptor 4 (TLR4), which recognizes gram-negative lipopolysaccharides (LPSs), has increased expression in preterm intestinal epithelium relative to adults. In preliminary animal studies, maternally fed preterm mice had less TLR4 expression than formula-fed mice. Thus, TLR4 is hypothesized to play a key role in the protective role of human breast milk.[30]

Increased amounts of NO are present in pathological intestinal specimens from preterm infants with NEC. NO synthase, the enzyme responsible for the formation of NO, exists in the gastrointestinal tract in both constitutive and inducible forms. At normal levels, NO likely plays an important physiological role by regulating vascular and mucosal integrity. However, it is produced in larger amounts in response to inflammatory cytokine release. At higher levels, NO creates oxidative compounds with cytopathic effects, such as peroxynitrite ($ONOO^-$).[31,32]

Ischemic damage in preterm NEC patients likely develops secondary to a hyperactive immune response, instead of being the event that initiates NEC. Since NEC presents much earlier in term infants and frequently occurs following hypoxic and hypoperfused states such as septic shock, congenital heart disease, and hypoxic-ischemic events, ischemia may play more of an inciting role in term infants.[30,32]

Genetics

Only a small fraction of age-matched preterm infants with similar clinical courses develop NEC. Thus, it is likely that some infants have a genetic susceptibility, and identifying genetic risk factors for NEC has become a research priority. For example, a recent study found higher surgery and mortality risks in preterm infants with NEC who had reduced H-antigen secretion secondary to a polymorphism in the gene for fucosyltransferase (FUT-2), an enzymatic component of glycosylation in innate immunity.[33]

CLINICAL PRESENTATION AND DIFFERENTIAL DIAGNOSIS

The physical examination remains a key component of evaluation for NEC. Abdominal distension is found in almost all patients with NEC. The abdomen may be initially soft to palpation but becomes firm and tender with disease progression. Palpable, distended bowel loops, decreased bowel sounds, abdominal wall erythema, or bluish discoloration may be noted. Abdominal wall erythema is highly predictive of NEC but is only present in 10% of patients (Figure 37-5).[34] Lethargy is noted in severe illness. Vital sign changes include tachycardia, hypotension, and apnea and oxygen desaturation with resulting bradycardic episodes. Respiratory failure requiring intubation occurs in severe illness.

In its most mild or early from, necrotizing enterocolitis presents subtly with nonspecific gastrointestinal symptoms, including feeding intolerance or increased bilious or nonbilious gastric residuals, and signs that include abdominal distention and irritability. Besides NEC, the differential diagnosis for a stable infant in this setting includes decreased bowel motility secondary to prematurity or enteral feeding intolerance of nonspecific cause. Other causes of abdominal distension include anatomical obstruction, which is typically readily distinguished from NEC, and gastric distention from improper nasogastric tube placement. Hematochezia in the clinically well premature infant is most commonly caused by anal fissure, milk-protein allergy, or swallowed maternal blood.

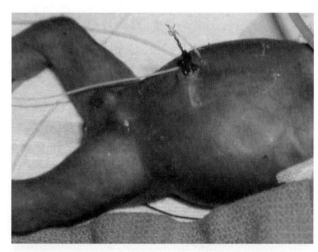

FIGURE 37-5 The abdomen of a child with bowel perforation shows distension and discoloration due to perforated bowel.

Clinical instability ensues as NEC progresses. In severe cases of NEC, sudden instability may be the first presenting symptom. Sepsis is the major diagnosis that presents with findings similar to severe NEC. Ileus secondary to sepsis causes abdominal distension that may mimic NEC. In both severe NEC and sepsis, infants develop lethargy, apnea, poor peripheral perfusion, and abdominal tenderness. Fortunately, the same medical therapy regimen of holding feedings, starting antibiotics, and providing supportive care are appropriate for both conditions.

DIAGNOSTIC TESTS

Complete blood cell counts (CBC), electrolytes, and abdominal radiographs aid the clinician in the diagnosis of NEC. Serial physical examination and testing facilitate monitoring of worsening disease. Laboratory findings are nonspecific but can include thrombocytopenia; increased or decreased white blood cell counts with bandemia; elevated acute-phase reactants (C-reactive protein [CRP], CD64, or erythrocyte sedimentation rate [ESR]); hypo- or hyperglycemia; electrolyte instability, including hyperkalemia and hyponatremia; and metabolic acidosis. These laboratory abnormalities become more prominent as the severity of NEC increases.

The plain abdominal radiograph remains the most important radiological modality for NEC diagnosis and severity assessment. The abdominal anteroposterior (AP) view and a second dependent view (left lateral decubitus or cross table) to aid in evaluation for pneumoperitoneum provide invaluable diagnostic information. Distended bowel loops, air-fluid levels, and thickened bowel walls are frequently found not only in early NEC but also in septic ileus and are thus nonspecific. Pneumatosis intestinalis is the most specific radiographic finding in NEC. Air bubbles are seen as lucencies within the bowel wall and are most often located in the right lower quadrant (Figures 37-6 and 37-7). Fixed bowel loops, portal venous air, and pneumoperitoneum are ominous signs. Pneumoperitoneum indicates perforation requiring surgical intervention (Figures 37-8 and 37-9). A gasless abdomen may be seen due to fluid-filled bowel loops but is nonspecific and can occur in sepsis or a patient receiving neuromuscular blockade.

Abdominal ultrasound is not indicated for most infants with suspected NEC, but it may be helpful in some circumstances, such as the deteriorating infant with abdominal distension and gasless bowel loops on plain films. Possible ultrasound findings include free intraperitoneal fluid with debris, increased bowel wall echogenicity, bowel wall thickening or narrowing, absent bowel perfusion, and portal venous air.[35,36]

Whenever there is a strong clinical suspicion for perforation or necrotic bowel but no clear radiological

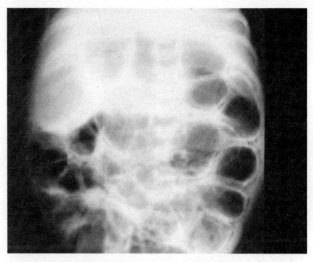

FIGURE 37-6 Abdominal x-ray showing pneumatosis intestinalis.

evidence, a paracentesis may aid in diagnosis. Bilious or brown fluid and bacteria on Gram stain or culture indicate the need for immediate intervention; sterile straw or pink fluid is found in the absence of perforation or necrosis.

MANAGEMENT

Prevention

Prevention is the ultimate goal in NEC management. NEC occurs more frequently in infants who have been

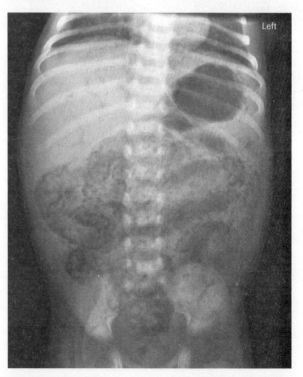

FIGURE 37-7 Abdominal x-ray showing extensive pneumatosis intestinalis and portal venous gas.

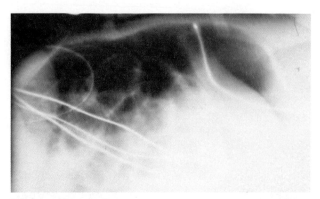

FIGURE 37-8 Lateral decubitus x-ray revealing free air secondary to bowel perforation.

fed,[18] and many of the recent advances in preventive research have been nutrition based. Clinicians once feared that early initiation of enteral feeding contributed to NEC. However, no association between early feeding and NEC has been demonstrated. The increased frequency of NEC in enterally fed infants may be confounded by the fact that the majority of preterm infants are fed by the time of average NEC onset at 2 weeks.

Human Milk

Maternal Milk

Maternal milk is the best source of neonatal nutrition. Due to ethical reasons, it is impossible to perform a

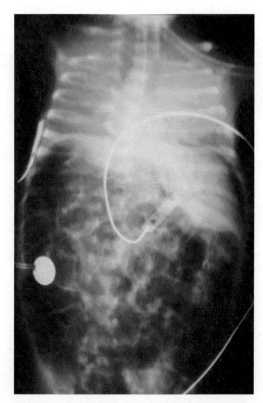

FIGURE 37-9 Abdominal x-ray showing extensive pneumatosis and free air within the peritoneum.

randomized controlled trial (RCT) to test the comparative effectiveness of breast milk vs infant formula to reduce NEC. A Cochrane review of RCTs comparing formula milk to maternal breast milk for feeding preterm or low birth weight infants was inconclusive due to lack of evidence.[37] However, limited observational evidence shows that breast milk may lead to a reduction in NEC incidence.[38,39] Therefore, all mothers should be encouraged to provide breast milk for their infants except in the rare occasion it is contraindicated for medical reasons.[38] Human milk contains protective immune compounds, including secretory immunoglobulin (Ig) A and phagocytes, as well as immune modulatory compounds such as CD14 and lactoferrin. It also contains compounds such as peptides and nondigestible oligosaccharides that play a role in development of normal bowel flora, as well as compounds such as EGF that stimulate bowel development.[40]

Lucas and Cole prospectively determined that human milk reduced the odds of NEC 10-fold compared to formula feedings only and 3.5 times when breast milk and formula were administered in combination.[39] The effect of human milk appears to be dose dependent. NEC appears to be proportionally reduced in neonates with birth weight less than 1000 g, as they receive incrementally larger volumes of human milk.[41]

Even VLBW infants who are exclusively fed their mother's milk usually receive fortification to increase caloric intake and aid their growth. Fortification does not appear to worsen NEC risk and improves growth. Within a randomized study of feeding strategies, Schanler et al prospectively determined that fortified maternal breast milk significantly reduced NEC when compared to preterm formula in infants born at 26–30 weeks' gestation. Fortified maternal milk had a protective impact independent of whether infants had early (postnatal day 4) vs late feeding initiation (postnatal day 14) and whether they received continuous vs bolus feeds.[42]

However, recent evidence showed that NEC risk may be potentially reduced further based on the type of milk fortifier used. Sullivan et al randomized VLBW preterm infants to fortification with commonly used cow's-milk-based fortifiers vs an exclusive human-milk-based diet including breast milk based fortifier. Those who received human-milk-based fortifier had both lower rates of NEC and NEC requiring surgical intervention.[43]

Pasteurized Milk From Human Donors

When maternal breast milk is unavailable, pasteurized donated human milk can be substituted. The pasteurization process affects the nutritional and immunological function of human milk. Still, meta-analyses have shown that unfortified pasteurized human milk is associated with a decreased risk of NEC compared to preterm formula.[44,45] Most of the RCTs that studied donated pasteurized milk were conducted with unfortified milk. The addition of fortifying agents to donor milk promotes preterm infant growth and is common practice. Therefore, further research is needed to determine if fortification alters the benefits of pasteurized human milk.[37,45]

Enteral Feeding Methods

Feeding rates and protocols have been studied to determine if certain feeding routines reduce NEC. Early trophic feedings of small amounts of milk to promote bowel development have not been shown to increase the risk of NEC and may be beneficial in NEC prevention. A study examining delayed enteral feeding onset showed no benefit in infants who were fed human milk or human milk in combination with formula. Delaying feedings did benefit infants who were solely formula fed.[46] Slowing feed advancement in VLBW infants has also been proposed as a mechanism to prevent NEC. However, a meta-analysis examining different rates of enteral feeding advancement showed no difference in NEC rates.[47]

Probiotics

Supplementation with probiotics will likely play an important role in NEC prevention. Probiotics are live microorganisms that colonize the gastrointestinal tract after being administered as food products. The most common strains include bifidobacteria and lactobacilli. It is hypothesized that they reduce NEC risk by promoting intestinal homeostasis and barrier function, as well as discouraging pathogenic bacteria by facilitating growth of beneficial commensal organisms.[48]

Randomized controlled trials of probiotic administration have shown an average of 30% relative risk reduction in the development of NEC and 40% relative risk reduction in all-cause mortality.[49–51] Despite the exciting potential of probiotic therapy, the methodology of many of the studies is subject to question, and various combinations of bacteria were used in the RCTs included in the meta-analyses.[49–51] A methodologically sound large multiple-center trial is needed. It is still unclear which species/combination of bacteria show the most promise for NEC prophylaxis. Concerns regarding possible long-term detrimental effects on the immune system and late development of metabolic syndrome are under study. Although reports of adverse events have been minimal in probiotic trials, the safety of probiotic administration to preterm neonates remains a concern, and future research goals include identification of dosage, determination of treatment length, and identifying the safest and most effective probiotic combinations.

Finally, the renewed emphasis on prematurity reduction research may prove to be the most effective NEC prevention. Preterm birth is the single greatest risk factor for NEC, and reduction in the preterm birth rate will be the ultimate NEC prophylaxis.

Supportive Management

Once necrotizing enterocolitis is diagnosed, transfer to a level 3 neonatal intensive care unit with continuous monitoring, experienced nursing care, and access to experienced pediatric surgeons is necessary. The infant should immediately not receive anything by mouth and a large-bore tube placed to suction for gastric decompression. Blood cultures should be drawn and antibiotics with gram-negative coverage started. Antibiotics with anaerobic coverage should also be prescribed should perforation or the need for surgical intervention appear imminent. Serial radiographs should be obtained to monitor for perforation, and serial laboratory tests should be ordered to monitor for acidosis, thrombocytopenia, anemia, and electrolyte abnormalities, including hyperkalemia and hyponatremia. Reliable intravenous access is mandatory for fluid, antibiotic, and nutrition administration. Perfusion, urine output, and blood pressure must be followed closely, and isotonic fluid boluses, pressors, and corticosteroids may be indicated if hypotension ensues. Hypoxemia and eventual respiratory failure develop in severe cases of NEC and caregivers should be prepared for intubation and mechanical ventilation.

The modified Bell staging criteria are used to stage the severity of NEC (Table 37-1). The stage I category consists of the nonspecific findings of suspected NEC, stage II infants have definite NEC, and stage III infants suffer the symptoms of severe NEC.[35,36] In many cases of NEC, infants recover with supportive treatment and should remain without oral feeding for 7–10 days. However, 42% of infants progress to surgery or death, making it both the most common gastrointestinal and the most common surgical emergency in neonates.[18] It is difficult to predict which infants with NEC will progress to surgery. Perforation is the only absolute indication for surgery. Under ideal conditions, surgical intervention would occur prior to perforation when the bowel has become necrotic and rupture is imminent. However, this is often difficult to determine, and prediction modeling based on clinical parameters has not been successful since most of the reliable predictors of poor outcomes in NEC patients are not present until NEC has already progressed to a severe state.[18,53] In a worsening infant with no clear radiographic indication of perforation, the surgeon must take multiple factors into account when deciding whether to operate. These include but are not limited to a worsening physical examination and increasing metabolic acidosis despite maximal medical therapy.

Surgical options for NEC treatment include laparotomy with resection of necrotic bowel and peritoneal

CHAPTER 37

Table 37-1 Modified Bell Staging Criteria for Necrotizing Enterocolitis (NEC)[a]

Stage	Systemic Signs	Intestinal Signs	Radiologic Signs
IA: Suspected NEC	Temperature instability, apnea, bradycardia, lethargy	Elevated pregavage residuals, mild abdominal distension, emesis, guaiac-positive stool	Normal or intestinal dilation, mild ileus
IB: Suspected NEC	Same as IA	Bright red blood from rectum	Same as above
IIA: Definite NEC Mildly ill	Same as IA	Same as 1A and/or 1B *plus* absent bowel sounds, ± abdominal tenderness	Intestinal dilation, ileus, pneumatosis intestinalis
IIB: Definite NEC Moderately ill	Same as 1A *us* mild metabolic acidosis, mild thrombocytopenia	Same as IIA *plus* absent bowel sounds, definite abdominal tenderness, ± abdominal cellulitis or right lower quadrant mass	Same as IIA *plus* portal venous gas ± ascites
IIIA: Advanced NEC Severely ill	Same as IIB *plus* hypotension, bradycardia, severe apnea, combined respiratory and metabolic acidosis, disseminated intravascular coagulation, neutropenia	Same as IIB *plus* signs of generalized peritonitis, marked tenderness, and distension of abdomen	Same as IIB *plus* definite ascites
IIIB: Advanced NEC Severely ill Perforated bowel	Same as IIIA	Same as IIIA	Same as IIB *plus* pneumoperitoneum

[a]Reproduced with permission from Walsh and Kliegman.[52]

drain placement (Figure 37-10). Two RCTs[54,55] by Moss et al and Rees et al and one large multicenter cohort study by Blakely et al[8,56] evaluated the comparative effectiveness of laparotomy to primary peritoneal drainage after previous retrospective research was not able to determine the relative merits of each procedure.[57] Both trials demonstrated no significant differences in mortality or requirement for long-term parental nutrition. An ongoing multicenter RCT by the NICHD neonatal network will attempt to determine if there is a difference in longer-term neurodevelopmental outcome between the 2 procedures.[58] Infants who receive either primary drain placement or laparotomy may need subsequent operations should stricture or bowel obstruction develop. When infants who received laparotomy with bowel resection and ostomy placement are stable with good weight gain, they should undergo reanastomosis to improve feed tolerance and absorption.

OUTCOME AND FOLLOW-UP

Mortality

Virtually all of the mortality from NEC is in those infants who require surgical intervention. Mortality increases with decreasing birth weight.[59] Among all patients with NEC, mortality averages 15%–16%.[1,60] In surgical patients,[1] mortality averages 25%–40% overall, and it is 51% in infants with birth weight less than 1000 g.[8]

Gastrointestinal Morbidity

Medically and surgically managed patients with NEC are at risk for stricture formation, with the left colon the most common site.[61–63] Intestinal strictures develop in 10%–35% of patients treated for NEC, regardless of whether they have been treated medically or surgically.[64,65] In addition, there does not appear to be a difference in stricture development among patients managed by laparotomy or peritoneal drainage.[56,66]

Short-bowel syndrome, inadequate capacity for caloric absorption secondary to loss of diseased bowel, affects 40% of patients with NEC who require surgical intervention and roughly one-quarter of all patients with NEC. The long-term prognosis for intact intestinal function is correlated with both the percentage of surviving bowel and the affected site.[67] The ileum has greatest adaptive capacity, and patients without ileal involvement have a higher likelihood of improved absorptive function. The benefit of ileocecal valve

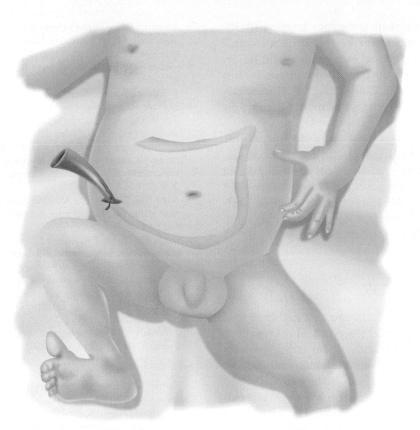

FIGURE 37-10 Illustration of a peritoneal drain.

preservation on nutritional outcomes is unclear, and the length of preserved distal ileum appears to have a much greater impact. Mortality, length of stay, and cost are significantly higher when the small intestine is affected, in isolation or in combination with the large intestine, as compared to the large intestine alone.[67]

All infants with NEC require at least 7–10 days of parenteral nutrition (PN) during their treatment course. However, postoperative patients often remain on PN for many weeks. A multicenter investigation that examined infants requiring surgical intervention for NEC found the incidence of parental nutrition–associated liver disease (PNALD) was 70%. Independent risk factors for PNALD were a history of small-bowel resection or jejunostomy placement, preoperative length of PN exposure, and total weeks of PN therapy.[68]

In addition to nutritional deficiencies and malabsorption, VLBW neonates with short-bowel syndrome are at increased risk of bloodstream infections during their hospitalizations.[69] These infections are probably due to a combination of translocation of intestinal bacteria and the presence of indwelling central venous catheters.

Long-Term Outcomes in Short-Bowel Syndrome

Within a multicenter cohort of infants in the NICHD NRN with birth weight less than 1000 g, those with short-bowel syndrome were more likely to still require tube feeding (33%) at 18 to 22 months of age and to have been rehospitalized (79%). These infants had delayed growth with shorter length and smaller head circumference than infants without short-bowel syndrome.[70]

When infants with intestinal failure are unable to achieve full enteral feedings, small-bowel transplantation becomes a consideration. Associated liver transplantation is also often required. A recent study found that patients with NEC with short-bowel syndrome comprised 19% of the patients listed for intestinal transplantation in the United Network for Organ Sharing (UNOS) database. Listed patients with NEC were 1.5 times more likely to die than to receive a transplant.[71] Those who receive a transplant face a 5-year mortality of up to 50% and lifelong immunosuppressive treatment.[72]

Neurodevelopmental Morbidity

We have known that the risk of neurodevelopmental delay in survivors of NEC is considerable since 1980 when Stevenson et al and Schulzke et al reported their findings from a prospective investigation of neurodevelopment in discharged patients with a history of NEC.[73,74] Shah et al prospectively followed a cohort of preterm infants born prior to 30 weeks and obtained

CHAPTER 37

nonsedated head magnetic resonance imaging (MRI) with blinded interpretation at 40 weeks' postmenstrual age and neurodevelopmental examination with Bayley Scales of Infant Development at 2 years of age. Infants with a diagnosis of stage 2 or greater NEC were significantly more likely to have white matter injury, gray matter injury, and neurodevelopmental delay.[75]

However, survivors of NEC who do not require surgery have outcomes similar to their gestational age-matched peers. Hintz et al and Rees et al found that at 18- to 22-month assessment, infants who required surgical treatment of NEC were nearly twice as likely to have neurodevelopmental delays, including both cognitive and psychomotor deficits.[76,77]

Outcomes Following Spontaneous Intestinal Perforation

Patients with a history of SIP are at a higher risk of mortality than their unaffected peers. However, their mortality risk is significantly lower than patients with NEC who required surgical intervention.[8,23,78] Gastrointestinal outcomes are better as well. SIP patients rarely lose more than 2 cm of bowel, and primary reanastomosis is sometimes possible.[77] Survivors of SIP also have significantly better neurodevelopmental outcomes at 1 year of age when compared to those with a history of surgical NEC.[79]

CONCLUSION

In conclusion, NEC remains a major cause of neonatal mortality and morbidity. This disease is especially devastating in VLBW infants, and the need for surgery greatly increases the risk of both death and subsequent gastrointestinal and neurodevelopmental impairment. Fortunately, we are slowly beginning to better understand the pathophysiology of NEC, and this knowledge is being used to design investigations of novel preventive therapies.

REFERENCES

1. Holman RC, Stoll BJ, Curns AT, et al. Necrotising enterocolitis hospitalisations among neonates in the United States. *Paediatr Perinat Epidemiol*. 2006;20:498–506.
2. Sankaran K, Puckett B, Lee DS, et al. Variations in incidence of necrotizing enterocolitis in Canadian neonatal intensive care units. *J Pediatr Gastroenterol Nutr*. 2004;39:366–372.
3. Stoll BJ, Hansen NI, Bell EF, et al. Neonatal outcomes of extremely preterm infants from the NICHD Neonatal Research Network. *Pediatrics*. 2010;126:443–456.
4. Berrington JE, Hearn RI, Bythell M, et al. Deaths in preterm infants: changing pathology over 2 decades. *J Pediatr*. 2012;160:49–53.e1.
5. Lambert DK, Christensen RD, Henry E, et al. Necrotizing enterocolitis in term neonates: data from a multihospital healthcare system. *J Perinatol*. 2007;27:437–443.
6. Gonzalez-Rivera R, Culverhouse RC, Hamvas A, et al. The age of necrotizing enterocolitis onset: an application of Sartwell's incubation period model. *J Perinatol*. 2011;31:519–523.
7. Meinzen-Derr J, Morrow AL, Hornung RW, et al. Epidemiology of necrotizing enterocolitis temporal clustering in two neonatology practices. *J Pediatr*. 2009;154:656–661.
8. Blakely ML, Lally KP, McDonald S, et al. Postoperative outcomes of extremely low birth-weight infants with necrotizing enterocolitis or isolated intestinal perforation. *Ann Surg*. 2005;241:984–994.
9. Sood BG, Lulic-Botica M, Holzhausen KA, et al. The risk of necrotizing enterocolitis after indomethacin tocolysis. *Pediatrics*. 2011;128:e54–e62.
10. Amin SB, Sinkin RA, Glantz JC. Metaanalysis of the effect of antenatal indomethacin on neonatal outcomes. *Am J Obstet Gynecol*. 2007;197:486.e1–10.
11. Paul DA, Mackley A, Novitsky A, et al. Increased odds of necrotizing enterocolitis after transfusion of red blood cells in premature infants. *Pediatrics*. 2011;127:635–641.
12. Blau J, Calo JM, Dozor D, et al. Transfusion-related acute gut injury: necrotizing enterocolitis in very low birth weight neonates after packed red blood cell transfusion. *J Pediatr*. 2011;158:403–409.
13. El-Dib M, Narang S, Lee E, et al. Red blood cell transfusion, feeding and necrotizing enterocolitis in preterm infants. *J Perinatol*. 2011;31:183–187.
14. Cotten CM, Taylor S, Stoll B, et al. Prolonged duration of initial empirical antibiotic treatment is associated with increased rates of necrotizing enterocolitis and death for extremely low birth weight infants. *Pediatrics*. 2009;123:58–66.
15. Alexander VN, Northrup V, Bizzarro MJ. Antibiotic exposure in the newborn intensive care unit and the risk of necrotizing enterocolitis. *J Pediatr*. 2011;159:392–397.
16. Madara J. Building an intestine—architectural contributions of commensal bacteria. *N Engl J Med*. 2004;351:1685–1686.
17. Jacquot A, Neveu D, Aujoulat F, et al. Dynamics and clinical evolution of bacterial gut microflora in extremely premature patients. *J Pediatr*. 2011;158:390–396.
18. Moss RL, Kalish LA, Duggan C, et al. Clinical parameters do not adequately predict outcome in necrotizing enterocolitis: a multi-institutional study. *J Perinatol*. 2008;28:665–674.
19. United States Food and Drug Administration. Simply Thick: Public Health Notification: Risk of Life-Threatening Bowel Condition. May 2011. http://www.fda.gov/Safety/MedWatch/SafetyInformation/SafetyAlertsforHumanMedicalProducts/ucm256257.htm.
20. Abrams SA. Be cautious in using thickening agents in preemies. AAP News. News.http://aapnews.aappublications.org/content/early/2011/06/03/aapnews.20110603-1.full.
21. Aschner JL, Deluga KS, Metlay LA, et al. Spontaneous focal gastrointestinal perforation in very low birth weight infants. *J Pediatr*. 1988;113:364–367.
22. Attridge JT, Clark R, Walker MW, Gordon PV. New insights into spontaneous intestinal perforation using a national data set: (1) SIP is associated with early indomethacin exposure. *J Perinatol*. 2006;26:93–99.
23. Attridge JT, Herman AC, Gurka MJ, et al. Discharge outcomes of extremely low birth weight infants with spontaneous intestinal perforations. *J Perinatol*. 2006;26:49–54.
24. Tatekawa Y, Muraji T, Imai Y, et al. The mechanism of focal intestinal perforations in neonates with low birth weight. *Pediatr Surg Int*. 1999;15:549–552.
25. Ballance WA, Dahms BB, Shenker N, Kliegman RM. Pathology of neonatal necrotizing enterocolitis: a ten-year experience. *J Pediatr*. 1990;117:S6–S13.

26. Shin CE, Falcone RA, Stuart L, et al. Diminished epidermal growth factor levels in infants with necrotizing enterocolitis. *J Pediatr Surg.* 2000;35:173–177.

27. Radulescu A, Zhang HY, Yu X, et al. Heparin-binding epidermal growth factor–like growth factor overexpression in transgenic mice increases resistance to necrotizing enterocolitis. *J Pediatr Surg.* 2010;45:1933–1939.

28. Hunter CJ, Upperman JS, Ford HR, Camerini V. Understanding the susceptibility of the premature infant to necrotizing enterocolitis (NEC). *Pediatr Res.* 2008;63:117–123.

29. Grave GD, Nelson SA, Walker WA, et al. New therapies and preventive approaches for necrotizing enterocolitis: report of a research planning workshop. *Pediatr Res.* 2007;62:510–514.

30. Lin PW, Nasr TR, Stoll BJ. Necrotizing enterocolitis: recent scientific advances in pathophysiology and prevention. *Semin Perinatol.* 2008;32:70–82.

31. Upperman JS, Potoka D, Grishin A, et al. Mechanisms of nitric oxide-mediated intestinal barrier failure in necrotizing enterocolitis. *Semin Pediatr Surg.* 2005;14:159–166.

32. Nankervis CA, Giannone PJ, Reber KM. The neonatal intestinal vasculature: contributing factors to necrotizing enterocolitis. *Semin Perinatol.* 2008;32:83–91.

33. Morrow AL, Meinzen-Derr J, Huang P, et al. Fucosyltransferase 2 non-secretor and low secretor status predicts severe outcomes in premature infants. *J Pediatr.* 2011;158:745–751.

34. Kosloske AM. Indications for operation in necrotizing enterocolitis revisited. *J Pediatr Surg.* 1994;29:663–666.

35. Silva CT, Daneman A, Navarro OM, et al. Correlation of sonographic findings and outcome in necrotizing enterocolitis. *Pediatr Radiol.* 2007;37:274–282.

36. Faingold R, Daneman A, Tomlinson G, et al. Necrotizing enterocolitis: assessment of bowel viability with color doppler US. *Radiology.* 2005;235:587–594.

37. Quigley MA, Henderson G, Anthony MY, McGuire W. Formula milk versus donor breast milk for feeding preterm or low birth weight infants. *Cochrane Database Syst Rev.* 2007;(4):CD002971.

38. Gartner LM, Morton J, Lawrence RA, et al. Breastfeeding and the use of human milk. *Pediatrics.* 2005;115:496–506.

39. Lucas A, Cole TJ. Breast milk and neonatal necrotising enterocolitis. *Lancet.* 1990;336:1519–1523.

40. Walker A. Breast milk as the gold standard for protective nutrients. *J Pediatr.* 2010;156:S3–S7.

41. Meinzen-Derr J, Poindexter B, Wrage L, et al. Role of human milk in extremely low birth weight infants' risk of necrotizing enterocolitis or death. *J Perinatol.* 2009;29:57–62.

42. Schanler RJ, Shulman RJ, Lau C. Feeding strategies for premature infants: beneficial outcomes of feeding fortified human milk versus preterm formula. *Pediatrics.* 1999;103:1150–1157.

43. Sullivan S, Schanler RJ, Kim JH, et al. An exclusively human milk-based diet is associated with a lower rate of necrotizing enterocolitis than a diet of human milk and bovine milk-based products. *J Pediatr.* 2010;156:562–567.e1.

44. Quigley M, Henderson G, Anthony M, McGuire W. Formula milk versus donor breast milk for feeding preterm or low birth weight infants. *Cochrane Database Syst Rev.* 2007;4:CD002971.

45. Boyd CA, Quigley MA, Brocklehurst P. Donor breast milk versus infant formula for preterm infants: systematic review and meta-analysis. *Arch Dis Child Fetal Neonatal Ed.* 2007;92:F169–F175.

46. Lucas A, Cole TJ. Breast milk and neonatal necrotising enterocolitis. *Lancet.* 1990;336:1519–1523.

47. Morgan J, Young L, McGuire W. Slow advancement of enteral feed volumes to prevent necrotizing enterocolitis in very low birth weight infants. *Cochrane Database Syst Rev.* 2013;3:CD001241.

48. Stenger MR, Reber KM, Giannone PJ, Nankervis CA. Probiotics and prebiotics for the prevention of necrotizing enterocolitis. *Curr Infect Dis Rep.* 2011;13:13–20.

49. Deshpande G, Rao S, Patole S, Bulsara M. Updated meta-analysis of probiotics for preventing necrotizing enterocolitis in preterm neonates. *Pediatrics.* 2010;125:921–930.

50. Alfaleh K, Anabrees J, Bassler D, Al-Kharfi T. Probiotics for prevention of necrotizing enterocolitis in preterm infants. *Cochrane Database Syst Rev.* 2011;(3):CD005496.

51. Alfaleh K, Anabrees J, Bassler D. Probiotics reduce the risk of necrotizing enterocolitis in preterm infants: a meta-analysis. *Neonatology.* 2010;97:93–99.

52. Walsh MC, Kliegman RM. Necrotizing enterocolitis treatment based on staging criteria. *Pediatr Clin North Am.* 1986;33:179.

53. Thompson A, Bizzarro M, Yu S, et al. Risk factors for necrotizing enterocolitis totalis: a case-control study. *J Perinatol.* 2011;31(11):730–738.

54. Moss RL, Dimmitt RA, Barnhart DC, et al. Laparotomy versus peritoneal drainage for necrotizing enterocolitis and perforation. *N Engl J Med.* 2006;354:2225–2234.

55. Rees CM, Eaton S, Kiely EM, et al. Peritoneal drainage or laparotomy for neonatal bowel perforation? A randomized controlled trial. *Ann Surg.* 2008;248:44–51.

56. Blakely ML, Tyson JE, Lally KP, et al. Laparotomy versus peritoneal drainage for necrotizing enterocolitis or isolated intestinal perforation in extremely low birth weight infants: outcomes through 18 months adjusted age. *Pediatrics.* 2006;117:e680–e687.

57. Moss RL, Dimmitt RA, Henry MC, et al. A meta-analysis of peritoneal drainage versus laparotomy for perforated necrotizing enterocolitis. *J Pediatr Surg.* 2001;36:1210–1213.

58. National Institutes of Health. ClinicalTrials.gov. October 2011. http://clinicaltrials.gov/ct2/show/NCT01029353?term=laparotomy+AND+necrotizing+AND+enterocolitis&rank=1.

59. Fitzgibbons SC, Ching Y, Yu D, et al. Mortality of necrotizing enterocolitis expressed by birth weight categories. *J Pediatr Surg.* 2009;44:1072–1075; discussion 1075–1076.

60. Clark RH, Gordon P, Walker WM, et al. Characteristics of patients who die of necrotizing enterocolitis. *J Perinatol.* 2012;32(3):199–204.

61. Bell MJ, Ternberg JL, Askin FB, et al. Intestinal stricture in necrotizing enterocolitis. *J Pediatr Surg.* 1976;11:319–327.

62. Kosloske AM, Burstein J, Bartow SA. Intestinal obstruction due to colonic stricture following neonatal necrotizing enterocolitis. *Ann Surg.* 1980;192:202–207.

63. Janik JS, Ein SH, Mancer K. Intestinal stricture after necrotizing enterocolitis. *J Pediatr Surg.* 1981;16:438–443.

64. Butter A, Flageole H, Laberge JM. The changing face of surgical indications for necrotizing enterocolitis. *J Pediatr Surg.* 2002;37:496–499.

65. Schimpl G, Höllwarth M, Fotter R, Becker H. Late intestinal strictures following successful treatment of necrotizing enterocolitis. *Acta Pediatr Suppl.* 1994;83:80–83.

66. Blakely ML, Lally KP, McDonald S, et al. Postoperative outcomes of extremely low birth-weight infants with necrotizing enterocolitis or isolated intestinal perforation. *Ann Surg.* 2005;241:984–994.

67. Zhang Y, Ortega G, Camp M, et al. Necrotizing enterocolitis requiring surgery: outcomes by intestinal location of disease in 4371 infants. *J Pediatr Surg.* 2011;46:1475–1481.

68. Duro D, Mitchell PD, Kalish LA, et al. Risk factors for parenteral nutrition-associated liver disease following surgical therapy for necrotizing enterocolitis. *J Pediatr Gastroenterol Nutr.* 2011;52:595–600.

69. Cole CR, Hansen NI, Higgins RD, et al. Bloodstream infections in very low birth weight infants with intestinal failure. *J Pediatr.* 2012;160(1):54–59.e2.

70. Cole CR, Hansen NI, Higgins RD, et al. Very low birth weight preterm infants with surgical short bowel syndrome: incidence, morbidity and mortality, and growth outcomes at 18 to 22 months. *Pediatrics.* 2008;122:e573–e582.

71. Lao OB, Healey PJ, Perkins JD, et al. Outcomes in children with intestinal failure following listing for intestinal transplant. *J Pediatr Surg.* 2010;45:100–107; discussion 107.

72. Duro D, Kamin D, Duggan C. Overview of pediatric short bowel syndrome. *J Pediatr Gastroenterol Nutr.* y;47(Suppl 1):S33–S36.

73. Stevenson DK, Kerner JA, Malachowski N, Sunshine P. Late morbidity among survivors of necrotizing enterocolitis. *Pediatrics.* 1980;66:925–927.

74. Schulzke SM, Deshpande GC, Patole SK. Neurodevelopmental outcomes of very low-birth-weight infants with necrotizing enterocolitis: a systematic review of observational studies. *Arch Pediatr Adolesc Med.* 2007;161:583–590.

75. Shah DK, Doyle LW, Anderson PJ, et al. Adverse neurodevelopment in preterm infants with postnatal sepsis or necrotizing enterocolitis is mediated by white matter abnormalities on magnetic resonance imaging at term. *J Pediatr.* 2008;153:170–175, 175.e1.

76. Hintz SR, Kendrick DE, Stoll BJ, et al. Neurodevelopmental and growth outcomes of extremely low birth weight infants after necrotizing enterocolitis. *Pediatrics.* 2005;115:696–703.

77. Rees CM, Pierro A, Eaton S. Neurodevelopmental outcomes of neonates with medically and surgically treated necrotizing enterocolitis. *Arch Dis Child Fetal Neonatal Ed.* 2007;92:F193–F198.

78. Buchheit JQ, Stewart DL. Clinical comparison of localized intestinal perforation and necrotizing enterocolitis in neonates. *Pediatrics.* 1994;93:32–36.

79. Adesanya OA, O'Shea TM, Turner CS, et al. Intestinal perforation in very low birth weight infants: growth and neurodevelopment at 1 year of age. *J Perinatol.* 2005;25:583–589.

Gastrointestinal Bleeding

Ann Ming Yeh and William Berquist

EPIDEMIOLOGY

In the population of healthy neonates, the incidence of upper gastrointestinal (GI) bleeding is uncommon but not rare. A case cohort series of 5180 infants indicated that approximately 1.2% of healthy infants experienced upper GI bleeding that was brought to medical attention.[1] Incidence is likely increased in populations of more acutely sick neonates, such as those in the intensive care unit; however, the exact incidence is unknown, as some may have a high prevalence of asymptomatic gastritis.[2] In the pediatric intensive care population, studies have shown that patients who receive acid-blocking prophylaxis have a lower incidence of upper GI bleeding,[3] but a similar study was not found in the neonatal intensive care population.

The incidence of lower GI bleeding in the healthy neonatal population is unknown. One study in the tertiary emergency room setting had an incidence of 0.3% of all pediatric visits ($n = 104$), where the chief complaint was rectal bleeding. Of these, half of the patients were younger than 1 year old, and the most common diagnoses were allergic colitis and anorectal fissure.[4] In the neonatal intensive care unit population, serious pathology such as neonatal necrotizing enterocolitis (NEC) and milk protein allergy has a higher prevalence than in the general population.[4]

DIFFERENTIAL DIAGNOSIS

The differential diagnosis, assessment, and treatment of GI bleeding in neonates, as in older children and adults, depend on identifying the location of the bleed. In neonates, it may be difficult to differentiate between upper tract and lower tract bleeding, as upper GI bleeding may be brisk and manifest as hematochezia due to the rapid intestinal transit time in infants.

The following are definitions used in this chapter:

- Upper GI bleeding: bleeding arising proximal to the ligament of Treitz
- Lower GI bleeding: bleeding distal to the ligament of Treitz
- Hematemesis: Vomiting of blood, which may be obviously red or the color of coffee grounds (Table 38-1)
- Hematochezia: Passage of fresh red blood per anus, usually in or with stools (Table 38-2)
- Melena: Passage of dark, tarry stools

Upper Gastrointestinal Bleeding

In healthy neonates, the most common causes of upper GI bleeding are swallowed maternal blood or a

Table 38-1 Neonatal Differential Diagnosis for Hematemesis[a]

Swallowed maternal blood
Stress ulcer
Gastritis
Duplication cyst
Vascular malformation
Vitamin K deficiency
Hemophilia
Maternal idiopathic thrombocytopenic purpura
Maternal nonsteroidal anti-inflammatory drugs
Trauma (nasogastric tube, nasal suction)

[a]Adapted from Friedlander and Mamula.[5]

Mallory-Weiss tear secondary to persistent vomiting. In tertiary care settings where infants may be more ill, other common causes of upper GI bleeding include gastric or duodenal ulcers, esophagogastroduodenitis, bleeding disorders, and nasogastric tube (NGT) trauma.

Maternal Blood

Swallowed maternal blood associated with childbirth usually manifests within the first few days of birth. There is a greater incidence in neonates delivered by cesarean section. Other sources of swallowed maternal blood may be from a maternal nipple fissure in a breast-fed baby. Typically, the baby is well appearing without any other signs of distress.

Ulcers and Gastritis

Gastric acid secretion begins shortly after birth, and this can cause ulcers or gastritis. Risk factors

Table 38-2 Neonatal Differential Diagnosis for Hematochezia[a]

Swallowed maternal blood
Dietary protein intolerance
Infectious colitis
Necrotizing enterocolitis
Hirschsprung disease and enterocolitis
Duplication cyst
Vascular malformation
Hemophilia
Maternal idiopathic thrombocytopenic purpura
Maternal nonsteroidal anti-inflammatory drugs
Anal fissure
Intussusception

[a]Adapted from Friedlander and Mamula.[5]

include stressed preterm babies in the critical care setting, mechanical ventilation, no or short duration of enteral nutrition, and medication administration[6] (Figure 38-1). Medications such as indomethacin, sulindac, tolazoline, and α-adrenergic agonists have been implicated, as well as maternal aspirin ingestion.[6–10] NGT trauma from forceful insertion or improper tube size or continuous suction resulting in a suction blister can also cause gastric irritation and bleeding.

Infection with *Helicobacter pylori* causes gastric inflammation and is associated with causing duodenal and gastric ulcers. The prevalence of *H. pylori* infection is much lower in developed countries than in developing countries. Although *H. pylori* infection is exceedingly rare in neonates in the United States, cross-sectional studies of disease prevalence in preschool children in the United States and Europe indicated prevalence ranging from 7% to 13%, with 60% at 60 years of age.[11] Ulcer disease from *H. pylori* is rare in children but has been reported to cause hematemesis.[12]

Bleeding Disorders

Hemorrhagic disease of the newborn from a deficiency in vitamin K may result in coagulopathy, especially in a patient who did not receive vitamin K at birth. Other causes of coagulopathy, such as maternal idiopathic thrombocytopenia purpura, neonatal thrombocytopenia, or congenital hemophilia, may

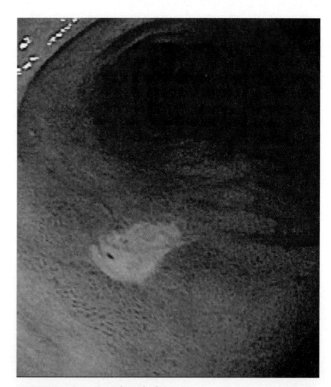

FIGURE 38-1 Duodenal ulcer.

also predispose the baby to increased bleeding risk. Significant renal failure may also cause platelet dysfunction from an acquired qualitative platelet defect, which may be treated best by dialysis but can also be remedied by desamino-D-arginine vasopressin (DDAVP)[13] (see chapter 33 for information on neonatal bleeding disorders).

Varices and Portal Hypertension

Portal hypertension from extrahepatic vascular disease or intrinsic liver disease is defined as elevated blood pressure above 5 mm Hg in the portal vein and its tributaries. Varices develop as the blood flow from the splanchnic system finds alternative pathways of portosystemic shunts back to the systemic system. Given the high blood flow and pressure in this system and the increased wall tension in the varices and abnormal blood vessel wall integrity, the rate of hemorrhage from variceal bleeding can be extremely brisk and life threatening. Varices may occur in the esophagus (Figure 38-2), stomach, or duodenum, though most sites of variceal bleeding originate from esophageal varices.

Extrahepatic vascular causes of portal hypertension include portal vein thrombosis and neonatal umbilical disorders. The most frequently reported risk factors for developing portal vein thrombosis in infancy and early childhood include intra-abdominal infections due to umbilical vein catheterization, neonatal omphalitis, and congenital malformations.[14,15] Intrinsic liver diseases in infancy, such as cirrhosis from biliary atresia,

hemochromatosis, and parenteral nutrition-induced liver disease, cause liver fibrosis and portal hypertension (see chapter 40 on congenital liver failure and neonatal hepatitis).

Obstructing Lesions and Mallory-Weiss Tears

Obstructing lesions such as pyloric stenosis, duodenal webs, and antral webs may cause vomiting significant enough to cause esophagitis and hematemesis. Mallory-Weiss tears, defined as a tear in the gastroesophageal mucosa, may be secondary to persistent emesis in infants.[16] Obstructing lesions should be considered when the patient has persistent and forceful emesis.[17] Intrinsic intestinal lesions (webs, stenosis, atresia, or duplication) and extrinsic lesions (annular pancreas or malrotation with congenital bands) mostly present in the first 24 hours of life with vomiting (66% bilious), weight loss, abdominal distension, and dehydration.[18] Pyloric stenosis typically presents at 3–4 weeks of age with poor weight gain, projectile vomiting, and electrolyte imbalances.

Other Causes

Allergic enteropathy can also present as hematemesis, but this is often also associated with mucoid bloody stools and allergic colitis.[19,20] Similarly, NEC (see chapter 37) often presents with blood in stool but may also manifest as an ileus with associated hematemesis.

Vascular malformations: Although rare, isolated cavernous hemangiomas of the stomach have been reported to cause extensive upper GI bleeding in infants and young children.[21–23] Arteriovascular malformations (AVMs) associated with blue rubber bleb nevus syndrome,[24] and Osler-Rendu-Weber syndrome[25–27] also may cause upper GI bleeding.

Gastric teratoma: Although gastric teratomas are extremely rare in infants and children, with only 51 cases reported in the literature, they can manifest as upper GI bleeding. On plain film radiographs, they appear as a calcified intra-abdominal mass, most often arising from the greater curvature of the stomach. This benign condition is treatable with surgical resection.[28,29]

Dieulafoy lesion: A Dieulafoy lesion is a large submucosal artery under the muscularis mucosa and protrudes into the gastric lumen. It appears with inflammation around the mucosal lesion. The majority of these lesions are located in the upper third of the stomach but can also be found in the small intestine. Given that the lesions are of arterial origin, they can manifest as large-volume bleeding. Reports of Dieulafoy lesions are rare in infants, but case reports cited Dieulafoy lesions in neonates as young as 1 month old.[30–33]

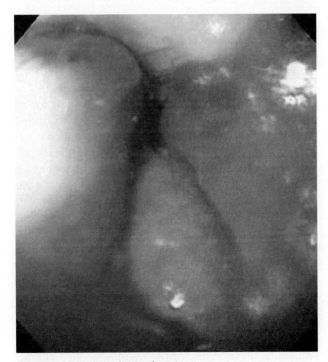

FIGURE 38-2 Esophageal varix.

Lower Gastrointestinal Bleeding

Anal Fissures

Anal fissures are the most common cause of rectal bleeding in the first 2 years of life. An anal fissure is a tear in the epithelium and squamous lining of the anal canal. Fissures can be classified as either acute or chronic. Acutely, the fissure may start as a simple crack in the anoderm; however, this may develop into a chronic fissure with infection and poor healing. A chronic fissure is where symptoms persist longer than 6 weeks after treatment and fibrosis is present at base of fissure. Skin tags may develop with chronic fissures. Most anal fissures are caused by constipation after the traumatic passage of a large, hard stool. Recent acute diarrhea may also irritate the epithelium sufficiently to cause a fissure. Irritation from a rectal thermometer may also cause minor bleeding. Typically, the bleeding associated with anal fissures appears as streaks of blood in the stool (not mucoid).[34] A large fissure with surrounding bruising should raise concern for child abuse.

Cow's Milk Protein Allergy/Allergic Colitis

The incidence of cow's milk protein allergy is estimated at approximately 1%–3% of the general population.[35,36] Cow's milk protein allergy is the most common form of enterocolitis caused by food allergies and is a leading cause of rectal bleeding in healthy children second to anal fissures. In a study of infants presenting with rectal bleeding, 46% had biopsy-proven allergic colitis.[37] Although it can rarely present in the first few days of life,[38] it usually presents in the first few months of life. Infants with allergic colitis typically have loose stools with varying amounts of mucus and gross or occult blood and may present with failure to thrive. Carbohydrate malabsorption may also cause abdominal distension, perianal erythema, and significant diaper dermatitis. Malabsorption may also cause micronutrient deficiency in iron and zinc. Further laboratory examinations may show peripheral eosinophilia, hypoalbuminemia, and anemia. Constipation as the primary symptom has also been reported.[39] Patients may also have concurrent atopic illnesses such as eczema and asthma.

Cow's milk contains the β-lactoglobulin protein, which is absent in human milk and may contribute to the development of cow's milk protein intolerance. Immunoglobulin (Ig) E–positive allergy responses are linked to the casein protein, and those with IgE-mediated allergy are less likely to outgrow their allergy.[40,41] Endoscopic examination of the colon often shows focal erythema, erosions, and nodular lymphoid hyperplasia. Histological examination reveals infiltration of the mucosa and lamina propria with eosinophils (>6–10/high-powered field) with eosinophilic degranulation or infiltrate of the crypt and surface epithelium and nodular lymphoid hyperplasia.[42]

The clinical course is usually self-limited, with most children tolerating antigen reintroduction by 2–3 years of life.[43,44]

Necrotizing Enterocolitis

It is important to exclude NEC (see chapter 37) in any neonate presenting with hematochezia, as patients with NEC may progress to significant morbidity. NEC is inflammatory bowel necrosis of portions of the small or large intestine. It typically affects premature infants, but neonates with a history of birth asphyxia, polycythemia, transfusions, intrauterine growth restriction, maternal cocaine use, cyanotic heart disease, or sepsis may also increase the risk for bowel ischemia.[9,45,46]

Symptoms may initially start with feeding intolerance and small amounts of blood in the stool or residuals from nasogastric feedings. This may progress with emerging signs of systemic instability, such as apnea, bradycardia, desaturations, temperature instability, and increased gastric residuals. Physical examination may reveal signs of abdominal distension, tenderness, erythema around the abdominal wall, and decreased bowel sounds. The classic radiological finding of NEC is pneumatosis intestinalis (gas in the bowel wall). Abdominal films may also show dilated loops of bowel, bowel wall thickening, and even free air in cases of frank perforation.

Infectious Colitis

Enteroinvasive infections cause lower GI bleeding via disrupting the mucosal integrity of the bowel. Bacterial pathogens include *Salmonella*, *Shigella*,[47] *Campylobacter*, *Yersinia enterocolitica*, *Clostridium difficile*, and *Escherichia coli* (in particular the O157:H7 variant). It is important to note that *Clostridium difficile* toxin can be found in 10%–36% of healthy neonates[48] due to microbial colonization, and 71% of neonates were stool culture–positive in a study in a special care nursery setting.[49] Therefore, a true *C. difficile* infection often requires a concomitant clinical picture of bloody diarrhea with mucus and, in the more severe forms, fever, leukocytosis, and hypoalbuminemia. Parasitic infections with *Entamoeba histolytica* can also cause infectious colitis. Viral infections with *Cytomegalovirus* (CMV) and herpes simplex virus can also cause significant lower GI hemorrhage, especially in immunodeficient patients.[50]

Meckel Diverticulum

Meckel diverticulum[51] (MD) is the most common congenital abnormality of the small intestine, with an incidence of approximately 2% of the population. It consists of a vestigial remnant of the vitelline duct that contains heterotopic gastric mucosa (80%) or pancreatic tissue (5%). The diverticulum is usually located within 100 cm of the terminal ileum. The acid-secreting mucosa causes ulceration of the adjacent mucosa and results in painless rectal bleeding and classically currant jelly stool but also may manifest as melena, hematochezia, or even frank perforation.[52]

Other Causes

Hirschsprung disease with enterocolitis: Hirschsprung disease is a congenital absence of the neural ganglia extending for a variable distance from the internal anal sphincter. Classic clinical presentation of Hirschsprung disease is of delayed passage of meconium and severe constipation and abdominal distension. However, about 10%–30% of patients with Hirschsprung disease may have enterocolitis that manifests with diarrhea, rectal bleeding, poor weight gain, and hypoalbuminemia.

Polyps: Juvenile polyps usually present with painless rectal bleeding in the toddler to preschool age but have been reported in infancy.[53]

Intestinal duplications: Intestinal duplications are congenital lesions either cystic or tubular, with muscular walls with GI mucosal lining. They may exist adjacent to the alimentary tract or may communicate with the lumen. Most commonly, these are located in the ileum. These become symptomatic when the ectopic mucosa of gastric or pancreatic tissue causes lower GI bleeding.[54,55]

Inflammatory bowel disease and chronic granulomatous disease: Inflammatory bowel diseases such as Crohn's colitis and ulcerative colitis are extremely rare in infancy. However, intractable ulcerating enterocolitis of infancy is a rare form that accounts for 0.5% of all diagnosed forms of inflammatory bowel disease. Onset is usually in the first few months of life; it responds poorly to immunosuppression, and often requires colectomy or bone marrow transplant if due to chronic granulomatous disease.[56,57]

Bowel obstruction with ischemic injury: Lower GI bleeding is a late finding in bowel ischemia that may be associated with intussusception or malrotation with volvulus. Clinically, this is also associated with vomiting, abdominal distension, pain, and peritoneal signs.

Bleeding disorder: Hematologic causes of bleeding coagulopathy also need to be considered in neonates with significant GI bleeding. Hemorrhagic disease of the newborn and other neonatal coagulopathies are discussed further in chapter 33, Bleeding Disorders.

Vascular malformations: Vascular malformations are uncommon causes of lower GI bleeding in infants and children. AVMs in children are usually small, single, and located in the rectum and descending colon and rarely in the small bowel.[58,59] Clinical presentation may be with gross lower GI bleeding or chronic iron deficiency anemia. Malformations associated with Klippel-Trenaunay syndrome (a triad of varicose veins, cutaneous capillary malformation, and hypertrophy of bone and [or] soft tissue) can also cause massive GI bleeding. GI vascular malformations such as colonic varices and cavernous hemangiomas in Klippel-Trenaunay syndrome may present with significant hematochezia or melena.[60,61] Blue rubber bleb nevus syndrome and its associated characteristic GI and cutaneous hemangiomas also may cause upper and lower GI bleeding.[24]

Anastomotic ulcers: In patients who have had prior abdominal surgeries and bowel resections (eg, for NEC) have a higher risk of anastomotic ulcers or stitch granulomas at the anastomosis sites.

EVALUATION

Initial assessment in a patient who presents with GI bleeding is the immediate evaluation of the degree and volume of blood loss and fluid resuscitation and hemodynamic stabilization if needed. Patient history, physical, and diagnostic studies may all assist in this assessment.

History
Patient History

Patient history should first elicit the quantity, volume, and location of bleeding. Questions should first ensure that the presentation is truly of GI bleeding from the patient. Food products and some medications may mimic hematochezia, such as the ingestion of food colorings, gelatin, tomato and fruit skins, and beets. Melena may also be confused with iron preparations, bismuth, spinach, grape juice, and blueberries.[62] Recent nose bleeding or nasal traumas may also appear as GI bleeding.

In the neonate, the birth history and cesarean section may predispose to swallowed maternal blood and cause hematemesis in the first days of life. A history of bleeding from the maternal nipple in a breast-fed baby can present as melena in the infant. Lack of vitamin K administration at birth may predispose to hemorrhagic disease of the newborn.

In an older infant, a history of omphalitis, sepsis, dehydration, umbilical catheterization, or prematurity in the neonatal period may predispose the patient to portal hypertension secondary to portal vein thrombosis. A history of recent frequent emesis may increase suspicion for a Mallory-Weiss tear, especially if the first few episodes of emesis were not bloody. Stooling pattern may also help determine a predilection toward constipation or diarrhea. Furthermore, exposure history to day care or contaminated foods may also increase risk for infectious etiologies. A recent introduction in the diet of formula or other new foods may point to cow's milk protein allergy or soy allergy.

Family History

A close family history of hemophilia, allergy, inflammatory bowel disease, or familial hemorrhagic telangiectasia would be suggestive of these diseases in the patient.

Physical Examination

Vital sign assessment is important in any infant for whom there is a concern for GI bleeding. Tachycardia may indicate early signs of hypovolemia and significant blood loss. Hypotension and delayed capillary refill are later signs of hemodynamic instability that would require prompt hemodynamic resuscitation. Fever will suggest an infectious process or inflammatory disorder. If the infant appears toxic or ill, NEC, infectious colitis, bowel ischemia, and food protein–induced enterocolitis should be considered over more benign conditions such as anal fissures or cow's milk protein allergy.

Measurements of height, weight, and weight for length are important in the older infant and can determine the chronicity of the disease. Growth delay and failure to thrive may be more indicative of chronic diseases such as Hirschsprung disease or inflammatory bowel disease.

Other physical examination findings may elucidate the cause of the bleeding. For the upper GI tract, a careful examination of nasopharynx and blood in nares may pinpoint this as the source. Skin findings of caput medusa, spider angiomas, and jaundice may indicate liver dysfunction. Hemangiomas and telangiectasias of the skin may suggest similar findings in the GI tract. Eczema may be associated with the atopic picture of cow's milk protein allergy. The abdominal examination may reveal hepatosplenomegaly or ascites, which would point to portal hypertension and varices or angiodysplasia as the cause of bleeding. Careful perianal area and rectal examination is imperative to pinpoint lower GI causes such as fissures and polyps.

Nasogastric tube aspirate: Gastric aspiration from an NGT is a simple indicator to distinguish between upper GI and lower GI bleeding. The presence of bloody aspirate indicates active bleeding, usually gastric or esophageal, but clear aspirate does not eliminate a duodenal source.

Diagnostic Tests

Initial lab tests such as the guaiac test can confirm that the appearance of blood in stool or vomitus is true blood rather than a substance that mimics the appearance of blood. Hemoccult tests are available to test for occult blood in the stool. Similar to the hemoccult, a gastroccult test can be sent for gastric aspirate or vomitus. Guaiac is a naturally occurring phenolic compound that can be oxidized to quinine by hydrogen peroxide in the hemoglobin with detectable color change. Iron preparations do not give false-positive tests in the newer preparations, but rarely false positives can be seen from hemoglobin or myoglobin in meat or peroxidase in certain uncooked vegetables. Newer immunochemical tests that are more specific to the hemoglobin A chain are now validated for the adult population to screen for fecal occult blood, and these are currently being validated for the neonatal population.

Apt Test

In a neonate, the Apt test distinguishes maternal blood from fetal blood and is based on the premise that the infant's hemoglobin is great than 60% fetal hemoglobin, which is alkali resistant. Maternal blood consists mostly of hemoglobin A. When maternal blood is mixed with an alkali reagent, maternal blood turns brownish yellow, whereas fetal blood remains pink. First, the specimen is mixed with 3–5 mL of tap water and centrifuged. The supernatant must have a pink color to proceed. To 5 parts of supernatant, 1 part 0.25 N (1%) NaOH is added. A pink color persisting over 2 minutes indicates fetal hemoglobin. Adult hemoglobin gives a pink color that becomes yellowish brown in 2 minutes or less, indicating denaturation of the adult hemoglobin.[63]

Laboratory Studies

Common laboratory studies in the initial evaluation of a bleeding infant include a complete blood count, reticulocyte count, coagulation panel, and chemistry and liver function panel. A type and crossmatch should also be obtained in case the need for transfusion arises. A blood gas may also be helpful in a patient with signs of shock or systemic illness. The serum urea nitrogen (BUN)/creatinine ratio may be useful for assessing the source of a GI bleed. A ratio BUN/creatinine ratio of 30 or above is 98% sensitive and 69% specific for upper GI bleeding in pediatric patients.[64]

Stool studies may also help to reveal the etiology of the GI bleeding. In patients with hematochezia, stool examination for bacterial culture, ova, and parasites and *C. difficile* toxin assay are diagnostic for infectious etiologies. CMV polymerase chain reaction (PCR) can also be sent, especially in the neonatal intensive care unit setting. An *H. pylori* stool antigen test before acid suppressant therapy may also be helpful for a patient with hematemesis, though the gold standard diagnostic test for this infection is still via endoscopy and biopsy.

Imaging Studies

Abdominal Radiographs

Abdominal films are important to evaluate the bowel gas pattern and to look for hallmark radiological findings for specific bleeding etiologies (Table 38-3). Emergently, an upright film and supine view may be helpful to look for air-fluid levels, which would be indicative of an ileus or obstruction. The presence of free air in the abdomen is concerning for perforation.

Infants with NEC may show evidence of pneumatosis intestinalis, or air bubbles within the bowel wall. The bowel wall may also be thickened, giving a railroad track appearance. Further, patients with Hirschsprung enterocolitis may show evidence of dilated proximal intestine and colon with paucity of air seen in the rectum. Prone films are helpful for this as air moves into the rectum in this position if there is no obstruction. NGT position can also be evaluated for proper positioning. Plain films may also be helpful in identifying unsuspected foreign bodies.

Table 38-3 Imaging Studies and Associated Indications[a]

Test	Indication
Abdominal x-ray	Constipation Foreign body Vomiting
Upper gastrointestinal series	Dysphagia Odynophagia Drooling Obstruction Vomiting
Barium enema	Suspected stricture Intussception Hirschsprung disease
Ultrasound (Doppler recommended for liver disease)	Suspected stricture Intussusception
Meckel scan	Meckel diverticulum
Tagged red blood cell scan	Obscure gastrointestinal bleeding
Magnetic resonance/ computed tomography/ direct angiography	Obscure gastrointestinal bleeding Suspected arteriovenous malformation

[a]Adapted from Friedlander and Mamula.[5]

Upper Gastrointestinal Series

An upper GI series is a series of radiographs taken after the patient ingests contrast to evaluate the anatomy of the stomach and small bowel. This is an important study to perform if there is suspicion for gastric outlet obstruction, malrotation, and midgut volvulus. If there is concern for obstruction or partial obstruction, the upper GI series may also be able to evaluate for a transition point. In the rare care of Crohn's disease, the upper GI series can also evaluate for small-bowel involvement. Of note, if endoscopy is needed for the diagnosis or management of a bleeding patient, this should be performed prior to contrast studies with barium, as the barium may obscure the visualization of the mucosa.

Abdominal Ultrasound

In upper GI bleeding, an abdominal ultrasound is useful in the assessment of portal hypertension and pyloric stenosis and if large vascular anomalies are suspected. In lower GI bleeding, an ultrasound could be diagnostic if there is concern for an acute abdominal disorder with obstruction, ischemia, or intussusception.

Nuclear Medicine Scans

Meckel scan: A Meckel scan involves using technetium Tc 99m pertechnetate, a radiolabeled isotope, to evaluate patients with lower GI bleeding suspicious of a Meckel diverticulum. The isotope is taken up by the gastric acid–producing cells and then secreted into the gut lumen. If the Meckel diverticulum contains ectopic gastric mucosa, this ectopic gastric mucosa is illuminated away from the stomach. Cimetidine, or another H_2 receptor antagonist, can be given prior to increase the sensitivity of the scan by cimetidine-mediated retention of pertechnetate in the gastric mucosa.[65]

Bleeding scan: Technetium-labeled red blood cell scintigraphy scans are sometimes helpful in the diagnosis and localization of obscure bleeding in the small bowel. This scan is typically performed in older children or adults but can sometimes be helpful in infants in rare circumstances. This scan involves injection of radioactive particles labeled by technetium Tc 99m. These particles pass through the mesenteric vascular bed, and if there is a leak or tear in these vessels, extravasation can be seen into the bowel. This test can detect a bleeding rate down to 0.05 mL/min for newer techniques of reference subtraction scintography and has a sensitivity of 79%–97%, but the patient must be bleeding actively during the scan.[66,67]

Computed Tomography and Magnetic Resonance Imaging

Computed tomographic (CT) scans and magnetic resonance imaging (MRI) can be especially helpful for detecting congenital GI tract duplications, mass lesions, and vascular malformations. Emerging angiographic techniques in both CT and MRI are proving to be promising first-line modalities to identify GI hemorrhage.[68] Diagnosis and localization of obscure GI bleeding, similar to a nuclear medicine bleeding scan or angiography, require active extravasation of contrast into the intestinal lumen during the scan.

Angiography

If bleeding is not detected on upper endoscopy or lower endoscopy, angiography may be considered. Angiography can be a useful tool in both upper and lower GI bleeding and can detect and localize a bleeding rate of at least 0.5 mL/min.[69] Angiography may also offer a therapeutic advantage to perform selective arterial embolization or other therapy for the potential bleeding site.[59]

Endoscopy and Colonoscopy

Upper endoscopy or esophagogastroduodenoscopy is the test of choice to evaluate and treat the underlying cause of hematemesis. Upper endoscopy can identify the cause of bleeding in up to 90% of cases in pediatrics (from ulceration, gastritis, variceal bleeding, or a Dieulafoy lesion). For neonates, there are endoscopes designed for babies as small as 0.9 kg. Emergency endoscopy is indicated if the rate of bleeding continues to be life threatening, requiring continuous transfusions with evidence of hemodynamic instability. Otherwise, the optimal timing for the upper endoscopy is when the patient has undergone fluid resuscitation and is hemodynamically stable for anesthesia and the procedure.

Colonoscopy, or the more limited protosigmoidoscopy, is also a useful tool to diagnose lower GI bleeding. NEC must first be ruled out prior to the procedure, as it is a definite contraindication to performing a lower endoscopy given the high risk of perforation in these patients. Lower endoscopies can detect anal fissures, polyps, and angiodysplasia and assess the intestinal mucosa for signs of inflammatory bowel disease. Video capsule endoscopy, though diagnostic in older children and adult patients, is contraindicated in infants and neonates given the size limitations.

MANAGEMENT

The management of a neonate or infant with GI bleeding depends on the severity of the bleeding and the patient's underlying illness. In severe bleeding, hemodynamic stabilization and treatment should be the first priority and then specific care given depending on the cause of the bleeding.

Supportive Care

Patients with significant bleeding require supportive care to maintain hemodynamic stability. Patients should have adequate intravenous access with placement of 1–2 larger-bore intravenous lines and be admitted to an intensive care unit setting. Fluid depletion should first be replaced with isotonic saline solution. If isotonic fluids are not sufficient, transfusion of blood products may be required, as well as drugs for resuscitation.[70] Patients who have poor tissue perfusion secondary to significant hemorrhage or shock should also receive oxygen. Infants younger than 1 year old with any significant upper GI or lower GI bleeding or significant heme-positive stool should be hospitalized for observation.

Gastric Lavage

Gastric lavage may help to diagnose upper GI bleeding. It involves placement of an NGT followed by sequential administration and removal of small volumes of warm or body temperature fluid, usually normal saline. The presence of blood during the gastric lavage diagnoses upper GI bleeding, including duodenal hemorrhage that may reflux into the stomach. If the aspirated fluid begins to clear after several lavages, the bleeding may have stopped.

Specific Care
Gastritis and Ulcers

Patients who are identified with bleeding secondary to gastric or duodenal ulcers by endoscopy should receive nothing by mouth for 24 to 48 hours or until significant bleeding subsides. Acid blockage should be addressed with an H_2 receptor agonist (such as cimetidine, ranitidine, or famotidine) or proton pump inhibitor (such as Protonix, esomeprazole, omeprazole, or lansoprazole), which are the first-line medications for gastritis and peptic ulcer disease. Initial medications for the first 48 hours should be administered intravenously and then transitioned to oral medications if the bleeding does not recur.[70] Since these patients can have nothing by mouth, intravenous pantoprazole is preferred at a dose of 1 mg/kg every 12–24 hours. (Of note, this is an off-label use for this drug for upper GI bleeding in neonates.) If a patient has an NGT, pH monitoring of the gastric contents can aid in the dosing of the acid-suppressive medication. The goal pH level should be maintained at greater than 4.5. Barrier agents, such as sucralfate, are also used as a topical agent to coat ulcers and to treat gastritis.

Variceal Bleeding

Somatostatin analogs such as octreotide or vasopressin act by decreasing the splanchnic flow to the mesenteric vasculature and decrease acid production in the stomach. Vasopressin has significant undesirable side effects, such as bowel ischemia. Therefore, octreotide, the longer-acting somatostatin analog, is the preferred medication of choice for significant upper GI bleeding. The dosing for octreotide is an initial bolus of 1 μg/kg up to 50 μg and 1–2 μg/kg/hour as a continuous infusion.

Surgical Conditions

Surgical evaluation and correction are indicated in patients who have GI bleeding from perforation, volvulus from malrotation, or other anatomical anomalies, such as duplications or vascular malformations.

Cow's Milk Protein Intolerance

Patients who are diagnosed with cow's milk protein intolerance or allergic colitis require a change in formula to a hypoallergenic, hydrolyzed, or elemental amino acid–based formula. Soy formulas are not indicated because of the cross-reactivity between the 30-kDa soy protein and cow's milk protein. Exclusively breast-fed infants may improve with strict elimination of dairy products from the maternal diet. With the change in diet, gross bleeding resolves in 3 weeks, although heme-positive stools may persist for 6–12 weeks. If the gross or occult bleeding is not resolved in this time frame, endoscopy is indicated to look for other etiologies of the bleeding. The prognosis of patients with cow's milk protein intolerance is good, with 56% of patients tolerating an unrestricted diet by 1 year, up to 77% by 2 years, and up to 87% at 3 years.[44]

Anal Fissures

Treatment of anal fissures is directed at treating constipation using stool softeners such as lactulose or polyethylene glycol or by fiber supplementation. Warm sitz baths may also help to reduce anal hypertonicity. Of these patients, 80% will heal the acute fissure with these measures. If on examination there is evidence of perianal erythema, the patient may have an α-hemolytic streptococcus infection, which can be diagnosed by an anal culture. Treatment of this would require appropriate antibiotics. For patients with persistent fissures and constipation, allergic colitis or cow's milk intolerance may be considered as a possible etiology.

Necrotizing Enterocolitis

Management of NEC may be medical or surgical depending on the severity of the disease (chapter 37).

Endoscopic Therapy

Endoscopic therapy offers various techniques to achieve hemostasis depending on the underlying disease. In patients with an identified bleeding site, thermal energy can be used for cautery. These techniques include argon plasma coagulation, mono- or bipolar cautery, heater probe, and laser techniques. An ulcer with a bleeding vessel can be injected with epinephrine in combination with a sclerosing agent to tamponade the bleeding. Hemostatic clips can be passed via the endoscopic channel, but these are typically too small for the instrument channels on the neonatal endoscopes.

Infants with esophageal varices may undergo sclerotherapy to inject sclerosant medications into the varix.

Endoscopic polypectomy is performed using electrocautery with bipolar snares. Most polyps in the pediatric population are isolated simple juvenile polyps that have no premalignant potential.

SUMMARY

Gastrointestinal hemorrhage is a relatively common problem seen in the neonatal and infant population. Prognosis of GI bleeding in the neonate and infant often depends on the severity of underlying disease etiology, as the bleeding can occur in any area of the GI tract. Patient presentation can vary from life threatening to benign and therefore requires systematic evaluation in all patients. Best outcomes require collaboration between the neonatologist, pediatrician, gastroenterologist, radiologist, and surgeon to diagnose and treat the underlying condition. Evaluation and therapeutic options continue to evolve and now involve multiple endoscopic and angiographic techniques.

REFERENCES

1. Lazzaroni M, Petrillo M, Tornaghi R, et al. Upper GI bleeding in healthy full-term infants: a case-control study. *Am J Gastroenterol*. 2002;97(1):89–94.
2. Mäki M, Ruuska T, Kuusela AL, Karikoski-Leo R, Ikonen RS. High prevalence of asymptomatic esophageal and gastric lesions in preterm infants in intensive care. *Crit Care Med*. 1993;21(12):1863–1867.
3. López-Herce J, Dorao P, Elola P, et al. Frequency and prophylaxis of upper gastrointestinal hemorrhage in critically ill children: a prospective study comparing the efficacy of almagate, ranitidine, and sucralfate. The Gastrointestinal Hemorrhage Study Group. *Crit Care Med*. 1992;20(8):1082–1089.

4. Teach SJ, Fleisher GR. Rectal bleeding in the pediatric emergency department. *Ann Emerg Med.* 1994;23(6):1252–1258.

5. Friedlander J, Mamula P. Gastrointestinal hemorrhage. In: Wyllie R, Hyams JS, eds. *Pediatric Gastrointestinal and Liver Disease,* 4th ed. New York, NY: Elsevier; 2011.

6. Abramo TJ, Evans JS, Kokomoor FW, Kantak AD. Occult blood in stools and necrotizing enterocolitis: Is there a relationship? *Am J Dis Child.* 1988;142(4):451–452.

7. Ojala R, Ruuska T, Karikoski R, Ikonen RS, Tammela O. Gastroesophageal endoscopic findings and gastrointestinal symptoms in preterm neonates with and without perinatal indomethacin exposure. *J Pediatr Gastroenterol Nutr.* 2001;32(2):182–188.

8. Ng PC, So KW, Fok TF, et al. Fatal haemorrhagic gastritis associated with oral sulindac treatment for patent ductus arteriosus. *Acta Paediatr.* 1996;85(7):884–886.

9. Telsey AM, Merrit TA, Dixon SD. Cocaine exposure in a term neonate. Necrotizing enterocolitis as a complication. *Clin Pediatr (Phila).* 1988;27(11):547–550.

10. Dillard RG. Fatal gastrointestinal hemorrhage in a neonate treated with tolazoline. *Clin Pediatr (Phila).* 1982;21(12): 761–762.

11. Lindkvist P, Asrat D, Nilsson I, et al. Age at acquisition of *Helicobacter pylori* infection: comparison of a high and a low prevalence country. *Scand J Infect Dis.* 1996;28(2):181–184.

12. Mitchell JD, Mitchell HM, Tobias V. Acute *Helicobacter pylori* infection in an infant, associated with gastric ulceration and serological evidence of intra-familial transmission. *Am J Gastroenterol.* 1992;87(3):382–386.

13. Zachée P, Vermylen J, Boogaerts MA. Hematologic aspects of end-stage renal failure. *Ann Hematol.* 1994;69(1):33–40.

14. Obladen M, Ernst D, Feist D, Wille L. Portal hypertension in children following neonatal umbilical disorders. *J Perinat Med.* 1975;3(2):101–104.

15. Seixas CA, Hessel G, Ribeiro CC, Arruda VR, Annichino-Bizzacchi JM. Factor V Leiden is not common in children with portal vein thrombosis. *Thromb Haemost.* 1997;77(2):258–261.

16. Cannon RA, Lee G, Cox KL. Gastrointestinal hemorrhage due to Mallory-Weiss syndrome in an infant. *J Pediatr Gastroenterol Nutr.* 1985;4(2):323–324.

17. Takeuchi S, Tamate S, Nakahira M, Kadowaki H. Esophagitis in infants with hypertrophic pyloric stenosis: a source of hematemesis. *J Pediatr Surg.* 1993;28(1):59–62.

18. Bailey PV, Tracy TF Jr, Connors RH, et al. Congenital duodenal obstruction: a 32-year review. *J Pediatr Surg.* 1993;28(1):92–95.

19. Heldenberg D, Abudy Z, Keren S, Auslaender L. Cow's milk-induced hematemesis in an infant. *J Pediatr Gastroenterol Nutr.* 1993;17(4):450–452.

20. el Mouzan MI, al Quorain AA, Anim JT. Cow's-milk-induced erosive gastritis in an infant. *J Pediatr Gastroenterol Nutr.* 1990;10(1):111–113.

21. Abrahamson J, Shandling B. Intestinal hemangiomata in childhood and a syndrome for diagnosis: a collective review. *J Pediatr Surg.* 1973;8(4):487–495.

22. Nagaya M, Kato J, Niimi N, et al. Isolated cavernous hemangioma of the stomach in a neonate. *J Pediatr Surg.* 1998;33(4):653–654.

23. Schettini ST, Ribeiro RC, Brito PL, et al. Gastric hemangioma in a 5-year-old boy. *J Pediatr Surg.* 2007;42(4):717–718.

24. Hansen LF, Wewer V, Pedersen SA, Matzen P, Paerregaard A. Severe blue rubber bleb nevus syndrome in a neonate. *Eur J Pediatr Surg.* 2009;19(1):47–49.

25. Abdalla SA, Geisthoff UW, Bonneau D, et al. Visceral manifestations in hereditary haemorrhagic telangiectasia type 2. *J Med Genet.* 2003;40(7):494–502.

26. Odell JM, Haas JE, Tapper D, Nugent D. Infantile hemorrhagic angiodysplasia. *Pediatr Pathol.* 1987;7(5–6):629–636.

27. Mestre JR, Andres JM. Hereditary hemorrhagic telangiectasia causing hematemesis in an infant. *J Pediatr.* 1982;101(4):577–579.

28. Cairo MS, Grosfeld JL, Weetman RM. Gastric teratoma: unusual cause for bleeding of the upper gastrointestinal tract in the newborn. *Pediatrics.* 1981;67(5):721–724.

29. Haley T, Dimler M, Hollier P. Gastric teratoma with gastrointestinal bleeding. *J Pediatr Surg.* 1986;21(11):949–950.

30. Karamanoukian HL, Wilcox DT, Hatch EI, Sawin R, Glick PL. Dieulafoy's disease in infants. *Pediatr Surg Int.* 1994;9(8). http://www.springerlink.com/content/w458378lk3333662/ (accessed August 11, 2011).

31. Lee Y, Walmsley R, Leong R. Dieulafoy's lesion. *Gastrointestinal Endoscopy.* 2003. http://usagiedu.com/articles/dl/dl.pdf.

32. Lilje C, Greiner P, Riede UN, Sontheimer J, Brandis M. Dieulafoy lesion in a one-year-old child. *J Pediatr Surg.* 2004;39(1):133–134.

33. Koo YH, Jang JS, Cho JH, et al. [Endoscopic injection treatment for gastric dieulafoy lesion in two newborn infants]. *Korean J Gastroenterol.* 2005;46(5):413–417.

34. Anveden-Hertzberg L, Finkel Y, Sandstedt B, Karpe B. Proctocolitis in exclusively breast-fed infants. *Eur J Pediatr.* 1996;155(6):464–467.

35. Høst A, Husby S, Osterballe O. A prospective study of cow's milk allergy in exclusively breast-fed infants. Incidence, pathogenetic role of early inadvertent exposure to cow's milk formula, and characterization of bovine milk protein in human milk. *Acta Paediatr Scand.* 1988;77(5):663–670.

36. Jakobsson I, Lindberg T. A prospective study of cow's milk protein intolerance in Swedish infants. *Acta Paediatr Scand.* 1979;68(6):853–859.

37. Xanthakos SA, Schwimmer JB, Melin-Aldana H, et al. Prevalence and outcome of allergic colitis in healthy infants with rectal bleeding: a prospective cohort study. *J Pediatr Gastroenterol Nutr.* 2005;41(1):16–22.

38. Kumar D, Repucci A, Wyatt-Ashmead J, Chelimsky G. Allergic colitis presenting in the first day of life: report of three cases. *J Pediatr Gastroenterol Nutr.* 2000;31(2):195–197.

39. Iacono G, Cavataio F, Montalto G, et al. Intolerance of cow's milk and chronic constipation in children. *N Engl J Med.* 1998;339(16):1100–1104.

40. Vila L, Beyer K, Järvinen KM, et al. Role of conformational and linear epitopes in the achievement of tolerance in cow's milk allergy. *Clin Exp Allergy.* 2001;31(10):1599–1606.

41. Järvinen K-M, Beyer K, Vila L, et al. B-cell epitopes as a screening instrument for persistent cow's milk allergy. *J Allergy Clin Immunol.* 2002;110(2):293–297.

42. Machida HM, Catto Smith AG, Gall DG, Trevenen C, Scott RB. Allergic colitis in infancy: clinical and pathologic aspects. *J Pediatr Gastroenterol Nutr.* 1994;19(1):22–26.

43. Chandra RK. Five-year follow-up of high-risk infants with family history of allergy who were exclusively breast-fed or fed partial whey hydrolysate, soy, and conventional cow's milk formulas. *J Pediatr Gastroenterol Nutr.* 1997;24(4):380–388.

44. Høst A, Jacobsen HP, Halken S, Holmenlund D. The natural history of cow's milk protein allergy/intolerance. *Eur J Clin Nutr.* 1995;49(Suppl 1):S13–S18.

45. De La Torre CA, Miguel M, Martínez L, et al. [The risk of necrotizing enterocolitis in newborns with congenital heart disease. a single institution-cohort study.] *Cir Pediatr.* 2010;23(2):103–106.

46. Singh R, Visintainer PF, Frantz ID 3rd, et al. Association of necrotizing enterocolitis with anemia and packed red blood cell transfusions in preterm infants. *J Perinatol.* 2011;31(3):176–182.

47. Huskins WC, Griffiths JK, Faruque AS, Bennish ML. Shigellosis in neonates and young infants. *J Pediatr.* 1994;125(1):14–22.

48. Donta ST, Myers MG. *Clostridium difficile* toxin in asymptomatic neonates. *J Pediatr.* 1982;100(3):431–434.

49. Al-Jumaili IJ, Shibley M, Lishman AH, Record CO. Incidence and origin of *Clostridium difficile* in neonates. *J Clin Microbiol.* 1984;19(1):77–78.

50. Daley AJ, Craven P, Holland AJA, et al. Herpes simplex virus colitis in a neonate. *Pediatr Infect Dis J.* 2002;21(9):887–888.

51. Brown RL, Azizkhan RG. Gastrointestinal bleeding in infants and children: Meckel's diverticulum and intestinal duplication. *Semin Pediatr Surg.* 1999;8(4):202–209.

52. Canty T, Meguid MM, Eraklis AJ. Perforation of Meckel's diverticulum in infancy. *J Pediatr Surg.* 1975;10(2):189–193.

53. Krishnegowda L, Mahajan JK, Rao KLN. Rectal polyp in a newborn leading to massive lower gastrointestinal bleed. *J Pediatr Surg.* 2008;43(6):E15–E16.

54. Bower RJ, Sieber WK, Kiesewetter WB. Alimentary tract duplications in children. *Ann Surg.* 1978;188(5):669–674.

55. Macpherson RI. Gastrointestinal tract duplications: clinical, pathologic, etiologic, and radiologic considerations. *Radiographics.* 1993;13(5):1063–1080.

56. Thapar N, Lindley KJ, Kiparissi F, et al. Treatment of intractable ulcerating enterocolitis of infancy by allogeneic bone marrow transplantation. *Clin Gastroenterol Hepatol.* 2008;6(2):248–250.

57. Thapar N, Shah N, Ramsay AD, Lindley KJ, Milla PJ. Long-term outcome of intractable ulcerating enterocolitis of infancy. *J Pediatr Gastroenterol Nutr.* 2005;40(5):582–588.

58. de la Torre L, Carrasco D, Mora MA, Ramírez J, López S. Vascular malformations of the colon in children. *J Pediatr Surg.* 2002;37(12):1754–1757.

59. Silveri M, Falappa P, Casciani E, Natali G, Rivosecchi M. Diagnostic and therapeutic tricks in a rare case of pediatric ileal congenital arteriovenous malformation. *J Pediatr Gastroenterol Nutr.* 51(1):90–92.

60. Servelle M, Bastin R, Loygue J, et al. Hematuria and rectal bleeding in the child with Klippel and Trenaunay syndrome. *Ann Surg.* 1976;183(4):418–428.

61. Parashette KR, Cuffari C. Sclerotherapy of rectal hemangiomas in a child with Klippel-Trenaunay-Weber syndrome. *J Pediatr Gastroenterol Nutr.* 2011;52(1):111–112.

62. Leung A. Lower gastrointestinal bleeding in children. *Pediatric Emergency Care.* 2002. http://journals.lww.com/pec-online/Abstract/2002/08000/Lower_gastrointestinal_bleeding_in_children.22.aspx.

63. Apt L, Downey WS Jr. Melena neonatorum: the swallowed blood syndrome; a simple test for the differentiation of adult and fetal hemoglobin in bloody stools. *J Pediatr.* 1955;47(1):6–12.

64. Urashima M, Toyoda S, Nakano T, et al. BUN/Cr ratio as an index of gastrointestinal bleeding mass in children. *J Pediatr Gastroenterol Nutr.* 1992;15(1):89–92.

65. Petrokubi RJ, Baum S, Rohrer GV. Cimetidine administration resulting in improved pertechnetate imaging of Meckel's diverticulum. *Clin Nucl Med.* 1978;3(10):385–388.

66. Currie GM, Towers PA, Wheat JM. Improved detection and localization of lower gastrointestinal tract hemorrhage by subtraction scintigraphy: phantom analysis. *J Nucl Med Technol.* 2006;34(3):160–168.

67. Currie GM, Kiat H, Wheat JM. Scintigraphic evaluation of acute lower gastrointestinal hemorrhage: current status and future directions. *J Clin Gastroenterol.* 2011;45(2):92–99.

68. Wu L-M, Xu J-R, Yin Y, Qu X-H. Usefulness of CT angiography in diagnosing acute gastrointestinal bleeding: a meta-analysis. *World J Gastroenterol.* 2010;16(31):3957–3963.

69. Afshani E, Berger PE. Gastrointestinal tract angiography in infants and children. *J Pediatr Gastroenterol Nutr.* 1986;5(2):173–186.

70. Ament ME. Diagnosis and management of upper gastrointestinal tract bleeding in the pediatric patient. *Pediatr Rev.* 1990;12(4):107–116.

Conjugated Hyperbilirubinemia

Johann Peterson and William Berquist

EPIDEMIOLOGY

Historical estimates place the incidence of cholestasis among all neonates at 1 in 2500 live births.[1] A recent retrospective data review found that among all infants cared for in a large hospital system in the United States who had at least 1 measured conjugated bilirubin level, 3 in 1000 had a peak conjugated (direct) bilirubin greater than 2.0 mg/dL[2]; however, in the majority of these patients a specific hepatobiliary disorder was not identified, and the peak bilirubin was relatively low (<5 mg/dL). The incidence of cholestasis in the neonatal intensive care unit (NICU) is significantly higher. In 1 series, cholestasis (defined as direct bilirubin > 1.0 mg/dL when total bilirubin is 5 mg or less or direct bilirubin > 20% of total bilirubin when the total bilirubin is above 5 mg/dL) was identified in 2% of all NICU patients.[3] Risk factors that are common in this population include prematurity, low birth weight, sepsis, shock, surgery, and parenteral nutrition.[4] Thus, although cholestatic liver disease is rare in general outpatient pediatrics, the neonatologist must be familiar with the initial triage and diagnostic evaluation, as well as supportive care, of the cholestatic infant.

PATHOPHYSIOLOGY

Cholestasis refers to any impairment in the hepatic excretion of bile. Bile is an aqueous solution of bile acids, cholesterol, conjugated bilirubin, proteins, phospholipids, toxins and xenobiotic substances, and electrolytes. Biochemically, an increase in serum conjugated bilirubin is the most commonly identified marker of cholestasis. The usual rule of thumb is that a direct-reacting fraction of bilirubin greater than 2 mg/dL or greater than 15% of total bilirubin should be regarded as evidence of cholestasis. However, it is helpful to remember that direct and conjugated bilirubin are not identical. Unconjugated bilirubin is the product of heme breakdown, which in the liver is conjugated with glucuronic acid prior to secretion into bile. The traditional assay relies on the fact that conjugated bilirubin (the "direct-reacting fraction") reacts much more readily with a diazo reagent than does unconjugated bilirubin (the "indirect-reacting fraction"), which is measured after the addition of an accelerating agent. Unconjugated bilirubin does participate, albeit more slowly, in the unaccelerated reaction, and when the concentration of unconjugated bilirubin is high, the direct bilirubin measurement will be spuriously elevated.[5,6] Laboratories that report conjugated and unconjugated fractions as such, rather than as direct and indirect fractions, are typically using a newer spectrophotometric method (Kodac BuBc), and some laboratories report measurements for both direct and conjugated bilirubin. The direct bilirubin measurement (ironically, an indirect estimate of the conjugated bilirubin concentration) is generally a higher number than the conjugated bilirubin measurement, and it also includes measuring the delta bilirubin or the bilirubin bound to albumin.

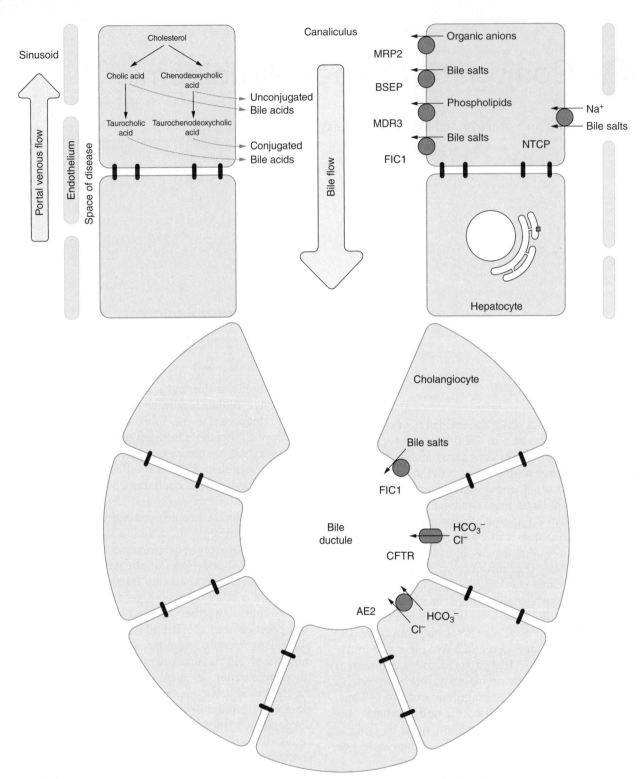

FIGURE 39-1 Basic anatomy of the hepatocytes and cholangiocytes as it relates to bile formation and enterohepatic circulation. The specific transporters are discussed in the text. BSEP, bile salt excretory protein; FIC1, familial intrahepatic cholestasis 1.

Physiology of Normal Bile Production and Excretion

Some understanding of bile acid physiology is necessary for an adequate description of cholestatic pathophysiology. The biochemistry and transport of bile acids is complex, and this discussion is restricted to the clinically salient points. Figure 39-1 provides a cartoon representation of the basic machinery of bile excretion.

Bile Acid Synthesis and Enterohepatic and Cholehepatic Circulation

Bile acids are synthesized from cholesterol within hepatocytes. Cholic acid and chenodeoxycholic acid are the bile acids synthesized by the liver and are referred to as "primary" bile acids. After conjugation with glycine or taurine, they are secreted with other normal bile constituents into the duodenum. Bacterial action within the small bowel converts cholic acid to deoxycholic acid and chenodeoxycholic acid to lithocholic acid, the "secondary" bile acids. The majority of intestinal bile acid is reabsorbed through an active transport mechanism in the ileum, transported to the liver via the portal vein, and again taken up by hepatocytes.[7] This cycle is referred to as the enterohepatic circulation.

Functions of Bile Acids

Bile acids perform myriad physiologic functions. Within the hepatocyte, they participate in the regulation of multiple genes by means of the farnesoid X receptor, a nuclear receptor also known as the bile acid receptor.[8] In bile, they form the major osmotic force driving the secretion of water, increasing bile volume and flow rate (so-called bile-acid-dependent flow), and thus an adequate pool of bile acids is required for normal bile excretion.[9] Fecal loss of bile acids provides a major route for the elimination of cholesterol in humans, and bile acids solubilize unmodified cholesterol in bile as well. Bile acids function within the intestine to promote diffusion and absorption of fatty acids and lipid-soluble vitamins (A, D, E, K). They have direct antimicrobial activity and appear to regulate other antimicrobial activity within the small intestine mediated by FXR receptors. In the colon, bile acids stimulate propulsive motility as well as modulate water and electrolyte transport. There is also intriguing evidence that bile acids act as endocrine factors via G protein-coupled receptors to modulate adipocyte thermogenesis and hepatic blood flow.[7]

Physiologic Cholestasis of the Neonate

The normal physiology of the neonatal liver differs from that of older children and adults in clinically important ways, particularly with regard to the processing and excretion of bile. Evidence collected from human and animal studies has led to the concept of a "physiologic cholestasis" of infancy.[10] Compared to older infants and adults, the neonate possesses a decreased total-body pool of bile acid, and this pool is relatively concentrated in the hepatic and circulating compartments rather than within the bowel lumen. After birth, the rates of bile acid synthesis and uptake

by hepatocytes increase rapidly, as does the intraluminal concentration of bile acids within the bowel. The concentrations of bile acids in serum decline more slowly to normal adult levels over the first 6–12 months of life.[11–13] These findings are thought to reflect immaturity in the uptake and synthesis of bile acids by hepatocytes and in the transport of bile acids across the ileal epithelium.

Consequences of Cholestasis

The result of cholestasis is retention of bile acids and bile products within the hepatocytes and liver. As the level of these products builds, damage to the hepatocytes results.

Hepatic Injury and Biliary Cirrhosis

As the intrahepatic level of bile salt and bile contents increases, there is activation of Kupffer cells and other cells to produce fibrosis.[14,15] Over time with chronic cholestasis, the typical periportal fibrosis accompanied by bile stasis and loss of bile ducts is characteristic of biliary cirrhosis. The fibrosis gradually increases within and between portal tracts.

Malabsorption and Malnutrition

Bile acids act as a detergent within the bowel lumen, solubilizing lipids and allowing their absorption by enterocytes. Because of the decreased concentration of bile acids in the bowel, some degree of steatorrhea is normal in neonates and is more pronounced in infants fed cow's milk–based formula because it lacks the lipase activity found in human milk.[16] Pathologic cholestasis exacerbates this fat malabsorption and predisposes the infant to fat-calorie malnutrition as well as deficiency in the fat-soluble vitamins (A, D, E, and K).[17] One patient series found a high prevalence of fat-soluble vitamin deficiency among children waiting for a liver transplant, with a majority of patients having a deficiency in at least 1 of the vitamins A, D, E, and K.[18]

In addition to malabsorption and secondary deficiencies in specific micronutrients, children with chronic liver disease are likely to have higher resting energy expenditure than their healthy age cohort.[19,20] Thus, supplemental enteral feeding is sometimes required in chronic liver disease to maintain normal growth.

Pruritus

Pruritus in chronic cholestasis presumably results from the activity of an unknown "pruritogen," which is normally excreted in bile and that at elevated levels can stimulate either peripheral or central itch pathways.[21] Although there do not appear to be any published data regarding pruritus in neonates, it is a widespread and sometimes-debilitating problem among older patients with cholestatic liver disease.[22]

DIFFERENTIAL DIAGNOSIS

Because of the unique susceptibility of the neonatal liver, cholestasis is often a nonspecific response to systemic stress, resulting in a self-limited "idiopathic neonatal hepatitis." However, it may also be the presenting sign of serious infectious or metabolic disease or of biliary tract anomalies that require surgical attention. To make matters more complicated, the neonatologist and gastroenterologist are often faced with an infant whose history includes prematurity, septic or ischemic insults, and recent or ongoing reliance on parenteral nutrition, all of which may contribute to cholestasis. In such cases, the decision regarding how extensively, and when, to search for other possible causes of cholestasis is a difficult one. Although it is almost impossible to enumerate all disorders that can result in neonatal cholestasis, a neonatologist is likely to find it helpful to know those entities that are common, require urgent diagnosis and treatment, or respond to specific therapy (Table 39-1).

As Figure 39-2 illustrates, the diagnostic categories of neonatal cholestasis have been refined over the past 4 decades. Research into the biochemistry and genetics of bile formation, often enabled by individual patients or families with inherited cholestatic disorders, has broken the previous majority diagnosis of "idiopathic neonatal hepatitis" into multiple specific genetic and metabolic entities.[23]

Obstructive Disorders

Extrahepatic

Biliary obstructive disorders, either intrahepatic or extrahepatic, make up the largest proportion (50%) of cases of conjugated hyperbilirubinemia in infants for which a single cause can be identified.[24] Biliary atresia is the most common diagnosis in this group, which includes other "anatomic" problems of the bile ducts, such as choledochal cysts, choledochoceles, inspissated bile syndrome, strictures, and cholelithiasis. Both intrahepatic and extrahepatic biliary obstruction may occur as a result of compression of bile ducts by an extrinsic mass, for example, in hepatoblastoma.

Intrahepatic

There are a number of possible intrahepatic causes. Alagille syndrome due to jagged 1 protein or NOTCH receptor mutations may have significant cholestasis with high cholesterol and γ-glutamyl transferase

(GGT) and with paucity of intralobular ducts on liver biopsy.[25] There are also some infants with a so-called nonsyndromic paucity of bile ducts. There are a number of cholestatic genetic syndromes that result in abnormal bile flow due to canalicular bile transport mechanisms. One group is the progressive familial intrahepatic cholestasis (PFIC) disorders (Figure 39-1). They are autosomal recessive disorders affecting various transporters. PFIC1 or Byler disease is due to an adenosine triphosphate (ATP)–dependent amino phospholipid transporter or FIC1 (familial intrahepatic cholestasis 1). PFIC2 involves bile salt excretory protein (BSEP), which is an ATP-dependent bile acid transport protein.[26] MDR3 defects involving an ATP-dependent phospholipid transport protein are found in PFIC3 patients, who are distinguished by having an elevated GGT and elevated triglycerides.[27] Benign recurrent intrahepatic cholestasis (BRIC) is a category of cholestasis also caused by defective BSEP or FIC1 protein function but due to different mutations than in PFIC1/2 and having a milder clinical course.[28] Other disorders of intrahepatic cholestasis include Dubin-Johnson syndrome and Rotor syndrome.[29] Caroli disease and congenital hepatic fibrosis with portal hypertension occur in patients with autosomal recessive polycystic kidney disease (ARPKD)[30] as a result of malformation of the ductal plate and embryologic stage in the formation of the liver.[31,32] Mutations in CFTR affect chloride and bicarbonate transport and may lead to inspissated bile and the cholangiopathy associated with cystic fibrosis.[33,34] Neonatal sclerosing cholangitis is another rare cause of intrahepatic obstruction.[35]

Hepatocellular Disorders

The other major category of cholestasis is related to hepatocellular injury and dysfunction. Although it is reasonable to categorize some disease as either hepatocellular or obstructive (eg, the PFICs), we have chosen to label them obstructive because they are due to a specific defect in bile transport rather than generalized hepatocellular dysfunction.

Infections

Viral hepatitis represents only 5% of neonatal cholestasis but is important to consider, as are other infectious hepatitides, since specific pharmacologic therapy may be necessary. A large list of viruses may cause neonatal cholestasis or hepatitis: cytomegalovirus (CMV), herpes simplex virus (HSV), human herpesvirus 6 (HHV-6), parvovirus B19, coxsackie virus, echovirus, and the classic hepatitis viruses A, B, C, and E.[24,36,37] Nearly any bacterial, protozoal, or fungal infection severe enough to provoke a systemic inflammatory

Table 39-1 A Somewhat Comprehensive List of Diagnoses That May Lead to Cholestasis in the Neonate

Obstructive disorders of bile flow
  Extrahepatic
    Biliary atresia
    Choledochal cyst
    Cholelithiasis
    Stenosis
Intrahepatic or extrahepatic duct obstruction
from compression
  Benign or malignant masses
Paucity of intrahepatic ducts
  Alagille syndrome
  Nonsyndromic paucity
Cannilicular transport defects
  Progressive familial intrahepatic cholestasis
    (PFIC 1–3)
  Benign recurrent intrahepatic cholestasis
    (BRIC)
  Dubin-Johnson and Rotor syndromes
Ductal malformations or ectasies
  Congenital hepatic fibrosis (autosomal polystic
    kidney disease)
  Caroli disease
Inspissation of bile
  Cystic fibrosis
Sclerosis of bile ducts
  Neonatal sclerosing cholangitis
Hepatocellular disorders
  Infections
    Viral
      Cytomegalovirus
      Herpes simplex Uipus
      Human herpesvirus
      Parvovirus B-19
      Coxsackievirus
      Echovirus
      Adenovirus
      Rubella
      Human immunodeficiency virus
      Paramyxovirus
      Hepatitis A, B, C, E
    Bacterial
      Sepsis
      Urinary tract infection (endotoxemia)
      Tuberculosis
      Syphilis
      Listeria
    Toxoplasmosis
    Fungal sepsis

Metabolic disorders
  Bile acid synthesis defect
    3-β-Hyrogenase deficiency
    5-β-Reductase deficiency
Peroxisomal defects (eg, Zellweger sydrome,
adrenoleukodystropy, D-bifunctional protein deficiency)
  α1 alpantitrypsin (AAT) deficiency
  Carbohydrate metabolism
    Galactosemia
    Hereditary fructose intolerance
    Glycogen storage disease type IV
Amino acid metabolism
  Tyrosinemia type I
  Citrin deficiency
  Arginosuccinate lyase deficiency
Lipids: Niemann-Pick type C, mucopolysaccharidosis,
Gaucher disease
  Niemann-Pick type **C**
  Mucopolysaccharidosis
  Gaucher disease
  Glycosylation disorders
  Mitochondrial disorders
Endocrine disorders
  Hypothyroidism
  Panhypopituitarism
Toxic
  Iatrogenic
  Maternal drugs and alcohol
  Intestinal failure associated with liver disease (sepsis,
  parenteral nutrition)
Immunologic
  Neonatal hemochromatosis (neonatal iron storage
  disease)
  Neonatal lupus erythematosus
  Hemophagocytic lymphohistiocytosis (HLH)
Chromosomal or dysmorphic syndromes
  Trisomy 18
  Trisomy 21
  Arthrogryposis-renal tubular dysfunction-cholestasis
  (ARC) syndrome
  Kabuki syndrome
Hypoxic or ishemic injury
  Cardio respiratory compromise events, shock
  Congenital cardiac lesions
  Budd-Chiari syndrome
Miscellaneous
  Aagenaes syndrome (lymphedema-cholestasis)
  North American Indian childhood cirrhosis

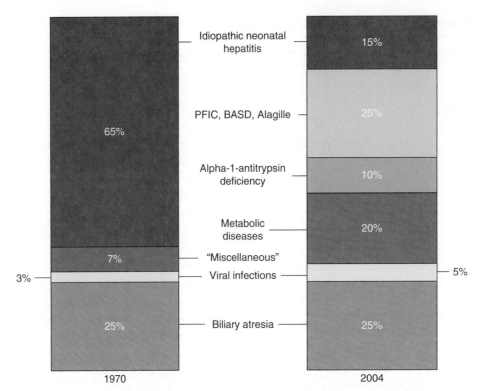

FIGURE 39-2 Major diagnoses resulting in neonatal cholestasis as of 1970 and 2004. Observe that the proportions of biliary atresia and viral hepatitis have remained constant. The previously large group of infants who were labeled with having "idiopathic neonatal cholestasis" has been broken down into multiple genetic disorders. The majority of these infants with chronic cholestasis can now be successfully diagnosed given sufficient time and resources. AAT, α_1-antitrypsin. (Adapted with permission from Balistreri WF, Bezerra JA. Whatever happened to "neonatal hepatitis"? *Clin Liver Dis.* 2006;10(1):27–53.)

response can cause cholestasis, but several in particular should be considered: occult urinary tract infection, gram-negative sepsis, tuberculosis, syphilis, and listeria; fungemia due to central line contamination; and toxoplasmosis.

Metabolic Disorders

Metabolic diseases as a group cause some 20% of neonatal cholestasis, but a large number of specific diagnoses fall into this category, each of which is rare. Thus, if a preliminary biochemical screening produces signs of an inborn error of metabolism, it is essential to involve a medical geneticist early in the workup. Some of the more common disorders are discussed here.

α_1-Antitrypsin (AAT) deficiency of the ZZ and SZ phenotypes predisposes to progressive liver injury and cholestasis, which can begin in infancy. AAT deficiency by itself is among the more common causes of neonatal cholestasis (20%).[38] Other common inborn errors of metabolism that can cause cholestasis include galactosemia, hereditary fructose intolerance, and tyrosinemia.[39] Galactosemia can present in the first days of life with lethargy, hepatic dysfunction, and lactic acidosis. Galactosuria can be identified by a positive test for urinary reducing substances. Hereditary fructose

intolerance produces hypoglycemia, gastrointestinal symptoms, and liver and renal tubular dysfunction but should not present until the introduction of fructose-containing foods, typically after weaning. Untreated tyrosinemia results in severe liver injury that can cause acute liver failure or rapidly progressive cirrhosis with cholestasis and portal hypertension within the first year. Older children may have recurrent bouts of severe pain, cirrhosis, and hepatocellular carcinoma. Because outcomes are significantly improved with medical treatment in all of these disorders, it is important to make the diagnosis promptly.

The remaining metabolic disorders that can lead to cholestasis are extremely numerous but can be divided into several broad categories: mitochondrial respiratory chain disorders; fatty acid oxidation disorders; peroxisomal disorders; disorders of amino acid metabolism, including urea cycle defects; bile acid synthetic defects; congenital disorders of glycosylation; and glycogen storage diseases (see Table 39-1).

Endocrine Disorders

Panhypopituitarism, isolated cortisol deficiency, and perhaps hypothyroidism can all cause neonatal cholestasis.[40,41] Since rapid medical treatment is beneficial, an endocrine screening is recommended early in the evaluation.

Toxic Causes

Toxic hepatic injury can be the result of maternal use of medications or illicit drugs, as well as an iatrogenic illness caused by medications given to the infant after birth. Perhaps the most important of the toxic etiologies is intestinal failure-associated liver disease (IFALD; total parenteral nutrition [TPN] cholestasis).[42] Infants with intestinal failure develop cholestasis and cirrhosis, probably due the combined effects of toxic elements in TPN (eg, lipid emulsion) and recurrent bacterial infection or translocation. IFALD is a major cause of end-stage liver disease requiring transplant, but new therapeutic approaches discussed in the management section can help to normalize liver function and may reduce the need for transplantation in the future. Cholestatic liver injury due to medications is often idiosyncratic and difficult to predict, but there has been a suggestion that fluconazole may predispose neonates to cholestasis.[43,44] Other agents more commonly associated with cholestatic liver injury in older patients should also be considered, such as amoxicillin-clavulanate, macrolides, and nonsteroidal anti-inflammatory drugs (NSAIDs).[45]

Prenatal exposure to certain agents, such as carbemazepine[46–48] and methamphetamine,[49] has also been associated with neonatal cholestasis.

Immunologic Causes

Immune-mediated injury to the hepatocytes is responsible for some causes of neonatal cholestasis. Examples include neonatal lupus erythematosus[50–52] and neonatal hemochromatosis (neonatal iron storage disorder),[53] caused by maternal antibodies, and hemophagocytic lymphohistiocytosis (HLH).[54]

Genetic Disorders

There are a number of genetic disorders that may present with cholestasis. Trisomy 18 and 21 are examples with dysmorphic features. Other examples are the ARC syndrome (arthrogryposis-renal dysfunction-cholestasis syndrome) and the Kabuki syndrome (associated with cleft palate).

Hypoxia or Hypoperfusion Injury

Infants who suffer hypoxic or hypoperfusion injury due to congenital or acquired cardiopulmonary disease,[55,56] shock, or hepatovenous obstruction (Budd-Chiari syndrome) will often present with jaundice. Frequently, these infants will have other evidence of end-organ injury, such as renal disease.

Other Causes

There are a few other disorders found in specific ethnic groups, such as Aagenaes syndrome (lymphedema with cholestasis syndrome)[57,58] and North American Indian childhood cirrhosis.[59]

Figure 39-3 presents some of the more important diagnoses leading to neonatal cholestasis according to anatomic location to illustrate the scheme used for organizing these disorders.

DIAGNOSTIC TESTS

Initial Evaluation of the Cholestatic Infant

In the general pediatric setting, cholestasis is usually first identified by the presence of visible jaundice. Although most otherwise-healthy term infants with jaundice have self-limited unconjugated hyperbilirubinemia of benign origin, it is important to identify those few with conjugated hyperbilirubinemia. A consensus guideline from the North American Society for Pediatric Gastroenterology, Hepatology, and Nutrition (NASPGHAN) recommends obtaining fractionated bilirubin levels in infants who remain visibly jaundiced past 2 weeks of age.[1] This is partly in response to the typical schedule of well-baby visits in the United States, according to which an infant who is healthy at 2 weeks of age may not normally be seen again by the pediatrician until 2 months of age. Two months is an unacceptably long delay for an infant who is subsequently found to have cholestatic jaundice, particularly given that the prevailing wisdom is that outcomes for surgical management of biliary atresia become significantly worse between 2 and 3 months of age.[60,61] Newly published evidence suggests that early elevation of direct bilirubin (within 48 hours of birth) may identify infants with biliary atresia.[62] However, it remains to be seen whether biliary atresia can reliably be excluded on the basis of a normal fractionated bilirubin level at such a young age. In the NICU, cholestasis is frequently identified by laboratory screening in the absence of visible jaundice. Occasionally, evidence of cholestasis is specifically sought because there is suspicion of a disease that may entail cholestasis, for example, if there are morphologic signs of Alagille syndrome or a positive screening test for cystic fibrosis.

After confirming the presence of cholestasis by conjugated and unconjugated (or direct and indirect) bilirubin levels, the clinician is faced with 2 immediate questions. The first relates to the degree of illness. Since cholestasis may be a sign of severe infection, shock, or metabolic disease, it is important to determine if the cholestatic infant is in need of immediate specific treatment. Usually, this triage can be made on the basis of

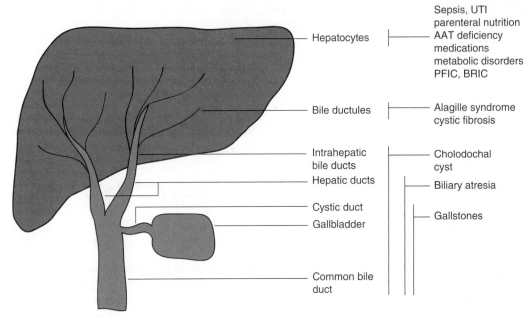

Sepsis, UTI
parenteral nutrition
AAT deficiency
medications
metabolic disorders
PFIC, BRIC

Alagille syndrome
cystic fibrosis

Cholodochal
cyst

Biliary atresia

Gallstones

Hepatocytes

Bile ductules

Intrahepatic
bile ducts
Hepatic ducts

Cystic duct
Gallbladder

Common bile
duct

FIGURE 39-3 Common disorders, arranged according to anatomic site, leading to neonatal cholestasis. AAT, α_1-antitrypsin; BRIC, benign recurrent intrahepatic cholestasis; PFIC, progressive familial intrahepatic cholestasis; UTI, urinary tract infection.

information already in hand, such as the clinical history, vital signs, and overall clinical assessment. Second, an initial assessment of liver function is important at this stage as well since an infant with impaired function is in need of more urgent diagnostic evaluation and possible listing for liver transplantation. Thus, it is important to obtain or review measures of blood glucose, ammonia, albumin, and coagulation times.

In an infant who is generally well, with preserved hepatic function, the clinician can then evaluate in a stepwise fashion. Table 39-2 presents a reference list of tests that the physician will need to consider ordering, arranged somewhat arbitrarily into stages according to when they might typically be appropriate. Of course, the severity of illness, the age of the infant, and the presence of diagnostic clues in the history and physical will influence the choice of tests in particular patients.

The initial step in the diagnostic workup usually will include a complete biochemical evaluation for liver injury (AST [aspartate aminotransferase], ALT [alanine aminotransferase], alkaline phosphatase, GGT), as well as selected specific diagnostic tests, such as ultrasound of the liver and gallbladder, and urinalysis and culture. Depending on the degree of suspicion, other serious bacterial infections will need to be ruled out in the initial phase.

History

The pertinent history will include questions of prematurity; sepsis; shock or asphyxia; cardiac disease or cyanosis; timing and content of feedings (lactose, fructose); parenteral nutrition; and surgeries. The stool color and pattern are important, as is the appearance of the urine. In severe cholestasis, the stools are typically beige, clay, or light colored (acholic stools) and the urine dark in color. Reports of the infant with bruising or poor coagulation ability and use of vitamin K as well as other fat-soluble vitamin supplementation should be obtained. The maternal and pregnancy history should include infections, chronic conditions such as lupus, medications, and episodes of jaundice during the pregnancy. A mother's history of cholelithiasis, thrombophilia,[63] and prior pregnancies is important. It can be helpful to search the infant's medication history for drugs that have been associated with cholestasis. (Several were mentioned previously.) The family history may offer additional information that would be helpful, such as consanguinity and ethnic background. (PFIC1, for example, is more common among the Amish.) The presence of early-onset emphysema or chronic lung disease in the immediate family may suggest AAT deficiency.

Physical

The general appearance of the infant may provide immediate clues to a genetic or dysmorphic syndrome such as the trisomies, Alagille syndrome, or Zellweger syndrome. Gestational age, head circumference, and growth pattern may signal the presence of a genetic disorder or infectious process in the immediate neonatal period.

Table 39-2 Tests Often Used in the Evaluation of Neonatal Cholestasis

Test or Procedure	Diagnosis or Information Sought
Immediate	
Physical examination Review clinical history	Evidence of infection, ischemia or shock, cardiac disease, neurologic or metabolic decompensation or other urgent condition; history of parenteral nutrition
Initial testing	
total and direct bilirubin	Confirm cholestatic jaundice
AST. ALT Alk Phos, GGT albumin and total protein	Ongoing liver or biliary injury Liver synthetic function
INR (PT, PTT), fibrinogen	Synthetic function, need for intensive support
glucose	Metabolic function, need for intensive support
ammonia, lactic acid, pyruvate	Liver metabolic function, mitochondrial hepatopathies
CBC with differential. ESR. CRP	Infection, hematologic disease
review newborn screen	Cystic fibrosis (IRT), galactosemia, fatty acid oxidation disorders
ultrasound with Doppler	Gailstones, choledochal cyst, presence of gallbladder (argues against biliary atreia), portal hypertension/splenomegaly, hepatic echotexture (cirrhosis, masses)
Urinalysis and culture	Occult urinary tract infection
Follow-up testing	
α_1-Antitrypsin phenotype (Pi type)	α_1-antitrypsin deficiency
fat-soluble vitamin levels	Fat malabsorption, chronicity of cholestasis, need for supplemental vitamins
1-25-Hydroxy vitamin D Retinol INR and/or factors V, VII, and VIII plasma α-tocopherol/total lipid ratio paracenteis if ascites exists	Vitamin D status Vitamin A status Vitamin K status Vitamin E status Infections, biliary leakage, portal hypertension
blood culture, CSF culture and examination	Serious bacterial infections
infectious studies: CMV, HHV-6, HSV, adenovirus, enteroviruses. HIV, toxoplasma titers	Intrauterine infections
TSH. T_A free and stimulated Cortisol urine reducing substances and/or erythrocyte galactose 1-phosphate uridyl transferase plasma amino acids; urine organic acids with succinyl acetone; α-fetoprotein serum iron and ferritin	Hypothyroidism, hypopituitarism Galactosemia Tyrosinemia Neonatal hemochromatosis
Further testing as indicated	
Cardiology consult and/or echocardiogram spinal x-rays skull x-ray for calcifications	Estaolish normal cardiac anatomy and function Alagille syndrome Butterfly vertebrae (Alagille syndrome) TORCH infection
liver biopsy with electron microscopy hepatobiliary scintigraphy (HIDA scan)	Proliferation vs paucity of bile ducts, hepatitis Demonstrate excretion of bile (rule out biliary atresia)
MRCP/ERCP	Precise biliary anatomy: strictures, choledochal cysts, stones
operative cholangiogram	Biliary atresia, choledochal cyst
ophthalmologic examination genetics consult and/or specific genetic testing	Posterior embryotoxon (Alagille syndrome): infectious retinitis

CHAPTER 39

(Continued)

Table 39-2 Tests Often Used in the Evaluation of Neonatal Cholestasis (*Continued*)

Test or Procedure	Diagnosis or Information Sought
CFTR mutation analysis and/or sweat chloride	Cystic fibrosis
comparative genomic hybridization (or karyotype and FISH analysis) serum and urine bile acids (while not on ursodeoxycholic)	Broad range of chromosomal anomalies Disorders of bile acid synthesis
acylcamitine profile plasma amino acids very long chain fatty acids glycosylated transferring Jaundice chip	Defects in fatty acid oxidation urea cycle defects (eg, citrullinemia) peroxisomal disorders (eg, adrenoleukodystrophy) Congenital disorders of glycosylation Alagille syndrome; PFIC 1, 2, and 3:A1AT deficiency

Abbreviations: Alk Phos, alkaline phosphatase; ALT, alanine aminotransferase; AST, aspartate aminotransferase; CBD, complete blood count; CMV, cytomegalovirus; CRP, C-reactiveprotein; CSF, cerebrospinal fluid; ERCP, endoscopic retrograde cholangiopancreatography; ESR, erythrocyte sedimentation rate; FISH, fluorescence in situ hybridization; GGT, γ-glutamyl transferase; HHV, human herpesvirus; HIDA, hepatobiliary iminodiacetic acid; HSV, herpes simplex virus; INR, international normalized ratio; MRCP, magnetic resonance cholangiopancreatography; PFIC, progressive familial intrahepatic cholestasis; PT, prothrombin time; PTT, partial thromboplastin time; T_4, thyroxine; TORCH, toxoplasmosis, rubella, cytomegalovirus, herpes simplex virus; TSH, thyroid-stimulating hormone.
The separation into distinct steps is of course arbitrary, but tests near the top of the table will almost always be performed as a matter of routine, while tests near the bottom will be ordered more selectively and often after discussing the case with consultants.

The ophthalmologic examination may also be helpful. Findings of chorioretinitis and cataracts can suggest congenital infection, optic nerve appearance consistent with septo-optic dysplasia may lead to the diagnosis of hypopituitarism, and posterior embryotoxon is a feature (though not a pathognomonic one) of Alagille syndrome.

The presence of a murmur or other cardiac abnormalities may provide clues that the cholestasis is due to cardiac disease or part of a syndrome such as trisomy 21 or Alagille syndrome (which may include peripheral pulmonic stenosis). Dextrocardia and situs inversus is associated with biliary atresia along with splenic malformation (absent spleen or polysplenia).

A careful abdominal examination to determine any masses or hepatosplenomegaly and the presence of ascites or caput medusa will assist in assessing possible causes (tumors, cysts) and degree of cirrhosis or portal hypertension. Disorders of the mitochondrial respiratory chain and some other genetic diseases, such as Niemann-Pick disease, may be suspected based on a careful neurological examination.

Ataxia and hypotonia with decreased deep tendon reflexes may also be features of vitamin E deficiency as a result of fat malabsorption and inadequate vitamin E supplementation. Bone fractures and radiologic abnormalities of bone are features of significant rickets due to vitamin D deficiency. The presence of rashes may signal a concern for congenital infections, and bruising may be a sign of coagulopathy due to vitamin K deficiency, disseminated intravascular coagulation (DIC), or hematologic abnormalities.

Icthyosis of the skin and abnormal joint mobility may suggest ARC syndrome. Lymphedema may be a feature of Aagenaes syndrome in an infant with Norwegian ethnicity. The infant with typical biliary atresia will often have normal weight gain and may present as an apparently healthy baby except for jaundice, acholic stools, and hepatomegaly. In fact, the parents have often either not noticed the child's jaundice or have assumed it to be physiologic and are therefore surprised at the diagnosis.

Laboratory Studies

Table 39-2 provides a list of possible diagnostic tests for cholestasis. The initial laboratory tests are used to confirm conjugated hyperbilirubinemia with both direct and total bilirubin. The AST and ALT are enzymes that appear in the blood if there is hepatocellular injury from metabolic dysfunction, inflammation, or apoptosis. They are not tests of liver synthetic function and may even be normal in some forms of end-stage liver disease when there are few remaining hepatocytes. Among NICU patients, this can, for example, be observed in neonatal hemochromatosis. These infants may have severely impaired liver synthetic function and yet only mildly elevated AST and ALT. Alkaline phosphatase and GGT are enzymes that not only reflect cholangiocyte and bile duct injury but also can be normal when the source of cholestasis is at a canalicular transport level, as in PFIC1 and PFIC2 (so-called low-GGT cholestasis).

There are a number of general laboratory tests that reflect liver synthetic function, such as those for glucose, ammonia, and cholesterol, since the liver participates in their metabolism and storage. Elevated ammonia may be due to urea cycle defects or portosystemic shunting, as well as to hepatocellular dysfunction.

Proteins synthesized by the liver include albumin and most of the coagulation factors (except for factor VIII), which have a short half-life in serum. Low levels of coagulation factors and coagulopathy may also be due to deficiency in vitamin K, especially in cholestatic patients, or to consumption by DIC. Therefore, some care is required in interpreting coagulation times. Due to its widespread availability, speed of measurement, and convention, the initial test is usually the international normalized ratio (INR). INR testing can be repeated several hours after an intravenous dose of vitamin K to assess the contribution of vitamin K deficiency to the coagulopathy. Since factor V is not dependent on vitamin K for synthesis, the next step may be to obtain quantitative coagulation factors levels (eg, of factors V, VII, and VIII). One must not forget to measure the other fat-soluble vitamins E, A, and D, which are not well absorbed in cholestatic conditions.

Infectious causes of cholestasis are most important to detect and treat as early as possible in infants. A complete blood cell count (CBC) with differential, erythrocyte sedimentation rate (ESR), and C-reactive protein (CRP) assessment followed by appropriate TORCH (toxoplasmosis, rubella, cytomegalovirus, HSV) titers and viral serology or polymerase chain reaction (PCR) as recommended in Table 39-2 should be obtained. Depending on the clinical status of the patient, blood and urine cultures are also necessary as endotoxemia and gram-negative sepsis, or even occult urinary tract infection,[64] are significant causes of conjugated hyperbilirubinemia.

Endocrine causes should be evaluated, as panhypopituitarism is a well-documented cause of cholestasis.[40,65,66] Screening with thyroid-stimulating hormone (TSH), free levorotatory thyroxine (T_4), and cortisol is usual.

Genetic and metabolic assessment begins with an AAT phenotype (Pi type in some laboratories) and level. Phenotype testing is performed by electrophoresis and is important since the blood level of AAT may vary in the perinatal period[67] or in response to inflammation.[68] Plasma amino acids and urine succinylacetone with urine organic acids and α-fetoprotein offer a means to screen for tyrosinemia. Urine reducing substances (while the infant is on lactose-containing formula) and erythrocyte galactose-1-phosphate uridyl transferase (GALT) will screen for galactosemia. The newborn screen or other testing (CFTR mutation analysis or sweat chloride) should be checked as well for cystic fibrosis. Serum or plasma lactate, pyruvate, and acylcarnitine panel screen for mitochondrial disorders. Quantitative serum bile salts may detect the possibility of a bile salt synthetic defect, in which case a urine bile salt analysis (while off ursodeoxycholate therapy) is warranted. Peroxisomal disorders may be screened with very long chain fatty acids, and disorders of glycosylation may be detected by a glycosylated

transferrin level. Specific genetic testing for the more common inherited causes of neonatal cholestasis is available from several laboratories (see GeneReviews. org or http://www.ncbi.nlm.nih.gov/gtr/), and several genes (*JAG1*, Alagille syndrome; *ATP8B1*, PFIC1; *ABCB11*, PFIC2; *ABCB4*, PFIC3; and *SERPINA1*, AAT deficiency) may be tested using a single sample with the Jaundice Chip assay[69] from Cincinnati Children's Hospital.

Radiological Studies

Ultrasound

Ultrasound is the most useful imaging modality for evaluating cholestasis, and every infant with newly identified or worsening cholestasis deserves an evaluation by ultrasound. Liver echotexture and size, ascites, or the presence of splenomegaly can help suggest cirrhosis and portal hypertension. Ultrasound may also document stones in the gallbladder or common bile duct, dilated bile ducts, intrahepatic mass lesions, presence of the gallbladder, choledochal cysts, and abnormal vascular anatomy or situs anomalies. Doppler measurement of blood flow can also demonstrate vascular occlusion or hepatofugal portal flow, which may be indicative of portal hypertension. Lack of a pancreas with fibrosis or calcifications may suggest cystic fibrosis. Extrahepatic masses that may impinge or compress the biliary tract and result in cholestasis may be found. Abnormal visceral anatomy suggestive of congenital syndromes or cystic kidney lesions may also contribute clues to the diagnosis.

Several ultrasonographic findings are useful in supporting the diagnosis of biliary atresia. The "triangular cord sign" refers to the finding of an echogenic tubular or triangular structure near the bifurcation of the portal vein. Observational studies suggest that the triangular cord is specific but not sensitive enough to use for making surgical decisions.[70–74] The presence and size of the gallbladder are also relevant, as an abnormally small or absent gallbladder is consistent with biliary atresia.[74] The absence of the triangular cord sign and the presence of a normal gallbladder are reassuring, but neither sign is sensitive enough to use in place of liver biopsy or cholangiogram when a diagnosis of biliary atresia is considered.

Hepatobiliary Scintigraphy

The hepatobiliary iminodiacetic acid (HIDA) scan (generically hepatobiliary scintigraphy) is a quantitative nuclear medicine technique used to assess liver function and biliary excretion. A radiolabeled analog of iminodiacetic acid (eg, technetium TC 99m

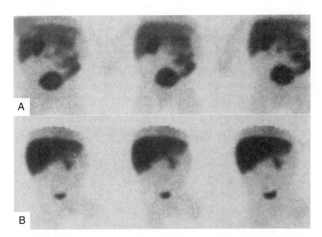

FIGURE 39-4 Hepatobiliary scintigraphy (hepatobiliary iminodiacetic acid, HIDA) images. A, Characteristic of an infant with a nonobstructive cause of cholestasis. Although it may take hours for the radiotracer to be excreted, ultimately the gallbladder and bowel are easily visualized. B, Typical image in biliary atresia. The liver has taken up the tracer, but the gallbladder and bowel are not visualized even after 24 hours. The density (right) on the image is the left kidney, and the lower density is the bladder. (Reproduced with permission from Nadel HR. Hepatobiliary scintigraphy in children. *Semin Nucl Med.* 1996;26(1):25–42.)

mebrofenin) is injected intravenously, and a series of 2-dimensional images is obtained by γ-camera over minutes to hours following the injection. The tracer is actively taken up by hepatocytes and secreted into bile. A HIDA scan can quantify the uptake of tracer by the liver, giving an indirect assessment of hepatocellular function, and in a normally functioning biliary system, subsequent images can demonstrate the gallbladder and bowel filling with tracer (Figure 39-4). In cholestatic infants, who may have slow excretion regardless of the diagnosis, images may be obtained as late as 24 hours after injection, though in a healthy patient the gallbladder can usually be visualized within minutes.[76] Hepatobiliary scintigraphy is highly sensitive for complete extrahepatic obstruction, in that it is (almost[77]) unheard-of for an infant with biliary atresia to show excretion by HIDA scan. However, it is nonspecific.[78,79] In our experience, many infants with nonsurgical causes for cholestasis fail to show excretion, especially when the conjugated bilirubin is high. Most institutions use a protocol in which the infant receives phenobarbital or ursodeoxycholate for 3–5 days prior to the scan. These agents increase the rate of bile excretion from hepatocytes and therefore may allow excretion to be visualized in infants with intrahepatic causes of cholestasis (improving the specificity of the study).[80,81]

Computed Tomography or Magnetic Resonance Imaging

Imaging with computed tomographic (CT) or magnetic resonance imaging (MRI) scans may allow better detection of detail than ultrasound, with the disadvantages of radiation or sedation and increased cost. In particular, magnetic resonance cholangiopancreatography (MRCP) is capable of detecting cholelithiasis and define pancreaticobiliary anatomy, including choledochal cysts. A few series have reported on the accuracy of MRCP in distinguishing biliary atresia from other causes of cholestasis.[82,83] Although the method currently does not appear to offer an alternative to biopsy or cholangiogram, it is an area of research, and new contrast agents may increase its utility.[84]

Cholangiography (Transhepatic or Operative) or Endoscopic Retrograde Cholangiopancreatography

Other means of determining biliary anatomy include percutaneous transhepatic cholangiogram or endoscopic retrograde cholangiopancreatography (ERCP). ERCP in infants requires proper equipment and expertise, but in experienced hands appears to be safe. Several large series showed ERCP had excellent sensitivity for biliary atresia with specificity better than noninvasive techniques such as MRCP and HIDA.[85–87] Therefore, it offers a viable alternative to operative cholangiogram in selected patients at certain centers. Ultimately, operative cholangiogram may be required to accurately diagnose biliary atresia or abnormalities of the biliary tract and guide appropriate therapy, such as hepatoportojejeunostomy or Kasai procedure.

Plain Radiographs

Plain radiographic films can provide valuable indirect information to guide the diagnosis of the cholestatic infant. Often, films of the chest and abdomen have already been obtained in the normal course of care of an infant by the time cholestasis is identified, and these films should be reviewed. Chest radiographs may confirm lung or cardiac disease and may show dextrocardia, which is associated with biliary atresia. A finding of butterfly vertebrae suggests Alagille syndrome. Abdominal radiographs may show calcifications from cholelithiasis or nephrocalcinosis. Other specific radiographic studies may be useful in selected cases. For example, skull films may detect calcifications due to congenital infections or have patterns suggestive of underlying neurologic disorder or hypopituitarism. Long-bone changes may signal rickets and vitamin D deficiency. Other genetic syndromes, such as Hurler syndrome, may be suggested by radiographic findings.

Liver Biopsy

One of the most helpful tests in the diagnosis of cholestasis is the liver biopsy. Biopsy can be performed percutaneously at the bedside, transvascularly in the interventional radiology suite, or operatively. When there is proliferation of bile ducts or bile plugging in ductules, biliary obstruction as in biliary atresia is most likely. A paucity of intralobular bile ducts suggests Alagille syndrome. Giant cell transformation or hepatitis refer to a nonspecific reaction in the neonatal liver and can be associated with multiple disorders. Deficiency of AAT may be suspected if there are multiple periodic acid–Schiff (PAS)–positive granules in hepatocytes. The liver biopsy may also be used for cultures, electron microscopic diagnosis, and other metabolic or genetic testing as appropriate, based on clinical evaluation. The most significant risk of liver biopsy is bleeding. Significant hemorrhage requiring transfusion is possible, though with ultrasound guidance percutaneous biopsy is relatively safe.[88–90] Often, the risk and pain involved in biopsy are weighed against the risk of delaying a diagnosis. In an infant older than about 2 months, in whom a delay in the diagnosis of biliary atresia can mean a higher likelihood of poor outcome, the decision to biopsy may be made sooner, saving the time required for less-invasive imaging studies such as HIDA.

MANAGEMENT

The first priority in the management of infants with conjugated hyperbilirubinemia is to diagnose and treat those causes that are rapidly life threatening, such as gram-negative sepsis, adrenal insufficiency, metabolic disease, or shock. The specific management of biliary atresia, acute liver failure, and various infectious causes of cholestasis are discussed in chapters 40 and 41. With that in mind, we focus here on problems common to chronic cholestatic liver disease in general and their management in infants. Good supportive care of these cholestatic infants is important and can often prevent the nutritional and other complications of liver disease. Several of the common agents used in the management of neonates with cholestatic liver disease are summarized in Table 39-3.

Nutrition

Patients with cholestasis have impaired fat absorption as a consequence of inadequate bile salts in the intestinal lumen. Medium-chain triglycerides (MCTs) do not require bile salts for absorption. Changing the primary feedings to a formula high in MCTs or supplementing the feedings with MCTs to provide 30%–50% of the total fat calories in the form of MCTs can be helpful.

With malabsorption of fat comes malabsorption of the fat-soluble vitamins A, D, E, and K. All cholestatic infants should receive prophylactic doses of the fat-soluble vitamins and periodic screening for deficiency. The treatment table (Table 39-3) summarizes typical dosing. Keep in mind that infants with cholestasis sometimes require much higher doses of the fat-soluble vitamins than are usually recommended; however, these vitamins can be toxic, and levels must be monitored during supplementation.

Besides specific fat and vitamin deficiencies, infants with liver disease can have elevated energy requirements[19,20] and may need up to 130% or more of the usual daily caloric requirement to meet growth needs. To achieve this goal, supplemental nutrition may need to be given by nasogastric, orogastric, or gastrostomy feeds. In some cases, parenteral nutrition should be considered.

Ascites

Ascites, the accumulation of intraperitoneal fluid, is a result of end-stage cirrhosis and portal hypertension exacerbated by hypoproteinemia. It may complicate respiration and limit feeding volumes. It also creates a risk of spontaneous bacterial peritonitis and can make children uncomfortable. Medical management includes fluid and salt restriction, albumin supplementation, and careful use of diuretics.[91] Oral spironolactone is often added to oral or intravenous furosemide to limit the potassium losses caused by furosemide.

Bleeding

In chronic liver disease with portal hypertension, varices form throughout the gastrointestinal tract, but the most dangerous are usually in the lower esophagus. The splenomegaly resulting from portal hypertension leads to thrombocytopenia, and hepatic dysfunction and vitamin K deficiency cause coagulopathy, both of which may worsen the bleeding from varices or portal hypertensive gastropathy.

Medical management with venous access, volume resuscitation, acid suppression, and octreotide is primary. The infant must be stabilized if at all possible prior to any attempt at endoscopic treatment. Banding, which is common in older patients, is difficult in infants due to the size of the equipment, so endoscopic therapy will often be sclerotherapy (endoscopic injection of a sclerosing agent into the variceal vessels). Occasionally, interventional radiology with TIPSS or vascular embolization may be helpful. Balloon tamponade or surgical intervention to perform a portosystemic shunt may be necessary in refractory bleeding until liver transplantation can be performed in appropriate cases. The role of nonselective β-blocker therapy for the prophylaxis of bleeding is controversial in infants.

Table 39-3 Medical Treatments That Are Frequently Useful in the Treatment of Infants With Cholestatic Liver Disease

Agent	Purpose	Usual Dose
Phenobarbital	Enhances bile excretion prior to biliary scintigraphy; antipruritic.	5–6 mg/kg divided twice daily for at least 3 days prior to scan
Fat-soluble vitamins Solubilized ADEK Multivitamin (AquADEK™)	Single-agent prophylactic dosing for cholestatic infant	1 mL/day
Vitamin A[a]	Treatment of vitamin A deficiency	5000–25,000 IU/day
Vitamin D[a]	Treatment of vitamin D deficiency	400–4000 IU/day cholecalciferol
Vitamin K[a]	Acute correction of vitamin K-deficiency coagulopathy; treatment of chronic vitamin K deficiency	2.5 mg IV daily × 3 days 2.5 mg PO weekly to 5 mg PO daily
Vitamin E[a]	Treatment of vitamin E deficiency	25–50 IU/kg/d α-tocopherol
	Water-soluble form (TPGS) enhances absorption of other fat-soluble vitamins	15–25 IU/kg/day TPGD (Liqui-E™)
Medium-chain triglyceride (MCT)	Enhances fat absorption in cholestasis and pancreatic insufficiency	30%–70% of total lipid intake
Ursodiol (UDCA)	Alters bile acid & cholesterol balance Antipruritic	10–15 mg/kg/dose 2–3 times daily
Rifampicin	Antipruritic	10 mg/kg/d divided once or twice daily
Cholestyramine		240 mg/kg/d divided 3 times daily
Furosemide	Loop diuretic, control of ascites	1 mg/kg/dose given 1–2 times daily
Spironolactone	Potassium-sparing diuretic, control of ascites	1–3 mg/kg/day divided 1–2 times daily
Lactulose	Hepatic encephalopathy/hyperammonemia Enhances excretion of ammonia	2–10 mL/day divided 4 times daily
Diphenhydramine	Antihistamine, antipruritic	5 mg/kg/d divided 4 times daily
naltrexone	Opioid antagonist, antipruritic	1–2 mg/kg/d

[a] The dosing and indications are for general information and cannot replace medical expertise. Consult a pharmacist. The fat-soluble vitamins in particular can be toxic and should never be supplemented without a plan for monitoring their levels.

Pruritus

Pharmacologic treatment of pruritus can include ursodeoxycholate; antihistamines (diphenhydramine, hydroxyzine); cholestyramine; rifampin; and naloxone. In severe cases, a combination of medications is often used.[21,22,92] Surgical approaches have included biliary diversion[93,94] or ileal exclusion,[95] which have had particular success reducing or eliminating pruritus (and xanthomas) in some patients with Alagille syndrome or PFIC. However, in the most refractory cases, pruritus can be an indication for liver transplantation.

Specific Management

Specific management of neonatal cholestasis depends on the diagnosis but is broadly divided into surgical and nonsurgical diseases. Biliary atresia, choledochal cyst, and the other extrahepatic obstructive disorders require surgical intervention, and once the diagnosis is reasonably certain, the patient will undergo operative cholangiogram proceeding to Kasai hepatoportoenterostomy. Various infections that can lead to cholestasis benefit from specific medical treatment, which is covered elsewhere in this volume.

Genetic Disorders

The bile salt synthetic defects sometimes benefit from bile salt analogs such as ursodeoxycholate.[96–98] Galactosemia, fructose intolerance, glycogen storage diseases, and urea cycle disorders are treated with dietary management. Tyrosinemia is now treated with 2-(2-nitro-4-trifluoromethyl-benzoyl)-1,3-cyclohexandione (NTBC).[99]

Parenteral Nutrition

Intestinal failure-associated liver disease should be thought of as multifactorial, and treatment should begin with optimizing enteral feeding, attempting to prevent septic complications, treating bacterial overgrowth when suspected, adding oral ursodeoxycholate, and minimizing intravenous soy-based lipid emulsions. Other intravenous fat emulsions, which are higher in omega-3 fatty acids, lower in phytosterols, and higher in vitamin E such as fish oil-based[100,101] (Omegaven) or combination soy, MCTs, olive oil, fish oil (SMOF)[102–104] lipid emulsion have also proven effective in decreasing cholestatic liver disease and the need for combined liver and small intestinal transplantation.[105]

Neonatal Hemachromatosis

Management of neonatal hemochromatosis has changed over the decade since the mid-2000s as our understanding of the pathophysiology has changed. This disease is now regarded as an alloimmune disorder[53] and is treated with exchange transfusion and intravenous immunoglobulin (IVIG).[106] It may be prevented in at-risk pregnancies by maternal IVIG therapy during pregnancy.[107] Some cases may still require liver transplantation.

OUTCOME AND FOLLOW-UP

As previously discussed, there has been remarkable progress in the diagnosis and management of neonatal cholestasis with fewer idiopathic "neonatal hepatitis" cases. It is difficult to generalize since outcomes depend on the specific etiology. The few published series point to the fact that severe cholestasis is often a sign of significant illness. In 1 report of 27 NICU patients with cholestasis, one-third died or underwent liver transplantation. Infants in this poor-outcome group had significantly higher conjugated bilirubin levels than those with good outcomes (6.32 ± 1.93 vs 2.64 ± 0.33).[3] However, most neonatal cholestasis is not severe and is nonspecific and self-limited. In the recent large series mentioned in the epidemiology section, almost 70% of infants with a direct bilirubin in the range of 2–5 mg/dL had no specific diagnosis associated with cholestasis.[2]

It is safe to say that in infants with ongoing extrahepatic illness, such as cardiac disease, prolonged dependence on parenteral nutrition, or severe metabolic defects, cholestasis is likely to be a poor prognostic sign. That said, remarkable improvements in the care of IFALD make short-bowel syndrome an increasingly survivable long-term diagnosis. And, in infants who have recovered from their primary disease and are otherwise doing well, residual cholestasis is likely to resolve over time.

POINTS

- The newborn liver is uniquely susceptible to cholestasis in the setting of inflammation or other systemic insults.
- Most neonatal cholestasis is of the mild, self-limiting, nonspecific variety.
- Sometimes, neonatal cholestasis can herald a life-threatening disease.
- The list of possible diagnoses is extremely long, and choosing a safe, cost-effective, efficient, and minimally invasive diagnostic algorithm is challenging.
- Attempts should be made to rule out biliary atresia or to proceed to surgery by 2 months of age.

REFERENCES

1. Moyer V, Freese DK, Whitington PF, et al. Guideline for the evaluation of cholestatic jaundice in infants: recommendations of the North American Society for Pediatric Gastroenterology, Hepatology and Nutrition. *J Pediatr Gastroenterol Nutr.* 2004;39(2):115–128.
2. Davis AR, Rosenthal P, Escobar GJ, Newman TB. Interpreting conjugated bilirubin levels in newborns. *J Pediatr.* 2011;158(4):562–565.e1.
3. Tufano M, Nicastro E, Giliberti P, et al. Cholestasis in neonatal intensive care unit: incidence, aetiology and management. *Acta Paediatr.* 2009;98(11):1756–1761.
4. Champion V, Carbajal R, Lozar J, Girard I, Mitanchez D. Risk factors for developing transient neonatal cholestasis. *J Pediatr Gastroenterol Nutr.* 2012. http://www.ncbi.nlm.nih.gov/pubmed/22684346 (accessed August 4, 2012).
5. Kirk JM. Neonatal jaundice: a critical review of the role and practice of bilirubin analysis. *Ann Clin Biochem.* 2008;45(Pt5):452–462.
6. Doumas BT, Wu TW. The measurement of bilirubin fractions in serum. *Crit Rev Clin Lab Sci.* 1991;28(5–6):415–445.
7. Hofmann AF. The enterohepatic circulation of bile acids in mammals: form and functions. *Front Biosci.* 2009;14:2584–2598.
8. Modica S, Gadaleta RM, Moschetta A. Deciphering the nuclear bile acid receptor FXR paradigm. *Nucl Recept Signal.* 2010;8:e005.
9. Hofmann AF, Hagey LR. Bile acids: chemistry, pathochemistry, biology, pathobiology, and therapeutics. *Cell Mol Life Sci.* 2008;65(16):2461–2483.
10. Suchy FJ, Balistreri WF, Heubi JE, Searcy JE, Levin RS. Physiologic cholestasis: elevation of the primary serum bile acid concentrations in normal infants. *Gastroenterology.* 1981;80(5 Pt 1):1037–1041.
11. Watkins JB. Neonatal cholestasis: developmental aspects and current concepts. *Semin Liver Dis.* 1993;13(3):276–288.
12. Watkins JB. Bile acid metabolism and fat absorption in newborn infants. *Pediatr Clin North Am.* 1974;21(2):501–512.
13. Balistreri WF, Heubi JE, Suchy FJ. Immaturity of the enterohepatic circulation in early life: factors predisposing to

"physiologic" maldigestion and cholestasis. *J Pediatr Gastroenterol Nutr.* 1983;2(2):346–354.

14. Scott-Conner CE, Grogan JB. The pathophysiology of biliary obstruction and its effect on phagocytic and immune function. *J Surg Res.* 1994;57(2):316–336.

15. Allen K, Jaeschke H, Copple BL. Bile acids induce inflammatory genes in hepatocytes: a novel mechanism of inflammation during obstructive cholestasis. *Am J Pathol.* 2011;178(1):175–186.

16. Murphy GM, Signer E. Bile acid metabolism in infants and children. *Gut.* 1974;15(2):151–163.

17. Ng VL, Balistreri WF. Treatment options for chronic cholestasis in infancy and childhood. *Curr Treat Options Gastroenterol.* 2005;8(5):419–430.

18. Chin SE, Shepherd RW, Thomas BJ, et al. The nature of malnutrition in children with end-stage liver disease awaiting orthotopic liver transplantation. *Am J Clin Nutr.* 1992;56(1):164–168.

19. Pierro A, Koletzko B, Carnielli V, et al. Resting energy expenditure is increased in infants and children with extrahepatic biliary atresia. *J Pediatr Surg.* 1989;24(6):534–538.

20. Greer R, Lehnert M, Lewindon P, Cleghorn GJ, Shepherd RW. Body composition and components of energy expenditure in children with end-stage liver disease. *J Pediatr Gastroenterol Nutr.* 2003;36(3):358–363.

21. Bunchorntavakul C, Reddy KR. Pruritus in chronic cholestatic liver disease. *Clin Liver Dis.* 2012;16(2):331–346.

22. Imam MH, Gossard AA, Sinakos E, Lindor KD. Pathogenesis and management of pruritus in cholestatic liver disease. *J Gastroenterol Hepatol.* 2012;27(7):1150–1158.

23. Balistreri W. Whatever happened to "neonatal hepatitis"? *Clin Liver Dis.* 2006;10(1):27–53.

24. Dick MC, Mowat AP. Hepatitis syndrome in infancy—an epidemiological survey with 10 year follow up. *Arch Dis Child.* 1985;60(6):512–516.

25. Spinner NB, Colliton RP, Crosnier C, et al. Jagged1 mutations in Alagille syndrome. *Hum Mutat.* 2001;17(1):18–33.

26. Davit-Spraul A, Fabre M, Branchereau S, et al. ATP8B1 and ABCB11 analysis in 62 children with normal gamma-glutamyl transferase progressive familial intrahepatic cholestasis (PFIC): phenotypic differences between PFIC1 and PFIC2 and natural history. *Hepatology.* 2010;51(5):1645–1655.

27. Davit-Spraul A, Gonzales E, Baussan C, Jacquemin E. Progressive familial intrahepatic cholestasis. *Orphanet J Rare Dis.* 2009;4:1.

28. Knisley A, Bull L, Schneider B. Low γ-GT familial intrahepatic cholestasis. In: Pagon R, Bird T, Dolan C, eds. *GeneReviews.* Seattle, WA: University of Washington, Seattle; 2001. http://www.ncbi.nlm.nih.gov/books/NBK1297/ (accessed August 3, 2012).

29. Strassburg CP. Hyperbilirubinemia syndromes (Gilbert-Meulengracht, Crigler-Najjar, Dubin-Johnson, and Rotor syndrome). *Best Pract Res Clin Gastroenterol.* 2010;24(5):555–571.

30. Srinath A, Shneider BL. Congenital hepatic fibrosis and autosomal recessive polycystic kidney disease. *J Pediatr Gastroenterol Nutr.* 2012;54(5):580–587.

31. Roskams T, Desmet V. Embryology of extra- and intrahepatic bile ducts, the ductal plate. *Anat Rec (Hoboken).* 2008;291(6):628–635.

32. Raynaud P, Tate J, Callens C, et al. A classification of ductal plate malformations based on distinct pathogenic mechanisms of biliary dysmorphogenesis. *Hepatology.* 2011;53(6):1959–1966.

33. Feranchak AP, Sokol RJ. Cholangiocyte biology and cystic fibrosis liver disease. *Semin Liver Dis.* 2001;21(4):471–488.

34. Moyer K, Balistreri W. Hepatobiliary disease in patients with cystic fibrosis. *Curr Opin Gastroenterol.* 2009;25(3):272–278.

35. Feldmeyer L, Huber M, Fellmann F, et al. Confirmation of the origin of NISCH syndrome. *Hum Mutat.* 2006;27(5):408–410.

36. Kimberlin DW. Herpes simplex virus infections in neonates and early childhood. *Semin Pediatr Infect Dis.* 2005;16(4):271–281.

37. Balistreri WF. Neonatal cholestasis. *J Pediatr.* 1985;106(2):171–184.

38. Nelson DR, Teckman J, Di Bisceglie AM, Brenner DA. Diagnosis and management of patients with α1-antitrypsin (A1AT) deficiency. *Clin Gastroenterol Hepatol.* 2012;10(6):575–580.

39. Hansen K, Horslen S. Metabolic liver disease in children. *Liver Transpl.* 2008;14(4):391–411.

40. Braslavsky D, Keselman A, Galoppo M, et al. Neonatal cholestasis in congenital pituitary hormone deficiency and isolated hypocortisolism: characterization of liver dysfunction and follow-up. *Arq Bras Endocrinol Metabol.* 2011;55(8):622–627.

41. Fahnehjelm KT, Fischler B, Martin L, Nemeth A. Occurrence and pattern of ocular disease in children with cholestatic disorders. *Acta Ophthalmol.* 2011;89(2):143–150.

42. Fulford A, Scolapio JS, Aranda-Michel J. Parenteral nutrition-associated hepatotoxicity. *Nutr Clin Pract.* 2004;19(3):274–283.

43. Aghai ZH, Mudduluru M, Nakhla TA, et al. Fluconazole prophylaxis in extremely low birth weight infants: association with cholestasis. *J Perinatol.* 2006;26(9):550–555.

44. Bhat V, Fojas M, Saslow JG, et al. Twice-weekly fluconazole prophylaxis in premature infants: association with cholestasis. *Pediatr Int.* 2011;53(4):475–479.

45. Padda MS, Sanchez M, Akhtar AJ, Boyer JL. Drug induced cholestasis. *Hepatology.* 2011;53(4):1377–1387.

46. Frey B, Braegger CP, Ghelfi D. Neonatal cholestatic hepatitis from carbamazepine exposure during pregnancy and breast feeding. *Ann Pharmacother.* 2002;36(4):644–647.

47. Frey B, Schubiger G, Musy JP. Transient cholestatic hepatitis in a neonate associated with carbamazepine exposure during pregnancy and breast-feeding. *Eur J Pediatr.* 1990;150(2):136–138.

48. Merlob P, Mor N, Litwin A. Transient hepatic dysfunction in an infant of an epileptic mother treated with carbamazepine during pregnancy and breastfeeding. *Ann Pharmacother.* 1992;26(12):1563–1565.

49. Dahshan A. Prenatal exposure to methamphetamine presenting as neonatal cholestasis. *J Clin Gastroenterol.* 2009;43(1):88–90.

50. Lee LA, Reichlin M, Ruyle SZ, Weston WL. Neonatal lupus liver disease. *Lupus.* 1993;2(5):333–338.

51. Lin S-C, Shyur S-D, Huang L-H, et al. Neonatal lupus erythematosus with cholestatic hepatitis. *J Microbiol Immunol Infect.* 2004;37(2):131–134.

52. Shahian M, Khosravi A, Anbardar M-H. Early cholestasis in neonatal lupus erythematosus. *Ann Saudi Med.* 2011;31(1):80–82.

53. Whitington PF. Neonatal hemochromatosis: a congenital alloimmune hepatitis. *Semin Liver Dis.* 2007;27(3):243–250.

54. Whaley BF. Familial hemophagocytic lymphohistiocytosis in the neonate. *Adv Neonatal Care.* 2011;11(2):101–107.

55. Gimeno-Díaz de Atauri A, Gil-Sánchez A, García-Parrón A, Murga-Herrero V. Neonatal cholestasis. A rare complication of fetal tachycardia. *Rev Esp Cardiol.* 2009;62(7):824–826.

56. Herzog D, Chessex P, Martin S, Alvarez F. Transient cholestasis in newborn infants with perinatal asphyxia. *Can J Gastroenterol.* 2003;17(3):179–182.

57. Aagenaes O. Hereditary cholestasis with lymphoedema (Aagenaes syndrome, cholestasis-lymphoedema syndrome). New cases and follow-up from infancy to adult age. *Scand J Gastroenterol.* 1998;33(4):335–345.

58. Drivdal M, Trydal T, Hagve T-A, Bergstad I, Aagenaes O. Prognosis, with evaluation of general biochemistry, of liver disease in lymphoedema cholestasis syndrome 1 (LCS1/Aagenaes syndrome). *Scand J Gastroenterol.* 2006;41(4):465–471.

59. Yu B, Mitchell GA, Richter A. Nucleolar localization of cirhin, the protein mutated in North American Indian childhood cirrhosis. *Exp Cell Res.* 2005;311(2):218–228.

60. Wong KKY, Chung PHY, Chan IHY, Lan LCL, Tam PKH. Performing Kasai portoenterostomy beyond 60 days of life is not necessarily associated with a worse outcome. *J Pediatr Gastroenterol Nutr.* 2010;51(5):631–634.

61. Mieli-Vergani G, Howard ER, Portman B, Mowat AP. Late referral for biliary atresia—missed opportunities for effective surgery. *Lancet.* 1989;1(8635):421–423.

62. Harpavat S, Finegold MJ, Karpen SJ. Patients with biliary atresia have elevated direct/conjugated bilirubin levels shortly after birth. *Pediatrics.* 2011;128(6):e1428–e1433.

63. Ernst LM, Grossman AB, Ruchelli ED. Familial perinatal liver disease and fetal thrombotic vasculopathy. *Pediatr Dev Pathol.* 2008;11(2):160–163.

64. Garcia FJ, Nager AL. Jaundice as an early diagnostic sign of urinary tract infection in infancy. *Pediatrics.* 2002;109(5):846–851.

65. Binder G, Martin DD, Kanther I, Schwarze CP, Ranke MB. The course of neonatal cholestasis in congenital combined pituitary hormone deficiency. *J Pediatr Endocrinol Metab.* 2007;20(6):695–702.

66. Karnsakul W, Sawathiparnich P, Nimkarn S, et al. Anterior pituitary hormone effects on hepatic functions in infants with congenital hypopituitarism. *Ann Hepatol.* 2007;6(2):97–103.

67. Kueppers F, Offord KP. Alpha-1 antitrypsin elevation in healthy neonates. *J Lab Clin Med.* 1979;94(3):475–480.

68. Perlmutter DH. Alpha-1-antitrypsin deficiency: diagnosis and treatment. *Clin Liver Dis.* 2004;8(4):839–859, viii–ix.

69. Liu C, Aronow BJ, Jegga AG, et al. Novel resequencing chip customized to diagnose mutations in patients with inherited syndromes of intrahepatic cholestasis. *Gastroenterology.* 2007;132(1):119–126.

70. Imanieh MH, Dehghani SM, Bagheri MH, et al. Triangular cord sign in detection of biliary atresia: is it a valuable sign? *Digest Dis Sci.* 2009;55(1):172–175.

71. Kanegawa K, Akasaka Y, Kitamura E, et al. Sonographic diagnosis of biliary atresia in pediatric patients using the "triangular cord" sign versus gallbladder length and contraction. *AJR Am J Roentgenol.* 2003;181(5):1387–1390.

72. Kim MJ, Park YN, Han SJ, et al. Biliary atresia in neonates and infants: triangular area of high signal intensity in the porta hepatis at T2-weighted MR cholangiography with US and histopathologic correlation. *Radiology.* 2000;215(2):395–401.

73. Kotb MA, Kotb A, Sheba MF, et al. Evaluation of the triangular cord sign in the diagnosis of biliary atresia. *Pediatrics.* 2001;108(2):416–420.

74. Park WH, Choi SO, Lee HJ. The ultrasonographic "triangular cord" coupled with gallbladder images in the diagnostic prediction of biliary atresia from infantile intrahepatic cholestasis. *J Pediatr Surg.* 1999;34(11):1706–1710.

75. Nadel HR. Hepatobiliary scintigraphy in children. *Semin Nucl Med.* 1996;26:25–42. http://www.sciencedirect.com/science/article/pii/S0001299896800146 (accessed August 8, 2012).

76. Krishnamurthy S, Krishnamurthy GT. Technetium-99m-iminodiacetic acid organic anions: review of biokinetics and clinical application in hepatology. *Hepatology.* 1989;9(1):139–153.

77. Williamson SL, Seibert JJ, Butler HL, Golladay ES. Apparent gut excretion of Tc-99m-DISIDA in a case of extrahepatic biliary atresia. *Pediatr Radiol.* 1986;16(3):245–247.

78. Shah I, Bhatnagar S, Rangarajan V, Patankar N. Utility of Tc99m-mebrofenin hepato-biliary scintigraphy (HIDA scan) for the diagnosis of biliary atresia. *Trop Gastroenterol.* 2012;33(1):62–64.

79. Spivak W, Sarkar S, Winter D, et al. Diagnostic utility of hepatobiliary scintigraphy with 99mTc-DISIDA in neonatal cholestasis. *J Pediatr.* 1987;110(6):855–861.

80. Poddar U, Bhattacharya A, Thapa BR, Mittal BR, Singh K. Ursodeoxycholic acid–augmented hepatobiliary scintigraphy in the evaluation of neonatal jaundice. *J Nucl Med.* 2004;45(9):1488–1492.

81. Majd M, Reba RC, Altman RP. Effect of phenobarbital on 99mTc-IDA scintigraphy in the evaluation of neonatal jaundice. *Semin Nucl Med.* 1981;11:184–204. http://www.sciencedirect.com/science/article/pii/S0001299881800049 (accessed August 8, 2012).

82. Jaw TS, Kuo YT, Liu GC, Chen SH, Wang CK. MR cholangiography in the evaluation of neonatal cholestasis. *Radiology.* 1999;212(1):249–256.

83. Norton KI, Glass RB, Kogan D, et al. MR cholangiography in the evaluation of neonatal cholestasis: initial results. *Radiology.* 2002;222(3):687–691.

84. Ryeom HK, Choe BH, Kim JY, et al. Biliary atresia: feasibility of mangafodipir trisodium–enhanced mr cholangiography for evaluation. *Radiology.* 2005;235(1):250–258.

85. Petersen C, Meier PN, Schneider A, et al. Endoscopic retrograde cholangiopancreaticography prior to explorative laparotomy avoids unnecessary surgery in patients suspected for biliary atresia. *J Hepatol.* 2009;51(6):1055–1060.

86. Shanmugam NP, Harrison PM, Devlin J, et al. Selective use of endoscopic retrograde cholangiopancreatography in the diagnosis of biliary atresia in infants younger than 100 days. *J Pediatr Gastroenterol Nutr.* 2009;49(4):435–441.

87. Shteyer E, Wengrower D, Benuri-Silbiger I, et al. Endoscopic retrograde cholangiopancreatography in neonatal cholestasis. *J Pediatr Gastroenterol Nutr.* 2012;55(2):142–145.

88. Amaral JG, Schwartz J, Chait P, et al. Sonographically guided percutaneous liver biopsy in infants: a retrospective review. *AJR Am J Roentgenol.* 2006;187(6):W644–W649.

89. Nobili V, Comparcola D, Sartorelli MR, et al. Blind and ultrasound-guided percutaneous liver biopsy in children. *Pediatr Radiol.* 2003;33(11):772–775.

90. Pietrobattista A, Fruwirth R, Natali G, et al. Is juvenile liver biopsy unsafe? Putting an end to a common misapprehension. *Pediatr Radiol.* 2009;39(9):959–961.

91. Giefer MJ, Murray KF, Colletti RB. Pathophysiology, diagnosis, and management of pediatric ascites. *J Pediatr Gastroenterol Nutr.* 2011;52:503–513.

92. Bergasa NV. Update on the treatment of the pruritus of cholestasis. *Clin Liver Dis.* 2008;12(1):219–234, x.

93. Yang H, Porte RJ, Verkade HJ, De Langen ZJ, Hulscher JBF. Partial external biliary diversion in children with progressive familial intrahepatic cholestasis and Alagille disease. *J Pediatr Gastroenterol Nutr.* 2009;49(2):216–221.

94. Arnell H, Papadogiannakis N, Zemack H, et al. Follow-up in children with progressive familial intrahepatic cholestasis after partial external biliary diversion. *J Pediatr Gastroenterol Nutr.* 2010;51(4):494–499.

95. Kaliciński PJ, Ismail H, Jankowska I, et al. Surgical treatment of progressive familial intrahepatic cholestasis: comparison of partial external biliary diversion and ileal bypass. *Eur J Pediatr Surg.* 2003;13(5):307–311.

96. Jacquemin E, Hermans D, Myara A, et al. Ursodeoxycholic acid therapy in pediatric patients with progressive familial intrahepatic cholestasis. *Hepatology.* 1997;25(3):519–523.

97. Gonzales E, Gerhardt MF, Fabre M, et al. Oral cholic acid for hereditary defects of primary bile acid synthesis: a safe and effective long-term therapy. *Gastroenterology.* 2009;137(4):1310–1320.e1-3.

98. Takahashi A, Hasegawa M, Sumazaki R, et al. Gradual improvement of liver function after administration of ursodeoxycholic acid in an infant with a novel ABCB11 gene mutation with phenotypic continuum between BRIC2 and PFIC2. *Eur J Gastroenterol Hepatol.* 2007;19(11):942–946.

99. Masurel-Paulet A, Poggi-Bach J, Rolland M-O, et al. NTBC treatment in tyrosinaemia type I: long-term outcome in French patients. *J Inherit Metab Dis.* 2008;31(1):81–87.

100. de Meijer VE, Gura KM, Le HD, Meisel JA, Puder M. Fish oil-based lipid emulsions prevent and reverse parenteral nutrition-associated liver disease: the Boston experience. *JPEN J Parenter Enteral Nutr.* 2009;33(5):541–547.

101. de Meijer VE, Le HD, Meisel JA, Gura KM, Puder M. Parenteral fish oil as monotherapy prevents essential fatty acid deficiency in parenteral nutrition-dependent patients. *J Pediatr Gastroenterol Nutr.* 2010;50(2):212–218.

102. Goulet O, Antébi H, Wolf C, et al. A new intravenous fat emulsion containing soybean oil, medium-chain triglycerides, olive oil, and fish oil: a single-center, double-blind randomized study on efficacy and safety in pediatric patients receiving home parenteral nutrition. *JPEN J Parenter Enteral Nutr.* 2010;34(5):485–495.

103. Rayyan M, Devlieger H, Jochum F, Allegaert K. Short-term use of parenteral nutrition with a lipid emulsion containing a mixture of soybean oil, olive oil, medium-chain triglycerides, and fish oil: a randomized double-blind study in preterm infants. *JPEN J Parenter Enteral Nutri.* 2012;36(1 Suppl):81S–94S.

104. Tomsits E, Pataki M, Tölgyesi A, et al. Safety and efficacy of a lipid emulsion containing a mixture of soybean oil, medium-chain triglycerides, olive oil, and fish oil: a randomised, double-blind clinical trial in premature infants requiring parenteral nutrition. *J Pediatr Gastroenterol Nutr.* 2010;51(4):514–521.

105. Peterson J, Kerner JA. New advances in the management of children with intestinal failure. *J Parenter Enteral Nutr.* 2012;36(1 Suppl):36S–42S.

106. Rand EB, Karpen SJ, Kelly S, et al. Treatment of neonatal hemochromatosis with exchange transfusion and intravenous immunoglobulin. *J Pediatr.* 2009;155(4):566–571.

107. Whitington PF, Kelly S. Outcome of pregnancies at risk for neonatal hemochromatosis is improved by treatment with high-dose intravenous immunoglobulin. *Pediatrics.* 2008;121(6):e1615–e1621.

Congenital Liver Failure and Neonatal Hepatitis

Jennifer Burgis and Melissa Hurwitz

EPIDEMIOLOGY

Neonatal hepatitis is a vague term that describes a heterogeneous group of disorders occurring in infants up to 3 months of age due to a variety of insults. It includes all forms of neonatal cholestasis not attributed to extrahepatic biliary tract obstruction. In many instances, a specific inciting event, infectious agent, or metabolic cause cannot be found. Approximately 40% of cases of neonatal cholestasis are due to neonatal hepatitis.[1]

Neonatal acute liver failure (ALF) is rare but often fatal. It is defined as the development of hepatic necrosis associated with hepatic encephalopathy and coagulopathy within 8 weeks of the onset of liver disease without evidence of chronic liver disease. This definition is challenging given prenatal liver disease is challenging to identify, and encephalopathy in neonates is difficult to distinguish. The Pediatric Acute Liver Failure study group defined ALF as hepatic-based coagulopathy defined as prothrombin time (PT) of 15 seconds or longer or international normalized ratio (INR) of 1.5 or more, not corrected by vitamin K, in the presence of clinical hepatic encephalopathy, or a PT of 20 or more or INR of 2 or more regardless of the presence or absence of clinical hepatic encephalopathy, along with biochemical evidence of acute liver injury and no known evidence of chronic liver disease.[2]

This chapter review focuses on known causes of neonatal hepatitis, concentrating on those that can progress to ALF. Please refer to the chapters on conjugated hyperbilirubinemia, congenital infections, and metabolic diseases for additional discussion.

PATHOPHYSIOLOGY

Sporadic neonatal hepatitis is often ascribed to a specific injury from infectious, ischemic, or environmental factors, whereas familial neonatal hepatitis is assumed to be caused by genetic defects in hepatic metabolic or excretory function. Idiopathic neonatal hepatitis is a generic name for indeterminate causes of ALF. Biopsies classically show formation of syncytial hepatic giant cells, variable inflammation, and lobular cholestasis. A review of 62 cases showed lobular extramedullary hematopoiesis was present in 74%, lobular cholestasis in 84%, and mild patchy chronic inflammation in 54%. Fibrosis was present in 30% of cases. Most cases (49%) remained idiopathic, but 16% of cases were diagnosed with hypopituitarism and 14% as having biliary atresia or Allagille syndrome. The biopsy findings did not readily distinguish between the specific etiologies.[3]

Neonatal Hepatitis

The classic pathology of neonatal hepatitis is characterized by predominantly parenchymal lobular inflammation with preservation of the zonal distribution of portal tracts and central veins. There is ballooning degeneration of hepatocytes. There can be intense giant cell transformation. Cholestatic features can also be seen, such as cytoplasmic feathery degeneration, formation of cholestatic rosettes, cholestatic plugs, and Kupffer cell activation. No obstructive pathology should be evident, and there are a normal number of bile ducts. Extramedullary hematopoiesis can be seen.[3]

CHAPTER 40

Neonatal Acute Liver Failure

The most common etiologies of liver failure present with classic features. Severe coagulopathy and normal aminotransferases are seen in neonatal hemochromatosis. Severe coagulopathy and high aminotransferases are typical of viral hepatitis. Moderate coagulopathy and hepatitis are consistent with metabolic disorders. Metabolic failure, such as hypoglycemia, is common. Presentation in the first weeks of life is an important consideration with neonatal hemochromatosis, mitochondrial hepatopathy, and disseminated herpesvirus infection. Galactosemia and tyrosinemia, in addition to infections, should be considered in the second and third weeks of life. After 3 weeks, disorders to consider include bile acid synthesis defects, vertically transmitted hepatitis B, and hemophagocytic lymphohistiocytosis.[4] The underlying mechanism for severe hepatic necrosis is multifactorial and is dependent on patient age, underlying susceptibility, and extent of injury. There should be a high index of suspicion in infants with elevated liver function tests, as well as infants with sepsis or recurrent hypoglycemia. Liver disease can be reversible with acute damage to hepatocytes without destruction of the liver's capacity to regenerate. In fulminant cases of severe hepatocyte necrosis or in end-stage cirrhotic disease, there are insufficient residual hepatocytes to maintain essential liver function, and the complications are irreversible.

DIFFERENTIAL DIAGNOSIS

Infectious Causes of Hepatitis

Bacteria and Septicemia

Hepatitis in neonatal sepsis typically presents with hepatomegaly and jaundice. Gram-negative bacteria are the most frequent etiologic agents, such as *Escherichia coli*. Other bacteria include *Staphylococcus aureus* or *Listeria monocytogenes*. Typical features include leukocytosis, conjugated hyperbilirubinemia with mild to moderately elevated serum aminotransferase levels, and coagulopathy if disseminated intravascular coagulation is present.

Toxoplasmosis, Rubella, Cytomegalovirus, and Herpes Simplex Virus: The TORCH Infections

Toxoplasmosis: Toxoplasmosis is an intracellular protozoan parasite. Maternal infection occurs by contact with oocytes in cat feces or ingestion of contaminated raw meat. Most newborns are asymptomatic but may present with hepatomegaly, prominent hepatitis, and neurologic findings such as microcephaly, intracranial calcifications, and chorioretinitis.

Rubella: Hepatic involvement is common in congenital rubella, including cholestasis, hepatosplenomegaly, and elevated serum alkaline phosphatase and aminotransferases. Other presenting symptoms include thrombocytopenia, congenital heart disease, cataracts, and neurologic impairments. Hepatic failure is rare. There has been a drastic (over 99%) decline in congenital rubella infections since introduction of the rubella vaccine.[5]

Cytomegalovirus (CMV): Approximately 10% of CMV-infected newborns have clinical evidence of disease in the neonatal period. More severely infected infants are associated with primary maternal infection in the first trimester. The mortality rate is approximately 20%. Classic symptoms include a petechial rash, hepatosplenomegaly, and jaundice. The hepatitis is typically mild and often resolves within weeks to months, but persistent neurodevelopmental abnormalities cause the most morbidity. CMV is an uncommon cause of ALF, with rare development of cirrhosis and cholestasis leading to liver transplantation. Infection can be treated with ganciclovir and CMV immunoglobulin.[6-8]

Herpes simplex virus (HSV): Both HSV-1 and HSV-2 cause neonatal infection. HSV is the most common infectious cause of ALF. It can result in severe multisystem infection with encephalopathy. Initial symptoms can be nonspecific, such as lethargy, poor feeding, and fever. Infants often develop a septic-like picture due to disseminated disease with jaundice, hepatomegaly, and ascites. Encephalitis with seizures is present in up to one-third of cases. A vesicular rash can be absent in up to 30% of cases. Laboratory findings include coagulopathy, elevated total and direct bilirubin, and transaminitis. Most neonatal infections are associated with a primary maternal infection late in gestation, but up to 60%–80% of maternal infections are unknown. Liver biopsy reveals necrosis and viral inclusions in intact hepatocytes.[9] Mortality is high.

Other congenital infections: Congenital syphilis causing severe infection can present with hepatosplenomegaly and jaundice, and milder cases can have anicteric hepatitis with elevated serum aminotransferases and poor weight gain with snuffles. It is a rare cause of fulminant hepatic failure, and chronic liver disease has not been reported in infants treated appropriately. Tuberculous hepatitis is rare in neonates but can occur through aspiration of infected amniotic fluid or placental spread from miliary tuberculosis. Hepatic lesions show typical caseating necrosis with surrounding giant cells, and the course is often fatal.

Hepatotropic Viruses

Hepatitis A: Hepatitis A is rare in neonates. Incidence in the United States is approximately 25,000 cases per year among all ages. It is a nonenveloped RNA virus, classified as a *Picornavirus*. The route of transmission is fecal-oral, and the incubation period is 15–50 days. Maternal symptoms and the highest viral titers occur 2 weeks before the illness and up to 1 week after delivery. Most infants and children are asymptomatic (>80%) but can develop fever, malaise, anorexia, nausea, abdominal discomfort, dark urine, and jaundice. Mild elevation in aspartate aminotransferase (AST) and alanine aminotransferase (ALT) and elevated total and direct bilirubin are seen. The clinical illness usually does not last longer than 2 months, although 10%–15% of persons have prolonged or relapsing signs and symptoms for up to 6 months. The virus may be excreted during a relapse. There is no chronic carrier state. Fulminant hepatitis A is rare.[10]

Hepatitis B: Hepatitis B virus (HBV) is a small, double-shelled virus in the Hepadnaviridae family. Over 90% of neonatal infections occur by vertical transmission through amniotic fluid, vaginal secretions, or maternal blood or postnatally via blood transfusion and prolonged household blood contact. The risk of transmission increases with the presence of hepatitis B e antigen (HBeAg), elevated HBV DNA viral load, acute maternal hepatitis in the third trimester, or a prior infant with chronic infection. As many as 90% of infants who acquire HBV infection via vertical transmission become chronically infected, compared to 30%–50% who become HBV infected when exposed between 1 and 5 years of age. Acute hepatitis B in the neonatal period is rare. The prodromal phase lasts from 3 to 10 days. It is characterized by malaise, anorexia, nausea, vomiting, right upper quadrant abdominal pain, fever, headache, myalgia, skin rashes, arthralgias and arthritis, and dark urine. The icteric phase is variable but usually lasts from 1 to 3 weeks and is characterized by jaundice, light or gray stools, hepatic tenderness, and hepatomegaly (splenomegaly is less common). During convalescence, malaise and fatigue may persist for weeks or months, while jaundice, anorexia, and other symptoms disappear. Fulminant HBV leading to ALF is rare but typically presents at 12 weeks of age. It has been associated with basic core promoter and precore mutants.[11]

Hepatitis C: Hepatitis C is a small enveloped RNA virus of the family Flaviviridae. Seroprevalence in children in the United States is 0.1%–0.2%. Vertical transmission from mother to fetus is the major route of HCV infection, and the risk is about 5%, with increased risk in maternal human immunodeficiency (HIV) coinfection (3- to 4-fold higher), specific genotypes, and high maternal viral titers. There is no difference in transmission by delivery mode, and transmission through breast milk has not been documented. Most infections are asymptomatic, but acute disease can be associated with jaundice and less transaminitis, as compared to hepatitis B. ALF in infants is rare.[12]

Hepatitis D: Delta hepatitis virus is a subviral satellite as it can only propagate in the presence of hepatitis B. Transmission is parenteral through blood exposure or illicit drug use. Vertical transmission is unusual. It is not a known cause of ALF.[13]

Hepatitis E: Hepatitis E is a small nonenveloped RNA virus, and it can cause acute hepatitis in newborns. A study by Khuroo et al revealed that in 15 of 19 babies born to mothers infected with hepatitis E who had positive polymerase chain reaction (PCR) at birth, 37% developed icteric hepatitis, 26% had hepatitis without jaundice, and 26% had high serum bilirubin and normal liver enzymes. Overall, 37% died within the first 7 days of life. The remainder of the infants had self-limited disease without prolonged viremia.[14]

Other Viral Infectious Causes

Enteroviruses cause mild disease, but immature immune systems create a higher risk for neonates. Multiorgan involvement occurs with encephalomyocarditis (most characteristic of group B coxsackie viruses) and hemorrhage-hepatitis syndrome (most characteristic of echovirus 11).[15] Other viruses that can cause neonatal hepatitis include adenovirus, parvovirus B19, human herpesvirus 6 (HHV-6), paramyxovirus, and HIV.

Metabolic and Genetic Causes

Carbohydrate Disorders

Among the carbohydrate disorders, hereditary fructose intolerance is an autosomal recessive disease from defective enzymatic activity of fructose 1,6-bisphosphate aldolase, which is active in the liver, renal cortex, and small intestine. Symptoms such as vomiting, diarrhea, abdominal distension, and failure to thrive develop with introduction of sucrose or fructose. This can progress to hepatomegaly, hemorrhagic disease, and seizures with metabolic acidosis, hyperuricemia, and renal Fanconi syndrome.[16]

Galactosemia has an incidence of 1:50,000 infants. Features include vomiting, diarrhea, jaundice, poor weight gain, and sometimes sepsis. Hypoglycemia is common. Eye findings can include cataracts and retinal detachment. Despite strict dietary restriction, affected children can have progressive declining cognitive function, speech delay, and other neurologic symptoms. It can lead to acute or chronic liver disease, which often improves after therapy. Most children recover and do well, surviving into adulthood.[13]

Other carbohydrate disorders, such as fructose 1,6-bisphosphatase deficiency, congenital disorders of glycosylation, glycogen storage disease types IV and IX, and transadolase deficiency, can also cause ALF.[17]

Amino Acid Disorders

Hereditary tyrosinemia type 1 is an autosomal recessive disorder due to lack of fumaryl acetoacetate hydrolase (FAH), which leads to an accumulation of succinylacetone that damages the liver and kidneys. ALF can present in infancy. Chronic liver disease in combination with rickets and renal Fanconi syndrome occurs with late presentation between 4 and 24 months of age. Significantly elevated α-fetoprotein (AFP) and a classic profile of plasma amino acids are diagnostic. These children are at ongoing risk of developing hepatocellular carcinoma. Other amino acid disorders, such as urea cycle defects, citrin defect, and S-adenosylhomocysteine-hydrolase deficiency can present with ALF.[17]

Other Genetic Disorders

Deficiency of α_1-antitrypsin is the most common genetic cause of neonatal hepatitis. Up to 90% of children with α_1-antritrypsin deficiency who develop liver disease present with neonatal hepatitis. Symptoms include severe cholestasis, hepatomegaly, and rarely severe coagulopathy. Approximately half of the infants with liver disease will have progression to cirrhosis. The duration of jaundice is a critical prognostic sign since infants in whom jaundice resolves by 6 months are likely to have a good outcome. A study by Francavilla and coworkers identified that persistence of elevated serum aminotransferases and γ–glutamyl transferase (GGT) through 6–12 months of age and pathologic evidence of bile duct proliferation and bridging fibrosis are markers of rapidly progressive liver disease.[18] This is discussed in more detail in the chapter on conjugated hyperbilirubinemia.

There are 3 known types of progressive familial intrahepatic cholestasis (PFIC) due to defects in different transporters in the hepatocyte bile canalicular membrane. All 3 types present with cholestasis and develop diarrhea, pruritis, and fat-soluble vitamin deficiencies. Classic distinguishing features include a normal GGT in PFIC1 and PFIC2 but elevated GGT in PFIC3. Cirrhosis often develops in early childhood, and liver transplantation is required. Please refer to the chapter on conjugated hyperbilirubinemia for more information.[13]

Trisomy 21 has a known association with transient myeloproliferative disorder. About 20% of patients with transient leukemia develop hepatic fibrosis. A study by Hirabayshi et al identified risk factors of reduced hepatic functional reserve (elevated direct bilirubin and PT and presence of ascites); elevated hyaluronic acid; respiratory failure associated with hepatosplenomegaly; and fibrosis on liver biopsy.[19]

Neonatal hepatitis is known to occur in trisomy 18 with intrahepatic cholestasis, but there are no clear reports of ALF. A study by Alpert et al examining autopsy cases of 19 infants found an association of neonatal hepatitis with cholestasis and trisomy 18. Of the 3 infants who survived beyond the immediate neonatal period, all had hepatic parenchymal damage with focal necrosis.[20]

Primary disorders of bile acid synthesis can produce neonatal cholestatic liver disease and progressive neurologic disease. Features include elevated transaminases with normal GGT and liver biopsy with giant cell hepatitis. Neurologic features include spastic paralysis. The most useful screening test is urinary cholanoids (bile acids and bile alcohols). Two inherited defects in the enzymes of bile synthesis include 3β-hydroxysteroid-Δ5-C27-steroid dehydrogenase deficiency and Δ4-3-oxosteroid 5β-reductase deficiency. Early diagnosis is important as these diseases can be treated effectively with supplementation of critical bile acids.[21]

Additional metabolic and genetic diseases that can be associated with ALF include fatty acid oxidation disorders, Niemann-Pick type C (a disorder of cholesterol esterification), cystic fibrosis, Zellweger syndrome (the reduction or absence of functional peroxisomes), Wolman disease (a deficiency of lysosomal acid lipase), Wilson disease, and neonatal adrenoleukodystrophy.[4,22]

Mitochondrial Disorders

Mitochondrial disorders should be suspected if there is an association of neuromuscular symptoms with liver dysfunction, multisystem involvement in acute or chronic liver disease, and the presence of lactic acidosis, hepatic steatosis, or ketonemia.[23] Mitochondrial hepatopathies involving respiratory chain defects can present as ALF. These can be caused by mutations in the *SCO1* gene (required for assembly of complex IV) and mutations in *BVS1L* (required for assembly of function of complex III). Features include cholestasis, hepatic steatosis, lethargy, hypotonia, vomiting, poor suck, apnea, and seizures. Low hepatic activity of respiratory chain complexes IV (most common), I, III, and occasionally II can be found in these infants. Liver failure progresses to death within weeks to months. Mitochondrial DNA depletion syndromes (MDSs) are other mitochondrial disorders occurring in 2 phenotypes, a myopathic form and a hepatocerebral form. The hepatocerebral form presents in the first weeks of life with vomiting, severe reflux, failure to thrive, developmental delay, and hepatomegaly. The progression of liver failure is less rapid than mitochondrial respiratory chain diseases. Other mitochondrial disorders that can present in infancy include Alpers-Huttenlocher syndrome, Pearson syndrome, and Navajo neurohepatopathy.[24]

Immunologic Causes

Neonatal hemachromatosis is a unique fetal liver disease and common cause of ALF.[25] Intrauterine growth restriction, oligohydramnios, and fetal distress have been documented. Affected infants demonstrate hypoglycemia, extreme cholestasis, severe synthetic dysfunction, and hypoalbuminemia. Serum AST and ALT are typically low, and ferritin and AFP are extremely elevated. Diagnosis rests on abnormally distributed iron deposition in both hepatic and extrahepatic tissues. Abdominal magnetic resonance imaging (MRI) can show abnormal iron signal in the heart, pancreas, spleen, and adrenal glands. The gold standard for diagnosis is to indentify siderosis in extrahepatic tissues, such as submucosal glands, on a buccal mucosal biopsy. Pathology reveals marked fibrosis and cirrhosis, supporting the hypothesis of fetal liver insult. The most likely pathogenic mechanism is a gestational alloimmune disease against a common fetal antigen, evidence exists of increased risk of recurrence in subsequent pregnancies and mothers with affected babies with different fathers.[26]

Neonatal lupus erythematosus (NLE) is a rare autoimmune disease classically presenting with cardiac disease, specifically congenital heart block, and cutaneous lesions. Maternal autoantibodies, anti-Ro/SSA or anti-La/SSB, are passed transplacentally. A review of a large national registry revealed 9% of infants with NLE had hepatobiliary disease in 3 variants: (1) severe liver failure similar to neonatal hemochromatosis, (2) conjugated hyperbilirubinemia with minimal hepatitis, and (3) mild hepatitis at 2 to 3 months of life. Outside the severe hepatic failure presentation, prognosis was excellent.[27] Mild hepatomegaly and splenomegaly can be seen. The hepatic abnormalities can be compounded by congestive heart failure in children with cardiac manifestations of NLE. Elevated liver function tests typically resolve within the first months of life. Pathology tends to resemble that of idiopathic neonatal giant cell hepatitis.[28]

Oncologic Causes

Hemophagocytic lymphohistiocytosis (HLH) is a life-threatening condition due a hyperinflammatory state from high levels of inflammatory cytokines related to impaired function of natural killer cells and cytotoxic T cells.[29] Primary familial HLH is inherited in an autosomal recessive pattern, and acquired HLH is thought to be triggered by infection, immune dysregulation, malignancy, or other insult. Clinical criteria include fever, splenomegaly, cytopenia, hypertriglyceridemia,

hypofibrinogenemia, and extremely elevated ferritin levels. Additional clinical features include lymphadenopathy, central nervous system (CNS) involvement, and rash. Hepatomegaly and hepatitis often occur early in the disease. Liver pathology is characterized by a variable degree of portal and sinusoidal lymphohistocytic infiltrate with bile duct damage and interface necrosis and inflammation.[30] HLH is rapidly progressive and often fatal in the neonatal period without chemotherapy and hematopoietic stem cell transplantation (overall survival 58%). Liver transplantation alone is not curative.[31]

Neonatal leukemia, neuroblastoma, and hepatic tumors (benign vascular tumors and mesenchymal hamartomas and hepatoblastoma) have also been associated with ALF.[13,32,33]

Vascular Causes

Shock-liver syndrome is related to reduced hepatic blood flow due to low cardiac output. The typical clinical phases include sudden and transient elevation in serum transaminase levels early in the course of circulatory failure with improvement as the hemodynamic condition is corrected. This is followed by persistent cholestatic jaundice that lasts several weeks. A case report suggested this could be related to the ductus venosus, which may remain patent in the setting of perinatal hypoxemia, leading to a significant reduction in blood flow to the right hepatic lobe, making it more susceptible to ischemia during cardiovascular stress.[34]

Additional cardiac or vascular abnormalities can lead to ALF, such as myocarditis or development of Budd-Chiari physiology with a portal vein obstruction from thrombotic disorders such as congenital disorders of glycosylation. Other inherited disorders of coagulation to consider in the case of thrombosis include antithrombin III, protein S, and protein C deficiencies and fibrinogen abnormalities.[35]

Miscellaneous Causes

Various other etiologies are known to cause hepatitis and liver failure in neonates. Medications shown to be hepatotoxic in neonates include valproate, isoniazid, and acetaminophen. Perinatal hypoxia can lead to abnormal liver function, but ALF is rare. Anatomic or structural abnormalities such as extrahepatic bile duct obstruction in biliary atresia and bile duct paucity in Alagille syndrome can cause mild hepatitis and cholestasis but rarely are present with ALF in the neonatal period. Up to 30%–40% of the causes of ALF are indeterminate.

Table 40-1 provides a list of common etiologies of ALF in infants aged 0–90 days.

Table 40-1 Etiologies of Acute Liver Failure in Infants Aged 0–90 Days (n = 148)[a]

Diagnosis	Number	%
Metabolic diseases	28	18.9
Galactosemia	12	8.1
Respiratory chain defect	5	3.4
Tyrosinemia	3	2.0
Neiman-Pick type C	3	2.0
Mitochondrial disorder	3	2.0
Urea cycle defect	1	0.7
Ornithine transcarbamylase deficiency	1	0.7
GALD, gestational alloimmune liver disease	20	13.5
Viral infections	24	16.2
Herpes simplex virus	19	12.8
Enterovirus	4	2.7
Cytomegalovirus infection	1	0.7
Other etiologies	19	12.8
Shock	6	4.1
Hemophagocytic syndrome	4	2.7
Escherichia coli sepsis	2	1.4
Hemangioendothelioma	2	1.4
Acetaminophen	1	0.7
Down syndrome	1	0.7
Leukemia	1	0.7
Intraventricular hemorrhage	1	0.7
Multiple diagnoses	2	1.4
Indeterminate	56	37.8

[a]Reproduced with permission from Sundaram et al.[53]

DIAGNOSTIC TESTS

History and Physical Examination

Important history features include consanguinity, onset and symptoms of possible antenatal or perinatal maternal illness, and previous miscarriages or neonatal deaths. Exposure history is important, including family history of tuberculosis, travel history, animal exposures, recent insect bites, and high-risk foods such as unpasteurized dairy food.

A thorough physical examination is critical. Dysmorphic features are important to identify. Irritability and fatigue may be signs of encephalopathy. Scleral icterus may be prominent. A murmur may herald cardiac disease or other genetic syndromes. Other findings, such as pulmonary rales, could indicate pulmonary edema suspicious for cardiac failure. An abdominal examination can reveal hepatomegaly, splenomegaly, or the presence of a fluid wave indicating ascites. An assessment of peripheral edema, wasting, clubbing, or poor peripheral perfusion is helpful. Jaundice, petechiae, ecchymosis, or spider angiomas are important to identify on a skin examination.

Laboratory Tests

First Tier

Laboratory: An initial workup should include basic hematology and chemistry tests, such as complete blood cell count (CBC) with differential, blood type, and Coombs; complete metabolic panel, including glucose, liver function tests such as total and direct bilirubin, AST, ALT, alkaline phosphatase, and GGT. Liver synthetic function should be evaluated in all infants with a coagulation profile, fibrinogen, factor levels (V, VII, and VIII), and albumin. Iron studies and ferritin should be also sent.

Microbiology: The key is to focus on direct identification of possible infectious agents through specific immunoglobulin (Ig) M antibodies, viral titers, PCR-based diagnostics, or culture. Key screening should include hepatotropic viruses with anti-HAV (anti-hepatitis A virus) IgM, hepatitis B surface antigen (HBsAg) and anti-HBs, and hepatitis B core antibody (anti-HBc) IgM. Maternal testing involves HBsAg, HBeAg, hepatitis B e antibody (anti-HBe), anti-HBc, anti-hepatitis C IgM, and hepatitis C PCR. Evaluation for HSV includes HSV PCR on cerebrospinal fluid (CSF) or culture of skin lesions plus eye, oropharyngeal, and rectal cultures. HIV enzyme-linked immunosorbent assay (ELISA) should be sent. CMV and Epstein-Barr virus (EBV) serology or quantitative PCR should also be considered. Other viruses may be identified by respiratory direct fluorescence assay (DFA).

Urine studies: Urine culture and urine CMV antigen test should be sent. An initial metabolic workup should include urine reducing substances (positive in galactosemia), urine succinylacetone (elevated in tyrosinemia), and urine organic acids. Urine toxicology is important to identify potential exposures.

Second Tier (Based on Suspected Diagnosis)

Metabolic and genetic: A basic metabolic workup may include assessment of lactate, pyruvate, ammonia, and a venous blood gas. Plasma acylcarnitine profile, serum amino acids, and α_1-antritypsin serum level and phenotype are also commonly sent. The initial screen for galactosemia is urine reducing substances, which are nonspecific and can be positive in prematurity or negative in infants too sick for oral feedings. Confirmation of galactosemia is made by a quantitative assay of erythrocyte galactose-1-phosphate uridyl transferase

(GALT) enzyme activity. This must be sent prior to blood transfusion. Diagnosis can also be confirmed by aldolase activity in a liver biopsy specimen. A traditional fructose tolerance test is contraindicated because of the risk of hypoglycemia. Hereditary tyrosinemia is often associated with an elevated AFP, between 40,000 and 70,000 µg/L. The plasma amino acid profile will show elevations in tyrosine, phenyalanine, and methionine. There is positive succinylacetone in the urine. Genetic diagnoses may be identified by karyotype or chromosomal genomic hybridization. Molecular resequencing arrays can be sent for known mutations in Alagille syndrome, PFIC, and α_1-antitrypsin deficiency. Urine quantitative bile acids determination by mass spectrometry can screen for disorders of bile synthesis.

Immunologic: Neonatal hemochromatosis is characterized by high serum ferritin and high serum AFP and confirmed by demonstrating extrahepatic iron deposits sparing the reticuloendothelial system.

Oncologic: The diagnosis of hemophagocytic lymphohistiocytosis can be made by fulfillment of 5 of 8 criteria: fever, splenomegaly, cytopenias, hypertriglyceridemia and/or hypofibrinogenemia, hemophagocytosis in the bone marrow, abnormal natural killer cell functional assay, elevated soluble interleukin (IL) 2R α level (>2400 U/mL), and elevated ferritin level (>50 µg/L). Molecular analysis for known mutations in familial HLH could also be performed.[36]

Mitochondrial: Mitochondrial disorders can be identified by a markedly elevated plasma lactate, an elevated molar ratio of plasma lactate to pyruvate (>20), and an elevated β-hydroxybutyrate. A distinguishing feature of MDS is a low ratio (<10%) of the normal amount of mitochondrial DNA (mtDNA) relative to nuclear DNA in the affected tissues and a normal mtDNA sequence.[24]

Table 40-2 provides additional details on laboratory testing.

Radiology Studies

Imaging studies for workup of hepatitis should include an abdominal ultrasound with Doppler to assess hepatic appearance, hepatosplenomegaly, bile duct anatomy, vascular patency, and hepatopedal flow. Abdominal MRI for sidersosis is important in neonatal hemochromatosis, as discussed previously. An echocardiogram is also part of a standard liver transplant evaluation to assess cardiac anatomy and function.

Pathology

A percutaneous liver biopsy will often provide key diagnostic information, but severe coagulopathy can thwart procedure safety. In the case of severe coagulopathy, a transjugular biopsy by interventional radiology may be considered. A buccal mucosal biopsy is an important diagnostic step in neonatal hemochromatosis. Bone marrow biopsies may be considered in HLH. Muscle biopsies may be pursued in suspected cases of mitochondrial disorders.

MANAGEMENT

General

Isolation precautions are paramount given the concern for possible infectious etiologies. Specific infections need to be reported to local health departments. Appropriate active or passive immunization for contacts should be considered.

Nutritional Interventions

Nutrition for these neonates may be affected by a presumed diagnosis. There has been no documented transmission of hepatitis B or hepatitis C from breastfeeding. Brief use of a restricted diet, such as a lactosefree and low-protein formula, is sometimes justifiable in an infant with severe neonatal hepatitis until testing results for galactossemia and tyrosinemia are available. All infants with severe, prolonged cholestasis will likely require elemental formulas containing medium-chain triglycerides, which can be absorbed without bile acids. Monitoring these infants for appropriate caloric intake and weight gain is necessary, including use of fortified formulas, nasogastric feedings, or parenteral nutrition.

Fat-soluble vitamin supplementation is often necessary. Oral vitamin A recommended doses range from 5000 to 25,000 IU per day of water-miscible vitamin A. Vitamin D needs range from 600 to 2000 IU per day of ergocaliferol. Cholestatic infants need vitamin E (α-tocopheral) 15–25 IU/kg per day in the form of tocopherol polyethylene glycol succinate (TPGS). Dosing for Vitamin K replacement is typically 2.5 mg for children less than 2 years of age but may increase to 5 mg per day in infants with severe coagulopathy. This additional supplementation is typically more than a combination preparation can provide, and the vitamins often have to be given individually. There is a risk of vitamin A toxicity, and all fat-soluble vitamin levels should be monitored every 3 to 6 months.

Pharmacologic Therapy

Pruritis due to severe cholestasis can be debilitating and difficult to treat. Use of traditional antihistamines as monotherapy is typically inadequate to control symptoms. Other agents with improved efficacy include rifampin, phenobarbital, ursodiol, opioid antagonists, and bile-binding resins.[37]

Table 40-2 General Investigation of Neonatal Liver Failure[a]

Blood
Hematology
Full blood count and peripheral smear, blood group, and Coombs test
Prothrombin time, partial thromboplastin time, fibrinogen
D dimers/fibrin degradation products
Biochemistry
Urea and electrolytes, creatine kinase, amylase
Bilirubin (unconjugated/conjugated), transaminases, γ–glutamyl transferase, alkaline phosphatase, albumin
Acid-base balance
Glucose, lactate, ammonia
Cholesterol, triglycerides, free fatty acids, β-hydroxybutyrate
Ferritin and transferrin saturation
Plasma amino acids
Galactose-1-phosphate uridyl transferase
Carnitine/acyl carnitines
Cortisol (9 AM)
Serum bile salts
Transferrin
α-Fetoprotein
Toxicology, including acetaminophen
Microbiology
Bacterial/viral culture and PCR detection
Viral serology: mother and infant (immunoglobulin M in infant may be negative for several weeks)
Other
Storage for DNA
Urine
Biochemistry
Amino acids; organic acids, including succinyl acetone, orotic acid
pH, ketones, reducing substances
Toxicology
Urinary bile salts
Microbiology
Bacterial/viral culture and PCR detection
Other samples for viral culture/PCR viral detection
Stool/rectal swab
Nasopharyngeal secretions
Vesicle fluid
Cerebrospinal fluid
Eye swab
Ascitic fluid
Radiology
Chest x-ray
Echocardiography
Doppler ultrasound scan of abdomen

Abbreviation: PCR, polymerase chain reaction.
[a]From McClean and Davison.[22]

Targeted Antiviral Treatment

Hepatitis A: If there is serologic confirmation of HAV infection by IgM anti-HAV testing in index patients, infants should receive postexposure treatment with a single dose of immune globulin (0.02 mL per kg) as soon as possible. Immunoglobulin and the hepatitis A vaccine should be administered to all previously unvaccinated household and sexual contacts of persons with serologically confirmed hepatitis. Earliest vaccine administration can occur after 12 months of age.

Hepatitis B: Infants born to women who are HBsAg positive are at high risk for HBV transmission and chronic HBV infection. HBV vaccine and a single dose of hepatitis B immunoglobulin (HBIG) administered within 24 hours after birth are 85%–95% effective in preventing both acute HBV infection and chronic HBV infection. HBV vaccine administered alone within 24 hours after birth is 70%–95% effective in preventing perinatal HBV infection. HBIG and HBV vaccine should be given intramuscularly at different sites within 12 hours of birth. Completion of the 3-dose HBV vaccine series is paramount. Testing for HBsAg and anti-HBs is recommended at 9 to 18 months of age (3 to 12 months after the third dose) to monitor success of therapy. If the mother's HBsAg status is unknown at the time of birth, the infant should be vaccinated within 12 hours of birth. If the mother is found to be HBsAg positive, the infant should received HBIG as soon as possible but no later than 7 days of age. Infants born to HBsAg-positive women and who weigh less than 2000 g at birth should receive the same postexposure prophylaxis and complete the HBV vaccine series, but the birth vaccine dose should not be counted in the 3-dose schedule. Lamivudine, a reverse-transcriptase inhibitor, is a possible therapeutic option in fulminant hepatitis B. Infants can survive without liver transplantation, but seroconversion to anti-HBs is rare.

Hepatitis C: No immune prophylaxis for hepatitis C is available. Infants born to infected mothers should be tested for anti-HCV at 12 months of age to assess for chronic infection. Spontaneous clearance can occur in up to 30% of children. Up to 60%–80% progress to chronic liver disease, and 20% will develop cirrhosis and remain at risk for hepatocellular carcinoma.[12,38]

Herpes simplex virus: High-dose intravenous acyclovir is a well-known effective therapy for HSV infection and should be initiated early in suspected infection. It has shown improved survival and long-term neurological outcome.[39] There are no standard recommendations for antenatal screening, but prophylaxis with oral acyclovir at 36 weeks of gestation for mothers with known HSV has been shown to reduce viral shedding. Data are unclear if it affects transmission rate.[40] Early antiviral therapy in neonates improves prognosis and has decreased the rate of disseminated neonatal infections.

Other Therapies

Tyrosinemia: Treatment with 2-(2-nitro-4-trifluoro-methyl-benzoyl)-1,3-cyclohexandione, also known as NTBC, which prevents the production of toxic metabolites in combination with a low-tyrosine and low-phenylalanine diet can dramatically extend survival.[41]

Mitochondrial disorders: There is no clear evidence to suggest benefit of any medical therapy in mitochondrial disorders. However, antioxidants (vitamins E and C) and electron acceptors and cofactors (coenzyme Q_{10}, thiamine, riboflavin) have been used.[42]

Neonatal hemochromatosis: The antioxidant cocktail of N-acetylcysteine, vitamin E, deferoxamine, selenium, and prostaglandin E_1 was historically given to remove excess iron and protect against iron-induced oxidant injury.[43] This chelation-antioxidant therapy is no longer recommended, and liver transplantation remains the treatment of choice.[44,45] For mothers with a previously affected infant, success for less-severe neonatal disease has been shown with prenatal maternal intravenous immunoglobulin (IVIG) infusions (1 g/kg weekly from week 18 of gestation until delivery).[46] Double-volume exchange transfusion in neonates in combination with prenatal maternal IVIG is gaining more attention.[47]

Management of Acute Liver Failure

Referral

Referral to a pediatric liver transplantation center and transfer to a critical care unit are paramount. Orthotopic liver transplantation may be the only definitive treatment of many severe neonatal ALF etiologies.

Supportive Care

Access

Adequate intravenous access is necessary at all times, with a minimum of 2 peripheral intravenous catheters.

Fluids and Electrolytes

Close monitoring of fluid balance is crucial as volume overload can have dangerous outcomes, such as cerebral edema. Infants rarely herniate given their pliable skull.

Hyponatremia in liver failure should be treated with fluid restriction as patients are total body sodium overloaded. Hyponatremia causes secondary hyperaldosteronism in liver failure. Due to poor synthetic function of the liver with low albumin and low oncotic pressure, low serum sodium contributes to third-spacing of fluids. Therefore, there is high extravascular sodium and low intravascular sodium. This leads to an increased production of aldosterone by the adrenal glands in an attempt to increase serum sodium. Hyponatremia should not be corrected rapidly given the risk of central pontine myelinosis. Additional sodium can also increase portal pressure and lead to gastrointestinal bleeding.

Hypoglycemia is common in ALF as glycogenolysis and gluconeogenesis are impaired. An infusion of dextrose-containing intravenous fluids with a goal glucose infusion rate (GIR) of 5–7mg of carbohydrate (CHO) per kilogram per minute is required. Acid suppression is important, and an intravenous proton pump inhibitor infusion is often initiated. The use of N-acetylcysteine in neonatal ALF has not been studied. Its use in non-acetaminophen-induced pediatric ALF also is controversial.[48]

The development of ascites often requires a diuretic regimen with a combination of furosemide and spironolactone, occasionally in conjunction with albumin infusions if hypoalbuminemia is significant. If ascites impedes respiratory effort, it may be necessary to perform a therapeutic paracentesis.

Closely monitor renal function as a considerable proportion of neonates required hemodialysis or continuous venovenous hemofiltration (CVVH), which is difficult to perform in such small patients. CVVH without heparin is started for renal insufficiency (oliguria, elevated creatinine, volume overload, or electrolyte imbalance), hyperammonemia resistant to treatment, and hepatorenal syndrome.

Respiratory

Usually, infants with severe coagulopathy and encephalopathy are intubated.

Cardiovascular

Circulatory changes can be similar to systemic inflammatory response syndrome. Depressed cardiac function can be evident. Support with inotropic agents may be necessary.

Hematologic

Thrombocytopenia, coagulopathy, and disseminated intravascular coagulation contribute to the risk of bleeding, and bleeding complications are more common in neonates than in older children. Monitor the coagulation profile and fibrinogen at least once daily. Patients should receive vitamin K 2.5 mg IV daily. To correct coagulopathy if the INR is more than 2.5–3, there is active bleeding, or a procedure is planned, give fresh-frozen plasma (FFP) 10 mL/kg over 30 minutes. Occasionally, a continuous infusion of fresh frozen plasma (FFP) is needed (10 mL/kg every 4 hours) to prevent bleeding. Cryoglobulin 5 mL/kg over 30 minutes (1 unit = 15–20 mL) is given if the fibrinogen value is less than 100. Consider collecting or storing blood specimens for further workup prior to administration of blood products.

Neurologic

Use sedation and pain medications only if absolutely necessary. Avoid benzodiazepines as clearance is dependent on liver function. Frequent neurologic assessments for excessive crying, poor feeding, and sleepiness are needed as these can be signs of cerebral irritation, which can progress to lethargy and coma. Encephalopathy can be a subtle finding, but it occurs commonly in neonates, especially in metabolic liver disease. It is important to monitor ammonia levels daily, as these correlate well with degree of liver dysfunction, although not with the degree of encephalopathy. Lactulose, an osmotic laxative (1–3 mL/kg per day in divided doses), can be given orally or by nasogastric tube to treat hyperammonemia. Bacteria degrade the lactulose, creating an acidic environment that inhibits diffusion of NH_3 into the blood and enhances diffusion of NH_3 into the gut lumen, where conversion from NH_3 to NH_4^+ occurs. Monitor for signs of cerebral edema. Noncontrast head computed tomography (CT) can assess for cerebral edema or intracranial bleeding. Mannitol remains the treatment of increased intracranial pressure.

Infectious

Consider starting broad-spectrum antibiotics, including acyclovir, for infectious processes. Antifungal prophylaxis should also be considered. Secondary infection and sepsis are common in ALF because of decreased hepatic clearance of bacteria and enhanced inflammatory processes due to hepatic dysfunction.[49] Malnutrition also contributes to their risk of bacterial infections.

Other

Other conditions that can occur in neonatal ALF include pancreatitis and depressed cardiac function.

Table 40-3 provides information on the medical management of cholestasis and liver failure.

Liver Transplant

A PELD (Pediatric End-Stage Liver Disease) score represents the score on a continuous severity scale to determine the need for a liver transplant for children less than 12 years of age. It is calculated by a formula incorporating serum bilirubin and albumin levels, INR, growth failure, and age at listing. The Organ Procurement and Transplantation Network website, which supervises the allocation of donor organs, has an online PELD calculator (http://optn.transplant.hrsa.gov/resources/MeldPeldCalculator.asp?index=99).

Absolute contraindications for liver transplantation include permanently fixed and dilated pupils,

Table 40-3 Medical Management of Neonatal Cholestasis and Liver Failure

Malabsorption/malnutrition	
Optimize caloric intake	
Feed fortification/concentration	
Fat supplementation (30%–50% as MCTs)	Consider pregestimil or MCT oil supplement
Ranitidine	2–4 mg/kg/d divided twice daily
Pantoprazole	0.5–1 mg/kg/d divided twice daily
Vitamin and micronutrients	
Monitor for fat-soluble vitamin deficiencies Check for response to replacement	Vitamin A 5000–25,000 IU/d Vitamin D 600–2000 IU/d Vitamin E 15–25 IU/kg/d Vitamin K 2.5–5 mg/d
Pruritis associated with cholestasis	
Ursodiol	10 mg/kg/dose 3 times daily
Rifampin	10–20 mg/kg/d
Ascites	
Sodium restriction	
Diuretic therapy Furosemide Spironolactone	0.5–2 mg/kg/dose up to 4 times daily 1–3 mg/kg/d divided twice daily
Therapeutic paracentesis	
Portal hypertension and variceal hemorrhage	
Fresh-frozen plasma if INR >2.5–3	Up to 10 mL/kg over 30 minutes every 4 hours
Cryoglobulin if fibrinogen < 100	5 mL/kg over 30 minutes
Endoscopic sclerotherapy	
Surgical shunt procedure	
Encephalopathy	
Lactulose	1–3 mL/kg/d in divided doses, goal 2–3 loose stools per day
Specific therapy	
NTBC (tyrosinemia)	0.5 mg/kg/dose twice daily
Acyclovir (suspected sepsis, HSV)	10–20 mg/kg/dose 3 times daily

Abbreviations: HSV, herpes simplex virus; NTBC, 2-(2-nitro-4-trifluoromethyl-benzoyl)-1,3-cyclohexandione; INR, international normalized ratio; MCT, medium-chain triglycerides.
[a]Data from Clayton P et al,[4] with permission; Nightingale S, Ng VL.[50,p739] Copyright Elsevier with permission.

uncontrolled sepsis, and multiorgan failure. Possible contraindications include metabolic disease that may respond to specific medical therapy or affect other organs, significant neurologic involvement, HLH, HIV, and neonatal leukemia.[51]

Donor organs for neonates are rarely full-size grafts. Grafts from donors less than 6 kg are associated with higher risk of graft failure. The most common graft is a left lateral segment allograft from infant and young child donors. These technical variant grafts such have longer cold ischemia times, higher risk of primary nonfunction, poor early function, and higher risk of postoperative bleeding and bile leaks. There is also a higher incidence of vascular thrombosis, specifically hepatic artery thrombosis. Neonates can receive ABO-incompatible donors since they lack prior sensitization to major blood group antigens. There is no decrease in graft survival with ABO-incompatible grafts at both 1 and 5 years posttransplantation.[52]

OUTCOMES

Neonatal ALF is rare, and the outcome is generally poor. There are many diagnostic considerations to make. The use of emergent orthotopic liver transplantation has improved outcomes in some of these children.

The Pediatric Acute Liver Failure study group, a multicenter prospective study of pediatric patients with ALF, analyzed 148 infants at less than 90 days of life with acute liver injury combined with either severe coagulopathy or encephalopathy with moderate coagulopathy. Follow-up of the patients was 3 weeks. The most common etiologies of ALF were indeterminate (38%), neonatal hemochromatosis (14%), and HSV (13%). Only 41% of infants with ALF were listed for transplantation, and 16% underwent liver transplantation. Infants with an indeterminate cause of liver failure were more likely to undergo liver transplantation. Spontaneous survival without liver transplantation occurred in 60% of infants, and 24% died without liver transplantation. Spontaneous survival and the rate of transplantation were lower in neonates compared to older children with ALF.[2] The mortality rate of young infants (≤90 days of life) was 24% compared to 10.5% of children. There was a significantly higher incidence of death in infants with viral ALF (64%) vs metabolic disease (20%), neonatal hemochromatosis (16%), or indeterminate causes (14%).[53]

Given their critical condition at transplantation, infants younger than 90 days are thought to experience high complication rates and prolonged hospital stays with poor graft and patient survival.

A review of 38 patients between 0 and 90 days of life at the time of transplant was conducted by Sundaram et al. Median follow-up was 12.5 months. The mean PELD score was 34.8 at the time of transplant. The 2 most common indications for transplantation were fulminant hepatic failure of unknown etiology (39%) and metabolic diseases (34%), including neonatal hemochromatosis (24%). These neonates had hospitalizations that were significantly more prolonged (50.9 ± 7.6 days), longer intensive care unit stays (22.1 ± 1.5 days), and longer needs for ventilation (16.2 ± 2.7 days) than older pediatric recipients. The reoperation rate (65%) and postoperative bacterial infection rate (52.6%) were significantly higher than for older pediatric patients. Reoperations occurred for bleeding, wound complications, biliary complications, and sepsis. The overall graft survival was 76.1%, and patient survival was 87.8% at 1 year, similar to older children.[54]

Neonatal hepatitis and ALF can be a diagnostic dilemma. It demands systematic evaluation to help guide treatment decisions. Many diagnoses can progress to chronic liver disease. ALF demands critical and comprehensive care. Liver transplantation in neonates at an experienced transplant center may be an option for improved survival, although complications are common.

REFERENCES

1. Suchy FJ, Sokol RJ, Balistreri WF. *Liver Diseases in Children*. 3rd ed. Cambridge, UK: Cambridge University Press; 2007.
2. Squires RH Jr, Shneider BL, Bucuvalas J, et al. Acute liver failure in children: the first 348 patients in the pediatric acute liver failure study group. *J Pediatr*. 2006;148(5):652–658.
3. Torbenson M, Hart J, Westerhoff M, et al. Neonatal giant cell hepatitis: histological and etiological findings. *Am J Surg Pathol*. 2010;34(10):1498–1503.
4. Clayton PT. Inborn errors presenting with liver dysfunction. *Semin Neonatol*. 2002;7(1):49–63.
5. Roush SW, Murphy TV. Historical comparisons of morbidity and mortality for vaccine-preventable diseases in the United States. *JAMA*. 2007;298(18):2155–2163.
6. Modlin JF, Grant PE, Makar RS, Roberts DJ, Krishnamoorthy KS. Case records of the Massachusetts General Hospital. Weekly clinicopathological exercises. Case 25-2003. A newborn boy with petechiae and thrombocytopenia. *N Engl J Med*. 2003;349(7):691–700.
7. Fowler KB, Stagno S, Pass RF, et al. The outcome of congenital cytomegalovirus infection in relation to maternal antibody status. *N Engl J Med*. 1992;326(10):663–667.
8. Vancíková Z, Kucerová T, Pelikán L, Zikmundová L, Priglová M. Perinatal cytomegalovirus hepatitis: to treat or not to treat with ganciclovir. *J Paediatr Child Health*. 2004;40(8):444–448.
9. Nazareth KM, Ngo PD. Neonatal herpetic hepatitis. *J Pediatr Gastroenterol Nutr*. 2011;52(6):645.
10. Fagan EA, Hadzic N, Saxena R, Mieli-Vergani G. Symptomatic neonatal hepatitis A disease from a virus variant acquired in utero. *Pediatr Infect Dis J*. 1999;18(4):389–391.
11. Delaplane D, Yogev R, Crussi F, Shulman ST. Fatal hepatitis B in early infancy: the importance of identifying HBsAg-positive pregnant women and providing immunoprophylaxis to their newborns. *Pediatrics*. 1983;72(2):176–180.
12. Recommendations for prevention and control of hepatitis C virus (HCV) infection and HCV-related chronic disease. Centers for Disease Control and Prevention. *MMWR Recomm Rep*. 1998;47(RR-19):1–39.
13. Roberts EA. Neonatal hepatitis syndrome. *Semin Neonatol*. 2003;8(5):357–374.
14. Khuroo MS, Kamili S, Khuroo MS. Clinical course and duration of viremia in vertically transmitted hepatitis E virus (HEV) infection in babies born to HEV-infected mothers. *J Viral Hepat*. 2009;16(7):519–523.
15. Increased detection and severe neonatal disease associated with coxsackievirus B1 infection—United States, 2007. *MMWR Morb Mortal Wkly Rep*. 2008;57(20):553–556.
16. Long WW, Pawel B, Morrow G 3rd. Pathological case of the month. Hereditary fructose intolerance. *Arch Pediatr Adolesc Med*. 1997;151(11):1165–1166.
17. Saenz MS, Van Hove J, Scharer G. Neonatal liver failure: a genetic and metabolic perspective. *Curr Opin Pediatr*. 2010;22(2):241–245.
18. Francavilla R, Castellaneta SP, Hadzic N, et al. Prognosis of alpha-1-antitrypsin deficiency-related liver disease in the era of paediatric liver transplantation. *J Hepatol*. 2000;32(6):986–992.
19. Hirabayashi K, Shiohara M, Takahashi D, et al. Retrospective analysis of risk factors for development of liver dysfunction in transient leukemia of Down syndrome. *Leuk Lymphoma*. 2011;52(8):1523–1527.
20. Alpert LI, Strauss L, Hirschhorn K. Neonatal hepatitis and biliary atresia associated with trisomy 17–18 syndrome. *N Engl J Med*. 1969;280(1):16–20.
21. Clayton PT. Disorders of bile acid synthesis. *J Inherit Metab Dis*. 2011;34(3):593–604.
22. McClean P, Davison SM. Neonatal liver failure. *Semin Neonatol*. 2003;8(5):393–401.
23. Sokol RJ, Treem WR. Mitochondria and childhood liver diseases. *J Pediatr Gastroenterol Nutr*. 1999;28(1):4–16.
24. Lee WS, Sokol RJ. Liver disease in mitochondrial disorders. *Semin Liver Dis*. 2007;27(3):259–273.
25. Whitington PF. Neonatal hemochromatosis: a congenital alloimmune hepatitis. *Semin Liver Dis*. 2007;27(3):243–250.

26. Whitington PF, Malladi P. Neonatal hemochromatosis: is it an alloimmune disease? *J Pediatr Gastroenterol Nutr.* 2005;40(5):544–549.

27. Lee LA, Sokol RJ, Buyon JP. Hepatobiliary disease in neonatal lupus: prevalence and clinical characteristics in cases enrolled in a national registry. *Pediatrics.* 2002;109(1):E11.

28. Silverman E, Jaeggi E. Non-cardiac manifestations of neonatal lupus erythematosus. *Scand J Immunol.* 2010;72(3):223–225.

29. Janka GE. Familial and acquired hemophagocytic lymphohistiocytosis. *Eur J Pediatr.* 2007;166(2):95–109.

30. Chen J-H, Fleming MD, Pinkus GS, et al. Pathology of the liver in familial hemophagocytic lymphohistiocytosis. *Am J Surg Pathol.* 2010;34(6):852–867.

31. Lindamood KE, Fleck P, Narla A, et al. Neonatal enteroviral sepsis/meningoencephalitis and hemophagocytic lymphohistiocytosis: diagnostic challenges. *Am J Perinatol.* 2011;28(5):337–346.

32. Makin E, Davenport M. Fetal and neonatal liver tumours. *Early Hum Dev.* 2010;86(10):637–642.

33. Isaacs H Jr. Fetal and neonatal hepatic tumors. *J Pediatr Surg.* 2007;42(11):1797–1803.

34. Bergounioux J, Franchi-Abella S, Monneret S, Essouri S, Jacquemin E. Neonatal ischemic liver failure: potential role of the ductus venosus. *J Pediatr Gastroenterol Nutr.* 2004;38(5):542–544.

35. Ernst LM, Grossman AB, Ruchelli ED. Familial perinatal liver disease and fetal thrombotic vasculopathy. *Pediatr Dev Pathol.* 2008;11(2):160–163.

36. Henter J-I, Horne A, Aricó M, et al. HLH-2004: diagnostic and therapeutic guidelines for hemophagocytic lymphohistiocytosis. *Pediatr Blood Cancer.* 2007;48(2):124–131.

37. Cies JJ, Giamalis JN. Treatment of cholestatic pruritus in children. *Am J Health-Syst Pharm.* 2007;64(11):1157–1162.

38. Arshad M, El-Kamary SS, Jhaveri R. Hepatitis C virus infection during pregnancy and the newborn period—are they opportunities for treatment? *J Viral Hepat.* 2011;18(4):229–236.

39. Verma A, Dhawan A, Zuckerman M, et al. Neonatal herpes simplex virus infection presenting as acute liver failure: prevalent role of herpes simplex virus type I. *J Pediatr Gastroenterol Nutr.* 2006;42(3):282–286.

40. Hollier LM, Wendel GD. Third trimester antiviral prophylaxis for preventing maternal genital herpes simplex virus (HSV) recurrences and neonatal infection. *Cochrane Database Syst Rev.* 2008;(1):CD004946.

41. Holme E, Lindstedt S. Tyrosinaemia type I and NTBC (2-(2-nitro-4-trifluoromethylbenzoyl)-1,3-cyclohexanedione). *J Inherit Metab Dis.* 1998;21(5):507–517.

42. Chinnery P, Majamaa K, Turnbull D, Thorburn D. Treatment for mitochondrial disorders. *Cochrane Database Syst Rev.* 2006;(1):CD004426.

43. Whitington PF, Kelly S, Ekong UD. Neonatal hemochromatosis: fetal liver disease leading to liver failure in the fetus and newborn. *Pediatr Transplant.* 2005;9(5):640–645.

44. Rodrigues F, Kallas M, Nash R, et al. Neonatal hemochromatosis—medical treatment vs transplantation: the king's experience. *Liver Transpl.* 2005;11(11):1417–1424.

45. Leonis MA, Balistreri WF. Neonatal hemochromatosis: it's OK to say "NO" to antioxidant-chelator therapy. *Liver Transpl.* 2005;11(11):1323–1325.

46. Whitington PF, Kelly S. Outcome of pregnancies at risk for neonatal hemochromatosis is improved by treatment with high-dose intravenous immunoglobulin. *Pediatrics.* 2008;121(6):e1615–e1621.

47. Rand EB, Karpen SJ, Kelly S, et al. Treatment of neonatal hemochromatosis with exchange transfusion and intravenous immunoglobulin. *J Pediatr.* 2009;155(4):566–571.

48. Kortsalioudaki C, Taylor RM, Cheeseman P, et al. Safety and efficacy of N-acetylcysteine in children with non-acetaminophen-induced acute liver failure. *Liver Transpl.* 2008;14(1):25–30.

49. Dhainaut JF, Marin N, Mignon A, Vinsonneau C. Hepatic response to sepsis: interaction between coagulation and inflammatory processes. *Crit Care Med.* 2001;29(7 Suppl):S42–S47.

50. Nightingale S, Ng VL. Neonatal hepatitis. In: Wyllie R, Hyams JS, eds. *Pediatric Gastrointestinal and Liver Diseases.* 4th ed. Boston, MA: Saunders; 2011:728–740.

51. Durand P, Debray D, Mandel R, et al. Acute liver failure in infancy: a 14-year experience of a pediatric liver transplantation center. *J Pediatr.* 2001;139(6):871–876.

52. Cacciarelli TV, Esquivel CO, Moore DH, et al. Factors affecting survival after orthotopic liver transplantation in infants. *Transplantation.* 1997;64(2):242–248.

53. Sundaram SS, Alonso EM, Narkewicz MR, Zhang S, Squires RH. Characterization and outcomes of young infants with acute liver failure. *J Pediatr.* 2011;159(5):813–818.e1

54. Sundaram SS, Alonso EM, Anand R. Outcomes after liver transplantation in young infants. *J Pediatr Gastroenterol Nutr.* 2008;47(4):486–492.

CHAPTER 40

41

Biliary Tract Anomalies

Amy Lightner and Waldo Concepcion

BILIARY ATRESIA

Epidemiology

Although biliary atresia is a rare disorder, it is the most common surgically correctable liver disorder in infancy. The most accurate estimates of national prevalence come from the United Kingdom and France, where 1 in 17,000–19,000 live-born infants are affected.[1,2] East Asian countries are most commonly affected, with a reported frequency of 1 in 5000 in Taiwan.[3] Other reported estimates are 1 in 15,000 in the southeastern United Sates[4] and 1 in 19,000 in the Netherlands.[5] Within these regions, there appears to be a higher incidence of the disease in non-white populations (African American, French Polynesian, and Chinese) and among females (1.25:1).[6,7]

Up to 20% of all cases of biliary atresia are associated with other anatomical abnormalities, suggesting that the pathologic process begins in the embryonic period. The most common congenital cluster of malformations is biliary atresia splenic malformation (BASM) syndrome, seen in approximately 10% of European and US series. BASM includes biliary atresia in association with polysplenia (90%), situs inversus (50%), and unusual vascular anomalies. In utero, there may also be an association with maternal diabetes and genetic anomalies such as trisomy 18 and 21.

In the other 80% of neonates with biliary atresia, the disorder appears to be a sporadic event with an unknown etiology, and the pathological obliterative process begins later in the perinatal period. Classic genetic inheritance is not supported by any clinical evidence as the disorder is rarely seen within families and, when seen in twins, is rarely concordant.[8] Some studies have suggested time-space clustering of cases and seasonal variation, with the majority of cases occurring in the fall and winter months (December–March),[9,10] but large population-based studies from France, Sweden, and Japan have failed to identify significant seasonal or time-space clustering.[9–12] After controlling for geographic and racial factors, associations have been made with advanced maternal age and increased parity, but not with smoking, maternal age, education, alcohol use, folic acid intake, gravidity, parental income, infant sex, preterm birth, infant birthweight, or plurality.[5,9,12]

Pathophysiology

Although histopathologic features of biliary atresia have been extensively studied in surgical specimens from excised extrahepatic biliary systems of infants, the pathogenesis of this disorder remains an unanswered question. Because some infants with biliary atresia are born with other congenital malformations, early studies postulated the etiology was a congenital malformation of the biliary ductal system. However, the majority of patients have isolated biliary atresia with progressive inflammatory lesions on histology occurring in the perinatal period. Therefore, it might be that biliary atresia represents a final common phenotypic pathway of neonatal liver injury caused by a diverse group of etiologies, including viral, inflammatory, immune dysregulation, or toxic exposure in genetically predisposed individuals[5] (Figure 41-1).

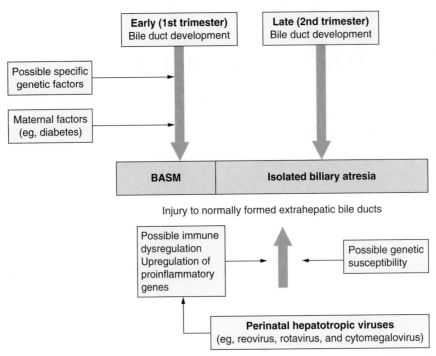

FIGURE 41-1 Possible causal relations in biliary atresia. BASM, biliary atresia splenic malformation. (Reprinted from *The Lancet*, Hartley, Davenport, and Kelly.[5])

Genetics

There is a growing body of evidence supporting the involvement of specific genes in both embryonic (somatic mutations of genes involved in morphogenesis of the biliary tree) and perinatal (genetic predisposition to an aberrant immune response to exogenous stimuli) biliary atresia. In the embryonic form, underlying genetic mutations may lead to morphologic abnormalities. In mice, a mutation of the *INVS* gene can cause morphologic change resembling biliary atresia.[13] In these mice, morphological analysis of the hepatobiliary system by Trypan blue cholangiography and technetium 99m-labeled tracer demonstrated a defect in patency of the extrahepatic ductular system and absent biliary excretion.[14] Inconsistent with the diagnosis, however, is the complete absence of inflammation or necrosis within hepatic parenchyma and absence of inflammation and fibrosis of the extrahepatic biliary tree.[14,15] In addition, human studies of the *INVS* gene did not support the finding of morphologic defects.[16] Other genetic etiologies of morphologic changes in mice have been proposed, including abnormalities in *(HNF)-6* and *HNF-1B*.[17,18] and constitutional or delayed inactivation of genes *Hes1*, *Foxf1*, and *Foxm1b*,[19–21] but these are still being investigated. In the perinatal form, genetics may be the foundation for further infectious or inflammatory insult. For example, alterations in genes, including CFC1, *ICAM1* (intercellular adhesion molecule 1), macrophage migration inhibitory factor gene, CD14 endotoxin receptor gene, and hepcidin antimicrobial peptide gene, can speed the progression of biliary fibrosis.[22–25]

Viral

The possibility of a viral infection acting as the initiating event for biliary atresia was first suggested by Landing, who saw biliary atresia along a continuum with choledochal cysts and neonatal intrahepatic cholestasis, all of which could be linked by a shared infectious insult.[26] Since the introduction of this concept, viral pathogenesis of nonsyndromic causes of biliary atresia has been studied in animals and humans. Inoculation of mice with rotavirus strains RRV and SA11-FM,[27] reovirus, and cytomegalovirus (CMV)[28,29] has resulted in jaundice with intrahepatic histology similar to biliary atresia. In humans, an interesting study of viral infection in biliary atresia was conducted by Rauschenfels and coworkers,[30] who used wedge liver biopsy samples obtained from 74 infants at Kasai portoenterostomy to look for a panel of DNA and RNA hepatotropic viruses and Mx protein, a marker of inflammation secondary to viruses. A third of infants had evidence of viruses, and this finding increased with age, suggesting that the viral component may be a secondary insult to the specific cause of biliary atresia. Ninety percent of infants expressed Mx protein, suggesting that there is ongoing inflammation secondary to the immune response, perhaps mounted from a viral infection.[30] Additional supporting evidence of a viral etiology are hepatitis B virus antigens detected in the liver of infants with biliary atresia in Japan,[31] prevalence of antibodies against reovirus type 3 and the detection of the virus in hepatobiliary specimens of patients with biliary atresia,[32-35] and a study demonstrating that reverse transcription–polymerase chain reaction (RT-PCR) identified reovirus in 55% of hepatobiliary samples from patients with biliary atresia.[36] Also suggestive of a viral role is that CMV infection in infants with biliary atresia has a severe clinical course, with low rates of jaundice clearance and raised rates of cholangitis and liver fibrosis.[37] However, negating this suggestion of viral etiology is that viral particles in the liver or biliary tract of infected infants have not been reproducible across studies conducted at different time points or in different locations. This inconsistency and lack of reproducibility may be due to the clearance of direct viral traces by an inflammatory reaction or simply lack of consistent viral etiology.[38]

Inflammation/Immunology

Interestingly, when an infant has biliary atresia, there is a pronounced inflammatory response in both the liver and circulation. In the liver, mononuclear cells infiltrate the periductal space, and the vascular and biliary epithelium have increased expression of HLA-DR and intracellular adhesion molecules such as ICAM1 and E selectin.[39] Simultaneously, the circulation has increased numbers of soluble inflammatory adhesion molecules and cytokines, even when a successful Kasai portoenterostomy has been performed. Although it appears that the bile duct damage is most likely lymphocyte-mediated biliary inflammation, the trigger for this response remains unknown.

Given the histologic features of progressive inflammation, various studies have implicated immune dysregulation, either as a primary disorder or as the result of infectious or genetic triggers, as a potential link with biliary atresia. In patients with biliary atresia, inflammatory cytokines such as interlukin 2, interleukin 12, interferon γ (IFN-γ), and tumor necrosis factor α (TNF-α) are upregulated along with Kuppfer cells, natural killer (NK) cells, CD3+ and CD8+ T cells, and CXCR3+ cells.[40] Of note, the oligoclonal expansion of CD4+ and CD8+ T cells within the liver and extrahepatic bile ducts is suggestive of a response to specific antigenic stimulation.[41] An example of a specific infectious trigger is the development of biliary atresia in mice after inoculation with rotavirus is increased when type I IFN receptor is inactivated.[42] and the tissue-specific hepatobiliary inflammation induced by dysregulation of gamma interferon after inoculation with rotavirus.[43] Genetic triggers of immune dysregulation may also play a role. Coordinated activation of genes involved with lymphocyte differentiation, particularly those associated with T helper 1 immunity, has been

identified in liver samples from infants with biliary atresia.[5] Polymorphisms that enhance expression of the CD14 gene, which plays a role in the recognition of bacterial endotoxin, have been associated with biliary atresia.[5] Gene expression microarrays of RNA from extrahepatic tissue and gallbladders in rotavirus-induced murine models of biliary atresia have shown upregulation of many genes regulating immunity.[44] Microarrays from human samples have also shown an overexpression of immune regulatory genes.[45]

Graft-vs-host issues may also play a role, as demonstrated by a high concentration of maternal chimeric cells that have been found in the portal and sinusoidal areas of patients with biliary atresia, suggesting that maternal lymphocytes cause bile duct injury through a graft-vs-host immune response.[46]

Toxic Insult

The only supportive patient-based evidence for the role of a toxic insult as a causative factor of biliary atresia is the time-space clustering of cases. In Australia between 1964 and 1988, there were unusual outbreaks of hepatobiliary injury in lambs and calves in New South Wales. However, despite localized outbreaks, there were no causative phytotoxins or myotoxins discovered through exhaustive investigation.[47]

Differential Diagnosis

There is a high degree of overlap in clinical, radiologic, and histologic characteristics of biliary atresia and other causes of hepatitis in the neonatal period. The differential is broad and includes structural, genetic, infectious, and metabolic conditions.[48] Some of these conditions include anatomic (choledochal cyst, bile duct stenosis, sclerosing cholangitis of the newborn, cholelithiasis, tumors/masses); infectious (viral, bacterial); metabolic/genetic (Alagille syndrome [AGS], disorders of amino acid metabolism, disorder of glucose metabolism, cystic fibrosis); and toxic insult (parenteral nutrition, drugs).

Infants with biliary atresia are typically born full term with normal birthweight. Shortly after birth, these infants present with persistent jaundice, pale stools, and dark urine. All premature and term infants who remain jaundiced after 21 and 14 days, respectively, should have serologic laboratory tests to evaluate potential liver disease. The cardinal biochemical feature of biliary atresia is conjugated hyperbilirubinemia. However, there is considerable overlap in the clinical, biochemical, radiologic, and histologic features of biliary atresia and other causes of neonatal jaundice on the differential. Radiologic tests are important in making an accurate and timely diagnosis, essential for timely surgical intervention. Prompt intervention is recommended as operative success is highest before 60 days, and efficacy declines as the infant ages.[48]

Diagnostic Tests

Initial diagnostic testing includes laboratory studies to identify cholestatic liver disease[5] (Figure 41-2). Of note, serum γ-glutamyltransferase (GGT) is usually higher in biliary atresia than in other causes of neonatal cholestasis, especially when correlated with age.[49]

Ultrasound is the first step in imaging and is useful for excluding other causes of neonatal jaundice. An abdominal ultrasound will show an enlarged liver, absence of biliary dilation due to the inflammatory process, an absent or contracted gallbladder after a 4-hour fast,[50] or a triangular cord sign (triangular or band-like echogenic density seen just above the porta hepatis).[51] The sensitivity and specificity of a small or absent gallbladder in detecting biliary atresia range from 73% to 100% and 67% to 100%, respectively, when combined with clinical, pathologic, and subsequent surgical evaluations. The triangular cord sign is highly suggestive of biliary atresia[52,53] but is operatordependent, with reported sensitivities varying from 49% to 73%[54] to 83%–100% and with specificity of 98%–100%.[55]

Hepatobiliary scintigraphy (hepatobiliary iminodiacetic acid [HIDA] scan) can help distinguish biliary atresia from other etiologies of conjugated hyperbilirubinemia that do not need early surgical intervention[56,57] by demonstrating the failure of bile excretion into the bowel. The reported sensitivity and specificity are 100% and 40%–100%, respectively.[48] Improved specificity and sensitivity have been reported if the patient is premedicated with phenobarbital 5 mg/kg for 5 days.[48] However, the specificity limits this radiographic tool in diagnosing biliary atresia.

Liver histology obtained on percutaneous biopsy is often considered the gold standard for the diagnosis of biliary atresia. One group reported accuracy of 96%–98% if the specimen contained at least 5–7 portal spaces,[58] while another review reported that biliary atresia was only diagnosed correctly in 50%–99% of cases.[55] Typical pathologic findings are extrahepatic biliary obstruction by varying degrees of portal tract

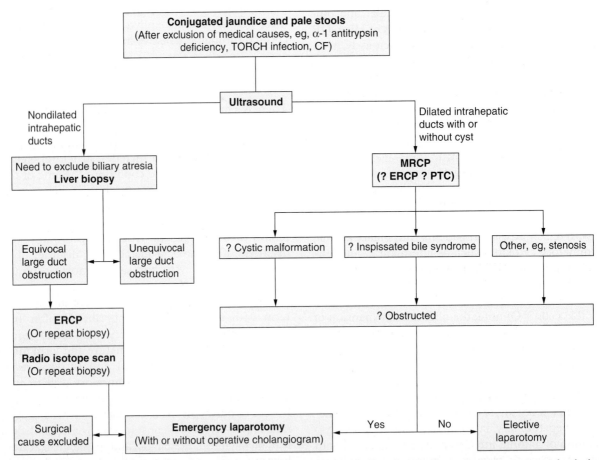

FIGURE 41-2 Suggested algorithm for investigation of infants. CF, cystic fibrosis; ERCP, endoscopic retrograde cholangiopancreatography; MRCP, magnetic resonance retrograde cholangiopancreatography; PTC, percutaneous transhepatic cholangiography; TORCH, toxoplasmosis, rubella, cytomegalovirus, herpes simplex virus. (Reprinted from *The Lancet*, Hartley, Davenport, and Kelly.[5])

fibrosis, edema, ductular proliferation, and cholestasis with the appearance of bile plugs. The possible presence of giant cell transformation may make the differentiation from other causes of neonatal hepatitis difficult. Of note, liver biopsy samples taken before 6 weeks of age, in the early development of biliary atresia, might not have the typical histologic features necessary for diagnosis.[59]

When the diagnosis is unclear, endoscopic retrograde cholangiopancreatography (ERCP) to visualize the biliary tract may be useful. Data supporting ERCP are that it is technically possible in 90% of infants and gives few false positives.[60] However, it is a technically challenging procedure in neonates and generally not an option unless in a large center. Also, data supporting the use of ERCP for the diagnosis of biliary atresia are sparse. Magnetic resonance retrograde cholangiopancreatography (MRCP) has been evaluated as another potentially helpful tool for diagnosing biliary atresia, and results from initial studies are promising. In 2 recent studies, the negative and positive predictive values of MRCP detecting biliary atresia were from 91% to 100% and from 75% to 96%, respectively.[61,62] The challenge with MRCP is the technical constraints in identification of luminal patency of the infantile bile ducts, which is often only 1 mm diameter or less.[63] However, this noninvasive test may become more useful as it becomes more commonplace for radiologists and as the technology improves.

The true diagnostic gold standard is the intraoperative cholangiogram, done laparoscopically if there is doubt regarding the diagnosis before proceeding with Kasai portoenterostomy. If the diagnosis is made at the time of the cholangiogram, the surgeon can then proceed with the portoenterostomy.

Management

Portoenterostomy and liver transplantation remain the cornerstones of treatment of biliary atresia. Portoenterostomy, or the Kasai portoenterostomy, named after the Japanese surgeon Morio Kasai, who described the technique in the 1950s, is a procedure in which the entire extrahepatic biliary tree is excised so that the porta hepatis is transected at the level of the liver capsule, and the ductules that remain are exposed. A jejunal Roux loop is then anastomosed to the cut surface, completing a reconstruction (Figure 41-3). If successful, any patent intrahepatic bile ducts will drain into the Roux limb, allowing relief of the biliary obstruction. If possible, the Kasai procedure should be performed before 60 days of age when its short-term success is 80%.[2,11,64] Efficacy of the procedure is thought to drop with age. However, this drop in efficacy may be limited to the less-common subgroups of patients with biliary atresia, including those with BASM syndrome or cystic

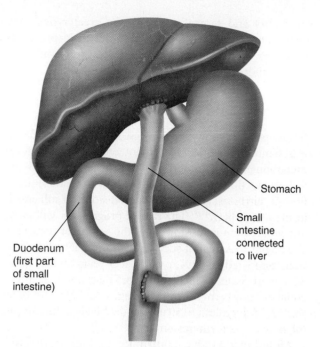

FIGURE 41-3 Kasai procedure. To perform the Kasai procedure, surgeons first carefully remove the damaged ducts outside the liver. They use a small segment of the patient's own intestine to replace the ducts at the spot where bile is expected to drain. This segment not only connects to the liver but also connects to the rest of the intestine. The Y-shaped passageway formed by the Kasai procedure allows bile to flow from the liver into the intestine.

biliary atresia. Supporting this notion is a large series that reported that children older than 100 days with isolated biliary atresia still had a native liver survival rate of 45% at 5 years.[5,65]

Because Kasai portoenterostomy is a palliative procedure and is not curative for biliary atresia, liver transplantation is the ultimate definitive therapy. Indications for liver transplantation depend on the success of the portoenterostomy and the rate of development of complications.[5] In those infants who do not achieve adequate bile drainage with portoenterostomy, transplantation is usually indicated within 6 months to 2 years of age. In those children who had a successful portoenterostomy, liver transplantation is considered when the child has persistent or progressive cholestasis, development of cirrhosis with hepatic dysfunction, or development of portal hypertension with ascites and variceal bleeding unresponsive to endoscopic management. Factors that may predict the need for a liver transplantation are the bilirubin value 30 days postportoenterostomy[66] and a score approaching 10 for pediatric end-stage liver disease assessment.[67]

In those children who have syndromic variants of biliary atresia rather than isolated biliary atresia, the associated anomalies increase the risk of early morbidity and mortality, creating a greater need for liver transplantation. Despite the increased potential for other anatomic anomalies, results are similar to those children with isolated biliary atresia.[68]

Outcome and Follow-up

Intrahepatic inflammatory processes will continue for at least 6 months after Kasai portoenterostomy.[37] Therefore, even though the procedure may provide relief of mechanical obstruction and restoration of bile flow, subsequent fibrosis, cirrhosis, and portal hypertension will still ensue in the native liver.[45,69] The rate of progression will vary, but progression is most likely in the setting of recurrent cholangitis.[70] Actuarial survival with the native liver has been estimated at 32% to 61% at 5 years and 27% to 54% at 10 years of life.[71-73] Factors that are most influential on long-term outcome are age (<60 days) and the size of the ductules (>150 μm) in the biliary remnants at the time of portoenterostomy.[71,74,75]

Other factors that contribute to long-term outcomes are episodes of cholangitis after surgery, the decade when surgery was performed, and the experience of the surgical team.[72,76] In Japan, the actuarial survival of 307 patients treated with portoenterostomy improved[71] from 20% before 1971 to 70% between 1971 and 1998. In the United Kingdom, a prospective study from 1993 to 1995 identified 93 cases of biliary atresia and showed that of 15 UK centers, only 2 operated on 5 or more cases per year, which resulted in a statistically significant difference in 5-year native liver survival (63% in centers with 5 or more cases and 14% in others) and overall survival.[1] The higher success rates in larger-volume centers was confirmed by studies in France, which had improved survival rates.[2]

Those countries using living-related transplantation are reporting excellent outcomes, with 98% recipient 5-year survival.[77] The largest follow-up study data from the United States reported 10-year actuarial graft survival of 73% and patient survival of 86% across 1976 patients.[78] Transplantation also improves long-term catchup growth, nutrition, and maintenance of healthy development.[79]

ALAGILLE SYNDROME

Epidemiology

Alagille syndrome, first described in 1967, is an autosomal dominant genetic disorder affecting 1 in 30,000 live births,[80] with variable expressivity of multisystem disease. The syndrome is characterized by a paucity of interlobular bile ducts with other associated features, including cholestasis (present in 96% of patients),

cardiac anomalies (97%), butterfly vertebrae (51%), posterior embryotoxin of the eye (78%), and dysmorphic facies (96%).[80] The dysmorphic facial features of AGS are described as a broad nasal bridge, triangular facies, and deep-set eyes. Renal anomalies, both functional and structural, and neurovascular accidents are much less common (15%) but can be associated with AGS.[80]

Pathophysiology

Microdeletion of the *20p12* gene corresponding to *JAG1* is thought to result in AGS.[81,82] The *JAG1* gene is involved in signaling between adjacent cells during embryonic development, which influences how the cells are used to build organ systems in the developing embryo. Thus, mutations in *JAG1* disrupt this signaling pathway, resulting in errors of development, especially of the heart, bile ducts in the liver, spinal column, and certain facial features.

When the bile ducts are narrowed and malformed, the bile produced in the liver is unable to be transported to the small intestine. Thus, the bile builds up in the liver and causes scarring and eventual cirrhosis.

Differential Diagnosis

As most infants present with cholestatic jaundice, 1 of the first differentials is biliary atresia. Other differentials considered include congenital hepatic fibrosis, cystic fibrosis, neonatal jaundice, polycystic kidney disease, progressive familial intrahepatic cholestasis, and tyrosinemia.

Diagnostic Testing

Clinical suspicion should drive the initial workup and evaluation of suspected AGS. Because AGS potentially involves many systems, ophthalmologic examination, echocardiogram, and imaging of the vertebrae are all useful in ascertaining the diagnosis. For those infants who present with cholestatic disease, initial evaluation should include liver function tests, prothrombin time, and levels of fat-soluble vitamins. In these patients, an ultrasound should also be considered to rule out biliary atresia. However, there are no ultrasound findings specific to AGS. Hepatobiliary scintigraphy, and intraoperative cholangiogram may also be useful in distinguishing AGS from biliary atresia or choledochal cysts. The challenge with a HIDA scan is that up to 61% of patients with AGS have been reported to have no evidence of tracer excretion from the liver, as would be expected with biliary atresia.[83] In these patients, cholangiogram, either percutaneous or intraoperative, may be useful. If infants with AGS have hypoplasia of the extrahepatic biliary tree,[83] liver biopsy can be useful for diagnosis.

The advent of genetic testing for AGS has led to an increase in diagnosis. Deletion or mutation of the *JAG1* gene on the short arm of chromosome 20 is present in 60% to 70% of patients with AGS.[84] Genetic testing should be conducted for any patient for whom there is suspicion of AGS.

Management

Management of AGS focuses on treatment of the individual components of the disease. Cholestasis is treated medically with choleretics, most commonly ursodiol. Debilitating pruritus from hyperbilirubinemia in AGS can be addressed with antihistamines, sedatives, and rifampin.[85] However, in refractory pruritus, a partial biliary diversion may be needed or even liver transplantation. Synthetic liver function is rarely affected in AGS unless it progresses to end-stage liver disease. Because AGS can be associated with cholestasis resulting in nutritional deficiencies, aggressive nutritional therapy and fat-soluble vitamin supplementation should be provided to prevent development delays in children.[86] Overall, surgical intervention is not recommended for AGS unless the patient progresses to end-stage liver disease, experiences intractable pruritis, has failure to thrive, or develops severe portal hypertension, at which time liver transplantation may be considered. But, for most cases of AGS, surgical intervention has been associated with worsened hepatic outcomes.[87]

Due to several similarities between biliary atresia and AGS, it is of utmost importance to be as certain of the diagnosis as possible before proceeding with portoenterostomy for a child with cholestasis since those with AGS have worsened outcomes after the operation.[87] Some studies have noted that up to 3%–5% of patients undergoing the Kasai procedure for biliary atresia are eventually diagnosed with nonsyndromic bile duct paucity or AGS.

Outcomes and Follow-up

Outcomes are largely affected by whether the patient undergoes liver transplantation and whether there are cardiac anomalies. Of those patients with AGS, 20% end up with end-stage liver disease secondary to chronic cholestasis, severe portal hypertension, or intractable pruritis,[80] each of which is an indication for liver transplantation.[88] For those with and without liver transplantation, 20-year survival is 60% and 80%, respectively,[83] significantly lower than those children who are transplanted for biliary atresia.[89] Prognosis in AGS has been associated with presence of complex heart disease,[83] and cardiac lesions play an important role in prognosis. Overall 20-year survival[83] for all patients with AGS is 75%; for those with significant intracardiac lesions, it is 40%, while those without intracardiac lesions have significantly higher survival at 80%.[83]

CHOLEDOCHAL CYSTS

Epidemiology

Choledochal cysts are a rare medical condition, occurring in 1 in 100,000 to 150,000 live births worldwide, except in Asia, where there appears to be an unexplained higher incidence of 1 in 1000 live births.[90,91] Although the typical presentation for choledochal cysts is a triad of jaundice, abdominal pain, and a right upper quadrant mass, younger children will rarely have all 3 components. Children most commonly present prior to the age of 2, but it is possible for the diagnosis to be made antenatally. There is a female predominance[90] with a female-to-male ratio of 3.5 to1.

Classifications

Choledochal cysts are currently classified by the Todani modification of the Alonzo-Lej classification into 1 of 5 categories depending on number of cysts, intrahepatic vs extrahepatic location, and type of bile duct dilation (Figure 41-4). Type I cysts have cystic dilation of the common bile duct (CBD) alone. Type II cysts have a cystic diverticulum of the extrahepatic CBD. Type III choledochal cysts, otherwise known as choledochoceles, have dilation of the distal CBD within the wall of the duodenum and involve the ampulla of Vater. Type IV choledochal cysts have multiple cystic dilations of the bile ducts (Figure 41-5). These are further classified into subtypes: Type IVA cysts involve multiple intra- and extrahepatic ductal dilations, whereas type IVB cysts involve multiple extrahepatic CBD dilations. Type V choledochal cysts, referred to as Caroli disease, consist of multiple intrahepatic dilations of the bile ducts.[91,92] Although there are many subtypes of choledochal cysts described, 80% to 90% of diagnosed choledochal cysts fall into the type I classification.

Pathophysiology

Several etiologies of choledochal cysts have been hypothesized. One proposed etiology is abnormal anatomy of the pancreaticobiliary junction proximal to the ampulla of Vater, resulting in an abnormally long common channel, allowing the reflux of pancreatic enzymes into the CBD. This can then result in inflammation and subsequent deterioration of the duct wall,

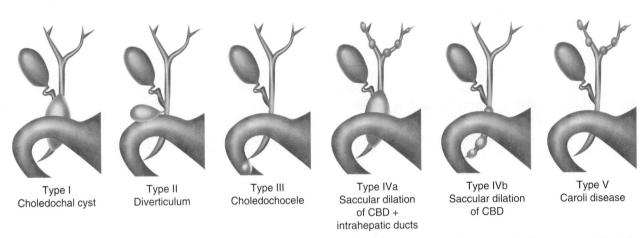

Type I	Type II	Type III	Type IVa	Type IVb	Type V
Choledochal cyst	Diverticulum	Choledochocele	Saccular dilation of CBD + intrahepatic ducts	Saccular dilation of CBD	Caroli disease

FIGURE 41-4 Classification of choledochal cysts. The Todani classification of bile duct cysts divides cysts of the bile duct into 5 groups. Type I, a true choledochal cyst, is characterized by fusiform dilation of the extrahepatic bile duct. Type II are true diverticula, or saccular outpouchings, arising from the supraduodenal extrahepatic bile duct or the intrahepatic bile ducts. Type III represent protrusion of a focally dilated, intramural segment of the distal common bile duct into the duodenum. Type IV is made up of multiple communicating intra- and extrahepatic duct cysts. Type V, otherwise known as Caroli disease, is characterized by cystic dilations of intrahepatic bile ducts. (From Dahnert WF. Liver, Bile Ducts, Pancreas and Spleen, 2007. Lippincott Williams & Wilkins, Philadelphia, PA.)

resulting in ductal dilation.[93] Supporting this etiology is the higher levels of pancreatic amylase found in choledochal cysts, suggestive of reflux of pancreatic fluid. However, only 50%–80% of choledochal cysts contain an abnormal pancreaticobiliary ductal connection, arguing there must be additional factors contributing to cyst formation.[91]

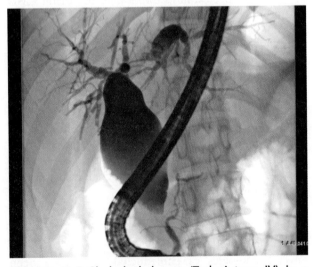

FIGURE 41-5 Choledochal cyst (Todani type IV) in a 1-year-old boy. Operative cholangiogram shows dilatation of intrahepatic biliary tree and common bile duct (arrow). Gallbladder (GB) is noted. (Liver imaging Atlas, www.liveratlas.org. Copyright @2010 University of Washington. Image used with permission from University of Washington.)

Another theory is that choledochal cysts are congenital in nature because of ductal obstruction with subsequent dilation of the CBD system. Distal obstruction may be due to sphincter of Oddi dysfunction or aganglionosis, such as seen in Hirschsprung disease. Both a decrease in elastin among infants prior to the age of 1 year and an increase in biliary tree pressure from distal obstruction could lead to proximal dilation of the ductal system.[94]

Differential Diagnosis

Most patients present with fevers, abdominal pain, nausea, and vomiting, which leaves many possible diagnoses. The classic triad of abdominal pain, jaundice, and vomiting is present in less than 20% of patients with choledochal cysts.[92] Since more than 80% of patients with choledochal cysts present[95] before the age of 10, the palpable abdominal mass, more often seen in children, can help make the diagnosis.[96] In 1 study, 53% of children with choledochal cysts presented with an abdominal mass, compared to only 21% of adults.[95]

In most cases, the presenting symptoms are due to secondary complications of choledochal cysts, such as ascending cholangitis, biliary stasis, inflammation, and pancreatitis. Thus, clinical suspicion must be raised in any pediatric patient who experiences recurrent bouts of pancreatitis or other symptoms consistent with biliary stasis. Recurrent infections and obstruction with choledochal cysts can lead to secondary biliary cirrhosis, which may lead to portal hypertension with splenomegaly and gastrointestinal bleeding.[94] Although uncommon to initially present with these symptoms, they are important to keep in mind.

Diagnostic Tests

The initial study is typically an abdominal ultrasound, which is the best choice of imaging for choledochal cysts, with a sensitivity of 71% to 97%.[92] The majority of choledochal cystic lesions are able to be seen by routine ultrasonography.[97] Ultrasound should confirm a cystic mass in the biliary tree and include information regarding the diameter of the bile duct and the degree of intrahepatic dilation. It is important to confirm the location of the cystic mass since there are many other abdominal cystic locations, including pancreatic pseudocysts. MRCP is another useful noninvasive test that is replacing computed tomography (CT) and ERCP for the diagnosis of choledocal cyst. The ability to identify surrounding anatomy without radiation or an invasive procedure makes this a preferred option.

A technetium 99m HIDA scan is helpful to view the continuity of bile ducts and distinguish choledochal cysts from biliary atresia in the newborn period. However, visualization of the intrahepatic ductal system is not optimal and in fact is inadequate for type IV or V choledochal cysts. Visualization of contrast in the small bowel rules out biliary atresia and points toward choledochal cysts. This can be helpful when needing to rapidly rule out the diagnosis of biliary atresia.

Due to the detailed visualization of the biliary tree, cholangiography has long been the goldstandard imaging modality for diagnosis and operative planning for choledochal cyst.[92] ERCP is another alternative to visualize the biliary tree and is less invasive. However, the administration of contrast and manipulation of the ampulla in those with choledochal cysts have an increased risk of cholangitis and pancreatitis. Therefore, MRCP, rather than ERCP, has become the preferred imaging modality for visualization of the biliary tree, thereby avoiding cholangiography. The limitation of MRCP is its inability to delineate subtle findings in the biliary tree, especially in children less than 3 years of age. But, evidence has been promising for its use in the diagnosis of choledochal cysts. In 2002, Kim et al[98] revealed that MRCP was able to accurately show aberrant pancreaticobiliary union in 60% of patients prior to intraoperative cholangiography. Park et al[99] in 2005 revealed that MRCP was able to detect choledochal cysts in 96% of their patient population and provided diagnostic images to determine the type of cystic lesion present in those patients. Given its ability to provide adequate diagnostic imaging of choledochal cysts while simultaneously minimizing risk to the patient, MRCP will likely replace both cholangiography and ERCP for diagnosis of choledochal cysts.[99]

Management

From the 1950s to the 1980s, before there was known evidence of malignancy due to retained cysts, treatment consisted of internal drainage with cystenterostomy to provide relief of symptoms. Subsequently, increasing amounts of evidence supported that retention of the cyst's mucosal layer increased the risk of biliary carcinoma. Therefore, the standard treatment of choledochal cyst disease has become total cyst excision with hepaticoenterostomy. By creating a Roux-en-Y hepaticojejunostomy for biliary drainage, the biliary tree is isolated from the pancreatic duct and the pancreatic duct drains into the native duodenum, thereby eliminating pancreatic reflux into the biliary tree. Some studies[100] have reported success rates of hepaticojejunostomy as high as 92%. If inflammation is present, there is an increased technical challenge due to the increased risk of injury to the underlying portal vein. When the inflammation and adhesions present a hazardous risk, a safe alternative is to perform partial cyst excision with mucosectomy.[94]

For type I, II, and IV cysts, regardless of previous surgery or other comorbidities, surgical intervention should always include cholecystectomy and cyst excision, most commonly with hepaticojejunostomy.[96,101] Some surgeons advocate for a hepaticoduodenostomy because it appears more physiologic, but this procedure has been associated with an increased complication rate (42%), including increased risk of biliary gastric reflux with resultant gastritis and esophagitis.[102] Therefore, several advise against a hepaticoduodenostomy for children with choledochal cysts.[102]

For type III cysts, management involves unroofing the cyst by an open duodenotomy or ERCP, thereby allowing internal drainage into the duodenum. For type V cysts (Caroli disease), hepaticojejunostomy is not effective because of the intrahepatic nature of the disease. Management for these cysts is still controversial. If the lesion is isolated to 1 lobe, some surgeons have advocated a partial hepatectomy,[96] while other surgeons have advocated Roux-en-Y cholangiojejunostomy, with placement of transhepatic stents.[96] Extensive disease may require hepatic transplantation.

Outcomes and Follow-up

The most common complication of a hepaticojejunostomy (done for type I, II, and IV cysts) immediately postoperatively is cholangitis. Later complications include bowel obstruction, chronic abdominal pain, and biliary cirrhosis. Overall, long-term complications from complete cyst excision are rare, and mortality in the pediatric population is as low as 0% in some studies.[103] Regardless of the surgical intervention chosen for choledochal cyst disease, long-term follow-up is

CHAPTER 41

required because of continued risk for the development of malignancy in the intrapancreatic CBD or the hepaticojejunostomy anastomotic site.

All types of choledochal cysts are at risk for malignant transformation. While the reason for this transformation is not entirely clear, cellular dysplasia due to chronic inflammation, recurrent infections, or the presence of pancreatic enzymes have all been suggested. Adenocarcinoma is responsible for 73% to 84% of tumors. If the cyst is not excised, the risk of malignancy has been reported as high as 75% in patients by the age of 70, whereas rates after cyst excision were only 0.70% in long-term follow-up.[104] These numbers clearly advocate cyst excision at an early age.

SPONTANEOUS PERFORATION OF BILE DUCTS

Epidemiology

Although spontaneous perforation of the bile duct (SPBD) is a rare condition affecting infants, it is the second-most-common surgical cause of jaundice in infancy after biliary atresia.[105] Since the first case report was published in 1932, only 150 additional cases have been reported. A recent review by Evans reported on all cases seen in the past 20 years. They found the condition is commonly seen in children less than 4 years of age, with the peak incidence in the first year of life; the ratio of male to female is 2:1, and previous history pertaining to biliary tract disease was usually absent.[106]

Pathophysiology

The etiology of SPBD is unknown, but proposed theories include congenital mural weakness of the CBD, ischemia, distal biliary obstruction, and pancreaticobiliary malunion (PBM).[106] Unlike biliary atresia, the etiology is not thought to be viral or inflammatory in nature as most infants are healthy prior to perforation, and investigations have not found abnormal viral titers or immunoglobulin levels.[106]

The idea of congenital mural weakness of the CBD was first proposed by Peterson in 1955 and later by Johnston in 1961 because most perforations occurred close to the junction of the cystic and hepatic ducts. The thought was that there was a developmental weakness in the wall of the duct that perforates once a certain intraductal pressure is reached.

An ischemic etiology was proposed by Northover and Terblanche[107] due to the posterolateral arterial supply making the anterior wall of the CBD susceptible to ischemia. The CBD receives its blood supply from 2 pairs of marginal arteries coming from the superior pancreaticoduodenal artery and the

right hepatic artery. These contribute 60% and 40%, respectively, of the vascular supply of the CBD. The junctional area between these 2 vascular territories is a potential ischemic watershed. This may predispose to focal ischemia of the CBD if there were a hypoperfusion event, resulting in perforation. A particular susceptibility to splanchnic ischemia in neonates may explain localized injury in infants with precarious bile duct blood supply.[108]

Distal biliary obstruction due to stones or stenosis can cause an increase in intraductal pressure and increase the susceptibility to perforation.

In the congenital anomaly PBM, the union of the pancreatic and biliary ducts is located outside the duodenal wall containing the sphincter of Oddi.[109,] This location causes the pancreatic juice to reflux into the bile duct, activating bile and causing it to become potentially destructive. This, in combination with distal bile duct stenosis, could potentially lead to SPBD due to acute inflammation and microabscess formation in the duct wall from bile stasis, eventually resulting in perforation.[110] Others have felt that SPBD in association with PBM is related to an abrupt increase in intraluminal pressure from impaction of a protein plug, which is likely to be associated with PBM and congenital dilation of the bile duct.[106]

Differential Diagnosis

The differential can be challenging if the only presenting symptom is jaundice. In that case, the differential is as broad as it is for biliary atresia. However, if the neonate has jaundice with abdominal distension, fever, pale-color stools, and sepsis, investigation for SPDB should be expedited to perform appropriate patient management.

Diagnostic Tests

Serum bilirubin and liver enzymes are often normal or only mildly elevated. There may be a mild leukocytosis. If an ascitic tap is performed to confirm the diagnosis, the concentration of bilirubin is higher in the peritoneal fluid than in the serum.

To make a rapid diagnosis in a neonate with insidious onset of jaundice and abdominal distension with alcoholic stools, an abdominal ultrasound and biliary radionuclide scan can be used. Ultrasound demonstrates either free ascitic fluid or loculated subhepatic fluid. The hepatobiliary scan can differentiate this condition from other causes of prolonged neonatal jaundice by demonstrating the flow of bile into the peritoneal cavity and not into the bowel.[106] In contrast, biliary atresia would show a complete lack of tracer excretion from the liver, and neonatal hepatitis would demonstrate delayed excretion, but excretion still going into the gastrointestinal tract.

Management

There are several methods of management reported, but it is important that management be dictated by the condition of the patient. Procedures performed are simple peritoneal drainage, repair of the perforation, T-tube drainage with or without cholecystectomy, Roux-en-Y intestinal anastomosis, and ERCP.[106] Ideally, intraoperative cholangiogram would be performed first to look at the biliary anatomy. If a distal obstruction is found, decompression will usually resolve the obstruction thought to be secondary to the perforation. Although some have suggested biliary bypass is the best initial therapy, recent reviews suggested that simple peritoneal drainage and T-tube drainage are the better alternatives due to the risk of exploring the porta hepatis with a significant amount of inflammation following perforation.[106] And, in the majority of patients, simple decompression is curative without the need to repair the perforation itself. In fact, repair of the perforation can be hazardous and creates a risk of postoperative stricture.[106] However, in the cases of PBM detected on cholangiography, biliary intestinal anastomosis is necessary to prevent biliary cirrhosis, portal hypertension, recurrent pancreatitis, and ultimately biliary carcinoma.[111] However, this can be done at a second laparotomy when the inflammation has decreased.

With recent advances in laparoscopic surgery, diagnosis and percutaneous drainage are definite alternatives.[112] In centers with appropriate equipment and expertise, ERCP is an alternative primary therapy, avoiding the need for surgery.[113]

Outcome/Follow-up

The postoperative course may be complicated with cholangitis or peritonitis, which requires prolonged antibiotic treatment.[114] There have also been a handful of reported cases with portal venous thrombosis postoperatively.[115,116] Four patients in the Charcot series had postoperative portal hypertension, and 2 of these were attributed to portal vein thrombosis. The etiology is assumed to be as simple as irritative bile or a biloma abutting onto the portal vein and is thought to occur more commonly with posterior perforations.[116]

TUMORS OF THE BILE DUCT

Epidemiology

Children almost never develop carcinoma of the biliary tree. However, when they do, the most common malignant tumor is rhabdomyosarcoma, sometimes referred to as boytroid rhabdomyosarcoma, which accounts for only 0.04% of childhood neoplasms.[117] The median age at presentation is 3 years, and there is a slight male predominance.[118] On discovery, the tumor can often exceed 8 cm and can invade the duodenum.[118] The tumor can arise from nearly anywhere along the biliary tree, including the liver, intrahepatic and extrahepatic biliary tree, gallbladder, ampulla, or even hepatic or choledochal cysts.[119]

Differential Diagnosis

The most common clinical features are jaundice and abdominal distention with pain, vomiting, and fever (less frequent).[118] Elevation in liver transaminases and bilirubin is often present. Although the previously discussed disorders are on the differential, if determined on imaging to be a tumor, a tumor arising from the biliary tree discovered in children over 1 year of age is most commonly an embryonal rhabdomyosarcoma. Other considerations include choledochal cysts, inflammatory pseudotumor, and cholangiocarcinoma arising within a choledocal cyst.[119] In older children, considerations would also include hepatoblastoma and hepatocellular carcinoma, which would be distinguished from embryonal rhabdomyosarcoma by elevated α-fetoprotein levels.[117]

Diagnostic Modalities

Following laboratory values of a liver panel and α-fetoprotein, ultrasound is good initial imaging test. Ultrasound typically shows biliary ductal dilation, an intraductal mass, or fluid-filled mass if the tumor has a cystic component.[117] These findings make it similar in appearance to a choledochal cyst, especially if there is no local invasion. Although CT may be useful to show a heterogeneous or hypoattenuating mass with biliary ductal dilatation, magnetic resonance imaging (MRI) has several advantages as an imaging modality due to its ability to define the extent of disease and relationship to hepatic vasculature.[117] Generally, definitive diagnosis is made by pathology from either percutaneous or intraoperative tissue sampling.[120]

Management

Surgical approach depends on the extent of the tumor burden. Different options include Roux-en-Y hepaticojejunostomy[121] and choledochojejunostomy with cholecystectomy and end-to-side jejunojejunostomy.[121,122] In a handful of select cases, neoadjuvant chemotherapy and radiation therapy may be useful to shrink the tumor burden prior to surgery.[121] Adjuvant therapy is useful in allowing for positive margins at surgical resection without an increase in mortality.[121]

Outcomes and Follow-up

With the combination of therapies, survival has increased significantly, and a recent study reported a survival rate of greater than 75%, compared to 25% in 1970.[122] However, other studies recommend longer-term follow-up studies because hepatobiliary rhabdomyosarcoma has been reported to recur up to 9 years after therapy.[119] Because of this potential for late recurrence, it is recommended that surveillance monitoring should be annually for several years with CT scans.[119,121,122]

OTHER DISORDERS

There are several other disorders that can result in neonatal jaundice due to conjugated hyperbilirubinemia. Although uncommon in the neonatal period, others at least worth mentioning are cholelithiasis and biliary dyskinesia.

Cholelithiasis

Cholelithiasis is very rare in children[123] and affects less than 0.2% of children under the age of 15. The most common causes of pediatric cholelithiasis are hemolytic diseases such as sickle cell anemia, thalassemia, and hereditary spherocytosis and nonhemolytic causes such as parenteral nutrition, cystic fibrosis, and metabolic disorders.[124] Although most children remain asymptomatic, cholelithiasis can be complicated by cholecystitis, pancreatitis, and biliary cholic. It has been reported that for those with clinically silent cholelithiasis, conservative management is both safe and appropriate.[125] For those children who are symptomatic, most commonly seen in patients with hemolytic disease, laparoscopic cholecystectomy is a safe and effective treatment.[125]

Biliary Dyskinesia

Biliary dyskinesia is a motility disorder causing irregular emptying from the gallbladder and sphincter of Oddi.[126] It most commonly affects children between the ages of 14 and 16[127,128] and presents with symptoms similar to gallstone disease, including right upper quadrant pain, fatty food intolerance, nausea, vomiting, and abdominal pain. Unfortunately, many patients are left undiagnosed due to several negative tests and a large differential.[128]

The diagnosis of gallbladder dyskinesia is usually made by cholecystokinin–diisopropyl iminodiacetic acid (CCK-DISIDA) scanning with a gallbladder ejection fraction of less than 35% or pain with administration of CCK, both suggestive of dyskinesia in the absence of cholelithiasis. The treatment of biliary dyskinesia is cholecystectomy. Kaye et al[128] showed that 77.3% of patients who were diagnosed with gallbladder dyskinesia and who had pain with CCK-DISIDA scan had resolution of symptoms after laparoscopic cholecystectomy. Similarly, Hofeldt et al[127] reported a 93% likelihood of resolution of symptoms in children with a known ejection fraction of less than 15% and associated right upper quadrant pain. The results of this study and numerous others suggest that laparoscopic cholecystectomy is the standard treatment for children with gallbladder dyskinesia when the diagnosis has been confirmed and other etiologies for their symptoms have been ruled out.

CONCLUSIONS

Biliary disease in children presents numerous challenges for both diagnosis and treatment. Because of the mortality associated with pediatric biliary diseases, such as biliary atresia and choledochal cysts, accurate diagnosis and timely appropriate treatment are essential to patient outcomes. Although the etiology and pathogenesis of several of biliary disease in children are still in question, several advances in diagnosis, medical treatment, and surgical intervention are helping improve patient outcomes.

REFERENCES

1. McKiernan PJ, Baker AJ, Kelly DA. The frequency and outcome of biliary atresia in the UK and Ireland. *Lancet.* 2000;355(9197):25–29.
2. Chardot C, et al. Prognosis of biliary atresia in the era of liver transplantation: French national study from 1986 to 1996. *Hepatology.* 1999;30(3):606–611.
3. Hsiao CH, et al. Universal screening for biliary atresia using an infant stool color card in Taiwan. *Hepatology.* 2008;47(4):1233–1240.
4. Yoon PW, et al. Epidemiology of biliary atresia: a population-based study. *Pediatrics.* 1997;99(3):376–382.
5. Hartley JL, Davenport M, Kelly DA. Biliary atresia. *Lancet.* 2009;374(9702):1704–1713.
6. Balistreri WF. Neonatal cholestasis. *J Pediatr.* 1985;106(2):171–184.
7. Davenport M, et al. Biliary atresia splenic malformation syndrome: an etiologic and prognostic subgroup. *Surgery* 1993;113(6):662–668.
8. Silveira TR, et al. Extrahepatic biliary atresia and twinning. *Braz J Med Biol Res.* 1991;24(1):67–71.
9. Danks DM, et al. Studies of the aetiology of neonatal hepatitis and biliary atresia. *Arch Dis Child.* 1977;52(5):360–367.
10. Strickland AD, Shannon K. Studies in the etiology of extrahepatic biliary atresia: time-space clustering. *J Pediatr.* 1982;100(5):749–753.
11. Chardot C, et al. Epidemiology of biliary atresia in France: a national study 1986–96. *J Hepatol.* 1999;31(6):1006–1013.
12. Fischler B, Haglund B, Hjern A. A population-based study on the incidence and possible pre- and perinatal etiologic risk factors of biliary atresia. *J Pediatr.* 2002;141(2):217–222.

13. Yokoyama T, et al. Reversal of left-right asymmetry: a situs inversus mutation. *Science*. 1993;260(5108):679–682.

14. Mazziotti MV, et al. Anomalous development of the hepatobiliary system in the Inv mouse. *Hepatology*. 1999;30(2):372–378.

15. Perlmutter DH, Shepherd RW. Extrahepatic biliary atresia: a disease or a phenotype? *Hepatology*. 2002;35(6):1297–1304.

16. Shimadera S, et al. The inv mouse as an experimental model of biliary atresia. *J Pediatr Surg*. 2007;42(9):1555–1600.

17. Clotman F, et al. The onecut transcription factor HNF6 is required for normal development of the biliary tract. *Development*. 2002;129(8):1819–1828.

18. Coffinier C, et al. Bile system morphogenesis defects and liver dysfunction upon targeted deletion of HNF1beta. *Development*. 2002;129(8):1829–1838.

19. Balistreri WF, et al. Intrahepatic cholestasis: summary of an American Association for the Study of Liver Diseases single-topic conference. *Hepatology*. 2005;42(1):222–235.

20. Li L, et al. Alagille syndrome is caused by mutations in human Jagged1, which encodes a ligand for Notch1. *Nat Genet*. 1997;16(3):243–251.

21. McCright B, Lozier J, Gridley T. A mouse model of Alagille syndrome: Notch2 as a genetic modifier of Jag1 haploinsufficiency. *Development*. 2002;129(4):1075–1082.

22. Arikan C, et al. Polymorphisms of the ICAM-1 gene are associated with biliary atresia. *Dig Dis Sci*. 2008;53(7):2000–2004.

23. Arikan C, et al. Positive association of macrophage migration inhibitory factor gene-173G/C polymorphism with biliary atresia. *J Pediatr Gastroenterol Nutr*. 2006;42(1):77–82.

24. Davit-Spraul, A, et al. CFC1 gene involvement in biliary atresia with polysplenia syndrome. *J Pediatr Gastroenterol Nutr*. 2008;46(1):111–112.

25. Shih HH, et al. Promoter polymorphism of the CD14 endotoxin receptor gene is associated with biliary atresia and idiopathic neonatal cholestasis. *Pediatrics*. 2005;116(2):437–441.

26. Landing BH. Considerations of the pathogenesis of neonatal hepatitis, biliary atresia and choledochal cyst—the concept of infantile obstructive cholangiopathy. *Prog Pediatr Surg*. 1974;6:113–139.

27. Volpert D, et al. Outcome of early hepatic portoenterostomy for biliary atresia. *J Pediatr Gastroenterol Nutr*. 2001;32(3):265–269.

28. Lee HC, et al. Dilatation of the biliary tree in children: sonographic diagnosis and its clinical significance. *J Ultrasound Med*. 2000;19(3):177–182; quiz 183–184.

29. Muise AM, et al. Biliary atresia with choledochal cyst: implications for classification. *Clin Gastroenterol Hepatol*. 2006;4(11):1411–1414.

30. Rauschenfels S, et al. Incidence of hepatotropic viruses in biliary atresia. *Eur J Pediatr*. 2009;168(4):469–476.

31. Balistreri WF, Tabor E, Gerety RJ. Negative serology for hepatitis A and B viruses in 18 cases of neonatal cholestasis. *Pediatrics*. 1980;66(2):269–271.

32. Glaser JH, Balistreri WF, Morecki R. Role of reovirus type 3 in persistent infantile cholestasis. *J Pediatr*. 1984;105(6):912–915.

33. Morecki R, et al. Detection of reovirus type 3 in the porta hepatitis of an infant with extrahepatic biliary atresia: ultrastructural and immunocytochemical study. *Hepatology*. 1984;4(6):1137–1142.

34. Morecki R, et al. Biliary atresia and reovirus type 3 infection. *N Engl J Med*. 1984;310(24):1610.

35. Richardson SC, Bishop RF, Smith AL. Reovirus serotype 3 infection in infants with extrahepatic biliary atresia or neonatal hepatitis. *J Gastroenterol Hepatol*. 1994;9(3):264–268.

36. Tyler KL, et al. Detection of reovirus RNA in hepatobiliary tissues from patients with extrahepatic biliary atresia and choledochal cysts. *Hepatology*. 1998;27(6):1475–1482.

37. Shen C, et al. Relationship between prognosis of biliary atresia and infection of cytomegalovirus. *World J Pediatr*. 2008;4(2):123–126.

38. Harada K, et al. Innate immune response to double-stranded RNA in biliary epithelial cells is associated with the pathogenesis of biliary atresia. *Hepatology*. 2007;46(4):1146–1154.

39. Davenport M, et al. Immunohistochemistry of the liver and biliary tree in extrahepatic biliary atresia. *J Pediatr Surg*. 2001;36(7):1017–1025.

40. Shinkai M, et al. Increased CXCR3 expression associated with CD3-positive lymphocytes in the liver and biliary remnant in biliary atresia. *J Pediatr Surg*. 2006;41(5):950–954.

41. Mack CL, et al. Oligoclonal expansions of CD4+ and CD8+ T-cells in the target organ of patients with biliary atresia. *Gastroenterology*. 2007;133(1):278–287.

42. Kuebler JF, et al. Type-I but not type-II interferon receptor knockout mice are susceptible to biliary atresia. *Pediatr Res*. 2006;59(6):790–794.

43. Shivakumar P, et al. Obstruction of extrahepatic bile ducts by lymphocytes is regulated by IFN-gamma in experimental biliary atresia. *J Clin Invest*. 2004;114(3):322–329.

44. Carvalho E, et al. Analysis of the biliary transcriptome in experimental biliary atresia. *Gastroenterology*. 2005;129(2):713–717.

45. Gyorffy A, et al. Promoter analysis suggests the implication of NFkappaB/C-Rel transcription factors in biliary atresia. *Hepatogastroenterology*. 2008;55(85):1189–1192.

46. Muraji T, et al. Maternal microchimerism in underlying pathogenesis of biliary atresia: quantification and phenotypes of maternal cells in the liver. *Pediatrics*. 2008;121(3):517–521.

47. Harper P, Plant JW, Unger DB. Congenital biliary atresia and jaundice in lambs and calves. *Aust Vet J*. 1990;67(1):18–22.

48. Bassett MD, Murray KF. Biliary atresia: recent progress. *J Clin Gastroenterol*. 2008;42(6):720–729.

49. Rendon-Macias ME, et al. Improvement in accuracy of gamma-glutamyl transferase for differential diagnosis of biliary atresia by correlation with age. *Turk J Pediatr*. 2008;50(3):253–259.

50. Humphrey TM, Stringer MD. Biliary atresia: US diagnosis. *Radiology*. 2007;244(3):845–851.

51. Farrant P, Meire HB, Mieli-Vergani G. Ultrasound features of the gall bladder in infants presenting with conjugated hyperbilirubinaemia. *Br J Radiol*. 2000;73(875):1154–1158.

52. Park WH, et al. A new diagnostic approach to biliary atresia with emphasis on the ultrasonographic triangular cord sign: comparison of ultrasonography, hepatobiliary scintigraphy, and liver needle biopsy in the evaluation of infantile cholestasis. *J Pediatr Surg*. 1997;32(11):1555–1559.

53. Kotb MA, et al. Evaluation of the triangular cord sign in the diagnosis of biliary atresia. *Pediatrics*. 2001;108(2):416–420.

54. Roquete ML, et al. Accuracy of echogenic periportal enlargement image in ultrasonographic exams and histopathology in differential diagnosis of biliary atresia. *J Pediatr (Rio J)*. 2008;84(4):331–336.

55. Moyer V, et al. Guideline for the evaluation of cholestatic jaundice in infants: recommendations of the North American Society for Pediatric Gastroenterology, Hepatology and Nutrition. *J Pediatr Gastroenterol Nutr*. 2004;39(2):115–128.

56. Howman-Giles R, et al. Hepatobiliary scintigraphy in infancy. *J Nucl Med*. 1998;39(2):311–319.

57. Majd M, Reba RC, Altman RP. Hepatobiliary scintigraphy with 99mTc-PIPIDA in the evaluation of neonatal jaundice. *Pediatrics*. 1981;67(1):140–145.

58. Lai MW, et al. Differential diagnosis of extrahepatic biliary atresia from neonatal hepatitis: a prospective study. *J Pediatr Gastroenterol Nutr*. 1994;18(2):121–127.

59. Azar G, et al. Atypical morphologic presentation of biliary atresia and value of serial liver biopsies. *J Pediatr Gastroenterol Nutr*. 2002;34(2):212–215.

60. Iinuma Y, et al. The role of endoscopic retrograde cholangiopancreatography in infants with cholestasis. *J Pediatr Surg*. 2000;35(4):545–549.

61. Han SJ, et al. Magnetic resonance cholangiography for the diagnosis of biliary atresia. *J Pediatr Surg.* 2002;37(4):599–604.

62. Norton KI, et al. MR cholangiography in the evaluation of neonatal cholestasis: initial results. *Radiology.* 2002;222(3):687–691.

63. Takaya J, et al. Usefulness of magnetic resonance cholangiopancreatography in biliary structures in infants: a four-case report. *Eur J Pediatr.* 2007;166(3):211–214.

64. Laurent J, et al. Long-term outcome after surgery for biliary atresia. Study of 40 patients surviving for more than 10 years. *Gastroenterology.* 1990;99(6):1793–1797.

65. Davenport M, et al. The outcome of the older (> or =100 days) infant with biliary atresia. *J Pediatr Surg.* 2004;39(4):575–581.

66. Toyoki Y, et al. Timing for orthotopic liver transplantation in children with biliary atresia: a single-center experience. *Transplant Proc.* 2008;40(8):2494–2496.

67. Cowles RA, et al. Timing of liver transplantation in biliary atresia-results in 71 children managed by a multidisciplinary team. *J Pediatr Surg.* 2008;43(9):1605–1609.

68. Varela-Fascinetto G, et al. Biliary atresia-polysplenia syndrome: surgical and clinical relevance in liver transplantation. *Ann Surg.* 1998;227(4):583–589.

69. Narayanaswamy B, et al. Serial circulating markers of inflammation in biliary atresia—evolution of the post-operative inflammatory process. *Hepatology.* 2007;46(1):180–187.

70. Wu ET, et al. Bacterial cholangitis in patients with biliary atresia: impact on short-term outcome. *Pediatr Surg Int.* 2001;17(5–6):390–395.

71. Ohi R, Biliary atresia. A surgical perspective. *Clin Liver Dis.* 2000;4(4):779–804.

72. Altman RP, et al. A multivariable risk factor analysis of the portoenterostomy (Kasai) procedure for biliary atresia: twenty-five years of experience from two centers. *Ann Surg.* 1997;226(3):348–353; discussion 353–355.

73. Chiba T, Mochizuki I, Ohi R. Postoperative gastrointestinal hemorrhage in biliary atresia. *Tohoku J Exp Med.* 1990;162(3):255–259.

74. Kasai M. Treatment of biliary atresia with special reference to hepatic porto-enterostomy and its modifications. *Prog Pediatr Surg.* 1974;6:5–52.

75. Howard ER. Extrahepatic biliary atresia: a review of current management. *Br J Surg.* 1983;70(4):193–197.

76. Schweizer P, Lunzmann K. Extrahepatic bile duct atresia: how efficient is the hepatoporto-enterostomy? *Eur J Pediatr Surg.* 1998;8(3):150–154.

77. Chen CL, et al. Living donor liver transplantation for biliary atresia: a single-center experience with first 100 cases. *Am J Transplant.* 2006;6(11):2672–2679.

78. Barshes NR, et al. Orthotopic liver transplantation for biliary atresia: the US experience. *Liver Transpl.* 2005;11(10):1193–1200.

79. van Mourik ID, et al. Long-term nutritional and neurodevelopmental outcome of liver transplantation in infants aged less than 12 months. *J Pediatr Gastroenterol Nutr.* 2000;30(3):269–275.

80. Kamath BM, Schwarz KB, Hadzic N. Alagille syndrome and liver transplantation. *J Pediatr Gastroenterol Nutr.* 2010;50(1):11–15.

81. Oda T, et al. Identification of a larger than 3 Mb deletion including JAG1 in an Alagille syndrome patient with a translocation t(3;20)(q13.3;p12.2). *Hum Mutat.* 2000;16(1):92.

82. Oda T, et al. Mutations in the human Jagged1 gene are responsible for Alagille syndrome. *Nat Genet.* 1997;16(3):235–242.

83. Emerick KM, et al. Features of Alagille syndrome in 92 patients: frequency and relation to prognosis. *Hepatology.* 1999;29(3):822–829.

84. Kamath BM, et al. Consequences of JAG1 mutations. *J Med Genet.* 2003;40(12):891–895.

85. Kamath BM, Loomes KM, Piccoli DA. Medical management of Alagille syndrome. *J Pediatr Gastroenterol Nutr.* 2010;50(6):580–586.

86. Novy MA, Schwarz KB. Nutritional considerations and management of the child with liver disease. *Nutrition.* 1997;13(3):177–184.

87. Kaye AJ, et al. Effect of Kasai procedure on hepatic outcome in Alagille syndrome. *J Pediatr Gastroenterol Nutr.* 2010;51(3):319–321.

88. Ling SC. Congenital cholestatic syndromes: what happens when children grow up? *Can J Gastroenterol.* 2007;21(11):743–751.

89. Arnon R, et al. Orthotopic liver transplantation for children with Alagille syndrome. *Pediatr Transplant.* 2010;14(5):622–628.

90. Singhavejsakul J, Ukarapol N. Choledochal cysts in children: epidemiology and outcomes. *World J Surg.* 2008;32(7):1385–1388.

91. Singham J, Yoshida EM, Scudamore CH. Choledochal cysts: part 1 of 3: classification and pathogenesis. *Can J Surg.* 2009;52(5):434–440.

92. Singham J, Yoshida EM, Scudamore CH. Choledochal cysts: part 2 of 3: Diagnosis. *Can J Surg.* 2009;52(6):506–511.

93. Todani T, et al. Anomalous arrangement of the pancreatobiliary ductal system in patients with a choledochal cyst. *Am J Surg.* 1984;147(5):672–676.

94. Goldman M, Pranikoff T. Biliary disease in children. *Curr Gastroenterol Rep.* 2011;13(2):193–201.

95. Huang CH, et al. Endoscopic retrograde cholangiopancreatography (ERCP) for intradiverticular papilla: endoclip-assisted biliary cannulation. *Endoscopy.* 2010;42(Suppl 2):E223–E224.

96. Lipsett PA, Pitt HA. Surgical treatment of choledochal cysts. *J Hepatobiliary Pancreat Surg.* 2003;10(5):352–359.

97. Dabbas N, Davenport M. Congenital choledochal malformation: not just a problem for children. *Ann R Coll Surg Engl.* 2009;91(2):100–105.

98. Kim MJ, et al. Using MR cholangiopancreatography to reveal anomalous pancreaticobiliary ductal union in infants and children with choledochal cysts. *AJR Am J Roentgenol.* 2002;179(1):209–214.

99. Park DH, et al. Can MRCP replace the diagnostic role of ERCP for patients with choledochal cysts? *Gastrointest Endosc.* 2005;62(3):360–366.

100. Tao KS, et al. Procedures for congenital choledochal cysts and curative effect analysis in adults. *Hepatobiliary Pancreat Dis Int.* 2002;1(3):442–445.

101. Shi LB, et al. Diagnosis and treatment of congenital choledochal cyst: 20 years' experience in China. *World J Gastroenterol.* 2001;7(5):732–734.

102. Shimotakahara A, et al. Roux-en-Y hepaticojejunostomy or hepaticoduodenostomy for biliary reconstruction during the surgical treatment of choledochal cyst: which is better? *Pediatr Surg Int.* 2005;21(1):5–7.

103. Huang CS, Huang CC, Chen DF. Choledochal cysts: differences between pediatric and adult patients. *J Gastrointest Surg.* 2010;14(7):1105–1110.

104. Watanabe Y, Toki A, Todani T. Bile duct cancer developed after cyst excision for choledochal cyst. *J Hepatobiliary Pancreat Surg.* 1999;6(3):207–212.

105. Stringel G, Mercer S. Idiopathic perforation of the biliary tract in infancy. *J Pediatr Surg.* 1983;18(5):546–550.

106. Evans K, Marsden N, Desai A. Spontaneous perforation of the bile duct in infancy and childhood: a systematic review. *J Pediatr Gastroenterol Nutr.* 2010;50(6):677–681.

107. Northover JM, Terblanche J. A new look at the arterial supply of the bile duct in man and its surgical implications. *Br J Surg.* 1979;66(6):379–384.

108. Lloyd JR. The etiology of gastrointestinal perforations in the newborn. *J Pediatr Surg.* 1969;4(1):77–84.

109. Hasegawa T, et al. Does pancreatico-biliary maljunction play a role in spontaneous perforation of the bile duct in children? *Pediatr Surg Int.* 2000;16(8):550–553.

110. Ohkawa H, Takahashi H, Maie M. A malformation of the pancreatico-biliary system as a cause of perforation of the biliary tract in childhood. *J Pediatr Surg.* 1977;12(4):541–546.

111. Murakami Y, et al. Anomalous arrangement of the pancreaticobiliary ductal system without dilatation of the biliary tract. *Surg Today.* 1992;22(3):276–279.

112. Banani SA, Bahador A, Nezakatgoo N. Idiopathic perforation of the extrahepatic bile duct in infancy: pathogenesis, diagnosis, and management. *J Pediatr Surg.* 1993;28(7):950–952.

113. Barnes BH, Narkewicz MR, Sokol RJ. Spontaneous perforation of the bile duct in a toddler: the role of endoscopic retrograde cholangiopancreatography in diagnosis and therapy. *J Pediatr Gastroenterol Nutr.* 2006;43(5):695–697.

114. Kanojia RP, et al. Spontaneous biliary perforation in infancy and childhood: clues to diagnosis. *Indian J Pediatr.* 2007;74(5):509–510.

115. Chardot C, et al. Spontaneous perforation of the biliary tract in infancy: a series of 11 cases. *Eur J Pediatr Surg.* 1996;6(6):341–346.

116. Livesey E, Davenport M. Spontaneous perforation of the biliary tract and portal vein thrombosis in infancy. *Pediatr Surg Int.* 2008;24(3):357–359.

117. Roebuck DJ, et al. Hepatobiliary rhabdomyosarcoma in children: diagnostic radiology. *Pediatr Radiol.* 1998;28(2):101–108.

118. Ruymann FB, et al. Rhabdomyosarcoma of the biliary tree in childhood. A report from the Intergroup Rhabdomyosarcoma Study. *Cancer.* 1985;56(3):575–581.

119. Geoffray A, et al. Ultrasonography and computed tomography for diagnosis and follow-up of pelvic rhabdomyosarcomas in children. *Pediatr Radiol.* 1987;17(2):132–136.

120. Chowdhury T, et al. Ultrasound-guided core needle biopsy for the diagnosis of rhabdomyosarcoma in childhood. *Pediatr Blood Cancer.* 2009;53(3):356–360.

121. Perera MT, et al. Embryonal rhabdomyosarcoma of the ampulla of Vater in early childhood: report of a case and review of literature. *J Pediatr Surg.* 2009;44(2):e9–e11.

122. Nemade B, et al. Embryonal rhabdomyosarcoma of the biliary tree mimicking a choledochal cyst. *J Cancer Res Ther.* 2007;3(1):40–42.

123. Punia RP, et al. Clinico-pathological spectrum of gallbladder disease in children. *Acta Paediatr.* 2010;99(10):1561–1564.

124. Chan S, et al. Paediatric cholecystectomy: shifting goalposts in the laparoscopic era. *Surg Endosc.* 2008;22(5):1392–1395.

125. Bogue CO, et al. Risk factors, complications, and outcomes of gallstones in children: a single-center review. *J Pediatr Gastroenterol Nutr.* 2010;50(3):303–308.

126. Toouli J. Biliary dyskinesia. *Curr Treat Options Gastroenterol.* 2002;5(4):285–291.

127. Hofeldt M, et al. Laparoscopic cholecystectomy for treatment of biliary dyskinesia is safe and effective in the pediatric population. *Am Surg.* 2008;74(11):1069–1072.

128. Kaye AJ, et al. Use of laparoscopic cholecystectomy for biliary dyskinesia in the child. *J Pediatr Surg.* 2008;43(6):1057–1059.

Part F: Genito-Urinary Tract

Acute Kidney Injury in Infants

Gia Oh and Paul Grimm

EPIDEMIOLOGY

Definition of Acute Kidney Injury

Acute kidney injury (AKI) is a condition defined by an acute decrease in the glomerular filtration rate (GFR), resulting in dysregulation of volume, electrolytes, acid-base balance and inability to excrete metabolic waste products. The term AKI has replaced the older term acute renal failure (ARF) to highlight the varying degrees of renal dysfunction, to enable clinicians to recognize renal dysfunction earlier in the patient's course, and to allow researchers to apply a uniform definition of acute renal dysfunction.[1] The Acute Dialysis Quality Initiative (ADQI) and Acute Kidney Injury Network (AKIN) groups standardized the definition of AKI in adult patients based on the increase in serum creatinine (Cr) or oligoanuria, and the pediatric community has adopted modified criteria based on the ADQI and AKIN definitions (Table 42-1).[2]

Definition of AKI in Neonates and Infants

There are additional important factors to consider in defining AKI in neonates using serum Cr and urine output criteria. First, neonatal serum Cr following birth reflects maternal Cr, and it decreases to a steady state over 1 to 2 weeks in term infants and over 3 to 4 weeks in preterm infants as the neonate's GFR steadily improves.[3,4] Tables 42-2 and 42-3 show the increasing GFR in preterm and term neonates.[5,6]

Second, unlike in critically ill adults or children, critically ill neonates may not have their serum Cr measured daily due to the concern for blood loss, and AKI may go unrecognized.[7] Elevated bilirubin levels can interfere with the Jaffe reaction assay, a common laboratory method used to measure serum Cr, and lead to an underestimation in the serum Cr if the laboratory does not correct for the bilirubin interferences.[8,9] Likewise, oliguria is not a sensitive marker for AKI in neonates because neonates commonly have nonoliguric AKI.[7,10] In spite of these limitations, serum Cr and urine output measurements currently remain the main clinical tools in identifying and diagnosing AKI in neonates. Jetton et al have proposed a standardized definition of neonatal AKI based on the AKIN criteria,[7] and recent studies in neonatal AKI have utilized modified RIFLE (risk injury failure loss end stage) criteria, pediatric RIFLE (pRIFLE), and the AKIN criteria to define AKI.[11–13] Table 42-4 shows the modified definitions used in these studies. The following modifications were made: (1) The upper cutoff Cr of 4.0 mg/dL in stage 3 (AKIN) and stage F failure (RIFLE) is lowered to 2.5 mg/dL to reflect the neonates' lower muscle mass and lower steady-state baseline Cr.[11] (2) The 6-hour period used in the urine output criteria is changed to an 8-hour period to be consistent with the pRIFLE definition of oliguria, which was validated in pediatric patients.[12] These proposed definitions of neonatal AKI are promising alternatives to the current practice of arbitrarily defining AKI, but these definitions need to be validated to determine their clinical utility.

Table 42-1 Acute Kidney Injury Definitions Using RIFLE, pRIFLE, and AKIN

	Stage	Serum Creatinine/GFR Criteria	Urine Output Criteria
RIFLE[a]	R	SCr increase 1.5 times or GFR decrease >25%	<0.5 mL/kg/h for 6 h
	I	SCr increase 2 times or GFR decrease >50%	<0.5 mL/kg/h for 12 h
	F	SCr increase 3 times or SCr ≥ 4mg/dL or GFR decrease >75%	<0.3 mL/kg/h for 24 h or anuria for 12 h
	L	Persistent failure > 4 weeks	
	E	Persistent failure >3 months	
Pediatric RIFLE[b]	R	eCCl[d] decrease > 25%	<0.5 mL/kg/h for 8 h
	I	eCCl decrease > 50%	<0.5 mL/kg/h for 16 h
	F	eCCl decrease > 75% or eCCl < 35 mL/min/1.73 m²	<0.3 mL/kg/h for 24 h or anuria for 12 h
	L	Persistent failure > 4 weeks	
	E	Persistent failure > 3 months	
AKIN[c]	1	SCr increase > 0.3 mg/dL or > 1.5–2 times baseline	<0.5 mL/kg/h for 6 h
	2	SCr increase > 2–3 times baseline	<0.5 mL/kg/h for 12 h
	3	SCr increase > 3 times baseline or SCr ≥ 4.0 mg/dL with acute increase ≥ 0.5 mg/dL	<0.3 mL/kg/h for 24 h or anuria for 12 h

Abbreviations: AKIN, Acute Kidney Injury Network; eCCl, estimated creatinine clearance; pRIFLE, pediatric RIFLE; RIFLE, risk injury failure loss end stage; SCr, serum creatinine
[a]Bellomo et al.[125]
[b]Akcan-Arikan et al.[120]
[c]Mehta et al.[126]
[d]Schwartz GJ et al.[127]

Incidence of AKI in Neonates and Infants

Acute kidney injury has been reported in 3.4%–24% of the neonates admitted to neonatal intensive care units (NICUs).[10,11,13] The true incidence of neonatal AKI is unknown, however, and it is believed to be higher than the reported values since most studies of neonatal AKI use a high serum Cr value or the need for dialysis to define AKI, thus failing to include those with mild and moderate forms of AKI.[14,15]

Prematurity

In a prospective study of very low birth weight (VLBW) neonates (birth weight 500–1500 g), AKI was found in 18% of the cohort using modified AKIN AKI criteria.[11] AKI was reported in 12.5% of extremely low birth weight (ELBW) neonates in a retrospective case-control study, but mild, moderate, and nonoliguric AKI were unidentified in this study because the study defined AKI as serum Cr greater than 1.5 mg/dL or oliguria of less than 1 mL/kg/h.[13]

Perinatal Asphyxia

Acute kidney injury is reported in 36.1%–56% of neonates with perinatal asphyxia, variously defined[15–17] as 1-minute Apgar score below 7 or 5-minute Apgar scores less than 6 to 7. The incidence of AKI increases with the severity of asphyxia: AKI was reported in 9.1% of infants with moderate asphyxia (1-minute Apgar score 4–6) and in 56% of infants with severe asphyxia (1-minute Apgar score < 3).[15]

Table 42-2 Glomerular Filtration Rate (GFR) by Inulin Clearance in Preterm and Term Infants[a]

Age	Mean GFR ± SD (mL/min/1.73 m²)
Preterm infants	
1–3 days	14.0 ± 5
1–7 days	18.7 ± 5.5
3–13 days	47.8 ± 10.7
1.5–4 months	67.4 ± 16.6
Term infants	
1–3 days	20.8 ± 5.0
4–14 days	36.8 ± 7.2
15–19 days	46.9 ± 12.5
1–3 months	85.3 ± 35.1
4–6 months	87.4 ± 22.3
7–12 months	96.2 ± 12.2

[a]From Schwartz and Furth.[5]

Table 42-3 Glomerular Filtration Rate (GFR) by Creatinine Clearance in Very Preterm Infants During First Month of Life

Age	GFR (mL/min/1.73m²) Median (3rd–97th percentile)
27 weeks' GA	
Day 7	13.4 (7.9–18.9)
Day 14	16.2 (10.7–21.7)
Day 21	18.0 (12.5–23.5)
Day 28	21.0 (15.5–26.5)
28 weeks' GA	
Day 7	16.2 (10.7–21.7)
Day 14	19.1 (13.5–24.6)
Day 21	20.8 (15.3–26.3)
Day 28	23.9 (18.3–29.4)
29 weeks' GA	
Day 7	19.1 (13.6–24.6)
Day 14	21.9 (16.4–27.4)
Day 21	23.7 (18.2–29.2)
Day 28	26.7 (21.2–32.2)
30 weeks' GA	
Day 7	21.9 (16.4–27.4)
Day 14	24.8 (19.3–30.3)
Day 21	26.5 (21.0–32.0)
Day 28	29.6 (24.0–35.0)
31 weeks' GA	
Day 7	24.8 (19.3–30.3)
Day 14	27.6 (22.1–33.1)
Day 21	29.4 (23.9–34.9)
Day 28	32.4 (26.9–37.9)

Abbreviation: GA, gestational age.
[a]From Vieux et al.[6]

Extracorporeal Membrane Oxygenation

In a large retrospective study using data from the Extracorporeal Life Support Organization (ELSO) Registry, AKI was found in 8% (638/7941) of infants who received extracorporeal membrane oxygenation (ECMO) for noncardiac reasons; AKI was defined as serum Cr greater than 1.5 mg/dL, diagnostic code for ARF, or procedural code for dialysis.[18] AKI, defined by modified RIFLE, was reported at a much higher rate of 71% (48/68) in a single-center retrospective study of neonates who received ECMO for congenital diaphragmatic hernia (CDH).[19] The large disparity in the AKI incidence in the 2 studies is likely due to the varying definitions of AKI.

Cardiac Surgery for Congenital Heart Disease

Two recent large studies showed that postoperative AKI, defined by the modified AKIN criteria, occurs commonly (52%–62%) in infants undergoing cardiac repair surgery for congenital heart disease.[12,20] The following factors were associated with postoperative AKI in multivariate analyses: single-ventricle physiology (odds ratio [OR] 1.6; 95% confidence interval [CI] 1.1, 2.4); the need for cardiopulmonary bypass (CPB) (OR 1.2; 95% CI 1.01, 1.5)[12]; CPB duration longer than 180 minutes (OR 5.63; 95% CI 1.13, 28); deep hypothermic circulatory arrest (DHCA) (OR 2.14; 95% CI 1.04, 4.43); and the presence of chromosome abnormality (OR 4.4; 95% CI 1.26, 15.4).[20]

PATHOPHYSIOLOGY

The pathophysiology of AKI is complex, and it involves an intricate interplay of various mechanisms involving exogenous and endogenous toxins, hemodynamic instability in renal macro- and microcirculation, hypoxia, ischemia-reperfusion injury, inflammation, and oxidative stress. A complete review of the various pathophysiologic mechanisms of AKI is beyond the scope of this chapter. A few key mechanisms pertinent to neonatal AKI are highlighted in this section.

Incomplete Nephrogenesis in Prematurity

Nephrogenesis begins at 4–5 gestational weeks and completes at 34–36 gestational weeks.[4,21] Importantly, autopsy studies have shown that nephrogenesis and glomerulogenesis do not continue normally in the extrauterine environment for prematurely born infants. Prematurely born infants (27 ± 3 gestational weeks) were autopsied at 63 ± 27 weeks postconceptual age. Their glomerulogenesis, as measured by radial glomerular counts (RGCs), was found to be significantly lower than in term infants autopsied at 40 ± 1 weeks postconceptual age, suggesting that extrauterine glomerulogenesis in prematurely born infants is suboptimal when compared to intrauterine glomerulogenesis seen in term infants.[22] Moreover, glomerulogenesis in premature infants with AKI was noted to be significantly less than in premature infants without AKI.[22]

Impaired Autoregulatory Mechanisms Increase the Risk of Prerenal Injury

Renal blood flow (RBF) is determined by cardiac output (CO) and renal perfusion pressure. Renal perfusion pressure is approximately equal to systemic arterial blood pressure (BP) and renal vascular resistance

CHAPTER 42

Table 42-4 Proposed Definitions and Classification of AKI in Neonates and Infants

	Stage	Serum Creatinine (SCr)	Urine Output Criteria[a]
RIFLE[b]	R	SCr increase 1.5 times	<0.5 mL/kg/h for 8 h
	I	SCr increase 2 times	<0.5 mL/kg/h for 16 h
	F	SCr increase 3 times or SCr > 2.5 mg/dL[c]	<0.3 mL/kg/h for 24 h or anuria for 12 h
	L	Persistent failure > 4 weeks	
	E	Persistent failure > 3 months	
AKIN[c]	1	SCr increase by 0.3 mg/dL or 1.5–2 times previous trough value	<0.5 mL/kg/h for 8 h
	2	SCr increase 2–3 times previous trough value	<0.5 mL/kg/h for 16 h
	3	SCr increase > 3 times previous trough value or SCr > 2.5 mg/dL or dialysis requirement	<0.3 mL/kg/h for 24 h or anuria for 12 h

Abbreviations: AKIN, Acute Kidney Injury Network; RIFLE, risk injury failure loss end stage.
[a]Data from Blinder et al.[12]
[b]Data from Gadepalli et al.[19]
[c]Data from Koralkar et al.[11]
[c]From Jetton and Askenazi.[7]

(RVR), which is largely determined by the afferent and efferent arterioles.[23] RBF can be expressed as RBF = BP/RVR.[23]

Renal blood flow and GFR change only modestly when the renal perfusion pressure (ie, BP) changes within the range that is commonly found in humans (Figure 42-1).[24] This tight regulatory control of RBF and GFR are due to autoregulatory mechanisms from the myogenic response and tubuloglomerular feedback, and these mechanisms maintain RBF and GFR in the setting of decreased renal perfusion.[23–25] When renal perfusion decreases, the afferent arteriole vasodilates, which lowers the RVR and maintains RBF.

Efferent arteriolar vasoconstriction maintains the glomerular pressure (and therefore filtration) in the face of reduced total glomerular blood flow. Decrease in renal perfusion stimulates the generation of prostaglandins (causing afferent vasodilation), catecholamine secretion, and renin-angiotensin system activation (both causing efferent constriction), which all contribute to maintenance of GFR.

In adults with intact autoregulation, GFR is maintained until the mean arterial pressure decreases below 80 mm Hg. In those with impaired autoregulation, however, GFR decreases even in the setting of normal BPs, resulting in normotensive AKI (Figure 42-2).[26]

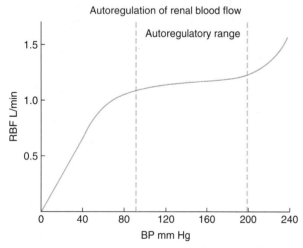

FIGURE 42-1 Autoregulation allows the renal blood flow (RBF) to be maintained at a relatively steady rate during changes in blood pressure within the common range. Glomerular filtration rate follows a similar pattern as the RBF. (Reproduced with permission from Kibble J, Halsey CR. Medical Physiology: The Big Picture. New York: McGraw-Hill; 2009.)

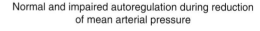
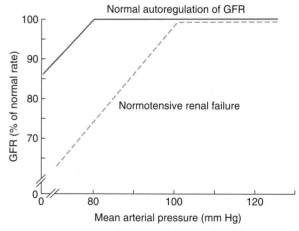

FIGURE 42-2 In normal autoregulation, glomerular filtration rate (GFR) is maintained until the mean arterial pressure decreases below 80 mm Hg. In patients with impaired autoregulation, however, GFR decreases even when the mean arterial pressure is within normal limits. (From Abuelo.[26])

Table 42-5 Factors That Impair Renal Autoregulation and Increase Susceptibility to Acute Kidney Injury

Inability to decrease arteriolar resistance
  Reduction in vasodilatory prostaglandins
    Nonsteroidal anti-inflammatory drugs (NSAIDs)
    Cyclooxygenase 2 inhibitors
  Afferent glomerular arteriolar vasoconstriction
    Sepsis
    Hypercalcemia
    Hepatorenal syndrome
    Cyclosporin or tacrolimus
    Radiocontrast agents
Failure to increase efferent arteriolar resistance
  Angiotensin-converting enzyme inhibitors (ACEIs)
  Angiotensin receptor blockers (ARBs)
Decreases tubuloglomerular feedback
  Furosemide
  ACEIs and ARBs
  Renal artery stenosis

ªFrom Abuelo.[26]

Therefore, in patients with impaired autoregulation, higher renal perfusion pressure (ie, systemic BP) is needed to maintain RBF and GFR. Table 42-5 lists conditions that may impair renal autoregulation and result in increased susceptibility to AKI even in settings of moderate hypoperfusion.[26] Neonates on indomethacin and furosemide therapies for persistent ductus arteriosus (PDA), for example, have impaired renal autoregulation due to indomethacin's inhibition of prostaglandin production as well as furosemide's inhibition of $Na^+/K^+/2Cl^-$ cotransporter, which is involved in the tubuloglomerular feedback mechanism.[25,27]

Inflammation and Oxidative Stress in AKI

Experimental AKI models in ischemia-reperfusion, sepsis-endotoxemia, and nephrotoxin injury have shed further light in the pathogenesis of AKI. The initial insult from ischemia, sepsis, and nephrotoxin results in morphologic and functional changes to endothelial cells and tubular epithelial cells, which in turn initiate the proinflammatory cascade.[28] In the endothelium, for example, ischemic injury disrupts the cell-to-cell border, leading to impaired barrier function and increased vascular permeability, which facilitates leukocyte infiltration into the injured parenchyma.[28] Injured proximal tubular epithelial cells express interferon regulatory factor 1 (IRF-1), a transcription factor that activates proinflammatory genes, including interferons and chemokines.[29] Injured cells and leukocytes produce proinflammatory cytokines/chemokines, such as

tumor necrosis factor α (TNF-α), interleukin (IL) 2, IL-6, IL-10, and monocyte chemoattractant protein-1 (MCP-1), which are important in the initiation and extension of inflammation in AKI.[28]

The combination of reactive oxygen species (ROS) and impaired antioxidant capacity are believed to contribute significantly to the pathogenesis in AKI. Under normal circumstances, ROS such as hydroxyl radical (HO^-), peroxynitrite ($ONOO^-$), and hyperchlorous acid (OCl^-) are generated in low concentrations and are neutralized by endogenous antioxidants, including catalase and glutathione. In hypoxemic and inflammatory settings, however, the homeostasis between the oxidants and antioxidants is altered to favor oxidants, leading to tissue injury.[25,30] These ROSs attack various cellular components and cause disruptions in the plasma membrane, cytoskeletal proteins, and cell-to-cell adhesions.[25,31] ROSs also scavenge nitric oxide and cause vasoconstriction.[25]

DIFFERENTIAL DIAGNOSES

The causes of AKI are classically divided into 3 categories: prerenal, intrinsic, and postrenal (obstructive) (Table 42-6). Prerenal azotemia is considered a functional response to renal hypoperfusion, and renal microstructure and parenchyma are preserved. Prerenal azotemia resolves within a few days of restoring adequate renal perfusion. Intrinsic AKI can be further subdivided into vascular (large vessels and microvascular), glomerular, and tubulointerstitial causes. Despite this classification system, it is important to recognize that AKI in the clinical setting is often multifactorial, and that the risk of AKI increases with the number of nephrotoxic insults.[27,32] A few specific causes of AKI commonly seen in neonates are discussed.

Aminoglycoside-Induced AKI

Kidneys are susceptible to drug-induced toxicity due to their high blood flow, their role in drug metabolism and elimination, and high concentrations of the drug in the tubular lumen and interstitium.[25] In aminoglycoside nephrotoxicity, the cationic amino groups on the drug bind to the anionic phospholipid residue on the proximal tubule. The drug is then internalized through endocytosis and sequestered in the lysosomes, where it causes lysosomal rupture and leads to mitochondrial dysfunction, impaired protein synthesis, and cell apoptosis.[33-35] Aminoglycoside-induced nephrotoxicity typically causes nonoliguric AKI with tubular dysfunction, which can lead to multiple electrolyte anomalies, such as hypokalemia, hypophosphatemia, and hypomagnesemia.[35] The risk factors for developing aminoglycoside-induced AKI

Table 42-6 Causes of Acute Kidney Injury in Neonates and Infants

Prerenal

Intravascular volume depletion
- Gastrointestinal losses: vomiting, diarrhea, nasogastric tube loss, ostomy loss
- Renal losses: diuretic use, osmotic diuresis, diabetes insipidus
- Hemorrhage: twin-twin transfusion, surgery
- Skin, mucous membrane losses
- Third-space loss: capillary leakage, sepsis

Decreased renal blood flow/perfusion
- Hypotension
- Cardiogenic shock
- ECMO
- Cardiopulmonary bypass surgery
- Congenital heart disease: persistent ductal arteriosus (large left-to-right shunt)
- Perinatal asphyxia
- Abdominal compartment syndrome

Renal vasoconstriction
- Hepatorenal syndrome
- Acute hypercalcemia
- Drugs: NSAIDs, norepinephrine, vasopressin
- Iodinated contrast agents

Intrinsic

Acute tubular necrosis/tubular injury
- Prolonged ischemia
- Endogenous toxins: myoglobin, hemoglobin, uric acid
- Exogenous toxins: antibiotics, radiocontrast agents, phosphate preparations

Acute tubulointerstitial nephritis
- Drugs: NSAIDs, antibiotics
- Infections: bacterial, viral, fungal infections

Vascular lesions
- Cortical necrosis
- Renal vein thrombosis
- Renal artery thrombosis

Congenital/Genetic

Hypoplasia
- Dysplasia with or without obstructive uropathy
- Cystic renal diseases
  - ARPKD
  - ADPKD (rare to have renal dysfunction in infancy)
  - Cystic dysplasia
- Congenital nephrotic syndrome

Postrenal/Obstructive

- Obstructive uropathy: posterior urethral valves, neurogenic bladder
- Obstruction of ureters, bladder, or urethra
- Retroperitoneal mass
- "Pseudo-AKI": urinary tract perforation

Abbreviations: AKI, acute kidney injury; ADPKD, autosomal dominant polycystic kidney disease; ARPKD, autosomal recessive polycystic kidney disease; ECMO, extracorporeal membrane oxygenation; NSAID, nonsteroidal anti-inflammatory drug.

in neonates include prolonged duration of therapy (>5–10 days), high trough and peak levels, concomitant nephrotoxic medications, and the presence of renal hypoperfusion.[35]

Nonsteroidal Anti-inflammatory Drug-Induced AKI

Nonsteroidal anti-inflammatory drugs (NSAIDs), such as indomethacin and ibuprofen, decrease RBF by inhibiting cyclooxygenase (COX) enzyme, thus inhibiting the production of prostaglandins, vasodilators in renal circulation. NSAIDs can also cause kidney injury independent of the cyclooxygenase inhibition. In vitro studies have shown that indomethacin causes renal epithelial cell injury by downregulating its antiapoptotic proteins and upregulating proapoptotic proteins.[36] Likewise, it is well known that NSAIDs can cause interstitial nephritis in humans.[37] In a Japanese postmarking surveillance study consisting of 2538 low birth weight infants, electrolyte and renal abnormalities (defined as Na < 125 mEq/L, K > 7 mEq/L, urine output decrease > 40%, serum urea nitrogen [BUN] > 40 mg/dL, or Cr > 1.7 mg/dL) were seen in 40% of the infants following indomethacin administration.[38] Risk factors associated with the development of electrolyte abnormality or renal insufficiency included maternal tocolysis with indomethacin (OR 1.4; 95% CI 1.01, 1.95); chorioamnionitis (OR 1.39; 95% CI 1.04, 1.86); and preexisting electrolyte or renal abnormalities (OR 1.23; 95% CI 1.23, 2.73).[38]

Some have hypothesized that furosemide may attenuate the nephrotoxic side effects of indomethacin as furosemide was found to stimulate COX-2, resulting in increased prostaglandin E_2 (PGE_2) production.[39–41] However, recent clinical studies have shown a higher incidence of AKI in neonates who received indomethacin with furosemide compared to those who received indomethacin alone for PDA.[42,43] In a single center, a randomized, prospective study of indomethacin plus furosemide vs indomethacin alone in preterm infants with PDA, AKI (defined as serum Cr > 1.6 mg/dL) was seen in 59% of those who received indomethacin and furosemide and in 10% of those who received indomethacin alone (OR 12.38; 95% CI 3.1, 49.0).[43] In fact, the study was terminated early due to the significantly higher risk of AKI in the indomethacin-plus-furosemide group. In these neonates, who often have multiple risk factors for AKI, such as prematurity, respiratory distress syndrome, exposure to nephrotoxic medications, and renal hypoperfusion due to large shunting via PDA, furosemide may act as an additive nephrotoxic insult by causing hypovolemia and further impairment in renal autoregulation.

Ibuprofen has fewer nephrotoxic side effects than indomethacin and a closure rate similar to PDA.[44] In a prospective, multicenter, randomized trial of indomethacin vs ibuprofen in 148 infants with PDA, oliguria (urine output < 1 mL/kg/h) occurred in 19% of the infants in the indomethacin group and in 7% of the infants in the ibuprofen group (P = .03). Serum Cr was 1.09 mg/dL in the indomethacin group and 0.95 mg/dL in the ibuprofen group (P = .04) 4 days following therapy.[45] A Cochrane database review in 2010 examined the efficacy and adverse effects of indomethacin vs ibuprofen in PDA closure in preterm infants and concluded that the PDA closure failure rate was similar between the 2 agents and that transient renal insufficiency was seen less in the ibuprofen group.[46] Although the mechanisms that differentiate the nephrotoxic effects of indomethacin and ibuprofen are unclear, 1 hypothesis is that indomethacin may inhibit COX-1, which is believed to have a more prominent role in the renal basal physiologic processes than COX-2, more than ibuprofen.[44,45]

DIAGNOSTIC TESTS

History and Physical Examination

Prenatal history, perinatal history, and physical examination are important in the workup of a neonate with AKI. Table 42-7 summarizes pertinent history and physical examination findings. A urethral Foley catheter not only can facilitate in the strict in-and-out fluid measurements but also can be used to diagnose obstructive AKI. In addition, intravesical pressure can be measured in clinically suspected cases of abdominal compartment syndrome. The World Society of Abdominal Compartment Syndrome (WSACS) defines abdominal compartment syndrome as sustained intra-abdominal pressure greater than 20 mm Hg associated with new organ dysfunction or failure.[47] In children and infants, however, abdominal compartment syndrome has been described in patients with lower intra-abdominal pressures (10–12 mm Hg).[48,49]

Table 42-7 Pertinent History and Physical Examination in Neonates/Infants With Acute Kidney Injury

Findings	Comments
History	
Prenatal ultrasound	• Oligohydraminios/anhydraminios in obstructive uropathy • Renal hypoplasia, dysplasia, and other structural abnormalities
Perinatal history	• Placenta abruption • Apgar score (perinatal asphyxia) • Twin-twin transfusion
Umbilical artery/vein catheterization?	• Increased risk for renal artery thrombosis/renal vein thrombosis
Exposure to nephrotoxic medications?	• Aminoglycosides, NSAIDs, other antimicrobials, chemotherapy agents
Physical examination	
Weight trend	• Volume status
Urine output	• Oliguria usually defined as < 0.5–1 mL/kg/h
Hypertension	• May suggest hypervolemia, renal artery thrombosis • Coarctation of aorta may cause renal hypoperfusion
Hypotension	• Renal hypoperfusion
Heart murmur	• Large left-to-right shunts may cause renal hypoperfusion
Abdominal examination	• Significant distention may suggest abdominal compartment syndrome or urine ascites causing "pseudo"-AKI (rare) • Tenderness may suggest renal vein thrombosis • Mass may suggest ARPKD/obstructive AKI
Potter syndrome	• Pulmonary insufficiency, flattened nasal bridge, low-set ears, joint contractures; seen in obstructive uropathy
Gross hematuria	• Renal artery thrombosis, infection, hemorrhage, cortical necrosis

Abbreviation: ARPKD, autosomal recessive polycystic kidney disease; NSAID, nonsteroidal anti-inflammatory drug.

Laboratory Evaluation

Serum Creatinine

Serum Cr is a marker of renal dysfunction and late consequence of injury, not a marker for injury itself. Serum Cr may not change until 25%–50% of the kidney function has been lost, thus relying only on serum Cr delays the diagnosis of true kidney injury. Also, at lower GFR levels, serum Cr overestimates the true GFR as tubular secretion of Cr increases.[14] Nonetheless, serum Cr is the most commonly used biomarker to identify AKI in the clinical setting.

Urine Studies

Fractional excretion of sodium (FeNa) is less than 2.5% in prerenal azotemia and more than 2.5% in intrinsic AKI in neonates.[50,51] FeNa is calculated as $[(U_{Na} \times P_{Na})/(U_{Cr} \times P_{Cr})] \times 100$. Fractional excretion of urea (FeUrea) less than 35% has been associated with prerenal azotemia in adult patients; however, this has not been studied in neonates.[52] Similar to FeNa, FeUrea is calculated as $[(U_{urea} \times P_{BUN})/(U_{Cr} \times P_{Cr})] \times 100$.

Plasma and Urine Biomarkers

Various biomarkers, including cystatin C (CysC), neutrophil gelatinase-associated lipocalin (NGAL), kidney injury molecule 1 (KIM-1), and IL-18 have been studied in neonates in attempts to identify kidney injury early and allow for earlier intervention with the ultimate goal of improving morbidity and mortality. These biomarkers have been studied in the clinical settings of asphyxia, cardiac surgery, sepsis, and nephrotoxic exposures. Although the majority of the results are promising for the biomarkers' ability to predict AKI earlier than serum Cr in the neonatal population, biomarkers continue to remain primarily a research interest and have not yet been widely incorporated into daily clinical use.

Cystatin C. CysC is an endogenous cysteine protease inhibitor produced by most nucleated cells at a constant rate. It is freely filtered by the glomerulus, not secreted by the renal tubules, and completely reabsorbed and catabolized in the proximal tubule.[53,54] Unlike serum Cr, serum CysC levels in term infants do not reflect maternal serum values, making CysC an attractive alternative for estimating GFR in neonates.[54] Although serum CysC has been shown to better estimate GFR in children, this remains to be seen in neonates.[55-57]

Urine CysC concentration has been found to be elevated in neonates with AKI. In a nested case-control study of neonates with 5-minute Apgar scores less than 7, urine CysC concentration in 9 neonates with AKI

was 1771% higher than in 24 neonates without AKI.[58] The area under the curve (AUC) was 0.82, indicating good positive prediction for AKI. Li et al prospectively collected urine biomarkers from nonseptic critically ill neonates and showed that urine CysC levels collected 0–48 hours prior to the clinical diagnosis of AKI was significantly higher in 11 neonates with AKI compared to 51 neonates without AKI.[59] For every 1000 ng/mg increase in urine CysC/urine Cr, the adjusted OR of developing AKI within 48 hours was 2.18 (95% CI 1.16, 4.12), with an excellent AUC of 0.92.

Neutrophil gelatinase-associated lipocalin. NGAL is a protein expressed in renal tubules after ischemic or toxic injury.[54] There is a rapid upregulation of NGAL messenger RNA (mRNA) in the proximal tubules and in the loop of Henle within a few hours of nephrotoxic stimuli.[60] Among 35 neonates (>37 gestational weeks) undergoing cardiac surgery, plasma and urine NGAL concentrations were elevated 2 hours following CPB initiation in 8 neonates who developed AKI compared to 27 neonates who did not develop AKI.[61] For every 10 ng/mL increase in the 2-hour post-CPB initiation plasma NGAL level, the odds of AKI increased by 47% (OR 1.47; 95% CI 1.29, 1.73). Likewise, for every 10 ng/mL increase in the 2-hour urine NGAL concentration, the odds of AKI increased by 32% (OR 1.32; 95% CI 1.17, 1.52). In a small case-control study of neonates with perinatal asphyxia with and without AKI, plasma and urine NGAL concentrations were noted to be significantly elevated in those with AKI when checked on day of life (DOL) 1, 3, and 10.[62] Urine NGAL has also been found to be elevated in VLBW infants with and without AKI.[63] For every 100 ng/mL increase in NGAL, the odds of having AKI increased by 20% (OR 1.2; 95% CI 1.0, 1.6; $P < .01$). It is important to note that the absolute NGAL cut-off values in the 3 studies mentioned differed notably from 18.6 ng/mL[62] to 985 ng/mL[63] using the enzyme-linked immunosorbent assay (ELISA) method. This may be due to the age of the infants at the time of the sampling, their gestational age, interassay variations between different commercial assays, and possibly the different underlying pathologic processes that led to the common clinical outcome of AKI as defined by serum Cr.

Kidney injury molecule 1. KIM-1 is a transmembrane glycoprotein expressed on renal tubules following ischemic or toxic injury. It confers on the epithelial cells the ability to recognize and phagocytose dead cells.[64] Urine KIM-1 levels were not significantly different in asphyxiated neonates with and without AKI on DOL 1 or 3, but the levels were higher on DOL 10.[62] Urine KIM-1 levels were not significantly different in VLBW infants with and without AKI, but urine KIM-1 level was higher in nonsurvivors than in survivors.[63]

Imaging Studies

Renal ultrasound is an important initial imaging study in evaluating neonates with AKI. It can identify congenital renal disease such as ARPKD or obstructive causes of AKI (Figure 42-3). Pertinent features of the parenchyma include kidney size and volume, echogenicity, corticomedullary differentiation, and cortical thickness.[65] The presence of severe bilateral urinary tract dilation and hydronephrosis may suggest obstructive causes of AKI. Patients with acute tubular necrosis or other causes of intrinsic AKI may have increased echogenicity of the cortex, but more commonly, the ultrasound is normal. Doppler study should also be obtained to evaluate the blood flow to the kidneys. Noncontrast MRI may be needed to more accurately characterize renal perfusion if there are strong clinical concerns for renal infarcts, renal vein thrombosis, or renal artery stenosis. Echocardiogram is important in neonates suspected to have congenital heart disease or heart failure as AKI can occur in the setting of cardiorenal syndrome.[66,67]

MANAGEMENT

The management of AKI, in most cases, depends on the etiology of AKI. In prerenal AKI, fluid resuscitation is required to restore renal perfusion and renal function. In obstructive AKI, the creation of a lower-resistance urinary flow tract by placing a urinary Foley catheter or pylostomy may be required. As the risk and the severity of AKI increase with the number of nephrotoxic insults, it is important to minimize these insults by removing nephrotoxic medications and preventing hypovolemia and hypotension to maintain renal perfusion. As discussed, many infants with AKI have decreased ability to autoregulate RBF; therefore, they often require higher BPs to maintain adequate renal perfusion.

Acute Management of Intrinsic AKI

There is no specific treatment of AKI; therefore, the management focus is interventions to prevent the

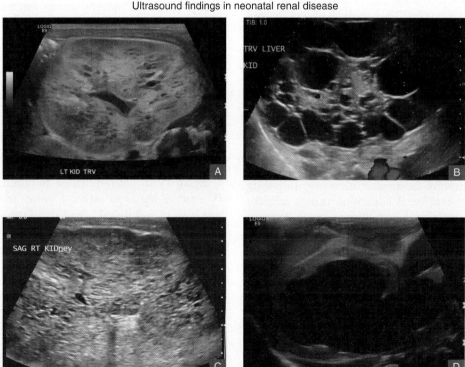

Ultrasound findings in neonatal renal disease

FIGURE 42-3 Ultrasound findings in renal disease. A, Renal ultrasound of a 2-day-old term girl with increasing serum creatinine and anuria. Renal ultrasound shows bilateral cystic dysplasia. She was started on peritoneal dialysis. B, Renal ultrasound of a day-old boy born at 29 gestational weeks with increasing serum creatinine and anuria. Renal ultrasound shows bilateral multicystic kidneys. He underwent bilateral nephrectomy and was started on peritoneal dialysis. C, Renal ultrasound of a day-old term boy with elevated serum creatinine and anuria. Renal ultrasound shows large echogenic kidneys with innumerable small cysts consistent with autosomal recessive polycystic kidney disease. D, Renal ultrasound of a few-day-old boy born at 36 gestational weeks with pulmonary hypoplasia and Potter syndrome. He was found to have posterior urethral valves. This ultrasound shows a large urinoma in the left kidney with little parenchymal tissue.

development of AKI and to minimize the degree of renal injury once AKI occurs. A few interventions have shown promising results in neonates with AKI.

Rasburicase

Recent data from animal model, clinical, and epidemiological studies have suggested a pathogenic role of uric acid in the development and progression of kidney disease.[68,69] Uric acid may cause vasoconstriction, impair autoregulation, decrease GFR, and stimulate proinflammatory responses.[70] Rasburicase is a recombinant urate oxidase enzyme that converts existing uric acid to allantoin, which is highly water soluble and readily excretable.[71] In a small retrospective study consisting of 7 neonates with AKI and hyperuricemia (serum uric acid > 8 mg/dL), a single intravenous dose of rasburicase (0.15–0.20 mg/kg) followed by normal saline flush was administered. The cause of AKI in these neonates included hypoxic ischemic event, sepsis with and without multiorgan failure, and acute tubular necrosis (ATN). Serum uric acid decreased significantly within 24 hours, mean serum Cr decreased from 3.2 ± 2 mg/ dL to 2.0 ± 1.2 mg/dL ($P < .05$) within 24 hours, and urine output increased from 2.4 ± 1.2 mL/kg/h to 5.9 ± 1.8 mL/kg/h ($P < 0.05$).[72] This study, however, lacked a control group. Although there are other case reports of hyperuricemic AKI improvement following rasburicase administration in pediatric patients, a prospective randomized study is needed.[73–75] Rasburicase should be avoided in patients with glucose-6-phosphate dehydrogenase deficiency, methemoglobinemia, and other conditions known to cause hemolytic anemia.[71]

Theophylline

Renal production of adenosine increases following ischemic injury, and renal adenosine causes afferent arteriolar vasoconstriction and efferent arteriolar vasodilation, leading to a decrease in GFR.[76] Theophylline and aminophylline are methylxanthine derivatives that act as nonspecific adenosine receptor antagonists and have been shown to decrease renal injury in animal models[77] and decrease contrast-induced nephropathy in patients.[78] A single dose of theophylline was shown to decrease the incidence of AKI in term infants with perinatal asphyxia in a randomized, double-blind, and placebo-controlled study.[79] Twenty-four infants were randomized to receive theophylline (8 mg/kg IV), and 27 infants were randomized to receive placebo within an hour of delivery. AKI developed in 4/24 (17%) infants in the theophylline group compared to 15/27 (55%) infants in the placebo group (relative risk [RR] 0.30; 95% CI 0.12, 0.78; $P < .001$). Serum Cr was similar between the 2 groups on day of life (DOL) 1, but it was higher in the placebo group during the remaining study period from DOL 2 to 5. Urine output was

significantly higher in the theophylline group during the first 4 DOL than in the placebo group. Serum theophylline level was 12.7 µg/mL (range 7.5–18.9 µg/mL) in the treatment group at 36–48 hours compared to 0.87 µg/mL in the placebo group. In a similar randomized, placebo-controlled study of 70 term infants with perinatal asphyxia, 40 infants received a single intravenous dose of theophylline (8 mg/kg), and 30 infants received a single dose of placebo within 1 hour of birth. AKI was seen in 10/40 (25%) of infants in the treatment group compared to 18/30 (60%) of infants in the placebo group (RR 0.41; 95% CI 0.22, 0.76; $P < .001$).[80] Urine output was significantly higher in the treatment group on DOL 2 and 3, and the fluid output/ input ratio was greater in the treatment group during the first 5 DOL. Serum Cr normalized by 6 weeks of life in all infants with AKI. At 1-year follow-up, serum Cr and Cr clearance were similar in both groups. In a randomized, double-blind, placebo-controlled study of 47 preterm (<32 gestational weeks) infants with respiratory distress syndrome requiring mechanical ventilation or nasal continuous positive airway pressure, the infants who received theophylline (1 mg/kg IV daily for 3 days) had higher urine output on DOL 1 than those in the placebo group, but there was no difference in the urine output between the 2 groups over the remaining 10 days of the study period.[81] Serum Cr was significantly lower in the theophylline group on DOL 2, but serum Cr levels were similar on DOL 5 and DOL 11. Current evidence shows that theophylline improves urine output and estimated GFR in the early course of the AKI. Long-term effects on clinically important outcomes such as mortality and hospital length of stay were not examined in these studies. At our center, we administer a single loading dose of 5 mg/kg IV of aminophylline followed by 1.8 mg/kg IV every 6 hours to target a serum trough theophylline level of 5–7 µg/mL. A study of the effectiveness of aminophylline treatment in prevention of AKI in high-risk newborns requiring CPB is ongoing in our center (Clinicaltrials.gov, NCT01245595).

Fenoldopam

Fenoldopam is a selective dopamine 1 receptor agonist that has been shown to induce renal vasodilation, diuresis, and natriuresis.[82] Randomized studies in critically ill adult patients have shown mixed results, with some showing reduction in the incidence of AKI[83,84] and some showing no benefit.[85,86] Recent meta-analyses showed that fenoldopam reduced AKI in adult patients undergoing cardiac surgery[87] and reduced AKI, the need for renal replacement therapy (RRT), and in-hospital mortality in critically ill adult patients.[88] A retrospective study of 13 critically ill pediatric patients showed that fenoldopam increased diuresis without adverse effects such as hypotension.[89] In a prospective, nonblinded clinical trial consisting of 40 neonates undergoing cardiac surgery requiring CPB, 20 neonates were assigned to receive fenoldopam at 0.1 µg/kg/min following anesthesia induction to 72 hours postoperatively; the control group received standard therapy.[90] There was a trend toward higher urine output and a fluid balance that was more negative in the fenoldopam group during the study period of 4 postoperative days, but this was not significantly different. Serum Cr was also not significantly different between the 2 groups. Hypotension rate and inotropic score were similar between the 2 groups. The authors hypothesized that the fenoldopam dose may have been too low to show clinical effect. The same group conducted a randomized, double-blinded, placebo-controlled study consisting of 80 infants undergoing CPB for cardiac repair surgery; high-dose fenoldopam (1 µg/kg/min) was used from CPB initiation to CPB weaning.[91] The fenoldopam group's urinary NGAL and CysC were significantly lower than for the control group immediately following the surgery. The incidence of AKI, as defined by pRIFLE, tended to be lower in the treatment group compared to the control group, 50% vs 72%, respectively ($P = .08$, OR 0.38; 95% CI 0.14, 1.02). Current evidence in the pediatric and neonatal literature does not support routine use of fenoldopam, but the results appear promising.

Maintenance Management of Intrinsic AKI

Fluid Management

It is important to maintain euvolemia in patients with AKI, particularly in the light of the recently emerging evidence that fluid overload is an independent mortality risk in critically ill children.[92,93] The most helpful clinical tool in assessing fluid status is daily weight measurement. Infants with AKI should receive daily to twice daily weight measurements.[3] Strict intake and output also need to be measured. A urethral Foley catheter is recommended to facilitate in strict urine output measurements.

Diuretics

Clinical studies in adult patients with AKI showed that diuretics do not reduce the need for RRT or the risk of hospital mortality.[94] However, inducing urine output with diuretics can facilitate fluid balance in patients with oliguric AKI and, importantly in infants, enable the administration of more nutrition. The most commonly used diuretics include loop diuretics (furosemide, bumetanide) and thiazide diuretics (hydrochlorothiazide, metolazone). Loop diuretics decrease sodium reabsorption by inhibiting the Na-K-2Cl transporter on the thick ascending limb of the loop of Henle, thereby decreasing water reabsorption. Loop diuretics are highly protein bound and therefore minimally filtered at the glomerulus. Organic acid transporters located in the proximal tubule actively secrete loop diuretics from the blood into the urine, and they reach the Na-K-2Cl transporters in the loop of Henle.[82] Hypoalbuminemia and the presence of other highly protein-bound drugs can decrease the tubular delivery of loop diuretics and lead to reduced diuretic effect.[82] Loop diuretic dose requirement in AKI is higher than in the non-AKI setting because these diuretics depend on RBF for adequate delivery to the tubules. Furosemide bolus dose ranges from 0.5 to 1 mg/kg in the non-AKI setting; therefore, the initial bolus dose in the AKI setting should be at least 2 mg/kg.[95] If furosemide induces diuresis in the patient, furosemide may be continued every 6–8 hours in term infants, every 12 hours in preterm infants older than 32 gestational weeks, and every 24 hours in preterm infants younger than 32 gestational weeks.[95] Alternatively, the patient can be placed on continuous infusion starting at 0.1 mg/kg/h. Bumetanide is an alternate to furosemide. In a retrospective study consisting of 35 preterm infants with AKI, bumetanide (0.01–0.06 mg/kg/dose every 12–24 hours) increased urine output from 0.6 ± 0.6 mL/kg/h to 3.0 ± 2.1 mL/kg/h.[96] Loop diuretics should be discontinued if adequate diuresis cannot be achieved following appropriately dosed diuretic trial to minimize the risk of adverse effects such as ototoxicity.[82,95] Thiazide diuretics show a synergistic diuretic effect with loop diuretics by inhibiting the Na-Cl channel in the distal convoluted tubule, thereby blocking reabsorption distal to the loop diuretic's site of action.[82] If a patient remains oliguric despite adequate diuretic challenge, the patient's fluid intake should be reduced to estimated insensible water loss plus output (urine output, stool output, ostomy output) to maintain fluid balance.

The infant's renal function recovery may be accompanied by a polyuric diuretic phase, especially following the initial relief of obstruction, caused by the excretion of volume and solute retained during the renal obstruction. Prolonged polyuria may also occur due to the delayed recovery of tubular function relative to GFR, which results in excretion of excessive solute and water.[97,98] Intravenous fluid may be needed during this phase to prevent the development of hypotension and prerenal AKI.

Hemodynamic Support

Patients with persistent hypotension despite adequate fluid resuscitation require systemic vasopressor support to minimize AKI. Current evidence in adult literature does not support the use of "renal-dose" or "low-dose" dopamine but emphasizes restoring BP in hypotensive patients to maintain end-organ perfusion and restore regional autoregulation.[99–102] Although there are several controlled and uncontrolled clinical experimental studies of low-dose dopamine in infants, well-powered, randomized, controlled clinical trials are lacking, and there is not enough evidence to justify the routine use of low-dose dopamine for "renal protection."[103–106]

Electrolyte Management

Hyponatremia, hyperkalemia, hyperphosphatemia, and metabolic acidosis can occur in AKI. Hyponatremia most often reflects hypervolemia and can be corrected with fluid restriction.[3] Hyponatremia in the setting of polyuric AKI may reflect total body sodium depletion due to impaired tubular reabsorption; therefore, increased sodium intake is needed. Serum sodium less than 120 mEq/L may increase the infant's risk of seizures, so correction with 3% saline should be considered.

Hyperkalemia may result secondary to decreased renal excretion due to reduced GFR and intracellular shift in AKI-induced metabolic acidosis. Hyperkalemia may result in cardiac arrhythmias and cardiac arrest; therefore, potassium should be monitored frequently in infants with AKI. Potassium should be removed from IVF and parenteral nutrition (PN) on identifying AKI to minimize the risk of hyperkalemia. Infants on formula should be placed on low-potassium nutrition such as maternal breast milk (MBM) or renal formula PM60/40. Depending on the degree of hyperkalemia, pharmaceutical interventions include (1) calcium chloride (via central line) or calcium gluconate to stabilize the cardiac resting membrane potential; (2) insulin/dextrose, sodium bicarbonate (if the patient is acidotic), and inhaled β-adrenergic agonist to shift potassium into the intracellular compartment; and (3) furosemide and sodium polystyrene sulfonate to remove potassium. Sodium polystyrene sulfonate (available as Kayexalate in the United States) is a cation exchange resin that binds potassium in exchange for sodium in the large intestine; therefore, hypernatremia can develop as a side effect. In addition, bowel necrosis has been reported in infants receiving sodium polystyrene sulfonate, particularly preterm infants, postoperative patients, patients with preexisting bowel obstruction, or patients receiving it administered as an enema.[107,108] If hyperkalemia persists despite changing the formula to a renal formula, potassium in the formula can be further decreased by pretreating it with sodium polystyrene sulfonate, then decanting it.[109–111]

Hyperphosphatemia may occur due to decreased renal excretion in AKI. Hyperphosphatemia can be managed by restricting phosphorus intake by removing phosphate from PN and by decreasing enteral feed phosphorus content by pretreating then decanting it with phosphate binder such as sevelamer.[112]

Metabolic acidosis may occur in AKI due to reduced renal excretion of acid generated by dietary intake and cellular metabolism. It is important to consider serum ionized calcium and correct low calcium when considering treatment of metabolic acidosis. Total serum calcium is present in protein-bound form and free ionized form, which exerts physiologic effects. Acidosis treatment can shift ionized calcium to bind to protein, leading to an acute decrease in ionized calcium, which can precipitate tetany or seizures.[27]

Nutrition

Infants with AKI require optimal nutrition because AKI is often associated with catabolism, and malnutrition can develop quickly in these patients, further delaying their recovery.[27] Enteral nutrition is preferred if the patient is stable enough to tolerate it. MBM is the preferred nutrition for infants with AKI. It may be helpful to fortify MBM to increase caloric intake. If MBM is not available, renal formula (PM60/40) is preferred in infants with hyperkalemia. Depending on the patient's fluid status, PN should be concentrated as much as possible without compromising the administered calories and protein. Potassium, phosphorus, and magnesium may need to be removed from PN on initial diagnosis of AKI and returned in smaller amounts if needed.

Renal Replacement Therapy

Indications for initiating RRT in AKI include hyperkalemia or metabolic acidosis not responsive to pharmaceutical interventions, complications of hypervolemia, or the need for increased fluid intake with inadequate ability to increase diuresis to match the increased intake (eg, infants with liver failure who require high volumes of fresh-frozen plasma or infants who require more fluid for nutrition). Available RRT for infants with AKI includes peritoneal dialysis (PD), intermittent hemodialysis (IHD), and continuous hemofiltration with or without dialysis. The preferred type of RRT depends on patient factors as well as the availability of local personnel and equipment resources.

Peritoneal Dialysis

The PD system consists of peritoneal capillary blood flow (peritoneal microcirculation); the peritoneal membrane, which serves as the semipermeable dialysis membrane; and the dialysis fluid.[113] Commercially available dialysis fluid contains an osmotic agent such as glucose or icodextrin, a buffer to correct the patient's metabolic acidosis, and balanced concentrations of electrolytes sodium, calcium, and magnesium. The major driving force for ultrafiltration, the bulk movement of water across the semipermeable membrane, comes from the osmotic gradient provided by glucose or icodextrin in the dialysis fluid. Glucose concentrations of 1.5%, 2.5%, and 4.25% are commercially available, and various combinations of the dialysis fluid bags can be used at bedside to provide intermediate glucose concentrations, if needed. Solute exchange occurs primarily through diffusive transport driven by the solute concentration gradient and secondarily by solute removal by convection in ultrafiltration. The major advantages of PD include relatively easier access to the peritoneal cavity compared to vascular access, there is no need for systemic heparinization, and it is well tolerated in small infants and hemodynamically unstable patients (Figures 42-4 and 42-5). Disadvantages include slower correction of metabolic derangements and the risk of peritonitis, which is higher in those with a temporary compared to a permanent tunneled PD catheter. Additional assessment of risks and benefits are required in infants with intra-abdominal pathologies such as massive organomegaly and ostomies.[27]

Intermittent Hemodialysis

Solute exchange through the semipermeable dialyzer membrane occurs primarily through diffusion driven by the concentration gradient and by convective solute removal in the ultrafiltrate. Hemodialysis (HD) corrects metabolic derangements rapidly, and it can be used successfully in the initial management of

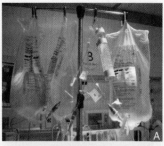
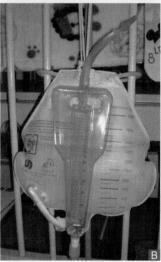

FIGURE 42-5 Manual peritoneal dialysis setup in the neonatal intensive care unit. Manual peritoneal dialysis. A, Bureterol device (sterile graduated cylinder), Y set, and a graduated drain. Peritoneal dialysis bags consisting of different dextrose concentrations (1.5%, 2.5%, 4.25%) are attached to 1 end of the bureterol device, and the other end is attached to the patient's peritoneal dialysis catheter via a Y set. B, The other limb of the Y set is connected to a graduated drain to measure the effluent.

hyperammonemia in urea cycle defects.[114,115] Blood circuit priming is recommended when the extracorporeal volume exceeds 10% of the patient's estimated blood volume (80 mL/kg × body weight) to prevent acute hypotension and anemia.[113,116]

Continuous Renal Replacement Therapy

Continuous renal replacement therapy (CRRT) can be delivered as continuous venovenous hemofiltration (CVVH), which utilizes convective clearance; continuous venovenous hemodialysis (CVVHD), which utilizes diffusive clearance; and continuous venovenous hemodiafiltration (CVVHDF), which utilizes both diffusive and convective clearance. Ultrafiltration and solute clearance occur gradually over time; thus, this modality is well tolerated in hemodynamically unstable patients. CRRT can be used effectively in small infants, even in patients less than 3 kg.[117] As with

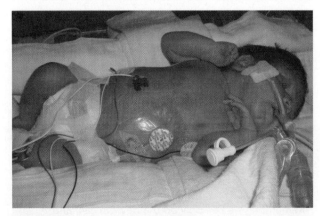

FIGURE 42-4 Peritoneal dialysis is well tolerated in small infants. This infant was started on peritoneal dialysis soon after birth at 1.7 kg of birth weight.

Table 42-8 Hemodialysis Catheter Size Based on Patient Size[a]

Patient Size	Catheter	Insertion Site
Neonate	Dual-lumen 7.0F catheter	Internal/external jugular, femoral vein
3–6 kg	Dual-lumen 7.0F catheter	Internal/external jugular, femoral vein
6–30 kg	Dual-lumen 8.0F catheter	Internal/external jugular, femoral vein
>15 kg	Dual-lumen 9.0F catheter	

[a]From Goldstein.[116]

intermittent HD, blood circuit priming is necessary when the extracorporeal volume exceeds 10% of the patient's blood volume. Good functional vascular access is required to deliver adequate CRRT and HD, and vascular access can be challenging in critically ill infants (Table 42-8). A double-lumen catheter can be placed in the internal jugular, femoral, or subclavian vein. The jugular vein is the preferred site as femoral vein catheters can experience complications from increased intra-abdominal pressure and subclavian catheters have been associated with stenosis at the subclavian-internal jugular junction.[113] We do not use subclavian access for dialysis at our center. The optimal site of catheter placement, however, should be assessed by the patient characteristics, the risk of complications, and the operator's skills and experience. Two 5F single-lumen catheters have been used to deliver CRRT, but we do not routinely recommend this method because the circuit survival has been shown to be poor at less than 20 hours.[116,118]

Ethical Considerations

An extensive discussion of the ethical considerations in dialysis in neonates with end-stage renal disease (ESRD), such as ARPKD and anuric dysplastic kidneys, is beyond the scope of this chapter. The decision to initiate or withhold dialysis in a neonate with AKI requires a thoughtful evaluation of many factors, including the patient's comorbidity, the risks and benefits of dialysis to the patient, and the parents' wishes. Shooter et al discussed cases for which the parents and the medical team might consider withholding or withdrawing dialysis (Table 42-9) and outlined general guidelines to consider particularly when different parties disagree on what may be the best interest of the child (Table 42-10).[119]

Table 42-9 Situations for Which Withholding or Withdrawal of Medical Treatment Might Be Considered[a]

The brain-dead child: In an older child if criteria of brainstem death are agreed by 2 practitioners in the usual way
The permanent vegetative state: The child who develops a permanent vegetative state following insults, is reliant on others for all care, and does not react or relate with the outside world
The "no chance" situation: The child has such severe disease that life-sustaining treatment simply delays death without significant alleviation of suffering
The "no purpose" situation: Although the patient may be able to survive with treatment, the degree of physical or mental impairment will be so great that it is unreasonable to expect the patient to bear it
The "unbearable" situation: The child or family feels that in the face of progressive and irreversible illness, further treatment is more than can be borne

[a]From Shooter and Watson.[119]

OUTCOME

Short-Term Follow-up

Recent studies of critically ill adults and children with AKI have consistently shown that AKI is an independent risk factor for mortality.[14,18] In a single-center prospective cohort study of 150 critically ill pediatric patients, those with a pRIFLE score of I (injury) or higher had an adjusted 28-day mortality OR of 3.0 (95% CI 1.1, 8.1) compared to those with lower level of AKI or no AKI.[120] The ELSO Registry data on neonates who required ECMO for noncardiac causes

Table 42-10 Ethical Decisions: Guidelines for Practice[a]

Always act in the child's best interest.
Never rush the decision. Continue treatment until it can be properly made.
Assemble all the available evidence.
Respect the opinions of everyone in the team.
Discuss the issues with the whole family.
Attempt a consensus whenever possible.
Make sure everyone appreciates the burden of care.
Try to avoid adding to the guilt of anyone involved.
Consider the child's palliative and terminal care.
Offer support for all those affected, parents and staff alike.
Remember, we can only do the best we can, and sometimes there is no ideal solution.

[a]From Shooter and Watson.[119]

showed that AKI and the need for RRT are independent risk factors for death.[18] The survival of neonates who developed AKI or required RRT was lower than for those who had neither (Table 42-11). The odds of death, even after adjusting for various clinical variables, in the neonates with AKI were 3 times higher than those without AKI (adjusted OR 3.2; 95% CI 2.6, 4.0; $P < .0001$). Likewise, the odds of death were 2 times higher in the neonates who received RRT compared to those who did not receive RRT (adjusted OR 1.9; 95% CI 1.6, 2.2; $P < .0001$). With the emergence of such evidence, the traditional belief that patients die "with" renal failure is now shifting to the notion that patients die "of" renal failure.[121] In fact, both clinical and in vitro studies have shown that injured kidneys activate inflammatory cascades that contribute to distant organ (lungs, heart, brain, liver) dysfunction via complex mechanisms of organ crosstalk.[122,123]

The prognosis and recovery of AKI in infants are dependent on the underlying etiology of AKI and comorbidities. In a retrospective study of 85 infants less than 10 kg who received CRRT, those with multiorgan dysfunction had the lowest survival (15%).[117] Infants weighing less than 3 kg also had lower survival rate (25%) than those weighing more than 3 kg (41%). Hypotension, need for vasopressors, need for mechanical ventilation, and oliguria have also been associated with increased mortality in infants with AKI.[13,27]

Long-Term Follow-up

There are few data on long-term follow-up of infants with AKI. In a retrospective case-control study of ELBW infants with AKI, follow-up data at the time of NICU discharge was available for 13 of 36 surviving infants with AKI.[13] Their serum Cr (0.35 ± 0.11 mg/dL), BP (systolic BP/diastolic BP 90 ± 8/51 ± 10), and weight (2.9 ± 1.7 kg) were similar to the control group of infants without AKI. Abitbol et al conducted a retrospective long-term follow-up study of 20 patients who were born prematurely with ELBW and experienced AKI during their neonatal course.[124] At a mean follow-up period of 7.5 + 4.6 years, 9 of the 20 (45%) patients had low estimated GFR, defined as estimated GFR less than 75 mL/min/1.73 m² using the Schwartz formula. Five of the 20 (25%) patients had ESRD as defined by estimated GFR less than 10 mL/min/1.73 m² or the need for RRT (dialysis or kidney transplantation). Urine protein/Cr ratio greater than 0.6 and serum Cr greater than 0.6 mg/dL at 1 year of age were predictive of developing chronic renal insufficiency.

REFERENCES

1. Mehta RL, Chertow GM. Acute renal failure definitions and classification: time for change? *J Am Soc Nephrol.* 2003;14(8):2178–2187.
2. Basu RK, Devarajan P, Wong H, Wheeler DS. An update and review of acute kidney injury in pediatrics. *Pediatr Crit Care Med.* 2011;12(3):339–347.
3. Gouyon JB, Guignard JP. Management of acute renal failure in newborns. *Pediatr Nephrol.* 2000;14(10–11):1037–1044.
4. Drukker A, Guignard JP. Renal aspects of the term and preterm infant: a selective update. *Curr Opin Pediatr.* 2002;14(2):175–182.
5. Schwartz GJ, Furth SL. Glomerular filtration rate measurement and estimation in chronic kidney disease. *Pediatr Nephrol.* 2007;22(11):1839–1848.
6. Vieux R, Hascoet JM, Merdariu D, Fresson J, Guillemin F. Glomerular filtration rate reference values in very preterm infants. *Pediatrics.* 2010;125(5):e1186–e1192.
7. Jetton JG, Askenazi DJ. Update on acute kidney injury in the neonate. *Curr Opin Pediatr.* 2012;24(2):191–196.
8. Lolekha PH, Jaruthunyaluck S, Srisawasdi P. Deproteinization of serum: another best approach to eliminate all forms of bilirubin interference on serum creatinine by the kinetic Jaffe reaction. *J Clin Lab Anal.* 2001;15(3):116–121.
9. Rajs G, Mayer M. Oxidation markedly reduces bilirubin interference in the Jaffe creatinine assay. *Clin. Chem.* 1992;38(12):2411–2413.
10. Agras PI, Tarcan A, Baskin E, Cengiz N, Gurakan B, Saatci U. Acute renal failure in the neonatal period. *Renal Failure.* 2004;26(3):305–309.
11. Koralkar R, Ambalavanan N, Levitan EB, McGwin G, Goldstein S, Askenazi D. Acute kidney injury reduces survival in very low birth weight infants. *Pediatr Res.* 2011;69(4):354–358.
12. Blinder JJ, Goldstein SL, Lee VV, et al. Congenital heart surgery in infants: effects of acute kidney injury on outcomes. *J Thorac Cardiovasc Surg.* 2012;143(2):368–374.
13. Viswanathan S, Manyam B, Azhibekov T, Mhanna MJ. Risk factors associated with acute kidney injury in extremely low birth weight (ELBW) infants. *Pediatr Nephrol.* 2012;27(2):303–311.
14. Askenazi DJ, Ambalavanan N, Goldstein SL. Acute kidney injury in critically ill newborns: what do we know? What do we need to learn? *Pediatr Nephrol.* 2009;24(2):265–274.
15. Kaur S, Jain S, Saha A, et al. Evaluation of glomerular and tubular renal function in neonates with birth asphyxia. *Ann Trop Pediatr.* 2011;31(2):129–134.
16. Gupta BD, Sharma P, Bagla J, Parakh M, Soni JP. Renal failure in asphyxiated neonates. *Indian Pediatr.* 2005;42(9):928–934.

Table 42-11 Extracorporeal Life Support Organization Registry: Survival of Noncardiac Neonates on Extracorporeal Membrane Oxygenation With and Without Acute Kidney Injury (AKI) and the Need for Renal Replacement Therapy (RRT)

Neonatal Population (n = 7941)	Percentage Survival
Neither AKI nor RRT	80.1
RRT without AKI	58.1
AKI without RRT	45.7
AKI and RRT	28.2

[a]Data from Askenazi et al.[18]

17. Aggarwal A, Kumar P, Chowdhary G, Majumdar S, Narang A. Evaluation of renal functions in asphyxiated newborns. *J Trop Pediatr.* 2005;51(5):295–299.

18. Askenazi DJ, Ambalavanan N, Hamilton K, et al. Acute kidney injury and renal replacement therapy independently predict mortality in neonatal and pediatric noncardiac patients on extracorporeal membrane oxygenation. *Pediatr Crit Care Med.* 2011;12(1):e1–e6.

19. Gadepalli SK, Selewski DT, Drongowski RA, Mychaliska GB. Acute kidney injury in congenital diaphragmatic hernia requiring extracorporeal life support: an insidious problem. *J Pediatr Surg.* 2011;46(4):630–635.

20. Morgan CJ, Zappitelli M, Robertson CM, et al. Risk factors for and outcomes of acute kidney injury in neonates undergoing complex cardiac surgery. *J Pediatr.* 2013;162(1):120–127.e1.

21. Schreuder MF. Safety in glomerular numbers. *Pediatr Nephrol.* 2012;27(10):1881–1887.

22. Rodriguez MM, Gomez AH, Abitbol CL, Chandar JJ, Duara S, Zilleruelo GE. Histomorphometric analysis of postnatal glomerulogenesis in extremely preterm infants. *Pediatr Dev Pathol.* 2004;7(1):17–25.

23. Avner ED, Harmon WE, Niaudet P, Yoshikawa N. *Pediatric Nephrology.* Vol 1. 6th ed. Berlin, Germany: Springer-Verlag; 2009.

24. Vander AJ, Pooler J, Eaton DC. *Vander's Renal Physiology.* Lange Physiology Series. New York, NY: Lange Medical Books/McGraw Hill, Medical Publishing Division; 2004:v.

25. Taal MW, Brenner BM, Rector FC. *Brenner and Rector's the Kidney.* 9th ed. Philadelphia, PA: Elsevier/Saunders; 2012.

26. Abuelo JG. Normotensive ischemic acute renal failure. *N Engl J Med.* 2007;357(8):797–805.

27. Andreoli SP. Acute renal failure in the newborn. *Semin Perinatol.* 2004;28(2):112–123.

28. Akcay A, Nguyen Q, Edelstein CL. Mediators of inflammation in acute kidney injury. *Mediators Inflamm.* 2009;2009:137072.

29. Wang Y, John R, Chen J, et al. IRF-1 promotes inflammation early after ischemic acute kidney injury. *J Am Soc Nephrol.* 2009;20(7):1544–1555.

30. Aksu U, Demirci C, Ince C. The pathogenesis of acute kidney injury and the toxic triangle of oxygen, reactive oxygen species and nitric oxide. *Contrib Nephrol.* 2011;174:119–128.

31. Heyman SN, Rosen S, Rosenberger C. A role for oxidative stress. *Contrib Nephrol.* 2011;174:138–148.

32. Moffett BS, Goldstein SL. Acute kidney injury and increasing nephrotoxic-medication exposure in noncritically-ill children. *Clin J Am Soc Nephrol.* 2011;6(4):856–863.

33. Sandoval RM, Molitoris BA. Gentamicin traffics retrograde through the secretory pathway and is released in the cytosol via the endoplasmic reticulum. *Am J Physiol Renal Physiol.* 2004;286(4):F617–F624.

34. Lopez-Novoa JM, Quiros Y, Vicente L, Morales AI, Lopez-Hernandez FJ. New insights into the mechanism of aminoglycoside nephrotoxicity: an integrative point of view. *Kidney Int.* 2011;79(1):33–45.

35. Fanos V, Cataldi L. Antibacterial-induced nephrotoxicity in the newborn. *Drug Saf.* 1999;20(3):245–267.

36. Ou YC, Yang CR, Cheng CL, et al. Indomethacin causes renal epithelial cell injury involving Mcl-1 down-regulation. *Biochem Biophys Res Commun.* 2009;380(3):531–536.

37. Maniglia R, Schwartz AB, Moriber-Katz S. Non-steroidal anti-inflammatory nephrotoxicity. *Ann Clin Lab Sci.* 1988;18(3):240–252.

38. Itabashi K, Ohno T, Nishida H. Indomethacin responsiveness of patent ductus arteriosus and renal abnormalities in preterm infants treated with indomethacin. *J Pediatr.* 2003;143(2):203–207.

39. Schnermann J. Juxtaglomerular cell complex in the regulation of renal salt excretion. *Am J Physiol.* 1998;274(2 Pt 2):R263–R279.

40. Yeh TF, Wilks A, Singh J, Betkerur M, Lilien L, Pildes RS. Furosemide prevents the renal side effects of indomethacin therapy in premature infants with patent ductus arteriosus. *J Pediatr.* 1982;101(3):433–437.

41. Reyes JL, Aldana I, Barbier O, Parrales AA, Melendez E. Indomethacin decreases furosemide-induced natriuresis and diuresis on the neonatal kidney. *Pediatr Nephrol.* 2006;21(11):1690–1697.

42. Andriessen P, Struis NC, Niemarkt H, Oetomo SB, Tanke RB, Van Overmeire B. Furosemide in preterm infants treated with indomethacin for patent ductus arteriosus. *Acta Paediatr.* 2009;98(5):797–803.

43. Lee BS, Byun SY, Chung ML, et al. Effect of furosemide on ductal closure and renal function in indomethacin-treated preterm infants during the early neonatal period. *Neonatology.* 2010;98(2):191–199.

44. Giniger RP, Buffat C, Millet V, Simeoni U. Renal effects of ibuprofen for the treatment of patent ductus arteriosus in premature infants. *J Matern Fetal Neonatal Med.* 2007;20(4):275–283.

45. Van Overmeire B, Smets K, Lecoutere D, et al. A comparison of ibuprofen and indomethacin for closure of patent ductus arteriosus. *N Engl J Med.* 2000;343(10):674–681.

46. Ohlsson A, Walia R, Shah SS. Ibuprofen for the treatment of patent ductus arteriosus in preterm and/or low birth weight infants. *Cochrane Database Syst Rev.* 2010(4):CD003481.

47. Malbrain ML, Cheatham ML, Kirkpatrick A, et al. Results from the International Conference of Experts on Intra-abdominal Hypertension and Abdominal Compartment Syndrome. I. Definitions. *Intensive Care Med.* 2006;32(11):1722–1732.

48. Steinau G, Kaussen T, Bolten B, et al. Abdominal compartment syndrome in childhood: diagnostics, therapy and survival rate. *Pediatr Surg Int.* 2011;27(4):399–405.

49. Akhobadze GR, Chkhaidze MG, Kanjaradze DV, Tsirkvadze I, Ukleba V. Identification, management and complications of intra-abdominal hypertension and abdominal compartment syndrome in neonatal intensive care unit (a single centre retrospective analysis). *Georgian Medical News.* 2011;(192):58–64.

50. Ellis EN, Arnold WC. Use of urinary indexes in renal failure in the newborn. *Am J Dis Child.* 1982;136(7):615–617.

51. Mathew OP, Jones AS, James E, Bland H, Groshong T. Neonatal renal failure: usefulness of diagnostic indices. *Pediatrics.* 1980;65(1):57–60.

52. Carvounis CP, Nisar S, Guro-Razuman S. Significance of the fractional excretion of urea in the differential diagnosis of acute renal failure. *Kidney Int.* 2002;62(6):2223–2229.

53. Grubb A. Diagnostic value of analysis of cystatin C and protein HC in biological fluids. *Clin Nephrol.* 1992;38(Suppl 1):S20–S27.

54. Argyri I, Xanthos T, Varsami M, et al. The role of novel biomarkers in early diagnosis and prognosis of acute kidney injury in newborns. *Am J Perinatol.* 2013;30(5):347–352.

55. Ylinen EA, Ala-Houhala M, Harmoinen AP, Knip M. Cystatin C as a marker for glomerular filtration rate in pediatric patients. *Pediatr Nephrol.* 1999;13(6):506–509.

56. Armangil D, Yurdakok M, Canpolat FE, Korkmaz A, Yigit S, Tekinalp G. Determination of reference values for plasma cystatin C and comparison with creatinine in premature infants. *Pediatr Nephrol.* 2008;23(11):2081–2083.

57. Treiber M, Pecovnik-Balon B, Gorenjak M. Cystatin C versus creatinine as a marker of glomerular filtration rate in the newborn. *Wien Klin Wochenschr.* 2006;118(Suppl 2):66–70.

58. Askenazi DJ, Koralkar R, Hundley HE, et al. Urine biomarkers predict acute kidney injury in newborns. *J Pediatr.* 2012;161(2):270–275.e271.

59. Li Y, Fu C, Zhou X, et al. Urine interleukin-18 and cystatin-C as biomarkers of acute kidney injury in critically ill neonates. *Pediatr Nephrol.* 2012;27(5):851–860.

60. Bolignano D, Donato V, Coppolino G, et al. Neutrophil gelatinase-associated lipocalin (NGAL) as a marker of kidney damage. *Am J Kidney Dis.* 2008;52(3):595–605.

61. Krawczeski CD, Woo JG, Wang Y, Bennett MR, Ma Q, Devarajan P. Neutrophil gelatinase-associated lipocalin concentrations predict development of acute kidney injury in neonates and children after cardiopulmonary bypass. *J Pediatr.* 2011;158(6):1009–1015.e1001.

62. Sarafidis K, Tsepkentzi E, Agakidou E, et al. Serum and urine acute kidney injury biomarkers in asphyxiated neonates. *Pediatr Nephrol.* 2012;27(9):1575–1582.

63. Askenazi DJ, Montesanti A, Hunley H, et al. Urine biomarkers predict acute kidney injury and mortality in very low birth weight infants. *J Pediatr.* 2011;159(6):907–912.e901.

64. Bonventre JV, Yang L. Kidney injury molecule-1. *Curr Opin Crit Care.* 2010;16(6):556–561.

65. Gordon I, Riccabona M. Investigating the newborn kidney: update on imaging techniques. *Semin Neonatol.* 2003;8(4):269–278.

66. Price JF, Goldstein SL. Cardiorenal syndrome in children with heart failure. *Curr Heart Failure Rep.* 2009;6(3):191–198.

67. Jefferies JL, Goldstein SL. Cardiorenal syndrome: an emerging problem in pediatric critical care. *Pediatr Nephrol.* 2013;28(6):855–862; erratum 989.

68. Lapsia V, Johnson RJ, Dass B, et al. Elevated uric acid increases the risk for acute kidney injury. *American J Med.* 2012;125(3):302.e309–317.

69. Obermayr RP, Temml C, Gutjahr G, Knechtelsdorfer M, Oberbauer R, Klauser-Braun R. Elevated uric acid increases the risk for kidney disease. *J Am Soc Nephrol.*. 2008;19(12):2407–2413.

70. Ejaz AA, Dass B, Kambhampati G, et al. Lowering serum uric acid to prevent acute kidney injury. *Med Hypotheses.* 2012;78(6):796–799.

71. Oldfield V, Perry CM. Rasburicase: a review of its use in the management of anticancer therapy-induced hyperuricaemia. *Drugs.* 2006;66(4):529–545.

72. Hobbs DJ, Steinke JM, Chung JY, Barletta GM, Bunchman TE. Rasburicase improves hyperuricemia in infants with acute kidney injury. *Pediatr Nephrol.* 2010;25(2):305–309.

73. Hooman N, Otukesh H. Single dose of rasburicase for treatment of hyperuricemia in acute kidney injury: a report of 3 cases. *Iran J Kidney Dis.* 2011;5(2):130–132.

74. Lin PY, Lin CC, Liu HC, et al. Rasburicase improves hyperuricemia in patients with acute kidney injury secondary to rhabdomyolysis caused by ecstasy intoxication and exertional heat stroke. *Pediatr Crit Care Med.* 2011;12(6):e424–e427.

75. Acosta AA, Hogg RJ. Rasburicase for hyperuricemia in hemolytic uremic syndrome. *Pediatr Nephrol.* 2012;27(2):325–329.

76. Yap SC, Lee HT. Adenosine and protection from acute kidney injury. *Curr Opin Nephrol Hypertens.* 2012;21(1):24–32.

77. Gouyon JB, Guignard JP. Theophylline prevents the hypoxemia-induced renal hemodynamic changes in rabbits. *Kidney Int.* 1988;33(6):1078–1083.

78. Dai B, Liu Y, Fu L, Li Y, Zhang J, Mei C. Effect of theophylline on prevention of contrast-induced acute kidney injury: a meta-analysis of randomized controlled trials. *Am J Kidney Dis.* 2012;60(3):360–370.

79. Jenik AG, Ceriani Cernadas JM, Gorenstein A, et al. A randomized, double-blind, placebo-controlled trial of the effects of prophylactic theophylline on renal function in term neonates with perinatal asphyxia. *Pediatrics.* 2000;105(4):E45.

80. Bhat MA, Shah ZA, Makhdoomi MS, Mufti MH. Theophylline for renal function in term neonates with perinatal asphyxia: a randomized, placebo-controlled trial. *J Pediatr.* 2006;149(2):180–184.

81. Cattarelli D, Spandrio M, Gasparoni A, Bottino R, Offer C, Chirico G. A randomised, double blind, placebo controlled trial of the effect of theophylline in prevention of vasomotor nephropathy in very preterm neonates with respiratory distress syndrome. *Arch Disease Child Fetal Neonatal Ed.* 2006;91(2):F80–F84.

82. Nigwekar SU, Waikar SS. Diuretics in acute kidney injury. *Semin Nephrol.* 2011;31(6):523–534.

83. Morelli A, Ricci Z, Bellomo R, et al. Prophylactic fenoldopam for renal protection in sepsis: a randomized, double-blind, placebo-controlled pilot trial. *Crit Care Med.* 2005;33(11):2451–2456.

84. Brienza N, Malcangi V, Dalfino L, et al. A comparison between fenoldopam and low-dose dopamine in early renal dysfunction of critically ill patients. *Crit Care Med.* 2006;34(3):707–714.

85. Tumlin JA, Finkel KW, Murray PT, Samuels J, Cotsonis G, Shaw AD. Fenoldopam mesylate in early acute tubular necrosis: a randomized, double-blind, placebo-controlled clinical trial. *Am J Kidney Dis.* 2005;46(1):26–34.

86. Bove T, Landoni G, Calabro MG, et al. Renoprotective action of fenoldopam in high-risk patients undergoing cardiac surgery: a prospective, double-blind, randomized clinical trial. *Circulation.* 2005;111(24):3230–3235.

87. Zangrillo A, Biondi-Zoccai GG, Frati E, et al. Fenoldopam and acute renal failure in cardiac surgery: a meta-analysis of randomized placebo-controlled trials. *J Cardiothorac Vasc Anesth.* 2012;26(3):407–413.

88. Landoni G, Biondi-Zoccai GG, Tumlin JA, et al. Beneficial impact of fenoldopam in critically ill patients with or at risk for acute renal failure: a meta-analysis of randomized clinical trials. *Am J Kidney Dis.* 2007;49(1):56–68.

89. Moffett BS, Mott AR, Nelson DP, Goldstein SL, Jefferies JL. Renal effects of fenoldopam in critically ill pediatric patients: A retrospective review. *Pediatr Crit Care Med.* 2008;9(4):403–406.

90. Ricci Z, Stazi GV, Di Chiara L, et al. Fenoldopam in newborn patients undergoing cardiopulmonary bypass: controlled clinical trial. *Interact Cardiovasc Thorac Surg.* 2008;7(6):1049–1053.

91. Ricci Z, Luciano R, Favia I, et al. High-dose fenoldopam reduces postoperative neutrophil gelatinase-associated lipocaline and cystatin C levels in pediatric cardiac surgery. *Crit Care.* 2011;15(3):R160.

92. Sutherland SM, Zappitelli M, Alexander SR, et al. Fluid overload and mortality in children receiving continuous renal replacement therapy: the prospective pediatric continuous renal replacement therapy registry. *Am J Kidney Dis.* 2010;55(2):316–325.

93. Selewski DT, Cornell TT, Lombel RM, et al. Weight-based determination of fluid overload status and mortality in pediatric intensive care unit patients requiring continuous renal replacement therapy. *Intensive Care Med.* 2011;37(7):1166–1173.

94. Ho KM, Power BM. Benefits and risks of furosemide in acute kidney injury. *Anaesthesia.* 2010;65(3):283–293.

95. Moghal NE, Shenoy M. Furosemide and acute kidney injury in neonates. *Arch Dis Child Fetal Neonatal Ed.* 2008;93(4):F313–F316.

96. Oliveros M, Pham JT, John E, Resheidat A, Bhat R. The use of bumetanide for oliguric acute renal failure in preterm infants. *Pediatr Crit Care Med.* 2011;12(2):210–214.

97. Boone TB, Allen TD. Unilateral post-obstructive diuresis in the neonate. *J Urol.* 1992;147(2):430–432.

98. Coar D. Obstructive nephropathy. *Del Medical J.* 1991;63(12):743–749.

99. Denton MD, Chertow GM, Brady HR. "Renal-dose" dopamine for the treatment of acute renal failure: scientific

rationale, experimental studies and clinical trials. *Kidney Int.* 1996;50(1):4–14.

100. Chertow GM, Sayegh MH, Allgren RL, Lazarus JM. Is the administration of dopamine associated with adverse or favorable outcomes in acute renal failure? Auriculin Anaritide Acute Renal Failure Study Group. *Am J Med.* 1996;101(1):49–53.

101. Bellomo R, Wan L, May C. Vasoactive drugs and acute kidney injury. *Crit Care Med.* 2008;36(4 Suppl):S179–S186.

102. Dellinger RP, Levy MM, Carlet JM, et al. Surviving Sepsis Campaign: international guidelines for management of severe sepsis and septic shock: 2008. *Crit Care Med.* 2008;36(1):296–327.

103. Emery EF, Greenough A. Efficacy of low-dose dopamine infusion. *Acta Paediatr.* 1993;82(5):430–432.

104. Cuevas L, Yeh TF, John EG, Cuevas D, Plides RS. The effect of low-dose dopamine infusion on cardiopulmonary and renal status in premature newborns with respiratory distress syndrome. *Am J Dis Child.* 1991;145(7):799–803.

105. Lynch SK, Lemley KV, Polak MJ. The effect of dopamine on glomerular filtration rate in normotensive, oliguric premature neonates. *Pediatr Nephrol.* 2003;18(7):649–652.

106. Prins I, Plotz FB, Uiterwaal CS, van Vught HJ. Low-dose dopamine in neonatal and pediatric intensive care: a systematic review. *Intensive Care Med.* 2001;27(1):206–210.

107. Rugolotto S, Gruber M, Solano PD, Chini L, Gobbo S, Pecori S. Necrotizing enterocolitis in a 850 gram infant receiving sorbitol-free sodium polystyrene sulfonate (Kayexalate): clinical and histopathologic findings. *J Perinatol.* 2007;27(4):247–249.

108. Vemgal P, Ohlsson A. Interventions for non-oliguric hyperkalaemia in preterm neonates. *Cochrane Database Syst Rev.* 2012;5:CD005257.

109. Bunchman TE, Wood EG, Schenck MH, Weaver KA, Klein BL, Lynch RE. Pretreatment of formula with sodium polystyrene sulfonate to reduce dietary potassium intake. *Pediatr Nephrol.* 1991;5(1):29–32.

110. Fassinger N, Dabbagh S, Mukhopadhyay S, Lee DY. Mineral content of infant formula after treatment with sodium polystyrene sulfonate or calcium polystyrene sulfonate. *Adv Peritl Dial.* 1998;14:274–277.

111. Rivard AL, Raup SM, Beilman GJ. Sodium polystyrene sulfonate used to reduce the potassium content of a high-protein enteral formula: a quantitative analysis. *JPEN J Parenter Enter Nutr.* 2004;28(2):76–78.

112. Ferrara E, Lemire J, Reznik VM, Grimm PC. Dietary phosphorus reduction by pretreatment of human breast milk with sevelamer. *Pediatr Nephrol.* 2004;19(7):775–779.

113. Warady BA. *Pediatric Dialysis.* New York: Springer; 2011.

114. Bunchman TE, Barletta GM, Winters JW, Gardner JJ, Crumb TL, McBryde KD. Phenylacetate and benzoate clearance in a hyperammonemic infant on sequential hemodialysis and hemofiltration. *Pediatr Nephrol.* 2007;22(7):1062–1065.

115. Picca S, Bartuli A, Dionisi-Vici C. Medical management and dialysis therapy for the infant with an inborn error of metabolism. *Semin Nephrol.* 2008;28(5):477–480.

116. Goldstein SL. Advances in pediatric renal replacement therapy for acute kidney injury. *Semin Dial.* 2011;24(2):187–191.

117. Symons JM, Brophy PD, Gregory MJ, et al. Continuous renal replacement therapy in children up to 10 kg. *Am J Kidney Dis.* 2003;41(5):984–989.

118. Hackbarth R, Bunchman TE, Chua AN, et al. The effect of vascular access location and size on circuit survival in pediatric continuous renal replacement therapy: a report from the PPCRRT registry. *Int J Artif Organs.* 2007;30(12):1116–1121.

119. Shooter M, Watson A. The ethics of withholding and withdrawing dialysis therapy in infants. *Pediatr Nephrol.* 2000;14(4):347–351.

120. Akcan-Arikan A, Zappitelli M, Loftis LL, Washburn KK, Jefferson LS, Goldstein SL. Modified RIFLE criteria in critically ill children with acute kidney injury. *Kidney Int.* 2007;71(10):1028–1035.

121. Kellum JA, Angus DC. Patients are dying of acute renal failure. *Crit Care Med.* 2002;30(9):2156–2157.

122. Li X, Hassoun HT, Santora R, Rabb H. Organ crosstalk: the role of the kidney. *Curr Opin Crit Care.* 2009;15(6):481–487.

123. Feltes CM, Van Eyk J, Rabb H. Distant-organ changes after acute kidney injury. *Nephron Physiol.* 2008;109(4):80–84.

124. Abitbol CL, Bauer CR, Montane B, Chandar J, Duara S, Zilleruelo G. Long-term follow-up of extremely low birth weight infants with neonatal renal failure. *Pediatr Nephrol.* 2003;18(9):887–893.

125. Bellomo R, Ronco C, Kellum JA, Mehta RL, Palevsky P. Acute renal failure—definition, outcome measures, animal models, fluid therapy and information technology needs: the Second International Consensus Conference of the Acute Dialysis Quality Initiative (ADQI) Group. *Crit Care.* 2004;8(4):R204R212.

126. Mehta RL, Kellum JA, Shah SV, et al. Acute Kidney Injury Network: report of an initiative to improve outcomes in acute kidney injury. *Crit Care.* 2007;11(2):R31.

127. Schwartz GJ, Brion LP, Spitzer A. The use of plasma creatinine concentration for estimating glomerular filtration rate in infants, children, and adolescents. *Pediatr Clin North Am.* 1987;34(3):571–590.

Congenital Renal Masses

Robert P. Payne and William A. Kennedy II

INTRODUCTION

Perinatally detected abdominal masses are a common clinical finding, and two-thirds originate from the kidney.[1] With the increased use of prenatal ultrasound evaluation, approximately 15% of congenital renal masses are detected prenatally. Of those diagnosed postnatally, nearly half present with a palpable abdominal mass. Congenital renal tumors, however, are exceedingly rare, representing only 7% of all neonatal tumors.[2] Abdominal ultrasound, whether done prenatally or postnatally, will often give an accurate description of these renal lesions. Congenital renal masses can be broadly divided into 2 main categories based on its sonographic appearance. Solid and cystic renal masses can be further subcategorized as either benign or malignant (Table 43-1).

Congenital cystic renal masses are far more frequently encountered and more likely to be benign when compared to solid renal masses. The most common cystic lesions include hydronephrosis, multicystic dysplastic kidney, and hereditary polycystic kidney diseases (PKDs).[3] The majority of congenital solid renal masses are also benign. Solid masses, however, can represent 1 of several rare neonatal neoplasms. During the first year of life, malignant Wilms tumor (WT) is the most common solid renal tumor, followed by congenital mesoblastic nephroma (CMN), rhabdoid tumor of the kidney (RTK), and clear cell sarcoma of the kidney (CCSK). However, during the neonatal period, two-thirds of all solid renal tumors are CMN, followed by WT, RTK, and CCSK[4] (Table 43-1).

CYSTIC RENAL MASSES OF THE NEWBORN

Hydronephrosis

Fortunately, the great majority of congenital renal masses are benign. Forty percent of all neonatal abdominal masses are due to hydronephrosis and renal cystic disease.[5] Depending on the onset and severity of hydronephrosis, a newborn child may warrant serial renal ultrasounds, voiding cystourethrograms (VCUGs), or renal scintigraphy in the early stages of life. The most common causes of antenatal hydronephrosis are ureteropelvic junction (UPJ) obstruction, ureterovesical junction obstruction, vesicoureteral reflux (VUR), primary megaureter, neurogenic bladder, posterior urethral valves, and prune-belly syndrome.[3] These clinical entities are discussed in greater detail in the chapter 44 on obstructive uropathies.

Multicystic Dysplastic Kidney

Unilateral multicystic dysplastic kidney (MCDK) is the most common cystic renal disease of the newborn, with an incidence of 1 in 4300 live births, occurring more frequently on the left-hand side.[6] Some have postulated that MCDK is a result of ureteral obstruction or atresia,[7] while others believe that aberrant or nonunion of the ureteric bud and metanephric blastema during the eighth week of gestation is the inciting event.[8] This embryologic error results in a nonfunctioning cystic mass resembling a bag of

Table 43-1 Differential Diagnosis of a Retroperitoneal Mass During the Neonatal Period

Cystic Renal Masses	Solid Renal Masses
Benign	*Benign*
Hydronephrosis	Renal vein thrombosis
Multicystic dysplastic kidney	Horseshoe kidney
Autosomal recessive polycystic kidney disease	Ectopic kidney (fused or nonfused)
Autosomal dominant polycystic kidney disease	
Malignant	*Malignant*
Multilocular cystic nephroma	Congenital mesoblastic nephroma
Cystic partially differentiated nephroblastoma	Wilms tumor and precursor lesions
	Rhabdoid tumor of the kidney
Cystic Wilms tumor	Clear cell sarcoma of the kidney
Extrarenal Retroperitoneal Masses	
Adrenal hemorrhage	
Neuroblastoma	

grapes that is typically devoid of any nephrons and composed of primitive ducts and immature glomeruli.[9] While a full description of MCDK can be found in chapter 44 on obstructive uropathies, Table 43-2

and Figure 43-1 outline the radiographic features that can help differentiate MCKD from hydronephrosis in the newborn.

Polycystic Kidney Disease (Recessive Type and Dominant Type)

Polycystic kidney disease (PKD) can present at any stage of life, but when detected in the neonate, the recessive-type predominates.[10] The severity of PKD varies with the age of disease onset and seems to appear in its most severe form earliest in life.[3] It is important to note that the terms *polycystic* and *multicystic* differ despite implying the same thing. As explained previously, *multicystic* refers to a dysplastic kidney that underwent abnormal nephrogenesis and contains little-to-no nephrons, while *polycystic* refers to a nondysplastic kidney that developed normally and contains nephrons. Both autosomal recessive polycystic kidney disease (ARPKD) and autosomal dominant polycystic kidney disease (ADPKD) can present as a congenital renal mass. In both the fetus and the newborn, the diagnosis is considered when ultrasound examination reveals very large, homogeneously hyperechogenic kidneys bilaterally with loss of corticomedullary differentiation. Oligohydramnios is often present in utero. As seen in Figure 43-2, newborns with ADPKD demonstrate diffuse and large cysts, whereas ARPKD rarely contains visible cysts because the dilated collecting ducts are tightly packed together and too small to be resolved on ultrasound.[3] Both ARPKD and ADPKD are discussed further in the chapter on acute renal failure in the newborn.

Table 43-2 Radiographic Features Distinguishing Multicystic Dysplastic Kidney (MCDK) From Severe Hydronephrosis

MCDK	Severe Hydronephrosis
Ultrasound	*Ultrasound*
Random distribution of cysts of various sizes without a large central or medial cyst	Cysts/calyces organized peripherally around a large central or medial cysts representing a dilated renal pelvis
No visible communications between cysts	Cysts/calyces communicate with each other
Minimal-to-no recognizable renal parenchyma	Renal parenchyma present but often thin
No evidence of renal sinus	Renal sinus surrounds the central or medial cyst
Congenital renal anomaly commonly found in contralateral kidney (ie, UPJO, VUR)	Contralateral renal anomalies are less frequent
Concomitant Wolfian duct anomalies commonly found on ipsilateral side	Rarely associated with anomalies of the Wolfian duct
Renal scintigraphy (DMSA scan)	*Renal scintigraphy (DMSA scan)*
No renal function or uptake of radionuclide	Renal function present with uptake of radionuclide

Abbreviations: DMSA, dimercaptosuccinic acid; UPJO, ureteropelvic junction obstruction; VUR, vesicoureteral reflux.

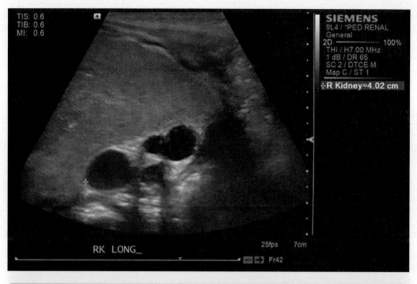

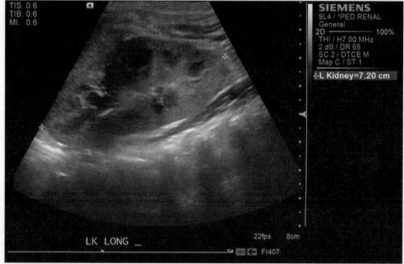

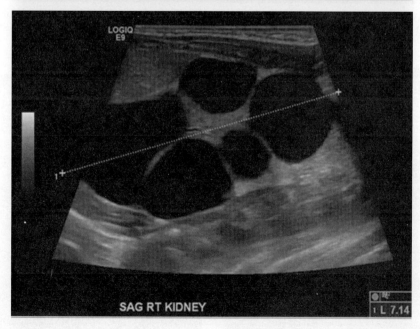

FIGURE 43-1 (*Continued*)

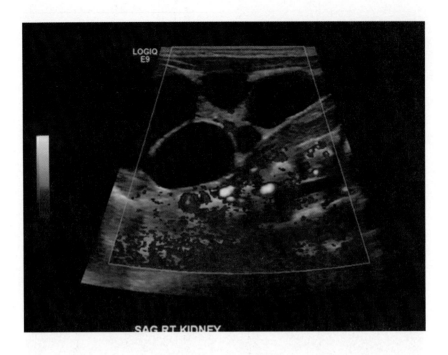

FIGURE 43-1

SOLID RENAL MASSES OF THE NEWBORN

Renal Vein Thrombosis

Renal vein thrombosis (RVT) is the most common non-catheter-related thrombotic event during the neonatal period. Two-thirds of all cases occur during the first 3 days of life, with only 7% detected in utero during routine ultrasound evaluation. There have been reports of in utero RVT being misdiagnosed as a congenital renal tumor and therefore must always be considered in a neonate with a renal mass.[11] Renal sonography typically reveals an enlarged kidney that is focally or diffusely echogenic, with loss of the normal corticomedullary junction and occasional calcifications. The thrombus can be seen extending from the renal vein into the inferior vena cava in about half of cases. However, when only the intrarenal vessels are involved, a thrombus may not be visible.[12] Doppler studies can be helpful in making an accurate diagnosis of RVT when the confirmatory thrombus is not visualized by demonstrating increased resistive indices and reversed diastolic flow through the renal vasculature.[13] Approximately one-third of cases are bilateral, which often carries a grave prognosis for the child[12] (Figure 43-3).

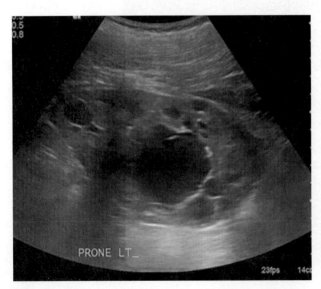

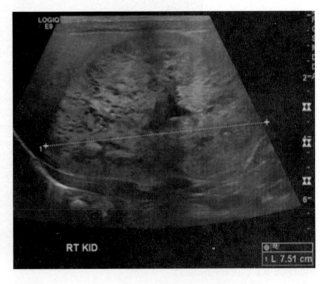

FIGURE 43-2

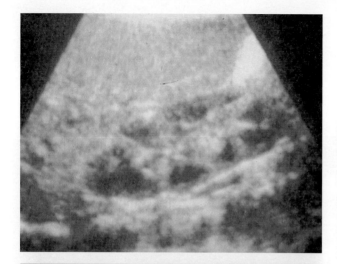
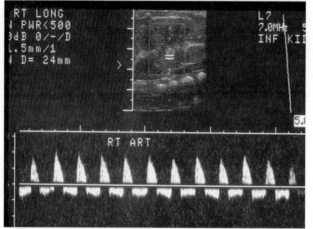
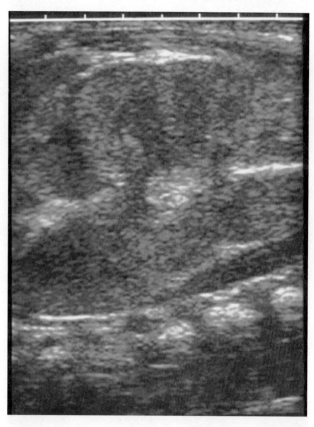

FIGURE 43-3

Horseshoe Kidney

Epidemiology

The horseshoe kidney (HSK) is the most common of all renal fusion anomalies, occurring between 1 in 400 and 1 in 666 people, or approximately 0.25% of the population, and has a 2-fold male predominance.[14] A HSK consists of 2 distinct renal units fused at their inferior poles by a fibrous or parenchymal isthmus that crosses the midplane of the body and lies anterior to the vertebral column at the L3–L4 level (Figure 43-4). Rarely, in less than 5% of cases, the fusion occurs superiorly between the upper poles of the kidney.[15]

Pathophysiology

This anomaly takes place early on in fetal development, likely during the fourth and sixth weeks of gestation. Normally, after the ureteric bud and metanephric blastema fuse, they begin their rotational ascent to their typical locations high in the retroperitoneum. In the

case of an HSK, a slight alteration in the orientation of the closely positioned fetal kidneys allows them to fuse. The fused metanephric mass then ascends en bloc until it is stopped in the midline by the inferior mesenteric artery as it exits the aorta, causing the horseshoe appearance. Due to the incomplete ascent, the HSK typically display aberrant vasculature with duplication or even triplication of the renal vessels, and the ureters often insert higher on the renal pelvis than in normal kidneys.[16] Extra renal vessels and high-inserting ureters can cause partial obstruction at the UPJ, leading to dilation of the renal pelvis and obstruction of urinary flow. Distally, the ureters insert normally into the trigone of the bladder and are rarely ectopic.[3]

Diagnostic Tests

In most cases, the diagnosis of an HSK can be reliably made with ultrasound examination in both the antenatal and postnatal periods.[17] The typical sonographic features of an HSK include low-lying kidneys

CHAPTER 43

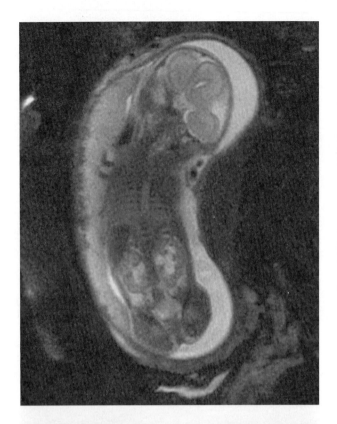

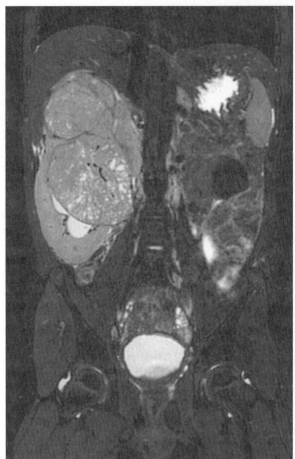

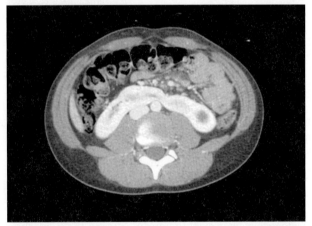

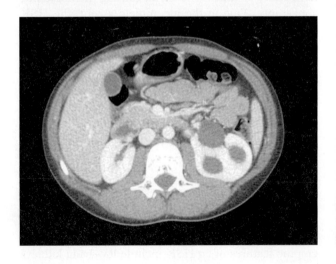

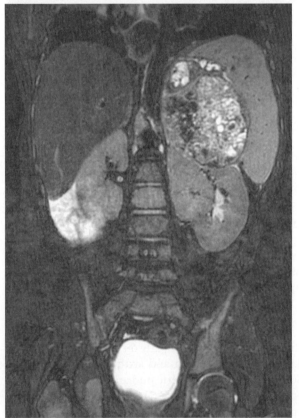

FIGURE 43-4

bilaterally, malrotation with anterior-facing renal pelvises and posterior-pointing calyces, and ill-defined inferior poles. The most confirmatory sign is visualization of the isthmus, which can be seen sonographically in approximately 80% of cases.[18] These features can be significantly altered due to various associated uropathies, such as hydronephrosis or multicystic dysplasia, making the diagnosis less clear. Historically, excretory urography was used to diagnose HSK, but this technology has been abandoned in lieu of newer and more reliable imaging modalities. When ultrasound evaluation is inconclusive, the diagnosis can be confirmed with computed tomography (CT), magnetic resonance imaging (MRI), or renal scintigraphy. Radionucleotide scans with technetium 99m dimercaptosuccinic acid (DMSA) have been reported to visualize the isthmus in 100% of children with HSK.[19] Cross-sectional imaging studies are often reserved to accurately assess the renal anatomy, vasculature, and associated uropathies prior to surgical intervention.

Associated Anomalies

When diagnosed in the newborn, HSKs are frequently associated with additional congenital anomalies that tend to be less compatible with long-term survival. In an autopsy series that examined 99 cases of HSK, additional malformations were found in 79% of stillborns and infants who died during the first year of life. These fatal anomalies primarily involved the gastrointestinal, skeletal, cardiovascular, and central nervous systems.[20] In another report, approximately one-third of all patients with HSK were found to have 1 or more additional congenital anomalies.[21]

Several chromosomal abnormalities have a predilection for HSK when compared to the general population. Trisomy 18 is associated with several renal anomalies, with HSK the most common and was seen in 21% of patients examined during an autopsy series.[22] Turner syndrome is also commonly associated with renal anomalies, which primarily include HSK and ureteral duplication.[23,24]

Genitourinary anomalies are frequently seen in patients with HSK (Table 43-3). VUR and UPJO are the most commonly encountered uropathies requiring surgical reconstruction.[24]

Management

In the newborn, there are no specific management recommendations for an HSK in an otherwise-healthy child. However, when associated congenital anomalies are present, supportive therapy may be required based on the degree and severity of their complications. Later in life, the most common indications for surgical management include UPJ obstruction, ZZVUR, kidney

Table 43-3 Genitourinary Anomalies Associated With Horseshoe Kidneys

Genital Anomalies	
Hypospadias	4%[a]
Undescended testes	4%[a]
Bicornuate uterus	7%[a]
Septate vagina	7%[a]
Urinary Collecting System Anomalies	
Ureteral duplication	10%[b]
Ureteropelvic junction dilation/ obstruction	23%[c] to 80%[d]
Vesicoureteral reflux	33%[c]

[a]Boatman et al.[21]
[b]Pitts and Muecke.[97]
[c]Cascio et al.[24]
[d]Segura et al.[98]

stone disease, and malignancy.[17] Concomitant fetal uropathies, such as UPJ obstruction or VUR, should be investigated and managed accordingly, as outlined in chapter 44 on obstructive uropathies. They do not warrant any special treatment related to the presence of an HSK.

Outcome and Follow-up

It has been observed that over 60% of patients with an HSK remain asymptomatic over a 10-year period, and when symptoms occur, they are generally related to hydronephrosis, urinary tract infections, or nephrolithiasis.[25]

Congenital Mesoblastic Nephroma

Epidemiology

Congenital mesoblastic nephroma is the most common solid renal tumor of the newborn, accounting for 66% of tumors identified during the first 2 months of life. There is a slight predilection for males (male/female = 1.5:1).[4] The proportion of CMN in relation to other congenital renal tumors is highest during the first month of life and quickly begins to decline as age increases, representing 54% of tumors diagnosed in the first month, 33% in the second month, 16% in the third, and less than 10% in the months thereafter.[26] The true incidence of CMN is difficult to ascertain given its nonmalignant nature and lack of reporting to population-based cancer registries.[27]

Pathophysiology

Historically, CMN was classified as a congenital variant of WT but is now considered a distinct entity due to its almost-exclusive occurrence during the first year of life, nonaggressive behavior with low malignant potential, and mesenchymal origin.[28] There are 3 histological variants: classic (49% of cases), cellular (30% of cases), and mixed (21% of cases). Classic histology tumors generally present earlier in life, with a median age at diagnosis of 17 days, compared to the mixed and cellular subtypes, which typically present after the neonatal period with a median age at diagnosis of 43 and 149 days, respectively.[27] Classic histology CMN are nonmalignant and do not metastasize but may recur locally if incompletely resected. Despite the general benign nature of all CMN, the mixed and cellular variants have been reported to recur distantly after surgical excision[29] and metastasize to the lung, liver, heart, bone, and brain.[30]

Recently, a chromosomal translocation at t(12;15) (p13;q25) has been identified in cellular CMN, which results in the ETV6-NTRK3 gene fusion (Rubin, Chen, et al, 1998). Infantile fibrosarcoma, another soft tissue tumor that generally behaves in a benign fashion despite aggressive histological features, shares this chromosomal translocation and establishes a genetic link between these neonatal neoplasms.[31] Interestingly, the classic subtype does not express the ETV6-NTRK3 gene product, which has been used to subclassify these tumors based on molecular markers.[32] However, the presence of this translocation does not clearly identify patients at risk of local or distant recurrence that may benefit from adjuvant chemotherapy.[27]

Clinical Presentation

Similar to all solid renal masses detected in the neonatal period, CMN most commonly presents with an abdominal mass detected by either physical examination or routine antenatal ultrasound. CMN are unilateral in nature and can be very large, affecting both left and right kidneys equally, and can result in hematuria (microscopic and macroscopic), nausea, and vomiting.[4] When detected in utero, these masses are frequently associated with fetal and labor-related complications that increase perinatal morbidity and mortality. Polyhydramnios was detected in 39% of prenatally diagnosed cases of CMN and was associated with a significantly increased risk of preterm labor, resulting in a 50% rate of premature delivery. Nonimmune fetal hydrops, acute fetal distress, dystocia, anemia, and respiratory distress of the newborn requiring mechanical ventilation have all been described in these patients, which underscores the high-risk nature of these pregnancies.[32] This strongly supports the recommendation for delivering children with antenatally detected renal tumors in a pediatric tertiary care center due to the high likelihood of

perinatal complications that often require immediate surgical delivery and supportive therapy.

Congenital mesoblastic nephroma is also commonly associated with paraneoplastic syndromes. Hypercalcemia is secondary to a tumor-secreted parathyroid hormone-like peptide and occurs in less than 10% of cases. It can be severe enough to warrant supportive medical therapy prior to surgical resection and may require postoperative supplementation until the depleted bone reservoirs are replenished.[33] Hypertension occurs in up to 22% of cases and is often related to elevated plasma renin activity and can thus be managed preoperatively with angiotensin-converting enzyme inhibitors.[34] In all cases, elevated blood pressure and calcium levels normalized with complete excision of the mass.[32]

Differential Diagnosis

The differential diagnosis of a congenital solid renal mass is outlined in Table 43-1 and should include all benign and malignant intrarenal and extrarenal masses. During the neonatal period, the most likely diagnosis of a solid renal mass is CMN, followed by WT, RTK, and CCSK. There is no radiological finding or study that can reliably distinguish these lesions from each other. For this reason, all solid congenital renal masses are initially investigated and often treated in the same manner, with the final diagnosis based on pathological assessment from surgical specimens.

Extrarenal masses found in the retroperitoneum, including neuroblastoma and adrenal hemorrhagic cysts, can resemble an intrarenal mass arising from the upper pole and must also be considered in the differential diagnosis. During infancy, neuroblastomas are much more common than renal tumors and infiltrate the neighboring kidney through direct invasion in 20% of cases, mimicking a primary renal mass. However, cross-sectional radiologic studies can usually differentiate intrarenal tumors from neuroblastomas based on an adrenal or paravertebral sympathetic ganglion origin, the absence of the claw sign (renal parenchyma stretched around and cupping the tumor suggesting a renal origin), and a tendency for invasion rather than capsule formation[35] (Figure 43-5).

Diagnostic Tests

When investigating a newborn with a suspected renal mass, a thorough metastatic workup is required because of the potential for malignant pathology and includes both laboratory and radiological studies. Laboratory investigations are performed preoperatively and should include a complete blood count with differential, liver function tests, electrolytes, serum creatinine, serum calcium, and routine urinalysis. Acquired von

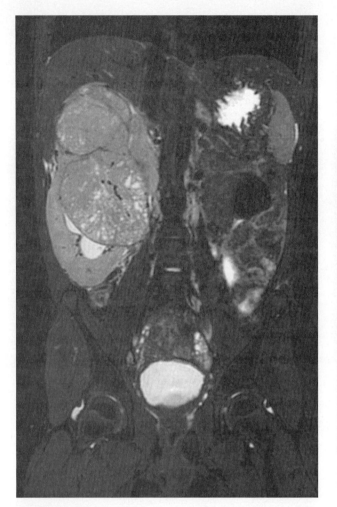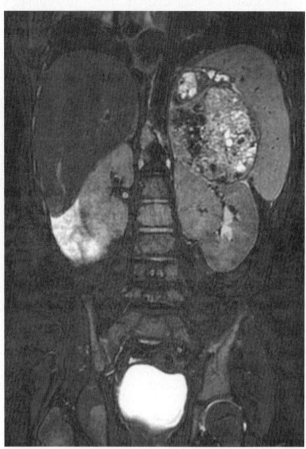

FIGURE 43-5

Willebrand disease occurs in approximately 4%–8% of WT patients and has been reported in CMN,[36] warranting the preoperative measurement of coagulation parameters (prothrombin time [PT], partial thromboplastin time [PTT], von Willebrand factor antigen, ristocetin cofactor, and factor VII levels) in most children prior to surgical resection[37] (Table 43-4).

The radiologic studies performed should confirm the origin of the mass and establish whether there is any evidence of contiguous spread to the regional lymph nodes or inferior vena cava. In addition, the presence of a contralateral kidney should be confirmed and assessed for possible involvement, the urinary tract should be evaluated for congenital anomalies (ie,

Table 43-4 Recommended Investigations for the Initial Workup of Neonatal Kidney Tumors

Laboratory tests	• Routine urinalysis • CBC with differential, LFTs, electrolytes, serum Cr, serum Ca²⁺ • Coagulation parameters: PT, PTT, vWF antigen, ristocetin cofactor, factor VII levels
Radiologic tests	• Abdominal ultrasoundᵃ • CT abdomen/pelvis (or MRI) • Chest x-ray or CT chest • Bone scan (clear cell sarcoma only) • MRI brain (clear cell sarcoma and rhabdoid tumor only)ᵇ

Abbreviations: CBC, complete blood cell count; Cr, creatinine; CT, computed tomography; LFT, liver function test; MRI, magnetic resonance imaging; PT, prothrombin time; PTT, partial thromboplastin time; vWF, von Willebrand factor.
ᵃAbdominal ultrasound is the first imaging study performed. If the mass has a solid component, then a full metastatic workup is required.
ᵇMRI of the brain should also be performed on any child presenting with neurological symptoms.

solitary, horseshoe, ectopic kidneys), and evidence of distant metastatic spread must be determined.

The initial imaging study of choice to evaluate a suspected neonatal renal mass is an abdominal ultrasound that focuses on both the kidneys and the bladder. On ultrasound, CMN appears as a large, solid, and heterogeneous renal mass that contains a cystic component in over 50% of patients. Cystic changes seen during sonographic evaluation correlated with cellular and mixed subtypes in over 80% of cases. CMN also often displays a hypoechoic ring that surrounds the periphery of the mass, which may help differentiate this mass from WT.[38]

Detection of a solid renal mass in a neonate mandates a full metastatic workup, which should include some type of contrast-enhanced cross-sectional imaging of the abdomen and, at a minimum, a chest radiograph. On CT, CMN appears as a large uniform mass with soft tissue attenuation that often replaces the majority of the kidney and occasionally extends beyond the renal capsule. Tumor extension into the renal vein has been reported but is exceedingly rare and should raise the suspicion of a WT.[39] These masses generally show heterogeneous uptake of contrast material, with the tumor itself enhancing less than the neighboring renal parenchyma.[40] Contrast-enhanced CT scanning of the chest provides the best means of detecting metastatic lung nodules as chest x-rays alone can miss a significant number of small lesions. These patients would therefore be understaged and receive suboptimal therapy, resulting in higher rates of recurrence.[41] However, in this age category, pulmonary lymphadenopathy is often related to benign conditions, such as fibrosis or infection, and there is some degree of controversy regarding the clinical relevance of these lesions detected only by CT.

Magnetic resonance imaging is being used more commonly to evaluate congenital renal masses because it does not expose patients to ionizing radiation, and in some centers, it has replaced CT scanning as the baseline abdominal imaging study of choice.[42] However, in this age group, MRI requires general anesthesia and is an inferior modality to assess the lungs for metastatic spread. MRI is the preferred imaging technique when assessing for intracranial metastases, typically seen with RTK and CCSK, and is recommended prior to initiation of treatment.[26]

Staging

There are 2 main staging systems used for pediatric renal tumors that were developed by the North American Children's Oncology Group (COG) and the European Society of Pediatric Oncology (SIOP). The COG classification is based on pathological findings from up-front nephrectomy and lymph node specimens and preoperative imaging studies that assess for distant metastatic spread (Table 43-5). SIOP protocols generally treat with neoadjuvant chemotherapy followed by nephrectomy, and staging is therefore based on prechemotherapy imaging studies and postchemotherapy surgical findings.[35]

In the largest North American series examining fetal and neonatal renal tumors, CMN typically presented with low-stage disease, and 88% of all cases were classified as stage I/II. Stage III and IV disease was found in 9% and 3% of cases, respectively, with no reports of bilateral or stage V tumors during the neonatal period.[4]

Management

The initial management of a neonatal renal tumor requires a multidisciplinary approach in which complete excision of the mass is paramount. During the neonatal period, standard therapy for a unilateral solid renal mass includes a radical nephrectomy with mandatory regional lymph node sampling via a

Table 43-5 Children's Oncology Group Staging System for Pediatric Renal Tumors[a]

Stage I	Tumor confined to the kidney and completely resected. The renal capsule is intact, and the tumor was not ruptured prior to removal. No renal sinus extension. There is no residual tumor.
Stage II	Extracapsular penetration, but tumor is completely resected. Renal sinus extension or extrarenal vessels may contain tumor thrombus or may be infiltrated by tumor.
Stage III	Residual nonhematogenous tumor confined to the abdomen, defined as • Regional lymph node involvement • Any tumor spillage or preoperative biopsy • Peritoneal implants • Tumor beyond surgical margin • Tumor incompletely resected
Stage IV	Hematogenous metastases to lung, liver, bone, brain, and so on
Stage V	Bilateral renal involvement at diagnosis

[a]Wein et al.[3]

transabdominal approach.[3] It is critical that the surgeon adhere to basic oncological principles due to the potential for malignant pathology and perform a complete en bloc excision of the mass and involved structures with careful handling of the mass to avoid tumor rupture and spillage. A formal retroperitoneal lymph node dissection is not recommended due to the morbidity associated with the procedure in the absence of any prognostic benefit.[43] Partial nephrectomy is not recommended because CMNs have a tendency to grow into the renal sinus and perirenal fat, increasing the risk of local recurrence.[44]

Postoperative complications are common and include hemorrhage, small-bowel obstruction, chylous ascites, and intussusception. Significant cardiovascular complications have also been reported, including intraoperative hypertensive crisis and cardiac arrest.[27]

In the setting of classic CMN, surgery alone has been associated with excellent outcomes, and there is no current role for adjuvant therapy with complete excision of the mass.[39] Chemotherapy is generally reserved for patients with recurrent or metastatic disease[45] or those with stage III cellular histology who are diagnosed beyond 3 months of age.[46] Historically, adjuvant therapy protocols used a combination of chemotherapy and external beam radiotherapy with varying success.[39] However, the recent identification of a chromosomal translocation and gene fusion product found in both CMN and congenital infantile fibrosarcoma has led some to believe that these 2 cancers are biologically similar and could be treated using sarcoma-based chemotherapeutic agents. However, the presence of the ETV6-NTRK3 translocation does not clearly identify patients who may benefit from adjuvant therapy.[47]

Outcome/Follow-up

Outcomes for all stages of CMN diagnosed during the first 7 months of life are excellent, with a 5-year overall survival rate of 96%.[26] In a large neonatal series, those classified as stage I and II treated with surgery alone had survival rates of 93% and 96%, respectively, whereas stage I/II patients treated with a combination of surgery followed by chemotherapy faired much worse, with only 53% surviving. Seventy-three percent of patients with stage III CMN survived, whereas all those classified as stage IV died. In the same series, neonates had better survival rates than fetuses, 84% and 76%, respectively, related to the high likelihood of perinatal complications associated with antenatally detected CMN as described previously.[4]

The rate of recurrence and metastases in neonates with CMN are 5% and 2%, respectively.[4] Risk factors for disease recurrence and metastases include positive surgical margins or tumor spillage (stage III), cellular histology, and advanced age at diagnosis (>3 months of age). Tumor recurrence often develops rapidly and almost exclusively during the first year of follow-up. The mean time from diagnosis to disease recurrence is 4 months, highlighting the need for close radiographic follow-up during this critical time period.[30] Table 43-6 outlines the follow-up schedule recommended for neonates with renal tumors.

Table 43-6 Follow-up Schedule and Imaging Studies Recommended for Neonatal Renal Tumors

Final Pathology	Imaging Study	Schedule
CMN (classic or cellular variants)	Abdominal US	Every 3 months × 4, then every 6 months × 2
Wilms tumor (favorable histology)	Abdominal US[a]	Postoperatively at 6 weeks and 3 months, then every 3 months × 8, then every 6 months × 4
	Chest x-ray or CT chest	Every 6 weeks until complete remission
Anaplastic Wilms' tumor or rhabdoid tumor of the kidney	Abdominal US and chest X-ray	Postoperatively at 6 weeks and 3 months, then every 3 months × 8, then every 6 months × 4
	CT abdomen and CT chest	Every 6 weeks until complete remission, then every 3months × 8, then every 6 months × 4
	MRI brain (rhabdoid tumor only)	Every 3 months × 4, then every 6 months × 2
Clear cell sarcoma	Chest x-ray or CT chest	Every 6 weeks until complete remission is documented; every 3 months × 8, then every 6 months × 6
	Abdominal US or CT abdomen	Every 6 weeks until complete remission is documented; every 3 months × 8, then every 6 months × 6
	Bone scan	Every 6 months × 6
	MRI brain	Every 6 months × 6

Abbreviations: CMN, congenital mesoblastic nephroma; CT, computed tomography; US, ultrasound.
[a]Patients with bilateral Wilms tumor or nephrogenic rests warrant abdominal US every 3 months for 8 years.

Wilms Tumor and Precursor Lesions

Epidemiology

Wilms tumor, or nephroblastoma, is an embryonal tumor that arises from the remnants of immature kidney. It is the most common primary renal malignancy of childhood, with an annual incidence between 7 and 10 cases per million children less than 15 years of age.[48] WT is mainly seen in young children, with more than 80% of cases presenting before 5 years of age. The median age at diagnosis is 38 months, although boys and those with bilateral disease tend to have occurrences earlier in life.[48] The worldwide sex ratio is close to 1, whereas in North America a slight female predilection exists.[3]

During the neonatal period, WT is the second most common solid renal mass after CMN, accounting for approximately 20% of all neonatal renal tumors in a large North American series.[4] By 1993, the National Wilms Tumor Study had only 11 cases of neonatal WT among the 6832 patients registered to the study, representing a 0.16% incidence.[49]

Approximately 10% of WTs are associated with developmental anomalies or malformation syndromes, and some have been linked to specific chromosomal abnormalities.[50] These syndromes are often associated with precursor lesions called nephrogenic rests (NRs) and can be broadly categorized into those associated with overgrowth and those without overgrowth (Table 43-4). Genitourinary abnormalities, such as renal fusion anomalies, hypospadias, and cryptorchidism, are present in 5% of patients with WT[51] (Table 43-7).

Pathophysiology

WTs develop from the remnants of immature kidney and were originally thought to occur following a "2-hit" genetic phenomenon proposed by Knudson, based on his previous work with retinoblastoma.[52] However, Wilms' tumorigenesis is a much more complex process that has been linked to several genetic alterations that can each lead to WT development.[53] In 1978, the first WT gene, *WT1*, was identified in patients with Wilms tumor, aniridia, genitourinary anomalies, retardation (WAGR) syndrome based on the discovery of a common chromosomal 11p13 germline deletion.[54] The *WT1* gene encodes a zinc-finger transcription factor that regulates growth factors involved in cellular growth and differentiation.[55] Both WAGR and Denys-Drash syndrome are the result of *WT1* gene mutations and subsequently share a strong predisposition toward WT development and renal failure.[56]

The second WT gene, *WT2*, was identified in patients with Beckwith-Wiedemann syndrome (BWS) who had a loss of heterozygosity (LOH) at the 11p15 locus.[57] The *WT2* locus contains several genes, including *IGF2*, which encodes for insulin-like growth factor

Table 43-7 Syndromes Commonly Associated With Wilms Tumor (WT)[a]

Syndrome	Gene (Locus)	Risk of WT	Precursor Lesion
Associated with Overgrowth			
Beckwith-Wiedemann (islet cell hyperplasia and neonatal hypoglycemia, omphalocele, macroglossia, visceromegaly, gigantism)	*WT2* (11p15)	5%–10%	Perilobar NR
Perlman (islet cell hyperplasia and neonatal hypoglycemia, fetal gigantism, facial dysmorphism, cryptorchism)	Unknown	33%	Multifocal nephroblastmatosis
Simpson-Golabi-Behmel (gigantism, macrosomia, bulldog facies, congenital heart defects, skeletal anomalies, mental retardation)	*GPC3* (Xq26)	10%	
No Overgrowth			
WAGR (Wilms tumor, aniridia, genitourinary anomalies, mental retardation, delayed-onset renal failure)	*WT1* (11p13)	30%	Intralobar NR
Denys-Drash (ambiguous genitalia, renal mesangial sclerosis, and Wilms tumor)	*WT1* (11p13)	50%–90%	Intralobar NR
Frasier (ambiguous genitalia, streak gonads, focal segmental glomerulosclerosis)	*WT1* (11p13)	8%	Intralobar NR
Bloom (constitutional dwarfism, photosensitivity, leukemia, characteristic facial features)	*BLM* (15q26)	3%	

Abbreviation: NR, nephrogenic rest.
[a]From Bove[50] and Pizzo and Poplack.[44]

2 (IGF-2), which promotes cellular proliferation and is highly expressed in the fetal kidney.[58] Recently, a third mutation, called *WTX*, has been identified at the Xq11.1 locus and is inactivated in approximately one-third of WTs.[59] Alterations in the *FTW1* and *FTW2* genes have been linked to familial WT, which represents 1%–2% of all cases and typically presents at a younger age with a propensity for bilateral involvement.[60] Several other chromosomal abnormalities have been linked to WT development, underlining the complex nature of Wilms' tumorigenesis.

Nephrogenic Rests and Nephroblastomatosis

Precursor lesions, known as nephrogenic rests (NRs), are found in over one-third of kidneys resected for WT. They occur when islands of the metanephric blastema persist after normal nephrogenesis, which is complete by 36 weeks of gestation. If these persistent fetal rests proliferate, they may evolve into WTs.[61] However, the majority of these lesions undergo involution and never differentiate into WTs.[62] NRs are generally divided into 2 distinct groups: perilobar nephrogenic rests (PLNRs) and intralobar nephrogenic rests (ILNR) based on their location within the renal lobe. PLNRs are sharply demarcated lesions restricted to the lobar periphery, containing blastema and tubules predominantly, and are often multiple. These lesions are typically found in children with BWS related to the *WT2* locus. Conversely, ILNRs are stroma rich and can be found anywhere within the kidney, including the renal sinus and collecting system. Interestingly, ILNRs are seen in children with aniridia, WAGR, and DDS due to mutations in the *WT1* gene. Patients with a *WT1* mutation or those associated with ILNRs generally present at a younger age.[3] The risk of developing contralateral disease is significantly increased when WTs are found in association with NRs, especially the perilobar variety.

Nephroblastomatosis occurs when multiple or diffuse NRs are present in 1 or both kidneys. Diffuse nephroblastomatosis presents with enlarged and often-palpable kidneys bilaterally and is often seen in association with congenital malformations. CT or MRI shows bilateral nephromegaly with a thick homogeneous rind that surrounds the normal parenchyma while preserving its normal reniform shape.[63] The diagnosis of nephroblastomatosis is based on either CT/MRI findings or open renal biopsy.[64]

Nephroblastomatosis has never been the focus of the cooperative pediatric oncology groups; therefore, there is no general consensus on its management. The behavior of these diffuse lesions is variable and multiple treatment regimes have been used, including active surveillance, prophylactic chemotherapy with vincristine (VCR) and dactinomycin (AMD), or surgical resection. Radiotherapy is not overly effective and is of little benefit in the absence of an associated WT. Typically, patients are either observed with serial ultrasounds every 3–4 months or receive up-front VCR and AMD. If the lesions progress in size or appearance, chemotherapy is started or surgical exploration is performed. A nephron-sparing approach is preferred due to the risk of developing WT in the contralateral kidney.[65]

Pathology

Grossly, WTs are often surrounded by an intrarenal pseudocapsule caused by the compression of neighboring renal parenchyma, which can help differentiate it from other solid renal masses or precursor lesions.[17] WT pathology has important implications regarding both patient management and prognosis due to the considerable histologic diversity and response to standard chemotherapeutic protocols.[66] Certain histopathological findings are considered *unfavorable* histology (UH) because they are associated with increased rates of recurrence and death. These are present in approximately 10% of cases and include lesions with anaplasia or tumors composed predominantly of sarcomatous stroma.[67] Anaplastic WT, which occurs almost exclusively in older children, is resistant to chemotherapy and carries a poor prognosis regardless of tumor stage.[68] When anaplasia is absent, the tumor is referred to as having *favorable* histology (FH) related to the better outcomes seen in these patients.[67] Practically all cases of neonatal WT have FH, and to date, anaplasia has not been described this age group.[49]

Most neonates with WT display the classic "triphasic" pattern with varying proportions of blastemal, stromal, and epithelial components. Other histological subtypes of WT more commonly encountered during infancy include the rhabdomyomatous variant, boytroid tumors of the renal pelvis, and cystic partially differentiated nephroblastoma.[69] Essentially, these atypical cellular variants are associated with the same prognosis and outcomes as the typical WT with FH.[5]

Clinical Presentation

During the neonatal period, WT typically presents as an asymptomatic abdominal mass detected on either physical examination (49%) or prenatal ultrasound (16%). The remaining cases are identified during the investigation of polyhydramnios (8%), hydrops fetalis (7%), or other congenital anomalies (7%).[4] Several nonspecific findings may also be appreciated postnatally, including pallor, anemia, vomiting, lethargy, fevers, abdominal distension, hematuria, and failure to thrive.[70] Hypertension is seen more commonly in older children and can affect approximately half of patients found to have a WT. This rise in blood pressure is often secondary to hyperreninemia, which resolves postoperatively following complete excision of the tumor.[34] These lesions are typically unilateral, although bilateral renal involvement (stage V) is seen in up to 12% of neonatal and fetal cases of WT and are often associated with NRs and the predisposing syndromes[4] listed in Table 43-4. Physical examination may also demonstrate findings consistent with these associated WT syndromes, such as aniridia, hemihypertrophy, and genitourinary defects (renal fusion anomalies, cryptorchidism, and hypospadias). Less commonly, a varicocele, hepatomegaly, ascites, or congestive heart failure may be present if the tumor extends into the renal vein or inferior vena cava.[3]

Extrarenal neonatal WTs have been reported and are exceedingly rare, often presenting in an atypical manner depending on the location of the tumor.[71] Extrarenal WTs are most commonly located within the retroperitoneum, although less-common sites include the inguinoscrotal area, sacrococcygeal region, mediastinum, spermatic cord, uterus, ovaries, and chest wall.[72]

Differential Diagnosis

The differential diagnosis of a congenital solid renal mass is outlined in Table 43-1 and should include all benign and malignant intrarenal and extrarenal masses. During the neonatal period, the most likely diagnosis of a unilateral solid renal mass is CMN, followed by WT, RTK, and CCSK. However, in the setting of bilateral neonatal renal masses, WT becomes the most likely diagnosis followed by RTK.[4] It is important to remember that there is no radiological finding or study that can reliably distinguish these lesions from each other; therefore, they must be managed with care due to the risk of harboring malignancy.

Diagnostic Tests

The initial workup of any solid renal mass includes a thorough history and physical examination, followed by laboratory and radiologic investigations (Table 43-4).

Ultrasound evaluation should be the first radiographic study performed in a newborn with an abdominal mass as it will demonstrate the solid or cystic nature of the lesion. Doppler studies can help identify tumor thrombus extending into the inferior vena cava (IVC), which occurs in 6% of WT patients.[73] If ultrasonography cannot exclude IVC thrombus extension, MRI is the modality of choice.[42] Contrast-enhanced cross-sectional imaging of the abdomen with CT or MRI should be performed next. This will provide the preoperative images needed to plan a major cancer operation and help to establish the presence and function of the contralateral kidney prior to nephrectomy. Cross-sectional imaging can sometimes demonstrate local extension of the tumor beyond the renal capsule or involvement of the retroperitoneal lymph nodes. However, the utility of preoperative imaging for tumor staging purposes remains controversial because children commonly have benign retroperitoneal adenopathy, and CT/MRI cannot accurately determine the malignant potential of an enlarged node.[3] Positron emission tomography (PET) has no clinical advantage over conventional imaging techniques in the preoperative assessment of WT.[74] A CT of the chest or chest radiograph is also recommended prior to surgery because the lungs are the most common site of distant metastasis in children with WT, although not all lesions identified represent metastatic spread.[75]

Staging

Fetal and neonatal WT primarily have low-stage disease, with 80% of cases presenting as either stage I/II. Stage III tumors represent a small proportion of cases, and there have been no documented reports of distant metastatic disease in a neonate (stage IV) in any North American series. Stage V, or bilateral WT, has been reported in neonates and can be found in 12% of cases, often in association with specific congenital syndromes.[49]

Management

The contemporary management of WT includes a stage-specific combination of surgery, chemotherapy, and radiotherapy. Neonatal WTs are generally low stage with FH and therefore receive an up-front nephrectomy followed by chemotherapy (VCR and AMD). Based on the review of Ritchey et al, neonates with stage I disease, FH, and tumors weighing less than 550 g can be managed by surgery alone without adjuvant chemotherapy or radiation. These patients must be followed closely with frequent imaging studies for disease recurrence.[49] A formal retroperitoneal lymph node dissection is not recommended, but selective nodal sampling is essential for accurate tumor staging and assessing the need for adjuvant therapy.[76] In North America, patients with stage II–V disease are treated with combination chemotherapeutic agents according to the COG protocol, which is ultimately based on the final pathological assessment.[70] It has also been recommended that all patients under 1 year of age requiring adjuvant chemotherapy receive a 50% dose reduction to minimize treatment toxicities while maintaining survival outcomes equivalent to full-dose therapy.[77] Radiotherapy is reserved for stage III–IV tumors.

Bilateral WTs are seen in approximately 5%–10% of fetal and neonatal cases and are associated with an increased frequency of congenital malformations and NRs.[4,78,79] The current COG protocol for the treatment in patients with stage V disease is directed toward preserving renal function to avoid renal insufficiency and need for dialysis. This is accomplished through an initial 6-week course of preoperative chemotherapy to allow for tumor shrinkage, followed by wedge resections of any residual tumor amenable to partial nephrectomy. SIOP investigators have noted late relapses in patients with bilateral WTs 4 years after treatment and recommend long-term follow-up.[80]

Outcome/Follow-up

Most newborns and infants with WTs present with lower-stage tumors that are of FH, which likely contributes to the excellent outcomes seen in this age group.[49,81] In the largest series of fetal and neonatal WTs, 91% of patients, stages I through V, who received treatment were still alive at last follow-up. The overall survival in this group, however, was only 78% related to associated conditions like polyhydramnios, fetal hydrops, and stillbirths that prevented the initiation of appropriate therapy.[4] Given the rarity of this tumor in the neonatal period and the small number of reported cases, it is difficult to quote stage-specific survival rates. In older children with WT, the overall 4-year survival rates have been reported as 96.5% (stage I/FH), 92.2% (stage II/FH), 86.9% (stage III/FH), and 73% (all stage IV and UH).[82] Risk factors related to local recurrence, which is associated with a 2-year survival rate of less than 50%, include tumor spillage, UH, incomplete tumor removal, and failure to sample regional lymph nodes.[76] LOH on chromosomes 16q and 1p has been noted in 20% of WTs and is an adverse prognostic factor that is associated with higher rates of relapse, independent of tumor histology and stage.[83]

Close follow-up is mandatory in all patients with WT and should include combination abdominal and chest imaging studies (Table 43-6). Surveillance should continue until age 8 years for patients with bilateral WTs or NRs.[44]

Rhabdoid Tumor of the Kidney

Epidemiology

Rhabdoid tumor of the kidney accounts for fewer than 2% of renal tumors registered to the National Wilms Tumor Study Group (NWTSG) (Tomlinson, Breslow, et al 2005). RTK is a highly malignant tumor, characterized by early metastasis and high mortality rate. Between 60% and 70% of all RTK occur during the newborn period.[84] It is the third-most-common solid renal tumor in the neonatal period, representing 11% of perinatal renal tumors, with a 3-fold male predominance.[4] Rhabdoid tumors can occur in extrarenal sites, including the central nervous system, skin, chest wall, and other soft tissue locations.[84]

Pathophysiology

The cellular origin of this aggressive tumor remains unknown despite its resemblance to rhabdomyoblasts. All rhabdoid tumors are associated with deletions and mutations in the tumor suppressor gene *hSNF5/INI1*, in the chromosomal region of 22q11, supporting a common genetic basis for renal and extrarenal rhabdoid tumors.[85]

Clinical Presentation

Rhabdoid tumors of the kidney present with a palpable or sonographically detected abdominal mass in over 50% of cases in addition to a variety of nonspecific findings, which include hematuria (gross or microscopic), fever, hypertension, anemia, and hypercalcemia. At the time of diagnosis, 47% of fetal and neonatal cases present with stage IV disease and harbor distant metastasis. Metastatic spread most frequently targets the regional lymph nodes and lungs, although the liver, bone, and brain can also be involved.[86] RTK is interestingly associated with a high incidence of concomitant primary brain tumors, including primitive neuroectodermal tumor, ependymoma, and cerebellar and brainstem astrocytomas.[87] These associated tumors tend to occur more commonly in neonates and can be found in 26% of perinatal cases.[4]

Differential Diagnosis

The differential diagnosis of a congenital renal mass is outlined in Table 43-1 and should include all benign and malignant intrarenal and extrarenal masses. Although CMN is the most common solid renal mass during the neonatal period, those presenting with distant metastatic disease (stage IV) are most likely RTK or CCSK. In the absence of an associated brain tumor, it is difficult to reliably distinguish RTK from other solid renal tumors, and the final diagnosis is ultimately based on pathological evaluation after surgical excision.

Diagnostic Tests

The workup for RTK is similar to all neonatal renal tumors and includes a thorough history and physical examination followed by blood work and routine imaging studies (Table 43-4). On ultrasound, RTK appears as a large heterogeneous and lobulated mass involving the renal hilum, which may extend into the renal vein or IVC.[88] CT or MRI generally shows areas of fat and calcifications within a heterogeneously enhancing mass and may demonstrate a peripheral crescent-shaped subcapsular fluid collection.[89] Radiological findings are typically nonspecific, and there are no pathognomonic findings for RTK. Once the diagnosis of RTK is confirmed pathologically, a MRI of the brain is required to rule out any intracranial pathology.

Management

The initial treatment of all neonatal renal tumors is essentially the same, consisting of a radical nephrectomy followed by chemotherapy or radiation therapy. Chemotherapeutic regimes for RTK have evolved over the years. The initial treatment strategies consisted of VCR, AMD, and doxorubicin, with or without cyclophosphamide, which yielded poor outcomes.[90] Newer regimens were adopted in NWTS-5, but this treatment arm of the study was closed prematurely because preliminary outcomes were equivocal to previous regimens. Currently, patients enrolled on the current COG protocol with RTK receive regimen UH-1, consisting of VCR, doxorubicin, carboplatin, cyclophosphamide, and etoposide.

Radiotherapy is currently standard treatment of patients with RTK. Patients generally receive 19.8 Gy (10.8 for patients ≤ 12 months) of irradiation to the whole abdomen regardless of stage.[44]

Outcome/Follow-up

The outcomes of fetal and neonatal RTK is dismal, with an overall 8% survival rate.[84] Outcomes improve in older children as their age at diagnosis increases. The 2-year event-free survival (EFS) in patients older than 27 months at diagnosis was 48%, compared to 15% for patients younger than 6 months of age.[91] In patients of all ages treated by the NWTSG, overall stage-specific survival rates are 33% for stage I, 47% for stage II, 22% for stage III, and 8% for stage IV.[92]

Close follow-up of these children is mandatory given their poor survival outcomes, as outlined in Table 43-6.

Clear Cell Sarcoma of the Kidney

Epidemiology

Clear cell sarcoma of the kidney is a rarely encountered renal malignancy in the newborn and accounted for only 3% of neonatal renal tumors reported in a large North American series.[4] Across all ages, approximately 20 new cases of CCSK are diagnosed annually in the United States, with individuals having a mean age at diagnosis of 36 months, ranging from 2 months to 14 years. Boys are more frequently affected, with a

2:1 gender distribution. Among the 351 patients registered to NWTSG with CCSK, only 1 tumor was associated with PLNR; there were no documented cases of familial inheritance, and CCSK is not associated with any predisposition syndromes as seen in WT.[93]

The stage distribution at presentation, based on data from the NWTSG, was 25% (stage I), 37% (stage II), 34% (stage III), 4% (stage IV), and no reported cases of bilateral involvement (stage V).[93]

Pathophysiology

Despite being called a sarcoma, ultrastructural and immunohistochemical findings do not support this, and the histogenesis of CCSK remains unknown. Most CCSK have a distinct histological appearance, but a number of variants exist that can mimic WT and cause diagnostic uncertainty. This rare neonatal tumor has a much higher rate of recurrence and death compared to WT, likely related to its propensity for both hematogenous and lymphatic spread. CCSK are recognized for their propensity to spread to bone; originally, CCSK was called the bone-metastasizing renal tumor of childhood. Other common sites of metastasis and relapse include the brain, lungs, abdomen, liver, and a number of bizarre soft tissues, such as the scalp, neck, nasopharynx, and orbit.[93]

Differential Diagnosis

The differential diagnosis of a congenital solid renal mass is outlined in Table 43-1 and should include all benign and malignant intrarenal and extrarenal masses.

Diagnostic Tests

The workup for CCSK is similar to that for all neonatal renal tumors and includes a thorough history and physical examination followed by blood work and imaging studies (Table 43-4).

Radiologic investigations are nonspecific and often will show a large, unicentric solid mass that distorts or almost completely replaces the normal kidney. Tumor necrosis is commonly seen, and most tumors will display cystic components that can easily be mistaken for benign cystic lesions, such as multiloculated cystic nephroma or segmental cystic dysplasia.[94] Renal vein involvement is seen in 5% of cases reported to the NWTSG. A large proportion of patients present with disseminated disease, with a 29% rate of lymph node involvement at the time of surgical resection. Ipsilateral renal hilar lymph nodes are the most common site of metastasis at presentation.[93]

The final diagnosis is completely dependent on tumor pathology and can only be accurately made following surgical resection. Once CCSK has been confirmed histologically, a bone scan and MRI of the brain are recommended due to its propensity to spread to bone and brain.[95]

Management

The management plan for all solid neonatal masses is a radical nephrectomy and should include sampling of the retroperitoneal lymph nodes for staging purposes. All patients, regardless of stage, receive adjuvant chemotherapy with a combination of VCR, AMD, and doxorubicin. The addition of doxorubicin to the chemotherapeutic regime for all stages of CCSK was initiated after the first 3 NWTS trials suggested that doxorubicin improved 6-year RFS rates.[96] Later trials eventually showed that doxorubicin therapy was associated with a 66% reduction in tumor-related mortality.[93]

Eighty-five percent of patients with CCSK in the NWTS trials from all age groups received radiotherapy to the tumor bed, compared to the 29% of neonates who received adjuvant radiation in Isaacs' series.[4,93]

Outcome/Follow-up

Clear cell sarcoma of the kidney has been associated with poor outcomes due to its tendency to metastasize to bone and brain. However, with the addition of doxorubicin therapy to all stages of disease, outcomes have improved significantly. In patients under the age of 2 years, the tumor-specific survival rose from 18% to 73% once doxorubicin became standard therapy. In neonates, the overall survival was 86% across all stages.[4] Currently, the 6-year survival rate for stage I patients is 98%, followed by 75% (stage II), 77% (stage III), and 50% (stage IV). Stage V has not been described in CCSK.[93]

Vigilant follow-up is mandatory for these patients given their likelihood for metastatic spread and late relapse (Table 43-6). Approximately 20% of metastatic cases occurred 3 years or more after diagnosis, with some patients relapsing as late as 10 years.[93]

REFERENCES

1. Pinto E, Guignard JP. Renal masses in the neonate. *Biol Neonate*. 1995;68(3):175–184.
2. Lakhoo K, Sowerbutts H. Neonatal tumours. *Pediatr Surg Int*. 2010;26(12):1159–1168.
3. Wein AJ, Kavoussi LR, et al. *Campbell-Walsh Urology*. Philadelphia, PA: Elsevier Saunders; 2012.
4. Isaacs H Jr. Fetal and neonatal renal tumors. *J Pediatr Surg*. 2008;43(9):1587–1595.
5. Isaacs H. *Tumors of the Fetus and Infant: An Atlas*. New York, NY: Springer; 2002.
6. Schreuder MF, Westland R, et al. Unilateral multicystic dysplastic kidney: a meta-analysis of observational studies on the incidence, associated urinary tract malformations and the contralateral kidney. *Nephrol Dial Transplant*. 2009;24:1810–1818.
7. Felson B, Cussen LJ. The hydronephrotic type of unilateral congenital multicystic disease of the kidney. *Semin Roentgenol*. 1975;10(2):113–123.
8. Mackie GG, Stephens FD. Duplex kidneys: a correlation of renal dysplasia with position of the ureteral orifice. *J Urol*. 1975;114:278–280.
9. Biscerglia M, Galliani CA, et al. Renal cystic disease: a review. *Adv Anat Pathol*. 2006;13(1):26–52.
10. Cole BR, Conley SB, et al. Polycystic kidney-disease in the 1st year of life. *J Pediatr*. 1987;111(5):693–699.
11. Fishman JE, Joseph RC. Renal vein thrombosis in utero: duplex sonography in diagnosis and follow-up. *Pediatr Radiol*. 1994;24:135–136.
12. Lau KK, Stoffman JM, et al. Neonatal renal vein thrombosis: review of the english-language literature between 1992 and 2006. *Pediatrics*. 2007;120(5):e1278–e1284.
13. Argyropoulou MI, Giapros VI, et al. Renal venous thrombosis in an infant. *Euro Radiol*. 2003;13(8):2027–2030.
14. Weizer AZ, Silverstein AD, et al. Determining the incidence of horseshoe kidney from radiographic data at a single institution. *J Urol*. 2003;170(5):1722–1726.
15. Love L, Wasserman D. Massive unilateral non-functioning hydronephrosis in horseshoe kidney. *Clin Radiol*. 1975;26(3):409–415.
16. Cho JY, Lee YH, et al. Prenatal diagnosis of horseshoe kidney by measurement of the renal pelvic angle. *Ultrasound Obstet Gynecol*. 2005;25(6):554–558.
17. Docimo SG, Kelalis PP, et al. *The Kelalis-King-Belman Textbook of Clinical Pediatric Urology*. Abingdon, UK; 2007.
18. Strauss S, Dushnitsky T, et al. Sonographic features of horseshoe kidney: review of 34 patients. *J Ultrasound Med*. 2000;19(1):27–31.
19. Kao PF, Sheih CP, et al. The 99mTc-DMSA renal scan and 99mTc-DTPA diuretic renogram in children and adolescents with incidental diagnosis of horseshoe kidney. *Nucl Med Commun*. 2003;24(5):525–530.
20. Zondek LH, Zondek T. Horseshoe kidney and associated congenital malformations. *Urol Int*. 1964;18:347–356.
21. Boatman DL, Kolln CP, et al. Congenital anomalies associated with horseshoe kidney. *J Urol*. 1972;107(2):205–207.
22. Warkany J, Passarge E, et al. Congenital malformations in autosomal trisomy syndromes. *Am J Dis Child*. 1966;112(6):502–517.
23. Lippe B, Geffner ME, et al. Renal malformations in patients with Turner syndrome: imaging in 141 patients. *Pediatrics*. 1988;82(6):852–856.
24. Cascio S, Sweeney B, et al. Vesicoureteral reflux and ureteropelvic junction obstruction in children with horseshoe kidney: treatment and outcome. *J Urol*. 2002;167(6):2566–2568.
25. Glenn JF. Analysis of 51 patients with horseshoe kidney. *N Engl J Med*. 1959;261:684–687.
26. van den Heuvel-Eibrink MM, Grundy P, et al. Characteristics and survival of 750 children diagnosed with a renal tumor in the first seven months of life: a collaborative study by the SIOP/GPOH/SFOP, NWTSG, and UKCCSG Wilms tumor study groups. *Pediatr Blood Cancer*. 2008;50(6):1130–1134.
27. England RJ, Haider N, et al. Mesoblastic nephroma: a report of the United Kingdom Children's Cancer and Leukaemia Group (CCLG). *Pediatr Blood Cancer*. 2011;56(5):744–748.
28. Bolande RP, Brough AJ, et al. Congenital mesoblastic nephroma of infancy. A report of eight cases and the relationship to Wilms' tumor. *Pediatrics*. 1967;40(2):272–278.
29. Santos LG, Carvalho Jde S, et al. Cellular congenital mesoblastic nephroma: case report. *J Bras Nefrol*. 2011;33(1):109–112.
30. Steinfeld AD, Crowley CA, et al. Recurrent and metastatic mesoblastic nephroma in infancy. *J Clin Oncol*. 1984;2(8):956–960.
31. Knezevich SR, Garnett MJ, et al. ETV6-NTRK3 gene fusions and trisomy 11 establish a histogenetic link between

mesoblastic nephroma and congenital fibrosarcoma. *Cancer Res.* 1998;58(22):5046–5048.

32. Leclair MD, El-Ghoneimi A, et al. The outcome of prenatally diagnosed renal tumors. *J Urol.* 2005;173(1):186–189.

33. Srivastava T, Kats A, et al. Parathyroid-hormone-related protein-mediated hypercalcemia in benign congenital mesoblastic nephroma. *Pediatr Nephrol.* 2011;26(5):799–803.

34. Maas MH, Cransberg K, et al. Renin-induced hypertension in Wilms tumor patients. *Pediatr Blood Cancer.* 2007;48(5):500–503.

35. Pizzo PA, Poplack DG. *Principles and Practice of Pediatric Oncology.* Philadelphia, PA: Lippincott Williams & Wilkins; 2006.

36. Mogilner JG, Fonseca J, et al. Congenital mesoblastic nephroma associated with acquired von Willebrand disease: a case report. *Isr J Med Sci.* 1995;31(7):441–443.

37. Blanchette V, Coppes MJ. Routine bleeding history and laboratory tests in children presenting with a renal mass. *Pediatr Blood Cancer.* 2009;52(3):314–315.

38. Chaudry G, Perez-Atayde AR, et al. Imaging of congenital mesoblastic nephroma with pathological correlation. *Pediatr Radiol.* 2009;39(10):1080–1086.

39. Howell CG, Othersen HB, et al. Therapy and outcome in 51 children with mesoblastic nephroma: a report of the National Wilms' Tumor Study. *J Pediatr Surg.* 1982;17(6):826–831.

40. Riccabona M. Imaging of renal tumours in infancy and childhood. *Eur Radiol.* 2003;13(Suppl 4):L116–L129.

41. Owens CM, Veys PA, et al. Role of chest computed tomography at diagnosis in the management of Wilms' tumor: a study by the United Kingdom Children's Cancer Study Group. *J Clin Oncol.* 2002;20(12):2768–2773.

42. Schenk J-P, Graf N, et al. Role of MRI in the management of patients with nephroblastoma. *Eur Radiol.* 2008;18(4):683–691.

43. Othersen HB Jr, DeLorimer A, et al. Surgical evaluation of lymph node metastases in Wilms' tumor. *J Pediatr Surg.* 1990;25(3):330–331.

44. Pizzo PA, Poplack DG. *Principles and Practice of Pediatric Oncology.* Philadelphia, PA: Wolters Kluwer Health/Lippincott Williams & Wilkins; 2011.

45. Gormley TS, Skoog SJ, et al. Cellular congenital mesoblastic nephroma: what are the options. *J Urol.* 1989;142(2 Pt 2):479–483; discussion 489.

46. Furtwaengler R, Reinhard H, et al. Mesoblastic nephroma—a report from the Gesellschaft fur Padiatrische Onkologie und Hamatologie (GPOH). *Cancer.* 2006;106(10):2275–2283.

47. Loeb DM, Hill DA, et al. Complete response of recurrent cellular congenital mesoblastic nephroma to chemotherapy. *J Pediatr Hematol Oncol.* 2002;24(6):478–481.

48. Breslow N, Olshan A, et al. Epidemiology of Wilms tumor. *Med Pediatr Oncol.* 1993;21(3):172–181.

49. Ritchey ML, Azizkhan RG, et al. Neonatal Wilms tumor. *J Pediatr Surg.* 1995;30(6):856–859.

50. Bove KE. Wilms' tumor and related abnormalities in the fetus and newborn. *Semin Perinatol.* 1999;23(4):310–318.

51. Breslow NE, Beckwith JB. Epidemiological features of Wilms' tumor: results of the National Wilms' Tumor Study. *J Natl Cancer Inst.* 1982;68(3):429–436.

52. Knudson AG Jr, Strong LC. Mutation and cancer: a model for Wilms' tumor of the kidney. *J Natl Cancer Inst.* 1972;48(2):313–324.

53. Strong LC. The two-hit model for Wilms' tumor: where are we 30 years later? *Genes Chromosomes Cancer.* 2003;38(4):294–299.

54. Riccardi VM, Sujansky E, et al. Chromosomal imbalance in the Aniridia-Wilms' tumor association: 11p interstitial deletion. *Pediatrics.* 1978;61(4):604–610.

55. Kreidberg JA, Sariola H, et al. WT-1 is required for early kidney development. *Cell.* 1993;74(4):679–691.

56. Breslow NE, Collins AJ, et al. End stage renal disease in patients with Wilms tumor: results from the National Wilms Tumor Study Group and the United States Renal Data System. *J Urol.* 2005;174(5):1972–1975.

57. Koufos A, Grundy P, et al. Familial Wiedemann-Beckwith syndrome and a second Wilms tumor locus both map to 11p15.5. *Am J Hum Genet.* 1989;44(5):711–719.

58. Bjornsson HT, Brown LJ, et al. Epigenetic specificity of loss of imprinting of the IGF2 gene in Wilms tumors. *J Natl Cancer Inst.* 2007;99(16):1270–1273.

59. Rivera MN, Kim WJ, et al. An X chromosome gene, WTX, is commonly inactivated in Wilms tumor. *Science (NY).* 2007;315(5812):642–645.

60. Ruteshouser EC, Huff V. Familial Wilms tumor. *Am J Med Genet C Semin Med Genet.* 2004;129C(1):29–34.

61. Beckwith JB, Kiviat NB, et al. Nephrogenic rests, nephroblastomatosis, and the pathogenesis of Wilms' tumor. *Pediatr Pathol.* 1990;10(1–2):1–36.

62. Beckwith JB. Nephrogenic rests and the pathogenesis of Wilms tumor: developmental and clinical considerations. *Am J Med Genet.* 1998;79(4):268–273.

63. Perlman EJ, Faria P, et al. Hyperplastic perilobar nephroblastomatosis: long-term survival of 52 patients. *Pediatr Blood Cancer.* 2006;46(2):203–221.

64. Rohrschneider WK, Weirich A, et al. US, CT and MR imaging characteristics of nephroblastomatosis. *Pediatr Radiol.* 1998;28(6):435–443.

65. Prasil P, Laberge JM, et al. Management decisions in children with nephroblastomatosis. *Med Pediatr Oncol.* 2000;35(4):429–432; discussion 433.

66. Weirich A, Leuschner I, et al. Clinical impact of histologic subtypes in localized non-anaplastic nephroblastoma treated according to the trial and study SIOP-9/GPOH. *Ann Oncol.* 2001;12(3):311–319.

67. Beckwith JB, Palmer NF. Histopathology and prognosis of Wilms tumors: results from the First National Wilms' Tumor Study. *Cancer.* 1978;41(5):1937–1948.

68. Dome JS, Cotton CA, et al. Treatment of anaplastic histology Wilms' tumor: results from the fifth National Wilms' Tumor Study. *J Clin Oncol.* 2006;24(15):2352–2358.

69. Ugarte N, Gonzalez-Crussi F, et al. Wilms' tumor: its morphology in patients under one year of age. *Cancer.* 1981;48(2):346–353.

70. Powis M. Neonatal renal tumours. *Early Hum Dev.* 2010;86(10):607–612.

71. Hussain S, Nizami S, et al. Neonatal extra-renal Wilm's tumour. *J Pak Med Assoc.* 2004;54(1):37–38.

72. Sastri J, Dedhia R, et al. Extra-renal Wilms' tumour—is it different? *Pediatr Nephrol.* 2006;21(4):591–596.

73. Shamberger RC, Ritchey ML, et al. Intravascular extension of Wilms tumor. *Ann Surg.* 2001;234(1):116–121.

74. Misch D, Steffen IG, et al. Use of positron emission tomography for staging, preoperative response assessment and post-therapeutic evaluation in children with Wilms tumour. *Eur J Nucl Med Mol Imaging.* 2008;35(9):1642–1650.

75. Ehrlich PF, Hamilton TE, et al. The value of surgery in directing therapy for patients with Wilms' tumor with pulmonary disease. A report from the National Wilms' Tumor Study Group (National Wilms' Tumor Study 5). *J Pediatr Surg.* 2006;41(1):162–167; discussion 162–167.

76. Shamberger RC. Pediatric renal tumors. *Semin Surg Oncol.* 1999;16(2):105–120.

77. Corn BW, Goldwein JW, et al. Outcomes in low-risk babies treated with half-dose chemotherapy according to the Third National Wilms' Tumor Study. *J Clin Oncol.* 1992;10(8):1305–1309.

78. Blute ML, Kelalis PP, et al. Bilateral Wilms tumor. *J Urol.* 1987;138(4 Pt 2):968–973.

79. Campbell AN, Chan HS, et al. Malignant tumours in the neonate. *Arch Dis Childhood.* 1987;62(1):19–23.

80. Coppes MJ, de Kraker J, et al. Bilateral Wilms' tumor: long-term survival and some epidemiological features. *J Clin Oncol.* 1989;7(3):310–315.

81. Marsden HB, Lawler W. Primary renal tumours in the first year of life. A population based review. *Virchows Arch A Pathol Anat Histopathol.* 1983;399(1):1–9.

82. D'Angio GJ, Breslow N, et al. Treatment of Wilms' tumor. Results of the Third National Wilms' Tumor Study. *Cancer.* 1989;64(2):349–360.

83. Grundy PE, Breslow NE, et al. Loss of heterozygosity for chromosomes 1p and 16q is an adverse prognostic factor in favorable-histology Wilms tumor: a report from the National Wilms Tumor Study Group. *J Clin Oncol.* 2005;23(29):7312–7321.

84. Isaacs H Jr. Fetal and neonatal rhabdoid tumor. *J Pediatr Surg.* 2010;45(3):619–626.

85. Biegel JA, Zhou JY, et al. Germ-line and acquired mutations of INI1 in atypical teratoid and rhabdoid tumors. *Cancer Res.* 1999;59(1):74–79.

86. Amar AM, Tomlinson G, et al. Clinical presentation of rhabdoid tumors of the kidney. *J Pediatr Hematol Oncol.* 2001;23(2):105–108.

87. Bonnin JM, Rubinstein LJ, et al. The association of embryonal tumors originating in the kidney and in the brain. A report of seven cases. *Cancer.* 1984;54(10):2137–2146.

88. Hugosson C, Nyman R, et al. Imaging of solid kidney tumours in children. *Acta Radiol.* 195;36(3):254–260.

89. Han TI, Kim MJ, et al. Rhabdoid tumour of the kidney: imaging findings. *Pediatr Radiol.* 2001;31(4):233–237.

90. Weeks DA, Beckwith JB, et al. Rhabdoid tumor of kidney. A report of 111 cases from the National Wilms' Tumor Study Pathology Center. *Am J Surg Pathol.* 1989;13(6):439–458.

91. van den Heuvel-Eibrink MM, van Tinteren H, et al. Malignant rhabdoid tumours of the kidney (MRTKs), registered on recent SIOP protocols from 1993 to 2005: a report of the SIOP renal tumour study group. *Pediatr Blood Cancer.* 2011;56(5):733–737.

92. Tomlinson GE, Breslow NE, et al. Rhabdoid tumor of the kidney in the National Wilms' Tumor Study: age at diagnosis as a prognostic factor. *J Clin Oncol.* 2005;23(30):7641–7645.

93. Argani P, Perlman EJ, et al. Clear cell sarcoma of the kidney: a review of 351 cases from the National Wilms Tumor Study Group Pathology Center. *Am J Surg Pathol.* 2000;24(1):4–18.

94. Glass RB, Davidson AJ, et al. Clear cell sarcoma of the kidney: CT, sonographic, and pathologic correlation. *Radiology.* 1991;180(3):715–717.

95. Feusner JH, Beckwith JB, et al. Clear cell sarcoma of the kidney: accuracy of imaging methods for detecting bone metastases. Report from the National Wilms' Tumor Study. *Med Pediatr Oncol.* 1990;18(3):225–227.

96. Green DM, Breslow NE, et al. Treatment of children with clear-cell sarcoma of the kidney: a report from the National Wilms' Tumor Study Group. *J Clin Oncol.* 1994;12(10):2132–2137.

97. Pitts WR, Muecke EC. Horseshoe kidneys: a 40-year experience. *J Urol.* 1975;113(6):743–746.

98. Segura JW. Observations on renal ectopia and fusion in children. *J Urol.* 1972;108(20):333–336.

99. Rubin BP, Chen CJ, et al. Congenital mesoblastic nephroma t(12;15) is associated with ETV6-NTRK3 gene fusion: cytogenetic and molecular relationship to congenital (infantile) fibrosarcoma. *Am J Pathol.* 1998;153(5):1451–1458.

CHAPTER 43

44 Obstructive Uropathies

Winifred A. Owumi and William A. Kennedy II

INTRODUCTION

The urinary system is essential for the elimination of metabolic wastes, maintenance of physiologic pH, and the preservation of fluid and electrolyte homeostasis. It also contributes to vital functions like erythropoiesis and blood pressure control. Obstruction in the upper or lower urinary tract system can lead to disruption in these vital body physiologies and can lead to significant morbidity, which may be irreversible and ultimately lead to mortality. In neonates and young children, reports have shown that obstruction of the urinary tract is the most common cause of renal insufficiency, especially in boys under the age of 1, as well as the number 1 cause of renal transplantation in children.[1,2] The majority of these obstructive uropathies are congenital in nature. The neonatal kidney is still developing, therefore obstruction can lead to alterations in the normal growth pattern and differentiation of the renal cells beginning in the intrauterine period and progressing postpartum, ultimately resulting in the development of fibrosis and renal failure. Obstruction can be limited to the upper urinary tract, the lower urinary tract, or a combination.

The main sign of obstructive uropathy is hydronephrosis, which involves dilation of the renal collecting system, including the renal pelvis and the renal calyces. Even the ureters may be dilated from the accumulation of urine in the collecting system. Genitourinary anomalies can be found in up to 0.2%–5% of pregnancies. Hydronephrosis comprises up to 87% of the identified anomalies. From prenatal ultrasound screening, varying degrees of hydronephrosis can be seen in up to 1.4% of fetuses, detected as early as the 12th week of pregnancy.

More than half of these resolve spontaneously after birth. It is estimated that 48% are transient in nature (ie, from fetal folds in the proximal ureter during organogenesis), 15% are normal physiologic findings, 11% are from ureteropelvic junction (UPJ) obstruction, 9% are from vesicoureteral reflux (VUR), 4% are associated with congenital megaureters, and the others derive from miscellaneous causes (ie, from ureteroceles, posterior urethral valve [PUV], prune-belly syndrome [PBS]). There is a 2:1 male-to-female predominance of hydronephrosis. It can also be bilateral in 20%–40% of neonates.

Prenatal sonogram is mostly the means by which obstruction in the urinary tract is picked up in the developed world. If prenatal ultrasound was not obtained, neonatal presentations can range from palpable abdominal mass, urinary tract infections (UTIs), hematuria, failure to thrive, and occasionally renal failure. The risk of postnatal pathology from a prenatal finding of hydronephrosis has been correlated with the degree of the hydronephrosis seen. One meta-analysis reported 11.9% in cases of mild hydronephrosis and 45.1% in moderate and 88.3% in severe antenatal hydronephrosis.[3] We examine some of the most common obstructive uropathies in neonates.

URETEROPELVIC JUNCTION OBSTRUCTION

Epidemiology

As the name suggests, UPJ obstruction is an obstruction in the urinary tract at the junction between the renal pelvis and the ureter. It is the most common cause of hydronephrosis in children. It can be seen in 1 in 1000–2000 neonates, with the majority of these diagnosed on prenatal ultrasound imaging of the fetus.[4,5] In the neonatal period, UPJ obstruction has a 2:1 predominance in boys compared to girls; and left-sided to right-sided lesions are also more than 2:1 predominant in the neonatal period, approaching 67%. The reason for this is not entirely clear.[6] It can be seen bilaterally in 10%–40% of neonatal presentations, although less than 5% of these patients will need bilateral repair.[7] There is a hypothesis suggesting that multicystic dysplastic kidneys may result from early complete upper ureter or UPJ obstruction.

Pathophysiology

The etiology of UPJ obstruction is still debatable, and there are many theories regarding the pathophysiology. It can be described as an intrinsic defect in the UPJ that produces functional obstruction that results from poor ureter and renal pelvis smooth muscle activity.[8] The development of fetal and rodent models of partial and complete UPJ obstruction has helped to shed more light on the pathophysiology.[9,10] In experimental models, defects in the development of the smooth muscles have led to UPJ obstruction-induced hydronephrosis. Smooth muscle cell defects, as well as defects in the innervation of the renal pelvis and proximal ureter, can also be seen in human specimens obtained from patients who undergo pyeloplasty.[11,12] Other mechanisms are anatomical anomalies, such as kinking of the UPJ from crossing vessels or even high insertion of the ureter into the renal pelvis.[13] Sometimes, it is a combination of both mechanisms, but by and large, the exact mechanism is still being investigated.

Fetal and neonatal kidneys are still under significant growth and development; therefore, obstruction in the urinary tract can have deleterious effects. UPJ obstructions have been reported to lead to decreased nephrogenesis, manifesting from destruction of already-formed glomeruli, halting new glomeruli development,[14,15] and phenotypic transformation of already-formed glomerular cells into mesenchymal cells.[10,16] It promotes dilation, atrophy, apoptosis, and necrosis of the renal tubules.[14,17–23] All of which leads to compensatory growth and hypertrophy of the non-obstructed contralateral kidney based on the degree and chronicity of the obstruction.[24] In the fetus, due to the placenta being involved in exchange of nutrients and fetal blood filtration, the demand on renal function is much less than in the neonate[25]; therefore, the sequelae of renal failure may not be evident until the postpartum period. It has also been reported that if obstruction continues after birth, the neonatally obstructed kidney develops marked inflammatory infiltrates and, subsequently, increased fibrosis.[26]

Differential Diagnosis

Intuitively, because hydronephrosis is the most common finding in UPJ obstruction, the differential diagnosis usually includes most of the obstructive uropathies that can also present with unilateral or bilateral hydronephrosis. Some of these include non-pathologic extrarenal pelvis, multicystic dysplastic kidney, ureteral fibroepithelial polyps, ureteral valves, ureterovesical junction (UVJ) obstruction, VUR, ureteroceles, congenital megaureter and PUVs (usually if bilateral hydronephrosis is seen), among others.

Diagnostic Tests

Ultrasound

Pre- and postnatal ultrasounds are usually the first diagnostic imaging used to investigate neonatal obstructive uropathy. In utero, the second and third trimesters give the best estimate of the severity of postnatal hydronephrosis. The Society of Fetal Urology has a standardized grading system based on the anterior-pelvic (AP) diameter on the transverse plane of the renal pelvis. Dilation of 4–7 mm is considered mild, 7–10 mm is moderate, and greater than 10 mm is severe hydronephrosis. Renal pelvis AP diameter greater than 15 mm in the third trimester has the highest risk of neonatal renal deterioration. When combined with findings of oligohydramnios and increased renal echogenicity, this was also highly predictive of urinary tract obstruction.[27] Late gestational and postnatal hydronephrosis can be graded from grade I to grade IV.[28] Grade I is mild dilation of the renal pelvis only, grade II is moderate dilation of the renal pelvis and a few calyces, grade III involves dilation of the renal pelvis with uniform dilation and visualization of all the calyces, and grade IV is a progression of grade III with evident thinning of the renal parenchyma.[29]

Prenatal and postnatal ultrasound offer the advantages of early detection of those cases of obstruction with potential postpartum health impact by identifying cases that will require further antenatal and postnatal evaluation. It helps limit the use of ionizing radiographic studies and can help mitigate parental distress and encourage timely referral to a pediatric urologist if possible interventions are needed to minimize adverse outcomes. Ideally, the first postnatal sonogram should be done at day of life 3 because of the physiologic oliguria that is experienced in neonates in the first 48 hours of life. This can temporarily decrease the dilation of the collecting system and give a false negative, especially if the hydronephrosis is not severe. If a negative study is obtained or only grade I to II hydronephrosis is seen, then repeating the ultrasound in 4–6 weeks is recommended for follow-up as this may remain normal or spontaneously resolve. If grade III–IV hydronephrosis is present, a more urgent workup and referral to a pediatric urologist is warranted.

Voiding Cystourethrogram

In neonates diagnosed with persistent hydronephrosis postpartum, voiding cystourethrogram (VCUG) is generally recommended. The American Urological Association (AUA) guidelines state that a VCUG should be done for children with grades 3 and 4 hydronephrosis, hydroureter, or an abnormal bladder on late-term prenatal or postnatal ultrasound or those neonates who develop a UTI postnatally while under observation.[30] In cases of low-grade hydronephrosis (grades I and II), a VCUG need not be done, and observation of the neonate with ultrasound alone is acceptable. When recommended, a VCUG can be obtained within the first few days of life, prior to discharge from the hospital. The fluoroscopic VCUG is preferred as it provides the physician with the grade of the VUR and details of any anomalies within the bladder or urethra. The radionuclear VCUG has the advantage of exposing the infant to less radiation: 1 to 5 mrad in radionuclear VCUG vs 27 to 1000 mrad in fluoroscopic VCUG, although more recent studies report doses as low as 1.7 to 5.2 mrad with the fluoroscopic VCUG utilizing digital equipment.[31] The radionuclear VCUG has more sensitivity in detecting VUR; however, it only answers whether there is reflux, but not the grade of vesicourethral reflux. Therefore, the nuclear VCUG would not be the imaging test of choice for the initial study given the desire to both grade the reflux and visualize any anatomic pathology. Fluoroscopic VCUGs can also be used to diagnose ureteroceles, ectopic ureter insertions, bladder diverticula, PUVs, among other neonatal genitourinary anomalies.

Diuretic Renogram

Due to immaturity of the neonatal kidneys, the best time to do a diuretic renogram is at 4 to 6 weeks after birth. The technetium 99 mercapto acetyl triglycine (^{99m}Tc MAG-3) renal scan done with Lasix is frequently used to assess renal perfusion, differential function, drainage, and the site of obstruction in the collecting system (UPJ vs UVJ). If differential function is normal and obstruction is mild, then the child can be observed with serial imaging until a time when spontaneous resolution is documented. If differential function of a kidney is diminished and high-grade obstruction is documented, then intervention may be required.

Computed Tomography–Intravenous Pyelogram

Computed tomography (CT)–intravenous pyelogram is not routinely used in the neonatal period for diagnosing obstruction in the urinary tract. This is due to the high amount of ionizing radiation associated with this study. Magnetic resonance imaging (MRI) under sedation is rapidly becoming the preferred anatomical and functional study of choice in the case of severe hydronephrosis.

Magnetic Resonance Urethrogram

Although the magnetic resonance urethrogram requires some degree of anesthetic sedation to keep the infant still during the image acquisition, it offers the advantage of not exposing the neonate to ionizing radiation and is able to dynamically assess renal parenchymal signal intensity changes deduced from the perfusion, filtration, and concentration of contrast. Compared to CT scan and renal scan, it has inherent superior contrast and spatial and temporal resolution.[32] We are able to assess both anatomic and functional information from this study. The study provides us with differential renal function. In addition to detecting hydronephrosis, it can diagnose the location and possible cause of obstruction within the collecting system (ie, ureteral kinking, aberrant vessels, strictures). Based on the quality of the renal parenchyma and the degree of preoperative uropathy, MRU can provide some prognostic information for the surgeon[32] and help guide the type and timing of intervention.

Management

One of the first things to determine in neonates with urinary tract obstruction is whether antibiotic prophylaxis is needed. The AUA 2010 guidelines recommended that in grade I to II hydronephrosis, no antibiotic prophylaxis is immediately needed unless the patient develops a UTI while being observed.[30] In the first 3 months, penicillins or first-generation cephalosporins are recommended for UTI prophylaxis, but after that nitrofurantoin or trimethoprim/sulfamethoxazole can be used. A quarter of the standard antibiotic treatment dose given once nightly is preferred for UTI prophylaxis.

Timing for optimal surgical intervention is still an issue of controversy as there are currently no effective markers for determining the degree and progressive uropathic potential of various degrees of urinary tract obstruction.[10,33] Pediatric urology experts advocate close follow-up, and it is recommended that intervention is warranted if there is continued compromise in renal function or progressive hydronephrosis.[34–37] It is estimated that 25%–50% of the children diagnosed with prenatal hydronephrosis will eventually need some kind of surgical intervention.[38,39]

In neonates with solitary kidneys, severe bilateral hydronephrosis, and renal function compromise, early workup plus prophylactic antibiotics and surgical intervention are usually indicated. For those under observation, repeat imaging as appropriate (sonogram, renogram, and VCUG) in 3, 6, or 12 months can help determine improvement, stability, or progressive deterioration, which will dictate whether to follow the path of continued observation or surgical repair. Occasionally, when there is severe hydronephrosis and suggestion of significant renal functional compromise, percutaneous drainage of the affected kidney for a few weeks and repeating the renogram may help give a better idea of the actual renal function. This may provide useful information regarding whether repair of the obstruction or removal of the kidney is the preferred surgical strategy.

Outcomes and Follow-up

Despite appropriate surgical intervention, studies have shown that UPJ obstruction can result in permanent modifications to the renal parenchyma.[40] Although studies looking at long-term postsurgical outcomes following repair of UPJ obstruction are limited, reports have shown that the reoperation rate can be up to 5%, and in some cases renal function improvement can be seen over time.[41,42]

RETROCAVAL URETER

Retrocaval ureter is a rare phenomenon that happens when the ureter travels posterior to the inferior vena cava (IVC). The embryologic event that precipitates it is the abnormal persistence of the subcardinal vein on the right side.[43] It is typically characterized by an S-shaped deformity on intravenous or retrograde pyelography. It can also be detected on CT. The IVC can result in extrinsic compression of the ureter, which may cause significant obstruction. The ureter is usually medially deviated around the area of the third lumbar vertebra. It usually becomes symptomatic in the third to fourth decade of life; however, there have been rare case reports in neonates.[44]

It is corrected surgically like a UPJ obstruction by performing a dismembered pyeloplasty. This involves transection of the ureter above the IVC and moving and reanastomosing the proximal and distal ureter end anterior to the vena cava.[45]

VESICOURETERAL REFLUX

Epidemiology

Vesicoureteral reflux is the retrograde flow of urine from the bladder into the upper urinary tract. It can be seen in about 1% of neonates and up to 30%–45% of children who are diagnosed with a UTI.[46-48] Statistically,

10%–15% of infants found to have UPJ obstruction do have ipsilateral VUR, hence the need to rule this out in neonates being worked up for UPJ obstruction. Girls are 2 times more likely to have VUR, although in patients who present with antenatal hydronephrosis, there tends to be a male predominance. Blacks are also more likely to have low-grade reflux as compared to Caucasian children, who have higher-grade and 3 times more VUR. Children younger than 2 years are also more likely to have VUR. There is about a 27% prevalence rate among siblings, and that rate is 36% for children with an affected parent. Among identical twins, there is up to 80% concordance as compared to 35% in fraternal twins.[30,49-50]

Pathophysiology

Primary VUR is most commonly due to an intrinsic defect in the vesicoureteral junction from improper insertion (ie, ectopic ureter insertion or inadequate tunneling of the intravesical ureter), leading to a loss of the natural antireflux mechanism. As the bladder fills with urine, the detrusor muscles compress and seal off the intravesical ureter, thereby preventing urine from refluxing backward into the ureter from the bladder. Secondary VUR can also result from anatomic defects (ie, PUVs or neurogenic bladder) affecting urine flow out of the bladder. According to the International Reflux Study Group (IRSG) who developed a classification system, VUR is classified based on the degree of retrograde filling of the ureter, calyceal and ureteral dilation seen on VCUG. Grade I involves reflux into the ureter without dilation. Grade II also is without dilation, but the urine fills retrograde into the renal collecting system. In grade III VUR, there is mild dilation of the ureter and the collecting system with mild blunting of the calyces. Grade IV shows gross dilation and tortuosity of the ureter and the collecting system with blunting of the calyces, while grade V is the most severe, with urine reflux grossly dilating the collecting system, severe tortuosity of the ureter, blunting of all the calyces with a loss of papillary impression and cortical thinning.[51] Grades I and II are considered mild VUR, grade III is moderate VUR, and grade IV and V are severe VUR.

Differential Diagnosis

Some differential diagnoses to consider include UVJ obstruction, ureteroceles, congenital megaureter, PUVs, urethral atresia, and PBS.

Diagnostic Tests

Workup for VUR is usually prompted by the prenatal screening ultrasound finding of hydronephrosis. In neonates in whom prenatal hydronephrosis is missed, febrile UTI may be the reason to consider an infant has VUR. VUR is primarily diagnosed when reflux can be demonstrated on either fluoroscopic or radionuclear VCUG.

Management, Outcomes, and Follow-up

In addition to physical examination, including blood pressure measurement, a metabolic panel should be checked to assess renal function and rule out any significant metabolic derangement. The AUA guidelines encourage that in the management algorithm for VUR, primary care providers and urologists must bear in mind the likelihood of spontaneous resolution, risk of recurrent UTI, and renal parenchymal scarring.[52] Spontaneous resolution can occur in cases of VUR. One retrospective study reported spontaneous resolution rates of 72%, 61%, 49%, and 32% for grades I, II, II, and IV/V, respectively by 5 years of age.[53] Up to 50% of children with VUR and on continuous antibiotic prophylaxis will have spontaneous resolution within 24 months. Renal parenchyma abnormalities can be seen in about 8.2% of infants with VUR. Based on a meta-analysis of the available literature on prenatal hydronephrosis and VUR, the AUA consensus panel on the management of VUR in children has given 2 primary recommendations: (1) Children less than 1 year of age with VUR and a history of a febrile UTI or (2) children who have grades III—V VUR should be placed on continuous antibiotic prophylaxis until resolution of the reflux. Continuous antibiotic prophylaxis is optional in an infant who has grade I–II VUR and no history of UTI. To also decrease the risk of UTI in infant boys, circumcision is an option that can be discussed with the parents. There is, however, insufficient data to evaluate the degree of an uncircumcised boy's increased risk of UTI and the protective duration of circumcision.[52] Surgery is usually the last option for management.

Some criteria used by urologists to determine whether surgical intervention to correct VUR is needed are as follows: persistent moderate-to-severe (III–V) VUR, recurrent UTIs while on continuous antibiotic prophylaxis, noncompliance with taking prophylactic antibiotics, or worsening renal function. Surgical options include endoscopic injection of a bulking agent into the suburothelial layer of the UVJ. This works best for low-grade VUR, with about a 70% success rate and a higher rate if a second injection is performed.[54,55] Open or laparoscopic ureteroneocystostomy (ureteral reimplant) can be done with over a 90% success rate for resolution of the VUR. In the case of secondary VUR, the primary pathology has to be addressed first. Correction of the primary insult may indeed lead to complete resolution of the reflux without need for further surgery. Once resolution of the VUR is documented, no further antibiotic prophylaxis, urological imaging, or clinical follow-up is needed unless clinically indicated.

URETEROCELES AND ECTOPIC URETER

Ureteroceles are structural cystic dilation of the distal end of the ureter. They have the appearance of a diverticulum bulging into the bladder, typically causing obstruction of the upper urinary tract. The incidence is as high as 1 in 500 births, with a preponderance for females (6:1). Ureteroceles occur more commonly in Caucasians. Up to 10% of the time, they can occur bilaterally.[56,57] Ureteroceles can be detected on prenatal ultrasound and are responsible for up to 2% of prenatal hydronephrosis.[58] They can be intravesicular or combined with an ectopic ureter insertion and extending beyond the bladder neck into the urethra. Ectopic ureteroceles can lead to urethral obstruction and sometimes present as a bulging urethral mass in girls. Occasionally, in girls only, ectopic ureters can present with urinary incontinence in childhood due to insertion of the distal end of the ureter to the sphincter. Of the ureteroceles, 80% are associated with the upper pole of a duplicated renal collecting system, of which 60% are ectopic.[58]

Postnatally, ureteroceles can be picked up on screening or diagnostic renal-bladder ultrasound for workup of hydronephrosis or UTI. After ultrasound diagnosis, a VCUG can be used to assess the presence of vesicoureteral reflux, which can extend into the ipsilateral lower pole in 50% of patients and into the contralateral side in 25% of patients.[58–60] Sometimes, ureteroceles missed on ultrasounds can be detected in the early bladder-filling phase of a VCUG study. In addition, MAG-3 renal scan can be obtained to determine renal function and rule out obstruction.[58,59] This may help guide the urologist on the best surgical intervention to perform.

Obstructive ureteroceles can be managed endoscopically by puncture with a cold knife, electrocautery, or laser. If endoscopic puncture fails or the child continues to have recurrent infections, definitive surgical treatment with ureteral reimplantation with or without partial nephrectomy or complete nephrectomy may be necessary. Endoscopic management of extravesical ureteroceles is challenging, but effective, in alleviating the initial obstruction, but often open surgical excision and ureteral reimplantation are required after the age of 1 year. For those children with no evidence of upper tract or bladder neck obstruction and no VUR, observation only can be done.[61,62] Prior to surgical intervention, these children are placed on continuous antibiotic prophylaxis to prevent UTIs.

URETEROVESICAL JUNCTION OBSTRUCTION

The main diagnostic finding in UVJ obstruction is hydroureter and hydronephrosis. This can usually be seen on prenatal ultrasound. There is dilation of the upper tract collecting system down to the insertion of the ureter into the bladder. Some congenital etiologies include ectopic ureter insertion or stenosis with normal insertion.[62] UVJ obstruction can also be due to urolithiasis, benign fibroepithelial polyps, or even scar tissue formed following UTIs. Definitive surgical management is usually required with open ureteral reimplantation. In neonates with renal compromise, temporal distal cutaneous ureterostomy (bringing the ureter to the skin surface to drain) can be performed before the final reimplant is done when the child is older (usually before toilet training).

POSTERIOR URETHRAL VALVES

Although a rare phenomenon, PUVs are the most common lower urinary tract obstruction seen in the male fetus and infant. It affects 1 in 4000–7500 infants and tends to be more disproportionately seen in children with Down syndrome and children of African descent. PUVs lead to end-stage renal disease in 30% of these patients and are responsible for 17% of all renal transplantations in children.[63,64] Although first described in 1802 by Langenbeck, it was not until 1919 that Hugh Young gave a detailed description and classification of the types of urethral valves.[65]

Young described 3 types of PUVs. Type I represents about 95% of PUVs; these PUVs are sail-like folds extending distally from the verumontanum into the urethra. Type II are hypertrophied urethral folds that are not usually clinically significant, and type III appear to be cannulated septa. The exact embryology of PUVs is still unclear but is usually present by the 14th week of gestation, at which time the fetal male urethra is developed. Recent descriptions believe that type I and II valves may actually be the same entity.[63] Cobb's collar has been used to describe a distinct urethral valve obstruction that occurs distal to the external urethral sphincter.[66]

Posterior urethral valves are now mostly detected through prenatal ultrasound, accounting for up to 10% of prenatal hydronephrosis. Up to 50% are diagnosed neonatally and up to 70% by the first year of life. In addition to ultrasound diagnosis, VCUG is the gold standard for diagnosing PUVs, as the filling linear defect in the posterior urethra can be seen in the voiding phase of the study. Postnatally, they may present with weak urinary stream, UTIs, or failure to thrive

and, in older boys, postvoid dribbling, urinary retention, diurnal enuresis, and even hematuria.

Posterior urethral valves result in high voiding pressures, which lead to varying degrees of lower and upper urinary tract destruction. The verumontanum becomes distorted, the ejaculatory ducts are dilated from reflux of urine, and the prostatic urethra can be severely distended to the point that its storage capacity can even exceed that of the bladder. The bladder neck is elevated, hypertrophied and rigid due to the distal obstruction. In many cases, after the obstruction is relieved, there is improved function of the bladder neck. The bladder itself is thickened and hypercontractile, and the high pressure generated can be transmitted upstream to the ureters through the UVJ, which in most cases loses its antireflux mechanism. The ureter walls become thickened as well and the lumen severely dilated, which affects the antegrade propulsion of urine from the kidneys to the bladder. Hydroureteronephrosis results and is a hallmark of PUVs.[67] Owing to either the obstruction or increased pressure, renal dysplasia can result due to maldevelopment of the renal parenchyma and cellular maturation, as well as obstructive uropathy leading to tubular and glomerular injury of the filtration system. Although dysplasia is an irreversible injury, the obstructive uropathy effect on renal filtration may be reversible if the obstructing insult is relieved in a timely manner. Renal tubular damage can lead to nephrogenic diabetes insipidus with inability to concentrate or acidify urine, and the high urine output can contribute to persistent dilation in the renal collecting system, as evidenced by persistent hydroureteronephrosis. As the child ages, the renal and bladder function can continue to deteriorate, ultimately leading to end-stage renal disease in 30% of these infants and to neurogenic bladders.[63,68,69]

Although the fate of the renal function is usually set at birth, prior to intervention, some features are considered prognostic factors to overall renal health and subsequent failure. Some of these are echogenic kidneys, multicystic kidney, diagnosis before the age of 1, creatinine staying above 1 at age 1, low glomerular filtration rate, elevated serum urea nitrogen (BUN), late diagnosis, proteinuria, distal renal tubular acidosis, or continued diurnal incontinence at age 5 years.[63,70,71] Craig Peters and colleagues also described the "valve bladder syndrome," which is a sequela of antenatal damage to the bladder and chronic distension, which can still progress postnatally from being hyperreflexic, which may be managed with anticholinergic therapy, to a small noncompliant bladder, which may require occasional catheterization or even bladder augmentation, and subsequently myogenic failure of the bladder. This may require a lifetime need for clean intermittent catheterizations.[72] Due to resulting bladder dysfunction and poor sphincter competence, up to 70% of these children, even at advanced ages, suffer from urinary incontinence.[63]

Postnatally, the first intervention is usually to relieve the obstruction with a catheter placed into the bladder. Once the infant or child has been stabilized, endoscopic valve ablation is then performed. If renal function improves after this, this may be all that is needed; however, if renal function remains unchanged and hydronephrosis persists, creation of a vesicostomy or placement of diverting nephrostomy tubes may be necessary to promote low-pressure drainage. If renal function still does not improve, then it means that the renal dysplasia is severe enough that there is not much renal functional reserve left.[63] In utero, if severe oligohydramnios develops, then consideration of early delivery of the fetus to allow for the appropriate interventions to drain the obstructed system may be necessary. Unfortunately, this is often complicated by poor lung development, and in severe cases, pulmonary hypoplasia results.[73] Although still under investigation, some physicians have advocated some highly complicated intrauterine interventions, like percutaneous fetal cystoscopy with valve ablation, vesicoamniotic shunting, and even open fetal surgery. The benefits of these are still not clear. While preliminary results from the PLUTO (Percutaneous Shunting in Lower Urinary Tract Obstruction) trial showed an improvement in perinatal survival in fetuses that underwent vesicoamniotic shunting, the final results are yet to be published.[63,74]

ANTERIOR URETHRAL VALVES

Anterior urethral valves are even rarer than PUVs, and unlike PUVs, the obstruction is due to more of a diverticulum causing extrinsic compression rather than the typical valve leaflets seen in PUVs.[75] These are typically seen in boys, and presentation is often past the neonatal period, with symptoms such as straining to void, incontinence, or UTIs. About a third present with antenatal hydronephrosis, a third voiding symptoms, and a third with a visible diverticulum on examination.[76] The diverticulum can be more evident during voiding as it expands with urine from the pooling of urine. There can also be varying degrees of obstructive uropathy, from mild to severe, even leading to spontaneous rupture of the fetal bladder.[77] Postnatally, due to the ballooning of the urethra, the diagnosis can be suspected on physical examination; however, the gold standard of diagnosis is by VCUG or via cystoscopy. A catheter can be passed to temporarily relieve the obstruction as in PUVs, but this can be difficult. In neonates or infants with severe uropathy, a temporary vesicostomy can be created as well until definitive surgical repair is done.[78] Anterior urethral valves can be corrected surgically through open excision of the

diverticulum or endoscopically through transurethral excision.[65,79] In general, the long-term nephropathy seen is not as severe as that seen in cases of PUVs, with less than 5% of children developing end-stage renal disease as compared to 30% of those with PUVs.[80,81]

URETHRAL ATRESIA

Urethral atresia is the most severe form of neonatal obstructive uropathy. It is an extremely rare condition, and in most cases, it is not compatible with extrauterine life. Usually, those affected are stillborn or succumb to respiratory failure from severe pulmonary hypoplasia. Fetal ultrasound findings of a distended bladder, bilateral hydroureteronephrosis, and oligohydramnios are characteristic. The infants most likely to survive are the ones who have a patent urachus, creating a pop-off valve for drainage of urine into the amniotic sac. In this case, oligohydramnios is usually not likely.

There have been a few case reports of boys who survived urethral atresia. One study reported the outcome in 6 boys born with urethral atresia. Three had vesicoamniotic shunts placed at 17 and 30 weeks (2 boys) of gestation, and the remaining 3 were born with a patent urachus or a vesicocutaneous fistula. All of them had high-grade VUR, and 5 had diagnosis of PBS. Five had renal failure before the age of 10 years, and 67% eventually required some form of supravesical urinary diversion.[82]

URETHRAL HYPOPLASIA

Urethral hypoplasia is also rare but is less severe than urethral atresia. The lumen is extremely small, making passage of a small urethral catheter nearly impossible. Cutaneous vesicostomy in the neonatal period is usually required to decompress the bladder. The effect on the upper urinary tract can be variable, with the most severe cases ending up with end-stage renal disease. Surgical interventions can vary from gradual urethral dilation, to urethral reconstruction, and even to continent urinary diversion.

URETHRAL DIVERTICULUM

In the neonatal period, urethral diverticulum uropathy is more common in males. It is an outpouching of the urethra due to distension of a segment of the urethra and attachment of a narrow neck structure to the urethra like a müllerian remnant. It can also occur from incomplete circumferential development of the ventral urethra, with the sheer voiding force leading to further distension of that segment of the urethra. The distal lip of the defect may become an obstructive valve, which further contributes to the enlargement of the diverticulum.[83] Although a urethral diverticulum can be detected by VCUG, it is more likely to be detected via cystourethroscopy or retrograde urethrogram. Unless it is large or symptomatic, it does not have to be treated.

PRUNE-BELLY SYNDROME

Prune-belly syndrome, also known as Eagle-Barrett syndrome, is a rare congenital disorder characterized by the triad of abdominal muscle deficiency, severe urinary tract abnormalities, and bilateral cryptorchidism. It is more common in males but can occur in females. Females are referred to as having pseudo-PBS as they lack the third triad of bilateral cryptorchidism in the original description of the syndrome. Although the pathophysiology of the disease is not known, it is believed to be either from an early urethral obstruction by the eighth week of gestation with subsequent recanalization or primarily from a mesenchymal developmental defect.[84] By 30 weeks of gestation, bladder distention, hydroureters, and irregular abdominal circumference dilation can be seen.[62] Prenatally, it can be difficult to tell on ultrasound whether the findings seen are due to the result of the presence of PUVs or severe VUR. It is usually confirmed at birth based on the clinical triad mentioned. Overall prognosis depends on the degree of renal damage that results from the obstruction. In severe cases of renal dysplasia, pulmonary hypoplasia can result and lead to acute respiratory distress and perinatal mortality. At birth, it is important to check serial metabolic panels, including serum creatinine. A creatinine nadir greater than 0.7 mg/dL is a prognostic sign of poor renal function continued deterioration that may ultimately require renal transplantation.[62,85]

In addition to renal-bladder ultrasound, a VCUG should be done postnatally to help assess the degree of dilation within the urinary tract.

Surgical treatment of the dilated urinary tract remains controversial. Excellent outcomes from appropriate surgical intervention, including temporary procedures to decompress the dilated system, such as urethrotomy, bilateral open nephrostomies, or early supravesical diversion by pyelostomy or cutaneous vesicostomy. Finally, a single-stage reconstruction consisting of bilateral tapered ureteroneocystostomy, reduction cystoplasty, bilateral orchiopexy, and abdominoplasty can be considered.[86]

REFERENCES

1. Seikaly MG, Ho PL, Emmett L, Fine RN, Tejani A. Chronic renal insufficiency in children: the 2001 Annual Report of the NAPRTCS. *Pediatr Nephrol.* 2003;18(8):796–804.

2. Benfield MR, McDonald RA, Bartosh S, Ho PL, Harmon W. Changing trends in pediatric transplantation: 2001 annual report of the North American Pediatric Renal Transplant Cooperative Study. *Pediatr Transplant.* 2003;7:321–335.

3. Lee RS, Cendron M, Kinnamon DD, Nguyen HT. Antenatal hydronephrosis as a predictor of postnatal outcome: a meta-analysis. *Pediatrics.* 2006;118(2):586–593.

4. Chang CP, McDill BW, Neilson JR, et al. Calcineurin is required in urinary tract mesenchyme for the development of the polyureteral peristaltic machinery. *J Clin Invest.* 2004;113:1051–1058.

5. Chevalier RL, Thornhill BA, Forbes MS, Kiley SC. Mechanisms of renal injury and progression of renal disease in congenital obstructive nephropathy. *Pediatr Nephrol.* 2010;25:687–697.

6. Morin L, Cendron M, Crombleholme TM, Garmel SH, Klauber GT, D'Alton ME. Minimal hydronephrosis in the fetus:clinical significance and implications for management. *J Urol.* 1996;155(6) 2047–2049.

7. Koff SA, Mutabagani KH. Anomalies of the kidney. In: Gillenwater JY, Grayhack JT, Howards SS, Mitchell ME, eds. *Adult and Pediatric Urology.* 4th ed. Philadelphia, PA: Lippincott Williams and Wilkins; 2002:2129.

8. Mendelsohn C. Functional obstruction: the renal pelvis rules. *J Clin Invest.* 2004;113:957–959.

9. Peters CA. Animal models of fetal renal disease. *Prenat Diagn.* 2001;21:917–923.

10. Thornbill BA, Burt LE, Chen C, Forbes MS, Chevalier RL. Variable chronic partial ureteral obstruction in the neonatal rat: a new model of ureteropelvic junction obstruction. *Kidney Int.* 2005;67:42–52.

11. Miyazaki Y, Tsuchida S, Nishimura H, et al. Angiotensin Induces the urinary peristaltic machinery during the perinatal perios. *J Clin Invest.* 1998;102:1489–1487.

12. Zhang PL, Peters CA, Rosen S. Ureteropelvic junction obstruction: morphological and clinical studies. *Pediatr Nephrol.* 2000;14:820–826.

13. Yiee JH, Johnson-Welch S, Baker LS, Wilcox DT. Histologic differences between extrinsic and intrinsic ureteropelvic junction obstruction. *Urology.* 2010;76:181–184.

14. Cachat F, Lange-Sperandio B, Chang AY, et al. Ureteral obstruction in neonatal mice elicits segment-specific tubular cell responses leading to nephron loss. *Kidney Int.* 2003;63:564–575.

15. Eskild-Jensen A, Thomsen K, Rungo C, et al. Glomerular and tubular function during AT1 receptor blockade in pigs with neonatal induced partial ureteropelvic junction obstruction. *Am J Physiol Renal Physiol.* 2007;292:F921–F929.

16. Chevalier RL. Chronic partial ureteral obstruction and the developing kidney. *Pediatr Radiol.* 2008;38(Suppl 1):S35–S40.

17. Norwood VF, Carey RM, Geary KM, Jose PA, Gomez RA, Chevalier RL. Neonatal ureteral obstruction stimulates recruitment of renin-secreting renal cortical cells. *Kidney Int.* 1994;45:1333–1339.

18. Chevalier RL, Chung KH, Smith CD, Ficenec M, Gomez RA. Renal apoptosis and clusterin following ureteral obstruction: the role of maturation. *J Urol.* 1996;156:1474–1479.

19. Chevalier RL, Thornhill BA, Wolstenholme JT, Kim A. Unilateral ureteral obstruction in early development alters renal growth: dependence on the duration of obstruction. *J Urol.* 1999;161:309–313.

20. Fern RJ, Yesko CM, Thornhill BA, Kim HS, Smithies O, Chevalier RL. Reduced angiotensinogen expression attenuates renal interstitial fibrosis in obstructive nephropathy in mice. *J Clin Invest.* 1999;103:39–46.

21. Malik RK, Thornhill BA, Chang AY, Kiley SC, Chevalier RL. Renal apoptosis parallels ceramide content after prolonged ureteral obstruction in the neonatal rat. *Am J Physiol Renal Physiol.* 2001;281:F56–F61.

22. Shi Y, Li C, Thomsen K., et al. Neonatal ureteral obstruction alters expression of renal sodium transporters and aquaporin water channels. *Kidney Int.* 2004;66:203–215.

23. Topcu SO, Pedersen M, Norregaard R, et al. Candesartan prevents long-term impairment of renal function in response to neonatal partial unilateral ureteral obstruction. *Am J Physiol Renal Physiol.* 2007;292:F736–F748.

24. Yoo KH, Thornhill BA, Forbes MS, Chevalier RL. Compensatory renal growth due to neonatal ureteral obstruction:implications for clinical studies. *Pediatr Nephrol.* 2006;21:368–375.

25. Peters CA. Obstruction of the fetal urinary tract. *J Am Soc Nephrol.* 1997;8:653–663.

26. Muire PY, Gelas T, Dijoud F, et al. Complete unilateral ureteral obstruction in the fetal lamb. Part II: long-term outcomes of renal tissue development. *J Urol.* 2006;175:1548–1558.

27. Kaefer M, Peters CA, Retik AB, et al. Increased renal echogenicity:a sonographic sign for differentiating between obstructive and nonobstructive etiologies of in utero bladder distention. *J Urol.* 1997;158:1026–1029.

28. Grignon A, Filion R, Filiatrault D, et al. Urinary tract dilatation in utero: classification and clinical application. *Radiology.* 1986;160:645–647.

29. Peters CA, Chevalier RL. Congenital urinary obstruction: pathophysiology and clinical evaluation. In: Wein AJ, Kavoussi LR, Partin A, Novick AC, Peters CA (eds). *Campbell-Walsh Urology.* 10th ed. Philadelphia, PA: Saunders Elsevier; 2011:3028–3046e.

30. Skoog SJ, Peters CA, Arant BS Jr, et al. Pediatric Vesicoureteral Reflux Guidelines Panel summary report: clinical practice guidelines for screening siblings of children with vesicoureteral reflux and neonates/infants with prenatal hydronephrosis. *J Urol.* 2010;184(3):1145–1151.

31. Canning DA, Lambert SM. Evaluation of the pediatric urology patient. In: Wein AJ, Kavoussi LR, Partin A, Novick AC, Peters CA (eds). *Campbell-Walsh Urology.* 10th ed. Philadelphia, PA: Saunders Elsevier; 2011:3067–3084e3.

32. Grattan-Smith JD, Little SB, Jones RA. MR urography evaluation of obstructive uropathy. *Pediatr Radiol.* 2008;38(Suppl 1):S49–S69.

33. Chevalier RL. Biomarkers of congenital obstructive nephropathy: past, present and future. *J Urol.* 2004;172(3):852–857.

34. Peters CA. Urinary obstruction in children. *J Urol.* 1995;154: 1874–1884.

35. Csaicsich D, Greenbaum LA, Aufricht C. Upper urinary tract: when is obstruction obstruction? *Curr Opin Urol.* 2004;14:213–217.

36. Eskild-Jensen A, Gordon I, Piepsz A, et al. Congenital unilateral hydronephrosis: a review of the impact of diuretic renography on clinical treatment. *J Urol.* 2005;173:1471–1476.

37. Koff SA, Campbell KD. The nonoperative management of unilateral neonatal hydronephrosis: natural history of poorly functioning kidneys. *J Urol.* 1994;152:593–595.

38. Chertin B, Pollack A, Koulikov D, et al. Conservative treatment of ureteropelvic junction obstruction in children with antenatal diagnosis of hydronephrosis: lessons learned after 16 years of follow-up. *Eur Urol.* 2006;49:734–739.

39. Ulman I, Jayanthi VR, Koff SA. The long-term followup of newborns with severe unilateral hydronephrosis initially treated nonoperatively. *J Urol.* 2000;164:1101–1105.

40. Klein J, Gonzalez J, Miravete M, et al. Congenital ureteropelvic junction obstruction: human disease and animal models. *Int J Exp Pathol.* 2011;92(3):168–192.

41. Braga LH, Lorenzo AJ, Bägli DJ, et al. Risk factors for recurrent ureteropelvic junction obstruction after open pyeloplasty in a large pediatric cohort. *J Urol.* 2008;180:1684–1687.

42. Chertin B, Pollack A, Koulikov D, et al. Does renal function remain stable after puberty in children with prenatal hydronephrosis and improved renal function after pyeloplasty? *J Urol.* 2009;182:1845.

43. Considine J: Retrocaval ureter. A review of the literature with a report on two new cases followed for 15 years and two years respectively. *Br J Urol.* 1966;38:412–423.

44. Yen T, Yeh S. Retrocaval ureter in newborn demonstrated by Tc-99m DTPA renal scintigram. *Clin Nucl Med.* 1993;18(11):941–1016.

45. Chung B, Gill I. Laparoscopic dismembered pyeloplasty of a retrocaval ureter: case report and review of the literature. *Eur Urol.* 2008;54(6):1433–1436.

46. Dillon MJ, Goonasekera CD. Reflux nephropathy. *J Am Soc Nephrol.* 1998;9(12):2377–2383.

47. Shah KJ, Robins DG, White RH. Renal scarring and vesicoureteric reflux. *Arch Dis Child.* 1978;5(3):210–217.

48. Smellie JM, Normand IC, Katz G. Children with urinary infection: a comparison of those with and those without vesicoureteric reflux. *Kidney Int.* 1981;20(6):717.

49. Chand DH, Rhoades T, Poe SA, et al. Incidence and severity of vesicoureteral reflux in children related to age, gender, race and diagnosis. *J Urol.* 2003;170(4):1548.

50. Kaefer M, Curran M, Treves ST, et al. Sibling vesicoureteral reflux in multiple gestation births. *Pediatrics.* 2000;105(4):800.

51. International Reflux Study Committee. Medical versus surgical treatment of primary vesicoureteral reflux: a prospective international reflux study in children. *J Urol.* 1981;125:277–283

52. Peters CA, Skoog SJ, Arant BS, et al. Summary of the AUA guideline on management of primary vesicoureteral reflux in children. *J Urol.* 2010;184:1134–1144.

53. Estrada CR Jr, Passerotti CC, Graham DA, et al. Nomograms for predicting annual resolution rate of primary vesicoureteral reflux: results from 2462 children. *J Urol.* 2009;182(4):1535–1541.

54. Läckgren G, Wählin N, Sköldenberg E, et al. Long-term follow-up of children treated with dextranomer/hyaluronic acid copolymer for vesicoureteral reflux. *J Urol.* 2001;166:1887–1892.

55. Kirsch AJ, Perez-Brayfield MR, Scherz HC. Minimally invasive treatment of vesicoureteral reflux with endoscopic injection of dextranomer/hyaluronic acid copolymer: the Children's Hospitals of Atlanta experience. *J Urol.* 2003;170:211–215.

56. Uson AC, Lattimer JK, Melicow MM. Ureteroceles in infants and children:a report based on 44 cases. *Pediatrics.* 1961;27:971–983.

57. Shokeir AA, Nijman RJ. Ureterocele:an ongoing challenge in infancy and childhood. *BJU Int.* 2002;90(8):777–783.

58. Coplen DE, Duckett JW. The modern approach to ureteroceles. *J Urol.* 1995;153(1):166–171.

59. Geringer AM, Berdon WE, Seldin DW, Hensle TW. The diagnostic approach to ectopic ureterocele and the renal duplication complex. *J Urol.* 1983;129(3):539–542.

60. Jesus LE, Farhat WA, Amarante AC, et al. Clinical evolution of vesicoureteral reflux following endoscopic puncture in children with duplex system ureteroceles. *J Urol.* 2011;186(4):1455–1458.

61. Hagg MJ, Mourachov PV, Snyder HM, et al. The modern endoscopic approach to ureterocele. *J Urol.* 2000;163(3):940–943.

62. Hubert KC, Palmer JS. Current diagnosis and management of fetal genitourinary abnormalities. *Urol Clin North Am.* 2007;34(1):89–101.

63. Hodges SJ, Patel B, McLorie G, Atala A. Posterior urethral valves. *SciWorld J.* 2009;9:1119–1126.

64. Seikaly M, Ho PL, Emmett L and Tejani A. The 12th Annual Report of the North American Pediatric Renal Transplant Cooperative Study:renal transplantation from 1987 through 1998. *Pediatr Transplant.* 2001;5:215–31.

65. Casale AJ. Posterior urethral valves. In: Wein AJ, Kavoussi LR, Partin A, Novick AC, Peters CA (eds). *Campbell-Walsh Urology.* 10th ed. Philadelphia, PA: Saunders Elsevier; 2011:3389–3410.e4.

66. Krishnan A, De Souza AM, Konijeti R, Baskin KS. The anatomy and embryology of posterior urethral valves. *J Urol.* 2006;175:1214–1220.

CHAPTER 44

67. Gearhart JP, Lee BR, Partin AW, et al. A quantitative histological evaluation of the dilated ureter of childhood: II. Ectopia, posterior urethral valves, and the prune belly syndrome. *J Urol.* 1995;153:172–176.

68. Parkhouse HF, Woodhouse CR. Long-term status of patients with posterior urethral valves. *Urol Clin North Am.* 1990;17:373–378.

69. Dinneen MD, Duffy PG, Barratt TM, Ransley PG. Persistent polyuria after posterior urethral valves. *Br J Urol.* 1995;75(2):236–240.

70. DeFoor W, Clark C, Jackson E, Reddy P, Minevich E, Shelton C. Risk factors for end stage renal disease in children with posterior urethral valves. *J Urol.* 2008;180:1705–1708.

71. Sarhan OM, El-Ghoneimi AA, Helmy TE, Dawaba MS, Ghali AM, Ibrahiem EI. Posterior urethral valves: multivariate analysis of factors affecting the final renal outcome. *J Urol.* 2011;185:2491–2496.

72. Peters CA, Bolkier M, Bauer SB, et al. The urodynamic consequences of posterior urethral valves. *J Urol.* 1990;144:122–126.

73. Lopez P, Martinez Urrutia MJ, Jaureguizar E. Initial and long-term management of posterior urethral valves. *World J Urol.* 2004;22:418–424.

74. Morris R, Kilby M. The PLUTO trial: percutaneous shunting in lower urinary tract obstruction [abstract]. *AJOG.* January 2012;(Suppl):S14.

75. Tank ES. Anterior urethral valves resulting from congenital urethral diverticula. *Urology.* 1987;30:467.

76. Van Savage JG, Khoury AE, McLorie GA. An algorithm for the management of anterior urethral valves. *J Urol.* 1997;158:1030.

77. Merrot T, Chaumoitre K, Shojai R, et al. Fetal bladder rupture due to anterior urethral valves. *Urology.* 2003;61:1259.

78. Rushton HG, Parrott TS, Woodard JR, Walther M. The role of vesicostomy in the management of anterior urethral valves in neonates and infants. *J Urol.* 1987;138:107.

79. Elder JS. Obstruction of the urinary tract. In: Kliegman RM, Stanton BF, St. Geme III JW, Schor NF, Behrman RE (eds). *Kliegman: Nelson Textbook of Pediatrics.* 19th ed. Philadelphia, PA: Saunders; 2011:1838–1847e1.

80. Rawat J, Khan TR, Singh S, et al. Congenital anterior urethral valves and diverticula:diagnosis and management in six cases. *Afr J Paediatr Surg.* 2009;6(2):102–105.

81. Kaplan GW, Scherz HC: Infravesical obstruction. In: Kelalis PP, King LR, Belman AB, eds. *Clinical Pediatric Urology.* 3rd ed. Philadelphia, PA: Saunders; 1992:821–864.

82. González R, De Filippo R, Jednak R, Barthold JS. Urethral atresia: long-term outcome in 6 children who survived the neonatal perios. *J Urol.* 2001;165(6):2241–2244.

83. Jordan GH, McCammon KA. Surgery of the penis and urethra. In: Wein AJ, Kavoussi LR, Partin A, Novick AC, Peters CA (eds). *Campbell-Walsh Urology.* 10th ed. Philadelphia, PA: Saunders Elsevier; 2011:956–1000.e5.

84. Stephens FD, Gupta D. Pathogenesis of the prune belly syndrome. *J Urol.* 1994;152(6):2328–2331.

85. Strand WR. Initial management of complex pediatric disorders: prune belly syndrome, posterior urethral valves. *Urol Clin North Am.* 2004;31:399–415.

86. Denes FT, Arap MA, Giron AM, et al. Comprehensive surgical treatment of prune belly syndrome: 17 years' experience with 32 patients. *Urology.* 2004;64:789–793.

CHAPTER 44

Part G: Endocrine

Hypoglycemia in the Newborn

Mark A. Sperling and Ram Menon

INTRODUCTION

This chapter outlines the epidemiology, etiology, pathophysiology, differential diagnosis, and management approach to the neonate with hypoglycemia, here defined as 40 mg/dL or less (≤2.2 mmol, the fifth percentile for age) during the first 2 days of life and 50 mg/dL or less (≤2.8 mmol) of whole blood glucose thereafter, with or without suggestive symptoms. Note that plasma glucose concentration is about 10%–15% greater than whole blood glucose concentration, so criteria for hypoglycemia based on plasma glucose measurements must be appropriately adjusted to be greater. Recent advances in our understanding of the biochemistry, physiology, and molecular biology regulating prenatal and postnatal glucose homeostasis combine to provide a rational basis for defining, identifying, diagnosing, and treating hypoglycemia in the newborn to enable normal neurodevelopment.[1,2] These considerations provide a systematic approach to the problem of neonatal hypoglycemia and argue for glucose measurements to become part of routine care in all neonates prior to discharge from the newborn nursery and in all sick neonates even after discharge from the newborn nursery.

EPIDEMIOLOGY

Hypoglycemia is a relatively common and highly important problem in the newborn.[3–5] Precise data on incidence are unavailable and depend in part on the definition of hypoglycemia, an area of ongoing discussion, as well as the degree of gestational maturity and condition of the newborn.[1–3] Based on a meta-analysis,[5] it has been proposed that, in full-term normal newborns, blood glucose of 40 mg/dL or less in the first 48 hours and 48 mg/dL or less between 48 and 72 hours represents less than the fifth percentile for age. A minor modification to these data permits defining hypoglycemia as 40 mg/dL or less in the first 2 days of life and 50 mg/dL or less thereafter. By the fourth day of life, normal infants usually maintain average blood glucose values greater than 60 mg/dL, approaching values of healthy children and adults. Using these criteria, the reported incidence of hypoglycemia in the first days of life varies from approximately 70% in infants who are small for gestational age (SGA),[6] 20%–50% in those large for gestational age (LGA) but otherwise-normal newborn infants born to nondiabetic mothers, and greater than 50% in those born to infants of diabetic mothers[7]; only about 2% of term infants born to nondiabetic mothers after normal pregnancy develop hypoglycemia.[8]

The importance of neonatal hypoglycemia lies in its association with potential impairment of neurocognitive development[6] because glucose is the preferential energy substrate of the newborn's brain, which normally utilizes greater than 90% of normal basal glucose turnover and has been shown to be about 4–8 mg/kg/min.[9] Although the brain of a neonate can use other energy substrates, such as lactate and β-hydroxybutyrate, in hypoglycemia secondary to hyperinsulinism (HI), the production of glucose (by glycogenolysis or gluconeogenesis) is suppressed, as is lipolysis and ketogenesis, while glucose utilization and storage are increased. Hence, in HI, the brain is effectively deprived of all sources of nutrients. The consequences of such hyperinsulinemic hypoglycemia, the most common form of persistent hypoglycemia of the newborn, include high rates of seizures, mental retardation, neuromuscular spasticity, and other disturbances in psychomotor development.[10-12]

In SGA and preterm infants, hypoglycemia that is recurrent or repetitive is a more predictable factor for long-term neurodevelopmental deficits than the severity of a single hypoglycemia episode.[6] Thus, the degree and duration of hypoglycemia, as well as associated conditions such as hypoxia and seizures, add to the risk of neural and intellectual impairment. Moreover, the younger the infant, the earlier and more persistent the hypoglycemia, and the greater the difficulty to control seizures by medical means alone, the more likely it is that long-term neural and intellectual development will be adversely affected.[10-12] There is some evidence that the neonatal brain may be more resistant than the adult brain to hypoglycemia, especially because of its ability to better use lactate and β-hydroxybutyrate as alternate fuels.[13] Precisely for these reasons, HI is the most concerning of the syndromes of hypoglycemia of the newborn because generation of alternate fuels also is diminished or abolished by the HI.

Based on these findings, we suggest that an operational threshold of whole blood glucose of 50 mg/dL or less should be viewed with concern for monitoring and intervention. In making this recommendation, we recognize that we are "raising the bar" from previous standards. However, it is now established that persistent hypoglycemia is harmful, even if a precise glucose concentration below which harm ensues cannot be individually determined.[10-12] Hence, we urge earlier investigation and intervention as a precautionary measure. When symptoms of hypoglycemia, especially seizures, accompany the low glucose measurements, adverse neurodevelopmental outcomes should be anticipated.

PATHOPHYSIOLOGY

Hypoglycemia

Neonatal hypoglycemia has its origins in utero and in the dramatic transition to independent existence following separation from the placenta. In utero, the fetus receives all of its nutrients from the mother via the umbilical vein, and gluconeogenesis is absent or minimal until birth.[1,2] During the third trimester, weight doubles from approximately 1700 g at 32 weeks' gestation to approximately 3500 g at term, representing in large part accretion and deposition of glycogen, fat, and muscle tissue. The degree of fetal insulin secretion,

though modest, is sufficient to stimulate cognate insulin receptors and permit partitioning of nutrients for immediate energy use and for tissue growth. Excessive nutrient transfer, as occurs to a variable degree in all diabetic pregnancies, promotes secretion of insulin, a growth-promoting hormone, which leads to macrosomia in utero.[14,15] Transient neonatal hypoglycemia, lasting 1-3 days, occurs after umbilical cord cutting, when glucose supply is interrupted, whereas excessive insulin continues for some time. Similar considerations determine macrosomia resulting from genetic defects causing HI in utero, but in these cases, postnatal hypoglycemia persists.[16,17] The severity of the hypoglycemia depends on the degree of HI and the duration between feedings, that is, "fasting."

The term *hyperinsulinism* denotes excessive insulin action relative to the prevailing blood glucose concentration. This is reflected in the metabolic profile of HI-associated hypoglycemia caused by suppressed glucose production concurrent with increased glucose utilization, exceeding the usual range of 4–8 mg/kg/min,[9] suppressed lipolysis leading to low circulating free fatty acids (FFAs), and suppressed ketogenesis leading to low circulating concentrations of β-hydroxybutyrate. The degree of HI may not be reflected in the circulating concentration of insulin, in part because insulin is secreted into the portal vein, and hepatic extraction may exceed the theoretical 50% reported in normal adults, and in part because activating mutations in elements of the insulin-signaling pathway will produce an identical clinical and biochemical phenotype (macrosomia, hypoglycemia, low FFA, low β-hydroxybutyrate) but with insulin levels that are low (<2 mIU/mL) or even below the limits of assay detection.[18] Thus, the key to differentiating and managing the causes of neonatal hypoglycemia is the metabolic profiles of glucose, FFAs, and β-hydroxybutyrate, which are more readily available in most laboratories than accurate ultra-sensitive assays for measurement of hormones such as insulin, cortisol, and growth hormone (GH).

Umbilical cord cutting at birth triggers a series of coordinated hormonal and enzymatic changes that mobilize the fuel stores deposited in utero to sustain energy needs until feeding is established.[19] Epinephrine and glucagon concentrations increase 3- to 5-fold within minutes and can act quickly via cyclic adenosine monophosphate (cAMP) to mobilize glucose by glycogenolysis. GH and cortisol concentrations in blood also are high in the initial hours after birth. Cortisol promotes gluconeogenesis, which takes several hours to be initiated and several days before it is fully established, whereas GH in concert with epinephrine acts to induce lipolysis with provision of fatty acids for oxidation, and the high concentrations of glucagon induce ketogenesis in mitochondria. A key enzyme for gluconeogenesis, phosphoenol pyruvate carboxykinase (PEPCK) is not expressed at birth and, under the influence of glucocorticoids, matures by about 24 hours.[19,20] Likewise, a key enzyme for ketogenesis, carnitine palmitoyl transferase 1 (CPT-1) is not expressed initially, and transcription is activated in part by long-chain fatty acids that are contained in colostrum, so that expression is evident by about 24 hours.[20,21]

Thus, immediately after birth, all infants initially must rely on glucose derived from glycogen and calories received from feedings of colostrum or milk. Moreover, whereas the four energy-mobilizing hormones are increased, insulin concentrations initially decline in the first few hours after delivery, and insulin secretion responds only sluggishly to glucose stimulation. As a result, the pattern in a normal full-term infant is for glucose to decrease to approximately 50 mg/dL in the first few hours after delivery and to return to average concentrations of 60 mg/dL or higher by day 2 and certainly by day 3 of life.[5] Thus, conditions that diminish nutrient reserves for mobilization, such as intrauterine growth retardation or premature birth, will impair the ability to maintain glucose concentration that is appropriate for a normal newborn and hence predispose to hypoglycemia.

It has long been known that, in the first 8 hours after birth, almost one-third of term infants who are adequate for gestational age (AGA) and almost one-half of preterm or immature infants will have blood glucose concentrations less than 50 mg/dL.[22] These are the normal adaptations in the transition from intrauterine life and dependence on maternal glucose supply to extrauterine existence with integration of glucose homeostasis during feeding and fasting that may be associated with "transitional" forms of hypoglycemia during adaptation. However, by day 3 of life, virtually no term AGA infant and less than 1% of all those in other categories have a plasma glucose concentration below 50 mg/dL.[5,22]

Hypoglycemia, as we have defined it, represents a mismatch between the ability to provide glucose either entirely by endogenous production or supplemented by feeding and factors that enhance its utilization. Hence, the ability to maintain glucose concentration may be impaired if feeding is delayed; if enzymatic pathways are not established fully, as occurs in the premature infant; or if there is transient persistence of excessive insulin secretion, as occurs in infants born to mothers with diabetes during pregnancy.[23] Hypoglycemia will persist if there are defects in the ability to metabolize glycogen to glucose, to initiate gluconeogenesis, or to convert fatty acids to ketones as a source of energy. Higher-than-normal glucose utilization rates can be anticipated with conditions such as sepsis, fever, or seizures, all of which also prevent normal feeding, or if hypoxia or other intrauterine stress

has depleted glycogen stores. However, a glucose utilization rate in excess of 10 mg/kg/min, as reflected in the glucose infusion rate needed to maintain blood glucose above 60 mg/dL, almost invariably indicates a state of HI.[1,2,16–18] In an otherwise-healthy full-term AGA infant, delay in initiating feeding via breast or bottle does not in itself cause hypoglycemia, but it hastens the unmasking of an underlying defect, such as HI, deficiency of cortisol or GH, or even more rarely, severe defects in gluconeogenesis or fatty acid oxidation.[23–25] Less-severe disorders of glycogen breakdown and gluconeogenesis are not likely to manifest while the baby is being fed at 2- to 4-hour intervals, and with rare exceptions the same holds for disorders of fatty acid oxidation. These tend to be manifested later when the interval between feedings is lengthened (eg, at weaning), and the increased period of fasting unmasks an inborn error of metabolism. GH deficiency and cortisol deficiency, either as isolated defects or as part of hypopituitarism,[26] also may be masked by frequent feedings and unmasked by fasting.[24–26] The same holds true for transient or permanent HI, the most important and frequent cause of persistent hypoglycemia in a newborn child.[1,2] The more severe the defect, the sooner the clinical manifestations will appear in an otherwise-normal full-term newborn even with a normal feeding schedule.

In the absence of predisposing factors such as diabetes mellitus in the mother, premature birth, or intrauterine growth retardation, hypoglycemia in the first hours or days of life is almost always caused by deficiencies of GH or cortisol,[24,25] HI associated with perinatal asphyxia/hypoxia,[27,28] or HI due to genetic defects in the regulation of insulin secretion, manifesting as "fasting hypoglycemia" when the baby cannot feed or the interval between feedings is lengthened.[29–31]

Mechanisms of Central Nervous System Damage

Neuroglycopenia of short duration may be reversible. However, prolonged severe hypoglycemia, when glucose concentration is 1 mM (18 mg/dL) or less, results in neuronal death from cellular energy failure and the release of the excitatory amino acid aspartate into the extracellular space. Interaction of aspartate with its receptor on central nervous system (CNS) cells leads to membrane disruption, influx of calcium, activation of enzymes such as phospholipase, changes in cellular redox state, and cell death primarily affecting the posterior cerebral cortex but sparing the cerebellum and brainstem.[32] In addition, hypoglycemia is reported to activate A1 adenosine receptors, permitting influx of calcium and activation of the proapoptotic enzyme caspase-3; blockade of adenosine A1 receptors ameliorated neuronal damage in the mouse model used.[33,34] These findings suggest the possible future use of adenosine A1 receptor antagonists to mitigate neuronal damage in newborns with severe hypoglycemia.[33,34] They also may explain the patterns of injury in severe hypoglycemia reported in magnetic resonance imaging (MRI) studies.

Magnetic Resonance Imaging in Neonatal Hypoglycemia

Some investigators reported specific patterns of MRI changes in newborns with severe hypoglycemia that differed from findings reported in hypoxic-ischemic brain injury. Diffuse cortical and subcortical white matter damage affecting primarily the parietal and occipital lobes is typically seen with severe hypoglycemia of less than 20 mg/dL and may be associated with bilateral occipital lobe cortical atrophy, a possible distinguishing feature not seen in hypoxic-ischemic brain injury. These changes may later manifest as cortical blindness. In some reports, changes observed initially seemed to resolve over time.[35–38]

Diagnostic Approach

The symptoms and signs of hypoglycemia in a newborn are predominantly neurological, due to neuroglycopenia, as listed in Table 45-1. Most are nonspecific and could be caused by other conditions, such as sepsis in the newborn. Hence, eternal vigilance and consideration for the possibility of hypoglycemia as the cause of the symptom are keys to early diagnosis and favorable outcome. Therefore, we recommend that hypoglycemia be considered in any newborn with the symptoms listed. A blood glucose concentration of less than 40 mg/dL on days 1–2 of life, less than 50 mg/dL on day 3, and less than 60 mg/dL thereafter should be followed at a minimum by a formal blood glucose measurement in a laboratory together with the concentration of FFAs and β-hydroxybutyrate. If all 3 are suppressed, HI is the most likely diagnosis. If glucose is low but β-hydroxybutyrate and FFAs are normal or elevated, a defect in the ability to produce glucose is most likely. If the concentrations of both glucose and β-hydroxybutyrate are low but that of FFA is elevated, then a defect in fatty acid oxidation should be suspected. Sufficient blood should be made available to measure insulin, GH, and cortisol; a more detailed analysis of the "critical sample" taken at the time of hypoglycemia is discussed in the section on the diagnostic approach and treatment.

CLASSIFICATION OF NEONATAL HYPOGLYCEMIA

A classification of neonatal hypoglycemia is presented in Table 45-2. Routine screening of blood glucose concentration is not indicated in a healthy term infant after a normal pregnancy and delivery and with no hint of perinatal asphyxia. Blood glucose measurements and monitoring are promptly indicated in any infant who manifests the signs and symptoms listed in Table 45-1. Such infants also require measurements of FFAs and β-hydroxybutyrate and determination of insulin, GH, and cortisol.

Transitional Hypoglycemia (Days)

Transitional hypoglycemia that resolves within days occurs in newborn infants who are SGA or born prematurely. Such newborns should be monitored for hypoglycemia (<40 mg/dL) within 4 hours of birth and treated by feeding and intravenous glucose as needed to maintain plasma glucose concentrations equal to or greater

Table 45-1 Symptoms and Signs of Hypoglycemia in the Neonate

Lethargy
Somnolence
Irritability: fussiness
Feeding difficulty
Jitteriness: myoclonic jerks
Wilting spells: hypotonia
Subnormal temperature
High-pitched cry
Apnea
Seizures
Coma

Table 45-2 Classification of Neonatal Hypoglycemia

Transitional (days)
• Developmental immaturity of fasting adaptation: premature and small-for-gestational-age infant
• Peripartum stress: glycogen depletion
• Hyperinsulinemia: infant of mother with poorly controlled diabetes mellitus
Transient-prolonged (weeks)
• Hyperinsulinism associated with perinatal stress (birth asphyxia, small-for-gestational-age infant, preeclampsia)
Persistent
• Congenital hyperinsulinism (see Table 45-3)
• Hypopituitarism
• Adrenal insufficiency
• Inborn errors
  – Glycogen breakdown defect
  – Gluconeogenesis defect
  – Fatty acid oxidation: defective ketogenesis
• Beckwith-Wiedemann syndrome
Other

than 45 mg/dL before each feeding. The target glucose should be greater than 45 mg/dL before routine feedings during the first 4 to 48 hours of life and greater than 50–60 mg/dL thereafter. Late preterm infants, defined as infants at 34 to 37 weeks' gestation, are likely to resolve their hypoglycemia within days as they have transitional hypoglycemia due to delay in enzyme maturation and diminished nutrient reserves.

Infants born to mothers with diabetes pre-dating pregnancy or developing during pregnancy also should be monitored as they are likely to need frequent feeding or continuous intravenous glucose infusion at rates of 5 to 7 mg/kg/min. These infants typically are LGA and have a surfeit of nutrients that they cannot mobilize due to hyperinsulinemia and diminished glucagon. Also glycogen may have been depleted if there was prolonged labor resulting in stress-activated epinephrine secretion. Meticulous glycemic control during pregnancy minimizes macrosomia, hypoglycemia, and other perinatal problems.[39,40] During labor and delivery of a pregnant woman with diabetes mellitus, intravenous glucose infusion should be avoided if possible as glucose crosses the placenta to the fetus and will stimulate insulin secretion that predisposes to hypoglycemia after placental separation. Treatment of such newborn infants also should avoid bolus glucose infusions; they stimulate surges of insulin secretion and cause rebound hypoglycemia. Most infants of diabetic mothers are stabilized within 3 to 5 days of birth using frequent feedings supplemented by intravenous glucose.

In the absence of a history of documented maternal diabetes, infants born LGA should be suspected of having HI and monitored accordingly. Such infants, along with infants who are SGA, should not be discharged from the hospital without demonstrating that their blood glucose is maintained at equal to or greater than 60 mg/dL at least 4 hours after a feeding for 3 feeding cycles. Blood glucose should be measured one-half hour before the next scheduled feeding. If feeding cannot be established and intravenous glucose infusion rates exceed 5–7 mg/kg/min to maintain a glucose concentration above 60 mg/dL, HI should be suspected. If glucose infusion rates of 10 to 12 mg/kg/min or greater are necessary to maintain blood glucose greater than 60 mg/dL, the cause is most likely HI.

Transient Hypoglycemia (Days–Weeks)

Transient hypoglycemia due to HI that lasts days to weeks is also reported in newborn infants with a history of perinatal stress, including maternal hypertension, preeclampsia, intrauterine growth retardation (IUGR), hypoxia, and cesarean delivery.[27,28] Onset may be sudden, unanticipated, and severe, with glucose concentrations plunging to levels below 20 mg/dL; these

concentrations are associated with subsequent neurological devastation. Onset may occur after discharge from the newborn nursery and may be heralded by the baby having "feeding difficulties." Insulin concentrations are modestly elevated but inappropriate for the degree of hypoglycemia; FFA and β-hydroxybutyrate concentrations are lower than normal. The majority of affected infants respond to diazoxide at a dose of 5–15 mg/kg/d, with the median effective dose 8 mg/kg/d in 1 reported series.[27] Some 20% of such affected newborns require frequent feedings or supplementation with intravenous glucose until hypoglycemia resolves. A variant of this hyperinsulinemic syndrome is associated with lactic acidosis and is thought to be associated with defects in the pyruvate dehydrogenase complex.[28] Diazoxide is the treatment of choice, and resolution usually occurs within 3–4 weeks. The mechanism responsible for malfunction of insulin secretion in these syndromes is unknown but likely involves the potassium channel regulated by adenosine triphosphate (K_{ATP}).

Persistent Hypoglycemia in Infancy

The causes of persistent hypoglycemia in infancy are listed in Tables 45-2 and 45-3. Their onset may be in the newborn period, but unlike the causes described previously, they persist if left untreated and can lead to neurological sequelae. Three separate reviews in the literature all pointed to early onset, prolonged hypoglycemia, and inability to achieve target blood glucose concentrations of greater than 60 mg/dL by medical means alone as poor prognostic signs.[10–12]

The persistent forms of hypoglycemia in infancy include deficiency of the counterregulatory hormones GH and cortisol, either alone or in combination, as occurs in hypopituitarism. Clues for the diagnosis of hypopituitarism include midline facial defects such as cleft palate, holoprosencephaly, and nystagmus as a manifestation of the septo-optic dysplasia syndrome.[26] Jaundice with both cholestatic and inflammatory features is frequently found in hypopituitarism and is likely due to GH and cortisol deficiency; treatment with GH plus cortisol reverses the hepatic defects.[41] In boys, micropenis and small undescended testes provide important clinical clues that gonadotropin deficiency also exists. In normal full-term boys, testosterone concentrations in the first few days of life are as high as they are in the midteen years, and GH concentrations average 30–40 ng/dL in the first days of life. Therefore, stimulation tests for GH or testosterone are unnecessary; low concentrations in association with hypoglycemia are strong clues to the existence of hypopituitarism. If prolactin is elevated while GH, cortisol, and testosterone are low, the primary defect is in the hypothalamus, which normally restrains prolactin

Table 45-3 Classification of Hyperinsulinemic Hypoglycemia of Newborns

Transient
  Days: Infant of mother who has poorly controlled diabetes mellitus
  Weeks: Peripartum asphyxia, preeclampsia, small-for-gestational-age neonate
Responds to diazoxide and feeding
Persistent
  K_{ATP} channel defects
    ABCC8 (sulfonylurea receptor 1, SUR1): inactivating mutations, dominant or recessive
    KCNJ11 (Kir6.2): inactivating mutations, dominant or recessive
  Glucokinase (GK): activating mutations, dominant
  Glutamate dehydrogenase (GDH): activating mutation, dominant
  Short-chain L-3-hydroxycacyl-coenzyme A dehydrogenase (HADH) mutation, recessive
  Uncoupling protein 2 (UCP2 mitochondrial mutation)
  Hepatic nuclear factor 4 alpha (HNF4α mutation), dominant
  Undefined
    Autosomal dominant
    Autosomal recessive
  β-Cell adenoma: multiple endocrine neoplasia type I
  Beckwith-Wiedemann syndrome
  Factitious insulin administration (Munchausen by proxy)
  Oral sulfonylurea drugs: pharmaceutical error
  Congenital disorders of glycosylation (CDGs)
    CDG-Ia
    CDG-Ib (phosphomannose isomerase deficiency)
    CDG-Id
  Other rare syndromes (see text)

through the secretion of dopamine, previously called prolactin-inhibiting factor (PIF). MRI with contrast may reveal an ectopic posterior pituitary bright spot with interruption or absence of the pituitary stalk.[26,42] The deficiencies of GH and cortisol permit the unopposed action of insulin so that hypoglycemia occurs during fasting, which may represent only brief periods beyond the customary 2 to 3 hours between feedings. Cortisol should be replaced at 10 to 15 mg/m²/d, and GH may be given at a dose of 20–40 µg/kg/d if hypoglycemia persists and GH deficiency is documented.

Clues to the existence of an adrenal disorder causing cortisol deficiency may include ambiguous genitalia, hyponatremia, hyperkalemia, and metabolic acidosis. These findings are secondary to lack of aldosterone, and abnormal patterns of steroid precursors define the site of the biosynthetic block in congenital adrenal hyperplasia, the most common of which is 21-OH deficiency.

Bilateral adrenal hemorrhage should be considered after difficult delivery; in boys, congenital adrenal hypoplasia, a contiguous gene defect on the X chromosome also associated with Duchenne muscular dystrophy, and deficiency of glycerol kinase should be considered. Elevated serum levels of creatine phosphokinase (CPK) and triglycerides rapidly identify this condition. Adrenoleukodystrophy, another X-linked condition, usually does not present in the newborn period. Congenital unresponsiveness to ACTH (corticotropin) and the triple A syndrome (alacrima, achalasia, adrenal insufficiency; also known as Allgrove syndrome) can affect both sexes and should be considered in the differential diagnosis of primary adrenal insufficiency (low cortisol with high ACTH) associated with hypoglycemia, although presentation does not generally occur in the newborn period.[43]

Inborn errors of metabolism affecting glycogen breakdown or synthesis, gluconeogenesis, and fatty acid oxidation are unlikely to become apparent unless feeding is delayed for periods of much longer than the customary schedule of feedings every 2 to 4 hours. These defects generally become apparent after 3 to 6 months when the feeding schedules are progressively delayed and the child is being weaned so that the interval between feedings becomes 4 to 6 hours rather than the previous 2 to 4 hours.[1,2] Fatty acid oxidation defects, unless severe, do not manifest in the immediate newborn period when feedings are frequent. Difficulties with initiating breast-feeding may unmask any of the aforementioned entities, including severe fatty acid oxidation defects that can result in hypoglycemia.[21,23] Moreover, enhanced neonatal genetic screening now identifies infants with defects in fatty acid oxidation so that the diagnosis is known within days after discharge from the newborn nursery. Note again that all these syndromes are manifestations of the inability to adapt to fasting, and that there is an inverse relationship between the duration of fasting necessary to provoke hypoglycemia and the severity of the defect(s) in counterregulatory hormones, in glycogen breakdown, in gluconeogenesis, in fatty acid oxidation defects, and in HI.

Persistent Hyperinsulinemic Hypoglycemia of Infancy

Persistent hyperinsulinemic hypoglycemia of infancy is now generally known as congenital HI and is the most common form of persistent hypoglycemia of infancy, caused by one of several genetic entities (Table 45-3). Understanding the biochemical and molecular basis has revolutionized the care of the newborn with HI and is essential for appropriate management and optimum outcome in affected newborns.[1,16,17,29–31] The biochemistry of HI, discussed in the previous material, is summarized in Table 45-4. The glycemic response to glucagon is a rapid means to confirm that the liver

Table 45-4 The Critical Sample: Blood and Urine Tests at Time of Hypoglycemia

Group A: Essential
 1. Glucose and bicarbonate
 2. β-Hydroxybutyrate, free fatty acids
 3. Insulin, cortisol, growth hormone
Group B: Desirable
 4. Lactate, ammonia
 5. Save tube of blood
Group C: Glycemic response 30 minutes after glucagon 0.5–1.0 mg IV or IM
Group D: If possible (may be obtained on another occasion)
 6. Total acyl carnitine profile and free carnitine (to rule out fatty acid oxidation defect)
 7. Save extra tube of blood for repeat or unplanned tests
Urine
 1. Ketones
 2. Organic acids

contains glycogen, whose breakdown is inhibited by the excess actions of insulin. This restraint can be overcome by the intravenous or intramuscular injection of 0.5–1.0 mg glucagon, resulting in a rise of glucose concentration greater than 30 mg/dL above the baseline 30 minutes after injection. In other fasting forms of hypoglycemia, liver glycogen stores are less responsive or unresponsive to glucagon due to a block in glycogenolysis, as occurs in glycogen storage disease, or because glycogen has been depleted by fasting, as occurs in defects of gluconeogenesis or fatty acid oxidation; hence, these entities respond with an increment in glucose less than 30 mg/dL.

A genetic basis for HI was suspected because of its familial nature, especially in certain ethnic groups, and distinct patterns of autosomal-recessive or autosomal-dominant transmission. Genetic linkage studies localized some forms of HI to chromosome 11.[44] In 1995, the sulfonylurea receptor 1 (SUR1) gene and its association with familial HI was discovered[45] and shortly thereafter was shown to be closely linked functionally to an inward-rectifying potassium channel (Kir6.2), which together constituted the K_{ATP} channel.[46] The genes for both the SUR1 (*ABCC8*) and Kir6.2 (*KCNJ11*) were closely associated on chromosome 11. Mutations in the K_{ATP} were rapidly shown to be responsible for several forms of HI, and several other genetic defects have subsequently been discovered,[47,48] permitting the construct of a model, summarized in Figure 45-1. As shown in Figure 45-1, the model explains the following:

1. It indicates the mechanism by which the chemical energy of glucose is converted to an electrical signal that acts like a rheostat to close channels and cause insulin secretion when ATP concentration rises after glucose or amino acids are metabolized and gradually decreases insulin secretion as ATP generation falls when glucose or amino concentration falls. Insulin secretion generally ceases altogether at glucose concentrations of less than 40–50mg/dL. The normal (active) state of the K_{ATP} channel is to be open; inability to close the channel results in diminished insulin secretion, which is responsible for neonatal diabetes or diabetes in later life depending on the severity of the defect. Thus, *inactivating* mutations of either ABCC8 or KCNJ11, which inappropriately maintain the channel closed even at low glucose concentrations, cause HI, whereas *activating* mutations in these genes, which keep the channel open despite high glucose concentration, cause neonatal diabetes.[47,48] Likewise, *activating* mutations of the enzyme glucokinase (GCK) will promote insulin secretion at low glucose concentrations and result in hypoglycemia.[49]

2. The model shows the site and potential mechanism by which drugs such as sulfonylurea act to close the channel causing insulin secretion, whereas diazoxide opens the channel and therefore limits insulin secretion. Somatostatin, a hormone that inhibits various secretory processes in tissues, including the endocrine pancreas, may be effective in the short term to inhibit insulin secretion in HI,[50] but it should be used with caution as a case of necrotizing enterocolitis (NEC) has been attributed to its use.[51]

3. The model shows the mechanisms of amino acid–stimulated insulin secretion, including leucine-stimulated insulin secretion, in which leucine acts as an allosteric positive stimulus for the enzyme glutamate dehydrogenase (GDH), enhancing the metabolism of amino acids and explaining the entity previously known as leucine-sensitive hypoglycemia.[52,53]

4. The model shows locations within the cell of some of the other recognized genetic defects responsible for HI.[54]

Despite these advances, the molecular basis for some 30% to 50% of HI remains unknown and under investigation.[1,16,17,31] It should be noted that there are different potassium channels in which mutations have been shown to be involved in neonatal human epilepsy,[55] in vasospastic angina,[56] and serving a protective role in hypoxia-induced generalized seizures.[57] The mechanisms responsible for hypoglycemia in mutations of short-chain hydroxyl-acyl dehydrogenase (SCHAD),[58] hepatic nuclear factor 4 alpha (HNF4α),[59] and mitochondrial uncoupling protein 2 (UCP2)[60] (Figure 45-1) are not completely defined, so these entities are only briefly mentioned. There is, however, evidence that the enzyme **L-3-hydroxycacyl-coenzyme A dehydrogenase**

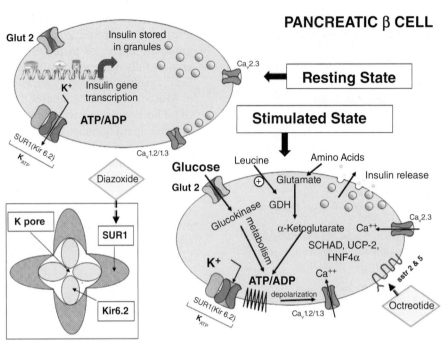

FIGURE 45-1 The regulation of insulin secretion by the pancreatic β cells at rest (top left), during feeding with glucose or amino acids (bottom right), and the heterotetramer structure of K$_{ATP}$ (potassium channel regulated by adenosine triphosphate [ATP]) composed of the 4 inward-rectifying potassium units (Kir6.2) that form the channel pore itself and its 4 surrounding regulatory subunits, the sulfonylurea receptor 1 (SUR1) (bottom left). In the resting (basal) state, a small amount of insulin secretion is constantly ongoing, mediated largely by factors that activate insulin gene transcription and, in part, stimulated by basal levels of glucose and other nutrients. Insulin synthesized within the β cell is stored in granules, some of which are aligned close to the cell membrane so that they can be secreted quickly in response to a stimulus such as a rise in glucose concentration, and constitutes the first-phase insulin response. A second set of granules is stored within the interior of the cytoplasm of the β cell and can be mobilized to constitute the second-phase insulin response. Because nutrient supply is at its basal rates, the ratio of ATP/ADP (adenosine diphosphate) is such that it permits the K$_{ATP}$ channel to remain open and allow potassium to freely exit the cell, thereby maintaining the plasma membrane in a hyperpolarized state. In the stimulated state that occurs during feeding (lower right panel), glucose enters the β cell via the non-insulin-dependent glut2 transporter, where it is phosphorylated by glucokinase to glucose 6-phosphate, permitting metabolism of glucose to ATP. The rise of ATP relative to ADP results in closure of the K$_{ATP}$ channel so that potassium cannot leave the intracellular space. The rise in potassium eventually causes membrane depolarization; this depolarization opens voltage-gated calcium channels as shown, allowing the influx of calcium to the intracellular space. This influx of calcium causes contraction of microtubular and microfilamentous structures, which results in insulin secretion as depicted. Amino acids also can increase insulin secretion via the K$_{ATP}$ channel through the oxidation of glutamate to α-ketoglutarate by the enzyme glutamate dehydrogenase (GDH). The amino acid L-leucine is an allosteric stimulus to GDH action. Also depicted in the lower right panel are 3 additional genetic loci (short-chain hydroxyacyl dehydrogenase, SCHAD; mitochondrial uncoupling protein 2, UCP2; hepatic nuclear factor 4 alpha, HNF4α), in which mutations also can result in hyperinsulinism (HI). Thus, there are at present 7 known loci associated with genetic forms of neonatal HI as listed in Table 45-3; more than half of infants with HI have unknown genetic defects. SCHAD, UCP2, and HNF4α are rare, leaving the 4 more common disorders as activating mutations in glucokinase, activating mutations in GDH, and inactivating mutations in SUR1 or Kir6.2, which together constitute the K$_{ATP}$ channel. The bottom left panel schematically depicts the 4 Kir6.2 units that define the boundaries of the actual potassium pore and their surrounding corresponding 4 regulatory subunits of SUR1. SUR1 is specified by the ABCC8 gene, and Kir6.2 is specified by the KCNJ11 gene, both of which are located on chromosome 11. Each β cell has thousands of K$_{ATP}$ channels, and a mutation in either component should result in a Gaussian distribution of 1, 2, 3, or all 4 subunits being normal or abnormal within each individual K$_{ATP}$ unit. The severity of the abnormal insulin secretion will depend, in part, on the random number of abnormal mutated components within each K$_{ATP}$ unit as well as other factors, such as the location of the mutation, that influence the channel's function. Note that, in the resting state, the channel normally is open; inactivating mutations in either ABCC8 or KCNJ11 determine that a K$_{ATP}$ channel may remain closed, hence resulting in insulin secretion despite the glucose being below the critical level above which glucose-stimulated insulin secretion occurs, normally approximately 50 mg/dL. Inactivating mutations in ABCC8 are the most common cause of HI hypoglycemia of the newborn and may result in focal or diffuse abnormalities of β cells within islets of the pancreas (see text for details). Diazoxide, used to treat HI, acts via binding to SUR1 and keeps the channel open. Long-acting somatostatin analogs (octreotide) act via the somatostatin receptor (ssrtr) family to inhibit insulin secretion by a variety of mechanisms, including keeping the potassium channel open, inhibiting the insulin gene promoter, and inhibiting mobilization of intracellular calcium.

(HADH) (shown in Table 45-3), which is mutated in the clinical entity SCHAD, normally restrains the activity of the enzyme GDH, so that mutations in SCHAD remove this restraint and result in activation similar to the constitutive activation of the GDH syndrome. Major clinical relevance resides in the K_{ATP} channel itself with mutations in the ABCC8 gene, which specifies the protein SUR1, and the KCNJ11 gene, which specifies the protein Kir6.2 (potassium inward-rectifying channel); ABCC8 mutations are more common in HI.

Familial forms of K_{ATP} channel defects are common in some defined populations, with an incidence that may be as high as 1:2500 to 1:3000 live births.[1,31] Among the general population, however, the incidence of K_{ATP} mutations is only 1:30,000 to 1:50,000 live births, and most are sporadic rather than familial. Most of the sporadic mutations for the recessive forms of HI occur in the ABCC8 gene responsible for SUR1; mutations are predominantly located within certain sites of the molecule, particularly the nuclear-binding fold-2 and some transmembrane domains.[48] In patients of Ashkenazi Jewish descent, almost 90% of reported cases had 1 of 2 mutations in the nuclear-binding fold-2 region (3993-9G>A; ΔF1388). The severity of clinical manifestations depends on the site of the mutation and the extent of impaired function, which may be in part caused by the chance distribution of normal and abnormal subunits because each K_{ATP} channel contains 4 SUR1 and 4 Kir6.2 subunits (48) (Figure 45-1).

Among the sporadic forms, 2 types of histopathological lesions, a focal and a diffuse form, are found in approximately equal distribution.[61] Distinguishing between the focal and diffuse forms is critical for guiding the surgeon preoperatively to perform a local excision of the focal form, which is curative for hypoglycemia, while retaining sufficient pancreatic endocrine tissue to enable normal insulin secretion and avoid hyperglycemia-diabetes in the future.[61,62] By contrast, the diffuse forms require near-total pancreatectomy to control hypoglycemia, which may not be curative of hypoglycemia and yet predispose to diabetes in later life.[61,62]

The focal forms of HI are characterized by focal adenomatous hyperplasia of islet-like cells with small β-cell nuclei packed closely together.[61] This focal defect results from a "2-hit" mechanism of molecular changes.[63] The first consists of a loss of a maternal allele in the p15 region of chromosome 11, with the loss expressed only in certain regions of the pancreas. This locus on the maternal allele contains an imprinted region containing H19 and p57[KIP], which normally suppress growth.[63] The paternal allele contains a mutation in the ABCC8 gene in a locus normally associated with the expression of insulinlike growth factor 2 (IGF-2), which promotes growth but

now is no longer balanced by the normal copy of the maternal allele that suppresses growth.[63] Hence, the focal lesion within the pancreas represents somatic reduction to homozygosity for a paternal ABCC8 mutation promoting growth within the affected β-cell area of the pancreas and causing focal hyperplasia. In the diffuse form of HI, heterozygosity is maintained within each cell because the lesion results from inheritance of both a paternal and a maternal mutation. Distinction between these two currently is made by positron emission tomographic (PET) scanning using ^{18}F-L-dopa, which is taken up by pancreatic β cells, providing a remarkably accurate picture when overlain on a computed tomographic (CT) image and pinpointing the site and size of a lesion as focal or as diffuse (Figure 45-2); however, occasional difficulties in resolving these forms of diffuse or focal lesions remain.[62]

Nevertheless, in most cases when a focal lesion is identified via PET scanning, the surgeon can be guided preoperatively with the extent of resection. Molecular diagnostic confirmation of the type of the lesion can be obtained by testing the surgical specimen for the presence of p57[KIP], the imprinted region of the maternal gene missing in the focal lesion, because it only contains the paternal allele with the ABCC8 mutation. The paternal copy of this region of chromosome 11 expresses the imprinted IGF-2 gene, which promotes growth without the restraint imposed by p57[KIP] and adjacent H19 regions of the maternally imprinted genes, thereby explaining the mechanism for the focal hyperplasia.[63,64]

Alterations in these imprinted gene regions, including abnormal methylation patterns, are also responsible for the various defects found in Beckwith-Wiedemann syndrome, which also may be associated with perinatal hyperinsulinemic hypoglycemia.[65,66] Beckwith-Wiedemann syndrome is characterized by other abnormalities, including macroglossia, hemihypertrophy, distinctive earlobe fissures, omphalocele or other umbilical anomalies, and a propensity for tumors.[65,66]

The ability to distinguish the localized from the diffuse form preoperatively has revolutionized the care of the newborn or infant with HI and may require the transfer of infants affected by HI to centers capable of performing the PET scans and with the requisite surgical and histopathology expertise to successfully treat affected infants.[67,68]

AUTOSOMAL-DOMINANT HYPERINSULINISM

Patients who have autosomal-dominant HI tend to have milder clinical presentations than those who have the autosomal-recessive or focal lesions; these autosomal

Focal   Diffuse

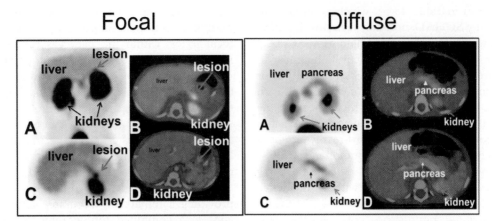

FIGURE 45-2 ^{18}F-L-dopa scans in the focal (left panels) and diffuse (right panels) forms of hyperinsulinemic hypoglycemia. In each, A and C represent the positron emission tomographic (PET) scans in the coronal and axial planes; B and D represent the axial computed tomographic (CT) images fused with the PET and color enhanced in D. Note the clearly delineated focal lesion in the tail of the pancreas, which would guide the surgeon to enable local excision, resulting in cure of hypoglycemia while retaining sufficient pancreas for normal endocrine and exocrine function. Near-total pancreatectomy would likely be required to control hypoglycemia in the diffuse form and may lead to exocrine pancreatic insufficiency or diabetes later in life. (Used with permission of Lisa J. States, MD, Division of Radiology, and Charles A. Stanley, MD, Division of Endocrinology, Children's Hospital of Philadelphia, University of Pennsylvania Perelman School of Medicine.)

forms include activating mutations of GCK and GDH, as well as inactivating mutations in ABCC8 and KCNJ11.[69] Macrosomia is less common at birth, and symptoms may occur only after the neonatal period when weaning has occurred and the duration of fasting between feedings is extended to 6 to 8 hours. Some of these mutations do involve the K_{ATP} channel, primarily the potassium pore itself (ie, the Kir6.2 protein encoded by KCNJ11). Note again that the mutations of the K_{ATP} channel involving ABCC8 and KCNJ11 are inactivating mutations. By contrast, activating mutations of GCK and GDH cause neonatal HI[69,70] (see Figure 45-1).

An activating mutation of GCK causes HI because GCK serves as the sentinel of the β-cell glucose-sensing apparatus. Thus, inactivating mutations of GCK require a higher glucose concentration before adequate phosphorylation of glucose can occur; therefore, in the heterozygous state, they cause a form of monogenic diabetes of youth termed MODY 2 (mature-onset diabetes of the young). *Homozygous inactivating* mutations of GCK cause permanent neonatal diabetes. However, activating mutations of GCK permit glucose to be phosphorylated and lead to closure of the K_{ATP} channel at lower-than-customary glucose concentrations. Most of the GCK mutations present after the age of 3 to 6 months because milder mutations will be masked by the frequent feeding patterns of infancy. Hence, it would require a severe activating mutation of GCK to manifest as neonatal hypoglycemia, an event that is rare but reported. These activating mutations decrease the threshold for insulin release to approximately 2 mM in comparison to the normal 4 to

5 mM in normal subjects. Marked clinical heterogeneity has been reported in families with several members affected by the same mutation, demonstrating that the mutation itself cannot be the entire explanation for the heterogeneity within families.[71]

Another form of autosomal-dominant HI involves an activating mutation of the GDH gene (Figure 45-1). Here, increased activity of the enzyme in β cells leads to increased glutamate oxidation, generating ATP, which induces insulin secretion, as illustrated in the figure. Leucine is an allosteric activator of this enzyme, whereas normally, guanosine triphosphate (GTP) inhibits its activity. This is the mechanism responsible for the previously termed condition leucine-sensitive hypoglycemia and could manifest in the newborn period if infants are fed formula milk.[72] Generally, such affected infants present in the first year of life with milder episodes of hypoglycemia that generally respond to diazoxide. A biochemical feature is the presence of moderate hyperammonemia, in the range of 80 to 200 μmol/L, but patients lack symptoms of hyperammonemia, such as lethargy and coma, found with the inborn errors of the urea cycle. A report of a patient with GDH mutation and with seizures in the absence of hypoglycemia suggests that this mutation may induce hyperexcitability of the CNS. Clearly, in leucine-sensitive hypoglycemia, dietary restriction of L-leucine-containing nutrients should be used in conjunction with diazoxide to avoid hypoglycemia.[72]

A third form of activating mutation responsible for HI in the newborn is HNF4α.[73] HNF4α is a transcription factor normally involved in the secretion of insulin, so that affected individuals present later in life with a form of monogenic diabetes, labeled MODY1. Nevertheless, a number of patients with this entity have been described as having both macrosomia and hypoglycemia at birth and only later in life proceeding to hyperglycemia and diabetes.[59] Hence, a family history of hypoglycemia in infancy followed by hyperglycemia later in life should alert the clinician to the possibility of this entity. A similar pattern of HI representing a dominant heterozygous mutation E1506K in the ABCC8 gene was described in a Finnish family; this pattern was characterized by hypoglycemia in infancy, loss of insulin secretory capacity in early adulthood, and diabetes in middle age.[74]

Recently, an activating mutation in the *AKT-2* component of the insulin-signaling pathway was reported in 3 subjects whose metabolic profile was consistent with a hyperinsulinemic effect but in whom insulin concentrations were below the limits of detection.[18,70] Thus, an activating mutation in the insulin receptor or its transduction-signaling cascade can result in the same phenotype as excessive insulin secretion.[17,18,70] The mechanism is fundamentally the same: increased insulin action, in this instance due to activation of the insulin receptor effect despite low insulin levels. It is likely that other similar patients will be described in the future.

OTHER CAUSES OF NEONATAL HYPOGLYCEMIA

Hypoglycemia is a feature of the hyperviscosity syndrome seen in neonates with a hematocrit of 65% or higher. Mechanisms are unclear, with excessive glycolysis in red blood cells implicated; treatment is symptomatic.[75,76] Hyperglycemia also occurs frequently in neonatal sepsis when increased metabolic rates require glucose production that cannot be sustained, especially in the absence of feeding, which may be limited by the ongoing septic process; treatment is symptomatic.[77] Maternal use of propranolol or salicylates may inhibit gluconeogenesis in the mother and fetus, hence leading to hypoglycemia in the newborn.[78,79] Drug-induced hypoglycemia with insulin, or oral hypoglycemic agents, is virtually unknown in the newborn infant but might result from a pharmaceutical therapeutic error.[80] Distinction between these possibilities relies on the fact that exogenous insulin administration suppresses endogenous insulin secretion so that C-peptide levels will be low, whereas with an insulin-stimulating agent such as a sulfonylurea, both insulin and C-peptide are elevated.[81]

A defect in the Glut-1 glucose transporter has been described in 2 newborn infants with a seizure disorder.[82] Their cerebrospinal fluid (CSF) glucose concentration was low despite normal plasma glucose concentration;

CSF lactate also was low, indicating that this was not a bacterial septic process.[82] By definition, these children did not have hypoglycemia, although they did have hypoglycorrhachia. These infants were successfully treated with a ketogenic diet, which reduced the severity of seizures by providing ketones to the brain as a fuel source capable of bypassing the metabolic effect of diminished glucose transport into the brain.[82]

Hyperinsulinism has been described as a presenting sign in phosphomannose isomerase deficiency.[83] However, this manifestation of a carbohydrate-deficient glycoprotein syndrome, treatable by oral mannose supplementation, did not present until 3 months of age and therefore is not, strictly speaking, a disorder of the newborn.

Galactosemia may be associated with hypoglycemia after milk feeding and can be diagnosed by the presence of reducing substances but not glucose in the urine, by the presence of hepatomegaly and jaundice, and by enzyme activity of Gal1P-uridyltransferase measured as part of neonatal screening programs.[84,85]

DIAGNOSTIC APPROACH AND TREATMENT

An algorithm for approaching the newborn with suspected hypoglycemia is shown in Figures 45-3 and 45-4. Clearly, the appropriate treatment of neonatal hypoglycemia depends on the establishment of the specific diagnosis, and making that diagnosis is facilitated by careful review of the history during labor and delivery; by noting any of the nonspecific symptoms or signs listed in Table 45-1 and considering hypoglycemia to be their cause; by obtaining a family history, which may provide clues to the diagnosis of a familial disorder; by appropriate physical examination (noting jaundice, midline facial defects, umbilical hernia/omphalocele, microphallus or cryptorchidism in a male); and by performing key laboratory investigations, including the metabolic fuel profile at the time of hypoglycemia and key hormone measurements. This constitutes the critical sample, with emphasis on the concentration of glucose, β-hydroxybutyrate, and FFAs as well as insulin, GH, and cortisol, as listed in Figure 45-5. A single low level of cortisol or GH in the absence of other confirmatory features may not be diagnostic of adrenal-pituitary disease, especially beyond the first few days of life.[86] In the newborn, GH is constitutively high, averaging approximately 40 ng/dL in the initial days of life, so values below 10 ng/mL suggest GH deficiency in the newborn.

When hypoglycemia is considered, a bedside point-of-care glucose measurement is performed, and values below 50 mg/dL on days 1 and 2 or less than 60 mg/dL thereafter are confirmed via a laboratory glucose

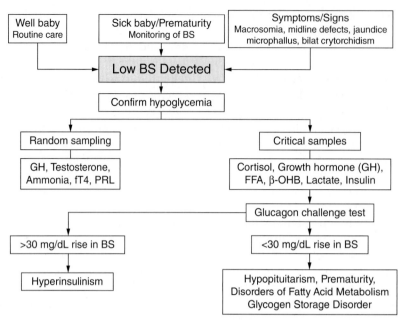

FIGURE 45-3 An algorithmic approach to detection and diagnosis of hypoglycemia in the newborn. See text for details. bilat, bilateral; BS, blood sugar; FFA, free fatty acids; fT4, free thyroxine; GH, growth hormone; β-OHB = beta-hydroxybutyrate; PRL, prolactin.

measurement before treatment is undertaken. In the absence of macrosomia, perinatal asphyxia, or features of hypopituitarism, it is reasonable to treat an infant, particularly if premature, with 0.5 g glucose per kilogram given as a bolus over 5 minutes in the form of 5 mL 10% dextrose in water per kilogram and retesting the infant 30 minutes later. Persistence of hypoglycemia should be treated via an infusion of intravenous glucose providing 4–8 mg/kg/min and glucose monitored hourly. Recurrence or persistence of hypoglycemia despite these measures or the need

to increase the glucose infusion rate to 10 mg/kg/min or greater to maintain blood glucose above 60 mg/dL should alert the clinician to the possibility of hypopituitarism or HI and require the performance of a critical sample as described previously and in Table 45-4.

A critical sample should be taken immediately from any infant with glucose below 50 mg/dL on day 3 of life; the metabolic profile and hormone measurements may define the problem as hypopituitarism, which can be treated with cortisol 10–15 mg/m^2/d in 3 divided doses or GH 20–40 µg/kg/d given by subcutaneous

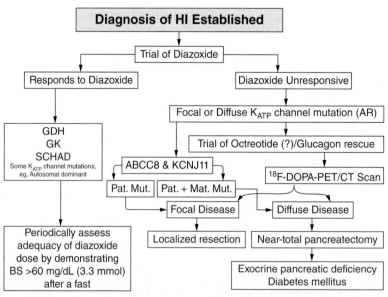

FIGURE 45-4 An algorithmic approach to the management of established hyperinsulinism (HI). See text for details and extended abbreviation definitions. AR, autosomal recessive; Mat, maternal; Mut, mutation; Pat, paternal.

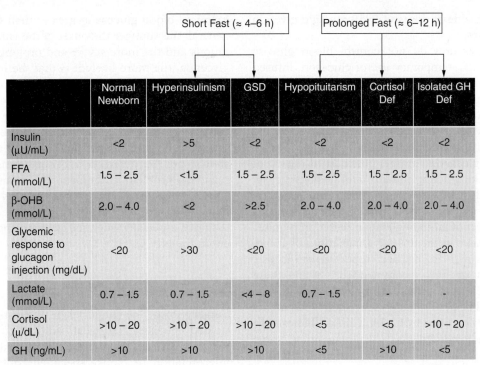

	Short Fast (≈ 4–6 h)			Prolonged Fast (≈ 6–12 h)		
	Normal Newborn	Hyperinsulinism	GSD	Hypopituitarism	Cortisol Def	Isolated GH Def
Insulin (μU/mL)	<2	>5	<2	<2	<2	<2
FFA (mmol/L)	1.5 – 2.5	<1.5	1.5 – 2.5	1.5 – 2.5	1.5 – 2.5	1.5 – 2.5
β-OHB (mmol/L)	2.0 – 4.0	<2	>2.5	2.0 – 4.0	2.0 – 4.0	2.0 – 4.0
Glycemic response to glucagon injection (mg/dL)	<20	>30	<20	<20	<20	<20
Lactate (mmol/L)	0.7 – 1.5	0.7 – 1.5	<4 – 8	0.7 – 1.5	-	-
Cortisol (μ/dL)	>10 – 20	>10 – 20	>10 – 20	<5	<5	>10 – 20
GH (ng/mL)	>10	>10	>10	<5	>10	<5

FIGURE 45-5 Key biochemical and hormonal values in normal newborn infants (>3 days of life) and in various forms of neonatal hypoglycemia typically found after short (~4–6 hours) or moderate (~6-12 hours) fasting. FFA, free fatty acid; GH, growth hormone; GSD, glycogen storage disease; β-OHB, beta-hydroxybutyrate.

injection once daily. MRI of the brain and pituitary should be performed to define the lesion(s),[26,87] and biochemical/genetic testing should be undertaken to examine the cause of primary adrenal insufficiency determined by the presence of high plasma concentrations of ACTH, in contrast to the low concentration of ACTH in hypopituitarism.[43] Consultation with a pediatric endocrinologist facilitates diagnosis and management.

Hyperinsulinism should be suspected as the likely cause of hypoglycemia in a full-tem infant without any predisposing factors and certainly if the infant is macrosomic without confirmed maternal diabetes, if the infant has a glucose level below 20 mg/dL at any time, or if there has been perinatal asphyxia. The critical sample should reveal low glucose plus low FFA plus low β-hydroxybutyrate. Defects in glucose production via glycogen breakdown or gluconeogenesis[88,89] will be revealed by normal or elevated β-hydroxybutyrate and lactate, whereas defects in fatty acid oxidation are likely if FFA levels are elevated while β-hydroxybutyrate is low; these should become apparent only in an infant who is not feeding well because normal feeding beyond day 2 of life should avoid these manifestations when there is available glucose from feedings every 2–3 hours. In these circumstances, the acylcarnitine profile and genetic testing become essential to establish the defect and manage accordingly.[21,90]

Hyperinsulinism, the most common cause of persistent neonatal hypoglycemia, is managed medically, with surgery reserved for those who do not respond to medical management.[31]

Medical Management

Initial medical management is the provision of glucose by intravenous infusion at rates to maintain a glucose level above 60 mg/dL; this may require a central line and rates of 10–20 mg/kg/min (occasionally higher) or supplemental milk feedings "thickened" with polycose to provide more than the customary 20 calories/ounce. Diazoxide, a drug that inhibits insulin secretion by maintaining the K_{ATP} channel in an open state, can be used at 5–20 mg/kg/d given orally in 3 divided doses; increments should be made at 2-day intervals to permit equilibration of the drug's long half-life and metabolic effects. Side effects include fluid retention, which may precipitate congestive heart failure if cardiac reserve is already impaired; thrombocytopenia, neutropenia, anemia, hyperuricemia, and pancreatitis also are described but occur only rarely. In long-term use, hirsutism most evident on the back and limbs as well as coarsening of facial features occur but are reversible with discontinuation of the drug. Doses above 15 mg/kg/d require more careful monitoring of electrolyte and hematological side effects. Fluid retention can be minimized by the concurrent use of oral chlorothiazide at doses of 7–10 mg/kg/d given in 2 divided doses.

If these measures do not control blood glucose above 60 mg/dL, temporary use of glucagon, infused intravenously or subcutaneously at a constant rate to deliver 1 mg per day (24 hours), may help to maintain the desired glucose concentration because glycogen is available for release and the restraint imparted by the excess insulin is overcome by the opposing glycogenolytic effect of glucagon. Another possibility is the use of octreotide, a long-acting somatostatin analogue given at a starting dose of 3–5 µg/kg/d divided into subcutaneous injections every 6–8 hours. Rapid desensitization to its effect of inhibiting insulin secretion requires gradual increases in the dose to a maximum of 15 µg/kg/d. In addition, NEC has been reported with its use, so caution is strongly recommended.[51] While these measures are being provided, molecular diagnostic testing should be performed on the patient and parents in a laboratory certified by CLIA (Clinical Laboratory Improvement Amendments)[91] while retaining some DNA for potential investigation in research laboratories for mutations yet to be discovered.

Mutations in GDH or GCK often can be managed medically and hence have a better prognosis for normal intellectual development; they may be new mutations or transmitted in an autosomal-dominant mode from a parent. Heterozygous mutations of the ABCC8 or KCNJ11 genes in both parents suggest the infant has homozygous or compound heterozygous mutations, which are associated with diffuse pancreatic hyperplasia and likely will require subtotal pancreatectomy as medical measures often fail. A paternal mutation without a maternal mutation raises the possibility that the infant may have focal disease, which needs to be confirmed by ^{18}F-L-dopa PET scanning, which may then permit curative local excision. Single-parental mutation also suggests the possibility of an autosomal-dominant form of HI resulting from these K_{ATP} genes, and these also tend to have milder features with good response to medical measures. There are only a limited number of centers capable of performing ^{18}F-L-dopa scans at present.

Success with medical management to enable discharge from the hospital is defined by the ability to maintain blood glucose above 60 mg/dL with diazoxide plus feeding of milk or fortified formula without the use of intravenous glucose infusion; the infant should be able to maintain glucose above 60 mg/dL even if a feeding is missed (ie, 4–8 hours of fasting on 2 occasions). The use of cornstarch in the management of HI is generally considered ineffective.

Failure of medical treatment is assumed if maximal doses of diazoxide with enhanced feeding and the use of temporary glucagon infusion fail to consistently maintain blood glucose at greater than 60 mg/dL. In general, the younger the onset of the clinical manifestations and the more severe and prolonged the hypoglycemia, the more likely it is that the infant will not respond to medical measures and will require definitive therapeutic surgery to avoid neurodevelopmental impairment. The decision regarding the need for surgery, or transfer to a unit capable of performing the requisite investigation and surgical management, should not be deferred if hypoglycemia remains a recurring problem in the neonatal intensive care unit (NICU). Medical approaches succeed in approximately 20%–30% of cases; surgery is required in the majority, especially when the cases first become apparent in the NICU.[31,71]

Surgical Management

Surgery must be undertaken in institutions with trained pediatric surgical and anesthesia teams together with requisite expertise in histopathological interpretation of biopsy specimens obtained during the operation, which may guide the extent of surgical resection.[64,67,68] Laparoscopic approaches enable resection of preoperatively defined focal lesions that result in cure of hypoglycemia and preservation of exocrine and endocrine function; traditional open abdominal approaches are needed for suspected diffuse lesions. Remarkably, despite wide resection of the pancreas in diffuse lesions, hypoglycemia may persist or recur, and pancreatic exocrine function remains paradoxically normal; these phenomena are not understood. Hyperglycemia or frank diabetes are more likely after extensive pancreatic resections but may not be apparent until puberty with its attendant resistance to insulin.[61]

FUTURE DIRECTIONS

Improvements in laparoscopic instrumentation, particularly in video magnification, may permit pancreatic biopsies as a means to more rapidly identify and distinguish focal as opposed to diffuse disease without the need for preoperative PET scanning via ^{18}F-L-dopa. The era of whole-genome or exome sequencing, soon to be ushered in to routine practice, will permit identification of the genetic defect(s) of the 50%–60% of newborns with HI in whom the cause is currently unknown.[92] It is conceivable that pancreatic β cells isolated from the resected pancreas of patients with diffuse hyperplasia could be cultured, stored, and reimplanted at some future date into the same patient to "cure" their diabetes because rejection of their own tissue would not be a consideration.

REFERENCES

1. Dekelbab BH, Sperling MA. Hypoglycemia in newborns and infants. *Adv Pediatr*. 2006;53:5.

2. Sperling MA, Menon RK. Differential diagnosis and management of neonatal hypoglycemia. *Pediatr Clin N Am*. 2004;51:703.

3. Hay WW Jr, Raju TN, Higgns RP, et al. Knowledge gaps and research needs for understanding and treating neonaltal hypoglycemia: workshop report from Eunice Kennedy Shriver National Institute of Child Health and Human Development. *J Pediatr*. 2009;155(5):612.

4. Committee on Fetus and Newborn, Adamkin DH. Postnatal glucose homeostasis in late-preterm and term infants. *Pediatrics*. 2011;127(3):575.

5. Alkalay AL, Sarnat HB, Flores-Sarnat L, et al. Population meta-analysis of low plasma glucose thresholds in full-term normal newborns. *Am J Perinatol*. 2006;23(2):115.

6. Duvanel CB, Fawer CL, Cotting J, et al. Long-term effects of neonatal hypoglycemia on brain growth and psychomotor development in small-for-gestational-age preterm infants. *J Pediatr*. 1999;134(4):389.

7. Schaefer-Graf UM, Rossi R, Buhrer C, et al. Rate and risk factors of hypoglycemia in large-for-gestational-age newborn infants of nondiabetic mothers. *Am J Obstet Gynecol*. 2002;187(4):913.

8. DePuy AM, Coassolo KM, Som DA, et al. Neonatal hypoglycemia in term, nondiabetic pregnancies. *Am J Obstet Gynecol*. 2009;200(5):e45.

9. Bier DM, Leake RD, Haymond MW. et al. Measurement of "true" glucose production rates in infancy and childhood with 6,6-dideuteroglucose. *Diabetes*. 1997;26(11):1016.

10. Menni F, de Lonlay P, Sevin C, et al. Neurologic outcomes of 90 neonates and infants with persistent hyperinsulinemic hypoglycemia. *Pediatrics*. 2001;107(3):476.

11. Meissner T, Wendel U, Bugard P, et al. Long-term follow-up of 114 patients with congenital hyperinsulinism. *Eur J Endocrinol*. 2003;149:43.

12. Steinkrauss L, Lipman TH, Hendell CD. Effects of hypoglycemia on developmental outcome in children with congenital hyperinsulinism. *J Pediatr Nurs*. 2005;20(2):109.

13. Yager JY. Hypoglycemic injury to the immature brain. *Clin Perinatol*. 2002;29(4):651.

14. Henriksen T. The macrosomic fetus: a challenge in current obstetrics. *Acta Obstet Gynecol Scand*. 2008;87(2):134.

15. Menon RK, Cohen RM, Sperling MA, et al. Transplacental passage of insulin in pregnant women with insulin-dependent diabetes mellitus. Its role in fetal macrosomia. *N Engl J Med*. 1990;323(5):309.

16. De Leon DD, Stanley CA. Mechanisms of disease: advances in diagnosis and treatment of hyperinsulinism in neonates. *Nat Clin Practice Endocrinol Metab*. 2007;3(1):57.

17. Kapoor RR, James C, Hussain K. Advances in the diagnosis and management of hyperinsulinemic hypoglycemia. *Nat Clin Practice Endocrinol Metab*. 2009;5(2):101.

18. Hussain K, Challis B, Rocha N, et al. An activating mutation of AKT2 and human hypoglycemia. *Science*. 2011:334(6055):474.

19. Menon RK, Sperling MA. Carbohydrate metabolism. *Semin Perinatol*. 1988;12(2):157.

20. Pegorier JP, Chatelain F, Thumelin S, et al. Role of long-chain fatty acids in the postnatal induction of genes coding for liver mitochondrial beta-oxidative enzymes. *Biochem Soc Trans*. 1998; 26(2):113.

21. Stanley CA. Dissecting the spectrum of fatty acid oxidation disorders. *J Pediatr*. 1998;132(3 Pt 1):384.

22. Lubchenco LO, Bard H. Incidence of hypoglycemia in newborn infants classified by birth weight and gestational age. *Pediatrics*. 1971;47(5):831.

23. Stanley CA, Baker L. The causes of neonatal hypoglycemia. *N Eng J Med*. 1999;340(15):1200.

24. Bell JJ, August GP, Blethen SL, et al. Neonatal hypoglycemia in a growth hormone registry: incidence and pathogenesis. *J Pediatr Endocrinol Metab*. 2004;17(4):629.

25. Pham L, Garot C, Brue T, et al. Clinical biological and genetic analysis of 8 cases of congenital isolated adrenocorticotrophic hormone (ACTH) deficiency. *PloS One*. 2011;6(10):e26516.

26. McCabe MJ, Alatzoglou KS, Dattani MT. Septo-optic dysplasia and other midline defects: the role of transcription factors: HESX1 and beyond. *Best Pract Res Clin Endocrinol Metab*. 2011; 25:115.

27. Hoe FM, Thornton PS, Wanner LA, et al. Clinical features and insulin regulation in infants with a syndrome of prolonged neonatal hyperinsulinsim. *J Pediatr*. 2006;258:207.

28. Hussain K, Thornton PS, Otonkoski T, et al. Severe transient neonatal hyperinsulinism associated with hyperlactataemia in non-asphyxiated infants. *J Pediatr Endocrinol Metab*. 2004; 17(2):203.

29. Kapoor RR, Flanagan SE, James C, et al. Hyperinsulinaemic hypoglycaemia. *Arch Dis Child*. 2009;94:450.

30. Arnoux J, Berkarre V, Saint-Martin C, et al. Congenital hyperinsulinism: current trends in diagnosis and therapy. *Orphanet J Rare Dis*. 2011;6:63.

31. Stanley CA, De Leon DD. *Monogenic Hyperinsulinemic Hypoglycemia Disorders*. Basel, Switzerland: Karger; 2012.

32. Auer RN. Hypoglycemic brain damage. *Metab Brain Dis*. 2004; 19(3–4):169.

33. Turner CP, Blackburn MR, Rivkees SA. A1 adenosine receptors mediate hypoglycemia-induced neuronal injury. *J Mol Endocrinol*. 2004;32:129.

34. Kim M, Yu ZX, Fredholm BB, et al. Susceptibility of the developing brain to acute hypoglycemia involving A1 adenosine receptor activation. *Am J Physiol Endocrinol Metab*. 2005; 289(4):E562.

35. Barkovich AJ, Ali FA, Rowley HA, et al. Imaging patterns of neonatal hypoglycemia. *AJNR Am J Neuroradiol*. 1998;19(3):592.

36. Alkalay AL, Flores-Sarnat L, Sarnat HB, et al. Brain imaging findings in neonatal hypoglycemia: case report and review of 23 cases. *Clin Pediatr*. 2005;44:783.

37. Caksen H, Guven AS, Yilmaz C, et al. Clinical outcome and magnetic resonance imaging findings in infants with hypoglycemia. *J Child Neurol*. 2011;26:25.

38. Tam EW, Haeusslein LA, Bonifacio SL, et al. Hypoglycemia is associated with increased risk for brain injury and adverse neurodevelopmental outcome in neonates at risk for encephalopathy. *J Pediatr*. 2012;161(1):88–93.

39. Sperling MA, Menon RK. Infant of the diabetic mother. *Curr Ther Endocrinol Metab*. 1997;6:405.

40. Vargas R, Repke JT, Ural SH. Type 1 diabetes mellitus and pregnancy. *Rev Obstet Gynecol*. 2010;3(3):92.

41. Karnsakul W, Sawathiparnich P, Nimkarn S, et al. Anterior pituitary hormone effects on hepatic functions in infants with congenital hypopituitarism. *Ann Hepatol*. 2007;6(2):97.

42. Raivio T, Avbelj M, McCabe MJ, et al. Genetic overlap in Kallmann syndrome, combined pituitary hormone deficiency, and septo-optic dysplasia. *J Clin Endocrinol Metab*. 2012;97(4):E694.

43. Hsieh S, White PC. Presentation of primary adrenal insufficiency in childhood. *J Clin Endocrinol Metab*. 2011;96(6):E925.

44. Glaser B, Chiu KC, Anker R, et al. Familial hyperinsulinism maps to chromosome 11p14–15.1, 30 cM centromeric to the insulin gene. *Nat Genet*. 1994;7(2):185.

45. Thomas PM, Cote GJ, Wohllk N, et al. Mutations in the sulfonylurea receptor gene in familial persistent hyperinsulinemic hypoglycemia of infancy. *Science*. 1995;268(5209):426.

46. Philipson LH, Steiner DF. Pas de deux or more: the sulfonylurea receptor and K+ channels. *Science*. 1995;268(5209):372.

CHAPTER 45

47. Sperling MA. ATP-sensitive potassium channels—neonatal diabetes mellitus and beyond. *N Engl J Med*. 2006;355(5):507.

48. Ashcroft FM. ATP-sensitive potassium channelopathies: focus on insulin secretion. *J Clin Invest*. 2005;115(8):2047.

49. Glaser B, Kesavan P, Heyman M, et al. Familial hyperinsulinism caused by an activating glucokinase mutation. *N Engl J Med*. 1998;338(4):226.

50. Thornton PS, Alter CA, Katz LE, et al. Short-and long-term use of octreotide in the treatment of congenital hyperinsulinism. *J Pediatr*. 1993;123(4):637.

51. Laje P, Halaby L, Adzick NS, et al. Necrotizing enterocolitis in neonates receiving octreotide for the management of congenital hyperinsulinism. *Pediatr Diabetes*. 2010;11(2):142.

52. Hsu BY, Kelly A, Thornton PS, et al. Protein-sensitive and fasting hypoglycemia in children with the hyperinsulinism/hyperammonemia syndrome. *J Pediatr*. 2001;138(3):383.

53. Stanley CA. Regulation of glutamate metabolism and insulin secretion by glutamate dehydrogenase in hypoglycemic children. *Am J Clin Nutr*. 2009;90(3):862S.

54. Mardquard J, Palladino AA, Stanley CA, et al. Rare forms of congenital hyperinsulinism. *Semin Pediatr Surg*. 2011;20(1):38.

55. Bockenhauer D, Feather S, Stanescu HC, et al. Epilepsy, ataxia, sensorineural deafness, tubulopathy, and KCNJ10 mutations. *N Engl J Med*. 2009;360(19):1960.

56. Chutkow WA, Pu J, Wheeler MT, et al. Episodic coronary artery vasospasm and hypertension develop in the absence of Sur2 K(ATP) channels. *J Clin Invest*. 2002;110(2):203.

57. Yamada K, Inagaki N. Neuroprotection by KATP channels. *J Mol Cell Cardiol*. 2005;38(6):945.

58. Li C, Chen P, Palladino A, et al. Mechanism of hyperinsulinism in short-chain 3-hydroxyacyl-CoA dehydrogenase deficiency involves activation of glutamate dehydrogenase. *J Biol Chem*. 2010; 285(41):31806.

59. Pearson ER, Boj SF, Steele AM, et al. Macrosomia and *Hyperinsulinaemic Hypoglycaemia in Patients with Heterozygous Mutations in* the HNF4A Gene. *PLoS Med*. 2007;4(4):e118.

60. Gonzalez-Barroso MM, Giurgea I, Bouillaud F. Mutations in UCP2 in congenital hyperinsulinism reveal a role for regulation of insulin secretion. *PLoS One*. 2008;3(12):e3850.

61. de Lonlay-Debeney P, Poggi-Travert F, Fournet JC, et al. Clinical features of 52 neonates with hyperinsulinism. *N Engl J Med*. 1999;340(15):1169.

62. Hardy OT, Hernandez-Pampaloni M, Saffer JR, et al. Accuracy of [18F]fluorodopa positron emission tomography for diagnosing and localizing focal congenital hyperinsulinism. *J Clin Endocrinol Metab*. 2007;92(12):4706.

63. Verkarre V, Fournet JC, de Lonlay P, et al. Paternal mutation of the sulfonylurea receptor (SUR1) gene and maternal loss of 11p15 imprinted genes lead to persistent hyperinsulinism in focal adenomatous hyperplasia. *J Clin Invest*. 1998;102(7):1286.

64. Suchi M, MacMullen CM, Thornton PS, et al. Molecular and immunohistochemical analyses of the focal form of congenital hyperinsulinism. *Mod Pathol*. 2006;19(1):122.

65. Poole RL, Leith DJ, Docherty LE, et al. Beckwith-Wiedemann syndrome caused by maternally inherited mutation of an OCT-binding motif in the IGF2/H19-imprinting control region, ICR1. *Eur J Hum Genet*. 2012;20(2):240.

66. Baple EL, Poole RL, Mansour S, et al. An atypical case of hypomethylation at multiple imprinted loci. *Eur J Hum Genet*. 2001;19(3):360.

67. Adzick NS, Thornton PS, Stanley CA, et al. A multidisciplinary approach to the focal form of congenital hyperinsulinism leads to successful treatment by partial pancreatectomy. *J Pediatr Surg*. 2004;39(3):270.

68. Laje P, Stanley CA, Palladino AA, et al. Pancreatic head resection and roux-en-Y pancreaticojejunostomy for the treatment of the focal form of congenital hyperinsulinism. *J Pediatr Surg*. 2012;47(1):130.

69. Thornton PS, Satin-Smith MS, Herold K, et al. Familial hyperinsulinism with apparent autosomal dominant inheritance: clinical and genetic differences from the autosomal recessive variant. *J Pediatr*. 1998;132(1):9.

70. Senniappan S, Shanti B, James C, et al. Hyperinsulinaemic hypoglycaemia: genetic mechanisms, diagnosis and management. *J Inherit Metab Dis*. 2012;35(4):589–601.

71. Sayed S, Langdon DR, Odili S, et al. Extremes of clinical and enzymatic phenotypes in children with hyperinsulinism caused by glucokinase activating mutations. *Diabetes*. 2009;58(6):1419.

72. Palladino AA, Stanley CA. The hyperinsulinism/hyperammonemia syndrome. *Rev Endocr Metab Disord*. 2010;11(3):171.

73. Flanagan SE, Kapoor RR, Mali G, et al. Diazoxide-responsive hyperinsulinemic hypoglycemia caused by HNF4A gene mutations. *Eur J Endocrinol*. 2010;162(5):987.

74. Vieira TC, Bergamin CS, Gurgel LC, et al. Hyperinsulinemic hypoglycemia evolving to gestational diabetes and diabetes mellitus in a family carrying the inactivating ABCC8 E1506K mutation. *Pediatr Diabetes*. 2010;11(7):505.

75. Hay WW Jr. Care of the infant of the diabetic mother. *Curr Diab Rep*. 2012;12(1):4.

76. Ozek E, Soll R, Schimmel MS. Partial exchange transfusion to prevent neurodevelopmental disability in infants with polycythemia. *Cochrane Database Syst Rev*. 2010;(1):CD005089.

77. Kermorvant-Duchemin E, Laborie S, Rabilloud M, Lapillonne A, et al. Outcome and prognostic factors in neonates with septic shock. *Pediatr Crit Care Med*. 2008;9(2):186.

78. Cissoko H, Jonville-Bera AP, Swortfiguer D, et al. Neonatal outcome after exposure to beta adrenergic blockers late in pregnancy. *Arch Pediatr*. 2005;12(5):543.

79. Pickering D, Ellis H. Neonatal hypoglycaemia due to salicylate poisoning. *Proc R Soc Med*. 1968;61(12):1256.

80. Green RP, Hollander AS, Thevis M, et al. Detection of surreptitious administration of analog insulin to an 8-week-old infant. *Pediatrics*. 2010;125(5):e1236.

81. Marks V. Murder by insulin: suspected, purported and proven—a review. *Drug Test Anal*. 2009;1(4):162.

82. Veggiotti P, Teutonico F, Alfei E, et al. Glucose transporter type 1 deficiency: ketogenic diet in three patients with atypical phenotype. *Brain Dev*. 2010;32(5):404.

83. de Lonlay P, Seta N, Barrot S, et al. A broad spectrum of clinical presentations in congenital disorders of glycosylation I: a series of 26 cases. *J Med Genet*. 2001;38(1):14.

84. Bosch AM. Classical galactosaemia revisited. *J Inherit Metab Dis*. 2006;29(4):516.

85. Hennermann JB, Schadewaldt P, Vetter B, et al. Features and outcome of galactokinase deficiency in children diagnosed by newborn screening. *J Inherit Metab Dis*. 2001;34(2):399.

86. Kelly A, Tang R, Becker S, et al. Poor specificity of low growth hormone and cortisol levels during fasting hypoglycemia for the diagnoses of growth hormone deficiency and adrenal insufficiency. *Pediatrics*. 2008;122(3):e522.

87. Kelberman D, Rizzoti K, Lovell-Badge R, et al. Genetic regulation of pituitary gland development in human and mouse. *Endocr Rev*. 2009;30(7):790.

88. Mayatepek E, Hoffmann B, Meissner T. Inborn errors of carbohydrate metabolism. *Best Pract Res Clin Gastroenterol*. 2010;(5):607.

89. Chou JY, Jun HS, Mansfield BC. Glycogen storage disease type I and G6Pase-β deficiency: etiology and therapy. *Nat Rev Endocrinol*. 2010;6(12):676.

90. Parini R, Corbetta C. Metabolic screening for the newborn. *J Matern Fetal Neonatal Med*. 2011;24(Suppl 2):6.

91. http://www.genetests.org.

92. Phimister EG, Feero WG, Guttmacher AE. Realizing genomic medicine. *N Engl J Med*. 2012;366:757.

Congenital Adrenal Hyperplasia

Jose Bernardo Quintos and Charlotte M. Boney

DEFINITION/CLASSIFICATION

Congenital adrenal hyperplasia (CAH) is a family of inherited, autosomal recessive disorders of adrenal steroidogenesis due to an abnormality in a step necessary for conversion of cholesterol to cortisol in the adrenal cortex (Figure 46-1). Of all CAH cases, 95% are caused by 21-hydroxylase deficiency. There are 2 forms of 21-hydroxylase deficiency: classic and nonclassic CAH (also called late-onset CAH). Classic CAH comprises the salt-wasting form (cortisol deficiency and aldosterone deficiency) and simple virilizing form. The salt-wasting form comprises 75% and simple virilizing form 25% of patients with 21-hydroxylase deficiency. The classic form is associated with severe enzyme deficiency, leading to prenatal virilization in girls; the nonclassic form has mild enzyme deficiency that causes postnatal hyperandrogenism but no prenatal virilization.

ETIOLOGY

The most common form of CAH is caused by mutations in *CYP21A2*, the gene encoding the adrenal steroid 21-hydroxylase enzyme (P450c21).[1] The steroid 21-hydroxylase enzyme catalyzes conversion of 17-hydroxyprogesterone (17-OHP) to 11-deoxycortisol and progesterone to deoxycorticosterone, which are precursors of cortisol and aldosterone, respectively. In 21-hydroxylase deficiency, because of deficient cortisol synthesis, progesterone and 17-hydroxyprogesterone are shunted to the androgen synthetic pathway

(androstenedione and testosterone). These adrenal androgens are oversecreted in utero, resulting in variable degrees of virilization in the female fetus.

EPIDEMIOLOGY

The incidence of classic CAH in the general population, as shown by newborn screening in different populations worldwide, ranges from 1:10,000 to 1:20,000, with an overall incidence of 1:15,000.[2,3] The incidence of CAH in specific populations ranges from 1 in 5000 live births in Saudi Arabia to 1 in 21,270 live births in New Zealand. The newborn screening incidence in the United States and Canada is 1 in 14,203 live births, with Brazil at 1 in 1863 live births and Japan at 1 in 18,827. A high frequency of CAH exists among Yupik Eskimos from western Alaska: 1 in 282 live births.

The prevalence of nonclassic 21-hydroxylase deficiency CAH in the general heterogeneous population of New York City was estimated to be 1 in 100. Ashkenazi Jews have the highest prevalence at 1/27. Other ethnic groups with a high prevalence of nonclassic CAH include Hispanics (1/40), Slavs (1/50), and Italians (1/300).[1]

CLINICAL MANIFESTATIONS

The cardinal feature of classic CAH in newborn females is ambiguous genitalia (Figure 46-2). Clitoromegaly occurs as a result of adrenal androgens binding to genital skin androgen receptors. Females may present with

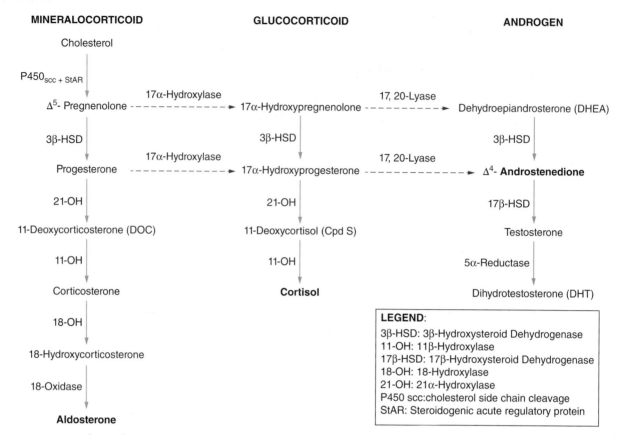

FIGURE 46-1 Adrenal biosynthesis pathway.

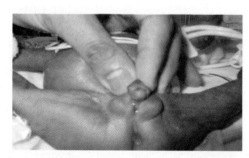

FIGURE 46-2 Ambiguous genitalia in a girl with classic congenital adrenal hyperplasia (CAH): scrotalization/pigmentation of the labia majora, labial fusion, and clitoromegaly.

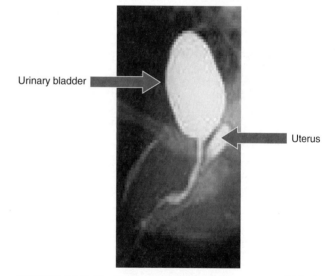

FIGURE 46-3 Genitogram showing the uterus and bladder in a girl with classical congenital adrenal hyperplasia (CAH).

a urogenital sinus (Figure 46-3). Urogenital sinus due to high levels of circulating adrenal androgens beginning at about 7 weeks' gestation prevent the formation of separate vaginal and urethral canals. Females with classic CAH have normal Müllerian structures (uterus, fallopian tubes). The girl with classic CAH has ambiguous or male-appearing external genitalia with perineal hypospadia, chordee, and cryptorchidism. The severity

of virilization is graded using Prader staging, a 5-point scale developed by Prader, with stage 1 indicating mild clitoromegaly and stage 5 representing a cryptorchid male with penile urethra.

Males with classic CAH do not have ambiguous genitalia but may present with subtle scrotal hyperpigmentation because of corticotropin (ACTH) hypersecretion or phallic enlargement because of excessive adrenal androgens in utero.

Neonates with classic salt-wasting CAH typically manifest salt-wasting crisis during the first 1–3 weeks of life. Salt-wasting crisis may occur as late as a few months of age. This manifests as poor feeding, vomiting, weak cry, failure to thrive, loose stools, dehydration, and lethargy. The biochemical *sine qua non* of salt-wasting crisis is hyponatremia, hyperkalemia, and metabolic acidosis with or without hypoglycemia. Without treatment, circulatory collapse, arrhythmias from hyperkalemia, and death may occur within days or weeks.

Postnatally in untreated boys and girls, excessive adrenal androgen secretion leads to rapid somatic growth, bone age advancement, progressive penile or clitoral enlargement, and premature appearance of pubic hair, axillary or facial hair, and acne. Without cortisol treatment, early epiphyseal closure occurs as a result of aromatization of adrenal androgens (androstenedione and testosterone to estrone and estradiol, respectively) and results in short adult height.

DIAGNOSIS

CAH is the most common cause of ambiguous genitalia in the newborn, especially if no gonads are palpable in the scrotum or inguinal canal. Timely diagnosis is needed to prevent sex misassignment of a female newborn as male. If gonads are palpable in the scrotum or inguinal canal, workup for 46 XY disorder of sex differentiation or other causes of ambiguous genitalia should be pursued.

Immediate steroid treatment is necessary to prevent salt-wasting crisis in the salt-wasting form of CAH. Karyotype will identify chromosomal sex, and pelvic ultrasonography will help identify Müllerian structures (ovaries and uterus). Consultation with an endocrinologist should be sought. Adrenal steroids should be measured by blood sample on day 2–3 of life. A markedly elevated level of 17-OHP (>10,000 ng/dL or > 300 nmol/L) in a virilized 46,XX female with nonpalpable gonads is most likely due to CAH.

Diagnosis of 21-hydroxylase deficiency is most accurately established by measuring 17-OHP before and 30 or 60 minutes after intravenous injection of 0.25 mg of Cosyntropin (ACTH1-24). Basal and 60-minute 17-OHP are plotted on a nomogram and distinguish normal individuals and patients with nonclassical and classical CAH.

In affected females, androstenedione and testosterone levels are high. In males, testosterone is usually elevated because of minipuberty in the first 6 months of life and is thus not helpful. ACTH levels are high but are not needed for diagnosis. In salt-wasting CAH, plasma renin is elevated and serum aldosterone is inappropriately low for the renin level.

TREATMENT

Cortisol deficiency is treated with glucocorticoids, usually in the form of hydrocortisone. Glucocorticoid treatment also suppresses high adrenal androgens, preventing further virilization, rapid somatic growth, and early epiphyseal fusion.[4]

Hydrocortisone tablets at a dose of 10–15 mg/m²/d in 2 or 3 divided doses are the preferred treatment. Infants with CAH require higher doses, 50 mg/m²/d divided in 2 to 4 doses during the first few weeks of life to suppress ACTH hypersecretion. Patients with salt-wasting CAH require mineralocorticoid replacement with fludrocortisone 0.1–0.3 mg daily in 1 or 2 divided doses and NaCl supplementation at 1–3 g/d. NaCl tablets are available, and a 1-g tablet is equivalent to 17 mEq of NaCl. Table salt (one-quarter teaspoon = 575 mg NaCl) can also be added to formula if NaCl tablets are not available.

Stress dosing (3–5 times the maintenance dose) is needed in febrile illness (>38.5°C), gastroenteritis with dehydration, surgery accompanied by general anesthesia, and major trauma. Parenteral Solu-Cortef® (hydrocortisone sodium succinate) 25 mg IM or IV should be given for severe vomiting, dehydration, surgery, or severe trauma.

Glucocorticoid treatment of CAH patients involves the delicate balance of adrenal androgen suppression against iatrogenic Cushing syndrome. Glucocorticoid excess suppresses growth hormone secretion and impairs growth. Inadequate glucocorticoid causes high 17-OHP, which is shunted to androstenedione and testosterone; the latter is aromatized to estradiol, the principal hormone that closes epiphyses. An acceptable 17-OHP range in the treated patient is 100–1000 ng/dL.

SURGERY

Surgery for significantly virilized females early in childhood is no longer considered conventional treatment in many tertiary care centers. Surgical procedures have traditionally included both vaginoplasty to repair the urogenital sinus and reduction clitoroplasty to feminize the appearance of the clitoris. Vaginoplasty should be individualized and performed by an experienced surgeon, usually before puberty. Numerous studies have revealed poor sexual functioning in adult women with CAH who underwent feminizing surgery as a child, suggesting that clitoroplasty should be restricted to fully informed patients.[5] A growing number of subspecialists are emphasizing functional outcome over cosmetic appearance. We recommend consideration of clitoroplasty be delayed until the age of consent, when the young woman can make an informed decision about the risks and benefits of surgery. In the meantime, parents can be assured that the severity of clitoromegaly will decrease with suppressive glucocorticoid therapy during the first 6–12 months of treatment.

PROGNOSIS

Untreated salt-wasting CAH can lead to circulatory collapse, arrhythmia, and death. Untreated nonclassical and simple virilizing CAH can lead to excessive adrenal androgen secretion, rapid bone age advancement, and short adult stature. The majority of females with classic CAH have female gender identity and behavior, and most women can bear healthy offspring, thus providing the rationale for female sex assignment.

PREVENTION

Because CAH is common and potentially fatal, it is a disease that is ideal for newborn screening. As of 2009, all 50 states in the United States and 12 other countries screened for CAH. Early recognition and treatment can prevent morbidity and mortality.

CAH is an autosomal recessive condition. If a mother has a previously affected child with CAH and is pregnant with a child from the same father, the fetus has a 1 in 4 chance of having CAH. Prenatal treatment of 21-hydroxylase deficiency with dexamethasone has been shown to prevent virilization should the fetus be an affected female.[6] Dexamethasone at a dose of 20 μg/kg/d in 3 divided doses is administered to the pregnant mother before 10 weeks' gestation. Dexamethasone does not bind cortisol-binding globulin in the maternal blood and is not metabolized by placental 11β-hydroxysteroid dehydrogenase; therefore, it crosses the placenta, suppresses fetal ACTH secretion, and reduces fetal androgen production. Prenatal therapy is considered experimental and should be pursued through protocols approved by institutional review boards at specialized centers.

ADRENAL INSUFFICIENCY IN THE PREMATURE INFANT

Hypocortisolemia in premature infants is related to immaturity of the hypothalamic-pituitary-adrenal (HPA) axis. Activation of the HPA axis with sufficient cortisol secretion is critical in maintaining hemodynamic homeostasis. Relative adrenal insufficiency (RAI) refers to inadequate cortisol production for the degree of stress or illness and has been described in acutely stressed adults, children, and premature and term newborns with cardiovascular instability and shock. RAI is a contributing factor to cardiovascular instability in the sick premature newborn. Many ill premature newborns have inadequate cortisol production due to immaturity of the HPA axis and lagging expression of adrenal steroidogenic enzymes.

Normal Adrenal Development

At 4–5 weeks' gestation in humans, cells from the intermediate mesoderm migrate retroperitoneally to the upper pole of the mesonephros and develop into adrenal cortex. At 7–8 weeks, neural crest-derived sympathetic cells infiltrate the adrenal gland and give rise to the adrenal medulla. By 7 weeks' gestation, the fetal hypothalamus is visible, and it contains releasing hormones by 8–10 weeks. ACTH secretion is evident in pituitary cells by 5–8 weeks. ACTH is suppressible by transplacental dexamethasone by 7–8 weeks, and the ACTH-adrenal feedback arc is functional by 9 weeks.

At 12 weeks, vascular connections to the pituitary are present, but the definitive portal system develops in the third trimester. ACTH is measurable in fetal plasma by 16 weeks. Corticotropin-releasing factor (CRF) from the hypothalamus stimulates pituitary ACTH release by 14 to 20 weeks. Therefore, the HPA axis has emerged by 20 weeks' gestation.[7]

Adrenal Function in the Fetus and Premature Infant

The adrenal cortex in preterm newborns does not express 3-β-hydroxysteroid dehydrogenase (3β-HSD) before 23 weeks and thus has limited capacity for de novo cortisol synthesis until 30 weeks.[8] However, prior to 30 weeks, the fetal adrenal gland uses placental progesterone to bypass 3β-HSD and produce cortisol. Adrenal steroid precursor concentrations are higher in premature infants compared to term infants, indicating the need for 3β-HSD and 11-β-hydroxylase for cortisol synthesis.

The serum cortisol concentrations in ill preterm infants are variable due to intrinsic and extrinsic factors; therefore, assessment of serum cortisol concentration and definition of normal and insufficient amounts are equally problematic. Intrinsic (eg, immaturity of the HPA axis, physiologic decline of serum cortisol in immediate postpartum period, effect of antenatal steroids on HPA axis) and extrinsic factors (eg, vaginal delivery, low Apgar scores, respiratory distress syndrome, mechanical ventilation, hypoglycemia, infection) affect serum cortisol concentrations during the first few weeks of life.[9]

Newborn infants lack mature circadian rhythm for cortisol regulation, but pulsatility of cortisol secretion exists, and random cortisol levels vary widely. Jett et al found cortisol levels of 2 to 54 μg/dL (55–1489 nmol/L) in extremely low birth weight (ELBW) infants less than 28 weeks, with minimal variability over time.[10]

For a more extensive discussion of the physiology and adrenal development of the fetus and premature newborn, see an excellent review by Watterberg.[11]

Definition of Relative Adrenal Insufficiency in the Premature Infant

Relative or transient adrenal insufficiency in premature infants was initially described in abstracts by Colasurdo in 1989 and Ward in 1991 in ELBW infants presenting with "Addisonian"-like crisis: hypotension, oliguria, hyponatremia, hyperkalemia, and cortisol less than 15 μg/dL (<413 nmol/L). Since these initial reports, several case series have been published describing clinical variables and response to glucocorticoid treatment.[12]

Most infants treated with steroids were less than 30 weeks' gestation and presented with volume and pressor-resistant hypotension either within a few hours of life or as late as 3 weeks of life. These infants rapidly responded to dexamethasone (0.25 mg/kg) or hydrocortisone (stress dose 25–60 mg/m^2/d). The rise in blood pressure occurred as early as 30 minutes and within 8 hours to maintain normal mean arterial pressure without needing pressor support. However, hydrocortisone treatment failure occurred in some infants, suggesting other causes of hypotension. In some infants, a second course of stress steroids was needed due to persistent hypotension.

ACTH Testing in Premature Infants

Adrenal function testing in the premature infant is complicated by lack of consensus about the appropriate dose of cosyntropin (ACTH), different gestational and postnatal ages of ACTH testing, severity of illness, and criteria of appropriate cortisol response after ACTH stimulation. Different ACTH (1-24 corticotropin) doses (0.1 μg/kg, 1 μg/1.73 m^2, 0.2 μg/kg, 1 μg/kg, up to 36 μg/kg) have been administered to premature infants at different postnatal ages using different criteria for adequate cortisol response, yielding a wide range (10%–56%) of reported RAI.[12]

Watterberg's study of cortisol response of 276 ELBW infants weighing 500–999 g comparing 1 μg/kg vs 0.1 μg/kg showed that the higher dose (1 μg/kg) yielded higher median cortisol values, 24.6 μg/dL (678 nmol/L) vs 17.4 μg/dL (480 nmol/L), and fewer negative responses (2% vs 21%).[13] The 1-μg/kg dose showed different responses for girls vs boys, infants receiving enteral nutrition vs not, infants exposed to chorioamnionitis vs not, and those receiving mechanical ventilation vs not. A response curve for the 1-μg/kg dose for infants receiving enteral nutrition (surrogate marker of clinically well infants) showed a cortisol response at the 10th percentile of 16.96 μg/dL (468 nmol/L). Infants who stimulated less than 17 μg/dL (468 nmol/L) showed an increased incidence of bronchopulmonary dysplasia (BPD) and length of hospital stay.

Based on Watterberg's study, we conclude that 1 μg/kg ACTH to test adrenal function is the most discriminating in neonates in whom adrenal insufficiency is suspected.

Management

There is presently no consensus and insufficient evidence to support the routine use of glucocorticoids in patients with suspected adrenal insufficiency of prematurity. Current therapy for refractory hypotension includes volume expanders and vasopressors.

Two randomized controlled trials showed the benefit of glucocorticoids for preventing and treating refractory hypotension during the first week of life.[14,15] These studies showed that this regimen effectively reduces the use of volume expansion, dopamine, and dobutamine for blood pressure support compared to placebo. Significantly more very low birth weight infants who were treated with hydrocortisone were weaned off pressors within 3 days.

A meta-analysis examined the relationship between hydrocortisone administration, hypotension, and vasopressor requirements and found that hydrocortisone significantly increased blood pressure and reduced vasopressor requirements in hypotensive and vasopressor-dependent preterm infants.[16]

A treatment algorithm has been proposed in critically ill infants with cardiovascular instability and hypotension[8] (Figure 46-4). If hydrocortisone treatment is being considered for treatment of refractory hypotension, a serum cortisol value should be obtained before administering empiric hydrocortisone. Caution should be taken not to administer hydrocortisone treatment with indomethacin or ibuprofen to avoid the risk of spontaneous gastrointestinal perforation. If a random cortisol value is high (>15 to 20 μg/dL; 413–551 nmol/L), discontinue glucocorticoid if there has been no cardiovascular response. If serum cortisol is less than 15 μg/dL and the patient responds to glucocorticoid treatment, reassessment of cardiovascular function after 3–5 days of hydrocortisone treatment should be done.

The goal is to minimize prolonged treatment with hydrocortisone because the long-term clinical benefit of hydrocortisone therapy has yet to be established.

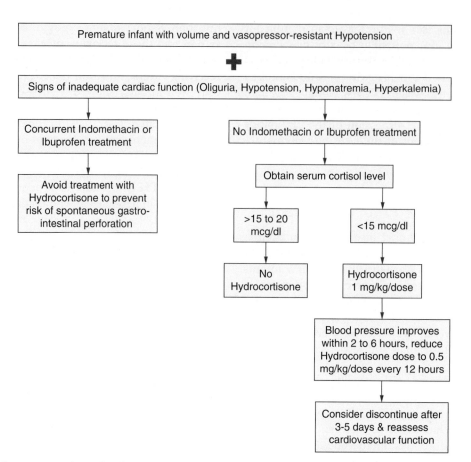

FIGURE 46-4 Therapeutic algorithm for treatment of adrenal insufficiency of prematurity.

Outcome and Follow-up

Adrenocortical insufficiency in the preterm infant is transient. The majority of preterm newborns respond to exogenous CRF and ACTH testing by 2–3 weeks of life, suggesting increased expression and activity of 3β-HSD and 11-β-hydroxylase enzymes and maturity of the HPA axis.[17]

An association between adrenocortical dysfunction, cardiovascular instability, and BPD has been reported and led to studies testing the hypothesis that hydrocortisone prophylaxis of early adrenal insufficiency prevents BPD.[18,19]

Watterberg's study of neurologic outcome at 18 to 22 months corrected age of 360 preterm infants at 25 weeks' gestational age showed that infants treated with prophylactic hydrocortisone compared to placebo did not have an increased incidence of neurologic impairment.[18] Peltoniemi et al reported follow-up data from a randomized trial of early hydrocortisone vs placebo given for 10 days and found neurological and neuropsychological examination at 2 years corrected age were similar.[19] However, more randomized, controlled studies with longer follow-up are needed.

REFERENCES

1. Nimkarn S, New MI. 21-Hydroxylase-deficient congenital adrenal hyperplasia. In: Pagon RA, Bird TC, Dolan CR, Stephens K, eds. *Gene Reviews* [Internet]. Seattle, WA: University of Washington, Seattle; 2010:1–28.
2. Pang S. Newborn screening for congenital adrenal hyperplasia. *Pediatr Ann.* 2003;32(8):516–523.
3. Pang SY, Wallace MA, Hoffman L, et al. Worldwide experience in newborn screening for classical congenital adrenal hyperplasia due to 21-hydroxylase deficiency. *Pediatrics.* 1988; 81(6):866–874.
4. Speiser PW, Azziz R, Baskin LS, et al. Congenital adrenal hyperplasia due to steroid 21-hydroxylase deficiency: an endocrine society clinical practice guideline. *J Clin Endocrinol Metab.* 2010;95(9):4133–4160.
5. Nordenskjold A, Holmdahl G, Frisen L, et al. Type of mutation and surgical procedure affect long-term quality of life for women with congenital adrenal hyperplasia. *J Clin Endocrinol Metab.* 2008;93(2):380–386.
6. New MI, Carlson A, Obeid J, et al. Prenatal diagnosis for congenital adrenal hyperplasia in 532 pregnancies. *J Clin Endocrinol Metab.* 2001;86(12):5651–5657.
7. Brosnan PG. The hypothalamic pituitary axis in the fetus and newborn. *Semin Perinatol.* 2001;25(6):371–384.
8. Fernandez EF, Watterberg KL. Relative adrenal insufficiency in the preterm and term infant. *J Perinatol.* 2009;29(Suppl 2): S44–S49.

9. Ng PC. Is there a "normal" range of serum cortisol concentration for preterm infants? *Pediatrics*. 2008;122(4):873–875.

10. Jett PL, Samuels MH, McDaniel PA, et al. Variability of plasma cortisol levels in extremely low birth weight infants. *J Clin Endocrinol Metab*. 1997;82(9):2921–2925.

11. Watterberg KL. Adrenocortical function and dysfunction in the fetus and neonate. *Semin Neonatol*. 2004;9(1):13–21.

12. Quintos JB, Boney CM. Transient adrenal insufficiency in the premature newborn. *Curr Opin Endocrinol Diabetes Obes*. 2010; 17(1):8–12.

13. Watterberg KL, Shaffer ML, Garland JS, et al. Effect of dose on response to adrenocorticotropin in extremely low birth weight infants. *J Clin Endocrinol Metab*. 2005;90(12): 6380–6385.

14. Ng PC, Lee CH, Bnur FL, et al. A double-blind, randomized, controlled study of a "stress dose" of hydrocortisone for rescue treatment of refractory hypotension in preterm infants. *Pediatrics*. 2006;117(2):367–375.

15. Efird MM, Heerens AT, Gordon PV, et al. A randomized-controlled trial of prophylactic hydrocortisone supplementation for the prevention of hypotension in extremely low birth weight infants. *J Perinatol*. 2005;25(2):119–124.

16. Higgins S, Friedlich P, Seri I. Hydrocortisone for hypotension and vasopressor dependence in preterm neonates: a meta-analysis. *J Perinatol*. 2010;30:373–378.

17. Ng PC, Lee CH, Lam CW, et al.. Transient adrenocortical insufficiency of prematurity and systemic hypotension in very low birthweight infants. *Arch Dis Child Fetal Neonatal Ed*. 2004;89(2):F119–F126.

18. Watterberg KL, Shaffer ML, Mishefske MJ, et al. Growth and neurodevelopmental outcomes after early low-dose hydrocortisone treatment in extremely low birth weight infants. *Pediatrics*. 2007;120(1):40–48.

19. Peltoniemi OM, Lano A, Puosi R, et al. Trial of early neonatal hydrocortisone: two-year follow-up. *Neonatology*. 2009;95(3): 240–247.

CHAPTER 46

Thyroid

Molly O. Regelmann, Evan Graber, Dennis Chia, and Robert Rapaport

INTRODUCTION

Disorders of the thyroid are one of the most common reasons for pediatric endocrinology consultations in the newborn period. Physical symptoms of thyroid disease are often absent, but the effects of thyroid dysfunction in the neonatal period could result in significant deleterious health effects later in life. This chapter reviews disorders of the thyroid most likely to be encountered in the newborn nursery and neonatal intensive care unit (NICU).

THYROID DEVELOPMENT AND FUNCTION

Prenatal Development of the Hypothalamic-Pituitary-Thyroid Axis

The hypothalamic-pituitary-thyroid system develops during the first trimester of gestation. The hypothalamus forms from the neural plate by gestational week 6.[1] The anterior pituitary is derived from oral ectodermal tissue that becomes Rathke's pouch. Studies have demonstrated formation of the pouch as early as 8.5 days and separation from the ectodermal tissue by 12.5 days of gestation.[2,3] Several transcription factors are responsible for formation of the anterior pituitary cells, including HESX1, sonic hedgehog (*SHH*), *SIX3*, *ZIC1*, and others. *HESX1* mutations have been reported in septo-optic dysplasia, which results in pituitary hypoplasia.[4] Mutations in *SHH*, *SIX3*, and *ZIC1* are associated with holoprosencephaly.[5-7] *Pit1* is

a major transcription factor responsible for formation of thyrotrophs (thyroid-stimulating hormone-producing cells), somatotrophs (growth hormone-producing cells), and lactotrophs (prolactin-producing cells).[8] This factor interacts with the promoter regions of genes responsible for production of the β subunit of thyroid-stimulating hormone (TSH) and the thyrotropin-releasing hormone (TRH) receptor and is involved in thyroid hormone receptor formation.[9,10]

The thyroid gland is derived from components of the pharyngeal floor and the fourth pharyngobronchial pouch.[1] Follicular cells migrate from the pharyngeal floor along the thyroglossal duct until they merge with the parafollicular C cells formed from the fourth pharyngobronchial pouch. The thyroid is fully formed and located in its normal position in the anterior neck by 50 days' gestation.[1,11] Morphologic errors that occur during these 50 days can result in ectopic thyroid tissue anywhere along the migratory tract, including sublingually, high in the neck, or even in the mediastinum or the heart.[1] Rarely, thyroid tissue may be found in a thyroglossal duct cyst, when the thyroid does not migrate appropriately and the thyroglossal duct simultaneously does not appropriately degenerate.

Multiple homeobox genes and transcription factors are involved in normal development and migration of the thyroid. Thyroid transcription factor 1 (TTF-1 or Nkx2.1) is necessary for survival and proliferation of primitive thyroid cells.[1] Thyroid transcription factor 2 (TTF-2 or FOXE-1) is responsible for proper migration of thyroid tissue to its normal position in the neck.[12,13] *Pax8* is important for follicular cell development.[13,14] Other genes, such as various *Hox, Hex,*

FOXE-2, and *Eya* subtypes, interact with TTF-1, TTF-2, and Pax8 to form the thyroid gland.[13] Although critically important in thyroid development, mutations in TTF-1, TTF-2, and Pax8 genes are responsible for only 2% of thyroid dysgenesis in newborns with congenital hypothyroidism (CH).[14]

Maturation of the Fetal Thyroid

The fetal thyroid gland begins to function at 14 weeks' gestation, which is when it is able to trap iodine. Thyroid hormone production is minimal until 18–20 weeks' gestation, when iodine uptake is increased and thyroxine (T_4) levels rise throughout the remainder of gestation.[15–18] Triiodothyronine (T_3) concentrations remain low until about 30 weeks' gestation and then rise slowly until term. This is due in part to low tissue concentrations of type I iodothyronine monodeiodinase, which converts T_4 to T_3, and high concentrations of type III monodeiodinase in the placenta and many fetal tissues, which converts T_4 to the inactive reverse T_3 (rT_3). As the fetal liver matures, hepatic type I monodeiodinase increases T_4 to T_3 conversion, resulting in rising T_3 levels.[19]

Pituitary secretion of TSH begins in the 14th week of gestation. TSH concentrations begin to rise significantly between 16 and 18 weeks' gestation until a TSH surge occurs immediately after birth.[20] The pituitary begins responding to TRH by 25 weeks' gestation. Pituitary production of TSH seems to initially occur independently of T_4 production, as the fetal TSH concentration continues to rise throughout gestation despite normal adult concentrations of T_4 by the third trimester.[18] However, the ratio of TSH to free T_4 progressively decreases into extrauterine life, suggesting that the negative-feedback system matures as TSH-producing cells in the pituitary become more sensitive to circulating T_4 concentrations.[21]

Thyroid Hormone Metabolism and Transport

Eighty percent of T_3 found in the body is derived from T_4 that undergoes deiodination in peripheral tissues.[22] T_4 is produced exclusively by the thyroid gland. The peripheral conversion of T_4 to T_3 is controlled by 2 enzymes, type I and type II monodeiodinase.[23,24] Type I monodeiodinase is found predominantly in the liver, kidney, and thyroid itself, whereas type II monodeiodinase is found in the brain, pituitary, placenta, skeletal muscle, heart, thyroid, and brown adipose tissue. Type I monodeiodinase can be inhibited by propylthiouracil (PTU), whereas type II cannot.[1,23] Type II monodeiodinase is the major enzyme involved in peripheral conversion of T_4 to T_3.[22–24] It is particularly important in making sure the brain is provided with sufficient T_3 for development.[25,26]

The thyroid hormones can also be irreversibly inactivated by deiodination of T_4 and T_3 into rT_3 and diiodothyronine (T_2), respectively, which are biologically inactive.[22] This inactivation can be catalyzed by type I monodeiodinase but is mostly controlled by a third enzyme, type III monodeiodinase. This enzyme is found in the brain, placenta, pregnant uterus, and most fetal tissues.[27] Type II and type III deiodinase work to regulate the amount of active thyroid hormone to which the fetus is exposed from the mother.[27,28] All 3 enzymes are regulated by the thyroid status of the fetus.[1]

T_3 and T_4 travel in the blood bound to proteins, primarily thyroid-binding globulin (TBG). Forty-nine to 64% of total T_4 and 80% of total T_3 are bound to TBG.[29] Fetal TBG production by the liver increases in the second half of gestation and is stimulated by placental estrogen.[23] TBG and other transport proteins are discussed in greater detail further in the chapter (in the section on disorders of thyroid hormone transport proteins).

At the time of birth in full-term infants, there is a large increase in TRH and TSH that results in the so-called TSH surge. TSH levels peak to as high as 100 mU/L by about 30 minutes after birth and then decrease progressively to normal levels by 3 to 5 days of life.[21,30,31] T_4 also rises, in response to this surge, and free T_4 levels remain elevated for up to 10 weeks after birth.[32] T_3 levels also rise due to increased thyroidal production in response to the surge and increased activity of hepatic type 1 monodiodinase.[28,33]

Placental Iodine and Thyroid Hormone Transport

The biologically active thyroid hormones T_3 and T_4 are formed by coupling of tyrosine rings and organification of iodide. The placenta transports iodide to the fetus via a Na^+/I^- symporter.[34,35] The iodide can then be used to synthesize thyroid hormones. Severe CH occurs in populations of mothers with insufficient iodine intake and may affect the brain development in the fetus.[13,36,37] The mechanism for hypothyroidism is 2-fold. In the first trimester, prior to the fetal thyroid gland functioning, the fetus is dependent on maternal T_4. When maternal iodine intake is insufficient, she becomes hypothyroid, and the fetus does not have sufficient T_4. The second is maternal and fetal thyroid competition for iodide.[38] When iodide concentrations are low in the maternal serum, the fetal thyroid is unable to increase its affinity for iodide despite upregulation of the Na^+/I^- symporter, resulting in underproduction of fetal T_4.[32,34]

Influence of Maternal Thyroid Function on the Fetus

While the fetal thyroid begins to function at 14 weeks' gestation, the fetal brain T_3 receptors are detectable by 10 weeks' gestation.[16,39] The placenta contains mono-deiodinases that convert most maternal T_4 and T_3 to the inactive thyroid hormones rT_3 and T_2, respectively.[13,27] However, T_4 and T_3 have been found in fetal tissues as early at 9 weeks' gestation, and by 13 weeks, T_3 concentrations in the cortex have been found to be 50%–60% of those found in adults.[40] Children born to mothers with undiagnosed hypothyroidism in the first trimester have been found to have cognitive impairment.[41–44] Newborns without functional thyroid glands have low levels of circulating T_4 at birth of maternal origin.[45,46] Presence of circulating maternal T_4 in utero is neuroprotective and in the newborn is, at least partially, responsible for the frequently asymptomatic nature of CH early in postnatal life. Figure 47-1 summarizes maternal-placental-fetal interactions with respect to the hypothalamic-pituitary-thyroid axis.[47]

DISORDERS OF THYROID HORMONE TRANSPORT PROTEINS

The majority of thyroid hormone, present in serum, is bound to proteins, including thyroid TBG, albumin, and T_4-binding prealbumin, also known as transthyretin (TTR).[48] Of these proteins, TBG carries the majority of T_4 and T_3.[49] In general, patients with defects of thyroid hormone transport proteins are euthyroid,

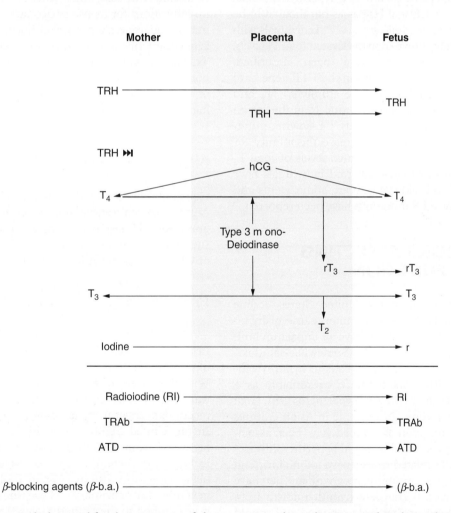

FIGURE 47-1 Maternal-placental-fetal transport of hormones and medications related to the hypothalamic-pituitary-thyroid axis. ATD, antithyroid drugs; β-b.a., β-blocking agents; hCG, human chorionic gonadotropin; I, iodine; RI, radioactive iodine; rT³, reverse triiodothyronine; T₂, diiodothyronine; T₃, triiodothyronine; T₄, thyroxine; TRAb, thyrotropin receptor antibodies; TRH, thyrotropin-releasing hormone; TSH, thyrotropin. (Adapted from Peter and Muzsnai.[47])

with normal measurement of free T_4 and TSH, but have measured abnormalities in the total T_4.

Both complete and partial TBG deficiency have been described. TBG deficiency is X linked; consequently, it is more common in male infants. However, due to variable X inactivation, female infants can also express TBG deficiency. Prevalence estimates range from 1 in 5000 to 1 in 12,000 newborns.[1]

Excess of TBG, which is also X linked, is less common, occurring in 1 in 6000 (Birmingham, UK) to 1 in 40,000 (New York, USA) newborns on screening. The variability in the reported prevalence may be related to transient TBG excess. Those with inherited forms of TBG excess have levels that are 3 to 4.5 times the normal range in affected males and intermediate between normal and affected males in female carriers.[50]

Familial dysalbuminemic hyperthyroxinemia (FDH), which is inherited in an autosomal dominant fashion, is the most common cause of euthyroid hyperthyroxinemia, occurring in up to 1.8% of Hispanics but thought to be less common in other ethnic groups.[48,51] Individuals with FDH are clinically euthyroid with elevated total T_4 levels.

Rarely, TTR variants have been described. Autosomal dominant mutations in the TTR gene have been described that increase the affinity for T_4 and lead to detection of low levels of total T_4 in the serum in otherwise-euthyroid individuals.[52] Likewise, mutations of the TTR gene that decrease the affinity for T_4 and lead to detection of elevated levels of total T_4 in the serum in otherwise-euthyroid individuals have been described. Individuals who are homozygous and heterozygous for TTR mutations have been reported.[53]

MEDICATIONS AFFECTING THYROID FUNCTION

Although uncommon in the United States, iodine deficiency remains the most common cause of hypothyroidism worldwide and can have an impact on both a pregnant mother and her fetus. Somewhat paradoxically, iodine excess also acutely leads to hypothyroidism via the Wolff-Chaikoff effect, presumably as a feedback mechanism to prevent hyperthyroidism. High levels of dietary iodine, for example in Asian cultures with heavy consumption of seaweed, have been associated with both hypothyroidism and hyperthyroidism.[54] Rare cases of CH related to excessive iodine intake in nutritional supplements by a pregnant mother have also been reported.[55] Transient hypothyroidism from topical iodine exposure has been reported and should be in the differential diagnosis but is not a common cause of transient neonatal CH in North America.[56] The premature infant is at particularly high risk because of the increased frequency of procedures and the immature skin that allows increased absorption.

Although there is the potential for iodinated contrast during computed tomographic (CT) studies also to negatively affect the developing thyroid gland of the fetus, a retrospective study of 21 pregnancies in which contrast CT studies were performed between 8 and 37 weeks' gestation (mean 23) revealed no evidence of hypothyroidism in the offspring.[57]

Dopamine and glucocorticoids interfere with TSH release from the pituitary and therefore could contribute to central hypothyroidism or mask TSH rise in primary CH. Antithyroid medications used in Graves disease are discussed further in the chapter (in the neonatal hyperthyroidism section).

Several other drugs are well known to have an impact on the thyroid axis; however, many are not routinely utilized in pregnancy or the neonatal period. For example, lithium is associated with thyroid dysfunction; however, it is a class D drug in pregnancy because of its link with congenital heart disease, and there are no indications for its use in neonates. The antiarrhythmic amiodarone alters thyroid hormone secretion but is uncommonly used in pregnant woman and neonates. Transient hypothyroidism has been reported in infants born to mothers treated with amiodarone.[58] The uses of other medications, such as interferon α, in pregnancy are at the case report level.[59]

NEONATAL HYPOTHYROIDISM

Congenital hypothyroidism is a common preventable cause of mental retardation. Newborn screening programs for CH have been a huge public health success, such that severe mental retardation as a consequence of CH has been essentially eliminated.

Primary Congenital Hypothyroidism

Epidemiology

Prior to the onset of newborn screening, the incidence of primary CH was estimated to be 1 in 7000 births.[60] With the advent of newborn screening, the incidence was initially lowered to the 1:3–4000 range.[61] More recent data suggest the incidence may be even higher. In the United States, the incidence of primary CH increased from 1:4098 in 1987 to 1:2370 in 2002. In New York State, the reported rates have been even higher,[62] with 1:2278 in 1978 to 1:1414 in 2005. The near doubling of primary CH over the past 2–3 decades is not limited to the United States.[63] Several proposed reasons likely together contribute to the increasing incidence of primary CH, including changing trends in ethnic populations, earlier screening, higher proportion of low birth weight infants, and possibly additional prenatal environmental exposures.[64,65]

Perhaps most significantly, lower TSH cutoffs have increased identification of mild hypothyroidism.[66,67]

Higher incidences of primary CH have been reported in Hispanic, Asian, and Native American ethnic groups, with lower incidences among whites and non-Hispanic blacks.[63,64,68] There is an unexplained higher incidence of females with primary CH. An odds ratio of 1.56 was reported in the United States from 1991 to 2000. The sex-specific odds ratio is increased in certain ethnic groups and has been reported as high as 2.6 in Hispanic newborns in California.[64]

Pathophysiology and Genetics

Congenital hypothyroidism can result from several distinct pathophysiological mechanisms. Primary hypothyroidism describes the condition in which there is inadequate thyroid hormone synthesis or release in response to TSH, leading to the distinctive laboratory feature of elevated TSH. The 2 major causes of primary hypothyroidism are thyroid dysgenesis, in which the thyroid gland does not properly form, and dyshormonogenesis, when the gland forms normally and in the correct location but does not function appropriately. Together, they make up the majority of primary CH cases.[69] Table 47-1 summarizes the known causative genes associated with primary CH.[47,70–72]

Thyroid Dysgenesis

Developmental disorders of the thyroid ranging from complete absence of thyroid gland development to hypoplasia to ectopic placement historically make up the majority of cases of primary CH. Thyroid dysgenesis is typically considered sporadic, such that the risk of recurrence in a future pregnancy is only modestly different from the general population. Familial cases have been shown to occur in 2%–3% of cases, and causative mutations in genes encoding transcription factors critical to thyroid development and differentiation, including PAX-8, TTF-1, TTF-2, and GL-153, have been identified.[71,73–75] While thyroid dysplasia has been estimated to constitute approximately 75% of CH cases, this may no longer hold true with the recent change in incidence driven by increasing identification of mild cases. An Italian study identified 435 cases of CH with a cutoff of 10 mU/L over a 7-year period, calculated as an incidence of 1:1446. They then grouped the cases by etiologies, athyreosis/profound hypoplasia, ectopy/hemiagenesis, or gland in situ and determined that 68% were classified as gland in situ, that is, not thyroid dysgenesis, conflicting with the long-held postulate about frequency of different etiologies of CH.[76]

Dyshormonogenesis

Disorders in which the thyroid gland fails to concentrate iodide, form thyroid hormone, and secrete it into the circulation collectively are referred to as thyroid dyshormonogenesis. Key steps in thyroid hormone synthesis and secretion have been reviewed previously; defects in any of these steps can lead to CH. Included among these are defects of the TSH receptor, sodium/iodide symporter, peroxidase system, thyroglobulin, and deiodinases.[77]

Transient and Mild Hypothyroidism

While thyroid dysgenesis and dyshormonogenesis are considered to have established pathophysiological mechanisms, the diagnoses of transient and mild hypothyroidism are somewhat controversial. Transient elevations in TSH can have identifiable etiologies, such as maternal antithyroid drugs, maternal thyrotropin receptor-blocking antibodies (TRAbs), or exposure to excessive iodine.[78,79] Genetic etiologies have rarely been described, but it is known that patients heterozygous for DUOX2 and THOX2 mutations can have transient or mild CH.[80,81] Most often, the cause of transient CH is not definitively determined. In addition, as one cannot always predict with certainty whether an infant has permanent or transient hypothyroidism, clinicians will often begin treatment in the neonatal period, thereby precluding the opportunity to observe the natural history. Meanwhile, the cutoff TSH value for upper range of normal is arbitrary, and no single feature reliably consistently distinguishes mild hypothyroidism from normal physiology.

Controversy exists regarding whether to treat infants with "borderline" or "subclinical" hypothyroidism: those with normal T_4 but TSH levels persistently above the upper limit of normal but less than 10 μIU/mL. As TSH is considered the most sensitive indicator for hypothyroidism, it is possible that the mild elevation is an indicator of insufficient T_4, even if the T_4 is within the normal reference range for the assay. There are no controlled studies in otherwise-healthy infants to evaluate outcomes in those treated with levothyroxine $(L-T_4)$ for mild TSH elevations vs those left untreated. A randomized, double-blind, placebo-controlled study of children with Down syndrome and borderline TSH values in the newborn period showed that those who received $L-T_4$ in the first 2 years of life had better motor development and a trend toward, but not significantly, better cognitive development. The $L-T_4$-treated group also had a better length at 2 years of age when compared to the placebo-treated group, suggesting that treatment may benefit growth.[82] TRH tests have been used to identify infants with mild elevations of TSH who are most likely to benefit from treatment.[83]

Newborn Screening

Newborn screening for CH to prevent the outcome of mental retardation fits Wilson and Jungener's 1968

Table 47-1 Genes Associated With Congenital Primary Hypothyroidism

Gene	Chromosome Location	Type of Protein	Role in Thyroid Formation/Function	Etiology of Primary CH	Associated disorders
TTF1 (Nkx2.1)	14q13.3	Transcription factor	Regulates transcription of TG, TPO, and TSHR genes; involved in proper formation of follicular cells	Dysgenesis	Neonatal respiratory distress, choreoathetosis
TTF2 (FOXE1)	9q22.3	Transcription factor	Involved in proper thyroid migration	Dysgenesis	Cleft palate, choanal atresia, spiky hair
PAX8	2q13	Transcription factor	Activates transcription of TPO, TG, and NIS; involved in proper formation of follicular cells	Dysgenesis	Renal agenesis
GNAS1	20q13.32	Signaling protein	Regulates TSH signaling	Dysgenesis	Albright hereditary osteodystrophy
TSHR	14q31.1	Receptor protein	Regulates TSH binding	Dysgenesis	
TPO	2p25.3	Enzyme	Iodide oxidation, organification, and iodotyrosine coupling	Dyshormonogenesis	
TG	8q24.22	Glycoprotein precursor to T_3 and T_4	Prohormone	Dyshormonogenesis	
SLC5A5	19p13.11	Transporter	Mediates active iodide uptake on basolateral membrane of follicular cell	Dyshormonogenesis	
SLC26A4	7q22.3	Transporter	Mediates iodide transport from the apical membrane of the follicular cell into the colloid space	Dyshormonogenesis	Pendred syndrome (sensorineural hearing loss and hypothyroidism)
IYD (DEHAL1)	6q25.1	Enzyme	Catalyzes deiodination of T_1 and T_2 for iodide recycling	Dyshormonogenesis	
DUOX1 (THOX1)	15q21.1	Enzyme	Catalyzes production of H_2O_2 for iodide oxidation	Dyshormonogenesis	
DUOX2 (THOX2)	15q21.1	Enzyme	Catalyzes production of H_2O_2 for iodide oxidation	Dyshormonogenesis	
GLIS3	9p24.3-p23	Transcription factor	Not described	Dyshormonogenesis	Neonatal diabetes mellitus, polycystic kidneys, glaucoma

Abbreviations: CH, congenital hypothyroidism; NIS, sodium iodide symporter; T_1, monoiodotyrosine; T_2, diiodothyronine; T_3, triiodothyronine; T_4, thyroxin; TG, thyroglobulin; TPO, thyroid peroxidase; TSH, thyroid-stimulating hormone; TSHR, TSH receptor.

classical principles for screening for a medical condition in every respect.[84]

Infants born with CH may be indistinguishable from those without CH on physical examination; however, a small sample of blood obtained by heel stick is sufficient to identify the condition. The most significantly affected newborn will achieve normal or near-normal cognitive outcomes when treatment is initiated early. Newborn screening for CH first became available in the 1970s with pilot programs originating in Quebec, Toronto, and Pittsburgh, Pennsylvania.[85] Since then, newborn screening for CH has been established as a mainstay of newborn care in the United States and the industrialized world.

Primary T$_4$ Screening

Using filter paper blood spots, an initially low or low-normal T$_4$ measurement is followed up with a TSH measurement. A major advantage of the primary T$_4$ screening test is that it has the potential to detect infants with both primary and central hypothyroidism. In addition, it will detect infants with TBG deficiency, and if high values are reported, T$_4$ screening can detect hyperthyroxinemia. A potential challenge with interpretation is with infants who have an initially normal T$_4$ concentration, especially if samples are collected close to birth, when the T$_4$ surge may give a false-negative result. For this reason, special consideration should be given to children with Down syndrome in regions with primary T$_4$ screens and a TSH sample should be obtained in the newborn period given the high incidence of primary CH in this population of children.[86] T$_4$ screening is also associated with a higher false-positive rate, generating additional recall visits.[61]

Primary TSH Screening

As the primary condition to identify by newborn screen is primary hypothyroidism, for which the most sensitive laboratory finding is hyperthyrotropinemia, it follows that screening by TSH has significant appeal. With improvement in the TSH assay on dried spot filter paper samples coupled with the recognition that a primary TSH screen has a lower false-positive rate than primary T$_4$ screening, there have been several newborn screening programs that have transitioned to the primary TSH screen since the beginning of the 2000s. Data from the National Newborn Screening and Genetics Resource Center revealed, in 1998, strictly a primary T$_4$ test was used by 75% of states. A decade later,[87] the percentage had decreased to 50%. Finally, a few states have programs that simultaneously assay both TSH and T$_4$, but such testing is considerably more expensive.[88]

Primary TSH screening has the disadvantage of failing to identify infants with central hypothyroidism. In addition, it creates a challenge to identify those with a late rise in TSH.[89] Some screening programs routinely collect a second newborn screening specimen at 1–3 weeks of age in all infants. The justification for a second screen is not restricted to identifying CH with late rise in TSH, as other metabolic diseases may have false-negative results on the initial newborn screen. The trend toward early discharge of uncomplicated term newborns, thereby shifting the collection time for the initial newborn screen sample, has driven the increasing use of a second newborn screen to maintain high sensitivity. With CH, the TSH surge shortly after birth leads to rapid changes in the normal reference interval, creating challenges in defining appropriate cutoffs for follow-up. Second screens are currently not routine, as it has yet to be definitively established that they improve outcomes to balance the increased cost.[90]

Follow-up Thyroid Function Testing

Results suspicious for CH by filter paper newborn screen require confirmatory serum testing. Therefore, individuals with the pattern of grossly elevated TSH (eg, > 40 mU/L) and low T$_4$ should immediately receive confirmatory serum testing and initiation of L-T$_4$. When the elevation in TSH is less pronounced, a repeat newborn screen is often helpful. Most screening programs have established protocols for contacting the provider to request a repeat newborn screen sample. If the time frame for receiving results from a repeat screen extends beyond the infant's second week, obtaining serum thyroid function tests to expedite the results may be more reasonable. Infants with prolonged stays in the NICU require routine monitoring of thyroid function tests.[91]

Imaging

Imaging studies of the thyroid gland can be useful for diagnosing the underlying etiology for primary CH, thereby allowing appropriate family counseling. It remains controversial whether imaging has an impact on clinical decision making or outcomes, and imaging studies have yet to be routinely recommended by the American Academy of Pediatrics (AAP).[61] One group has promoted a treatment paradigm factoring in the etiology for CH that thus requires imaging[92]; however, it could be argued that severity could be assessed by TSH alone. Two complementary modalities are routinely available for imaging: radionuclide scans and ultrasound.

Radionuclide Scans

There are 2 commonly used radionuclide scans for the evaluation of primary CH, sodium technetium 99m pertechnetate (^{99m}Tc) and iodine 123 (^{123}I). ^{123}I and ^{99m}TC scan can identify thyroid aplasia, hypoplasia, and an ectopic thyroid gland. A large gland with increased early ^{123}I uptake can be consistent with dys-hormonogenesis.[68] Current guidelines from the AAP state that radionuclide imaging is optional, at least in part because of potential risks from exposure to low doses of ionizing radiation.[61]

Ultrasound

Thyroid ultrasound can be useful as both a primary diagnostic test and in conjunction with a radionuclide scan. In the absence of radionuclide uptake, an ultra-sound would confirm thyroid aplasia or dysplasia. If the thyroid gland is noted to be in a normal location with normal size by ultrasound, the absence of radio-nuclide uptake suggests TSH receptor-inactivating mutations, iodine-trapping defects, maternal thyroid-blocking antibodies, and TSH-β gene mutations as possible underlying etiologies.[68]

As a primary diagnostic tool for detecting an ecto-pic thyroid gland, color Doppler ultrasonography is reported to be less sensitive than radionuclide scan, detecting only 90% of ectopic thyroid glands at 1 cen-ter.[93] The advantages of ultrasound are that it is not impacted by exogenous thyroid treatment and there is no ionizing radiation exposure.

Treatment, Management, and Outcomes

To ensure the best neurodevelopmental outcome, once the diagnosis of CH has been made, treatment with L-T$_4$ should be started immediately. L-T$_4$ is the treatment choice for hypothyroidism because of its longer half-life and local conversion to T$_3$ by deiodination. The goal of therapy is to normalize thyroid function tests as soon as possible, with AAP policy goals of normalization of T$_4$ by 2 weeks of life and TSH within 1 month.[61] An initial dose of 10–15 μg/kg/day of L-T$_4$ is recommended, with a higher initial dose for those with severely low T$_4$ values less than 5 μg/dL. At 4 years, children treated with an ini-tial dose of 10–15 μg/kg had higher IQ than those treated with either 6–8 or 8–10 μg/kg/d.[94] In a randomized-controlled trial, full-scale IQ testing was significantly higher in those treated with high initial dose (average 14.5 μg/kg/d) compared with those treated with a lower dose (average 10.5 μg/kg/d); a nonsignificant trend for verbal and performance IQ was also reported.[95] Synthetic L-T$_4$ should be administered in the form of a pill crushed and suspended in a few milliliters of formula, breast milk, or water. L-T$_4$ should not be administered with soy, iron, calcium, or fiber as they can interfere with absorption. Suspensions of L-T$_4$ and alternative thyroid hormone replacement that are not regulated by the US Food and Drug Administration are unreliable and should not be used.[61]

After initiation of treatment with L-T$_4$, the AAP, American Thyroid Association, and Pediatric Endocrine Society joint statement recommends infants

have repeat TSH and serum T$_4$ or free T$_4$ measurements at 2 and 4 weeks, then every 1 to 2 months during the first 6 months of life and every 3 to 4 months between 6 months and 3 years of life.[61] Repeat TSH and serum T$_4$ or free T$_4$ should be tested 4 weeks following dose adjustments or changes in medication source. More frequent testing is also recommended if there are con-cerns for compliance.[61] A more recent study suggested monthly monitoring continue until 12 months of life.[96]

At 3 years of age, once the critical period of neuro-development dependent on thyroid hormone is com-plete, if a child does not have evidence of permanent CH, a trial without L-T$_4$ can be undertaken. TSH and free T$_4$ should be measured 4 weeks following the trial.[97] Evidence for permanent hypothyroidism, including thyroid scan revealing agenesis or an ecto-pic thyroid gland and rise in TSH above 10 mIU/mL after the first year of life, can be taken as evidence of permanent hypothyroidism, and such a trial should be deferred.

Infants with CH appropriately identified and treated achieve near-normal cognitive function. Gruters et al reviewed 8 prospective studies with IQ scores in patients with CH and controls.[98] Small differences of global IQ scores ranging from 2 to 10 were reported, although in only 2 of these studies did the difference reach statistical significance. The IQ scores of the patients with CH in all studies were in the normal range. Current guidelines are more aggressive in tar-geting early correction than in the past. While there is a rationale that this will lead to better prognoses, it may be difficult to demonstrate a difference in studies given the already-normal IQ scores. It should be recognized that up to 10% of appropriately identified patients with CH demonstrate developmental and neurological symptoms. Potential explanations include more severe hypothyroidism leading to a greater impact during fetal development, genetic etiologies that also influ-ence central nervous system development indepen-dent of the thyroid, suboptimal treatment, and poor compliance.

The Premature and Ill Infant

Prematurity presents an additional challenge in the interpretation of thyroid function tests and the decision about whether to intervene with L-T$_4$. As discussed in the previous section, the hypothalamic-pituitary-thyroid axis continues to mature throughout gesta-tion and into the early neonatal period. Therefore, the normal values for preterm infants are different from those in term infants. While the incidence of perma-nent CH is not different in preterm infants, transient primary hypothyroidism and late rise in TSH are both seen more frequently in preterm and low birth weight infants.[99]

Hypothyroxinemia of Prematurity and Sick Euthyroid Syndrome

Preterm infants have a blunted TSH surge after birth and consequently blunted T_4 and T_3 rise as well.[100] In general, levels of both T_4 and T_3 are low in preterm infants, hence the term *hypothyroxinemia of prematurity*. The difference in biologically active free thyroid hormones is attenuated as levels of TBG are also low in premature infants. For that reason, measurements of free T_4, preferably by equilibrium dialysis, are recommended. On the other hand, TSH levels are typically normal or low in preterm infants; therefore, elevations of TSH are still interpreted as evidence of primary hypothyroidism.

There has been interest in whether infants with typical hypothyroxinemia of prematurity benefit from exogenous thyroxine to achieve thyroid hormone levels typical of term infants. To date, there is no conclusive evidence for a clinical benefit of thyroxine treatment, and it has been recommended that such treatment only be performed in the setting of a clinical trial, although a significant proportion of neonatologists reported treating regularly in the past.[101-103] While a persistently low T_4 level with normal TSH can simply be consistent with hypothyroxinemia of prematurity, it is the same pattern of thyroid function tests seen with central hypothyroidism. Central hypothyroidism without other pituitary hormone deficits is exceedingly uncommon, and the clinical picture should shape the level of concern for central hypothyroidism.

Sick euthyroid syndrome (SES), a condition in which the peripheral conversion of T_4 to T_3 is inhibited and TSH is low, is more common in ill preterm infants. Infants with a history of birth trauma, hypoxia, acidosis, infection, hypoglycemia, and hypocalcemia are at increased risk for SES.[104] There is no benefit to treating SES as the cause is generally nonthyroidal in nature.[105]

Late Rise in TSH

The phenomenon in which an infant initially has a low T_4 and normal TSH that later evolves to an elevated TSH is referred to as late rise in TSH. The mechanism producing the delayed rise is not well defined, but late rise in TSH is much more frequent in low birth weight or critically ill infants.[89] A single newborn screen may miss this diagnosis; therefore, protocols have been adjusted to monitor for it. In a retrospective NICU study of 736 patients, Hyman et al reported the frequency of late rise of TSH, as defined as a TSH greater than 10 μIU/mL following a normal TSH, was 1.4%. Of those with late rise in TSH, 54% required treatment, at least transiently, with L-T_4. Risk factors associated with late rise in TSH were surgery, sepsis evaluation, dopamine treatment, gastrointestinal disorders, low birth weight, and prematurity.[89] While there is no standard protocol for repeating thyroid screening tests in premature infants,

it has been suggested that routine serial thyroid screening tests be performed in premature and sick infants to detect late rise in TSH.[91] With a primary T_4 screen, the T_4 value is characteristically low, triggering measurement of TSH, which returns normal. This in turn should prompt an additional newborn screen sample to be sent. A primary TSH screen would not identify an abnormal result and therefore requires specific plans to rescreen those at high risk.

Central (Secondary and Tertiary) Congenital Hypothyroidism

Epidemiology

Central CH (CCH) is much less common than primary CH,[106] with prevalence rates ranging from 1:16,000 to as high as 1:160,000. Reports from the Dutch screening program indicated rates of CCH are 1:21,000–22,000 in an iodine-replete population.[107]

Pathophysiology, Genetics, and Clinical Manifestations

Central CH is caused by a dysfunction of either the hypothalamus or the pituitary gland, which leads to inadequate stimulation of the normal thyroid gland by TSH. CCH is frequently associated with genetic mutations, which are summarized in Table 47-2.[106,108] Noninherited causes of CCH can be caused by insult to the hypothalamus or pituitary gland, such as can occur with hypoxic events. Patients with CCH, when untreated, present similarly to those with primary CH, with prolonged jaundice, coarse cry, poor growth, hypotonia, umbilical hernia, macroglossia, temperature instability, constipation, and skin mottling.[106] In addition, they may also exhibit symptoms of other pituitary hormone deficiencies, including growth failure and hypoglycemia.

Laboratory Evaluations

In the setting of CCH, free T_4 will be low with an inappropriately low TSH. TRH stimulation testing allows distinguishing hypothalamic from pituitary causes of central hypothyroidism.[109,110] In addition to evaluating thyroid function, infants should be screened for other pituitary hormone deficiencies. In the newborn period, secondary adrenal insufficiency and growth hormone deficiency should be evaluated in any infant with suspected CCH. Gonadotropins may also be evaluated in the first few months of life.[111]

Imaging

Infants with the diagnosis of CCH should have imaging of the hypothalamus and pituitary gland

CHAPTER 47

Table 47-2 Genes Associated With Central Congenital Hypothyroidism

Gene	Chromosome Location	Mode of Inheritance	Hormone Deficiency(ies)	Phenotype
TSHβ	1p13.2	Recessive	TSH	Severe isolated central hypothyroidism, pituitary hyperplasia
TRH-R	8q23.1	Recessive	TSH	Isolated central hypothyroidism with uneventful infant development but growth retardation in childhood
POU1F1	3p11.2	Dominant or recessive	TSH, GH, PRL	Moderate-to-severe central hypothyroidism with GH and PRL defects present in the neonate or infant; prominent forehead, midface hypoplasia and depressed nose
PROP1	5q35.3	Recessive	TSH, GH, LH/FSH, PRL	Moderate-to-severe central hypothyroidism with GH, prolactin, and LH/FSH deficits in the neonate or infant; also delayed ACTH deficiency and pituitary hypo- or hyperplasia
HESX1	3p14.3	Dominant or recessive	TSH, GH, LH/FSH, PRL, ACTH	Severe multiple pituitary hormone deficiencies associated with septo-optic dysplasia, supernumerary/hypoplastic digits
LHX3	9q34.3	Recessive	TSH, GH, LH/FSH, PRL	ACTH function intact and pituitary hypo- or hyperplasia; cervical spine is short/rigid; there are vertebral abnormalities and variable deafness or mental retardation
LHX4	1q25.2	Dominant	TSH, GH, LH/FSH, PRL, ACTH	Variable anterior pituitary defects associated with cerebellar and small sella turcica abnormalities; ectopic posterior pituitary gland variably found
LEPR	1p31.3	Recessive	TSH, LH/FSH	Severe obesity, hyperphagia, hypogonadotropic hypogonadism, and mild thyrotropin defect

Abbreviations: ACTH, corticotropin; GH, growth hormone; LH/FSH, luteinizing hormone/follicle-stimulating hormone; PRL, prolactin; TSH, thyroid-stimulating hormone.

to assess for structural abnormalities. The preferred technique for evaluation is magnetic resonance imaging (MRI).[112] An ectopic pituitary gland or other midline defects, such as absence of the corpus callosum, can help confirm the diagnosis of CCH; however, the absence of pathology on MRI does not exclude the diagnosis.

Treatment

As with primary CH, infants should be treated with L-T_4. Prior to starting treatment, secondary adrenal insufficiency should be excluded. If adrenal insufficiency is present, hydrocortisone replacement should be initiated prior to starting L-T_4. For neonates, the initial starting dose of L-T_4 is 10–15 µg/kg/day.[61] Monitoring the dose is more challenging than in primary CH because TSH is not a good marker for adequacy of dose. Measurements of free T_4 should ideally be just prior to the daily dose of L-T_4. The goal should be to keep the free T_4 in the central part of the reference range for the patient's age. In adult studies, an unsuppressed TSH above 1 mU/L may be associated with insufficient L-T_4, but this has not been studied specifically in infants or children.[113] The L-T_4 dose may need to be increased when treatment with recombinant human growth hormone is indicated.[114]

NEONATAL HYPERTHYROIDISM

Neonatal hyperthyroidism is most commonly due to maternal active or inactive Graves disease. Rarely, neonatal hyperthyroidism is associated with mutations leading to activation in the TSH receptor or resistance to the negative feedback of T_4 on the hypothalamus and pituitary.

Neonatal Graves Disease

Epidemiology

Neonatal Graves disease occurs in 1% to 5% of newborns born to mothers with Graves disease. As Graves disease is relatively rare in the pregnant population, the occurrence is estimated to be between 1:25,000 and 50,000 births.[47]

Pathophysiology and Clinical Manifestations

Neonatal Graves disease is caused by the transplacental passage of maternal TSH receptor-stimulating antibodies (TRAb). During the second and third trimesters, TRAb can stimulate the fetal thyroid gland. This leads to excess fetal thyroxine, ultimately causing symptoms of fetal hyperthyroidism, which is manifest most commonly as fetal tachycardia and enlargement of the fetal thyroid gland. Women with an intact thyroid gland can exhibit symptoms of hyperthyroidism, including tachycardia, poor weight gain, goiter with or without bruit, fine tremor, exophthalmos, and hyperemesis. Symptoms may be worse during the first trimester due to high levels of human chorionic gonadotropin (hCG). Mothers with a history of Graves disease who had ablative therapy prior to pregnancy remain at risk for having a child with neonatal Graves disease as the TRAb can remain elevated for months following ablation.[115] Table 47-3 lists the potential complications associated with maternal Graves disease.[116,117] Maternal hyperthyroidism, alone, has been associated with a 13% increased risk of congenital anomalies in the United States.[118] Both methimazole (MMI) and PTU, the medications used to treat maternal Graves disease, have been implicated in congenital anomalies. MMI, in the first trimester, has been shown to have a rare but significantly increased risk for cutis aplasia. PTU has been

Table 47-3 Complications Associated With Maternal Graves Disease

Maternal	Obstetric	Fetal	Neonatal
Miscarriages	Premature delivery	Congenital malformations	Central hypothyroidism
Gestational hypertension	Placenta abruption	Hip dysplasia (associated with first trimester)	Neonatal Graves disease
Preeclampsia	Premature rupture of membranes	Tachycardia	Craniosynostosis
Hyperemesis gravidum	Gestational hypertension	Goiter	Advanced bone age
Congestive heart failure	Postpartum bleeding	Hypothyroidism (from maternal medications or blocking antibodies)	Small for gestational age
Exophthalmos		Intrauterine growth retardation	Goiter (can obstruct airway)
"Thyroid storm"		Prematurity	Congestive heart failure
		Hydrops	Tachycardia/ tachyarrhythmia
			Liver dysfunction
			Poor feeding/weight gain

associated with an increased risk for maternal hepatotoxicity.[119] The American Thyroid Association recommends that pregnant women requiring treatment with antithyroid medications receive PTU during the first trimester and then MMI during the second and third trimesters due to the risk for maternal liver dysfunction associated with PTU.[120]

Neonatal Graves disease onset can vary from shortly after birth to up to a few months after birth. The timing of the development of symptoms is dependent on the presence of maternal thyroid-blocking antibodies, as well as the presence of antithyroid hormone medication, which can take days to dissipate. In infants whose mothers are not on treatment with antithyroid medications, symptoms typically develop shortly after birth. Most commonly, symptoms develop in the second week of life in those infants born to mothers treated with antithyroid medications.[1] In the rare cases of mothers with thyroid-blocking antibodies, it can take up to several weeks until symptoms of neonatal Graves disease develop in the infant.[121,122] Symptoms of neonatal Graves disease include tachycardia (heart rate > 160 beats/minute), goiter, tachyarrhythmias, congestive heart failure, hyperactivity, restlessness, hyperreflexia, insomnia/poor sleep, jaundice, hyperphagia, vomiting, poor weight gain, exophthalmos, hepatosplenomegaly, liver dysfunction, thrombocytopenia, and lymphadenopathy.[47] In addition, infants can have an advanced bone age, craniosynostosis, frontal bossing, and triangular facies. Neonatal Graves disease typically resolves in 3 to 12 weeks as maternal TRAbs degrade. The half-life of TRAb is approximately 12 days.

Laboratory Evaluations

When neonatal Graves disease is suspected, thyroid function tests should be obtained. Serum T_4 and T_3 will be higher than normal, and the TSH will be lower than normal for age. Obtaining TRAb can be helpful to confirm diagnosis. The newborn TRAb titer has been reported to predict the likelihood of symptoms developing.[123] Maternal TRAb titers are not as predictive of onset, but elevations of more than 3 to 5 times the upper limit of normal in the third trimester have been associated with neonatal Graves disease as well.[124,125]

Imaging

Thyroid ultrasound may help to confirm enlargement of the thyroid gland and can be useful for assessing the potential impact of a goiter on the other structures in the neck, particularly the trachea. A consultation with a pediatric cardiologist and an echocardiogram are also recommended to assess for congestive heart failure.

Treatment

Prompt initiation of treatment can be lifesaving once the diagnosis of neonatal Graves disease has been confirmed. MMI is the first-line medication in the newborn period because of the relatively less-severe side effect profile when compared to PTU, which has higher rates of hepatotoxicity.[126] MMI is dosed at 0.5–1 mg/kg divided into 3 doses, every 8 hours, daily. If, after 24–36 hours, a therapeutic response is not observed, then the dose should be titrated up. Iodide can also be added to the treatment to inhibit thyroid hormone release. Iodide is administered as Lugol solution (126 mg iodine/mL) 1 drop (8 mg) by mouth every 8 hours.[1] Anti-inflammatory doses of glucocorticoids can also be added to inhibit thyroid hormone secretion and decrease peripheral conversion of T_4 to T_3. The infant's thyroid function tests should be monitored frequently, and in the event the infant is overtreated and develops hypothyroidism, L-T_4 should be added temporarily to prevent side effects of hypothyroidism. TRAb titers should also be monitored, and when normalized, treatment can be weaned.

As the antithyroid medications can take several days to correct the hyperthyroidism, tachycardia should be treated with a β-adrenergic blocker, such as propranolol, which is dosed at 2 mg/kg divided into 3 doses daily, every 8 hours. Once the infant is euthyroid, treatment with the β-blocker can usually be discontinued. If the infant already has signs of congestive heart failure, digitalization, with or without sedation, is indicated.

Outcomes

When treatment is appropriately started, most infants become euthyroid within a few days. There are few studies that evaluated long-term outcomes in children with neonatal Graves disease. A study of 9 children diagnosed with hyperthyroidism in the newborn period and followed up at 5 months to 10 years of age reported 3 of the children had borderline intelligence, 1 had moderately severe psychomotor retardation, 1 had above-average intelligence, and the remaining children were reported as average.[127]

Infants Born to Mothers Treated for Hyperthyroidism During Pregnancy

The majority of infants born to mothers diagnosed with hyperthyroidism do not develop neonatal Graves disease. However, there are other potential complications associated with maternal hyperthyroidism in the newborn. Children born to mothers with inadequate treatment of gestational Graves disease have been noted to have higher rates of central hypothyroidism and thyroid gland dysmorphology, mainly decreased gland volume. The cause is speculated to be secondary to excess fetal exposure to thyroid hormone, which led to inhibition of fetal TSH during a critical period of development of the pituitary-thyroid axis.[128] Infants born to mothers with thyroid-blocking antibodies and mothers treated during pregnancy with antithyroid medication are also at risk for hypothyroidism and goiter development.[129] At times, the goiter can become so large that it compromises the airway, presenting a medical emergency.

REFERENCES

1. Fisher DA, Grueters A. Disorders of the thyroid in the newborn and infant. In: Sperling MA, ed. *Pediatric Endocrinology.* 3rd ed. Philadelphia, PA: Saunders Elsevier; 2008:198–204.

2. Dasen JS, Rosenfeld MG. Signaling and transcriptional mechanisms in pituitary development. *Annu Rev Neurosci.* 2001;24:327.

3. Sheng HZ, Moriyama K, Yamashita T, et al. Multistep control of pituitary organogenesis. *Science.* 1997;278:1809.

4. Dattani MT, Martinez-Barbera JP, Thomas PQ, et al. Molecular genetics of septo-optic dysplaisa. *Horm Res.* 2000;53(Suppl 1):26.

5. Roessler E, Belloni E, Gaudenz K, et al. Mutations in the human *Sonic Hedgehog* gene cause holoprosencephaly. *Nat Genet.* 1996;14:357.

6. Wallis DE, Roesslr E, Hehr U, et al. Mutations in the homeodomain of the human *SIX3* gene cause holoprosencephaly. *Nat Genet.* 1999;22:196.

7. Brown SA, Warburton D, Brown LY, et al. Holoprosencephaly due to mutations in *ZIC2*, a homologue of *Drosophila odd-paired. Nat Genet.* 1998;20:180.

8. Li S, Crenshaw III B, Rawson EJ, et al. Dwarf locus mutants lacking three pituitary cell types result from mutations in the POU-domain gene *pit-1. Nature.* 1990;347:528.

9. Andersen B, Rosenfeld MG: POU domain factors in the neuroendocrine system: lessons from developmental biology provide insights into human disease. *Endocr Rev.* 2001;22(1):2.

10. Palomino T, Sanchez-Pacheco A, Pena P, Aranda A. A direct protein-protein interaction is involved in the cooperation between thyroid hormone and retinoic acid receptors and the transcription factor GHF-1. *FASEB J.* 1998;12:1201.

11. Salvatore D, Davies TF, Schlumberger MJ, Larsen PR. Thyroid physiology and diagnostic evaluation of patients with thyroid disorders. In: Melmed S, Polonsky KS, Larsen PR, Kronenberg HM, eds. *Williams Textbook of Endocrinology.* 12th ed. Philadelphia, PA: Elsevier Saunders; 2011:327–330.

12. Delange FM. Endemic cretinism. In: Braverman LE, Utiger RD, eds. *Werner and Ingbar's The Thyroid: A Fundamental and Clinical Text.* 9th ed. Philadelphia, PA: Lippincott Williams and Wilkins; 2005:736–739.

13. DeFelice M, DiLauro R. Thyroid development and its disorders: genetics and molecular mechanisms. *Endocr Rev.* 2004;25(5):722.

14. Mansouri A, Chowdhury K, Gruss P. Follicular cells of the thyroid gland require Pax8 gene function. *Nat Genet.* 1998;19(1):87.

15. Brown RS, Huang SA, Fisher DA. The maturation of thyroid function in the perinatal period and during childhood. In: Braverman LE, Utiger RD, eds. *Werner and Ingbar's The Thyroid: A Fundamental and Clinical Text.* 9th ed. Philadelphia, PA: Lippincott Williams and Wilkins; 2005:1015–1016.

16. Santisteban P. Development and anatomy of the hypothalamic-pituitary-thyroid axis. In: Braverman LE, Utiger RD, eds. *Werner and Ingbar's The Thyroid: A Fundamental and Clinical Text.* 9th ed. Philadelphia, PA: Lippincott Williams and Wilkins; 2005:8–25.

17. Hume R, Simpson J, Delahunty C, et al. Human fetal and cord serum thyroid hormones: developmental trends and interrelationships. *J Clin Endocrinol Metab.* 2004;89(8):4097.

18. Thorpe-Beeston JG, Nicolaides KH, McGregor AM. Fetal thyroid function. *Thyroid.* 1992;2(3):207.

19. Santini F, Chiovato L, Ghirri P, et al. Serum iodothyronines in the human fetus and the newborn: evidence for an important role of placenta in fetal thyroid hormone homeostasis. *J Clin Endocrinol Metab.* 1999;84(2):493.

20. Ballabio M, Nicolini U, Jowett T, et al. Maturation of thyroid function in normal human foetuses. *Clin Endocrinol (Oxf).* 1989;31:565.

21. Fisher DA, Nelson JC, Carlton EI. Maturation of human hypothalamic-pituitary-thyroid function and control. *Thyroid.* 2000;10(3):229.

22. Bianco AC, Larsen PR. Intracellular pathways of iodothyronine metabolism. In: Braverman LE, Utiger RD, eds. *Werner and Ingbar's The Thyroid: A Fundamental and Clinical Text.* 9th ed. Philadelphia, PA: Lippincott Williams and Wilkins; 2005:110–113.

23. Kuiper GGJM, Kester MHA, Peeters RP, et al. Biochemical mechanisms of thyroid hormone deiodination. *Thyroid.* 2005;15(8):787.

24. Maia AL, Kim BW, Huang SA, et al. Type 2 iodothyronine deiodinase is the major source of plasma T_3 in euthyroid humans. *J Clin Invest.* 2005;115(9):2524.

25. Burrow GN, Fisher DA, Larsen PR. Maternal and fetal thyroid function. *New Engl J Med.* 1994;331(16):1072.

26. Kester MHA, Martinez de Mena R, Obregon MJ, et al. Iodothyronine levels in the human developing brain: major regulatory roles of iodothyronine deiodinases in different areas. *J Clin Endcrinol Metab.* 2004;89(7):3117.

27. Huang SA. Physiology and pathophysiology of type 3 deiodinase in humans. *Thyroid.* 2005;15(8):875.

28. Richard K, Hume R, Kaptein E, et al. Ontogeny of iodothyronine deiodinases in human liver. *J Clin Endocrinol Metab.* 1998;83(8):2868.

29. Benvenga S, Lapa D, Trimarchi F. Thyroxine binding to members and non-members of the serine protease inhibitor family. *J Endocrinol Invest.* 202;25:32.

30. DeZegher F, Vanhole C, Vandenberghe G, et al. Properties of thyroid-stimulating hormone and cortisol secretion by the human newborn on the day of birth. *J Clin Endocrinol Metab.* 1994;79(2):576.

31. Fisher DA, Odell WD. Acute release of thyrotropin in the newborn. *J Clin Invest.* 1969;48:1670.

32. Schroder-Van Der Elst JP, Van Der Heide D, Kastelijn J, et al. The expression of the sodium/iodide symporter is up-regulated in the thyroid of fetuses of iodine-deficient rats. *Endocrinology.* 2001;142(9):3736.

33. Wu S, Green WL, Huang W. Alternate pathways of thyroid hormone metabolism. *Thyroid.* 2005;15(8):943.

34. Mitchell AM, Manley SW, Morris JC, et al. Sodium iodide symporter (NIS) gene expression in human placenta. *Placenta.* 2001;22:256.

35. Manley SW, Li H, Mortimer RH. The BeWo choriocarcinoma cell line as a model of iodine transport by placenta. *Placenta.* 2005;26:380.

36. Roti E, Gnudi A, Braverman LE. The placental transport, synthesis and metabolism of hormones and drugs which affect thyroid function. *Endocr Rev.* 1983;4(2):131.

37. Buttfield JH, Hetzel BA. Endemic cretinsim in eastern New Guinea. *Astralas Ann Med*. 969;18(3):217.

38. Versloot PM, Schroder-Van Der Elst JP, Van Der Heide D, et al. Effects of marginal iodine deficiency during pregnancy: iodide uptake by the maternal and fetal thyroid. *Am J Physiol Endocrinol Metab*. 1997;273:E1121.

39. Bernal J, Pekonon F: Ontogenesis of the nuclear 3,5,5' triiodothyronine receptors in the human fetal brain. *Endocrinology*. 1984;114(2):677.

40. Calvo RM, Jauniaux E, Gulbis B, et al. Fetal tissues are exposed to biologically relevant free thyroxine concentrations during early phases of development. *J Clin Endocrinol Metab*. 2002;87(4):1768.

41. Haddow JE, Palomaki GE, Allan EC, et al. Maternal thyroid deficiency during pregnancy and subsequent neuropsychological development of the child. *N Engl J Med*. 1999;341(8):549.

42. Pop VJ, Kuijpens JL, vanBaar AL, et al. Low maternal free thyroxine concentrations during early pregnancy are associated with impaired psychomotor development in infancy. *Clin Endocrinol (Oxf)*. 1999;50:149.

43. Pop VJ, Brouwers EP, Vader HL, et al. Maternal hypothyroxinaemia during early pregnancy and subsequent child development: a 3-year follow-up study. *Clin Endocrinol (Oxf)*. 2003;59:282.

44. Freire C, Ramos R, Amaya E, et al. Newborn TSH concentration and its association with cognitive development in healthy boys. *Eur J Endocrinol*. 2010;163:901.

45. Contempre B, Juaniaux E, Calvo R, et al. Detection of thyroid hormones in human embryonic cavities during the first trimester of pregnancy. *J Endocrinol Metab*. 1993;77(6):1719.

46. Vulsma T, Gons MH, de Vijlder JJ. Maternal-fetal transfer of thyroxine in congenital hypothyroidism due to a total organification defect or thyroid agenesis. *N Engl J Med*. 1989;321(1):13.

47. Peter F, Muzsnai A. Congenital disorders of the thyroid: hypo/hyper. *Endocrinol Metab Clin North Am*. 2009;38(3):491.

48. Benvenga S. Thyroid hormone transport proteins and the physiology of hormone binding. In: Braverman LE, Utiger RD, eds. *Werner and Ingbar's the Thyroid: A Fundamental and Clinical Text*. 9th ed. Philadelphia, PA: Lippincott Williams and Wilkins; 2005:97–108.

49. Oppenheimer JH. Role of plasma proteins in the binding, distribution, and metabolism of the thyroid hormones. *N Engl J Med*. 1968;278(21):1153.

50. Refetoff S. Inherited thyroxine binding globulin abnormalities in man. *Endocr Rev*. 1989;10(3):275.

51. DeCosimo DR, Fang SL, Braverman LE. Prevalence of familial dysalbuminemic hyperthyroxinemia in Hispanics. *Ann Intern Med*. 1987;107(5):780.

52. Moses AAC, Lawlor JF, Haddow JE, et al. Familial euthyroid hyperthyroxinemia resulting from increased immunoreactive thyroxinemia resulting from increased immunoreactive thyroxine-binding prealbumin (TBPA). *N Engl J Med*. 1982;306(16):966.

53. Refetoff S, Marinov VS, Tunca H, et al. A new family with hyperthyroxinemia caused by transthyretin Val109 misdiagnosed as thyrotoxicosis and resistance to thyroid hormone—a clinical research center study. *J Clin Endocrinol Metab*. 1996;81(9):3335.

54. Kundra P, Burman KD. The effect of medications on thyroid function tests. *Med Clin North Am*. 2012;96(2):283.

55. Connelly KJ, Boston BA, Pearce EN, et al. Congenital hypothyroidism caused by excess prenatal maternal iodine ingestion. *J Pediatr*. 2012;161(4):760.

56. Brown RS, Bloomfield S, Bednarek FJ, et al. Routine skin cleansing with providone-iodine is not a common cause of transient neonatal hypothyroidism in North America: a prospective controlled study. *Thyroid*. 1997;7(3):395.

57. Atwell TD, Lteif AN, Brown DL, et al. Neonatal thyroid function after administration of IV iodinated contrast agent to 21 pregnant patients. *AJR Am J Roentgenol*. 2008;191(1):268.

58. Lomenick JP, Jackson WA, Backeljauw PF. Amiodarone-induced neonatal hypothyroidism: a unique form of transient early-onset hypothyroidism. *J Perinatol*. 2004;24(6):397.

59. Hiratsuka M, Minakami H, Koshizuka S, et al. Administration of interferon-alpha during pregnancy: effects on fetus. *J Perinat Med*. 2000;28(5):372.

60. Alm J, Larsson A, Zetterstrom R. Congenital hypothyroidism in Sweden. Incidences and age at diagnosis. *Acta Paediatr Scand*. 1978;67:1.

61. American Academy of Pediatrics, Section on Endocrinology and Committee on Genetics; Rose SR; American Thyroid Association, Public Health Committee; Brown RS; Lawson Wilkins Pediatric Endocrine Society. Update of newborn screening and therapy for congenital hypothyroidism. *Pediatrics*. 2006;117(6):2290.

62. Harris KB, Pass KA. Increase in congenital hypothyroidism in New York State and in the United States. *Mol Genet Metab*. 2007;91(3):268.

63. LaFranchi SH. Increasing incidence of congenital hypothyroidism: some answers, more questions. *J Clin Endocrinol Metab*. 2011;96(8):2395.

64. Hinton CF, Harris KB, Borgfeld L, et al. Trends in incidence rates of congenital hypothyroidism related to select demographic factors: data from the United States, California, Massachusetts, New York, and Texas. *Pediatrics*. 2010;125(S2):S37.

65. Hershman JM. Perchlorate and thyroid function: what are the environmental issues? *Thyroid*. 2005;15(5);427.

66. Mitchell ML, Hsu HW, Sahai I; Massachusetts Pediatric Endocrine Work Group. The increased incidence of congenital hypothyroidism: fact or fancy? *Clin Endocrinol (Oxf)*. 2011;75(6):806.

67. Rapaport R. Congenital hypothyroidism: an evolving common clinical conundrum. *J Clin Endocrinol Metab*. 2010;95(9):4223.

68. LaFranchi SH. Approach to the diagnosis and treatment of neonatal hypothyroidism. *J Clin Endocrinol Metab*. 2011;96(10):2959.

69. Rastogi MV, LaFranchi SH. Congenital hypothyroidism. *Orphanet J Rare Dis*. 2010;5:17.

70. Park SM, Chatterjee VK. Genetics of congenital hypothyroidism. *J Med Genet*. 2005;42(5):379.

71. Senée V, Chelala C, Duchatelet S, et al. Mutations in GLIS3 are responsible for a rare syndrome with neonatal diabetes mellitus and congenital hypothyroidism. *Nat Genet*. 2006;38(6):682.

72. Taha D, Barbar M, Kanaa H, et al. Neonatal diabetes mellitus, congenital hypothyroidism, hepatic fibrosis, polycystic kidneys, and glaucoma: a new autosomal recessive syndrome? *Am J Med Genet A*. 2003;122A(3):269.

73. Tonacchera M, Banco ME, Montanelli L, et al. Genetic analysis of PAX8 gene in children with congenital hypothyroidism and dysgenetic or eutopic thyroid glands: identification of a novel sequence variant. *Clin Endocrinol*. 2007;67:34.

74. Krude H, Schutz B, Biebermann H, et al. Choreoathetosis, hypothyroidism, and pulmonary alterations due to human NKX2–1 haploinsufficiency. *Clin Invest*. 2002;109:475.

75. Castanet M, Park SM, Smith A. A novel loss-of-function mutation in TTF-2 is associated with congenital hypothyroidism, thyroid agenesis, and cleft palate. *Hum Mol Genet*. 2002;11:2051.

76. Corbetta C, Weber G, Cortinovis F. A 7-year experience with low blood TSH cutoff levels for neonatal screening reveals an unsuspected frequency of congenital hypothyroidism (CH). *Clin Endocrinol (Oxf)*. 2009;71(5):739.

77. Grasberger H, Refetoff S. Genetic causes of congenital hypothyroidism due to dyshormonogenesis. *Curr Opin Pediatr.* 2011;23(4):421.

78. Bhavani N. Transient congenital hypothyroidism. *Indian J Endocrinol Metab.* 2011;15(Suppl 2):S117.

79. Evans C, Gregory JW, Barton J, et al. Transient congenital hypothyroidism due to thyroid-stimulating hormone receptor blocking antibodies: a case series. *Ann Clin Biochem.* 2011;48(Pt 4):386.

80. Moreno JC, Bikker H, Kempers MJ. Inactivating mutations in the gene for thyroid oxidase 2 (THOX2) and congenital hypothyroidism. *N Engl J Med.* 2002;347(2):95.

81. Moreno JC, Visser TJ. New phenotypes in thyroid dyshormonogenesis: hypothyroidism due to DUOX2 mutations. *Endocr Dev.* 2007;10:99.

82. van Trotsenburg AS, Vulsma T, van Rozenburg-Marres SL, et al. The effect of thyroxine treatment started in the neonatal period on development and growth of two-year-old Down syndrome children: a randomized clinical trial. *J Clin Endocrinol Metab.* 2005;90(6):3304.

83. Rapaport R, Sills I, Patel U, et al. Thyrotropin-releasing hormone stimulation tests in infants. *J Clin Endocrinol Metab.* 1993;77(4):889.

84. Wilson JMG, Jungner G. Principles and practice of screening for disease. World Health Organization public health papers, No. 34. http://whqlibdoc.who.int/php/WHO_PHP_34.pdf. Published 1968. Accessed January 20, 2013.

85. Newborn Committee of the American Thyroid Association. Recommendations for screening programs for congenital hypothyroidism. *Can Med Assoc J.* 1977;116(6):631.

86. Bull MJ, Committee on Genetics. Clinical report—health supervision for children with Down syndrome. *Pediatrics.* 2011;128(2):393.

87. LaFranchi SH. Newborn screening strategies for congenital hypothyroidism: an update. *J Inherit Metab Dis.* 2010;33(Suppl 2):S225.

88. Pass KA, Neto EC. Update: newborn screening for endocrinopathies. *Endocrinol Metab Clin N Am.* 2009;38(4):827–837.

89. Hyman SJ, Greig F, Holzman I, et al. Late rise of thyroid stimulating hormone in ill newborns. *J Pediatr Endocrinol Metab.* 2007;20(4):501.

90. Bijarnia S, Wilcken B, Wiley VC. Newborn screening for congenital hypothyroidism in very-low-birth-weight babies: the need for a second test. *J Inherit Metab Dis.* 2011;34(3):827.

91. Rapaport R. Evaluation of thyroid status of infants in intensive care settings: recommended an extension of newborn screening. *J Pediatr.* 2003;143(5):556.

92. Mathai S, Cutfield WS, Gunn AJ. A novel therapeutic paradigm to treat congenital hypothyroidism. *Clin Endocrinol (Oxf).* 2008;69(1):142.

93. Ohnishi H, Sato H, Noda H. Color Doppler ultrasonography: diagnosis of ectopic thyroid gland in patients with congenital hypothyroidism caused by thyroid dysgenesis. *J Clin Endocrinol Metab.* 2003;88(11):5145.

94. Salerno M, Militerni R, Bravaccio C, et al. Effect of different starting doses of levothyroxine on growth and intellectual outcome at four years of age in congenital hypothyroidism. *Thyroid.* 2002;12(1):45.

95. Selva KA, Harper A, Downs A, et al. Neurodevelopmental outcomes in congenital hypothyroidism: comparison of initial T_4 dose and time to reach target T_4 and TSH. *J Pediatr.* 2005;147(6):775.

96. Balhara B, Misra M, Levitsky L. Clinical monitoring guidelines for congenital hypothyroidism: laboratory outcome data in the first year of life. *J Pediatr.* 2011;158(4):532.

97. Eugster EA, LeMay D, Zerin JM, et al. Definitive diagnosis in children with congenital hypothyroidism. *J Pediatr.* 2004;144(5):643.

98. Gruters A, Jenner A, Krude H. Long-term consequences of congenital hypothyroidism in the era of screening programmes. *Best Pract Res Clin Endocrinol Metab.* 2002;16(2):369.

99. Srinivasan R, Hariqopal S, Turner S, et al. Permanent and transient congenital hypothyroidism in preterm infants. *Acta Paediatr.* 2012;101(4):e179.

100. Murphy N, Hume R, van Toor H, et al. The hypothalamic-pituitary-thyroid axis in preterm infants; changes in the first 24 hours of postnatal life. *J Clin Endocrinol Metab.* 2004;89(6):2824.

101. Osborn DA, Hunt RW. Postnatal thyroid hormones for preterm infants with transient hypothyroxinaemia. *Cochrane Database Syst Rev.* 2007;24(1):CD005945.

102. Rapaport R, Rose SR, Freemark M. Hypothyroxinemia in the preterm infant: the benefit and risk of thyroxine treatment. *J Pediatr.* 2001;139(2):182.

103. La Gamma EF, Paneth N. Clinical importance of hypothyroxinemia in the preterm infant and a discussion of treatment concerns. *Curr Opin Pediatr.* 2012;24(2):172.

104. Kratzch J. Thyroid gland development and defects. *Best Pract Res Clin Endocrinol Metab.* 2008;22(1):57.

105. Hyman SJ, Novoa Y, Holzman I. Perinatal endocrinology: common endocrine disorders in the sick and premature newborn. *Pediatr Clin North Am.* 2011;58(5):1083.

106. Persani L. Central hypothyroidism: pathogenic, diagnostic, and therapeutic challenges. *J Clin Endocrinol Metab.* 2012;97(9):3068.

107. Kempers MJ, Lanting CI, van Heijst AF, et al. Neonatal screening for congenital hypothyroidism based on thyroxine, thyrotropin, and thyroxine-binding globulin measurement: potentials and pitfalls. *J Clin Endocrinol Metab.* 91:3370.

108. Cohen LE. Genetic disorders of the pituitary. *Curr Opin Endocrinol Diabetes Obes.* 2012;19(1):33.

109. Rapaport R, Akler G, Regelmann MO, et al. Time for thyrotropin releasing hormone to return to the United States of America. *Thyroid.* 2010;20(9):947.

110. Van Tijn DA, de Vijlder JJ, Vulsma T. Role of the thyrotropin-releasing hormone stimulation test in diagnosis of congenital central hypothyroidism in infants. *J Clin Endocrinol Metab.* 2008;93(2):410.

111. Van Tijn DA, Schroor EJ, Delemarre-van de Waal HA, et al. Early assessment of hypothalamic-pituitary-gonadal function in patients with congenital hypothyroidism of central origin. *J Clin Endocrinol Metab.* 2007;92(1):104.

112. Delman BN. Imaging of pediatric pituitary abnormalities. *Endocrinol Metab Clin North Am.* 2009;38(4):673.

113. Shimon I, Cohen O, Lubetsky A, et al. Thyrotropin suppression by thyroid hormone replacement is correlated with thyroxine level normalization in central hypothyroidism. *Thyroid.* 2002;12:823.

114. Beck-Peccoz P. Treatment of central hypothyroidism. *Clin Endocrinol (Oxf).* 2011;74(6):671.

115. Laurberg P, Bournaud C, Karmisholt J, et al. Management of Graves' hyperthyroidism in pregnancy: focus on both maternal and foetal thyroid function, and caution against surgical thyroidectomy in pregnancy. *Eur J Endocrinol.* 2009;160:1.

116. Mestman JH. Hyperthyroidism in pregnancy. *Curr Opin Endocrinol Diabetes Obes.* 2012;19(5):394.

117. Franklyn JA, Boelaert K. Thyrotoxicosis. *Lancet.* 2012;379(9821):1115.

118. Korelitz JJ, McNally DL, Masters MN, et al. Prevalence of thyrotoxicosis, anti-thyroid medication use, and complications

among pregnant women in the United States. *Thyroid.* 2013;23(6):758–765.

119. Hackmon R, Blichowski M, Koren G. The safety of methimazole and propylthiouracil in pregnancy: a systematic review. *J Obstet Gynaecol Can.* 2012;34(11):1077.

120. Stagnaro-Green A, Abalovich M, Alexander E, et al. Guidelines of the American Thyroid Association for the diagnosis and management of thyroid disease during pregnancy and postpartum. *Thyroid.* 2011;21(10):1081.

121. Zakarija M, McKenzie JM, Munro DS. Studies on multiple thyroid cell membrane directed antibodies in Graves' disease. *J Clin Invest.* 1983;76:1885.

122. Zakarija M, McKenzi JM, Hoffman WH. Prediction and therapy of intrauterine and late-onset neonatal hyperthyroidism. *J Clin Endocrinol Metab.* 1986;62(2):368.

123. Skuza KA, Sill IN, Stene M, et al. Prediction of neonatal hyperthyroidism in infants born to mothers with Graves disease. *J Pediatr.* 1996;128(2):264.

124. Zakarija M, McKenzie JM. Pregnancy-associated changes in the thyroid-stimulating antibody of Graves' disease and the relationship to neonatal hyperthyroidism. *J Clin Endocrinol Metab.* 1986;62:368.

125. De Groot L, Abalovich M, Alexander EK, et al. Management of thyroid dysfunction during pregnancy and postpartum: an Endocrine Society clinical practice guideline. *J Clin Endocrinol Metab.* 2012;97(8):2543.

126. Rivkees SA, Szarfman A. Dissimilar hepatotoxicity profiles of propylthiouracil and methimazole in children. *J Clin Endocrinol Metab.* 2010;95(7):3260.

127. Daneman D, Howard NJ. Neonatal thyrotoxicosis: intellectual impairment and craniosynostosis in later years. *J Pediatr.* 1980;97(2):257.

128. Kempers MJE, van Trotsenburg ASP, van Rijn RR, et al. Loss of integrity of thyroid morphology and function in children born to mothers with inadequately treated Graves' disease. *J Clin Endocrinol Metab.* 2007;92(8):2984.

129. Gallagher MP, Schachner HC, Levine LS, et al. Neonatal thyroid enlargement associated with propylthiouracil therapy of Graves' disease during pregnancy: a problem revisited. *J Pediatr.* 2001;139(6):896.

48 Disorders of Sexual Differentiation

Romano T. DeMarco and H. Eugene Hoyme

INTRODUCTION

Normal sexual development requires a series of sequential and highly regulated events early in fetal development. This sexual differentiation process is regulated through complex interactions from both genetic and hormonal signals. Any disruption in this developmental pathway can lead to a disorder of sex differentiation (DSD).

Neonates born with ambiguous genitalia present a daunting challenge to all involved in health care delivery to the individual patient. An urgent evaluation by appropriate disciplines with discrete and delicate interaction with the family is mandatory. Older and potentially negative and confusing terminology has been replaced and should not be used. A new nomenclature for disorders of sex development, introduced at the 2005 Chicago Consensus Conference,[1] is more precise, integrates better the progress in our understanding of the molecular basis of development, and is more sensitive to the concerns of the family and patients (Table 48-1).

NORMAL SEXUAL DIFFERENTIATION AND DEVELOPMENT

Undifferentiated Stage of Sexual Differentiation

Normal fetal development of the gonads and the genitalia proceed through 3 sequential stages. The first stage involves the formation of the bipotential gonads

from the adrenogonadal ridge at approximately 4 to 5 weeks' gestation. During this undifferentiated stage, identical structures form in both the XY and XX embryo (Figure 48-1). These structures emanate from the mesonephros and coelomic epithelium. They are the wolffian (precursors to the formation of the seminal vesicles, epididymis, and vas deferens) and müllerian ducts (precursors to the fallopian tubes, uterus, and vagina).

During this phase, the cloaca, which is the terminal portion of the hindgut limited by the cloacal membrane, is partitioned into an anterior urogenital sinus and a posterior anorectal canal. Subsequently, the urogenital sinus becomes the bladder in both sexes and is the precursor for the prostate and proximal urethra in males and the entire urethra and vagina in females.

Gonadal Differentiation

Testis Formation

By the seventh week of gestation, the undifferentiated gonads in a male embryo develop into a testis under the influence of the *SRY* (sex determining region of the Y chromosome) gene located on the short arm of the Y chromosome. The *SRY* gene expression causes the primitive sex cords to differentiate into Sertoli cells, which when organized form the seminiferous cords. Primordial germ cells populate near the basement membrane of the cords, while Leydig cells appear in the interstitium between the cords around 8 weeks.

Table 48-1 Proposed Revised Nomenclature

Previous	Proposed
Intersex	Disorders of sex development (DSD)
Male pseudohermaphrodite	
Undervirilization of an XY male	46,XY DSD
Undermasculinization of an XY male	
Female pseudohermaphrodite	
Overvirilization of an XX female	46,XX DSD
Masculinization of an XX female	
True hermaphrodite	Ovotesticular DSD
XX male or XX sex reversal	46,XX testicular DSD
XY sex reversal	46,XY complete gonadal dysgenesis

[a]Reproduced with permission from Hughes IA, Houk C, Ahmed SF, et al.[1]

Ovary Formation

In the female embryo, the undifferentiated gonad does not contain the Y chromosome. Thus, there is no *SRY* gene production with no resultant differentiation of cells into Sertoli cells. The primitive sex cords degenerate, and secondary sex cords formed from the genital ridge join with primordial germ cells to form the ovarian follicles. At this time, the germ cells differentiate into oogonia and become oocytes following the first meiotic division. Many oocytes at this time are surrounded by a single layer of granulosa cells, becoming primary follicles at around 15 weeks' gestation. Further meiosis is arrested under puberty when under hormonal influence meiosis resumes. The total population of germ cells reaches an apex of several million by 5 months' gestation. However, by the time of birth, most cells have undergone apoptosis, leaving approximately 150,000 oocytes in each ovary at birth.

Other Genes Involved in Gonadal Differentiation

DAX1

The *DAX1* gene has been implicated in several cases of XY sex reversal.[2] Screening of XY females with a normal SRY gene detected the presence of a submicroscopic duplication of a region designated DDS (dosage-sensitive sex reversal). Within this region, the *DAX1* gene was identified. Investigation using a transgenic, XY genotype mouse carrying extra copies of the *DAX1* gene led to a phenotypically female mouse in the setting of low expression of the SRY gene.[3]

SOX9

The *SOX9* gene was found to play a role in sex determination through investigation of patients with campomelic dysplasia (CD).[4] In this rare skeletal disorder, a high preponderance of patients were found to have male-to-female sex reversal. Loss-of-function mutations of *SOX9* were found in XY females with CD, pointing to a critical role *SOX9* likely plays in sex determination.[5] While the exact targets of *SOX9* are

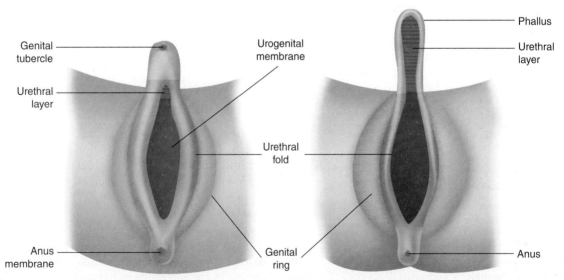

FIGURE 48-1 Diagram of the external genitalia in the undifferentiated period. (Reproduced with permission from Diamond.[29])

unclear, it is structurally similar to *SRY* and has been proposed to be responsible for an *SRY*-negative, XX male patient.[6]

SF-1

Steroidogenic factor 1 (*SF-1*) is a transcription factor that plays a key role in the regulation of endocrine function and development of the adrenal glands and the gonads in both sexes. The results of *SF-1* knockout mice models demonstrated a failure of adrenal and gonadal development with XY sex reversal with persistence of the müllerian ducts in males. Ovaries fail to develop in XX female mice lacking the *SF-1* gene.[7] Clinically, there has been a report of an XY female who was found to have adrenal failure at 2 weeks with a poorly differentiated testis, normal female genitalia, and the presence of a uterus. On evaluation, she was found to have a heterozygous mutation in the DNA-binding domain of *SF-1*, which was likely the cause of the clinical findings.[8]

WT1

The Wilms tumor 1 (*WT1*) gene was originally discovered on chromosome 11p13 during efforts to find the oncogene responsible for Wilms tumor.[9] Following its discovery, further investigation of *WT1* expression in humans and mice models demonstrated a significant relationship between *WT1* protein secretion and sex determination. *WT1* expression has been found to have a complex role with multiple sites of action, including modulating *SF-1* expression, regulating *SRY* gene actions, and competing with *DAX1*.[10–12]

Mutations involving *WT1* expression are linked to urinary and genital abnormalities in 3 syndromes: WAGR (Wilms tumor, aniridia, genitourinary anomalies, and mental retardation) syndrome, Denys-Drash syndrome, and Frazier syndrome. Denys-Drash syndrome is a rare genetic disorder associated with gonadal and genital abnormalities, Wilms tumor, and renal failure due to mesangial sclerosis. Frasier syndrome is characterized by male-to-female sex reversal, focal segmental glomerular sclerosis, and Wilms tumor.

Differentiation of the Genital Ducts and External Genitalia

Male Genital Duct Development

By the eighth week of gestation, the developing Sertoli cells secrete müllerian-inhibiting substance (MIS), which causes the müllerian ducts to regress rapidly by the 10th week of gestation. Between the 8th and 12th weeks, Leydig cells secrete testosterone, which stimulates the cranial aspect of the wolffian duct to transform into the epididymis and vas deferens. The caudal portion of the wolffian duct develops into the ejaculatory ducts and seminal vesicles (Figure 48-2).

Female Genital Duct Development

In the female fetus, müllerian duct formation proceeds in the absence of MIS secretion. The müllerian ducts give rise to the fallopian tubes and uterus by the 12th week of gestation. Historically, it was accepted that the upper two-thirds of the vagina originated from the müllerian ducts, with the lower third developing from the posterior urogenital sinus and fusing around 12 weeks' gestation. Recent small-animal studies have called into question this theory, with genetic molecular work pointing to a complete müllerian vagina.[13]

Development of the External Genitalia

The early development of the external genitalia is similar in both sexes. Around the fifth week of gestation, a pair of swellings called the cloacal folds joins anterior to the cloacal membrane to form the genital tubercle. The urogenital and labioscrotal folds then appear shortly on either side of the genital tubercle.

Development of Male External Genitalia

In the male fetus, the undifferentiated stage of genital development ends around the ninth week with secretion of testosterone and local conversion to dihydrotestosterone causing an increase in distance between the genital tubercle and anal folds (Figure 48-3). The genital tubercle elongates to become the penis, with the urethral groove forming over the ventrum of the penis. Urethral folds, which are extensions of the urogenital folds, form the lateral margins of the urethral groove. The urethra is then created with the fusion of the urethral folds over the urethral groove. The labioscrotal folds then fuse in the midline to create the scrotum. The urogenital folds fuse over the newly created urethra to provide skin coverage for the penis. This process is completed by the 14th week. The phallus will continue to grow throughout the remainder of gestation. Testicular descent occurs through multiple mechanisms and is typically complete by the third trimester.

Development of Female External Genitalia

In the absence of testosterone, the genital tubercle bends inferiorly and forms the clitoris in the female fetus (Figure 48-4). The labioscrotal folds do not fuse in the midline and develop primarily in the caudal portions, forming the labia majora. The urethral folds do not fuse and become the labia minora. The anterior urethral meatus and posterior vaginal orifice form

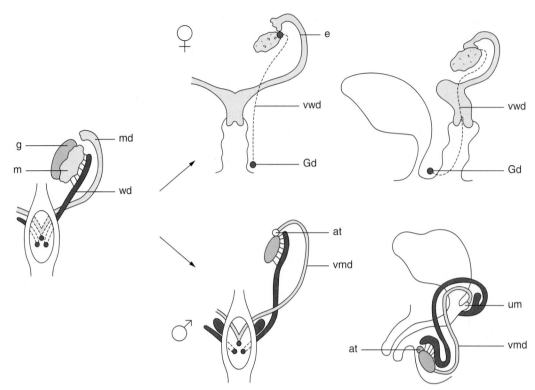

FIGURE 48-2 Fate of the wolffian and müllerian ducts. In the male, the wolffian ducts form the epididymis, vas, and seminal vesicle. In the female, the müllerian ducts form the fallopian tubes, uterus, and upper third of the vagina. at, appendix testis; e, epoöphoron; G, gonad; Gd, Gartner duct; m, mesonephros; md, müllerian duct; um, utriculus masculinus; vmd, vestigial müllerian duct; vwd, vestigial wolffian duct; wd, wolffian duct. (Reproduced with permission from Kelalis P, King LR, Belman AB, et al: The Kelalis-King-Belman textbook of clinical pediatric urology. 5th ed. Abingdon, UK: Informa Healthcare; 2007.)

between the labia minora, with this process complete by 14 weeks.

Psychosexual Differentiation

Our understanding of human psychosexual differentiation is limited and appears complex and multifactorial. The previously accepted view that humans are psychosexually neutral at birth[14] has more recently been questioned by those who support the opposing view that a "neural bias" exists determined primarily by prenatal hormonal exposure.[15] Studies in mammals demonstrated a significant role of both testosterone and estrogen exposure prenatally and sexual differentiation of the brain and behavior in utero.[16,17] This relationship between hormone exposure in utero and psychosexual differentiation is less clear in humans. However, the accumulated evidence demonstrates that androgen exposure prenatally has more influence on gender role (aspects of behavior in which males and

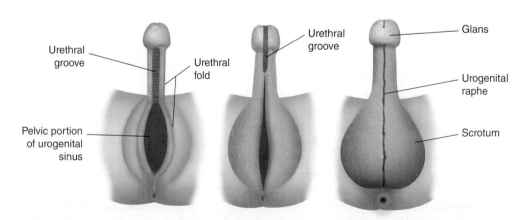

FIGURE 48-3 Differentiation of the male external genitalia. (Reproduced with permission from Diamond.[29])

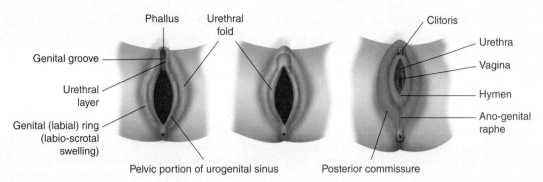

Phallus

Urethral
fold

Clitoris

Genital groove

Urethra

Vagina

Urethral
layer

Hymen

Genital (labial) ring
(labio-scrotal
swelling)

Ano-genital
raphe

Pelvic portion of urogenital sinus

Posterior commissure

FIGURE 48-4 Differentiation of the female external genitalia. (Reproduced with permission from Diamond.[29])

females appear to differ) than gender identity (identification of oneself as either male or female).[18]

CLINICAL EVALUATION OF INFANTS WITH AMBIGUOUS GENITALIA

Prenatal Findings

Prenatal suspicion of a DSD occurs most commonly when abnormalities of the genitalia are found on prenatal sonography or when there is a suspected genotype-phenotype mismatch with the karyotype and visualized genitalia or uterus.[19] Characteristic findings are seen with ultrasound allowing for accurate prenatal sexual determination. Normal male genital findings on ultrasound include the penis, which is initially visualized as an upwardly projected phallic structure, in contrast to the clitoris, which will have a downward bend.[19] Also, fetal penile length can then be measured in terms of a range throughout development.[20] The scrotum can also be detected as a distinct structure by the second trimester[21] and is sonographically distinct from the developing labia.[22] In addition, a nomogram exists for uterine width and circumference measurements, which allows for assessment of normal female genital tract development from the second trimester until birth.[23]

In the rare situations for which genital abnormalities are suspected prenatally, it is important to follow the fetus longitudinally throughout the pregnancy. Fetal ultrasounds at 13–15 weeks are not good predictors of external genital development.[19] The presence of a uterus after 19 weeks is a reliable predictor of internal reproductive organs. Karyotypic or external genital discrepancies based on the presence of a uterus should lead to cautious antenatal counseling, which can include the disciplines of neonatology, pediatric endocrinology, genetic counseling, pediatric urology, and psychology. Certainly, the assignment of sex for the child would be withheld until appropriate postnatal evaluation.

Postnatal Evaluation

Every newborn must have a careful and complete genital examination. The importance of the examination includes not only assignment of the appropriate gender, but also the accurate diagnosis of more common abnormalities, such as hypospadias, chordee, and undescended testes.

Optimal management of neonates with a suspected DSD as recommended by the Lawson Wilkins Pediatric Endocrine Society (LWPES) and the European Society for Paediatric Endocrinology (ESPE) includes the following: (1) Avoidance of gender assignment before expert evaluation is complete. (2) Evaluation and long-term management must be carried out at center with an experienced multidisciplinarian team. (3) All neonates should receive a gender assignment. (4) Open communication with patients and families is essential, and participation in decision making is encouraged. (5) Patient and family concerns should be respected and addressed in strict confidence.

Physical Examination

In the apparent male neonate, the palpability, location, and size of the testis (or ovotestis) should be noted. Ovaries do not descend. The length and diameter of the penis should be measured. Penile length is measured as the stretched length following the reduction of the prepubic fat from the pubic ramus to the tip of glans. Boys with a stretched penile length at term of less than 2 cm in an otherwise physically normal phallus have a micropenis. The location of the urethral meatus should be properly identified. The presence of ventral congenital curvature (chordee) should be documented. Neonates with severe chordee can make obtaining a true stretched penile length difficult. A flat, symmetric scrotum typically indicates bilateral undescended testes. A cleft or bifid scrotum usually occurs in conjunction with a severe penoscrotal or scrotal hypospadias and can look similar to labia.

In the apparent female neonate, the clitoris should be assessed for general size. Clitoromegaly can be dramatic, and in these patients, a stretched length and width should be measured. The urethral location and relationship to a separate vaginal orifice should be carefully assessed. In female fetuses exposed to high levels of testosterone in utero, a common distal stem off the vagina and urethra can occur (urogenital sinus). The os of the urogenital sinus can be located on the perineum or associated with the masculinized clitoris. The labia are normally unfused in females. Fusion, anterior placement of the labia with hyperpigmentation, and absence of labia minora are also signs of in utero androgen exposure. The uterus may be palpable on rectal examination as a cord-like structure anterior to the rectum.

A DSD evaluation should proceed in neonates with the physical findings of (1) overt genital ambiguity; (2) apparent female genitalia with an enlarged clitoris, posterior labial fusion, or an inguinal or labial mass; or (3) apparent male genitalia with bilateral undescended testes, micropenis, isolated perineal hypospadias, or hypospadias (Figure 48-5).

Laboratory Evaluation

Immediate laboratory evaluation of a neonate with a suspected DSD consists of measurement of serum electrolytes, testosterone, and dihydrotestosterone levels and karyotype. Serum 17-hydroxyprogesterone should not be measured until day of life 3 or 4 because elevated levels of this corticosteroid precursor can be found in normal neonates during the first few days of life due to the stress of delivery.[24] If 17-hydroxyprogesterone is elevated, 11-deoxycortisol and deoycorticosterone levels are required. LH (luteinizing hormone) levels or a hCG (human chorionic gonadotropin) stimulation test can be performed

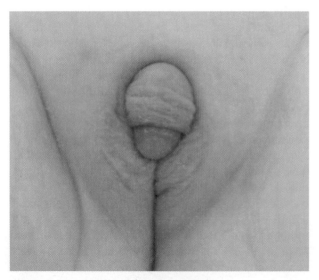

FIGURE 48-5 Virilized female genitalia.

to determine if functioning testicular tissue is present in the neonate with bilateral nonpalpable testes.

Radiographic Evaluation

An abdominal and pelvic ultrasound is recommended as the first-line imaging study in the neonate with ambiguous genitalia. The presence of a uterus is accurately seen with pelvic ultrasound.[25] Gonads may be seen, but the specificity and sensitivity of ultrasound is poor for nonpalpable testes and the presence of ovaries.[26] The absence of visible gonads does not confirm their absence. In experienced hands, adrenal sonography is an accurate adjunct for the diagnosis of congenital adrenal hyperplasia (CAH).[27] Studies, such as pelvic magnetic resonance imaging (MRI), flush genitogram, and retrograde urethrogram, are necessary in certain situations, typically dependent on physical examination findings.

CLASSIFICATION OF DISORDERS OF SEXUAL DIFFERENTIATION

Sex Chromosome Disorder of Sex Development

45,X/46,XY (Mixed Gondal Dysgenesis)

Mixed gonadal dysgenesis (MGD) is a group of disorders characterized by a unilateral testis, which is typically undescended; an intra-abdominal contralateral streak gonad, persistent müllerian duct structures; and varying degrees of virilization of the external genitalia.[28] Infants typically present with ambiguous genitalia as this condition is the second-most-common cause of a DSD in the newborn period.[29] The unilateral testis may be descended but usually is palpable in the groin or nonpalpable when located abdominally.

The uterus is typically rudimentary with bilateral fallopian tubes. In those patients with a well-differentiated testis, the ipsilateral fallopian is commonly absent. A urogenital sinus is present in about one-half of patients.

When the unilateral testis is palpable, it is typically more normal. However, the testicular cellular architecture is consistently abnormal in the adult patient, demonstrating few germ cells and sclerosis of the tubules.[30] Wolffian structures are more commonly found on the side of the unilateral testis and usually include only the epididymis, with a well-differentiated vas deferens rarely present.

47,XXY (Klinefelter Syndrome and Variants)

Klinefelter syndrome is the most common abnormality of sexual differentiation, occurring in approximately 1 in every 600 live newborn males.[31] The syndrome is classically characterized by gynecomastia, small testes, absent spermatogenesis, normal-to-moderately reduced Leydig cell function, and increased secretion of follicle-stimulating hormone (FSH).[32] It is most commonly associated with the 47,XXY karyotype, but upward of 20% of patients will have higher-grade chromosome aneuploidies, 46XY/47XXY mosaicism, or structurally abnormal X chromosomes.[33]

The diagnosis is made prenatally in approximately 10% of patients because of genetic screening programs.[31] Neonatal diagnosis is rare but can occur during an evaluation for micropenis, severe hypospadias, and undescended or small testes. Typically, the diagnosis is made following puberty when androgen deficiency becomes apparent. Young men with Klinefelter syndrome have sparse body and facial hair. Approximately half of the patients will develop gynecomastia. Adult men have small testes, which rarely exceed 2 cm in length and are atrophic on microscopic examination.

45,X (Turner Syndrome and Variants)

Turner syndrome is associated with an immature female phenotype with short stature, streak gonads, and various congenital anomalies. It is classically and most frequently associated with a missing X chromosome. Variant forms occur less commonly and include partial deletions of the second X chromosome. Various mosaicisms do occur and typically involve the X chromosome. In approximately 5% of patients, a 45,X/46XY mosaicism is found.

Neonates with Turner syndrome do not have ambiguous genitalia but have other somatic features that are noted both antenatally and perinatally, which can lead to the diagnosis (Table 48-2). A clinical guideline pathway exists for those children with a new diagnosis of Turner syndrome. The workup includes a cardiology evaluation, renal ultrasound, hearing testing, and referral to the appropriate support groups. Those patients with a diagnosis missed early in life are typically diagnosed later because of short stature, primary amenorrhea, or lack of secondary sexual development.

Müllerian structures are well differentiated but remain small. The ovaries are streaks by birth with rare surviving oocytes by adolescence. A small number of pregnancies have been reported. Those children with 45,X/46XY mosaicism and occult Y chromosome material have a 7% to 30% risk of developing a gonadoblastoma.

46,XX/46,XY Chimerism or Ovotesticular Development

Ovotesticular disorder, formerly known as true hermaphroditism, is defined as an individual who has both testicular tissue with seminiferous tubules and ovarian tissue with primordial follicles. The combination of

Table 48-2 Antenatal and Neonatal Features of Turner Syndrome[a]

Frequency	Findings
Greater than 50%	Low posterior hairline
	Lymphedema
	Nail dysplasia
	Prominent ears
	Retrognathia
	Narrow palate
	Webbed neck
25%–50%	Cubitus valgus
	Short fourth metacarpals
	Ptosis
	Strabismus
	Multiple nevi
	Epicanthal folds
10%–25%	Scoliosis
	Kyphosis
	Pectus excavatum
	Single palmar crease
	Inverted nipples
	Genu valgum
Less than 10%	Madelung deformity
	Patellar dislocation

[a]Reproduced with permission from Davenport.[68]

gonads in this disorder includes an ovotestis and ovary (40%), bilateral ovotestes (34%), ovotestis and testis (15%), and ovary and testis (10%).[34]

Patients predominantly are born with ambiguous genitalia and can have varying karyotypes. Approximately 60% of patients are 46,XX, 33% are either a 46,XX/46,XY chimerism or a 46,XX/46XXY mosaicism, and 7% are 46,XY. Understanding of the signaling pathway for testicular formation in patients with a 46,XX karyotype is not completely elucidated but likely involves an X-linked or autosomal mutation, which causes testicular differentiation downstream of the SRY gene.[29]

Most have more masculinized genitalia and are raised as males following hypospadias and chordee repair. Children raised as females usually have clitoromegaly and a urogenital sinus. Ovaries are typically in a normal location with an associated fallopian tube and usually found on the left side. Testes or ovotestes are more commonly found on the right and can be found anywhere in the normal testicular descent pathway.[35] Testes or an ovotestis with predominantly testicular tissue are more likely to descend. A vas deferens and epididymis are almost always present with a testis.

In ovotestes, a fallopian tube is found two-thirds of the time as compared to either a vas deferens or both internal ducts in a third.

Histologically, ovarian tissue is typically normal in the ovotestis with the exception of a reduced number of primordial follicles. In contrast, the testicular component of an ovotestis has tubular atrophy with absent spermatogenesis. Gonadal tumors occur in 2%–3% of these patients.[36]

46,XY Disorders of Sexual Development

Disorders of Testicular Development

Complete Gonadal Dysgenesis

Children with complete gonadal dysgenesis have a 46,XY karyotype, female-appearing external genitalia, normal müllerian structures, and bilateral streak gonads similar to Turner syndrome.[37] The majority of patients present in their teens with absent breast development and amenorrhea. Some patients demonstrate clitoromegaly, thought to be due to the elevated levels of gonadotropins.[29] The diagnosis is usually made from the karyotype ordered during the evaluation. Patients with complete gonadal dysgenesis have a 30% risk of developing malignant tumors in their gonads by age 30.[38]

Partial Gonadal Dysgenesis

Patients with partial gonadal dysgenesis (PGD) present similarly to those patients with MGD except that those with PGD have 2 dysgenetic testes rather than 1 dysgenetic testis and a streak gonad. The genital phenotype can range from ambiguous to either normal male or female. This variance is due to the ability and timing of secretion of testosterone from the dysgenetic testes. Usually, persistent müllerian structures are present, but to varying degrees related to MIS secretion. Similar to patients with complete gonadal dysgenesis, those with PGD are at a high risk for gonadal malignancy.[38]

Testis Regression and Bilateral Vanishing Testes Syndromes

The testis regression and bilateral vanishing testes syndromes encompass a wide spectrum of phenotypes that occur due to testes that "vanish" antenatally, causing varying degrees of abnormalities of both the external genitalia and internal duct development. Testis regression syndrome usually refers to a loss of testicular tissue within the first trimester, resulting in genital ambiguity. In contrast, bilateral vanishing testes syndrome is thought to occur later in utero, after male sexual differentiation of both the internal ducts and external genital anatomy.[39]

The etiology of the vanishing testis is not elucidated, but hypotheses include bilateral torsion, a genetic mutation, or a teratogen. Neonates with bilateral vanishing testes syndrome present typically with phallic abnormalities, such as a micropenis or severe chordee, or as a phenotypically normal male with an empty scrotum.[40] Newborns have castrate levels of testosterone in the setting of elevated serum LH and FSH and a 46,XY karotype.

Patients with bilateral vanishing testes syndrome present with ambiguous genitalia or as a phenotypically normal female, depending on the in utero timing of the insult. In severe cases, a 46,XY female is diagnosed at puberty with no müllerian or wolffian structures. This is thought to occur due to the secretion of MIS from the testes prior to regression before androgen secretion.

Disorders in Androgen Synthesis or Action

Androgen Biosynthesis Defect

A defect in any of the steps involved in the synthesis of testosterone from cholesterol will result in absent or decreased production of androgens and resultant 46,XY DSD. There are 6 specific steps involved in this process, 5 involving enzymes (Figure 48-6). Three of these enzymes are required also for cortisol production (cholesterol side-chain cleavage enzyme, 17α-hydroxylase, 3β-hydroxysteroid dehydrogenase), and their defect will lead to impaired cortisol and possibly mineralocorticoid production. All 5 of these enzyme deficiencies are inherited in an autosomal recessive pattern.

StAR Deficiency (Congenital Lipoid Adrenal Hyperplasia). The first step in steroidogenesis involves the transport of cholesterol into the mitochondria. This defect in steroidogenic acute regulator (StAR) protein leads to significant feminization of the genitalia with either completely female features or ambiguous genitalia. Patients have testes located in the abdomen, inguinal canal, or labia. Rudimentary wolffian structures are present with an absence of müllerian ducts. Neonates develop adrenal insufficiency. In some cases, this is life-threatening, affecting newborns as young as 1–2 days old. Other newborns have a milder presentation and present at an older age (2–4 weeks). Patients with this disorder have an enormous accumulation of lipid in the adrenal gland as seen on abdominal imaging, alternatively giving the name congenital lipoid adrenal hyperplasia.

Cholesterol Side-Chain Cleavage Enzyme Deficiency. The second step in steroid hormone synthesis is the conversion of cholesterol to pregnenolone by cholesterol side-chain cleavage enzyme. A deficiency in this enzyme leads to ambiguous genitalia in affected

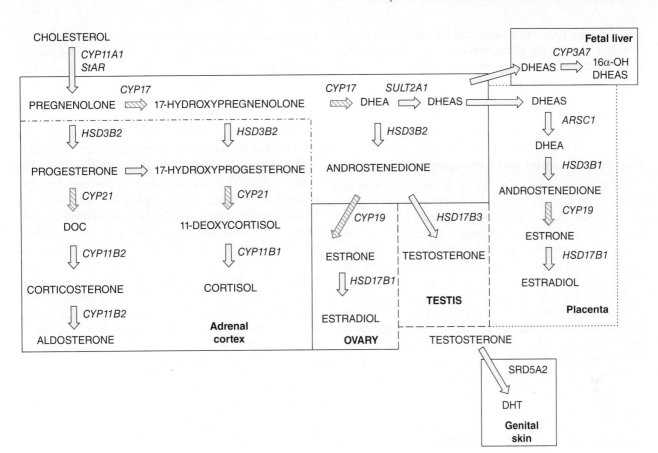

FIGURE 48-6 Steroidogenic pathways. Substrates, products, and genes involved in adrenal, ovarian, testicular, and placental steroidogenesis. Genes are 17α-hydroxylase/17,20-lyase (CYP17), 3β-hydroxysteroid dehydrogenase (HSD3B2), 21-hydroxylase (CYP21), 11β-hydroxylase (CYP11B1), aldosterone synthase (CPY11B2), aromatase (CYP19), 17β-hydroxysteroid dehydrogenase type 1 (HSD17B1), 17β-hydroxysteroid dehydrogenase type 3 (HSD17B3), 5α-reductase type 2 (SRD5A2), sulfotransferase (SULT2A1), and steroid sulfatase/arylsulfatase C (ARSC1). CYP3A7 is a cytochrome P450 enzyme expressed in fetal liver, where it catalyzes the 16α-hydroxylation of estrone (E1) and DHEA (dehydroepiandrosterone). Its expression decreases postnatally. Steroidogenic enzymes that utilize P450 oxidoreductase to transfer electrons are indicated by hatched arrows. DHEAS, dehydroepiandrosterone sulfate; DHT, dihydrotestosterone; DOC, 11-deoxycortisol. (Reproduced from Witchel and Lee.[68])

XY males. Corticosteroid and mineralocorticoid production is also impaired, requiring prompt identification and treatment.

3β-Hydroxysteroid Dehydrogenase Deficiency. The 3β-hydroxysteroid dehydrogenase enzyme is found early in the pathway for steroidogenesis and is required for formation of all steroids. Its deficiency affects production of glucocorticoids, mineralocorticoids, and the sex steroids. Boys with 3β-hydroxysteroid dehydrogenase insufficiency have incomplete masculinization of the external genitalia, with findings of a small phallus with hypospadias, a urogenital sinus with blindending vaginal pouch, and scrotal testes on examination. Patients have normal wolffian and no müllerian ducts. Salt wasting occurs because of the impaired production of cortisol and aldosterone.

17α-Hydroxylase Deficiency. Patients with 17α-hydroxylase deficiency disorder have absent or only slight masculinization of the external genitalia.

Many have normal female genitalia with a blindending vaginal pouch and intra-abdominal testes. The deficiency of 17α-hydroxylase leads to the accumulation of desoxycorticosterone, corticosterone, and 18-hydroxycorticosterone in the adrenals, which leads to salt and water retention, hypokalemia, and hypertension.

17,20-Lyase Deficiency. Newborns with deficiency of 17,20-lyase can have a wide spectrum of genital abnormalities, but usually present with ambiguous genitalia. If the diagnosis is not made as an infant, patients present at puberty because of a lack of secondary sexual characteristics.

17β-Hydroxysteroid Oxireductase Deficiency. Newborns with deficiency of 17β-hydroxysteroid oxireductase appear to have a normal phenotype and are typically raised female. These patients have intra-abdominal, inguinal, or labial located testes with normal wolffian and absent müllerian ducts. The diagnosis may be made during repair of an inguinal hernia but typically is made at puberty when there is significant phallic growth and development of male secondary sexual characteristics. Pubertal increases in gonadotropin production lead to a spike in androstenedione production, which overcomes the enzymatic defect and raises testosterone levels into the low-normal range.

Androgen Receptor and Postreceptor Defects

Androgen Insensitivity Syndromes. Patients with both complete and partial androgen receptor defects characteristically have a 46,XY karyotype with bilateral testes. Abnormalities of androgen receptor function represent the most common definable cause of the undervirilized male and are transmitted as an X-linked trait.[29] Those with complete androgen insensitivity syndrome have no associated or limited derivatives of wolffian structures.[41] These patients have a female phenotype and no müllerian structures. Diagnosis is rare before puberty unless a karyotype is performed during pregnancy or if testes are found in the groin or labia on physical examination or during repair of an inguinal hernia. Otherwise, these patients present at puberty with primary amenorrhea and development of secondary female sexual characteristics due to the conversion of testosterone to estradiol.

Newborns with partial androgen insensitivity syndrome have incomplete masculinization of their external genitalia. On examination, there is a wide spectrum of findings, but patients usually have hypospadias, bilateral undescended testes, and rudimentary wolffian structures. Multiple mutations of the androgen receptor gene exist, but in general, the abnormality exists as a reduced number of normally functioning receptors or a normal receptor number but decreased binding affinity.[42]

Disorders of Androgen Action. 5α-Reductase is an enzyme that converts testosterone to dihydrotestosterone. The absence of the enzyme is transmitted in an autosomal recessive pattern, with only homozygous males affected. These children have normal formation of testes and male internal genital duct through the action of testosterone. However, without dihydrotestosterone, normal male external genitalia do not occur. Neonates with this condition present with severe hypospadias or more commonly with ambiguous genitalia. Patients undiagnosed as newborns with bilateral nonpalpable testes can present in a very unusual fashion at puberty with significant phallic development and subsequent gender reversal due to markedly high levels of testosterone.[43]

Luteinizing Hormone Receptor Abnormality. LH receptor abnormality or Leydig cell aplasia is found typically during an evaluation for a delay in puberty in an adolescent girl. Younger patients may present with this condition with a palpable testis in the inguinal canal or labia. This disorder is characterized by a normal 46,XY karyotype with no wolffian or müllerian structures and a short vagina. It is transmitted as an autosomal recessive trait. Laboratory examination is classic for a low basal level of testosterone, which does not respond to hCG stimulation. Testicular cellular architecture demonstrates an absence or severe reduction in the number of Leydig cells but normal Sertoli cells.

Antimüllerian Hormone and Receptor Abnormality. The condition of antimüllerian hormone and receptor (AMR) abnormality, also known as persistent müllerian duct syndrome or as classically described hernia uteri inguinale,[44] has characteristic features of a normal-appearing 46,XY male with internal müllerian structures. Patients usually have bilateral fallopian tubes, a uterus, a vagina draining into a prostatic utricle, and either unilateral or bilateral undescended testes. Most frequently, this condition is found during an inguinal hernia repair or orchiopexy when müllerian structures are encountered.

Antimüllerian hormone and receptor abnormality appears to be a heterogeneous genetic disorder affecting the production of either AMH or its receptor. Its transmission occurs as a sporadic mutation or as an X-linked trait. Several clinical forms have been described. The majority of patients (60%–70%) have bilateral intra-abdominal testes similar in location to ovaries. The next-most-common presentation (20% to 30%) is when 1 testis is partially descended and a uterus and fallopian tube are encountered during the inguinal hernia repair, the classic hernia uteri inguinale presentation. The least commonly seen group (10%) is when both testes are found in the same hernia sac with fallopian tubes and uterus due to transverse testicular ectopia.[45]

46,XX Disorders of Sex Development

Disorders of Ovarian Development

Gonadal Dysgenesis

Children with 46,XX gonadal dysgenesis have findings similar to Turner syndrome: bilateral streak gonads, normal müllerian structures with absence of wolffian structures, and normal external genitalia. They differ as these patients have a normal karyotype and stature without other classic physical findings seen in Turner syndrome. Familial cases do occur, which may include include renal disorders, neurologic abnormalities, and sensorineural hearing loss.[46]

Testicular Disorder of Sex Development (46,XX Male)

The classic presentation of an individual with testicular disorder of sex development (46,XX male) is a normal male phenotype with a 46,XX karyotype. Nonclassic forms occur around 10%–20% percent of the time in neonates with varying degrees of sexual ambiguity and a 46,XX karyotype.[47] Patients with this condition have normal testes at birth that under the influence of the second X chromosome, deteriorate by adulthood as demonstrated by small testicular volume, an absence of spermatogonia, and hyalinization of the seminiferous tubules. Approximately 90% of boys of with this disorder result from an abnormal Y-to-X translocation involving the SRY gene during meiosis.[48] Those with more SRY gene material are typically more virilized.

46,XX Ovotesticular Disorder

For discussion of 46,XX ovotesticular disorder, refer to the previous section on 46,XX/46,XY (chimerism or ovotesticular disorder).

Androgen Excess

Congenital Adrenal Hyperplasia

Congenital adrenal hyperplasia is the leading cause for a masculinized female and most common DSD in general. Of the 5 enzymatic deficiencies that cause CAH, only abnormalities in 21-hydroxylase (21HD), 11β-hydroxylase, and to a lesser extent 3β-hydroxysteroid dehydrogenase lead to virilization of the female genitalia.

21-Hydroxylase Deficiency. By far the most common cause of CAH is a deficiency of 21HD, which catalyzes the conversion of 17-OH progesterone to 11-deoxycortisol, a precursor of cortisol. It is transmitted in an autosomal recessive pattern and occurs in approximately 1:15,000 live births. 21HD deficiency is responsible for 95% of CAH cases.[49]

There are 2 forms of 21HD deficiency. The most common classic presentation is an infant with both salt wasting and virilization (75%). Twenty-five percent of newborns only virilize.[50] The nonclassic form

is milder, with patients presenting in adolescence and adulthood with androgen excess.

Newborns present with varying degrees of virilization. Girls have enlargement of their clitoris, labia fusion, and a common urogenital sinus. In severe cases, the clitoris appears completely phallic. Prader classified the degrees of masculinization of the external genitalia in females with CAH[51] (Figure 48-7). Müllerian structures and ovaries are typically normal. Without treatment, progressive virilization of the genitalia will continue, with early development of secondary sexual characteristics, premature epiphyseal closure, and short stature.

In neonates with the salt-wasting variant, symptoms become evident within the first several weeks of life. These include nausea, vomiting, dehydration, and progressive weight loss. In some patients, adrenal crisis can occur. Often, this condition is confused with pyloric stenosis. Without rapid and appropriate resuscitation, death can occur due to hyperkalemia, dehydration, and shock.

Affected males, without the salt variant, present with sexual precocity. Characteristic signs can be seen as early as 2 years and include significant phallic enlargement, pubic hair, deepening of the voice, acne, and advanced bone age. The term *little Hercules* has been used to physically describe these boys.

11β-Hydroxylase Deficiency. 11β-Hydroxylase deficiency is the second-most-likely enzymatic deficiency leading to virilization in patients with CAH.[52] Both classic and nonclassic forms are seen. The classic presentation of 11β-hydroxylase deficiency is similar to the classic presentation of 21HD deficiency with marked virilization. In contrast to 21HD deficiency, hypertension is found in the classic form due to the increased serum levels of desoxycorticosterone. Patients with the nonclassic variant present in childhood or adolescence with early virilization. Similar to 21HD, 11β-hydroxylase deficiency is inherited as an autosomal recessive disorder.

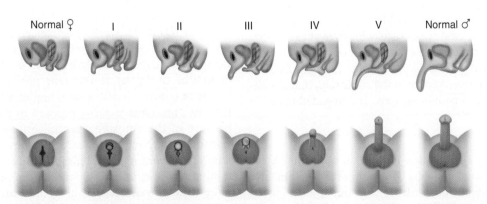

FIGURE 48-7 Classification of masculinization of genitalia in girls with congenital adrenal hyperplasia as described by Prader. (Reproduced with permission from Incidence of congenital adrenogenital syndrome. *Helv Paediatr Acta.* 1958;13(5):426–431.)

3β-Hydroxysteroid Dehydrogenase Deficiency. 3β-Hydroxysteroid dehydrogenase deficiency is the least-common enzyme deficiency causing virilization in CAH. Similar to 21HD deficiency, neonates present with virilization and can have issues with salt wasting. However, genital virilization is usually less in this condition than in children with 21HD deficiency.[53]

Cytochrome P450 Oxidoreductase Deficiency. The cytochrome P450 oxidoreductase enzyme acts as a cofactor for the P450 microsomal enzymes, which include 17α-hydroxylase, 17,20-lyase, and 21HD. Deficiencies in this enzyme can lead to a wide spectrum of both genital abnormalities and cortisol insufficiency.[54] Most neonates with this condition also have Antley-Bixler syndrome (craniosynostosis, hydrocephalus, distinct facies, low-set ears, multiple skeletal anomalies, renal abnormalities, and developmental delay).

Maternal Androgen Excess. Maternal androgen excess is a rare cause of masculinization of the female fetus. Historically, the administration of exogenous androgens or progestational agents during pregnancy caused virilization of the female fetus. Maternal ovarian or adrenal tumors during pregnancy are also rare causes of masculinization. Normal cytochrome P450 aromatase in the placenta converts weak fetal adrenal androgens to estrogens. Its deficiency can lead to virilization of both mother and the female, fetus which resolves following birth.

Unclassified Forms

Exstrophy-Epispadias Complex

The exstrophy-epispadias complex of birth defects is considered a spectrum of embryologic malformations that include abnormalities of the genitalia in both sexes. Boys in particular can have a wide variability in genital anatomy, at times looking ambiguous. In males with epispadias, the urethra is open partially or completely over the dorsum of the penis. The penis is small with significant dorsal chordee. Boys with classic bladder exstrophy similarly have short, dorsally tethered penises but have no urethra, with the bladder opening on the lower abdominal wall. Male newborns with cloacal exstrophy have widely divergent, short corporal bodies, which may be asymmetric or absent unilaterally, giving a bizarre genital appearance. Adding to the confusion, males with cloacal exstrophy commonly have undescended testes.

Hypospadias

Hypospadias is a common congenital abnormality of the male external genitalia. It occurs in approximately 1 in 250 male newborns. Boys with hypospadias usually have 3 anomalies of the penis: (1) abnormal ventral opening of the urethra; (2) abnormal ventral curvature of the penis; and (3) deficient ventral shaft skin with

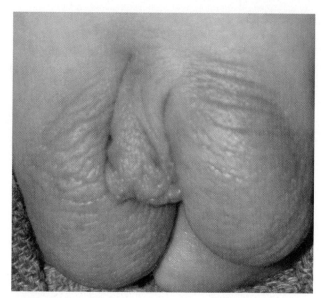

FIGURE 48-8 Boy with severe hypospadias and bifid scrotum.

a redundant prepuce over the dorsum (dorsal hood). Most males have a mild form. Patients with severe hypospadias may have a perineal or scrotal meatus with severe foreshortening and dorsal curvature of the penis giving an ambiguous appearance to the genitalia (Figure 48-8). Undescended testes are common (7%–9%) in boys with hypospadias and can make sexual determination difficult.

MANAGEMENT

Prenatal Therapy

Prenatal treatment with dexamethasone is available for those fetuses at high risk for CAH and is aimed at reducing congenital virilization of the female genitalia. This therapy is initiated in pregnant mothers with a history of a previous child with CAH and is highly successful at preventing virilization in 85% of female fetuses.[55] Because genital differentiation occurs between 8 and 12 weeks postconception, oral dexamethasone should be started as soon as pregnancy is determined. Unfortunately, because sex determination cannot be made before this time period with routine methods (chorionic villus sampling at 10 weeks), 7 of 8 fetuses are unnecessarily exposed to corticosteroids because of the autosomal recessive nature of genetic transmission. New noninvasive testing using cell-free fetal DNA from maternal plasma is accurate at determining fetal sex as early 5 weeks postconception and once widely available will likely become part of the workup prior to corticosteroid therapy.[56]

Prenatal administration of dexamethasone may lead to growth retardation, disruption of the hypothalamic-pituitary-adrenal axis, behavioral issues, and developmental delays in children.[57] Maternal exposure may cause abnormal glucose tolerance, hypertension, osteoporosis, cataracts, and increased risk for infection during treatment.[58] Because of these factors and other ethical and sociological concerns, prenatal treatment with dexamethasone continues to be a controversial subject and is considered experimental therapy.[59]

Postnatal Therapy

The management of a newborn with ambiguous genitalia requires great sensitivity. An experienced group of physicians from the disciplines of neonatology, endocrinology, medical genetics, pediatric urology, and psychiatry/psychology is best from an experienced center in managing these patients. It is paramount that the team works collectively to make a precise and appropriate diagnosis and includes the parents in this process. In addition, all caregivers and ancillary staff should be made aware of the sensitive aspect of the situation.

When treating children with a DSD, it is good to consider the parameters of optimal gender policy as described by Meyer-Bahlburg.[60] These include (1) reproductive potential (if attainable at all); (2) good sexual function; (3) minimal medical procedures; (4) an overall gender-appropriate appearance; (5) a stable gender identity; and (6) contentment in life.

Medical Management

Once the diagnosis of a DSD is made, stabilization of the neonate is the priority during the evaluation. Particular attention should be paid to the newborn's general condition, feeding status, heart rate, blood pressure, and urine output. Daily electrolyte testing is recommended until screening studies return in those neonates with concerns for having CAH.

In neonates in an acute salt-wasting crisis, aggressive fluid replacement with 0.9% saline at 20 mL/kg body weight is initiated with administration of both glucocorticoids (50–100 mg/m² of hydrocortisone) and mineralocorticoids (Florinef® acetate 0.1 to 0.2 mg orally every 12 to 24 hours).[61] Electrolyte and metabolic derangements are commonly seen in these patients and should be corrected aggressively.

Once stabilized, cortisol replacement should be decreased to a range to suppress corticotropin (ACTH) secretion, usually between 12 and 20 mg/m² daily. Florinef dosing often can be titrated downward based on the child's blood pressure and renin levels. Routine salt administration is rarely required after the newborn period. Information on the dosing of hydrocortisone during periods of illness or stress should be explained in detail to the parents prior to discharge.

Testosterone therapy may be administered in infant males with a micropenis or those with a small penis prior to reconstructive surgery. However, in the vast majority of patients with hypogonadism, exogenous hormonal therapy is initiated to induce puberty at a time determined by the patient, family, and endocrinologist. Hormonal therapy then leads to a cascade of both physical and emotional changes that requires routine adherence for a lifetime.

Gender Assignment

Gender uncertainty is stressful for families of the newborn. Gender assignment requires a thorough evaluation and discussion with the multidisciplinary team. Factors involved in the decision include diagnosis, genital appearance, surgical options, need for lifelong replacement therapy, potential for fertility, views of the family, and cultural practices.[62] Family participation is essential in the decision-making process. While the decision should be made deliberately, gender assignment should be made as early as possible, preferably in the newborn period. Some have advocated for the deferment of the decision until the patient can provide informed consent. However, cultural norms and practices make this approach difficult.

Surgical Management

Surgery in patients with DSD can be complex and challenging. Only surgeons with specific training in genital reconstruction surgery should perform these procedures.

It is generally accepted that clitoroplasty is best performed in the first few months of life. Waiting several months allows for stabilization of the child from an endocrine and metabolic standpoint. Corticosteroid replacement therapy typically leads to some improvement of the virilization of the external genitalia. All current techniques have preservation of the clitoral sensation and function as their cornerstone.

In contrast to timing of clitoral reconstruction, the optimal age for vaginal reconstruction is more controversial. Benefits of proceeding at a younger age include improved tissue transfer and reduced scarring secondary to estrogen stimulation, minimization of parental anxiety over the child's condition, and earlier self-acceptance of the child's gender identity and genital anatomy.[63] Others have advocated a delayed approach because of the need for subsequent surgery for vaginal stenosis in children who had early vaginal reconstruction.[64]

One of the major factors in determining gender assignment is potential phallic adequacy in adulthood. Today, most genital reconstruction is performed with respect to genetic sex. However, in some situations with severe phallic insufficiency, gender conversion may be appropriate. Reasonable and expected outcomes following surgery are an important part of the discussion with the parents.

Penile surgery should occur around 6 months of age or older and may proceed as part of a staged procedure.[65] Preoperative testosterone is a useful adjunct in boys with small penises and is typically administered intramuscularly about a month prior to surgery. Persistent müllerian remnants are usually not excised unless the child becomes clinically symptomatic.

Prophylactic gonadectomy or removal of streak goads is generally recommended to prevent malignancy in patients raised as girls with Y genetic material. This is usually performed at the time of reconstructive surgery or within the first year of life. In girls with complete androgen insensitivity, gonadectomy may be deferred until the teenage years or not be performed because of the low malignant potential of the testes.[66] Children raised as males with MGD or PGD should in general have streak gonads and intra-abdominal gonads removed. Testes with mostly normal architecture can be brought down into the scrotum and can be managed with close surveillance.[29]

REFERENCES

1. Hughes IA, Houk C, Ahmed SF, et al. Consensus statement on management of intersex disorders. *Arch Dis Child.* 2006;91(7):554.
2. Ogata T, Hawkins JR, Taylor A, et al. Sex reversal in a child with a 46,X,Yp+ karyotype: support for the existence of a gene(s), located in distal Xp, involved in testis formation. *J Med Genet.* 1992;29(4):226.
3. Swain A, Narvaez V, Burgoyne P, et al. Dax1 antagonizes Sry action in mammalian sex determination. *Nature.* 1998;391(6669):761.
4. Kwok C, Weller PA, Guioli S, et al. Mutations in *SOX9*, the gene responsible for campomelic dysplasia and autosomal sex reversal. *Am J Hum Genet.* 1995;57(5):1028.
5. Wagner T, Wirth J, Meyer J, et al. Autosomal sex reversal and campomelic dysplasia are caused by mutations in and around the SRY-related gene *SOX9*. *Cell.* 1994;79(6):1111.
6. Huang B, Wang S, Ning Y, et al. Autosomal XX sex reversal caused by duplication of SOX9. *Am J Med Genet.* 1999;87(4):349.
7. Luo X, Ikeda Y, Parker KL. A cell-specific nuclear receptor is essential for adrenal and gonadal development and sexual differentiation. *Cell.* 1994;77(4):481.
8. Achermann JC, Ito M, Ito M, et al. A mutation in the gene encoding steroidogenic factor-1 causes XY sex reversal and adrenal failure in humans. *Nat Genet.* 1999;22(2):125.
9. Call KM, Glaser T, Ito CY. Isolation and characterization of a zinc finger polypeptide gene at the human chromosome 11 Wilms' tumor locus. *Cell.* 1990;60(3):509.
10. Nachtigal MW, Hirokawa Y, Enyeart-VanHouten DL. Wilms' tumor 1 and Dax-1 modulate the orphan nuclear receptor SF-1 in sex-specific gene expression. *Cell.* 1998;93(3):445.
11. Hossain A, Saunders GF. The human sex-determining gene SRY is a direct target of WT1. *J Biol Chem.* 2001;276(20):16817.
12. Bruening W, Bardeesy N, Silverman BL, et al. Germline intronic and exonic mutations in the Wilms' tumour gene (WT1) affecting urogenital development. *Nat Genet.* 1992;1(2):144.
13. Cai Y. Revisiting old vaginal topics: conversion of the müellerian vagina and origin of the "sinus" vagina. *Int J Dev Biol.* 2009;53(7):925.
14. Money J. The development of sexuality and eroticism in humankind. *Q Rev Biol.* 1981;56(4):379.
15. Reiner WG, Kropp BP. A 7-year experience of genetic males with severe phallic inadequacy assigned female. *J Urol.* 2004;172(6 Pt 1):2395.
16. Gorski RA. Hypothalamic imprinting by gonadal steroid hormones. *Adv Exp Med Biol.* 2002;511:57.
17. McEwen BS. Invited review: estrogens effects on the brain: multiple sites and molecular mechanisms. *J Appl Physiol.* 2001;91(6):2785.
18. Gooren L. The biology of human psychosexual differenation. *Horm Behave.* 2006;50(4):589.
19. Pinhas-Hamiel O, Zalel Y, Smith E, et al. Prenatal diagnosis of sex differentiation disorders: the role of fetal ultrasound. *J Clin Endocrinol Metab.* 2002;87(10):4547.
20. Zalel Y, Pinhas-Hamiel, Lipitz S, et al. The development of the fetal penis—an in utero sonographic evaluation. *Ultrasound Obstet Gynecol.* 2001;17(2):129.
21. Odeh M, Granin V, Kais M, et al. Sonographic fetal sex determination. *Obstet Gynecol Surv.* 2009;64(1):50.
22. Katorza E, Pinhas-Hamiel O, Mazkereth R, et al. Sex differentiation disorders (DSD) prenatal sonographic diagnosis, genetic and hormonal work-up. *Pediatr Endocrinol Rev.* 2009;7(1):12.
23. Soriano D, Lipitz S, Seidman DS, et al. Development of the fetal uterus between 19 and 38 weeks of gestation: in-utero ultrasonographic measurements. *Hum Reprod.* 1999;14(1):215.
24. Migeon CJ, Donohue PA. Congenital adrenal hyperplasia caused by 21-hydroxylase deficiency. Its molecular basis and its remaining therapeutic problems. *Endocrinol Metab Clin North Am.* 1991;20(2):277.
25. Gassner I, Geley TE. Ultrasound of female genital anomalies. *Eur Radiol.* 2004;14(Suppl 4):107.
26. Tasian Ge, Copp HL. Diagnostic performance of ultrasound in nonpalpable cryptorchidism: a systematic review and meta-analysis. *Pediatrics.* 2011;127(1):119.
27. Al-Alwan I, Navarro O, Daneman O, et al. Clinical utility of adrenal ultrasonography in the diagnosis of congenital adrenal hyperplasia. *J Pediatr.* 1999;135(1):71.
28. Zäh W, Kalderon AE, Tucci JR. Mixed gonadal dysgenesis. *Acta Endocrinol Suppl.* 1975;197:1.
29. Diamond DA. Sexual differentiation: normal and abnormal. In: Wein AJ, Kavoussi LR, Novick AC, Partin AW, Peters CA, eds. *Campbell-Walsh Urology.* 9th ed. Philadelphia, PA: Saunders Elsevier; 2007.
30. Robboy SJ, Jaubert E. Neoplasms and pathology of sexual development disorders (intersex). *Pathology.* 2007;39(1):147.
31. Bojesen A, Juul S, Gravholt CH. Prenatal and postnatal prevalence of Klinefelter syndrome: a national registry study. *J Clin Endocrinol Metab.* 2003;88(2):622.
32. Klinefelter HF, Reifenstein EC, Albright F. Syndrome characterized by gynecomastia, aspermatogenesis without a-Leydigism, and increased secretion of follicle-stimulating hormone. *Am J Clin Dermatol.* 1942;2:615.
33. Lanfranco F, Kamischke A, Zitzmann M, et al. Klinefelter's syndrome. *Lancet.* 2004;364(9430):273.
34. Walker AM, Walker J, Adams S, et al. True hermaphroditism. *J Paediatr Child Health.* 2000;36(1):69.
35. Mittwoch U. Genetics of sex determination: exceptions that prove the rule. *Mol Genet Metab.* 2000;71(1–2):405.
36. Pleskacova J, Hersmus R, Oosterhuis JW, et al. Tumor risk in disorders of sex development. *Sex Dev.* 2010;4(4–5):259.

37. Wilhelm D, Koopman P. The makings of maleness: towards an integrated view of male sexual development. *Nat Rev Genet.* 2006;7(8):620.

38. Manuel H, Katavama PK, Jones HW Jr. The age of occurrence of gonadal tumors in intersex patients with a Y chromosome. *Am J Obstet Gynecol.* 1976;124(3):293.

39. Marcantonio SM, Fechner PY, Migeon CJ, et al. Embryonic testicular regression sequence: a part of the clinical spectrum of 46,XY gonadal dysgenesis. *Am J Med Genet.* 1994;49(1):1.

40. Edman CD, Winters AJ, Porter JC, et al. Embryonic testicular regression. A clinical spectrum of XY agonadal individuals. *Obstet Gynecol.* 1977;49(2):208.

41. Hannema SE, Scott IS, Hodapp J, et al. Residual activity of mutant androgen receptors explains wolffian duct development in the complete androgen insensitivity syndrome. *J Clin Endocrinol Metab.* 2004;89(11):5815.

42. Brinkmann AO. Molecular mechanisms of androgen action—a historical perspective. *Methods Mol Biol.* 2011;776:3.

43. Cheon CK. Practical approach to steroid 5alpha-reductase type 2 deficiency. *Eur J Pediatr.* 2011;170(1):1.

44. Nilson O. Hernis uteris inguinalis beim Manne. *Acta Chir Scand.* 1939;83:231.

45. Brandli DW, Akbal C, Eugsster E, et al. Persistent mullerian duct syndrome with bilateral abdominal testis: surgical approach and review of the literature. *J Pediatr Urol.* 2005;1(6):423.

46. Jacob JJ, Paul TV, Mathews SS, et al. Perrault syndrome with Marfanoid habitus in two siblings. *J Pediatr Adolesc Gynecol.* 2007;20(5):305.

47. Boucekkine C, Toublanc JE, Abbas N, et al. Clinical and anatomical spectrum in XX sex-reversed patients: relationship to the presence of Y-specific DNA sequences. *Clin Endocrinol.* 1994;40(6):733.

48. Braun A, Kammerer S, Cleve A, et al. True hermaphroditism in a 46 XY individual caused by postzygotic somatic point mutation in the male gonadal sex-determing locus (SRY): molecular genetics and histological findings in a sporadic ase. *Am J Hum Genet.* 1993;52(3):578.

49. Therrell BLG, Berenbaum SA, Manter-Kapanke V, et al. Results of screening 1.9 million Texas newborns for 21-hydroxylase-deficient congenital adrenal hyperplasia. *Pediatrics.* 1998;101(4 Pt 1):583.

50. Kohn B, Day D, Alemzadeh R, et al. Splicing mutation in CYP21 associated with delayed presentation of salt-wasting congenital adrenal hyperplasia. *Am J Med Genet.* 1995;57(3):450.

51. Prader A. Die Haufigkeit der kongenitalen androgenitalen Syndroms. *Helv Pediatr Acta.* 1958;13:426.

52. Rösler A, Leiberman E, Cohen T. High frequency of congenital adrenal hyperplasia (classic 11-β-hydroxylase deficiency) among Jews from Morocco. *Am J Med Genet.* 1992;42(6):827.

53. Simard J, Mosian AM, Morel Y. Congenital adrenal hyperplasia due to 3β-hydroxysteroid dehydrogenase/D⁵-D⁴ isomerase deficiency. *Semin Reprod Med.* 2002;20(3):255.

54. Huang N, Pandey AV, Agrawal V, et al. Diversity and function of mutations in P450 oxioreductase in patients with Antley-Bixler syndrome and disorded steroidogenesis. *Am J Hum.* 2005;76(5):729.

55. Vos AA, Bruinse HW. Congenital adrenal hyperplasia: do the benefits of prenatal treatment defeat the risks? *Obstet Gynecol Surv.* 2010;65(3):196.

56. Speiser PW, Assiz R, Baskin LS, et al. Congenital adrenal hyperplasia due to steroid 21-hydroxylase deficiency: an Endocrine Society clinical practice guideline. *J Clin Endocrinol Metab.* 2010;95(11):4133.

57. Lajic S, Nordenstrom A, Hirvikoski T. Long-term outcome of prenatal treatment of congenital adrenal hyperplasia. *Endocr Dev.* 2008;13:82.

58. Hui L, Bianchi DW. Prenatal pharmacotherapy for fetal anomalies: a 2011 update. *Prenat Diagn.* 2011;31(7):735.

59. Kamenova K. Politics and persuasion in medical controversies. *Am J Bioeth.* 2010;10(9):68.

60. Meyer-Bahlburg HF. Gender assignment and reassignment in intersexuality: controversies, data, and guidelines for research. *Adv Exp Med Biol.* 2002;511:199.

61. Claahsen-van der Grinten HL, Stikkelbroeck NMML, Otten BJ, et al. Congenital adrenal hyperplasia—pharmacologic interventions from the prental phase to adulthood. *Pharmacol Ther.* 2011;132(1):1.

62. Lee PA, Houk CP, Ahmed SF, et al. Consensus statement on management of intersex disorders. International Consensus Conference on Intersex. *Pediatrics.* 2006;118(2):488.

63. Adams MC, DeMarco RT. Surgery for intersex disorders and urogenital sinus. In: Docimo SG, Canning DA, Khoury AE, eds. *Clinical Pediatric Urology.* 5th ed. London, UK: Informa Healthcare; 2008:1187–1204.

64. Alizai NK, Thomas DF, Lilford RJ, et al. Feminizing genitoplasty for congenital adrenal hyperplasia: what happens at puberty? *J Urol.* 1999;161(5):1588.

65. Section on Urology. Timing of elective surgery on the genitalia of male children with particular reference to the risks, benefits, and psychological effects of surgery and anesthesia. *Pediatrics.* 1996;97:590.

66. Barbaro M, Wedell A, Nordenström A. Disorders of sex development. *Semin Fetal Neonatal Med.* 2011;16(2):119.

67. Davenport M. Approach to the patient with Turner syndrome. *J Clin Endocrinol Metab.* 2010;95(4):1487–1495.

68. Witchel SF, Lee PA. Ambiguous genitalia. In: Sperling MA, ed. *Pediatric Endocrinology.* 3rd ed. Philadelphia, PA: Saunders Elsevier; 2008.

Part H: Immune System

Ontogeny of the Immune System

David B. Lewis

INTRODUCTION

The fetus and neonate are more vulnerable than older children and adults to severe infection with pathogens, including pyogenic bacteria, fungi, viruses, and intracellular protozoa.[1] Although this vulnerability indicates substantial limitations in innate and adaptive immunity in prenatal and early postnatal life, the mechanistic basis for these is only partially understood. Hematopoietic stem cell transplantation also provides compelling evidence for impairment of neonatal T-cell and natural killer (NK) cell immunity: Allogeneic hematopoietic cell transplantation with cord blood is associated with a significantly lower risk of acute graft-vs-host disease—a disease that is mainly mediated by donor-derived naïve T cells—compared to bone marrow and peripheral blood transplants containing adult T cells.[2]

DENDRITIC CELLS AND ANTIGEN PRESENTATION

CD11c+ dendritic cells (DCs) are myeloid-derived cells that participate in antigen presentation to T cells and B cells and also produce critical cytokines that shape adaptive immune responses. For example, the cytokines interleukin (IL)-12 p70, a heterodimer of the IL-12/IL-23 p40 subunit and IL-12 p35, and IL-15, which are produced by DCs, not only provide early innate immune protection but also promote the development of an adaptive immune response dominated by T helper 1 (Th1)–type effector CD4 T cells that produce interferon (IFN)-γ. Plasmacytoid dendritic cells

(pDCs) are a distinct DC population that, at rest, lacks the characteristic dendrite-like protrusions of CD11c+ DCs and is found in lymphoid tissue, the circulation, and certain sites of tissue inflammation (eg, the skin in herpes simplex virus [HSV] infection). Activated pDCs are an important source of type I IFNs, which include multiple types of IFN-α and a single type of IFN-β. These type I IFNs are an important source of early and systemic innate antiviral immunity and enhance the later adaptive immune response, including Th1 differentiation from naïve CD4 T-cell precursors. DCs are activated by their recognition of conserved structures of microbial pathogens by toll-like receptors (TLRs), C-lectin-type receptors (CLRs), retinoic acid inducible gene-I (RIG-I)-like receptors (RLRs), and nucleotide binding domain and leucine-rich repeat-containing receptors (NLRs)[3] as well as other stimuli.

DCs in Tissues

The colonization of CD11c+ DCs in extralymphoid and lymphoid tissues is developmentally regulated and occurs independently of exposure to inflammatory mediators. Immature CD11c+ DC lineage cells are found in the interstitial regions of solid organs, including the kidney, heart, pancreas, and lung, but not the brain, by 12 weeks of gestation; their numbers progressively increase through 21 weeks' gestation.[3] Epidermal DC-like cells that express the human MHC (major histocompatibility complex) class II isotype, HLA-DR (human leukocyte antigen DR), are found in the skin earlier, at 7 weeks' gestation, and are probably derived from CD45+ HLA-DR+ cells that enter the epidermis, extensively proliferate, and then acquire the characteristic features of Langerhans DCs, including CD1c, langerin, and CD1a in a stepwise manner.[4]

Circulating and Monocyte-Derived DCs

Most phenotypic and functional studies of primary human DCs have for practical reasons analyzed circulating DCs, although a major caveat is whether these results also apply to tissue DCs.[3] Circulating CD11c+ DCs are typically CD11c[high] and HLA-DR[high] but are lineage-negative (Lin−), that is, lacking markers for other cell lineages, such as T cells, monocytes/macrophages, B cells, NK cells, granulocytes, and erythroid cells. Human pDCs are CD11c[low]Lin− and express high levels of CD123 (the IL-3 receptor α-chain) and blood-derived dendritic cell antigen (BDCA)-2 (CD303 or C-type lectin-like receptor 4C [CLEC4C]), a type II transmembrane C-type lectin. Cord blood and adult peripheral blood have similar concentrations of CD11c+ DCs that are also phenotypically similar.[3] An exception is CD86 (B7–2), a protein that engages CD28 on the T cell and provides it costimulation and that is lower on cord blood CD11c+ DCs. In contrast, the concentration of pDCs in cord blood is significantly higher than in adult peripheral blood and gradually declines after birth.[3]

Circulating neonatal DCs have selective limitations in the TLR-mediated upregulation of expression of molecules involved in T-cell costimulation by CD28 engagement (CD80 and CD86) and other DC–T-cell interactions (HLA-DR and CD40) compared to those of the adult.[3] For example, cord blood CD11c+ DCs have reduced CD40 expression after exposure in vitro to ligands for TLR-2/6 (*Mycoplasma fermentans*), TLR-3 (polyinosine-cytosine (I:C), TLR-4 (lipopolysaccharide [LPS]), and TLR-7 (imiquimod) and have reduced CD80 in response to TLR-3 and TLR-4 ligands. In contrast, CD11c+ DCs of neonates and adults similarly increase CD40 in response to GU-rich single-stranded RNA, a TLR-8 ligand, and MHC class II and CD86 after stimulation with TLR-3 and TLR-4 ligands. The pDCs of cord blood and adult peripheral blood also similarly upregulate HLA-DR, CD80, and CD86 after stimulation with TLR-9 ligands, such as DNA phosphothioate oligonucleotides lacking methylation of CpG residues (CpG DNA).[3]

Th1 immunity may be particularly limited in the neonate and young infant compared to older individuals because of decreased IL-12 p70 production by CD11c+ DCs, such as in response to LPS plus IFN-γ.[1] However, this limitation is likely pathogen dependent, as decreased IL-12 production by cord blood CD11c+ DCs is similar to adult CD11c+ DCs after stimulation with certain gram-positive and gram-negative bacteria or meningococcal outer-membrane proteins.[1] Circulating DCs from cord blood can also stimulate allogeneically (ie, in a MHC mismatched context) cord blood T cells in vitro,[1] but it is unclear if they are as effective as adult DCs in promoting Th1 differentiation under these conditions.

The production of type I IFNs by cord blood CD11c+ DCs and pDCs is also reduced compared to those of adult peripheral blood and could contribute to the limited ability of the neonate to control pathogens such as HSV. For example, IFN-α production by cord blood CD11c+ DCs in response to a TLR-3 ligand and by cord blood pDCs in response to TLR-9 ligands—such as live or inactivated HSV or CpG DNA—is reduced compared to adult DCs.[3] This decreased production of type I IFNs is not attributable to diminished TLR-9 expression by cord blood pDCs but appears to be due to reduced nuclear translocation of interferon regulatory factor 7 (IRF7), a transcription factor that is essential for type I IFN gene expression.[3]

A number of studies have compared the function and phenotype of monocyte-derived dendritic cells (MDDCs), which are produced by culturing monocytes from cord blood or adult peripheral blood in vitro with granulocyte-macrophage colony-stimulating factor (GM-CSF) and IL-4; these MDDCs are typically evaluated for function after their activation by incubation with tumor necrosis factor (TNF)-α or other stimuli. Although cord blood MDDCs have reduced IL-12 p70 expression after stimulation, it is unclear if these and other functional and phenotypic differences apply to fetal and neonatal DCs of the tissues. Gene expression profiling analysis suggested that MDDCs may best model inflammatory DCs, which are generated from monocytes in vivo at sites of marked tissue inflammation, such as during Th1-driven reversal reactions of infection with *Mycobacterium leprae*.[3] It remains unclear regarding the extent these inflammatory DCs are generated in the fetus and neonate in response to infection or other proinflammatory stimuli.

Postnatal DC Maturation

HLA-DR expression and CD80 expression induced by LPS (a TLR-4 ligand), which, as noted, is significantly reduced in cord blood CD11c+ DCs, reaches the levels of circulating adult CD11c+ DCs by 3 months of age.[5] In a longitudinal study of infants from the Gambia, TNF-α, IL-6, and IL-12/IL-23 p40 expression by CD11+ DCs in response to LPS were significantly greater at 1 year and 2 years of age than at birth or compared to their expression by these cells in adult peripheral blood.[6] In contrast, CD11c+ DCs of newborns, 1-year-olds, and 2-year-olds all had higher levels of production of these cytokines in response to a TLR-2 agonist (PAM 3Cys) and a TLR-7/8 agonist (3M-003). For pDCs, adult levels of HLA-DR and CD80 expression induced by a TLR-9 agonist

(CpG DNA) were not achieved until 6–9 months of age.[6] The production by pDCs of TNF-α and IL-6 and in response to either TLR-7/8 or TLR-9 agonists at 1 year of age was similar to those of adult pDCs. Thus, the maturation of DC function after birth is not uniform for all functions but rather occurs in a TLR-specific manner. The maturation of responses to non-TLR ligands has largely not been explored.

T CELLS

Ontogeny of Thymic Development

Initial colonization of the fetal thymus anlage by pro-thymocytes occurs at 8.5 weeks of gestation. This is followed by dramatic increases in thymic cellularity during the second and third trimesters. Transient thymic involution, with a prominent loss of cortical double-positive (CD4^{high}CD8^{high}) thymocytes, appears to occur at the end of the third trimester due to a prenatal surge in the circulating glucocorticoid levels.[1] This involution is followed by recovery of thymocyte cellularity at 1 month of age. Peak thymocyte cellularity in relation to body size and, presumably, output of recent thymic emigrants (RTEs), occurs between 6 and 12 months of age.[1,7]

Repertoire of αβ-T-Cell Receptors

T-cell receptor diversity is generated by the process of V(D)J recombination in developing thymocytes and involves the joining variable (V), diversity (D), and joining (J) segments in the case of the T-cell receptor (TCR)-β chain and V and J segments in the case of the TCR-α chain. The usage of TCR-β D and J gene segments in the thymus is initially less diverse than subsequently. The complementarity determinant region 3 (CDR3) region of the TCR-β chain transcripts, which is encoded at the 3′ end of the V segment and the adjacent D and J segments, is also reduced in length and sequence diversity between 8 and 15 weeks of gestation. This is likely due to decreased activity of the terminal deoxytransferase (TdT) enzyme, which performs random N-nucleotide addition during V(D)J recombination. An impact of limitations in αβ-TCR diversity on the ability of the fetus to respond to congenital infection would be expected to be most pronounced in the first trimester of pregnancy, as intrathymic TdT activity, CDR3 length, and V segment diversity by the second trimester are similar to that of postnatal thymic tissue.[1] A low-resolution analysis (ie, not direct DNA or messenger RNA [mRNA] sequencing) of the TCR repertoire expressed on cord blood T cells indicates that the diversity of TCR usage and CDR3 length are similar to that of antigenically naïve T cells in adults

and infants. Together, these observations suggest that the functional preimmune repertoire is well formed by birth.

Signal joint TCR excision circles (sjTRECs) are generated as a part of TCR-α gene rearrangement of thymocytes and may persist for long periods in T-lineage cells that do not proliferate. sjTREC levels in cord blood are relatively high compared to adult peripheral blood, consistent with the expected predominance of naïve (CD45RA^{high}CD45R0^{low}) T cells and RTEs in cord blood (see "Fetal T-Cell Development and Phenotype" section below).[1,8]

Fetal T-Cell Development and Phenotype

By 14 weeks' gestation, CD4 and CD8 T cells are found in the fetal circulation, liver, and spleen, and T cells are detectable in lymph nodes. The percentage of circulating T cells increases during the second and third trimesters of pregnancy until about 6 months of age, followed by a gradual decline to adult levels. The ratio of CD4 to CD8 T cells in the circulation is high during fetal life (about 3.5) and gradually declines with postnatal age.

Most circulating CD4 T cells in the term and preterm neonate and in the second- and third-trimester fetus express a CD45RA^{high}CD45R0^{low}CCR7$^+$CD25$^-$CD95$^-$ surface phenotype, which is similar to that of antigenically naïve CD4 T cells of the adult circulation. However, second-trimester naïve CD4 T cells have high basal levels of Foxp3, a key transcription factor for regulatory T-cell (Treg) development and function, and, upon allogeneic stimulation, are highly skewed toward differentiation into Tregs, which potently suppress effector T-cell function. In contrast, adult peripheral blood naïve CD4 T cells have lower basal levels of Foxp3 and preferentially differentiate into effector cells with allogeneic stimulation.[9] Tregs are also more abundant in fetal peripheral lymphoid tissue compared to that of the adult.[10] This tendency for Treg skewing by fetal CD4 T cells appears to be a characteristic of T cells that are derived from fetal hematopoietic stem cells (HSCs) rather than adult HSCs and is likely an important mechanism for fetal-maternal tolerance.[9] It remains unclear at what age this fetal HSC program of T-cell differentiation is replaced with an adult-type HSC program favoring effector cell rather than Treg differentiation.

Protein tyrosine kinase 7 (PTK7), a surface protein and member of the receptor tyrosine kinase superfamily, identifies RTEs among human adult naïve CD4 T cells and is also expressed uniformly at high levels by cord blood T cells and postnatal thymocytes.[8] These observations are consistent with the fetal and neonatal peripheral T-cell compartment being enriched in

RTEs, an idea that is also supported by the high level of thymic cellularity in the newborn and young infant.[7] Cord blood T cells may be more prone than adult naïve T cells to undergo homeostatic proliferation because of a greater sensitivity to the mitogenic effects of IL-7, and this may also be a reflection of their enrichment in RTEs, which also have this propensity.[1,8] In contrast, CD38, a cell surface ectoenzyme involved in intracellular calcium mobilization, is found on virtually all peripheral fetal and neonatal T cells as well as fetal and postnatal thymocytes but is absent on adult naïve T cells, including adult RTEs.[1,8] Together, these observations suggest that peripheral T cells in the fetus and neonate have a distinct thymocyte-like immature phenotype beyond that attributable to their enrichment in RTEs.

CD4 T-Cell Responses

Herpesvirus Infections

A striking limitation in neonatal T-cell immunity is the reduced and delayed HSV-specific CD4 T-cell cytokine (IL-2, IFN-γ, and TNF-α) production and proliferation in neonates compared to adults after primary HSV infection.[11] CD4 T-cell help for HSV-specific antibody production is also likely reduced in neonates.[1] Older infants and young children also have reduced CD4 T-cell immunity (antigen-specific IL-2, IFN-γ, and CD40-ligand [CD154] expression) after primary infection with cytomegalovirus (CMV), another herpesvirus, compared to adults.[12] This reduced CD4 T-cell response is associated with persistent CMV shedding in the urine and saliva of young children following primary infection.[12] This reduced response also likely applies to the neonate and young infant with congenital, perinatal, or postnatally acquired CMV infection, all of whom persistently shed CMV for years following its acquisition.

Vaccines

The robustness and quality of the CD4 T-cell response of the neonate and young infant to live vaccines varies with the particular agent. BCG vaccination at birth is as effective as vaccination at 2 or 4 months of age for inducing mycobacterial-specific CD4 T-cell proliferation and IFN-γ production and is not associated with increased Th2 skewing (ie., IL-4, IL-5, or IL-13 production) and reduced levels of IFN-γ.[1] However, the Th1 responses of infant BCG vaccine recipients have not been directly compared with those of older children and adults. In contrast to BCG, newborns given oral poliovirus vaccine (OPV) at birth, 1, 2, and 3 months of age have lower OPV-specific CD4 T-cell proliferation and IFN-γ production compared to adults who were immunized later in childhood.[1] Interestingly, the neonate's and infant's antibody titers are higher than those of adults, suggesting that CD4 follicular T-cell help for B cells is not impaired by early OPV immunization. OPV may be less effective at inducing a Th1 response than BCG in neonates and young infants because of its limited replication (BCG vaccination results in persistent infection), its site of inoculation, or a more limited ability to stimulate antigen-presenting cells (APCs) in a manner conducive to Th1 immunity. In contrast to BCG, the administration of pertussis vaccine to neonates may result in a skewing of pertussis antigen-specific T cells toward a Th2 cytokine profile.[13]

Mechanisms for Reduced Immunity

Normal CD4 T-cell activation by engagement of the αβ-TCR and the CD28 molecule on the T-cell surface results in the activation of transcription factors, including NFAT (nuclear factor of activated T cells), AP-1 (activated protein-1), and NF-κB (nuclear factor-κB), resulting in the de novo transcription of genes such as IL-2 and CD154. IL-2 promotes CD4 T-cell proliferation in an autocrine and paracrine fashion. CD154 engages CD40 on CD11c+ DCs to increase their surface expression of CD80 and CD86 and their production of IL-12 p70. In addition to the limitations in DC function discussed, several other potential mechanisms intrinsic to the neonatal CD4 T cell may limit its ability to expand into memory/effector Th1 cells. These impairments include reduction in neonatal CD4 T-cell NFAT proteins, which is mediated by microRNA-184,[14] IL-2 and CD154 expression,[15] and IL-12p70-induced activation of signal transducer and activator of transcription 4 (STAT4) by tyrosine phosphorylation,[15] and decreased early Th1 differentiation, as indicated by reduced IFN-γ mRNA and protein expression.[1,15] The IFN-γ gene locus is also more highly methylated in neonatal compared to adult naïve CD4 T cells,[1] which may limit its accessibility to transcription factors required for its efficient expression. Reduced CD154 expression, in turn, may decrease the CD40 engagement of CD11c+ DCs and their IL-12p70 production.[1] Decreased STAT4 signaling, which normally enhances IFN-γ gene transcription, may also impair Th1 differentiation in neonatal CD4 T cells.[1]

CD8 T-Cell and γδ-T-Cell Responses

CD8 T-cell responses to herpesviruses, such as CMV, that is acquired congenitally or in infancy or early childhood, are similar to those of adults.[1] Congenital CMV infection also elicits a robust fetal γδ-T-cell response that includes IFN-γ production and cytotoxin expression.[16] Neonates with congenital Chagas disease, which is due to infection by *Trypanosoma cruzii*, also have readily detectable CD8 T-cell responses to this pathogen.[1] Interestingly, this infection also appears to influence the subsequent quality of immune responses to vaccination with unrelated antigens. However, these apparently robust responses do not rule out a relatively brief, but potentially important, lag in the onset of CD8 or γδ-T-cell immunity that might compromise the early immune control of these pathogens. Studies of CD8 T-cell responses to human immunodeficiency virus type 1 (HIV-1) in perinatally or in utero-infected infants also indicates that CD8 T cells capable of mediating cytotoxicity are also typically generated in vivo in the fetus.[17] However, CD8 T-cell-mediated cytotoxicity may be reduced and delayed in appearance compared to that of adults following highly active antiretroviral therapy.[1] The maintenance of HIV-1-specific CD8 T cells with effector function depends on HIV-1-specific CD4 T cells, which tend to be selectively depleted by the virus. However, the role of age-related impairments in HIV-specific CD4 T-cell immunity in limiting HIV-specific CD8 T-cell immunity remains poorly understood. Interestingly, the suppressive effects of HIV-1 on CD8 T-cell responses appear to be relatively specific, in that HIV-1-infected infants with poor HIV-specific CD8 T-cell responses maintain robust CD8 T-cell responses to herpesviruses.[1]

B CELLS

Ontogeny of B Cells

Pre-B cells are first detected in the fetal liver and omentum by 8 weeks of gestation and in the fetal bone marrow by 13 weeks of gestation. The bone marrow becomes the predominant site of pre-B-cell development by midgestation, and by 30 weeks' gestation, it is the sole site.

By 16 weeks' gestation, all heavy-chain isotypes (ie, immunoglobulin (Ig) M, IgG, IgA, and IgE) are detectable in fetal bone marrow B cells, although the stimulus for this fetal isotype switching remains unclear. The frequency of B cells in tissues rapidly increases, and by 22 weeks' gestation, the proportion of B cells in the spleen, blood, and bone marrow is similar to that in adults. Cord blood B cells expressing surface IgG or IgA are usually rare (ie, < 1% of circulating B cells). True germinal centers in the spleen and lymph nodes are normally absent during fetal life but appear during the first months after birth as a result of postnatal antigenic stimulation.

A distinct feature of fetal and cord blood B cells is their high frequency of markers, including CD5, CD10, CD24, and CD38, that are found on transitional and prenaïve B cells in healthy adults, which are relatively low-frequency subsets. These markers also predominate during early immune reconstitution of B-lineage cells following hematopoietic stem cell transplantation.[18] The predominance of transitional B-cell markers on neonatal B cells is consistent with the rapid expansion of the B-cell compartment during late fetal and early postnatal development. Cord blood B cells, particularly of those prematurely born, also have significantly reduced expression of CD40, CD80, CD86, and B-cell activating factor of the TNF family (BAFF)-receptor and a reduced ability to proliferate in response to BAFF and a B-cell receptor (BCR) signal or to produce IgM, IgG, and IgA in response to CD154 and IL-10.[19] It is unclear how long postnatally this reduction in surface expression and function of naïve B cells in the preterm infant persists. However, the similar level of antibody responses to most T-dependent (TD) antigens in vaccines in 2-month-old preterm vs term infants suggests that this functional impairment is largely resolved by this chronological age (see "Ontogeny of Responsiveness to T-Dependent and T-Independent Antigens" section below).

Immunoglobulin Repertoire

The preimmune immunoglobulin repertoire consists of antibodies that can be expressed prior to an encounter with antigen. It is determined by the number of different B-cell clones with distinct antigen specificity.[20] During early to midgestation, this preimmune repertoire is limited by less-diverse usage of immunoglobulin gene V segments but by the third trimester is as diverse as that of the adult. Both an over- and underrepresentation of certain V(D)J segments have been reported for the neonate, but the importance of such skewing in limiting the neonatal humoral immune response remains unclear. The length of the CDR3 region of the immunoglobulin heavy chain, which is located at the center of the antigen-combining site, is shorter in B cells from the midgestation fetus compared to these cells at birth or in the adult. This reduced CDR3 region length is most likely due to decreased TdT activity. As the CDR3 region is the most hypervariable portion of immunoglobulins, a short CDR3 region may significantly reduce fetal immunoglobulin repertoire diversity[20] and could potentially compromise the antibody response of the fetus (eg, in response to congenital infection). CDR3 length of the immunoglobulin heavy chain progressively increases during the third trimester and reaches the length found in adult B cells (12–13 amino acids) by about 2 months postnatally.[20] Somatic hypermutation is limited or absent for neonatal B-cell responses to protein antigens (eg, encoded by respiratory syncytial virus [RSV]), but by age 3 months becomes similar to those of adult B cells.[21]

B1 B Cells

B1 B cells, which constitute 4% of cord blood B cells, have a CD20+CD27+CD43+ surface phenotype.[22]

They exhibit tonic intracellular signaling, are highly effective at stimulating allogeneic CD4 T cells, and spontaneously secrete IgM. This IgM is encoded by heavy-chain immunoglobulin genes with minimal somatic hypermutation but a substantial amount of N-region additions performed by the TdT enzyme.[22] Like murine B1 B cells, those of adult peripheral blood are enriched for certain specificities, such as phosphorylcholine, a component of certain bacteria, such as *Streptococcus pneumoniae*. Thus, human B1 B cells appear to act as part of the innate immune system in providing protection against pathogens, such as certain encapsulated bacteria.

ONTOGENY OF RESPONSIVENESS TO T-DEPENDENT AND T-INDEPENDENT ANTIGENS

The chronology of the adequacy of the antibody response to different antigens differs depending on the need for cognate CD4 T-cell help (Table 49-1). Antigens that depend on help involving direct CD4 T-cell–B-cell interactions include most proteins and polysaccharide–protein conjugates, which are collectively called T-dependent (TD) antigens. The response to TD antigens is characterized by the

generation of memory B cells that express somatically mutated, high-affinity immunoglobulin that often has also undergone switching from IgM to other isotypes. Antigens that are partially or completely independent of CD4 T-cell help, which are also known as T-independent antigens, can be divided into T-independent type 1 (TI-1) and type 2 (TI-2) antigens. TI-1 antigens directly bind to B cells and activate them to produce antibodies. Examples of TI-1 antigens include fixed *Brucella abortus* bacteria and CpG DNA. TI-2 antigens include unconjugated bacterial capsular polysaccharides, such as those contained in the 23-valent pneumococcal vaccine. TI-2 antigens require additional signals for optimal antibody production, such as TLR ligands that are directly recognized by B cells or cytokines produced by non-B cells (eg, NK cells, NK T cells, γδ-T cells, or DCs). The response to TI-2 antigens is characterized by a lack of B-cell memory, which accounts for the requirement for relatively frequent revaccination of the 23-valent pneumococcal polysaccharide vaccine. The TI-2 response is also much more limited compared to the response to TD antigens in terms of somatic hypermutation and isotype expression.

The capacity of the neonate and young infant to respond to TD antigens is well established at birth, and this allows immunization to begin for most protein and polysaccharide-conjugate vaccines by 6 weeks of age (Table 49-2). Nevertheless, there are clear differences between neonates and older infants in the magnitude of the antibody response to protein antigens: In the case of hepatitis B surface antigen (HBsAg), the initial antibody response in term neonates immunized shortly after birth is substantially lower than if primary immunization is delayed until 1 month of age.[1] However, in the case of neonatal vaccination, the ultimate anti-HBsAg titers achieved after secondary and tertiary immunizations are similar to those of older children, indicating that neonatal immunization does not result in tolerance. Thus, the developmental limitations responsible for reduced antibody responses are transient, although the precise mechanisms remain undefined.

Antibody production by human neonatal B cells in vitro to a TI-1 antigen (*Brucella abortus*) is only modestly reduced (Table 49-1), but it is unclear if this reduction also applies following in vivo immunization or infection.

The response to TI-2 antigen is the last to appear chronologically and accounts for the neonate's poor antibody response to infection with encapsulated bacteria (eg, group B streptococci [GBS]) or vaccination with unconjugated polysaccharide antigens, such as for *Haemophilus influenzae* and *Streptococcus pneumoniae* (Table 49-2). The response to some unconjugated polysaccharide antigens can be demonstrated

Table 49-1 Ontogeny After Birth of Competence for Antibody Responses to CD4 T-Cell-Dependent (TD) and CD4 T-Cell Independent Type 1 (TI-1) and Type 2 (TI-2) Antigens

Antigen Type	Nature of Antigen	Age by Which Response Is Established
TD	Proteins and protein-conjugated polysaccharides	At birth
TI-1	Certain microbial-derived products that directly activate B cells (eg, *Brucella abortus*, CpG DNA)	At birth
TI-2	Unconjugated polysaccharides, such as those from bacterial capsules of *Streptococcus pneumoniae*, *Haemophilus influenzae*, and *Neisseriae meningitidis*	Delayed until 6 to 24 months of age—varies with specific antigen

Table 49-2 Postnatal Antibody Responses of Infants 6 Months of Age or Younger to Vaccines

Vaccine	Antigen Type	Antibody Response in Neonate and Young Infant
Diphtheria toxoids	TD	Immunogenic at birth but response superior when vaccination series delayed until 1 month of age
Haemophilus influenzae type b polysaccharide-conjugate vaccine	TD	Immunogenic at birth but response superior when vaccination series delayed until 2 months of age
Haemophilus influenzae type b polysaccharide unconjugated vaccine	TI-2	Not reliably immunogenic until 18–24 months of age
Hepatitis B surface antigen	TD	Moderately decreased with vaccination at birth compared to 1 month of age; decreased response in premature compared to term neonate; delay of vaccination series recommended for premature infants of HBsAg⁻ mothers
Meningococcal polysaccharide, conjugated vaccine (types A, C, Y, W-135)	TD	Increased antibody titers in response to vaccination beginning at 2 months of age, with evidence of priming—efficacy?
Meningococcal polysaccharide vaccine, unconjugated (types A, C, Y, W-135)	TI-2	Serotype A immunogenic as early as 3 months of age; other serotypes not reliably immunogenic until 24 months of age; vaccination with type C induces tolerance to subsequent immunization in adults and presumably all age groups
Pertussis vaccine, acellular	TD	Immunogenic when series begun at 2 months of age; Th2 skewing when given at birth
Pertussis vaccine, whole cellular	TD	Possible tolerance to pertussis toxin after vaccination at birth but not at 1 month—controversial
Pneumococcal polysaccharide, conjugated vaccines (7, 11, or 13 valent)	TD	Protective to immunity (>2.0 µg/mL of anticapsular antibody) for majority of serotypes after 3 doses when series is begun at 2 months of age
Pneumococcal polysaccharide, unconjugated vaccine (23 valent)	TI-2	Not reliably immunogenic until 18–24 months of age for the majority of serotypes
Tetanus toxoid	TD	Protective antibody response following vaccination in neonatal period but relatively delayed compared to immunization begun at 2 months of age

Abbreviations: TD, T-cell-dependent antigen; TI-1, CD4 T-cell-independent type 1 antigen; TI-2, CD4 T-cell-independent type 2 antigen.

by 6 months of age (eg, *Neisseriae meningitidis* type A), but the response to vaccination with the capsular polysaccharides of *H. influenzae* type b and *Neisseriae meningitidis* type C or to most unconjugated pneumococcal polysaccharides, such as those contained in the 23-valent Pneumovax vaccine, is poor until approximately 18–24 months of age. This poor response in children less than 2 years of age is associated with a lack of circulating memory (CD27^high) B cells that express IgM and have not undergone isotype switching, a cell type that is also absent in adults after splenectomy. These observations suggest that CD27^high IgM⁺ B cells that react with polysaccharide antigens depend on the spleen microenvironment for their generation or long-term survival. It is unclear whether decreased TI-2 antigen responses of children less than 2 years of age are due to an intrinsic immaturity in splenic B cells or APCs or both or to other limitations in the spleen microenvironment.

ANTIBODY RESPONSES OF THE PREMATURE INFANT

The antibody response of premature infants to immunization with protein antigens is reduced during the first month of life compared to term infants, but this resolves by 2 months of age (Table 49-2). Thus, postnatal age is a more important determinant of antibody responses to TD antigens than is gestational age.[1] This may be of particular clinical relevance for hepatitis B vaccination (ie, with the HBsAg protein), which in term neonates but not premature infants is effective when given immediately after birth. As in term infants, the antibody responses of premature infants to TI-2 antigen are delayed until 6–24 months of age, depending on the particular antigen.

Maternal-Fetal Transfer of IgG

Maternal IgG is transported to the fetus by transcytosis and is detectable in the fetal circulation by 17 weeks of gestation. Circulating concentrations of IgG in the fetus rise steadily thereafter and often exceed those of the mother after 34 weeks of gestation, consistent with the IgG transfer being actively transported. The fetus synthesizes minimal amounts of IgG, with the concentration in utero almost entirely maternally derived.[1] As expected, the degree of prematurity is reflected in proportionately lower neonatal IgG concentrations.

Fetal and Postnatal Immunoglobulin Synthesis

Immunoglobulin G is the predominant isotype of immunoglobulin at all ages.[1] The half-life of IgG in the plasma is about 21 days, so maternally derived IgG levels fall rapidly after birth. The amount of IgG synthesized by the neonate and that passively derived from the mother are approximately equal when the neonate reaches 2 months of age. By 10–12 months of age, nearly all of the IgG is infant derived. IgG values reach a nadir of approximately 400 mg/dL in term infants at 3–4 months of age and rise thereafter.[1] The premature infant at birth has a lower IgG concentration, and this reaches a nadir at 3 months of age. The slow onset of IgG synthesis in the neonate is apparently an intrinsic limitation of the neonate rather than an inhibitory effect of maternal antibody. This is suggested by the observation that a similar slow onset pattern of IgG development is observed in neonates born to mothers with untreated severe hypogammaglobulinemia.

Immunoglobulin M, which does not cross the placenta, increases from a mean of 6 mg/dL in premature infants less than 28 weeks of gestation to a mean level at term of 11 mg/dL (approximately 8% of the maternal serum IgM level). This IgM, which is likely to be preimmune or "natural," is enriched for polyreactive antibodies produced by B1 cells and may play a role in the innate defense against infection. Postnatal IgM concentrations rise rapidly in premature and term infants in the first month and then more gradually thereafter, presumably in response to antigenic stimulation.[1] Although elevated (>20 mg/dL) IgM concentrations in cord blood suggest possible intrauterine infections, this is not a sensitive screen for congenital infections.

Immunoglobulin A, which also does not cross the placenta, has a concentration in cord blood of about 0.1–5.0 mg/dL (approximately 0.5% of the levels in maternal sera). Concentrations are similar in term and premature neonates and increase to approximately 20% of those in adults by 1 year of age.[1] Increased cord blood IgA concentrations are observed in some infants with congenital infection, with elevated IgA a common feature of young infants infected by vertical transmission with HIV-1. IgA has a plasma half-life of only about 5 days. Secretory IgA is present in the saliva in substantial amounts by 10 days after birth.

The serum IgE concentration of cord blood is typically only about 0.5% of maternal levels. The rate of postnatal increase varies, with a greater increase in infants predisposed to allergic disease or experiencing greater allergen environmental exposure. Although the level of cord blood IgE has been reported to also predict the risk of the subsequent development of atopy, elevated serum IgE levels at birth may also reflect maternally derived IgE in a substantial number of cases, which may obscure the predictive value of this measurement.[23] The mechanisms by which maternal IgE can be transferred to the fetus remain unclear.

NATURAL KILLER CELLS

Natural killer cells are produced by the human fetal liver as early as 6 weeks of gestation. The bone marrow is the major site for NK-cell production from late in the first trimester of gestation onward. NK cells are present in greatest numbers in the circulation during the second trimester of fetal development. They make up about 15% of total lymphocytes in the neonatal circulation, which is typically equal to or greater than the percentage of NK cells in adult blood. IL-15 plays a central role in NK-cell development, suggesting that NK-lineage cells in the fetus and neonate have normal IL-15 responsiveness and that IL-15 synthesis (mainly by nonhematopoietic cells) is also adequate.

Natural killer cells can be divided into CD56^{high} and CD56^{low} populations that are respectively specialized for cytokine production and cell-mediated cytotoxicity.[1] Cord blood CD56^{low} NK cells have a distinct surface phenotype in that they display markedly higher levels of expression of the CD94/NKG2A inhibitory receptor and significantly lower expression of several types of inhibitory receptors (multiple killer inhibitory receptors [KIRs] and leukocyte inhibitory receptor [LIR]-1/immunoglobulin-like transcript 2 [ILT2]), and the NKG2D activating receptor than adult peripheral blood NK cells.[24] The functional consequences of these differences in receptor expression by neonatal vs. adult CD56^{low} NK cells remain unclear. Cord blood NK cells overall have a markedly reduced capacity to release cytotoxic granules, to kill by natural cytotoxicity K562 erythroleukemia cells, and to kill by antibody-dependent cellular cytotoxicity (ADCC) anti-CD20 monoclonal antibody-coated Raji cells, compared to adult NK cells.[24] Full cytotoxic function is not probably achieved until at least 9–12 months of age and possibly longer.[1] NK cells from the premature infant have more pronounced reductions in killing by natural cytotoxicity or ADCC than those of the term neonate. In contrast, cytokine-stimulated killing of K562 cells by cord blood NK cells using IL-2 is comparable to that by adult NK cells. This suggests a potential cytokine immunotherapeutic strategy for augmenting NK cell activity in the newborn. CD56[low] cord blood NK cells also have a markedly greater capacity to produce IFN-γ in response to IL-12 p70 and IL-18 stimulation than their adult NK cell counterparts.[24] Taken together, these observations suggest that neonatal NK cells do not have generalized immaturity in function compared to adult NK cells but rather have a distinct functional capacity profile.

PHAGOCYTES-NEUTROPHILS

Mature neutrophils are first detected between 14 and 16 weeks of gestation. At midgestation, postmitotic neutrophils constitute only 10% of circulating leukocytes. Postmitotic neutrophils are also in markedly lower numbers in the bone marrow compared to term newborns and adults. Sepsis and other perinatal complications frequently cause neutropenia, and severe or fatal sepsis is often associated with persistent neutropenia, particularly in the premature infant. Neutropenia is frequently associated with increased margination of circulating neutrophils, which occurs early in response to infection, whereas sustained neutropenia often reflects depletion of the neonate's limited postmitotic neutrophil storage pool. Importantly, neonates with sepsis and neutropenia in whom the neutrophil storage pool is depleted are more likely to die than are those with normal storage pools. Reduced granulocyte colony-stimulating factor (G-CSF) production may also be a factor in neutropenia complicating sepsis in the newborn, but this does not appear to be a major general mechanism.

Neonatal phagocytic function in the tissues is also limited by reduction or delays in neutrophil migration from the blood to sites of infection and inflammation.[1] This delay in neutrophil accumulation in the tissues may explain why the early inflammatory response in neonatal skin often contains a larger number of eosinophils than in adult skin and why the transition from a neutrophil-predominant to a mononuclear cell–predominant tissue inflammatory response is delayed. The combination of a deficiency in the abundance of CD62-L (L-selectin) and ability to shed this protein from the surface of neonatal neutrophils and decreased binding of neonatal neutrophils to CD62-P (P-selectin) may contribute to defective cell adhesion to activated endothelium. Neonatal neutrophil chemotaxis to leukotrienes, such as LTB4, IL-8, and other

stimuli, may also be impaired. In contrast, phagocytosis and killing by neonatal neutrophils, including by the phagocyte oxidase and nonoxidative mechanisms, are largely intact. Such killing mechanisms can be compromised when opsonins, such as IgG and complement, are limiting or the bacterial density is high; such deficits in uptake and killing are greater in preterm neonates. The phagocyte oxidase pathway of signaling is also involved in the neutrophil extracellular trap (NET) generation. NETs are lattices of extracellular DNA, chromatin, and antibacterial proteins that serve to eliminate extracellular bacteria in the tissues. Cord blood neutrophils of premature and term infants have impaired NET formation compared to adult peripheral blood neutrophils, and this may compromise neonatal antibacterial defenses.[25]

PHAGOCYTES-MONONUCLEAR PHAGOCYTES

Circulating monocytes from neonates are normal in number and in phagocytic and microbicidal activity compared to adult monocytes. In contrast, the migration of neonatal monocytes into sites of inflammation, such as induced by delayed-type hypersensitivity reactions, is reduced.[1] The capacity of mononuclear phagocytes to produce proinflammatory cytokines, such as IL-1β, IL-6, IL-8, and IL-12/IL-23 p40, is substantially reduced in premature neonates[1,26]; this is associated with decreased expression of signaling molecules involved in TLR and IL-1 receptor signaling, such as MyD88.[26] These limitations in mononuclear cell function may be further compromised by a concomitant deficiency in IFN-γ production by neonatal T cells and NK cells and, to a more limited extent, by impaired responsiveness of neonatal mononuclear phagocytes to IFN-γ and a reduced capacity for TNF-α production in response to TLR ligands.[1] In contrast, cord blood monocytes of term neonates have a significantly greater capacity than adult peripheral monocytes to express IL-12/IL-23 p40, again emphasizing that the term neonatal innate immune response is not quantitatively deficient across the board compared to that of adults but rather is qualitatively different.

HUMORAL MEDIATORS OF INFLAMMATION AND OPSONIZATION

Humoral factors that participate in the response to infection and inflammation include complement components, mannan-binding lectin, fibronectin, surfactant apoproteins, and C-reactive protein, a member of the pentraxin family. Compared with adults, neonates have moderately diminished alternative complement pathway activity and slightly diminished classic complement pathway activity. Fibronectin and mannanbinding lectin concentrations are also slightly lower. Consistent with these findings, neonatal sera are less effective than adult sera in opsonization either in the absence of antibody or at low titers of antibody. Generation of complement-derived chemotactic activity is also moderately diminished. These differences are greater in preterm than in term neonates. Preterm neonates may also have compromised lung defenses as a result of reduced abundance of surfactant apoprotein A. These deficiencies, in concert with the phagocyte deficits described, may contribute to delayed inflammatory responses and impaired bacterial and fungal clearance in neonates.

HOST DEFENSE MECHANISMS AGAINST SPECIFIC PATHOGENS

Herpes Simplex Virus

Herpes simplex virus infection is severe in term infants infected at birth or postnatally up to 4 weeks of age. Characteristically, HSV infection in the neonate results in disseminated disease, with liver involvement and disseminated intravascular coagulation or central nervous system disease in approximately 60%–65% of cases.[11] Deficiencies in innate immune function mediated by neonatal NK cells, CD11c+ DCs, and pDCs may all contribute to the poor early control of infection. Reduced pDC function, including for type I IFN secretion and the activation by pDCs of CD4 T cells in the tissues may be particularly important in the vulnerability of the neonate to severe HSV infection.[3] Fetal and neonatal NK cells ex vivo have reduced natural and antibody-dependent cytotoxicity against HSV-infected target cells. These decreased NK cell responses are likely important, as older children and adults with selective NK cell deficiency are also highly susceptible to severe and disseminated infection with HSV and other herpesviruses.

As discussed, HSV-specific neonatal CD4 T-cell responses are diminished and delayed compared to those of adults following primary HSV infection. Neonates typically do not achieve adult levels of these responses until 3–6 weeks after clinical presentation, whereas adults develop robust responses by 1 week postpresentation.[11] Since CD4 T cells provide multiple effector functions that may be critical for the resolution of HSV infection, this marked lag could be an important contributor to the tendency of the neonate to develop disseminated disease and severe organ damage. The basis for the delayed development of HSV

antigen-specific CD4 T cells in neonates is not known. It is plausible that it could reflect limitations in DC function or intrinsic limitations in the ability of neonatal naïve CD4 T cells to be activated and differentiate into effector cells or both. The age at which primary HSV infection in children results in a CD4 T-cell response of similar kinetics to that of adults is unknown, but severe or disseminated infection in otherwise-healthy infants is extremely rare after 4 weeks of age.

The postinfection kinetics of HSV-specific CD8 T-cell responses in the fetus, neonate, or young infant is unknown, and particularly, it is unclear if there is any lag compared to that of the adult. Neonates have a reduced HSV-specific antibody response following infection compared to adults with primary infection,[11] and it is plausible that this could also reflect reduced and delayed HSV-specific CD4 T-cell function, as the follicular helper CD4 T-cell subset is essential for the generation of antibody responses to TD antigens, such as HSV proteins. Passively transferred maternal antibody to HSV may also play a role in decreasing transmission or ameliorating disease severity in neonatal HSV, although it is unclear if the administration of γ-globulin to neonates has a beneficial impact on established disease.

Group B Streptococci

In the absence of maternally derived type-specific opsonizing antibody, the neonate is at risk for GBS infection. The cumulative effect of individual limitations in a number of other host defense mechanisms may account for the marked susceptibility of the neonate to GBS infection[1]: Neonates lack secretory IgA and have reduced amounts of secreted fibronectin compared to older individuals. In the lungs of preterm neonates, decreased levels of surfactant apoprotein A, reduced numbers of alveolar macrophages, and diminished phagocytosis and killing of GBS by these cells may allow invasion through the respiratory tract. Limitations in the generation of chemotactic factors or chemotactic responses of neonatal neutrophils may delay recruitment of neutrophils to tissue sites of infection. Neonatal neutrophils that do reach infected tissues may kill bacteria less efficiently because of limited amounts of opsonins available. The microbicidal activity of neutrophils from certain neonates, particularly those who are the sickest, may also be decreased. Rapidly progressive infection often depletes the limited bone marrow neutrophil reserve, which contributes further to this problem. GBS may compound these developmental limitations in phagocyte function by its β protein engaging Siglec (sialic acid binding Ig-like lectin)-5 of neutrophils and of mononuclear phagocytes. This engagement impairs phagocytosis, the oxidative burst, and NET production.[27]

Once GBS infection is established, the adequacy of neutrophil production is likely critical for preventing morbidity and mortality. Severe or fatal sepsis from GBS is often associated with neutropenia, particularly in preterm neonates, and when persistent most likely reflects the depletion of the postmitotic neutrophil storage pool in the bone marrow.

The use of intravenous immunoglobulin or subcutaneously administered colony-stimulating factors in the prevention or treatment of neonatal GBS and other pyogenic infections is attractive from a theoretical standpoint. However, an analysis of multiple clinical trials suggested that this approach or using white blood cell transfusions in cases of established sepsis does not consistently reduce mortality.[1] Monoclonal antibody therapy for neonatal sepsis still holds promise. For example, there have been encouraging results from a study using an antilipotechoic humanized monoclonal antibody for the prevention of staphylococcal sepsis in prematurely born neonates.[28]

SUMMARY

A careful evaluation of components of the innate and acquired immune systems of the human fetus and neonate reveals both quantitative and qualitative deficiencies as well as skewing of innate immune response toward particular effector functions. Increased bacterial infections of the neonate, as seen in neonatal nurseries and intensive care units throughout the world, result from impaired production or function of soluble factors that serve as opsonins and defective mobility and chemotaxis of phagocytes. An inability of phagocytes to be produced at high levels under stress is also important in many cases. Increased viral infections in neonates obtains from functional deficiencies of NK cells, CD11c[+] DCs, and pDCs as well as diminished and delayed CD4 T-cell responses, which have been best documented for HSV infection. Whether diminished and delayed cytolytic CD8 T-cell responses also contribute remains unclear. Better countermeasures are needed for the protection of newborns and infants from infection, particularly those born prematurely. Specific immunotherapy is an intriguing prospect for achieving such protection.

REFERENCES

1. Lewis DB, Wilson CB. Developmental immunology and role of host defenses in the fetal and neonatal susceptibility to infection. In: Remington JS, Klein JO, Wilson CB, et al, eds. *Infectious Diseases of the Fetus and Newborn Infant.* 7th ed. Philadelphia, PA: Elsevier; 2010:80–191.
2. Merindol N, Charrier E, Duval M, Doudeyns H. Complimentary and contrasting roles of NK cells and T cells in pediatric umbilical cord blood transplantation. *J Leuk Biol.* 2011;90(1):49–60.
3. Lewis DB. Neonatal T-cell immunity and its regulation by innate immunity and dendritic cells. In: Ohls R, Yoder MC, eds. *Hematology, Immunology, and Infectious Diseases: Neonatology, Questions and Controversies.* Philadelphia, PA: Elsevier; 2011:189–217.
4. Schuster C, Vaculik C, Fiala C, et al. HLA-DR[+] leukocytes acquire CD1 antigens in embryonic and fetal human skin and contain functional antigen-presenting cells. *J Exp Med.* 2009;206(1):169–181.
5. Nguyen M, Leuridan E, Zhang T, et al. Acquisition of adult-like TLR4 and TLR9 responses during the first year of life. *PLoS One.* 2010;5(4):e10407.
6. Corbett NP, Blimkie D, Ho KC, et al. Ontogeny of toll-like receptor mediated cytokine responses of human blood mononuclear cells. *PLoS One.* 2010;5(11):e15041.
7. Weerkamp F, de Haas E, Naber B, et al. Age-related changes in the cellular comparison of the thymus in children. *J Allergy Clin Immunol.* 2005;115(4):834–840.
8. Haines CJ, Giffon TD, Lu LS, et al. Human CD4[+] T cell recent thymic emigrants are identified by protein tyrosine kinase 7 and have reduced immune function. *J Exp Med.* 2009;206(2):275–285.
9. Mold JE, Venkatasubrahmanyam S, Burt TD, et al. Fetal and adult hematopoietic stem cells give rise to distinct T cell lineages in humans. *Science.* 2010;330(6011):1695–1699.
10. Michaelsson J, Mold JE, McCune JM, Nixon DF. Regulation of T cell response in the developing fetus. *J Immunol.* 2006;176(10):5741–5748.
11. Muller WJ, Jones CA, Koelle DM. Immunobiology of herpes simplex virus and cytomegalovirus infections of the fetus and newborn. *Curr Immunol Rev.* 2010;6(1):38–55.
12. Tu W, Chen S, Sharp M, et al. Persistent and selective deficiency of CD4[+] T cell immunity to cytomegalovirus in immunocompetent young children. *J Immunol.* 2004;172(5):3260–3267.
13. White OJ, Rowe J, Richmond P, et al. Th2-polarisation of cellular immune memory to neonatal pertussis vaccination. *Vaccine.* 2010;28(14):2648–2652.
14. Weitzel RP, Lesniewski ML, Haviernik P, et al. microRNA 184 regulates expression of NFAT1 in umbilical cord blood CD4[+] T cells. *Blood.* 2009;113(26):6648–6657.
15. Chen L, Cohen AC, Lewis DB. Impaired allogeneic activation and T-helper 1 differentiation of human cord blood naïve CD4 T cells. *Biol Blood Marrow Transplant.* 2006;12(2):160–171.
16. Vermijlen D, Brouwer M, Donner C, et al. Human cytomegalovirus elicits fetal γδ T cell responses in utero. *J Exp Med.* 2010;207(4):807–821.
17. Thobakgale CF, Ramduth D, Reddy S, et al. Human immunodeficiency virus-specific CD8[+] T-cell activity is detectable from birth in the majority of in utero-infected infants. *J Virol.* 2007;81(23):12775–12784.
18. Suryani S, Tangye SG. Therapeutic implications of advances in our understanding of transitional B-cell development in humans. *Exp Rev Clin Immunol.* 2010;6(5):765–775.
19. Kaur K, Chowdhury S, Greespan NS, et al. Decreased expression of tumor necrosis factor family receptors involved in humoral immune responses in preterm neonates. *Blood.* 2007;110(8):2948–2954.
20. Schroeder HW Jr. Similarity and divergence in the development and expression of the mouse and human antibody repertoires. *Dev Comp Immunol.* 2006;30(1-2):118–135.
21. Williams JV, Weitkamp J-H, Blum DL, et al. The human neonatal B cell response to respiratory syncytial virus uses a biased antibody variable gene repertoire that lacks somatic mutations. *Mol Immunol.* 2009;47(2-3):407–414.
22. Griffin DO, Holodick NE, Rothstein TL. Human B1 cells in umbilical cord and adult peripheral blood express the

novel phenotype CD20⁺CD27⁺CD43⁺CD70⁻. *J Exp Med.* 2011;208(1):67–80.

23. Bennelykke K, Pipper CB, Bisgaard H. Transfer of maternal IgE can be a common cause of increased IgE levels in cord blood. *J Allergy Clin Immunol.* 2010;126(3):657–663.

24. Le Garff-Tavernier M, Veziat V, Decocq J, et al. Human NK cells display major phenotypic and functional changes over the life span. *Aging Cell.* 2010;9(4):527–535.

25. Yost CC, Cody MJ, Harris ES, et al. Impaired neutrophil extracellular trap (NET) formation: a novel innate immune deficiency of human neonates. *Blood.* 2009;113(25):6419–6427.

26. Lavoie PM, Huang Q, Jolette E, et al. Profound lack of interleukin (IL)-12/IL-23–40 in neonates born early in gestation is associated with an increased risk of sepsis. *J Infect Dis.* 2010;202(11):1754–1763.

27. Carlin AF, Chang Y-C, Areschoug T, et al. Group B streptococcus suppression of phagocyte functions by protein-mediated engagement of human Siglec-5. *J Exp Med.* 2009;206(8):1691–1699.

28. Weisman LE, Thrackray HM, Steinhorn RH, et al. A randomized study of a monoclonal antibody (pagibaximab) to prevent staphylococcal sepsis. *Pediatrics.* 2011;128(2):271–279.

CHAPTER 49

Thymic Aplasia and T-Cell Disorder

Yu-Lung Lau and Pamela Lee

INTRODUCTION

As detailed in chapter 49, host defense mechanisms against pathogens are defective in the newborn as a result of immature immunity. Preterm infants are particularly vulnerable to infections associated with prematurity-related complications and medical interventions. The recognition of inborn errors of immunity and differentiation from functional immaturity of the immune system pose a diagnostic challenge. An organized clinical approach is essential to facilitate early diagnosis, which has a significant impact on prognosis and survival.

To date, more than 150 monogenic primary immunodeficiency disorders (PIDs) have been described.[1] They can be classified into (1) combined T- and B-cell immunodeficiencies, (2) predominantly antibody deficiencies, (3) immune dysregulatory syndromes, (4) phagocytic disorders, (5) defects in innate immunity, (6) diseases of immune dysregulation, (7) complement deficiencies, and (8) other well-defined disorders, such as Wiskott-Aldrich syndrome (WAS) and DNA repair defects. Among them, combined T- and B-cell deficiencies constitute the most clinically important group of disorders in neonates and infants. The lack of cell-mediated immunity results in susceptibility to opportunistic infections, which is the principle manifestation leading to diagnosis in most infants with severe combined immunodeficiency (SCID). In addition, defective T-cell homeostasis may lead to immune dysregulation and lymphoproliferation, which are less commonly encountered in the neonatal period.

EPIDEMIOLOGY

Primary immunodeficiency disorders are rare disorders. SCID is estimated to occur in 1:50,000 to 1:100,000 live births, but the exact incidence is unknown as some affected infants might have died before a diagnosis could be made.[2] In addition, atypical SCID caused by hypomorphic mutations may be underdiagnosed. The implementation of newborn screening (NBS) for SCID is expected to provide epidemiological data on the true incidence rate.

The spectrum of immunological phenotypes and genetic etiology vary with ethnic background and consanguinity rate of the population. In the United States, interleukin (IL) 2 receptor γ chain (γc) deficiency of T^-B^+ immunophenotype inherited in an X-linked manner accounts for 45%–50% of SCID.[2] However, T^-B^- SCID of autosomal recessive (AR) inheritance predominates in the Athabascan-speaking Navajo and Apache native Americans because of the high frequency of *DCLRE1C* (Artemis) founder mutation (2.1%), giving rise to an incidence as high as 1:2000 live births in these ethnic groups.[3] AR-SCIDs are also more common in populations with a high prevalence of consanguineous marriage, such as North Africa and the Middle East.[4–6]

Other types of T-cell disorders presenting in the neonatal and infancy period, such as WAS and familial hemophagocytic lymphohistiocytosis, are much rarer, and the incidence varies from 1:100,000 to 1:1,000,000.[7,8]

PATHOPHYSIOLOGY

The immune response is a complex host defense network that functions to protect the body against pathogens, recognize self- and non-self-antigens, sense DNA damage, and eliminate malignant clones. To achieve these tasks, the system requires a functional repertoire consisting of optimal numbers of immune cells that can generate specific immune response to a diversity of pathogens, effectively remove the pathogen, and elicit recall memory response. The immune system must also recognize and reject alloantigens while sustaining immune tolerance to self-antigens and harmless environmental antigens. Finally, effective immune surveillance toward DNA damage is required to prevent malignancy. The immune response is tightly regulated to maintain homeostasis and prevent tissue damage from overreactivity.

Disorders of Lymphocyte Development and Differentiation

Disorders of T-cell development and differentiation constitute the most important category of T-cell disorder in neonates and infants. Molecular defects leading to numerical and functional T-cell deficiencies can be classified into 6 main categories (Table 50-1).[9]

Cytokine Signaling

The development, proliferation, survival, and differentiation of T cells take place in the thymus and are supported by cytokines, including IL-2, IL-4, IL-7, IL-9, and IL-15.[10] Receptors of these cytokines share γc as a common component. Cytokines bind to their receptors and activate the JAK-STAT signaling pathway, leading to transcription of specific genes. IL-2 promotes T-cell growth, immunoglobulin (Ig) production, and natural killer (NK) cell cytotoxicity. Therefore, SCID caused by defects in γc and JAK3 are characterized by severe depletion of T cells and NK cells. The B cells are present but are functionally abnormal due to the lack of T-cell help and defective IL-4- and IL-21-mediated signaling. In IL-7 receptor α -chain (IL7Rα) deficiency, T cells are absent but B cells and NK cells are present.[11]

V(D)J Recombination

Normal maturation of T cells and B cells depends on successful somatic recombination of variable (V), diversity (D), and joining (J) gene segments that encode the variable regions of the T-cell receptors (TCRs) and immunoglobulin receptors, respectively. V(D)J recombination is initiated by the introduction of site-specific DNA double-strand breaks (DSBs) to regions flanking the V, D, and J gene segments,

Table 50-1 Genetic Etiology and Immunophenotype of Severe T-Cell Defects Manifesting in Neonatal or Early Infancy Period

Functional Defect	Examples of Gene Defects	Immunophenotype
Cytokine signaling	IL-2RG, JAK3, IL-7R	T⁻B⁺SCID/Omenn syndrome
V(D)J recombination	RAG1, RAG2, DCLRE1C (Artemis), LIG4, DNAPKcs, Cernunnos	T⁻B⁻SCID/Omenn syndrome
Basic cellular processes	ADA, PNP	SCID with severe T/B/NK-cell deficiency, Omenn syndrome
	RMRP, SMARCAL1	Immuno-osseous dysplasia with T lymphopenia/SCID
	AK2	Reticular dysgenesis
Antigen presentation	MHC class I deficiency: TAP1, TAP2, TAPBP	CD8 lymphopenia, normal CD4
	MCH class II deficiency: CIITA, RFX5, RFXAP, RFXANK	CD4 lymphopenia, normal CD8
T-cell receptor and surface antigen signaling	Defects in the components of T-cell receptor–CD3 complex (CD3γ, CD3δ, CD3ε, CD3ζ)	T⁻B⁺SCID
	ZAP70	CD8 lymphopenia, normal CD4
	CD45	T⁻B⁺SCID
Absent/hypoplastic thymus	22q11 deletion syndrome, CHARGE association	T⁻B⁺SCID/Omenn syndrome
Defective thymic egress	CORO1A	T⁻B⁺SCID

Abbreviations: CHARGE, coloboma, heart defects, choanal atresia, mental retardation, genitourinary, and ear anomalies; IL, interleukin; MHC, major histocompatibility complex and the broken ends are rejoined by the nonhomologous end-joining (NHEJ) pathway. V(D)J recombination defects lead to a block of T-cell and B-cell maturation, while NK lineage is spared, giving rise to a T⁻B⁻NK⁺ immunophenotype. The ubiquitously expressed NHEJ pathway is also an important DNA repair mechanism for maintaining genomic integrity; hence, tissue cells with dysfunctional NHEJ DSB repair machinery are prone to mutagenesis induced by ionizing radiation.[12]

Defects in Basic Cellular Processes

A number of PIDs are caused by disorders in various housekeeping processes, such as purine salvage pathways and ribosome biogenesis. Adenosine deaminase (ADA) and purine nucleoside phosphorylase (PNP) are enzymes of the purine salvage pathway expressed in all tissues of the body, with the highest expression in lymphoid cells. Purine metabolites are toxic to the lymphocyte progenitors, and they interfere with V(D)J recombination. Apoptosis of the immature thymocytes results in profound lymphopenia.[13] Both ADA and PNP deficiencies are associated with neurological deficits, such as developmental delay, learning disability, and sensorineural hearing loss.[14] ADA deficiency has additional organ involvement, including pulmonary interstitial inflammation, skeletal abnormalities, and hepatic and renal dysfunction.

Dysfunction of ribosomal biogenesis accounts for several congenital bone marrow failure syndromes, among which cartilage-hair hypoplasia (CHH) exhibits severe T-cell defects. CHH is caused by mutation of the ribonuclease mitochondrial RNA-processing endonuclease (RMRP), which is involved in ribosomal RNA cleavage. Affected neonates displays short-limb dwarfism related to underlying metaphyseal chondrodysplasia. The immunological defect is thought to be related to disturbed cell cycle control.[15]

Reticular dysgenesis is caused by a defect of adenylate kinase 2, a mitochondrial enzyme involved in cellular energy generation by oxidative phosphorylation. It manifests early in the neonatal period with SCID and profound neutropenia as a result of developmental arrest in myeloid and lymphoid lineages, especially T and NK cells. Affected infants also have severe sensorineural deafness.[16,17]

Defect of T-Cell Receptor Signaling

The response of T lymphocytes to antigens is mediated through signaling via the antigen receptor complex, which consists of the TCRαβ or TCRγδ and the associated invariant accessory proteins collectively called CD3 (CD3δε, CD3γε, CD3ζζ). Signaling through the multimeric TCR/CD3 complex

determines the development, survival, and effector functions of T lymphocytes.[18] CD3δ, CD3ε, CD3ζ deficiencies are known to cause SCID with T⁻B⁺NK⁺ phenotype. CD3γ deficiency leads to partial T lymphopenia, and clinical severity is more variable.[19,20] Deficiency of other molecules involved in TCR signaling, such as CD45[21] and ζ-associated protein, 70kd (ZAP70), were also reported in young infants with SCID manifestations. Characteristically, patients with ZAP70 deficiency exhibit very low or total absence of CD8⁺ T-cells.[22]

Defects of Antigen Presentation

The CD8⁺ T lymphocytes recognize viral particles associated with major histocompatibility complex (MHC) class I molecules and CD4⁺ T lymphocytes recognize antigens presented by MHC class II molecules. Deficiencies of MHC class I or class II molecules are collectively known as bare lymphocyte syndrome.[23] Patients with MHC class II deficiency present in infancy with protracted opportunistic infections as they fail to mount CD4⁺ T-cell-mediated response to specific pathogens and display severe CD4⁺ lymphopenia and impaired humoral immunity.[24] Unlike MHC class II deficiency, the age of onset of MHC class I deficiency varies from childhood to adulthood, and clinical features include recurrent sinopulmonary bacterial infections, bronchiectasis, and granulomatous skin inflammations.[25]

Disorder of Thymic Development and Functions

The thymus provides an architecturally and functionally organized microenvironment for T-cell development. Immature thymocytes undergo successive stages of TCR gene rearrangement, positive selection, lineage commitment to single-positive (CD4 or CD8) T cells, negative selection, and finally exit the thymus to the circulation as peripheral T-cell repertoire.[26] T-cell deficiency occurs in developmental defects of the thymus, such as 22q11.2 deletion syndrome (DiGeorge syndrome, DGS) and CHARGE (coloboma, heart defects, choanal atresia, mental retardation, genitourinary and ear anomalies) association. Abnormal migration of neural crest cells into pouch ectoderm forms the basis of thymic hypoplasia, hypoparathyroidism, and conotruncal cardiac defects in 22q11.2 deletion. Thymic aplasia ("complete" DGS) occurs in less than 0.5% patients with 22q11.2 deletion and manifests as SCID. The majority have impaired thymic development, leading to variable defects in T-cell numbers, T-regulatory cell function, and central tolerance with increased predisposition to infections and autoimmunity.[27,28]

Haploinsufficiency of the CHD7 gene was identified as a cause of CHARGE syndrome. CHD7 is expressed in the mesenchyme of the pharyngeal arches, and a small number of patients were found to have thymic aplasia or hypoplasia.[29] The prevalence of immunodeficiency in patients with CHARGE syndrome is unknown, but a few cases of T⁻B⁺NK⁺ SCID were reported.[30]

Immunological Consequence of Defects in T-Cell Development

Profound numerical and functional deficits of T and B lymphocytes severely compromise the host's defense against infections. If residual protein expression or activity is permitted by hypomorphic mutation, impairment of the adaptive immune response is variable, and some function may be retained. Hypomorphic mutations of SCID-causing genes, such as *RAG1, RAG2, Artemis, LIG4, IL2RG, IL7R, ADA, RMRP, CHD7,* and 22q11.2 deletion, are known to cause Omenn syndrome, which is characterized by generalized erythroderma, lymphadenopathy, eosinophilia, and increased IgE in addition to severe immunodeficiency.[9,31-33] The thymus is dysplastic, but the residual, yet aberrant, thymic function allows maturation of a limited number of T cells, which manage to exit the thymus to the periphery, where they expand on activation by antigens. Therefore, T-cell count may be slightly reduced or even increased, but they exhibit an oligoclonal TCR repertoire and fail to mount effective cell-mediated immune response against pathogens.[34] Impaired central tolerance as well as abnormal development and function of T-regulatory cells account for the emergence of autoreactive T cells, which cause uncontrolled tissue inflammation and autoimmunity.[35,36]

Immune Dysregulatory Disorders

Naturally arising regulatory T cells (CD4⁺CD25⁺FOXP3⁺ Tregs) is a specialized T-cell subset defined by high intracellular levels of Foxp3 protein expression. FOXP3 is a transcription factor required for the development and function of Treg cells, which are critical mediators of peripheral tolerance. Treg cells downregulate activated effector T cells by suppressing their production of proinflammatory cytokines and by secreting inhibitory cytokines such as IL-10 and transforming growth factor β (TGF-β).[37] The absence of FOXP3-expressing Tregs leads to immune dysregulation, polyendocrinopathy, enteropathy, X-linked (IPEX) syndrome, which is characterized by multiple organ-specific autoimmunity, such as type I diabetes mellitus, thyroiditis, severe enteropathy and villous atrophy, immune cytopenia, dermatitis, and recurrent infections.[38,39]

When regulatory mechanisms of natural termination of immune response are disrupted, uncontrolled activation and proliferation of immune cells will cause systemic hyperinflammation. Hemophagocytic lymphohistiocytosis (HLH) is a group of disorders caused by ineffective cytotoxic T-cell and NK-cell response secondary to defects in granule-mediated cytotoxicity. Cytotoxic T cells and NK cells kill infected cells by forming an immunological synapse, through which cytolytic granules containing perforin, granzyme, and other serine-specific proteases are released into the target cells.[40] Genetic defects of vesicle transport, priming, docking, fusion, and pore formation at the cytotoxic cell–target cell interface result in familial HLH.[41] In the majority of cases, though, HLH is secondary to known triggers, such as infections (especially Epstein-Barr virus), malignancy, rheumatic diseases, and metabolic conditions.[42] While infected target cells fail to be cleared, the activated inflammatory cells continue to proliferate and infiltrate various organs, causing massive tissue damage. Cytopenia occurs as activated macrophages spontaneously phagocytose blood cells and platelets. The majority of familial HLH present before 1 year of age, and approximately 10% are symptomatic in the neonatal period.

Autoimmune lymphoproliferative syndrome (ALPS) is a disorder of programmed cell death. In normal circumstances, proliferation and activation of lymphocytes after antigenic stimulation is kept in check by the process of activation-induced cell death, which is mediated by the interaction between Fas and Fas ligand expressed on activated lymphocytes. This triggers the intracellular caspase cascade and subsequent proteolysis, DNA degradation, and apoptosis.[43,44] Molecular defects along the apoptotic pathway lead to ALPS, which presents as lymphadenopathy, splenomegaly, hepatomegaly, lymphocytosis, and autoimmunity. ALPS of neonatal or prenatal onset is often severe.[45,46] In general, most patients with ALPS do not have intrinsic susceptibility to infection. There is an increased risk of malignancy.

CLINICAL INDICATORS OF PRIMARY IMMUNODEFICIENCIES AND DIFFERNTIAL DIAGNOSES

The suspicion of potential primary immunodeficiencies relies on the recognition of clinical pointers, such as protracted sepsis with unusual severity and suboptimal response to appropriate antimicrobials, opportunistic infections, inflammatory manifestations such as skin rash and enterocolitis, and autoimmunity such as cytopenia and endocrinopathies. Initiation of immunological investigations should be considered after thorough clinical review for maternal, peripartum, and neonatal risk factors for infections and the source of infection and rule out secondary causes of immunodeficiencies (Table 50-2). Maternal human immunodeficiency virus (HIV) status should be ascertained, and HIV testing of the infant should be considered as appropriate. Awareness of the early signs and laboratory features that indicate a potential underlying immunodeficiency is crucial to facilitate early diagnosis, minimize infection or immune-mediated damage to vital organs, and optimize transplant outcome.

Opportunistic Infections

Infections commonly occurring in patients with T-cell defects and other categories of PIDs are listed in Table 50-3. An infant with SCID classically presents with cough, tachypnea, wheezing, and oxygen desaturation, often with a history of chronic diarrhea, persistent oral candidiasis, poor feeding, and suboptimal weight gain.[47] Chest x-ray often shows diffuse interstitial shadowing or ground glass appearance typical of *Pneumocystis jiroveci* pneumonia (PCP), and absence of thymic shadow may be evident. Identification of *P. jiroveci* requires a sample obtained by bronchoalveolar lavage, which is also useful to identify other coexisting pathogens, such as cytomegalovirus (CMV), adenovirus, and bacille Calmette-Guérin (BCG) if vaccinated.[48] PCP is regarded as an indicator disease for PIDs and HIV infection, though isolated nursery outbreaks of PCP were reported in resource-poor settings.[49]

Systemic viral dissemination, such as of CMV and adenovirus, can lead to significant morbidities and mortalities. In addition to bronchopneumonia, infants with disseminated adenovirus infection may develop hepatitis, meningoencephalitis, pancytopenia, and disseminated intravascular coagulation.[50] Similar features are also present in disseminated CMV, but chorioretinitis, sensorineural hearing loss, and long-term neurological deficits are special concerns.[51] Antiviral agents can provide some degree of control over viral replication, but clearance requires immunoreconstitutive procedures such as hematopoietic stem cell transplantation (HSCT).

Disseminated candidiasis is a frequent infection in infants born under the gestational age of 32 weeks and those with very low birth weight.[52] Invasive aspergillosis is uncommon among neonates, but together with candidiasis their incidences have increased since the mid-1990s, coinciding with the increased survival of premature infants.[49,52] The occurrence of these fungal infections in infants without obvious risk factors, especially when there are other concurrent opportunistic infections, should raise suspicions for PIDs.

Infants with PIDs undiagnosed at birth may suffer from live vaccine-related illness as they are vaccinated according to schedule. In countries where live-attenuated BCG vaccine is routinely given at birth, regional or disseminated BCG commonly occurs in infants with major primary immunodeficiencies such as SCID, chronic granulomatous disease (CGD), and inborn defects of IL-12-interferon-γ axis.[53,54] They present with persistent discharge and ulceration at the BCG inoculation site; ipsilateral axillary lymphadenopathy; and distant and systemic dissemination, including pneumonia, hepatosplenomegaly, multifocal lymphadenopathy, skin nodules, osteomyelitis, and bone marrow involvement. Chronic rotavirus gastroenteritis and disseminated chickenpox has also been reported in infants with undiagnosed SCID who received rotavirus and varicella vaccines.[55,56]

Table 50-2 Causes of Recurrent Infections and Secondary Immunodeficiencies in Neonates

Breach of physical barrier
  Pulmonary
  Central nervous system
  Urinary tract
  Skin
	Ciliary dysfunction, cystic fibrosis, aspiration pneumonia secondary to oromotor
	  dysfunction, tracheoesophageal fistula or esophageal fistula
	Spinal dysraphism (eg, myelomeningocele, congenital dermal sinus tract, basal skull
	  defect)
	Vesicoureteric reflux, pelvic-ureteric obstruction, urethral stenosis
	Skin fragility and breakdown associated with prematurity, bullous disorders

Environmental	Nosocomial infections in nursery/intensive care unit Personal/contacts of chronic carriage of pathogenic organisms (eg, *Staphylococcus aureus*)
Foreign bodies	Endotracheal intubation and prolonged ventilation, indwelling catheters
Secondary immunodeficiencies	Malnutrition Protein-losing states (nephrotic syndrome, enteropathy) Renal failure Diabetes mellitus Immunosuppressive therapy

Table 50-3 Common Pathogens in Primary Immunodeficiencies

Defects	Organisms	Types of Infections/Organs Involved
T-cell deficiencies	Respiratory viruses such as respiratory syncytial virus, adenovirus, influenza virus, parainfluenza virus, rhinovirus Rotavirus, norovirus Adenovirus, cytomegalovirus, Epstein-Barr virus *Mycobacteria* species *Salmonella* species *Pneumocystis jiroveci* Fungi (eg, candida, aspergillus)	Bronchiolitis, pneumonitis Chronic enteritis Viremia, systemic dissemination Bacille Calmette-Guérin (BCG)-itis/disseminated BCG, *Mycobacterium tuberculosis* infection Chronic enteritis, bacteremia, osteomyelitis, meningitis Pneumonitis Mucocutaneous candidiasis, aspergillosis
Antibody deficiencies	Encapsulated bacteria: *Streptococcus pneumoniae, Haemophilus influenzae* *Giardia lamblia* *Ureaplasma urealyticum* *Mycoplasma* Echovirus Poliovirus	Sinopulmonary infections, meningitis, bacteremia Chronic diarrhea Chronic arthritis Chronic arthritis, pneumonia Meningoencephalitis Vaccine-associated polio (oral live-attenuated polio vaccine)
Phagocytic defects	Catalase-positive bacteria (eg, *Staphylococcus aureus*) Gram-negative bacteria (eg, *Klebsiella* species, *Escherichiacoli, Enterobacter, Serratia marcescens, Salmonella* species, *Pseudomonas* species) Fungi (eg, *Candida, Aspergillus*) Mycobacteria species	Skin abscess, pneumonia, osteomyelitis Recurrent diarrhea, bacteremia, musculoskeletal infections Candidiasis, pulmonary/disseminated aspergillosis BCG-itis/disseminated BCG, *M. tuberculosis* infection
Complement deficiencies	*Neisseria meningitidis* Encapsulated bacteria (eg, *S. pneumoniae, H. influenzae*)	Meningitis Sinopulmonary infections, bacteremia, meningitis

Skin Eruptions

Infants with various PIDs can present with generalized erythroderma or diffuse exfoliative skin rash. As described in a previous section, erythroderma and secondary alopecia and loss of eyebrows is characteristic of Omenn syndrome, in which activated, oligoclonal T cells infiltrate the skin and elicit an inflammatory response. The skin is thickened and leathery, and skin biopsy typically shows acanthosis and parakeratosis, with an inflammatory infiltrate prominent at the dermis consisting of CD3+ T cells, eosinophils, and some macrophages. Hypoproteinemia and generalized edema often occur because of protein loss through the skin, as well as chronic diarrhea, which often coexists.[34]

An infant with SCID lacks the ability to reject allogeneic cells. Maternal T lymphocytes are not uncommonly detectable in the infant's peripheral blood and may cause a graft-vs-host reaction manifesting as diffuse skin erythema, neutropenia, eosinophilia, and increased liver enzymes. The skin eruption resembles atopic dermatitis but preferentially affects the palms and soles.[31] Maternofetal engraftment is usually mild or asymptomatic in most cases; in contrast, transfusion of nonirradiated blood products can cause fatal graft-vs-host disease (GVHD) with diffuse necrotizing erythroderma, severe mucosal inflammation of the gut, and biliary tract destruction.[57]

Other causes of neonatal erythroderma include staphylococcal scalded skin syndrome, congenital cutaneous candidiasis, hereditary ichthyoses such as congenital ichthyosiform erythroderma and harlequin ichthyosis, Netherton syndrome, psoriasis, and drug eruptions. Skin biopsy is helpful to reach the definitive diagnosis.[58]

Eczematous skin rash also occurs in other forms of PIDs, such as WAS, Job syndrome (autosomal dominant hyper-IgE syndrome), and IPEX.[59]

Enteropathy

Enteropathy associated with PIDs can be infective, inflammatory, or both. Immunodeficiencies with gastrointestinal symptoms presenting in the neonatal and early infancy period include SCID, CGD, IPEX, ALPS, and defect of NF-κB regulation (NF-κB essential modulator [NEMO] deficiency).[60,61] Chronic viral or bacterial enteritis also leads to mucosal damage and villus atrophy. Infants with IPEX may develop auto-immune enteropathy within the first few days of life, and diagnostic clues are provided by evidence of multiorgan autoimmunity, such as type 1 diabetes mellitus and hypothyroidism.[62]

Congenital Malformations and Dysmorphisms

Some forms of PIDs are associated with a characteristic group of structural anomalies or organ dysfunction. In such syndromic PIDs, somatic features are often the presenting manifestations that lead to further investigations. Recognizable syndromes include 22q11.2 deletion syndrome, CHARGE syndrome, immuno-osseous dysplasia such as CHH, and microcephaly syndromes such as Nijmegen breakage syndrome. While the severity of a cellular defect is often variable, some of them may manifest as classical SCID with life-threatening infections and autoimmunity.

For an infant with congenital heart malformation, facial dysmorphism, and palatal defect, it is important to look for hypocalcemia and lymphopenia, which suggest 22q11.2 deletion syndrome or CHARGE syndrome.[63] Further immunological investigations, including for lymphocyte subset and Ig levels, should be initiated. As blood transfusion and platelet support are often required when these infants undergo cardiac operation, the blood bank should be notified to provide irradiated, CMV-negative blood products if lymphopenia is apparent.

Table 50-4 summarizes the various forms of syndromic immunodeficiencies that can be recognized at birth because of body dysmorphisms and susceptibility to infections. In some forms of syndromic immunodeficiencies, immune aberrations progress with age and susceptibility to infections occurs later in childhood, such as ataxia telangiectasia. Review of the full spectrum of syndromic PID is beyond the scope of this chapter, and readers can refer to a few excellent reviews by Ming et al[64,65] and Kersseboom et al.[66]

Cytopenia

A number of PIDs are associated with cytopenia caused by immune-mediated destruction or bone marrow failure.[67] As described in a previous section, patients with leaky SCID may develop immune cytopenia. Infants with WAS commonly present with petechial rash and eczematous skin lesions, and in severe cases, major bleeding such as intracranial hemorrhage may result from profound thrombocytopenia. Autoimmune hemolytic anemia and neutropenia may coexist.[68] Autoimmune cytopenia affects more than 70% of patients with ALPS, and hypersplenism may cause consumptive thrombocytopenia, which is often severe and refractory to treatment.[44,45] In reticular dysgenesis, arrest in myeloid differentiation leads to neutropenia,[16] while patients with dyskeratosis congenita develop aplastic anemia.[69] Fever unresponsive to antimicrobials, hepatosplenomegaly, and cytopenia are cardinal signs of HLH, and further laboratory investigations are required to fulfill the diagnostic criteria.[42] Infants with cytopenia are often brought to the attention of hematologists, and the constellation of infectious and autoimmune complications should prompt the consideration of respective PID syndromes.

Family history

Family history of recurrent infections, autoimmune disease, malignancy, and unexplained infant deaths should be elicited to determine the pattern of inheritance. Presence of affected male relatives on the maternal side is particularly relevant, as X-linked SCID accounts for more than 50% of all forms of SCID.[70] Other X-linked PIDs are listed in Table 50-5.[71] The risk of AR disorders is increased in consanguineous families, which are prevalent in the Middle East; northern and sub-Saharan African; and western, central, and southern Asia. Some PIDs are also more prevalent in certain ethnic populations due to founder mutations, such as Artemis-deficient SCID in Athabascan-speaking native Americans[72] and CHH in the Amish population.[73]

INVESTIGATIONS

Diagnostic investigations of an infant with suspected PID follow a stepwise approach, from initial screening, immunophenotyping, functional characterization, to molecular diagnosis.[74] It should be noted that age-specific reference range, ideally locally derived, has to be used.

Complete Blood Cell Count

Complete blood cell count provides useful information as an initial evaluation. It has to be emphasized that infants have high levels of total lymphocytes, and an age-specific reference range should be used. The reference interval for absolute lymphocyte count (ALC) is 3.4–7.6 × 10^9/L for healthy newborns, and T cells normally make up 70% of circulating lymphocytes.[74] An infant with an ALC less than 3.0 × 10^9/L is lymphopenic, and immediate immunologic evaluation is warranted if confirmed on a repeat test. It should be noted that ALC can be normal or increased in Omenn syndrome and maternal T-cell engraftment.[75]

Table 50-4 Somatic and Immunological Features of Syndromic Primary Immunodeficiencies

Disease	Somatic Features	Other Organ Dysfunction	Immunophenotype	Molecular Defect/ Inheritance
Skeletal dysplasia				
Cartilage-hair hypoplasia	Metaphyseal chondrodysplasia, fine sparse hair, growth failure	Hirschsprung disease, intestinal malabsorption, macrocytic anemia	Lymphopenia, impaired lymphocyte proliferation, may have humoral deficiency, autoimmunity, malignant predisposition, may present with SCID/Omenn phenotype	RMRP, AR
Schimke immune-osseous syndrome	Spondyloepiphyseal dysplasia, lumbar lordosis, hyperpigmented macules, thin hair, facial dysmorphism, IUGR, growth failure	Glomerulosclerosis, end-stage renal failure, cerebral ischemia, bone marrow failure	Lymphopenia (particularly CD4⁺), impaired lymphocyte proliferation, abnormal immunoglobulin pattern	SMARCAL1, AR
Facial dysmorphism				
22q11.2 deletion syndrome	Facial dysmorphism, cleft palate/ velopharyngeal insufficiency, conotruncal anomalies, renal anomalies	Hypoparathyroidism (neonatal hypocalcemic tetany), developmental delay	Thymic aplasia/ hypoplasia, SCID/Omenn phenotype in < 0.5%; majority have partial T-cell defects, predisposition to autoimmunity	22q11.2 deletion, 10% familial (AD)
CHARGE syndrome	Coloboma, heart defects, atresia of the choanae, retardation of growth and development, genital hypoplasia, and ear anomalies or deafness	Hypoparathyroidism, cranial nerve defect (IX, X, XI, V), tracheoesophageal fistula, developmental delay	Lymphopenia, rarely manifests as SCID/ Omenn phenotype with absent thymus	CHD7, sporadic
Immunodeficiency, centromeric instability, and facial anomalies (ICF) syndrome	Facial dysmorphism, micrognathia, macroglossia	Psychomotor impairment, developmental delay	T lymphopenia, humoral deficiency	ICF1: DNMT3B, AR ICF2: ZBTB24, AR
Microcephaly				
DNA ligase IV deficiency	Microcephaly, facial dysmorphism, skin anomalies, growth retardation	Pancytopenia, radiosensitivity, malignant predisposition, developmental delay	SCID/Omenn phenotype	LIG4, AR
Nijmegen breakage syndrome	Microcephaly, facial dysmorphism ("bird-like" facies), limb anomalies (polydactyly/syndactyly), growth retardation	Radiosensitivity, malignant predisposition, progressive mental retardation	Progressive T lymphopenia (particularly CD4⁺), impaired lymphocyte proliferation, humoral deficiency, predisposition to lymphoid malignancy	NBS1, AR
Hoyeraal-Hreidarsson syndrome (X-linked dyskertosis congenita)	Microcephaly, cerebellar hypoplasia, enteropathy (classical mucocutaneous abnormalities absent in infancy), intrauterine growth retardation	Bone marrow failure with pancytopenia, developmental delay	Progressive lymphopenia may have SCID-like manifestations with opportunistic infections (eg, PCP, CMV); relatively preserved T cells with near absence of B cells and NK cells is characteristic	DKC1, X-linked

Abbreviations: AD, autosomal dominant; AR, autosomal recessive; CMV, cytomegalovirus; IUGR, intrauterine growth retardation; NK, natural killer; PCP, *Pneumocystis jiroveci* pneumonia; RMRP, ribonuclease mitochondrial RNA-processing endonuclease; SCID, severe combined immunodeficiency.

Table 50-5 X-Linked Primary Immunodeficiencies (PIDs)

PID Category	Disease
Combined T- and B-cell immunodeficiency	Common γ-chain-deficient severe combined immunodeficiency (SCID)
Predominantly antibody deficiencies	X-linked agammaglobulinemia (XLA, BTK defect) X-linked hyperimmunoglobulin M syndrome (X-HIM, CD40L defect)
Phagocytic defects	X-linked chronic granulomatous disease (X-CGD, gp91phox defect)
Immune dysregulatory disorders	X-linked lymphoproliferative (XLP) disorder XLP1: SH2D1A defect XLP2: XIAP defect Immune dysregulation, polyendocrinopathy, X linked (IPEX, FOXP3 defect)
Innate immune defects	Anhidrotic ectodermal dysplasia with immunodeficiency (EDA-ID, NEMO defect)
Complement deficiencies	Properdin deficiency
Other well-defined disorders	Wiskott-Aldrich syndrome Hoyeraal-Hreidarsson syndrome (X-linked dyskeratosis congenita, dyskerin defect)

Abbreviations: IPEX, immune dysregulation, polyendocrinopathy, enteropathy, X-linked syndrome; NEMO, nuclear factor κB essential modulator.

Chest X-ray

The normal thymus is visualized on the chest x-ray as a prominent soft-tissue density in the anterosuperior mediastinum up to the age of 3 years.[76] Narrowing of the anterior mediastinum is suggestive of thymic hypoplasia. The chest x-ray of an infant with severe T-cell deficiency often shows features of interstitial pneumonia commonly caused by respiratory viruses or PCP. Cupping and flaring of the costochondral junction of the ribs characteristic of ADA deficiency may be appreciated.[48]

Lymphocyte Subset

The total number and percentage of T cells (CD3+) and their major subsets (CD4+ and CD8+), B cells (CD19+), and NK cells (CD16+/CD56+) in the peripheral blood are determined by flow cytometry. This provides information on the degree of numerical deficiency and immunophenotype that provides clues to the underlying molecular diagnosis.[75,77] T−B+ phenotype suggests defects in the signaling pathway mediated by cytokines belonging to the γc family, while T−B− phenotype indicates V(D)J recombination defects. Lymphopenia is more profound in ADA SCID and reticular dysgenesis and may exhibit near absence of all T, B, and NK cells. Selective absence of CD4+ T cells suggests MHC class II deficiency, while ZAP70 deficiency should be considered when CD8+ T cells are absent.[75,78] IPEX is diagnosed by the absence of FOXP3-expressing CD4+CD25+ T cells. CD3+TCRαβ+CD4−CD8− double-negative T cells are increased in ALPS.[75]

Antibody Assays

The level of serum IgG in infants under the age of 6 months reflects passive transfer of maternal IgG across the placenta. Therefore, infants with SCID have apparently normal serum IgG despite their intrinsic failure of immunoglobulin production. IgA and IgM levels are normally low at birth. Immune dysregulation may lead to aberrant production of IgM. Serum IgE is elevated in Omenn syndrome, hyper-IgE syndrome, and IPEX.[79]

Older infants who have received routine vaccination can be tested for functional antibodies toward vaccine antigens, such as tetanus, diphtheria, and pneumococcus. These are absent in severe T-cell deficiency due to the lack of T-cell help for specific antibody response and primary B-cell deficiency.

These tests are the basic initial investigations that should be performed for infants suspected to have T-cell deficiencies. Pediatric immunologists should be consulted for clinical evaluation and specialized investigations to further delineate the immunophenotype and confirm the molecular etiology.

Lymphocyte Function

The ability of lymphocytes to proliferate in response to mitogens (phytohemagglutinin [PHA], concanavalin A [ConA], pokeweed mitogen [PWM]); antigens to which the individual is previously sensitized (eg, candida, purified protein derivative [PPD]); or monoclonal antibodies specific to T-cell surface antigens mediating signal transduction (eg, anti-CD3, anti-CD28) is evaluated by lymphocyte proliferation assay. Peripheral blood mononuclear cells are cultured with standard concentrations of stimulants, and incorporation of radiolabeled DNA precursor (tritiated thymidine) into the proliferating lymphocytes is evaluated at the end of the incubation period by a scintillation counter.[75,78]

Lymphocyte proliferation is typically absent in SCID and other severe T-cell deficiencies.

Analysis of T-Cell Origin and Clonality

Omenn syndrome and maternal engraftment can be distinguished by studying the origin of the T cells. Maternal engraftment can be confirmed by X/Y fluorescence in situ hybridization (FISH) if the patient is a boy, HLA typing, or analysis of short-tandem repeats. Maternal T cells can be detected in 50% of B⁻SCID and 80% of B⁺SCID. Most of them have a mature T-cell phenotype (CD45RO⁺).[31,34]

Clonality of T cells can be studied by analyzing the distribution of different TCR β-chains (Vβ) by flow cytometry or quantitative polymerase chain reaction (PCR). A restricted TCR repertoire can be observed in B⁻SCID with residual V(D)J recombination capacity.[80] These oligoclonal T cells are activated and express activation markers such as HLA-DR and CD25.

Evaluation of Thymic Output

The majority of T cells (>90%) in newborns are naïve cells that are able to respond to neoantigens. They bear the surface marker CD45RA. After antigen encounter, a proportion of T cells differentiates into memory T cells that express CD45RO. The generation of naïve CD4⁺ and CD8⁺ T cells is a measurement of thymic output.[81]

Naïve T cells that exit the thymus contain circular DNA fragments generated during V(D)J recombination, known as T-cell receptor excision circles (TRECs). TRECs can be quantified by real-time quantitative PCR and is a reliable surrogate marker for enumerating recent thymic T-cell emigrants. Naïve T cells and TRECs are diminished in severe T-cell deficiency regardless of underlying molecular etiology. The assessment of TRECs together with TCR clonal distribution provides valuable information to the severity of T-cell defect and peripheral T-cell homeostasis.[82] TRECs assay is also applied in NBS for SCID.[83,84]

Other Specialized Tests

Diagnosis of ADA and PNP deficiency can be established by measuring enzyme activity and concentrations of dATP (deoxyadenosine triphosphate) or dGTP (deoxyguanosine triphosphate) in red blood cells, respectively. Urine for deoxyadenosine is also useful for diagnosis of ADA SCID.[85] It should be noted that these tests become invalid if the patient has received a red cell transfusion.

Patients with B⁻SCID may have DNA repair defects (Artemis, ligase IV, DNA-PKcs, Cernunnos deficiencies) leading to radiosensitivity. This can be evaluated by radiosensitivity assay and the capacity of

Table 50-6 Diagnostic Criteria for Hemophagocytic Lymphohistiocytosis (HLH)

The following parameters should be evaluated in all patients with HLH:
1. Fever
2. Splenomegaly
3. Cytopenias (affecting 2 of 3 lineages in the peripheral blood):
   Hemoglobin < 9.0 g/dL (in infants < 4 weeks: hemoglobin < 100 g/L)
   Platelets < 100 × 10⁹/L
   Neutrophils < 1.0 × 10⁹/L
4. Hypertriglyceridemia or hypofibrinogenemia:
   Fasting triglycerides ≥ 3.0 mmol/L (ie, 265 mg/dL)
   Fibrinogen ≤ 1.5 g/L
5. Hemophagocytosis in bone marrow, spleen, or lymph nodes without evidence of malignancy
6. Low or absent natural killer cell activity (according to local laboratory reference)
7. Ferritin > 500 µg/L
8. Soluble CD25 (interleukin 2 receptor) ≥ 2400 U/mL

The diagnosis of HLH is made if 5 of 8 of these criteria are fulfilled or if a molecular diagnosis consistent with HLH is established.

DSB repair induced by γ-irradiation of cultured skin fibroblasts obtained by skin biopsy.[86] These tests are performed in specialized laboratories and may not be widely available.

Specific laboratory tests are needed to establish the diagnoses of HLH and ALPS according to consensus diagnostic criteria, as summarized in Table 50-6[87] and Table 50-7,[88] respectively.

Diagnostic Molecular Studies

Diagnostic confirmation of the molecular defect can be performed by protein expression (immunoblotting or flow cytometry)[76] and sequencing of target genes guided by the cellular phenotype.[89] Genetic diagnosis also provides useful information for carrier screening, prenatal diagnosis, and identification of affected family members who are presymptomatic.

MANAGEMENT

Infants with primary immunodeficiency often present with life-threatening infections, and admission to an intensive care unit is not infrequent. As soon as acute medical issues are managed and the patient is stabilized, urgent referral to a pediatric immunologist is warranted. The definitive treatment of the various T-cell deficiencies mentioned in this chapter, including SCID, WAS, familial HLH, and IPEX, is HSCT. The majority of infants with SCID will not survive beyond the age of 1 year if a corrective procedure is not performed.

Table 50-7 Diagnostic Criteria for Autoimmune Lymphoproliferative Syndrome (ALPS)

Major criteria
1. Chronic nonmalignant lymphoproliferation: splenomegaly or lymphadenopathy of ≥ 2 nodal groups for more than 6 months
2. Marked elevation of peripheral blood double-negative (CD4⁻CD8⁻) T cells ≥ 5%
3. Defective in vitro Fas-mediated apoptosis
4. Germline or somatic pathogenic mutation in FAS, FASLG, CASP10, or NRAS

Minor criteria
1. Autoimmune cytopenia
   Thrombocytopenia, neutropenia, or hemolytic anemia, and
   Proven to be immune mediated by the presence of autoantibody (eg, direct antiglobulin test) or response to immunosuppressive treatment
2. Moderate elevation in double-negative T cells
   Elevated double-negative T cells in spleen or lymph node biopsy, or
   Peripheral blood double-negative T cells < 5% but > 2 SD above the mean of laboratory reference
3. Elevated serum immunoglobulin G
4. Elevated serum interleukin 10
5. Elevated serum vitamin B$_{12}$
6. Elevated plasma Fas ligand level

The diagnosis of ALPS is made if 3 major criteria or 2 major plus 2 minor criteria are fulfilled.

Supportive Treatment

All infants with severe immunodeficiency should be nursed in protective isolation, and contact with persons having infective symptoms should be strictly avoided. Hand washing should be reinforced for all clinical staff and carers. The source and identity of infectious agents should be established by culture, PCR, or histological studies of appropriate tissue specimens, and screening for other potential opportunistic organisms should be carried out. Infections should be treated promptly with broad-spectrum antimicrobials, and inputs from microbiologists will be beneficial. Nutritional support should be optimized. Breast-feeding is discouraged if the mother is CMV positive. Infants with SCID should receive prophylaxis against PCP, fungus, and virus. Immunoglobulin replacement, which can be given intravenously or subcutaneously, will be commenced. As blood products may contain viable lymphocytes that can elicit graft-vs-host reaction, only irradiated blood products should be used. To prevent transmission of CMV, blood products should be CMV negative or leukodepleted. Live vaccines should not be given.[47]

Enzyme replacement therapy with pegylated ADA (PEG-ADA) is available for ADA deficiency. It serves to clear the accumulated purine metabolites and leads to improvement in metabolic and immunological parameters. Although it is not a curative treatment, it serves an important role of optimizing the clinical status before transplantation or gene therapy by improving feeding, weight gain, and lung function. The trough plasma ADA activity level is monitored to evaluate the efficiency of detoxification and guides dosage adjustment.[90]

Infants with Omenn syndrome require special attention. Extensive inflammation of the skin and gut predispose the young infant to dehydration, hypoalbuminemia, and generalized edema. Fluid and electrolyte balance has to be carefully maintained. Systemic immunosuppressants, such as prednisolone and cyclosporin, are used to control inflammation caused by the activated T-cell clones.[34]

Autoimmune manifestations in ALPS are treated by immunosuppressants. Satisfactory treatment response is usually achieved by corticosteroid, but more aggressive immunosuppression may be required for severe cytopenia, such as mycophenolate mofetil (MMF) and sirolimus. Rituximab may be considered for immune cytopenia not responsive to these agents. Splenectomy should be avoided, except in the case of refractory thrombocytopenia caused by hypersplenism. The role of HSCT is unclear.[44,45]

Hemophagocytic lymphohistiocytosis is rapidly fatal without specific intervention. It is treated by a chemotherapy-based regimen consisting of corticosteroids, etoposide, and cyclosporin A, which aims to suppress hypercytokinemia, interrupt cellular proliferation, and remove the ongoing stimulus for inflammation by eliminating activated macrophages and histiocytes. Infections should be treated aggressively. A donor search should be initiated for patients with familial HLH, and continuation treatment should be given until a suitable donor is available for HSCT.[42,87]

Hematopoietic Stem Cell Transplantation and Gene Therapy

Allogeneic hematopoietic stem cell transplantation is a curative procedure for a broad range of malignant and nonmalignant diseases, including hematological malignancies, PIDs, bone marrow failure syndromes, hemoglobinopathies, and metabolic disorders. Cure of PID is achieved by adoptive transfer of healthy donor stem cells, which replace the faulty immune system of the host, thereby attaining long-term immunoreconstitution.[91] The source of donor cells includes HLA-genoidentical siblings, matched related donors (mostly in consanguineous families), mismatched related donors (including haploidentical parents), match-unrelated donors, and unrelated cord blood units.[92] Stem cells can be collected from bone marrow or peripheral blood after macrophage colony-stimulating factor (G-CSF) mobilization from the donor.

The need for conditioning, which consists of myeloablative and immunosuppressive medications to create "space" for donor stem cell engraftment, and the choice of the regimen vary with the type of PID and the immunophenotype.[91] Reduced-intensity conditioning provides the advantage of decreasing treatment-related toxicities, especially for children who have preexisting organ damage.[91,93] The outcome is influenced by the age at transplantation, disease type, stem cell source, and degree of HLA matching, conditioning-related toxicities, infections, donor cell engraftment, and GVHD.[94,95] At present, long-term survival of greater than 90% can be achieved for SCID infants receiving matched-sibling transplantation, especially when performed before the age of 3 months.[96,97] With improvement of supportive care, conditioning regimens, HLA typing, and expansion of unrelated donor registry and cord blood banks, long-term survival after unrelated donor transplantation is now approaching 80%.[98]

Since the mid-2000s, gene therapy has emerged as a promising curative procedure for treating PIDs.[99–101] It provides an important therapeutic alternative for patients without suitable donors. Such an approach is based on ex vivo transfer of the therapeutic gene into the patient's own hematopoietic stem cells using nonreplicating retroviral vectors. Long-term immunoreconstitution is achieved by the selective survival advantage of transduced lymphocytes conferred by the therapeutic genes. The use of autologous stem cells alleviates the risk of GVHD. Gene therapy has been clinically applied to treat X-SCID, ADA-SCID, CGD, and WAS.[99] Cure with sustained immunoreconstitution has been achieved in patients with X-SCID[102] and ADA-SCID.[103] Due to the nature of the γ-retroviral vectors used to deliver the corrective transgene in earlier clinical trials, leukemic transformation related to insertional mutagenesis occurred in some patients. Strategies have been developed to improve the safety and efficacy of gene therapy procedures by optimizing vector design and transgene expression.[104]

Newborn Screening

The importance of early diagnosis for SCID cannot be emphasized enough. The infective and immune complications associated with SCID are life threatening, and they also lead to organ damage, which may compromise the outcome of transplantation. A study by Brown et al showed that patients with SCID who were investigated and diagnosed in the neonatal period because of previous affected siblings have a much higher survival rate (90%) compared with the probands (40%), irrespective of donor choice, conditioning regimen, or underlying diagnosis.[105] The reasons were obvious, as protective measures against infections, immunoglobulin replacement therapy, nutritional support, clinical monitoring, and donor search can be instituted early. Better transplantation outcome can be expected when performed in a relatively well child at a younger age.[106]

Newborn screening is an ideal approach to facilitate early diagnosis of SCID in the presymptomatic stage. It utilizes the detection of TRECs on dried blood spots on filter paper (Guthrie card).[107] TRECs is a surrogate marker for recent thymic emigrants, and its absence indicates failure to generate functional T lymphocytes regardless of the molecular etiology. At present, population-based NBS for SCID is implemented in Wisconsin,[107] Massachusetts,[108] and California in the United States. In Massachusetts, the first case of SCID was identified in 2010 after screening 100,597 infants since February 1, 2009.[109] The program employs a high-throughput DNA-based assay to quantify TRECs with an internal quality control for proof of DNA integrity and amplifiability. Infants who have 2 out-of-range screening results from independently obtained specimens will undergo further testing by flow cytometric enumeration of T cells (including markers for naïve T cells), B cells, and NK cells. If T lymphopenia or low naïve T cells are present, the infant will be referred for diagnostic evaluation by an immunologist. Once the diagnosis of SCID is confirmed, specific treatment will be given immediately.[108] In May 2010, SCID was added to the Department of Health and Human Services' (HHS) core panel of 29 genetic disorders recommended for inclusion in state NBS programs.[110] Neonatologists and care providers should familiarize themselves with their respective state's NBS program and screening algorithms.

REFERENCES

1. Notarangelo LD, Fischer AF, Geha RS, et al. Primary immunodeficiencies: 2009 update. *J Allergy Clin Immunol.* 2009;124:1161–1178.
2. Griffith LM, Cowan MJ, Kohn DB, et al. Allogeneic hematopoietic cell transplantation for primary immune deficiency diseases: current status and critical needs. *J Allergy Clin Immunol.* 2008;122:1087–1096.
3. Li L, Moshous D, Zhou Y, et al. A founder mutation in Artemis, an SNM1-like protein, causes SCID in Athabascan-speaking Native Americans. *J Immunol.* 2002;168(12):6323–6329.
4. Suliaman F, Al-Ghonaium A, Harfi H. High incidence of severe combined immune deficiency in the Eastern Province of Saudi Arabia. *Pediatr Asthma, Allergy Immunol.* 2006;19(1):14–18.
5. Shabestari MS, Maljaei SH, Baradaran R, et al. Distribution of primary immunodeficiency diseases in the Turk ethnic group, living in the northwestern Iran. *J Clin Immunol.* 2007;27(5):510–516.
6. Yeganeh M, Heidarzade M, Pourpak Z, et al. Severe combined immunodeficiency: a cohort of 40 patients. *Pediatr Allergy Immunol.* 2008;19(4):303–306.

7. Ochs HD, Filipovich AH, Veys P, Cowan MJ, Kapoor N. Wiskott-Aldrich syndrome: diagnosis, clinical and laboratory manifestations, and treatment. *Biol Blood Marrow Transplant.* 2009;15(1 Suppl):84–90.

8. Freeman HR, Ramanan AV. Review of haemophagocytic lymphohistiocytosis. *Arch Dis Child.* 2011;96(7):688–693.

9. Liston A, Enders A, Siggs OM. Unravelling the association of partial T-cell immunodeficiency and immune dysregulation. *Nat Rev Immunol.* 2008;8(7):545–558.

10. Rochman Y, Spolski R, Leonard WJ. New insights into the regulation of T cells by gamma(c) family cytokines. *Nat Rev Immunol.* 2009;9(7):480–490.

11. Gaspar HB, Gilmour KC, Jones AM. Severe combined immunodeficiency–molecular pathogenesis and diagnosis. *Arch Dis Child.* 2001;84(2):169–173.

12. Dvorak CC, Cowan MJ. Radiosensitive severe combined immunodeficiency disease. *Immunol Allergy Clin North Am.* 2010;30(1):125–142.

13. Gaspar HB. Bone marrow transplantation and alternatives for adenosine deaminase deficiency. *Immunol Allergy Clin North Am.* 2010;30(2):221–236.

14. Camici M, Micheli V, Ipata PL, Tozzi MG. Pediatric neurological syndromes and inborn errors of purine metabolism. *Neurochem Int.* 2010;56(3):367–378.

15. Notarangelo LD, Roifman CM, Giliani S. Cartilage-hair hypoplasia: molecular basis and heterogeneity of the immunological phenotype. *Curr Opin Allergy Clin Immunol.* 2008;8(6):534–539.

16. Pannicke U, Hönig M, Hess I, et al. Reticular dysgenesis (aleukocytosis) is caused by mutations in the gene encoding mitochondrial adenylate kinase 2. *Nat Genet.* 2009;41(1):101–105.

17. Lagresle-Peyrou C, Six EM, Picard C, et al. Human adenylate kinase 2 deficiency causes a profound hematopoietic defect associated with sensorineural deafness. *Nat Genet.* 2009;41(1):106–111.

18. Dave VP. Hierarchical role of CD3 chains in thymocyte development. *Immunol Rev.* 2009;232(1):22–33.

19. Recio MJ, Moreno-Pelayo MA, Kiliç SS, et al. Differential biological role of CD3 chains revealed by human immunodeficiencies. *J Immunol.* 2007;178(4):2556–2564.

20. Roberts JL, Lauritsen JP, Cooney M, et al. T-B+NK+ severe combined immunodeficiency caused by complete deficiency of the CD3zeta subunit of the T-cell antigen receptor complex. *Blood.* 2007;109(8):3198–3206.

21. Kung C, Pingel JT, Heikinheimo M, et al. Mutations in the tyrosine phosphatase CD45 gene in a child with severe combined immunodeficiency disease. *Nat Med.* 2000;6(3):343–345.

22. Fischer A, Picard C, Chemin K, Dogniaux S, le Deist F, Hivroz C. ZAP70: a master regulator of adaptive immunity. *Semin Immunopathol.* 2010;32(2):107–116.

23. Gadola SD, Moins-Teisserenc HT, Trowsdale J, Gross WL, Cerundolo V. TAP deficiency syndrome. *Clin Exp Immunol.* 2000;121(2):173–178.

24. Picard C, Fischer A. Hematopoietic stem cell transplantation and other management strategies for MHC class II deficiency. *Immunol Allergy Clin North Am.* 2010;30(2):173–178.

25. Zimmer J, Andrès E, Donato L, Hanau D, Hentges F, de la Salle H. Clinical and immunological aspects of HLA class I deficiency. *QJM.* 2005;98(10):719–727.

26. Poliani PL, Vermi W, Facchetti F. Thymus microenvironment in human primary immunodeficiency diseases. *Curr Opin Allergy Clin Immunol.* 2009;9(6):489–495.

27. McLean-Tooke A, Spickett GP, Gennery AR. Immunodeficiency and autoimmunity in 22q11.2 deletion syndrome. *Scand J Immunol.* 2007;66(1):1–7.

28. Sullivan KE. The clinical, immunological, and molecular spectrum of chromosome 22q11.2 deletion syndrome and DiGeorge syndrome. *Curr Opin Allergy Clin Immunol.* 2004;4(6):505–512.

29. Zentner GE, Layman WS, Martin DM, Scacheri PC. Molecular and phenotypic aspects of CHD7 mutation in CHARGE syndrome. *Am J Med Genet A.* 2010;152A(3):674–686.

30. Gennery AR, Slatter MA, Rice J, et al. Mutations in CHD7 in patients with CHARGE syndrome cause T-B+ natural killer cell + severe combined immune deficiency and may cause Omenn-like syndrome. *Clin Exp Immunol.* 2008;153(1):75–80.

31. Niehues T, Perez-Becker R, Schuetz C. More than just SCID—the phenotypic range of combined immunodeficiencies associated with mutations in the recombinase activating genes (RAG) 1 and 2. *Clin Immunol.* 2010;135(2):183–192.

32. Ege M, Ma Y, Manfras B, et al. Omenn syndrome due to ARTEMIS mutations. *Blood.* 2005;105(11):4179–4186.

33. Felgentreff K, Perez-Becker R, Speckmann C, et al. Clinical and immunological manifestations of patients with atypical severe combined immunodeficiency. *Clin Immunol.* 2011;141(1):73–82.

34. Villa A, Notarangelo LD, Roifman CM. Omenn syndrome: inflammation in leaky severe combined immunodeficiency. *J Allergy Clin Immunol.* 2008;122(6):1082–1086.

35. Cassani B, Poliani PL, Moratto D, et al. Defect of regulatory T cells in patients with Omenn syndrome. *J Allergy Clin Immunol.* 2010;125(1):209–216.

36. Somech R, Simon AJ, Lev A, et al. Reduced central tolerance in Omenn syndrome leads to immature self-reactive oligoclonal T cells. *J Allergy Clin Immunol.* 2009;124(4):793–800.

37. Li L, Boussiotis VA. Molecular and functional heterogeneity of T regulatory cells. *Clin Immunol.* 2011;141(3):244–252. doi:10.1016/j.clim.2011.08.011.

38. Bennett CL, Christie J, Ramsdell F, et al. The immune dysregulation, polyendocrinopathy, enteropathy, X-linked syndrome (IPEX) is caused by mutations of FOXP3. *Nat Genet.* 2001;27(1):20–21.

39. Gambineri E, Perroni L, Passerini L, et al. Clinical and molecular profile of a new series of patients with immune dysregulation, polyendocrinopathy, enteropathy, X-linked syndrome: inconsistent correlation between forkhead box protein 3 expression and disease severity. *J Allergy Clin Immunol.* 2008;122(6):1105–1112.e1.

40. Filipovich AH. Hemophagocytic lymphohistiocytosis (HLH) and related disorders. *Biol Blood Marrow Transplant.* 2010;16(1 Suppl):S82–S89.

41. Pachlopnik Schmid J, Côte M, et al. Inherited defects in lymphocyte cytotoxic activity. *Immunol Rev.* 2010;235(1):10–23.

42. Freeman HR, Ramanan AV. Review of haemophagocytic lymphohistiocytosis. *Arch Dis Child.* 2011;96(7):688–693.

43. Madkaikar M, Mhatre S, Gupta M, Ghosh K. Advances in autoimmune lymphoproliferative syndromes. *Eur J Haematol.* 2011;87(1):1–9.

44. Teachey DT, Seif AE, Grupp SA. Advances in the management and understanding of autoimmune lymphoproliferative syndrome (ALPS). *Br J Haematol.* 2010;148(2):205–216.

45. Woods CW, Bradshaw WT, Woods AG. Hemophagocytic lymphohistiocytosis in the premature neonate. *Adv Neonatal Care.* 2009;9(6):265–273.

46. Turbyville JC, Rao VK. The autoimmune lymphoproliferative syndrome: a rare disorder providing clues about normal tolerance. *Autoimmun Rev.* 2010;9(7):488–493.

47. Griffith LM, Cowan MJ, Notarangelo LD, et al. Improving cellular therapy for primary immune deficiency diseases: recognition, diagnosis, and management. *J Allergy Clin Immunol.* 2009;124(6):1152–1160.e12.

48. Gennery AR, Cant AJ. Diagnosis of severe combined immunodeficiency. *J Clin Pathol.* 2001;54(3):191–195.

CHAPTER 50

49. Maldonado YA. Pneumocystis and other less common fungal infections. In: Klein JO, Wilson CB, Nizet V, Maldonado Y, eds. *Infectious Diseases of the Fetus and Newborn Infant.* 7th ed. Philadelphia, PA: Saunders/Elsevier; 2011:1078–1123.

50. Hierholzer JC. Adenoviruses in the immunocompromised host. *Clin Microbiol Rev.* 1992;5(3):262–274.

51. Boeckh M, Geballe AP. Cytomegalovirus: pathogen, paradigm, and puzzle. *J Clin Invest.* 2011;121(5):1673–1680.

52. Bendel CM. Candidiasis. In: Klein JO, Wilson CB, Nizet V, Maldonado Y, eds. *Infectious Diseases of the Fetus and Newborn Infant.* 7th ed. Philadelphia, PA: Saunders/Elsevier; 2011:1055–1077.

53. Santos A, Dias A, Cordeiro A, et al. Severe axillary lymphadenitis after BCG vaccination: alert for primary immunodeficiencies. *J Microbiol Immunol Infect.* 2010;43(6):530–537.

54. Galkina E, Kondratenko I, Bologov A. Mycobacterial infections in primary immunodeficiency patients. *Adv Exp Med Biol.* 2007;601:75–81.

55. Bakare N, Menschik D, Tiernan R, Hua W, Martin D. Severe combined immunodeficiency (SCID) and rotavirus vaccination: reports to the Vaccine Adverse Events Reporting System (VAERS). *Vaccine.* 2010;28(40):6609–6612.

56. Ghaffar F, Carrick K, Rogers BB, Margraf LR, Krisher K, Ramilo O. Disseminated infection with varicella-zoster virus vaccine strain presenting as hepatitis in a child with adenosine deaminase deficiency. *Pediatr Infect Dis J.* 2000;19(8):764–766.

57. Sebnem Kilic S, Kavurt S, Balaban Adim S. Transfusion-associated graft-versus-host disease in severe combined immunodeficiency. *J Investig Allergol Clin Immunol.* 2010;20(2):153–156.

58. Fraitag S, Bodemer C. Neonatal erythroderma. *Curr Opin Pediatr.* 2010;22(4):438–444.

59. Sillevis Smitt JH, Wulffraat NM, Kuijpers TW. The skin in primary immunodeficiency disorders. *Eur J Dermatol.* 2005;15(6):425–432.

60. Agarwal S, Mayer L. Gastrointestinal manifestations in primary immune disorders. *Inflamm Bowel Dis.* 2010;16(4):703–711.

61. Kobrynski LJ, Mayer L. Diagnosis and treatment of primary immunodeficiency disease in patients with gastrointestinal symptoms. *Clin Immunol.* 2011;139(3):238–248.

62. Blanco Quirós A, Arranz Sanz E, Bernardo Ordiz D, Garrote Adrados JA. From autoimmune enteropathy to the IPEX (immune dysfunction, polyendocrinopathy, enteropathy, X-linked) syndrome. *Allergol Immunopathol (Madr).* 2009;37(4):208–215.

63. Jyonouchi S, McDonald-McGinn DM, Bale S, Zackai EH, Sullivan KE. CHARGE (coloboma, heart defect, atresia choanae, retarded growth and development, genital hypoplasia, ear anomalies/deafness) syndrome and chromosome 22q11.2 deletion syndrome: a comparison of immunologic and nonimmunologic phenotypic features. *Pediatrics.* 2009;123(5):e871–e877.

64. Ming JE, Stiehm ER, Graham JM Jr. Immunodeficiency as a component of recognizable syndromes. *Am J Med Genet.* 1996;66(4):378–398.

65. Ming JE, Stiehm ER, Graham JM Jr. Syndromic immunodeficiencies: genetic syndromes associated with immune abnormalities. *Crit Rev Clin Lab Sci.* 2003;40(6):587–642.

66. Kersseboom R, Brooks A, Weemaes C. Educational paper: syndromic forms of primary immunodeficiency. *Eur J Pediatr.* 2011;170(3):295–308.

67. Notarangelo LD. Primary immunodeficiencies (PIDs) presenting with cytopenias. *Hematology Am Soc Hematol Educ Program.* 2009:139–143.

68. Ochs HD, Thrasher AJ. The Wiskott-Aldrich syndrome. *J Allergy Clin Immunol.* 2006;117(4):725–738.

69. Walne AJ, Dokal I. Advances in the understanding of dyskeratosis congenita. *Br J Haematol.* 2009;145(2):164–172.

70. Buckley RH. Molecular defects in human severe combined immunodeficiency and approaches to immune reconstitution. *Annu Rev Immunol.* 2004;22:625–655.

71. Pessach IM, Notarangelo LD. X-linked primary immunodeficiencies as a bridge to better understanding X-chromosome related autoimmunity. *J Autoimmun.* 2009;33(1):17–24.

72. Li L, Moshous D, Zhou Y, et al. A founder mutation in Artemis, an SNM1-like protein, causes SCID in Athabascan-speaking Native Americans. *J Immunol.* 2002;168(12):6323–6329.

73. Ridanpää M, Jain P, McKusick VA, Francomano CA, Kaitila I. The major mutation in the RMRP gene causing CHH among the Amish is the same as that found in most Finnish cases. *Am J Med Genet C Semin Med Genet.* 2003;121C(1):81–83.

74. Shearer WT, Rosenblatt HM, Gelman RS, et al. Lymphocyte subsets in healthy children from birth through 18 years of age: the Pediatric AIDS Clinical Trials Group P1009 study. *J Allergy Clin Immunol.* 2003;112(5):973–980.

75. Oliveira JB, Fleisher TA. Laboratory evaluation of primary immunodeficiencies. *J Allergy Clin Immunol.* 2010;125(2 Suppl 2):S297–S305.

76. Williams H. The normal thymus and how to recognize it. *Arch Dis Child Educ Pract Ed.* 2006;91:ep25–ep28.

77. O'gorman MR. Role of flow cytometry in the diagnosis and monitoring of primary immunodeficiency disease. *Clin Lab Med.* 2007;27(3):591–626.

78. Folds JD, Schmitz JL. Clinical and laboratory assessment of immunity. *J Allergy Clin Immunol.* 2003;111: S702–S11.

79. Ozcan E, Notarangelo LD, Geha RS. Primary immune deficiencies with aberrant IgE production. *J Allergy Clin Immunol.* 2008;122(6):1054–1062.

80. de Saint-Basile G, Le Deist F, de Villartay JP, et al. Restricted heterogeneity of T lymphocytes in combined immunodeficiency with hypereosinophilia (Omenn's syndrome). *J Clin Invest.* 1991;87(4):1352–1359.

81. Beverley PC. Functional analysis of human T cell subsets defined by CD45 isoform expression. *Semin Immunol.* 1992;4(1):35–41.

82. Somech R. T-cell receptor excision circles in primary immunodeficiencies and other T-cell immune disorders. *Curr Opin Allergy Clin Immunol.* 2011;11(6):517–524. doi:10.1097/ACI.0b013e32834c233a.

83. Comeau AM, Hale JE, Pai SY, et al. Guidelines for implementation of population-based newborn screening for severe combined immunodeficiency. *J Inherit Metab Dis.* 2010;33(Suppl 2):S273–S281.

84. Baker MW, Grossman WJ, Laessig RH, et al. Development of a routine newborn screening protocol for severe combined immunodeficiency. *J Allergy Clin Immunol.* 2009;124(3):522–527.

85. Carlucci F, Tabucchi A, Aiuti A, et al. Capillary electrophoresis in diagnosis and monitoring of adenosine deaminase deficiency. *Clin Chem.* 2003;49(11):1830–1838.

86. Slatter MA, Gennery AR. Primary immunodeficiencies associated with DNA-repair disorders. *Expert Rev Mol Med.* 2010;12:e9.

87. Henter JI, Horne A, Aricó M, et al. HLH-2004: diagnostic and therapeutic guidelines for hemophagocytic lymphohistiocytosis. *Pediatr Blood Cancer.* 2007;48:124–131.

88. Oliveira JB, Bleesing JJ, Dianzani U, et al. Revised diagnostic criteria and classification for the autoimmune lymphoproliferative syndrome: report from the 2009 NIH International Workshop. *Blood.* 2010;116:e35–e40.

89. Morra M, Geigenmuller U, Curran J, et al. Genetic diagnosis of primary immune deficiencies. *Immunol Allergy Clin North Am.* 2008;28(2):387–441.

90. Booth C, Gaspar HB. Pegademase bovine (PEG-ADA) for the treatment of infants and children with severe combined immunodeficiency (SCID). *Biologics.* 2009;3:349–358.

CHAPTER 50

91. Szabolcs P, Cavazzana-Calvo M, Fischer A, Veys P. Bone marrow transplantation for primary immunodeficiency diseases. *Pediatr Clin North Am.* 2010;57(1):207–237.

92. Hough R, Cooper N, Veys P. Allogeneic haemopoietic stem cell transplantation in children: what alternative donor should we choose when no matched sibling is available? *Br J Haematol.* 2009;147(5):593–613.

93. Satwani P, Cooper N, Rao K, Veys P, Amrolia P. Reduced intensity conditioning and allogeneic stem cell transplantation in childhood malignant and nonmalignant diseases. *Bone Marrow Transplant.* 2008;41(2):173–182.

94. Gennery AR, Slatter MA, Grandin L, et al. Transplantation of hematopoietic stem cells and long-term survival for primary immunodeficiencies in Europe: entering a new century, do we do better? *J Allergy Clin Immunol.* 2010;126(3):602–610. e1–11.

95. Buckley RH. Transplantation of hematopoietic stem cells in human severe combined immunodeficiency: longterm outcomes. *Immunol Res.* 2011;49(1–3):25–43.

96. Buckley RH, Schiff SE, Schiff RI, et al. Hematopoietic stem-cell transplantation for the treatment of severe combined immunodeficiency. *N Engl J Med.* 1999;340:508–516.

97. Myers LA, Patel DD, Puck JM, Buckley RH. Hematopoietic stem cell transplantation for severe combined immunodeficiency in the neonatal period leads to superior thymic output and improved survival. *Blood.* 2002;99: 872–878.

98. Grunebaum E, Roifman CM. Bone marrow transplantation using HLA-matched unrelated donors for patients suffering from severe combined immunodeficiency. *Hematol Oncol Clin North Am.* 2011;25(1):63–73.

99. Fischer A, Hacein-Bey-Abina S, Cavazzana-Calvo M. Gene therapy for primary immunodeficiencies. *Hematol Oncol Clin North Am.* 2011;25(1):89–100.

100. Fischer A, Hacein-Bey-Abina S, Cavazzana-Calvo M. Gene therapy for primary adaptive immune deficiencies. *J Allergy Clin Immunol.* 2011;127(6):1356–1359.

101. Booth C, Gaspar HB, Thrasher AJ. Gene therapy for primary immunodeficiency. *Curr Opin Pediatr.* 2011;23(6):659–666. doi:10.1097/MOP.0b013e32834cd67a.

102. Hacein-Bey-Abina S, Hauer J, et al. Efficacy of gene therapy for X-linked severe combined immunodeficiency. *N Engl J Med.* 2010;363(4):355–364.

103. Gaspar HB, Cooray S, Gilmour KC, et al. Hematopoietic stem cell gene therapy for adenosine deaminase-deficient severe combined immunodeficiency leads to long-term immunological recovery and metabolic correction. *Sci Transl Med.* 2011;3(97):97ra80.

104. Kay MA. State-of-the-art gene-based therapies: the road ahead. *Nat Rev Genet.* 2011;12(5):316–328.

105. Brown L, Xu-Bayford J, Allwood Z, et al. Neonatal diagnosis of severe combined immunodeficiency leads to significantly improved survival outcome: the case for newborn screening. *Blood.* 2011;117: 3243–3246.

106. Railey MD, Lokhnygina Y, Buckley RH. Long-term clinical outcome of patients with severe combined immunodeficiency who received related donor bone marrow transplants without pretransplant chemotherapy or post-transplant GVHD prophylaxis. *J Pediatr.* 2009;155:834–840.

107. Chase NM, Verbsky JW, Routes JM. Newborn screening for T-cell deficiency. *Curr Opin Allergy Clin Immunol.* 2010;10: 521–525.

108. Comeau AM, Hale JE, Pai SY, et al. Guidelines for implementation of population-based newborn screening for severe combined immunodeficiency. *J Inherit Metab Dis.* 2010;33(Suppl 2):S273–S281.

109. Hale JE, Bonilla FA, Pai SY, et al. Identification of an infant with severe combined immunodeficiency by newborn screening. *J Allergy Clin Immunol.* 2010;126:1073–1074.

110. SCID added to national newborn screening standards. *Am J Med Genet A.* 2010;152A(8):ix.

Phagocytic Disorder

Yu-Lung Lau and Pamela Lee

INTRODUCTION

Phagocytosis is the process by which leukocytes internalize particles larger than 1 μm, such as microbes, apoptotic cells, and chemical substances.[1] It is an essential component of the innate and adaptive immune response, as well as tissue remodeling and repair.[2] Neutrophils, macrophages, and dendritic cells are professional phagocytes that are derived from the common myeloid progenitor.[3] As the invading microbes cross the skin and mucosal barrier and enter the tissue, they are recognized by resident macrophages and dendritic cells through germline-encoded pattern recognition receptors. The release of proinflammatory cytokines activates local endothelial and epithelial cells, which express chemoattractants and adhesion molecules. Circulating neutrophils adhere to the endothelium and migrate through the endothelial lining into the tissues.[4,5]

Phagocytosis is a receptor-mediated process. Apart from pattern recognition receptors, foreign particles bound by complements and immunoglobulins in the circulation and interstitial fluid are recognized by phagocytes through the opsonic receptors.[6,7] The ingested microorganism is degraded in the phagolysosome, and the presentation of antigenic peptide on the surface of the phagocytes leads to lymphocyte activation. The mechanism of killing is accomplished by de novo synthesis of reactive oxygen species and release of proteases stored in lysosomal granules into the phagolysosome.

Phagocytosis is the first line of defense against infection and forms the link between innate and adaptive immunity.[8] Phagocytic defects commonly present in the neonatal period and early infancy.

The spectrum of disorders includes numerical deficiency and functional defects such as impaired adhesion, chemotaxis, ingestion, degranulation, and intracellular killing.

PATHOPHYSIOLOGY

Neutrophil Count in the Neonates

The absolute neutrophil count (ANC) is calculated by multiplying the total white blood cell count (WCC) by the percentage of bands and mature neutrophils. The ANC of the newborn varies with gestational age, postnatal age, birth weight, geographical factors such as altitude, and clinical factors, including intrapartum oxytocin administration and maternal hypertension.[9–11] The commonly used ANC reference range in term and near-term neonates was established in 1979 by Manroe et al.[12] At birth, the ANC ranges from 1800 to 5500/mm^3, which subsequently increases 3- to 5-fold and peaks at 12–18 hours of life. Gradual fall in ANC occurs by 24 hours, ranging from 1800 to 7200/mm^3 at 60 hours and remaining at 1800 to 5400/mm^3 within the first 28 days. The ANC reference range in very low birth weight (VLBW) neonates was published in 1994 by Mouzinho et al.[13] In their study of 193 premature infants born at mean gestational age of 29.5 weeks with mean birth weight of 1157 g, the lower boundary of ANC was found to be 500/mm^3 at birth, rose less steeply to 2200/mm^3 at 18–20 hours, then decreased to 1100/mm^3 at 60 hours. From 60 hours to 28 days of life, the normal range of ANC is 1100–6000/mm^3.

Subsequent studies showed that both neutropenia and neutrophilia occur more commonly in premature neonates compared with those born near or at term, reflecting their immature granulopoietic regulation.[14] The reported prevalence of neutropenia in preterm infants varies from 6% to 58%, depending on the reference range used and the specific population risk factors.[15–18] Rebound neutrophilia is commonly observed in the second week of life in the absence of infections. Idiopathic neutropenia of prematurity refers to neutropenia that occurs after 3 weeks of life. It was reported in 26% of preterm neonates whose birth weights were appropriate for gestational age (AGA) and generally resolves spontaneously without complications.[19–21]

Neutropenia

Neutropenia is the absolute reduction in the number of neutrophils in the circulation. It is usually defined as an ANC of less than 1500/mm^2, but in neonates factors such as age and maturity, as mentioned, should be taken into account. The peripheral neutrophil count reflects the equilibrium between the intra- and extramedullary compartments. Neutropenia can be caused by (1) decreased production; (2) increased consumption or destruction; (3) excessive margination; (4) excessive apoptosis, or a combination of these causes. Acquired or secondary neutropenia are much more common than congenital neutropenia (Table 51-1). Frequently identified causes include maternal hypertension, sepsis, immune-mediated destruction, and drug exposure.

Maternal preeclampsia, birth asphyxia, and sepsis are common perinatal events associated with neutropenia presenting in the first few days of life. It was reported that up to half of premature infants born to hypertensive mothers are neutropenic, attributable to a placenta-derived granulopoiesis inhibitor.[22,23] Association of neutropenia and early-onset sepsis (<48 hours) caused by group B streptococcus

and other bacterial infections has been well demonstrated.[24–26] Circulating neutrophils and platelets are diminished as a result of depleted reserve in the bone marrow. It is important to realize the significance of neutropenia and potential sepsis within the first day of life, when the ANC should normally be rising to its peak. Viral infections, such as cytomegalovirus (CMV), Epstein-Barr virus (EBV), and parvovirus, can lead to bone marrow suppression and neutropenia, which may be accompanied by anemia or thrombocytopenia.

Immune-mediated neutrophil destruction can be caused by transplacental passage of maternal immunoglobulin (Ig) G antineutrophil antibodies in maternal autoimmune neutropenia and neonatal alloimmune neutropenia.[27] Neonatal alloimmune neutropenia is mediated by maternal antibodies against fetal neutrophil antigens inherited from the father, analogous to hemolytic disease of the newborn (HDN) caused by rhesus isoimmunization. Unlike HDN, alloimmune neutropenia can occur in the firstborn child.[28] Sensitization occurs when fetal neutrophils enter the maternal circulation during pregnancy, and antibody-mediated neutrophil destruction occurs in utero and after delivery. In most cases, maternal alloantibodies are directed toward neutrophil-specific antigens, human neutrophil antigen (HNA) 1a and HNA-2a, and less commonly HNA-1b or others.[29] Antibodies against human leukocyte antigens (HLA) may also cause alloimmune neutropenia.[30] The incidence is estimated to be 1 in 1000 newborns.[31] Affected infants are neutropenic at birth. Most of them are asymptomatic; some may present with omphalitis, delayed separation of the umbilical cord, mild skin infections, fever, or pneumonia, but severe infections are rare.[32,33]

Idiosyncratic drug-induced neutropenia is uncommon in neonates and children. The overall population incidence is 2.4–15.4 per million per year.[34] The incidence increases with age, and only 10% of cases occur in children and young adults. Among the long list of medications associated with neutropenia,[35–37] drugs that are more commonly encountered in neonatal practice include antimicrobials, antiepileptic agents, antithyroid drugs, and cardiovascular and some gastrointestinal medications (Table 51-2). Neutropenia is usually profound, often below 200/mm^3. Neutropenia associated with carbimazole, propylthiouracil, phenytoin, hydralazine, and procainamide is immune mediated, whereas sulfonamides, trimethoprim-sulfamathoxazole, carbamazepine, sodium valproate, and antivirals such as ganciclovir cause neutropenia by suppressing granulopoiesis. Idiosyncractic neutropenia caused by penicillin is mediated by both mechanisms.[37]

Neutropenia with underlying genetic defects are rare. They include severe chronic neutropenia (SCN), bone marrow failure syndromes, metabolic disorders,

Table 51-1 Acquired or Secondary Causes of Neutropenia in Neonates

Maternal or Materno-Fetal Factors
Maternal hypertension
Maternal autoimmune neutropenia
Neonatal alloimmune neutropenia
Postnatal Factors
Birth asphyxia
Bacterial sepsis
Viral infections
Drug-induced agranulocytosis
Autoimmune neutropenia
Hypersplenism
Nutritional deficiency

Table 51-2 Idiosyncratic Drug-Induced Neutropenia[a]

Category	Examples
Antimicrobials	
Antibiotics	β-Lactams: penicillin, cephalosporins Cotrimoxazole Chloramphenicol Others: metronidazole, clindamycin, vancomycin, linezolid
Antimycobacterials Antimalarials Antivirals	Isoniazid, rifampicin Quinine, atovaquone Aciclovir; antiretrovirals, including nucleoside reverse transcriptase inhibitors and protease inhibitors
Cardiovascular Antihypertensives	Propranolol, ACE inhibitors, hydralazine, nifedipine
Diuretics	Furosemide, thiazide diuretics, spironolactone
Antiarrhythmics	Amiodarone, procainamide, propafenone
Antiepileptic	Carbamazepine, phenytoin, sodium valproate
Gastrointestinal drugs	H_2 antagonists (eg, ranitidine) Proton pump inhibitors (eg, omeprazole, lansoprazole)
NSAIDs	Ibuprofen, indomethacin
Antithyroid	Carbimazole

Abbreviations: ACE, angiotensin-converting enzyme; NSAID, nonsteroidal anti-inflammatory drug.
[a]The medications listed in this table are more commonly administered in neonatal practice. Other medications implicated in drug-induced neutropenia include antipsychotics, antidepressants, analgesics, antithyroid drugs, immunosuppressants, and chemotherapeutics.[35–37]

and neutropenia associated with cellular and humoral immunodeficiencies (Table 51-3).[38–42] SCN involves a genetically heterogeneous group of disorders characterized by maturation arrest of myelopoiesis at the level of the promyelocyte/myelocyte stage in the bone marrow, resulting in profound neutropenia.[43] Mutation of the neutrophil elastase 2 (ELA2) gene inherited in an autosomal dominant manner accounts for 50%–60% of patients with SCN. Mutations of other genes, such as GFI1, HAX1, SBDS, WAS, and G6PC3, altogether account for less than 5% of SCN, so the genetic basis in 40% of cases remains unknown.[44]

While loss-of-function mutation in the WAS gene causes classical Wiskott-Aldrich syndrome or X-linked thrombocytopenia, mutations in the guanosine triphosphatase (GTPase)–binding domain of WAS abrogates the autoinhibitory conformation and produces a constitutively activated form, resulting in enhanced actin polymerization and cellular apoptosis.[45]

As neutrophils have a short half-life with high cellular turnover, they are most susceptible to derangements in cellular metabolism. The pathogenesis of congenital bone marrow failure syndromes involves various basic cellular processes, including ribosome biogenesis, mitochondrial metabolism, and DNA repair.[46,47] Infants with congenital bone marrow failure syndromes often have pancytopenia. Skeletal malformations are common, and some are associated with lymphocyte abnormalities and increased risk of malignancy. Neutropenia also occurs in metabolic disorders such as glycogen storage type 1b[48,49] and organic aciduria.[50]

Some forms of humoral and cellular immunodeficiencies are associated with neutropenia,[51] such as reticular dysgenesis[52,53] and hyper-IgM syndrome.[54–56] Disorders of abnormal lysosomal trafficking such as Chediak-Higashi syndrome, Griscelli syndrome type 2, and Hermansky-Pudlak syndrome type 2 are characterized by partial oculocutaneous albinism, bleeding tendency, neutropenia, and hemophagocytic lymphohistiocytosis.[57,58] Immune cytopenia occurs in autoimmune lymphoproliferative syndrome (ALPS) and is discussed in Chapter 60. Other forms of primary immunodeficiencies associated with neutropenia include humoral deficiencies that include X-linked agammaglobulinemia,[59,60] common variable immunodeficiency,[61,62] and WHIM (warts, hypogammaglobulinemia, infections, and myelokathexis),[63] but they do not present in the neonatal period.

Susceptibility to infections depends on the ANC, adequacy of neutrophil reserve pool in the bone marrow, and other factors, such as integrity of mucosal barriers and coexisting cellular immune deficiencies. Patients with ANC below 500/mm[3] or neutropenia secondary to chemotherapy, marrow failure, or marrow exhaustion are at the greatest risk of overwhelming bacterial and fungal infections.[64]

Disorders of Phagocyte Function

Defects of Neutrophil Adhesion and Chemotaxis

To reach the focus of infection in the extravascular space, circulating neutrophils must leave the bloodstream by migrating through the vascular endothelium. Tissue trauma or inflammation leads to activation of endothelial cells, which express adhesion molecules such as selectins and integrins.[65] Selectin binding brings leukocytes into contact with the endothelium,

Table 51-3 Neutropenia with Single-Gene Defects: Inheritance, Pathogenetic Mechanisms, and Clinical Features

Condition	Genetic Defect and Inheritance	Mechanism	Phenotypic Features
Severe congenital neutropenia (SCN)	ELA2; AD	Accelerated apoptosis of neutrophil precursors	Accounts for 50%-60% of SCN; mutation of ELA2 gene also causes cyclical neutropenia in older infants and children
	HAX1; AR	Accelerated apoptosis of neutrophil precursors	Identified in the descendants of the family originally described by Kostmann; may have neurologic involvement
	G6PC3; AR	Accelerated apoptosis of neutrophil precursors	Associated cardiac and urogenital anomalies
	GFI1; AD	Defective hematopoietic stem cell differentiation	Associated lymphoid immune defects
	WAS; X-linked	X-linked neutropenia (XLN): Activating mutation in the GTPase-binding domain disrupts the autoinhibited conformation and enhances actin-polymerizing activity	Associated with impaired lymphocyte survival and genomic stability
Bone marrow failure syndromes			
Fanconi syndrome	FANC; AR	DNA repair defect	Pancytopenia, dysplastic thumbs
Dyskeratosis congenital (DKC)	DKC1; X linked TREC, TERT; AD NOP10; AR	Molecular defects of the components in the telomerase complex	Pancytopenia, skin pigmentation, leukoplakia, dystrophic nails, cerebellar hypoplasia, pulmonary fibrosis, gastrointestinal and urinary tract abnormalities, osteoporosis, risk of malignancy X-linked DKC is the severe infantile form associated with deficiency of B and NK cells
Diamond-Blackfan syndrome	>10 genes involved in ribosomal synthesis; AD, AR	Defective ribosome biogenesis	Macrocytic anemia, short stature, thumb abnormalities, craniofacial defects, increased risk of malignancy
Schwachman-Diamond syndrome	SBDS; AR	Defective ribosome biogenesis and RNA processing	Ineffective hematopoiesis causing pancytopenia, exocrine pancreatic insufficiency, short stature, skeletal abnormalities, increased risk of myelodysplasia, and malignant transformation
Cartilage-hair hypoplasia	RMRP; AR	Defective ribosomal RNA synthesis	Hypoplastic hair, short-limb dwarfism, gastrointestinal dysfunction, macrocytic anemia, T-cell immunodeficiency, increased risk of malignancies
Pearson's syndrome	Sporadic	Mitochondrial respiratory chain dysfunction	Refractory sideroblastic anemia, neutropenia, thrombocytopenia, exocrine pancreatic insufficiency,

Disease	Gene; Inheritance	Mechanism	Clinical features
Metabolic disorders			
Glycogen storage disease type 1b	SLC37A4; AR	Defective glucose-6-phosphate translocase; hypocellular bone marrow with increased granulocyte apoptosis	Neutropenia, defective oxidative burst and chemotaxis, hypoglycemia, lactic acidosis, dyslipidemia, hyperuricemia, hepatomegaly
Organic aciduria - Isovaleric acidemia - Methylmalonic aciduria - Propionic aciduria	IVD; AR MUT, MMAA, MMAB; AR PCCA, PCCB; AR	Accumulation of organic acids inhibits proliferation and differentiation of myeloid stem cells	Progressive neurological deterioration, seizures, encephalopathy
- Barth syndrome	TAZ; X-linked	Defective remodeling of cardiolipin essential for mitochondrial integrity	Cardiomyopathy, skeletal myopathy, 3-methylglutaconic aciduria
Primary immunodeficiencies			
Reticular dysgenesis	AK2; AR	Defective energy production in mitochondria	Pancytopenia, severe combined immunodeficiency, sensorineural hearing loss
WHIM syndrome	CXCR4; AR	Neutrophil apoptosis	Warts, hypogammaglobulinemia, recurrent infections, myelokathexis (retention of mature neutrophils in the bone marrow)
Hyper-IgM syndrome	CD40L; X-linked CD40, AID, UNG; AR	Defective CD40-mediated stimulation of myeloid precursors	Recurrent sinopulmonary infections, opportunistic infections, such as cytomegalovirus (CMV), Pneumocystis jiroveci pneumonia (PCP), cryptosporidiosis, cholangiopathy, liver cirrhosis and failure, autoimmunity, increased risk of malignancy
Chediak-Higashi syndrome	LYST; AR	Disorder of lysosomal trafficking, impaired vesicle transport, and exocytosis in cytotoxic T and NK cells	Intermittent neutropenia, oculocutaneous albinism, bleeding tendency, neuropathy, hemophagocytic lymphohistiocytosis
Griscelli syndrome type 2	RAB27A; AR	Defective vesicle transport	Intermittent neutropenia, thrombocytopenia, partial albinism, hemophagocytic lymphohistiocytosis
Hermansky-Pudlak syndrome type 2	AP3B1; AR	Disorder of lysosomal trafficking, abnormal subcellular targeting of neutrophil elastase	Chronic neutropenia, bleeding tendency, , oculocutaneous albinism, facial dysmorphism noticeable in late childhood
p14 deficiency	p14; AR	Disorder of lysosomal trafficking	Chronic neutropenia, oculocutaneous albinism, short stature, coarse facial features

Abbreviations: AD, autosomal dominant; AR, autosomal recessive; GTPase, guanosine triphosphatase; NK, natural killer; WHIM, warts, hypogammaglobulinemia, infections, and myelokathexis.

on which leukocyte rolling is followed by integrin-mediated adhesion and transendothelial migration via paracellular or transcellular paths to the site of inflammation guided by chemotactic factors.[66]

At present, 3 forms of leukocyte adhesion deficiency (LAD) are known, and all are autosomal recessive disorders.[67] LAD type I is caused by a defect of the common chain (CD18) of β2 integrins, which serve as receptors for the opsonic complement fragment C3b and intercellular adhesion molecules 1 and 2 (ICAM-1 and ICAM-2, respectively) expressed on endothelial cells and leukocytes. The β2-integrin molecule is a heterodimer of α chains (CD11a, CD11b, or CD11c) and β chain (CD18). Defective heterodimer formation leads to profound impairment of leukocyte emigration from the bloodstream to the site of inflammation in the extravascular space. As CD11b/CD18 is the predominant receptor for the complement fragment C3bi, ingestion of C3bi-opsonized microbes and C3bi-mediated phagocytic activities is also affected.[68]

Patients with LAD exhibit marked leukocytosis, and the ANC may reach up to 100,000/mm³ during acute infections. The lack of pus formation at the site of inflammation despite persistent granulocytosis is characteristic. Impaired local control of infection predisposes to systemic spread. Bacterial infections and skin abscesses are often apparent in the early neonatal period. Delayed separation of the umbilical cord and omphalitis with persistent discharge are pathognomic of LAD. Common causative organisms include *Staphylococcus aureus* and gram-negative enteric bacteria. Fungal infections are also common. Infant and children with LAD often have severe gingivitis and periodontitis. In addition, healing of traumatic or surgical wound is significantly impaired.[69] Clinical severity correlates with the residual surface expression of CD18.[70]

Leukocyte adhesion deficiency type II is a disorder of fucose metabolism caused by defective guanosine diphosphate (GDP)–fucose transporter.[71] Neutrophils fail to roll on the vascular endothelium because of the absence of SLeX, a fucosylated ligand for selectins expressed on the surface of leukocytes. Infective and inflammatory manifestations are similar to LAD I, but additional features in LAD II include coarse facial features, short stature, moderate-to-severe mental retardation, and absence of H antigen on erythrocytes (Bombay phenotype). LAD II is extremely rare and has been reported in fewer than 10 patients in the literature.[72]

Leukocyte adhesion deficiency type III is caused by defect of Kindlin-3, a hematopoietic structural protein that mediates integrin activation.[73] In addition to leukocyte adhesion defect, platelet aggregation is abnormal and causes severe bleeding tendency.[74,75] Other features of LAD III include increased bone density resembling osteopetrosis and neurodevelopmental disabilities.[76]

Defects of Phagocyte Killing

Chronic Granulomatous Disease

Chronic granulomatous disease (CGD) is a disorder of phagocytic oxidative burst as a result of impaired nicotinamide adenine dinucleotide phosphate (NADPH) oxidase activity.[77] The NADPH oxidase is a multimeric enzyme complex that catalyzes the transfer of electrons from cytoplasmic NADPH to molecular oxygen. The membrane-bound flavocytochrome b558 of NADPH oxidase consists of gp91phox and p22phox.[78] Phagocytosis of microorganisms triggers the translocation of 4 cytosolic factors (p47phox, p67phox, p40phox, and Rac2) to the cell membrane, where they associate with gp91phox and p22phox (Figure 51-1). Electrons transported from cytoplasmic NADPH via the activated NADPH oxidase convert molecular oxygen to superoxide anion in the phagosome, generating bactericidal oxidants such as hydrogen peroxide and hypohalous acid. At the same time, the activation of antimicrobial proteases and release of neutrophil extracellular traps (NETs) further augments antimicrobial defense. Granular proteases such as neutrophil elastase and cathepsin G sequestered in the azurophilic granules enhance killing within the phagolysosomes,[79] and NETs entrap bacteria and fungi and facilitates extracellular killing.[80]

Molecular defects of various components of the NADPH oxidase complex have been identified to cause CGD. X-linked mutations in the *CYBB* gene encoding gp91phox account for 60%–70% of CGD.[81] Genetic defects of p22phox (*CYBA*), p47phox (*NCF1*), p67phox (*NCF2*), and p40phox (*NCF4*) are inherited in an autosomal recessive manner.[82]

Chronic granulomatous disease affects 1 in 200,000 to 250,000 individuals. Most patients present in early infancy, but CGD with attenuated phenotypes is increasingly diagnosed in adulthood. Patients with CGD are susceptible to *S. aureus*; *Nocardia* species; gram-negative bacteria such as *Salmonella* species, *Serratia marcescens*, and *Burkholderia cepacia*; fungal infections such as *Aspergillus*; and mycobacteria, including *M. tuberculosis* and *M. bovis* BCG (bacillus Calmette-Guérin.[83] Common presentations in the neonatal period and early infancy include recurrent skin and perianal abscesses, suppurative adenitis, and pneumonia. Bacterial and fungal dissemination by the hematogenous route may lead to septicemia, liver abscess, osteomyelitis, meningitis, and brain abscess. Infants often have a history of prolonged antibiotic use as well as multiple incision and drainage procedures for recurrent abscesses. Those who receive BCG vaccine at birth may present with ulceration at the site of inoculation and enlargement of ipsilateral axillary lymph nodes, and some may develop systemic dissemination.[84,85]

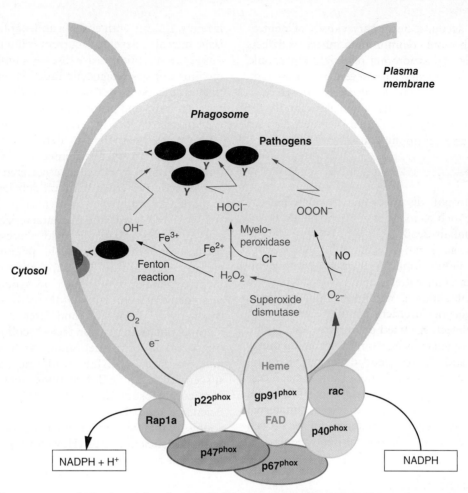

FIGURE 50-1 Components of nicotinamide adenine dinucleotide phosphate (NADPH) oxidase and respiratory burst.

Patients with CGD have a unique susceptibility to *Chromobacterium violaceum*, which is a soil and water saprophyte mostly confined to tropical and subtropical areas.[86] *Chromobacterium violaceum* infection was first reported to occur at unusually high frequency among patients with CGD living in the southeastern United States, such as in Florida and Louisiana.[87]

Children and adults with CGD may have hyperinflammatory manifestations such as colitis, granuloma, and excessive inflammatory reaction at the site of trauma.[88] The mechanisms of exaggerated inflammatory response in CGD include reduced degradation of phagocytosed materials causing persistent phagocytic activation, induction of Th17 cells, impaired neutrophil apoptosis, dysregulation of the redox-sensitive antiinflammatory molecule Nrf2, and activation of NLRP3 inflammasome.[88,89] Hyperinflammatory lesions may affect any part of the gastrointestinal tract, from the oral cavity to anus. Granulomatous colitis can mimic Crohn disease and manifests as bloody diarrhea, malabsorption, anemia, and failure to thrive.[90] Granuloma may obstruct hollow viscera such as the gastric outlet and urethral orifices.

Myeloperoxidase Deficiency

Myeloperoxidase is a component of the azurophilic granules in phagocytes. It catalyzes the reaction of hydrogen peroxide with chloride ion to form hypochlorous acid, which is then converted to chlorine.[79] As superoxide is generated normally, intracellular killing of pathogens is only minimally affected, except impaired candida killing, which can be demonstrated by in vitro assays. In general, individuals with myeloperoxidase deficiency are asymptomatic, but those who have concomitant diabetes mellitus are susceptible to severe candidiasis.[91,92]

DIFFERENTIAL DIAGNOSIS

The main clinical presentations of phagocytic disorders in the neonatal period are infections and abnormal wound healing. Sepsis can be the cause or result of neutropenia and should be treated aggressively with broad-spectrum antimicrobial therapy. Neutrophil count should be interpreted with caution and serially monitored, and factors including gestational age, postnatal age, perinatal events, and drug exposure should be taken into account. Secondary causes of neutropenia are much more common than inherited defects of myelopoiesis and syndromal disorders but should be considered if neutropenia is severe and persistent, when other cell lineages are involved, and in the presence of coexisting congenital anomalies. Studies of phagocytic functions are warranted if clinical features are suggestive and neutrophil count is normal.

Family History

Inherited neutrophil disorders can be suggested by family history, such as recurrent infections and unexplained early infant deaths. Family history of hematological malignancy may be elicited in patients with bone marrow failure syndromes or severe congenital neutropenia. The pattern of inheritance may be apparent by obtaining a detailed family pedigree. X-linked phagocytic disorders include CGD caused by gp91phox defect, X-linked dyskeratosis congenita, X-linked neutropenia arising from an activating mutation in WAS, and CD40 ligand deficiency. Parental consanguinity increases the chance of autosomal recessive disorders. Infants with neonatal lupus syndrome can have severe neutropenia, and relevant maternal history should be sought.[93,94] Maternal full blood cell count should be reviewed to look for neutropenia.

Physical Examination

On physical examination, the clinician should aim to identify the sites of infection and features suggestive of syndromal disorders. The oral cavity should be inspected for candidiasis. In older infants, gingivostomatitis may be apparent. Cutaneous pyogenic infections include impetigo, cellulitis, and abscess. The perianal region should be examined for induration, abscess, fistula formation, and scars. There may be persistent inflammation and discharge from the umbilicus or features suggestive of abnormal healing. Clinical signs of invasive infections, such as meningitis, osteomyelitis, and deep organ abscess should be sought. Failure to thrive is common in infants with chronic recurrent infections. Skeletal anomalies and growth retardation are often identified in patients with congenital bone marrow failure syndromes, such as dysplastic thumbs in Fanconi anemia and short-limb dwarfism in cartilage-hair hypoplasia. Cutaneous hypopigmentation is a feature common to various disorders of lysosomal trafficking, such as Chediak-Higashi syndrome and Griscelli syndrome type 2.

Recurrent Skin Abscess

Neutropenia and functional phagocytic disorders are the most important causes for recurrent skin abscess in infancy. Infants with eczema and staphylococcal carriage may also develop recurrent cellulitis and cutaneous abscesses, but invasive disease is unlikely. Diabetes mellitus impairs phagocytic function and predisposes to skin infections, but neonatal diabetes mellitus is a rare condition and primarily presents with intrauterine growth retardation, hyperglycemia, and dehydration. Humoral and complement deficiencies also increase susceptibility to pyogenic infections. Other primary immunodeficiency disorders associated with pyogenic skin infections include humoral deficiencies, complement defects, and hyper-IgE syndrome.[95]

Hyper-IgE syndrome is characterized by eczematous eruption, cutaneous cold abscesses, recurrent pneumonia and pneumatocele, pneumothorax, and elevated serum IgE.[96,97] Infants with autosomal dominant hyper-IgE syndrome (Job syndrome) characteristically present with erythematous skin rash in the neonatal period[98,99] and later develop somatic features, including coarse facies, scoliosis, bone fractures, and abnormal dentition. Patients with autosomal recessive hyper-IgE syndrome have additional susceptibility to viral infections, including molluscum contagiosum and warts.[100,101] T-cell immunodeficiency should always be considered and ruled out in young infants with recurrent infections, and human immunodeficiency virus (HIV) testing should be performed as appropriate.

Perianal Abscess and Fistula

Perianal sepsis is not an uncommon condition in young infants and has a male preponderance. Most initially present with perianal abscess, subsequently progress to or recur as fistula-in-ano. The etiology appears to be related to congenital anomalies of anal crypts that predispose to abscess and fistula formation. In most healthy children, long-term or serious complications from perianal abscess or fistula are rare. Recurrence of perianal abscess is likely if a coexisting fistula is not identified and resected at the time of primary drainage.[102,103] Phagocytic disorders should be considered if there is frequent recurrence and poor healing. Persistent perianal fistula and diarrhea are also presenting symptoms of neonatal/infantile-onset inflammatory bowel disease, which was recently identified as a group of genetic disorders in interleukin (IL) 10 signaling.[104,105]

Omphalitis and Delayed Separation of the Umbilical Cord

Separation of the umbilical cord normally occurs between 5 and 8 days after birth. The incidence of omphalitis in developed countries is estimated to be 0.5%–1.0%.[106] Omphalitis delays the process of umbilical vessel obliteration and hence cord separation.

Common risk factors for omphalitis include nonsterile delivery, maternal genital tract infection, prolonged rupture of membrane, prematurity, low birth weight, procedural complications such as umbilical cord catheterization, and improper handling and care of the umbilical cord stump.[107,108] Omphalitis commonly occurs in neonates with neutropenia and phagocytic disorders, and delayed separation of the umbilical cord is characteristic of LAD.

BCG Complications

BCG vaccine complications such as ulceration, persistent discharge, and scarring are well recognized in infants who receive BCG vaccine in the neonatal period. Some of them may develop abscess at the site of inoculation, and the incidence of regional lymphadenitis is estimated to be 1 in 2800 vaccinations.[109] Occurrence of BCG-related complications depends on external factors such as vaccine strains and technique of administration, and most affected infants are otherwise healthy.[110–112] However, distant spread and systemic dissemination raise the alert for primary immunodeficiencies.[113–117] T-cell deficiency and HIV infection should be excluded in such conditions. BCG complications also occur in genetic defects of the IL12–interferon-γ axis, collectively known as Mendelian susceptibility to mycobacterial diseases (MSMD).[118,119] In addition to mycobacterial infections, patients with MSMD are prone to extraintestinal disease caused by nontyphoidal salmonella.

Neutrophilia

Neutrophilia is a characteristic of LAD. Other conditions associated with neutrophilia are listed in Table 51-4. Leukemoid reaction, defined as an ANC greater than 10 standard deviations above the mean for gestational age or more than $50 \times 10^3/\text{mm}^3$ during the first week of life, occurs in 1.3% to 15% of infants admitted to neonatal intensive care units.[120,121] It is characterized by significantly elevated numbers of early neutrophil precursors, such as myelocyte, metamyelocyte, and band forms in the peripheral blood; occasionally, promyelocytes and myeloblasts may be present. Normal proliferation, maturation, and morphology of all myeloid elements distinguish leukemoid reaction from leukemia. Toxic granules, Döhle bodies, and cytoplasmic vacuoles may be observed in the peripheral blood film in leukemoid reactions secondary to sepsis.[64] Conditions associated with leukemoid reactions include prematurity,[121,122] infections,[123,124] severe anemia, chromosomal anomalies,[125,126] exposure to antenatal corticosteroids,[127,128] persistent pulmonary hypertension of the newborn,[129] and bronchopulmonary dysplasia.[130–132]

Table 51-4 Conditions Associated with Neutrophilia in the Newborn Infant

Perinatal complications
- Infection
- Stressful labor
- Birth asphyxia
- Meconium aspiration
- Pneumothorax
- Periventricular hemorrhage
- Seizure
- Symptomatic hypoglycemia
Hematological disorders
- Hemolysis (eg, ABO incompatibility)
Leukemoid reaction
- Persistent pulmonary hypertension of the newborn (PPHN)
- Bronchopulmonary dysplasia
Chromosomal anomalies (eg, trisomy 21, trisomy 18, trisomy 13)
Leukocyte adhesion deficiency

DIAGNOSTIC TESTS

Neutropenia

Full blood cell count with differentials and direct blood smear provide valuable clues to underlying disorders. An increase in the proportion of immature neutrophils suggests active proliferation and differentiation from the myeloid progenitors in response to peripheral consumption, such as sepsis. Pancytopenia suggests bone marrow failure syndromes, infiltrative diseases, or reticular dysgenesis. Pathognomonic features for specific disorders may be present, such as giant neutrophil granules in Chediak-Higashi syndrome and lymphocyte cytoplasmic vacuolation in metabolic diseases.[133]

Paucity of mature neutrophils is evident in both SCN and neonatal alloimmune neutropenia; the former is caused by maturation arrest of myeloid precursors, and the latter is caused by destruction mediated by antibodies against antigens expressed on myelocytes, metamyelocytes, and band and segmented forms of neutrophils. Relative or absolute monocytosis may be seen, representing a compensatory response especially when there is concurrent sepsis. Diagnosis of alloimmune neutropenia requires the demonstration of IgG antineutrophil antibodies in the serum of mother and baby, which react with paternal neutrophils. Commonly used assays include granulocyte agglutination (GAT), granulocyte immunofluorescence (GIFT) or flow cytometry, and monoclonal antibody immobilization of granulocyte antigens (MAIGA). The combination of GAT and GIFT is regarded as the standard approach for detecting antineutrophil antibodies. The MAIGA assay allows confirmation of antibody specificity to various human neutrophil antigens.[134–136]

Full sepsis workup should be performed. Viral causes for neutropenia in the neonatal setting include CMV; parvovirus and disseminated herpes simplex virus can be ruled out by serology and polymerase chain reaction (PCR) assays. Persistent neutropenia necessitates inputs from pediatric hematologists. Bone marrow examination should be considered when congenital bone marrow failure syndromes, SCN, and malignancy are suspected.[137] Bone marrow smear of SCN is characterized by maturation arrest at the promyelocyte or myelocyte stage and monocytosis but normal erythropoietic and thombopoietic lineages.[43] The lack of mature forms of neutrophils may also be caused by immune-mediated destruction in autoimmune neutropenia. Screening for autoantibodies should be considered.

Evaluation of Phagocytic Functions

Chronic granulomatous disease is diagnosed by functional assays of superoxide production. Nitroblue tetrazolium (NBT) test evaluates the ability of stimulated neutrophils to reduce NBT from yellow to blue-black formazan deposits in the cytoplasm, which are visible on microscopic inspection. The result is quantified by the percentage of neutrophils containing the formazan black deposits in the cytoplasm compared with a normal control.[138] The dihydrorhodamine-1,2,3 (DHR) oxidation test is a flow-cytometry-based method that detects oxidation of DHR in activated neutrophils. DHR is oxidized by hydrogen peroxide to a highly fluorescent rhodamine-1,2,3. The result is expressed as a ratio of the fluorescence in stimulated cells to the fluorescence observed in unstimulated cells and is compared with a normal control.[139] The DHR assay is more sensitive and reliable than NBT; in addition, the shape of the DHR assay histogram can distinguish X-linked from autosomal recessive forms of CGD.[140,141] Both tests can be utilized for carrier detection in X-linked CGD.

Leukocyte adhesion deficiency type I can be diagnosed by flow cytometric analysis of CD11/CD18 complex expression on activated neutrophils.[142] Very low expression of less than 1% of normal levels predicts severe disease and poor survival. Patients with reduced expression of 1%–10% have moderate disease and often survive into adulthood. Carriers with 50% expression of CD18 are clinically asymptomatic.[141,143]

MANAGEMENT

Prevention of Infections

The primary goal of management is prevention and early treatment of infections. Oral and dental hygiene and skin and perineal care should be emphasized.

Infants with phagocytic disorders should receive routine vaccinations, except BCG vaccine, which should be avoided in CGD because of the risk of dissemination.

Long-term prophylactic antibiotic therapy is indicated for SCN, CGD, and LAD.[144] Prophylactic trimethoprim/sulfamethoxazole reduces the frequency of major infections, especially staphylococcal and skin infections.[145–147] It is concentrated inside the host cells and therefore targets intracellular pathogens. In addition to staphylococcus, it is active against *Serratia marcescens* and *Burkholderia* spp., to which patients with CGD are susceptible. Because of the risk of kernicterus, trimethoprim/sulfamethoxazole prophylaxis should be commenced after the age of 6 weeks. Glucose-6-phosphate dehydrogenase (G-6-PD) deficiency should be excluded. Antifungal prophylaxis should be given to patients with CGD and LAD. Itraconazole is the drug of choice as it has good activity against aspergillus.[148,149] Caution is given when used in infants younger than 1 month because of potential hepatotoxicity.

Prophylactic use of interferon γ has been shown to be beneficial in patients with CGD by reducing the number and severity of infections.[150,151] Interferon γ is administered 3 times per week as a subcutaneous injection. Some experts recommend its continuous use as prophylaxis, but in some centers, interferon γ is only used as rescue therapy in the presence of severe infections.[152]

Treatment of Acute Infections

Infections should be treated promptly. The threshold for starting antibiotic treatment should be lowered in neonates and young infants because symptoms and signs of sepsis are often subtle, and deterioration can be rapid. In general, a combination of a β-lactam drug such as third-generation cephalosporin and aminoglycoside for broad-spectrum coverage is recommended, but the specific protocol depends on the prevalence and antibiotic susceptibility of organisms in the community and hospital setting. If initial response to empirical antibiotics is suboptimal and fever persists, antifungal coverage should be added.

In children and adults with CGD, a regimen consisting of teicoplanin and ciprofloxacin is recommended as initial treatment as both drugs are actively concentrated within neutrophils and have good intracellular activity against gram-positive and gram-negative bacteria, particularly *S. aureus*.[152] However, ciprofloxacin is uncommonly prescribed to neonates because of the concern about potential cartilage toxicity and remains as an off-label application in treatment-resistant bacterial sepsis.[153]

Administration of antifungal therapy is especially important for patients with CGD. Conventional amphotericin B is the standard treatment of all forms of aspergillosis in neonates. Second-generation azoles, such as voriconazole, are commonly used in treating fungal infections in children with CGD,[152] but they have not been evaluated in neonates for pharmacokinetics, efficacy, and safety and therefore are not recommended.[154] Adjustment of the antimicrobial regimen is guided by culture and sensitivity results. The focus of infections, such as soft tissue and deep organ abscess, may need to be eradicated by surgical drainage or debridement.

Granulocyte Transfusion

Granulocyte transfusion was first given in the 1930s to patients with neutropenia.[155] Granulocyte concentrates are prepared by leukapheresis or centrifugation of whole blood, known as buffy coats. Although effectiveness was demonstrated in some patients, its clinical application remains controversial because of the lack of prospective trials. A recent Cochrane systematic review on randomized studies evaluating the efficacy of granulocyte transfusion for neonates with confirmed or suspected sepsis and neutropenia did not show significant difference in all-cause mortality compared with placebo or no transfusion. The evidence to support or refute the use of granulocyte transfusion in neutropenic neonates with sepsis is inconclusive.[156] Granulocyte transfusion has also been used in selected CGD patients with life-threatening bacterial and fungal infections.[157,158] It should be noted that granulocyte transfusion is associated with a number of complications, including fluid overload, transmission of blood-borne infection, graft-vs-host disease (GVHD) caused by mature donor lymphocytes, respiratory complications secondary to leukocyte aggregation and sequestration in the pulmonary circulation, and sensitization to donor erythrocyte and leukocyte antigens.[159] Granulocyte concentrates require technical expertise for preparation and are not universally available, and they are costly.[156] At present, guidelines for the application of granulocyte transfusion for neutropenic and phagocytic defects are lacking.

Granulocyte Colony-Stimulating Factors

Granulocyte colony-stimulating factor (G-CSF) and granulocyte-macrophage colony-stimulating factor (GM-CSF) are granulocyte growth factors that stimulate differentiation and maturation of neutrophils. They also promote the survival and proliferation of neutrophil progenitors.[160] G-CSF is commonly used for treating febrile neutropenia in patients undergoing chemotherapy for cancer and has been shown to reduce the duration of parenteral antibiotic treatment and hospitalization.[161] Translating these

benefits to neonates with neutropenia appears to be attractive. Earlier studies in the late 1990s showed that G-CSF or GM-CSF, when administered as prophylaxis for up to 5 days, could reduce the incidence of sepsis in small-for-gestational age neonates[162] and those with early postnatal neutropenia attributable to maternal pre-eclampsia.[163] However, both studies involved small sample size, and a Cochrane review in 2003 concluded that there was inadequate evidence for adopting prophylactic colony-stimulating factors in the management of neonates with neutropenia.[164]

Results from recent studies on prophylactic colony-stimulating factors in preterm infants remain controversial. A multicenter, randomized, double-blind, placebo-controlled trial involving 25 neonatal intensive care units in France evaluated the use of G-CSF for 3 days in 200 preterm infants less than 32 weeks' gestation with ANC less than 1.5×10^9/L. There was no difference in infection-free survival between the treatment and placebo groups at 4 weeks after treatment, but a transient effect at 2 weeks was observed.[165]

Another multicenter, single-blind, randomized controlled trial in 26 centers in the United Kingdom recruited 280 neonates less than 31 weeks' gestation and below the 10th centile for birth weight to receive GM-CSF for 5 days or standard management. Although ANC rose significantly more rapidly in infants treated with GM-CSF, that did not result in reduction of sepsis-free survival, including the subgroup with neutropenia (ANC < 1100/mm³).[166]

At present, there is still no conclusive evidence on the routine use of colony-stimulating factors as prophylaxis for or treatment of established sepsis in neutropenic infants without specific underlying causes.[167]

Neonatal alloimmune neutropenia is often severe and prolonged for weeks or months, and G-CSF is an effective treatment. The usual starting dose of G-CSF for immune-mediated neutropenia is 5–10 μg/kg/day. In most cases, response is evident within 24–48 hours,[168] and subsequent doses are titrated to maintain ANC above 1000/mm³. Apart from promoting granulocyte differentiation and maturation, G-CSF also downregulates the expression of some neutrophil antigens, rendering them less susceptible to degradation by circulating antibodies.[169]

Usually, 2 to 3 weeks of treatment are sufficient, and stabilization of neutrophil count would be expected as maternal alloantibodies are cleared from the baby's circulation. However, there are variations in treatment response, such as latency and magnitude of increment,[168] dose of G-CSF required to maintain the desired neutrophil count,[170] and complete failure of response to G-CSF.[171] Neonatal alloimmune neutropenia refractory to G-CSF has been reported. Development of thrombocytopenia related to G-CSF use has also been described.[172]

Intravenous immunoglobulin (IVIG) is also used to treat neonatal alloimmune neutropenia, but treatment failure has been reported in several cases that subsequently responded to G-CSF. Because of the rarity of neonatal alloimmune neutropenia, there is a lack of randomized controlled trials providing evidence for the comparative efficacy of IVIG vs G-CSF. For autoimmune neutropenia in children, G-CSF is considered the standard of care as first-line treatment, and IVIG is not recommended as routine treatment.[173]

Lifelong G-CSF administration is the mainstay of treatment of SCN. G-CSF acts by stimulating neutrophil production and delaying apoptosis. Before the availability in 1987 of G-CSF, 42% of children with SCN died within the first 2 years of life.[174] Long-term G-CSF therapy dramatically reduces the incidence, duration of infection-related events, and mortality rate. According to data from the Severe Congenital Neutropenia International Registry (SCNIR) on more than 700 patients with SCN, over 90% responded well to G-CSF therapy and required significantly fewer antibiotics and days of hospitalization.[175–179] Cumulative incidence of death from sepsis was 8% after receiving 10 years of G-CSF treatment.[180] G-CSF can be administered by the subcutaneous route. The usual starting dose is 5 μg/kg/day, and the dose is adjusted to target at maintaining an ANC of 1.0–2.5 × 10^9/L.[43]

Hematopoietic Stem Cell Transplantation

Hematopoietic stem cell transplantation (HSCT) is the definitive treatment of SCN, CGD, and LAD type I and type III.[181] Timing and indications for transplantation in these conditions are variable, depending on individual clinical course, availability of suitable donor, center experience, and views of the patient and family. Nevertheless, early initiation for donor search and counseling is crucial. Guidelines and transplant protocols are constantly evolving, and it is essential for the patients and their family to be well informed of the options.

The current recommendations for HSCT in patients with SCN are refractoriness to G-CSF therapy or development of malignant transformation. However, once myelodysplastic syndrome (MDS) or leukemia develops, the success rate of HSCT is poor.[182–184] It is suggested that early HSCT with the best-available donor should be considered in patients who acquire cytogenetic abnormalities or require a high dose of G-CSF.[185]

Leukocyte adhesion deficiency type I is associated with high mortality in early life, and affected children should undergo early HSCT if a suitable HLA-matched family donor can be identified. In a recent multicenter cohort consisting of 36 children with LAD type I, the overall long-term survival was 75%.[186] The median age at the time of transplant was 8 months. Survival rates in matched family donor and unrelated donor transplants were similar. The study also demonstrated the success of reduced-intensity conditioning with good safety profile and outcome. Mixed chimerism in donor neutrophil engraftment was sufficient for preventing infections. In a more recent single-center study of 11 children with LAD type I in Saudi Arabia, an excellent overall survival rate of 91% was achieved, and all patients who received matched family donor and unrelated cord blood transplants had long-term event-free survival.[187]

Hematopoietic stem cell transplantation is recommended for selected patients with CGD. A risk-stratified approach has been suggested.[188] Patients with 1 life-threatening infection in the past, severe granulomatous disease with progressive organ dysfunction, limited access to specialist care or noncompliance to prophylactic therapy belong to the standard-risk category, and HSCT is recommended if an HLA-matched family or unrelated donor can be identified. High-risk patients are those with active treatment-refractory infections and steroid-dependent granulomatous disease, such as inflammatory colitis. In such situations, "salvage" HSCT is considered after clinical improvement is attained after maximal antimicrobial or immunosuppressive therapy. Successful HSCT results in normalized neutrophil function, clearance of preexisting infections, resolution of inflammatory complications, and catchup growth.[189,190] Morbidity and mortality can be reduced by using a non-myeloablative conditioning regimen.[191] HSCT is only considered for patients with uncomplicated CGD if an HLA-genoidentical sibling donor is available.[188]

OUTCOME AND FOLLOW-UP

Most infants with neutropenia associated with prematurity, neonatal alloimmune neutropenia, and secondary neutropenia do not have life-threatening infections, and neutropenia is transient. Neonatal alloimmune neutropenia usually resolves by 2–3 months when maternal IgG is cleared from the baby's circulation but may take up to 7 months.[31]

Congenital neutropenia and inherited phagocytic defects require specialist follow-up by hematologists or immunologists. Patients with SCN require lifelong monitoring as they are at risk for developing MDS and leukemia. Malignant transformation is associated with acquired genetic abnormalities, such as mutations in the G-CSF receptor gene (*CSF3R*), monosomy 7, and trisomy 21. The cumulative incidence of mortality from sepsis was 10% and 22% for MDS and leukemia, respectively, after 15 years of G-CSF therapy.[192] The need for a higher dose of G-CSF to maintain normal neutrophil count predicted a higher risk of developing leukemia.[193] Bone marrow examination and cytogenetic studies should be performed annually or whenever cytopenia develops to identify morphological and clonal abnormalities (eg, monosomy 7) suggestive of malignant transformation. An acquired mutation in the G-CSF receptor gene (*CSF3R*) is a strong predictor of leukemic development and is a useful marker for diagnostic monitoring.[194,195]

With good medication compliance and prompt treatment of infections, an increasing number of patients with CGD can now live into adulthood.[77] Still, survival is limited, and quality of life is adversely affected by organ dysfunction, medication side effects, and frequent hospitalizations. The clinical outcome is influenced by the underlying molecular defect, amount of residual NADPH oxidase activity, the patient's own history of infections, inflammatory manifestations, compliance with medications, and access to medical care.[83] The clinical course of autosomal recessive CGD is usually less severe than X-linked CGD.

Fungal infections are difficult to eradicate completely despite prolonged antifungal treatment. Residual lesions often contain both fungal and inflammatory elements and may cause space-occupying effects on vital organs and harbor the nidus for recurrence. Patients with hyperinflammatory conditions requiring immunosuppressants are at even higher risks for bacterial and fungal infections, posing a treatment dilemma for clinicians. Invasive fungal infections and inflammatory conditions such as colitis are the main causes of mortality in CGD.

REFERENCES

1. Jutras I, Desjardins M. Phagocytosis: at the crossroads of innate and adaptive immunity. *Annu Rev Cell Dev Biol.* 2005;21:511–527.

2. Flannagan RS, Jaumouillé V, Grinstein S. The cell biology of phagocytosis. *Annu Rev Pathol.* 2011. doi:10.1146/annurev-pathol-011811–132445.

3. Stuart LM, Ezekowitz RA. Phagocytosis: elegant complexity. *Immunity.* 2005;22: 539–550.

4. Williams MR, Azcutia V, Newton G, Alcaide P, Luscinskas FW. Emerging mechanisms of neutrophil recruitment across endothelium. *Trends Immunol.* 2011;32: 461–469.

5. Schmidt EP, Lee WL, Zemans RL, Yamashita C, Downey GP. On, around, and through: neutrophil-endothelial interactions in innate immunity. *Physiology (Bethesda).* 2011;26: 334–347.

6. Vidarsson G, van de Winkel JG. Fc receptor and complement receptor-mediated phagocytosis in host defence. *Curr Opin Infect Dis.* 1998;11:271–278.

7. van Lookeren Campagne M, Wiesmann C, Brown EJ. Macrophage complement receptors and pathogen clearance. *Cell Microbiol.* 2007;9:2095–2102.

8. Mantovani A, Cassatella MA, Costantini C, Jaillon S. Neutrophils in the activation and regulation of innate and adaptive immunity. *Nat Rev Immunol.* 2011;11:519–531.

9. Weinberg GA, D'Angio CT. Laboratory aids for diagnosis of neonatal sepsis. In: Remington JS, Klein JO, Wilson CB,
Nizet V, Maldonado YA, eds. *Infectious Diseases of the Fetus and Newborn Infant.* 7th ed. Philadelphia, PA: Elsevier Saunders; 2011:1144–1160.

10. Koenig JM, Christensen RD. Incidence, neutrophil kinetics, and natural history of neonatal neutropenia associated with maternal hypertension. *N Engl J Med.* 1989;321:557–562.

11. Schmutz N, Henry E, Jopling J, Christensen RD. Expected ranges for blood neutrophil concentrations of neonates: the Manroe and Mouzinho charts revisited. *J Perinatol.* 2008;28:275–281.

12. Manroe BL, Weinberg AG, Rosenfeld CR, Browne R. The neonatal blood count in health and disease. I. Reference values for neutrophilic cells. *J Pediatr.* 1979;95:89–98.

13. Mouzinho A, Rosenfeld CR, Sanchez PJ, Risser R. Revised reference ranges for circulating neutrophils in very-low-birth-weight neonates. *Pediatrics.* 1994;94:76–82.

14. Juul SE, Hayes JW, McPherson RJ. Evaluation of neutropenia and neutrophilia in hospitalized preterm infants. *J Perinatol.* 2004;24:150–157.

15. Christensen RD, Henry E, Wiedmeier SE, Stoddard RA, Lambert DK. Low blood neutrophil concentrations among extremely low birth weight neonates: data from a multihospital health-care system. *J Perinatol.* 2006;26:682–687.

16. Engle WD, Rosenfeld CR. Neutropenia in high-risk neonates. *J Pediatr.* 1984;105:982–986.

17. Baley JE, Stork EK, Warkentin PI, Shurin SB. Neonatal neutropenia: clinical manifestation, cause and outcome. *Am J Dis Child.* 1988;142:1161–1165.

18. Gessler P, Luders R, Konig S, Haas N, Lasch P, Kachel W. Neonatal neutropenia in low birth weight premature infants. *Am J Perinatol* 1995;12:3412–3438.

19. Juul SE, Calhoun DA, Christensen RD. "Idiopathic neutropenia" in very low birthweight infants. Acta Paediatr 1998;87:963–968.

20. Omar SA, Salhadar A, Wooliever DE, Alsgaard PK. Late-onset neutropenia in very low birth weight infants. *Pediatrics.* 2000;106:E55.

21. Juul SE, Christensen RD. The effect of recombinant granulocyte colony stimulating factor on blood neutrophil concentrations among patients with "idiopathic neonatal neutropenia": a randomized, placebo-controlled trial. *J Perinatol.* 2003;23:493–497.

22. Doron MW, Makhlouf RA, Katz VL, Lawson EE, Stiles AD. Increased incidence of sepsis at birth in neutropenic infants of mothers with preeclampsia. *J Pediatr.* 1994;125:452–458.

23. Koenig JM, Christensen RD. The mechanism responsible for diminished neutrophil production in neonates delivered of women with pregnancy-induced hypertension. *Am J Obstet Gynecol.* 1991;165:467–473.

24. Faden HS. Early diagnosis of neonatal bacteremia by buffy-coat examination. *J Pediatr.* 1976;88:1032–1034.

25. Manroe BL, Rosenfeld CR, Weinberg AG, Browne R. The differential leukocyte count in the assessment and outcome of early-onset neonatal group B streptococcal disease. *J Pediatr.* 1977;91:632–637.

26. Payne NR, Burke BA, Day DL, Christenson PD, Thompson TR, Ferrieri P. Correlation of clinical and pathologic findings in early onset neonatal group B streptococcal infection with disease severity and prediction of outcome. *Pediatr Infect Dis J.* 1988;7:836–847.

27. Black LV, Maheshwari A. Immune-mediated neutropenia in the neonate. *NeoReviews.* 2009;10:446–453.

28. Lalezari P, Murphy GB, Allen FH Jr. NB1, a new neutrophil-specific antigen involved in the pathogenesis of neonatal neutropenia. *J Clin Invest.* 1971;50:1108–1115.

29. Trivedi DH, Bussel JB. Immunohematologic disorders. *J Allergy Clin Immunol.* 2003;111:S669–S676.

30. Bedu A, Baumann C, Rohrlich P, Duval M, Fenneteau O, Cartron J. Failure of granulocyte colony-stimulating factor in alloimmune neonatal neutropenia. *J Pediatr.* 1995;127:508–509.

31. Bux J, Jung KD, Kauth T, Mueller-Eckhardt C. Serological and clinical aspects of granulocyte antibodies leading to alloimmune neonatal neutropenia. *Transfus Med.* 1992;2:143–149.

32. Lakshman R, Finn A. Neutrophil disorders and their management. *J Clin Pathol.* 2001;54:7–19.

33. Palmblad JE, von dem Borne AE. Idiopathic, immune, infectious, and idiosyncratic neutropenias. *Semin Hematol.* 2002;39:113–120.

34. Strom BL, Carson JL, Schinnar R, Snyder ES, Shaw M. Descriptive epidemiology of agranulocytosis. *Arch Intern Med.* 1992;152:1475–1480.

35. Andersohn F, Konzen C, Garbe E. Systematic review: agranulocytosis induced by nonchemotherapy drugs. *Ann Intern Med.* 2007;146:657–665.

36. Andrès E, Zimmer J, Affenberger S, Federici L, Alt M, Maloisel F. Idiosyncratic drug-induced agranulocytosis: update of an old disorder. *Eur J Intern Med.* 2006;17:529–535.

37. Dinauer MC, Newburger PE. The phagocyte system and disorders of granulopoiesis and granulocyte function. In: Orkin SH, Nathan DG, Ginsburg D, Look AT, Fisher DE, Lux IV SE, eds. *Nathan and Oski's Hematology of Infancy and Childhood.* 7th ed. Philadelphia, PA: Saunders; 2008:1137–1221.

38. Segel GB, Halterman JS. Neutropenia in pediatric practice. *Pediatr Rev.* 2008;29:12–23.

39. Boztug K, Welte K, Zeidler C, Klein C. Congenital neutropenia syndromes. *Immunol Allergy Clin North Am.* 2008;28:259–275, vii–viii.

40. Klein C. Congenital neutropenia. *Hematology Am Soc Hematol Educ Program.* 2009:344–350.

41. Boztug K, Klein C. Novel genetic etiologies of severe congenital neutropenia. *Curr Opin Immunol.* 2009;21:472–480.

42. Klein C, Welte K. Genetic insights into congenital neutropenia. *Clin Rev Allergy Immunol.* 2010;38:68–74.

43. Welte K, Zeidler C. Severe congenital neutropenia. *Hematol Oncol Clin North Am.* 2009;23:307–320.

44. Xia J, Bolyard AA, Rodger E, et al. Prevalence of mutations in ELANE, GFI1, HAX1, SBDS, WAS and G6PC3 in patients with severe congenital neutropenia. *Br J Haematol.* 2009;147:535–542.

45. Westerberg LS, Meelu P, Baptista M, et al. Activating WASP mutations associated with X-linked neutropenia result in enhanced actin polymerization, altered cytoskeletal responses, and genomic instability in lymphocytes. *J Exp Med.* 2010;207:1145–1152.

46. Ganapathi KA, Shimamura A. Ribosomal dysfunction and inherited marrow failure. *Br J Haematol.* 2008;141:376–387.

47. Narla A, Ebert BL. Ribosomopathies: human disorders of ribosome dysfunction. *Blood.* 2010;115:3196–3205.

48. Chou JY, Jun HS, Mansfield BC. Neutropenia in type Ib glycogen storage disease. *Curr Opin Hematol.* 2010;17:36–42.

49. Visser G, de Jager W, Verhagen LP, et al. Survival, but not maturation, is affected in neutrophil progenitors from GSD-1b patients. *J Inherit Metab Dis.* 2012;35:287–300.

50. Ogier de Baulny H, Saudubray JM. Branched-chain organic acidurias. *Semin Neonatol.* 2002;7:65–74.

51. Rezaei N, Moazzami K, Aghamohammadi A, Klein C. Neutropenia and primary immunodeficiency diseases. *Int Rev Immunol.* 2009;28:335–366.

52. Pannicke U, Hönig M, Hess I, et al. Reticular dysgenesis (aleukocytosis) is caused by mutations in the gene encoding mitochondrial adenylate kinase 2. *Nat Genet.* 2009;41:101–105.

53. Lagresle-Peyrou C, Six EM, Picard C, et al. Human adenylate kinase 2 deficiency causes a profound hematopoietic defect associated with sensorineural deafness. *Nat Genet.* 2009;41:106–111.

54. Rezaei N, Aghamohammadi A, Ramyar A, Pan-Hammarstrom Q, Hammarstrom L. Severe congenital neutropenia or hyper-IgM syndrome? A novel mutation of CD40 ligand in a patient with severe neutropenia. Int Arch Allergy Immunol 2008;147:255–259.

55. Levy J, Espanol-Boren T, Thomas C, et al. Clinical spectrum of X-linked hyper-IgM syndrome. *J Pediatr.* 1997;131:47–54.

56. Winkelstein JA, Marino MC, Ochs H, et al. The X-linked hyper-IgM syndrome: clinical and immunologic features of 79 patients. *Medicine (Baltimore).* 2003;82:373–384.

57. Huizing M, Anikster Y, Gahl WA. Hermansky-Pudlak syndrome and Chediak-Higashi syndrome: disorders of vesicle formation and trafficking. *Thromb Haemost.* 2001;86:233–245.

58. Pachlopnik Schmid J, Côte M, Ménager MM, et al. Inherited defects in lymphocyte cytotoxic activity. *Immunol Rev.* 2010;235:10–23.

59. Farrar JE, Rohrer J, Conley ME. Neutropenia in X-linked agammaglobulinemia. *Clin Immunol Immunopathol.* 1996;81:271–276.

60. Winkelstein JA, Marino MC, Lederman HM, et al. X-linked agammaglobulinemia: report on a United States registry of 201 patients. *Medicine (Baltimore).* 2006;85:193–202.

61. Ogershok PR, Hogan MB, Welch JE, Corder WT, Wilson NW. Spectrum of illness in pediatric common variable immunodeficiency. *Ann Allergy Asthma Immunol.* 2006;97:653–656.

62. Lemos S, Jacob CM, Pastorino AC, et al. Neutropenia in antibody-deficient patients under IVIG replacement therapy. *Pediatr Allergy Immunol.* 2009;20:97–101.

63. Dotta L, Tassone L, Badolato R. Clinical and genetic features of warts, hypogammaglobulinemia, infections and myelokathexis (WHIM) syndrome. *Curr Mol Med.* 2011;11:317–325.

64. Dinauer MC, Coates TD. Disorders of phagocyte function and number. In: Hoffman R, Benz EJ Jr, Shattil SJ, et al, eds. *Hematology: Basic Principles and Practice.* 5th ed. London, UK: Churchill Livingstone; 2008:687–720.

65. Smith CW. Adhesion molecules and receptors. *J Allergy Clin Immunol.* 2008;121:S375–S379.

66. Langer HF, Chavakis T. Leukocyte-endothelial interactions in inflammation. *J Cell Mol Med.* 2009;13:1211–1220.

67. Etzioni A. Defects in the leukocyte adhesion cascade. *Clin Rev Allergy Immunol.* 2010;38:54–60.

68. Arnaout MA. Structure and function of the leukocyte adhesion molecules CD11/CD18. *Blood.* 1990;75:1037–1050.

69. Etzioni A. Leukocyte adhesion deficiencies: molecular basis, clinical findings, and therapeutic options. *Adv Exp Med Biol.* 2007;601:51–60.

70. Dimanche-Boitrel MT, Le Deist F, Quillet A, Fischer A, Griscelli C, Lisowska-Grospierre B. Effects of interferon-gamma (IFN-gamma) and tumor necrosis factor-alpha (TNF-alpha) on the expression of LFA-1 in the moderate phenotype of leukocyte adhesion deficiency (LAD). *J Clin Immunol.* 1989;9:200–207.

71. Lübke T, Marquardt T, Etzioni A, Hartmann E, von Figura K, Körner C. Complementation cloning identifies CDG-IIc, a new type of congenital disorders of glycosylation, as a GDP-fucose transporter deficiency. *Nat Genet.* 2001;28:73–76.

72. Gazit Y, Mory A, Etzioni A, et al. Leukocyte adhesion deficiency type II: long-term follow-up and review of the literature. *J Clin Immunol.* 2010;30:308–313.

73. Kinashi T, Aker M, Sokolovsky-Eisenberg M, et al. LAD-III, a leukocyte adhesion deficiency syndrome associated with defective Rap1 activation and impaired stabilization of integrin bonds. *Blood.* 2004;103:1033–1036.

74. Etzioni A, Alon R. Leukocyte adhesion deficiency III: a group of integrin activation defects in hematopoietic lineage cells. *Curr Opin Allergy Clin Immunol.* 2004;4:485–490.

75. Pasvolsky R, Feigelson SW, Kilic SS, et al. A LAD-III syndrome is associated with defective expression of the Rap-1 activator CalDAG-GEFI in lymphocytes, neutrophils, and platelets. *J Exp Med.* 2007;204:1571–1582.

76. Kilic SS, Etzioni A. The clinical spectrum of leukocyte adhesion deficiency (LAD) III due to defective CalDAG-GEF1. *J Clin Immunol.* 2009;29:117–122.

77. Holland SM. Chronic granulomatous disease. *Clin Rev Allergy Immunol*. 2010;38:3–10.

78. Lam GY, Huang J, Brumell JH. Lam GY, Huang J, Brumell JH. The many roles of NOX2 NADPH oxidase-derived ROS in immunity. *Semin Immunopathol*. 2010;32:415–430.

79. Faurschou M, Borregaard N. Neutrophil granules and secretory vesicles in inflammation. *Microbes Infect*. 2003;5:1317–1327.

80. Medina E. Neutrophil extracellular traps: a strategic tactic to defeat pathogens with potential consequences for the host. *J Innate Immun*. 2009;1:176–180.

81. Roos D, Kuhns DB, Maddalena A, et al. Hematologically important mutations: X-linked chronic granulomatous disease (third update). *Blood Cells Mol Dis*. 2010;45:246–265.

82. Roos D, Kuhns DB, Maddalena A, et al. Hematologically important mutations: the autosomal recessive forms of chronic granulomatous disease (second update). *Blood Cells Mol Dis*. 2010;44:291–299.

83. Kang EM, Marciano BE, DeRavin S, Zarember KA, Holland SM, Malech HL. Chronic granulomatous disease: overview and hematopoietic stem cell transplantation. *J Allergy Clin Immunol*. 2011;127:1319–1326.

84. Lau YL, Chan GC, Ha SY, Hui YF, Yuen KY. The role of phagocytic respiratory burst in host defense against Mycobacterium tuberculosis. *Clin Infect Dis*. 1998;26:226–227.

85. Lee PP, Chan KW, Jiang L, et al. Susceptibility to mycobacterial infections in children with X-linked chronic granulomatous disease: a review of 17 patients living in a region endemic for tuberculosis. *Pediatr Infect Dis J*. 2008;27:224–230.

86. Sirinavin S, Techasaensiri C, Benjaponpitak S, Pornkul R, Vorachit M. Invasive *Chromobacterium violaceum* infection in children: case report and review. *Pediatr Infect Dis J*. 2005;24:559–561.

87. Macher AM, Casale TB, Fauci AS. Chronic granulomatous disease of childhood and Chromobacterium violaceum infections in the southeastern United States. *Ann Intern Med*. 1982;97:51–55.

88. Schäppi MG, Jaquet V, Belli DC, Krause KH. Hyperinflammation in chronic granulomatous disease and anti-inflammatory role of the phagocyte NADPH oxidase. *Semin Immunopathol*. 2008;30:255–271.

89. Rieber N, Hector A, Kuijpers T, Roos D, Hartl D. Current concepts of hyperinflammation in chronic granulomatous disease. *Clin Dev Immunol*. 2012;2012:252–460. doi:10.1155/2012/252460.

90. Schäppi MG, Smith VV, Goldblatt D, Lindley KJ, Milla PJ. Colitis in chronic granulomatous disease. *Arch Dis Child*. 2001;84:147–151.

91. Lanza F. Clinical manifestation of myeloperoxidase deficiency. *J Mol Med*. 1998;76:676–681.

92. Lekstrom-Himes JA, Gallin JI. Immunodeficiency diseases caused by defects in phagocytes. *N Engl J Med*. 2000;343:1703–1714.

93. Silverman E, Jaeggi E. Non-cardiac manifestations of neonatal lupus erythematosus. *Scand J Immunol*. 2010;72:223–225.

94. Zuppa AA, Fracchiolla A, Cota F, et al. Infants born to mothers with anti-SSA/Ro autoantibodies: neonatal outcome and follow-up. *Clin Pediatr (Phila)*. 2008;47:231–236.

95. Johnston SL. Clinical immunology review series: an approach to the patient with recurrent superficial abscesses. *Clin Exp Immunol*. 2008;152:397–405.

96. Freeman AF, Holland SM. Clinical manifestations of hyper IgE syndromes. *Dis Markers*. 2010;29:123–130.

97. Woellner C, Gertz EM, Schäffer AA, et al. Mutations in STAT3 and diagnostic guidelines for hyper-IgE syndrome. *J Allergy Clin Immunol*. 2010;125:424–432.e8.

98. Chamlin SL, McCalmont TH, Cunningham BB, et al. Cutaneous manifestations of hyper-IgE syndrome in infants and children. *J Pediatr*. 2002;141:572–575.

99. Eberting CL, Davis J, Puck JM, et al. Dermatitis and the newborn rash of hyper-IgE syndrome. *Arch Dermatol*. 2004;140:1119–1125.

100. Chu EY, Freeman AF, Jing H, et al. Cutaneous manifestations of DOCK8 deficiency syndrome. *Arch Dermatol*. 2011. doi:10.1001/archdermatol.2011.262.

101. Zhang Q, Davis JC, Dove CG, Su HC. Genetic, clinical, and laboratory markers for DOCK8 immunodeficiency syndrome. *Dis Markers*. 2010;29:131–139.

102. Murthi GV, Okoye BO, Spicer RD, Cusick EL, Noblett HR. Perianal abscess in childhood. *Pediatr Surg Int*. 2002;18:689–691.

103. Ezer SS, Ouzkurt P, Ince E, Hiçsönmez A. Perianal abscess and fistula-in-ano in children: aetiology, management and outcome. *J Paediatr Child Health*. 2010;46:92–95.

104. Glocker EO, Kotlarz D, Boztug K, et al. Inflammatory bowel disease and mutations affecting the interleukin-10 receptor. *N Engl J Med*. 2009;361:2033–2045.

105. Glocker EO, Frede N, Perro M, et al. Infant colitis—it's in the genes. *Lancet*. 2010;376:1272.

106. Fraser N, Davies BW, Cusack J. Neonatal omphalitis: a review of its serious complications. *Acta Paediatr*. 2006;95:519–522.

107. Sawardekar KP. Changing spectrum of neonatal omphalitis. *Pediatr Infect Dis J*. 2004;23:22–26.

108. Mason WH, Andrews R, Ross LA, Wright HT. Omphalitis in the newborn infant. *Pediatr Infect Dis J*. 1989;8:521–525.

109. Lotte A, Wasz-Hockert O, Poisson N, et al. BCG complications. Estimates of risks among vaccinated subjects and statistical analysis of their main characteristics. *Adv Tuberc Res*. 1984;21:107–193.

110. Allerberger F. An outbreak of suppurative lymphadenitis connected with BCG vaccination in Austria 1990/1. *Am Rev Respir Dis*. 1991;144:469.

111. Vitkova E, Galliova J, Krepela K, et al. Adverse reactions to BCG. *Cent Eur J Public Health*. 1995;3:138–141.

112. Bolger T, O'Connell M, Menon A, Butler K. Complications associated with the bacille Calmette-Guérin vaccination in Ireland. *Arch Dis Child*. 2006;91:594–597.

113. Hesseling AC, Rabie H, Marais BJ, et al. Bacille Calmette-Guerin vaccine-induced disease in HIV-infected and HIV-uninfected children. *Clin Infect Dis*. 2006;42:548–558.

114. Talbot EA, Perkins MD, Silva SF, Frothingham R. Disseminated bacille Calmette-Guerin disease after vaccination: case report and review. *Clin Infect Dis*. 1997;24:1139–1146.

115. Casanova JL, Jouanguy E, Lamhamedi S, Blanche S, Fischer A. Immunological conditions of children with BCG disseminated infection. *Lancet*. 1995;346:581.

116. Casanova JL, Blanche S, Emile JF, et al. Idiopathic disseminated bacillus Calmette-Guérin infection: a French national retrospective study. *Pediatrics*. 1996;98:774–778.

117. Bernatowska EA, Wolska-Kusnierz B, Pac M, et al. Disseminated bacillus Calmette-Guérin infection and immunodeficiency. *Emerg Infect Dis*. 2007;13:799–801.

118. Al-Muhsen S, Casanova JL. The genetic heterogeneity of mendelian susceptibility to mycobacterial diseases. *J Allergy Clin Immunol*. 2008;122:1043–1051.

119. Qu HQ, Fisher-Hoch SP, McCormick JB. Molecular immunity to mycobacteria: knowledge from the mutation and phenotype spectrum analysis of Mendelian susceptibility to mycobacterial diseases. *Int J Infect Dis*. 2011;15:e305–e313.

120. Calhoun DA, Kirk JF, Christensen RD. Incidence, significance and kinetic mechanism responsible for leukemoid reactions in patients in the neonatal intensive care unit: a prospective evaluation. *J Pediatr*. 1996;129:403–409.

121. Rastogi S, Rastogi D, Sundaram R, Kulpa J, Parekh AJ. Leukemoid reaction in extremely low-birth-weight infants. *Am J Perinatol* 1999;16:93–97.

122. Hsiao R, Omar SA. Outcome of extremely low birth weight infants with leukemoid reaction. *Pediatrics*. 2005;116:e43–e51.

123. Zanardo V, Vedovato S, Trevisanuto DD, et al. Histological chorioamnionitis and neonatal leukemoid reaction in low-birth-weight infants. *Hum Pathol.* 2006;37:87–91.

124. Duran R, Ozbek UV, Ciftdemir NA, Acuna B, Süt N. The relationship between leukemoid reaction and perinatal morbidity, mortality, and chorioamnionitis in low birth weight infants. *Int J Infect Dis.* 2010;14:e998–e1001.

125. Cantù-Rajnoldi A, Cattoretti G, Caccamo ML, et al. Leukaemoid reaction with megakaryocytic features in newborns with Down's syndrome. *Eur J Haematol.* 1988;40:403–409.

126. Seibel NL, Sommer A, Miser J. Transient neonatal leukemoid reactions in mosaic trisomy 21. *J Pediatr.* 1984;104:251–254.

127. Zachman RD, Bauer CR, Boehm J, Korones SB, Rigatto H, Rao AV. Effect of antenatal dexamethasone on neonatal leukocyte count. *J Perinatol.* 1988;8:111–113.

128. Barak M, Cohen A, Herschkowitz S. Total leukocyte and neutrophil count changes associated with antenatal beta-methasone administration in premature infants. *Acta Paediatr.* 1992;81:760–763.

129. Engmann C, Donn SM. Severe neutrophilia in an infant with persistent pulmonary hypertension of the newborn. *Am J Perinatol* 2003;20:347–351.

130. Zanardo V, Magarotto M, Rosolen A. Neonatal leukemoid reaction and early development of bronchopulmonary dysplasia in a very low-birth-weight infant. *Fetal Diagn Ther.* 2001;16:150–152.

131. Zanardo V, Savio V, Giacomin C, Rinaldi A, Marzari F, Chiarelli S. Relationship between neonatal leukemoid reaction and bronchopulmonary dysplasia in low-birth-weight infants: a cross-sectional study. *Am J Perinatol.* 2002;19:379–386.

132. Zanardo V, Vedovato S, Trevisanuto D, Chiarelli S. Leukemoid reaction and bronchopulmonary dysplasia: a primary inflammatory mechanism? *Pediatrics.* 2000;116:1260–1261.

133. Bain BJ. Morphology of blood cells. In: Bain BJ, ed. *Blood Cells: A Practical Guide.* 4th ed. New York, NY: Wiley-Blackwell; 2006:61–174.

134. Verheugt FW, von dem Borne AE, Décary F, Engelfriet CP. The detection of granulocyte alloantibodies with an indirect immunofluorescence test. *Br J Haematol.* 1977;36:533–544.

135. Bux J, Kober B, Kiefel V, Mueller-Eckhardt C. Analysis of granulocyte-reactive antibodies using an immunoassay based upon monoclonal antibody-specific immobilization of granulocyte antigen (MAIGA). *Transfus Med.* 1993;3:157–162.

136. Bux J, Chapman J. Report on the second international granulocyte serology workshop. *Transfusion.* 1997;37:977–983.

137. Shimamura A. Clinical approach to marrow failure. *Hematology Am Soc Hematol Educ Program.* 2009:329–337.

138. Levinsky RJ, Harvey BA, Rodeck CH, Soothill JF. Phorbol myristate acetate stimulated NBT test: a simple method suitable for antenatal diagnosis of chronic granulomatous disease. *Clin Exp Immunol.* 1983;54:595–598.

139. O'Gorman MRG, Corrochano V. Rapid whole-blood flow cytometry assay for diagnosis of chronic granulomatous disease. *Clin Diagn Lab Immunol.* 1995;2:227–232.

140. Vowells SJ, Fleisher TA, Sekhsaria S, et al. Genotype-dependent variability in flow cytometric evaluation of reduced nicotinamide adenine dinucleotide phosphate oxidase function in patients with chronic granulomatous disease. *J Pediatr.* 1996;128:104–107.

141. O'gorman MR. Role of flow cytometry in the diagnosis and monitoring of primary immunodeficiency disease. *Clin Lab Med.* 2007;27:591–626.

142. O'Gorman MRG, McNally AC, Anderson DC, et al. A rapid whole blood lysis technique for the diagnosis of moderate or severe leukocyte adhesion deficiency (LAD). *Ann NY Acad Sci.* 1993;677:427–430.

143. Dimanche-Boitrel MT, Le Deist F, Quillet A, et al. Effects of interferon-gamma (IFNgamma) and tumor necrosis factor-alpha (TNF-alpha) on the expression of LFA-1 in the moderate phenotype of leukocyte adhesion deficiency (LAD). *J Clin Immunol.* 1989;9:200–207.

144. Bonilla FA, Bernstein IL, Khan DA, et al. Practice parameter for the diagnosis and management of primary immunodeficiency. Practice parameter for the diagnosis and management of primary immunodeficiency. *Ann Allergy Asthma Immunol.* 2005;94:S1–S63.

145. Weening RS, Kabel P, Pijman P, Roos D. Continuous therapy with sulfamethoxazole-trimethoprim in patients with chronic granulomatous disease. *J Pediatr.* 1983;103:127–130.

146. Mouy R, Fischer A, Vilmer E, Seger R, Griscelli C. Incidence, severity, and prevention of infections in chronic granulomatous disease. *J Pediatr.* 1989;114:555–560.

147. Margolis DM, Melnick DA, Alling DW, Gallin JI. Trimethoprim-sulfamethoxazole prophylaxis in the management of chronic granulomatous disease. *J Infect Dis.* 1990; 162:723–726.

148. Mouy R, Veber F, Blanche S, et al. Long-term itraconazole prophylaxis against *Aspergillus* infections in thirty-two patients with chronic granulomatous disease. *J Pediatr.* 1994;125, 998–1003.

149. Gallin JI, Alling DW, Malech HL, et al. Itraconazole to prevent fungal infections in chronic granulomatous disease. *N Engl J Med.* 2003;348:2416–2422.

150. International Chronic Granulomatous Disease Cooperative Study Group. A controlled trial of interferon gamma to prevent infection in chronic granulomatous disease. *N Engl J Med.* 1991;324:509–516.

151. Marciano BE, Wesley R, De Carlo ES, et al. Long term interferon-gamma therapy for patients with chronic granulomatous disease. *Clin Infect Dis.* 2004;39:692–699.

152. Seger RA. Modern management of chronic granulomatous disease. *Br J Haematol.* 2008;140:255–266.

153. Kaguelidou F, Turner MA, Choonara I, Jacqz-Aigrain E. Ciprofloxacin use in neonates: a systematic review of the literature. *Pediatr Infect Dis J.* 2011;30:e29–e37.

154. Maldonado YA. Pneumocystis and other less common fungal infections. In: Remington JS, Klein JO, Wilson CB, Nizet V, Maldonado YA, eds. *Infectious Diseases of the Fetus and Newborn Infant.* 7th ed. Philadelphia, PA: Elsevier Saunders; 2011:1079–1123.

155. Strumia MM. The effect of leukocytic cream injections in the treatment of the neutropenias. *Am J Med Sci.* 1934;187:527–544.

156. Pammi M, Brocklehurst P. Granulocyte transfusions for neonates with confirmed or suspected sepsis and neutropenia. *Cochrane Database Syst Rev.* 2011;5(10):CD003956.

157. von Planta, M, Ozsahin H, Schroten H, Stauffer UG, Seger RA. Greater omentum flaps and granulocyte transfusions as combined therapy of liver abscess in chronic granulomatous disease. *Eur J Pediatr Surg.* 1997;7:234–236.

158. Ozsahin H, von Planta M, Muller I, et al. Successful treatment of invasive aspergillosis in chronic granulomatous disease by bone marrow transplantation, granulocyte colony-stimulating factor-mobilized granulocytes, and liposomal amphotericin-B. *Blood.* 1998;92:2719–2724.

159. Hill HR. Granulocyte transfusions in neonates. *Pediatr Rev.* 1991;12:298–302.

160. Heuser M, Ganser A. Colony-stimulating factors in the management of neutropenia and its complications. *Ann Hematol.* 2005;84:697–708.

161. Heuser M, Ganser A, Bokemeyer C; American Society of Clinical Oncology; National Comprehensive Cancer Network; European Organization for Research and Treatment of Cancer. Use of colony-stimulating factors for chemotherapy-associated neutropenia: review of current guidelines. *Semin Hematol.* 2007;44:148–156.

162. Carr R, Modi N, Doré CJ, El-Rifai R, Lindo D. A randomized, controlled trial of prophylactic granulocyte-macrophage colony-stimulating factor in human newborns less than 32 weeks gestation. *Pediatrics.* 1999;103:796–802.

163. Kocherlakota P, La Gamma EF. Preliminary report: rhG-CSF may reduce the incidence of neonatal sepsis in prolonged preeclampsia-associated neutropenia. *Pediatrics*. 1998;102:1107–1111.

164. Carr R, Modi N, Doré C. G-CSF and GM-CSF for treating or preventing neonatal infections. *Cochrane Database Syst Rev*. 2003;(3):CD003066.

165. Kuhn P, Messer J, Paupe A, et al. A multicenter, randomized, placebo-controlled trial of prophylactic recombinant granulocyte-colony stimulating factor in preterm neonates with neutropenia. *J Pediatr*. 2009;155:324–330.e1.

166. Carr R, Brocklehurst P, Doré CJ, Modi N. Granulocyte-macrophage colony stimulating factor administered as prophylaxis for reduction of sepsis in extremely preterm, small for gestational age neonates (the PROGRAMS trial): a single-blind, multicentre, randomised controlled trial. *Lancet*. 2009;373:226–233.

167. Shann F. Sepsis in babies: should we stimulate the phagocytes? *Lancet*. 2009;373:188–190.

168. Rodwell RL, Gray PH, Taylor KM, Minchinton R. Granulocyte colony stimulating factor treatment for alloimmune neonatal neutropenia. *Arch Dis Child Fetal Neonatal Ed*. 1996;75:F57–F58.

169. Gilmore MM, Stroncek DF, Korones DN. Treatment of alloimmune neonatal neutropenia with granulocyte colony-stimulating factor. *J Pediatr*. 1994;125:948–951.

170. Maheshwari A, Christensen RD, Calhoun DA. Resistance to recombinant human granulocyte colony-stimulating factor in neonatal alloimmune neutropenia associated with anti-human neutrophil antigen-2a (NB1) antibodies. *Pediatrics*. 2002;109:e64.

171. Bedu A, Baumann C, Rohrlich P, Duval M, Fenneteau O, Cartron J. Failure of granulocyte colony-stimulating factor in alloimmune neonatal neutropenia. *J Pediatr*. 1995;127:508–509.

172. Wiedl C, Walter AW. Granulocyte colony stimulating factor in neonatal alloimmune neutropenia: a possible association with induced thrombocytopenia. *Pediatr Blood Cancer*. 2010;54:1014–1016.

173. Anderson D, Ali K, Blanchette V, et al. Guidelines on the use of intravenous immune globulin for hematologic conditions. *Transfus Med Rev*. 2007;21:S9–S56.

174. Zeidler C, Boxer L, Dale DC, Freedman MH, Kinsey S, Welte K. Management of Kostmann syndrome in the G-CSF era. *Br J Haematol*. 2000;109:490–495.

175. Dale DC, Bonilla MA, Davis MW, et al. A randomized controlled phase III trial of recombinant human granulocyte colony-stimulating factor (filgrastim) for treatment of severe chronic neutropenia. *Blood*. 1993;81:2496–2502.

176. Freedman MH. Safety of long-term administration of granulocyte colony-stimulating factor for severe chronic neutropenia. *Curr Opin Hematol*. 1997;4:217–224.

177. Welte K, Dale D. Pathophysiology and treatment of severe chronic neutropenia. *Ann Hematol*. 1996;72:158–165.

178. Welte K, Boxer L. Severe chronic neutropenia: pathophysiology and therapy. *Semin Hematol*. 1997;34:267–278.

179. Welte K, Zeidler C, Dale DC. Severe congenital neutropenia. *Semin Hematol*. 2006;43:189–195.

180. Rosenberg PS, Alter BP, Bolyard AA, et al. The incidence of leukemia and mortality from sepsis in patients with severe congenital neutropenia receiving long-term G-CSF therapy. *Blood*. 2006;107:4628–4635.

181. Griffith LM, Cowan MJ, Notarangelo LD, et al. Improving cellular therapy for primary immune deficiency diseases: recognition, diagnosis and management. *J Allergy Clin Immunol*. 2009;124:1152–1160.

182. Zeidler C, Welte K, Barak Y, et al. Stem cell transplantation in patients with severe congenital neutropenia without evidence of leukemic transformation. *Blood*. 2000;95:1195–1198.

183. Ferry C, Ouachée M, Leblanc T, et al. Hematopoietic stem cell transplantation in severe congenital neutropenia: experience of the French SCN register. *Bone Marrow Transplant*. 2005;35:45–50.

184. Choi SW, Boxer LA, Pulsipher MA, et al. Stem cell transplantation in patients with severe congenital neutropenia with evidence of leukemic transformation. *Bone Marrow Transplant*. 2005;35:473–477.

185. Connelly JA, Choi SW, Levine JE. Hematopoietic stem cell transplantation for severe congenital neutropenia. *Curr Opin Hematol* 2011. DOI:10.1097/MOH.0b013e32834da96e

186. Qasim W, Cavazzana-Calvo M, Davies EG, et al. Allogeneic hematopoietic stem-cell transplantation for leukocyte adhesion deficiency. *Pediatrics* 2009;123:836–840.

187. Al-Dhekri H, Al-Mousa H, Ayas M, et al. Allogeneic hematopoietic stem cell transplantation in leukocyte adhesion deficiency type 1: a single center experience. *Biol Blood Marrow Transplant*. 2011;17:1245–1249.

188. Seger RA. Hematopoietic stem cell transplantation for chronic granulomatous disease. *Immunol Allergy Clin North Am*. 2010;30:195–208.

189. Seger RA, Gungor T, Belohradsky BH, et al. Treatment of chronic granulomatous disease with myeloablative conditioning and an unmodified hemopoietic allograft: a survey of the European experience, 1985–2000. *Blood*. 2002;100:4344–4350.

190. Soncini E, Slatter MA, Jones LB, et al. Unrelated donor and HLA-identical sibling haematopoietic stem cell transplantation cure chronic granulomatous disease with good long-term outcome and growth. *Br J Haematol*. 2009;145:73–83.

191. Güngör T, Albert M, Schanz U, et al. Successful low-dose busulfan/ full-dose fludarabine based reduced intensity conditioning in high risk pediatric and adult chronic ganulomatous disease patients. Paper presented at: XIVth Meeting of the European Society for Immunodeficiencies; 2010; Istanbul, Turkey.

192. Rosenberg PS, Zeidler C, Bolyard AA, et al. Stable long-term risk of leukaemia in patients with severe congenital neutropenia maintained on G-CSF therapy. *Br J Haematol*. 2010;150:196–199.

193. Rosenberg PS, Alter BP, Bolyard AA, et al. The incidence of leukemia and mortality from sepsis in patients with severe congenital neutropenia receiving long-term G-CSF therapy. *Blood*. 2006;107:4628–4635.

194. Ancliff PJ, Gale RE, Liesner R, et al. Long-term follow-up of granulocyte colony stimulating factor receptor mutations in patients with severe congenital neutropenia: implications for leukaemogenesis and therapy. *Br J Haematol*. 2003;120:685–690.

195. Germeshausen M, Ballmaier M, Welte K. Incidence of CSF3R mutations in severe CN and relevance for leukemogenesis: results of a long-term survey. *Blood*. 2007;109:93–99.

52 Sepsis Neonatorum

Vladana Milisavljevic

INTRODUCTION

Neonatal sepsis or sepsis neonatorum is an important cause of morbidity and mortality among newborns 28 days of life or younger. It presents with the systemic signs of infection or isolation of a bacterial pathogen from the bloodstream.[1] According to the infant's age at the onset of symptoms, sepsis is classified as early or late.

Early-onset sepsis (EOS), discussed in this chapter, has the onset of symptoms within the first days of the newborn's life. Perinatally acquired bacterial neonatal sepsis is a low-incidence, high-risk disease that can be defined as a bloodstream infection at 72 hours of age or less[2] or, in the case of early-onset group B streptococcal (GBS) disease, as infection with the onset of symptoms through day 6 of life.[3] Presentation of EOS is within 24 hours of life in 85%, in 24–48 hours in 5%, and within 48–72 hours in the rest of the neonates. Infections present earlier in preterm neonates.

EPIDEMIOLOGY

Neonatal sepsis incidence is 1–5 cases/1000 live births. In term neonates, incidence is lower than in preterm, with 1–2 cases/1000 live births.[4]

Risk factors for neonatal sepsis include chorioamnionitis, intrapartum maternal fever (temperature ≥ 38°C [100.4°F]); rupture of membranes for 18 hours or longer[5]; delivery at less than 37 weeks' gestation; 5-minute Apgar score 6 or less; maternal GBS colonization; maternal GBS or gram-negative bacteriuria during the current pregnancy; and prior delivery of neonate with GBS disease. Additional risk factors are

the use of instrumentation, such as forceps, or placement of electrodes for intrauterine monitoring during labor and delivery.[6] Black race is a risk factor for both early- and late-onset GBS sepsis, and the reasons behind this are not fully understood.[7]

PATHOPHYSIOLOGY

Sepsis is a clinical syndrome that complicates severe infection, characterized by systemic inflammation and widespread tissue injury. Tissues remote from the original insult display the signs of inflammation, including vasodilation, increased microvascular permeability, and leukocyte accumulation. "Dysregulation" of the normal inflammatory response, with a massive and uncontrolled release of proinflammatory mediators, initiates a chain of events leading to widespread tissue injury. This host response, not the primary disease, is typically responsible for multiple-organ failure.

In an EOS, the most common route of transmission is vertical transmission by ascending contaminated amniotic fluid or bacteria colonizing or infecting the mother's lower genitourinary tract.[8]

Clinical picture and outcome of neonatal sepsis depend on time of onset, maturity of the host defense mechanisms, associated complications, timing of initiation of appropriate antibiotics, and supportive therapy.

Factors contributing to neonatal susceptibility to bacterial infections are the following:

- Anatomic and biochemical immaturity of skin and mucosal barriers (eg, lung, gut epithelia),

- Reduced numbers or function of macrophages and dendritic cells in peripheral tissues (eg, lung),
- Lower numbers of neutrophils in the bone marrow,
- Decreased immunoglobulin (Ig) G and complement levels, especially in premature infants, and
- Inability to respond to bacterial carbohydrate antigens.

During microbial invasion, the immune system produces cytokine to protect the host, but overproduction may have deleterious effects, resulting in multiple-organ injury. Cytokines, phospholipid-derived mediators, and coagulation factors produce widespread vascular endothelial injury, with increased vascular permeability, thrombosis, disseminated intravascular coagulopathy (DIC), and hypotension. Vascular endothelium is a target of tissue injury, where loss of tight junctions allows capillary leakage. In the case of gram-negative sepsis, endotoxins cause global depression of mitochondrial function, as well as damage to endothelium.

The following are the major lung lesions associated with sepsis:

- Pulmonary hypertension (early and late onset)
- Pulmonary parenchymal disease secondary to vascular injury

Pulmonary capillary endothelial cells are damaged by leukocyte-induced pulmonary microvascular injury. Increasing alveolar capillary permeability results in transudation of proteins, infiltration of inflammatory cells, and increased lung water, leading to parenchymal injury. The clinical picture is characterized with decreased pulmonary compliance and pulmonary edema, systemic hypoxemia, and tissue oxygen deprivation.

Increased mean airway pressure, required for maintaining ventilation in wet and noncompliant lungs, increases resistance to venous return and reduces cardiac output. In addition, pulmonary hypertension may impair right ventricular output, resulting in a negative impact on left ventricular output, causing reduction of overall cardiac output, potentially leading to heart and renal failures.

Clinical Presentation

The septic neonate can have a dramatic clinical presentation characterized by respiratory failure, persistent pulmonary hypertension of the newborn, DIC, hypotension, or multiorgan failure. However, signs and symptoms may be subtle and nonspecific, and considering severity of potential consequences, a high index of suspicion should be used in evaluation of neonates for potential sepsis.

Presentation may start as early as labor and delivery; the signs and symptoms may be intrapartum fetal tachycardia, meconium-staining of amniotic fluid (2-fold increase in sepsis if the mother did not receive intrapartum antibiotics[9]), and low Apgar scores (neonates with an Apgar score ≤ 6 or less at 5 minutes had a 36-fold higher likelihood[10] of sepsis than those with Apgar scores ≥ 7).

After delivery, clinical signs of sepsis can be nonspecific and subtle. They include:

- Temperature instability (fever or hypothermia, with fever more common in term and hypothermia in preterm neonates[11]),
- Apnea, tachypnea, respiratory distress (flaring, grunting, retractions or decreased breath sounds), pulmonary hemorrhage,
- Tachycardia or bradycardia, hypotension, prolonged capillary refill time, cool and clammy skin,
- Lethargy or irritability, hypotonia, weak cry, poor suck, seizures,
- Cyanosis, pallor, jaundice, mottled appearance, petechiae, purpura,
- Abdominal distension, feeding intolerance, emesis, diarrhea, bloody stools, hepatomegaly, and
- Oliguria.

Etiology

The most common causes of early-onset sepsis are Group B Streptococcus (GBS) and *Escherichia coli* (*E. coli*). In the National Institute of Child Health and Human Development (NICHD) Neonatal Network study of 396,586 neonates, those affected with GBS sepsis were mostly term (73%) infants and with *E. coli* sepsis mostly preterm (81%).[8] In this study, overall mortality was 16% of all infected infants, and it was the most frequent with *E. coli* sepsis (33%). Other, less-frequent, causes of EOS are *Listeria monocytogenes*, usually seen during listeriosis outbreaks,[12] and *Staphylococcus aureus*. A culture-independent, molecular-based study detected previously unrecognized, uncultivated, or difficult-to-cultivate species as causes of EOS.[13]

Prevention

Currently, the most important intervention in prevention of neonatal sepsis is the use of intrapartum antibiotic prophylaxis (IAP) in mothers with documented GBS colonization, GBS bacteriuria during the current pregnancy, or a previous birth of an infant with GBS disease. The 2010 revised GBS prevention guidelines of the Centers for Disease Control and Prevention (CDC) recommended chemoprophylaxis for women with risk factors at delivery who have unknown GBS colonization status at the time of labor onset, even with negative intrapartum screening cultures.[14] The use of IAP decreased the incidence of early-onset GBS by 80%, and it appeared to reduce the risk of early-onset *E. coli* infection in term infants as well.[15–19] However, if the mother received intrapartum antibiotics, it does not mean that the neonate cannot become infected and septic, as the 2011 NICHD study showed that in 53% of infants with EOS, mothers received intrapartum antibiotics within 72 hours prior to delivery (38% of infants with GBS, 79% with *E. coli* sepsis). Other interventions include prevention of preterm births, as well as early detection and treatment of urinary tract infection in mothers.

DIFFERENTIAL DIAGNOSIS

History, physical examination, laboratory evaluation, clinical course, microorganism cultures, or serology can distinguish bacterial neonatal sepsis from other diagnoses with similar clinical presentation.

Differential diagnosis includes:

1. Infections caused by organisms other then bacteria:
   - Viral infections: herpes simplex virus (HSV), cytomegalovirus (CMV), enteroviruses, and others,
   - Fungal infection: candidiasis, particularly in preterm neonates,
   - Parasitic infections: congenital toxoplasmosis,
   - Spirochetal infections: syphilis,
   - Nonbloodstream bacterial infections, including osteomyelitis, congenital pneumonia, septic arthritis, myositis, pericarditis, and urinary tract infection (frequently associated with congenital genitourinary tract malformation)
2. Neonatal asphyxia
3. Inborn errors of metabolism
4. Congenital heart disease, such as transposition of great vessels (TGV), total anomalous pulmonary venous return (TAPVR), pulmonary atresia (PA), hypoplastic left heart syndrome (HLHS), etc.
5. Neonatal respiratory distress: respiratory distress syndrome (RDS), especially in infants of diabetic mothers; transient tachypnea of the newborn (TTN); idiopathic persistent pulmonary hypertension of the newborn (PPHN); meconium aspiration syndrome (MAS); congenital diaphragmatic hernia (CDH); pulmonary hypoplasia; etc.
6. Necrotizing enterocolitis (NEC), malrotation with volvulus, bowel obstruction
7. Hemolytic disease of newborn

EVALUATION AND DIAGNOSTIC TESTS

The evaluation of the neonate includes a review of the pregnancy course, labor and delivery, maternal laboratory values, the use and timing of maternal IAP, determination of the risk factors for sepsis,[20] and a detailed physical examination. This includes overtly symptomatic septic infants who are admitted after delivery directly to the neonatal intensive care unit (NICU) because of the severity of their presentation, neonates with subtle signs and symptoms suggestive of infection, as well as initially well-appearing infants with identifiable risk factors. In a 2012 clinical report, the American Academy of Pediatrics (AAP) Committee on the Fetus and Newborn proposed a management approach for infants with suspected or proven EOS.[21]

The "gold standard" for diagnosis of neonatal sepsis is still a positive blood culture growing a pathogen. Currently, it may still take 24 hours or more for conventional culture to provide a result, and as many as 10% of neonates with sepsis can have false-negative cultures (for various reasons, the most frequent is an inadequate specimen). Therefore, a careful history and physical examination and use of clinical judgment in conjunction with currently available laboratory tests can identify neonates with likely sepsis for which empiric antibiotic treatment and close monitoring should be started in a timely fashion while waiting for the results of blood culture.

The criteria used in evaluation for sepsis should be broad, ensuring that all infected infants are identified and treated; however, a significant number of uninfected infants will end up being tested and treated.[22] Therefore, vigilance should be used by close follow-up of bacterial cultures and timely discontinuation of the antibiotics to avoid using antibiotics in well-appearing infants for extended periods of time.

Laboratory Evaluation

The laboratory evaluation includes bacterial cultures and polymerase chain reaction (PCR) tests of body fluids to determine the presence or absence of a pathogen, as well as other studies used to evaluate the likelihood of infection.

Blood Culture

The sensitivity of a blood culture is approximately 90%; the recommended volume obtained is a minimum of 1 mL. At least 1 culture should be obtained prior to initiating empirical antibiotic therapy. In a symptomatic infant who has a negative blood culture, however, if the clinical course and other tests are strongly suggestive of sepsis, a diagnosis of clinical sepsis can be made and the patient treated with a complete course of antibiotic therapy. With automated systems for continuous monitoring of blood cultures in most cases of neonatal sepsis, a blood culture will become positive within 24 to 36 hours.[23] In a study by Garcia-Prats et al, 97% and 99% of cultures were positive by 24 and 36 hours, respectively, if common bacterial pathogens were detected.[24]

Cerebrospinal Fluid Analysis and Culture

As clinical signs of meningitis and a positive blood culture can be absent in a neonate with meningitis,[25–27] the decision whether to perform a lumbar puncture (LP) for examination of cerebrospinal fluid (CSF) has to be made early in the evaluation and management course. The 2012 AAP report recommended that LP be performed for an infant with any of the following clinical conditions[20]:

- A positive blood culture,
- Clinical findings highly suggestive of sepsis,
- Laboratory data strongly suggestive of sepsis,
- Clinical status that is worsening on antibiotic therapy

Once obtained, CSF is sent for bacterial culture, Gram stain, cell count with differential, and protein and glucose concentrations. If in the differential diagnosis there is a possibility of viral or metabolic etiology, those studies should be sent as well.

If an infant has a severe clinical presentation and may have cardiovascular or respiratory compromise from the procedure, LP should be postponed until the patient's status has stabilized.

Tracheal Culture and Gram Stain

If tracheal aspirate is obtained immediately after endotracheal intubation, culture and Gram stain can identify the organisms present in amniotic fluid that are likely causes of the infection; however, these may only represent colonization.[28]

Urine Culture

Urine culture is not a part of the recommended EOS workup as a positive urine culture would likely represent seeding from the kidneys in bacteremia.[21]

Other Sites

In infants with early-onset infection, Gram stains of gastric aspirates and body surface (axilla, groin, and external ear canal) bacterial cultures are not routinely recommended.[21]

Complete Blood Cell Count

A complete blood cell count (CBC) is commonly used in the evaluation of infections and is usually obtained at 6–12 hours of age. Findings associated with sepsis are elevated white blood cell (WBC) count with a predominance of immature granulocytes (polymorphonuclear leukocytes [PMN]) or depressed WBC count with absolute neutropenia (<1500 PMN/μL). However, a normal WBC count is not infrequent

(it may be initially observed in as many as 50% of cases of culture-proven sepsis). Serial studies at 6-hour intervals may be more useful. Thrombocytopenia can also be observed, especially in association with septic shock.

Total Neutrophil Count

Factors affecting neutrophil count are gestational age (decrease with lower gestational age), type of delivery (lower in cesarean delivery), site of sampling (lower in arterial than in venous samples), maternal hypertension (neutropenia), altitude (higher at elevated altitudes), timing after delivery, periventricular or intraventricular hemorrhage, and severe birth asphyxia.

Ratio of Immature-to-Total Neutrophil Count

The immature-to-total neutrophil (I/T) ratio has a wide range of normal values, reducing its positive predictive value, especially in asymptomatic patients.[29] An elevated I/T ratio has a value in predicting likelihood of neonatal sepsis. For exclusion of sepsis, the maximum acceptable I/T ratio in the first 24 hours is 0.16. In most newborns, the ratio falls to 0.12 within 60 hours of birth. If the bone marrow is exhausted, band count can be low, and the ratio will be falsely low. The high negative predictive value (96%–100%) of the I/T ratio in combination with other tests or the presence of risk factors may be useful as an initial screen for neonatal sepsis.[30–33] The value of both absolute neutrophil count and I/T ratio is more in determining that an infant is not likely to be septic than diagnosing the infants with sepsis.

Two large multicenter studies have found that low WBC count (<5000/μL), absolute neutropenia (<1000 neutrophils/μL), relative neutropenia (<5000 neutrophils/μL), and an I/T ratio greater than 0.3 were associated with an increased probability of blood culture-proven, early-onset disease.[34,35]

C-Reactive Protein

C-reactive protein (CRP) is an acute-phase reactant that is increased in inflammatory conditions. It has limited ability to predict outcome or distinguish sepsis from other conditions, such as fetal distress, perinatal asphyxia, maternal fever, meconium aspiration, and intraventricular hemorrhage.[36] A CRP value greater than 1.0 mg/dL is 90% sensitive in detecting neonatal sepsis. Testing for CRP is not sensitive right at birth because it requires an inflammatory response to increase its level,[20] so a single CRP value soon after birth is not recommended. Monitoring serial CRP values is useful in supporting a diagnosis of sepsis, as neonatal bacterial sepsis is unlikely if the CRP level remains normal.[21] This test can also aid in evaluating the success of therapy. If elevated CRP levels decrease to less than

1.0 mg/dL 24 to 48 hours after the start of antibiotics, the neonate is probably not infected; however, if the CRP value is 1 mg/dL or greater, there is a high likelihood that the infant is septic, and the CRP value should not be used to guide the length of treatment.[37]

Cytokines

Although both pro- (interleukin [IL] 2, IL-6, interferon γ, and tumor necrosis factor α) and anti-inflammatory cytokines (IL-4 and IL-10) are increased in sepsis, because of insufficient sensitivity they are not routinely used in diagnostics of neonatal sepsis.[38]

Procalcitonin

The peptide precursor of calcitonin, procalcitonin, is released by parenchymal cells in response to bacterial toxins, and its serum levels are elevated in bacterial infections. It cannot be used as the only marker in sepsis and is not routinely available.[39]

MANAGEMENT

Management of sepsis includes antibiotics, as well as supportive therapy. Careful monitoring for early signs and symptoms of sepsis of asymptomatic newborns with risk factors for infection and full cardiopulmonary monitoring of symptomatic infants are crucial because the clinical condition can deteriorate rapidly.

The main goal of the therapy is to increase the delivery of substrates to meet tissue demand:

- Oxygen: Provide oxygen and, if respiratory distress is present, provide adequate support (from nasal cannula to endotracheal intubation and mechanical ventilation).
- Fluid: Initiate rapid fluid resuscitation with crystalloid or colloid parenteral solutions as needed to correct circulatory derangements. An adequate circulating blood volume is necessary to maintain right ventricular filling and cardiac output. However, repeated bolus administration of crystalloid and colloid solutions does not provide additional benefit. Underlying problems, such as peripheral vasodilation, have to be addressed.
- Correct metabolic abnormalities (hypoglycemia, hypocalcemia, etc). Management of fluid and electrolytes is extremely important. Metabolic acidosis and respiratory acidosis require timely correction.
- Initiate antibiotics as soon as possible, according to the most likely pathogens.
- Provide appropriate temperature control.
- Initiate inotropes as needed to maintain adequate blood pressure.
- Reverse abnormal blood clotting with transfusions and drugs.

- iNO (inhalation of nitric oxide): Use iNO in patients with severe hypoxic respiratory failure unable to maintain PaO_2 greater than 80 mm Hg despite maximal respiratory support or in ventilated patients with a significant (>50%) O_2 requirement and echocardiographic evidence of pulmonary artery pressures close to or above systemic pressure, especially if there is evidence of poor cardiac output (<150 mL/kg/min). The appropriate starting dose is 20 ppm.
- ECMO (extracorporeal membrane oxygenation) is used if other means of respiratory and cardiovascular support fail to be sufficient.

Antibiotic Therapy

In suspected sepsis, initial antibiotic therapy is empiric, covering the most likely pathogens, and needs to be initiated as soon as possible, preferably after the cultures have been obtained. Once a pathogen is identified, antibiotic therapy has to be adjusted based on the susceptibility of the organism. The duration of therapy depends on the organisms isolated and clinical course.

Recommended empiric antibiotics for the neonate with suspected EOS are ampicillin and gentamicin.[40] The NICHD Network study and other reports have shown the efficacy of this combination.[41,42] Our recommendation is to start meningitic doses of ampicillin if the suspicion for meningitis is strong enough that it warranted an LP for evaluation, even if the patient is not symptomatic. The same goes for the critically sick infant when LP was deferred. If treatment is continued longer than 48 hours, meningitis has been excluded, and clinical status is improving, ampicillin can be changed to a nonmeningitic dose.

An alternative regimen of ampicillin and a third-generation cephalosporin (eg, cefotaxime) is not more effective than the combination of ampicillin and gentamicin. Routine use of cefotaxime is not recommended due to the emergence of cephalosporin-resistant strains (eg, *Enterobacter cloacae*, *Klebsiella*, and *Serratia* species).[43] A large study found that in patients receiving ampicillin, the concurrent use of cefotaxime during the first 3 days after birth may be associated with an increased risk of death compared with the concurrent use of gentamicin.[44]

Specific Therapy

After the isolation of a pathogen and obtaining results for its antimicrobial susceptibility, antibiotics therapy has to be changed to specific therapy.

- Group B streptococcus: If GBS is the only identified organism, antibiotics can be changed to penicillin G alone because GBS is susceptible to penicillin.
- *Escherichia coli*: If *E. coli* is sensitive to ampicillin, the patient has improved clinically, and meningitis

was excluded, ampicillin alone can be continued for 10–14 days. In patients with ampicillin-resistant *E. coli*, therapy should be changed based on sensitivity and is likely to include an aminoglycoside, such as gentamicin, or cefotaxime. Meropenem is used for the treatment of systemic infections caused by extended-spectrum β-lactamase-producing organisms.

- Other gram-negative organisms: It is recommended that treatment includes both a β-lactam antimicrobial agent (eg, ampicillin or piperacillin-tazobactam) and an aminoglycoside for systemic infections.
- *Listeria monocytogenes*: In the initial therapy, a combination of ampicillin and gentamicin is more effective than ampicillin alone. Once the patient has clinically improved, a 10- to 14-day course can be completed with ampicillin alone.
- *Staphylococcus* species: The specific therapy for staphylococcal infection is determined by antibiotic sensitivity. For *S. aureus* infections, initial treatment should include both vancomycin and nafcillin until the susceptibility is available; therapy for methicillin-susceptible *S. aureus* should be completed with nafcillin. Coagulase-negative staphylococcal infection is treated with vancomycin.

Duration of Therapy

In neonates with culture-proven sepsis, the duration of therapy is generally 10 days. With appropriate management, symptomatic infants with proven sepsis clinically improve within 24 to 48 hours. The CBC differential and I/T ratio should begin to normalize by 72 hours.[45] Serum CRP initially rises within the first 24 to 48 hours and begins to decrease after 48 to 72 hours in responsive infants.[46] Blood culture needs to be repeated 24–48 hours after therapy was initiated. If the culture remains positive, this suggests inefficiency of the current antibiotic choice or the existence of another source of infection (osteomyelitis, septic arthritis, brain abscess, etc).

Because automated blood culture systems identify 97% of pathogens at 24 hours and 99% at 36 hours,[24] in well-appearing neonates with a negative culture empiric antibiotic therapy should be discontinued after 48 hours.[21]

If cultures are negative and the clinical condition remains concerning for a systemic infection, antibiotic therapy can be extended to complete a 10-day course of antibiotics unless another diagnosis explains the clinical findings.

Adjunctive Therapies

Routine use of adjunctive immunotherapeutics, such as white cell transfusions, intravenous immunoglobulin, granulocyte and granulocyte-macrophage colony-stimulating factors administration, and lactoferrin is not recommended; studies failed to show improved outcomes in neonatal sepsis.

OUTCOME AND FOLLOW-UP

Mortality from neonatal sepsis may be as high as 50% in nontreated infants. Overall mortality from GBS neonatal sepsis after the introduction of IAP and the routine use of empirical antibiotic therapy is 5%–10%. Increased mortality in early-onset GBS infection was found in infants with a birth weight less than 2500 g, absolute neutrophil count less than 1500 cells/mL, hypotension, apnea, and pleural effusion.[47] The mortality rate in neonates with early-onset *E. coli* sepsis is higher (up to 16%), especially if infected with an ampicillin-resistant organism or born prematurely.[48–50] Infection/inflammation in sepsis may have a negative impact on brain development in preterm neonates.[51,52] In a large study of over 6000 premature infants who weighed less than 1000 g at birth, neonatal infections were associated with poor neurodevelopmental and growth outcomes in early childhood.[53] Septic meningitis in neonates, including term infants, is associated with residual neurologic damage in 15%–30% of cases. Close follow-up for several years for neurodevelopmental assessment and, if needed, early intervention services and therapies are crucial for the achievement of the best possible outcome.

REFERENCES

1. Edwards MS, Baker CJ. Sepsis in the newborn. In: Gershon AA, Hotez PJ, Katz SL, eds. *Krugman's Infectious Diseases of Children.* 11th ed. Philadelphia, PA: Mosby; 2004:545.
2. Bizzarro MJ, Dembry LM, Baltimore RS, Gallagher PG. Changing patterns in neonatal *Escherichia coli* sepsis and ampicillin resistance in the era of intrapartum antibiotic prophylaxis. *Pediatrics.* 2008;121:689.
3. Committee on Infectious Disease, American Academy of Pediatrics. Group B streptococcal infections. In: Pickering LK, Baker CJ, eds. *Red Book: 2012 Report of the Committee on Infectious Diseases.* 29th ed. Elk Grove Village, IL: American Academy of Pediatrics; 2012:680.
4. Bailit JL, Gregory KD, Reddy UM, et al. Maternal and neonatal outcomes by labor onset type and gestational age. *Am J Obstet Gynecol.* 2010;202:245.e1.
5. Herbst A, Källén K. Time between membrane rupture and delivery and septicemia in term neonates. *Obstet Gynecol.* 2007;110:612.
6. Nizet V, Klein JO. Bacterial sepsis and meningitis. In: Remington JS, et al, eds. *Infectious Diseases of the Fetus and Newborn Infant.* 7th ed. Philadelphia, PA: Elsevier Saunders; 2010:222.
7. Phares CR, Lynfield R, Farley MM, et al. Epidemiology of invasive group B streptococcal disease in the United States, 1999–2005. *JAMA.* 2008;299:2056.
8. Stoll BJ, Hansen NI, Sánchez PJ, et al. Early onset neonatal sepsis: the burden of group B streptococcal and *E. coli* disease continues. *Pediatrics.* 2011;127:817.
9. Escobar GJ, Li DK, Armstrong MA, et al. Neonatal sepsis workups in infants ≥ 2000 grams at birth: a population-based study. *Pediatrics.* 2000;106:256.

10. Soman M, Green B, Daling J. Risk factors for early neonatal sepsis. *Am J Epidemiol*. 1985;121:712.

11. Osborn LM, Bolus R. Temperature and fever in the full-term newborn. *J Fam Pract*. 1985;20:261.

12. Gottlieb SL, Newbern EC, Griffin PM, et al. Multistate outbreak of Listeriosis linked to turkey deli meat and subsequent changes in US regulatory policy. *Clin Infect Dis*. 2006;42:29.

13. Wang X, Buhimschi CS, Temoin S, Bhandarani V, Han YW, Buhimschi IA. Comparative microbial analysis of paired amniotic fluid and cord blood from pregnancies complicated by preterm birth and early-onset neonatal sepsis. *PLoS One*. 2013;8(2):e56131.

14. Verani JR, McGee L, Schrag SJ; Division of Bacterial Diseases, National Center for Immunization and Respiratory Diseases, Centers for Disease Control and Prevention (CDC). Prevention of perinatal group B streptococcal disease: revised guidelines from CDC, 2010. *MMWR Recomm Rep*. 2010;59(RR-10):1–32.

15. Cohen-Wolkowiez M, Moran C, Benjamin DK, et al. Early and late onset sepsis in late preterm infants. *Pediatr Infect Dis J*. 2009;28:1052.

16. Bizzarro MJ, Raskind C, Baltimore RS, Gallagher PG. Seventy-five years of neonatal sepsis at Yale: 1928–2003. *Pediatrics*. 2005;116:595.

17. van den Hoogen A, Gerards LJ, Verboon-Maciolek MA, et al. Long-term trends in the epidemiology of neonatal sepsis and antibiotic susceptibility of causative agents. *Neonatology*. 2010;97:22.

18. Puopolo KM, Eichenwald EC. No change in the incidence of ampicillin-resistant, neonatal, early-onset sepsis over 18 years. *Pediatrics*. 2010;125:e1031.

19. Schrag SJ, Hadler JL, Arnold KE, et al. Risk factors for invasive, early-onset Escherichia coli infections in the era of widespread intrapartum antibiotic use. *Pediatrics*. 2006;118:570.

20. Puopolo KM, Draper D, Wi S, et al. Estimating the probability of neonatal early-onset infection on the basis of maternal risk factors. *Pediatrics*. 2011;128:e1155.

21. Polin RA, Committee on Fetus and Newborn. Management of neonates with suspected or proven early-onset bacterial sepsis. *Pediatrics*. 2012;129:1006.

22. Escobar GJ, Li DK, Armstrong MA, et al. Neonatal sepsis workups in infants ≥ 2000 grams at birth: a population-based study. *Pediatrics*. 2000;106:256.

23. Kurlat I, Stoll BJ, McGowan JE Jr. Time to positivity for detection of bacteremia in neonates. *J Clin Microbiol*. 1989;27:1068.

24. Garcia-Prats JA, Cooper TR, Schneider VF, et al. Rapid detection of microorganisms in blood cultures of newborn infants utilizing an automated blood culture system. *Pediatrics*. 2000;105:523.

25. Baker MD, Bell LM. Unpredictability of serious bacterial illness in febrile infants from birth to 1 month of age. *Arch Pediatr Adolesc Med*. 1999;153:508.

26. Stoll BJ, Hansen N, Fanaroff AA, et al. To tap or not to tap: high likelihood of meningitis without sepsis among very low birth weight infants. *Pediatrics*. 2004;113:1181.

27. Garges HP, Moody MA, Cotten CM, et al. Neonatal meningitis: what is the correlation among cerebrospinal fluid cultures, blood cultures, and cerebrospinal fluid parameters? *Pediatrics*. 2006;117:1094.

28. Sherman MP, Goetzman BW, Ahlfors CE, Wennberg RP. Tracheal aspiration and its clinical correlates in the diagnosis of congenital pneumonia. *Pediatrics*. 1980;65(2):258–263.

29. Jackson GL, Engle WD, Sendelbach DM, et al. Are complete blood cell counts useful in the evaluation of asymptomatic neonates exposed to suspected chorioamnionitis? *Pediatrics*. 2004;113:1173.

30. Cohen-Wolkowiez M, Benjamin DK Jr, Capparelli E. Immunotherapy in neonatal sepsis: advances in treatment and prophylaxis. *Curr Opin Pediatr*. 2009;21:177.

31. Gerdes JS. Diagnosis and management of bacterial infections in the neonate. *Pediatr Clin North Am*. 2004;51:939.

32. Russell GA, Smyth A, Cooke RW. Receiver operating characteristic curves for comparison of serial neutrophil band forms and C reactive protein in neonates at risk of infection. *Arch Dis Child*. 1992;67:808.

33. Murphy K, Weiner J. Use of leukocyte counts in evaluation of early-onset neonatal sepsis. *Pediatr Infect Dis J*. 2012;31:16.

34. Newman TB, Puopolo KM, Wi S, et al. Interpreting complete blood counts soon after birth in newborns at risk for sepsis. *Pediatrics*. 2010;126:903.

35. Hornik CP, Benjamin DK, Becker KC, et al. Use of the complete blood cell count in early-onset neonatal sepsis. *Pediatr Infect Dis J*. 2012;31:799.

36. Pourcyrous M, Bada HS, Korones SB, et al. Significance of serial C-reactive protein responses in neonatal infection and other disorders. *Pediatrics*. 1993;92:431.

37. Ehl S, Gering B, Bartmann P, et al. C-reactive protein is a useful marker for guiding duration of antibiotic therapy in suspected neonatal bacterial infection. *Pediatrics*. 1997;99:216.

38. Arnon S, Litmanovitz I. Diagnostic tests in neonatal sepsis. *Curr Opin Infect Dis*. 2008;21:223.

39. Maniaci V, Dauber A, Weiss S, et al. Procalcitonin in young febrile infants for the detection of serious bacterial infections. *Pediatrics*. 2008;122:701.

40. American Academy of Pediatrics. In: Pickering LK, Baker CJ, Kimberlin DW, Long SS, eds. *Red Book: 2009 Report of the Committee on Infectious Diseases*. 28th ed. Elk Grove Village, IL: American Academy of Pediatrics; 2009.

41. Maayan-Metzger A, Barzilai A, Keller N, Kuint J. Are the "good old" antibiotics still appropriate for early-onset neonatal sepsis? A 10 year survey. *Isr Med Assoc J*. 2009;11:138.

42. Muller-Pebody B, Johnson AP, Heath PT, et al. Empirical treatment of neonatal sepsis: are the current guidelines adequate? *Arch Dis Child Fetal Neonatal Ed*. 2011;96:F4.

43. Pickering LK, ed. *Red Book: 2009 Report of the Committee on Infectious Diseases*. Elk Grove Village, IL: American Academy of Pediatrics; 2009.

44. Clark RH, Bloom BT, Spitzer AR, Gerstmann DR. Empiric use of ampicillin and cefotaxime, compared with ampicillin and gentamicin, for neonates at risk for sepsis is associated with an increased risk of neonatal death. *Pediatrics*. 2006;117:67.

45. Gerdes JS. Diagnosis and management of bacterial infections in the neonate. *Pediatr Clin North Am*. 2004;51:939.

46. Pourcyrous M, Bada HS, Korones SB, et al. Significance of serial C-reactive protein responses in neonatal infection and other disorders. *Pediatrics*. 1993;92:431.

47. Payne NR, Burke BA, Day DL. Correlation of clinical and pathologic findings in early onset neonatal group B streptococcal infection with disease severity and prediction of outcome. *Pediatr Infect Dis*. 1998;7:836.

48. Alarcon A, Peña P, Salas S, et al. Neonatal early onset *Escherichia coli* sepsis: trends in incidence and antimicrobial resistance in the era of intrapartum antimicrobial prophylaxis. *Pediatr Infect Dis J*. 2004;23:295.

49. Schrag SJ, Hadler JL, Arnold KE, et al. Risk factors for invasive, early-onset *Escherichia coli* infections in the era of widespread intrapartum antibiotic use. *Pediatrics*. 2006;118:570.

50. Stoll BJ, Hansen NI, Sánchez PJ, et al. Early onset neonatal sepsis: the burden of group B streptococcal and *E. coli* disease continues. *Pediatrics* 2011;127:817.

51. Adams-Chapman I, Stoll BJ. Neonatal infection and long-term neurodevelopmental outcome in the preterm infant. *Curr Opin Infect Dis*. 2006;19(3):290–297.

52. Volpe JJ. Postnatal sepsis, necrotizing entercolitis, and the critical role of systemic inflammation in white matter injury in premature infants. *J Pediatr*. 2008;153(2):160–163.

53. Stoll BJ, Hansen NI, Adams-Chapman I, et al. Neurodevelopmental and growth impairment among extremely low-birth-weight infants with neonatal infection. *JAMA*. 2004;292(19):2357–2365.

53 Health Care-Associated Infections in the NICU

Vladana Milisavljevic

INTRODUCTION

Health care-associated infection (HCAI), also referred to as nosocomial or hospital-acquired infection, is an infection that a patient acquires and becomes evident 48 hours or more after admission to a hospital, it was not present or incubating at the time of admission to the hospital, and develops while the patient is receiving treatment of other conditions. These infections are associated with more serious illness, prolongation of stay in a health care facility, increased long-term disability, excess deaths, and high additional financial burden on health care and patients and their families.

The HCAIs commonly encountered in the neonatal intensive unit (NICU) are as follows:

1. Bloodstream infection (BSI), primarily catheter-associated bloodstream infection (CABSI), the most common HCAI in the NICU

2. Ventilator-associated pneumonia (VAP)

3. Catheter-associated urinary tract infection (CAUTI)

4. Surgical site infection (SSI)

5. Ventricular shunt-associated infection

EPIDEMIOLOGY

Incidence

According to the World Health Organization, the incidence rate of HCAIs in the United States is 4.5%; prevalence in the European countries is 7.1%; and in the low- and middle-income countries it varies from 5.7% to 19.1%. The overall annual direct medical costs of HCAI to US hospitals ranges from $28.4 to $45 billion, and the benefits of prevention range from $5.7 to $31.5 billion.[1] In 2002, the estimated number of HCAIs in US hospitals, adjusted to include federal facilities, was approximately 1.7 million, of that number, there were 33,269 among newborns in high-risk nurseries and 19,059 among newborns in well-baby nurseries; an estimated 98,987 deaths were associated with HCAIs.[2]

The Pediatric Prevention Network Study showed that of the 827 NICU patients surveyed, 11.4% had 116 hospital-acquired infections: 52.6% bloodstream, 12.9% lower respiratory tract, 8.6% ear-nose-throat, and 8.6% urinary tract infections (UTIs).[3] The National Healthcare Safety Network (NHSN) reported the highest incidence of device-associated infections (DAIs) was in neonates weighing 750 g or less.[4]

Hands are the most common vehicles to transmit health care-associated pathogens (Table 53-1). Transmission of pathogens from one patient to another via health care workers' hands requires 5 sequential steps:

1. Germs are present on the patient's skin and surfaces in the patient's surroundings.

2. By direct and indirect contact, the patient's germs contaminate health care workers' hands.

3. Germs survive and multiply on health care workers' hands.

4. Inadequate hand cleansing results in hands remaining contaminated.

759

Table 53-1 Modes of Transmission Within the Neonatal Intensive Care Unit

Mode of Transmission	Reservoir/Source	Transmission	Organism (Examples)
Direct contact	Patients, health care workers	Direct physical contact	CONS, *Staphylococcus aureus*, gram-negative organisms, viruses
Indirect contact	Medical devices, equipment (gloves, stethoscopes, soap dispensers, pumps)	Passive via an intermediate object	Gram-negative organisms, respiratory syncytial
Droplet	Patients, health care workers	Via large-particle droplets (>5 μm) transferring the germ through the air when the source and patient are close (sneezing, suctioning)	*Bordetella pertussis*, influenza virus, *Neisseria meningitidis*
Airborne	Patients, health care workers, dust	Germs contained within nuclei (<5 μm) evaporated from droplets or within dust particles, through air, within the same room or over a long distance (breathing)	*Mycobacterium tuberculosis, Legionella* spp.
Common vehicle	Food, water, or medication	Contaminated inanimate vehicle is a vector for transmission of the microbial agent to multiple patients (contaminated water, infusions, feedings)	Hepatitis B virus, gram-negative organisms, *Candida*

5. Microorganisms are cross transmitted between two patients via a health care worker's hands.

Risk factors for HCAI in the NICU are the following:

1. Patient-related factors contribute to neonatal susceptibility to bacterial infections:
   - Anatomically and biochemically immature, as well as frequently compromised, skin and mucous membranes
   - Reduced numbers or function of macrophages and dendritic cells in peripheral tissues (eg, lung)
   - Lower numbers of neutrophils in the bone marrow
   - Decreased immunoglobulin (Ig) G and complement levels, especially in premature neonates
   - Inability to respond to bacterial carbohydrate antigens
   - Nature of the illness requiring NICU admission

2. Use of indwelling medical devices during hospitalization:
   - Intravascular catheters (UAC [umbilical artery catheter], UVC [umbilical venous catheter], PICC [peripherally inserted central catheter], PIV [peripheral intravenous] catheter, PAL [peripheral arterial line] catheter)
   - Transmucosal medical devices (endotracheal tubes, oro-/nasogastric tubes, urinary catheters)
   - Ventricular shunts
   - Surgical drains, chest tubes

3. Use of medications, such as the following:
   - Broad-spectrum antibiotics: Antibiotics use modifies developing neonatal microflora. In addition, microorganisms have natural as well as acquired mechanisms of antibiotic resistance (eg, *Pseudomonas aeruginosa* efflux pumps pump antibiotics out, *S. marcescens amp C* gene can be induced by exposure to antibiotics), with the former representing microbial adaptation to antibiotics exposure. Judicious use, including narrowing antibiotic use after sensitivity is obtained, and timely discontinuation of antibiotics are essential.
   - Histamine$_2$-receptor antagonists.[5]

4. Total parenteral nutrition (TPN)[6]

5. Severity of underlying illness

6. Overcrowding and poor staffing ratio

PATHOGENESIS

Microorganisms causing HCAI can come from the patient's own microflora (eg, skin, nasopharynx, gastrointestinal or genitourinary tract) or from the environment/people in contact with the patient (family, visitors, health care workers). Most of the patients with bacterial or fungal HCAIs have indwelling medical devices used in their management (endotracheal tubes, intravascular lines, urinary catheters). In a study describing the epidemiology of 6290 nosocomial infections in pediatric intensive care units, BSIs, pneumonia, and UTIs were almost always associated with the use of an invasive device.[7]

Bloodstream Infections

Bloodstream infections are the most common HCAIs in the NICU. The highest rate of BSIs in the NICU is in the extremely low birth weight (ELBW) infants. However, even at a birth weight greater than 2.5 kg, BSI is still the most common infection. BSIs can be any of the following:

- Primary BSIs: These are the majority (64%) of all BSIs, primarily CABSIs. According to the Centers for Disease Control and Prevention (CDC) definitions, BSI can be
  - Laboratory-confirmed infection, or
  - Clinical sepsis (5% of BSIs). The CDC definition of clinical sepsis (introduced in 1986) was intended principally for infants because of its rarity in other patient groups.
- Secondary BSIs: These are related to infections at other sites (such as the urinary tract, lung, postoperative wounds, skin).

Catheter-Associated Bloodstream Infections

The majority of serious CABSIs are associated with central venous catheters (CVCs). CABSI is likely if a primary BSI develops in a patient who had a CVC within 48 hours before the development of the infection. If the time interval was longer than 48 hours since CVC placement, there must be compelling evidence that the infection was related to the vascular access device.

Potential routes for catheter contamination are the following:

1. Migration of skin organisms at the insertion site into the cutaneous catheter tract and along the surface of the catheter with colonization of the catheter tip;
2. Direct contamination of the catheter or catheter hub by contact with hands or contaminated fluids or devices;
3. Hematogenous seeding from another infection focus; or
4. Infusate contamination.

The major determinants of infection risk with intravenous catheters are:

1. Type of catheter
2. Location of catheter placement: Femoral catheterization was associated with increase in overall infection (20 vs 3.7 per 1000 catheter-days), clinical sepsis with or without documented BSI (4.5 vs 1.2/1000 catheter-days), and thrombotic complications.[8]

3. Duration of catheter placement: In one of the studies, the incidence rate of CABSIs increased by 14% per day during the first 18 days after PICC insertion; from days 36 through 60, the incidence rate again increased by 33% per day.[9]

Ventilator-Associated Pneumonia

Ventilator-associated pneumonia can be diagnosed in a patient who is on mechanical ventilation through an endotracheal or tracheostomy tube for at least 48 hours. Surveillance studies reported the incidence of pneumonia in the NICU was from 6.8% to 32.3% of HCAIs. The rate varied by birth weight category as well as by institution[10-13] due to the definition used, the people doing surveillance, and the frequency of surveillance. CDC definitions for VAP exist for infants less than 1 year of age, but there are no specific definitions for low or very low birth weight infants. Lower respiratory tract infections mostly occur by aspiration of bacteria that colonize the oropharynx or the upper gastrointestinal tract, which is facilitated by the presence of endotracheal tubes.[14-16] The aspiration can frequently be subclinical (microaspiration), and pepsin, a marker of aspiration, was detected in 91.4% of tracheal aspirates of preterm neonates.[17]

Biofilms

Biofilms have been found to be involved in a wide variety of microbial infections in the body. They are aggregates of microorganisms in which cells adhere to each other on a surface, frequently embedded within a self-produced matrix of extracellular polymeric substance. These formations of microbes lead to persistent infections resistant to conventional antimicrobial treatment and can be a major cause of treatment failure. In addition, antibiotic exposure can stimulate biofilm formation. According to the National Institutes of Health, up to 80% of human bacterial infections involve biofilm-associated microorganisms. HCAIs in the NICU in which biofilms have been implicated include catheter infections, UTI, endocarditis, and infections of permanent indwelling devices such as ventricular or cardiovascular shunts and grafts. Endotracheal tubes become coated with bacterial polysaccharide biofilms containing microbial flora, and during suctioning, these bacterial aggregates are dislodged and moved to the lower airways. Bacteria frequently involved in biofilm-associated infections include the gram-positive pathogens, such as *Staphylococcus epidermidis*, *Staphylococcus aureus*, and *Streptococcus* species, and gram-negative organisms, such as *P. aeruginosa* and Enterobacteriaceae (eg, *Escherichia coli*). Frequently, biofilm-associated infections are polymicrobial, with interaction between microbes increasing persistence.

Pathophysiology

Pathophysiology and clinical presentation of sepsis, a clinical syndrome complicating severe infection, is addressed in detail in chapter 52.

Etiology

Overall, the leading causes of HCAIs in the NICU are coagulase-negative staphylococci (CONS). In the first 30 days after birth, other frequent pathogens are *S. aureus*, Enterococcus species, and gram-negative enteric bacteria; after 30 days of age, fungi, especially *Candida* species and *Malassezia furfur*, are increasingly found.

The most frequent organisms causing BSIs in the NHSN study were CONS (28%), *S. aureus* (19%), and *Candida* species (13%).[10]

In a study looking at VAP in extremely preterm neonates in a NICU, most of the tracheal isolates grew polymicrobial cultures; the most commonly isolated organisms were *P. aeruginosa* (38.4%), *Enterobacter* spp. (38.4%), *S. aureus* (23%), and *Klebsiella* spp. (23%).[18] In the NHSN study, the most frequent pathogens in VAP were *Pseudomonas* species (16%), *S. aureus* (15%), and *Klebsiella* species (14%).[10]

The most frequent organisms causing UTIs are gram-negative enteric bacteria, and the leading pathogens are *E. coli*, *Candida albicans*, and *P. aeruginosa*.

Surgical site infections are most frequently caused by *S. aureus*, *P. aeruginosa*, and CONS.

The major problem is that up to 50%–60% of HCAIs are caused by multiresistant organisms. In the NHSN report, of 673 *S. aureus* isolates with susceptibility results, 33% were methicillin resistant; the incidence of methicillin-resistant *S. aureus* (MRSA) CABSIs has decreased in recent years, perhaps as a result of prevention efforts. Gram-negative organisms have significantly increased resistance to third-generation cephalosporins (eg, *Klebsiella pneumoniae* and *E. coli*), as well as imipenem and ceftazidine (*P. aeruginosa*). *Candida* spp. are found to be increasingly fluconazole resistant.

Prevention

The hospital-based programs of surveillance, prevention, and control can significantly reduce the rate of HCAIs.[19–21] In 2005, the NHSN succeeded and integrated previous surveillance systems at the CDC: National Nosocomial Infections Surveillance (NNIS), Dialysis Surveillance Network (DSN), and National Surveillance System for Healthcare Workers (NaSH). It is estimated that at least 50% of HCAIs could be prevented.

The single most effective measure to reduce HCAIs is hand hygiene.[22] Hand hygiene should be performed

Table 53-2 Prevention of Catheter-Associated Bloodstream Infections

The following are 5 evidence-based procedures strongly recommended by the Centers for Disease Control and Prevention for prevention of central catheter-associated blood stream infections (BSIs):

1. Hand washing
2. Full-barrier precautions during insertion of central venous catheters
3. Chlorhexidine for skin disinfection
4. Avoidance of the femoral insertion site
5. Removal of catheters when no longer indicated

with antimicrobial soap and water when hands are visibly dirty or soiled with blood and other body fluids; if not visibly soiled, alcohol-based hand rub may be used for routine decontamination of hands.

The following are 5 moments for hand hygiene (World Health Organization):

1. Before touching a patient;
2. Before a clean/aseptic procedure;
3. After body fluid exposure risk;
4. After touching a patient; and
5. After touching patient surroundings.

Validated and standardized prevention strategies have been shown to reduce HCAIs.[23,24] Prevention measures can be divided into the following:

1. General measures:
   - Surveillance
   - Standard precautions: hand hygiene, gloves, gowns, masks, and so on
   - Isolation precautions: contact, droplet, and airborne
2. Measures targeted against specific infections: BSIs (Table 53-2),[25] respiratory infections (Table 53-3),[26] UTIs, and so on.

Table 53-3 Prevention of Ventilator-Associated Pneumonia

1. Hand washing
2. Wearing gloves when suctioning
3. Avoiding intubation
4. Preventing accidental extubation
5. Aggressively weaning, discontinuation of mechanical ventilation as soon as possible
6. Limiting the amount of sedation
7. Limiting suctioning
8. Limiting exposure to resistant bacteria, isolating patients with resistant organisms
9. Elevating the head of the bed

3. Antibiotic control: Index of suspicion for HCAI should be high, ensuring that all infected neonates are recognized and treated; however, a significant number of uninfected infants end up being tested and treated. Therefore, vigilance should be used by close follow-up of bacterial cultures and timely adjustment and discontinuation of the antibiotics to avoid using antibiotics for extended periods of time.

Currently, no guidelines, definitions, or benchmark data exist for NICU patients with respect to CAUTIs.[27] Data on neonatal UTIs in general are limited and inconsistent.

The CDC recommendation for prevention of CAUTIs in hospitals in general include insertion of catheters only when appropriately indicated and leaving them in place only as long as needed, education of personnel in proper techniques of catheter insertion and care, and use of aseptic technique for catheter insertion and maintenance.[28]

DIFFERENTIAL DIAGNOSIS

Health care-associated infections can be distinguished from other diagnoses with similar clinical presentation based on history, physical examination, laboratory evaluation, clinical course, microbial cultures, or serology.

The differential diagnosis of HCAIs in the NICU includes the following:

- Late-onset sepsis caused by maternally transmitted organisms, such as late-onset group B streptococci (GBS) sepsis;
- Abdominal emergencies such as necrotizing enterocolitis (NEC), malrotation with volvulus, bowel obstruction, and the like; and
- Acute clinical deterioration that can be explained by the initial diagnosis (respiratory disease, cardiovascular disease, etc).

EVALUATION AND DIAGNOSTIC TESTS

The evaluation of the neonate for suspected HCAI includes a careful review of the clinical course, detailed physical examination, and determination of the patient's risk factors for infection. This includes overtly sick patients presenting with the septic picture, as well as neonates with subtle signs and symptoms suggestive of infection.

When culture results are interpreted, health care providers should remember that not all positive bacterial or fungal cultures are pathogenic, as they may represent microbial colonization, especially when respiratory cultures are interpreted. In the same time, growth of common commensal skin organisms (CONS, viridans streptococci, *Micrococcus*, *Corynebacterium*, *Propionibacterium*, and *Bacillus*) should not always be

treated as contamination, particularly in cultures of normally sterile body fluids (eg, blood, joint fluid, cerebrospinal fluid [CSF]), or in patients at high risk for infections (extremely premature neonates, the ones with intravascular catheters or ventricular shunts, etc). Repeat cultures may be necessary. Fungal growth on a blood culture should always be treated as a real infection.

Current CDC Definitions for Diagnosing Health Care-Associated Infections

Laboratory-Confirmed Central Line-Associated Bloodstream Infection[29]

A patient 1 year of age or younger has to have at least 1 of the following signs or symptoms (asterisks indicate with no other recognized cause):

Fever (>38°C core), hypothermia (<36°C core), apnea*, or bradycardia*,

and

Positive laboratory results not related to an infection at another site,

and

Recognized pathogen (eg, *E. coli*) growing from 1 or more blood culture,

or

Common skin commensal, such as CONS, including *S. epidermidis*), *Corynebacterium* spp. (not *C. diphtheriae*), *Bacillus* spp. (not *Bacillus anthracis*), *Propionibacterium* spp., viridans group streptococci, *Aerococcus* spp., *Micrococcus* spp. cultured from 2 or more blood cultures drawn on separate occasions; criterion elements must occur within a time frame that does not exceed a gap of 1 calendar day.

Blood Culture

Blood cultures should be sent from all the central lines that the patient has, as well as from peripheral blood (vein or artery), prior to initiating empirical antibiotic therapy. The recommended volume to obtain is a minimum of 1 mL for each culture. The sensitivity of a blood culture is approximately 90%. In a symptomatic infant who has a negative blood culture, however, with the clinical course and other tests strongly suggestive of sepsis, diagnosis of clinical sepsis can be made, and the patient should be treated with a complete course of antibiotic therapy. With automated systems for continuous monitoring of blood cultures in most cases of neonatal sepsis, a blood culture will become positive within 24 to 36 hours.[30]

Ventilator-Associated Pneumonia

Currently, there is a lack of a gold standard for the diagnosis of VAP in both adults and children, making comparison of the studies and their interpretation difficult.[31] The CDC/NHSN clinical criteria for the diagnosis of VAP are as follows[32]:

Two or more serial chest radiographs with at least 1 of the following:

- New or progressive and persistent infiltrate,
- Consolidation,
- Cavitation, or
- Pneumatoceles, in infants 1 year old or less.

Note: In patients without underlying pulmonary or cardiac disease (eg, respiratory distress syndrome, bronchopulmonary dysplasia, pulmonary edema, or chronic obstructive pulmonary disease), one definitive chest radiograph is acceptable.

There are alternate criteria for infants less than 1 year old: worsening gas exchange (eg, oxygen desaturations [pulse oximetry < 94%], increased oxygen requirements, or increased ventilator demand) *and* at least 3 of the following:

- Temperature instability;
- Leukopenia (<4000 WBC/mm³) or leukocytosis (≥15,000 WBC/mm³) and left shift (≥10% band forms);
- New onset of purulent sputum or change in character of sputum, increased respiratory secretions, or increased suctioning requirements;
- Apnea, tachypnea, nasal flaring with retraction of chest wall or grunting;
- Wheezing, rales, or rhonchi;
- Cough;
- Bradycardia (<100 beats/min) or tachycardia (>170 beats/min).

Tracheal aspirate culture and Gram stain may identify the organisms likely causing the infection; however, findings may represent just colonization, so correlation with the clinical picture and radiological findings has to be made. A Gram stain showing the presence of polymorphonuclear neutrophils, in addition to bacteria or fungi, suggests inflammation; however, it does not distinguish between pneumonia and tracheitis. A meta-analysis found that VAP is unlikely with a negative Gram stain; however, the positive predictive value of Gram stain was only 40%, concluding that a positive Gram stain should not be used to narrow anti-infective therapy until culture results become available.[33]

Catheter-Associated Urinary Tract Infection[34]

For CAUTI, the patient had to have an indwelling urinary catheter at the time of, or within 48 h before, onset of the event.

For a symptomatic UTI in a patient 1 year of age or younger, the guidelines are the following:

- At least 1 of the following signs or symptoms with no other recognized cause: fever (>38°C core), hypothermia (<36°C core), apnea, bradycardia, dysuria, lethargy, or vomiting;

and

- Positive urine culture of 10⁵ CFU/mL or greater with less than 2 species of microorganisms;

or

- At least 1 of the following: (1) positive dipstick for leukocyte esterase or nitrite; (2) pyuria (≥10 WBC/mm³ of unspun urine or ≥ 3 WBC/high-power field of spun urine); (3) microorganisms on Gram stain of unspun urine,

In addition to

- A positive urine culture of between 10³ or more and less than 10⁵ CFU/mL with 2 or fewer species of microorganisms;

Asymptomatic UTI in a patient 1 year of age or younger without signs or symptoms but with

- Positive urine culture of more than 10⁵ CFU/mL with 2 or fewer species of uropathogen microorganisms

and

- Positive blood culture with 1 or more matching the uropathogen to the urine culture or 2 or more matching blood cultures drawn on separate occasions if the matching pathogen is a common skin commensal.

Urine Culture

A catheterized specimen should be sent for urine culture as a part of the initial workup, as well as for urine analysis.

CSF Analysis and Culture

Initial workup of the patient who presents with signs and symptoms of infection may need to include CSF analysis, especially, but not exclusively, if the patient has a ventricular shunt. As clinical signs of meningitis and a positive blood culture can be absent in a neonate with meningitis,[35-37] the decision whether to perform a lumbar puncture (LP) or send shunt cultures has to be made prior to start of antibiotics. If a blood culture is positive, clinical findings or laboratory results are highly suggestive of sepsis, or clinical status is worsening on antibiotic therapy, an LP has to be done after the start of antibiotics. Once obtained, CSF is sent for bacterial culture, Gram stain, cell count with differential, and protein and glucose concentrations. If an infant may have cardiovascular or respiratory compromise from the procedure due to clinical status, the LP should be postponed until the patient's status has stabilized.

Other Laboratory Tests

Other laboratory tests, such as complete blood cell count (CBC) with manual differential, immature-to-total neutrophil count ratio (I/T ratio), C-reactive protein (CRP), procalcitonin, and so on and their interpretation are discussed in detail in chapters 64, 120, and 121.

MANAGEMENT

Medical management includes timely initiation of empiric broad-spectrum antimicrobials as well as supportive therapy. Full cardiopulmonary monitoring of symptomatic infants is crucial because the clinical condition can deteriorate rapidly.

Empiric broad-spectrum antimicrobials should cover against gram-positive and gram-negative bacteria, with the possible addition of antifungal therapy (if the patient has risk factors or clinical picture and laboratory finding suggestive of fungal infection). In addition, choice of initial antibiotics may be guided by the previous organisms isolated from the patient and the pattern of antibiotic resistance in the patient's NICU. Antibiotic coverage should consequently be adjusted according to susceptibility pattern of isolated organisms.

In neonates with culture-proven infection, the duration of antibiotic therapy varies, depending on source, isolated microorganism, clinical picture, or presence of complications (eg, endocarditis, meningitis, sepsis).

In CABSI, antibiotics should be continued for 7 days from the first negative blood culture. Antibiotics should be administered through a central catheter unless the catheter is removed. Catheter removal should be considered if it is no longer needed or the patient is critically ill, continues to have positive blood cultures, clinical status is not improving, and endocarditis or septic thrombophlebitis is present. In VAP, as clinical status is improving, the patient should be aggressively weaned, with the goal of extubation. In UTI, indwelling catheters should be removed if possible. In SSIs, a combination of surgical care (such as debridement) with antibiotic therapy is important.

More details on the antibiotic management and supportive care can be found in chapters 64, 120, and 121.

OUTCOME AND FOLLOW-UP

It was reported that very low birth weight neonates who developed late-onset sepsis had a significantly prolonged hospital stay (mean length of stay 79 vs 60 days) and were significantly more likely to die (18% vs 7%) than infected ones, especially in sepsis caused by gram-negative organisms (36%) or fungi (32%).[38]

Infection/inflammation in sepsis may have a negative impact on brain development in preterm neonates.[39,40] In neonates weighing less than 1000 g at birth, infections are associated with poor neurodevelopmental and growth outcomes in early childhood.[41] Septic meningitis in neonates, including term infants, is associated with residual neurologic damage in 15%–30% of cases. Close follow-up for several years for neurodevelopmental assessment and early intervention services and therapies as needed are crucial for the achievement of the best possible outcome.

REFERENCES

1. Scott RD. The direct medical costs of healthcare-associated infections in U.S. hospitals and the benefits of prevention. 2009. http://www.cdc.gov/hai/pdfs/hai/scott_costpaper.pdf. Updated November 2, 2011.
2. Klevens RM, Edwards JR, Richards, CL Jr, et al. Estimating health care-associated infections and deaths in U.S. hospitals, 2002. *Public Health Rep.* 2007;122:160–166.
3. Sohn AH, Garrett DO, Sinkowitz-Cochran RL, et al; Pediatric Prevention Network. Prevalence of nosocomial infections in neonatal intensive care unit patients: results from the first national point-prevalence survey. *J Pediatr.* 2001;139(6): 821–827.
4. Hocevar SN, Edwards JR, Horan TC, Morrell GC, Iwamoto M, Lessa FC. Device-associated infections among neonatal intensive care unit patients: incidence and associated pathogens reported to the National Healthcare Safety Network, 2006–2008. *Infect Control Hosp Epidemiol.* 2012;33(12):1200–1206.
5. Terrin G, Passariello A, De Curtis M, et al. Ranitidine is associated with infections, necrotizing enterocolitis, and fatal outcome in newborns. *Pediatrics.* 2012;129(1):e40–e45.
6. Perlman SE, Saiman L, Larson EL. Risk factors for late-onset health care-associated bloodstream infections in patients in neonatal intensive care units. *Am J Infect Control.* 2007;35:177–182.
7. Richards MJ, Edwards JR, Culver DH, Gaynes RP. Nosocomial infections in pediatric intensive care units in the United States. National Nosocomial Infections Surveillance System. *Pediatrics.* 1999;103(4):e39.
8. Merrer J, De Jonghe B, Golliot F, et al. Complications of femoral and subclavian venous catheterization in critically ill patients: a randomized controlled trial. *JAMA.* 2001;286(6):700–707.
9. Sengupta A, Lehmann C, Diener-West M, Perl TM, Milstone AM. Catheter duration and risk of CLA-BSI in neonates with PICCs. *Pediatrics.* 2010;125:648–653.
10. Edwards JR, Peterson KD, Mu Y, et al. National Healthcare Safety Network (NHSN) report: data summary for 2006 through 2008, issued December 2009. *Am J Infect Control.* 2009;37(10):783–805.
11. Drews MB, Ludwig AC, Leititis JU, Daschner FD. Low birth weight and nosocomial infection of neonates in a neonatal intensive care unit. *J Hosp Infect.* 1995;30:65–72.
12. Ford-Jones EL, Mindorff CM, Langley JM, et al. Epidemiologic study of 4684 hospital-acquired infections in pediatric patients. *Pediatr Infect Dis J.* 1989;8:668–675.
13. Hemming VG, Overall JC Jr, Britt MR. Nosocomial infections in a newborn intensive-care unit. Results of forty-one months of surveillance. *N Engl J Med.* 1976;294:1310–1316.
14. Polin RA, Denson S, Brady MT; Committee on Fetus and Newborn; Committee on Infectious Diseases. Epidemiology

CHAPTER 53

and diagnosis of health care-associated infections in the NICU. *Pediatrics.* 2012;129(4):e1104–e1109.

15. Goodwin SR, Graves SA, Haberkern CM. Aspiration in intubated premature infants. *Pediatrics.* 1985;75(1):85–88.

16. Hopper AO, Kwong LK, Stevenson DK, et al. Detection of gastric contents in tracheal fluid of infants by lactose assay. *J Pediatr.* 1983;102(3):415–418.

17. Farhath S, He Z, Nakhla T, et al. Pepsin, a marker of gastric contents, is increased in tracheal aspirates from preterm infants who develop bronchopulmonary dysplasia. *Pediatrics.* 2008;121(2):e253–e259.

18. Apisarnthanarak A, Holzmann-Pazgal G, Hamvas A, Olsen MA, Fraser VJ. Ventilator-associated pneumonia in extremely preterm neonates in a neonatal intensive care unit: characteristics, risk factors, and outcomes. *Pediatrics.* 2003;112:1283.

19. Hughes JM. Study on the efficacy of nosocomial infection control (SENIC Project): results and implications for the future. *Chemotherapy.* 1988;34(6):553–561.

20. Vital Signs: Central line-associated blood stream infections—United States, 2001, 2008, and 2009. *MMWR Morb Mortal Wkly Rep.* 2011;60(8):243–248.

21. Schulman J, Stricof R, Stevens TP, et al. Statewide NICU central-line-associated bloodstream infection rates decline after bundles and checklists. *Pediatrics.* 2011;127(3):436–444.

22. Larson E. Skin hygiene and infection prevention: more of the same or different approaches? *Clin Infect Dis.* 1999;29(5):1287–1294.

23. Payne NR, Finkelstein MJ, Liu M, Kaempf JW, Sharek PJ, Olsen S. NICU practices and outcomes associated with 9 years of quality improvement collaboratives. *Pediatrics.* 2010;125(3):437–446.

24. Bizzarro MJ, Sabo B, Noonan M, Bonfiglio MP, Northrup V, Diefenbach K; Central Venous Catheter Initiative Committee. A quality improvement initiative to reduce central line-associated bloodstream infections in a neonatal intensive care unit. *Infect Control Hosp Epidemiol.* 2010;31(3):241–248.

25. O'Grady NP, Alexander M, Dellinger EP, et al. Healthcare Infection Control Practices Advisory Committee. Guidelines for the prevention of intravascular catheter–related infections. *Infect Control Hosp Epidemiol.* 2002;23:759–769.

26. Garland JS. Strategies to prevent ventilator-associated pneumonia in neonates. *Clin Perinatol.* 2010;37(3):629–643.

27. Bizzaro MJ. Health care-associated infections in the neonatal intensive care unit: barriers to continued success. *Semin Perinatol.* 2012;36(6):437–444.

28. Gould CV, Umscheid CA, Agarwal RK, et al. Guideline for prevention of catheter-associated urinary tract infections 2009. CDC.

http://www.cdc.gov/hicpac/pdf/CAUTI/CAUTIguideline2009 final.pdf.

29. Horan TC, Andrus M, Dudeck MA, et al. CDC/NHSN surveillance definition of health care-associated infection and criteria for specific types of infections in the acute care setting. *Am J Infect Control.* 2008;36:309–332.

30. Kurlat I, Stoll BJ, McGowan JE Jr. Time to positivity for detection of bacteremia in neonates. *J Clin Microbiol.* 1989;27:1068.

31. Foglia E, Meier MD, Elward A. Ventilator-associated pneumonia in neonatal and pediatric intensive care unit patients. *Clin Microbiol Rev.* 2007;20(3):409–425.

32. CDC/NHSN surveillance definition of healthcare-associated infection and criteria for specific types of infections in the acute care setting, January 2013.

33. O'Horo JC, Thompson D, Safdar N. Is the Gram stain useful in the microbiologic diagnosis of VAP? A meta-analysis. *Clin Infect Dis.* 2012;55(4):551–561.

34. Centers for Disease Control and Prevention Device associated module catheter associated urinary tract infection event 7.1–7.13, January 2012.

35. Baker MD, Bell LM. Unpredictability of serious bacterial illness in febrile infants from birth to 1 month of age. *Arch Pediatr Adolesc Med.* 1999;153:508.

36. Stoll BJ, Hansen N, Fanaroff AA, et al. To tap or not to tap: high likelihood of meningitis without sepsis among very low birth weight infants. *Pediatrics.* 2004;113:1181.

37. Garges HP, Moody MA, Cotten CM, et al. Neonatal meningitis: what is the correlation among cerebrospinal fluid cultures, blood cultures, and cerebrospinal fluid parameters? *Pediatrics.* 2006;117:1094.

38. Stoll BJ, Hansen N, Fanaroff AA, et al. Late-onset sepsis in very low birth weight neonates: the experience of the NICHD Neonatal Research Network. *Pediatrics.* 2002;110(2 Pt 1):285–291.

39. Adams-Chapman I, Stoll BJ. Neonatal infection and long-term neurodevelopmental outcome in the preterm infant. *Curr Opin Infect Dis.* 2006;19(3):290–297.

40. Volpe JJ. Postnatal sepsis, necrotizing enterocolitis, and the critical role of systemic inflammation in white matter injury in premature infants. *J Pediatr.* 2008;153(2):160–163.

41. Stoll BJ, Hansen NI, Adams-Chapman I, et al. Neurodevelopmental and growth impairment among extremely low-birth-weight infants with neonatal infection. *JAMA.* 2004;292(19):2357–2365.

Congenital and Perinatal Human Cytomegalovirus Infections

Masako Shimamura and William J. Britt

EPIDEMIOLOGY OF CONGENITAL HUMAN CYTOMEGALOVIRUS INFECTIONS

Introduction

The natural history of congenital human cytomegalovirus (HCMV) infection has been studied exhaustively for nearly 4 decades, yet critical features of this intrauterine infection continue to be redefined as contemporary methodologies are employed to further investigate the biology of the virus and the disease. Perhaps this is most strikingly illustrated by the surprising findings that have been obtained from the application of next-generation nucleic acid sequence technologies to studies of the genetic diversity of viruses isolated from infants with congenital infections.[1] These studies have confirmed earlier studies that utilized comparatively crude methodologies to define genetic variation among viruses isolated from infants with congenital HCMV infections as well from viruses isolated from different sites in a single infant.[2–6]

Together, these studies have documented that individuals, including fetuses infected in utero, are not infected with a single strain of virus but a collection of genetically distinct viruses that in some cases approaches the genetic sequence diversity that closely resembles that found in RNA viruses.[1] These findings coupled with a more complete understanding of the limited protection afforded by preexisting maternal immunity prior to conception in the prevention of superinfection/reinfection during pregnancy have challenged many long-held concepts of the natural history of congenital HCMV infections and argued that the natural history of this congenital infection must in some populations be redefined.

Case Definition and Incidence

The case definition of congenital HCMV infection that has been used in most large natural history studies of this infection has remained unchanged for decades and requires the isolation of replicating HCMV from the urine of an infant within the first 2 weeks of life.[7] Since the early 2000s, the widespread use of polymerase chain reaction (PCR) in diagnostic laboratories has resulted in the increasing utilization of this technology in the diagnosis of congenital HCMV infections. Although PCR detection of HCMV is viewed by most investigators as equivalent to isolation of replicating virus, the possibility of false positives must be considered when samples such as saliva from breast-feeding infants are assayed. Positive PCR reactions in such cases can be confirmed by tissue culture isolation of virus from the urine of the infant or, alternatively, PCR analysis of urine from the infant.[7] Using either tissue culture isolation of HCMV or PCR detection, investigators have reported that HCMV is the most common virus infection in the newborn infant that is acquired in utero, with reported rates between 0.5% and 2.0% in different populations throughout the world[8] (Table 54-1). A large screening study of approximately 100,000 newborn infants in the United States that is nearing completion has reported that congenital HCMV infection occurs in about 0.5% of live births[7] (Table 54-1).

Table 54-1 Incidence of Congenital Human Cytomegalovirus Infection in Different Geographic Locations

Location	Incidence (per 1000)	Maternal Seroprevalence (%)	Reference
United States	5	60	7
Brazil	11	>96	19
India	21	>99	20
Ivory Coast	14	100	18
Gambia	39	100	300
United Kingdom	3	56	301
Israel	6	82	332
Denmark	4	52	302
Korea	12	96	303

Previous studies from several institutions in the United States have reported rates of about 1%, primarily in urban, lower-socioeconomic populations.[9] These rates are considerably higher than the rate of congenital HCMV infection in white middle- and upper-middle-class populations, a finding that suggests differences in both the risk of maternal infection and the nature of the maternal infection in women of different racial and socioeconomic groups.[9–13] Congenital HCMV infections are common throughout most areas of the world, with rates between 1% and 5%, depending on the region of the world and the case definition of congenital HCMV infection[8] (Table 54-1). However, in studies carried out using methodologies and case definitions consistent with currently accepted definitions, the rate of congenital HCMV infections in most populations appears to be approximately 1%.

A unique and incompletely understood feature of congenital HCMV infection is that it can occur in infants born to women who experienced a HCMV infection prior to pregnancy and have developed lasting serological immunity to the virus to HCMV, a characteristic that distinguishes congenital HCMV infections from other congenital infections, such as rubella and toxoplasmosis, but parallels the natural history of congenital syphilis.[14,15] In fact, there is nearly a linear relationship between the rate of maternal HCMV seroprevalence and the rate of congenital HCMV infections, such that the highest rates of congenital HCMV infection can be found in maternal populations with near-universal HCMV seroreactivity.[16] This finding is of great interest because maternal populations in most regions of the world, particularly the Southern Hemisphere, have very high rates of seroreactivity for HCMV, which in many populations approach 100%.[17–21] These observations clearly demonstrate that existing maternal immunity does not prevent intrauterine HCMV infection and raises several issues that must be

considered in the design and testing of vaccines that have been formulated for the prevention of congenital HCMV infections.

Clinical Features and Classification of Infection

The overwhelming majority of infants (90%) with congenital HCMV infections will exhibit no abnormal clinical findings in the perinatal period and will not be identified unless a newborn screening program is in place. These infants have been defined as asymptomatically infected for purposes of epidemiological studies. This classification also carries prognostic information because this population of infected infants has a lower overall incidence of neurologic sequelae associated with this intrauterine infection.[11,22] The remaining 10% of infants with congenital HCMV infections will exhibit symptoms characteristic of perinatal infections but not diagnostic of congenital HCMV infection. These infants have been classified as symptomatically infected and have an increased risk of long-term sequelae.[23,24] Physical findings can include hepatosplenomegaly; jaundice; microcephaly; petechial rashes; in rare cases cutaneous extramedullary hematopoiesis (blueberry muffin rash); neurological deficits, including seizures; and chorioretinitis[23–25] (Table 54-2). Laboratory and imaging findings can include thrombocytopenia, direct hyperbilirubinemia with evidence of hepatitis, and abnormal findings in imaging studies of the brain of infected infants[22,23] (Table 54-2).

It is important to note that the initial case definitions of congenital CMV infection were based on clinical findings with additional laboratory studies prompted by clinical findings of petechiae and jaundice. Studies, including central nervous system (CNS) imaging, were not routinely carried out. Thus, more

Table 54-2 Findings in Infants With Symptomatic Congenital Human Cytomegalovirus Infection

Finding	Frequency of Finding	Respective Reference
Hepatosplenomegaly	60% (63/105)	304
Petechiae	76% (80/106); 75.6% (31/42); 38.7% (24/62)	24, 298, 304
Jaundice	67% (69/103); 41.5% (17/42)	24, 304
Microcephaly	53% (54/102); 19.5% (8/42); 22.6% (14/62)	24, 298, 304
Seizures	7% (7/105); 12.9% (8/62); 7.3% (3/42)	24, 298, 304
Chorioretinitis	13% (7/56); 10% (6/62) raw; 17% (7/42); 22% (20/91)	24, 304, 305
Hearing loss	40% (85/209)	36
Imaging abnormalities[a]	70% (39/56); 78% (32/42)	24, 245
Intrauterine growth restriction[a]	50% (56/106); 29% (18/62); 26.8% (17/42)	24, 298, 304

[a] Intracranial calcifications, white matter abnormalities, ventricular dilatation, cortical atrophy.

recent reports that include patients identified by studies other than clinical examination may not be completely comparable to the findings reported in the older literature. Severe infections have a mortality rate of 5%–11%, and long-term neurologic sequelae are frequent in infants with severe infections, reportedly occurring in up to 60% of symptomatically infected infants.[23–27] Long-term sequelae are almost exclusively limited to the CNS, although poorly documented anecdotal reports of chronic liver disease were discussed in several reviews.

Several laboratory parameters have been identified that can further quantify the likelihood of long-term neurologic sequelae in a congenitally CMV-infected infant. Perhaps the most predictive of these but least well studied is the finding of encephalitis as defined by abnormalities in the cerebrospinal fluid (CSF) of infected infants.[23,24,28,29] Similarly, imaging (ultrasound, computed tomography [CT], magnetic resonance imaging [MRI]) abnormalities of the CNS of infected infants, such as intracranial calcifications, including periventricular calcifications; evidence of migration deficits leading to lissencephaly and polymicrogyria; cerebellar hypoplasia; and white matter abnormalities all point to CNS involvement and a substantially increased risk of long-term neurologic deficits in the infected infant. These are discussed in the following sections.

The finding of chorioretinitis has been associated with an increased rate of neurodevelopmental abnormalities in infected infants and likely also reflects the involvement of the CNS in this infection.[24,30] Attempts to utilize viral load measurements to identify infants at risk for neurodevelopmental sequelae, including hearing loss, have been disappointing when studied in screened populations of newborn infants primarily because of considerable variation in viral loads among individual infants.[31–33] Overall, infants with symptomatic infections, particularly those with

hepatosplenomegaly and thrombocytopenia, have increased levels of viral DNA in blood, urine, and other body fluids when compared to infants with asymptomatic infections, but these findings have not significantly refined the predictive value of the clinical findings in the individual patient.[31,32] As an example, when blood viral load was investigated as a potential approach for early identification of infected infants with hearing loss, it appeared to lack sufficient positive predictive value for routine use in a screening program.[33] Its negative predictive value was considered sufficient by some investigators, although many investigators believe such use in early infancy is unwarranted because up to 50% of congenitally infected infants with hearing loss will not exhibit evidence of hearing loss until after 6 months of age.[34–38]

Importance of Maternal Immunity in Transmission of CMV to the Fetus

Early studies of congenital HCMV infection reported that maternal immunity to HCMV played a critical role in limiting virus transmission to the fetus as well as in dramatically reducing severity of the ensuing intrauterine infection.[11] Thus, maternal immunity to HCMV prior to pregnancy is widely believed to be a major determinant in decreasing the risk of transmission of virus to the fetus as well as decreasing the likelihood of a severe fetal infection in pregnant women infected with CMV. This concept remains a useful paradigm, but in the face of newer findings of reinfection of previously immune women with new strains of virus and the occurrence of symptomatic congenitally infected infants born to previously CMV-immune women, it cannot be viewed with the same level of certainty as in the past.

Maternal HCMV infections during pregnancy that occur in women without preconceptional seroimmunity to HCMV are classified as primary maternal

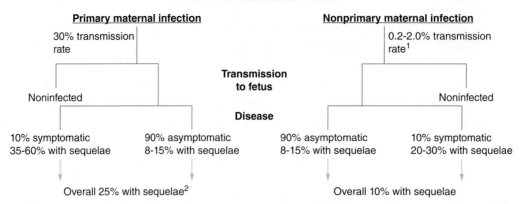

FIGURE 54-1 Natural history of congenital human cytomegalovirus (HCMV) infections in women without preconceptional serological immunity (primary) and those with preconceptional immunity and prior infection with HCMV (nonprimary). Intrauterine transmission rates and rates of disease and long-term sequelae are provided. [1]Rate of transmission following nonprimary maternal infection is unknown but estimated from rates of congenital HCMV infections in immune maternal populations. This rate likely underestimates the true rate of transmission following maternal nonprimary infection. [2]Rate of sequelae based on population of infants from screened cohort and referral population. As a result, the rate and severity of sequelae could represent an overestimate of true incidence.

infection, whereas those infections that occur during pregnancy in women with preconceptional immunity to HCMV are classified as nonprimary infections (Figure 54-1). Intrauterine transmission to the developing fetus occurs in about 30% of women undergoing primary infection during pregnancy as compared to somewhere between 1% and 2% of offspring born to women with nonprimary infection (Figure 54-1).[11,19,26] However, it is important to note that the true rate of transmission in women undergoing nonprimary infection is unknown because it is unclear if all women with preconceptional seroimmunity to HCMV have the same risk (or mechanism) for transmission to their fetus or a similar rate of reinfection following exposure to a new strain of virus (see next section). Importantly, in most natural history studies, the ratio of congenital HCMV-infected infants born following nonprimary maternal infection as compared to primary maternal infection is at least 4:1 in many populations and likely higher in others, indicating that the congenitally infected infants delivered to women undergoing nonprimary infections represent the vast majority of infants with congenital HCMV infection.[11,26] Thus, even if the incidence of symptomatic disease and long-term sequelae are less in infected infants following a nonprimary maternal infection as compared to that seen in infected offspring of mothers undergoing primary infection during pregnancy, infants infected following nonprimary maternal infection represent the major contributor to the disease burden associated with congenital HCMV infections.[26]

Several studies have demonstrated that primary maternal infections that occur during the late first and early second trimester are more commonly associated with more severe manifestations in the infected newborn than those that occur in the third trimester, a finding consistent with the developmental status of the fetus at these different gestational ages.[39–45] From studies of women undergoing primary infection, it also appears that the rate of transmission increases in the third trimester and occurs about twice as frequently as transmission in early gestation, a finding that parallels findings from studies of congenital toxoplasmosis, rubella, and syphilis.[39,46,47]

A caveat from these studies of congenital HCMV infections is that in most cases, the conclusions from these studies have been based on the gestational age of the fetus at the time of maternal seroconversion and not actual determination of intrauterine transmission in women undergoing seroconversion. Thus, it remains a possibility that the risk of intrauterine transmission (and disease) is related to the duration of exposure of the fetus to maternal infection and perhaps less of a function of a limited interval during the primary maternal infection. Such a distinction could be critical in intervention strategies, such as the use of passively transferred virus-neutralizing antibodies.

The virologic characteristics of primary maternal infection and virus transmission to the fetus have been detailed in a limited number of publications, whereas similar studies have not been accomplished in women with nonprimary infections during pregnancy. In women undergoing primary infection, the level of virus replication as measured by PCR analysis of the amount of viral DNA in peripheral blood failed to correlate with intrauterine transmission.[42,43] Using maternal anti-HCMV antibody responses as indirect evidence of the level of virus replication, Alford et al. suggested that increased virus replication was associated with virus transmission.[48] The limitations of this study, including the assumption that antibody responses in these women was a surrogate of virus replication, are readily apparent but do suggest that the virologic or immunologic characteristics of a maternal infection could influence the likelihood of transmission.

Finally, studies have demonstrated that women who deliver congenitally infected infants more commonly excrete virus in the postpartum period when compared to women who do not deliver an infected infant, regardless of the type of maternal HCMV infection.[49] Sites of virus excretion include urine, cervical secretions, saliva, and breast milk.[49,50]

These results do not speak to a specific relationship between virus replication and intrauterine transmission of HCMV in some women but suggest the possibility that intrauterine transmission of HCMV could include the altered capacity of a subpopulation of women to control virus replication and dissemination. The variations in host-derived responses to HCMV in normal pregnant women as an explanation for differing rates of intrauterine transmission and the severity of the ensuing fetal infections have not been rigorously investigated.

Importance of Maternal Immunity and the Outcome of Fetal HCMV Infection

Studies of primary maternal CMV infections linked to congenital HCMV infections have failed to identify specific immunologic features of the maternal infection that could be directly related to intrauterine transmission of the virus. Studies in women undergoing primary infection during pregnancy failed to find a correlation between anti-HCMV CD4+ and CD8+ T-lymphocyte responses and virus transmission to the developing fetus.[51] Studies that quantified maternal anti-HCMV antibody responses in relation to virus transmission to the fetus have demonstrated that women who transmit virus to their fetus often have higher levels of antiviral antibodies as compared to women who fail to transmit virus.[52] When these studies quantified virus-neutralizing antibodies, a biologically more relevant antibody response, a correlation was found between the level of virus-neutralizing antibodies and protection from intrauterine transmission.[52] Interestingly, this specific response was also directly correlated with the avidity of the antibodies reactive with the virus and a major viral envelope glycoprotein, gB, in that women with primary infection that failed to transmit virus to their offspring had, as a group, higher avidity antibodies.[52]

Finally, it is of interest to note that women in this study who transmitted virus to their offspring as a group had lower avidity antibodies and in some cases

did not exhibit the expected avidity maturation with time that was observed in women who did not transmit virus to their offspring.[52] This finding suggested a potential deficit in a maternal immune response associated with intrauterine transmission of HCMV.[52] However, it is important to note that these older studies were done using only a single envelope protein, glycoprotein B (gB), and thus must be viewed as incomplete because of the more contemporary understanding of the importance of antibodies reactive with the HCMV pentameric gH/gL/Ul128–131 glycoprotein complex, a glycoprotein complex that determines epithelial cell tropism and one that is likely critical for the in vivo cellular tropism of HCMV.

The presence of preexisting maternal immunity has also been argued to be a major factor in the outcome of intrauterine HCMV infections.[8,11,26,53,54] Early studies of congenital HCMV infections strongly supported an association between primary maternal infections and severe, clinically apparent congenital HCMV infections.[11] This dogma continues and is firmly established in the literature even though early studies from Sweden and, more recently, studies from the United States, Sweden, and Brazil have demonstrated that the incidence of severe, clinically apparent newborn infections is similar between congenitally infected offspring of primary and nonprimary maternal infections.[19,55-58] Some investigators have argued the most severely affected congenitally infected infants only result from intrauterine infection following a primary maternal infection and that infants with less-severe neurodevelopmental consequences of this intrauterine infection are more likely born to women with nonprimary infections.[54,59,60] This difference in the views of investigators and findings that described severe infections with neurodevelopmental sequelae in infants born to women with nonprimary HCMV infections cannot be ascribed to misidentification of cases because in most reports these infected infants were identified by clinical findings that were consistent with standard case definitions.

Although this important aspect of the epidemiology of congenital HCMV infection continues to be contentious, ongoing screening studies that will enroll large numbers of infected infants should resolve this issue. It is also worth noting that in at least 1 of the larger series of patients in which the association between significant neurological damage with long-term sequelae and primary maternal infection was described contained a potential enrollment bias secondary to inclusion of infants from nonscreened populations who were identified secondary to clinically apparent infections at nonscreening sites. More thorough review of the original findings in this often-referenced study has raised the possibility that little difference in terms of neurodevelopmental sequelae exists between infants infected following primary and nonprimary maternal infections (S. Ross, 2012). Finally, in recent newborn screening studies of infants born to maternal populations with near-universal seroimmunity to HCMV prior to pregnancy, the rates of clinically apparent congenital infections and long-term sequelae, including hearing loss, appears similar to the rates reported in infants infected in utero following primary maternal infection.[19,58]

Maternal Infection and Congenital HCMV Infections: Sources of Maternal Infection

Human cytomegalovirus establishes a persistent infection in its host that is characterized by both reservoirs of latently infected CD34[+] myeloid cells and a chronic productive infection in a number of different tissues (see following sections). During primary infection, infectious virus can be isolated from a number of sites, including the oropharynx, genital tract, urine, and blood. Virus excretion is prolonged in most acutely infected adults, and depending on the frequency and site of sampling, infectious virus can be recovered for months. In congenitally infected infants and in infants infected perinatally either during delivery or following exposure to infected breast milk, significant amounts of virus (10^{2-3} infectious units/mL) can be detected in the urine and saliva for years.[61-63] Thus, infants infected in utero and in the perinatal period represent an important reservoir of infectious virus that can serve to infect parents and other caretakers of HCMV-infected infants as well as other children, such as children in group care settings. CMV is readily transmitted during close and intimate contact and is considered a sexually transmitted infection (STI) (Table 54-3).

Epidemiological studies have consistently identified 2 sources of HCMV infection in pregnant women. Exposure to young children is thought to represent perhaps the most consistent risk factor for acquisition of HCMV that has been identified through epidemiological

Table 54-3 Sources of Human Cytomegalovirus Infections

Source	Mode
Transplacental	Hematogenous
Saliva	Mucosal exposure
Urine	Mucosal exposure
Genital secretions	Mucosal exposure
Breast milk	Mucosal exposure
Blood products	Hematogenous
Transplanted organ	Hematogenous; graft

studies of community-acquired HCMV infections.[64-68] Contact with young children in the home has been shown to represent a higher risk than does occupational exposure, suggesting that rigorous attention to hygienic precautions can limit virus acquisition by caretakers of young children.[69-71] As noted, a second major route of HCMV infection is through sexual contact. High rates of HCMV infection have been documented in sexually active populations, including homosexual men, sex workers, and women attending STI clinics.[72-76] Consistent with these observations, risk factors for the delivery of congenitally HCMV-infected infant include STIs such as gonorrhea and trichomonas.[77]

The relative contributions of exposure to young children and sexual transmission of HCMV to the incidence of maternal HCMV infection remain incompletely defined because of the difficulty of ascertainment of accurate exposure histories in most individuals, particularly sexual histories. However, several studies have documented the efficacy of counseling in preventing maternal infections with HCMV during pregnancy, with reductions in rates of maternal infections nearing 50%, an effect similar to the efficacy reported for a candidate HCMV vaccine.[78-80] These studies have further reinforced the arguments of public health officials that an effective education program could have a significant impact on the incidence of HCMV infection in many populations.[79]

PATHOGENESIS

Introduction

A definitive understanding of the pathogenesis of CMV infections, in particular congenital CMV infections, has remained elusive for many reasons, including the genetic complexity of the virus, the paucity of informative animal models secondary to the strict species tropism of the HCMV, and ubiquity of infection with this virus in most populations in the world. Extensive efforts in studies of human infections associated with CMV have produced a large body of descriptive and correlative findings. Although these studies have led to greater understanding of the natural history of HCMV infections, definitive understanding of the mechanism of disease associated with HCMV infection is lacking. Clinical observations and studies in animal models have clearly documented the importance of the immune system in the control of the replication of HCMV in the infected host.

In no case was this more obvious than the spectrum of clinical infections observed in patients infected with human immunodeficiency virus (HIV).[81] Yet, even in the immunocompetent normal host, a unique relationship between HCMV and the host allows persistence of the virus in the face of a robust immune response. In the normal, persistently infected host, a considerable proportion (up to 15%) of the peripheral CD8+ T-lymphocyte response can be directed at HCMV.[82] Although a definitive explanation for the persistence of virus infection in the presence of such an overwhelming host immune response is not available, it has been argued that the myriad virus-encoded immune evasion functions could enable virus persistence in the normal host.[83–87]

A second and as yet incompletely defined characteristic of this virus that could contribute to its persistence is the extensive genomic diversity of the virus. Recent studies have demonstrated that HCMV circulates in the infected individual as a quasi-species with extreme genetic diversity.[1] The relationship between this genetic diversity and virus persistence in the individual host remains unknown. Furthermore, the importance of the extensive genetic diversity of the virus to its transmission between hosts and its spread within populations is unknown. In almost all instances, attempts to define mechanisms of disease associated with HCMV infection have relied on relating disease with virus replication. It is unclear if a linear relationship between virus replication and disease exists in most cases, and without adequate definition of the host contribution to disease, thorough understanding of HCMV disease will likely remain elusive.

Sources of Virus and Routes of Transmission

The pathogenesis of CMV infections has been investigated in human subjects as well as in animal models. As discussed, infected individuals can shed HCMV from numerous body fluids, including saliva, urine, breast milk, and genital tract secretions. HCMV DNA has been identified in hepatocytes, renal epithelium, and pancreatic acinar cells from adults experiencing sudden demise from trauma or cardiac arrest.[88,89] HCMV DNA has also been identified in epithelial tissues of salivary glands, breast, and prostate tissue from normal asymptomatic hosts, and infectious virus has been recovered from saliva, urine, breast milk, and prostatic secretions from healthy hosts, suggesting that the epithelium in these sites can serve as a reservoir for the production of infectious virus that is released intermittently from asymptomatically infected individuals.[8]

It then becomes obvious how secretions/excretions from these sites can readily promote the spread of HCMV throughout populations. Young children excrete large quantities of infectious virus asymptomatically in saliva and urine, promoting person-to-person spread by close contact among young children and their caregivers. Nonepithelial reservoirs include mononuclear cells and endothelial cells, which more often serve as sources of virus in noncommunity infections, such as those acquired through blood transfusions or organ allograft transplantation.

In medical settings, in addition to transmission through conventional pathways, alternative modes of HCMV transmission include blood transfusion and transplantation of infected organs or stem cells. Because monocytes may serve as reservoirs of latent infection, use of irradiated blood and blood filtered to deplete leukocytes decreases the likelihood of virus transmission via blood transfusion.[90–95] However, cell-free virus may also exist in human blood products; thus, even though the risk of HCMV transmission through transfusion of leukocyte-reduced blood products remains low, it cannot completely be excluded by current practices.[95] The potential risk of blood transfusion-acquired HCMV infection in neonates has been recognized for over 3 decades.[96–98] Early studies demonstrated that term infants born to HCMV-seronegative women and premature infants were at risk for HCMV infection and disease from transfusion of blood from HCMV-seropositive donors.[97] HCMV can also be transmitted via transplantation of an infected solid organ or via stem cell transplantation. Reservoirs of infection are likely to include epithelial and endothelial cell reservoirs in solid organs and CD34+ myeloid progenitor cells in stem cell transplantation.[99–102] To date, strategies have not been devised or tested that could prevent reactivation from infected donor tissues, but the use of antiviral agents as prophylaxis against viral dissemination have significantly reduced the incidence of HCMV disease in seronegative transplant recipients receiving infected donor organs.[103–105] This last clinical observation is consistent with reactivation of latent infection as a significant source of HCMV infection in allograft recipients.

Transmission in normal individuals in a community setting is thought to occur via contact with infected secretions in the oropharynx or following sexual contact and exposure to genital secretions. HCMV envelope glycoproteins appear to determine attachment and entry of infectious virions into susceptible cells. Thus far, glycoproteins B (gB), H (gH), and L (gL) have been shown to be essential for infectivity in human fibroblasts under laboratory conditions, whereas the pentameric envelope glycoprotein complex of HCMV UL 128–131 (consisting of UL128, 130, 131a, gH, and gL) is required for entry into epithelial, endothelial, and mononuclear cells in vitro.[106–108] The role of gO, a component of gH/gL, in entry remains incompletely defined because of conflicting findings from a number of laboratories.[109–113] Entry in fibroblasts is pH independent and has been reported to occur by virion envelope fusion at the cell membrane, whereas entry in epithelial cells utilizes a receptor-mediated endocytosis followed by a pH-dependent fusion event.[107,114–116]

Recent findings have suggested that HCMV enters fibroblasts through an actin-dependent step that resembles macropinocytosis that has been described in phagocytic cells. The cellular receptor(s) mediating entry of HCMV remains undefined, although low-affinity interactions with cell surface proteoglycans have been shown to contribute to the initial attachment of the particle.[114]

Following entry into the host cell, a number of intracellular signaling events have been documented.[116–120] In most cases, the contributions of signaling through these pathways to the biology of the virus infection have yet to be fully determined. Similarly, intercellular events in these proximally infected, presumably epithelial, cells remain uncharacterized; however, based on animal models of cytomegalovirus infection, virus most likely passes through the mucosal surfaces and replicates in regional lymph nodes, resulting in primary viremia, and is followed by secondary replication in the liver and spleen. Thereafter, a secondary viremia develops, which is asymptomatic in most individuals but occasionally produces clinically observable symptoms, including fever, malaise, pharyngitis, and lymphadenopathy. Recent studies in a murine model of CMV dissemination in immunocompetent animals suggested that dissemination likely occurs during the primary viremia, and the seeding of end organs is less dependent on the amplification of virus titer in organs such as the liver and secondary viremia.[121,122]

Although these findings potentially could explain the lack of a linear relationship between viral loads in blood/plasma and disease in individual patients at risk for end-organ disease, they also fail to account for observations made in immunocompromised patients, such as transplant recipients and HIV-infected hosts who develop end-organ disease after prolonged periods of viremia.[123–125] Perhaps an explanation for the apparent differences in the pathogenesis of CMV dissemination is related to primarily a finite period of cell-associated viremia in the immunocompetent host vs a prolonged combination of cell-free and cell-associated viremia in the immunocompromised host. Viremia appears to be limited by host immune responses that control viral replication in diseased organs and curtail ongoing dissemination. In HIV-infected hosts, this control has been most convincingly associated with HCMV-specific CD4+ T-lymphocyte responses.[126,127]

Cells of monocyte/macrophage lineage can support productive infection.[99,128–131] In vitro and animal studies have suggested that recruitment of infected mononuclear cells to sites of inflammation can promote transfer of virus to local end organs, providing a mechanism for dissemination of virus to distant sites by hematogenous cell-associated spread in humans.[101,132,133] In experimental mouse models, investigators have demonstrated that expression of virus-encoded functions that share sequence similarities with chemokines but do not signal through known G-protein coupled receptors can increase recruitment of myeloid cells into sites of initial virus replication and therefore increase the efficiency of dissemination from sites of primary replication.[132] Viral gene products of HCMV have been characterized to share sequence and functional homology with human interleukin (IL) 8, a cytokine that has been associated with recruitment of myeloid cells.[134] Alternatively, during primary infection, cell-free virus may circulate in blood and directly infect susceptible cells in almost every organ.

In the normal host, HCMV likely establishes a persistent infection, replicating at low levels and entering what has been termed a quiescent state or, like other herpesviruses, may enter true latency. During latency, viral genomes within infected cells exhibit restricted viral gene expression without the production of late gene products or infectious virions. Reservoirs of persistence and latency in humans have been proposed based on in vitro analysis of human cell types in cell culture and from animal models, in particular CMV infection in mice (murine CMV, MCMV). Sites of latency are thought to include monocytes, endothelial cells, epithelial cells of the lung, spleen, kidney, prostate, cervix, and salivary glands. Several in vitro studies have demonstrated latent infection of CD34+ myeloid progenitor cells, and it is believed that these cells could be responsible for dissemination of HCMV following mobilization of this cell population for stem cell transplantation and reactivation of HCMV replication.[101] The nature of latency, including establishment, maintenance, and reactivation of latent infection in CD34+ cells, remains poorly understood and has been investigated primarily using in vitro systems. More recently, elegant systems utilizing humanized mice models to study HCMV infection in vivo have provided a platform that could permit a more definitive understanding of this complex virus-host interaction.

Perinatal HCMV Infection: Breast Milk Transmission

Human cytomegalovirus has been demonstrated to be present in breast milk of lactating women, primarily as cell-free virus.[135–137] Asymptomatic infection of term neonates via breast feeding has been demonstrated in approximately 60% of breast-fed infants of HCMV-seropositive women and almost certainly represents the most common mode of transmission of this virus in the world.[50,136] Although HCMV can be transmitted to premature infants via oral ingestion of infected breast milk, postnatal infection by this route has not been reported to be associated with CNS damage or other adverse late outcomes that are seen following congenital infection.[138] The pathogenesis underlying these observations has not been characterized but may be caused by differences in the mode of transmission (oral vs hematogenous), host maturity at time of infection, or perhaps potential differences in timing of damaging congenital infection in utero (first and second trimester) compared to infection of an infant at the age of viability. The lack of reported CNS disease in premature infants acquiring CMV following breast feeding must be interpreted in the context that less than 10% of congenitally infected infants exhibit CNS involvement, raising the possibility that results from studies of the role of breast feeding in premature infants could have been underpowered to document the true incidence of long-term sequelae following breast milk transmission of HCMV. Of considerable clinical importance, preterm infants can develop severe acute CMV infection, including pneumonitis, colitis, and viral sepsis.[139-142]

Intrauterine Transmission of HCMV: Placenta Infection

In congenital infection, the virus must pass through the placenta to enter the fetus, presumably by hematogenous spread to the placenta. Analysis by in situ DNA hybridization, PCR, and immunohistochemistry of placentas from women who delivered HCMV-infected infants have demonstrated evidence of HCMV infection in epithelial cells, cytotrophoblasts, syncytiotrophoblasts, placental fibroblasts, and endothelial cells.[143-150] In placentas with chorioamnionitis, HCMV DNA has been detected in maternal macrophages.[149] Immunohistochemical staining for HCMV proteins showed the presence of HCMV gB in fetal neutrophils, macrophages, and dendritic cells in the villus core.[148,151] In vitro studies suggested that cytotrophoblasts and syncytiotrophoblast cells are permissive for HCMV infection.[143-145,152,153] Interestingly, placental cells infected with HCMV in vitro can produce proinflammatory cytokines IL-6 and IL-8, and more recently, a proinflammatory signature of cytokines was found in the amniotic fluid of fetuses ultimately shown to be infected with HCMV in utero.[154,155] However, these in vitro studies have not yet been extended to studies of HCMV-infected placental tissues in vivo, and mechanisms of transmission and protection from intrauterine transmission remain undefined.

Studies of placentas derived from women delivering infected and noninfected newborn infants have suggested that antiviral antibodies could play a major role in limiting virus transmission to the fetus and could account for the protective functions of passively acquired immunoglobulins.[54,156,157] In vitro infection of human umbilical vein endothelial cells showed induction of αVβ6-integrin-mediated activation of transforming growth factor β, a potent fibrogenic cytokine,

as well as collagen synthesis, suggesting an effect of HCMV infection on extracellular matrix remodeling in the infected placenta.[158]

More recently, investigators have begun to suggest that HCMV-induced placental dysfunction could be an important comorbid event during maternal HCMV infection during pregnancy that could account for several of the more significant findings in infants with symptomatic congenital HCMV infection. These include disruption of normal placental architecture, a vasculopathy, and as noted, the creation of an inflammatory mileu.[54,146,159] This topic is rapidly evolving and extremely important for a more complete understanding of the pathogenesis of congenital HCMV infections. For those interested, several excellent reviews of the interactions between placental infection and HCMV are available.[148,160]

Establishment of animal models for congenital CMV infection have been hampered by lack of transplacental passage of CMVs in murine models, thought to be related to the number of cell layers at the maternal-fetal interface in these animal placentas.[161,162] The guinea pig placenta, like the human placenta, has only 1 cell layer at the maternal-fetal interface; thus, this model has been used as a model for congenital CMV infection to examine correlates of protective maternal immunity against damaging congenital disease.[163-171] However, the guinea pig model has some limitations, including a high incidence of severe disease and mortality among infected pups secondary to the extremely fulminant nature of this model of congenital infection. From reports that have described the guinea pig model of congenital HCMV infection, it is clear that congenital infection takes place, but the data are less compelling that disease in congenitally infected guinea pigs is secondary to virus infection of the developing guinea pig and could be secondary to significant placental dysfunction in the infected dam, as was suggested by studies in humans.[172]

Immune Control of HCMV Infection: Intrinsic and Innate Responses

The initial control of acute HCMV infection in the normal host is initiated by what have been described as intrinsic and extrinsic innate responses that include responses of the infected cell and innate immune responses, including the antiviral activity of natural killer (NK) cells and cells of the myeloid lineage, including tissue macrophages (Table 54-4). Cellular intrinsic responses have been identified primarily through studies that have described the capacity of virus-encoded gene products to modulate these responses in infected cells. An example of a viral function that limits cellular intrinsic responses is the virion tegument protein, pp71, which has been demonstrated

Table 54-4 Mechanisms of Resistance to Human Cytomegalovirus Replication

Response	Mechanism	Reference	Reference: Impairment in Fetus
Cellular intrinsic	Viral DNA degradation; apoptosis	178, 306–308	Unknown
Innate immunity	NK cells, interferons, γΔ-T cells	83, 181, 309, 310	Unknown
Adaptive immunity	CD8⁺ cytotoxic T cells; CD4 T cells; antiviral antibodies (virus-neutralizing antibodies), ADCC	82, 190, 210, 223, 293, 311–315	5, 63, 212, 316–318

Abbreviations: ADCC, antibody-dependent cellular cytotoxicity; NK, natural killer.

to function as an inhibitor of the cellular protein Daxx, a nuclear protein that targets exogenous nucleic acids of degradation[173,174] (Table 54-4).

Additional viral functions have been described that limit intrinsic responses, including the formation of promyelocytic leukemia (PML) bodies, a host response that sequesters nucleic acids in the nucleus and limits transcription from the HCMV genome, induction of interferon (IFN) responses, blocks programmed cell death through either apoptosis and necrosis, and increases the autophagic activity in infected cells.[174–178] Together, these viral functions are thought to enhance the capacity of the virus to establish infection, initiate viral gene expression, and permit productive infection in target cells. In the case of HCMV, the virus encodes an IL-10-like molecule that does not share structural or antigenic relatedness to the host IL-10 yet retains IL-10 function.[179] The production of the viral IL-10 early in infection has been postulated to inhibit the differentiation of myeloid cells into dendritic cells in the local sites of infection and potentially block early recognition of virus-infected cells by host responses.[180] The importance of extrinsic cellular responses such as NK cells in early control of herpesvirus infections has been shown in case reports describing severe herpesvirus infections in patients lacking NK cell function and a large number of studies in murine models.[181–184]

Additional evidence of the critical role of natural immunity in the control of CMV infections is perhaps best illustrated by the détente that appears to have been reached by the virus and host antiviral responses in normal individuals.[87] The genomes of both HCMV and MCMV encode numerous open reading frames (ORFs) that express proteins that can modulate surface host protein expression to evade host NK recognition of virus-infected cells, including downmodulation of major histocompatibility complex (MHC) class I, production of decoy MHC class I homologs, and downregulation of surface expression of ligands for the activating NK group 2 receptor (such as MICA/B, MULT-1, RAE-1, and H60).[185] The evasion of specific host responses following expression of virus-encoded genes illustrates a viral strategy for persistence but not virulence in the normal host. It is likely that such viral

immunoevasins developed during the coevolution of CMVs with their natural hosts.[87]

Immune Control of HCMV Infection: T-Lymphocyte Responses

Long-term control of HCMV infection is achieved by an adaptive immune response to HCMV, primarily through the activities of HCMV-specific T-lymphocyte responses. Expansion of cytotoxic effector CD8⁺ T lymphocytes terminates productive primary infection in animal models of human disease.[183,186–188] Interestingly, in these models CD4⁺ T cells were also capable of rescuing infected immunodeficient mice from lethal infection.[183] Establishment of HCMV-specific memory T cells limits viral shedding and may limit reactivation from latency.[189] Similar findings have been approximated in human studies. Adoptive transfer of HCMV-specific T cells in patients after hematopoietic stem cell transplantation was pioneered as a potential strategy to prevent HCMV disease in these immunodeficient patients but has not evolved into standard therapy for high-risk patients.[190,191] Interestingly, in these pivotal studies, reconstitution of HCMV-specific CD8⁺ CTL (cytotoxic lymphocyte) responses were associated with early control of virus replication, but long-term control of HCMV infection required the reconstitution of HCMV-specific CD4⁺ T-lymphocyte responses.[190]

Perhaps a unique aspect of the immunobiology of CMV infections is the magnitude and breadth of the T-lymphocyte response to this virus. Early studies readily detected both HCMV-specific CD4⁺ and CD8⁺ T-lymphocyte responses to crude antigens and virus-infected cells. As technology advanced, the distinctive characteristics of this response were cataloged. Once assays for intracellular cytokine production following antigen stimulation of T lymphocytes from immune individuals became routinely employed for measurement of T-lymphocyte responses to HCMV, many laboratories reported unsuspected features of this response.

As noted previously, some studies included the finding that, in healthy immunocompetent individuals, up to 10%–20% of peripheral blood T lymphocytes were specific for HCMV.[82] This finding was mirrored in mice infected with MCMV, and the phenomenon of memory inflation of the CD8$^+$ T-lymphocyte response became a distinctive characteristic of the CD8$^+$ T-lymphocyte response to CMVs.[82,192] The commitment of such a significant proportion of the host's CD8$^+$ T-lymphocyte response to 1 agent has been argued by some investigators as an explanation for immune senescence in older individuals leading to decreasing T-lymphocyte function in the elderly.[192–194]

A second finding that was somewhat unexpected was that normal immunocompetent individuals infected with HCMV generated T-lymphocyte responses to a large number of viral-encoded proteins, including a large number of virion structural proteins.[82] This finding provided support for the argument that HCMV likely persists in the infected host as a chronic productive infection with the expression of late gene products that can induce a measurable T-lymphocyte response.[82]

Finally, the availability of fluorochrome-conjugated tetramers (peptide epitopes folded with MHC class I molecules) have enabled investigators to precisely interrogate the viral antigen-specific CD8$^+$ T-lymphocyte response in a variety of patient populations in real time. This approach has allowed the enumeration of CD8$^+$ T-lymphocyte responses during acute, chronic, and reactivated infections and has provided prognostic information on patient outcome in patients at risk for severe infections with HCMV.[195,196] Together, these technological advances have advanced our understanding of the immunology of HCMV infections as well as providing a solid foundation for future studies of the role of T-cell immunity in the natural history of HCMV infections.

Adaptive Immune Responses: Antiviral Antibodies

Infection with HCMV induces a diverse and readily detectable antibody response that also includes the production of rheumatoid factor-like antibodies. Virus-specific antibodies are made shortly after infection and include an initial IgM response followed quickly by IgG antibodies. Rarely can an individual be identified with only IgM anti-HCMV antibodies and undetectable levels of IgG antibodies reactive with HCMV, thus making it difficult to accurately ascertain seroconversion with patient specimens provided during the early period after infection. However, several laboratories have demonstrated that the IgG antibody response undergoes an avidity maturation that can be easily measured in antibody-binding assays.[197] The avidity maturation of the IgG anti-HCMV antibody response forms the basis of diagnostic assays widely used in Europe to assess the duration of a serologically detected HCMV

infection. The utility of such assays when combined with screening for HCMV-specific IgM antibodies has permitted new insight into the natural history of maternal infections during pregnancy.

A broad repertoire of antiviral antibodies is produced against a large number of structural and nonstructural proteins produced within infected cells. In terms of antiviral antibodies that are thought to function in protective responses, most studies have indicated that antibodies directed at the envelope proteins of the virus are most consistently associated with protection in vivo. A detailed explanation of the antienvelope protein antibody response is likely beyond the scope of this discussion, but suffice it to say that the envelope of HCMV is extraordinarily complex and antibodies against most of the major protein components of the virion envelope have been shown to exhibit some virus-neutralizing activity assayed in vitro, a surrogate for in vivo protection (Table 54-4). In some cases, this activity appears to be limited to virus infection of human fibroblast cells, whereas in other cases antiviral antibodies against specific virion envelope proteins are more effective in neutralizing virus infection of epithelial cells.[198–207]

It is unclear at this time whether a single-antibody specificity is critical for protective responses in vivo, but it seems unlikely in view of the large numbers of antienvelope antibodies produced during infection. Data from a large number of studies have suggested that antiviral antibodies with virus-neutralizing activity as measured in vitro can modify disease associated with HCMV infections in a number of populations, including solid-organ transplant recipients, HIV-infected individuals, and in the infected newborn.[52,54,63,208–212] In many of these studies, protection from disease and not infection was achieved by the passive transfer of antiviral antibodies prepared from HCMV-immune donors.[54,210–212] Similarly, support for a protective role of antiviral antibodies has been provided from studies in a number of animal model systems.[167,213–215] However, it must also be noted that a detailed understanding of the mechanism of antiviral antibody protection in humans infected with HCMV and in most animal models is lacking. In addition to virus neutralization, data from animal model systems have suggested that cellular effector functions such as antibody-dependent cellular cytotoxicity (ADCC) participate in these protective responses.[216]

An important aspect of the proposed protective activities of antiviral antibodies, in particular virus-neutralizing antibodies, is that the virus-neutralizing antibody responses have been suggested as possible surrogates for the protective activity of candidate prophylactic vaccines. In fact, 1 of the most extensively tested vaccine candidates is a glycoprotein (gB) found in the envelope of the virus and a well-described target of virus-neutralizing antibodies.[217,218] Early studies argued for an association between the amount of antibodies reactive with gB and outcome of infection. Moreover, recently a small vaccine trial in renal transplant recipients utilizing an adjuvanted gB vaccine provided provocative data that was interpreted as evidence for a role in virus-neutralizing antibodies in limiting disease in these immunocompromised hosts.[219]

Last, an initial study that was uncontrolled and unfortunately has been followed with several observational studies that were also flawed either because of the lack of controls or biased enrollment have argued that congenital HCMV and its sequelae can be prevented by the administration of pooled human intravenous immunoglobulin (IVIG) in women undergoing primary HCMV infection during pregnancy (see following sections).[212] The quality of these studies is such that most investigators believe the data impossible to interpret; however, the possibility that such treatment could be efficacious has prompted additional trials using IVIG following documentation of primary maternal infections during pregnancy. The results of these studies should be available sometime during the next several years. Interestingly, a well-designed and controlled trial using the same preparation of the IVIG as was used in the initial trial failed to show any protection from fetal infection.[330]

From these data and studies in animal models, several pharmaceutical programs have initiated the development of systems that will permit production of large quantities of either human or humanized monoclonal antibodies that have potent in vitro neutralizing activities. It is anticipated that these antibody preparations will be used in either prophylactic or treatment protocols to limit disease secondary to HCMV infection in a number of different clinical settings, ranging from transplant recipients to fetuses exposed to HCMV in utero.

Immune Responses in the Congenitally Infected Infant

Immune responses in congenital CMV infection have been studied in a limited number of patients. In 8 neonates with congenital CMV infection, determination of postnatal CD8[+] T-cell responses revealed higher proportions of activated CD8[+] T cells which expressed surface markers including HLA-DR and CD95 but lower levels of CD62L, suggesting antigen exposure.[220] In addition, these investigators demonstrated that these CD8[+] T lymphocytes expressed differentiation markers, including CD45RO but low levels of CD28 and CD27, suggesting these cells represented an effector-memory population, a finding that contrasted to CD8[+] T lymphocytes isolated from uninfected newborns.[220]

Spectratyping analysis suggested oligoclonal expansion of antigen-experienced clones, compared to the naïve phenotype of CD8[+] cells from control uninfected newborns.[220] CD8[+] T cells from infants with congenital HCMV infection also demonstrated cytotoxic and cytokine production when compared to cells from uninfected neonates. These findings suggested that damaging intrauterine HCMV infection associated with congenital HCMV infection may not be prevented by establishment of antiviral CD8[+] T-lymphocyte responses in the fetus.[220]

Similar findings have been described in a study of 16 fetuses, although these authors suggested that overall the responses exhibited a slight decrease in IFN-γ responses following in vitro stimulation.[221] In a later study, Gibson and colleagues also documented HCMV-specific CD8[+] T-lymphocyte responses in the first day of life in congenitally infected infants and at later time points in young infants, indicating that young infants were capable of generating these adaptive responses.[222] In addition, these authors correlated the presence of these responses in infants with a decrease in the viral load in peripheral blood, suggesting a role of this response in control of HCMV replication.[222] Altogether, these studies have argued that CD8[+] T cells have the capacity to expand and differentiate in response to intrauterine viral infection such that by the time of birth, circulating CD8[+] T cells can exhibit a mature and antigen-specific phenotype.

In contrast, other investigators have argued that adaptive immune responses, specifically CD4[+] T-lymphocyte responses to HCMV, are depressed in HCMV-infected infants compared to adults.[223,224] Similar results that described decreased CD4[+] T-lymphocyte responses to HCMV in HCMV-infected infants were reported following studies carried out nearly 3 decades ago.[63,225,226] However, advances in the analysis of HCMV-specific T-lymphocyte responses that were described previously have made the extrapolation of results from these early studies to current findings somewhat difficult. Thus, the relationship between results from these early studies and those from more recent studies to the natural history of congenital HCMV infections remains undefined. However, it is interesting that a more recent study suggested that neonatal dendritic cells exhibit deficient IL-12 and IFN-γ production following exposure to HCMV.[227] This finding could potentially explain the previously described deficits in CD4[+] T-lymphocyte responses in infected infants.

The study of fetal and neonatal adaptive immune responses to infectious agents is an active area of research, and HCMV-infected infants offer an ideal opportunity to further define these responses in young infants. For more details, those are referred to recent reviews in the immunobiology of CMV infection in the fetus and neonate.[228]

DISEASES IN INFANTS WITH CONGENITAL HCMV INFECTION

Introduction

Although almost infants with congenital HCMV infection are asymptomatic in the newborn period, as noted previously some 10% will present with physical findings readily detectable on routine physical examination. Clinically apparent infections were originally designated as symptomatic infections as a category in natural history studies of congenital HCMV infection. Infants with symptoms attributable to congenital HCMV infection exhibited long-term neurological sequelae more frequently when compared to infected infants without symptoms in the newborn period. Thus, this simple clinical classification provided prognostic information for infants with congenital HCMV infections.

More recently, investigators have extended the definition of symptomatic infection to include laboratory evidence of end-organ disease, imaging abnormalities, and evidence of hearing loss. It is important to note that such criteria have not been validated in large-scale epidemiological studies such as those that originally defined the spectrum of disease and long-term sequelae in congenitally infected infants based on their presentation in the newborn period.

Congenital HCMV infection can involve almost every organ system in the newborn. Manifestations of end-organ disease in the liver, spleen, lungs, bone marrow, gastrointestinal tract, genitourinary tract, CNS, and skin have been described (Table 54-2).[23,229] In addition, evidence of HCMV infection has been reported in the salivary glands, pancreas, thyroid, and adrenal glands.[22] Thus, symptomatic infection in the newborn infant is characterized by multiple-organ involvement, with the most common physical findings being hepatosplenomegaly, jaundice, petechiae, and microcephaly (Table 54-2).[23] Although end-organ disease by definition is not present in infants with asymptomatic infection, HCMV can replicate in nearly every organ, raising the possibility that HCMV could be present in most organ systems even if disease is not evident. Thus, the unexpected finding of HCMV during histopathological examination of tissues from infants can suggest the possibility of an unrecognized congenital HCMV infection. Although a linear relationship between the absolute level of virus replication and end-organ disease has not been established, it is clear that the quantity of virus in the urine and the number of viral genome copies in the peripheral blood of symptomatically infected infants far exceeds the levels found in infants with asymptomatic infections.[32,33,35,230,231]

Based on these studies, it has been argued that end-organ disease associated with congenital HCMV infection is directly related to virus replication, a postulate that would suggest that antiviral therapy leading to a decrease in HCMV replication would be efficacious in infants with congenital HCMV infection. This relationship appears consistent with findings in some organ systems, but in other organs, a clear relationship between the level of virus replication and end-organ disease is not readily apparent.[33] Such observations suggest that multiple mechanisms of disease could be operative in fetuses/infants with congenital HCMV infections, some of which may only be indirectly related to virus replication and therefore less amenable to treatment with antiviral agents.

A unique characteristic of congenitally infected infants is prolonged replication of HCMV that has been observed in these patients. Virus replication and excretion routinely persist through the first 2 years of life and in some young children can persist until 3–4 years of age.[232] The duration of virus excretion has not been directly related to the severity of the congenital HCMV infection or the peak of virus replication, but interestingly, it has been shown to be similarly prolonged in infants infected during the perinatal period, including infants acquiring HCMV through breast milk exposure.

Previous studies have suggested a relationship between acquisition of HCMV-specific CD4$^+$ T-cell responses and cessation of virus excretion in congenitally infected infants.[63] This finding has not been confirmed in studies utilizing more contemporary technologies but still suggests a relationship between maturation of the immune response to HCMV and control of virus replication. Infection of newborn mice with MCMV is also associated with prolonged replication as compared to similar infections in adult mice, a finding that suggests a unique relationship between the development of the immune system and control of HCMV replication.[215]

Prolonged excretion of virus in congenitally infected infants remains an interesting experimental question, but its practical significance is in the transmission of HCMV to adults and other infants. Congenitally HCMV-infected infants represent a significant exposure risk for acquisition of HCMV and serve as viral reservoirs that promote the maintenance of the virus in populations.

Non-CNS Manifestations of Symptomatic Congenital HCMV Infection

Hepatomegaly has been reported as 1 of the most common manifestations of symptomatic congenital HCMV infection[23,24] (Table 54-2). Histopathologic findings include viral inclusions in epithelial cells lining bile ducts, hepatocyte necrosis, periportal mononuclear cell infiltrates, areas of hematopoiesis, and bile duct dilation with cholestasis.[233] Extramedullary hematopoiesis can be demonstrated in the liver.[233] Laboratory findings consistent with hepatic involvement include direct hyperbilirubinemia, elevations of hepatic transaminases, and increased levels of γ-glutamyl transpeptidase. Anecdotal reports have described cases of hepatic failure secondary to cirrhosis in patients with symptomatic congenital HCMV infection, but this outcome must be considered an extremely rare sequela in infants with congenital HCMV infection. Splenomegaly was associated with congestion and extramedullary hematopoiesis.

Petechial rashes and less commonly evidence of cutaneous extramedullary hematopoiesis are findings associated with symptomatic congenital HCMV infection.[23,24] Petechiae are associated with thrombocytopenia and, together with decreased red blood cell numbers, suggest involvement of the bone marrow, although consumption of platelets secondary to splenic enlargement likely contributes to the severity of thrombocytopenia in some infants. Most infants with congenital HCMV infection do not suffer hemorrhagic events secondary to thrombocytopenia or require transfusions secondary to their anemia. In most instances, abnormalities in hepatic and bone marrow function resolve within the first 2 months of life, whereas splenomegaly can persist during the first year of life.

HCMV infection of other organ systems has been reported. Perhaps the most significant is the presence of pneumonia in congenitally infected infants, which is often documented in infants who succumb to their infection in the immediate postnatal period.[23,234] Viral inclusions can be documented in cells in the air space, but viral inclusions are not reportedly found in bronchial or bronchiolar epithelium.[233] Renal involvement is common, with viral inclusions present in the epithelium of the tubules and lymphocyte infiltrations in the interstitial space. Viral inclusions can be found in the secretory epithelium of endocrine glands, including the pancreas, adrenals, and thyroid.[233] HCMV-infected cells are frequently detected in the salivary glands of congenitally infected infants. There seems to be little definitive evidence of congenital HCMV infections being associated with abnormalities in cardiac development.

As discussed previously, the level of virus replication as measured by detection of viral DNA in the peripheral blood of congenitally infected infants correlates with the presence of hepatitis and thrombocytopenia in symptomatically infected infants.[35] Furthermore, treatment with the antiviral ganciclovir (GCV) has been shown to decrease the level of virus replication and normalized abnormalities in liver function and platelet counts.[235,236] These results strongly argued that a direct relationship existed between virus replication, virus-induced cytopathology, and end-organ disease in the case of the liver and the bone marrow in infants

with symptomatic HCMV infections. In contrast, a linear relationship between virus replication and microcephaly, hearing loss, and other CNS manifestations of congenital HCMV infections was not found in the analysis of another series of patients.[33,35]

CNS Disease Following Congenital HCMV Infection

Congenital HCMV infection involving the CNS can result in a variety of abnormalities in CNS structures and neurologic functions. Morphologic abnormalities associated with congenital HCMV infection include the loss of the intermediate zone layer of the white matter, focal necrosis, hemorrhage, gliosis, and ventricular dilation.[233,237–241] Maldevelopment of normal brain architecture has also been well described, including abnormal sulcations, hypoplastic corpus callosum, polymicrogyria, lissencephaly, porencephaly, and schizencephaly[24,242–245] (Table 54-5). Cortical and periventricular calcifications may also be seen in infants with congenital HCMV infection, and in the not too distant past were considered as radiologic findings diagnostic of congenital HCMV infection (Figure 54-2). Ocular involvement in infants with congenital HCMV infection is not an infrequent finding in infants with symptomatic infections.[23,24,246,247] Although chorioretinitis is perhaps the most well-described eye finding in infants with congenital HCMV infection, other findings, including areas of retinal depigmentation, optic atrophy, and pigmented retinopathy have been reported.[246,247]

The cell types of the CNS infected by HCMV have been described in both animal models and in vitro

Table 54-5 Central Nervous System Imaging Findings From Various Techniques in Infants With Congenital Human Cytomegalovirus Infections

Technique	Findings	Reference
Ultrasound	Calcifications, ventriculomegaly, cysts, lenticulostriate vasculopathy	243, 299, 319–323
Computed tomography (CT)	Calcifications, ventriculomegaly, cortical atrophy, white matter abnormalities	24, 245
Magnetic resonance imaging	Migration deficits (lissencephaly, pachygyria; polymicrogyria), cerebellar hypoplasia, cysts, ventriculomegaly	244, 321, 324–330

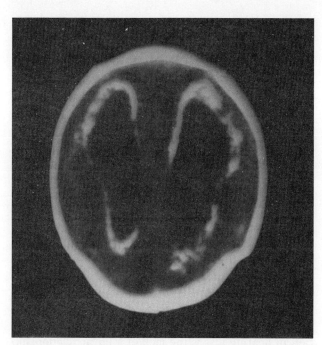

FIGURE 54-2 Computerized tomographic findings of infant with symptomatic (microcephaly) congenital human cytomegalovirus (HCMV) infection. Prominent periventricular calcifications, ventriculomegaly, and loss of cortical tissue are evident.

systems derived from cells from the human CNS.[248-252] Cell types infected in vitro include brain microvascular endothelial cells, astrocytes, neuronal cells and neural progenitor cells, oligodendrocytes, and microglia. However, not all of these cell types support productive infection. A more recent study using peripheral viral infection of neonatal mice, with subsequent hematogenous spread to the CNS, demonstrated infection of neurons, astroglial cells, cerebellar Bergman glia, meningeal cells, and rare vascular endothelial cells.[251]

A novel study describing infection of the developing primate CNS was reported by Tarantal and colleagues.[253] In this study, investigators, utilizing ultrasound guidance, inoculated rhesus macaque fetuses intraperitoneally during the late second trimester of gestation.[253] The spectrum of disease in infected animals ranged from lissencephaly to focal encephalitis, suggesting that under these experimental conditions other undetermined parameters of infection contributed to the phenotype of disease in infected animals.[253] Furthermore, disease manifestations were not directly correlated with virus replication, a finding suggesting that other factors, such as the host response to CNS infection could contribute to the overall phenotype of disease following intrauterine infection.[253]

Results from this experimental model and findings from imaging studies of infected fetuses in utero and in newborn infants with congenital HCMV infections have suggested that 1 mechanism of CNS damage in congenitally infected infants could result from infection of neural stem cells in the subventricular zone and subsequent loss of neuronal population or altered migration during cortical development.[24,242–245] Studies carried out in vitro with neural progenitor cells have also yielded results consistent with these findings.[248] Results from studies in small-animal models that have often utilized direct intracranial inoculation of CMV have also argued that the infection of neural progenitor cells is a critical feature of CNS damage following congenital HCMV infection secondary to the loss of a population of cells that populate the cortex of the brain.[249] Although these findings in animal models are provocative and consistent with findings in some human infants with congenital HCMV infection, they must also be tempered by the route of infection and the amount of virus inoculated into the experimental animal.

HCMV infects the fetus via the placenta and presumably spreads hematogenously to end organs, including the brain. The risk of neurologic sequelae appears to increase with earlier maternal infection, and presumably intrauterine transmission. Ex vivo infection of murine fetal and neonatal brain slices has indicated that susceptible cell types include subventricular zone neural progenitor cells and immature glial cells.[254] Murine neural progenitor cells are permissive for MCMV infection in vitro, although viral replication in this cell type is lower than in fibroblasts.[249,255] As noted in the immediately previous discussion, similar findings have been reported in studies using neural progenitor cells and HCMV.[248] Interestingly, it has been reported that more primitive stem cells are relatively resistant to infection with CMVs.[248] In vivo neonatal mouse infection with MCMV results in infection of neurons, astroglial cells, cerebellar Bergman glia, meningeal cells, and rare vascular endothelial cells throughout the brain.[251] One striking finding from these in vivo infections was the presence of widespread inflammation and global aberrations of morphogenesis, despite the focality of infected cells shown by immunohistochemical staining suggesting an indirect effect of virus infection on CNS developmental abnormalities.[251]

More recent studies in this same model have clearly demonstrated that inflammation in the CNS following this infection was a significant contributor to the observed disease in infected animals.[331] In addition, defects in granular neuron proliferation and migration were observed in MCMV-infected brains compared to uninfected controls.[251] In these studies in mice, antiviral CD8+ T lymphocytes were critical to control MCMV infection in the CNS of neonatal mice.[256]

In contrast to clinical findings in infants with congenital infection, CMV has not been reported to lead to neurologic manifestations during acute infection of immunocompetent children and adults. However, in the severely immune-compromised host, such as patients with acquired immunodeficiency syndrome (AIDS) or those patients undergoing hematopoietic stem cell transplantation, HCMV encephalitis has been well described, albeit with a relatively low incidence. In AIDS, CMV encephalitis can develop during severe immunosuppression, manifested by CD4+ cell counts below 50 cells/mL.[257] Cytomegalic inclusions can be observed within neurons, astrocytes, and endothelial cells.[258,259] Parenchymal necrosis, microglial nodules, and periventriculitis are observed with HCMV expression in histologically normal cells as well as in cytomegalic cells lining the ventricles.[258,259]

It has been argued that HCMV encephalitis in this setting is a disease of HCMV reactivation rather than acute infection; however, this remains a postulated mechanism of disease. Furthermore, the cellular reservoirs of HCMV in the CNS remain undefined, with candidates including neuronal cells, glial cells, and endothelial cells.

Other neurologic manifestations of HCMV disease in patients with AIDS patients include polyradiculopathies, retinitis, and multifocal neuropathy, with HCMV retinitis representing the most well described and frequent CNS manifestation of HCMV infections in such patients.[257,260,261] HCMV retinitis is a relatively unusual manifestation of disseminated HCMV infection in hematopoietic cell transplant recipients but interestingly has been in reported in patients receiving biological immune response modifiers such as anti–tumor necrosis factor (anti-TNF) antibody therapy as well as being a well-described entity in patients with advanced HIV infection.

Hearing Loss Following Congenital HCMV Infection

Sensorineural hearing loss is the most frequent long-term sequela of congenital CMV infection. Acquired CMV infection, even if acquired early in infancy, has not been associated with hearing loss. Because of the logistical challenges of characterizing the pathogenesis of hearing loss, few studies have evaluated CMV infection of inner ear structures during pre- and postnatal development. A recent study evaluating 6 inner ears from fetuses terminated for severe congenital CMV infection identified CMV infection of cochlear structures, particularly the stria vascularis, and vestibular structures, in particular the nonsensory epithelia.[239] Inflammatory infiltrates were demonstrated by immunohistochemical staining in affected structures. These results are consistent with other histologic studies of the CNS and peripheral organs demonstrating extensive inflammation surrounding foci of infected cells. As in other sites of persistent infection, epithelial cells

appear to be particularly susceptible to ongoing infection. However, pathogenesis of late-onset hearing loss has not been investigated, and the relative contributions of direct viral cytolysis and the host inflammatory response remain undefined.

An uncontrolled (treated infants compared to historical controls) trial utilizing GCV for treatment of infants at risk for hearing loss together with several anecdotal case reports and smaller series have reported improvement in hearing following treatment, findings that raised the possibility that ongoing viral replication may contribute to the destruction of infected inner ear cells or recruitment of leukocytes to areas of cochlear and vestibular infection.[236] The findings from this treatment trial as well as other reports suggesting a benefit from GCV treatment will need to be confirmed by controlled trials. From available data, it is not possible to state that virus replication has a direct line with HCMV-associated hearing loss. Adding to the uncertainty surrounding the contribution of virus replication to hearing loss is the lack of a linear relationship between peripheral virus burden as measured by PCR assays of viral genomes in blood and hearing loss.[33]

Studies of MCMV infection of murine auditory structures after direct intracerebral inoculation of virus demonstrated the presence of MCMV-positive cells in perilymphatic compartments, including the scala tympani and scala vestibule but not endolymphatic compartments, inner or outer hair cells, or the organ of Corti.[262] Labyrinthitis was observed, with infiltration of CD45+/CD3+ lymphocytes and CD45+/CD11b+ mononuclear cells. In this model, transcription of proinflammatory cytokines such as TNF-α, IL-6, and IFN-γ were elevated in MCMV-infected mice compared to saline-treated controls.

This was a fulminant model of CNS infection by CMV, with 100% of infected mice developing hearing loss within the first 3 weeks of life and almost all mice succumbing to the infection by about 4 weeks of life.[262] The route of CNS infection in this model does not resemble the presumably hematogenous mode of CNS infection in human fetuses with congenital infection; similar to other studies in murine models that have utilized direct inoculation of the CNS, the inflammatory response detailed in these studies may fail to model the response in human infants with congenital CMV infection and hearing loss. Furthermore, this model presumably included fatal encephalitis, a finding rarely observed in the infected human fetus. However, these studies supported the probability that CMV can directly infect cells of the inner ear and that a host inflammatory response can accompany this viral infection. Several studies utilizing the guinea pig and guinea pig CMV have provided results that are consistent with these interpretations.[263–269] In addition, findings from these studies also suggested the possibility that ongoing inflammation within a CMV-infected cochlea could contribute to progressive hearing loss in congenitally infected infants.

DIFFERENTIAL DIAGNOSIS

Introduction

The differential diagnosis of symptomatic congenital HCMV infection includes perinatal infections that decades ago were designated as the TORCH complex (toxoplasmosis, rubella, CMV, and herpes simplex virus [HSV]) as well as enteroviral infections in the perinatal period. Although congenital HCMV infection is more frequent than either toxoplasmosis or HSV, infants with congenital toxoplasmosis or HSV can present in the newborn period with signs and symptoms similar to infants with congenital HCMV infection. Because infections associated with toxoplasmosis or HSV have effective therapy, it is imperative that these infections be excluded immediately. Rubella is rarely seen in the Western world, where most women are rubella immune prior to conception, but continues to exist in regions without population-based rubella immunization programs. Similarly, congenital infection with lymphocytic choriomeningitis virus (LCMV) is rarely reported in the developed world. Disseminated enteroviral infections can present initially with findings similar to congenital HCMV infection, but the progressive and often-fulminant nature of this viral infection distinguishes it on clinical grounds from HCMV infections.

Congenital CMV Infection

The differential diagnosis of congenital HCMV infection includes many of the other described perinatal infections. Patients with congenital toxoplasmosis may also present with chorioretinitis, microphthalmia, microcephaly or macrocephaly, and cerebral calcifications. Unlike periventricular distribution of calcifications, which are often associated with congenital HCMV infection, the calcifications found in patients with congenital toxoplasmosis have been consistently described as scattered throughout the cerebral parenchyma. However, it is important to note that imaging abnormalities of the brain other than periventricular calcifications are more frequently seen in infants with congenital HCMV infections. The rash of toxoplasmosis is most often maculopapular, unlike the petechial and purpuric lesions of congenital CMV. Finally, the findings present in the chorioretinitis of infants with congenital HCMV infections are distinct from those of infants with congenital toxoplasmosis and can be readily recognized by an experienced ophthalmologist.

Congenital rubella syndrome may present with a blueberry muffin rash and hearing loss but, unlike congenital HCMV infection, may also demonstrate cardiac lesions, such as a patent ductus arteriosus, and cataracts. Congenital syphilis also can present with blueberry muffin-type rash, hepatomegaly, and long-bone abnormalities; however, many other findings of congenital syphilis are absent in congenital HCMV infection. Congenital LCMV infection can manifest with chorioretinitis, either microcephaly or hydrocephalus, or intracranial calcifications.[270–272] Hearing deficits and hepatosplenomegaly may be observed in a minority of infants with congenital LCMV infection, as well as rare nonimmune hydrops fetalis.[272]

In terms of noninfectious conditions, Aicardi-Goutières syndrome can also mimic congenital HCMV infection. This autosomal recessive genetic disorder is characterized by microcephaly, cerebral calcifications, leukodystrophy, and cerebral atrophy (reviewed in references 273 and 274). Some infants have no indications at birth and manifest these findings over time, but 20% of affected infants present at birth. Associated findings may include hepatosplenomegaly with transaminitis, anemia and thrombocytopenia, and seizures. Calcifications are often located in the basal ganglia but may also occur in the white matter, including the periventricular areas bilaterally. Interestingly, this syndrome is secondary to mutation in a host gene (*Trex*), which leads to the failure of the host to limit the activity of intracellular sensors of nucleic acids.[275,276] In the absence of this gene, the host responds to endogenous nucleic acids by the production of α-IFNs and inflammation in affected organ systems as part of the patterned responses.[275] Other metabolic encephalopathies presenting with basal ganglia calcifications include parathormone disorders, biotinidase deficiency, 3-hydroxy-isobutyric aciduria, Hoyeraal-Hreidarsson syndrome, and cerebroretinal microangiopathy with calcifications and cysts.[273] However, these entities would not exhibit other findings of patients with congenital CMV infection (Table 54-6).

Acquired CMV Infection

A number of infections resemble acute mononucleosis caused by acute CMV infection. Etiologies include Epstein-Barr virus, human herpes virus (HHV) 6, HSV-1, group A streptococcus, toxoplasmosis, acute retroviral syndrome caused by HIV, enterovirus, and adenovirus. CMV febrile syndrome seen in immunocompromised hosts and preterm infants may resemble bacterial, viral, or fungal sepsis. Localizing features of the febrile syndrome may assist with diagnosis, such as the presence of interstitial pneumonitis or colitis with CMV infection, but definitive diagnosis may require culture, nucleic acid testing, or biopsy.

Table 54-6 Differential Diagnosis of Symptomatic Congenital Human Cytomegalovirus (HCMV) Infection

Diagnosis	Similarities	Distinguishing Features
Toxoplasmosis	Chorioretinitis, microcephaly, cerebral calcifications, intrauterine growth retardation, abnormal neurological exam	Incidence low; pattern of intracranial calcifications; chorioretinitis pattern
Herpes simplex virus	Hepatitis, thrombocytopenia	Clinical onset; lack of more common findings in congenital HCMV such as hepatosplenomegaly, petechiae
Syphilis	Blueberry muffin rash, hepatomegaly, thrombocytopenia, hepatitis, anemia	Maternal serology; maternal risk factors; syphilis cases in community
Rubella	Blueberry muffin rash	Incidence extremely low; maternal immunization history; cardiac findings
Enterovirus	Hepatitis, thrombocytopenia, anemia, neurological findings	Age at presentation; rapidly progressive course
Aicardi-Goutières syndrome	Microcephaly, central nervous system calcifications, neurological findings	Lack of hepatosplenomegaly; jaundice; cutaneous lesions (acrocyanosis); white matter and basal ganglia calcifications

LABORATORY DIAGNOSIS

Introduction

A number of approaches have been used in the diagnosis of congenital HCMV infection, but today most laboratories utilize nucleic acid amplification assays and follow up a positive result with a confirmatory PCR or, in some centers, virus isolation. Serology can be used to rule out congenital infection because if the mother has no antibody reactivity to HCMV, it is likely that the infant was not exposed in utero. In contrast, serological assays that estimate the timing of maternal infection (avidity assays) are standard of care in some centers in Italy and Israel. Although of limited use in the United States secondary to differences in practices of pregnancy termination between the United States and these countries, as the development of therapeutics to treat intrauterine infections continues to mature, these assays will likely become more widely employed

Serology

Serology can be useful for determining whether a subject has been infected with HCMV in the past. The IgM response to HCMV was initially used to define a recent infection and more recently as a screen for primary infections; however, the IgM can persist for months after a primary infection; often, false-positive tests have been reported. Interestingly, HCMV infection has been associated with the production of rheumatoid factor, a biological response that can result in the detection of IgM antibodies directed at IgG antibodies and not HCMV antigens. Once established,

this finding requires additional measures to limit false positivity in IgM assays.

The detection of HCMV-specific IgM antibodies in the newborn infant was at 1 time utilized for the diagnosis of congenital CMV infections.[277] The assay for CMV-specific antibodies in cord blood or blood from newborn infants was technically demanding and required sensitivity that was only achievable in a research setting. It is of interest to note that the assay of HCMV-specific IgM antibodies in cord blood offered prognostic information in that high antibody titers were associated with more severe disease and an increased likelihood of long-term sequelae.[9,61] In contrast to the technical challenges associated with IgM measurements, the presence of HCMV-specific IgG antibodies indicates that an individual has been infected with HCMV.

In some studies, IgG avidity has been utilized to determine whether a subject has recent or distant infection, based on the premise that low-avidity IgG antibodies are present within the first few months after de novo infection, with later maturation of the IgG response to high-avidity antibodies. However, these tests have not become a standard of care in the United States, in contrast to many areas in Europe, and are primarily used for research in the United States. European centers routinely utilize IgG avidity testing in the prenatal care of women with HCMV IgM antibodies to help assess the risk of primary maternal HCMV infections during pregnancy.[197,278,279] Large clinical series from European investigators have detailed the use of prenatal HCMV-specific IgM testing followed by IgG avidity measurements and, if indicated based on results from these assays, amniocentesis and testing of amniotic fluid for the presence of HCMV DNA.[197] However, because some congenital infections may be caused by either maternal reinfections or reactivations, the maternal serologic IgG avidity status may not delineate the true risk to the fetus.

Serologic testing has also been used in the setting of solid-organ and stem cell transplantation to determine donor and recipient serostatus and risk of acute HCMV disease in the immunosuppressed recipient after transplantation. In general, risk of acute CMV disease is thought to be highest among patients with donor-positive/recipient-negative CMV serostatus, with other donor/recipient serostatus combinations conferring progressively lower risk of CMV disease posttransplant (Table 54-7).

Viral Culture

Historically, viral culture was utilized to detect HCMV infection in human subjects. Technical modifications to early tissue culture protocols coupled with the use of monoclonal antibody detection of immediate early gene products of HCMV in an immunofluorescence assay to identify infected cells in culture have permitted rapid culture diagnosis within 24–72 hours, whereas conventional cell culture isolation of HCMV often required 10–21 days to obtain interpretable results.[280–283] Culture of body fluids or tissue continues to be utilized if limited amounts of virus are present in the samples or there is a need to recover infectious virus for additional assays, such as drug sensitivity testing. Infectious virions can be recovered from saliva, urine, prostatic and vaginal secretions, fluid from bronchioalveolar lavage, and biopsy tissues of infected lesions, such as in the lung or the colon.

Antigen Detection

The HCMV antigen testing of blood (antigenemia) from patients suspected of having HCMV infection has been utilized to detect viral infection prior to onset of HCMV disease in high-risk, immunocompromised hosts, such as transplant recipients, and is utilized to initiate preemptive antiviral therapy for patients with antigenemia but without clinically apparent HCMV disease.[209,284–288] This assay utilizes a monoclonal antibody to detect HCMV proteins in circulating cells of the myeloid lineage, presumably detecting a systemic manifestation of an invasive infection. One limitation of this assay is the requirement for an adequate number of leukocytes to perform a valid test, which may be relevant in stem cell transplant populations prior to engraftment. Viral antigen staining by immunohistochemistry is also utilized to assess biopsies for virus-infected cells. Interpretation of the significance of immunohistochemical staining evidence of viral infection requires consideration of the clinical scenario for likelihood of HCMV end-organ disease, as infected cells have been described to express antigens in the setting of inflammation without the presence of HCMV-associated disease (eg, biopsies of inflamed intestinal lesions from patients with inflammatory bowel disease). Antigen testing is not routinely utilized for diagnosis of congenital HCMV infection.

Table 54-7 Diagnostic Approaches for Detection of Congenital Human Cytomegalovirus Infections

Diagnostic Approach	Advantages	Disadvantages
Virus isolation	Sensitive, specific	Time and labor intensive, maintenance of primary cells, specimens must be processed shortly after collection
Rapid culture with antibody detection of IE-1 protein	Rapid, specific, sensitivity approaches for virus isolation	Limited capacity for high throughput, requires maintenance of primary cells, specimens must be processed shortly after collection
Antigen detection in peripheral leukocytes (antigenemia)	Specific, quantifiable	Insensitive, dependent on sufficient number of leukocytes, specimens must be processed shortly after collection, takes time and expertise to complete assay
Nucleic acid detection (polymerase chain reaction)	Specific, sensitive, quantifiable, high throughput, specimens can be stored prior to assay	Sensitivity dependent on source of sample, contamination from specimens containing noninfectious virus, rigorous quality control, expensive
Cord blood cytomegalovirus-specific immunoglobulin M antibody assay	Rapid, simple assay, prognostic value	Limited sensitivity

Viral Nucleic Acid Detection (Polymerase Chain Reaction)

The PCR has replaced other techniques for nucleic acid detection and has been utilized to identify CMV infection in a wide variety of clinical settings. Currently, PCR assays represent the most commonly used approach for the diagnosis of HCMV infections. PCR testing has been shown to have similar sensitivity as rapid viral culture of saliva and urine for congenital HCMV infection in newborns.[7,289] Unfortunately, efforts to use PCR testing of dried blood spots for diagnosis of congenital HCMV infection have not demonstrated sufficient sensitivity in population-based screening to justify the use of this methodology for primary diagnosis of congenital HCMV infection.[289] PCR has also been used as an alternative to antigenemia testing in transplant recipients at risk for HCMV infection and disease as a monitoring strategy to initiate preemptive antiviral treatment. A number of variations of assay platforms, primers, and sample selection have been described; in general, most assays have similar specificity and sensitivity, with the source and type of clinical specimen the greatest cause of variability in assay performance.

Interferon-γ Release Assays

Recent interest has developed in assessing virus-specific lymphocyte responses as a correlate of protective immunity in immunocompromised patients. IFN-γ release assays, such as the Elispot® and the Quantiferon-CMV®, stimulate patient peripheral blood lymphocytes with viral proteins followed by measurement of IFN-γ production attributable to virus-specific lymphocytes. Such assays have been tested in research protocols for evidence of protective immunity in transplant populations but are not widely commercially available for clinical use at this time. These assays have not been utilized in the setting of congenital HCMV infection in a clinical study sufficiently powered to allow an assessment of their value.

MANAGEMENT

Introduction

The management of maternal and congenital CMV infections continues to be a contentious area among investigators, with limited data supporting the efficacy of therapeutic interventions and the natural history of this intrauterine infection arguing that many approaches may be limited by the delay in identification of patients who could benefit from treatment. Two approaches have been championed for the prevention of long-term neurological damage from this virus: (1) treatment of pregnant women undergoing a primary infection with goals of preventing fetal infection or limiting disease in the fetus and (2) treatment of the congenitally infected infant to limit the progression of CNS damage, a concept supported primarily by the high incidence of progressive hearing loss (and in some cases delayed hearing loss) in congenitally infected infants.

Treatment of congenitally infected infants with antiviral chemotherapeutic agents such as GCV has been accomplished and is justified by the rationale that reduction of virus replication could improve outcome, particularly in infants who could experience progressive CNS impairment. Conversely, treatment of pregnant women with currently available antiviral agents has not been universally accepted because of the uncertain efficacy of these agents in the developing fetus and, perhaps more important, the potential teratogenic effects of these agents in the developing fetus, including the possibility of fetal loss.

These possibilities must be considered in light of the excellent outcome of most maternal infections acquired during pregnancy, which is a likelihood that only 4%–7% of infected infants will develop sequelae secondary to a congenital HCMV infection. Thus, universal treatment of pregnant women undergoing a primary HCMV infection with a toxic agent such as GCV could result in significant disease unrelated to the congenital infection, perhaps with an incidence that exceeds that of congenital HCMV infection.

An alternative strategy that has been proposed involves identification of pregnant women undergoing primary HCMV infection using antibody screening and anti-CMV IgG avidity testing followed by invasive sampling around 20 weeks of gestation to identify infected fetuses.[41,43,46,47,197,290] Although such an approach does provide a rationale for the identification of infected fetuses for subsequent treatment, the delay in identification of an infected fetus until nearly the beginning of the third trimester of gestation could limit the efficacy of any treatment, especially when viewed in light of data that argue that the most damaging intrauterine HCMV infections appear to be associated with maternal seroconversions that take place in the early second trimester.[39]

More recently, attempts that have employed immunoglobulins and proposed treatments using human and humanized monoclonal antibodies directed at envelope glycoproteins of HCMV have been undertaken, with both treatment and prophylactic (prevention of infection) end points.

Treatment of Congenital CMV Infections During Pregnancy

Early studies demonstrated the potentially beneficial effects of antiviral antibodies that could be detected prior to conception in the outcome of the natural history of congenital HCMV infection.[11,291] These observational studies provided a framework for investigations of the role of protective antibodies in animal models of congenital and perinatal HCMV infections. As discussed previously, studies in the guinea pig model of congenital CMV infection and a more recent study in a mouse model of CNS infection following MCMV infection have clearly demonstrated that antiviral antibodies can limit infection and damage from intrauterine and perinatal CMV infection. Although the precise mechanism of such protection has not been defined, protection was correlated with the presence of virus-neutralizing antibodies.[214] In studies that pre-dated the studies of the role of antibodies in animal models of congenital CMV infections by decades, investigators demonstrated the protective activity of pooled human immunoglobulins containing substantial titers of antibodies reactive with HCMV in solid-organ transplant recipients.[292,293]

Together, these studies provided a strong rationale for the use of IVIG preparations in pregnant women with primary CMV infections to both interrupt transmission and possibly to treat established infections. The initial trial that studied the effects of IVIG treatment of pregnant women undergoing a primary CMV infection indicated that such treatment was both preventive and protective; however, this study was confounded by numerous methodological flaws, including lack of patient randomization.[212] As a result, the findings of the study have been viewed as provocative but far from definitive.

Recently, a well-controlled trial utilizing the same IVIG preparation used in the initial study was completed. This study was rigorous in its design, including its randomization at enrollment of study patients. The results of this study revealed no differences in the incidence of CMV infection in offspring between pregnant women with primary CMV infection who were treated with IVIG or left untreated (M. Grazi-Revello, personal communication). Whether the use of IVIG in these women will be associated with the modification of disease in infected infants has not been determined because of the need for additional follow-up patient visits. However, given the variability of disease in infected infants, it is unclear if this study was sufficiently powered to definitively address these questions.

The apparent lack of efficacy in the study described could be attributable to several possibilities, including the lack of a sufficiently potent virus-neutralizing response provided by the passively acquired antibodies. To circumvent this possibility, a number of potent virus-neutralizing monoclonal antibodies, including both humanized and human, have been developed. These antibodies have extraordinary virus-neutralizing activity and can be purified to near homogeneity. Although the activity of these antibodies in vitro has been extensively studied, their activity in vivo remains undefined and will likely require human trials as currently available animal models appear unsuitable to adequately establish the efficacy of individual antibodies.

Treatment with antiviral agents during pregnancy could represent an ideal strategy to limit virus replication in the pregnant women, thus limiting transmission and virus replication in the developing fetus infected in utero. Moreover, currently available antiviral agents are not licensed for use during pregnancy, and the agents with most activity against HCMV, including GCV, have documented teratogenic effects in animals. Thus, there is limited interest in this strategy. However, it should be noted that antiviral agents with some activity against HCMV have been given to pregnant women as treatment of HSV and varicella-zoster virus infections without evidence of adverse effects in the newborn infant.

A study carried out by investigators in France utilized valacyclovir in a maternal treatment protocol of fetuses determined to be HCMV infected by prenatal diagnosis.[294] Intrauterine infection was determined around 20 weeks of gestation, and treatment was begun at 28 weeks of gestation. The outcome was compared to a similar cohort of fetuses/infants who were diagnosed in utero with HCMV infection in women but who had received no treatment. The results suggested that therapeutic levels of drug could be achieved in the fetuses, and that outcome appeared similar in both groups, with about 50% of infants reported to have normal postnatal development without evidence of sequelae of the intrauterine infection. The authors argued that treatment had a favorable effect on the number of pregnancy terminations in the treated group as compared to the untreated group and suggested this could be evidence of some level of efficacy provided by this treatment.[294]

Treatment of Congenital HCMV Infection in the Perinatal Period and Infancy

The treatment of congenital HCMV infection has evolved from early studies utilizing acyclovir to a more recent clinical trial to determine the if the antiviral GCV could limit end-organ disease in symptomatically infected newborns with extension into an analysis of the effect of treatment on hearing loss in congenitally infected infants. Although the findings from the latter study suggested that treatment of infected infants with GCV during the perinatal period could limit end-organ disease and stabilize hearing loss, this study was not a controlled trial.[236] As a result, there continues to be reasonable skepticism of the validity of the findings from these studies, skepticism that it is hoped be eliminated when the results of a larger and more well-controlled trial using an oral formulation of GCV to treat congenitally infected infants becomes available.

However, widespread GCV treatment of congenitally infected infants has become routinely utilized at some institutions, and treatment continues to be instituted at the discretion of individual physicians. Fortunately, toxicity (primarily neutropenia) during treatment with GCV can be monitored and dosages modified to limit significant adverse events. Long-term toxicity, however, remains undefined, and risk-benefit comparisons should be considered when instituting treatment with this drug that has described teratogenic activity.

Treatment of infants with symptomatic congenital HCMV infections for 6 weeks with GCV administered by an intravenous route was shown to significantly reduce the quantity of virus excreted into the urine and in some infants result in clinical and laboratory improvement of end-organ disease such as hepatitis.[235] The follow-up evaluation of similarly treated infants revealed stabilization of hearing and improvement in auditory function in some patients.[236] These findings were based on comparison to the outcomes in a historical group of patients that served as the controls because the trial did not have a concomitantly enrolled control group. Even though this study can be criticized for the lack of control group, the small number of patients that necessitated treating the findings from individual ears as independent events, and the enrollment of only patients with symptomatic infections, the results from this study were pivotal and suggested that such an approach could modify the natural history of the most common long-term sequelae of this infection.

Subsequently, a larger and more well-controlled trial was initiated utilizing an oral formulation of valganciclovir to treat congenitally infected infants. Enrollment has been completed, and it is hoped there will be definitive information generated from this trial that can help guide the rational treatment of infants with congenital HCMV infections. GCV has also been used to treat infants with symptomatic infections associated with perinatally acquired HCMV, such as infections acquired from blood products, infections acquired in the intrapartum period, or those acquired from breast milk. Treatment of infants infected in the perinatal period with GCV has been shown to decrease levels of virus replication and in some cases has clearly limited the severity of end-organ disease. These are represented as case reports in the literature.

A limited number of newer antivirals with activity against HCMV have been developed, including analogues of cidovir, an inhibitor of the viral kinase, maribavir, and more recently an inhibitor of the viral terminase UL96. These agents have been tested primarily in immunocompromised adults, and at this time, it is uncertain if they will be evaluated for the treatment of infants with congenital HCMV infections.

PROGNOSIS

As has been described in previous sections, the prognosis of infants with congenital HCMV infections is often dictated by the infant's clinical presentation in the newborn period. Clinical evidence of symptomatic congenital infection increases risk for long-term sequelae. In previous studies and reviews, several authors have stated that over 60% of infants with symptomatic infections will develop long-term sequelae.[23,24,26,295] This rate is likely an overestimation secondary to a selection bias of infants with symptomatic infection who populated many of the early natural history studies of congenital HCMV infection. A more critical review of data from these studies has suggested that a significantly smaller number of infants with symptomatic HCMV infection detected by newborn screening and not through referral will develop long-term sequelae from this intrauterine infection (Ross, unpublished). Long-term sequelae are almost always secondary to CNS involvement, including abnormalities of vision and hearing.[36,38,246,247,296–298]

To date, there are no objective criteria that can be derived from routine laboratory examinations or from quantitative virologic studies that have allowed the identification of an individual infant who could be at risk for long-term sequelae. In contrast, several clinical findings and results from imaging studies of the CNS of congenitally infected infants have provided useful prognostic information (Table 54-8). Limited data suggest that infants with encephalitis as defined by abnormal findings in CSF are at higher risk for long-term neurological dysfunction.[23,24,28,29] Interestingly, the finding of chorioretinitis also increases the likelihood

Table 54-8 Prognostic Indicators of Long-Term Central Nervous System Sequelae in Infants With Congenital Human Cytomegalovirus Infections

Finding	Predictive Value (PV)
Symptomatic infection	Increased likelihood of developmental abnormalities and hearing loss
Microcephaly	Moderate PPV, strong NPV
Chorioretinitis	Moderate PPV, moderate-strong NPV
Seizures, motor deficits	Moderate PPV, strong NPV
Central nervous system imaging abnormalities	Moderate PPV, strong NPV

NPV, negative predictive value; PPV, positive predictive value.

of long-term sequelae in congenitally infected infants, a finding that likely reflects CNS involvement.[24,30]

Imaging findings, including CT and ultrasound, that demonstrate intracranial calcifications or structural abnormalities in the CNS have a moderate positive predictive value for abnormal long-term outcome in congenitally infected infants, but if normal, they have a very high negative predictive value.[24,245,299] Reported findings of MRI have been detailed previously and include pachygyria, cerebellar hypoplasia, ventriculomegaly secondary to thinning of the cortex, and less consistently white matter abnormalities. To date, these findings have been reported in studies of infants with an increased incidence of long-term sequelae but studies comparing outcomes in these infants to a screened population of infants who did not receive MRI for clinical indications is not available. Finally, high-resolution imaging of the temporal bone has been of limited value for identification of infants at risk for the development of hearing loss.

Since the beginning of the 2000s, there has been great interest in utilizing viral load measurements in the peripheral blood of congenitally infected infants to identify infants at risk for the development of sequelae following this intrauterine infection. Early studies argued that higher levels of viral DNA in the peripheral blood were more frequently detected in infants with symptomatic congenital infection, a finding that mirrored studies that were carried out over 3 decades ago.[61] Interestingly, similar results have been reported in studies that have described the viral load in blood of fetuses diagnosed in utero during prenatal evaluation of suspected HCMV infection. In both situations, there was selection bias for patients included in these studies because of the presence of symptoms in the infected newborn infant and, in the case of infected fetuses, secondary to the identification of primary maternal infection during pregnancy and diagnosis of an intrauterine infection. When the peripheral blood viral load was quantified in a large group of infected infants derived from a screened population, viral loads were indeed higher in symptomatic infants than infants with asymptomatic congenital infections; however, an absolute level of viral DNA in the peripheral blood could not be established that allowed identification of infants at risk for hearing loss.[33] Although several explanations could account for these findings, the viral burden in the peripheral blood may not reflect the severity of damage to the hearing apparatus. Alternatively, damage to the hearing apparatus could be secondary to host immune responses and be only indirectly related to viral burden in the cochlea. If so, it may be necessary to develop additional biomarkers that are directly related to cochlear damage.

REFERENCES

1. Renzette N, Bhattacharjee B, Jenson JD, Gibson L, Kowalik TF. Extensive genome-wide variability of human cytomegalovirus in congenitally infected infants. *PLoS Pathog.* 2011;7(5):e1001344.
2. Ross SA, Novak Z, Ashrith G, et al. Association between genital tract cytomegalovirus infection and bacterial vaginosis. *J Infect Dis.* 2005;192(10):1727–1730.
3. Ross SA, Novak Z, Pati S, et al. Mixed infection and strain diversity in congenital cytomegalovirus infection. *J Infect Dis.* 2011;204(7):1003–1007.
4. Yamamoto AY, Mussi-Pinhata MM, Boppana SB, et al. Human cytomegalovirus reinfection is associated with intrauterine transmission in a highly cytomegalovirus-immune maternal population. *Am J Obstet Gynecol.* 2010;202(3):297.e291–e298.
5. Boppana SB, Rivera LB, Fowler KB, Mach M, Britt WJ. Intrauterine transmission of cytomegalovirus to infants of women with preconceptional immunity. *N Engl J Med.* 2001;344(18):1366–1371.
6. Bale JF Jr, Petheram SJ, Souza IE, Murph JR. Cytomegalovirus reinfection in young children. *J Pediatr.* 1996;128(3):347–352.
7. Boppana SB, Ross SA, Shimamura M, et al. Saliva polymerase-chain-reaction assay for congenital cytomegalovirus screening in newborns. *N Engl J Med.* 2011;364:2111–2118.
8. Britt WJ. Cytomegalovirus. In: Remington JS, Klein JO, Wilson CB, Nizet V, Maldonaldo Y, eds. *Infectious Diseases of the Fetus and Newborn Infant.* 7th ed. Philadelphia, PA: Elsevier Saunders; 2010:706–755.
9. Stagno S, Pass RF, Dworsky ME, Alford CA. Congenital and perinatal cytomegaloviral infections. *Semin Perinatol.* 1983;7:31–42.
10. Stagno S, Dworsky ME, Torres J, Mesa T, Hirsh T. Prevalence and importance of congenital cytomegalovirus infection in three different populations. *J Pediatr.* 1982;101(6):897–900.
11. Stagno S, Pass RF, Dworsky ME, et al. Congenital cytomegalovirus infection: The relative importance of primary and recurrent maternal infection. *N Engl J Med.* 1982;306(16):945–949.
12. Stagno S, Pass RF, Dworsky ME, Alford CA. Maternal cytomegalovirus infection and perinatal transmission. *Clin Obstet Gynecol.* 1982;25:563–576.
13. Fowler KB, Stagno S, Pass RF. Maternal age and congenital cytomegalovirus infection: screening of two diverse newborn populations, 1980–1990. *J Infect Dis.* 1993;168:552–556.
14. Rubella and congenital rubella syndrome—United States, January 1, 1991–May 7, 1994. *MMWR Morb Mortal Wkly Rep.* 1994;43:391–401.
15. Alford CA. Chronic intrauterine and perinatal infections. In: Galasso GJ, Merigan TC, Buchanan RA, eds. *Antiviral Agents and Viral Diseases of Man.* 2nd ed. New York, NY: Raven Press; 1984:433–486.
16. Stagno S, Pass RF, Dworsky ME, Alford CA. Congenital and perinatal cytomegalovirus infections. *Semin Perinatol.* 1983;7(1):31–42.
17. Schopfer K, Lauber E, Krech U. Congenital cytomegalovirus infection in newborn infants of mothers infected before pregnancy. *Arch Dis Child.* 1978;53:536–539.
18. van der Sande MAB, Kaye S, Miles DJC, et al. Risk factors for and clinical outcome of congenital cytomegalovirus infection in a peri-urban West-African birth cohort. *PLoS One.* 2007;2(6):e492.
19. Mussi-Pinhata MM, Yamamoto AY, Moura-Britto RM, Lima-Issacs M, Boppana S, Britt WJ. Birth prevalence and natural history of congenital cytomegalovirus (CMV) infection in highly seroimmune population. *Clin Infect Dis.* 2009;49:522–528.
20. Dar L, Pati SK, Patro AR, et al. Congenital cytomegalovirus infection in a highly seropositive semi-urban population in India. *Pediatr Infect Dis J.* 2008;27(9):841–843.

21. Yamamoto AP, Mussi-Pinhata MM, Pinto PC, Figueiredo LT, Jorge SM. Congenital cytomegalovirus infection in preterm and full-term newborn infants from a population with a high seroprevalence rate. *Pediatr Infect Dis J.* 2001;20(2):188–192.

22. Britt W. Cytomegalovirus. In: Remington JS, Klein JO, Wilson C, Nizet V, Maldonado YA, eds. *Infectious Diseases of the Fetus and Newborn Infant.* 7th ed. Philadelphia, PA: Elsevier Saunders; 2010:706–756.

23. Boppana SB, Pass RF, Britt WJ, Stagno S, Alford CA. Symptomatic congenital cytomegalovirus infection: neonatal morbidity and mortality. *Pediatr Infect Dis J.* 1992;11:93–99.

24. Noyola DE, Demmler GJ, Nelson CT, et al. Early predictors of neurodevelopmental outcome in symptomatic congenital CMV infection. *J Pediatr.* 2001;138(3):325–331.

25. Stagno S. Cytomegalovirus infection: a pediatrician's perspective. *Curr Probl Pediatr.* 1986;16(11):629–667.

26. Kenneson A, Cannon MJ. Review and meta-analysis of the epidemiology of congenital cytomegalovirus (CMV) infection. *Rev Med Virol.* 2007;17(4):253–276.

27. Pass RF, Stagno S, Myers GJ, Alford CA. Outcome of symptomatic congenital cytomegalovirus infection: results of long-term longitudinal follow-up. *Pediatrics.* 1980;66(5):758–762.

28. Alarcon A, Garcia-Alix A, Cabanas F, et al. Beta2-microglobulin concentrations in cerebrospinal fluid correlate with neuroimaging findings in newborns with symptomatic congenital cytomegalovirus infection. *Eur J Pediatr.* 2006;165(9):636–645.

29. Troendle Atkins J, Demmler GJ, Williamson WD, McDonald JM, Istas AS, Buffone GJ. Polymerase chain reaction to detect cytomegalovirus DNA in the cerebrospinal fluid of neonates with congenital infection. *J Infect Dis.* 1994;169(6):1334–1337.

30. Conboy TJ, Pass RF, Stagno S, et al. Early clinical manifestations and intellectual outcome in children with symptomatic congenital cytomegalovirus infection. *J Pediatr.* 1987;111:343–348.

31. Boppana SB, Fowler KB, Pass RF, et al. Congenital cytomegalovirus infection: association between virus burden in infancy and hearing loss. *J Pediatr.* 2005;146(6):817–823.

32. Lanari M, Lazzarotto T, Venturi V, et al. Neonatal cytomegalovirus blood load and risk of sequelae in symptomatic and asymptomatic congenitally infected newborns. *Pediatrics.* 2006;117(1):e76–e83.

33. Ross SA, Novak Z, Fowler KB, Arora N, Britt WJ, Boppana SB. Cytomegalovirus blood viral load and hearing loss in young children with congenital infection. *Pediatr Infect Dis J.* 2009;28(7):588–592.

34. Williamson WD, Demmler GJ, Percy AK, Catlin FI. Progressive hearing loss in infants with asymptomatic congenital cytomegalovirus infection. *Pediatrics.* 1992;90:862–866.

35. Rivera LB, Boppana SB, Fowler KB, Britt WJ, Stagno S, Pass RF. Predictors of hearing loss in children with symptomatic congenital cytomegalovirus infection. *Pediatrics.* 2002;110(4):762–767.

36. Dahle AJ, Fowler KB, Wright JD, Boppana SB, Britt WJ, Pass RF. Longitudinal investigation of hearing disorders in children with congenital cytomegalovirus. *J Am Acad Audiol.* 2000;11(5):283–290.

37. Fowler KB, Dahle AJ, Boppana SB, Pass RF. Newborn hearing screening: will children with hearing loss caused by congenital cytomegalovirus infection be missed? *J Pediatr.* 1999;135(1):60–64.

38. Fowler KB, McCollister FP, Dahle AJ, Boppana S, Britt WJ, Pass RF. Progressive and fluctuating sensorineural hearing loss in children with asymptomatic congenital cytomegalovirus infection. *J Pediatr.* 1997;130(4):624–630.

39. Enders G, Daiminger A, Bader U, Exler S, Enders M. Intrauterine transmission and clinical outcome of 248 pregnancies with primary cytomegalovirus infection in relation to gestational age. *J Clin Virol.* 2011;52(3):244–246.

40. Stagno S, Pass RF, Cloud G, et al. Primary cytomegalovirus infection in pregnancy. Incidence, transmission to fetus, and clinical outcome. *JAMA.* 1986;256:1904–1908.

41. Revello MG, Lilleri D, Zavattoni M, Furione M, Middeldorp J, Gerna G. Prenatal diagnosis of congenital human cytomegalovirus infection in amniotic fluid by nucleic acid sequence-based amplification assay. *J Clin Microbiol.* 2003;41(4):1772–1774.

42. Revello MG, Zavattoni M, Furione M, Lilleri D, Gorini G, Gerna G. Diagnosis and outcome of preconceptional and periconceptional primary human cytomegalovirus infections. *J Infect Dis.* 2002;186(4):553–557.

43. Revello MG, Gerna G. Diagnosis and management of human cytomegalovirus infection in the mother, fetus, and newborn infant. *Clin Microbiol Rev.* 2002;15(4):680–715.

44. Gindes L, Teperberg-Oikawa M, Sherman D, Pardo J, Rahav G. Congenital cytomegalovirus infection following primary maternal infection in the third trimester. *BJOG.* 2008;115(7):830–835.

45. Pass RF, Fowler KB, Boppana SB, Britt WJ, Stagno S. Congenital cytomegalovirus infection following first trimester maternal infection: symptoms at birth and outcome. *J Clin Virol.* 2006;35(2):216–220.

46. Bodeus M, Kabamba-Mukadi B, Zech F, et al. Human cytomegalovirus in utero transmission: follow-up of 524 maternal seroconversions. *J Clin Virol.* 2009;47(2):201–202.

47. Bodeus M, Hubinont C, Bernard P, Bouckaert A, Thomas K, Goubau P. Prenatal diagnosis of human cytomegalovirus by culture and polymerase chain reaction: 98 pregnancies leading to congenital infection. *Prenat Diagn.* 1999;19(4):314–317.

48. Alford CA, Hayes K, Britt WJ. Primary cytomegalovirus infection in pregnancy: comparison of antibody responses to virus encoded proteins between women with and without intrauterine infection. *J Infect Dis.* 1988;158:917–924.

49. Pass RF, Stagno S, Dworsky ME, Smith RJ, Alford CA. Excretion of cytomegalovirus in mothers: observations after delivery of congenitally infected and normal infants. *J Infect Dis.* 1982;146(1):1–6.

50. Stagno S, Reynolds DW, Pass RF, Alford CA. Breast milk and the risk of cytomegalovirus infection. *N Engl J Med.* 1980;302:1073–1076.

51. Lilleri D, Fornara C, Furione M, Zavattoni M, Revello MG, Gerna G. Development of human cytomegalovirus-specific T cell immunity during primary infection of pregnant women and its correlation with virus transmission to the fetus. *J Infect Dis.* 2007;195(7):1062–1070.

52. Boppana SB, Britt WJ. Antiviral antibody responses and intrauterine transmission after primary maternal cytomegalovirus infection. *J Infect Dis.* 1995;171:1115–1121.

53. Stagno S, Reynolds DW, Huang E-S, Thames SD, Smith RJ, Alford CA. Congenital cytomegalovirus infection: occurrence in an immune population. *N Engl J Med.* 1977;296:1254–1258.

54. Adler SP, Nigro G, Pereira L. Recent advances in the prevention and treatment of congenital cytomegalovirus infections. *Semin Perinatol.* 2007;31(1):10–18.

55. Boppana SB, Fowler KB, Britt WJ, Stagno S, Pass RF. Symptomatic congenital cytomegalovirus infection in infants born to mothers with preexisting immunity to cytomegalovirus. *Pediatrics.* 1999;104(1 Pt 1):55–60.

56. Ross SA, Fowler KB, Guha A, et al. Hearing loss in children with congenital cytomegalovirus infection born to mothers with preexisting immunity. *J Pediatr.* 2006;148:332–336.

57. Ahlfors K, Ivarsson SA, Harris S. Secondary maternal cytomegalovirus infection—a significant cause of congenital disease. *Pediatrics.* 2001;107(5):1227–1228.

58. Yamamoto AY, Mussi-Pinhata MM, Isaac MDL, et al. Congenital cytomegalovirus infection as a cause of sensorineural hearing loss in a highly seropositive population. *Ped Infect Dis J*. 2011;30(12):1043–1046.

59. Pass RF, Johnson J, Anderson B. Congenital cytomegalovirus infection: impairment and immunization. Prevention of maternal and congenital cytomegalovirus infection. *J Infect Dis*. 2007;195(6):767–769.

60. Nigro G, Adler SP. Cytomegalovirus infections during pregnancy. *Curr Opin Obstet Gynecol*. 2011;23(2):123–128.

61. Stagno S, Reynolds DW, Tsiantos A, Fuccillo DA, Long W, Alford CA. Comparative serial virologic and serologic studies of symptomatic and subclinical congenitally and natally acquired cytomegalovirus infections. *J Infect Dis*. 1975;132(5):568–577.

62. Pass RF, Hutto C, Reynolds DW, Polhill RB. Increased frequency of cytomegalovirus in children in group day care. *Pediatrics*. 1984;74:121–126.

63. Pass RF, Stagno S, Britt WJ, Alford CA. Specific cell-mediated immunity and the natural history of congenital infection with cytomegalovirus. *J Infect Dis*. 1983;148(6):953–961.

64. Pass RF, Kinney JS. Child care workers and children with congenital cytomegalovirus infection. *Pediatrics*. 1985;75:971–973.

65. Fowler KB, Pass RF. Risk factors for congenital cytomegalovirus infection in the offspring of young women: exposure to young children and recent onset of sexual activity. *Pediatrics*. 2006;118(2):e286–e292.

66. Fowler KB, Pass RF, Stagno S. Young children as a source of maternal cytomegalovirus infection in young nonwhite urban women. Paper presented at Society for Pediatric Epidemiological Research 10th annual meeting; June 10–11, 1997; Edmonton, Alberta, Canada.

67. Fowler KB, Pass RF, Stagno S. Pre-school children as a source of maternal cytomegalovirus infection in young black women [abstract]. *Pediatr Res*. 1998;43(4):145A.

68. Adler SP. Cytomegalovirus and child day care: risk factors for maternal infection. *Pediatr Infect Dis J*. 1991;10:590.

69. Dworsky ME, Welch K, Cassady G, Stagno S. Occupational risk for primary cytomegalovirus infection among pediatric health-care workers. *N Engl J Med*. 1983;309(16):950–953.

70. Pass RF, Little EA, Stagno S, Britt WJ, Alford CA. Young children as a probable source of maternal and congenital cytomegalovirus infection. *N Engl J Med*. 1987;316:1366–1370.

71. Balcarek KB, Bagley R, Cloud GA, Pass RF. Cytomegalovirus infection among employees of a children's hospital: no evidence for increased risk associated with patient care. *JAMA*. 1990;263:840–844.

72. Chandler SH, Holmes KK, Wentworth BB, et al. The epidemiology of cytomegaloviral infection in women attending a sexually transmitted disease clinic. *J Infect Dis*. 1985;152:597–605.

73. Collier AC, Handsfield HH, Roberts PL, et al. Cytomegalovirus infection in women attending a sexually transmitted disease clinic. *J Infect Dis*. 1990;162:46–51.

74. Handsfield HH, Chandler SH, Caine VA, et al. Cytomegalovirus infection in sex partners: evidence for sexual transmission. *J Infect Dis*. 1985;151:344–348.

75. Drew WL, Mintz L. Cytomegalovirus infection in healthy and immune-deficient homosexual men. In: Ma P, Armstrong D, eds. *The Acquired Immune Deficiency Syndrome and Infections of Homosexual Men*. New York, NY: Yorke Medical Books; 1984:117–123.

76. Drew WL, Mintz L, Miner RC, Sands M, Ketterer B. Prevalence of cytomegalovirus infection in homosexual men. *J Infect Dis*. 1981;143:188–192.

77. Fowler KB, Pass RF. Sexually transmitted diseases in mothers of neonates with congenital cytomegalovirus infection. *J Infect Dis*. 1991;164:259–264.

78. Vauloup-Fellous C, Picone O, Cordier AG, et al. Does hygiene counseling have an impact on the rate of CMV primary infection during pregnancy? Results of a 3-year prospective study in a French hospital. *J Clin Virol*. 2009;46(Suppl 4):S49–S53.

79. Cannon MJ, Davis KF. Washing our hands of the congenital cytomegalovirus disease epidemic. *BMC Public Health*. 2005;5:70.

80. Adler SP, Starr SE, Plotkin SA, et al. Immunity induced by primary human cytomegalovirus infection protects against secondary infection among women of childbearing age. *J Infect Dis*. 1995;171:26–32.

81. Gallant JE, Moore RD, Richman DD, Keruly J, Chaisson RE. Incidence and natural history of cytomegalovirus disease in patients with advanced human immunodeficiency virus disease treated with zidovudine. The Zidovudine Epidemiology Study Group. *J Infect Dis*. 1992;166(6):1223–1227.

82. Sylwester AW, Mitchell BL, Edgar JB, et al. Broadly targeted human cytomegalovirus-specific CD4+ and CD8+ T cells dominate the memory compartments of exposed subjects. *J Exp Med*. 2005;202(5):673–685.

83. Jonjic S, Babic M, Polic B, Krmpotic A. Immune evasion of natural killer cells by viruses. *Curr Opin Immunol*. 2008;20(1):30–38.

84. Scalzo AA, Corbett AJ, Rawlinson WD, et al. The interplay between host and viral factors in shaping the outcome of cytomegalovirus infection. *Immunol Cell Biol*. 2007;85(1):46–54.

85. Lemmermann NA, Bohm V, Holtappels R, et al. In vivo impact of cytomegalovirus evasion of CD8 T-cell immunity: facts and thoughts based on murine models. *Virus Res*. 2007;157(2):161–174.

86. Pyzik M, Gendron-Pontbriand EM, Fodil-Cornu N, et al. Self or nonself? That is the question: sensing of cytomegalovirus infection by innate immune receptors. *Mamm Genome*. 2008;22(1–2):6–18.

87. Babic M, Krmpotic A, Jonjic S. All is fair in virus-host interactions: NK cells and cytomegalovirus. *Trends Mol Med*. 2011;17(11):677–685.

88. Hendrix MG, Daemen M, Bruggeman CA. Cytomegalovirus nucleic acid distribution within the human vascular tree. *Am J Pathol*. 1991;138(3):563–567.

89. Hendrix MG, Dormans PH, Kitslaar P, Bosman F, Bruggeman CA. The presence of cytomegalovirus nucleic acids in arterial walls of atherosclerotic and nonatherosclerotic patients. *Am J Pathol*. 1989;134(5):1151–1157.

90. Bowden RA, Slichter SJ, Sayers MH, Mori M, Cays MJ, Meyers JD. Use of leukocyte-depleted platelets and cytomegalovirus-seronegative red blood cells for prevention of primary cytomegalovirus infection after marrow transplant. *Blood*. 1991;78(1):246–520.

91. Pietersz RN, van der Meer PF, Seghatchian MJ. Update on leucocyte depletion of blood components by filtration. *Transfus Sci*. 1998;19(4):321–328.

92. Theiler RN, Caliendo AM, Pargman S, et al. Umbilical cord blood screening for cytomegalovirus DNA by quantitative PCR. *J Clin Virol*. 2006;37(4):313–316.

93. Thiele T, Kruger W, Zimmermann K, et al. Transmission of cytomegalovirus (CMV) infection by leukoreduced blood products not tested for CMV antibodies: a single-center prospective study in high-risk patients undergoing allogeneic hematopoietic stem cell transplantation (CME). *Transfusion*. 2011;51(12):2620–2626.

94. Josephson CD, Castillejo MI, Caliendo AM, et al. Prevention of transfusion-transmitted cytomegalovirus in low-birth weight infants (≤1500 g) using cytomegalovirus-seronegative and leukoreduced transfusions. *Transfus Med Rev*. 2011;25(2):125–132.

95. Smith D, Lu Q, Yuan S, Goldfinger D, Fernando LP, Ziman A. Survey of current practice for prevention of transfusion-transmitted cytomegalovirus in the United States: leucoreduction vs. cytomegalovirus-seronegative. *Vox Sang*. 2009;98(1):29–36.

96. Yeager AS. Transfusion-acquired cytomegalovirus infection in newborn infants. *Am J Dis Child*. 1974;128:478–483.

97. Yeager AS, Grumet FC, Hafleigh EB, Arvin AM, Bradley JS, Prober CG. Prevention of transfusion-acquired cytomegalovirus infections in newborn infants. *J Pediatr*. 1981;98:281–287.

98. Adler SP. Transfusion-associated cytomegalovirus infections. *Rev Infect Dis*. 1983;5:977–993.

99. Goodrum F, Jordan CT, Terhune SS, High K, Shenk T. Differential outcomes of human cytomegalovirus infection in primitive hematopoietic cell subpopulations. *Blood*. 2004;104(3):687–695.

100. Goodrum F, Reeves M, Sinclair J, High K, Shenk T. Human cytomegalovirus sequences expressed in latently infected individuals promote a latent infection in vitro. *Blood*. 2007;110(3):937–945.

101. Smith MS, Goldman DC, Bailey AS, et al. Granulocyte-colony stimulating factor reactivates human cytomegalovirus in a latently infected humanized mouse model. *Cell Host Microbe*. 2010;8(3):284–291.

102. Mendelson M, Monard S, Sissons P, Sinclair J. Detection of endogenous human cytomegalovirus in CD34+ bone marrow progenitors. *J Gen Virol*. 1996;77(Pt 12):3099–3102.

103. Khoury JA, Storch GA, Bohl DL, et al. Prophylactic versus preemptive oral valganciclovir for the management of cytomegalovirus infection in adult renal transplant recipients. *Am J Transplant*. 2006;6(9):2134–2143.

104. Witzke O, Hauser IA, Bartels M, Wolf G, Wolters H, Nitschke M. Valganciclovir prophylaxis versus preemptive therapy in cytomegalovirus-positive renal allograft recipients: 1-year results of a randomized clinical trial. *Transplantation*. 2012;93(1):61–68.

105. Razonable RR. Cytomegalovirus infection after liver transplantation: current concepts and challenges. *World J Gastroenterol*. 2008;14(31):4849–4860.

106. Hahn G, Revello MG, Patrone M, et al. Human cytomegalovirus UL131-128 genes are indispensable for virus growth in endothelial cells and virus transfer to leukocytes. *J Virol*. 2004;78(18):10023–10033.

107. Ryckman BJ, Jarvis MA, Drummond DD, Nelson JA, Johnson DC. Human cytomegalovirus entry into epithelial and endothelial cells depends on genes UL128 to UL150 and occurs by endocytosis and low-pH fusion. *J Virol*. 2006;80(2):710–722.

108. Ryckman BJ, Rainish BL, Chase MC, et al. Characterization of the human cytomegalovirus gH/gL/UL128–131 complex that mediates entry into epithelial and endothelial cells. *J Virol*. 2008;82(1):60–70.

109. Huber MT, Compton T. Characterization of a novel third member of the human cytomegalovirus glycoprotein H-glycoprotein L complex. *J Virol*. 1997;71(7):5391–5398.

110. Huber MT, Compton T. The human cytomegalovirus UL74 gene encodes the third component of the glycoprotein H-glycoprotein L-containing envelope complex. *J Virol*. 1998;72(10):8191–8197.

111. Huber MT, Compton T. Intracellular formation and processing of the heterotrimeric gH-gL-gO (gCIII) glycoprotein envelope complex of human cytomegalovirus. *J Virol*. 1999;73(5):3886–3892.

112. Li L, Nelson JA, Britt WJ. Glycoprotein H related complexes of human cytomegalovirus: identification of a third protein in the gCIII complex. *J Virol*. 1997;71:3090–3097.

113. Ryckman BJ, Chase MC, Johnson DC. Human cytomegalovirus TR strain glycoprotein O acts as a chaperone promoting gH/gL incorporation into virions but is not present in virions. *J Virol*. 2010;84(5):2597–2609.

114. Compton T. Receptors and immune sensors: the complex entry path of human cytomegalovirus. *Trends Cell Biol*. 2004;14(1):5–8.

115. Compton T, Nepomuceon RR, Nowlin DM. Human cytomegalovirus penetrates host cells by pH-independent fusion at the cell surface. *Virology*. 1992;191:387–395.

116. Netterwald JR, Jones TR, Britt WJ, Yang SJ, McCrone IP, Zhu H. Postattachment events associated with viral entry are necessary for induction of interferon-stimulated genes by human cytomegalovirus. *J Virol*. 2004;78(12):6688–6691.

117. Zhu H, Cong JP, Mamtora G, Gingeras T, Shenk T. Cellular gene expression altered by human cytomegalovirus: global monitoring with oligonucleotide arrays. *Proc Natl Acad Sci USA*. 1998;95(24):14470–14475.

118. Simmen KA, Singh J, Luukkonen BG, et al. Global modulation of cellular transcription by human cytomegalovirus is initiated by viral glycoprotein B. *Proc Natl Acad Sci USA*. 2001;98(13):7140–7145.

119. DeFilippis VR, Sali T, Alvarado D, White L, Bresnahan W, Fruh KJ. Activation of the interferon response by human cytomegalovirus occurs via cytoplasmic double-stranded DNA but not glycoprotein B. *J Virol*. 2010;84(17):8913–8925.

120. Browne EP, Wing B, Coleman D, Shenk T. Altered cellular mRNA levels in human cytomegalovirus-infected fibroblasts: viral block to the accumulation of antiviral mRNAs. *J Virol*. 2001;75(24):12319–12330.

121. Sacher T, Podlech J, Mohr CA, et al. The major virus-producing cell type during murine cytomegalovirus infection, the hepatocyte, is not the source of virus dissemination in the host. *Cell Host Microbe*. 2008;3(4):263–272.

122. Sacher T, Andrassy J, Kalnins A, et al. Shedding light on the elusive role of endothelial cells in cytomegalovirus dissemination. *PLoS Pathog*. 2011;7(11):e1002366.

123. Bowen EF, Wilson P, Atkins M, et al. Natural history of untreated cytomegalovirus retinitis. *Lancet*. 1995;346(8991–8992):1671–1673.

124. Bowen EF, Wilson P, Cope A, et al. Cytomegalovirus retinitis in AIDS patients: influence of cytomegaloviral load on response to ganciclovir, time to recurrence and survival. *AIDS*. 1996;10(13):1515–1520.

125. Spector SA, Wong R, Hsia K, Pilcher M, Stempien MJ. Plasma cytomegalovirus (CMV) DNA load predicts CMV disease and survival in AIDS patients. *J Clin Invest*. 1998;101(2):497–502.

126. Komanduri KV, Viswanathan MN, Wieder ED, et al. Restoration of cytomegalovirus-specific CD4+ T-lymphocyte responses after ganciclovir and highly active antiretroviral therapy in individuals infected with HIV-1. *Nat Med*. 1998;4(8):953–956.

127. Autran B, Carcelain G, LiTS, et al. Positive effects of combined antiretroviral therapy on CD4+ T cell homeostasis and function in advanced HIV disease. *Science*. 1997;277(5322):112–116.

128. Sinclair J, Sissons P. Latent and persistent infections of monocytes and macrophages. *Intervirology*. 1996;39(5–6):293–301.

129. Taylor-Wiedeman J, Sissons JG, Borysiewicz LK, Sinclair JH. Monocytes are a major site of persistence of human cytomegalovirus in peripheral blood mononuclear cells. *J Gen Virol*. 1991;72(Pt 9):2059–2064.

130. Soderberg-Naucler C, Fish KN, Nelson JA. Reactivation of latent human cytomegalovirus by allogeneic stimulation of blood cells from healthy donors. *Cell*. 1997;91(1):119–126.

131. Kondo K, Xu J, Mocarski ES. Human cytomegalovirus latent gene expression in granulocyte-macrophage progenitors in culture and in seropositive individuals. *Proc Natl Acad Sci USA*. 1996;93(20):11137–11142.

132. Noda S, Aguirre SA, Bitmansour A, et al. Cytomegalovirus MCK-2 controls mobilization and recruitment of myeloid progenitor cells to facilitate dissemination. *Blood*. 2006;107(1):30–38.

133. Stoddart CA, Cardin RD, Boname JM, Manning WC, Abenes GB, Mocarski ES. Peripheral blood mononuclear phagocytes mediate dissemination of murine cytomegalovirus. *J Virol.* 1994;68(10):6243–6253.

134. Luttichau HR. The cytomegalovirus UL146 gene product vCXCL1 targets both CXCR1 and CXCR2 as an agonist. *J Biol Chem.* 2009;285(12):9137–9146.

135. Hamprecht K, Vochem M, Baumeister A, Boniek M, Speer CP, Jahn G. Detection of cytomegaloviral DNA in human milk cells and cell free milk whey by nested PCR. *J Virol Method.* 1998;70:167–176.

136. Dworsky M, Yow M, Stagno S, Pass RF, Alford CA. Cytomegalovirus infection of breast milk and transmission in infancy. *Pediatrics.* 1983;72:295–299.

137. Jobe AH. CMV transmission in human milk. *J Pediatr.* 2009;154(6):A1.

138. Neuberger P, Hamprecht K, Vochem M, et al. Case-control study of symptoms and neonatal outcome of human milk-transmitted cytomegalovirus infection in premature infants. *J Pediatr.* 2006;148(3):326–331.

139. Miron D, Brosilow S, Felszer K, et al. Incidence and clinical manifestations of breast milk-acquired Cytomegalovirus infection in low birth weight infants. *J Perinatol.* 2005;25(5):299–303.

140. Capretti MG, Lanari M, Lazzarotto T, et al. Very low birth weight infants born to cytomegalovirus-seropositive mothers fed with their mother's milk: a prospective study. *J Pediatr.* 2009;154(6):842–848.

141. Fischer C, Meylan P, Bickle Graz M, et al. Severe postnatally acquired cytomegalovirus infection presenting with colitis, pneumonitis and sepsis-like syndrome in an extremely low birthweight infant. *Neonatology.* 2009;97(4):339–345.

142. Hamprecht K, Maschmann J, Jahn G, Poets CF, Goelz R. Cytomegalovirus transmission to preterm infants during lactation. *J Clin Virol.* 2008;41(3):198–205.

143. Halwachs-Baumann G, Wilders-Truschnig M, Desoye G, et al. Human trophoblast cells are permissive to the complete replicative cycle of human cytomegalovirus. *J Virol.* 1998;72(9):7598–7602.

144. Fisher S, Genbacev O, Maidji E, Pereira L. Human cytomegalovirus infection of placental cytotrophoblasts in vitro and in utero: implications for transmission and pathogenesis. *J Virol.* 2000;74(15):6808–6820.

145. Hemmings DG, Kilani R, Nykiforuk C, Preiksaitis J, Guilbert LJ. Permissive cytomegalovirus infection of primary villous term and first trimester trophoblasts. *J Virol.* 1998;72(6):4970–4979.

146. Iwasenko JM, Howard J, Arbuckle S, et al. Human cytomegalovirus infection is detected frequently in stillbirths and is associated with fetal thrombotic vasculopathy. *J Infect Dis.* 2011;203(11):1526–1533.

147. Ozono K, Mushiake S, Takeshima T, Nakayama M. Diagnosis of congenital cytomegalovirus infection by examination of placenta: application of polymerase chain reaction and in situ hybridization. *Pediatr Pathol Lab Med.* 1997;17(2):249–258.

148. Pereira L, Maidji E, McDonagh S, Tabata T. Insights into viral transmission at the uterine-placental interface. *Trends Microbiol.* 2005;13(4):164–174.

149. Kumazaki K, Ozono K, Yahara T, et al. Detection of cytomegalovirus DNA in human placenta. *J Med Virol.* 2002;68(3):363–369.

150. Sinzger C, Muntefering H, Loning T, Stoss H, Plachter B, Jahn G. Cell types infected in human cytomegalovirus placentitis identified by immunohistochemical double staining. *Virchows Arch A Pathol Anat Histopathol.* 1993;423(4):249–256.

151. McDonagh S, Maidji E, Chang HT, Pereira L. Patterns of human cytomegalovirus infection in term placentas: a preliminary analysis. *J Clin Virol.* 2006;35(2):210–215.

152. Maidji E, Percivalle E, Gerna G, Fisher S, Pereira L. Transmission of human cytomegalovirus from infected uterine microvascular endothelial cells to differentiating/invasive placental cytotrophoblasts. *Virology.* 2002;304(1):53–69.

153. Maidji E, Genbacev O, Chang HT, Pereira L. Developmental regulation of human cytomegalovirus receptors in cytotrophoblasts correlates with distinct replication sites in the placenta. *J Virol.* 2007;81(9):4701–4712.

154. Kovacs IJ, Hegedus K, Pal A, Pusztai R. Production of proinflammatory cytokines by syncytiotrophoblasts infected with human cytomegalovirus isolates. *Placenta.* 2007;28(7):620–623.

155. Scott GM, Chow SS, Craig ME, et al. Cytomegalovirus infection during pregnancy with maternofetal transmission induces a proinflammatory cytokine bias in placenta and amniotic fluid. *J Infect Dis.* 15;205(8):1305–1310.

156. Nozawa N, Fang-Hoover J, Tabata T, Maidji E, Pereira L. Cytomegalovirus-specific, high-avidity IgG with neutralizing activity in maternal circulation enriched in the fetal bloodstream. *J Clin Virol.* 2009;46(Suppl 4):S58–S63.

157. Maidji E, McDonagh S, Genbacev O, Tabata T, Pereira L. Maternal antibodies enhance or prevent cytomegalovirus infection in the placenta by neonatal Fc receptor-mediated transcytosis. *Am J Pathol.* 2006;168(4):1210–1226.

158. Tabata T, Kawakatsu H, Maidji E, et al. Induction of an epithelial integrin alphavbeta6 in human cytomegalovirus-infected endothelial cells leads to activation of transforming growth factor-beta1 and increased collagen production. *Am J Pathol.* 2008;172(4):1127–1140.

159. La Torre R, Nigro G, Mazzocco M, Best AM, Adler SP. Placental enlargement in women with primary maternal cytomegalovirus infection is associated with fetal and neonatal disease. *Clin Infect Dis.* 2006;43(8):994–1000.

160. Pereira L, Maidji E. Cytomegalovirus infection in the human placenta: maternal immunity and developmentally regulated receptors on trophoblasts converge. *Curr Top Microbiol Immunol.* 2008;325:383–395.

161. Medearis DN. Observations concerning human cytomegalovirus infection and disease. *Bull Johns Hopkins Med J.* 1964;114:181–211.

162. Medearis DN. Viral infections during pregnancy and abnormal human development. *Am J Obstet Gynecol.* 1964;90:1140–1148.

163. Bia FJ, Griffith BP, Fong CK, Hsiung GD. Cytomegaloviral infections in the guinea pig: experimental models for human disease. *Rev Infect Dis.* 1983;5(2):177–195.

164. Griffith BP, McCormick SR, Booss J, Hsiung GD. Inbred guinea pig model of intrauterine infection with cytomegalovirus. *Am J Pathol.* 1986;122(1):112–119.

165. Griffith BP, McCormick SR, Fong CK, Lavallee JT, Lucia HL, Goff E. The placenta as a site of cytomegalovirus infection in guinea pigs. *J Virol.* 1985;55:402–409.

166. Griffith BP, Aquino-de Jesus MJ. Guinea pig model of congenital cytomegalovirus infection. *Transplant Proc.* 1991;23:29–31.

167. Chatterjee A, Harrison CJ, Britt WJ, Bewtra C. Modification of maternal and congenital cytomegalovirus infection by anti-glycoprotein b antibody transfer in guinea pigs. *J Infect Dis.* 2001;183(11):1547–1553.

168. Harrison CJ, Britt WJ, Chapman NM, Mullican J, Tracy S. Reduced congenital cytomegalovirus (CMV) infection after maternal immunization with a guinea pig CMV glycoprotein before gestational primary CMV infection in the guinea pig model. *J Infect Dis.* 1995;172(5):1212–1220.

169. Bernstein DI, Bourne, N. Animal models for cytomegalovirus infection: guinea-pig CMV. In: Sande MA, Zak O, eds. *Handbook of Animal Models of Infection.* London, UK: Academic Press; 1999:935–941.

170. Bourne N, Schleiss MR, Bravo FJ, Bernstein DI. Preconception immunization with a cytomegalovirus (CMV) glycoprotein vaccine improves pregnancy outcome in a guinea pig model of congenital CMV infection. *J Infect Dis*. 2001;183(1):59–64.

171. Schleiss MR. Nonprimate models of congenital cytomegalovirus (CMV) infection: gaining insight into pathogenesis and prevention of disease in newborns. *ILAR J*. 2006;47(1):65–72.

172. Schleiss MR. Comparison of vaccine strategies against congenital CMV infection in the guinea pig model. *J Clin Virol*. 2008;41(3):224–230.

173. Hwang J, Kalejta RF. Proteasome-dependent, ubiquitin-independent degradation of Daxx by the viral pp71 protein in human cytomegalovirus-infected cells. *Virology*. 2007;367(2):334–338.

174. Kalejta RF. Functions of human cytomegalovirus tegument proteins prior to immediate early gene expression. *Curr Top Microbiol Immunol*. 2008;325:101–115.

175. Hakki M, Marshall EE, De Niro KL, Geballe AP. Binding and nuclear relocalization of protein kinase R by human cytomegalovirus TRS1. *J Virol*. 2006;80(23):11817–11826.

176. Upton JW, Kaiser WJ, Mocarski ES. Virus inhibition of RIP3-dependent necrosis. *Cell Host Microbe*. 22;7(4):302–313.

177. Goldmacher VS. Cell death suppression by cytomegaloviruses. *Apoptosis*. 2005;10(2):251–265.

178. Brune W. Inhibition of programmed cell death by cytomegaloviruses. *Virus Res*. 2011;157(2):144–150.

179. Jones BC, Logsdon NJ, Josephson K, Cook J, Barry PA, Walter MR. Crystal structure of human cytomegalovirus IL-10 bound to soluble human IL-10R1. *Proc Natl Acad Sci USA*. 2002;99(14):9404–9409.

180. Chang WL, Barry PA, Szubin R, Wang D, Baumgarth N. Human cytomegalovirus suppresses type I interferon secretion by plasmacytoid dendritic cells through its interleukin 10 homolog. *Virology*. 2009;390(2):330–337.

181. Biron CA, Byron KS, Sullivan JL. Severe herpesvirus infections in an adolescent without natural killer cells. *N Engl J Med*. 1989;320(26):1731–1735.

182. Biron CA, Brossay L. NK cells and NKT cells in innate defense against viral infections. *Curr Opin Immunol*. 2001;13(4):458–464.

183. Krmpotic A, Bubic I, Polic B, Lucin P, Jonjic S. Pathogenesis of murine cytomegalovirus infection. *Microbes Infect*. 2003;5(13):1263–1277.

184. Jonjic S, Bubic I, Krmpotic A. Innate immunity to cytomegaloviruses. In: Reddehase MJ, ed. *Cytomegaloviruses: Molecular Biology and Immunology*. Norfolk, UK: Caister; 2006:285–321.

185. Jonjic S, Krmpotic A, Arapovic J, Koszinowski UH. Dissection of the antiviral NK cell response by MCMV mutants. *Methods Mol Biol*. 2008;415:127–149.

186. Koszinowski UH, Reddehase MJ, Jonjic S. The role of CD4 and CD8 T cells in viral infections. *Curr Opin Immunol*. 1991;3(4):471–475.

187. Podlech J, Holtappels R, Wirtz N, Steffens HP, Reddehase MJ. Reconstitution of CD8 T cells is essential for the prevention of multiple-organ cytomegalovirus histopathology after bone marrow transplantation. *J Gen Virol*. 1998;79(Pt 9):2099–2104.

188. Reddehase MJ. The immunogenicity of human and murine cytomegaloviruses. *Curr Opin Immunol*. 2000;12(4):390–396.

189. Reddehase MJ, Simon CO, Seckert CK, Lemmermann N, Grzimek NK. Murine model of cytomegalovirus latency and reactivation. *Curr Top Microbiol Immunol*. 2008;325:315–331.

190. Walter EA, Greenberg PD, Gilbert MJ, et al. Reconstitution of cellular immunity against cytomegalovirus in recipients of allogeneic bone marrow by transfer of T-cell clones from the donor. *N Engl J Med*. 1995;333:1038–1044.

191. Cobbold M, Khan N, Pourgheysari B, et al. Adoptive transfer of cytomegalovirus-specific CTL to stem cell transplant patients after selection by HLA-peptide tetramers. *J Exp Med*. 2005;202(3):379–386.

192. Seckert CK, Griessl M, Buttner JK, et al. Viral latency drives "memory inflation": a unifying hypothesis linking two hallmarks of cytomegalovirus infection. *Med Microbiol Immunol*. 2012;201(4):551–566.

193. Pawelec G, Derhovanessian E. Role of CMV in immune senescence. *Virus Res*. 2011;157(2):175–179.

194. Wills M, Akbar A, Beswick M, et al. Report from the second cytomegalovirus and immunosenescence workshop. *Immun Ageing*. 2011;8(1):10.

195. Gratama JW, Boeckh M, Nakamura R, et al. Immune monitoring with iT Ag MHC tetramers for prediction of recurrent or persistent cytomegalovirus infection or disease in allogeneic hematopoietic stem cell transplant recipients: a prospective multicenter study. *Blood*. 2010;116(10):1655–1662.

196. Lacey SF, Gallez-Hawkins G, Crooks M, et al. Characterization of cytotoxic function of CMV-pp65-specific CD8⁺ T-lymphocytes identified by HLA tetramers in recipients and donors of stem-cell transplants. *Transplantation*. 2002;74(5):722–732.

197. Lazzarotto T, Guerra B, Lanari M, Gabrielli L, Landini MP. New advances in the diagnosis of congenital cytomegalovirus infection. *J Clin Virol*. 2008;41(3):192–197.

198. Macagno A, Bernasconi NL, Vanzetta F, et al. Isolation of human monoclonal antibodies that potently neutralize human cytomegalovirus infection by targeting different epitopes on the gH/gL/UL128-131A complex. *J Virol*. 2010;84(2):1005–1013.

199. Genini E, Percivalle E, Sarasini A, Revello MG, Baldanti F, Gerna G. Serum antibody response to the gH/gL/pUL128-131 five-protein complex of human cytomegalovirus (HCMV) in primary and reactivated HCMV infections. *J Clin Virol*. 2011;52(2):113–118.

200. Lilleri D, Kabanova A, Lanzavecchia A, Gerna G. Antibodies against neutralization epitopes of human cytomegalovirus gH/gL/pUL128-130-131 complex and virus spreading may correlate with virus control in vivo. *J Clin Immunol*. 2012;32(6):1324–1331.

201. Cui X, Meza BP, Adler SP, McVoy MA. Cytomegalovirus vaccines fail to induce epithelial entry neutralizing antibodies comparable to natural infection. *Vaccine*. 2008;26(45):5760–5766.

202. Gerna G, Sarasini A, Patrone M, et al. Human cytomegalovirus serum neutralizing antibodies block virus infection of endothelial/epithelial cells, but not fibroblasts, early during primary infection. *J Gen Virol*. 2008;89(Pt 4):853–865.

203. Mach M. Antibody-mediated neutralization of infectivity. In: Reddehase MJ, ed. *Cytomegaloviruses: Molecular Biology and Immunology*. Norfolk, UK: Caister; 2006:265–283.

204. Burkhardt C, Himmelein S, Britt W, Winkler T, Mach M. Glycoprotein N subtypes of human cytomegalovirus induce a strain-specific antibody response during natural infection. *J Gen Virol*. 2009;90(Pt 8):1951–1961.

205. Pati SK, Novak Z, Purser M, et al. Strain-specific neutralizing antibody responses against human cytomegalovirus envelope glycoprotein N. *Clin Vaccine Immunol*. 2012;19(6):909–913.

206. Potzsch S, Spindler N, Wiegers AK, et al. B cell repertoire analysis identifies new antigenic domains on glycoprotein B of human cytomegalovirus which are target of neutralizing antibodies. *PLoS Pathog*. 2011;7(8):e1002172.

207. Simpson JA, Chow JC, Baker J, et al. Neutralizing monoclonal antibodies that distinguish three antigenic sites on human cytomegalovirus glycoprotein H have conformationally distinct binding sites. *J Virol*. 1993;67(1):489–496.

208. Boppana SB, Polis MA, Kramer AA, Britt WJ, Koenig S. Virus specific antibody responses to human cytomegalovirus (HCMV) in human immunodeficiency virus type 1-infected individuals with HCMV retinitis. *J Infect Dis*. 1995;171:182–185.

209. Gerna G, Lilleri D, Chiesa A, et al. Virologic and immunologic monitoring of cytomegalovirus to guide preemptive therapy in solid-organ transplantation. *Am J Transplant.* 2011;11(11):2463–2471.

210. Snydman DR, Werner BG, Dougherty NN, et al. Cytomegalovirus immune globulin prophylaxis in liver transplantation. A randomized, double-blind placebo-controlled trial. *Ann Intern Med.* 1993;119:984–991.

211. Snydman DR, Werner BG, Heinze-Lacey B, et al. Use of cytomegalovirus immune globulin to prevent cytomegalovirus disease in renal-transplant recipients. *N Engl J Med.* 1987;317(17):1049–1054.

212. Nigro G, Adler SP, La Torre R, Best AM. Passive immunization during pregnancy for congenital cytomegalovirus infection. *N Engl J Med.* 2005;353(13):1350–1362.

213. Bratcher DF, Bourne N, Bravo FJ, et al. Effect of passive antibody on congenital cytomegalovirus infection in guinea pigs. *J Infect Dis.* 1995;172(4):944–950.

214. Cekinovic D, Golemac M, Pugel EP, et al. Passive immunization reduces murine cytomegalovirus-induced brain pathology in newborn mice. *J Virol.* 2008;82(24):12172–12180.

215. Jonjic S, Pavic I, Polic B, Crnkovic I, Lucin P, Koszinowski UH. Antibodies are not essential for the resolution of primary cytomegalovirus infection but limit dissemination of recurrent virus. *J Exp Med.* 1994;179:1713–1717.

216. Klenovsek K, Weisel F, Schneider A, et al. Protection from CMV infection in immunodeficient hosts by adoptive transfer of memory B cells. *Blood.* 2007;110(9):3472–3479.

217. Britt WJ, Vugler L, Butfiloski EJ, Stephens EB. Cell surface expression of human cytomegalovirus (HCMV) gp55–116 (gB): use of HCMV-vaccinia recombinant virus infected cells in analysis of the human neutralizing antibody response. *J Virol.* 1990;64:1079–1085.

218. Marshall GS, Rabalais GP, Stout GG, Waldeyer SL. Antibodies to recombinant-derived glycoprotein B after natural human cytomegalovirus infection correlate with neutralizing activity. *J Infect Dis.* 1992;165:381–384.

219. Griffiths PD, Stanton A, McCarrell E, et al. Cytomegalovirus glycoprotein-B vaccine with MF59 adjuvant in transplant recipients: a phase 2 randomised placebo-controlled trial. *Lancet.* 2011;377(9773):1256–1263.

220. Marchant A, Appay V, Van Der Sande M, et al. Mature CD8(+) T lymphocyte response to viral infection during fetal life. *J Clin Invest.* 2003;111(11):1747–1755.

221. Pedron B, Guerin V, Jacquemard F, et al. Comparison of CD8+ T Cell responses to cytomegalovirus between human fetuses and their transmitter mothers. *J Infect Dis.* 2007; 196(7):1033–1043.

222. Gibson L, Piccinini G, Lilleri D, et al. Human cytomegalovirus proteins pp65 and immediate early protein 1 are common targets for CD8+ T cell responses in children with congenital or postnatal human cytomegalovirus infection. *J Immunol.* 2004;172(4):2256–2264.

223. Chen SF, Tu WW, Sharp MA, et al. Antiviral CD8 T cells in the control of primary human cytomegalovirus infection in early childhood. *J Infect Dis.* 2004;189(9):1619–1627.

224. Tu W, Chen S, Sharp M, et al. Persistent and selective deficiency of CD4+ T cell immunity to cytomegalovirus in immunocompetent young children. *J Immunol.* 2004;172(5):3260–3267.

225. Gehrz RC, Markers SC, Knorr SO, Kalis JM, Balfour HH. Specific cell-mediated immune defect in active cytomegalovirus infection of young children and their mothers. *Lancet.* 1977;2:844–847.

226. Starr SE, Glazer JP, Friedman HM, Farquhar JD, Plotkin SA. Specific cellular and humoral immunity after immunization with live Towne strain cytomegalovirus vaccine. *J Infect Dis.* 1981;143:585–589.

227. Renneson J, Dutta B, Goriely S, et al. IL-12 and type I IFN response of neonatal myeloid DC to human CMV infection. *Eur J Immunol.* 2009;39(10):2789–2799.

228. Muller WJ, Jones CA, Koelle DM. Immunobiology of herpes simplex virus and cytomegalovirus infections of the fetus and newborn. *Curr Immunol Rev.* 2010;6(1):38–55.

229. Boppana S, Britt W. Cytomegalovirus. In: Newton VE, Vallely PJ, eds. *Infection and Hearing Impairment.* Sussex, UK: Wiley; 2006:67–93.

230. Halwachs-Baumann G, Genser B, Pailer S, et al. Human cytomegalovirus load in various body fluids of congenitally infected newborns. *J Clin Virol.* 2002;25(Suppl 3):S81–S87.

231. Revello MG, Zavattoni M, Baldanti F, Sarasini A, Paolucci S, Gerna G. Diagnostic and prognostic value of human cytomegalovirus load and IgM antibody in blood of congenitally infected newborns. *J Clin Virol.* 1999;14(1):57–66.

232. Cannon MJ, Hyde TB, Schmid DS. Review of cytomegalovirus shedding in bodily fluids and relevance to congenital cytomegalovirus infection. *Rev Med Virol.* 2011;21(4):240–255.

233. Becroft DMO. Prenatal cytomegalovirus infection: epidemiology, pathology, and pathogenesis. In: Rosenberg HS, Bernstein J, eds. *Perspective in Pediatric Pathology.* Vol 6. New York, NY: Masson Press; 1981:203–241.

234. McCracken GJ, Shinefield HR, Cobb K, Rausen AR, Dische MR, Eichenwald HF. Congenital cytomegalic inclusion disease. A longitudinal study of 20 patients. *Am J Dis Child.* 1969;117:522–539.

235. Bradford RD, Cloud G, Lakeman AD, et al. Detection of cytomegalovirus (CMV) DNA by polymerase chain reaction is associated with hearing loss in newborns with symptomatic congenital CMV infection involving the central nervous system. *J Infect Dis.* 2005;191(2):227–233.

236. Kimberlin DW, Lin CY, Sanchez PJ, et al. Effect of ganciclovir therapy on hearing in symptomatic congenital cytomegalovirus disease involving the central nervous system: a randomized, controlled trial. *J Pediatr.* 2003;143(1):16–25.

237. Gabrielli L, Bonasoni MP, Lazzarotto T, et al. Histological findings in foetuses congenitally infected by cytomegalovirus. *J Clin Virol.* 2009;46(Suppl 4):S16–S21.

238. Gabrielli L, Bonasoni MP, Santini D, et al. Congenital cytomegalovirus infection: patterns of fetal brain damage. *Clin Microbiol Infect.* 2012;18(10):E419-E427.

239. Teissier N, Delezoide AL, Mas AE, et al. Inner ear lesions in congenital cytomegalovirus infection of human fetuses. *Acta Neuropathol.* 2011;122(6):763–774.

240. Perlman JM, Argyle C. Lethal cytomegalovirus infection in preterm infants: clinical, radiological, and neuropathological findings. *Ann Neurol.* 1992;31:64–68.

241. Marques Dias MJ, Harmant-van Rijckevorsel G, Landrieu P, Lyon G. Prenatal cytomegalovirus disease and cerebral microgyria: evidence for perfusion failure, not disturbance of histogenesis, as the major cause of fetal cytomegalovirus encephalopathy. *Neuropediatrics.* 1984;15(1):18–24.

242. Malinger G, Lev D, Lerman-Sagie T. Imaging of fetal cytomegalovirus infection. *Fetal Diagn Ther.* 2011;29(2)117–126.

243. Malinger G, Lev D, Zahalka N, et al. Fetal cytomegalovirus infection of the brain: the spectrum of sonographic findings. *AJNR Am J Neuroradiol.* 2003;24(1):28–32.

244. Barkovich AJ, Lindan CE. Congenital cytomegalovirus infection of the brain: imaging analysis and embryologic considerations. *Am J Neuroradiol.* 1994;15:703–715.

245. Boppana SB, Fowler KB, Vaid Y, et al. Neuroradiographic findings in the newborn period and long-term outcome in children with symptomatic congenital cytomegalovirus infection. *Pediatrics.* 1997;99:409–414.

246. Amos CS. The ocular manifestations of congenital infections produced by toxoplasma and cytomegalovirus. *J Am Optom Assoc.* 1977;48(4):532–538.

247. Amos CS. Posterior segment involvement in selected pediatric infectious diseases. *J Am Optom Assoc.* 1979;50:1211–1220.

248. Luo MH, Schwartz PH, Fortunato EA. Neonatal neural progenitor cells and their neuronal and glial cell derivatives are fully permissive for human cytomegalovirus infection. *J Virol.* 2008;82(20):9994–10007.

249. Tsutsui Y, Kosugi I, Kawasaki H. Neuropathogenesis in cytomegalovirus infection: indication of the mechanisms using mouse models. *Rev Med Virol.* 2005;15(5):327–345.

250. Tsutsui Y, Kosugi I, Kawasaki H, et al. Roles of neural stem progenitor cells in cytomegalovirus infection of the brain in mouse models. *Pathol Int.* 2008;58(5):257–267.

251. Koontz T, Bralic M, Tomac J, et al. Altered development of the brain after focal herpesvirus infection of the central nervous system. *J Exp Med.* 2008;205(2):423–435.

252. Cheeran MC, Lokensgard JR, Schleiss MR. Neuropathogenesis of congenital cytomegalovirus infection: disease mechanisms and prospects for intervention. *Clin Microbiol Rev.* 2009;22(1):99–126, Table of Contents.

253. Tarantal AF, Salamat MS, Britt WJ, Luciw PA, Hendrickx AG, Barry PA. Neuropathogenesis induced by rhesus cytomegalovirus in fetal rhesus monkeys (*Macaca mulatta*). *J Infect Dis.* 1998;177(2):446–450.

254. Kawasaki H, Tsutsui Y. Brain slice culture for analysis of developmental brain disorders with special reference to congenital cytomegalovirus infection. *Congenit Anom (Kyoto).* 2003;43(2):105–113.

255. Kosugi I, Shinmura Y, Kawasaki H, et al. Cytomegalovirus infection of the central nervous system stem cells from mouse embryo: a model for developmental brain disorders induced by cytomegalovirus. *Lab Investig.* 2000;80(9):1373–1383.

256. Bantug GR, Cekinovic D, Bradford R, Koontz T, Jonjic S, Britt WJ. CD8+ T lymphocytes control murine cytomegalovirus replication in the central nervous system of newborn animals. *J Immunol.* 2008;181(3):2111–2123.

257. Gallant JE, Moore RD, Richman DD, Keruly J, Chaisson RE. Incidence and natural history of cytomegalovirus disease in patients with advanced human immunodeficiency virus disease treated with zidovudine. *J Infect Dis.* 1992;166:1223–1227.

258. Arribas JR, Storch GA, Clifford DB, Tselis AC. Cytomegalovirus encephalitis. *Ann Intern Med.* 1996;125(7):577–587.

259. Anders HJ, Goebel FD. Neurological manifestations of cytomegalovirus infection in the acquired immunodeficiency syndrome. *Int J STD AIDS.* 1999;10(3):151–159; quiz 160–151.

260. Jabs DA, Green R, Fox B, Polk BF, Bartlett JG. Ocular manifestations of acquired immune deficiency syndrome. *Ophthalmology.* 1989;96:1092–1099.

261. Dunn JP, Holland GN. Human immunodeficiency virus and opportunistic ocular infections. *Infect Dis Clin North Am.* 1992;6:909–923.

262. Schachtele SJ, Mutnal MB, Schleiss MR, Lokensgard JR. Cytomegalovirus-induced sensorineural hearing loss with persistent cochlear inflammation in neonatal mice. *J Neurovirol.* 2011;17(3):201–211.

263. Fukuda S, Keithley EM, Harris JP. Experimental cytomegalovirus infection: viremic spread to the inner ear. *Am J Otolaryngol.* 1988;9(3):135–141.

264. Harris JP, Fan JT, Keithley EM. Immunologic responses in experimental cytomegalovirus labyrinthitis. *Am J Otolaryngol.* 1990;11:304–308.

265. Harris S, Ahlfors K, Ivarsson S, Lemmark B, Svanberg L. Congenital cytomegalovirus infection and sensorineural hearing loss. *Ear Hear.* 1984;5:352–355.

266. Woolf NK, Harris JP, Ryan AF, Butler DM, Richman DD. Hearing loss in experimental cytomegalovirus infection of the guinea pig inner ear: prevention by systemic immunity. *Ann Otol Rhinol Laryngol.* 1985;94:350–356.

267. Woolf NK, Koehrn FJ, Harris JP, Richman DD. Congenital cytomegalovirus labyrinthitis and sensorineural hearing loss in guinea pigs. *J Infect Dis.* 1989;160:929–937.

268. Woolf NK, Ochi JW, Silva EJ, Sharp PA, Harris JP, Richman DD. Ganciclovir prophylaxis for cochlear pathophysiology during experimental guinea pig cytomegalovirus labyrinthitis. *Antimicrob Agents Chemother.* 1988;32(6):865–872.

269. Park AH, Gifford T, Schleiss MR, et al. Development of cytomegalovirus-mediated sensorineural hearing loss in a Guinea pig model. *Arch Otolaryngol Head Neck Surg.* 2010;136(1):48–53.

270. Jamieson DJ, Kourtis AP, Bell M, Rasmussen SA. Lymphocytic choriomeningitis virus: an emerging obstetric pathogen? *Am J Obstet Gynecol.* 2006;194(6):1532–1536.

271. Wright R, Johnson D, Neumann M, et al. Congenital lymphocytic choriomeningitis virus syndrome: a disease that mimics congenital toxoplasmosis or Cytomegalovirus infection. *Pediatrics.* 1997;100(1):E9.

272. Barton LL, Mets MB, Beauchamp CL. Lymphocytic choriomeningitis virus: emerging fetal teratogen. *Am J Obstet Gynecol.* 2002;187(6):1715–1716.

273. Orcesi S, La Piana R, Fazzi E. Aicardi-Goutieres syndrome. *Br Med Bull.* 2009;89:183–201.

274. Rice G, Patrick T, Parmar R, et al. Clinical and molecular phenotype of Aicardi-Goutieres syndrome. *Am J Hum Genet.* 2007;81(4):713–725.

275. Stetson DB, Ko JS, Heidmann T, Medzhitov R. Trex1 prevents cell-intrinsic initiation of autoimmunity. *Cell.* 2008;134(4):587–598.

276. Yan N, Lieberman J. Gaining a foothold: how HIV avoids innate immune recognition. *Curr Opin Immunol.* 2011;23(1):21–28.

277. Reynolds DW, Stagno S, Stubbs KG, et al. Inapparent congenital cytomegalovirus infection with elevated cord IgM levels. Casual relation with auditory and mental deficiency. *N Engl J Med.* 1974;290(6):291–296.

278. Lazzarotto T, Spezzacatena P, Pradelli P, Abate DA, Varani S, Landini MP. Avidity of immunoglobulin G directed against human cytomegalovirus during primary and secondary infections in immunocompetent and immunocompromised subjects. *Clin Diagn Lab Immunol.* 1997;4(4):469–473.

279. Bodeus M, Beulne D, Goubau P. Ability of three IgG-avidity assays to exclude recent cytomegalovirus infection. *Eur J Clin Microbiol Infect Dis.* 2001;20(4):248–252.

280. Griffiths PD. Diagnostic techniques for cytomegalovirus infection. *Clin Hematol.* 1984;13:631–644.

281. Griffiths PD, Panjwani DD, Stirk PR, et al. Rapid diagnosis of cytomegalovirus infection in immunocompromised patients by detection of early antigen fluorescent foci. *Lancet.* 1984;2:1242–1245.

282. Boppana SB, Smith R, Stagno S, Britt WJ. Evaluation of a microtiter plate fluorescent antibody assay for rapid detection of human cytomegalovirus infections. *J Clin Microbiol.* 1992;30:721–723.

283. Warren WP, Balcarek K, Smith R, Pass RF. Comparison of rapid methods of detection of cytomegalovirus in saliva with virus isolation in tissue culture. *J Clin Microbiol.* 1992;30:786–789.

284. Boeckh M, Bowden RA, Goodrich JM, Pettinger M, Meyers JD. Cytomegalovirus antigen detection in peripheral blood leukocytes after allogeneic marrow transplantation. *Blood.* 1992;80:1358–1364.

285. Boeckh M. Rising CMV PP65 antigenemia and DNA levels during preemptive antiviral therapy. *Haematologica.* 2005;90(4):439.

286. Boeckh M, Boivin G. Quantitation of cytomegalovirus: methodologic aspects and clinical applications. *Clin Microbiol Rev.* 1998;11(3):533–554.

287. Gerna G, Zavattoni M, Percivalle E, Grossi P, Torsellini M, Revello MG. Rising levels of human cytomegalovirus (HCMV) antigenemia during initial antiviral treatment of solid-organ transplant recipients with primary HCMV infection. *J Clin Microbiol.* 1998;36(4):1113–1116.

288. The TH, van der Bij W, van den Berg AP, et al. Cytomegalovirus antigenemia. *Rev Infect Dis.* 1990;12(S):734–744.

289. Boppana SB, Ross SA, Novak Z, et al. Dried blood spot real-time polymerase chain reaction assays to screen newborns for congenital cytomegalovirus infection. *JAMA.* 2010;303(14):1375–1382.

290. Lazzarotto T, Guerra B, Spezzacatena P, et al. Prenatal diagnosis of congenital cytomegalovirus infection. *J Clin Microbiol.* 1998;36(12):3540–3544.

291. Fowler KB, Stagno S, Pass RF, Britt WJ, Boll TJ, Alford CA. The outcome of congenital cytomegalovirus infection in relation to maternal antibody status. *N Engl J Med.* 1992;326(10):663–667.

292. Snydman DR. Cytomegalovirus immunoglobulins in the prevention and treatment of cytomegalovirus disease. *Rev Infect Dis.* 1990;12(S):839–848.

293. Snydman DR. Review of the efficacy of cytomegalovirus immune globulin in the prophylaxis of CMV disease in renal transplant recipients. *Transplant Proc.* 1993;25(5 Suppl 4):25–26.

294. Jacquemard F, Yamamoto M, Costa JM, et al. Maternal administration of valaciclovir in symptomatic intrauterine cytomegalovirus infection. *BJOG.* 2007;114(9):1113–1121.

295. Pass RF, Stagno S, Myers GJ, Alford CA. Outcome of symptomatic congenital CMV infection: results of long-term longitudinal follow-up. *Pediatrics.* 1980;66:758–762.

296. Kashden J, Frison S, Fowler K, Pass RF, Boll TJ. Intellectual assessment of children with asymptomatic congenital cytomegalovirus infection. *J Dev Behav Pediatr.* 1998;19(4):254–259.

297. McCollister FP, Simpson LC, Dahle AJ, et al. Hearing loss and congenital symptomatic cytomegalovirus infection: a case report of multidisciplinary longitudinal assessment and intervention. *J Am Acad Audiol.* 1996;7:57–62.

298. Munro SC, Trincado D, Hall B, Rawlinson WD. Symptomatic infant characteristics of congenital cytomegalovirus disease in Australia. *J Paediatr Child Health.* 2005;41(8):449–452.

299. Ancora G, Lanari M, Lazzarotto T, et al. Cranial ultrasound scanning and prediction of outcome in newborns with congenital cytomegalovirus infection. *J Pediatr.* 2007;150(2):157–161.

300. Kaye S, Miles D, Antoine P, et al. Virological and immunological correlates of mother-to-child transmission of cytomegalovirus in The Gambia. *J Infect Dis.* 2008;197(9):1307–1314.

301. Peckham CS, Chin KS, Coleman JC, Henderson K, Hurley R, Preece PM. Cytomegalovirus infection in pregnancy: preliminary findings from a prospective study. *Lancet.* 1983;1:1352–1355.

302. Andersen HK, Brostrom K, Hansen KB, et al. A prospective study on the incidence and significance of congenital cytomegalovirus infection. *Acta Paediatr Scand.* 1979;68(3):329–336.

303. Sohn YM, Park KI, Lee C, Han DG, Lee WY. Congenital cytomegalovirus infection in Korean population with very high prevalence of maternal immunity. *J Korean Med Sci.* 1992;7(1):47–51.

304. Boppana SB, Fowler KB, Pass RF, Britt WJ, Stagno S, Alford CA. Newborn findings and outcome in children with symptomatic congenital CMV infection. *Pediatr Res.* 1992;31:158A.

305. Anderson KS, Amos CS, Boppana S, Pass R. Ocular abnormalities in congenital cytomegalovirus infection. *J Am Optom Assoc.* 1996;67(5):273–278.

306. Isler JA, Skalet AH, Alwine JC. Human cytomegalovirus infection activates and regulates the unfolded protein response. *J Virol.* 2005;79(11):6890–6899.

307. Yew KH, Carsten B, Harrison C. Scavenger receptor A1 is required for sensing HCMV by endosomal TLR-3/-9 in monocytic THP-1 cells. *Mol Immunol.* 2010;47(4):883–893.

308. Boehme KW, Singh J, Perry ST, Compton T. Human cytomegalovirus elicits a coordinated cellular antiviral response via envelope glycoprotein B. *J Virol.* 2004;78(3):1202–1211.

309. Couzi L, Pitard V, Sicard X, et al. Antibody-dependent anticytomegalovirus activity of human gammadelta T cells expressing CD16 (FcgammaRIIIa). *Blood.* 2012;119(6):1418–1427.

310. Fornara C, Lilleri D, Revello MG, et al. Kinetics of effector functions and phenotype of virus-specific and gammadelta T lymphocytes in primary human cytomegalovirus infection during pregnancy. *J Clin Immunol.* 2011;31(6):1054–1064.

311. Quinnan GV Jr, Kirmani N, Rook AH, et al. Cytotoxic t cells in cytomegalovirus infection: HLA-restricted T-lymphocyte and non-T-lymphocyte cytotoxic responses correlate with recovery from cytomegalovirus infection in bone-marrow-transplant recipients. *N Engl J Med.* 1982;307(1):7–13.

321. Sester M, Sester U, Gartner BC, Girndt M, Meyerhans A, Kohler H. Dominance of virus-specific CD8 T cells in human primary cytomegalovirus infection. *J Am Soc Nephrol.* 2002;13(10):2577–2584.

313. Gibson L, Dooley S, Trzmielina S, et al. Cytomegalovirus (CMV) IE1- and pp65-specific CD8⁺ T cell responses broaden over time after primary CMV infection in infants. *J Infect Dis.* 2007;195(12):1789–1798.

314. Boppana SB, Britt WJ. Antiviral antibody responses and intrauterine transmission after primary maternal cytomegalovirus infection. *J Infect Dis.* 1995;171(5):1115–1121.

315. Urban M, Klein M, Britt WJ, Hassfurther E, Mach M. Glycoprotein H of human cytomegalovirus is a major antigen for the neutralizing humoral immune response. *J Gen Virol.* 1996;77(Pt 7):1537–1547.

316. Reynolds DW, Dean PH, Pass RF, Alford CA. Specific cell-mediated immunity in children with congenital and neonatal cytomegalovirus infection and their mothers. *J Infect Dis.* 1979;140:493–499.

317. Hayashi N, Kimura H, Morishima T, Tanaka N, Tsurumi T, Kuzushima K. Flow cytometric analysis of cytomegalovirus-specific cell-mediated immunity in the congenital infection. *J Med Virol.* 2003;71(2):251–258.

318. Elbou Ould MA, Luton D, Yadini M, et al. Cellular immune response of fetuses to cytomegalovirus. *Pediatr Res.* 2004;55(2):280–286.

319. Guerra B, Simonazzi G, Puccetti C, et al. Ultrasound prediction of symptomatic congenital cytomegalovirus infection. *Am J Obstet Gynecol.* 2008;198(4):380.e381–e387.

320. Amir J, Schwarz M, Levy I, Haimi-Cohen Y, Pardo J. Is lenticulostriated vasculopathy a sign of central nervous system insult in infants with congenital CMV infection? *Arch Dis Child.* 2011;96(9):846–850.

321. de Vries LS, Gunardi H, Barth PG, Bok LA, Verboon-Maciolek MA, Groenendaal F. The spectrum of cranial ultrasound and magnetic resonance imaging abnormalities in congenital cytomegalovirus infection. *Neuropediatrics.* 2004;35(2):113–119.

322. Duranovic V, Krakar G, Mejaski-Bosnjak V, Lujic L, Gojmerac T, Marn B. Lenticulostriatal vasculopathy—a marker for congenital cytomegalovirus infection? *Coll Antropol.* 2011;35(Suppl 1):149–153.

323. Lanari M, Capretti MG, Lazzarotto T, et al. Neuroimaging in CMV congenital infected neonates: how and when. *Early Hum Dev.* 2012;88(Suppl 2):S3–S5.

CHAPTER 54

324. Benoist G, Salomon LJ, Mohlo M, Suarez B, Jacquemard F, Ville Y. Cytomegalovirus-related fetal brain lesions: comparison between targeted ultrasound examination and magnetic resonance imaging. *Ultrasound Obstet Gynecol*. 2008;32(7):900–905.

325. Bosnjak VM, Dakovic I, Duranovic V, Lujic L, Krakar G, Marn B. Malformations of cortical development in children with congenital cytomegalovirus infection—a study of nine children with proven congenital cytomegalovirus infection. *Coll Antropol*. 2011;35(Suppl 1):229–234.

326. Hayward JC, Titelbaum DS, Clancy RR, Zimmerman RA. Lissencephaly-pachygyria associated with congenital cytomegalovirus infection. *J Child Neurol*. 1991;6(2):109–114.

327. Manara R, Balao L, Baracchini C, Drigo P, D'Elia R, Ruga EM. Brain magnetic resonance findings in symptomatic congenital cytomegalovirus infection. *Pediatr Radiol*. 2011;41(8): 962–970.

328. Picone O, Simon I, Benachi A, Brunelle F, Sonigo P. Comparison between ultrasound and magnetic resonance imaging in assessment of fetal cytomegalovirus infection. *Prenat Diagn*. 2008;28(8):753–758.

329. Sugita K, Ando M, Makino M, Takanashi J, Fujimoto N, Niimi H. Magnetic resonance imaging of the brain in congenital rubella virus and cytomegalovirus infections. *Neuroradiology*. 1991;33(3):239–242.

330. Revello MG, Lazzarotto T, Guerra B, Spinillo A, Ferrazzi E, Kusterman A. et al. *NEJM*. 2014;370(14):1316–1326. doi:10.1056/NEJM 09131214. PMID 24693891.

331. Kosmac K, Britt WJ. PLOS Pathogens. 2013;9(3):e1003200. doi: 1371/journal.ppat. 1003200. PMID 23505367.

332. Schlesinger Y, Reich D, Eldelman AI, et al. Congenital cytomegalovirus infection in Israel: screening in different populations. *Isr Med Assoc J*. 2005;7(4):237–240.

55 Herpes Simplex Virus

Kathleen Gutierrez

INTRODUCTION

Neonatal herpes simplex virus (HSV) infection refers to any HSV infection occurring in infants within the first 28 days of life. Most infants present with symptoms within the first 2–3 weeks of life, and some cases are recognized as late as 4–6 weeks of age (rare cases recognized up until 8 weeks of age). Both HSV-1 and HSV-2 cause serious infection in the neonate. If infection is unrecognized and untreated, 50% of infants with central nervous system (CNS) HSV disease and 85% of infants with disseminated HSV infection die by 1 year of age.[1] Advances in the diagnosis and treatment of neonatal HSV infection since the mid-1980s have improved the outcomes of infected infants.[2] Despite advances in care, there is no evidence that the incidence of infection has decreased. Delay in diagnosis persists, and some infants who survive infection suffer devastating long-term sequelae.[2]

EPIDEMIOLOGY

Neonatal HSV infection is an uncommon disease, but early recognition and treatment are crucial in preventing mortality and long-term morbidity. Most neonatal HSV infections are in infants born to mothers with genital HSV-1 or HSV-2 infection. The remaining cases occur in infants exposed shortly after birth to a family member or health care worker with mouth or skin HSV-1 lesions. Based on serologic data from the National Health and Nutrition Examination Survey (NHANES), it is estimated that 22% of pregnant women in the United States are HSV-2 positive, 63% are HSV-1 positive, and 13% are seropositive for both viruses.[3] Non-Hispanic white women were more likely to be seronegative for HSV compared to other racial and ethnic groups. HSV-2 causes most cases of genital herpes in the United States; however, genital infections with HSV-1 are increasing, and recent studies suggested that HSV-1 has now surpassed HSV-2 as a cause of genital herpes in college-age individuals.[4] Women infected with HSV-2 are more likely to have recurrent symptomatic and asymptomatic shedding of virus compared to those with HSV-1.[5]

Most persons (70%–80%) with genital HSV have no symptoms; therefore, a history of no lesions during pregnancy does not rule out risk for neonatal HSV infection (Table 55-1). Some women with primary infection or recurrent disease have only nonspecific symptoms, such as fever or genital burning with urination that is mistaken for a urinary tract infection. Recurrence of genital herpes during pregnancy is common. Asymptomatic reactivation of genital HSV associated with short episodes of viral shedding and rapid clearance of virus likely occurs more frequently than previously thought.[6]

There are approximately 1500 cases of neonatal HSV infection in the United States each year.[7,8] The exact number of cases is unknown because reporting of neonatal HSV infection to health departments is not required in most states.[9] The rate of neonatal HSV infection in the United States varies depending on geographic area, study population, and study methodology.[10] Studies utilizing state surveillance systems or hospital discharge data showed incidence rates

Table 55-1 Fiction and Fact Regarding Neonatal Herpes Simplex Virus (HSV) Infection[a]

Fiction	Fact
Infants with neonatal HSV infection are always born to women with a history of recurrent HSV genital lesions.	In most cases, genital lesions are not present at times of viral shedding. Mothers may have no symptoms or may relate nonspecific symptoms of fever, burning, vaginal discomfort.
Skin vesicles are always present on an infant with neonatal HSV infection.	Of infants with neonatal HSV infection, 30%–40% do not have skin lesions at the time of diagnosis.
A well-appearing infant with only skin, eye, or mucous membrane lesions can be treated with oral acyclovir.	The bioavailability of oral acyclovir is poor. Infants have an impaired immune response to neonatal HSV infection and are at risk for serious disseminated or CNS disease. **Intravenous therapy for all types of neonatal HSV infection is recommended.**
A negative CSF HSV PCR rules out with certainty neonatal HSV CNS infection.	The sensitivity of PCR varies depending on the laboratory and the timing of specimen collection. HSV PCR obtained from CSF early in the course of illness may be falsely negative. If clinical, laboratory, EEG, or radiology findings are suspicious for HSV CNS infection, the infant should be treated and PCR repeated.
The best test for diagnosing neonatal HSV infection is a serum HSV IgM.	The IgM response to HSV infection in the neonate is delayed. Serological testing of the infant is not useful in the acute phase of illness.
If a skin lesion culture is positive for *Staphylococcus aureus*, HSV infection is ruled out.	Occasionally, vesicular or pustular skin lesions are culture positive for both bacteria and virus.

Abbreviations: CNS, central nervous system; CSF, cerebrospinal fluid; EEG, electroencephalogram; HSV, herpes simplex virus; Ig, immunoglobulin; PCR, polymerase chain reaction.
[a]Data from Corey and Wald.[10]

of infection that range between 6 and 13 cases per 100,000 births.[10–14] Hospital *International Classification of Diseases, Ninth Revision* (*ICD-9*) coding appears to be reasonably sensitive but not specific in identifying infants discharged with HSV infection.[15] Use of *ICD-9* codes in conjunction with chart review and confirmatory laboratory testing found the incidence of confirmed or probable neonatal HSV infection in 2 managed care organizations was 12.9/100,000 live births.[15] One study utilizing *ICD-9* coding found a substantially higher rate of infection in a large managed care population.[16]

There are several factors that may explain a difference in incidence rates. One important factor is that there are currently no *ICD-9* codes specific for neonatal HSV infection. Investigators who utilize *ICD-9* coding choose codes that, based on their clinical experience, are likely to identify neonatal infection and vary with each study.[16] Standardization of coding or development of codes specific to neonatal HSV infection will improve the validity of future analyses. Many experts argue that neonatal HSV infection should be a reportable disease given its devastating effects in the most vulnerable of patients and their families and its comparable prevalence and increased morbidity in comparison to other reportable diseases.[9]

The only large prospective analysis[8] of neonatal HSV infection was performed in Seattle, Washington,

between 1982 and 1999. During the study period, the incidence of neonatal HSV infection was 31/100,000 births. The rate of transmission of infection was dependent on maternal serostatus. Infants born to mothers who were seronegative for both HSV-1 and HSV-2 during pregnancy were at highest risk (54/100,000 births) of infection, and those born to mothers who were seropositive for both viruses were at lowest risk (12/100,000 births).

Nonimmune pregnant women have an approximately 2% risk for developing a primary HSV infection during pregnancy.[17] The most significant risk factor for neonatal HSV infection is maternal primary HSV infection around the time of delivery.[17] As is typical with most primary genital HSV infections, the mother often has no symptoms but sheds significant amounts of virus from her cervix. The diagnosis of primary HSV infection in pregnancy cannot be based on clinical signs alone. A first HSV lesion may be reactivation of a previously asymptomatic infection. The diagnosis of primary HSV requires laboratory confirmation of HSV shedding (by viral culture or polymerase chain reaction [PCR]) plus either a negative antibody test with onset of symptoms or evidence of a change in serologic status over several weeks. An infant born to a mother with primary infection at the time of delivery has the highest (about 50%) risk of developing HSV infection.[8,17] The reasons for higher risk in this scenario include exposure

Table 55-2 Risk Factors for Neonatal Herpes Simplex Virus (HSV) Infection

1. Primary maternal HSV-1 or HSV-2 genital infection during pregnancy
2. Premature infant
3. Prolonged rupture of membranes
4. Vaginal delivery
5. Known maternal viral shedding, particularly cervical shedding
6. Use of fetal scalp monitors
7. Infant contact with caregiver with active HSV-1 skin or mouth lesions

of the infant to the larger amounts of virus shed during a primary infection and little or no exposure to HSV type-specific neutralizing antibody.

Infants born to mothers with new infections that are first episodes but nonprimary appear to be at lower risk. An example of this situation would be an infant born to a mother who was previously seropositive for HSV-1 but then develops a first episode of genital HSV-2 around the time of delivery. In cases such as this, transmission rates are estimated to be 25%–30% or higher.

The lowest risk of neonatal acquisition occurs when the mother has a known history of genital HSV-1 or HSV-2 prior to or earlier in pregnancy and then is found to reactivate and shed the same type virus around the time of delivery.[18] The estimated attack rate for neonatal herpes among these infants is less than 5%.

Other factors that increase the risk of neonatal infection if a mom is shedding HSV include use of fetal scalp electrode,[19] prolonged rupture of membranes (>6 hours),[20] known viral shedding at the time of delivery, cervical shedding, vaginal birth, and prematurity[21] (Table 55-2). If maternal HSV lesions are noted at the time of labor, delivery of the infant by cesarean section is protective; however, neonatal HSV infection after cesarean section does occur.[8]

Neonatal HSV infection is often diagnosed after an initially well-appearing infant has been discharged home from the nursery. One recent retrospective study found the prevalence of neonatal HSV infection in febrile infants admitted to the hospital from the emergency department similar to that of bacterial meningitis (0.2% vs 0.4%, respectively) but lower than that of serious bacterial infections (4.6%).[22]

PATHOPHYSIOLOGY

Etiology

Etiologically, HSV-1 and HSV-2 are enveloped, double-stranded DNA viruses in the family of Herpesviridae,

subfamily alphaherpesvirinae.[23] Typically, HSV-1 causes infection in the upper part of the body, including HSV gingivostomatitis, recurrent HSV oral lesions (cold sores), HSV keratitis, or herpetic whitlow. HSV-2 classically causes infection in the genital area. However, either virus can cause oral or genital infection.

Infection occurs when virus penetrates abraded skin or mucosa, replicates in the epidermis and dermis, and infects peripheral sensory nerve endings. HSV-1 and HSV-2 have the ability to establish latency and persist in sensory ganglion neurons for a patient's entire lifetime.[23] With infection of the oral mucosa, the site of viral latency is the trigeminal ganglia, and after genital infection, the site of latency is the sacral ganglia. The virus remains in a latent state with intermittent episodes of reactivation, causing virus excretion at mucosal or other sites. When reactivation is triggered, virus is transported back down axons to mucocutaneous sites, where replication and shedding of infectious HSV occurs. When epithelial cells are infected and destroyed, lesions are visible. However, excretion of infectious virus is often asymptomatic. As a result, infants with neonatal HSV infection are frequently born to mothers with no history of genital lesions at the time of delivery.

A number of HSV glycoproteins are required for infectivity and are targets of neutralizing antibodies. The amino acid sequence of 1 of these glycoproteins, glycoprotein G (gG) is varied enough that the antibody response to the molecule is different for HSV-1 (gG1) and HSV-2 (gG2).[24] Because there is minimal cross-reactivity in antibody response to the gG for each virus, serological methods have been developed that are used to differentiate infection with HSV-1 or HSV-2.[25] Use of type-specific testing has enhanced our understanding of the epidemiology and clinical presentation of each of these viruses.

Transmission

Infants may become infected with HSV in utero, intrapartum (most cases), and postnatally. In utero infection results from transplacental transmission of HSV or ascending infection from the cervix[26,27] and is considered rare, accounting for fewer than 5% of cases.[28] In instances of presumed transplacental infection, necrosis of the placenta has been documented, and viral inclusions have been identified in placental trophoblasts. Acquisition of infection in utero has caused spontaneous abortion of the fetus. In some cases, an infant is born with signs of congenital infection. HSV DNA has been detected in the amniotic fluid of women who later gave birth to healthy infants.[29] Risk factors for in utero transmission of virus from mother to infant are unclear because both primary and recurrent maternal infection have resulted in infection in utero. Ascending infection from the cervix through either ruptured or apparently intact membranes causing chorioamnionitis is an alternative cause of in utero infection.[30]

Most neonatal HSV infections occur at the time of birth when an infant's mucosa or abraded skin comes in contact with HSV-1- or HSV-2-infected maternal genital secretions. HSV-1 causes 27%–45% of cases of neonatal infection.[2,8] Although genital shedding with HSV-2 occurs more frequently than shedding of HSV-1, transmission of HSV-1 to the infant appears to be more efficient.[8] Presenting symptoms in the neonate infected with either virus are similar. According to 1 study, approximately 9% of infants have clinical findings of infection on the first day of life,[2] and some of these may reflect in utero acquisition of virus. Most infants appear well at birth, and it is not until viral replication at the site of infection occurs that symptoms appear. Infants with disseminated disease or skin, eye, and mucous membrane (SEM) disease typically present earliest (10–12 days of age), and some may develop symptoms within the first week of life. Infants with HSV infection localized to the CNS present later, at about 2–3 weeks of age.[2,31] In some with isolated CNS disease, symptoms are not recognized until 4–6 weeks (and rarely as late as 8 weeks) of age. The reasons for later presentation of isolated CNS disease are unclear, but most of these babies have transplacental HSV antibody. The pathogenesis of disease is possibly retrograde axonal transport of virus to the CNS, rather than hematogenous spread of virus to the brain, as is seen in CNS involvement with disseminated HSV infection.

Approximately 10% of infants acquire HSV infection postnatally.[31-33] An increase in the proportion of neonatal infection caused by HSV-1 may be in some part because of acquisition of virus in the days following birth. Postnatal infection can result from contact of the infant with infected secretions from the mother's mouth or lesions on the skin. Infants have developed infection after nursing from a breast with HSV lesions or after ritual circumcision.[33-35] Family members or hospital personnel with orolabial or skin lesions may also transmit infection to the newborn.[36] The seroprevalence of HSV-1 in the general population is approximately 58% (30% to 90% depending on age and race/ethnicity).[37] Many individuals have asymptomatic viral shedding, and those with close contact can unwittingly expose newborns to the virus. In addition, parents or family members may not realize that "cold sores" are caused by HSV and therefore pose a risk of infection to the newborn.

Immune Response

Because of an immature neonatal immune system, infants exposed to HSV in utero or within the first month of life have unique risks for viral dissemination. Neonates develop severe HSV disease that is not seen in older infants and children; therefore, early diagnosis and treatment are crucial. The developmental limitations in the neonatal immune response to HSV have not been fully elucidated but likely include deficiencies in both the early nonspecific innate and later antigen-specific adaptive immune response to HSV. Deficiencies in the function of neonatal natural killer and dendritic cells and decreased interferon-α (INF-α) production probably contribute to poor initial control of HSV infection.[38] A key component in the immune response to HSV infection is development of adaptive cellular immunity to the virus. Newborns with HSV infections have a delayed T-lymphocyte proliferative response, and most infants have no detectable T-lymphocyte responses to HSV when evaluated 2 to 4 weeks after the onset of clinical symptoms.[39,40] The delayed T-lymphocyte response to viral antigens in infants whose initial disease is localized to the skin, eye, or mouth likely explains the higher risk of progression to more severe disease in untreated infants.

Infants who receive transplacentally acquired neutralizing antibodies from the mother have a lower attack rate if exposed to virus.[18] Infants who lack neutralizing antibody are more likely to have early onset or disseminated disease.[39] The presence of passive antibody in the newborn, however, is not totally protective, and infants who have antibody at the onset of clinical symptoms and localized disease can develop disseminated or CNS infection if they do not receive antiviral treatment. Immunoglobulin (Ig) M antibody to HSV may be detected in some children 2–4 weeks after onset of symptoms. In previous studies, IgM was more often positive in infants with CNS disease and HSV-2, compared to those infants with SEM disease and infection with HSV-1.[39]

Finally, infants with higher titers of antibodies that mediate antibody-dependent cellular cytotoxicity (ADCC) appear to be at lower risk for disseminated infection than those with lower titers of ADCC antibodies.[41]

CLINICAL FINDINGS

Clinical findings in intrapartum and postnatal neonatal HSV-1 and HSV-2 infection are classified into 3 categories: (1) SEM disease; (2) CNS infection (encephalitis); and (3) disseminated disease, with or without CNS involvement. These clinical categories are assigned based on information learned from prospective studies performed by the National Institute of Allergy and Infection Diseases (NIAID) Collaborative Antiviral Study Group (CASG) in the

1980s and 1990s.[2] The prevalence of each clinical category is reported to occur with approximately equal frequency[2] but may vary depending on the time period and population studied.[42,43] In addition, utilization of PCR analysis has identified infants with CNS disease who would previously have been categorized as having only SEM infection.[44] Prognosis and treatment differ depending on the pattern of infection. Intrauterine HSV infection is discussed as a separate category.

Skin, Eye, and Mucous Membrane Disease

Infants with infection localized to the SEM typically present in the second week of life. Most infants with localized SEM disease are afebrile[2,42] and appear well. Skin lesions are often identified on the presenting part or at sites of trauma (fetal scalp monitors). Skin lesions are small (usually < 0.5 cm) vesicles that appear individually or grouped on an erythematous base (Figures 55-1 and 55-2). Vesicles may coalesce into larger (>1 cm) bullous lesions (Figure 55-3). If infection is untreated, new lesions will appear in close proximity to initial lesions or distant to initial lesions, probably as a result of viremic spread. In some cases, primary vesicles crust to resemble staphylococcal or streptococcal impetigo. Approximately 17% of children with SEM disease do not have skin lesions initially and present with eye (Figure 55-2) or other mucous membrane involvement.[2] HSV infection involving the eye causes keratoconjunctivitis and can progress to cause cataracts, corneal scarring, retinal necrosis, scarring, and detachment.[45] HSV keratoconjunctivitis must always be considered in the infant with conjunctival injection, tearing, and discharge. Oral mucous membrane involvement with neonatal HSV can manifest

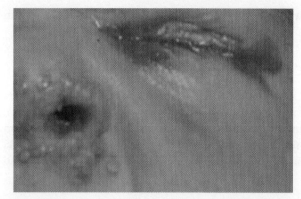

FIGURE 55-2 Typical vesicular lesions on the face of an infant with neonatal herpes simplex virus (HSV) infection. (Used with permission from Dr Ann Arvin.)

as ulcerative lesions of the oral mucosa and tongue. In some cases, the presence of oral lesions is not noted, even with positive oral cultures. It is not clear whether this is because of poor physical examination techniques or whether oral secretions in the neonate are sometimes positive in the absence of obvious oral ulcers. Untreated neonatal SEM HSV is associated with high risk of progression to CNS or disseminated disease.[46] Even after SEM disease is treated, infants have recurrent outbreaks of skin lesions throughout early childhood.[47]

The differential diagnosis of neonatal HSV skin lesions includes both infectious and noninfectious causes of vesicular or pustular skin eruptions (Table 55-3). Of note, even if a lesion is found to be culture positive for a bacterial organism such as *Staphylococcus aureus*, testing for HSV should be performed if clinical suspicion is high because both pathogens may be present. Bacterial organisms such as *Francisella tularensis*[48] and *Listeria*

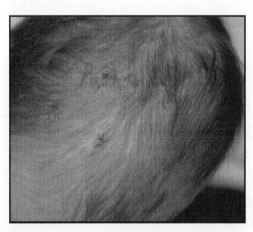

FIGURE 55-1 Typical vesicular lesions on the top of the head of an infant with neonatal herpes simplex virus (HSV) infection. (Used with permission from Dr Ann Arvin.)

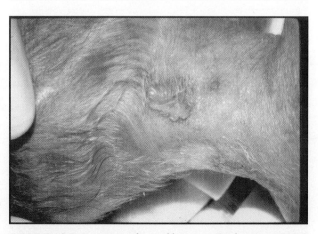

FIGURE 55-3 Larger coalesced herpes simplex virus (HSV) vesicular/bullous lesion, premature infant with neonatal HSV infection. (Used with permission from Dr Ann Arvin.)

monocytogenes can cause vesicular or pustular lesions in an infant.

Disseminated HSV Infection

Disseminated HSV infection carries the highest mortality of the different types of neonatal infection. Infants with disseminated HSV-1 or HSV-2 infection may become symptomatic within the first week of life, and almost all present by 3 weeks of age. Infants who are born prematurely are at higher risk for disseminated disease.[43] Diagnosis of disseminated infection is often delayed because the signs and symptoms are frequently nonspecific and similar to those seen in babies with bacterial sepsis.[42] Clinical features of disseminated neonatal HSV infection include temperature instability (fever or hypothermia), irritability, lethargy, shock, jaundice, bleeding, and respiratory distress. Progression of disease is rapid. Infection may involve any organ, including liver, lungs, gastrointestinal tract,

Table 55-3 Differential Diagnosis of Vesicular or Pustular Skin Lesions in the Newborn

Etiology	Characteristics
Infectious	
Viral	
Herpes simplex virus (See chapter text)	
Varicella zoster virus	Maternal or other exposure history
Enteroviruses	Season, maternal enterovirus illness
CMV	Usually petechial or purpuric
Bacterial	
Staphylococcal aureus (bullous impetigo, SSSS)	Larger lesions, positive bacterial culture
Treponema pallidum (syphilis)	Positive syphilis serology, hemorrhagic bullae, ulcers
Listeria monocytogenes	Associated with sepsis, meningitis
Francisella tularensis (vesicular tularemia)	Lesion may look similar to HSV[48]
Fungal	
Congenital cutaneous candidiasis	Patchy erythema, papules, pustules, vesicles
Parasitic	
Scabies	Not seen until > 3 weeks of age
Noninfectious	
Benign	
Erythema toxicum neonatorum	1- to 3-mm pustules on red base, trunk, and extremities
	Rash waxes and wanes; eosinophils seen on Tzanck smear
Neonatal pustular melanosis	More common in darker-skinned infants
	Hyperpigmented macules and pustules
In utero sucking blister	Sterile fluid-filled bullae/vesicles, hands/fingers
Neonatal acne	1- to 3-mm white or red follicular comedones
Infantile acropustulosis	Pruritic vesiculo/pustular lesions, hands and feet
	New crops of lesions every 2–4 weeks
Congenital	
Incontentia pigmenti	X-linked, multiple-organ involvement, linear lesions
Epidermolysis bullosa	Bullae at sites of minor trauma
Aplasia cutis congenita	Congenital absence of skin, often involving scalp
Other	
Drug eruption, neonatal mastocytosis	

Abbreviations: CMV, cytomegalovirus; SSSS, staphylococcal scalded skin syndrome.

adrenal glands, and brain. Fulminant hepatic failure is a complication of disseminated infection[42] and likely is caused by high levels of circulating virus.[49] Because CNS involvement is common in infants with disseminated HSV, seizures can occur. Laboratory abnormalities include elevated hepatic enzymes, thrombocytopenia, and a cerebrospinal fluid (CSF) pleocytosis, usually with a predominance of mononuclear cells, although polymorphonuclear neutrophil (PMN) cells may be present in the CSF.[50] Skin lesions are present in about 60% of cases of disseminated infection. Lesions are often not noted at the beginning of illness but develop later, even after antiviral therapy has been initiated.[2] One study found that a history of maternal fever was more common in mothers of infants with disseminated disease, compared to those with other categories of disease, and may be a surrogate marker for primary maternal infection.[43]

Differential Diagnosis

The differential diagnosis of disseminated neonatal HSV includes bacterial sepsis with typical neonatal bacterial pathogens and disseminated neonatal enterovirus infection.

Central Nervous System Infection

Infants with HSV-1 or HSV-2 encephalitis without disseminated disease typically present later, usually in the second or third week of life and occasionally as late as 4–6 weeks of age. In retrospect, history may reveal the presence of a skin lesion that pre-dated CNS symptoms. Clinical findings include fever, irritability, lethargy, poor feeding, seizures, a bulging fontanelle, or focal neurologic findings. Skin lesions may or may not be present at the time of diagnosis. In contrast to HSV encephalitis in adults, which is often localized to the temporal lobes, CNS-associated HSV infections in the neonate often involve multiple foci in the brain (Figure 55-4),

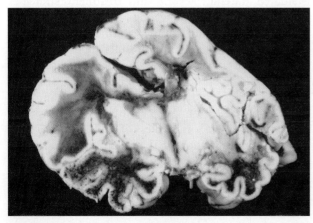

FIGURE 55-4 Postmortem findings of extensive herpes simplex virus (HSV) infection, cerebral cortex.

including rare case reports of brainstem or cerebellar involvement.[51] Extensive cortical involvement may be present. Children may present with relatively few CNS symptoms, but mortality and morbidity are high if infection is not recognized early and treated. Encephalitis caused by HSV-1 has less long-term morbidity compared to CNS infection with HSV-2.[2,47]

Differential Diagnosis

Differential diagnosis includes bacterial meningitis caused by usual newborn pathogens, such as *Streptococcus agalactiae*, *Escherichia coli*, *L. monocytogenes*, or *Enterococcus* spp., or enterovirus meningitis or encephalitis.

Intrauterine Infection

Intrauterine infection (Table 55-4) accounts for 5% or less of all cases of neonatal HSV infection. Case definitions of intrauterine infection have generally required

Table 55-4 Clinical Findings Reported With Intrauterine Herpes Simplex Virus (HSV) Infection[a]

Clinical Manifestations	Comment
Intrauterine demise[53]	
Fetal hydrops	Uncommon cause of nonimmune hydrops[52]
Premature birth	
Skin lesions	Reported to include vesicles in various healing stages, pustules, skin erosion, plaques, scars, erythema, hypopigmentation
Opthalmologic	Herpetic keratitis, chorioretinitis, optic atrophy, vitreal hemorrhage
Central nervous system	Intracranial calcifications, ventriculomegaly, microcephaly, encephalomalacia, seizures, hypertonicity
Limb and bone abnormalities	Metaphyseal lucencies of long bones, digit abnormalities, limb hypoplasia, synechiae
Other organ involvement	Hepatomegaly and hepatitis, lung and adrenal involvement noted postmortem

[a]Case definitions for the diagnosis of intrauterine HSV vary[26–28], but include evidence of disease within the first 24–48 hours of birth, virologic confirmation of HSV infection, placental involvement, older or evolving lesions noted at birth, evidence of abnormalities in embryogenesis, and exclusion of other diagnoses.

a triad of symptoms at birth (cutaneous, ophthalmologic, and CNS findings) plus virologically confirmed evidence of infection within the first 48 hours of life and the exclusion of other diseases.[26,28] Recent analysis of cases published over 45 years suggested that only about one-third of cases have the classic triad of symptoms.[27] Cutaneous lesions seen at birth include vesicobullous lesions, skin erosions, pustules, plaques, and hypopigmented scars. CNS abnormalities include porencephaly, microcephaly, ventriculomegaly, and intracranial calcifications. Clinical signs of seizures, meningoencephalitis, hypertonicity, and hepatomegaly may be present. Retinal disease, microphthalmia, and cataracts are the most common ophthalmological findings. Some infants have limb and bone abnormalities. Because of the variability of cutaneous findings, the diagnosis is often not considered initially. Intrauterine HSV infection is a rare case of nonimmune hydrops[52] and fetal demise.[53]

Differential Diagnosis

The differential diagnosis of intrauterine HSV infection includes other infectious causes of congenital infection, such as cytomegalovirus, rubella, and toxoplasmosis.

DIAGNOSIS

The diagnosis (Table 55-5) of neonatal HSV infection requires a solid understanding of epidemiologic and clinical factors of disease and a high index of suspicion in the ill neonate. It is essential that the proper viral cultures are obtained prior to initiation of antiviral therapy. Table 55-5 outlines appropriate specimens for HSV testing.

Laboratory Testing

Culture remains key in diagnosis of HSV infection. HSV grows rapidly in tissue culture, and 95% of positive isolates show cytopathic effect (CPE) within 5 days after specimen submission. Only 5% of isolates require longer (5–14 days) of inoculation.[54] Culture isolates should be typed to determine if an isolate is HSV-1 or HSV-2. Knowledge of virus type carries important epidemiologic and prognostic information. In general, the more sites cultured, the higher the likelihood that virus will be isolated if present. CSF viral culture may be positive if the infant has disseminated as well as CNS infection.

If skin lesions are present, immunofluorescent staining or polymerase chain reaction (PCR) testing (if available) for HSV from cells obtained from the base of the lesion for HSV has replaced testing by Tzanck smear. The Tzanck smear is relatively insensitive and cannot distinguish infection with HSV-1, HSV-2, or varicella.[55] A Tzanck smear remains useful in assisting with the diagnosis of other neonatal vesicular or pustular skin conditions.[56] The sensitivity of HSV immunofluorescent staining depends on the quality of the sample and whether an adequate number of cells are submitted.[57] It is important that a skilled technician read the slides to differentiate staining consistent with viral antigen vs nonspecific staining.[54] A concurrent viral culture of the specimen should also be obtained because of increased sensitivity of viral testing compared to direct fluorescence assay (DFA) and for confirmation of results. Immunofluorescent staining on samples other than vesicular skin lesions may be associated with decreased sensitivity or specificity of results.

Polymerase chain reaction testing for HSV DNA has improved and expanded diagnostic capabilities and is the gold standard for diagnosis of CNS HSV infection. Patients who were previously believed to have only SEM disease were later found to have CSF samples positive for HSV by PCR.[44] The reported sensitivity of PCR testing for diagnosis of neonatal HSV infection is variable (75%–100%); however, when performed by a reliable laboratory, the test is highly sensitive and specific. Early in the course of infection, PCR may not be sensitive enough to detect small amounts of viral DNA.[58] Therefore, the test should be repeated several days later if clinical suspicion remains high. A negative CSF PCR in conjunction with consistent symptoms does not rule out CNS HSV encephalitis. HSV PCR is frequently detected in peripheral blood mononuclear cells or plasma from patients with disseminated HSV infection.[59]

In the diagnosis of neonatal HSV encephalitis, CSF HSV PCR testing is a valuable tool; however, its use can be associated with a significantly longer hospitalization and hospital costs for infants who do not have neonatal HSV infection. These costs are because of the cost of secondary care provided infants while awaiting test results.[60] One cost-effectiveness analysis that evaluated different testing and treatment strategies determined that routine testing of febrile infants with CSF pleocytosis and empiric treatment pending test results may be cost effective if results are expeditiously available and those without disease are discharged by day 3 of hospitalization.[61] Therapeutic decisions should always be based on clinical findings, and acyclovir would be continued in an infant with symptoms consistent with HSV regardless of PCR results.

Serologic testing for HSV is of limited clinical utility in the infant. A positive IgG antibody for HSV-1 or HSV-2 reflects transplacental acquisition of maternal antibody. HSV IgG antibody may be negative in both baby and mother if the mother has a primary HSV infection and has not yet developed an antibody response. The development of IgM to HSV infection

Table 55-5 Laboratory Diagnosis of Suspected Neonatal Herpes Simplex Virus (HSV) Infection

Specimen	Test	Comment
Mucosal surface cultures: conjunctivae, nose, oropharynx, rectum	Viral culture	Most cultures for HSV are positive within 5–7 days, although cultures will be held for 10–14 days. Immunofluorescent staining techniques are not recommended for mucosal specimens.
Skin lesion (if present)	Immunofluorescent staining Viral culture Bacterial culture HSV DNA PCR if available	Immunofluorescent staining should be confirmed with viral culture. Positive culture for bacteria in a skin lesion does not rule out coinfection with HSV.
Blood	HSV DNA PCR Complete blood cell count Liver function studies Coagulation profile Blood culture (bacteria)	Positive in approximately two-thirds of cases of disseminated neonatal HSV[59] Thrombycytopenia seen with disseminated HSV infection Elevated transaminases seen with disseminated HSV infection Evaluate for DIC, seen with disseminated HSV infection Rule out other causes of infection in ill appearing infants.
Cerebrospinal fluid	HSV-1 and HSV-2 DNA PCR Enterovirus RNA PCR Viral culture Bacterial culture Cell count, glucose, and protein	HSV DNA PCR may be negative early in course of illness.[58] More often positive with disseminated neonatal HSV disease Typical findings with HSV include elevated protein, mildly decreased glucose, mononuclear cell predominance. Red blood cells are seen with hemorrhagic HSV encephalitis. *Listeria monocytogenes* meningitis may also present with a proportion of mononuclear cells in the CSF.
Ancillary tests		
Electroencephalogram (EEG)		Abnormal EEG findings seen in approximately 80% of infants with central nervous system disease[2]
Computed tomography (CT) or Magnetic resonance imaging (MRI)		Findings early in course of illness may be subtle. In neonatal HSV, multiple areas of brain can be involved.
Chest radiograph		Interstitial infiltrates or pleural effusion seen with HSV pneumonitis

Abbreviations: DIC, disseminated intravascular coagulation; PCR, polymerase chain reaction.

in the infant is delayed; therefore, testing for an IgM response does not assist with acute diagnosis and management. Serial antibody testing can be of value in long-term follow-up if the diagnosis of HSV was suspected but not confirmed initially and seroconversion is demonstrated.

Additional recommended laboratory testing includes a complete blood cell count (CBC) with differential, which may reveal thrombocytopenia; a coagulation panel; electrolytes; and liver function studies (LFTs). Thrombocytopenia and elevated LFTs are associated with disseminated infection.[43] Lumbar puncture (LP) should be performed. CSF typically shows a normal or modestly decreased glucose, normal or elevated protein,

and pleocytosis with a predominance of mononuclear cells, although PMN cells may be present.[50] CSF red blood cells are noted to be elevated in adult or childhood cases of HSV encephalitis[62]; however, their association with neonatal HSV encephalitis is less clear.[43] HSV encephalitis has been documented in children in whom the initial CSF parameters were normal.[50]

Ancillary Diagnostic Testing

Electroencephalograms (EEGs) are abnormal in approximately 78%–85% of infants with CNS involvement (disseminated disease with CNS involvement and localized CNS disease).[2] EEGs can show a pattern of

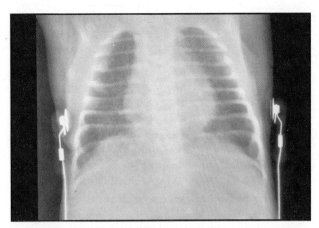

FIGURE 55-5 Chest radiograph showing herpes simplex virus (HSV) pneumonitis in a newborn.

paroxysmal lateralizing epileptiform discharges localized to the temporal region of the brain, nonspecific diffuse slowing, or multifocal epileptiform activity.[50]

Head imaging plays an important role in the early diagnosis of neonatal HSV infection and is abnormal in 75% of patients with CNS disease during the acute phase of illness. The imaging modalities used include computed tomography (CT) and magnetic resonance imaging (MRI). Imaging abnormalities may involve the temporal, frontal, parietal, subcortical areas, and occasionally brainstem and cerebellum.[51] Additional findings on CT include areas of edema, necrosis, or white matter hypoattenuation. CT may be negative early in the course of illness in a substantial (26%) number of patients with CNS disease. MRI is more sensitive, and MRI diagnosis is enhanced when diffusion-weighted imaging is used to assess for areas of disease and restricted diffusion.[63]

Interstitial pneumonitis and in rare cases pleural effusions may be seen on chest x-rays in infants with disseminated disease[64] (Figure 55-5).

TREATMENT

Empiric antiviral therapy (Tables 55-6 and 55-7) should be initiated promptly in any infant suspected of having neonatal HSV infection. There is debate among experts regarding whether all ill-appearing infants less than 21 days of age would benefit from empiric antiviral as well as antibiotic therapy pending results of diagnostic testing.[65, 66] Some argue that given the potential risk of HSV in an ill-appearing infant (with either fever without a source or hypothermia), early initiation of antiviral therapy is reasonable pending results of diagnostic tests and that a short course of empiric acyclovir carries little risk.[66] Others observe that neonatal HSV infection is a rare disease and recommend diagnostic evaluation and

Table 55-6 Treatment of Neonatal Herpes Simplex Virus Infection

Category of Disease	Drug/Dose	Duration[a]
Skin, eye, or mucous membrane	Acyclovir[b] 20 mg/kg/ day IV[c] every 8 hours	14 days
Disseminated disease	Acyclovir 20 mg/kg/ day IV every 8 hours	21 days
Central nervous system disease	Acyclovir 20 mg/kg/ day IV every 8 hours	21 days

Abbreviation: IV, intravenous.
[a]Durations given are minimum duration. If cerebrospinal fluid at end of therapy is positive for HSV DNA by polymerase chain reaction (PCR), most experts would extend duration of therapy until PCR is negative.
[b]Dose is for infant with normal renal function.
[c]Oral treatment is not recommended.

treatment with a sufficiently high index of suspicion, relying on additional clinical factors, such as hypothermia, respiratory distress, skin lesions, hepatitis, coagulopathy, seizures, or when, in a clinician's opinion, the infant appears septic or more ill than expected.[65]

If the clinician chooses to begin empiric therapy, it is imperative that comprehensive diagnostic testing by performed prior to initiation of acyclovir. Treatment is continued until HSV is reasonably ruled out by PCR and multiple surface cultures and the patient is doing well clinically. Growth of virus in culture generally takes 3–5 days. Cultures may occasionally become positive later than this.[54]

The drug used for treatment of neonatal HSV infection is the nucleoside analogue acyclovir (Zovirax). Acyclovir is monophosphorylated by HSV-specific thymidine kinases and then converted to its di- and triphosphate forms by cellular enzymes. Acyclovir acts as a competitive inhibitor of HSV DNA polymerase and terminates DNA chain elongation. Viruses with mutations in thymidine kinase or DNA polymerase are resistant to acyclovir and can be rarely identified in neonates.[67]

Table 55-7 Acyclovir Dosing in Infants With Renal Insufficiency

Creatinine Clearance	Dose	Interval
25 to 50 mL/ minute/1.73m2	20 mg/kg/dose	Every 12 h
10-25 mL/ minute/1.73m2	20 mg/kg/dose	Every 24 h
0-10 mL/ minute/1.73m2	10 mg/kg/dose	Every 24 h

From Pediatric and Neonatal Lexi-Drugs- Manufacturer's labeling recommends dose adjustment based on creatinine clearance.

All categories of neonatal HSV infection must be treated with intravenous acyclovir, even if the infant appears well and has only localized SEM. The bioavailability of oral acyclovir is poor, and neonates, by virtue of an immature immune system, are immunocompromised in their response to HSV. The current recommended standard dose of acyclovir for neonatal HSV is 60 mg/kg/day in 3 divided doses.[68] Infants with disseminated HSV and CNS infection require at least 21 days of therapy. Infants with SEM disease may be treated for 14 days, provided CNS involvement has been definitely ruled out. These dosing regimens are based on studies performed by the CASG in the 1980s and 1990s. Initial treatment trials of acyclovir for neonatal HSV utilized lower doses and a shorter duration of therapy(30 mg/kg/day for 10 days). Subsequent studies showed that higher doses and longer duration therapy were associated with improvement in outcomes.[69] Data regarding optimal acyclovir dosing in preterm infants remain sparse.

Infants with ocular infection should receive parenteral acyclovir as well as a topical antiviral ophthalmic solution (eg, 1% trifluridine). All infants suspected of having ocular infection should be managed in conjunction with an ophthalmologist.

It is recommended that an LP be performed at the end of therapy for patients with suspected or documented CNS disease and that the duration of therapy be extended if the CSF HSV PCR remains or has become positive.[2,7,88] Persistence of a positive HSV PCR in the CSF is associated with an increased risk of neurodevelopmental impairment.[70]

Acyclovir is generally well tolerated in the newborn. Side effects while on therapy include nausea, vomiting, diarrhea, neutropenia, elevated transaminases, skin rash (including hives), intravenous phlebitis, elevated serum urea nitrogen (BUN) and creatinine, and hematuria. Renal dysfunction is caused partly by crystallization of drug in the renal tubules and is not usually seen if the infant is well hydrated. Dose adjustment is necessary if the infant has impaired renal function (Table 55-7). No long-term side effects in treated infants have been reported to date.

Some infants with disseminated HSV infection have severe hemodynamic instability and respiratory compromise. Those neonates who require extracorporeal membrane oxygenation (ECMO) have poor outcomes according to 1 retrospective analysis, with only 25% of infants surviving.[71] Neonatal HSV hepatitis may result in liver failure, and rare cases of survival after liver transplant are reported.[72]

Treatment with high-dose acyclovir in conjunction with technological advances in neonatal intensive care have substantially decreased mortality from neonatal HSV infection and, to some extent, have decreased morbidity of infection.[73] Approximate mortality from disseminated infection at 2 years of age is 31% and for CNS infection is 6%.[69] Virtually all infants with SEM disease survive, and fewer than 2% have developmental impairment, as compared to 38% in the preantiviral era.[1] Most treated surviving children with disseminated disease have normal development. Unfortunately, only about one-third of infants with CNS disease have normal development following treatment. It is important that the diagnosis is considered early with prompt initiation of treatment because onset of seizures prior to therapy is associated with poorer outcomes.[2]

Suppressive Therapy

Despite appropriate diagnosis and timely initiation of therapy, a subset of infants continues to have recurrent skin lesions or recurrent positive HSV PCR in the CSF.[74] Studies performed by the NIAID CASG showed a correlation between frequency of recurrent skin lesions and neurologic impairment in patients with HSV-2 SEM disease.[47] All children who had fewer than 3 recurrences of skin lesions within the first 6 months of life developed normally, compared to 79% of children with 3 or more recurrences.[47] As a result of this information, the NIAID CASG conducted trials to evaluate the safety and efficacy of oral suppressive acyclovir therapy after an appropriate course of parenteral therapy in infants with neonatal HSV CNS or SEM disease. Recently published results of 2 parallel phase 3 trials reported that infants randomized to receive treatment with oral acyclovir 300 mg/m²/dose 3 times daily had higher mean Bayley Scales of Development Mental scores at 1 year compared to infants who received placebo ($P= .046$).[75] The benefits of 6 months of oral acyclovir to improve neurodevelopmental outcomes in infants with CNS disease and to suppress skin lesions appear to outweigh the risks of drug toxicity.[68,76]

One additional small cohort study using even higher-dose oral acyclovir for a period of 2 years described improved long-term neurologic outcomes in children compared to results reported from early NIAID CASG trials (for which suppressive therapy was not utilized).[77]

Complications of oral suppressive therapy include neutropenia and, rarely, selection of acyclovir-resistant viruses.[78] Oral acyclovir therapy has in some instances failed to prevent CNS HSV infection or reactivation.[79,80] The bioavailability of oral acyclovir is poor (10%–20%) and decreases with increasing doses. CSF concentrations are about 50% of serum concentration. Oral antivirals such as valacyclovir or famciclovir, with improved bioavailability and decreased dosing frequency, may be more suitable options for suppression in older infants in the future.[81,82]

PROGNOSIS

In general, there are no differences in mortality between infections caused by HSV-1 and HSV-2, although in the early lower-dose (30 mg/kg/day) NIAID CASG studies, mortality for HSV-1 disseminated disease was higher.[69]

Many infants with CNS disease develop deficits in cognitive function, speech, attention, or spastic cerebral palsy. Despite antiviral therapy, two-thirds of infants in the NIAID CASG studies with CNS disease had some developmental delay (ranging from mild to severe) at 12 months.[2] Infants with neonatal HSV-1 CNS infection fared better than those with HSV-2 CNS infection. Only 17.5% of those with HSV-2 infection had normal developmental evaluations compared to 57% of infants with HSV-1 CNS infection. However, CNS infection with either HSV-1 and HSV-2 can result in severe neurologic impairment.

Head imaging (CT) performed in the first week to month after diagnosis is not helpful in providing prognostic information. In 1 descriptive cohort study for which CT was the predominant radiologic modality utilized, infants with relatively subtle radiologic deficits had significantly poor neurologic outcome documented at long-term follow-up. Others with more significant CT abnormalities appeared to have near-normal development.[80] Children in this study received the lower dose of acyclovir, 30 mg/kg/day, which was standard during the time period they were diagnosed. Progressive abnormalities on CT could reflect either the natural history of resolving infection or evidence of intermittent continued CNS reactivation.

PREVENTION

It is recommended that women who develop primary or first-episode HSV infection during pregnancy be treated with either oral antivirals or intravenous acyclovir if they have severe genital disease or disseminated HSV infection.[83,84] Maternal prophylaxis with either acyclovir or valacyclovir beginning at 36 weeks of gestation is recommended for women with a history of recurrent genital HSV. Prophylaxis decreases symptomatic recurrences and decreases the need for cesarean section. Data are insufficient to prove that this approach decreases the incidence of neonatal HSV infection. In studies included in a recent Cochrane analysis, no infant in either the maternal treated or untreated groups developed HSV infection; however, the total number of infants included was insufficient to see differences between treatment-exposed and nonexposed groups. HSV (by PCR or culture) was detected from surface specimens of 2 treated and 1 untreated infant.[85] Therefore, there is still a potential risk of

neonatal infection in infants born to treated mothers. The history of maternal treatment should not preclude an evaluation of a symptomatic infant. The safety of antiviral therapy during pregnancy has not been definitely established; however, no increased risk of birth defects have yet been associated with prenatal exposure to acyclovir.[84] The American College of Obstetricians and Gynecologists (ACOG) currently recommends cesarean section for women with symptomatic genital lesions or prodromal symptoms of burning or pain at the time of delivery.[83] Cesarean section decreases the risk of neonatal HSV infection from 7.7% to 1.2% in infants born to mothers from whom HSV is isolated at the time of delivery.[8]

The ACOG does not recommend routine antepartum cultures for viral shedding.[83] Antepartum cultures do not predict shedding at the time of delivery. A rapid PCR test that is capable of detecting virus in vaginal secretions within 2 hours has been developed.[86] Clinical studies of this technology in informing clinical decision making are pending. Routine serologic screening for HSV during pregnancy is not currently recommended based on cost-benefit analysis[83]; however, there are some women who may benefit from this information and counseling regarding safe sex practices.

Proposed strategies for prevention of neonatal HSV infection are complex and include recommendations for abstinence from any sexual contact during pregnancy, serologic testing to identify "at-risk" women, and serologic testing of pregnant women and their partners to identify higher-risk women.[87] The last approach has the advantage of identifying a smaller group of high-risk women who are seronegative for HSV and have a seropositive partner. Intensive counseling regarding methods to prevent primary infection in the woman or consideration of suppressive antiviral therapy for the seropositive partner may be considered, although the effectiveness of this approach remains unproven.

Women with HSV infections may breast-feed their infants as long as the infant is protected from infectious secretions and there are no lesions on the breast. If a mother has orolabial lesions, she should wear a disposable surgical mask while in close contact with her infant until her lesions have crusted and dried. If the mother has skin lesions, these should be covered. The mother and all caregivers should be instructed regarding excellent hand hygiene.[68]

Management of asymptomatic infants who are known to be exposed to HSV infected lesions at the time of delivery has not been systematically evaluated. Detailed guidance on the management of asymptomatic infants born to mothers with genital herpes lesions has been published.[68,88] (Table 55-8). The risk to the infant varies depending on whether the maternal lesions reflect recurrent or primary disease, and recommendations vary accordingly. Infants born by either vaginal delivery or cesarean section to a mother

Table 55-8 Initial Management of Asymptomatic Infants Exposed to Herpes Simplex Virus (HSV) at Delivery[a,b]

Exposure	Management
Suspected or confirmed maternal primary infection	Surface viral cultures (and HSV PCR if available), blood HSV PCR, CSF studies including CSF and HSV PCR; at approximately 24 hours of age, serum ALT; initiate empiric acyclovir pending HSV study results. If cultures are positive or baby is ill, remainder of evaluation should be performed (see Table 55-5).
Recurrent genital lesions at delivery	Surface viral cultures (and HSV PCRs if available), HSV blood PCR, close observation, empiric acyclovir not generally recommended unless infant symptomatic.
History of recurrent genital HSV; no lesions at delivery	Baby should be evaluated clinically; surface cultures and empiric acyclovir are not recommended for well-appearing infant.

[a]Parents and caregivers of any infant with potential known exposure to HSV should be educated regarding signs and symptoms of disease and the need for immediate empiric antiviral therapy if the infant becomes ill.
[b]Data from the American Academy of Pediatrics Committee on Infectious Diseases *Redbook* 2012, and Committee on Infectious Diseases and Committee on Fetus and Newborn.[68,88]

with active lesions noted at delivery should have HSV cultures (and PCR if available) from mouth, nasopharynx, conjunctivae, scalp electrode site and rectum sent at approximately 24 hours of age, prior to initiation of any antiviral treatment. In addition, for infants born to mothers with a lesion but no preceding maternal HSV history (ie concern for primary infection), HSV blood PCR and CSF studies including HSV PCR are also recommended by the recent management document.[88] The sensitivity of viral cultures from infants whose mothers received prophylactic acyclovir from 36 weeks until delivery is unknown.

If the mother is experiencing her first symptomatic genital infection, culture and HSV PCR of the maternal lesion and reliable type-specific serologic testing of the mother are recommended. New guidelines recommend initiation of IV acyclovir pending results of maternal sero-status and viral diagnostic testing from infant. If the maternal lesion is positive for HSV by culture or PCR and the mother has no antibody to the virus isolated, it is likely that she is experiencing a primary infection. In this situation, the risk to the baby of acquiring neonatal HSV with a primary infection ranges from 30% to 60%.[8,17]

If the mother has a known history of genital HSV, the risk to the asymptomatic baby of acquiring infection is low (<5%), and most experts would not treat with acyclovir while awaiting test results, but would educate the infant's parents or caregivers regarding signs of disease during the first 6 weeks of life. It is important to educate both the parents and the primary care physician following the infant that if the child develops any clinical findings suggestive of neonatal HSV infection that diagnostic evaluation and empiric acyclovir therapy must be initiated immediately. It is also important to note that signs of infection are often subtle and nonspecific.[42]

If the surface cultures or PCR obtained from the infant at 24 hours of life become positive, the rest of the diagnostic workup outlined in the section on diagnosis must be performed. If surface cultures are positive (indicating infection) but no evidence of disease is found, the American Academy of Pediatrics (AAP) recommends treatment for at least 10 days in an attempt to prevent HSV disease.[68,88] See reference 88 for specific guidance. An infant with evidence of CNS, SEM, or disseminated disease is treated as discussed in the section on treatment.

INFECTION CONTROL

For infection control (Table 55-9), infants with HSV infection should be placed in contact isolation unless they have no clinical or laboratory evidence of SEM disease. If they have evidence of pulmonary disease, respiratory isolation is also recommended. Infants born to mothers with active HSV lesions should also be managed with contact precautions. Infants born to mothers with a history of recurrent lesions but no lesions at birth do not need to be placed in isolation. Infants who are well at birth and who have been exposed can be allowed to continuously room in with the mother.[68]

Health care personnel with herpetic whitlow should refrain from contact with infants until lesions are dry and crusted. Whether to allow health care personnel with orolabial herpes to care for an infant requires careful consideration of risk of exposing an infant to HSV vs excluding essential personnel from the nursery.[68] Recommendations particular to a specific nursery may vary but should be reviewed and there should be adherence. Because all individuals with latent HSV infection shed virus intermittently and often asymptomatically, meticulous hand hygiene is always necessary.

Table 55-9 Isolation Recommendations for Selected Scenarios[a]

Scenario	Type of Isolation
Infant born to mother with history of recurrent genital HSV, no lesions and no prodromal symptoms at the time of delivery	Standard precautions
Infant born to mother with lesions at delivery (primary or recurrent infection)	Vaginal delivery: Contact precautions, and encourage rooming in with mother Cesarean section: Contact precautions or if no prolonged ROM some experts would suggest standard precautions
Neonatal HSV disease	SEM or disseminated disease: Contact precautions. If pulmonary disease is present some would recommend addition of respiratory precautions. Isolated CNS disease: Standard precautions
Symptomatic maternal HSV infection	Skin lesions: cover lesions. Do not breast-feed from breast if lesions are present. Orolabial lesions: Disposable mask until lesions dried and crusted Genital lesions: Meticulous hand hygiene
Health care worker with herpetic whitlow	Do not allow direct care of infants until lesions resolved.
Health care worker with orolabial lesions	Adhere to institutional infection control guidelines—may weigh risk/benefit of excluding essential personnel to low risk of infant exposure (if lesions are covered by a mask and not touched).
Health care worker with genital HSV	Transmission unlikely, meticulous hand hygiene

[a]Data from American Academy of Pediatrics Committee on Infectious Disease, 2012 Redbook.[68]

REFERENCES

1. Whitley RJ, Nahmias AJ, Soong SJ, Galasso GG, Fleming CL, Alford CA. Vidarabine therapy of neonatal herpes simplex virus infection. *Pediatrics.* 1980;66(4):495–501.

2. Kimberlin DW, Lin CY, Jacobs RF, et al. Natural history of neonatal herpes simplex virus infections in the acyclovir era. *Pediatrics.* 2001;108(2):223–229.

3. Xu F, Markowitz LE, Gottlieb SL, Berman SM. Seroprevalence of herpes simplex virus types 1 and 2 in pregnant women in the United States. *Am J Obstet Gynecol.* 2007;196(1):43.e1–e6.

4. Roberts CM, Pfister JR, Spear SJ. Increasing proportion of herpes simplex virus type 1 as a cause of genital herpes infection in college students. *Sex Transm Dis.* 2003; 30(10):797–800.

5. Engelberg R, Carrell D, Krantz E, Corey L, Wald A. Natural history of genital herpes simplex virus type 1 infection. *Sex Transm Dis.* 2003;30(2):174–177.

6. Mark KE, Wald A, Magaret AS et al. Rapidly cleared episodes of herpes simplex virus reactivation in immunocompetent adults. *J Infect Dis.* 2008;198(8):1141–1149.

7. Thompson C, Whitley R. Neonatal herpes simplex virus infections: where are we now? *Adv Exp Med Biol.* 2011;697: 221–230.

8. Brown ZA, Wald A, Morrow RA, Selke S, Zeh J, Corey L. Effect of serologic status and cesarean delivery on transmission rates of herpes simplex virus from mother to infant. *JAMA.* 2003;289(2):203–209.

9. Handsfield HH, Waldo AB, Brown ZA, et al. Neonatal herpes should be a reportable disease. *Sex Transm Dis.* 2005;32(9): 521–525.

10. Corey L, Wald A. Maternal and neonatal herpes simplex virus infections. *N Engl J Med.* 2009;361(14):1376–1385.

11. Flagg EW, Weinstock H. Incidence of neonatal herpes simplex virus infections in the United States, 2006. *Pediatrics.* 2011; 127(1):e1–e8.

12. Gutierrez KM, Falkovitz Halpern MS, Maldonado Y, Arvin AM. The epidemiology of neonatal herpes simplex virus infections in California from 1985 to 1995. *J Infect Dis.* 1999;180(1):199–202.

13. Mark KE, Kim HN, Wald A, Gardella C, Reed SD. Targeted prenatal herpes simplex virus testing: can we identify women at risk of transmission to the neonate? *Am J Obstet Gynecol.* 2006;194(2):408–414.

14. Morris SR, Bauer HM, Samuel MC, Gallagher D, Bolan G. Neonatal herpes morbidity and mortality in California, 1995–2003. *Sex Transm Dis.* 2008;35(1):14–18.

15. Xu F, Gee JM, Naleway A, et al. Incidence of neonatal herpes simplex virus infections in two managed care organizations: implications for surveillance. *Sex Transm Dis.* 2008;35(6):592–598.

16. Whitley R, Davis EA, Suppapanya N. Incidence of neonatal herpes simplex virus infections in a managed-care population. *Sex Transm Dis.* 2007;34(9):704–708.

17. Brown ZA, Selke S, Zeh J, et al. The acquisition of herpes simplex virus during pregnancy. *N Engl J Med.* 1997;337(8):509–515.

18. Prober CG, Sullender WM, Yasukawa LL, Au DS, Yeager AS, Arvin AM. Low risk of herpes simplex virus infections in neonates exposed to the virus at the time of vaginal delivery to mothers with recurrent genital herpes simplex virus infections. *N Engl J Med.* 1987;316(5):240–244.

19. Parvey LS, Ch'ien LT. Neonatal herpes simplex virus infection introduced by fetal-monitor scalp electrodes. *Pediatrics.* 1980;65(6):1150–1153.

20. Nahmias AJ, Josey WE, Naib ZM, Freeman MG, Fernandez RJ, Wheeler JH. Perinatal risk associated with maternal genital herpes simplex virus infection. *Am J Obstet Gynecol.* 1971; 110(6):825–837.

21. O'Riordan DP, Golden WC, Aucott SW. Herpes simplex virus infections in preterm infants. *Pediatrics*. 2006;118(6): e1612–e1620.

22. Caviness AC, Demmler GJ, Almendarez Y, Selwyn BJ. The prevalence of neonatal herpes simplex virus infection compared with serious bacterial illness in hospitalized neonates. *J Pediatr*. 2008;153(2):164–169.

23. Roizman B, Knipe DM, Whitley RJ. Neonatal herpes simplex virus infection. In: Knipe DM, Howley PM, eds. Fields Virology. Vol 2. 6th ed. Philadelphia: Lippincott Williams & Wilkins; 2013.

24. Sullender WM, Yasukawa LL, Schwartz M, et al. Type-specific antibodies to herpes simplex virus type 2 (HSV-2) glycoprotein G in pregnant women, infants exposed to maternal HSV-2 infection at delivery, and infants with neonatal herpes. *J Infect Dis*. 1988;157(1):164–171.

25. Wald A, Ashley-Morrow R. Serological testing for herpes simplex virus (HSV)-1 and HSV-2 infection. *Clin Infect Dis*. 2001;35(Suppl 2):S173–S182.

26. Hutto C, Arvin A, Jacobs R, et al. Intrauterine herpes simplex virus infections. *J Pediatr*. 1987;110(1):97–101.

27. Marquez L, Levy ML, Munoz FM, Palazzi DL. A report of three cases and review of intrauterine herpes simplex virus infection. *Pediatr Infect Dis J*. 2011;30(2):153–157.

28. Baldwin S, Whitley RJ. Intrauterine herpes simplex virus infection. *Teratology*. 1989;39(1):1–10.

29. Alanen A, Hukkanen V. Herpes simplex virus DNA in amniotic fluid without neonatal infection. *Clin Infect Dis*. 2000; 30(2):363–367.

30. Chatterjee A, Chartrand SA, Harrison CJ, Felty-Duckworth A, Bewtra C. Severe intrauterine herpes simplex disease with placentitis in a newborn of a mother with recurrent genital infection at delivery. *J Perinatol*. 2001;21(8):559–564.

31. Kimberlin DW. Herpes simplex virus infections of the newborn. *Semin Perinatol*. 2007;31(1):19–25.

32. Light IJ. Postnatal acquisition of herpes simplex virus by the newborn infant: a review of the literature. *Pediatrics*. 1979; 63(3):480–482.

33. Sullivan-Bolyai JZ, Fife KH, Jacobs RF, Miller Z, Corey L. Disseminated neonatal herpes simplex virus type 1 from a maternal breast lesion. *Pediatrics*. 1983;71(3):455–457.

34. Dunkle LM, Schmidt RR, O'Connor DM. Neonatal herpes simplex infection possibly acquired via maternal breast milk. *Pediatrics*. 1979;63(2):250–251.

35. Rubin LG, Lanzkowsky P. Cutaneous neonatal herpes simplex infection associated with ritual circumcision. *Pediatr Infect Dis J*. 2000;19(3):266–268.

36. Yeager AS, Arvin AM. Reasons for the absence of a history of recurrent genital infections in mothers of neonates infected with herpes simplex virus. *Pediatrics*. 1984;73(2):188–193.

37. Xu F, Sternberg MR, Kottiri BJ, et al. Trends in herpes simplex virus type 1 and type 2 seroprevalence in the United States. *JAMA*. 2006;296(8):964–973.

38. Lewis DB, Wilson CB. Developmental immunology and role of host defenses in fetal and neonatal susceptibility to infection. In: Infectious Diseases of the Fetus and Newborn Infant. 7th ed. Remington JS, Klein JO, Wilson CB, Nizet V, Maldonado YA. Philadelphia, PA: Elsevier Saunders; 2011:162–169.

39. Sullender WM, Miller JL, Yasukawa LL, et al. Humoral and cell-mediated immunity in neonates with herpes simplex virus infection. *J Infect Dis*. 1987;155(1):28–37.

40. Kohl S. The neonatal human's immune response to herpes simplex virus infection: a critical review. *Pediatr Infect Dis J*. 1989;8(2):67–74.

41. Kohl S, West MS, Prober CG, Sullender WM, Loo LS, Arvin AM. Neonatal antibody-dependent cellular cytotoxic antibody levels are associated with the clinical presentation of neonatal herpes simplex virus infection. *J Infect Dis*. 1989;160(5):770–776.

42. Long SS, Pool TE, Vodzak J, Daskalaki I, Gould JM. Herpes simplex virus infection in young infants during 2 decades of empiric acyclovir therapy. *Pediatr Infect Dis J*. 2011;30(7):556–561.

43. Caviness AC, Demmler GJ, Selwyn BJ. Clinical and laboratory features of neonatal herpes simplex virus infection: a case-control study. *Pediatr Infect Dis J*. 2008;27(5):425–430.

44. Kimberlin DW, Lakeman FD, Arvin AM, et al. Application of the polymerase chain reaction to the diagnosis and management of neonatal herpes simplex virus disease. National Institute of Allergy and Infectious Diseases Collaborative Antiviral Study Group. *J Infect Dis*. 1996;174(6):1162–1167.

45. el Azazi M, Malm G, Forsgren M. Late ophthalmologic manifestations of neonatal herpes simplex virus infection. *Am J Ophthalmol*. 1990;109(1):1–7.

46. Whitley RJ, Corey L, Arvin A, et al. Changing presentation of herpes simplex virus infection in neonates. *J Infect Dis*. 1988;158(1):109–116.

47. Whitley R, Arvin A, Prober C, et al. Predictors of morbidity and mortality in neonates with herpes simplex virus infections. The National Institute of Allergy and Infectious Diseases Collaborative Antiviral Study Group. *N Engl J Med*. 1991;324(7):450–454.

48. Byington CL, Bender JM, Ampofo K, et al. Tularemia with vesicular skin lesions may be mistaken for infection with herpes viruses. *Clin Infect Dis*. 2008;47(1):e4–e6.

49. Kimura H, Ito Y, Futamura M, et al. Quantitation of viral load in neonatal herpes simplex virus infection and comparison between type 1 and type 2. *J Med Virol*. 2001;67(3):349–353.

50. Arvin AM, Yeager AS, Bruhn FW, Grossman M. Neonatal herpes simplex infection in the absence of mucocutaneous lesions. *J Pediatr*. 1982;100(5):715–721.

51. Pelligra G, Lynch N, Miller SP, Sargent MA, Osiovich H. Brainstem involvement in neonatal herpes simplex virus type 2 encephalitis. *Pediatrics*. 2007;120(2): e442–e446.

52. Anderson MS, Abzug MJ. Hydrops fetalis: an unusual presentation of intrauterine herpes simplex virus infection. *Pediatr Infect Dis J*. 1999;18(9):837–839.

53. Barefoot KH, Little GA, Ornvold KT. Fetal demise due to herpes simplex virus: an illustrated case report. *J Perinatol*. 2001;22(1):86–88.

54. Versalovic J, et al, eds. *Manual of Clinical Microbiology*. 10th ed, Vol. 2. Washington, DC: ASM Press; 2011.

55. Nahass GT, Goldstein BA, Zhu WY, Serfling U, Penneys NS, Leonardi CL. Comparison of Tzanck smear, viral culture, and DNA diagnostic methods in detection of herpes simplex and varicella-zoster infection. *JAMA*. 1992;268(18):2541–2544.

56. Johr RH, Schachner LA. Neonatal dermatologic challenges. *Pediatr Rev*. 1997;18(3):86–94.

57. Caviness AC, Oelze LL, Saz UE, Greer JM, Demmler-Harrison GJ. Direct immunofluorescence assay compared to cell culture for the diagnosis of mucocutaneous herpes simplex virus infections in children. *J Clin Virol*. 2010;49(1):58–60.

58. Weil AA, Glaser CA, Amad Z, Forghani B. Patients with suspected herpes simplex encephalitis: rethinking an initial negative polymerase chain reaction result. *Clin Infect Dis*. 2001;34(8):1154–1157.

59. Diamond C, Mohan K, Hobson A, Frenkel L, Corey L. Viremia in neonatal herpes simplex virus infections. *Pediatr Infect Dis J*. 1999;18(6):487–489.

60. Shah SS, Volk J, Mohamad Z, Hodinka RL, Zorc JJ. Herpes simplex virus testing and hospital length of stay in neonates and young infants. *J Pediatr*. 2010;156(5):738–743.

61. Caviness AC, Demmler GJ, Swint JM, Cantor SB. Cost-effectiveness analysis of herpes simplex virus testing and treatment strategies in febrile neonates. *Arch Pediatr Adolesc Med*. 2008;162(7):665–674.

62. Elbers JM, Bitnun A, Richardson SE, et al. A 12-year prospective study of childhood herpes simplex encephalitis: is

there a broader spectrum of disease? *Pediatrics.* 2007;119(2): e399–e407.

63. Vossough A, Zimmerman RA, Bilaniuk LT, Schwartz EM. Imaging findings of neonatal herpes simplex virus type 2 encephalitis. *Neuroradiology.* 2008;50(4):355–366.

64. Bennett RE Jr, Barnett DW. Perinatal herpes simplex infection presenting with pneumonia and pleural effusions. *Pediatr Infect Dis J.* 2001;20(2):228–230.

65. Kimberlin DW. When should you initiate acyclovir therapy in a neonate? *J Pediatr.* 2008;153(2):155–156.

66. Long SS. In defense of empiric acyclovir therapy in certain neonates. *J Pediatr.* 2008;153(2):157–158.

67. Levin MJ, Weinberg A, Leary JJ, Sarisky RT. Development of acyclovir-resistant herpes simplex virus early during the treatment of herpes neonatorum. *Pediatr Infect Dis J.* 2001;20(11):1094–1097.

68. American Academy of Pediatrics. Herpes simplex virus. In: *American Academy of Pediatrics Red Book: 2012 Report of the Committee on Infectious Diseases.* 29th ed. Pickering LK, Baker CJ, Kimberlin DW, Long SS, eds. Elk Grove Village, IL: American Academy of Pediatrics; 2012:398.

69. Kimberlin DW, Lin CY, Jacobs RF, et al. Safety and efficacy of high-dose intravenous acyclovir in the management of neonatal herpes simplex virus infections. *Pediatrics.* 2001;108(2):230–328.

70. Mejias A, Bustos R, Ardura MI, Ramirez C, Sanchez PJ. Persistence of herpes simplex virus DNA in cerebrospinal fluid of neonates with herpes simplex virus encephalitis. *J Perinatol.* 2009;29(4):290–296.

71. Prodhan P, Wilkes R, Ross A, et al. Neonatal herpes virus infection and extracorporeal life support. *Pediatr Crit Care Med.* 2010;11(5):599–602.

72. Verma A, Dhawan A, Zuckerman M, Hadzic N, Baker AJ, Mieli-Vergani G. Neonatal herpes simplex virus infection presenting as acute liver failure: prevalent role of herpes simplex virus type I. *J Pediatr Gastroenterol Nutr.* 2006;42(3):282–286.

73. Jones CA, Walker KS, Badawi N. Antiviral agents for treatment of herpes simplex virus infection in neonates. *Cochrane Database Syst Rev.* 2009;(3):CD004206.

74. Kimura H, Aso K, Kuzushima K, Hanada N, Shibata M, Morishima T. Relapse of herpes simplex encephalitis in children. *Pediatrics.* 1992;89(5 Pt 1):891–894.

75. Kimberlin DW, Whitley RJ, Wan W, et al. Oral acyclovir suppression and neurodevelopment after neonatal herpes. *N Engl J Med.* 2011;365(14):1284–1292.

76. Gershon AA. Neonatal herpes simplex infection and the Three Musketeers. *N Engl J Med.* 2011;365(14):1338–1339.

77. Tiffany KF, Benjamin DK, Jr., Palasanthiran P, O'Donnell K, Gutman LT. Improved neurodevelopmental outcomes following long-term high-dose oral acyclovir therapy in infants with central nervous system and disseminated herpes simplex disease. *J Perinatol.* 2005;25(3):156–161.

78. Kimberlin D, Powell D, Gruber W, et al. Administration of oral acyclovir suppressive therapy after neonatal herpes simplex virus disease limited to the skin, eyes and mouth: results of a phase I/II trial. *Pediatr Infect Dis J.* 1996;15(3):247–254.

79. Fonseca-Aten M, Messina AF, Jafri HS, Sanchez PJ. Herpes simplex virus encephalitis during suppressive therapy with acyclovir in a premature infant. *Pediatrics.* 2005;115(3):804–809.

80. Engman ML, Adolfsson I, Lewensohn-Fuchs I, Forsgren M, Mosskin M, Malm G. Neuropsychologic outcomes in children with neonatal herpes encephalitis. *Pediatr Neurol.* 2008;38(6): 398–405.

81. Kimberlin DW, Jacobs RF, Weller S, et al. Pharmacokinetics and safety of extemporaneously compounded valacyclovir oral suspension in pediatric patients from 1 month through 11 years of age. *Clin Infect Dis.* 2010;50(2):221–228.

82. Blumer J, Rodriguez A, Sanchez PJ, Sallas W, Kaiser G, Hamed K. Single-dose pharmacokinetics of famciclovir in infants and population pharmacokinetic analysis in infants and children. *Antimicrob Agents Chemother.* 2010;54(5):2032–2041.

83. ACOG Practice Bulletin. Clinical management guidelines for obstetrician-gynecologists. No. 82 June 2007. Management of herpes in pregnancy. *Obstet Gynecol.* 2007;109(6):1489–1498.

84. Centers for Disease Control and Prevention. Sexually Transmitted Diseases Treatment Guidelines 2010. Genital HSV Infections MMWR 2010; 59 (RR-12):20-27

85. Hollier LM, Wendel GD. Third trimester antiviral prophylaxis for preventing maternal genital herpes simplex virus (HSV) recurrences and neonatal infection. *Cochrane Database Syst Rev.* 2008;(1):CD004946.

86. Gardella C, Huang ML, Wald A, et al. Rapid polymerase chain reaction assay to detect herpes simplex virus in the genital tract of women in labor. *Obstet Gynecol.* 2010;115(6):1209–1216.

87. Gardella C, Brown Z. Prevention of neonatal herpes. BJOG. 2011;118(2):187–192.

88. Kimberlin DW, Baley J, Committee on Infectious Diseases and Committee on Fetus and Newborn. Guidance on management of asymptomatic neonates born to women with active genital herpes lesions. *Pediatrics* 2013;131;e635-e645.

56 Parvovirus B19 Infection

Natali Aziz and Mary E. Norton

INTRODUCTION

Human parvovirus B19, a single-stranded DNA virus, is a member of the erythrovirus genus within the Parvoviridae family and the only erythrovirus that is a pathogen in humans.[1] Human parvovirus was first identified by electron microscopy in 1975 and was associated with clinical disease approximately a decade later.[2] It is the etiologic organism that manifests clinically as erythema infectiosum (fifth disease), a common childhood viral exanthem. In immunocompetent adults, infection with B19 is generally asymptomatic or mild. It is most commonly transmitted through respiratory droplets, and primary B19 infection in pregnant women can also result in vertical transmission to the fetus. Although most commonly asymptomatic for both mother and fetus, in some cases primary or acute infection in pregnancy may lead to adverse perinatal outcomes, including spontaneous abortion, hydrops fetalis, and fetal demise.

EPIDEMIOLOGY

Parvovirus B19 infection occurs worldwide, and cases may be sporadic or may occur in clustered outbreaks and even as epidemics.[3,4] The infection is easily transmitted from person to person via the respiratory route. In the United States, B19 infection occurs more frequently between late winter and early summer. Cycles of local epidemics have also been reported, with case numbers peaking approximately every 4 years.[5,6] Hematogenous transmission can also occur from administration of blood or blood products containing B19. Individuals requiring regular infusions of blood products that are made from large plasma pools are at greater risk for acquiring the virus compared to those individuals receiving single units.[7]

Seroprevalence rates of parvovirus B19 vary based on age and geographic location. The percentage of people with measurable levels of B19-specific immunoglobulin (Ig) G increases with increasing age, with most individuals becoming infected during their school years. Seroprevalence is approximately 15% of preschool children, 50% in adults, and 85% in the elderly[3,8] and is high (82%–89%) in women who live or work with young children.[9] The secondary attack rate for household contacts may be as high as 50%.[3] Immunity is lifelong in immunocompetent individuals.[10]

Nonimmune pregnant women have the same susceptibility to B19 infection as other immunocompetent adults. In the United States, 50%–75% of women in the reproductive age group are immune and demonstrate antibodies to human parvovirus B19.[11–13] Therefore, approximately 30%–50% of pregnant women are susceptible to B19 infection, which then places their fetus at risk of infection. The incidence of acute B19 infection in pregnancy may range from 1% to 3.8% and may be as high as 10% during epidemics.[14–17]

PATHOPHYSIOLOGY

Parvoviridae are small, nonenveloped DNA viruses that infect a variety of animals, usually in a species-specific fashion; only parvovirus B19 is known to cause disease in humans. The virus replicates in erythroid progenitor cells (late erythroid cell precursors and burst-forming erythroid progenitors) of the bone marrow and blood leading to inhibition of erythropoiesis, which can result in symptoms of anemia. B19 also may stimulate a cellular process initiating apoptosis; this characteristic may attribute to the minimal inflammatory response noted in infected tissues.[18]

The pathophysiology of adverse fetal effects is primarily a result of the anemia caused by destruction of red blood cell precursors.[19] Cardiac failure leading to fetal hydrops and fetal death may result from severe fetal anemia but can also be due to hypoalbuminemia, hepatitis, myocarditis, and placental inflammation.[20,21] Risks to the fetus are higher in the second trimester than the third for a number of reasons. Transmission across the placenta is higher in the second trimester because of the far greater second vs third trimester expression of the globoside receptor in the trophoblast that allows transplacental transfer of B19.[22] In addition, in the second trimester the fetus undergoes a rapid increase in red cell mass while experiencing a significant reduction in red cell life span. These factors combine to make the second-trimester fetus particularly vulnerable to the impact of B19 infection on erythropoiesis.[3]

The humoral immune system is responsible for the development of the antibody response, which results in viral clearance and subsequent protection from disease. Parvovirus B19 infection also elicits an inflammatory cell-mediated immune response, including the production of tumor necrosis factor (TNF) α, interferon (IFN) γ, and interleukin (IL) 2 or IL-6. CD8 T cells may also play a role in the control of parvovirus, as a significant CD8 T-cell response may be maintained and eventually increased over several months after the resolution of illness.[23]

Clinical Features

Parvovirus may be transmitted via respiratory, hematogenous, and vertical routes, with respiratory transmission the most common. Although B19 is primarily associated with nonrespiratory symptoms, it is transmitted through close person-to-person contact, fomites, and respiratory secretions or saliva. Young children are the main source of respiratory acquired B19. Therefore, individuals at highest risk for acquiring the virus include household contacts, day care workers, and those in a crowded environment. Nonimmune pregnant women with young children at home are therefore at high risk of becoming infected. Health care workers may also be at increased risk of transmission depending on the degree of contact that they have with infected patients.

The incubation period for human parvovirus B19 infection usually ranges from 4 to 14 days but may last up to 3 weeks. Infected individuals are most contagious during the phase of active viral replication. Viremia occurs approximately 7 to 10 days after the exposure and usually lasts for 5 days.[24] Parvovirus B19-specific IgM antibodies are detected at days 10 through 12 and can persist for 3–4 months or longer; specific IgG antibodies are detectable approximately 2 weeks following infection and persist lifelong.

The clinical presentation associated with B19 infection may vary. Manifestations may depend on the infected individual's age, as well as hematologic and immunologic status. Most immunocompetent individuals are asymptomatic or only mildly ill. Approximately 25% of infected individuals will be completely asymptomatic during their infection; 50% will have only nonspecific flu-like symptoms of malaise, muscle pain, and fever. The remaining 25% of infected individuals will present with the classic symptoms of B19 infection, including rash, arthralgia, or edema.

In the first week after exposure, intense viremia may be accompanied by a nonspecific flu-like illness, including fever, malaise, myalgia, coryza, headache, and pruritus. Hematologic abnormalities, including reticulocytopenia, reduced hemoglobin concentration, leukopenia, or thrombocytopenia may also be present. In the following week, the more specific symptoms of rash or arthralgia occur. The rash in adults is less characteristic than the rash seen in children. During the second phase of parvovirus infection, which generally occurs 2 weeks after infection, a person may develop additional symptoms or signs (eg, arthralgia, arthritis, or an exanthem) of B19 infection. This is also the phase in which B19-specific antibody production and B19 antigen-antibody immune complex formations occur. Individuals are generally no longer infectious when exhibiting these clinical characteristics.

Maternal Infection and Fetal Disease

Vertical transmission to the fetus can occur if a nonimmune woman becomes infected during her pregnancy. Although 30%–50% of pregnant women are susceptible, a relatively small percentage of them will become infected with the virus.[11-13] Of those that do become infected, as many as half will be asymptomatic, so infection may not be recognized.[21] If maternal infection does occur, there is a reported 30% rate of transmission to the fetus,[25,26] although in the majority of cases the fetus is unaffected. The chance of fetal loss in cases of fetal infection is reported to be about 5%–10%.[15-17] Overall, B19 infection is thought to account for 8%–20% of fetal nonimmune hydrops (Figure 56-1).[22,26]

The risk of a poor outcome for the fetus varies depending on the gestational age of the fetus and appears to be greatest when the congenital infection occurs in the early second trimester (before 20 weeks

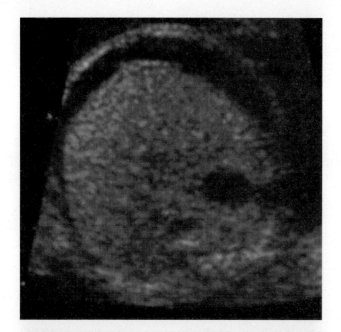

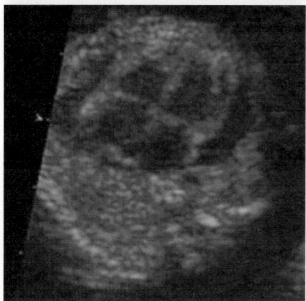

FIGURE 56-1 Ultrasound images of fetus with hydrops fetalis due to parvovirus B19 infections. A, Cross section through the fetal abdomen demonstrating fetal ascites. B, Cross section through the fetal chest demonstrating a pericardial effusion.

of gestation).[3,16,17] The risk of fetal death has been reported to be 15% at 13–20 weeks of gestation and 6% after 20 weeks.[27] As described, this difference is thought to be caused by both increased transplacental transmission in the second trimester and increased vulnerability of the fetus because of differences in hematopoiesis in the second vs the third trimesters. Fetal death can occur without evidence of hydrops, and it is also known that spontaneous resolution of hydrops because of B19 fetal infection occurs.[25]

The association of B19 with first-trimester fetal demise is unclear. B19 has been reported in association with enlarged sonographic nuchal translucency measurement,[28] but it is unclear if the infection was truly causative as the data are limited.

DIFFERENTIAL DIAGNOSIS

The differential diagnosis of maternal clinical parvovirus infection includes other viral exanthems, such as mumps, measles, and rubella, as well as nonspecific viral infections, such as cytomegalovirus (CMV). All of these disorders can result in a febrile illness, which in a pregnant woman should prompt investigation to determine if there is a risk of fetal disease as is the case with many viral illnesses. Detection of acute maternal parvovirus infection should prompt further evaluation and surveillance as outlined in the following discussion.

As discussed, parvovirus B19 is thought to be responsible for 8%–20% of cases of fetal hydrops.[22,26] The differential diagnosis of hydrops is extensive and beyond the scope of this chapter, but includes both immune causes, such as red cell alloimmunization, and nonimmune causes. Many nonimmune causes of fetal hydrops share a common underlying pathophysiology and are caused by fetal anemia; this is commonly assessed through evaluation of the middle cerebral artery (MCA) blood flow using Doppler velocimetry. Increase in the peak systolic velocity of the MCA, particularly in a fetus with hydrops, is indicative of severe fetal anemia and should prompt urgent referral to a tertiary center for further care (Figure 56-2). Parvovirus infection is an important cause of hydrops in this setting.

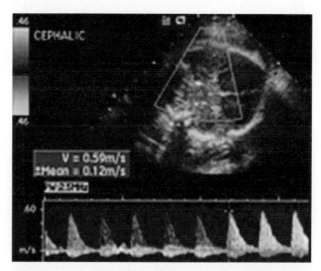

FIGURE 56-2 Ultrasound image demonstrating measurement of the peak systolic velocity of the middle cerebral artery, which in this case measures 0.59 m/s. Corrected for gestational age, this is an abnormal value consistent with severe fetal anemia.

DIAGNOSTIC TESTS

In immunocompetent individuals, acute infection is routinely diagnosed using serologic testing to identify B19-specific IgM and IgG antibodies. IgM may be detected within approximately 10 days of virus exposure and may persist for several months.[3,29] IgG antibodies are typically detected several days after IgM and usually provide lifelong protection.[10] Active infection is suspected when IgM antibodies are present, either with or without concurrent B19-specific IgG antibodies. Acute infection can also be diagnosed by demonstrating a 4-fold or greater rise in serum B19-specific IgG antibody titers. Follow-up serologic testing should be performed again in 4 weeks from exposure, or approximately 2–3 weeks since initial serologic testing, in individuals in whom exposure or infection is suspected but who are initially nonimmune.

The sensitivity of IgM antibody detection after maternal infection is reported to be relatively low, at 63%–70%.[30,31] If clinical suspicion is high, DNA testing of amniotic fluid or fetal cord blood with polymerase chain reaction (PCR) can be helpful in making a diagnosis as this method was reported to identify over 96% of cases in a recent series.[32] Such testing is considered the most sensitive approach for direct detection of virus within a specimen, and is the test of choice for diagnosing acute infection in the immunocompromised or immunosuppressed patient, including the fetus and neonate.

MANAGEMENT

Unlike some other viral infections, there is no specific antiviral therapy or vaccine available for B19 infection. Frequent hand washing and avoidance of infected individuals are therefore the only options for prevention of transmission. Management of potential exposure involves investigation with serologic testing of women with possible exposure and surveillance following confirmed B19 infection in pregnancy (Figure 56-3).

Following maternal B19 exposure, diagnostic evaluation as described is indicated. If maternal infection is confirmed, the fetus is at risk for severe anemia, leading to hydrops fetalis and fetal demise. Fetal anemia and intrauterine fetal demise (IUFD) typically occur between 2 and 6 weeks after maternal infection, although these have been reported as long as 20 weeks later.[29] Anemia, hydrops, and IUFD most commonly occur at 20–24 weeks of gestation, when the fetus is particularly susceptible because of the shorter half-life of erythrocytes at this stage of hematopoiesis.[21] Again, however, IUFD caused by B19 has been reported as early as 10 weeks and as late as 41 weeks of gestation.[33]

After confirmation of maternal B19 infection, fetal surveillance should be initiated. Such surveillance should include ultrasound examination to assess for the presence of fetal hydrops (Figure 56-1A and 56-1B) and Doppler interrogation of the MCA (Figure 56-2). With severe fetal anemia, the fetus can develop hydrops caused by cardiac decompensation; the most common

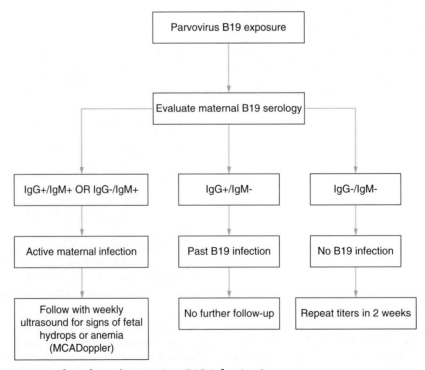

FIGURE 56-3 Management of confirmed parvovirus B19 infection in pregnancy.

early sonographic signs include cardiomegaly and ascites.[3,34] Ascites may also be a manifestation of hepatitis and hypoalbuminemia.[35] Assessment of the peak systolic velocity of the MCA is useful in surveillance for fetal anemia, as this will increase because of the increased cardiac output and decreased plasma viscosity associated with anemia.[36] Evaluation of the MCA Doppler peak systolic velocity is corrected for gestational age, and measurements are converted to multiples of the median (MoM). A peak systolic velocity in the MCA of more than 1.5 MoM indicates a high likelihood of severe fetal anemia.

If hydrops is detected or the MCA Doppler indicates likely fetal anemia, intrauterine transfusion (IUT) of red cells is performed in most cases. Although some fetuses will recover and the anemia and resultant hydrops will resolve spontaneously, it is difficult to predict, and in most cases, IUT is recommended.[32] Typically, one IUT is sufficient for correction of fetal anemia, after which fetal recovery with mounting of an immune response and resumption of normal erythropoiesis occurs. Despite successful transfusion with correction of anemia, it may take several weeks for complete resolution of all sonographic signs of hydrops.[29]

OUTCOME AND FOLLOW-UP

In 2 of the largest series of B19 infection in pregnancy, 1018 cases of documented maternal infection were reported. The fetal death rate was 6.8% (64/1018), and all fetal deaths occurred at less than 20 weeks' gestational age (64/579). In this series, 40/1018 cases (3.9%) developed hydrops. Of those that received IUT for hydrops, 85% survived; the few fetuses with hydrops that did not receive IUT died.[17]

The optimal timing of fetal intervention vs expectant management is unknown, and data on preferred management are conflicting. In a large survey study completed through the Society of Perinatal Obstetricians, respondents reported that 30% of fetuses hydropic because of B19 infection died when managed expectantly; only 6% of those who underwent IUT died in utero.[37] However, this study design is subject to reporting bias. In a study completed in the Netherlands, 30% of hydropic fetuses with B19 who underwent IUT died, and 32% of the survivors had delayed psychomotor development at long-term follow-up.[38] The neurodevelopmental outcome in this series did not correlate with the fetal hemoglobin at the time of IUT, and the authors hypothesized that the B19 infection itself may have caused central nervous system (CNS) damage. In another more recent study of 28 children, 11% were found to have neurodevelopmental impairment, a smaller percentage, yet still greater than the background risk.[39] A similar risk of neurodevelopmental impairment has been seen after IUT for isoimmunization.[40]

CONCLUSIONS

Parvovirus B19 infection is common in women of childbearing age; therefore, exposure or maternal infection often complicate pregnancy. Although most fetuses will remain asymptomatic, there is a risk for severe anemia, hydrops, and fetal death. Women with documented infection should be followed closely because intervention with in utero transfusion can be lifesaving for the affected fetus. A risk of long-term neurologic damage in surviving infants has been reported, but at this time, there are insufficient data to allow a precise estimate of risk.

REFERENCES

1. International Committee on Taxonomy of Viruses. Master Species List 2009—version 4. http://www.ictvonline.org/virusTaxonomy.asp?bhcp=1 (Accessed October 12, 2012.)
2. Cossart YE, Field AM, Cant B, Widdows D. Parvovirus-like particles in human sera. *Lancet.* 1975;1(7898):72–73.
3. Lamont RF, Sobel JD, Vaisbuch E et al. Parvovirus B19 infection in human pregnancy. *BJOG.* 2011;118(2):175–186.
4. Okochi K, Mori R, Miyazaki M, Cohen BJ, Mortimer PP. Nakatani antigen and human parvovirus (B19). *Lancet.* 1984;1 (8369):160–161.
5. Kooistra K, Mesman HJ, de Waal M, et al. Epidemiology of high-level parvovirus B19 viraemia among Dutch blood donors. *Vox Sang.* 2011;100(3):261–266.
6. Naides SJ. Erythema infectiosum (fifth disease) occurrence in Iowa. *Am J Public Health.* 1988;78(9):1230–1231.
7. Mortimer PP, Cohen BJ, Buckley MM, et al. Human parvovirus and the fetus. *Lancet.* 1985;2(8462):1012.
8. Röhrer C, Gärtner B, Sauerbrei A, et al. Seroprevalence of parvovirus B19 in the German population. *Epidemiol Infect.* 2008;136(11):1564–1575.
9. Kelly HA, Siebert D, Hammond R, Leydon J, Kiely P, Maskill W. The age-specific prevalence of human parvovirus immunity in Victoria, Australia compared with other parts of the world. *Epidemiol Infect.* 2000;124(3):449–457.
10. Beigi RH, Wiesenfeld HC, Landers DV, Simhan HN. High rate of severe fetal outcomes associated with maternal parvovirusb19 infection in pregnancy. *Infect Dis Obstet Gynecol.* 2008; 2008:524–601.
11. Kinney JS, Anderson LJ, Farrar J, et al. Risk of adverse outcomes of pregnancy after human parvovirus B19 infection. *J Infect Dis.* 1988;157(4):663–667.
12. Harger JH, Adler SP, Koch WC, Harger GF. Prospective evaluation of 618 pregnant women exposed to parvovirus B19: risks and symptoms. *Obstet Gynecol.* 1998;91(3):413–420.
13. Valeur-Jensen AK, Pedersen CB, Westergaard T, et al. Risk factors for parvovirus B19 infection in pregnancy. *JAMA.* 1999;281(12):1099–1105.
14. Ozawa K, Kurtzman G, Young N. Replication of the B19 parvovirus in human bone marrow cell cultures. *Science.* 1986;233 (4766):883–886.
15. Young N, Harrison M, Moore J, Mortimer P, Humphries RK. Direct demonstration of the human parvovirus in erythroid progenitor cells infected in vitro. *J Clin Invest.* 1984;74(6):2024–2032.
16. Garcia AG, Pegado CS, Cubel RC, Fonseca ME, Sloboda I, Nascimento JP. Feto-placentary pathology in human parvovirus B19 infection. *Rev Inst Med Trop Sao Paulo.* 1998;40(3):145–150.

17. Chisaka H, Morita E, Yaegashi N, Sugamura K. Parvovirus B19 and the pathogenesis of anaemia. *Rev Med Virol*. 2003; 13(6):347–359.

18. Jordan JA, DeLoia JA. Globoside expression within the human placenta. *Placenta*. 1999;20(1):103–108.

19. Isa A, Norbeck O, Hirbod T, et al. Aberrant cellular immune responses in humans infected persistently with parvovirus B19. *J Med Virol*. 2006;78(1):129–133.

20. Kishore J, Srivastava M, Choudhury N. Serological study on parvovirus B19 infection in multitransfused thalassemia major patients and its transmission through donor units. *Asian J Transfus Sci*. 2011;5(2):140–143.

21. Kroes ACM. Parvoviruses. In: Cohen J, Powderly WG, Opal SM, eds. pp. 1573-1577. *Infectious Diseases*. 3rd ed. London, UK: Mosby Elsevier; 2010.

22. Anand A, Gray ES, Brown T, Clewley JP, Cohen BJ. Human parvovirus infection in pregnancy and hydrops fetalis. *N Engl J Med*. 1987;316(4):183–186.

23. Yaegashi N, Niinuma T, Chisaka H, et al. The incidence of, and factors leading to, parvovirus B19-related hydrops fetalis following maternal infection; report of 10 cases and meta-analysis. *J Infect*. 1998;37(1):28–35.

24. Miller E, Fairley CK, Cohen BJ, Seng C. Immediate and long term outcome of human parvovirus B19 infection in pregnancy. *Br J Obstet Gynaecol*. 1998;105(2):174–178.

25. Enders M, Klingel K, Weidner A, et al. Risk of fetal hydrops and non-hydropic late intrauterine fetal death after gestational parvovirus B19 infection. *J Clin Virol*. 2010; 49(3):163–168.

26. Enders M, Weidner A, Zoellner I, Searle K, Enders G. Fetal morbidity and mortality after acute human parvovirus B19 infection in pregnancy: prospective evaluation of 1018 cases. *Prenat Diagn*. 2004;24(7):513–518.

27. Centers for Disease Control and Prevention (CDC). Risks associated with human parvovirus B19 infection. *MMWR Morb Mortal Wkly Rep*. 1989;38(6):81–88, 93–97.

28. Souka A, Kaisenberg C, Hyett J. Increased nuchal translucency with normal karyotype. *Am J Obstet Gynecol*. 2005;192(4): 1005–1021.

29. Dijkmans AC, de Jong EP, Dijkmans BA, et al. Parvovirus B19 in pregnancy: prenatal diagnosis and management of fetal complications. *Curr Opin Obstet Gynecol*. 2012;24(2):95–101.

30. Bredl S, Plentz A, Wenzel JJ, Pfister H, Möst J, Modrow S. False-negative serology in patients with acute parvovirus B19 infection. *J Clin Virol*. 2011;51(2):115–120.

31. Enders M, Helbig S, Hunjet A, Pfister H, Reichhuber C, Motz M. Comparative evaluation of two commercial enzyme immunoassays for serodiagnosis of human parvovirus B19 infection. *J Virol Methods*. 2007;146(1–2):409–413.

32. Bonvicini F, Puccetti C, Salfi C, et al. Gestational and fetal outcomes in B19 maternal infection: a problem of diagnosis. *J Clin Microbiol*. 2011;49(10):3514–3518.

33. Norbeck H, Papadogiannakis N, Petersson K, et al. Revised clinical presentation of parvovirus B19 associated intrauterine fetal death. *Clin Infect Dis*. 2002; 35(9):1032–1038.

34. Bond PR, Caul EO, Usher J, et al. Intrauterine infection with human parvovirus. *Lancet*. 1986;327(8478):448–449.

35. Brown T, Anand A, Ritchie LD, Clewley JP, Reid TM. Intrauterine parvovirus infection associated with hydrops fetalis. *Lancet*. 1984; 2(8410):1033–1034.

36. Mari G, Deter RL, Carpenter RL, et al. Noninvasive diagnosis by Doppler ultrasonography of fetal anemia due to maternal red-cell alloimmunization. Collaborative Group for Doppler Assessment of the Blood Velocity in Anemic Fetuses. *N Engl J Med*. 2000;342(1):9–14.

37. Rodis JF, Borgida AF, Wilson M, et al. Management of parvovirus infection in pregnancy and outcomes of hydrops: a survey of members of the Society of Perinatal Obstetricians. *Am J Obstet Gynecol*. 1998;179(4):985–988.

38. Nagel HT, de Haan TR, Vandenbussche FP, Oepkes D, Walther FJ. Long-term outcome after fetal transfusion for hydrops associated with parvovirus B19 infection. *Obstet Gynecol*. 2007;109(1):42–47.

39. De Jong EP, Lindenburg IT, van Klink JM, et al. Intrauterine transfusion for parvovirus B19 infection: long-term neurodevelopmental outcome. *Am J Obstet Gynecol*. 2012;206(3): 204.e1–e5.

40. Lindenburg IT, Smits-Wintjens VE, van Klink JM, et al; LOTUS study group. Long-term neurodevelopmental outcome after intrauterine transfusion for hemolytic disease of the fetus/newborn: the LOTUS study. *Am J Obstet Gynecol*. 2012;206(2):141.e1–e8.

Toxoplasmosis in the Fetus and Newborn Infant

Rima McLeod, Daniel Lee, Fatima Clouser, and Kenneth Boyer

INTRODUCTION AND EPIDEMIOLOGY

First identified in 1929 in a[1] human and as intrauterine in origin in 1942 in the United States,[2] congenital toxoplasmosis is now considered by neonatologists primarily when they encounter a TORCH (toxoplasmosis, rubella, cytomegalovirus, herpes simplex virus) infection, most often with chorioretinitis, intracerebral calcifications, and hydrocephalus. However, a much broader range of signs and symptoms and additional factors should be considered in the approach to this disease.

The causative agent, *Toxoplasma gondii*, is a ubiquitous protozoan parasite. It is estimated that more than 30% of the world's population has been infected, with varying frequencies of infections in different parts of the world and within countries as well. With rare exceptions, first infections of a pregnant woman acquired during gestation cause congenital toxoplasmosis. Primary gestational infections are generally unrecognized and may be asymptomatic or mild and self-limited and therefore go undiagnosed; fetal infections range in severity from asymptomatic at birth to devastating. Congenital toxoplasmosis is both treatable and preventable. Once established, however, infection is lifelong, with risk of recurrence.

Toxoplasma gondii is a 3 × 5 μm parasite in the apicomplexan family. Related apicomplexan parasites that also are pathogenic for humans include *Plasmodia*, which cause malaria; *Cryptosporidia*; and *Babesia*. *Toxoplasma gondii* exists in 3 primary life-cycle stages as it interfaces with the human host: tachyzoite, bradyzoite, and in the cat intestine, developing stages that mature into sporozoites in oocysts.[3-6] These life-cycle stages are shown in Figure 57-1.[4]

The rapidly growing tachyzoite form is present in acute postnatal infection (eg, in a pregnant woman), in active congenital infection, and when the infection recrudesces from encysted bradyzoites in recurrent eye disease or with immune suppression.[7-67] Tachyzoites evolve into the bradyzoite form when all infected persons and other animal hosts have a competent immune response. Bradyzoites then encyst and remain for the duration of an infected person's (or animal's) life, particularly in brain and muscle and in some instances in the eye. Types of immune suppression that lead to recrudescence of *Toxoplasma* tachyzoites include suppression related to AIDS, transplantation, autoimmune disease or malignancies, or treatment of these diseases or other medical problems with immunosuppressive agents.[62-65] Pregnant women who are chronically infected and have immunosuppressive conditions can also transmit their infection to their fetus. The fetus and newborn infant are immunologically immature, and there also appears to be immune unresponsiveness that is selective for *T. gondii* epitopes in this congenital infection in some instances, the mechanism of which is not yet established.[66,67] Oocysts develop in the cat intestine when cats eat cysts in meat, prey animals that they consume, or oocysts excreted by other cats. Oocysts are excreted in cat feces and then become infectious after sporulation in the environment during the next approximately 4 days.

The parasite is acquired by humans through consumption of oocysts contaminating food or water[44,50,57,71] or cysts in uncooked or undercooked meat (ie, not cooked to "well done").[71-77] Acquisition of infection and exposure are often unrecognized.[35,50,52]

CHAPTER 57

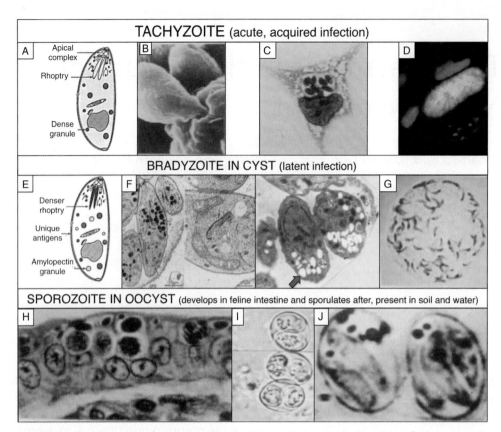

FIGURE 57-1 A, Schematic diagram of a tachyzoite. B, Transmission and scanning of electron micrographs of a tachyzoite invading a host cell. C, Light micrograph of tachyzoites replicating within a parasitophorous vacuole in the host cell cytoplasm. D, Immunofluorescence assay (IFA) (E Mui) with green fluorescent protein expressing tachyzoites in a parasitophorous vacuole. E, Schematic diagram of a bradyzoite. F, Transmission electron micrographs of a cyst containing bradyzoites. Red arrow in right panel indicates amylopectin granules. G, Light micrograph of a cyst containing bradyzoites. H, Development of oocysts in cat intestine. I, Oocysts in the lumen of a cat intestine. J, Sporulating oocysts that contain sporozoites. (Individual images reproduced with permission from A, McLeod et al[133]; B, Aikawa et al[135]; C, E, Long et al[132]; F, Weiss et al[136]; G, Remington,[137]; H, Gardiner et al[138]; J, Dubey et al.[139])

Oocysts are excreted by acutely infected members of the cat family for a period of about 20 days in extremely large numbers (up to 500 million oocysts from a single cat). Even 1 oocyst can be infectious.[3–6] The oocysts can be ubiquitous in the environment and isolated from soil and water.[71] For example, in 37 grammar schools in São Paulo, Brazil, oocysts were isolated from soil from 31 schoolyards.[72] Oocysts can remain viable and infectious in warm moist soil or sea or fresh water for up to a year.[73] They can contaminate raw fruits and vegetables.[74] Mussels can concentrate oocysts from seawater and thereby become a source of infection.[71,75] Dogs roll in cat feces, and oocysts can be acquired from contact with their fur by petting the dogs.[76] Further, dogs also eat cat feces, so even though oocysts do not form in the dog intestine, they can pass through the dog intestine and remain infectious in dog feces.[76] Animals that are a source of meat for humans also can be infected by ingestion of oocysts excreted by cats or by cysts acquired from eating other animals (prey or meat) that are infected (Figure 57-2A).[78] When humans eat infected meat that is not cooked to well done, they can become infected. The appearance of these different life-cycle stages; the means of transmission are shown in Figures 57-1 and 57-2.

Means to prevent infection based on this epidemiology are summarized in Figure 57-3. An educational pamphlet emphasizing these means for prevention for pregnant women can be downloaded (http://toxoplasmosis.org/pamphlet.pdf). Education about these means of prevention potentially can eliminate some infections (Tables 57-1 and 57-2). However, because sources of infection are so ubiquitous and often go unrecognized, such educational programs have only partial effectiveness.[79,80] Serologic testing for an antibody to an 11-kDa sporozoite protein has been used to identify acquisition of oocysts in the preceding 6 months in livestock animals and humans.[50] This assay

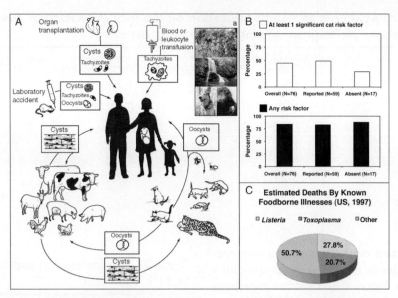

FIGURE 57-2 A, The life cycle of *Toxoplasma gondii*. The cat appears to be the definitive host. ªIn color, more recently identified vehicles of *T. gondii* infection (blueberries, water, dogs from infections of oocysts passing through intestine, and mussels that have filtered oocysts and been eaten by sea otters, which have then become ill or died). B, Significant cat exposure is defined as cleaning a cat's litter box; gardening; coming into contact with a sandbox; very close, sustained contact with a kitten. Any risk factor is defined as owning an indoor cat fed dry or canned food; preparing or consuming raw or undercooked meat or other foods that may have harbored the parasite, such as raw eggs or unpasteurized dairy products. C, Estimated deaths by known food-borne illnesses (United States, 1997). (A, Reproduced with permission from Remington and McLeod[140]; B, data from Boyer et al[52]; C, data from Mead et al.[141])

Prevention: Each woman should know if her unborn child is protected against *Toxoplasma*. Non-immune mothers should follow these precautions.

Eat meat and fish only when it is cooked to "well done" Avoid mussels and raw seafood and shellfish.

For example, do not eat meat tartare or "rare" meat

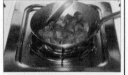

Wash foods,

Such as green salads and fruits, especially if it is to be eaten undercooked.

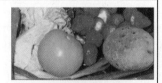

Avoid contact with materials potentially contaminated with cat excrement.

Have someone else dispose of the contents of your cat's litterbox and have them clean the litterbox immediately with boiling water. Do not feed your cat raw meat. Wear gloves while gardening.

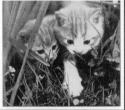

Follow your blood antibody test,

For Toxoplasma in conjunction with your doctor. If acute infection occurs, detection and treatment can protect your baby.

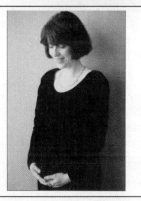

Wash your hands,

After handling bloody (raw) meat and before eating. Keep your hands away from your eyes while preparing undercooked meat.

FIGURE 57-3 Methods of prevention of *Toxoplasma gondii* infection. Available at the web page of the Toxoplasmosis Research Institute (http://www.toxoplasmosis.org/pamphlet.pdf)

Table 57-1 Effect of Attempts at Health Education on the Incidence Rate of *Toxoplasma* Infection in Selected Populations of Pregnant Women in the Paris Area[a]

Hospital	Period	Instruction	Seroconversion	Incidence/1000/Year
Hospitals Pinard and Baudelocque	Pre-1960	None	11/356	60
Centres Medico-Sociaux CPCAM	1961–1970	None	73/2, 496	64
Hospital X	1973–1975	None	18/710	59
Saint Antoine	1973	Verbal	7/463	37
	1974	Drawings	3/658	11
Longjumeau	1974–1981	Verbal	20/1938	22

[a]Reproduced with permission Roux et al.[79]

was used in a study that demonstrated that unrecognized ingestion of oocysts has occurred in epidemics in North and South America and caused a preponderance of the cases of congenital toxoplasmosis seen in a cohort study in North America during the past 3 decades, most without recognition of the risk factor (Figure 57-2B).[50,52] The Centers for Disease Control and Prevention found that toxoplasmosis is the second-most-frequent single cause of food-borne associated death in the United States (Figure 57-2C).

When an immunologically normal woman is acutely infected for the first time while pregnant, she may transmit the infection to her fetus in utero transplacentally. Rates of transmission by month of gestation are shown in Table 57-3. Infections acquired early in gestation are least often transmitted but most often severe.[16,17,51] By the end of gestation, infections are most often transmitted, but the infant may appear superficially normal. However, virtually all such infants who are untreated will develop manifestations of eye or central nervous system (CNS) infection later

Table 57-2 Epidemiology of Infection of National Collaborative Chicago-based Congenital Toxoplasmosis Study (NCCCTS), 1981–1998: Risk Factors Mothers Thought They Had

Risk Factor	Percentage
Exposure to cats	65
Exposure to meat	50
Exposure to cats or meat	75
Exposure to cat litter or rare uncooked meat	39
Toxoplasmosis-like illness during pregnancy	48
Exposure to cat litter or rare or uncooked meat or toxoplasmosis-like illness during pregnancy	48

Table 57-3 Transmission and Severity of Disease in Each Trimester[a]

Maternal Acquisition			Congenital Toxoplasmosis Present[b]		
Trimester	No.	%	No.	%	Relative Severity of Disease
First	29	20	5	17	Severe
Second	79	54	20	25	Intermediate severity
Third	37	26	24	65	Milder or asymptomatic
Total	145	100	49	84	

[a]Adapted with permission from Desmonts and Couvreur.[12]
[b]Infected, regardless of disease.

in life.[8,14,15,19] If the infants are evaluated carefully at birth (see further discussion in text), manifestations such as cerebrospinal fluid (CSF) abnormalities, intracranial calcifications, or retinal scars may be found in up to half the infants.[13,14,27,29,30] In pregnant women who have chronic, latent infection and immune compromise, transmission also may occur. Otherwise, it is extremely rare for infection acquired before the current pregnancy to be transmitted to the fetus.[51]

An acutely infected pregnant woman may be asymptomatic (most commonly) or occasionally have a flu-like illness or lymphadenopathy. Only occasionally are there signs and symptoms referable to involvement of brain, heart, muscle, eye, or other organ systems. The term *toxoplasmosis* refers to clinically overt diseases caused by this parasite.

Infection occurs commonly throughout the world (Figure 57-4). Infection rates may vary widely within a country and between countries. Based on age-specific seroprevalence in a population, the incidence of acquisition during childbearing years can be estimated.[81]

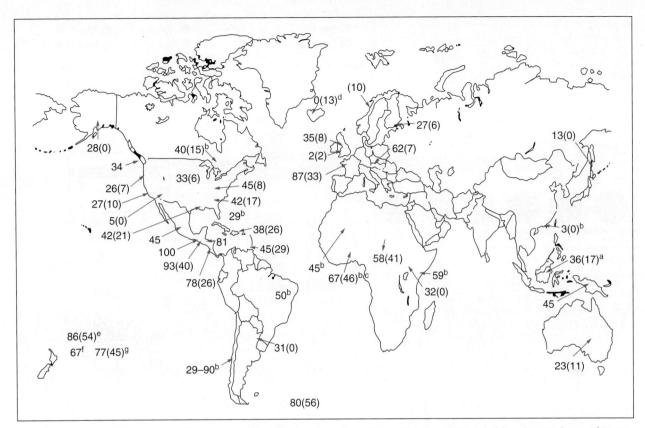

FIGURE 57-4 Prevalence of antibodies against *Toxoplasma gondii* in persons in selected locales. Unless otherwise specified, figures outside parentheses represent the percentage of seropositive adults approximately 30 to 40 years of age; figures inside parentheses are the percentage of seropositive children younger than 10 years. [a]Indirect hemagglutination antibodies; others were the indirect fluorescent antibody or dye test. [b]Adults with either age range not clearly specified or a wider age range than approximately 30 to 40 years. [c]Juveniles. [d]Fourteen individuals aged 30 to 39 years with no *Toxoplasma* antibody; 4 of 14 individuals 40 to 49 years of age with *Toxoplasma* antibody. [e]Society Island. [f]American Somoa. [g]Tahiti. (Reproduced with permission from Remington and McLeod.[142])

The infections occur in persons of all demographics in North America.[27,37,56] Variables that may influence these rates include climate, environmental hygiene, agricultural practices, and animal exposures.

There are different genetic types of parasites, which vary with geographic locale (Figure 57-5A,B)[56] and which can be distinguished by serological typing for certain alleles and by genotyping the parasites if they are isolated.[56] Certain serologic types are more frequently associated with differing demographics, frequency of prematurity, severity, severity of retinal disease, and patterns of neurologic disease (Figure 57-5C,D), and there is considerable genetic variability of parasites worldwide (Figure 57-5E). However, all types of parasites seem to respond favorably to treatment.[56] The best outcomes occur with the most prompt treatment of the fetus and newborn infant.[41–43] Host genetics also play a role in manifestations of disease.[41,82–91]

Infections may occur in family clusters or in other settings where exposures are similar.[50,52] There have been a number of family epidemics (eg, see Reference 50),

epidemics associated with drinking water,[68] epidemics associated with exposure to dust and oocysts in a riding stable,[92] and epidemics associated with contaminated meat.[77,78]

PATHOGENESIS AND PATHOLOGY

The parasite is acquired postnatally, usually through ingestion or rarely through blood or leukocyte transfusion or laboratory accident. An epidemic in a riding stable was associated with oocysts, but exactly how those were acquired (possibly ingestion or inhalation) was not established.[92] The parasite is acquired by the fetus after infection of the placenta.[20,51] There appears to be a time delay between acquisition during gestation and transplacental transmission to the fetus, but the reasons for this are not defined. The infant can be infected at birth during delivery as well. Following ingestion, the sporozoite or bradyzoite invades the intestinal cells.[93] In murine models, the distal small

CHAPTER 57

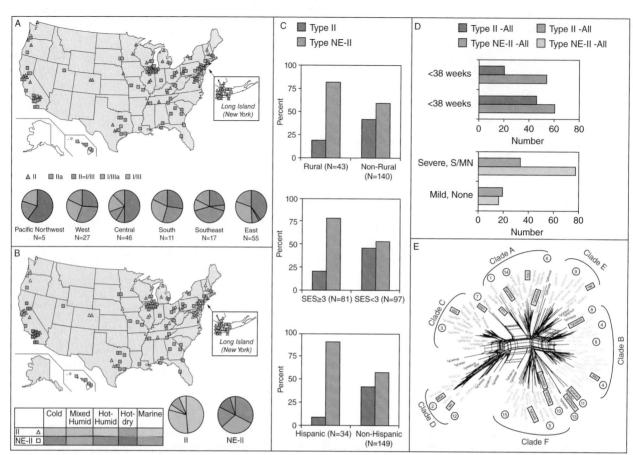

FIGURE 57-5 A, Distribution of parasite serotypes in the United States with locations mapped according to birthplace. (Climate regions, following designations of the Pacific Northwest National Laboratory and Oak Ridge National Library.[143] Map adapted from http://apps1.eere.energy.gov/buildings/publications/pdfs/building_america/ba_climateguide_7_1.pdf.) **B,** Serotypes and US regions. US regions were derived from the 10 standard federal regions as established by the Office of Management and Budget: East (regions I, II, and III); Southeast (region IV); South (region VI); Central (regions V, VII, and VIII); West (region IX); and Pacific Northwest (region X). The serotypes II, IIa, II = I/III, I/IIIa, I/III, and NE-II serotypes are defined elsewhere.[56] Pie graphs: Percentage = (Number of persons born in climate or geographic region with parasite serotype/Total number of persons with parasite serotype) × 100. **C,** NE-II serotype had greater proportions of persons residing in rural locales. Lower socioeconomic status was associated with NE-II serotype. Hispanic ethnicity was associated with NE-II serotype. *SES* indicates socioeconomic status calculated by the Hollingshead 4-factor socioeconomic score. SES of 4 persons with II and one person with NE-II serotype were not calculated because data were not available. SES of 4 persons with the II serotype and 1 person with the NE-II serotype was not calculated because data were not available. Rural: hometown population size, 1900 at the time of first visit to National Collaborative Chicago-based Congenital Toxoplasmosis Study (NCCCTS). **D,** Prematurity was associated with NE-II serotype, but not exclusively. Severe disease at birth was associated with NE-II serotype, but not exclusively. There were severely involved children diagnosed at birth with II and NE-II serotypes. *Rx* indicates persons in the NCCCTS cohort who were diagnosed in the perinatal period and treated during the first year of life.[24,25,27,30,35,37,39,41,51,83,84,98] *No Rx* indicates persons in the NCCCTS cohort who missed being treated in the first year of life and were referred to the NCCCTS after that time.[28,41,129] *All* indicates persons in the Rx plus No Rx cohorts. S, severe; S/MN, severe/moderate neurologic disease, as defined in Reference 27. **E,** NeighborNet phylogenetic network of *Toxoplasma gondii* isolates. Isolates from animals in the United States are in red letters. RH88, PTG, CTG, TgCgCa1 (also known as Cougar1, COUGAR), MAS, and TgCatBr5 are used as reference strains. Numeric number in parentheses following each isolate's identification number is the number of strains with the identical genotype from the same states. (A, B, reproduced with permission from McLeod et al[56]; C, D, data from McLeod et al[56]; E, reproduced with permission from Dubey and Se.[144])

A	Pathogenesis

Ingestion

Transport across intestine

Dissemination lymphohematogenously (transplacental)

Competent immune response:

• CD4 and CD8+ T cells

• Cytokines (especially IL-12 and IFNγ)

• Cyst form - parasites contained but persist

B	Pathology

Lymph node: Distinctive, no *Toxo*, no giant cells
Eye: Tachyzoites, necrosis, cysts, retinochoroidities
CNS: Meningoencephalitis (focal, diffuse), microglial nodules, perivascular inflammation, calcification
Congenital: Periaqueductal, periventricular vasculitis
Lung: Interstitial pneumonitis, other organisms
Immunocompromised: Granulomas, necrosis
Heart: Tachyzoites, necrosis, cysts - glomeruli, tubules
Glomerulonephritis - IgM, Ag-Ab, fibrinogen
Myositis
Immunocompromised: Pancreas
Congenital: Monoclonal gammopathy (IgG), + IgM

C   Ocular histopathology

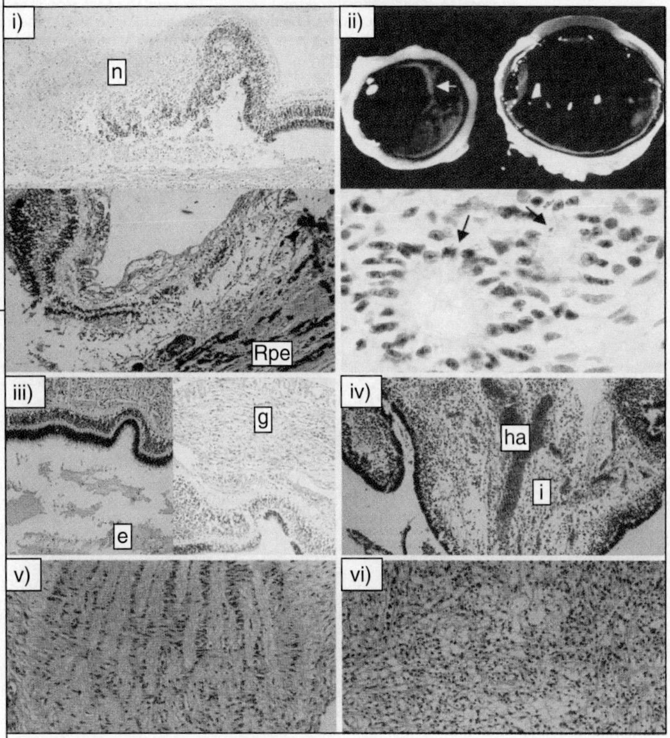

FIGURE 57-6 A, Overview of pathogenesis of infection. B, Specific pathology. C, Ocular histopathology in congenital toxoplasmosis: i, Top, a well-demarcated area of retinal necrosis (n) at the posterior pole in the eye of a fetus at 22 weeks' gestation (hematoxylin-eosin, original magnification ×3250). i, Bottom, the edge of a large retinochoroidal scar from the eye of a 2-year-old child. The scar is well demarcated with tubuloacinar proliferation of the retinal pigment epithelium (Rpe) at the edge of the scar. The center of the scar is devoid of retina (hematoxylin-eosin, original magnification ×3250). ii, Top, eye from a fetus at 32 weeks' gestation showing a large hyperpigmented scar, with a white rim, in the superotemporal region of the eye (arrow). ii, Bottom, the retina from the edge of the scar shows disorganization with formation of Flexner-Wintersteiner rosettes (arrows) (hematoxylin-eosin, original magnification ×3400). iii, Left, retina from a 5-day-old infant's eye showing retinal detachment with an exudate (e) between the retina and choroid. The inner retinal layer is edematous and inflamed (hematoxylin eosin, original magnification ×3100). iii, Right, retina from the eye of a fetus at 22 weeks' gestation showing gliosis (g) of the inner retinal layers (hematoxylin-eosin, original magnification ×3250). iv, Eye from a fetus at 23 weeks' gestation showing a moderate inflammatory infiltrate (i) within the primary vitreous and surrounding the hyaloid artery (ha) (hematoxylin-eosin, original magnification ×320). v, Optic nerve from the eye of an uninfected fetus at 24 weeks' gestation showing normal nerve architecture (hematoxylin-eosin, original magnification ×3100). vi, Optic nerve from the eye of a fetus at 23 weeks' gestation with congenital toxoplasmosis. The nerve architecture is disrupted with an inflammatory cell infiltrate (hematoxylin-eosin, original magnification ×3100). Ag-Ab, antigen-antibody; IFN, interferon; Ig, immunoglobulin; IL-12 (interleukin-12). (Reproduced with permission from Roberts et al.[145])

intestine is most commonly the more heavily infected part of the intestine following infection with oocysts.[93] The parasite multiplies locally in the intestine, spreads to mesenteric lymph nodes, and then disseminates systemically in white blood cells lymphohematogenously over the next days (Figures 57-6 and 57-7). At this time, it is found in the peripheral lymph nodes, lungs, heart, eyes, and brain (Figure 57-6). Parasites that differ genetically and hosts that differ genetically can cause or have infections of varying severity. Figure 57-7 shows the components of the innate and adaptive immune system important in a protective immune response

and some of the genes that have been associated with protective immunity in experimental models and in humans.[94]

Monozygotic twins usually have identical manifestations, and dizygotic twins may be discordant in whether they are infected at all and in their clinical manifestations.[95,96] These observations, as well as the identification of susceptibility and resistance genes associated with congenital toxoplasmosis and its manifestations, illustrate the importance of host genetics in acquisition of congenital infection and outcomes.[82–91,95,96]

CHAPTER 57

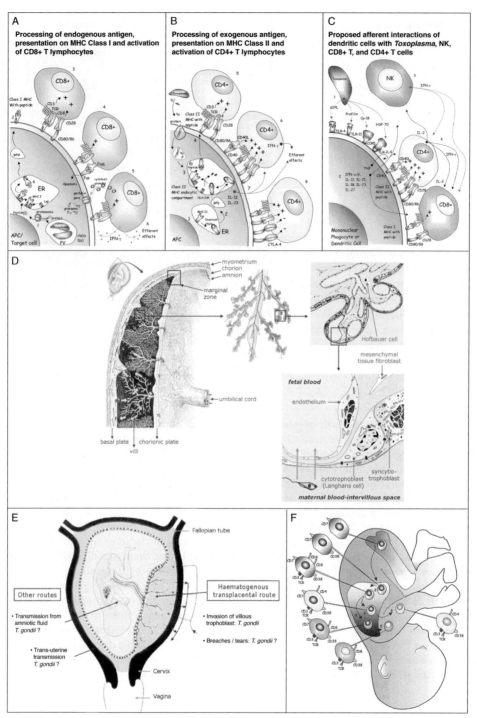

FIGURE 57-7 A, Processing of endogenous antigen presentation on major histocompatibility complex (MHC) class I and activation of CD8+ T lymphocytes to kill *Toxoplasma gondii*-infected cells. 1, Proteins escaping or released from the *T. gondii* parasitophorous vacuole are proteolytically cleaved in the proteosome and enter the endoplasmic reticulum (ER) via TAP (translocator associated with antigen processing) molecules. These peptides are loaded onto class I MHC (MHC I) molecules in the ER. 2, The class I MHC peptide complex is exported from the ER, through the Golgi, and ultimately to the surface of the cell. 3, Peptides presented on MHC I are recognized by CD8+ T lymphocytes via their surface α/β-TCR and CD8 molecules. The CD3 complex associated with α/β-TCRs acts as a docking site for tyrosine kinases that provide activating intracellular signals. CD28 on the surface of T cells interacts with CD80 or CD86 to provide costimulation for T cells. CD40 is expressed constitutively on dendritic cells and on ligation with CD40 ligand (CD40L), expressed on the surface of activated cells, increases CD80-86 expression on dendritic cells, and enhances T-cell costimulation. Engagement of CD40

(Continued)

activates the dendritic cell to produce cytokines such as interleukin (IL) 12 (see Figure 57-7B). Dendritic cells use a process called *cross presentation* to transfer proteins taken up as part of necrotic or apoptotic debris into the class I endogenous processing pathway. 4, Cytolytic CD8$^+$ T cells recognize specific *T. gondii*-derived peptides presented by MHC I molecules. Ligation of FasL on the surface of CD8$^+$ T cells with Fas on the surface of target cells induces apoptosis of target cells. 5, Following recognition of specific *T. gondii*-derived peptides presented by MHC I molecules, CD8$^+$ T cells can also kill target cells by release of perforin and granzyme. 6, CD8$^+$ T cells also receive interferon (IFN) γ, which can induce IDO (indoleamine-2,3-dioxygenase) and inducible nitric oxide synthase (iNOS) in target cells, which are effective in killing T. gondii tachyzoites. 7, At the later stages of activation, T cells express cytotoxic T-lymphocyte antigen (CTLA) 4, which, when engaged with CD80/86, delivers negative signals to the T cell that favor termination of activation (see Figure 57-7B). (Includes concepts from McLeod et al,[146] and Figure 4.1 in Lewis and Wilson.[147]) B, Processing of exogenous *T. gondii* antigen, presentation on MHC II and activation of CD4$^+$ T lymphocytes. 1, In the ER, MHC II molecules are bound by the invariant chain. 2, Export of the class II MHC-invariant chain complex from the ER, through the Golgi, and to MHC II endocytic compartments. 3, Endosomes containing *T. gondii*-derived proteins fuse with the MHC II endocytic compartments. The invariant chain is proteolytically cleaved, allowing internalized peptides to bind MHC II molecules. In humans, human leukocyte antigen (HLA-DM) molecules facilitate peptide loading. 4, MHC II molecules carrying peptide cargo are exported to the surface of the antigen-presenting cell (APC). 5, Peptides are presented on MHC II to CD4$^+$ T lymphocytes, which interact via their surface α/β-TCR and CD4 molecules. The CD3 complex becomes associated with α/β-TCRs and act as a docking site for tyrosine kinases that transmit activating intracellular signals. CD28 on the surface of T cells interacts with CD80 or CD86 on the APC to provide costimulation for the T cell. 6, CD40 is constitutively expressed on dendritic cells and interacts with CD40L expressed on the surface of activated T cells. This increases expression of CD80-86 on dendritic cells and enhances T-cell costimulation. C, Proposed afferent interactions of dendritic cells with Toxoplasma, natural killer (NK), CD8$^+$ T, and CD4$^+$ T cells. 1, *Toxoplasma gondii* releases a number of molecules that have immunological effects. GIPL binds TLR-4, profiling binds TLR-11, and Cp-18 binds CCR5 and HSP70, which induces dendritic cell maturation through an unknown mechanism (not all of these interactions may happen in all mammals, and TLR-11 apparently is not functional in humans). 2, The net effect of these molecules is dendritic cell activation and maturation with the likely production of IFN, IL-12, IL-15, IL-18, IL-23, and IL-27. These mediators act on NK cells and CD4$^+$ and CD8$^+$ T cells. 3, NK cells produce IFN-γ, which, together with IL-12, favors Th1-cell as opposed to Th2-cell maturation. 4, CD4$^+$ T-cell production of IL-2 further activates NK cells and favors the expansion of cytolytic CD8$^+$ T cells that can kill *T. gondii*-infected cells by a number of methods (see Figure 57-7A). (Includes concepts from McLeod et al,[145] and Figure 4.2 in Lewis and Wilson.[147]) D, Possible routes of maternal-fetal transmission of *T. gondii*. E, Hematogenous transplacental route of parasite transmission. F, Putative stages of human $\alpha\beta$-T-cell receptor-positive ($\alpha\beta$-TCR$^+$) thymocyte development. Prothymocytes express CD7 and are produced in the bone marrow or fetal liver. These enter the thymus via vessels at the junction between the thymic cortex and medulla. In the thymus, these cells differentiate to more mature $\alpha\beta$-TCR$^+$ thymocytes (defined by their pattern of the α/β-TCR-CD3 complex, CD4, CD8, and CD38). Rearrangement of the TCR–α and TCR-β chain genes occurs in the outer cortex. Positive selection occurs mainly in the central thymic cortex and involves the interaction of thymic epithelial cells. Negative selection occurs mainly in the medulla and involves the interaction of thymic dendritic cells. Medullary thymocytes emigrate into the circulation and colonize the peripheral lymphoid organs. These T cells are CD4$^+$ and CD8$^+$ with high levels of the $\alpha\beta$-TCR-CD3 complex. These cells are referred to as *recent thymic emigrants* (RTEs) and probably lack CD38 surface expression. CCR, chemokine receptor; DM, HLA-DM is a specific MHC class II molecule; GIPL, glycoinositolphospholipids; HSP, heat shock protein; IDO, indoleamine-2,3-dioxygenase; TCR, T-cell receptor; TLR, toll-like receptor; TNF, tumor necrosis factor. (A, B, C, Reproduced with permission from McLeod et al.[148] D, Reproduced with permission from Carlier et al.[149] E, Reproduced with permission from Benirschke et al.[150] F, Modified with permission from Remington et al.[167])

In the presence of a competent immune system characterized by the production of interferon γ, the parasite becomes a slowly growing bradyzoite, encysts, and remains for the rest of an infected person's or animal's life[97] (Figure 57-7). The parasite may recrudesce with immune compromise or at other times, particularly in untreated congenitally infected persons.[27,30,37,39,40]

Examples of destruction of the brain and eye in the congenitally infected fetus or infant are shown in Figures 57-8 to 57-13.[7,51,98] Often in the United States, disease is severe at birth because prenatal serologic screening and treatment are not practiced regularly (clinical manifestations at birth are shown in Tables 57-4 to 57-8).

DIFFERENTIAL DIAGNOSIS

Toxoplasma gondii infection and toxoplasmosis mimic many other clinical illnesses in the fetus and newborn infant. Some of the manifestations of this infection

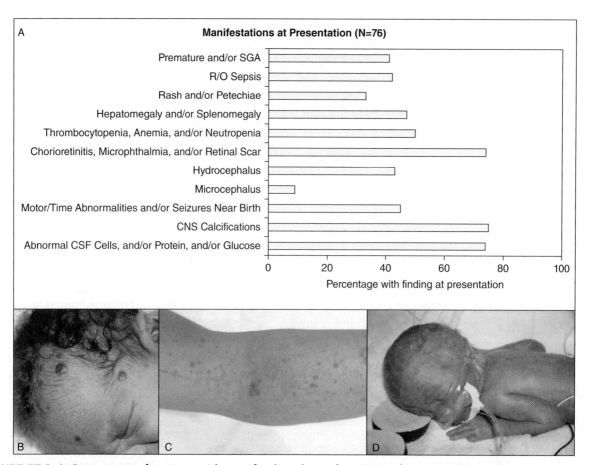

FIGURE 57-8 A, Percentage of patients with specific clinical manifestations of congenital toxoplasmosis at the time of presentation in our study. **B,** Blueberry muffin rash. The infant shown has Cytomegalovirus (CMV) but the "bluberry muffin" appearance of the rash is similar to those with congenital toxoplasmosis. **C,** Petechial Skin rash resulting from low platelets. **D,** Baby born prematurely caused by *Toxoplasma* infection. CNS, central nervous system; CSF, cerebrospinal fluid; R/O, rule out; SGA, small for gestational age. (A, Adapted with permission from McAuley et al.[27] B, Reproduced with permission from Mehta et al.[101] C, Reproduced with permission from National Heart, Lung, and Blood Institute.[151])

are given in Tables 57-4 to 57-7, and selected findings are shown in Figures 57-8 to 57-13.[51] Any of these manifestations should prompt an evaluation for congenital toxoplasmosis, including tests that suggest or that establish the diagnosis of toxoplasmosis. *Common findings that should alert the neonatologist to this infection include prematurity, intrauterine growth retardation, visceral abnormalities such as hepatosplenomegaly or conjugated hyperbilirubinemia, hematologic abnormalities such as thrombocytopenia or findings consistent with "culture-negative" sepsis, meningitis, or birth to an acutely infected mother.* The differential diagnosis for these manifestations is broad. Chorioretinal lesions (Figures 57-12 and 57-13), intracerebral calcifications, and hydrocephalus are the "classic triad" of findings present in some infants with congenital toxoplasmosis.[51] The differential diagnosis of these abnormalities often includes congenital cytomegalovirus infection, syphilis, and other TORCH infections and lymphochoriomeningitis virus (LCMV) infection. Aicardi-Goutières

syndrome can mimic the intracerebral calcifications of congenital toxoplasmosis,[51] although often the calcifications are more bilaterally symmetrical in that syndrome.

Treatment during gestation may eliminate manifestations at birth in a congenitally infected newborn[22,23,28,31–33,41–43,45,51,98–100] (Tables 57-8 to 57-19). This emphasizes the manner in which treatment of the fetus can complicate diagnosis at birth because of the efficacy of such treatment, when the newborn infant is infected but appears normal.

DIAGNOSIS: MANIFESTATIONS AND DIAGNOSTIC TESTS

General Nonspecific Clinical Abnormalities

As discussed, congenital toxoplasmosis may mimic the findings of many other etiologies of diseases with

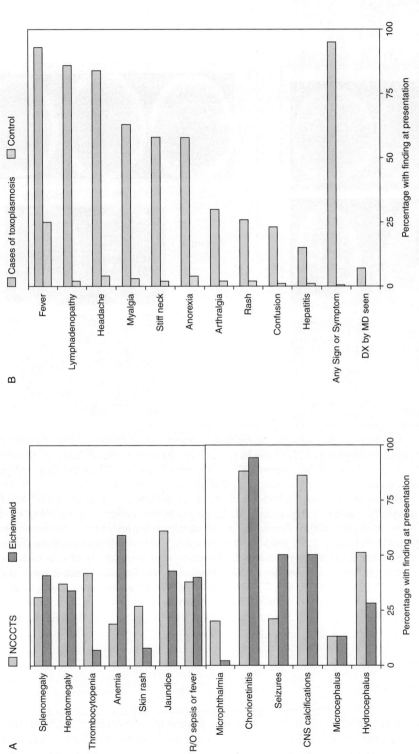

FIGURE 57-9 A, Percentage of patients who had a finding at presentation compared with the percentage from a study by Eichenwald.[8] Top: All children in our cohort were compared with the children with generalized or neurologic disease in the Eichenwald study. Four children from the Eichenwald study with only serologic or parasitologic evidence of infection were not included. Bottom: Children in our cohort with moderate or severe neurologic disease were compared with children from Eichenwald's neurologic disease cohort. We defined anemia as having a hemoglobin level less than 11 g/dL (26–39 weeks' preterm), 13.5 g/dL (at term), or 10.7 g/dL (in infants 1 month old or older) and thrombocytopenia as having platelet counts below 180,000 platelets/mL (26–30 weeks' preterm) or 150,000 platelets/mL (at term). Note that, in many categories, more children in our study had certain, very severe manifestations at presentation (ie, the time their illness was initially diagnosed). B Signs and symptoms in 37 cases of toxoplasmosis and 48 controls at a riding stable in Atlanta, Georgia, in October 1977. CNS, central nervous system; DX, diagnosis; NCCCTS, National Collaborative Chicago-based Congenital Toxoplasmosis Study; R/O, rule out. (A, Data from McLeod et al.[37] B, Data from Teutsch et al.[152])

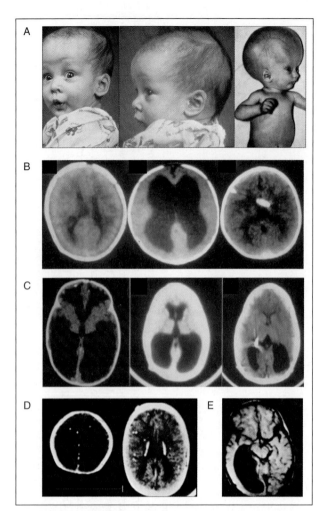

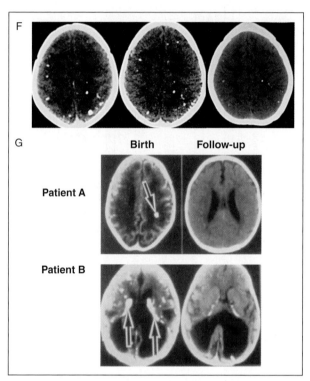

FIGURE 57-10 A, Infant with congenital toxoplasmosis. Note the bulging anterior fontanelle, sunset sign, and marked hydrocephalus. **B,** Computed tomography (CT) of the brain. Left, patient at birth. Middle, CT showing development of hydrocephalus at 3 months of age. Right, normal CT at 1 year of age. **C,** CT of the brain of patient at 2 months of age, before shunt placement (left); at 4 months, after shunt placement (middle); and at 14 months (right). **D,** Brain CT scans in the early newborn period (middle) and of the same child at 1 year of age (right). The child was developmentally and neurologically normal at 1 year of age. **E,** Magnetic resonance imaging (MRI) study of the brain demonstrating unilateral hydrocephalus (left). **F,** Cranial CT scans obtained for an infant in the newborn period, January 1993 (left) and at follow-up in February 1993 (middle) and January 1994 (right) demonstrate diminution or resolution of calcifications. This child has developed normally. **G,** Resolution or diminution of size of intracerebral calcifications during treatment of congenital toxoplasmosis in the first year of life. Cranial CT scans were obtained in the neonatal period and at 1 year of age. Each cranial CT scan was reviewed by the same study neuroradiologist. (B, C, Reproduced with permission from McAuley et al.[27] D, Reproduced with permission from Remington et al.[51] E, Reproduced with permission from McAuley et al.[27] F, Reproduced with permission from Patel et al.[98] G, Reproduced with permission from McLeod et al.[41])

similar manifestations. Manifestations such as intrauterine growth retardation, prematurity, thrombocytopenia, blueberry muffin rash (Figure 57-8),[101] hepatosplenomegaly, meningitis or meningoencephalitis, and eye or CNS abnormalities are all consistent with toxoplasmosis and other infections, such as those due to cytomegalovirus.[101]

Thus, diagnostic evaluation includes the general history, including maternal history, exposures, and travel; general physical examination of the infant, including examination of the retina; complete blood cell count with differential and quantitative platelet count (noting whether there is thrombocytopenia, anemia, neutropenia or neutrophilia, atypical lymphocytes,

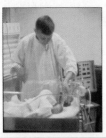

Sensorineural hearing outcomes			
Hearing impairment	Present	Wilson	Eichenwald
None	120	14	N/A
Mild	0	3	N/A
Moderate	0	2	N/A
Severe	0	0	N/A
Profound	0	0	15 "deaf"
Total	120	19	105

FIGURE 57-11 Testing for sensorineural hearing loss in infants and children has demonstrated no hearing loss ascribed to *Toxoplasma* infection. (Data from McGee et al.[153])

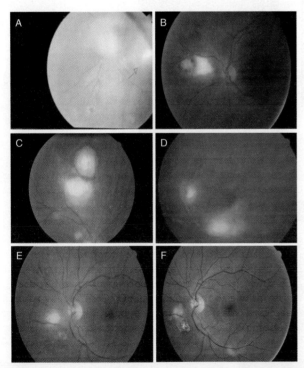

FIGURE 57-12 A, Vitritis seen as typical "headlight in fog." B, Typical form of ocular toxoplasmosis. Active white retinochoroiditis, satellite of a pigmented scar. C, Scarred and active ocular toxoplasmosis with contiguous vasculitis. D, Ocular toxoplasmosis with retinal artery occlusion. E, Active toxoplasmic lesion at presentation. F, Scarred toxoplasmic lesion. (A–F, Reproduced with permission from Delair et al.[7])

monocytosis or eosinophilia); liver function tests (noting direct bilirubin and transaminases); quantitative serum immunoglobulin (Ig) M (noting elevation); and lumbar puncture, including cell count, protein and glucose concentration (noting elevated white blood cell count, protein, or diminished glucose). A brain computed tomographic scan to evaluate ventricular size, presence of calcifications, and cortical thickness (Figure 57-10) is part of the evaluation of the infant when congenital toxoplasmosis is suspected. Similarly, evaluation of sensorineural hearing is part of the evaluation (Figure 57-11). This evaluation is summarized in Tables 57-9 and 57-10 (please also see Chapter 116). Abnormal CSF (especially elevated white blood cell count or protein concentration) is one of the most common manifestations and is present in approximately half of infected infants even though they may otherwise appear normal at birth. Elevated CSF protein greater than 1 g/dL is also seen in this infection when severe disease, especially with hydrocephalus, is present. A dilated fundoscopic examination can lead to identification of chorioretinitis or chorioretinal scars, which are characteristic in appearance (Figures 57-12 and 57-13).

As mentioned, effective treatment of the mother during gestation to treat the exposed/infected fetus can lead to prevention of infection or resolution of all manifestations of infection that might otherwise be present at birth. This effective treatment of the fetus may not completely eliminate the infection. Specific and nonspecific laboratory findings of infection also often are eliminated by such prenatal treatment (Tables 57-11 to 57-19).

Specific Clinical Abnormalities

Classical manifestations of toxoplasmosis (especially but not exclusively associated with first- and second-trimester infections) include chorioretinitis, chorioretinal scars, intracerebral calcifications, and hydrocephalus (Figures 57-10, 57-12, and 57-13). A baby infected later in gestation may have no manifestations at birth but develop manifestations later in life, especially eye disease in adolescence.

Other manifestations affecting the eye are shown in Figures 57-12 and 57-13 and Tables 57-20 and 57-21.[7,27,30] Additional manifestations may encompass those affecting other organ systems, including the CNS, heart, lungs, kidneys, liver, spleen, lymph nodes, skin, and placenta.

Infants may be asymptomatic and without signs at birth and develop symptoms and signs, especially retinal disease, later in life (Figures 57-12 and 57-13).[30,39,40] CNS findings are shown in Table 57-8 and Figures 57-10 and 57-11. Blueberry muffin rash and petechial rash are shown in Figure 57-8.[101]

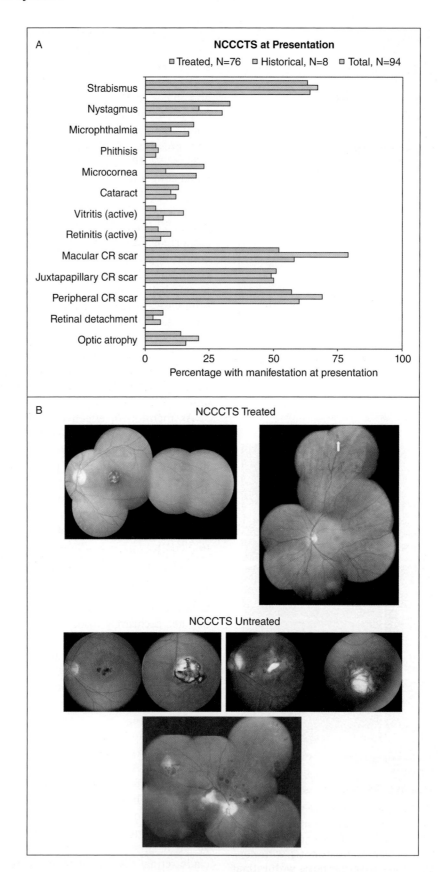

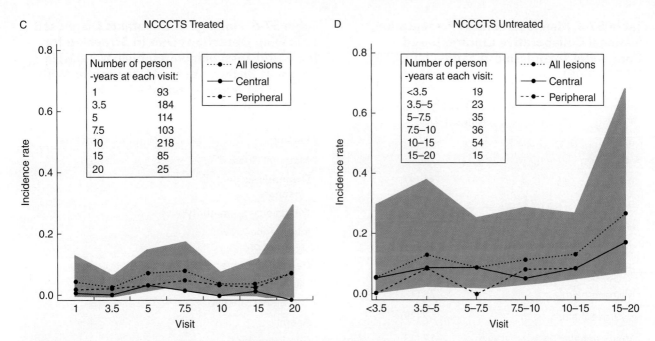

FIGURE 57-13 A, Ophthalmologic manifestations of congenital toxoplasmosis. *Treated* indicates persons in the National Collaborative Chicago-based Congenital Toxoplasmosis Study (NCCCTS) cohort who were diagnosed in the perinatal period and treated during the first year of life.[24,25,27,30,35,37,39,41,51,83,84,98] *Historical* indicates persons in the NCCCTS cohort who missed being treated in the first year of life and were referred to the NCCCTS after that time.[28,41,129] *Total* indicates persons in the Treated plus Historical cohorts. B, Treated: left, fundus photograph before development of new central chorioretinal lesion at age 5 years. The child received pyrimethamine, sulfadiazine, and leucovorin for the first 6 months of life. Right, fundus photograph of another child with a peripheral pigmented chorioretinal lesion noted for the first time during follow-up examination at the age of 11 years. It is not certain whether this peripheral lesion was new or had occurred while he was in utero or earlier in childhood but was undetected because of its far peripheral location. Untreated: representative examples of new toxoplasmic chorioretinal lesions. Top left, at age 19 years in right eye (left) and left eye (right) of patient. Top right, at age 13 years in left eye, at 2 different angles, of another patient. Bottom, at age 18 years in right eye of another patient. C, Left: new eye lesions in children treated in the first year of life. Right: new eye lesions in children who missed treatment in the first year of life. Incidence rate is the number of patients with new lesions per person-year. Blue shaded area is confidence interval. CR, chorioretinal. (A, Data from Mets et al.[154] B, Treated: reproduced with permission from Phan et al.[39] Untreated: reproduced with permission from Phan et al.[40] C, Reproduced with permission from McLeod et al.[41])

Specific Diagnostic Testing

Figures 57-14 to 57-16; Tables 57-9, 57-10, 57-11 to 57-19, and 57-22 to 57-24 offer an overview of manifestations in neonates and associated diagnostic testing.

Isolation, Polymerase Chain Reaction, and Lymphocyte Responses

Amniotic Fluid

The presence of *T. gondii* DNA in amniotic fluid, especially when obtained during gestation and determined in a reliable reference laboratory, can be key in establishing the diagnosis of congenital toxoplasmosis in the fetus and newborn infant.[26,46,51,102] The sensitivity and specificity of the polymerase chain reaction (PCR) to detect *T. gondii* DNA in amniotic fluid for the diagnosis of congenital toxoplasmosis (Figures 57-14 and 57-15) can be seen in Figure 57-16.[26,34,46,51,102,103]

Placenta

A useful test to establish the diagnosis of congenital toxoplasmosis has been isolation of the parasite by subinoculation of placenta from the fetal side into mice.[20,51] In Chapter 116 of this book, there are specific instructions for handling the placenta prior to subinoculation.

The placenta should not be placed in formalin but should be stored at standard refrigerator temperature (4°C) and should not be frozen. PCR has more recently complemented isolation for diagnosis.

Buffy Coat, Red Blood Cell Clot

Newborn infants who are congenitally infected are most often parasitemic in the first month of life. This can be detected with either subinoculation (buffy coat and red blood cell [RBC] clot)[51] or PCR (buffy coat).

Table 57-4 Manifestations at Presentation,[a] National Collaborative Chicago-based Congenital Toxoplasmosis Study (NCCCTS) (1981–2009)

Finding	Number of Infants (Percentage)
Premature (<37 weeks' gestation)	64 (43)
Rule out sepsis	55 (37)
Rash	37 (25)
Hepatomegaly	57 (39)
Splenomegaly	46 (31)
Chorioretinitis	110 (73)
Microphthalmia	23 (15)
Hydrocephalus	59 (39)
Microcephalus	19 (13)
Seizures	21 (14)
Central nervous system calcifications	106 (70)
Thrombocytopenia	58 (40)
Anemia	25 (17)
Abnormal cerebrospinal fluid (CSF) cells or protein or glucose[b]	51 (74)

[a]Infants diagnosed with congenital toxoplasmosis in the newborn period and referred to the NCCCTS in the first year of life.
[b]With CSF studies, value is 69.

Table 57-6 Findings in US Infants Diagnosed Following Detections Due to Screening for Increased Total Immunoglobulin M (IgM) in Serum at Birth: Data for 10 Newborns With Congenital *Toxoplasma* Infection by the Presence of IgM *Toxoplasma* Antibodies[a]

Finding	Number of Infants
Maternal Illness ("flu")	2
Diagnosis suspected (neonate)	1
Gestational prematurity[b]	5
Intrauterine growth retardation[c]	2
Hepatosplenomegaly	1
Jaundice	1
Thrombocytopenia	1
Anemia	1
Chorioretinitis	2
Abnormal head size	0
Hydrocephalus	1
Microcephaly	0
Abnormal cerebrospinal fluid	8[d]
Abnormalities on neurologic examination	1
Serum IgM elevated	9
Serum IgM *Toxoplasma* antibody	10

[a]Reproduced with permission from Alford et al.[10]
[b]Less than 37 weeks' gestation.
[c]Lower 10th percentile (Grunewald).
[d]Only 8 were examined.

Table 57-5 Details of Stratification of Randomized and Feasibility Cohorts, National Collaborative Chicago-based Congenital Toxoplasmosis Study (NCCCTS; 1981–2004): Most Disease Recognized in the United States at Birth Is Severe[a]

	Presence of Chorioretinitis			
	Patients With "None/Mild" Findings		Patients With "Severe" Findings	
Cohort	No	Yes	No	Yes
Randomized	15	4	7	59
Feasibility/ observational	4	1	3	27
Total	19	5	10	86

[a]Reproduced with permission McLeod et al.[37]

Table 57-7 New England Screening Program: Manifestations in Newborn Infants[a]

Site of Abnormality	Incidence, No. Affected/No. Examined (%)
Central nervous system	14/48 (29)[b]
Increased spinal fluid protein (≥100 mg/dL)[c]	8/32 (25)
Intracranial calcifications on CT scan	9/46 (20)
Enlarged lateral ventricles on CT scan or ultrasonogram	1/47 (2)
Retina	9/48 (19)
Active chorioretinitis	2/48 (4)
Retinal scars without active inflammation	7/48 (15)
Either site	19/48 (40)[d]

Abbreviation: CT, computed tomographic.
[a]Reproduced with permission from Guerina et al.[29]
[b]Three infants had increased protein levels and intracranial calcifications, 1 had intracranial calcifications and enlarged lateral ventricles, and 1 underwent cerebrospinal fluid evaluation but not intracranial imaging. Infants with more than 1000 red cells per cubic millimeter because of trauma due to lumbar puncture were excluded from this category.
[c]Protein levels ranged from 100 to 569 mg/dL in cerebrospinal fluid samples obtained at 3 to 6 weeks of age, when the normal mean (±SD) concentration is 59 ± 25 mg/dL.[164]
[d]Four infants had both central nervous system and retinal abnormalities.

Cerebrospinal Fluid

Isolation or PCR of parasites from CSF is most often found with severe infection and high parasite burden.

Other Tissues

Isolation or PCR of *T. gondii* DNA from tissues is most often seen with terminations of pregnancies or spontaneous abortions.

Urine

There is a small case series that indicated PCR from urine has been useful in the diagnosis of congenital toxoplasmosis.[104] This has not yet been established to be useful in large series.

Lymphocyte Blastogenesis and Interferon-γ Production

Lymphocyte blastogenesis in response to T. gondii antigens was initially reported to be a useful diagnostic test,[105] but this could not be confirmed in a larger series to have high sensitivity, although it is specific.[67] Perhaps this was because of differences in patient population, parasite type, severity of infections, or timing of acquisition.[66,67] Severely involved infants and those infected at the end of gestation most often tested negatively in this test.[66,67] Recently, there was a report from a single group that interferon-γ production in response to *T. gondii* antigens was a sensitive and specific test for congenital toxoplasmosis for a cohort of such infants in France.[106] This is consonant with an earlier observation that, with fetal blood sampling, the production of interferon γ in response to *Toxoplasma* lysate, antigens can be of diagnostic value.[107] The earlier observation of selective unresponsiveness to *T. gondii* antigens[66,67] potentially could also affect the value of an assay system based on detection of interferon-γ production in response to *T. gondii* antigens.

Serologic Tests in the Context of History of Infection or Illness

Mother

History, Recognized Exposures, Symptoms, and Signs A history of a febrile lymphadenopathic illness or new chorioretinitis may be suggestive of acquisition of the infection during gestation. A significant exposure or travel into a highly endemic area is another important part of the history. Physical examinations that demonstrate lymphadenopathy should suggest the diagnosis may be possible. Serologic tests would confirm this. A biopsy that demonstrates the classical histopathology in lymph nodes occasionally leads to detection of infection in the mother.[108]

An immune-compromised, chronically infected pregnant woman, such as a woman with AIDS and a CD4+ count below 200 may transmit the infection to her fetus.[51]

Serologic Tests
Serum *Toxoplasma*-Specific IgG: Figure 57-14 presents an optimized approach to diagnosis of acute acquired infection in the pregnant woman based on serologic screening monthly to detect seroconversion. This approach then facilitates treatment of the

Table 57-8 Treatment of *Toxoplasma gondii* Infection in the Pregnant Woman and Congenital *Toxoplasma* Infection in the Fetus, Infant, and Older Children[a]

Infection	Medication
In pregnant women infected during gestation	
First 18 weeks of gestation or until term if fetus found not to be infected by amniocentesis at 18 weeks or clinical findings	Spiramycin[b]
If fetal infection confirmed after week 18 of gestation and in all women infected after week 24	Pyrimethamine[c] *plus*
	Sulfadiazine *plus*
	Leucovorin (folinic acid)[c]
Congenital *T. gondii* infection in infant[d]	Pyrimethamine[c,e] *plus*
	Sulfadiazine[f] *plus*
	Leucovorin[c]
	Corticosteroids[g] (prednisone) have been used when CSF protein is ≥ 1 g/dL and when active chorioretinitis threatens vision
Active chorioretinitis in older children	Pyrimethamine[c] *plus*
	Sulfadiazine[d] *plus*
	Leucovorin[c]
	Corticosteroids[f] (prednisone)

Abbreviation: CSF, cerebral spinal fluid.
Please see dosages and comments in Chapter 116.
For detailed information on the dosage of medication and duration of therapy, see Table 116-1.
[a]Reproduced with permission from Remington et al.[51]
[b]In the United States, available only on request from the US Food and Drug Administration (telephone 301-443-5680), then, with this approval, by the physician's request to Aventis (908-231-3365).
[c]Adjusted for granulocytopenia; complete blood cell counts, including platelets, should be monitored each Monday and Thursday.
[d]Alternative medicines for patients with atopy or severe intolerance of sulfonamides have included pyrimethamine and leucovorin with clindamycin, or azithromycin, or atovaquone, with standard dosages as recommended according to weight. In the unusual circumstance that medicines cannot be administered orally or by intraintestinal tube feeding, trimethoprim, sulfamethoxazole, and clindamycin have been administered intravenously.
[e]Both regimens, a higher and lower dose, appear to be feasible and relatively safe. The duration of therapy is unknown for infants and children, especially those with AIDS.
[f]Corticosteroids should be used only in conjunction with pyrimethamine, sulfadiazine, and leucovorin treatment and should be continued until signs of inflammation (high CSF protein, ≥ 1 g/dL) or active chorioretinitis that threatens vision have subsided; dosage can then be tapered and the steroids discontinued.

Table 57-9 Samples Obtained From Mother and Infant[a]

	Sample	Use
Reference laboratory[b]		
Placenta obtained at the time of or after birth of infant	1. Obtain 200 g from near the insertion cord on the fetal side (approximately 14 × 3 × 3 cm = 100 g) or whole placenta	PCR, subinoculation Do NOT freeze or put in formalin; keep cool
	2. Obtain 10–20 mL amniotic fluid, if available (subinoculation)	PCR
Mother	1. Use 2 mL maternal serum	IgG, IgM, IgA
Infant subsequent to delivery	1. Two 1.0-mL sterile purple-top tubes, infant peripheral blood and clot underlying serum in the following *step 2* (2 mL blood)	PCR, subinoculation
	2. Obtain 1 mL serum	Sabin-Feldman dye test, IgM, ISAGA, IgA

(Continued)

Table 57-9 Samples Obtained From Mother and Infant[a] *(Continued)*

	Sample	Use
	3. Obtain 0.5 mL cerebrospinal fluid (PCR)	IgG, IgM
	4. Obtain 5 mL urine (PCR)	PCR (investigational)
Delivery hospital		
Infant subsequent to delivery	1. CBC with differential and platelet count	
	2. Serum	Total IgM, IgG, IgA (quantitative immunoglobulin), albumin
	3. Serum	SGPT, SGOT, total and direct bilirubin, creatine
	4. Urinalysis	
	5. Lumbar puncture	Cell count, glucose protein, and total IgG

Abbreviations: CBC, complete blood cell count; Ig, immunoglobulin; ISAGA, immunosorbent agglutination assay; PCR, polymerase chain reaction; SGOT, aspartate aminotransferase; SGPT, alanine aminotransferase.
[a]For detailed information on the storage, shipping, and use of samples, see Table 116-2.
[b]Samples should be kept cold (NOT FROZEN). If physician wishes to discuss results with Toxoplasmosis Center physicians, include permission form for the Palo Alto Medical Foundation to release serologic and isolation results to the Toxoplasmosis Research Institute and Center/Dr. McLeod.

Table 57-10 Examinations and Evaluations of Baby Following Birth

Examination/Evaluation	Comment
1. General examination	
2. Pediatric ophthalmologist	
3. Pediatric neurologist	
4. Computed tomographic scan of the brain	• Baby should not be sedated and may be gently swaddled. • This examination is done without contrast. • Examine for ventricular size and brain calcifications.
5. Auditory acoustic emissions or BAER (brainstem auditory evoked response, a hearing test)	

Table 57-11 Contrasting Transmission at Birth With and Without Treatment With Spiramycin: Attempts to Isolate *Toxoplasma*[a] **From Placenta at Delivery in Women Who Acquired** *Toxoplasma* **Infection During Pregnancy**[b]

	Infection Acquired During First Trimester		Infection Acquired During Second Trimester		Infection Acquired During Third Trimester		Total	
	No. Examined	No. Positive (%)	No. Examined	No. Positive (%)	No. Examined	No. Positive (%)	No. Examined	No. Positive (%)
None	16	4 (25)	13	7 (54)	23	15 (65)	52	26 (50)
Spiramycin	89	7 (8)	144	28 (19)	36	16 (44)	269	51 (19)
Total	105	11 (10)	157	35 (22)	59	31 (53)	321	77 (24)

[a]By mouse inoculation.
[b]Reproduced with permission from Desmonts and Couvreur.[165]

Table 57-12 Contrasting Transmission and Findings at Birth With and Without Treatment With Spiramycin: Outcome of 542 Pregnancies in which Maternal *Toxoplasma* Infection Was Acquired during Gestation[a]

Outcome of Offspring	No. of Affected Infants (%)	
	No Treatment	Treatment
No congenital *Toxoplasma* infection	60 (39)	297 (77)
Congenital toxoplasmosis		
Subclinical	64 (41)	65 (17)
Mild	14 (9)	13 (3)
Severe	7 (5)	10 (2)
Stillbirth or perinatal death	9 (6)	3 (1)
Total	154 (100)	388 (100)

[a]Reproduced with permission from Desmonts and Couvreur.[165]

fetus by prompt administration of medicines to the pregnant woman. This method begins with a prenatal serum that excludes presence of chronic infection in the mother by determining that she does not have *Toxoplasma*-specific IgG or IgM. This test can be performed using a number of different methods (Tables 57-9 and 57-10) and is reliable in most clinical laboratories in the United States. Seroconversion documents acquisition of the parasite. In the presence of a positive IgG specific for *Toxoplasma*,[51] acute infection is either confirmed or excluded using a test for *T. gondii*-specific IgM, avidity of *T. gondii*-specific IgG, and a differential agglutination test as described in the following material. The gold standard test for IgG specific for *Toxoplasma* is the Sabin-Feldman dye test,[109] which detects complement-dependent lysis of tachyzoites and their exclusion of the vital dye, methylene blue. Other IgG assays include the immunofluorescence assay (IFA), enzyme-linked immunosorbent assay (ELISA), direct agglutination, and Western blot. The dye test usually takes 6–8 weeks to reach a high, stable titer during the acute infection. In some cases, this observation can be used to help date the time of acquisition of infection by the pregnant woman, which may be especially useful.[110]

Serum *Toxoplasma*-Specific IgM: IgM specific for *T. gondii* is present in the acute acquired infection and may persist for varying amounts of times, up to several years (Figure 57-15). The tests may be less reliable when performed outside reference laboratories (reference laboratory information is listed in Tables 57-23 and 116-7).[111–113] Thus, a positive IgM result should always be confirmed by a reference laboratory.[111–113] Methodologies include IFAs and ELISAs[111–113] (Table 57-22). An IgM ISAGA (immunosorbent agglutination assay) is more sensitive and should be used to establish the diagnosis for infants under the age of 6 months.[111,112]

Serum *Toxoplasma*-Specific IgA: IgA specific for *T. gondii* tests performed by ELISA in a reference laboratory also indicate acute, acquired infection.[114]

Serum *Toxoplasma*-Specific IgE: IgE specific for *T. gondii* tests performed by ELISA in a reference laboratory are also indicators of acute acquired infection.[115]

Serum Differential Agglutination Test: The differential agglutination (AC/HS) test for *T. gondii* measures the antibody response to acetone-fixed parasites in serum (AC) and to formalin-fixed parasites (HS). This test can help to date acquisition of infection to 9 months or more earlier. The interpretation of the test is shown in Figure 57-15D.[51,111,116]

Serum Avidity Test: The avidity of *T. gondii*-specific IgG increases with time of infection; this observation has been used to date the infection to within the prior 12–16 weeks.[117–125] A high-avidity result indicates the infection was acquired more than 12–16 weeks earlier. Low-avidity antibodies may persist longer than this time. Thus, it is the high presence of avidity antibodies that is most useful in excluding recent infection. The Food and Drug Administration recently approved a commercial test for measuring IgG avidity. The US reference laboratories also perform this test.

Infant Not Treated In Utero

General Considerations
Manifestations and considerations concerning diagnosis for the infant not treated in utero are those discussed previously. Factors that influence those manifestations include the time when infection is acquired during gestation, genetics and other health parameters of mother and child, genetics of parasite, and probably magnitude (inoculum) of infecting parasite.

Serologic Tests
Serum *Toxoplasma*-Specific IgG: IgG specific for *T. gondii* at birth is primarily due to the mother's passively transplacentally passaged IgG from her infection and does not establish the diagnosis in the infant.

Serum *Toxoplasma*-Specific IgM: A test for IgM specific for *T. gondii* performed by IgM ISAGA in a

Table 57-13 Outcome of In Utero Treatment of Congenitally Infected Fetuses With Spiramycin or Spiramycin Followed by Pyrimethamine and Sulfadiazine[a]

| In Utero Treatment | No. of Patients | Dates of Study | Dates of Maternal Infection[b] | Duration of Follow-up | Isolates from Placenta, No. (%) | Immune Load of IgG | | IgM Prevalence, No. (%) | Subclinical Infections, No. (%) |
						At Birth	At 6 Months		
Spiramycin	51	1972–1982	22.8 (10–35)	Mean 46.7 months (2 months to 11 years)	23 (77)	139	137	18 (69)	17 (33)
Spiramycin + pyrimethamine + sulfadiazine	52	1983–1989	22.6 (10–30)	Mean 16 months (1-46 months)	16[c] (42)	86	70	8 (17)[d]	30 (57)

Abbreviation: Ig, immunoglobulin.
[a]Data from Couvreur et al.[166]
[b]Weeks' gestation.
[c]p < .01.
[d]p < .001.

Table 57-14 Transmission of *Toxoplasma gondii* Infection to Fetus, Appearance of Sequelae, and Severity of Sequelae According to Whether Prenatal Antibiotic Therapy Was Given[a]

	No. of Mothers	Time of Infection (weeks)		Transmission		Global Sequelae[b]		Severe Sequelae[b]	
		Mean	Range	No.	Percentage	No.	Percentage	No.	Percentage
Prenatal treatment	119[b]	18.7	3–34	46	38.7	12	10	4	3.5
No prenatal treatment	25	29	6–38	18	72[c]	7	28[d]	5	20[e]
Total	144	20.5	3–38	64	44	19	13	9	6

[a]Reproduced with permission from Foulon et al.[31]
[b]Four aborted fetuses are not included in the assessment of sequelae in the treated group.
[c]$p > .05$, by multivariate analysis and controlled for gestational age.
[d]$p = .026$, by multivariate analysis and controlled for gestational age.
[e]$p = .007$, by multivariate analysis and controlled for gestational age.

Table 57-15 Contrasting Outcomes With Fetal Diagnosis and Treatment: Prospective Study of Infants Born to Women Who Acquired *Toxoplasma* Infection During Pregnancy[a]

Finding	No. Examined	Positive, No. (%)
Prematurity	210	
Birth weight < 2500 g		8 (3.8)
Birth weight 2500–3000 g		5 (7.1)
Dysmaturity (intrauterine growth retardation)		13 (6.2)
Postmaturity	108	9 (8.3)
Icterus	201	20 (10)
Hepatosplenomegaly	210	9 (4.2)
Thrombocytopenia purpura	210	3 (1.4)
Abnormal blood cell count (anemia, eosinophelia)	102	9 (4.4)
Microcephaly	210	11 (5.2)
Hydrocephalus	210	8 (3.8)
Hypotonia	210	2 (5.7)
Convulsions	210	8 (3.8)
Psychomotor retardation	210	11 (5.2)
Intracranial calcifications on radiography	210	24 (11.4)
Abnormal ultrasound examination	49	5 (10)
Abnormal computed tomographic scan of brain	13	11 (84)
Abnormal electroencephalographic result	191	16 (8.3)
Abnormal cerebrospinal fluid	163	56 (34.2)
Microphthalmia	210	6 (2.8)
Strabismus	210	11 (5.2)
Chorioretinitis	210	
Unilateral		34 (16.1)
Bilateral		12 (5.7)

Signs and symptoms in 210 infants with proven congenital infection.
[a]Reproduced with permission from Remington et al.[51]

Table 57-16 Transmission With Treatment With Spiramycin and Pyrimethamine and Sulfadiazine Treatment: Incidence of Congenital *Toxoplasma gondii* Infection by Gestational Age at Time of Maternal Infection[a,b]

Weeks of Gestation	Infected Fetuses/Total No. Fetuses	Incidence (%)
0–2	0/100	0
3–6	6/384	1.6
7–10	9/503	1.8
11–14	37/511	7.2
15–18	49/392	13
19–22	44/237	19
23–26	30/116	26
27–30	7/32	22
31–34	4/6	67
Unknown	8/351	
Total	194/2632	7.4

[a]Adapted with permission from Hohlfeld et al.[26]
[b]Maternal infection was treated with spiramycin in a dose of 9 million IU (3 g) daily.

Table 57-17 Transmission With Treatment With Spiramycin and Pyrimethamine and Sulfadiazine: Fetal *Toxoplasma* Infection as a Function of Duration of Pregnancy[a,b]

Time of Maternal Infection	No. of Women	Percentage Infected
Periconception	182	1.2
6–16 weeks	503	4.5
17–20 weeks	116	17.3
21–35 weeks	88	28.9
Close to term	41	75

[a]Reproduced with permission from Forestier et al.[23]
[b]Women were treated during gestation as soon as feasible after diagnosis of the acute acquired infection was established or strongly suspected. If prenatal diagnosis was made in the fetus, treatment was with pyrimethamine-sulfadiazine; otherwise, it was spiramycin.

Table 57-19 Findings at Birth in 55 Live Infants Born of 52 Pregnancies With Prenatal Diagnosis of Congenital Toxoplasmosis[a]

	N[b]	Percentage
Subclinical infection	44/54	81
Multiple intracranial calcifications	5/54	9
Single intracranial calcification	2/54	4
Chorioretinal scar	3/54	6
Abnormal lumbar puncture	1/54	2
Evidence of infection on inoculation of placenta	23/46	50
Positive cord blood immunoglobulin M antibody	8/53	15

[a]Reproduced with permission from Hohlfeld et al.[22]
[b]Numerator is the number of abnormalities present at birth; denominator is the total number of infants examined for abnormalities.

Table 57-20 Ophthalmologic Manifestations of Congenital Toxoplasmosis[a]

	Number of Treated Patients With Finding (%) (N = 76)	Treated Patients With Bilateral Finding (N = 76)
Strabismus	26 (34)	–
Nystagmus	20 (26)	–
Microphthalmia	10 (13)	3/10 (30)[b]
Phthisis	4 (5)	2/4 (50)
Microcornea	15 (20)	8/15 (53)
Cataract	7 (9)	1/7 (14)
Vitritis (active)	3 (4)[c]	3/3 (100)[c]
Retinitis (active)	6 (8)	2/6 (33)
Chorioretinal scars (active)	56 (74)	38/56 (68)
Retinal detachment	7 (9)	4/7 (57)
Optic atrophy	14 (18)	8/14 (57)

[a]Adapted with permission from Mets et al.[30] [b]Numerator represents number of patients with bilateral finding; denominator is total number with finding. Number in parentheses is percentage.
[c]Two additional patients, not included in this table, were receiving treatment and retinochoroiditis had resolved, but vitreous cells and veils persisted at time of examination.

Table 57-18 Contrast Between Congenital Toxoplasmosis in France in 2007 With Treatment (Rx) and Earlier Studies of Those Without Treatment

France 2007 (Rx), Villena[45]		Desmonts/Couvreur[17] (No Rx)		Foulon et al[31] (No Rx)	
Asymptomatic	206/234 = 88%	Subclinical	64/94 = 68%	Other not specified	13/25 = 52%
Symptoms	21/234 = 8.9%	Mild	14/94 = 15%	Global sequelae	7/25 = 28%
Severe symptoms	7/234 = 3%	Severe	7/94 = 7%	Severe sequelae	5/25 = 20%
Death/stillborn	11/272 = 4%	Death/stillborn	9/94 = 10%	Death/stillborn	0/25 = 0%

Table 57-21 Chorioretinal Scars of Treated Patients[a]

	Number With Finding (N = 76) (%)	Number With Bilateral Finding (%)
Chorioretinal scars	56 (74)	38/56 (68)
Macular	39/72 (54)[b]	16/39 (41)
Juxtapapillary	37/72 (51)	17/37 (46)
Peripheral	43/72 (58)	17/43 (40)

[a]Adapted with permission from Mets et al.[30]
[b]Numerator represents the number of patients with finding; the denominator is the total number, unless otherwise specified. Patients with bilateral retinal detachment in whom the location of scars was not possible were excluded from the denominator.

reference laboratory also indicates that there is congenitally acquired infection in the infant.[112] This test was positive in 50% of infected babies in one series,[123] but sensitivity of results may be laboratory specific. Occasionally, maternal IgM might cross the placental barrier. Because of the short half-life of IgM, a serum sample from the infant at 8 days of life would then no longer have maternal IgM.

Serum *Toxoplasma*-Specific IgA: A test for IgA specific for *T. gondii* performed by ELISA in a reference laboratory is also diagnostic for congenital infection if present after 8 days of life and can be helpful in excluding serum from the mother having reached the infant at delivery ("placental leak"). This is because the half-life of IgA is brief, and it will be eliminated by the eighth day of life.[51,114]

Infant Treated In Utero

General Considerations

Treatment in utero can obscure all findings of congenital toxoplasmosis. This includes signs of infection on physical examinations, ability to isolate the parasite from placenta, and serologic evidence of infection, such as serum *Toxoplasma*-specific IgM antibody. Spiramycin treatment delays transmission and thereby can attenuate signs of infection, although it does not treat the infant. Pyrimethamine and sulfadiazine treat the infection in the infant and can thereby modify symptoms and signs, isolation results, and serologic test results.

Serologic Tests

Serum *Toxoplasma*-Specific IgG: IgG specific for *T. gondii* will reflect the mother's IgG at birth, and half will be lost each month (the half-life for IgG).[51] In some instances, antigens are recognized differentially, as demonstrated through IgG isotype specifically or differentiated reactivity in Western blots (Figure 57-15).

Serum *Toxoplasma*-Specific IgM: A test for IgM specific for *T. gondii* performed by ISAGA in a reference laboratory is also an indicator of congenital infection. With treatment of the fetus in utero by treating the pregnant woman, *T. gondii*-specific IgM is often absent at birth.[22] When serum IgM specific for *T. gondii* is present in the newborn infant, it is helpful in establishing the diagnosis of congenital toxoplasmosis.

Serum *Toxoplasma*-Specific IgA: A test for IgA specific for *T. gondii* performed by ELISA in a reference laboratory is also an indicator of congenital infection, but it may not be present in the infant who was treated in utero.

Cerebrospinal Fluid: Nonspecific abnormalities in CSF protein, glucose, cell count, or IgM specific for *T. gondii* are helpful in establishing the diagnosis of *T. gondii* infection in the newborn infant. Again, treatment of the fetus by treatment of the pregnant woman with pyrimethamine and sulfadiazine also often leads to normalization of such abnormalities.[22,41,42]

Infant Serum Antibody Load

In some instances, it is highly unlikely that an infant born to a mother who was infected during gestation is infected, and a decision is made not to treat the infant. Because it is not absolutely certain the infant escaped infection, one approach to determine whether infection of the infant has not occurred is to follow the infant's *T. gondii*-specific serum "antibody load" (Table 57-24).[51] (Also please see Table 116-8 in Chapter 116 for further information on this topic.) Physicians observe that passively transferred *T. gondii*-specific IgG, transferred from mother to infant, will decrease by 50% per month (the half-life of IgG) while the infant begins to synthesize his or her own total quantitative IgG (mg/dL), measured in the local hospital laboratory. A variety of different patterns of time exists in which the infant's immune system matures, and the infant begins to synthesize his or her own specific IgG during the first year of life; these patterns are shown in Figure 57-17. In this case, once each month after birth, the infant's serum is obtained for *T. gondii*-specific IgG (also including IgM and IgA specific for *T. gondii* for follow-up sera for each of the first 2 months). These sera are tested in parallel with the previous month's sample with 2-fold dilution in the Sabin-Feldman dye test. Sensitivity of the dye test is noted, which is a value obtained through comparison with a reference standard that allows comparison of amounts of *T. gondii*-specific IgG tested on different days. This is performed in a reference laboratory. Information on quantitative IgG is also obtained in the local hospital

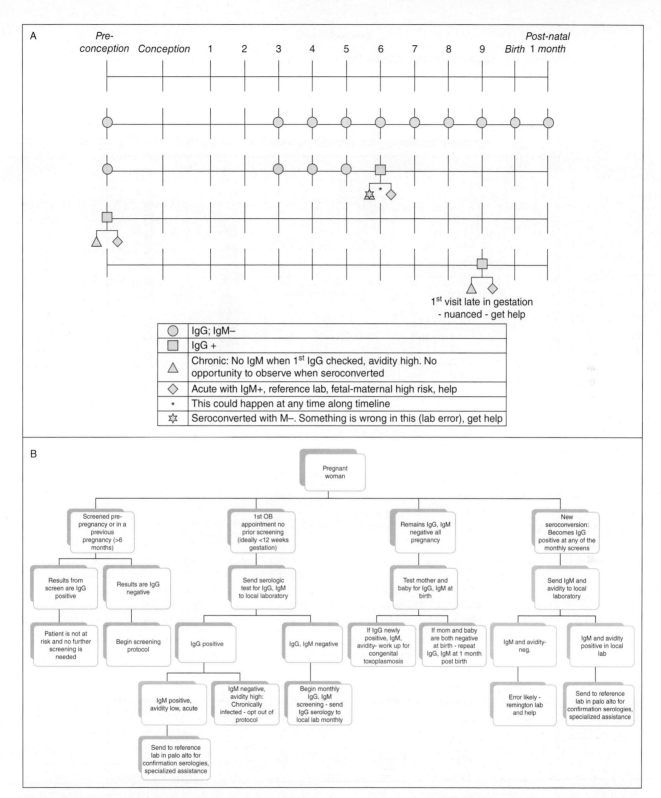

FIGURE 57-14 A, Schematic diagram of screening for *Toxoplasma* infection during gestation. **B,** Algorithm for screening for *Toxoplasma* infection during gestation. Blue box indicates help is needed from High-Risk Maternal Fetal Medicine, Toxoplasmosis Palo Alto Medical Foundation, *Toxoplasma* Serology Laboratory. Ig, immunoglobulin; OB, obstetrics. Multiplex IgG, IgM assays are being developed.

CHAPTER 57

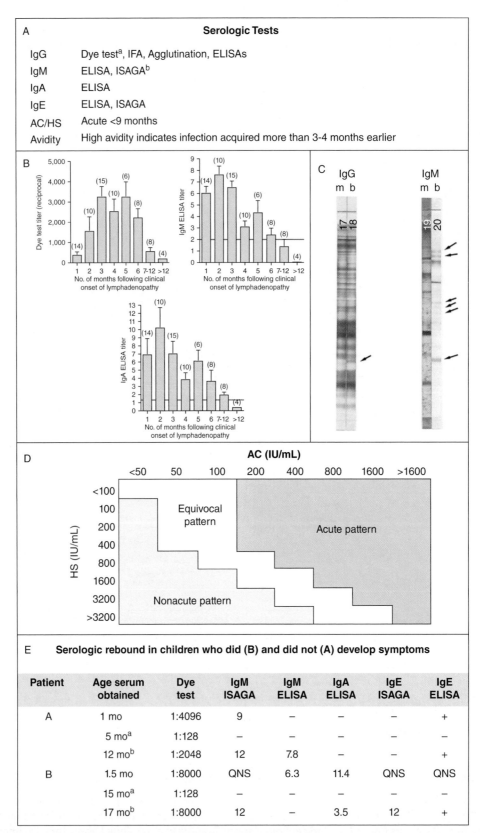

A Serologic Tests

IgG	Dye test[a], IFA, Agglutination, ELISAs
IgM	ELISA, ISAGA[b]
IgA	ELISA
IgE	ELISA, ISAGA
AC/HS	Acute <9 months
Avidity	High avidity indicates infection acquired more than 3-4 months earlier

E Serologic rebound in children who did (B) and did not (A) develop symptoms

Patient	Age serum obtained	Dye test	IgM ISAGA	IgM ELISA	IgA ELISA	IgE ISAGA	IgE ELISA
A	1 mo	1:4096	9	–	–	–	+
	5 mo[a]	1:128	–	–	–	–	–
	12 mo[b]	1:2048	12	7.8	–	–	+
B	1.5 mo	1:8000	QNS	6.3	11.4	QNS	QNS
	15 mo[a]	1:128	–	–	–	–	–
	17 mo[b]	1:8000	12	–	3.5	12	+

FIGURE 57-15 A, Serological tests. B, Serological test results (mean titers ± standard error of the mean [SEM]) for 75 serum samples from 40 consecutive patients with biopsy-proven toxoplasmic lymphadenitis. Left, geometric mean ± SEM of the reciprocal of the highest positive serum dilution in the Sabin-Feldman dye test. Right, mean ± standard

error (SE) of immunoglobulin (Ig) M enzyme-linked immunosorbent assay (ELISA). Bottom, IgA ELISA. Numbers in parentheses indicate the number of serum samples tested. Vertical bars = SE. Horizontal lines = cutoff for positive value (see text). C, IgG and IgM Western blots of serum from a mother (m) and her newborn son (b). Sera were drawn from mother and baby when the baby was 2 days old. Arrows point to bands in the blot of the serum of the baby that were not present in the corresponding blot of the serum from the mother. Serologic test results in the mother were as follows (results in the baby are in parentheses): dye test, 600 IU (300 IU); IgM ELISA, 2.9 (IgM immunosorbent agglutination assay [ISAGA], 3), both positive; IgA ELISA, 1.8 (1.3), both positive; IgE ELISA, negative (positive); polymerase chain reaction (PCR) assay in placental tissue, negative. *Toxoplasma* was isolated from the placental tissue. D, Interpretation of differential agglutination (AC/HS) test results. This test was performed as described in the text. (Data from Dannemann et al.[155]) E, Serologic rebound in children who did (B) and did not (A) develop symptoms. [a]Samples obtained while patient was still taking pyrimethamine and sulfadiazine. [b]Samples obtained after pyrimethamine and sulfadiazine were stopped. QNS, quality not sufficient. (B, Reproduced with permission from Montoya and Remington.[156] C, Reproduced with permission from Remington et al.[157] D, Reproduced with permission from Remington et al.[51] E, Adapted with permission from Remington et al.[51])

laboratory. The equation used for this calculation is as follows:

$$\textit{Infant serum antibody load} = \textit{Reciprocal of the Sabin-Feldman dye test} \times \textit{Sensitivity of the dye test} / \textit{Quantitative IgG (mg/dL)}$$

T. gondii saliva IgG from infants correlated well with results of serial IgG testing, which may be an alternate mode of testing in the future.

CSF Antibody Load

Calculation of antibody load in CSF has also been performed in a similar manner. In this case, the ratio of antibody load in serum and CSF is compared, and a ratio of 4 or greater has been found to be associated with CNS infections.[126] This test is only reliable for diagnoses of infection of the CNS when *T. gondii*-specific IgG in serum is less than 1:1024 (= 300 IU). This method was established by Georges Desmonts.[51,126,127]

MANAGEMENT

Abundant and convincing evidence demonstrated that available medicines block transmission to the fetus when given to the pregnant women, kill tachyzoites that are causing active disease, reduce or eliminate parasite burden, reduce or eliminate eye disease, reduce or eliminate brain disease, reduce severity of disease, eliminate meningitis, treat meningoencephalitis, and lower immune markers of infection (reviewed in the work of Kieffer et al[41,51]). Earlier, there was some controversy in the literature (discussed in Reference 100). However, current evaluations of in vitro and experimental animal data, attention to older publications that demonstrated efficacy, combined with several recent studies describing clinical experiences in which a shorter time interval between diagnoses and treatment led to better outcomes,[42,43] have demonstrated that treatment is

effective and beneficial (Figures 57-10, 57-13, and 57-18 to 57-27), and there is consensus about this now for those familiar with each of those aspects of recent work.[41-43,53] Recent data demonstrated how important it is to establish the correct diagnosis quickly because the time when the acute infection is diagnosed and treated is critical[41-43]: The earlier the infection is treated, the better the outcomes will be.[41-43] An algorithm for diagnosis of the acute acquired infection in the pregnant woman and treatment initiated quickly is in Figures 57-14, 57-23, and 116-1.[41-43,51]

Medical Treatment During Gestation to Prevent or Treat Infection in the Fetus

Types of treatment of the pregnant woman to prevent congenital infection and to treat the infected fetus, as well as medicines and dosages for their use in the treatment of the newborn infant, are summarized in Tables 57-8 and 116-1.

Spiramycin has been administered to pregnant women who acquired infections early in gestation to block transmission. This is continued until the time the infant is born if amniocentesis and ultrasound results indicate the infection has not been transmitted to the fetus. This approach has been used most widely for infections acquired before 18 weeks' gestation.[51]

After 21 weeks' gestation, medicines used to treat this infection include pyrimethamine (given with folinic acid, also called calcium leucovorin) and sulfadiazine. If significant sulfonamide hypersensitivity makes continued treatment of the pregnant woman impossible, second-line replacement medicines include clindamycin and azithromycin. There is little experience documenting their efficacy in the same manner as the use of pyrimethamine and sulfonamides. Pyrimethamine inhibits dihydrofolate reductase (DHFR) of the parasite and cannot be rescued by therapeutic amounts of leucovorin (Figure 57-18), whereas the effect on the

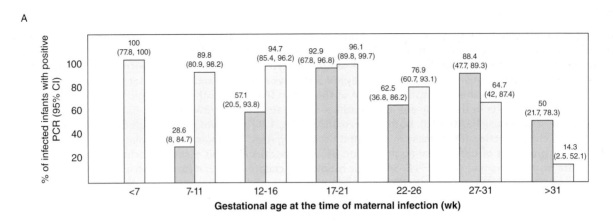

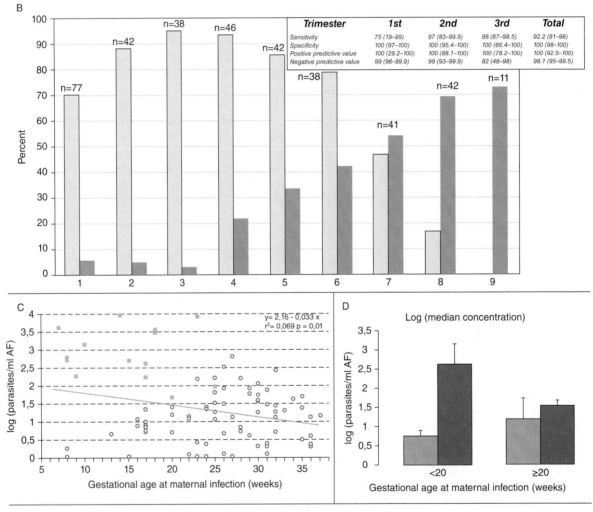

FIGURE 57-16 A, Prenatal diagnosis of congenital toxoplasmosis using polymerase chain reaction (PCR) assay in amniotic fluid (AF) according to gestational age at maternal infection. Light blue bars indicate sensitivity of PCR assay in AF; Darker blue bars indicate negative predictive value of PCR assay in AF; the 95% confidence interval (CI) is shown within parentheses at the top of the bars. These data were derived from three centers in France, with substantial variability in the time during gestation at which maternal infection was acquired, the time between maternal infection and amniocentesis, and the duration of treatment preceding amniocentesis. B, Percentage of patients undergoing amniocentesis and cases of congenital *Toxoplasma* infection according to gestational age at maternal seroconversion (inset shows sensitivity, specificity, and positive and negative predictive value estimates for PCR analysis). Inset data are percentage (95% CI). Light grey histogram bar is amniocentesis; Dark blue histogram bar is congenital toxoplasmosis. C, Correlation between *Toxoplasma* concentrations in AF samples and gestational age at maternal infection for the 86 cases. Severity of the infection is represented in each case by shaded block if severe signs of infection were recorded

or by open red circle if no or mild signs were observed. In general, the earlier the mother was infected, the higher the parasite numbers in AF. However, some babies who had relatively low numbers of parasites were severely infected, and many babies who had relatively high numbers of parasites were not severely infected. D, Comparison of median (interquartile range) parasite concentrations in AF between cases with subclinical infection (blue bars) and cases with infectious sequelae (red bars) for maternal infections acquired before or after 20 weeks of gestation. Clinical status was recorded either at birth or following fetal death (at fetopathologic examination). (A, Reproduced with permission from Remington et al.[51] B, Reproduced with permission from Wallon et al.[46] C, Reproduced with permission from Romand et al.[34] D, Reproduced with permission from Romand et al.[34])

Table 57-22 Immunoglobulin G Antibody Responses to *Toxoplasma* Infection as Measured by Different Serologic Methods[a,b]

Serologic Method	Uninfected Person	Recent (Acute) Infection	Chronic (Latent) Infection
Dye test	Negative (<1:4)	Rising from a negative or low titer (1:4) to a high titer (1:256 to 1:128,000)	Stable or slowly decreasing titer; titers usually are low (1:4 to 1:256) but may remain high (≥1:1024) for years
Agglutination test (after treatment of sera with 2-mercaptoethanol)	Negative (<1:4)	Rising slowly from a negative or low titer (1:4) to a high titer (1:512); if a high-sensitivity antigen is used, the titer may reach 1:128,000	Stable or slowly decreasing titer; titers usually are higher than in the dye test if a high-sensitivity antigen is used; striking differences between dye test and agglutination test titers observed in some patients
IHA test (after treatment of sera with 2-mercaptoethanol)	Negative (<1:16)	Rising very slowly from a negative or low titer (1:16) to a high titer (1:1024); it may take 6 months before a high titer is reached; in some patients, high titers are never observed	Stable or slowly decreasing high or low titer
Conventional IFA test (conjugated antiserum to IgG)	Negative (<1:20)	Rise in titer is parallel to rise in dye test titer, but decrease in titer might be slower than that in dye test	

Abbreviations: ELISA, enzyme-linked immunosorbent assay; IFA, immunofluorescent antibody test; IgG, immunoglobulin G; IHA, indirect hemagglutination test.
[a]Reproduced with permission from Remington et al.[167]
[b]Similar data for the IgG ELISA have not been published.

Table 57-23 Resources for Management of Congenital Toxoplasmosis[a]

Resource	Services Provided
Reference laboratory	Testing for serology, isolation, and PCR assay
FDA (United States)	IND number to obtain spiramycin for treatment for a pregnant woman (United States)
NIH (United States)	Educational pamphlet: "Toxoplasmosis," No. 83-308
Toxoplasmosis.org (http://www.toxoplasmosis.org)	Educational information available via Internet
NCCCTS (United States)	Longitudinal study evaluating persons with congenital toxoplasmosis

Abbreviations: FDA, US Food and Drug Administration; IND, Investigational New Drug; NIH, National Institutes of Health; NCCCTS, National Collaborative Chicago-based Congenital Toxoplasmosis Study; PCR, polymerase chain reaction.
[a]Adapted with permission from Remington et al.[167]

Table 57-24 Serum Antibody Load

	Sample	Date (month/day/year)	Dye Test	Sensitivity	Quantitative IgG (mg/dL)	Ab Load
Patient A	Serum	6/29/06	384	0.075	—	—
	Serum	7/11/06	192	0.075	—	—
	Serum	8/16/06	75	0.075	330	0.017
	Serum	10/4/06	24	0.075	178	0.01
	Serum	11/8/06	8	0.1	133	0.006
	Serum	1/31/07	0	0.1	199	0
	Serum	6/13/07	0	0.075	348	0
Patient B	Serum	7/11/06	256	0.075	899	0.021
	Serum	8/16/06	96	0.075	330	0.022
	Serum	10/4/06	16	0.075	—	—
	Serum	11/8/06	8	0.1	246	0.003
	Serum	1/31/07	2	0.1	334	0.0006
	Serum	6/13/07	0	0.075	583	0

Abbreviations: Ab, antibody; Ig, immunoglobulin.
Serum Antibody Load = (Reciprocal Dye Test × Sensitivity)/Quantitative IgG (mg/dL)

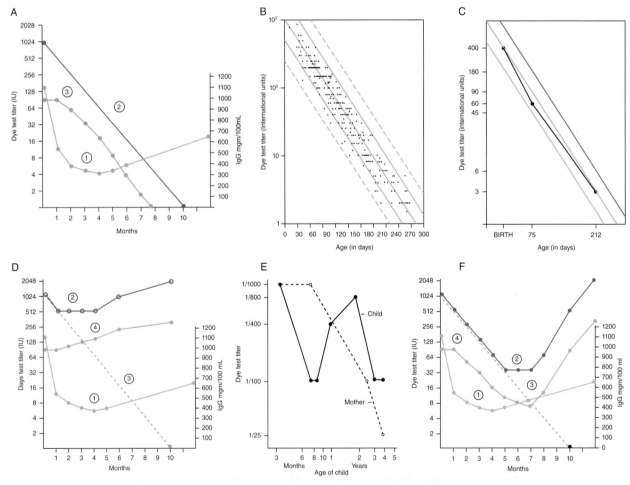

FIGURE 57-17 A, Immunoglobulin (Ig) G and *Toxoplasma* antibodies: uninfected child. Curve 1, milligrams of IgG per deciliter; curve 2, international units of *Toxoplasma* antibody per milliliter; curve 3, international units of *Toxoplasma* antibody per milligram of IgG. **B,** Decrease in maternally transmitted *Toxoplasma* antibodies (dye test) in uninfected infants.

The 2 parallel lines indicate one-half and twice the titer, plus or minus a 2-fold dilution. The result in 1 serum sample of each pair is on the theoretical line and is not represented by a dot. The result in the other serum sample of each pair is represented by a dot. C, Evolution of maternally transmitted antibody (dye test) in an uninfected infant from birth to the age of 212 days. D, Antibodies in congenital toxoplasmosis (cases with early synthesis of antibodies). Curve 1, milligrams of IgG per deciliter; curve 2, international units of *Toxoplasma* antibody per milliliter; curve 3, expected titer if antibodies were maternal in origin; curve 4, international units of *Toxoplasma* antibody per milligram of IgG. E, Example of antibody development (dye test) in a child with congenital toxoplasmosis in relation to time since birth. F, Antibodies in congenital toxoplasmosis (cases with delayed synthesis of antibodies). (Synthesis usually is not delayed more than 3 or 4 months if the child receives no treatment. It may be delayed up to the sixth or ninth months, or more, if treatment is given.) Curve 1, milligrams of IgG per deciliter; curve 2, international units of *Toxoplasma* antibody per milliliter; curve 3, expected titer if antibodies were maternal in origin; curve 4, international units of *Toxoplasma* antibody per milligram of IgG. (A–F, Reproduced with permission from Remington et al.[51])

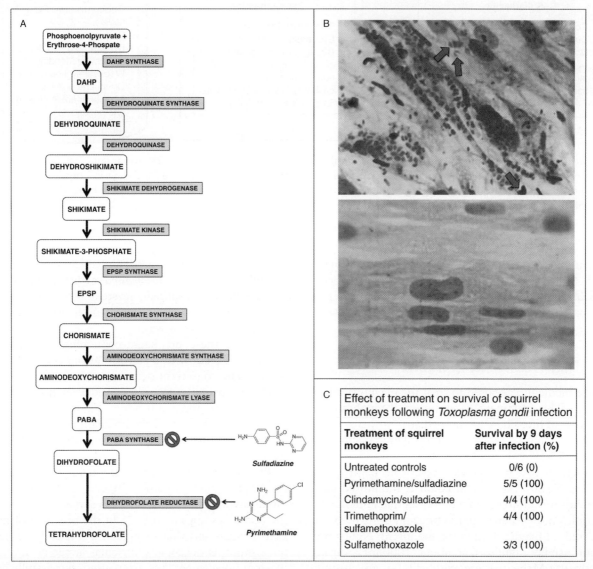

FIGURE 57-18 A, Synthesis of tetrahydrofolate and enzymes that sulfadiazine and pyrimethamine inhibit. **B, top:** *Toxoplasma gondii* tachyzoites in tissue culture with medium alone. Bottom: with antimicrobial agent. Note growth of parasite and destruction of host cells. **C,** Infection was with Beverly strain of *Toxoplasma* administered orally. Systemic disease that is almost always fatal in squirrel monkeys within 7–9 days was produced by oral inoculation of a brain suspension made from mice chronically infected with the Beverly strain of *T. gondii.* Dose regimens used in this study did not allow determination whether addition of PYR or TMP changed protection of sulfonamide alone and did not address comparative efficacy of sulfadiazine, clindamycin or pyrimethamine alone.[159] Other studies have demonstrated less efficacy of TMP/SMZ than pyrimethamine and sulfadiazine.[160] (B, Reproduced with permission from Zuther et al,[161]; provides an example of antimicrobials or novel compounds inhibiting the parasite in tissue culture. C, Data from McLeod et al.[41])

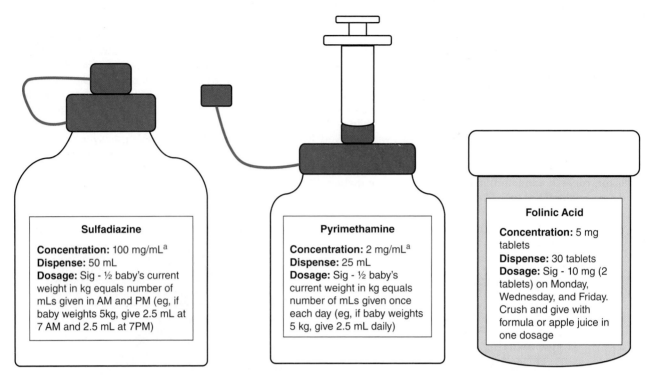

FIGURE 57-19 Medications used to treat congenital toxoplasmosis. ªSuspended in 2% sugar solution. Suspension at usual concentration must be made each week. Store refrigerated. First loading dose for 2 days is 1 mg/kg twice daily. For the third day, the dose is 1 mg/kg/d with in utero treatment; no loading dose postnatally is used. (Reproduced with permission from McAuley et al.[27])

human DHFR enzyme can be rescued with folinic acid. Sulfadiazine inhibits para-amino benzoic acid (PABA) synthase. The combination of the 2 medicines demonstrates 8-fold synergy compared to the use of either one alone.[51]

Medical Treatment in Infancy

These medicines are used to treat the newborn infant as well. This treatment is continued throughout the first year of life. There are no pediatric suspensions of these medicines. A method for formulation is shown in Figures 57-19 and 116-4.[24,27,37,51]

Potential toxicities include reversible neutropenia (Figure 57-20). Neutrophil count is monitored each Monday and Thursday in a blood sample obtained by heel stick rather than venipuncture and using 0.25 mL to avoid iatrogenic anemia for the infant. Neutrophil count usually stabilizes at about 1000/mL³ during treatment. Medicines are withheld for an absolute neutrophil count (ANC) of 500–600 or less and begun again when ANC is greater than 1000–1500. There has been no long-term toxicity associated with this treatment.

Granulocyte colony-stimulating factor (GCSF) has been used in a few instances recently when neutropenia occurs repeatedly over many weeks and precludes

administration of medicines. This has allowed continued administration of anti-*Toxoplasma* medicines when neutropenia has been especially severe or recurrent. There is no long-term follow-up of treatment-associated neutropenia managed in this way.

Because these are sugar-containing suspensions, cleaning of teeth with a soft toothbrush or washcloth is important to prevent dental carries.

Hypersensitivity to sulfonamides is not uncommon in the nonpregnant adult (Figure 57-20) but is relatively uncommon in the pregnant woman and rare in the infant. We have observed this only once during treatment of about 200 infants.

Prompt treatment of hydrocephalus may result in remarkably good outcomes (Figure 57-10). The more rapidly hydrocephalus is corrected surgically, the better the outcomes appear to be.[55] In the presence of high CSF protein and due to inflammation and the need for a shunt, endoscopic ventricular lavage at the time of shunt placement has been used successfully.[55] If there is a cavum septum pellucidum or obstruction of the foramen magnum so that both ventricles cannot be effectively decompressed with a single shunt, there can be a need for a Y shaped shunt with each end of the "Y" in one of the ventricles joining the reservoir of the stem subcutaneously.[55] Because there can be remarkable decompression of ventricles, placement of shunts far

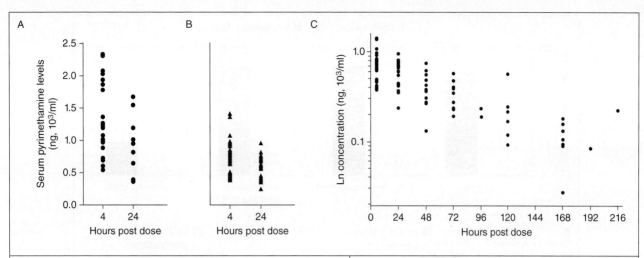

D	Pyrimethamine Pharmacokinetics and Toxicity	Toxicity and Complications

- Pyrimethamine half life = 64±12 hours
- Serum levels with 1 mg/kg/d dose = 1.3±0.5/ugm/ml 4 hrs after dose
- CSF levels are approximately 10%–25% concomitant serum levels
- Phenobarbital shortens pyrimethamine 1/2 life (33±12 hrs) lowering levels
- Serum and CSF levels in potentially therapeutic range (in vitro studies)
- Toxicity: reversible neutropenia, discoloration teeth (sugar suspensions)
- Similar incidence of reversible neutropenia for high and low dose

- Reversible neutropenia requiring temporary withholding of medications did not differ for treatment groups

- Eleven deaths, not related to treatment

E   **Episodes of Reversible Neutropenia Requiring Temporary Withholding of Medications for the US National Collaborative Study**

	No. of Episodes Medication Withheld (Mean ± S.D. [RANGE])	No. of Patients Who Stopped Medication/ No. in Cohort Who Have Completed 1 Year of Therapy (%)			No. Who Discontinued Medications Due To Neutropenia ≥4 Times
		Feasibility	Randomized	All	
Treatment A	2 ± 1 [1–4]	6/14 (43)	13/36 (36)	21/57 (37)	2
Treatment C	3 ± 3 [1–11]	6/11 (55)	10/28 (36)	20/59 ()	7

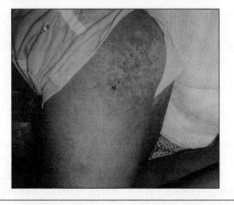

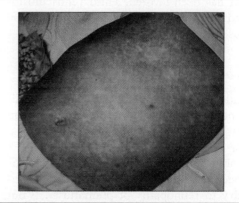

FIGURE 57-20 A, Pyrimethamine serum levels (4 and 24 hours after a dose) of children given 1 mg pyrimethamine per kilogram daily. B, Pyrimethamine serum levels (4 and 24 hours after a dose) of children given 1 mg pyrimethamine per milliliter on Monday, Wednesday, and Friday of each week. Values for children taking phenobarbital are not included. C, Pyrimethamine levels in sera of the entire population of infants taking 1 mg pyrimethamine per kilogram on Monday, Wednesday, and Friday of each week. Values for children taking phenobarbital are not included. D, Pyrimethamine pharmacokinetics and toxicity. E, Toxicity of treatments 1 and 2 was measured as episodes of reversible neutropenia requiring temporary withholding of medications. Although there were no significant differences, there was a trend (*p* = .09, Fisher exact test, 1 tailed) toward more infants with multiple episodes of reversible neutropenia in the higher-dose group (treatment 2). F, Sulfadiazine hypersensitivity causing skin rash. CSF, cerebrospinal fluid. (A–D, Reproduced with permission from McLeod et al.[23] E, Data from McLeod et al.[37] F, Reproduced with permission from McLeod et al.[162])

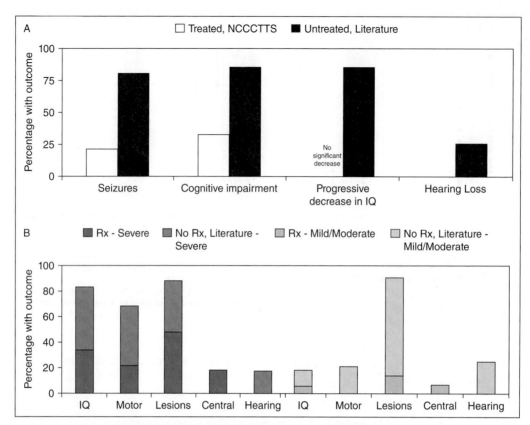

FIGURE 57-21 A, Outcomes in the National Collaborative Chicago-based Congenital Toxoplasmosis Study (NCCCTS) compared to those of Eichenwald.[8] **B,** Outcomes in the NCCCTS compared to those of Eichenwald[8] (No Rx [drug]–Severe) and Wilson et al.[14]

anteriorly can be complicated by entrapment into the brain parenchyma. Thus, somewhat more distal shunt tip placement has been favored. Third ventriculostomies have had a substantial failure rate in this disease and are not used.

Adjunctive Treatment

Active choroidal neovascular membranes in older children have responded rapidly and well to administration of intraocular LUCENTIS® (∝-vascular endothelial growth factor [∝-VEGF) with restoration of vision[129] and with resolution of bleeding (Figure 57-22). Anti-VEGF has been used in infants with neovascularization secondary to retinopathy of prematurity,[130] but there is no experience we are aware of describing its successful use for choroidal neovascular membranes due to *T. gondii* in infants.

Prednisone (1 mg/kg divided twice daily) has been used when CSF protein is 1000 mg/dL or greater or for active chorioretinitis threatening vision with severe vitritis or disease in the posterior pole and macula. This was adapted from early recommendations from France and has not been studied in a rigorous way. Stopping steroid treatment as quickly as the substantial

inflammatory process subsides (usually within weeks) is recommended. A perispinal cord lipoma has been associated with neonatal steroid administration along with the other more usual complications of steroid administration, reinforcing the need to limit the duration of steroid administration to as short a time as possible (usually a few weeks).[27,54]

OUTCOMES AND FOLLOW-UP

Untreated infection is often associated with a variety of disabilities (Tables 57-25 to 57-40), with more severe disease at birth and more prematurity with certain genetic types of parasites (Tables 57-35 to 57-39). When treatment of this infection is initiated as soon as the diagnosis is made for the pregnant woman according to the French algorithm shown in Figure 57-23, the outcome is usually good. There is a low incidence of peripheral retinal disease, and neurologic disabilities are infrequent, with follow-up into early adult life now available for more than 100 such children (Figure 57-24).[41,45,48] The more rapidly treatment is initiated for the pregnant woman to treat the fetus, the better the outcome is[41–43] as measured for both eyes (Figure 57-24 and Tables 57-25 to 57-30) and neurologic findings (Tables 57-31 to 57-34). These findings indicate that to be most effective in preventing retinal and neurologic disease, gestational screening should be performed monthly and treatment initiated promptly.

For the newborn infant whose mother has not been part of a systematic gestational serologic screening program, as this disease is diagnosed in symptomatic infants currently in the United States, 70%–80% of those children have retinal disease, and many have CNS findings at birth when the diagnosis is made. Often, it is too late to reverse the damage done by retinal scarring (Tables 57-20 and 57-21). Nonetheless, in contrast to earlier literature, when such infants were either not treated or treated only for 1 month, outcomes are quite good for the majority of those children who are treated during their first year of life (Figure 57-21). Comparison of outcomes for children who were not treated or treated for only 1 month with children in a US national collaborative treatment study is shown in Tables 57-25 to 57-40.

All outcomes for those children with no or mild involvement at birth and those with moderate or severe involvement were significantly better than that shown in the literature. This was the case when considering children treated with a lower dose of pyrimethamine after an initial dose of 1 mg/kg/day after 2 or after 6 months and those children considered together (Figure 57-26).

Recrudescence of infection, usually retinal, most often occurs around the age of school entry or in puberty, although it can occur at any time (Figure 57-13). When diagnosed and treated promptly, this usually resolves rapidly without loss of visual acuity with a short course of treatment with pyrimethamine and sulfadiazine (Figure 57-26). Azithromycin or clindamycin have replaced sulfadiazine when hypersensitivity occurs. Oral suspension formulations for pyrimethamine and sulfadiazine are shown in Table 57-41. No recurrences have occurred during treatment in the first year of life. Pyrimethamine and sulfadiazine do not eliminate the encysted bradyzoite form. No medicines available today are known to do so. This means that there is risk for recurrence, although in treated children this is relatively uncommon (<10% for children with no or mild symptoms at birth, 30% for those with severe disease at birth; Figure 57-13).

Although prognosis is good for most children with treated congenital toxoplasmosis, there are children whose treatment began after substantial damage had occurred, and outcomes have been poor for some of these children, with lifelong disabilities and medical problems. At the time an infant presents with severe involvement, our approach is to proceed expectant for a favorable outcome as it is not possible to predict with absolute certainty which child will respond well vs which child will have ongoing and severe difficulties. Earlier, prompt diagnosis and initiation of medical treatment and ventriculoperitoneal shunting, when needed, facilitate better outcomes.

THE FUTURE AND HOW PHYSICIANS CAN IMPROVE OUTCOMES

In France, gestational screening and treatment of the congenitally infected fetus have largely eliminated severe congenital toxoplasmosis (Tables 57-42 and 57-43), which is the primary way this disease is encountered in newborn infants in the United States.[41-43,45,48] Implementation of a gestational screening and prompt treatment program for pregnant women in the United States likely would improve outcomes considerably. In the absence of gestational screening, inclusion of *T. gondii* infection in newborn screening programs would allow prompt detection of this treatable infection in newborn infants at birth, both for those with no or mild manifestations obvious at birth (50% of whom would have meningoencephalitis that would otherwise go undetected or retinal disease) and those who have symptoms or signs that are not quickly ascribed to *T. gondii* infection and treated. An economic analysis performed recently[53] found that gestational screening would be cost minimizing within the broad range of parameters that exist in the United States (Tables 57-43 to 57-46)[53] and certainly in Brazil[131] and other countries where the incidence of disease is even higher. For example, in Belo Horizonte, Brazil, up to 50% of the approximately 1/700 newborns with toxoplasmosis have active retinal disease.[131]

Prompt diagnosis and treatment, including considering this infection for all newborns who are born prematurely, who have intrauterine growth retardation (IUGR), who are small for gestational age, who have thrombocytopenia not explained otherwise, who have meningitis not otherwise explained, who have been considered for ruling out sepsis, or who have unexplained direct hyperbilirubinemia or abnormal liver function tests—not just those with the classical triad of calcifications, hydrocephalus, and chorioretinitis—would be an improvement. A vaccine that prevents this infection and nontoxic medicines that do not have associated hypersensitivity that could promptly and completely eliminate the active and dormant parasite stages would be substantial improvements.

A simple point-of-service diagnostic test to identify all acutely infected women during gestation and the infant at birth would also be useful.

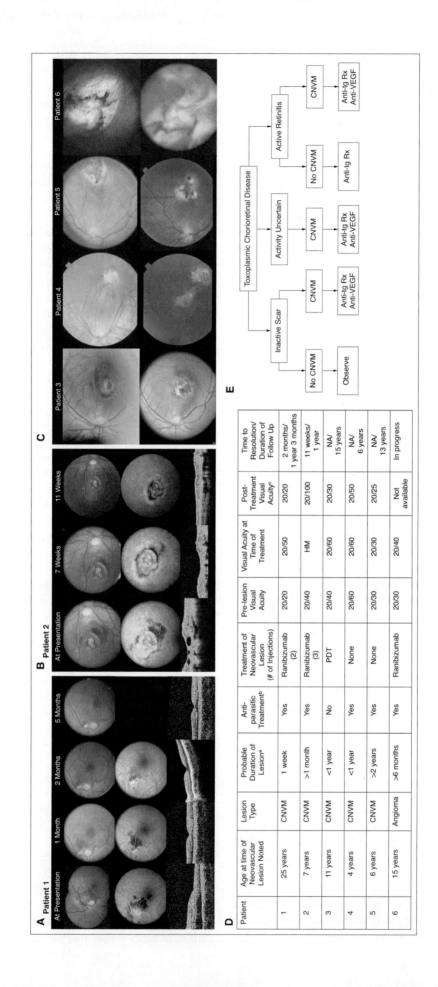

FIGURE 57-22 A Patient 1 fundus photographs, fluorescein angiography, and optical coherence tomography at presentation and 1, 2, and 5 months after the first ranibizumab injection. B Patient 2 fundus photograph, fluorescein angiography, and optical coherence tomography at first presentation and 7 and 11 weeks after the first ranibizumab injection. C Fundus photographs of patients 3, 4, 5, and 6. Patient 3 before choroidal neovascular membrane (CNVM) (top row) and 4 years after photodynamic therapy (PDT; bottom row). Patient 4 with CNVM (top row) and 3 months later (bottom row). Patient 5 with CNVM (top row) and 4 years later (bottom row). Patient 6 before (top row) and after developmental of angiomatous proliferation (bottom row). D, Brief description of children with ocular toxoplasmosis and CNVM. HM, hand motions; NA, data not available; VEGF, vascular endothelial growth factor. [a]The duration of symptoms noted by the patient suggested presence of neovascular lesions. Actual duration is especially imprecise in younger patients, who may not have perceived or complained of any symptoms. In these cases, the durations are given as an interval greater than the time between the lesion's first appearance on clinical examination and the date of treatment or an interval less than the time between the date of the last normal examination and the first time the lesion first was noted on clinical examination. [b]Antiparasitic treatment was given before and throughout and at least 1 week after treatment with anti-VEGF. Treatment was initially with pyrimethamine, sulfadiazine, and leucovorin; then, after 6 weeks in some instances, clarithromycin was substituted for sulfadiazine. Leucovorin was administered throughout and for 1 week after the time pyrimethamine was administered. Treatment with these medicines was continued for about 1 month beyond resolution of the CNVM and at least 1 week after toxoplasmic retinitis activity. [c]Visual acuity is best-corrected visual acuity unless otherwise stated in the case report. These measurements do not reflect defects in visual field that also impaired vision and were larger with larger scars. In some instances, these defects were the major morbidity of the lesions and their treatment (eg, with PDT). In prior reports, surgical excision in 2 patients[4, 5] and PDT in 4 small series have been reported as treatments for CNVM in ocular toxoplasmosis. With surgical excision, 2 patients had vision improved to 20/20 and 20/30, respectively. With PDT, for 14 reported patients, 3 patients worsened, 5 had partial improvement in vision but not to baseline, 1 improved to baseline, and 5 stabilized or improved with treatment but baseline visions were not provided. Cryotherapy or endophotocoagulation resulted in resorption of exudative fluid in 5 of 7 eyes with angiomatous lesions associated with Toxoplasma scars. In many instances, defects in visual field were the major morbidity of the lesions and their treatment with PDT and were not quantified or mentioned. E, Algorithm used to manage toxoplasmic retinal disease and active CNVM with extravasation of serous fluid or hemorrhage. Treatment of active toxoplasmic chorioretinitis (anti-tg Rx) or when a diagnosis of active toxoplasmic chorioretinitis cannot be excluded or activity might be induced by trauma, in the context of an active CNVM: pyrimethamine, 1 mg/kg/d (maximum dose 50–75 mg/d) following loading dose of 1 mg/kg twice a day for 2 days; leucovorin 10 mg each Monday, Wednesday, and Friday or adjusted based on absolute neutrophil count. Continued 1 week beyond resolution of active infection. Sulfadiazinc 100 mg/kg divided twice per day; maximum dose 4 g/d. Clindamycin or clarithromycin have been used in place of sulfadiazine when there is sulfonamide hypersensitivity. Complete blood cell count to monitor neutrophil count is obtained during pyrimethamine therapy twice weekly during and in the week after stopping pyrimethamine therapy. This treatment should be supervised with a pediatrician, an internal medicine physician, or infectious disease specialist. Additional suggestions concerning treatment of toxoplasmic chorioretinitis can be obtained by calling 773-834-4131. Anti-VEGF Rx indicates treatment of active CNVM, which in our experience has been with 0.5 mg in 0.05 mL ranizumab once a month. This is continued for at least 1 to 2 treatments beyond resolution of activity of CNVM. (A–E, Reproduced with permission from Benevento et al.[129])

CHAPTER 57

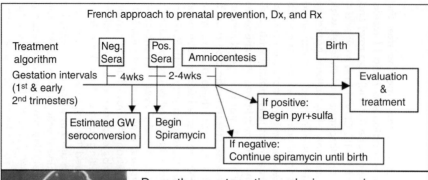

French approach to prenatal prevention, Dx, and Rx

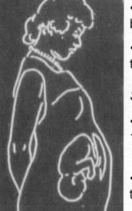

- Dx mother: systematic serologic screening, before conception & intrapartum

- Rx mother: if acute serology, spiramycin reduces transmission
  Untreated 94 (60%) of 154 vs treated 91 (23%) of 388 [a]

- Dx fetus: ultrasounds; amniocentesis, PCR at ≥ 18 weeks gestation
  Sensitivity 37 (97%) of 38: specificity 301 of 301 [b]

- Rx fetus: pyrimethamine, sulfadiazine or termination *N=54 livebirths; 34 terminations* [c]

Outcomes

- Hohlfeld [d]: All 54 normal development; 19% subtle findings *7 (13%) intracranical calcifications, 3 (6%) chorioretinal scars; follow-up of 18 children (median age 4.5 yr; range, 1-11yr): 39% retinal scars, most scars were peripheral.*

- Kieffer [e]: Shorter interval between diagnosis and treatment reduces subsequent retinal disease.

- Syrocot [f]: Shorter interval beteween diagnosis and treatment reduces subsequent neurologic disease.

- Favorable outcomes with treatment *in utero* in France and as French Algorithm applied in U.S. [g,h]

FIGURE 57-23 Top, Parisian algorithm for diagnosis (Dx) and treatment (Rx) of congenital toxoplasmosis. Middle, French approach to diagnosis and treatment of congenital toxoplasmosis in earlier decades and outcomes using this approach. Neg., negative; PCR, polymerase chain reaction; Pos., positive; pyr, person-year. [a]Data from Desmonts and Couvreur.[17] [b]Data from Hohlfeld et al.[26] [c]Data from Daffos et al.[21] [d]Data from Hohlfeld et al.[22] [e]Data from Kieffer et al.[42] [f]Data from Systematic Review on Congenital Toxoplasmosis (SYROCOT) Study Group et al.[163] [g]Data from Peyron et al.[48] [h]Data from Stillwaggon et al.[53] (Reproduced with permission from McLeod et al.[41])

ACKNOWLEDGMENTS

This work was supported by the National Institutes of Health (NIH), National Institute of Allergy and Infectious Diseases (NIAID) R01 AI027530-21 and gifts from the Mann and Cornwell, Taub, Cussen-Kapnick, Rooney-Alden, Engel, Pritzker, Harris, Zucker, Samuel, and Mussilami families, and NIH U01 5 U01 AI077887-05 and 2R01AI027530-18A2. We thank those families and physicians who have worked with us to help us learn more about how to diagnose, manage, and treat this disease and those who have taught us about it, especially George Desmonts, Jacques Couvreur, Philippe Thulliez, and Jack Remington.

This chapter is especially in honor of Dana, Chad, Dani Jo, Elena, Graham, Grant, Joshua, Lucky, Margaret, Miguel, Nicky, Robbie, Roxanne, and many others and their families who understand with special poignancy Edward Young's statement "who would not give a trifle to prevent what they would give a thousand worlds to cure."

A

Fetus   Birth   Infant   Child   Adolescent   Adult   Older Age

Rx of fetus
Rx *in utero* and/or infancy
Childhood and adolescence
Adult

Age of endpoint evaluations (B, C): 18-35

B

Quality of Life in Our Cohort Compared With That in an Age-matched General Population

	Study Cohort (n=102)		General Population (Age-matched)[a]	
	Mean	Standard Deviation	Mean	Standard Deviation
Anxiety	71.2	19.3	72.2	19.6
Positive well-being	64.7	17.0	64.0	18.7
Vitality	64.7	15.2	68.0	18.6
Depressed mood	85.9	17.9	83.5	17.1
Self-control	80.7	16.0	82.5	17.2
General health	84.7	16.1	78.4	18.4
Global score	74.7	14.2	73.7	15.3

C

Ophthalmological Characteristics and Neurological Problems of the Patients

	Absolute Number (%)
No. ocular lesions	
None	42 (41.2%)
1	25 (24.5%)
2	17 (16.7%)
3 or more	18 (17.6%)
Lesions in both eyes[b]	26 (25.5%)
Persons with reduced visual acuity[c]	13 (12.7%)
Localization of lesion (independent of eye)	
Fovea	16 (15.7%)
Other region	44 (43.1%)
None	42 (41.2%)
Recurrences	
Without recurrences	90 (88.2%)
One recurrence	12 (11.8%)
Squinting	6 (5.9%)
Microphthalmia	3 (2.9%)
Cataract	1 (0.9%)
Neurological findings	
Intracranial calcifications	11 (10.8%)
Hydrocephalus	2 (1.9%)

FIGURE 57-24 [a]European general population according to MAPI Institute; none of the differences attained statistical significance (*p*>.05). [b]One person had central lesions in both eyes. [c]As defined by a best-corrected Snellen score below 16 of 20. Rx, treatment. (B, C, Reproduced with permission from Peyron et al.[48])

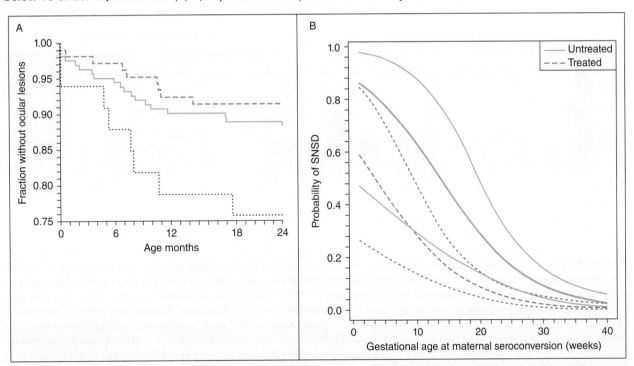

FIGURE 57-25 A, New eye lesions in children who had less than 8 or 8 or more weeks delay from diagnosis in utero to treatment. Kaplan-Meier plots showing the age at diagnosis of a first retinochoroiditis according to the delay between maternal infection and first treatment; less than 4 weeks (solid line), 4–8 weeks (dashed line), and more than 8 weeks (dotted line). B, Probability of severe neurological sequelae (SNSD). Probability of SNSD according to inputed gestational age at seroconversion and 95% Bayesian credible limits; dotted lines denote treated pregnancies; solid lines denote untreated pregnancies. (A, Reproduced with permission from Kieffer et al.[42] B, Reproduced with permission from Cortina-Borja et al.[43])

Endpoint 1: Neurologic outcomes (motor/tone abnormality)

A

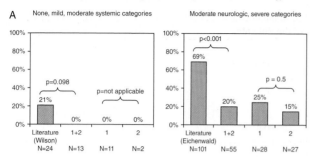

Wilson: Mean age at evaluation = 8 years
Eichenwald: Mean age at evaluation = 4 years
Ages at Chicago evaluation ≥5 years
Note: p values for literature vs 1+2, one sided; 1 vs 2, two sided

Endpoint 2: IQ < 70

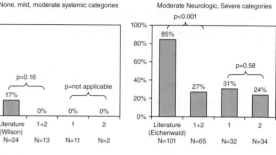

Wilson: Mean age at evaluation = 8 years
Eichenwald: Mean age at evaluation = 4 years
Ages at Chicago evaluation ≥3.5 years
Note: p values for literature vs 1+2, one sided; 1 vs 2, two sided

Endpoint 3: Decrease in IQ ≥15

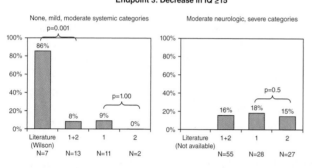

Wilson: Mean age at evaluation = 8 years
Ages at Chicago evaluation ≥5 years
Note: p values for literature vs 1+2, one sided; 1 vs 2, two sided

Endpoint 4: Vision <20/30

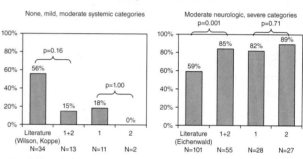

Wilson: Mean age at evaluation = 8 years
Koppe: Mean age at evaluation = 20 years
Eichenwald: Mean age at evaluation = 4 years
Ages at Chicago evaluation ≥5 years
Note: p values for literature vs 1+2, one sided; 1 vs 2, two sided

Endpoint 5: New eye lesions

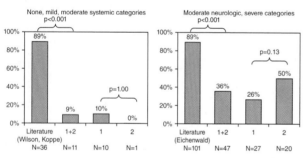

Wilson: Mean age at evaluation = 8 years
Koppe: Mean age at evaluation = 20 years
Eichenwald: Mean age at evaluation = 4 years
Ages at Chicago evaluation ≥75 years
Note: p values for literature vs 1+2; one sided; 1 vs 2, two sided

Endpoint 6: Hearing loss > 30dB

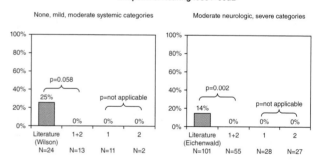

Wilson: Mean age at evaluation = 8 years
Eichenwald: Mean age at evaluation = 4 years
Ages at Chicago evaluation ≥5 years
Note: p values for literature vs 1+2; one sided; 1 vs 2; two sided

FIGURE 57-26 A, Improved outcomes in treated children contrasted with earlier cohorts and comparing a higher- and lower-dose regimen in a randomized controlled trial. Frequency of outcomes for each end point for patients in our study compared with the frequency in the literature.[8,14,15,19,38] There was no visible trend for superiority or statistically significant superiority for treatment arm 1 or treatment arm 2 at this time. Results may differ in the future because the majority of the children enrolled are entering adolescence and early adulthood, a critical time when outcomes may vary. It is also important that outcomes of offspring of the treated children be established in the following years of this study. 1, treatment arm 1 (daily doses of pyrimethamine [1 mg/kg] for 2 months); 2, treatment arm 2 (daily doses of pyrimethamine [1 mg/kg] for 6 months; following daily dosing with pyrimethamine, this dose was administered on each Monday, Wednesday, and Friday. Sulfadiazine 50 mg/kg was administered throughout, as was

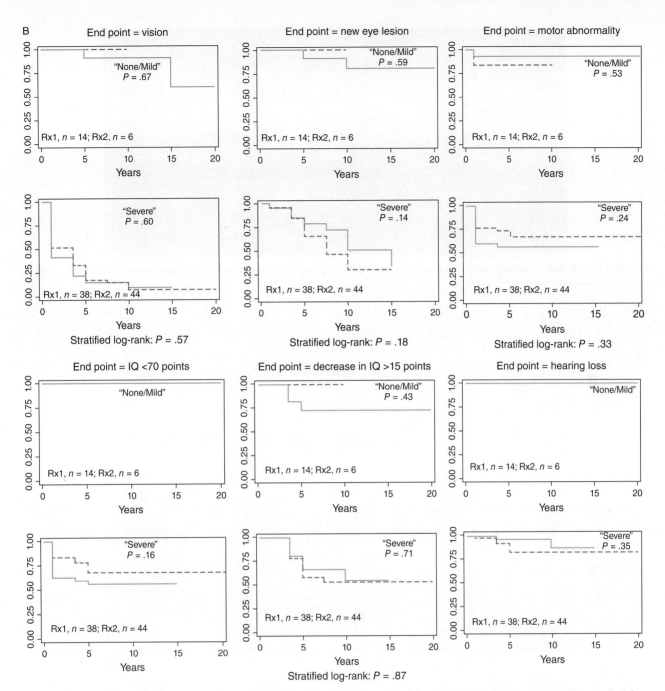

calcium leucovorin). B, Kaplan-Meier curves showing the outcomes for each end point for patients in the pooled feasibility/observational phase and the randomized phase who received treatment 1 (solid line) or treatment 2 (dotted line). There is no visible trend for superiority or statistically significant superiority at this time. Results may differ in the future because the majority of the children enrolled are entering adolescence and early adulthood, a critical time when outcomes may vary. It is also important that outcomes of offspring of the treated children be established in the following years of this study. IQ, intelligence quotient; Rx1, treatment arm 1; Rx2, treatment arm 2. (A, Reproduced with permission from McLeod et al.[41] B, Reproduced with permission from McLeod et al.[37])

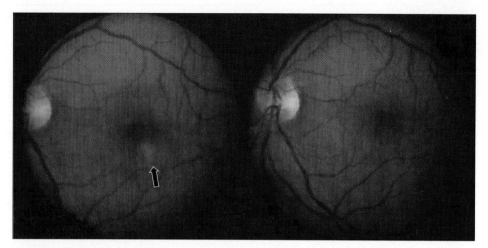

FIGURE 57-27 Active retinal lesion before (left) and within a month of initiating treatment (right). (Reproduced with permission from McLeod et al.[41])

Table 57-25 Quantitative Visual Acuity in Patients With Macular Lesions (m), National Collaborative Chicago-based Congenital Toxoplasmosis Study (NCCCTS) (1981–1996)[a]

Group[b]	Patient No.	Right Eye	Left Eye
Treated in the first year of life	7	20/20	20/20 (m)
	13	6/400 (m)	**20/50 (m)**[c]
	15	4/30 (m)	**20/30 (m)**[c]
	19	20/200[d]	20/20 (m)
	21	1/30 (m)	1/30 (m)
	26	3/30 (m)	1/30 (m)
	28	20/30 (m)	15/30 (m)
	30	1/30 (m)	12/30[e]
	36	20/30	8/30 (m)
Historical (not treated in the first year of life)	20	20/400 (m)	20/25
	25	20/400 (m)	20/30
	27	5/30 (m)	1/30[f]
	31	20/25	3/200 (m)
	38	20/400 (m)	**20/25**[f]
	41	20/30	20/200 (m)
	42	20/70 (m)	**20/30 (m)**[c]
	46	20/200 (m)	20/60 (m)
	47	3/30 (m)	3/30[f]
	82	20/400 (m)	20/15
	89	20/100 (m)	20/25

[a]Adapted with permission from Mets et al.[30]
[b]Treated: *n* = 39 (30 too young or with cognitive limitations that made it impossible for the child to cooperate with quantitative vision); historical: *n* = 13 (2 too young for quantitative vision).
[c]**Bold** type indicates surprisingly good vision in spite of foveal lesion.
[d]Strabismus, microphthalmia, and amblyopia present.
[e]Poor cooperation; patient was 4 years old.
[f]Peripheral lesion with dragging of the macula.

Table 57-26 Quantitative Visual Acuity in Treated Patients With Macular Lesions, National Collaborative Chicago-based Congenital Toxoplasmosis Study (NCCCTS) (1981–1996)[a]

Eye Status (Most Recent Examination) (N = 76)[b]	Number (%)
No disease	18 (24)
Lesion: normal visual acuity	19 (25)
Unilateral visual impairment	17 (22)
Bilateral visual impairment	22 (29)
New lesions	7/54 (13)[c]

[a]Adapted with permission from Mets et al.[30]
[b]Mean age at most recent examination: 45 ± 56 months, range 0.4–123 months.
[c]Developed after 1 year of therapy; eye disease quiescent during therapy in the first year of life for all children.

Table 57-27 New or Recrudescent Retinal Lesions After Therapy Stopped, National Collaborative Chicago-based Congenital Toxoplasmosis Study (NCCCTS) (1981–1996)[a]

Ages at which lesions noted	3, 4, 5, 6, 7, 8, and 10 years
Percentage with active lesions	4 (57%) of 7
Percentage with previously normal retina	3 (43%) of 7 initially
Percentage satelliting older lesion	5 (83%) of 6
Associated with change in visual acuity	1 (14%) of 7

[a]Data from Mets et al.[30]

Table 57-28 Characteristics of New Chorioretinal Lesions: Correlation With Development of New Chorioretinal Lesions, National Collaborative Chicago-based Congenital Toxoplasmosis Study (NCCCTS) (1981–2006)[a]

	Development of Any New Lesions	p Value	Development of New Central Lesions	p Value
Severity of overall disease		.074		.18
None (N = 10)	1 (10%)		0 (0%)	
Mild (N = 10)	2 (20%)		1 (10%)	
Severe (N = 88)	31 (35%)		14 (16%)	
Impaired vision near birth		.21		.59
Yes (N = 50)	19 (38%)		8 (16%)	
No (N = 58)	15 (26%)		7 (12%)	
Gestational treatment		.17		.35
Yes (N = 10)[b]	1 (10%)		0 (0%)	
No (N = 98)	33 (34%)		15 (15%)	

[a]Reproduced with permission from Phan et al.[39]
[b]Although 18 mothers were treated, only 10 patients currently have data regarding development of new chorioretinal lesions.

Table 57-29 Characteristics of New Chorioretinal Lesions: Numbers of Patients With and Locations of New Chorioretinal Lesions and Eyes in Which They Occur in Each Patient at Any Time by Treatment Group, National Collaborative Chicago-based Congenital Toxoplasmosis Study (NCCCTS) (1981–2006)[a]

	RA (*N* = 38; *n* = 32)	RC (*N* = 38; *n* = 32)	Feasibility[b] (*N* = 45; *n* = 38)	Total (*N* = 132; *n* = 108)
New lesion of any kind	10 (26%)	11 (34%)	13 (34%)	34 (31%)
Central[c]	5 (13%)	4 (13%)	6 (16%)	15 (14%)
Right eye only	2	2	4	8
Left eye only	1	0	1	2
OU	2	2	1	5
Peripheral[d]	7 (18%)	10 (31%)	10 (26%)	27 (25%)
Right eye only	2	2	4	8
Left eye only	3	5	3	11
OU	2	3	3	8

Abbreviations: n, number of patients who had return visits and were evaluated for new lesions; OU, both eyes; RA, patients randomized into the lower dose of pyrimethamine; RC, patients randomized into the higher dose of pyrimethamine.
[a]Reproduced with permission from Phan et al.[39]
[b]Nonrandomized patients treated with either the lower or the higher dose of pyrimethamine.
[c]In the macula and peripapillary area.
[d]Outside the macula and peripapillary area.

Table 57-30 Numbers and Locations of New Toxoplasmic Chorioretinal Lesions and Eyes in Which They Occur in Each Patient, National Collaborative Chicago-based Congenital Toxoplasmosis Study (NCCCTS) (1981–2005)[a]

	Number (%) With Findings	
	All Pts[b]	Patients Prob CT[c]
Findings	*N* = 38 (*n* = 31)	*N* = 28 (*n* = 25)
Chorioretinal lesions of any kind	22 (71%)	18 (72%)
Central chorioretinal lesions	16 (52%)	13 (52%)
OD	10	8
OS	6	5
OU	4	3
Peripheral chorioretinal lesion	14 (45%)	11 (44%)
OD	8	7
OS	8	6
OU	2	2

Abbreviations: CT, congenital toxoplasmosis; N, total number of patients in each group; n, number of patients who had return visits and were evaluated for new lesions; OD, right eye; OS, left eye; OU, both eyes. Central lesions are lesions in the macula and peripapillary area; a peripapillary lesion is defined as a lesion within 1 disc diameter of the optic nerve; peripheral lesions are lesions outside the macula and peripapillary area.
Note that patients were counted multiple times when tabulating the numbers in the OD, OS, and OU rows of the table if they had lesions at multiple visits.
[a]Adapted with permission from Phan et al.[40]
[b]Patients (Pts): There were 38 persons who were children at the time of diagnosis who were not treated during the first year of life.
[c]Patients with probable congenital toxoplasmosis (Pts Prob CT): There were 28 patients in whom congenital infection was likely attributable to the presence of serum antibody to *Toxoplasma gondii*, indicative of chronic infection at age 24 months or less and who had central nervous system calcifications or hydrocephalus or illness compatible with congenital toxoplasmosis perinatally but not diagnosed as congenital toxoplasmosis at that time.

Table 57-31 Contrasts of Neurologic and Developmental Outcomes[a]

Signs Neonatally	Study-Author (Year, N)	Seizures, N (%)	Abnormal Motor/ Tone, N (%)	IQ < 70, N (%)	Sequentially Lower IQ, N (%)
Generalized/ Neurological (Gen/neur)	Eichenwald[8] (1959, 101) NCCCTS (1991, 33)	82 (81) 4 (12)	71 (70) 8 (24)	87 (86) 8 (24)	n/a 3[b]/13 (0)
Subclinical	Wilson et al[14] (1980, 24) NCCCTS (1991, 3)	4 (17) 0 (0)	5 (21) 0 (0)	4 (17) 0 (0)	6/7 (86) 0/2 (0)

Abbreviations: NA, not available; NCCCTS, National Collaborative Chicago-based Congenital Toxoplasmosis Study. Number affected/number tested if different from N (%).
[a]Adapted with permission from Remington et al.[167]
[b]Three children had a more than 15-point diminution and 2 children had a more than 15-point increase in IQ score. The differences over time for the entire group were not statistically significant ($p > .05$).

Table 57-32 Comparison of Developmental Outcomes in Treated Children 1 and 3.5 Years of Age in the National Collaborative Chicago-based Congenital Toxoplasmosis Study (NCCCTS) (1981–1994)[a,b]

Test	Parameter Measured	Age, years	
		1	≥3.5
Bayley/WPPSI-R	Psychomotor	100 ± 15 (23)[c,d]	4 with abnormalities, 13 normal
	Cognitive	102 ± 22 (23)[d]	88 ± 13 (13)[d]
Vineland	Communication	92 ± 13 (21)[d]	92 ± 21 (14)[d]
	Daily living	94 ± 11 (21)[d]	87 ± 22 (14)[d]
	Socialization	98 ± 14 (21)[d]	94 ± 22 (14)[d]
	Motor	94 ± 16 (21)[d]	79 ± 24 (11)[d]
	3-Factor	93 ± 15 (21)[d]	89 ± 23 (14)[d]

[a]Adapted with permission from Roizen et al.[168]
[b]Measure for Bayley Psychomotor Developmental Index (PDI) and Mental Development Index (MDI) is DQ (Developmental Quotient). Measure for Stanford-Binet, Wechsler Preschool and Primary Scale of Intelligence–Revised (WPPSI-R), or Wechsler Intelligence Scale for Children (WISC-R) is IQ. Stanford-Binet was used in the initial part of the study for some children. Measure for Vineland is a standard score. No significant difference ($p > .05$) was found in scores over time.
[c]Mean ± standard deviation (n).
[d]Children with scores less than 50 were excluded.

Table 57-33 Outcomes of Treated Group vs Sibling Controls, National Collaborative Chicago-based Congenital Toxoplasmosis Study (NCCCTS) (1981–1992)[a]

	Measure	N	Mean IQ ± SD	Range
Treated	MDI, WPPSI-R, or WISC-R	7	87 ± 11[b]	68–97
	Vineland	5	86 ± 21[c]	49–103
Siblings	WPPSI-R, WISC-R, or Stanford Binet	7	112 ± 15[b]	85–132
	Vineland	5	108 ± 12[b]	93–126

Abbreviations: MDI, Mental Development Index; WISC-R, Wechsler Intelligence Scale for Children; WPPSI-R, Wechsler Preschool and Primary Scale of Intelligence–Revised.
[a]Data from Roizen et al.[168]
[b]By paired t test, $p < .05$.
[c]By paired t test, $p > .05$.

CHAPTER 57

Table 57-34 Outcomes of Repeated Testing of Treated Children, National Collaborative Chicago-based Congenital Toxoplasmosis Study (NCCCTS) (1981–1994)[a]

Patient	IQ First Evaluation	IQ Second Evaluation
2	100	100
4	140	115
7	96	97
9	130	96
12	91	111
13[b]	102	117
15[b]	99	82
19[b]	96	95
22[b]	73	60
23	96	92
Mean	102	97
SD	19	17

Not significant by paired t test, $p > .05$.
[a]Data from Roizen et al.[168]
[b]Visually impaired.

Table 57-35 Serotypes in US-Born, National Collaborative Chicago-based Congenital Toxoplasmosis Study (NCCCTS) (1981–2009), Contrasted With Literature Data for France and Brazil[a]

	II	NE-II	p Value
United States, NCCCTS	62/161 (39)[b]	99/161 (61)	<.001
France[c]	72/86 (84)	14/86 (16)	
Brazil[d]	0/20 (0)	20/20 (100)	

II and NE-II serotypes as defined previously.[56]
The p values are from chi-square tests or Fisher exact tests.
[a]Reproduced with permission from McLeod et al.[56]
[b]For numbers outside parentheses, the numerator represents number of persons with this parasite serotype residing in the country; the denominator represents the total number of persons residing in the country. The number within the parentheses represents the percentage of persons with this parasite serotype residing in the country.
[c]Data from Ajzenberg et al[169] and Peyron et al.[170]
[d]Data from Ferreira et al.[171]

Table 57-36 Serotypes in National Collaborative Chicago-based Congenital Toxoplasmosis Study (NCCCTS) (1981–2009) Analyzed in Two Cohorts and With Reference to Host Susceptibility Alleles and Gestational Illness[a]

	II	NE-II	p Value
Cohorts			
Treated	52/66 (79)[b]	93/117 (79)	.91
Untreated	14/66 (21)	24/117 (21)	
Host susceptibility alleles			
≥1 SNP[c] COL2A1, ABC4A	33/59 (56)	42/106 (40)	.04
Gestational Illness			
≥1 symptom[d]	15/52 (29)	45/92 (49)	.02

II and NE-II serotypes as defined previously.[56]
The p values reported are from chi-square tests or Fisher exact tests.
[a]Reproduced with permission from McLeod et al.[56]
[b]For the numbers outside parentheses, the numerator represents the number of persons who had characteristics with this parasite serotype; the denominator represents the total number of persons with this parasite serotype. The number within parentheses represents the percentage of persons with this parasite serotype who had characteristics.
[c]SNP indicates single-nucleotide polymorphisms genotyped with significant associations with congenital toxoplasmosis and brain or eye diseases: COL2A1: rs2276455, rs1635544, and ABCA4: rs952499.
[d]Symptoms were flu-like symptoms, fever, night sweats, headache, or lymphadenopathy. Only mothers of infants treated during the first year of life were included.

Table 57-37 Associations With Prematurity (Gestational Age < 38 Weeks), National Collaborative Chicago-based Congenital Toxoplasmosis Study (NCCCTS) (1981–2009)[a]

	II	NE-II	p Value
All	20/66 (30)[b]	54/114 (47)	.03
Rx	18/52 (35)	43/92 (47)	.16
No Rx	2/14 (14)	11/22 (50)	.04

Abbreviation: Rx, treatment.
II and NE-II serotypes as defined previously.[56]
Rx and No Rx as defined previously.[24,25,27,30,35,39,41,51,84,98]
The p values are from chi-square tests or Fisher exact tests.
[a]Reproduced with permission from McLeod et al.[56]
[b]For the numbers outside parentheses, the numerator represents the number of persons born at less than 38 weeks' gestation with this parasite serotype in the NCCCTS cohort; the denominator represents the total number of persons with this parasite serotype in the NCCCTS cohort. The number within the parentheses represents the percentage of persons with this parasite serotype in the NCCCTS cohort who were born at less than 38 weeks' gestation.

Table 57-38 Associations With Disease Severity at Birth and Other Manifestations for Those Who Were Treated during the First Year of Life, National Collaborative Chicago-based Congenital Toxoplasmosis Study (NCCCTS) (1981–2009)[a]

	II	NE-II	p Value
Severe, S/MN	33/52 (63)[b]	77/93 (83)	<.01
Eye severity score at birth ≥ 2	18/46 (39)	59/88 (67)	<.01
Systemic			
Splenomegaly	9/51 (18)	37/91 (41)	<.01
Hepatomegaly	14/51 (27)	42/91 (46)	.03
Thrombocytopenia	18/50 (36)	39/89 (44)	.37
Anemia	7/52 (13)	18/87 (21)	.28
Skin rash	8/51 (16)	29/91 (32)	.04
Jaundice	28/48 (58)	59/86 (69)	.23
R/O sepsis	16/52 (31)	38/93 (41)	.23
Neurologic/ophthalmologic			
Hydrocephalus	19/52 (37)	35/93 (38)	.90
Microcephalus	5/52 (10)	13/93 (14)	.60
CNS calcifications	32/52 (62)	69/93 (74)	.11
Seizures	8/52 (15)	12/93 (13)	.68
Chorioretinal scars	32/52 (62)	72/93 (77)	.04
Microphthalmia	10/52 (19)	13/92 (14)	.42

Abbreviations: CNS, central nervous system; R/O, rule out.
II and NE-II serotypes as defined previously.[56]
S indicates severe, S/MN indicates severe/moderate neurologic disease as defined previously.[27]
The p values reported are from chi-square tests or Fisher exact tests.
[a]Reproduced with permission from McLeod et al.[56]
[b]For the numbers outside parentheses, the numerator represents the number of persons in the NCCCTS cohort who were treated during the first year of life who had this manifestation at birth and this parasite serotype; the denominator represents the total number of persons in the NCCCTS cohort who were treated during the first year of life with this parasite serotype. The number within parentheses represents the percentage of persons in the NCCCTS cohort who were treated during the first year of life who had this manifestation and this parasite serotype.

CHAPTER 57

Table 57-39 Outcomes Later in Life Based on Parasite Serotype and Treatment Group, National Collaborative Chicago-based Congenital Toxoplasmosis Study (NCCCTS) (1981–2009)[a]

	II		NE-II		
	A[b]	C[c]	A	C	p Value
Vision < 20/30	10/19 (53)[d]	5/10 (50)	19/27 (70)	28/31 (90)	.17
New eye lesions	5/17 (29)	4/7 (57)	9/24 (38)	19/27 (70)	.85
New eye lesions: central only	2/17 (12)	2/7 (29)	6/24 (25)	7/27 (26)	.42
Motor/tone abnormality	3/19 (16)	2/10 (20)	6/27 (22)	3/31 (10)	.32
IQ < 70	2/19 (11)	4/13 (31)	10/30 (33)	8/37 (22)	.08
Decrease in IQ ≥ 15	3/19 (16)	2/10 (20)	6/27 (22)	6/31 (19)	.70
Hearing loss > 30 db	There was no hearing loss in any group.				

II and NE-II serotypes as defined previously.[56]
The p values reported are based on a test of the treatment group by parasite serotype interaction from a logistic regression model. A statistically significant interaction would indicate that the effect of treatment on outcome depends on parasite serotype.
These data are for both randomized and feasibility phases combined and include severely and mildly involved persons. The end points were determined at the following ages: Vision < 20/30, motor/tone abnormality, decrease in IQ ≥ 15, hearing loss > 30 db ≥ 5 years, new eye lesions: central + peripheral, new eye lesions: central only ≥ 7.5 years, IQ < 70 ≥ 3.5 years.
[a]Reproduced with permission from McLeod et al.[56]
[b]Treatment group A = treatment of daily pyrimethamine and sulfadiazine for 2 months, followed by pyrimethamine on Monday, Wednesday, and Friday and continued daily sulfadiazine for the remainder of the year of therapy.
[c]Treatment group C = treatment with daily pyrimethamine and sulfadiazine for 6 months, followed by pyrimethamine on Monday, Wednesday, and Friday and continued daily sulfadiazine for the remainder of the year.
[d]For the numbers outside parentheses, the numerator represents the number of persons in the NCCCTS treatment cohort with the end point who had this parasite serotype; the denominator represents the total number of persons in the NCCCTS treatment cohort who had this parasite serotype. The number within parentheses represents the percentage of persons in the NCCCTS cohort of treated persons who had this parasite serotype with this outcome.

Table 57-40 Findings in Those With Subclinical Infection at Birth by Age 9 Years: Adverse Sequelae With Subclinical Infection at Birth for Children Treated 1 Month or Less[a]

	Group I[b] (N = 13)	Group II[b] (N = 10)[c]
Ophthalmologic finding		
No sequelae (7.6, 10)[d]	2	0
Chorioretinitis		
Bilateral		
Bilateral blindness[e]	0	5
Unilateral blindness	3	3
Moderate unilateral visual loss	0	1[f]
Minimal or no visual loss	5	1
Unilateral		
Minimal or no visual loss	3	0
Mean age at onset (years)	3.67	0.42
Range	0.08–9.33	0.25–1.00
Recurrences of active chorioretinitis	3	2
Neurologic finding		
No sequelae	8	3
Major sequelae[g]		

(Continued)

Table 57-40 Findings in Those With Subclinical Infection at Birth by Age 9 Years: Adverse Sequelae With Subclinical Infection at Birth for Children Treated 1 Month or Less[a] (*Continued*)

	Group I[b] (*N* = 13)	Group II[b] (*N* = 10)[c]
Hydrocephalus	0	1[g]
Microcephaly	1[i]	1
Seizures	1	3[j]
Severe psychomotor impairment	1	2[k]
Minor sequelae		
Mild cerebellar dysfunction	2	4
Transiently delayed psychomotor development	2	2

[a]Reproduced with permission from Wilson et al.[14]
[b]Group I included children for whom serologic tests were performed either because *Toxoplasma* infection was diagnosed in the mother during pregnancy or at term or because the children were screened for nonspecific findings in the newborn period. Group II included children in whom no signs of congenital infection were found during the newborn period. Diagnosis was first suspected when they presented with signs suggestive of congenital *Toxoplasma* infection.
[c]One of the 11 children in group II was excluded because an adequate follow-up ophthalmologic examination was not performed.
[d]Age (years) at most recent examination.
[e]Blindness = vision not correctable to > 20/200.
[f]Macular involvement but vision correctable to 20/40.
[g]Microcephaly was diagnosed when the head circumference was below the third percentile; hydrocephalus was diagnosed on the basis of pneumoencephalography.
[h]The same child had a seizure disorder and severe psychomotor retardation and was included in the figures under those categories in group II.
[i]The same child had a seizure disorder and severe psychomotor retardation and was included in the figures under those categories in group I.
[j]One of these children had mild cerebellar dysfunction and was included in the figures under that category in group II.
[k]One of these 2 children first exhibited transiently delayed psychomotor development and was included in the figures under that category in group II.

Table 57-41 Oral Suspension Formulations for Pyrimethamine and Sulfadiazine

Pyrimethamine: 2-mg/mL suspension	1. Crush FOUR 25-mg pyrimethamine tablets in a mortar to a fine powder.
	2. Add 10 mL syrup vehicle.
	3. Transfer mixture to an amber bottle.
	4. Rinse mortar with 10 mL sterile water and transfer.
	5. Add enough of the syrup vehicle to bring to a 50-mL final volume.
	6. Shake well until this is a fine suspension.
	7. Label and give a 7-day expiration.
	8. Store refrigerated.
Sulfadiazine: 100-mg/mL suspension	1. Crush TEN 500 mg sulfadiazine tablets in a mortar to a fine powder.
	2. Add enough sterile water to make a smooth paste.
	3. Slowly triturate the syrup vehicle close to the final volume of 50 mL.
	4. Transfer the suspension to a larger amber bottle.
	5. Add sufficient syrup vehicle to bring to a 50-mL final volume.
	6. Shake well.
	7. Label and give a 7-day expiration.
	8. Store refrigerated.
Materials	
1. Pyrimethamine 25-mg tablets (Daraprim, Burroughs-Wellcome), NDC 0081-0201-55. 2. Sulfadiazine 500-mg tablets (Eon Labs). 3. Syrup vehicle: Suggest 2% sugar suspension for pyrimethamine. If the infant is not lactose intolerant, 2% sugar suspension can be 2 g lactose per 100 mL distilled H_2O. Suggest using simple syrup or alternatively with flavored cherry syrup for sulfadiazine suspension.	

Table 57-42 Outcomes of Parisian Children Born to Mothers Who Acquired Their Infection in the First or Early Second Trimesters and Who Were Treated In Utero[a]

Child Number	GW Seroconversion	Current Age (Years)	Boy (1)/ Girl (2)	Prenatal Spiramycin	GW Spiramycin Started	Amniocentesis	GW Amniocentesis	PCR Result	Pyr + Sulfa Prenatally	GW Pyr + Sulfa Started	GW at Birth	Calcifications	Chorioretinitis	Last Ophthalmic Examination (Months)
1	2	9	1	1[b]	8	0	ND	ND	0	b	39	0	0	27
2	11	5	1	1	14	1	17	0[c]	0	2.5 pb	37	0	0	36
3	13	6	2	1	16	1	19	1	1	19.5	38.5	0	0	25
4	13	9	2	1	15	1	19	0	0	20 pb	36.4	0	0	33
5	13	8	1	1	16	1	20	1	1	20.5	41	0	0	37
6	14	9	1	1	17	1	18	0	0	A.[c]	38	1[d]	0	22
7	15	5	2	1	19	1	21	1	1	21.5	40	1[e]	0	19
8	16	10	1	1	18	1	23	0	0	b	40	0	0	28
11	17	2	2	1	20	1	24	1	1	24	40	1	0	19
9	18	9	1	1	20	1	25	1	1	25.5	38.1	1[f]	1[g]	25
10	18	5	1	1	20.5	1	27	1	1	28	41.1	1[h]	0	55

Abbreviations: b, birth; GW, gestational week; Ig, immunoglobulin; MRI, magnetic resonance imaging; ND, not done; pb, weeks postbirth; PCR, polymerase chain reaction.

Note that none of the children had hydrocephalus in utero.

[a]Data from Kieffer et al 2008.[172]

[b]Spiramycin prenatally for only 1 month.

[c]For the children with negative amniocentesis, 3 had specific IgM at birth. The remaining two had rising specific IgG titers.

[d]Two very small (1- to 2-mm) calcifications on brain ultrasound.

[e]Left parietal macrocalcifications with a porencephalic cavity (brain ultrasound only).

[f]One small right parietal calcification on brain ultrasound.

[g]Two peripheral retinal scars 2 disc diameters, 1 disc diameter; visual acuity normal.

[h]Three large left parietal and 1 left frontal calcifications (antenatal MRI, neonatal ultrasound, and brain computed tomography); severe speech delay. This child experienced the longest time between diagnosis of maternal infection and treatment (10 weeks compared to 6–7 weeks). **Bold** indicates that this child had more severe symptoms.

Table 57-43 Eye Disease and Central Nervous System Findings in Infants With Untreated Congenital Toxoplasmosis in the United States[a]

Age[b]	Number of Infants With Clinical Signs/Number of Infants Evaluated (%)			
	E	C	H	E + C + H
0–30	61/70 (87.1)	52/64 (81.2)	39/53 (73.6)	31/46 (67.4)
31–90	35/36 (97.2)	28/33 (84.8)	21/29 (72.4)	16/24 (66.7)
91–180	23/23 (100)	14/21 (66.7)	7/17 (41.2)	6/16 (37.5)
Total	119/129 (92.2)	94/118 (79.6)	67/99 (67.7)	53/86 (61.6)

Abbreviations: C, calcifications; E, eye disease; H, hydrocephalus.
[a]Reproduced with permission from Olariu et al.[49]
[b]Age in days when first serum was drawn for testing.

Table 57-44 Cost/Benefit Analysis of Prenatal Screening by Country

Country	Year	Conclusions
United States	1990	If there are 407 to 9500 congenitally infected children born each year, then $369 to $8758 million in medical costs arise due to death, severe illness, retardation, vision, and hearing loss.
United Kingdom	1984	Consider impact of false positives.
Scotland	Early 1990s	Positive cost benefit.
Norway	Early 1990s	Positive cost benefit.
Finland	Early 1990s	Positive cost benefit.

Table 57-45 Cost Estimates for Outcomes of Congenital Toxoplasmosis (RTI Estimates Adjusted to 2010 Dollars)[a]

Developmental Disorder	Costs (2010 Dollars) at 3% Discount Rate
Fetal death (any cause)	$6,957,043
Visual, mild	$537,187
Visual, severe	$962,003
Cognitive, mild	$1,109,776
Cognitive, severe	$2,732,816
Hearing, mild	$383,635
Visual + cognitive, mild	$1,646,963
Visual + cognitive, severe	$2,910,003
Visual + cognitive + hearing, mild	$2,030,598
Visual + cognitive + hearing, severe	$3,293,638

Abbreviation: RTI, response to intervention
Based on costs in Honeycutt et al.[173]
[a]Reproduced with permission from Stillwaggon et al,[53] with permission.

Table 57-46 Costs Utilized in Calculations With Cost-Minimizing Equations for Prenatal Screening and Treatment[a]

Category	Test	Cost
Screening	Serological test for immunoglobulin (Ig) G, IgM	$12.00
	Toxoplasmosis serological profile (TSP)	$385.00
	Amniocentesis (polymerase chain reaction, PCR)	$1,300.00
Blood work	Complete blood count	$10.00
Treatment	Spiramycin	$0.00
	Pyrimethamine	$1.56 per day
	Sulfadiazine	$12.48 per day
	Folinic acid	$0.10 per day
	One-year pediatric PSF treatment	$210.00
	Drug compounding	$20.00 per week

[a]Reproduced with permission from Stillwaggon et al.[53]

REFERENCES

1. Jankü J. [Pathogenesis and pathologic anatomy of the "congenital coloboma" of the macula lutea in an eye of normal size, with microscopic detection of parasites in the retina.] *Cesk Parasitol.* 1923;62:1021–1027, 1052–1059, 1081–1085, 1111–1115, 1138–1143.

2. Wolf A, Cowen D. Granulomatous encephalomyelitis due to an encephalitozoon (encephalitozoic encephalomyelitis). A new protozoan disease of man. *Bull Neur Inst NY.* 1937;6:306–371.

3. Dubey JP. Advances in the life cycle of *Toxoplasma gondii. Int J Parasitol.* 1998;28(7):1019–1024.

4. Dubey JP, Beattie CP. *Toxoplasmosis of Animals and Man.* Boca Raton, FL: CRC Press; 1988.

5. Frenkel JK, Dubey JP, Miller NL. *Toxoplasma gondii* in cats: fecal stages identified as coccidian oocysts. *Science.* 1970;167(3919):893–896.

6. Hutchison WM, Dunachie JF, Siim JC, Work K. Coccidian-like nature of *Toxoplasma gondii. Br Med J.* 1970;1:142–144.

7. Delair E, Latkany P, Noble AG, et al. Clinical manifestations of ocular toxoplasmosis. *Ocul Immunol Inflamm.* 2011; 19(2):91–102.

8. Eichenwald HF. A study of congenital toxoplasmosis, with particular emphasis on clinical manifestations, sequelae and therapy. In: Siim J, ed. *Human Toxoplasmosis.* Munksgaard, Copenhagen: 1960:41–49.

9. Couvreur J, Desmonts G. Congenital and maternal toxoplasmosis. A review of 300 congenital cases. *Dev Med Child Neurol.* 1962;4:519–530.

10. Alford Jr C, Stagno S, Reynolds DW. Congenital toxoplasmosis: clinical, laboratory, and therapeutic considerations, with special reference to subclinical disease. *Bull NY Acad Med.* 1974; 50:160–181.

11. Kimball A, Kean BH, Fuchs F. Congenital toxoplasmosis: a prospective study of 4,048 obstetric patients. *Am J Obstet Gynecol.* 1971;111:211–218.

12. Desmonts G, Couvreur J. Toxoplasmosis in pregnancy and its transmission to the fetus. *Bull NY Acad Med: J Urban Health.* 1974;50:146–159.

13. Stagno S, Reynolds DW, Amos CS, et al. Auditory and visual defects resulting from symptomatic and subclinical congenital cytomegaloviral and *Toxoplasma* infections. *Pediatrics.* 1977;669–678.

14. Wilson C, Remington JS, Stagno S, Reynolds DW. Development of adverse sequelae in children born with subclinical congenital *Toxoplasma* infection. *Pediatrics.* 1980;66:767–774.

15. Koppe JG, Kloosterman GJ. Congenital toxoplasmosis: long-term follow-up. *Padiatr Padol.* 1982;17:171–179.

16. Desmonts G. Acquired toxoplasmosis in pregnant women. Evaluation of the frequency of transmission of *Toxoplasma* and of congenital toxoplasmosis. *Lyon Medical.* 1982;248:115–123.

17. Desmonts G, Couvreur J. Congenital toxoplasmosis. Prospective study of the outcome of pregnancy in 542 women with toxoplasmosis acquired during pregnancy. *Ann Pediatr* (Paris). 1984; 31:805–809.

18. Couvreur J, Desmonts G, Aron-Rosa D. Le prognostic oculare de la toxoplasmose congenitale: role du traitement [Ocular prognosis in congenital toxoplasmosis: the role of treatment. Preliminary communication]. *Ann Pediatr* (Paris). 1984;31(10): 855–858.

19. Koppe JG, Loewer-Sieger DH, de Roever-Bonnet H. Results of 20-year follow-up of congenital toxoplasmosis. *Lancet.* 1986;1(8475): 254–256.

20. Couvreur J, Desmonts G, Thulliez P. Prophylaxis of congenital toxoplasmosis. Effects of spiramycin on placental infection. *J Antimicrob Chemother.* 1988;22:193–200.

21. Daffos F, Forestier F, Capella-Pavlovsky M, et al. Prenatal management of 746 pregnancies at risk for congenital toxoplasmosis. *N Engl J Med.* 1988;318:271–275.

22. Hohlfeld P, Daffos F, Thulliez P, et al. Fetal toxoplasmosis: outcome of pregnancy and infant follow-up after in utero treatment. *J Pediatr.* 1989;115(5 Pt 1):765–769.

23. Forestier F, Daffos F, Hohlfeld P, Lynch L. [Infectious fetal diseases. Prevention, prenatal diagnosis, practical measures.] *Presse Med.* 1991;1448–1454.

24. McLeod R, Mack D, Foss R, et al. Levels of pyrimethamine in sera and cerebrospinal and ventricular fluids from infants treated for congenital toxoplasmosis. *Antimicrob Agents Chemother.* 1992;36:1040–1048.

25. Swisher CN, Boyer K, McLeod R, The Toxoplasmosis Study Group. Congenital toxoplasmosis. *Semin Pediatr Neurol.* 1994; 1(1):4–25.

26. Hohlfeld P, Daffos F, Costa J-M, et al. Prenatal diagnosis of congenital toxoplasmosis with a polymerase-chain-reaction test on amniotic fluid. *N Engl J Med.* 1994;695–699.

27. McAuley J, Boyer KM, Patel D, et al. Early and longitudinal evaluations of treated infants and children and untreated historical patients with congenital toxoplasmosis: the Chicago Collaborative Treatment Trial. *Clin Infect Dis.* 1994;18:38–72.

28. Foulon W, Naessens A, Derde MP. Evaluation of the possibilities for preventing congenital toxoplasmosis. *Am J Perinatol.* 1994;11:57–62.

29. Guerina NG, Hsu HW, Meissner HC, et al. Neonatal serologic screening and early treatment for congenital *Toxoplasma gondii* infection. *N Engl J Med.* 1994;330:1858–1863.

30. Mets M, Holfels E, Boyer KM, et al. Eye manifestations of congenital toxoplasmosis. *Am J Ophthalmol.* 1996;122:309–324.

31. Foulon W, Villena I, Stray-Pedersen B, et al. Treatment of toxoplasmosis during pregnancy: amulticenter study of impact on fetal transmission and children's sequelae at age 1 year. *Am J Obstet Gynecol.* 1999;180:410–415.

32. Naessens A, Jenum PA, Pollak A, et al. Diagnosis of congenital toxoplasmosis in the neonatal period: amulticenter evaluation. *J Pediatr.* 1999;135:714–719.

33. Wallon M, Kodjikian L, Binquet C, et al. Long-term ocular prognosis in 327 children with congenital toxoplasmosis. *Pediatrics.* 2004;113:1567–1572.

34. Romand S, Chosson M, Franck J, et al. Usefulness of quantitative polymerase chain reaction in amniotic fluid as early prognostic marker of fetal infection with *Toxoplasma gondii. Am J Obstet Gynecol.* 2004;190:797–802.

35. Boyer KM, Holfels E, Roizen N, et al. Risk factors for *Toxoplasma gondii* infection in mothers of infants with congenital toxoplasmosis: Implications for prenatal management and screening. *Am J Obstet Gynecol.* 2005;192:564–571.

36. Kodjikian L, Wallon M, Fleury M, et al. Ocular manifestations in congenital toxoplasmosis. *Graefes Arch Clin Exp Ophthalmol.* 2006;244:14–21.

37. McLeod R, Boyer K, Karrison T, et al. Outcomes of treatment for congenital toxoplasmosis, 1981–2004: the national collaborative Chicago-based, congenital toxoplasmosis study. *Clin Infect Dis.* 2006;42(10):1383–1394.

38. Berrebi A, Bardou M, Bessieres M, et al. Outcome for children infected with congenital toxoplasmosis in the first trimester and with normal ultrasound findings: a study of 36 cases. *Eur J Obstet Gynaecol Reprod Biol.* 2007;135:53–57.

39. Phan L, Kasza K, Jalbrzikowski J, et al. Longitudinal study of new eye lesions in treated congenital toxoplasmosis. *Ophthalmology.* 2008;115:553–559.

40. Phan L, Kasza K, Jalbrzikowski J, et al. Longitudinal study of new eye lesions in children with toxoplasmosis who were not treated during the first year of life. *Am J Ophthalmol.* 2008;146(3):375–384.

41. McLeod R, Kieffer, F, Sautter M, Hosten T, Pelloux H. Why prevent, diagnose and treat congenital toxoplasmosis? *Mem Inst Oswaldo Cruz.* 2009;104:320–344.

42. Kieffer F, Wallon M, Garcia P, et al. Risk factors for retinochoroiditis during the first 2 years of life in infants with treated congenital toxoplasmosis. *Pediatr Infect Dis J.* 2008;27(1):27–32.

43. Cortina-Borja M, Tan HK, Wallon M, et al. Prenatal treatment for serious neurological sequelae of congenital toxoplasmosis: an observational prospective cohort study. *PLoS Med.* 2010; 7(10):1–11.

44. Vaudaux JD, Muccioli C, James ER, et al. Identification of an atypical strain of *Toxoplasma gondii* as the cause of a waterborne outbreak of toxoplasmosis in Santa Isabel do Ivai, Brazil. *J Infect Dis.* 2010;202:1226–1233.

45. Villena I, Ancelle T, Delmas C, et al. Congenital toxoplasmosis in France in 2007: first results from a national surveillance system. *Eur Surveill.* 2010;15(25): pii: 19600.

46. Wallon M, Franck J, Thulliez P, et al. Accuracy of real-time polymerase chain reaction for *Toxoplasma gondii* in amniotic fluid. *Obstet Gynecol.* 2010;115:727–733.

47. Noble, AG, Latkany, P, Kusmierczyk, et al. Chorioretinal lesions in mothers of children with congenital toxoplasmosis in the National Collaborative Chicago-based, Congenital Toxoplasmosis Study. *Sci Med.* 2010;20(1):20–26.

48. Peyron F, Garweg JG, Wallon M, et al. Long-term impact of treated congenital toxoplasmosis on quality of life and visual performance. *Pediatr Infect Dis J.* 2011;30(7):597–600.

49. Olariu T, Remington S, McLeod R, Alam A, Montoya J. Severe congenital toxoplasmosis in the United States: clinical and serologic findings in untreated infants. *Pediatr Infect Dis J.* 2011;30(12):1056–1061.

50. Hill D, Coss C, Dubey JP, et al. Identification of a sporozoite-specific antigen from *Toxoplasma gondii.* *J Parasitol.* 2011; 97(2):328–337.

51. Remington JS, McLeod R, Thulliez, P, Desmonts G. *Toxoplasmosis.* In: Remington J, Klein J, eds. *Infectious Diseases of the Fetus and Newborn Infant.* 7th ed. Philadelphia, PA: Saunders; 2011;918–1040.

52. Boyer K, Hill D, Mui E, et al. Unrecognized ingestion of *Toxoplasma gondii* oocysts leads to congenital toxoplasmosis and causes epidemics in North America. *Clin Infect Dis.* 2011;53(11):1081.

53. Stillwaggon E, Carrier CS, Sautter M, McLeod R. Maternal serologic screening to prevent congenital toxoplasmosis: a decision-analytic economic model. *PLoS Negl Trop Dis.* 2011;5(9):e1333.

54. Burrowes D, Boyer K, Swisher CN, et al. Spinal cord lesions in congenital toxoplasmosis demonstrated with neuroimaging, including their successful treatment in an adult. *J Neuroparasitol.* 2012;3(2012): pii: 235533.

55. Hutson SL, McLeod R. Hydrocephalus caused by congenital toxoplasmosis responds to ventriculoperitoneal shunting. Unpublished manuscript.

56. McLeod R, Boyer KM, Lee D, et al. Prematurity and severity are associated with *Toxoplasma gondii* alleles (NCCCTS, 1981–2009). *Clin Infect Dis.* 2012;54(11):1595–1605.

57. Hutson S, McLeod R. Patterns of hydrocephalus caused by congenital *Toxoplasma gondii* infection and association with parasite genotype. Unpublished manuscript.

58. Noble G, Latkany P, Boyer K, et al. Retinal detachment in congenital toxoplasmosis. Unpublished manuscript.

59. Menon N, Noble AG, Ksiazek S, et al. Impact on vision and optimization of management of macular scars in patients with congenital toxoplasmosis. Unpublished manuscript.

60. Cinalli G, Sainte-Rose C, Chumas P, et al. Failure of third ventriculostomy in the treatment of aqueductal stenosis in children. *Neurosurg Focus.* 1999:6(4):e3.

61. Noble AG, Ksiazek S, Latkany P, et al. Patterns of retina disease and parasite genetics. Unpublished manuscript.

62. McLeod R, Berry PF, Marshall WH Jr, et al. Toxoplasmosis presenting as brain abscesses. Diagnosis by computerized tomography and cytology of aspirated purulent material. *Am J Med.* 1979;67(4):711–714.

63. Luft BJ, Conley F, Remington JS, et al. Outbreak of central-nervous-system toxoplasmosis in western Europe and North America. *Lancet.* 1983;1(8328):781–784.

64. Levin M, McLeod R, Young Q, et al. Pneumocystis pneumonia: importance of gallium scan for early diagnosis and description of a new immunoperoxidase technique to demonstrate *Pneumocystis carinii. Am Rev Respir Dis.* 1983;128:182–185.

65. Kovacs JA. Toxoplasmosis in AIDS: keeping the lid on. *Ann Intern Med.* 1995;123(3):230–231.

66. McLeod R, Beem MO, Estes RG. Lymphocyte anergy specific to *Toxoplasma gondii* antigens in a baby with congenital toxoplasmosis. *J Clin Lab Immunol.* 1985;17:149–153.

67. McLeod R, Mack DG, Boyer K, et al. Phenotypes and functions of lymphocytes in congenital toxoplasmosis. *J Lab Clin Med.* 1990;116(5):623–635.

68. Benenson MW TE, Lemon SM, Greenup RL, Sulzer AJ. Oocyst-transmitted toxoplasmosis associated with ingestion of contaminated water. *N Engl J Med.* 1982;307:666–669.

69. Isaac-Renton J, Bowie WR, King A, et al. Detection of *Toxoplasma gondii* oocysts in drinking water. *Appl Environ Microbiol.* 1998;64:2278–2280.

70. Jones JL, Kruszon-Moran D, Wilson M, et al. *Toxoplasma gondii* infection in the United States: seroprevalence and risk factors. *Am J Epidemiol.* 2001;154:357–365.

71. Jones JL, Dargelas V, Roberts J, et al. Risk factors for *Toxoplasma gondii* infection in the United States. *Clin Infect Dis.* 2009;49(6): 878–884.

72. dos Santos TR, Nunes CM, Luvizotto MC, et al. Detection of *Toxoplasma gondii* oocysts in environmental samples from public schools. *Vet Parasitol.* 2010;171(1–2):53–57.

73. Shapiro K, Conrad PA, Mazet JA, et al. Effect of estuarine wetland degradation on transport of *Toxoplasma gondii* surrogates from land to sea. *Appl Environ Microbiol.* 2010;76(20):6821–6828.

74. Alvarado-Esquivel C, Estrada-Martinez S, Liesenfeld O. *Toxoplasma gondii* infection in workers occupationally exposed to unwashed raw fruits and vegetables: a case control seroprevalence study. *Parasit Vectors.* 2011;4(1):235.

75. Conrad PA, Miller MA, Kreuder C, et al. Transmission of *Toxoplasma*: clues from the study of sea otters as sentinels of *Toxoplasma gondii* flow into the marine environment. *Int J Parasitol.* 2005; 35(11–12):1155–1168.

76. Frenkel JK, Parker BB. An apparent role of dogs in the transmission of *Toxoplasma gondii.* The probable importance of xenosmophilia. *Ann NY Acad Sci.* 1996;791:402–407.

77. Desmonts G, Couvreur J, Alison F, et al. Etude épidémiologique sur la toxoplasmose: de l'Influence de la cuisson des viandes de boucherie sur la fréquence de l'Infection Humaine. *Rev Franc Etud Clin Biol.* 1965;10:952–958.

78. Masur H, Jones TC, Lempert JA, Cherubini TD. Outbreak of toxoplasmosis in a family and documentation of acquired retinochoroiditis. *Am J Med.* 1978;64(3):396–402.

79. Roux C, Desmont G, Mulliez N, et al. [Toxoplasmosis and pregnancy. Evaluation of 2 years of prevention of congenital toxoplasmosis in the maternity ward of Hôpital Saint-Antoine (1973–1974).] *J Gynecol Obstet Biol Reprod* (Paris). 1976; 5(2):249–264.

80. Gollub EL, Leroy V, Gilbert R, Chêne G, Wallon M; European Toxoprevention Study Group (EUROTOXO). Effectiveness of health education on *Toxoplasma*-related knowledge, behaviour, and risk of seroconversion in pregnancy. *Eur J Obstet Gynecol Reprod Biol.* 2008;136(2):137–145.

81. Papoz L, Simondon F, Saurin W, Sarmini H. A simple model relevant to toxoplasmosis applied to epidemiologic results in France. *Am J Epidemiol.* 1986:154–161.

82. Mack DG, Johnson JJ, Roberts F, et al. HLA-class II genes modify outcome of *Toxoplasma gondii* infection. *Int J Parasitol.* 1999;29(9):1351–1358.

83. Jamieson SE, de Roubaix LA, Cortina-Borja M, et al. Genetic and epigenetic factors at COL2A1 and ABCA4 influence clinical outcome in congenital toxoplasmosis. *PLoS One.* 2008;3(6):e2285.

84. Jamieson SE, Cordell H, Petersen E, et al. Host genetic and epigenetic factors in toxoplasmosis. *Mem Inst Oswaldo Cruz.* 2009;104(2):162–169.

85. Jamieson SE, Peixoto-Rangel AL, Hargrave AC, et al. Evidence for associations between the purinergic receptor P2X(7) (P2RX7) and toxoplasmosis. *Genes Immun.* 2010;11(5):374–383.

86. Lees MP, Fuller SJ, McLeod R, et al. P2X7 receptor-mediated killing of an intracellular parasite, *Toxoplasma gondii*, by human and murine macrophages. *J Immunol.* 2010;184(12):7040–7046.

87. Witola WH, Mui E, Hargrave A, et al. NALP1 influences susceptibility to human congenital toxoplasmosis, proinflammatory cytokine response, and fate of *Toxoplasma gondii*-infected monocytic cells. *Infect Immun.* 2011;79(2):756–766.

88. Tan TG, Mui E, Cong H, et al. Identification of *T. gondii* epitopes, adjuvants, and host genetic factors that influence protection of mice and humans. *Vaccine.* 2010;28(23):3977–3989.

89. Belo S, Montpetit A, Mui E, Dutra M. Role of IRAK 4 in protection against *T. gondii*. Unpublished manuscript.

90. Witola WH, Liu SR, Montpetit A, Welti R, Hypolite M, Roth M, McLeod R. ALOX12 in Human Toxoplasmosis. *Infection and Immunity.* 2014;82(7):2670–2679. doi:10.1128/IAI.01505-13.

91. Hargrave A, Melo, Miller, et al. Role of TLR9 and TIRAP9 and their *Toxoplasma* ligands in protection. Unpublished manuscript.

92. Dubey JP, Sharma SP, Juranek DD, Sulzer AJ, Teutsch SM. Characterization *of Toxoplasma gondii* isolates from an outbreak of toxoplasmosis in Atlanta, Georgia. *Am J Vet Res.* 1981; 42(6):1007–1010.

93. Dubey JP, Ferreira LR, Martins J, McLeod R. Oral oocyst-induced mouse model of toxoplasmosis: effect of infection with *Toxoplasma gondii* strains of different genotypes, dose, and mouse strains (transgenic, out-bred, in-bred) on pathogenesis and mortality. *Parasitology.* 2012;139(1):1–13.

94. Weiss LM, Dubey JP. Toxoplasmosis: a history of clinical observations. *Int J Parasitol.* 2009;39(8):895–901.

95. Couvreur J, Desmonts G, Girre JY. Congenital toxoplasmosis in twins: a series of 14 pairs of twins: absence of infection in one twin in two pairs. *J Pediatr.* 1976;89(2):235–240.

96. Peyron F, Ateba AB, Wallon M, et al. Congenital toxoplasmosis in twins: a report of fourteen consecutive cases and a comparison with published data. *Pediatr Infect Dis J.* 2003;22:695–701.

97. Hermes G, Ajioka JW, Kelly KA, et al. Neurological and behavioral abnormalities, ventricular dilatation, altered cellular functions, inflammation, and neuronal injury in brains of mice due to common, persistent, parasitic infection. *J Neuroinflammation.* 2008;5:48.

98. Patel DV, Holfels EM, Vogel NP, et al. Resolution of intracranial calcifications in infants with treated congenital toxoplasmosis. *Radiology,* 1996;199(2):433–440.

99. Brezin AP, Thulliez P, Couvreur J, et al. Ophthalmic outcome after prenatal and postnatal treatment of congenital toxoplasmosis. *Am J Ophthalmol.* 2003;138:779–784.

100. Thulliez P. Commentary: efficacy of prenatal treatment for toxoplasmosis: a possibility that cannot be ruled out. *Int J Epidemiol.* 2001;30:1315–1316.

101. Mehta V, Balachandran C, Lonikar V. Blueberry muffin baby: a pictoral differential diagnosis. *Dermatol Online J.* 2008;14(2):8.

102. Grover CM, Thulliez P, Remington JS, Boothroyd JC. Rapid prenatal diagnosis of congenital *Toxoplasma* infection by using polymerase chain reaction and amniotic fluid. *J Clin Microbiol.* 1990;28(10):2297–2301.

103. Reischl U, Bretagne S, Krüger D, Ernault P, Costa JM. Comparison of two DNA targets for the diagnosis of toxoplasmosis by real-time PCR using fluorescence resonance energy transfer hybridization probes. *BMC Infect Dis.* 2003;3:7.

104. Fuentes I, Rodriguez M, Domingo CJ, et al. Urine sample used for congenital toxoplasmosis diagnosis by PCR. *J Clin Microbiol.* 1996;34(10):2368–2371.

105. Wilson CB, Desmonts G, Couvreur J, Remington JS. Lymphocyte transformation in the diagnosis of congenital toxoplasma infection. *N Engl J Med.* 1980;302(14):785–788.

106. Chapey E, Wallon M, Debize G, Rabilloud M, Peyron F. Diagnosis of congenital toxoplasmosis by using a whole-blood gamma interferon release assay. *J Clin Microbiol.* 2010; 48(1):41–45.

107. Raymond J, Poissonnier MH, Thulliez PH, et al. Presence of gamma interferon in human acute and congenital toxoplasmosis. *J Clin Microbiol.* 1990;28(6):1434–1437.

108. Vogel N, Kirisits M, Michael E, et al. Congenital toxoplasmosis transmitted from an immunologically competent mother infected before conception. *Clin Inf Dis.* 1996;23:1055–1060.

109. Sabin AB, Feldman HA. Dyes as microchemical indicators of a new immunity phenomenon affecting a protozoon parasite (*Toxoplasma*). *Science.* 1948;108(2815):660–663.

110. Montoya JG, Remington JS. Management of *Toxoplasma gondii* infection during pregnancy. *Clin Infect Dis.* 2008;47(4):554–566.

111. Montoya JG. Laboratory diagnosis of *Toxoplasma gondii* infection and toxoplasmosis. *J Infect Dis.* 2002;185(Suppl 1):S73–S82.

112. Naot Y, Remington JS. An enzyme-linked immunosorbent assay for detection of IgM antibodies to *Toxoplasma gondii*: use for diagnosis of acute acquired toxoplasmosis. *J Infect Dis.* 1980;142(5):757–766.

113. Liesenfeld O, Montoya JG, Tathineni NJ, et al. Confirmatory serologic testing for acute toxoplasmosis and rate of induced abortions among women reported to have positive *Toxoplasma* immunoglobulin M antibody titers. *Am J Obstet Gynecol.* 2001;184(2):140–145.

114. Stepick-Biek P, Thulliez P, Araujo FG, Remington JS. IgA antibodies for diagnosis of acute congenital and acquired toxoplasmosis. *J Infect Dis.* 1990;162(1):270–273.

115. Wong SY, Hajdu MP, Ramirez R, et al. Role of specific immunoglobulin E in diagnosis of acute *Toxoplasma* infection and toxoplasmosis. *J Clin Microbiol.* 1993;31(11):2952–2959.

116. Suzuki Y, Thulliez P, Desmonts G, Remington JS. Antigen(s) responsible for immunoglobulin G responses specific for the acute stage of *Toxoplasma* infection in humans. *J Clin Microbiol.* 1988;26(5):901–905.

117. Hedman K, Lappalainen M, Seppäiä I, Mäkelä O. Recent primary *Toxoplasma* infection indicated by a low avidity of specific IgG. *J Infect Dis.* 1989;159(4):736–740.

118. Liesenfeld O, Montoya JG, Kinney S, Press C, Remington JS. Effect of testing for IgG avidity in the diagnosis of *Toxoplasma gondii* infection in pregnant women: experience in a US reference laboratory. *J Infect Dis.* 2001;183(8):1248–1253.

119. Jenum PA, Stray-Pedersen B, Gundersen AG. Improved diagnosis of primary *Toxoplasma gondii* infection in early pregnancy by determination of antitoxoplasma immunoglobulin G avidity. *J Clin Microbiol.* 1997;35(8):1972–1977.

120. Lappalainen M, Koskela P, Koskiniemi M, et al. Toxoplasmosis acquired during pregnancy: improved serodiagnosis based on avidity of IgG. *J Infect Dis.* 1993;167(3):691–697.

121. Flori P, Tardy L, Patural H, et al. Reliability of immunoglobulin G anti-*Toxoplasma* avidity test and effects of treatment on avidity indexes of infants and pregnant women. *Clin Diagn Lab Immunol.* 2004;11(4):669–674.

122. Sensini A, Pascoli S, Marchetti D, et al. IgG avidity in the serodiagnosis of acute *Toxoplasma gondii* infection: a multicenter study. *Clin Microbiol Infect.* 1996;2(1):25–29.

123. Petersen E, Borobio MV, Guy E, et al. European multicenter study of the LIAISON automated diagnostic system for determination of *Toxoplasma gondii*-specific immunoglobulin G (IgG) and IgM and the IgG avidity index. *J Clin Microbiol.* 2005;43(4):1570–1574.

124. Lefevre-Pettazzoni M, Bissery A, Wallon M, et al. Impact of spiramycin treatment and gestational age on maturation of *Toxoplasma gondii* immunoglobulin G avidity in pregnant women. *Clin Vaccine Immunol.* 2007;14(3):239–243.

125. Meroni V, Genco F, Tinelli C, et al. Spiramycin treatment of *Toxoplasma gondii* infection in pregnant women impairs the production and the avidity maturation of *T. gondii*-specific immunoglobulin G antibodies. *Clin Vaccine Immunol.* 2009; 16(10):1517–1520.

126. Couvreuer J, Desmonts G. [Late evolutive outbreaks of congenital toxoplasmosis.] *Cah Coll Med Hop Paris.* 1964; 115:752–758. French.

127. Remington JS, Desmonts G. Congenital Toxoplasmosis. In: Remington JS, Klein JO, eds. *Infectious Diseases of the Fetus and Newborn Infant.* Philadelphia, PA: Saunders; 1976:297–299.

128. Wallon M, Kodjikian L, Binquet C, et al. Long-term ocular prognosis in 327 children with congenital toxoplasmosis. *Pediatrics.* 2004;113(6):1567–1572.

129. Benevento JD, Jager RD, Noble AG, et al. Toxoplasmosis-associated neovascular lesions treated successfully with ranibizumab and antiparasitic therapy. *Arch Ophthalmol.* 2008; 126:1152–1156.

130. Capone A Jr. Treatment of neovascularization in infants with retinopathy of prematurity with anti-VEGF: vitreous surgery for retinopathy of prematurity. Paper presented at annual meeting of the American Academy of Ophthalmology, November 13, 2006, Las Vegas, NV.

131. Vasconcelos-Santos DV, Machado Azevedo DO, Campos WR, Oréfice F, Queiroz-Andrade GM, et al. Congenital toxoplasmosis in southeastern Brazil: results of early ophthalmologic examination of a large cohort of neonates. *Ophthalmology.* 2009;116: 2199–2205.

132. Long SS, Pickering LK, Prober CG, ed. *Principles and Practice of Pediatric Infectious Diseases.* 3rd ed. Philadelphia, PA: Elsevier; 2008.

133. McLeod R, Mack D, Brown C. *Toxoplasma gondii*—new advances in cellular and molecular biology. *Exp Parasitol.* 1991; 72:109–121.

134. Dubey JP. *Toxoplasma gondii.* In: Baron S, ed. *Medical Microbiology.* 4th ed. Galveston, TX: University of Texas Medical Branch at Galveston; 1996: chap 84.

135. Aikawa M, Komata Y, Asai T, Midorikawa O. Transmission and scanning electron microscopy of host cell entry by *Toxoplasma gondii*. *Am J Pathol.* 1977;87:285–296.

136. Weiss LW, LaPlace D, Takvorian P, et al. A cell culture system for study of development of *Toxoplasma gondii* bradyzoites. *J Eukaryot Microbiol.* 1995;42(2):150–157.

137. Remington JS. In discussion, Lainson R. Observations on the nature and transmission of *Toxoplasma gondii* in light of its wide host and geographical range. Toxoplasmosis. *Surv Ophthmal.* 1961;6:721–758.

138. Gardiner CH, Fayer R, Dubey JP. *An Atlas of Protozoan Parasites in Animal Tissues.* Agricultural Handbook No. 651. Washington, DC: US Department of Agriculture; 1988.

139. Dubey JP Miller NL, Frenkel JK. The *Toxoplasma gondii* oocyst from cat feces. *J Exp Med.* 1970;132:636–662.

140. Remington JS, McLeod R. Toxoplasmosis. In: Braude Al, ed. *International Textbook of Medicine, Medical Microbiology and Infectious Disease.* Vol. 2. Philadelphia, PA: Saunders; 1981;1818.

141. Centers for Disease Control and Prevention, National Center for Infectious Diseases. Food-related illness and death in the United States. *Emerg Infect Dis.* 1999;5(5).

142. Remington JS, McLeod R. Toxoplasmosis. In: Braude IA, Davis CE, Fierer J, eds. *Infectious Diseases and Medical Microbiology.* 2nd ed. Philadelphia, PA: Saunders; 1986;1521–1535

143. Pacific Northwest National Laboratory and Oak Ridge National Library. *Guide to Determining Climate Regions by County.* Building America Best Practices Series (7.1). Washington, DC: US Department of Energy; 2010.

144. Dubey JP, Su C. Population biology of *Toxoplasma gondii*: what's out and where did they come from. *Mem Inst Oswaldo Cruz.* 2009;104:190–195.

145. Roberts F, Mets MB, Ferguson DJ, et al. Histopathological features of ocular toxoplasmosis in the fetus and infant. *Arch Ophthalmol.* 2001;119:51–58.

146. McLeod R, Johnson J, Estes R, Mack D. Immunogenetics in pathogenesis of and protection against toxoplasmosis. *Curr Top Microbiol Immunol.* 1996;219:95–112.

147. Wilson C, Lewis D. Basis and implications of selectively diminished cytokine production in neonatal susceptibility to infection. *Clin Infect Dis.* 1990;12(suppl 4):S410–S420.

148. McLeod R et al. In: Weiss LM, Kim K, eds. Adaptive immunity and genetics of the host immune response. Toxoplasma gondii *The Model Apicomplexan: Perspectives and Methods.* London, UK: Elsevier; 2007:609–697.

149. Carlier Y, Truyens C, Deloron P, Peyron F. Congenital parasitic infections: a review. *Acta Trop.* 2012;121:55–70.

150. Benirschke K, Kaufmann P, Baergen R. *Pathology of the Human Placenta.* 5th ed. New York, NY: Springer Science + Business Media; 2006.

151. National Heart, Lung, and Blood Institute. What is immune thrombocytopenia? March 14, 2012. http://www.nhlbi.nih.gov/health/health-topics/topics/itp/.

152. Teutsch SM, Juranek DD, Sulzer A, Dubey JP, Sikes RK. Epidemic toxoplasmosis associated with infected cats. *N Engl J Med.* 1979;300:695–699.

153. McGee T, Wolters C, Stein L, et al. Absence of sensorineural hearing loss in treated infants and children with congenital toxoplasmosis. *Otolaryngol Head Neck Surg.* 1992;106:75.

154. Mets MB, Holfels E, Boyer KM, et al. Eye manifestations of congenital toxoplasmosis. *Am J Ophthalmol.* 1997; 123(1):1–16.

155. Dannemann BR, Vaughan WC, Thulliez P, et al. Differential agglutination test for diagnosis of recently acquired infection with *Toxoplasma gondii*. *J Clin Microbiol.* 1990;28:1928–1933.

156. Montoya JG, Remington JS. Studies on the serodiagnosis of toxoplasmic lymphadenitis. *Clin Infect Dis.* 1995;20:781–789.

157. Remington JS, Thulliez P, Montoya JG. Recent developments for diagnosis of toxoplasmosis. *J Clin Microbiol.* 2004;42:941–945.

158. Desmonts G, Couvreur J. Toxoplasmosis: epidemiologic and serologic aspects of perinatal infection. In: Krugman S, Gersbon AA, eds. *Infections of the Fetus and the Newborn Infant. Progress in Clinical and Biological Research.* Vol 3. New York, NY: Liss; 1975;115–132.

159. Harper JS, 3rd, London WT, Sever JL. Five drug regimens for treatment of acute toxoplasmosis in squirrel monkeys *Am J Trop Med Hyg.* 1985;34:50–57.

160. Grossman PL, Remington JS. The effect of trimethoprim and sulfamethoxazole on *Toxoplasma gondii* in vitro and in vivo. *Am J Trop Med Hyg.* 1979;28:445–455. Grossman and Remington 1979.

161. Zuther E, Johnson JJ, Haselkorn R, McLeod R, Gornicki P. Growth of *Toxoplasma gondii* is inhibited by aryloxyphenoxypropionate herbicides targeting acetyl-CoA carboxylase. *Proc Natl Acad Sci U S A.* 1999;96:13387–13392.

162. McLeod R, Khan AR, Noble GA, et al; Toxoplasmosis Study Group. Severe sulfadiazine hypersensitivity in a child with reactivated congenital toxoplasmic chorioretinitis. *Pediatr Infect Dis J.* 2006;25(3):270–272.

163. Systematic Review on Congenital Toxoplasmosis (SYROCOT) Study Group, Thiébaut R, Leproust S, Chêne G, Gilbert R. Effectiveness of prenatal treatment for congenital toxoplasmosis: a meta-analysis of individual patients' data. *Lancet.* 2007;369(9556):115–122.

164. Bonadio WA, Stanco L, Bruce R, Barry D, Smith D. Reference values of normal cerebrospinal fluid composition in infants ages 0 to 8 weeks. *Pediatr Infect Dis J.* 1992;11:589–591.

165. Desmonts G, Couvreur J. Congenital toxoplasmosis: a prospective study of the offspring of 542 women who acquired toxoplasmosis during pregnancy: pathophysiology of congenital disease. In: Thalhammer O, Baumgarten K, Pollak A, eds. *Perinatal Medicine.* Sixth European Congress, Vienna. Stuttgart, Germany: Thieme; 1979;51–60.

166. Couvreur J, Thulliez P, Daffos F, et al. In utero treatment of toxoplasmic fetopathy with the combination pyrimethamine-sulfadiazine. *Fetal Diagn Ther.* 1993;8(1):45–50.

167. Remington JS, McLeod R, Thulliez P, Desmonts G. Toxoplasmosis. In: Remington JS, Klein JO, Wilson CB, Baker CJ, eds. *Infectious Diseases of the Fetus and Newborn Infant.* 6th ed. Philadelphia, PA: Elsevier Saunders; 2006;947–1091

168. Roizen N, Swisher CN, Stein MA, et al. Neurologic and developmental outcome in treated congenital toxoplasmosis. *Pediatrics.* 1995;95(1):11–20.

169. Ajzenberg D, Cogné N, Paris L, et al. Genotype of 86 *Toxoplasma gondii* isolates associated with human congenital toxoplasmosis, and correlation with clinical findings. *J Infect Dis.* 2002;186(5):684–689.

170. Peyron F, Lobry JR, Musset K, et al. Serotyping of *Toxoplasma gondii* in chronically infected pregnant women: predominance of type II in Europe and types I and III in Colombia (South America). *Microbes Infect.* 2006;8(9–10):2333–2340.

171. Ferreira Ade M, Vitor RW, Gazzinelli RT, Melo MN. Genetic analysis of natural recombinant Brazilian *Toxoplasma gondii* strains by multilocus PCR-RFLP. *Infect Genet Evol.* 2006; 6(1):22–31.

172. Kieffer F, Wallon M, Garcia P, Thulliez P, Peyron F, Franck J. Risk factors for retinochoroiditis during the first 2 years of life in infants with treated congenital toxoplasmosis. *Pediatr Infect Dis J.* 2008;27:27–32

173. Honeycutt A, Dunlap L, Chen H, al Homsi G. *The Cost of Developmental Disabilities: Task Order No. 0621-09.* Research Triangle Institute and US Bureau of Labor Statistics. 2000. http://data.bls.gov/cgi-bin/cpicalc.pI.

CHAPTER 57

HIV Infection

Avinash K. Shetty and Yvonne A. Maldonado

INTRODUCTION

Perinatal transmission is the most common route of human immunodeficiency virus type 1 (HIV-1) infection among infants and children.[1] Since the first reports of pediatric acquired immune deficiency syndrome (AIDS) cases more than 3 decades ago,[2] extraordinary advances have occurred in the prevention and treatment of pediatric HIV infection.[3–9] The epidemiology of the perinatal HIV epidemic has dramatically changed in the United States and other resource-rich countries because of effective implementation of strategies to prevent vertical transmission.[7–9] Improved survival of HIV-infected children into adolescence and adulthood because of the availability of highly active antiretroviral therapy (HAART) has significantly improved the health and longevity of HIV-infected children.[3–6]

Preventing perinatal HIV transmission became a reality in 1994 when the Pediatric AIDS Clinical Trials Group (PACTG) 076 published data showing that a long complex course of zidovudine (ZDV) prophylaxis given to an HIV-1-infected mother during early gestation and labor and then postnatally to the baby reduced perinatal HIV-1 transmission by almost two-thirds.[10] In 1995, the US Public Health Service (USPHS) issued guidelines recommending universal counseling and testing for pregnant women and use of ZDV to reduce perinatal transmission.[11] Since then, rates of perinatal HIV transmission in the United States and Europe have decreased to less than 1%–2% because of widespread implementation of universal antenatal HIV testing, combination antiretroviral

treatment (ART) during pregnancy, elective cesarean section, and avoidance of breast-feeding through the use of formula milk.[1,12–14] Currently, new pediatric HIV infections are rare in the United States and occur primarily because of missed prevention opportunities.[15] In recent years, remarkable progress has occurred in the prevention of mother-to-child HIV transmission (PMTCT) during breast-feeding.[16–18] However, translation of research into policy and practice remains a major challenge in many low- and middle-income countries (LMIC).[16–20]

This chapter reviews the epidemiology of perinatal HIV infection; discusses the pathophysiology of transmission; reviews the diagnosis, differential diagnosis, and clinical manifestations; describes the treatment and outcomes; and briefly summarizes the current perinatal HIV preventive strategies focusing primarily in the United States. Review of the global advances in PMTCT is outside the scope of this chapter, and they are not discussed; excellent reviews have been published on this topic.[1,8,16–18]

EPIDEMIOLOGY

Global Scope of the Problem

The World Health Organization (WHO) progress report in 2011 estimated that 34 million (31.6–35.2 million) adults worldwide were living with HIV/AIDS.[20] Approximately 2.7 million (2.4–2.9 million) adults had become newly infected with HIV in 2010 and 1.8 million (1.6–1.9 million) HIV-infected individuals died. In sub-Saharan Africa, approximately 22.9 million inhabitants were living with HIV.[20] In South and Southeast Asia, roughly 4 million people are living with HIV, followed by the Americas, including the Caribbean, where approximately 3 million HIV-infected individuals reside.[20]

The global pediatric HIV epidemic is driven by high levels of endemic HIV infection in women living in sub-Saharan Africa. Worldwide, 49% (46%–51%) of HIV-positive adults are women of childbearing age. In sub-Saharan Africa, 6 in 10 adults living with HIV in 2011 were women.[21] Seroprevalence rates among pregnant women have exceeded 35% in some antenatal clinics in several countries in sub-Saharan Africa, including South Africa, Swaziland, Lesotho, and Botswana.[20] Roughly 80% of HIV-infected women reside in sub-Saharan Africa.[20] HIV/AIDS is a major cause of morbidity and mortality among women of childbearing age in sub-Saharan Africa.

In 2011, approximately 3.4 million (3.1–3.9 million) children younger than 15 years were living with HIV; around 330,000 (280,000–380,000) infants became newly infected with HIV in 2011 alone, and an estimated 230,000 (200,000–270,000) children died from AIDS-related illness in the same year.[21] On a daily basis, roughly 1068 babies become infected with HIV, primarily through mother-to-child HIV transmission (MTCT) during pregnancy, labor, and delivery or postnatally during breastfeeding.[16,17] Roughly 90% of HIV-infected children live in sub-Saharan Africa.[20]

HIV/AIDS in Women

Since the beginning of the HIV epidemic in the United States, men accounted for the majority of new HIV infection and AIDS diagnoses. However, the incidence of HIV infection among women increased gradually until the late 1980s, but then declined in the early 1990s and has remained relatively stable over the past decade.[22,23] Of reported AIDS cases in adults, women accounted for 8% in 1985, 13% in 1993, 20% in 1995, 23% in 1999, 27% in 2000, and 25% in 2010.[22] Currently, approximately 1.2 million individuals in the United States are living with HIV/AIDS, including nearly 280,000 women (Table 58-1).[24,25] One in 5 (20%) of HIV-positive individuals are unaware of their infection. In 2009, there were 11,200 new HIV infections, and in 2010, there were 8422 new AIDS diagnoses among women.[22,23,26] In 2009, among women with AIDS, 4,693 deaths occurred.[22] HIV infection was among the top 10 leading causes of death for black/African American females aged 10–54 and Hispanic/Latino females aged 15–54.

Women of color, especially black/African American and Hispanic/Latino women are disproportionately affected by the HIV/AIDS epidemic. In 2010, of the total number of new HIV diagnoses, 64% occurred in black/African American females (representing 12% of the

Table 58-1 US Epidemiology of Adult and Pediatric HIV Infection[a]

Total number of people estimated to be living with HIV infection	1.2 million
New HIV infections annually	>55,000
Women living with HIV	280,000
New AIDS diagnosis among women (2010)	8422
Deaths among women with AIDS (2009)	4693
Rate of new diagnosis among black women	33.7 per 100,000
MTCT rate among African American women (2004–2007)	12.3 per 100,000
MTCT rate among Caucasian women (2004–2007)	0.5 per 100,000
Estimated HIV/AIDS diagnosis in children < 13 years through 2009	9448
Estimated perinatally transmitted AIDS cases diagnosed through 2009	8640
Number of infants infected with HIV via MTCT in 2009	131

Abbreviation: MTCT, mother-to-child transmission.
[a]Data from references 6 and 22–26.

US female population), followed by 16% in Hispanic/Latino females (representing ~ 14% of the female population). In contrast, white females (representing 68% of the female adult and adolescent population) accounted for only 18% of new HIV diagnoses among females. More than 75% of women with AIDS are in the reproductive age group at the time of diagnosis.

At the end of 2009, areas with the highest estimated rates (per 100,000 population) of adult and adolescent females living with a diagnosis of HIV infection were the US Virgin Islands (497.2), New York State (464.9), Florida (353.3), Puerto Rico (337.6), and New Jersey (330.8). Regional HIV seroprevalence rates vary, with the highest rates found among women residing in the northeastern and southern states. In 2009, the top 10 states with the highest number of women/girls living with AIDS were New York ($n = 23,859$) followed by Florida ($n = 15,081$), California ($n = 7817$), Texas ($n = 6795$), New Jersey ($n = 6312$), Maryland ($n = 6080$), Pennsylvania ($n = 4961$), Georgia ($n = 4679$), Illinois ($n = 3638$), and Puerto Rico ($n = 3326$).[25,26] During 2010, the highest rates of new AIDS diagnoses (per 100,000 population) among adult and adolescent females were in the District of Columbia (79.9), Maryland (18.5), and Louisiana (15.5), followed by

Florida (14.7), the US Virgin Islands (14.3), New York (14.1), New Jersey (11.6), Delaware (10.9), and Mississippi (10.3).[25,26]

For women living with HIV, the most common mode of transmission is high-risk heterosexual exposure and injection drug use. Among black and Latino women, heterosexual transmission accounts for 85% and 82% of new HIV/AIDS diagnoses, respectively, compared to white women (72%).[24] Injection drug use accounts for a greater proportion (28%) of new infections among white women.[24] Although dramatic decline (<2%) in the rate of perinatal HIV transmission has been documented in the United States and the relatively stable incidence of HIV among women, perinatal HIV infection will continue to occur each year, primarily among young black women warranting close surveillance.[1,22] A number of social factors, such as poverty, tight social networks, and assortative mixing as well as lack of prenatal care, antenatal HIV testing, and early access to combination ART contribute to the high rates of HIV infection among black women in the United States.[27]

HIV/AIDS in Children and Adolescents

Since the mid-1990s, the annual number of diagnoses of perinatally acquired HIV/AIDS cases has declined by more than 96% in the United States as a result of routine antenatal HIV testing in conjunction with implementation of effective interventions to prevent transmission.[28,29] In 1991, the annual number of infants with perinatal-acquired HIV peaked at 1650 infants but significantly declined to an estimated 215–370 cases in 2005, to 182 cases in 2008, and to 131 cases in 2009 (Table 58-1).[6,29-31] Cases of AIDS in children have accounted for less than 1% of all reported AIDS cases in the United States.[6]

The racial and ethnic and geographic distribution of AIDS cases in children parallels that of women with AIDS. Racial/ethnic disparities in perinatal HIV/AIDS incidence have persisted since the early part of the epidemic; 78% of children with AIDS were black or Hispanic[30] in 1981–1986. From 2004 through 2007, the Centers for Disease Control and Prevention (CDC) estimated that the overall annual rate of diagnosis of perinatal HIV infection in the 34 states was 2.7 per 100,000 infants aged less than 1 year.[31] Perinatally acquired HIV infection has occurred more frequently (85%) among black or Hispanic children during the same time period.[31] Compared to white children, rates were 23 times higher among black and 4 times higher among Hispanic children. However, there was a noted decrease in the racial/ethnic disparity during 2004–2007, as the annual rate of diagnosis of perinatal HIV infection decreased from 14.8 to 10.2 per 100,000 population for black infants.[31] Likewise, the

rate of diagnosis of perinatal infection decreased from 2.9 to 1.7 per 100,000 population for Hispanic infants during the same time period.[31]

The rate of acquisition of HIV/AIDS among adolescents and young adults continues to increase in the United States, occurring primarily among populations of minority race or ethnicity. Young black men who have sex with men (MSM) are at highest risk; during 2006–2009, new HIV cases increased by 48% in young US MSM.[23] Infection among adolescent women is acquired primarily through heterosexual contact.[23] In 2007, of adolescents and youth aged 13–19 years of age diagnosed with HIV, 31% were females, compared with 23% of individuals aged 20–24 years and 26% of adults aged 25 years or older.[6] In 2007, cases of AIDS in adolescents and young adults aged 13–24 years accounted for 4% of people living with HIV infection in the United States.[6]

Other modes of transmission of HIV, such as exposure to contaminated blood products, have been virtually eliminated because of effective screening methods since 1985 in the United States.[6] Probable HIV transmission from HIV-infected caregivers to their infants via feeding blood-tinged premasticated food has been reported, but no transmission of HIV infection to household contacts through casual contact has been documented.[6]

PATHOPHYSIOLOGY

Virus Biology

Regarding virus biology, HIV-1 is an enveloped cytopathic virus belonging to the Lentiviridae family of retroviruses and has a complex genomic structure, closely related to the simian immunodeficiency viruses (agents in African green monkeys and sooty mangabeys).[32,33] HIV-1 variants are classified into 3 distinct genetic groups: group M (main), group O (outlier), and group N (non-M/non-O). Group M accounts for the majority of HIV-1 infections globally and is further divided into 10 subtypes or clades (A to K). Individuals who acquire HIV-1 infection in the United States, Western Europe, and Australia are most frequently infected with subtype B.[32] Other HIV-1 subtypes circulate globally. Subtypes C and D predominate in southern and eastern Africa, subtype C on the Indian subcontinent, and subtype E is common in Southeast Asia.

Like all retroviruses, HIV-1 contains 3 principal genes: (1) *gag*, which encodes the core nucleocapsid polypeptides (gp24, p17, p9); (2) *env*, which encodes the surface-coat proteins of the virus (gp120 and gp41); and (3) *pol*, which codes for the viral reverse transcriptase and other enzymatic activities (ie, integrase and protease).

There are 2 regulatory (*tat* and *rev*) and 4 accessory genes (*vif, vpr, vpu,* and *nef*) that are essential for viral assembly and release. The retroviral core also contains 2 copies of the viral single-stranded RNA that requires the activity of a viral enzyme, reverse transcriptase, to convert the viral RNA to DNA.[34] A double-stranded DNA copy of the viral genome then incorporates into the host cell genome, where it persists as provirus.

The life cycle of HIV-1 is characterized by several distinct stages.[33,34] The first step in the entry process of HIV into a cell is the binding of the virion envelope glycoproteins (gp120 and gp41) to CD4 on resting or activated T cells. This results in conformation change in the envelope, interaction with a coreceptor, and fusion of the viral and cell membranes, allowing the viral genome to gain entry into the cell. Members of the chemokine receptor family are coreceptors for HIV. Human cord blood mononuclear cells are preferentially infected by macrophage-tropic (M-tropic) strains of HIV-1 using the CC chemokine receptor CCR5. T cell–tropic strains replicate in CD4$^+$ T cells and macrophages and use the chemokine receptor CXCR4, a member of the CXC chemokine family.[33,34]

Rates, Timing, and Mechanisms of Transmission

Mother-to-child transmission of HIV can occur during pregnancy, during labor and delivery, or postnatally through breast-feeding.[1,16,17,35] In the absence of antiretroviral (ARV) and obstetric interventions, the perinatal HIV transmission rate is estimated to be 15% to 25% in a resource-rich setting (eg, United States, Europe).[35] In contrast, without intervention, MTCT rates of 25%–45% has been observed among breast-feeding populations in Africa.[35] Knowledge about the precise timing of transmission is crucial for developing innovative preventive interventions.[36] Data based on cord blood or newborn HIV polymerase chain reaction (PCR) testing indicate that most (50% to 60%) of the perinatal HIV transmission occurs around the time of labor and delivery.[37] An infant is considered to have been infected in utero if the HIV-1 genome can be detected by PCR or be cultured from blood within 48 hours of birth. In contrast, a child is considered to have intrapartum infection if diagnostic assays such as culture, PCR, and serum p24 antigen were negative in blood samples obtained during the first week of life but became positive during the period from day 7 to day 90 and the infant had not been breast-fed.[38] In the breast-fed infant, 20%–25% of HIV transmission occurs during pregnancy, 35%–50% during labor and delivery, and another 25% to 35% of transmission during lactation.[35]

Intrauterine Infection

Early reports using PCR and in situ hybridization technology indicated the possibility of in utero transmission because the HIV was detected in aborted fetal tissues and amniotic fluid obtained during the first and second trimesters of pregnancy.[39] However, subsequent studies in animals and human fetuses reported almost no transmission during the first and second trimesters of pregnancy.[40,41] Based on viral detection during the first 48 hours of birth, intrauterine transmission occurs in about 20%–25% of infections.[35] Statistical modeling data also suggest that most in utero HIV transmission occurs during the last few weeks before delivery when the vascular integrity of the placenta is disrupted.[1,42]

Intrapartum Infection

Intrapartum transmission may occur in a variety of ways, including direct exposure of the infant with infected maternal blood and cervicovaginal secretions during birth, ascending infection after rupture of membranes, or maternal-fetal microtransfusions during uterine contractions.[43,44] Intrapartum transmission is supported by studies failing to detect HIV in infants born to HIV-infected women in the first month of life but subsequent detection of virus after 1 to 3 months of life.[45] Additional evidence to support exposure to maternal virus during delivery as a likely route of transmission include findings of increased HIV infection rates in first-born twins, increased risk associated with prolonged rupture of membranes, and the protective effect of elective cesarean delivery before onset of labor.[46–49] Some reports have documented an increased risk of MTCT associated with placental malaria infection, but not others.[50,51]

Postnatal Infection

In LMIC, where breast-feeding is the cultural norm and safe replacement feeding is not affordable, feasible, sustainable, or safe, postnatal transmission of HIV during breast-feeding remains a significant concern.[16–18,52,53] The exact mechanisms of breast milk HIV transmission are poorly understood. HIV genomes have been isolated from cellular and cell-free fractions of human milk from HIV-infected women and have been detected by culture or PCR in varying frequencies (39%–89%) in many studies.[54,55] Cell-associated virus may be a stronger predictor for transmission of HIV to the infant than cell-free virus.[54] Transmission of HIV through breast-feeding accounts for up to one-third to one-half of all new pediatric HIV infections. An estimated transmission risk of 10%–15% of all HIV-exposed infants exists; infants are infected through prolonged breast-feeding.[35,53] A large individual patient data meta-analysis from sub-Saharan Africa suggested that the risk of postnatal HIV transmission (after 4 weeks of life) is substantial and relatively constant (~0.7% per month of breast-feeding).[56]

Premastication

Anecdotal case reports from the United States have described probable HIV transmission by caregivers who premasticated food for infants.[6] Transmission in the reported cases was likely caused by blood-borne virus in the saliva (and not salivary virus) because bleeding gums or sores were described in 2 of the caregivers. Because safe alternative feeding methods are available in the United States, the CDC recommends physicians to counsel HIV-infected caregivers not to premasticate food for infants.[6]

Risk Factors

Many risk factors for perinatal HIV transmission have been identified, including maternal, obstetric, infant, genetic, and viral-related characteristics (Table 58-2).[36,57,58] The most critical factor associated with increased risk of intrauterine and intrapartum transmission is the maternal plasma HIV viral load.[13,57,58] However, perinatal transmission can occur across the entire range of maternal viral load among pregnant women (including those with low or undetectable serum levels of HIV around the time of labor and delivery).[59] Other maternal risk factors for perinatal HIV transmission include advanced clinical disease, acute HIV infection during pregnancy, and low CD4 T-lymphocyte counts. HIV viral load in cervicovaginal secretions is an independent risk factor for perinatal HIV transmission.[60] Genital ulcer diseases, especially herpes simplex virus (HSV), and syphilis, and other coinfections (such as hepatitis C virus, hepatitis B virus, malaria, tuberculosis) may increase the risk.[8,61–63] Behavioral risk factors, including maternal substance abuse, cigarette smoking during pregnancy, and noncompliance to ART, may also increase the risk of transmission.[64] Obstetric risk factors associated with increased risk of transmission include vaginal delivery, prolonged rupture of membranes, chorioamnionitis, and invasive obstetric procedures.[65] Premature infants born to HIV-infected women have a higher rate of perinatal HIV infection than full-term infants.[48]

Besides maternal viral load, other viral intrinsic factors affecting transmission include viral subtype, recombinant forms, resistant viral strains, and replication fitness.[16,52] Genetic and phylogentic studies indicated that infant quasi species are highly homogeneous and generally represent minor maternal variants, confirming that vertical transmission of clade B HIV transmission occurs across a selective bottleneck.[66]

Table 58-2 Risk Factors for Perinatal HIV Transmission

Maternal

- High maternal HIV viral load in plasma (and breast milk in breast-feeding populations)
- Low maternal CD4 T-lymphocyte count
- High vaginal/cervical shedding of HIV
- Advanced maternal clinical disease
- Concurrent STIs (syphilis, genital HSV)
- Coinfections (TB, malaria, HBV, HCV)
- Behavioral (cigarette smoking, substance abuse, poor adherence to combination ART)
- Genetic and immunologic characteristics (maternal HLA-A2301, upregulation of CCR5 receptor expression in placenta)

Obstetric

- Invasive procedures (amniocentesis, invasive monitoring)
- Chorioamnionitis
- Prolonged rupture of membranes
- Vaginal delivery (VL > 1000 copies/mL)

Fetal/Infant

- Prematurity (<34 weeks)
- Twin gestation (higher infection rate in first-born twin)
- Low birth weight
- Infant feeding choice (breast-feeding duration, mixed infant feeding)
- Maternal breast disease (mastitis, cracked or bleeding nipples)
- Genetic and immunologic characteristics (innate immunity/β-defensin polymorphisms, mannose-binding lectin gene polymorphisms, genetic variants of chemokine and chemokine receptors)

Abbreviations: ART, antiretroviral therapy; HBV, hepatitis B virus; HCV, hepatitis C virus; HSV, herpes simplex virus; STI, sexually transmitted infection; TB, tuberculosis; VL, viral load.

In this study, infant clones did not differ from the maternal clones in *env* length or glycosylation, and all infant variants utilized the CCR5 coreceptor but were not M-tropic.[66] Preferential in utero transmission of HIV subtype C compared to subtype A or D has been reported.[67] Host factors, including maternal-infant HLA concordance and maternal HLA homozygosity have been associated with increased transmission risks in MTCT, whereas genetic variants of chemokine and chemokine receptors have yielded conflicting results.[68,69]

Risk factors for breast milk HIV transmission include viral factors (high HIV DNA or RNA level in plasma and breast milk, maternal primary infection during lactation, decreased maternal CD4 cell count, maternal symptomatic disease/AIDS, virus subtype, and recombination forms); maternal clinical or immunological factors (bleeding or cracked nipples, subclinical/clinical mastitis, breast abscesses, malnutrition, micronutrient deficiencies); type of infant feeding (prolonged breast-feeding, mixed infant feeding); and maternal and infant host factors (oral candidiasis, oral ulcers).[57,58]

Pathogenesis of Perinatal HIV Infection

Recent studies have improved our understanding of the molecular mechanisms of MTCT. Although progress has been made in the understanding of the viral and immunopathogenesis of perinatal HIV infection, the true correlates of immune protection and immune failure and mechanisms of infection in neonatal target cells in the context of extreme viral and HLA diversity are unknown.[70-72] Compared to adult cells, HIV replicates more readily in neonatal T lymphocytes and monocytes or macrophages.[72] The *env* glycoprotein (gp160) engages the HIV receptor and coreceptors, facilitating the entry of the virus into cells, and represents the primary target for neutralizing antibodies. Viruses isolated in early vertical infection predominantly use the CCR5 coreceptor, although use of other receptors has been reported. The activation and direct infection of CD4 T cells result in high rates of viral production and dissemination throughout the body.

Perinatal HIV infection is characterized by high levels of plasma RNA (often exceeding 10^5–10^7/mL), decreasing only slowly to a "set point" by approximately 2 years of age, and may be related to many factors, including the increased HIV gene expression and replication in neonatal target cells, a large and renewable CD4 cell pool size, presence of an active thymus, and delayed or ineffective HIV-specific immune responses.[70-72] High viral loads correlate with more rapid disease progression in neonates or infants than adults, while lower levels of plasma HIV RNA with HAART are associated with clinical benefit. Regardless of the route of infection, the gastrointestinal lymphoid tissues are a major site of viral replication, persistence, and loss of CD4 T lymphocytes throughout infection.[73]

Immune disturbances in HIV infection lead to severe deficiencies in cell-mediated and humoral immunity resulting from quantitative and qualitative defects. In infants, thymic injury from HIV infection may have a significant impact on the developing immune system, resulting in progressive depletion of thymic CD4 T-lymphocyte cells, dramatic decrease in cortical CD4/CD8 double-positive cells, and an increased percentage of CD8 cells.[72] Other immune abnormalities noted include an inverted ratio of CD4/CD8, polyclonal B cell activation resulting in hypergammaglobulinemia (especially IgG and IgA), decreased lymphocyte proliferation in response to an antigen, and altered function of monocytes and neutrophils.[72] Panhypogammaglobulinemia is noted in fewer than 10% of patients and is associated with poor prognosis.[6]

HIV-Specific Immune Response

Vertically infected infants face considerable challenges in generating a specific immune response to HIV.[70] First, HIV transmission occurs before the immune system is fully developed in the infant, allowing for more efficient viral replication and less-efficient immunologic containment of the virus.[70] Second, infected infants carry a high frequency of maternally inherited HLA class I alleles (such as HLA-B*1801 and B*5802) associated with poor control of HIV. Third, transmitted maternal escape mutants are adapted to maternal HLA alleles and therefore preadapted to an infant's HLA.[74] Fourth, passive transfer of maternal, nonneutralizing antibodies could inhibit development of HIV-specific immune responses.[75]

CD8 cytotoxic T lymphocytes (CTLs) play a critical role in generation of HIV-specific immune response in acute adult infection. Many CTL epitopes are identified in various HIV genes that are conserved in HIV mother-infant sequences, indicating a role in perinatal transmission.[72] Although HIV-specific CTL activity can be demonstrated at a very early age, even in the fetus, the response is weak, less broad, and not associated with reduction in viral load and clinical outcomes compared to adults with primary infection.[76] HIV-specific CTL responses become more frequent and broad in infected infants after 6 months of life.[76] Some CTL responses in infants can select for viral escape variants very early in life.[77] In addition, disease progression is slower in children who express HLA-B*27 or HLA-B*57, indicating that CTL responses can have an important role in suppression of HIV in pediatric infection.[70] After the decline of passively transferred maternal antibody-dependent cellular cytotoxicity (ADCC) antibodies, the production of HIV-envelope cytotoxic antibodies is delayed in vertically infected infants.[78] Although neutralizing antibodies can be generated during early infection, the precise role of neutralizing antibodies in limiting MTCT is unclear.[70]

Several studies indicated that HIV-infected children have reduced antibody responses to certain childhood vaccines (eg, diphtheria, acellular pertussis vaccine).[78] Reduced antibody responses following immunization and vaccine failures in HIV-infected infants may result from a poor primary immune response, failure to generate memory responses, or loss of memory cells.[78] The majority of vertically infected infants who receive HAART before 3 months of age develop antibody and lymphproliferative responses to routine infant vaccines, although persistent HIV-specific immune responses are not detected.[78]

DIFFERENTIAL DIAGNOSIS

Human immunodeficiency virus (HIV) infection in children and adolescents causes a wide range of clinical manifestations, from asymptomatic infection to marked immunodeficiency. HIV infection must be included in the differential diagnosis of a wide spectrum of pediatric disorders (Table 58-3).

Clinical Manifestations

The clinical features of HIV infection in infants are highly variable and often nonspecific. Infants with perinatally acquired HIV infection are often asymptomatic, and physical examination is usually normal in the neonatal period. Growth delay can be an early sign of untreated perinatal HIV infection. Other features of infection in early infancy could include unexplained persistent or recurrent fevers or generalized lymphadenopathy, often associated with hepatosplenomegaly and recurrent or persistent otitis media (Table 58-4). Also commonly encountered are oral or diaper candidiasis, developmental delay, parotitis, and dermatitis.[6]

HIV encephalopathy is a well-described AIDS-defining complication of HIV in infants and children and can affect 10% to 25% of cases.[79,80] Encephalopathy can be either static or progressive, characterized by a classic triad of developmental delay, impaired brain growth or acquired microcephaly, and acquired symmetric motor deficits (hyperreflexia, hypertonia, ataxia, or gait disturbances).[81] Characteristic computed tomographic findings characteristic of HIV encephalopathy include cerebral atrophy (85% of cases) and bilateral symmetric calcification of the basal ganglia (15% of cases). Criteria for the definitive diagnosis of HIV encephalopathy are listed in Table 58-5. The onset of HIV encephalopathy is in the first year of life and was associated with increased mortality in the pre-ART era.[82] In the current era of HAART, the incidence of HIV encephalopathy decreased by 50%, but infected

Table 58-3 Differential Diagnoses of HIV Infection

- Anemia, chronic
- Autoimmune and chronic benign neutropenia
- Primary immune deficiency syndromes (Bruton agammaglobulinemia, common variable immunodeficiency, severe combined immunodeficiency, transient hypogammaglobulinemia of infancy)
- Constitutional growth delay
- Failure to thrive/malnutrition
- Lymphadenopathy
- Malabsorption syndromes

Table 58-4 Clinical Manifestations of HIV Infection in Infants Ages 1 to 2 Years

Failure to thrive, HIV wasting syndrome[a]
HIV encephalopathy[a]
Hepatosplenomegaly, lymphadenopathy
Pneumocystis jiroveci pneumonia[a]
Multiple or recurrent bacterial infections (especially *Streptococcus pneumoniae*)[a]
Refractory thrush or candida diaper dermatitis
Other opportunistic infections (eg, cytomegalovirus disease, severe herpes simplex virus)[a]
Lymphoid interstitial pneumonia or pulmonary lymphoid hyperplasia complex[a]

[a]AIDS-defining condition.

infants may present with more subtle and insidious central nervous system (CNS) manifestations.[79,83,84]

In the pre-ART era, *Pneumocystis jiroveci* pneumonia (PCP) (previously known as *Pneumocystis carinii*) was the leading AIDS-defining illness diagnosed during the first year of life and was associated with a high mortality rate. Other common AIDS-defining conditions in US children with vertically acquired infection include lymphoid interstitial pneumonitis, multiple or recurrent invasive bacterial infections caused by encapsulated bacteria, HIV encephalopathy, wasting syndrome, candida esophagitis, cytomegalovirus (CMV) disease, and *Mycobacterium avium* complex (MAC) infection.[81] With early infant HIV diagnosis and linkage to care and an ART program, the frequency of historically reported AIDS-defining illness and opportunistic infections (OIs) have dramatically decreased among children living with HIV in the United States and other resource-rich countries.[85] In the post-ART era, the rate of OIs decreased from 12.5 to 0.8 cases per 100,000 person-years pre- and post-ART, respectively.[85]

Table 58-5 Clinical and Neuroimaging Features of HIV Encephalopathy in Infants[a]

Clinical Manifestations

- Acquired microcephaly
- Developmental delay or regression
- Spasticity
- Pathologic reflexes
- Dystonia
- Gait abnormalities
- Expressive language impairment

Neuroimaging Features

- Cerebral atrophy
- Symmetric calcifications in basal ganglia

[a]Data from reference 81.

Pediatric AIDS Case Definition

The AIDS case definitions published by the CDC in 1987, and subsequently revised in 1993, 1994, and 2008, are intended primarily for public health surveillance and reporting purposes for monitoring the HIV epidemic.[86-89] The revised 1994 CDC classification system for HIV infection in children less than 13 years of age is based on (1) HIV infection status, (2) clinical disease, and (3) immunologic status.[88] Clinical categories are stratified from N, indicating no signs or symptoms, through A, B, and C, for mild, moderate, and severe (AIDS-defining) symptoms, respectively. The revised 2008 Pediatric AIDS case definitions did not make any changes in the HIV infection classification system, the 24 AIDS-defining conditions for children aged less than 13 years, or the AIDS case definition for children aged less than 18 months.[89] The case definitions are similar for adults and children with some important exceptions.[88] Lymphoid interstitial pneumonia (LIP) and multiple or recurrent serious bacterial infections are AIDS-defining illnesses only for children. Also, certain herpes virus infections (CMV, HSV) and toxoplasmosis of the CNS are AIDS-defining conditions only for adults and children older than 1 month of age.[88]

The immunologic categories place emphasis on the CD4 T-cell lymphocyte count and percentages for age, and include stage 1, no evidence of immunosuppression; stage 2, moderate immunosuppression; and stage 3, severe immunosuppression.[88,89] Once classified, a child cannot be reclassified into a less-severe category, even if the child's clinical status or immune function improves in response to ART or resolution of clinical events. HIV-exposed infants whose HIV infection status is indeterminate (unconfirmed) are classified by placing a prefix E (for perinatally exposed) before the appropriate classification code (eg, EN2).[89]

DIAGNOSTIC TESTS

Early Infant Diagnosis

Many advances have been made in the area of laboratory diagnosis of HIV infection.[90-92] Routine HIV antibody testing is not informative for early infant diagnosis because of transplacental passage of maternal IgG antibodies to the virus that are present in infants up to 18 months of age.[6] The diagnosis of HIV infection in infants warrants the use of PCR-based DNA or RNA assays (referred to as HIV nucleic acid amplification tests, NAATs) that are highly sensitive and specific and now widely available in developed countries.[90]

The HIV DNA PCR assay detects cell-associated proviral DNA and in the United States remains the preferred test for early infant HIV diagnosis; approximately, 93% of HIV-infected infants will test positive by HIV DNA PCR assay by 2 weeks of age, and approximately 95% of infected infants will test positive by DNA PCR assay by 1 month of age.[6] However, the HIV DNA PCR assay is less sensitive for identifying non-B-subtype virus and has been associated with false-negative tests in patients with non-B-subtype HIV infection.[90]

The HIV RNA PCR assay detects plasma viral RNA and can also be used for early infant diagnosis.[90] The newer HIV RNA assay is as sensitive or more sensitive and as specific for detection of HIV subtype B compared to HIV DNA PCR.[93] However, a false-negative result can occur in neonates receiving ARV prophylaxis.[6] HIV RNA PCR may be more sensitive than HIV DNA PCR test for detection of non-B-subtype virus.[94] Therefore, it is prudent to use HIV RNA PCR for diagnosis of infants born to women known or suspected to have non-B-subtype HIV infection.[90]

HIV DNA or RNA PCR testing is recommended at 14-21 days of age, and if test results are negative, repeat testing should be performed at 1-2 months of age and again at 4-6 months of age.[6,90] Virologic testing is recommended at birth by some experts to diagnose in utero infection if mothers did not receive ART or prophylaxis during pregnancy or in other high-risk scenarios, but a cord blood specimen should not be used because of possible contamination with maternal blood. It is assumed that children who have a positive HIV PCR result within the first 48 hours after birth were infected in utero, whereas those who are infected during the intrapartum period might become positive 2 to 6 weeks after birth.[38] An infant is diagnosed with HIV infection if 2 separate blood samples test positive for HIV DNA or RNA PCR.[90]

HIV isolation by culture is not recommended for routine diagnosis because culture is less sensitive, is more expensive, and needs a specialized laboratory, and results are not available for up to 28 days. Use of HIV-1 p24 antigen detection is not recommended for diagnosis of infant HIV-1 because of its poor sensitivity compared to HIV DNA PCR or culture.[6]

Hypergammaglobulinemia is a nonspecific but early finding of HIV infection. CD4 counts must be interpreted within the bounds of the age-dependent normal range, and changes in counts may result in a decrease in the normal ratio of more than 1.0 of CD4 to CD8 T-lymphocyte count.[6]

HIV infection can be *presumptively excluded* in non-breast-feeding HIV-exposed children younger than 18 months of age if there are (1) 2 negative HIV DNA or RNA PCR test results from separate specimens, both of which were obtained at greater than 2 weeks of age and 1 of which was obtained at greater than 4 weeks of age; *or* (2) 1 negative HIV RNA or DNA PCR test result from a specimen obtained at greater than 8 weeks of age; *or* (3) 1 negative HIV antibody test obtained at greater than 6 months of age; *and* no other laboratory (eg, no subsequent positive PCR test results if performed) or clinical (eg, no AIDS-defining illness) evidence of HIV infection.[6,90]

HIV infection can be *definitively excluded* in non-breast-feeding HIV-exposed children younger than 18 months of age if there are (1) 2 negative HIV DNA or RNA PCR test results from separate specimens, both of which were obtained at greater than 1 month of age and 1 of which was obtained at greater than 4 months of age; (2) 2 negative HIV antibody tests from separate specimens, both of which were obtained at greater than 6 months of age; *and* no other laboratory (eg, no subsequent positive PCR test results if performed) or clinical (eg, no AIDS-defining illness) evidence of HIV infection.[6,90]

In children with 2 negative HIV DNA PCR test results, many physicians confirm the absence of HIV infection by documenting a negative HIV antibody test result at 12 to 18 months of age ("seroreversion").[90] A non-breast-fed infant is considered HIV negative if 2 antibody test samples drawn at least 1 month apart and both obtained after 6 months of age are negative.[6] If HIV antibody testing is performed at 12 months of age in an HIV-exposed infant not known to be infected, and if the infant is still antibody positive, repeat testing at 18 months of age is recommended. Detection of HIV antibody in a child older than 18 months of age is diagnostic of HIV infection. Documentation of seroreversion may be more important when non-subtype-B HIV is possible or present.

MANAGEMENT

Early Antiretroviral Therapy

If infection is confirmed, the infant should be promptly referred to a pediatric HIV specialist for consideration of HAART and care.[95–99] Combination ART for HIV-infected infants and children is associated with improvement in growth and development; reduction in the risk of OIs, HIV encephalopathy, and other complications; and improvements of virologic and immunologic parameters. In the United States and other developed nations, use of HAART has resulted in dramatic reductions in mortality and morbidity of over 80%–90% in children.[5,83,99] HAART has evolved from simple nucleoside reverse transcriptase inhibitor (NRTI) regimens of the 1980s and early 1990s to current complex regimens of NRTI in combination with protease inhibitors (PIs) or nonnucleoside reverse transcriptase inhibitors (NNRTIs).

Most HIV-infected children need HAART based on age, clinical, immunologic, and virologic criteria.[96]

The consideration of early treatment of asymptomatic infants is based on the rationale that infants are at highest risk of rapid disease progression to AIDS or death, even when immune degradation and virus replication are moderately well contained.[98] Recent studies indicated that early initiation of combination ART within the first 3 months of life reduces morbidity and mortality compared with initiating therapy when symptomatic or immune suppressed.[6,98] Early treatment can result in complete cessation of viral replication and the preservation of normal immune function.

Treatment Guidelines

Panels of experts have developed guidelines for the use of ARV therapy in children (available on line at http://www.aidsinfo.nih.gov).[96] Pediatric HIV experts agree that infected infants with clinical symptoms of HIV disease or with evidence of immune suppression should receive HAART. Recently, a South African clinical trial (Children with HIV Early Antiretroviral Therapy [CHER] study) found that initiation of therapy at less than 12 weeks of age in asymptomatic infants with normal immune function resulted in 76% reduction in mortality and 75% reduction in HIV disease progression compared to waiting to initiate treatment of such infants until they met standard criteria for initiation of therapy.[98] Based on the results of the CHER study, current US guidelines recommend initiation of ART for all HIV-infected infants younger than 12 months regardless of clinical status, CD4 T-cell count, CD4 percentage, or HIV RNA level (Table 58-6).[96]

Choice of Initial ART Regimen

A 3-drug combination ART, consisting of a 2 NRTIs plus either a PI or an NNRTI as the initial regimen, provides the best opportunity to preserve immune function and to prevent disease progression.[96] Suppression of virus to undetectable levels and long-term preservation of immune function are the desired goals.[6] ARV resistance testing (viral genotyping) should be considered before starting ARV therapy in newly diagnosed infants under age 12 months, especially if the mother has known or suspected infection with drug-resistant virus.[96] A change in ART regimen should be considered if there is evidence of disease progression (clinical, immunologic, and virologic); adverse effects related to ARV therapy; or a new superior regimen becomes available.[96]

Antiretroviral Drugs

The most commonly used ARVs in newborns and infants, the NRTIs ZDV, lamivudine (3TC), abacavir

Table 58-6 Indications for Initiation of Pediatric Antiretroviral Therapy[a]

HIV-Infected Infants
ART is indicated regardless of clinical symptoms, immune status, or HIV RNA level. 4 > 500 cells/mm³ and an HIV RNA ≥ 100,000 copies/mL

Children From 1 to Less Than 5 Years of Age
• ART is recommended for all children with AIDS or significant HIV-related symptoms (CDC clinical categories C and B [except for the following category B condition: single episode of serious bacterial infection]), regardless of CD4 T-lymphocyte counts or HIV RNA level; CD4 < 25%, regardless of symptoms or HIV RNA level *or* Asymptomatic or mild clinical symptoms (CDC clinical categories A or N or the following category B condition: single episode of serious bacterial infection) *and* CD4 ≥ 25% and an HIV RNA ≥ 100,000 copies/mL

Children 5 Years and Older
• Therapy is recommended for all children with AIDS or significant HIV-related symptoms (CDC clinical categories C and B [except for the following category B condition: single episode of serious bacterial infection]); CD4 ≤ 500 cells/mm³ *or* Asymptomatic or mild clinical symptoms (CDC clinical categories A or N or the following category B condition: single episode of serious bacterial infection) and CD

Abbreviations: ART, antiretroviral treatment; CDC, Centers for Disease Control and Prevention.
[a]Data from reference 96.

(ABC), didanosine (ddI), the NNRTI nevirapine (NVP), and the PIs lopinavir/ritonavir (LPV/r) and nelfinavir (NLV) are briefly reviewed in Table 58-7. More extensive reviews are available in specific textbooks or the current recommendations from the CDC and the federal guidelines website (http://aidsinfo.nih. gov).[96] Because the standards of care are evolving, collaboration between the child's primary health care provider and an HIV treatment center is strongly suggested. Whenever possible, children should be enrolled in clinical trials; access and information can be obtained by calling 1-800-TRIALS-A (AIDS Clinical Trials Group [ACTG]), or 1-301-402-0696 (HIV and AIDS Malignancy Branch, National Cancer Institute). Several promising second-generation agents as well as new classes of ARV agents are currently being evaluated in adult clinical trials, but pharmacokinetic and safety data are limited in children.[96] These agents include duranavir (PI), maraviroc (CCR5 antagonist), raltegravir (integrase inhibitor), and etravirine (newer NNRTI). Data are insufficient to recommend these agents as initial therapy for infants.[96]

Challenges

Antiretroviral treatment of infected infants is complicated by poor adherence related to complex and demanding regimens, unpleasant tasting suspensions (eg, ritonavir), limited availability of pediatric liquid formulations, and adverse events such as nausea and vomiting.[95] Other issues include the need for refrigeration (eg, lopinavir), drugs with short shelf life (eg, didanosine), immature drug metabolism, and the lack of age-specific pharmacokinetic data to guide pediatric dosing. In addition, toxicity and development of drug resistance are other serious concerns.[95] Other unresolved ART management issues include long-term effects on growth and development, neurocognitive function, bone growth, metabolic abnormalities, and relationship between pediatric HAART and interventions for malaria, tuberculosis, and malnutrition.[100]

Chemoprophylaxis

All HIV-infected infants younger than 12 months of age should be started on PCP prophylaxis at 4 to 6 weeks of age and the treatment continued for the first year of life, regardless of their CD4 T-cell counts.[97] Given the high mortality caused by PCP, all HIV-exposed infants with indeterminate HIV infection status should receive PCP prophylaxis starting at 4 to 6 weeks of age.[90] Infants meeting criteria for presumptive or definitive HIV-uninfected status do not need PCP prophylaxis. The recommended prophylactic regimen is trimethoprim-sulfamethoxazole (TMP-SMX) with 150 mg/m²/day of TMP and 750 mg/m²/day of SMX given orally in divided doses twice each day during 3 consecutive days per week. The alternative regimen are TMP-SMX given once daily for 3 days/week or twice daily 7 days/week. If TMP-SMX is not tolerated, alternative regimens are dapsone taken orally (2 mg/kg once daily or 4 mg/kg once weekly) or intravenous pentamidine (4 mg/kg every 2–4 weeks) or atovaquone (30 mg/kg once daily for infants 1–3 months of age and 45 mg/kg once daily for infants aged 4 months to 24 months).[90] However, breakthrough infections can occur with every regimen and appear to be most frequent with intravenous pentamidine and least common with TMP-SMX. The CDC has published guidelines for prevention and treatment of OIs (MAC, CMV, *Toxoplasma gondii*, and other organisms) among HIV-infected infants and children.[97]

Table 58-7 Antiretroviral Drugs for Treatment of HIV Infection in Infants[a]

Antiretroviral Drug	Formulations	Dose	Side Effects
Nucleoside Reverse Transcriptase Inhibitors (NRTI)s			
Zidovudine (ZDV)	Syrup: 10 mg/mL	*Premature babies:* 1.5 mg/kg of body weight (IV) or 2 mg/kg of body weight by mouth every 12 hours, increased to every 8 hours at 2 weeks of age (neonates $\geq$ 30 weeks' GA) or at 4 weeks (neonates < 30 weeks' GA) *Neonatal/infant dose (age < 6 weeks):* 1.5 mg/kg of body weight (IV) or 2 mg/kg of body weight by mouth every 6 hours *Pediatric dose (6 weeks to < 18 years):* 180–240 mg/m^2 of BSA by mouth every 12 hours *or* 160 mg/m^2 by mouth every 8 hours; twice-daily dosing preferred in clinical practice *Body weight-based dosing:* 12 mg/kg by mouth every 12 hours (4 kg to < 9 kg); 9 mg/kg by mouth every 12 hour (9 kg to < 30 kg)	Macrocytic anemia, neutropenia, nausea, vomiting, headache, hepatotoxicity, myopathy, nail pigmentation, hyperlipidemia, insulin resistance/diabetes mellitus, lipoatrophy, lactic acidosis, hepatomegaly with steatosis
Lamivudine (3TC)	Pediatric oral solution: 10 mg/mL	*Neonatal/infant dose (age < 4 weeks):* 2 mg/kg of body weight by mouth every 12 hours *Pediatric dose (age $\geq$ 4 weeks):* 4 mg/kg of body weight by mouth every 12 hours	Headache, fatigue, reduced appetite, nausea, diarrhea, rash, pancreatitis, peripheral neuropathy, anemia, neutropenia, lactic acidosis, hepatomegaly with steatosis
Didanosine (ddl)	Pediatric powder for oral solution: 10 mg/mL (reconstituted)	*Premature:* no data *Neonatal/infant dose (aged 2 weeks to < 3 months of age):* 50 mg/m^2 of BSA every 12 hours *Infant dose (>3 months to 8 months of age):* 100 mg/m^2 of BSA by mouth every 12 hours *Pediatric dose (age > 8 months of age):* 120 mg/m^2 (range 90–150 mg/m^2) of BSA by mouth every 12 hours	Peripheral neuropathy, electrolyte abnormalities, diarrhea, abdominal pain, nausea, vomiting, lactic acidosis, hepatomegaly with steatosis (risk increased with combination of d4T with ddl), pancreatitis, retinitis, insulin resistance/diabetes mellitus
Stavudine (d4T)	Solution: 1 mg/mL	*Neonatal/infant dose (aged birth to 13 days):* 0.5 mg/kg of body weight by mouth every 12 hours *Pediatric dose (age 14 days up to weight of 30 kg):* 1 mg/kg of body weight by mouth every 12 hours	Headache, gastrointestinal upsets, rash, lipoatrophy peripheral neuropathy, pancreatitis, mitochondrial toxicity, lactic acidosis, hepatomegaly with steatosis (combination of d4T with ddl may result in enhanced toxicity), increased liver enzymes, insulin resistance/diabetes mellitus, ascending neuromuscular weakness (unusual)

(Continued)

Table 58-7 Antiretroviral Drugs for Treatment of HIV Infection in Infants[a] (*Continued*)

Antiretroviral Drug	Formulations	Dose	Side Effects
Abacavir (ABC)	Solution: 20 mg/mL	*Neonatal/infant dose (aged < 3 months of age):* Not approved for infants less than 3 months of age *Pediatric dose (age > 3 months of age):* 8 mg/kg by mouth twice daily	Hypersensitivity reaction (HSR) that may be fatal; HSR symptoms may include fever, rash, nausea, vomiting, malaise or fatigue, loss of appetite, respiratory symptoms (eg, sore throat, cough, dyspnea)[b]
Nonnucleoside Reverse Transcriptase Inhibitors (NNRTIs)			
Nevirapine (NVP)	Suspension: 10 mg/mL	*Neonatal/infant dose (aged < 14 days):* Treatment dose not defined in this age group *Pediatric dose (age < 8 years):* 200 mg/m^2 of BSA twice daily (start treatment once daily for the first 14 days; if no rash or adverse effects, give the drug twice daily)	Skin rash, including Stevens-Johnson syndrome and toxic epidermal necrolysis; fever; headache; nausea; symptomatic hepatitis, including fatal hepatic necrosis; severe systemic HSRs
Protease Inhibitors (PIs)			
Lopinavir-ritonavir (LPV/r)	Pediatric oral solution: 80 mg/20 mg LPV/r per milliliter	*Neonatal/infant dose (aged < 14 days):* No safety/dosing data available; not recommended for use *Neonatal/infant dose (aged 14 days to 12 months):* 300 mg/75 mg LPV/r per square meter of BSA *or* 16 m/4 mg LPV/r per kilogram body weight twice daily; because dosage data are not available for LPV/r administered with NVP in infants ≤ 6 months of age, LPV/r should not be administered in combination with NVP in these infants	Diarrhea, nausea, vomiting, headache, skin rash in patients receiving other antiretroviral agents, lipid abnormalities, fat redistribution, new-onset diabetes mellitus, hyperglycemia, ketoacidosis, hemolytic anemia, pancreatitis, life-threatening hepatitis Risk of cardiac toxicity, adrenal dysfunction and overdose, especially in premature infants

Abbreviations: BSA, body surface area; GA, gestational age; IV, intravenous.
[a]Data from reference 96.
[b]Before starting ABC, patients must be tested for the HLA-B*5701 allele to screen for risk of hypersensitivity; patients with the HLA-B*5701 allele should not receive ABC. Patients with no prior HLA-B*5701 testing who are tolerating ABC do not need to be tested.

Primary Care

HIV-infected children are at highest risk for developing vaccine-preventable diseases compared to HIV-uninfected children. Therefore, the American Academy of Pediatrics (AAP) recommends routine immunizations with some modifications for all HIV-exposed infants, whether they are infected or not.[6] Similar to other newborns, children born to HIV-infected mothers should receive hepatitis B vaccinations, but if the mother is positive for hepatitis B surface antigen (HBsAg), the child should also receive hepatitis B immunoglobulin (HBIG) within 12 hours after birth. Refer to the 2012 edition of the *Red Book* for guidance regarding immunization practices in HIV-infected children.[6]

Infants infected with HIV should be vaccinated at the appropriate age with inactivated vaccines (diphtheria, tetanus toxoids and acellular pertussis, *Haemophilus influenzae* type b, hepatitis B, hepatitis A, and pneumococcal conjugate vaccine) as well as the trivalent influenza vaccine annually. Live virus vaccine (oral poliovirus) or live bacterial vaccines (BCG) should not be given to patients with HIV infection. The exception is measles-mumps-rubella (MMR) vaccine and varicella zoster immunization, which can be given to asymptomatic HIV-infected children (1 through 5 years of age) with CD4 T-cell percentage greater than 15%. The oral rotavirus vaccine may be given for HIV-exposed and HIV-infected infants regardless of CD4 T-cell count. HIV-infected children should also receive a single dose of 23-valent polysaccharide pneumococcal vaccine after 24 months of age, with a minimum interval of 8 weeks since the last pneumococcal conjugate vaccine.[6] Postexposure passive immunization of children with HIV infection is recommended in certain circumstances, especially after exposure to measles, varicella, or tetanus.[6]

Other aspects of HIV management include careful monitoring of growth and development, assessment of organ system involvement, development and psychosocial assessments and intervention.[95] A family-centered approach involving a specialist pediatric HIV multidisciplinary team in collaboration with a primary care physician is crucial for long-term successful management.

Prevention of Perinatal HIV Transmission

A landmark trial published in 1994 by the PACTG (076 study) showed that a long course of ZDV prophylaxis given to an HIV-infected mother at 14 weeks of gestation and labor and to her newborn infant reduced perinatal HIV transmission by nearly 70% in a non-breast-feeding population.[10] Following the PACTG 076 study, remarkable progress has occurred in the United States with development and implementation of efficacious antepartum, intrapartum, and postpartum PMTCT interventions, leading to an extraordinary decline (to less than 2%) in rates of perinatal HIV transmission.[1,6–8,11–13] Highly successful approaches to prevent perinatal HIV transmission in resource-rich countries have included widespread implementation of routine antenatal HIV testing (opt-out approach) for all pregnant women, use of triple ARV prophylaxis or HAART, elective cesarean delivery, and avoidance of breast-feeding (Table 58-8).[6–8,12] Guidelines and recommendations for use of ARV in pregnant women for maternal health and perinatal HIV prevention are available from the USPHS (http://www.aidsinfo.nih.gov) and other professional societies (AAP, American College of Obstetricians and Gynecologists).[12]

Routine Antenatal (Opt-Out) HIV Testing

HIV testing during pregnancy is the gateway to access effective interventions to prevent perinatal HIV transmission and link HIV-positive women to care and treatment.[1] In 1995, following the publication of the PACTG 076 study, the CDC recommended universal HIV counseling and voluntary prenatal HIV testing.[11]

Table 58-8 Strategies to Prevent Perinatal HIV Transmission in the United States

- Primary prevention of HIV infection in reproductive age women
- Prevention of unintended pregnancies in HIV-infected women
- Prevention of perinatal HIV infection
  - Routine antenatal ("opt-out") HIV testing
  - Combination antiretroviral therapy
  - Elective cesarean delivery[a]
  - Avoidance of breast-feeding
- Provision of treatment, care, and support to HIV-positive women and their families

[a]Before labor and before rupture of membranes and if maternal viral load > 1000 copies/mL near the time of delivery.

In 1999, the US Congress provided target funding for prevention of perinatal HIV infection in high-prevalence states.[1] In 2001, the CDC issued revised HIV counseling and testing guidelines for pregnant women, recommending strategies to reduce barriers to offering antenatal HIV testing, including routine opt-out HIV screening for all pregnant women, offering rapid HIV testing during the labor/delivery period for women with unknown HIV status.[101] In 2003–2006, the CDC reported high uptake of screening of pregnant women using the opt-out strategy. In 2006, the CDC expanded the use of the opt-out strategy to include routine HIV testing in health care facilities to all patients aged 13–64 years as well as all pregnant women as part of a routine panel of antenatal tests, a second HIV test in the third trimester for women living in areas with a high incidence of HIV or those at high risk (eg, history of injection drug use, exchange of sex for money or drugs, multiple sex partners, or a partner known to be HIV infected), and rapid testing for women in labor with undocumented HIV infection status.[11,102] In some states, routine HIV testing during pregnancy is mandated by law.[6] Health care providers should provide routine education about HIV infection and testing as part of comprehensive care for all women of reproductive age.

Combination Antiretroviral Therapy During Pregnancy

Since the mid-2000s, innovative clinical trials conducted in both resource-rich and resource-limited countries have yielded important observations.[1,7,8,12,16–18] First, observational studies have demonstrated that combination ARV regimens during pregnancy are more effective for prevention of perinatal HIV transmission than ZDV alone.[12,13] Second, combination ARVs are effective in reducing perinatal transmission, even among women with advanced disease. Third, a longer duration of maternal antepartum ARV prophylaxis (starting at 28 weeks' gestation or earlier) is more effective than shorter-duration ARV prophylaxis (starting at 36 weeks' gestation). Finally, adding single-dose intrapartum NVP to HIV-positive women who are already receiving combination ARVs during pregnancy for prophylaxis or treatment does not offer any additional benefit among non-breast-feeding women in the United States and may increase the risk of resistance; therefore, it is not recommended.[12]

Current USPHS task force recommendations regarding ARVs for prevention of perinatal HIV transmission are summarized in Table 58-9. All HIV-infected

Table 58-9 US Public Health Service Guidelines for Preventing Perinatal HIV Transmission in Selected Clinical Circumstances[a]

HIV-Positive Women Currently on ART Who Became Pregnant

Mother
- Continue current combination ART during antepartum and intrapartum period if the regimen is safe and effective in achieving optimal viral suppression.
- ARV resistance testing if maternal viral load > 500–1000 copies/mL.
- Continuous intravenous ZDV infusion during labor for women with viral load > 400 copies/mL (or unknown viral load) near delivery regardless of antepartum regimen or mode of delivery.
- Scheduled cesarean delivery at 38 weeks' gestation if maternal plasma viral load is > 1000 copies/mL near the time of delivery.

Neonate
- Oral ZDV should be prescribed to the neonate as soon as possible after delivery (preferably within 6–12 hours of birth) and then continued for 6 weeks.

HIV-Positive Pregnant Women Who Have Never Received ART

Mother
- ARV resistance testing before starting ARV prophylaxis or therapy, but treatment must not be delayed pending results of resistance testing if maternal HIV diagnosis is made late in pregnancy.
- Combination ART during antepartum and intrapartum period.
- Continuous intravenous ZDV infusion during labor for women with viral load > 400 copies/mL (or unknown viral load) near delivery regardless of antepartum regimen or mode of delivery.
- Scheduled cesarean delivery at 38 weeks' gestation if maternal plasma viral load is > 1000 copies/mL near the time of delivery.
- Linkage to care and treatment program to evaluate the need for continuation of combination ART postpartum.
- Neonate
- Oral ZDV should be prescribed to the neonate as soon as possible after delivery (preferably within 6–12 hours of birth) and then continued for 6 weeks.

HIV-Positive Pregnant Women Who Are ART Experienced But Not Currently on ART

Mother
- ARV resistance testing before restarting ARV prophylaxis or therapy, but treatment must not be delayed pending results of resistance testing if maternal HIV diagnosis is made late in pregnancy.
- Combination ART during antepartum and intrapartum period.
- Continuous intravenous ZDV infusion during labor for women with viral load > 400 copies/mL (or unknown viral load) near delivery regardless of antepartum regimen or mode of delivery.
- Scheduled cesarean delivery at 38 weeks' gestation if maternal plasma viral load is > 1000 copies/mL near the time of delivery.
- Linkage to care and treatment program to evaluate the need for continuation of combination ART postpartum.
Neonate
- Oral ZDV should be prescribed to the neonate as soon as possible after delivery (preferably within 6–12 hours of birth) and then continued for 6 weeks.

HIV-Positive Women Who Have Received No ART Before Labor

Mother
- Continuous intravenous ZDV infusion during labor.
Neonate
- Combination ARV drug regimen as soon as possible after birth (oral ZDV for 6 weeks to the infant) plus 3 doses of oral NVP in the first week of life (at birth, 48 hours later, and 96 hours after the second dose).

Abbreviations: ARV, antiretroviral; ART, antiretroviral therapy; NVP, nevirapine; ZDV, zidovudine.
[a]Data from references 12 and 106.

pregnant women must receive fully suppressive combination ARV regimens (including at least 3 ARV agents) either for the treatment of maternal HIV infection or for PMTCT.[12] Drug resistance testing should be performed for all women before starting ART and for women who are already receiving ART without fully suppressed viral load (>500–1000 copies/mL). However, decisions regarding initiating ARV prophylaxis must not be delayed, especially when women present late in pregnancy. The guidelines also recommend that ZDV (used in the PACTG 076 study) should be included in the maternal ARV regimen, although a woman already receiving combination ART with suppressed viral load need not have her regimen altered.[6,12] Reduction of viral load in maternal blood and genital secretions is an important mechanism of action of ZDV in PMTCT.[60,103] In the PACTG 076 study, ZDV only modestly reduced maternal HIV RNA, and change in maternal HIV RNA levels accounted for only 17% of the reported efficacy of ZDV. Because transmission has been noted at all levels of maternal HIV RNA levels, other mechanisms of action of ARVs in PMTCT such as infant preexposure prophylaxis or infant postexposure prophylaxis may also offer a substantial component of protection.[7,103]

A 3-drug combination ART, consisting of a 2 NRTIs plus either a PI or an NNRTI is recommended (Table 58-10). Use of single or dual NRTIs alone is not recommended for therapy for HIV infection.[12] Based on clinical trials and other studies, the preferred dual-NRTI regimen of choice includes ZDV and 3TC; LPV/r is the preferred PI. Although NVP is the preferred NNRTI during pregnancy, the drug is not recommended for pregnant HIV-positive women with CD4 counts greater than 250 cells/μL because of the increased risk of potentially life-threatening hepatic toxicity noted in women with higher CD4 counts.[12] Another NNRTI, efavirenz is a class D teratogen and therefore is not recommended during the first trimester of pregnancy as part of the maternal ARV regimen but may be considered in later stages of pregnancy if other agents are not appropriate.[6,12] No data exist currently on the use of the newer agents, including PIs (darunavir, fosamprenavir, tipranavir); entry inhibitors (enfuvirtide and maraviroc); and integrase inhibitor (raltegravir). Limited experience exists for the newer NNRTI etravirine and NRTI tenofovir.[12]

Adverse events related to the use of ARV agents during pregnancy must be closely monitored. Hyperglycemia, new-onset diabetes mellitus, exacerbation of existing diabetes mellitus, and ketoacidosis may be associated with PI therapy, requiring standard glucose screening at 24–28 weeks' gestation.[12] PI-based combination ARV regimens during pregnancy may be associated with a small increased risk of preterm births, but data

are inconclusive, and PIs should not be withheld given the proven benefits.[12] Health care providers who treat maternal/pediatric patients should report instances of prenatal exposure to ARVs to the Antiretroviral Pregnancy Registry (1-800-258-4263 or http://www.apregistry.com). Long-term outcomes of infants exposed to ARVs in utero are unknown, warranting long-term follow-up.[6,12]

Maternal combination ART must be continued postpartum if indicated for maternal health or discontinued if ARVs were used solely for PMTCT, but these decisions must be made in close consultation with an HIV specialist.[6,12] Many factors must be taken into consideration about continuing ART postpartum, including current recommendations for initiating ART, current and nadir CD4 T-lymphocyte count and trends, maternal viral load, adherence issues, seronegative sexual partner, and patient preference.[12] Expert guidelines recommend continuation of ART postpartum in women with nadir CD4 counts less than the currently recommended threshold for initiation of ART or symptomatic HIV infection.[12] The risks vs benefits of discontinuing ART in postpartum women with HIV with higher CD4 counts is unknown and is the subject of future research (Promise Study, clinical trial NCT00955968). A recent landmark study (HPTN 052) involving serodiscordant couples demonstrated that starting HIV-infected individuals with ART early resulted in a significant reduction in sexual transmission of HIV to uninfected partners.[104] Therefore, in serodiscordant couples, continued administration of ARVs may be recommended in postpartum HIV-positive women with CD4 counts between 350 and 550 cells/μL and can be considered for women with CD4 counts greater than 550 cells/μL to prevent sexual transmission of HIV to the uninfected male partner.[12]

Elective Cesarean Delivery

The role of elective cesarean section delivery in reducing perinatal HIV transmission was recognized before the advent of combination ARV therapy during pregnancy.[47,48] Data from a large international meta-analysis of 15 prospective cohort studies and a randomized controlled trial from Europe have shown that cesarean section performed before labor and rupture of membranes reduces perinatal transmission of HIV-1 by 50%–80% independent of the use of ART or ZDV prophylaxis.[47,48] Both these studies were performed prior to the advent of HAART during pregnancy, and there was no information on maternal serum HIV RNA level. Although the level of maternal serum HIV RNA level is an important predictor of perinatal HIV-1 transmission,[58] no studies have demonstrated that suppression of viral load eliminates the risk of perinatal HIV transmission.[8] A recent observational

Table 58-10 Preferred and Alternative Antiretroviral (ARV) Drugs During Pregnancy[a]

Drug	FDA Pregnancy Category	Experience During Pregnancy and PK Data	Adverse Effects and Concerns
Preferred Nucleoside/Nucleotide Reverse Transcriptase Inhibitors (NRTIs): Zidovudine, Lamivudine			
Zidovudine (ZDV), azidothymidine (AZT)	C	Extensive experience; PK not significantly altered in pregnancy; no change in dosing indicated; high placental transfer to the fetus	Anemia, neutropenia, mitochondrial toxicity (neuropathy, myopathy, cardiomyopathy, pancreatitis, lactic acidosis, hepatomegaly with steatosis) No evidence of human teratogenicity Well tolerated during pregnancy and safe for mothers and infants in the short term
Lamivudine (3TC)[b]	C	Extensive experience; PK not significantly altered in pregnancy; no change in dosing indicated; high placental transfer to the fetus	Headache, fatigue, reduced appetite, nausea, diarrhea, rash, anemia, neutropenia mitochondrial toxicity (neuropathy, myopathy, cardiomyopathy, pancreatitis, lactic acidosis, hepatomegaly with steatosis) No evidence of human teratogenicity Well tolerated during pregnancy and safe for mothers and infants in the short-term
Alternative NRTIs: abacavir (ABC),[c] emtricitabine (FTC), tenofovir (TDF)[d] Use in special circumstances because of toxicity concerns: didanosine (ddI),[b] stavudine (d4T)[b]			
Preferred Nonnucleoside Reverse Transcriptase Inhibitors (NNRTIs)			
Nevirapine (NVP)	B	Extensive experience; PK not significantly altered; no change in dosing indicated; high placental transfer to the fetus	Skin rash, including Stevens-Johnson syndrome and toxic epidermal necrolysis, fever, headache, nausea, and abnormal liver enzymes Severe life-threatening hepatotoxicity and rash in women with a CD4 T-cell count > 250 cells/mL, hypersensitivity reactions For pregnant HIV-positive women with CD4 T-cell count > 250, NVP should be started only if benefit clearly outweighs the risk of rash associated hepatotoxicity Women who are already receiving NVP at the beginning of pregnancy and are tolerating the drug may continue NVP regardless of CD4 count Elevated baseline liver enzymes may increase risk of NVP toxicity No evidence of human teratogenicity

Use in special circumstances: efavirenz (EFV), classified as FDA pregnancy class D; case reports of neural tube defects with first-trimester exposure; relative risk unclear

Insufficient data to recommend use in pregnancy: etravirine (ETR), rilpivirine (RPV)

Protease Inhibitors (PIs)

Lopinavir-ritonavir (LPV/r)	C	AUC decreased in second and third trimester with standard dosing PK studies suggest increase in dosing to 600 mg/150 mg twice a day in second and third trimester, especially in PI-experienced patients Low placental transfer to the fetus	*More frequent:* diarrhea, nausea, vomiting, headache, skin rash in patients receiving other ARVs, lipid abnormalities *Less frequent:* fat redistribution *Rare:* new-onset diabetes mellitus, hyperglycemia, ketoacidosis, hemolytic anemia, pancreatitis, life-threatening hepatitis No evidence of human teratogenicity Well tolerated during pregnancy and safe for mothers and infants in the short-term
Atazanavir boosted with low-dose ritonavir (ATV/r)	C	Standard dosing of ATV/r results in decreased plasma concentrations of the drug in pregnancy Low placental transfer to the fetus	Generally safe Hyperbilirubinemia may need to be monitored No evidence of human teratogenicity

Alternative PIs: darunavir/ritonavir (DRV/r), saquinavir/ritonavir (SQV/r)
Use in special circumstances: indinavir/ritonavir (IDV/r), nelfinavir (NLV)
Insufficient data to recommend use in pregnancy: fosamprenavir (FPV), tipranavir (TPV)

Entry inhibitors: enfuvirtide (T20), maraviroc (MVC)
Insufficient data to recommend use in pregnancy

Integrase inhibitors: raltegravir (RAL)
Use in special circumstances

Abbreviations: AUC, area under the curve; FDA, Food and Drug Administration; PK, pharmacokinetics.
[a]From reference 12.
[b]Combinations of ddI and 3TC and ddI and d4T should not be used with one another because of the association with severe life-threatening lactic acidosis during pregnancy.
[c]Risk of hypersensitivity reaction with ABC (5%–8% of nonpregnant individuals; check HLA-B*5701 before starting ABC).
[d]Limited experience in pregnancy; potential fetal bone effects; tenofovir plus 3TC or FTC are the preferred NRTI pair for HIV-infected women with chronic hepatitis B coinfection.

cohort study demonstrated a significantly lower risk of transmission in women with delivery viral load of less than 400 copies/mL who underwent elective cesarean section compared with vaginal delivery.[105] Currently, scheduled cesarean section at 38 weeks' gestation is recommended for women with viral load greater than 1000 copies/mL or unknown viral load near the time of delivery to reduce the risk of perinatal HIV transmission.[12] Given the low rate of transmission in women receiving ART with plasma viral load below 1000 copies/mL, it is unclear if elective cesarean section would offer any additional benefit; therefore, it is not routinely recommended.[12] The USPHS task force recommendations regarding mode of delivery to

reduce perinatal HIV transmission are summarized in Table 58-11.

Neonatal ARV Prophylaxis

Neonatal ARV prophylaxis must begin as soon as possible after birth, preferably within 12 hours after delivery.[6,12] When the mother has received combination ARV during pregnancy, neonatal ZDV for 6 weeks is the recommended prophylaxis regimen of choice in the United States. When the mother has not received any ARV drugs during pregnancy or during the labor and delivery period, observational data suggest that administration of oral ZDV for 6 weeks to the infant,

Table 58-11 US Public Health Service Guidelines Related to Mode of Delivery for Preventing Perinatal HIV Transmission in Selected Clinical Circumstances[a]

HIV-positive women presenting late in pregnancy (>36 weeks' gestation) not currently on ART and results of viral load and CD4 T-lymphocyte count are unavailable before delivery
- Start combination ART
- Counsel women on the beneficial effect of scheduled cesarean delivery in reducing perinatal HIV transmission if viral suppression cannot be documented before 38 weeks' gestation
- Schedule cesarean delivery at 38 weeks' gestation, as determined by best obstetric dating
- Administer a loading dose of intravenous ZDV followed by continuous intravenous infusion before scheduled cesarean section
- Continue other ARV drugs per schedule during the perioperative period
- Follow standard cesarean delivery management procedures, including use of prophylactic antibiotics

HIV-positive women presenting in the third trimester currently on ART but viral load remains > 1000 copies/mL at 36 weeks' gestation
- Consult HIV specialist for recommendations regarding appropriate ART regimen
- Continue the current combination ART regimen if optimal virus suppression is achieved
- Recommend scheduled cesarean section if optimal viral load suppression not documented by 38 weeks' gestation given the additional beneficial effect in reducing perinatal HIV transmission; discuss the potential risks of operative delivery with woman (eg, anesthesia, surgery, and postoperative infection)
- Perform scheduled cesarean delivery at 38 weeks' gestation as determined by best obstetric dating
- Administer a loading dose of intravenous ZDV followed by continuous intravenous infusion before scheduled cesarean section
- Continue other ARV drugs per schedule during the perioperative period
- Follow standard cesarean delivery management procedures, including use of prophylactic antibiotics

HIV-positive pregnant women who are currently receiving combination ART and have undetectable viral load at 36 weeks' gestation
- Counsel mothers on the very low risk (<1%) of perinatal HIV with undetectable viral load, even with a vaginal delivery and lack of evidence of additional benefit of scheduled cesarean section in such circumstances
- Discuss the potential risks and uncertain benefits of cesarean delivery compared to vaginal delivery in women with undetectable viral load

HIV-positive pregnant women with viral load > 1000 copies/mL who have opted for scheduled cesarean delivery but present after membrane rupture or onset of labor at > 37 weeks' gestation
- Immediate initiation of intravenous ZDV
- Decisions regarding mode of delivery should be individualized, taking into consideration several factors affecting perinatal transmission of HIV, including duration of membrane rupture or labor, maternal viral load, and current ART regimen
- Vaginal delivery management (if selected) should be individualized; invasive procedures (such as scalp electrodes, invasive monitoring, and operative delivery); if clinically indicated, some experts recommend oxytocin to expedite delivery
- Cesarean section (if selected), if feasible, loading dose of intravenous ZDV must be administered and completed prior to the procedure

Abbreviations: ARV, antiretroviral; ART, antiretroviral therapy; ZDV, zidovudine.
[a]Data from reference 12.

when started within 24 hours after birth, may provide some benefit against transmission.[106] A recent multicountry study (NICHD-HPTN 040) of 1735 formula-fed infants whose mothers did not receive any ARV drugs during pregnancy and before labor demonstrated that combination infant ARV prophylaxis regimens consisting of ZDV for 6 weeks plus a 3-dose NVP treatment during the first week of life (birth and 48 and 96 hours of life) or ZDV plus 3TC plus NLV given from birth to 2 weeks of life reduced intrapartum transmission by approximately 50% compared with a ZDV-only infant prophylaxis regimen.[107] Because the 3-drug regimen is relatively toxic, current guidelines recommend the equally effective 2-drug neonatal prophylaxis regimen.[6,12]

Avoidance of Breast-Feeding

Because of the documented risk of postnatal HIV transmission through breast-feeding, HIV-infected mothers should be advised not to breast-feed their infants in the United States and other resource-rich countries where infant formulas are safe and readily available.

Success, Challenges, and Opportunities

Despite significant advances in perinatal HIV prevention, around 150 HIV-infected babies are born annually in the United States, primarily because of missed prevention opportunities, resulting from inadequate prenatal care, lack of antenatal HIV testing, and low maintenance of care for some subpopulations.[108] Knowledge of a woman's HIV status during labor is crucial for providing ARV prophylaxis for those who test positive and their babies to prevent perinatal transmission.[109] Routine antenatal HIV testing (opt-out approach) is recommended for all women as soon as pregnancy is confirmed. To reduce missed prevention opportunities, repeat testing in the third trimester of pregnancy is recommended for high-risk women to detect new infections as well as rapid HIV testing of women who present in labor with unknown HIV status.[101,102] Other challenges include preventing new-incident HIV infections in women of childbearing age, especially adolescent girls of minority race or ethnicity, and delayed diagnosis of HIV in some pregnant women.[1] The CDC has collaborated with 4 national organizations to form the National Organizations' Collaborative to Eliminate Perinatal HIV in the United States to end perinatal HIV transmission. Finally, development of a safe and effective vaccine and the use of passive immunization strategies to prevent MTCT, especially during breast-feeding, remain a top priority for perinatal HIV prevention in resource-limited settings.[110]

Table 58-12 **Factors Associated With Rapid Disease Progression in HIV-Infected Infants and Children**[a]

- Intrauterine transmission
- High HIV RNA concentrations in infants
- Specific HLA genotypes (HLA-DR3, C4A, DQB1*0604)
- Presence and maintenance of HIV-specific CD4 responses
- Thymic dysfunction
- Lack of receipt of perinatal zidovudine prophylaxis
- Enhanced viral fitness
- Poorer maternal health

[a]Data from reference 95.

OUTCOME AND FOLLOW-UP

Without ART, the risk of mortality[70] in HIV-infected children residing in the United States and Europe is 10%–20% but access to combination ART including PIs has significantly improved survival.[111] In contrast, data from Africa showed that about a third of children with HIV infection died by their first birthday and more than half by the age of 2 years.[112] The clinical course of HIV infection in children differs greatly from infected adults.[70] Studies from developed countries and sub-Saharan Africa indicated that HIV disease often progresses more rapidly in infants than in adults.[112]

Infants with perinatally acquired HIV infection have widely variable clinical courses and durations of survival. Early reports suggested a bimodal disease expression with 20%–25% of untreated HIV-infected infants rapidly progressing to AIDS or death over the first year of life, while others had a more slowly developing illness with a better prognosis, some now surviving into young adulthood.[113] These studies of the natural history of perinatal HIV infection were performed before the routine use of ART.

Infants with intrauterine or intrapartum acquisition of infection have the fastest disease progression (Table 58-12).[95,112] Factors associated with poor prognosis for untreated vertically infected infants include a high virus load (>100,000 copies/mL), severe immunosuppression, and early onset of AIDS-defining conditions (such as PCP and HIV encephalopathy or severe wasting).[6] In contrast, slow loss of CD4 count, late onset of clinical symptoms, and occurrence of LIP are associated with improved survival. Children born to mothers with advanced disease, low CD4 counts, and high viral load tend to progress more rapidly to category C disease or death, emphasizing the importance of diagnosis and adequate treatment of HIV-infected pregnant women.[114]

With the introduction of HAART, the natural history of HIV infection in children has changed significantly in resource-rich settings. Early initiation of ART in HIV-infected children leads to dramatic decreases in the morbidity and mortality rates.[3,5] In the United States, mortality in HIV-infected children decreased from 7.2/100 person-years in 1993 to 0.8/100 person-years in 2006. Although deaths related to OIs have decreased significantly, non-AIDS-defining infections and multiorgan failure remain major causes of death.[6] Other challenges for physicians are related to provision of lifelong care to HIV-infected children, addressing issues related to ART compliance and toxicity, resistance and treatment failure, transition through adolescence and adult care, and quality of life.

REFERENCES

1. Fowler MG, Gable AR, Lampe MA, Etima M, Owor M. Perinatal HIV and its prevention: progress towards an HIV-free generation. *Clin Perinatol.* 2010;37(4):699–719.

2. Centers for Disease Control. Unexplained immunodeficiency and opportunistic infections in infants—New York, New Jersey, California. *MMWR Morb Mortal Wkly Rep.* 1982;31(49):665–667.

3. Hazra R, Siberry GK, Mofenson LM. Growing up with HIV: children, adolescents and young adults with perinatally acquired HIV infection. *Annu Rev Med.* 2010;61:169–185.

4. De Cock KM, Jaffe HW, Curran JW. The evolving epidemiology of HIV/AIDS. *AIDS.* 2012;26(10):1205–1213.

5. Brady MT, Oleske JM, Williams PL, et al. Decline in mortality rates and changes in causes of death in HIV-1 infected children during the HAART era. *J Acquir Immune Defic Syndr.* 2010;53:86–94.

6. American Academy of Pediatrics. Human immunodeficiency virus infection. In: Pickering LK, Baker CJ, Kimberlin DW, Long SS, eds. *Red Book.* 28th ed. Elk Grove Village, IL: American Academy of Pediatrics; 2012:418–437.

7. Read JS. Prevention of mother-to-child transmission of HIV: antiretroviral strategies. *Clin Perinatol.* 2010;37(4):765–776.

8. Mepham SO, Bland RM, Newell ML. Prevention of mother-to-child transmission of HIV in resource-rich and -poor settings. *BJOG.* 2011;118(2):202–218.

9. Forbes JC, Alimenti AM, Singer J, et al. A national review of vertical HIV transmission. *AIDS.* 2012;26(6):757–763.

10. Connor EM, Sperling RS, Gelber R, et al. Reduction of maternal-infant transmission of human immunodeficiency virus type 1 with zidovudine treatment. *N Engl J Med.* 1994;331(18):1173–1180.

11. Centers for Disease Control and Prevention. US Public Health Service recommendations for human immunodeficiency virus counseling and voluntary testing for pregnant women. *MMWR Morb Mortal Wkly Rep.* 1995;44(RR-7):1–15.

12. Panel on Treatment of HIV-Infected Pregnant Women and Prevention of Perinatal Transmission. Recommendations for use of antiretroviral drugs in pregnant HIV-1 infected women for maternal health and interventions to reduce HIV-1 transmission. December 2011:1–117. http://aidsinfo.nih.gov/guidelines. Accessed July 29, 2012

13. Cooper ER, Charurat M, Mofenson LM, et al. Combination antiretroviral strategies for treatment of pregnant HIV-infected women and prevention of perinatal HIV-1 transmission. *J Acquir Immune Defic Syndr.* 2002; 29(5):484–494.

14. Townsend CL, Cortina-Borja M, Peckham CS, de Ruiter A, Lyall H, Tookey PA. Low rates of mother-to-child transmission of HIV following effective pregnancy interventions in the United Kingdom and Ireland, 2000–2006. *AIDS.* 2008;22(8):973–981.

15. Centers for Disease Control and Prevention. *HIV/AIDS Surveillance Report.* Vol. 21. 2009. http://www.cdc.gov/hiv/surveillance/resources/reports/2009report/#commentary. Accessed July 29, 2012

16. Fowler MG, Kourtis AP, Aizire J, Onyango-Mukumbi C, Bulterys M. Breastfeeding and transmission of HIV-1: epidemiology and global magnitude. *Adv Exp Med Biol.* 2012;743:3–25.

17. Mofenson LM. Antiretroviral drugs to prevent breastfeeding HIV transmission. *Antivir Ther.* 2010;15(4):537–553.

18. Mofenson LM. Prevention in neglected subpopulations: prevention of mother-to-child transmission of HIV infection. *Clin Infect Dis.* 2010;50(Suppl 3):S130–S148.

19. Tudor Car L, Van Velthoven MH, Brusamento S. Integrating prevention of mother-to-child HIV transmission programs to improve uptake: a systematic review. *PLoS One.* 2012;7(4):e35268. Epub 2012 Apr 27.

20. WHO, UNAIDS, and UNICEF. *Global HIV/AIDS Response: Epidemic Update and Health Sector Progress Towards Universal Access: Progress Report 2011.* Geneva, Switzerland: WHO; 2011. http://whqlibdoc.who.int/publications/2011/9789241502986_eng.pdf. Accessed July 29, 2012.

21. Joint United Nations Program on HIV/AIDS (UNAIDS). *Together We Will End AIDS.* Geneva, Switzerland: UNAIDS; 2012. http://whqlibdoc.who.int/publications/2011/9789241502986_eng.pdf. Accessed July 29, 2012.

22. Centers for Disease Control and Prevention (CDC). HIV surveillance-United States, 1981–2008. *MMWR Morb Mortal Wkly Rep.* 2011;60(21):689–693.

23. Prejean J, Song R, Hernandez A, Ziebell R, Green T, et al. Estimated HIV incidence in the United States, 2006–2009. *PLoS ONE.* 2011;6(8):e17502.

24. Fauci AS, Folkers GK. Towards an AIDS-free generation. *JAMA.* 2012;308(4):343–344.

25. Centers for Disease Control and Prevention (CDC). *Fact Sheet: HIV in the United States: At a Glance.* March 2012. http://cdc.gov/hiv/resources/factsheets/us.htm. Accessed July 15, 2012.

26. Centers for Disease Control and Prevention. *Fact Sheet: Estimates of New HIV Infections in the United States, 2006–2009.* Atlanta, GA: US Department of Health and Human Services, Centers for Disease Control and Prevention; August 2011.

27. Aral SO, Adimora AA, Fenton KA. Understanding and responding to the HIV and other sexually transmitted infections in African Americans. *Lancet.* 2008;372(9635):337–340.

28. Centers for Disease Control and Prevention. *HIV/AIDS Surveillance Report.* 2007:19. Atlanta, GA: US Department of Health and Human Services, Centers for Disease Control and Prevention; 2009. http:www.cdc.gov/hiv/topics/surveillance/resources/reports/. Accessed July 30, 2012.

29. Lindegren ML, Steinberg S, Byers RH Jr. Epidemiology of HIV/AIDS in children. *Pediatr Clin N Am.* 2000;47(1):1–20.

30. Zhang X, Rhodes P, Blair J. Estimated number of perinatal HIV infections in the United States, 2005–2009. In: Programs and Abstracts of the National HIV Prevention Conference 2009; August 23–29, 2009; Atlanta, GA.

31. Centers for Disease Control and Prevention (CDC). Racial/ethnic disparities among children with diagnoses of perinatal HIV infection-34 states, 2004–2007. *MMWR Morb Mortal Wkly Rep.* 2010;59(4):97–101.

32. Buonaguro L, Tornesello ML, Buonaguro FM. Human immunodeficiency virus type 1 subtype distribution in the worldwide epidemic: pathogenetic and therapeutic implications. *J Virol.* 2007;81(19):10209–10219.

33. Engelman A, Cherepanov P. The structural biology of HIV-1: mechanistic and therapeutic insights. *Nat Rev Microbiol.* 2012;10(4):279–290.

34. Fauci AS, Pantaleo G, Stanley S, Weissman D. Immuno-pathogenic mechanisms of HIV infection. *Ann Intern Med.* 1996;124(7):654–663.

35. DeCock KM, Fowler MG, Mercier E, et al. Prevention of mother-to-child transmission of HIV infection in resource-poor settings. Translating research into policy and practice. *JAMA.* 2000;283(9):1175–1182.

36. Cavarelli M, Scarlatti G. Human immunodeficiency virus type 1 mother-to-child transmission and prevention: successes and controversies. *J Intern Med.* 2011;270(6):561–579.

37. Simonon A, Lepage P, Karita E, et al. An assessment of the timing of mother-to-child transmission of human immunodeficiency virus type 1 by means of polymerase chain reaction. *J Acquir Immune Defic Syndr.* 1994;7(9):952–957.

38. Bryson YJ, Luzuriaga K, Sullivan JL, et al. Proposed definitions for in utero versus intrapartum transmission of HIV-1. *N Engl J Med.* 1992;327:1246–1247.

39. Lewis SH, Reynolds-Kohler C, Fox HE, Nelson JA. HIV-1 in trophoblastic and villous Hofbauer cells, and haematological precursors in eight-week fetuses. *Lancet.* 1990;335(8689):565–568.

40. Brossard Y, Aubin JT, Mandelbrot L, et al. Frequency of early in utero HIV-1 infection: a blind DNA polymerase chain reaction study on 100 fetal thymuses. *AIDS.* 1995;9(4):359–366.

41. Van Dyke RB, Korber BT, Popek E, et al. The Ariel Project: a prospective cohort study of maternal-child transmission of human immunodeficiency virus type 1 in the era of maternal antiretroviral therapy. *J Infect Dis.* 1999;179(2):319–328.

42. Kourtis AP, Lee FK, Abrams EJ, et al. Mother-to-child transmission of HIV-1: timing and implications for prevention. *Lancet Infect Dis.* 2006;6(11):726–732.

43. Newell ML. Mechanisms and timing of mother-to-child transmission of HIV-1. *AIDS.* 1998;12:831–837.

44. Kaneda T, Shiraki K, Hirano K, et al. Detection of maternofetal transfusion by placental alkaline phosphatase levels. *J Pediatr.* 1997;130(5):730–735.

45. Rogers MF, Ou CY, Rayfield M, et al. Use of the polymerase chain reaction for early detection of the proviral sequences of human immunodeficiency virus in infants born to seropositive mothers. *N Engl J Med.* 1989;320:1649–1654.

46. Goedert JJ, Duliege AM, Amos CI, Felton S, Biggar RJ. High risk of HIV-1 infection for firstborn twins. *Lancet.* 1991;338(8781):1471–1475.

47. European Mode of Delivery Collaboration. Elective caesarean-section versus vaginal delivery in prevention of vertical HIV-1 transmission: a randomised clinical trial. *Lancet.* 1999;353(9158):1035–1039.

48. The International Perinatal HIV Group. The mode of delivery and the risk of vertical transmission of human immunodeficiency virus type 1—a meta-analysis of 15 prospective cohort studies. *N Engl J Med.* 1999;340(13):977–987.

49. Boer K, England K, Godfried MH, et al. Mode of delivery in HIV-infected pregnant women and prevention of mother-to-child transmission: changing practices in Western Europe. *HIV Med.* 2010;11(6):368–378.

50. Brahmbhatt H, Sullivan D, Kigozi G, et al. Association of HIV and malaria with mother-to-child transmission, birth outcomes, and child mortality. *J Acquir Immune Defic Syndr.* 2008;47(4):472–476.

51. Inion I, Mwanyumba F, Gaillard P, et al. Placental malaria and perinatal transmission of human immunodeficiency virus type 1. *J Infect Dis.* 2003;188(11):1675–1678.

52. Bulterys M, Ellington S, Kourtis AP. HIV-1 and breastfeeding: biology of transmission and advances in prevention. *Clin Perinatol.* 2010;37(4):807–824.

53. Fowler MG, Kourtis AP, Aizire J, Makumbi, Bulterys M, Ellington S. HIV-1 and breastfeeding: biology of transmission and advances in prevention. *Clin Perinatol.* 2010;743:807–824.

54. Rousseau CM, Nduati RW, Richardson BA, et al. Longitudinal analysis of HIV-1 RNA in breast milk and its relationship to infant infection and maternal disease. *J Infect Dis.* 2003;187(5):741–747.

55. Koulinska IN, Villamor E, Chaplin B, Msamanga G, Fawzi W, Renjifo B, Essex M. Transmission of cell-free and cell-associated HIV-1 through breastfeeding. *Virus Res.* 2006;41(1)120:93–99.

56. Coutsoudis A, Dabis F, Fawzi W, et al. Late postnatal transmission of HIV-1 in breastfed children: an individual patient data meta-analysis. *J Infect Dis.* 189(12):2154–2166.

57. Magder LS, Mofenson L, Paul ME, et al. Risk factors for in utero and intrapartum transmission of HIV. *J Acquir Immune Defic Syndr.* 2005;38(1):87–95.

58. Garcia P, Kalish LA, Pitt J, et al. Maternal levels of plasma human immunodeficiency virus type-1 RNA and the risk of perinatal transmission. *N Engl J Med.* 1999;341(6):394–402.

59. Tubiana R, Le Chenadec J, Rouzioux C, et al. Factors associated with mother-to-child transmission of HIV-1 despite a maternal viral load <500 copies/ml at delivery: a case-control study nested in the French perinatal cohort (EPF-ANRS CO1). *Clin Infect Dis.* 2010;50(4):585–596.

60. Chuachoowong R, Shaffer N, Siriwasin W, et al. Short-course antenatal zidovudine reduces both cervicovaginal human immunodeficiency virus type 1 RNA levels and risk of perinatal transmission. Bangkok Collaborative Perinatal HIV Transmission Study Group. *J Infect Dis.* 2000;181(1):99–106.

61. Cowan FM, Humphrey JH, Ntozini R, Mutasa K, Morrow R, Iliff P. Maternal herpes simplex virus type 2 infection, syphilis and risk of intra-partum transmission of HIV-1: results of a case control study. *AIDS.* 2008;22(2):193–201.

62. England K, Thorne C, Newell M. Vertically acquired paediatric coinfection with HIV and hepatitis C virus. *Lancet.* 2006;6(2):83–90.

63. Vogler MA, Singh R, Wright R. Complex decisions in managing HIV infection during pregnancy. *Curr HIV/AIDS Rep.* 2011;8:122–131.

64. Galli L, Puliti D, Chiappini E, Gabiano C, Ferraris G, Mignone F, et al. Is the interruption of antiretroviral treatment during pregnancy an additional major risk factor for mother-to-child transmission of HIV type 1? *Clin Infect Dis.* 2009;48:1310–1317.

65. Mofenson LM, Lambert JS, Stiehm ER, et al. Pediatric AIDS Clinical Trials Group Study 185 Team. Risk factors for perinatal transmission of human immunodeficiency virus type 1 in women treated with zidovudine. *N Engl J Med.* 1999;341(6):385–393.

66. Kishko M, Somasundaran M, Brewster F, Sullivan JL, Clapham PR, Luzuriaga K. Genotypic and functional properties of early infant HIV-1 envelopes. *Retrovirology.* 2011;15;8:67.

67. Renjifo B, Gilbert P, Chaplin B, Msamanga G, Mwakagile D, Fawzi W, Essex M. Preferential in-utero transmission of HIV-1 subtype C as compared to HIV-1 subtype A or D. *AIDS.* 2004;18:1629–1636.

68. Mackelprang RD, John-Stewart G, Carrington M, et al. Maternal HLA homozygosity and mother-child HLA concordance increase the risk of vertical transmission of HIV-1. *J Infect Dis.* 2008;197:1156–1161.

69. Contopoulos-Ioannidis DG, O'Brien TR, Goedert JJ, Rosenberg PS, Ioannidis JP. Effect of CCR5-delta32 heterozygosity on the risk of perinatal HIV-1 infection: a meta-analysis. *J Acquir Immune Defic Syndr.* 2003,32(1):70–76.

70. Prendergast A, Tudor-Williams G, Jeena P, et al. International perspectives, progress, and future challenges of paediatric HIV infection. *Lancet.* 2007;370(9581):68–80.

71. Kourtis AP, Bulterys M. Mother-to-child transmission of HIV: pathogenesis, mechanisms and pathways. *Clin Perinatol.* 2010;37(4):721–737.

72. Ahmad N. Molecular mechanisms of HIV-1 mother-to-child transmission and infection in neonatal target cells. *Life Sci.* 2011;88(21–22):980–986.

73. Mehandru S, Poles MA, Tenner-Racz K, et al. Primary HIV-1 infection is associated with preferential depletion of CD4⁺ T lymphocytes from effector sites in the gastrointestinal tract. *J Exp Med.* 2004;200(6):761–770.

74. Kuhn, L, Abrams EJ, Palumbo P, et al. Maternal versus paternal inheritance of HLA class I alleles among HIV-infected children: consequences for clinical disease progression. *AIDS.* 2004;18(9):1281–1289.

75. Luzuriaga, K., Newell ML, Dabis F, Excler JL, Sullivan JL. Vaccines to prevent transmission of HIV-1 via breastmilk: scientific and logistical priorities. *Lancet.* 2006;368(9534):511–521.

76. Lohman BL, Slyker JA, Richardson BA, et al. Longitudinal assessment of human immunodeficiency virus type-1 (HIV-1)-specific gamma interferon responses during the first year of life in HIV-1 infected infants. *J Virol.* 2005;79(13):8121–8130.

77. Feeney ME, Tang Y, Pfafferott K, et al. HIV-1 viral escape in infancy followed by emergence of a variant-specific CTL response. *J Immunol.* 2005;174(12):7524–7530.

78. Obaro SK, Pugatch D, Luzuriaga K. Immunogenicity and efficacy of childhood vaccines in HIV-1-infected children. *Lancet Infect Dis.* 2004;4(8):510–518.

79. Lobato MN, Caldwell MB, Ng P, Oxtoby MJ. Encephalopathy in children with perinatally acquired human immunodeficiency virus infection. *J Pediatr.* 1995;126(5 Pt 1):710–715.

80. Chiriboga CA, Fleishman S, Champion S, Gaye-Robinson L, Abrams EJ. Incidence and prevalence of HIV encephalopathy in children with HIV infection receiving highly active anti-retroviral therapy (HAART). *J Pediatr.* 2005;146(3):402–407.

81. Mitchell CD. HIV-1 encephalopathy among perinatally infected children: Neuropathogenesis and response to highly active antiretroviral therapy. *Ment Retard Dev Disabil Res Rev.* 2006;12(3):216–222.

82. Cooper ER, Hanson C, Diaz C, et al. Encephalopathy and progression of human immunodeficiency virus disease in a cohort of children with perinatally acquired human immunodeficiency virus infection. Women and Infants Transmission Study Group. *J Pediatr.* 1998;132(5):808–812.

83. Patel K, Ming X, Williams PL, et al. Impact of HAART and CNS-penetrating antiretroviral regimens on HIV encephalopathy among perinatally infected children and adolescents. *AIDS.* 2009;23(14):1893–1901.

84. Van Rie A, Harrington PR, Dow A, Robertson K. Neurologic and neurodevelopmental manifestations of pediatric HIV/AIDS: a global perspective. *Eur J Paediatr Neurol.* 2007;11(1):1–9.

85. Nesheim SR, Kapogiannis BG, Soe MM, et al. Trends in opportunistic infections in the pre- and post-highly active antiretroviral therapy eras among HIV-infected children in the Perinatal AIDS Collaborative Study, 1986–2004. *Pediatrics.* 2007;120(1):100–109.

86. Centers for Disease Control and Prevention Revision of the CDC surveillance case definition for acquired immunodeficiency syndrome. *MMWR Morb Mortal Wkly Rep.* 1987;36(Suppl 1):1–15.

87. Centers for Disease Control and Prevention. 1993 Revised classification system for HIV infection and expanded surveillance case definition for AIDS among adolescents and adults. *MMWR Morb Mortal Wkly Rep.* 1992;41(RR-17):1–19.

88. Centers for Disease Control and Prevention. 1994 Revised classification system for human immunodeficiency virus infection in children less than 13 years of age. *MMWR Morb Mortal Wkly Rep.* 1994;43(RR-12):1.

89. Centers for Disease Control and Prevention. Revised surveillance case definitions for HIV infection among adults, adolescents, and children aged <18 months and for HIV Infection and

AIDS among children aged 18 months to < 13 years—United States, 2008. *MMWR Morb Mortal Wkly Rep.* 2008;57:1.

90. Havens PL, Mofenson LM and American Academy of Pediatrics, Committee on Pediatric AIDS. HIV testing and prophylaxis to prevent mother-to-child transmission in the United States. *Pediatrics.* 2008;122(5):1127–1134.

91. Read JS and American Academy of Pediatrics, Committee on Pediatric AIDS. Diagnosis of HIV infection in children younger than 18 months in the United States. *Pediatrics.* 2007;120:(6): e1547–e1562.

92. King SM; American Academy of Pediatrics, Committee on Pediatric AIDS. Evaluation and treatment of the human immunodeficiency virus-1-exposed infant. *Pediatrics.* 2004;114(2):497–505.

93. Lambert JS, Harris DR, Stiehm ER, et al. Performance characteristics of HIV-1 culture and HIV-1 DNA and RNA amplification assays for early diagnosis of perinatal HIV-1 infection. *J Acquir Immune Defic Syndr.* 2003;34(5):512–519.

94. Kline NE, Schwarzwald H, Kline MW. False negative DNA polymerase chain reaction in an infant with subtype C human immunodeficiency virus 1 infection. *Pediatr Infect Dis J.* 2002;21(9):885–886.

95. Camacho-Gonzalez AF, Ross AC, Chakraborty R. The clinical care of the HIV-1 infected infant. *Clin Perinatol.* 2010;37(4):873–885.

96. Panel on Antiretroviral Therapy and Medical Management of HIV-Infected Children. Guidelines for the use of antiretroviral agents in pediatric HIV infection. August 11, 2011:1–268.

97. Mofenson LM, Brady MT, Danner ST, et al. Guidelines for prevention and treatment of opportunistic infections among HIV-exposed and HIV-infected children. Recommendations from CDC, the National Institutes of Health, the HIV Medicine Association of the Infectious Diseases Society of America, the Pediatric Infectious Disease Society, and the American Academy of Pediatrics. *MMWR Recomm Rep.* 2009;58(RR-11):1–166.

98. Violari A, Cotton MF, Gibb DM, et al. Early antiretroviral therapy and mortality among HIV-infected infants. *N Engl J Med.* 2008;359(21):2233–2244.

99. Peacock-Villada E, Richardson BA, John-Stewart GC. Post-HAART outcomes in pediatric populations: comparison of resource-limited and developed countries. *Pediatrics.* 2011;127(2):e423–e441.

100. Heidari S, Mofenson LM, Hobbs CV, Cotton MF, Marlink R, Katabira E. Unresolved antiretroviral treatment management issues in HIV-infected children. *J Acquir Immune Defic Syndr.* 2012;59(2):161–169.

101. Branson BM, Handsfield HH, Lampe MA, et al. Revised recommendations for HIV testing of adults, adolescents, and pregnant women in health-care settings. *MMWR Recomm Rep.* 2006;55(RR-14):1–17.

102. Centers for Disease Control and Prevention. Revised guidelines for HIV counseling, testing, and referral and revised recommendations for HIV screening of pregnant women. *MMWR Morb Mortal Wkly Rep.* 2001;50(RR-19):1–110.

103. Sperling RS, Shapiro DE, Coombs RW, et al. Maternal viral load, zidovudine treatment, and the risk of transmission of human immunodeficiency virus type 1 from mother to infant. Pediatric AIDS Clinical Trials Group Protocol 076 Study Group. *N Engl J Med.* 1996;335(22):1621–1629.

104. Cohen MS, Chen YQ, McCauley M, et al; HPTN 052 Study Team. Prevention of HIV-1 infection with early antiretroviral therapy. *N Engl J Med.* 2011;365(6):493–505.

105. Boer K, England K, Godfried HM, Thorne C. Mode of delivery in HIV-infected pregnant women and prevention of mother-to-child transmission: changing practices in Western Europe. *HIV Med.* 2010;11(6):368–378.

106. Wade NA, Birkhead GS, Warren BL, et al. Abbreviated regimens of zidovudine prophylaxis and perinatal

transmission of the human immunodeficiency virus. *N Engl J Med*. 1998;339(20):1409–1414.

107. Nielsen-Saines K, Watts DH, Veloso VG, et al. Three postpartum antiretroviral regimens to prevent intrapartum HIV infection. *N Engl J Med*. 2012;366(25):2368–2379.

108. Peters V, Liu K, Dominiguez K, et al. Missed opportunities for perinatal HIV prevention among HIV-exposed infants born 1996–2000, pediatric spectrum of HIV disease cohort. *Pediatrics*. 2003;111(5):1186–1191.

109. Bulterys M, Jameison DJ, O'Sullivan MJ, et al. Rapid HIV-1 testing during labor: a multicenter study. *J AMA*. 2004;292(2):219–233.

110. Mofenson LM. Prevention of mother-to-child HIV-1 transmission—why we still need a preventive HIV immunization strategy? *J Acquir Immune Defic Syndr*. 2011;58(4):359–362.

111. Gortmaker SL, Hughes M, Cervia J, et al. Effect of combination therapy including protease inhibitors on mortality among children and adolescents infected with HIV-1. *N Engl J Med*. 2001;345(21):1522–1528.

112. Newell ML, Coovadia H, Cortina-Borja M, et al. Mortality of infected and uninfected infants born to HIV-infected mothers in Africa: a pooled analysis. *Lancet*. 2004.364(9441):1236–1243.

113. Gray L, Newell ML, Thorne C, et al. Fluctuations in symptoms in human immunodeficiency virus-infected children: the first 10 years of life. *Pediatrics*. 2001;108(1):116–122.

114. Abrams EJ, Wiener J, Carter R, et al. Maternal health factors and early pediatric antiretroviral therapy influence the rate of perinatal HIV-1 disease progression in children. *AIDS*. 2003;17(6):867–877.

Part J: Metabolic-Genetic

59 Neonatal Hyperammonemia

Brendan Lanpher, Uta Lichter-Konecki, Marshall Summar, and Mark L. Batshaw

INTRODUCTION

The most common concern for neonates who present with poor feeding, tachypnea, hypothermia, and lethargy during the first days of life is sepsis; in fact, this is the most likely cause of severe illness. However, it is important to also consider the possibility of an inborn error of metabolism. Although individually these are rare disorders, as a group they probably are present in more than 1 in 5000 live births[1]; if they are not identified early, most die or are left with severe brain damage.

Many inborn errors that present in the newborn period with a catastrophic illness have elevated ammonia levels as a presenting symptom. It is our recommendation that every neonate who is worked up for sepsis should also have a plasma ammonia level drawn. While expanded newborn screening has been helpful in diagnosing a number of causes of neonatal hyperammonia, the results are often not available until the outcome of the disease is unalterable. At best, they become available when the child is showing symptoms and may aid in making the diagnosis. In this chapter, we discuss the clinical presentation, laboratory evaluation, and clinical effects of neonatal hyperammonemia. Chapter 106 provides a clinical management template for intervention in neonatal hyperammonemia.

DEFINING HYPERAMMONEMIA AND OBTAINING A SPECIMEN

Typical plasma ammonia levels in neonates are less than 40 μmol/L, similar to that in older children and adults. Premature infants may have somewhat higher levels (in the range of 40–60 μmol/L) because of the immaturity of their liver function and lower production of arginine during the first few weeks of life.[2] Clinical symptoms attributable to hyperammonemia in the newborn generally occur above levels of 150 μmol/L, and it is not uncommon for neonates with urea cycle disorders to have plasma ammonia levels in the 1000–2000 μmol/L range.

The measurement of plasma ammonia can be affected by the collection technique, so a free-flowing sample is recommended. Plasma, once obtained, should immediately be placed on ice, taken to the laboratory, and analyzed within 30 minutes. With delayed measurement after sample collection, glutamine is deaminated to glutamate, which can lead to false elevation of plasma ammonia. Levels of plasma ammonia over 200 μmol/L in the neonate are highly suggestive of an underlying inborn error of metabolism and require immediate intervention.

CLINICAL PRESENTATION OF HYPERAMMONEMIA IN THE NEONATE

The classic presentation of neonatal hyperammonemia is as a catastrophic illness in the first week of life. Signs and symptoms of hyperammonia in the neonate depend on the proximate cause and the rapidity of ammonia accumulation. In patients with rapidly accumulating ammonia, presentation may occur in the first 2–3 days of life with lethargy and poor feeding. This may progress over a matter of hours to temperature instability, coma, and evidence of increased intracranial pressure.

With more indolent ammonia accumulation, initial presentation may be a poor suck, vomiting, intermittent encephalopathy, and seizures. The symptoms of hyperammonemia may be cryptic and nonspecific early in the course, so assessment of plasma ammonia is critical in any neonate with systemic symptoms without a known or obvious cause.[3-5]

The electroencephalographic (EEG) pattern during hyperammonemic coma is one of low voltage with slow waves and asymmetric delta and theta waves. It may show a burst suppression pattern, and the duration of the interburst interval may correlate with the height of ammonium levels.[6] Neuroimaging studies show cerebral edema with small ventricles, flattening of cerebral gyri, and diffuse low density of white matter; there may also be intracranial hemorrhage.[7]

DIFFERENTIAL DIAGNOSIS OF NEONATAL HYPERAMMONEMIA

Hyperammonemia is the result of either primary or secondary failure of nitrogen clearance. Ammonia is generated by the breakdown of amino acids and is converted into urea via the urea cycle (Figure 59-1). Hyperammonemia can result from primary failure of the urea cycle (urea cycle disorders); secondary impairment of the urea cycle by other inborn errors of metabolism (eg, organic acidemias, fatty acid oxidation [FAO] defects, mitochondrial disorders); generalized liver failure; or mechanical or clinical disease that increases protein breakdown that overwhelms the urea cycle (eg, port-systemic shunt, sepsis, crush injuries, and status epilepticus).

In the newborn period, hyperammonemia due to an inborn error of metabolism has a similar presentation to a number of acquired conditions, including sepsis, intracranial hemorrhage, congenital heart disease, and acute gastrointestinal events such as intussusception or volvulus. As noted, the measurement of plasma ammonia levels is critical for distinguishing between these conditions. The acquired disorders generally do not have significant elevations in ammonium levels, but the inborn errors of metabolism do. On the other hand, elevated lactate levels may be seen at initial presentation in all of these conditions other than urea cycle disorders.

A number of inborn errors of metabolism can cause hyperammonemia; these include urea cycle disorders, organic acidemias, nonketotic hyperglycinemia, congenital lactic acidoses, lysinuric protein intolerance, and FAO disorders. Lysinuric protein intolerance, however, rarely presents in the newborn period, and only rare severe long-chain FAO disorders present with hyperammonemia in the newborn.

Once hyperammonemia is identified, widely available tests with rapid turnaround times help narrow the differential diagnosis and guide initial intervention. First-line tests that should be collected after hyperammonemia is identified include a comprehensive metabolic panel, urinalysis, and arterial blood gas. If coagulopathy and elevated transaminases are present, then generalized hepatic failure is likely the cause. If not, then a specific inherited metabolic disease or structural anomaly leading to hyperammonemia must be considered.

Often, the first available laboratory data are the blood gas results. Respiratory alkalosis in the setting

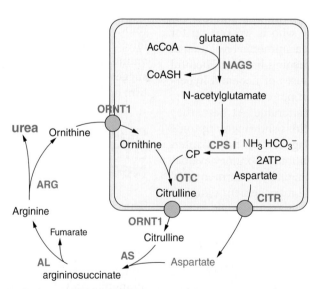

FIGURE 59-1 The urea cycle. AcCoA, acetyl-coenzyme A; AL, argininosuccinate lyase; Arg, arginase; AS, argininosuccinate synthetase; CITR, citrin; CoASh, coenzyme A; CPSI, carbamylphosphate synthetase I; NAGS, *N*-acetylglutamate synthetase; ORN1, ornithine translocase; OTC, ornithine transcarbamylase.

of hyperammonemia is specific and typical for primary urea cycle disorders. Acidosis would be consistent with an organic academia, congenital lactic acidosis, sepsis, or other causes of hyperammonemia. An elevated anion gap is typical in organic acidemias. Urinalysis for ketone measurement is fast and useful as ketones are unusual in neonates, even when critically ill. Significant ketone accumulation is suggestive of an organic acidemia. Standard electrolyte measurement can provide information about an elevated anion gap (which would suggest an organic acidemia or lactic acidosis). A low or absent serum urea nitrogen (BUN) may be seen with impaired urea cycle function. Liver function tests (coagulation profiles and transaminases) may reveal global hepatic dysfunction.[8]

Additional laboratory tests to be collected immediately include plasma amino acid (PAA) analysis, urine organic acid analysis, and plasma acylcarnitine profile. The results for these tests will not likely be available until after intervention has begun, but they will help identify the underlying cause for the hyperammonemia and guide more specific treatment.

Other clinical signs and symptoms may help narrow the differential diagnosis. In the organic acidemias (eg, propionic acidemia, methylmalonic acidemia, isovaleric acidemia, glutaric acidemia type II, and multiple carboxylase deficiency), hypoglycemia and pancytopenia may also be present. Mass spectrometric analysis of urine organic acids or blood acylcarnitine profile will yield the specific diagnosis. In these disorders, PAA analysis (but not cerebrospinal fluid [CSF]) may show an elevated glycine level, from which the initial name, ketotic hyperglycinemia, was derived. This is contrasted with nonketotic hyperglycinemia, in which there is the absence of ketosis, elevated glycine levels in both plasma and CSF, and an increased CSF/plasma glycine ratio.[9]

Fatty acid oxidation defects are caused by different chain length acyl-coenzyme A dehydrogenase deficiencies. Patients with these disorders typically present with hypoglycemia and no or little ketosis. There may be signs of liver disease and often heart involvement. Patients with severe long-chain FAO disorders occasionally present with hyperammonemia in the newborn period. Urinary organic acids show a dicarboxylic aciduria; plasma carnitine levels may be low, and abnormal acylcarnitine species are found.[10]

Congenital lactic acidosis can be the result of a primary deficiency of pyruvate carboxylase or pyruvate dehydrogenase or can be secondary to a defect within the mitochondrial respiratory chain. The principal biochemical finding is lactic acidosis. In pyruvate dehydrogenase deficiency and mild pyruvate carboxylase deficiency, the ratio of lactate to pyruvate is maintained at 10–20:1. In severe pyruvate carboxylase deficiency, mitochondrial respiratory chain defects, and secondary lactic acidosis, however, this ratio is significantly increased.[11] In these oxidative phosphorylation defects and in other mitochondrial diseases, the 3-hydroxybutyrate/acetoacetate ratio is also elevated.

Patients with primary urea cycle disorders show a normal urinary organic acid profile, and the plasma lactate level is generally normal or mildly increased. Although peak plasma ammonium levels are typically in the range of 100–500 μmol/L in organic acidemia and congenital lactic acidosis, in neonatal onset urea cycle disorders they are generally above 500 μmol/L.

Plasma amino acid patterns are also distinct in urea cycle disorders (Figure 59-2), with low levels of arginine and abnormal (low or high) levels of citrulline. Citrulline is the product of carbamyl phosphate synthetase (CPSI) and ornithine transcarbamylase (OTC) and the substrate for argininosuccinate synthetase (AS) and argininosuccinate lyase (AL). Thus, its level is absent in *N*-acetyl-glutamate synthetase (NAGS), CPSI, and OTC deficiencies, and it is markedly elevated in AS and AL deficiencies.[12] Differentiation of AS from AL deficiencies depends on finding argininosuccinic acid (ASA) in plasma and urine in AL deficiency. In ornithine translocase deficiency (HHH syndrome), there is accumulation of homocitrulline in the urine, and in argininemia, very high arginine levels are observed. HHH syndrome, however, has not been described as causing neonatal illness, and argininemia rarely presents in the neonatal period.[13]

Distinction of CPSI from OTC deficiency is dependent on detecting excessive urinary orotic acid excretion in OTC deficiency and normal or decreased excretion in CPSI deficiency. A deficiency of NAGS is biochemically similar to CPSI deficiency, with low or normal orotic acid excretion.[14]

In summary, it is likely that measurement of ammonium, amino acids, and lactate in blood and of amino acids, organic acids, and orotic acid in urine will identify almost all genetic causes of neonatal hyperammonemia. Confirmation of the diagnosis may require enzymatic or mutation analyses but is not necessary prior to beginning treatment.

TREATMENT OF NEONATAL HYPERAMMONEMIC COMA

The treatment of neonatal hyperammonemic coma requires a highly coordinated team of specialists.[15,16] Emergency management is based on 3 interdependent principles: (1) physical removal of the ammonia by dialysis; (2) reversal of the catabolic state

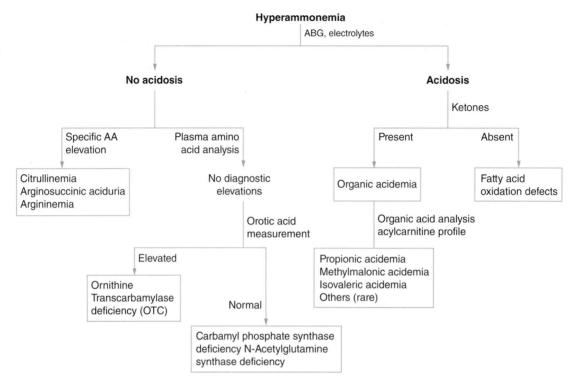

FIGURE 59-2 Urea cycle disorders. AA, amino acid; ABG, arterial blood gas.

through caloric supplementation, aided by insulin as needed to maintain high-set-point normoglycemia; and (3) reduction of nitrogen intake as well as pharmacologic scavenging of waste nitrogen. These are not to be implemented consecutively but should be pursued independently and in parallel as rapidly as possible.[8–10] (Table 59-1). A detailed approach to the treatment of hyperammonemia can be found in chapter 106.

Table 59-1 Treatment and Organization

- Fluids, dextrose, and interlipid to mitigate catabolism and dehydration
- Antibiotics and septic workup to treat potential triggering events or primary sepsis (continue through treatment course)
- Contract and transport to treatment-capable institution as soon as possible
- Remove protein from intake (by mouth or total parenteral nutrition [TPN])
- Establish central venous access
- Provide physiologic support (pressors, buffering agents, etc). (Renal output is critical to long-term success.)
- Stabilize airway as cerebral edema may result in sudden respiratory arrest.

OUTCOMES

Rapid response to the hyperammonemia is indispensable for an optimal outcome.[17–19] Acute symptomatology centers around cerebral edema, disruptions in neurochemistry, and pressure on the brainstem. Hyperammonemia affects the central nervous system (CNS) in a number of ways. Ammonia freely diffuses across the blood-brain barrier. Once in the CNS, it combines with glutamate to form glutamine via glutamine synthase. Glutamine accumulation leads to osmotic changes and astrocyte swelling. This may result in decreased blood flow, cerebral swelling, and uncal herniation. The cerebral edema and resulting mental status changes do not reverse immediately after plasma ammonia normalizes.[20]

Patients with organic acidemias may have neurologic effects from other metabolic disturbances beyond those directly attribute to hyperammonia. Stroke-like episodes are common, with the basal ganglia most susceptible. Severe metabolic acidosis may also cause or exacerbate CNS injury.[5]

Although mortality from neonatal hyperammonemic coma has improved, morbidity remains high. A significant percentage of affected children have intellectual and other developmental disabilities. Even in patients who escape severe brain damage, there is a significantly increased risk for milder neurologic deficits.[19]

There appears to be a correlation between intellectual function and duration of hyperammonemic coma, so rapid and effective therapy is essential to obtain the best outcome. Children in coma for less than 3 days had a far better outcome than those in coma for longer periods of time.[18]

REFERENCES

1. Wilcken B, Wiley V, Hammond J, Carpenter K. Screening newborns for inborn errors of metabolism by tandem mass spectrometry. *N Engl J Med.* 2003;348(23):2304–2312.

2. Zschocke J, Hoffman GF. *Vendemecum Metabolicum: Manual of Metabolic Paediatrics.* 2nd ed. Friedrichsdorf, Germany: Schattauer, 2004:8–12, 24, 57–70, 75–78, 86–99.

3. Tuchman M, Lee B, Licher-Koneki U, et al. Cross-sectional multicenter study of patients with urea cycle disorders in the United States. *Mol Genet Metab.* 2008;94:397–402.

4. Summar ML, Dobbelaere D, Brusilow S, Lee B. Diagnosis, symptoms, frequency and mortality of 260 patients with urea cycle disorder from a 21-year, multicenter study of acute hyperammonaemic episodes. *Acta Paediatr.* 2008;97:420–425.

5. Pena L, Franks J, Chapman KA, et al. Natural history of propionic acidemia. *Mol Genet Metab.* 2012;105(1):5–9. Epub 2011 Sep 22.

6. Clancy RR, Chung HJ. EEG changes during recovery from acute severe neonatal citrullinemia. *Electroencephalogr Clin Neurophysiol.* 1991;78(3):222–227.

7. Gropman AL. Brain imaging in urea cycle disorders. *Mol Genet Metab.* 2010;100(Suppl 1):S20–S30.

8. Burton BK. Inborn errors of metabolism in infancy: a guide to diagnosis. *Pediatrics.* 1998;102(6):E69.

9. Tada K, Hayasaka K. Non-ketotic hyperglycinaemia: clinical and biochemical aspects. *Eur J Pediatr.* 1987;146:221–227.

10. Roe DR, Ding J. Mitochondrial fatty acid oxidation disorders. In: *The Metabolic and Molecular Bases of Inherited Diseases.* Scriver C, Beaudet A, Sly W, Valle D, Childs B, Kinzler K, Vogelstein B. New York, NY: McGraw-Hill; 2001:2297–2326.

11. Zeviani M, Bonilla E, DeVivo DC, DiMauro S. Mitochondrial diseases. *Neurol Clin.* 1989;7:123–156.

12. Lanpher BC, Gropman A, Chapman KA, et al. Urea cycle disorders overview. In: Pagon RA, Bird TD, Dolan CR, Stephens K, Adam MP, eds. *GeneReviews™* [Internet]. Seattle, WA: University of Washington, Seattle; 1993–2003 [updated September 1, 2001].

13. Jain-Ghai S, Nagamani SC, Blaser S, Siriwardena K, Feigenabaum A. Arginase I deficiency: severe infantile presentation with hyperammonemia: more common than reported? *Mol Genet Metab.* 2011;104(1–2):107–111.

14. Caldovic L, Ah Mew N, Shi D, Morizono H, Yudkoff M, Tuchaman M. N-Acetylglutamate synthase: structure, function and defects. *Mol Genet Metab.* 2010;100(Suppl 1):S13–S19.

15. Zeviani M, Bonilla E, DeVivo DC, and DiMauro S. Mitochondrial diseases. *Neurol Clin.* 1989;7:123–156.

16. Chapman KA, Gropman A, MacLeod E, et al. Acute management of propionic academia. *Mol Genet Metab.* 2012;138 (1 Suppl):S30–S39.

17. Bachmann C. Outcome and survival of 88 patients with urea cycle disorders: a retrospective evaluation. *Eur J Pediatr.* 2003;162:410–416.

18. Msall M, Batshaw ML, Suss R, Brusilow SW, and Mellits ED. Neurologic outcome in children with inborn errors of urea synthesis. Outcome of urea-cycle enzymopathies. *N Engl J Med.* 1984;310:1500–1505.

19. Krivitzky L, Babikian T, Lee HS, Thomas NH, Burk-Paull KL, Batshaw ML. Intellectual, adaptive, and behavioral functioning in children with urea cycle disorders. *Pediatr Res.* 2009;66(1):96–101.

20. Norenberg MD, Jayakumar AR, Rama Rao KV, Panickar KS. New concepts in the mechanism of ammonia-induced astrocyte swelling. *Metab Brain Dis* 2007:22(3–4):219–234.

Metabolic Acidosis in the Newborn

Kristina Cusmano-Ozog and Kimberly Chapman

INTRODUCTION

Metabolic acidosis in the neonate can be caused by several reasons, including increased acid intake from exogenous sources; increased endogenous production of an acid, such as seen in an inborn error of metabolism (IEM); inadequate excretion of acid by the kidneys; or excessive loss of bicarbonate in urine or stool. Presence or absence of an anion gap (AG) can help to distinguish the underlying etiology.

In general, with a pure or uncompensated metabolic acidosis, every 10 mEq/L fall in bicarbonate (HCO_3) results in an average pH fall of 0.15. Neonates have an average arterial pH of 7.37 (range of 7.35–7.45). The average bicarbonate level in a neonate is 20 mEq/L. A diagnosis of metabolic acidosis can be made when the pH is less than 7.35 and a base deficit greater than 5 exists.[1]

The AG is calculated by subtracting the serum concentrations of the measured anions (bicarbonate and chloride) from the cation sodium (Figure 60-1). The AG equation can be written as AG = ($[Na^+]$) − ($[Cl^-] + [HCO_3^-]$). A normal AG is typically less than 12 mEq/L.[1] If the AG is elevated (ie, > 15 mEq/L), then there are anions that have not been accounted for, and an investigation must be performed to search for the culprit. Common anions that result in an elevated AG include lactate and the ketone bodies β-hydroxybutyrate and acetoacetate. Neonates with intoxication IEMs usually have elevated AGs from accumulation of the toxic organic acid, such as isovaleric acid in isovaleric acidemia (IVA), in addition to lactate and ketone bodies secondary to clinical decompensation.

Infants will try to correct metabolic acidosis by a reflex respiratory alkalosis using hyperventilation and Kussmaul respirations. More severe uncompensated acidosis can decrease peripheral vascular resistance and cardiac ventricular function, leading to hypotension, pulmonary edema, and tissue hypoxia, which will further complicate the picture by increasing lactate production because of hypoxia and poor perfusion.

Infants with IEMs are usually normal at birth. They develop nonspecific findings similar to sepsis, such as poor feeding, vomiting, lethargy, hypotonia, hypothermia, seizures, and coma. In any child less than 4 weeks old who presents with sepsis, consider additional testing to look for an IEM. Although expanded newborn screening to look for IEMs is regular practice in the United States, remember that this is just a screen; it is neither comprehensive nor diagnostic. If there is a clinical concern for an IEM, additional testing should be done regardless of the result of the newborn screen.

Clues that increase the likelihood of identifying an IEM include a family history of consanguinity or history of a neonatal or sibling death. Occasionally, maternal history of acute fatty liver of pregnancy (AFLP) may be solicited. In addition, physical findings of Kussmaul respirations, hepatomegaly, or unusual odor may be seen. For example, individuals with untreated IVA can smell like sweaty socks.

Treatment of the metabolic acidosis depends on cause. Although sodium bicarbonate can be given to improve the pH, it will not treat the underlying cause of the acidosis, especially if the underlying etiology is an IEM. The typical dose of sodium bicarbonate is 1 mEq/kg per dose. If too much bicarbonate is given,

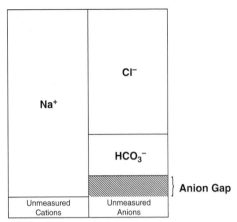

FIGURE 60-1 Anions are molecules that contain a negative charge. Cations are molecules that contain a positive charge. Generally, the total amount of anions and cations in plasma, serum, or urine are equivalent. The anion gap (AG) is the difference between the measured anions and cations and can be calculated by subtracting the concentrations of bicarbonate and chloride from sodium. The AG equation can be written as AG = ([Na$^+$]) − ([Cl$^-$] + [HCO$_3^-$]). A normal AG is less than 12 mEq/L. If the AG is elevated, then there are anions in the bodily fluid that have not been accounted for in the equation. Common anions that result in an elevated AG include lactate and the ketone bodies β-hydroxybutyrate and acetoacetate. Organic acids that accumulate in inborn errors of metabolism (IEMs) can also lead to an increased anion gap.

calcium and potassium levels will fall and can lead to complications like tetany, seizures, and arrhythmias.

CAUSES OF METABOLIC ACIDOSIS WITH NORMAL ANION GAP

Metabolic acidosis with a normal AG is usually the result of intestinal or renal loss of bicarbonate. In this situation, an increase in chloride compensates for the loss of bicarbonate. For this reason, this is also known as hyperchloremic metabolic acidosis.

Intestinal loss of bicarbonate can result from diarrhea, fistulas, or a pancreatic ileostomy. Renal loss of bicarbonate can occur from renal tubular acidosis and renal Fanconi syndrome. Medications, including arginine hydrochloride, which is used for the growth hormone stimulation test, as well as carbonic anhydride inhibitors such as the antiepileptic drug topiramate and the diuretic acetazolamide, can lead to hyperchloremic metabolic acidosis. This type of acidosis can also be seen in individuals with hyperkalemia and those recovering from diabetic ketoacidosis because of shifts in electrolytes and osmolarity.

Renal Fanconi syndrome can be caused by IEMs as well as other causes but does not present with an AG like most of the other IEMs. Infants will have dehydration, failure to thrive, and rickets due to urine loss of phosphate. Diagnostic laboratory investigations include findings of elevation of multiple amino acids on urine amino acids analysis (known as generalized aminoaciduria), glucosuria in the presence of normoglycemia, and hyperphosphaturia.[1]

Cystinosis, galactosemia, glycogen storage disorders (especially types I and III), hereditary fructose intolerance, tyrosinemia I, Fanconi-Bickel (glycogen storage disorder XI), Wilson disease, Lowe syndrome, mitochondrial disorders, and osteopetrosis can all manifest as renal Fanconi syndrome. Consequently, other testing is necessary to identify the underlying cause.

Medications, including antibiotics such as tetracycline and the aminoglycosides; chemotherapeutic agents such as cisplatin, ifosfamide, 6-mercaptopurine; the common seizure medication valproate, and some human immunodeficiency virus (HIV) medications, including tenofovir, can all lead to renal Fanconi syndrome. Other causes include heavy metal exposure to cadmium, lead, mercury, platinum, and uranium and several Chinese herbs. More commonly seen in adults, the dysproteinemias, including multiple myeloma, amyloidosis, light-chain nephropathy, and benign monoclonal gammopathy, can also lead to renal Fanconi syndrome. Finally, immunologic injury resulting from interstitial nephritis, renal transplantation, or malignancy can be a cause of renal Fanconi syndrome.[1]

CAUSES OF METABOLIC ACIDOSIS WITH ELEVATED/INCREASED ANION GAP

The differential for metabolic acidosis includes a number of disorders that increase the AG with free acids or decreased buffering by bicarbonate. The memory aid MUDPILES can be used to remember the possible sources that increase the AG (Table 60-1). Although some of the conditions in the MUDPILES list may not be relevant in the neonate, do not forget to consider the maternal contribution to the current clinical state of the neonate, especially if the child is less than 48 hours old or is consuming breast milk.

An important source of free acid in neonates is lactate, which is included in the MUDPILES mnemonic. Lactic acidosis is a common finding in the neonate and can result from primary or secondary causes. Secondary causes are numerous and include seizure, infection, sepsis, shock, hypoxia, anoxia, hypovolemia, hemorrhage, poor perfusion or circulation, congenital heart defects, and the necessity for resuscitation in addition to several of the IEMs.[1] If lactic acidosis is identified, testing for secondary causes such

Table 60-1 Causes of Metabolic Acidosis With Elevated Anion Gap

MUDPILES
  Methanol, metformin
  Uremia
  Diabetic ketoacidosis
  Paraldehyde, propylene glycol, phenformin
  Iron, isoniazid, inborn errors of metabolism (see
    separate section this table)
  Lactic acid
  Ethanol, ethylene glycol (antifreeze)
  Salicylates
Ketosis
  Diabetic ketoacidosis
  Starvation
  Inborn errors of metabolism (see separate section
    this table)
Lactic acidosis
  Sepsis
  Shock
  Tissue hypoxia and poor perfusion
  Congenital heart defect
  Inborn errors of metabolism (see separate section
    this table)
Inborn errors of metabolism
  Disorders of amino acid metabolism
    Propionic acidemia
    Methylmalonic acidemia
    Isovaleric acidemia
    Maple syrup urine disease
    Multiple carboxylase deficiency
    Betaketothiolase deficiency
  Disorders of carbohydrate metabolism
    Pyruvate carboxylase deficiency
    Pyruvate dehydrogenase deficiency
    Fructose-1,6-bisphosphatase deficiency
    Glycogen storage disease type I
  Disorders of fatty acid metabolism
    Very long-chain acyl-CoA dehydrogenase
      deficiency
    Long-chain hydroxyacyl-CoA dehydrogenase
      deficiency
    Carnitine palmitoyltransferase I
    Carnitine palmitoyltransferase II and carnitine
      translocase deficiency

Abbreviation: CoA, coenzyme A.

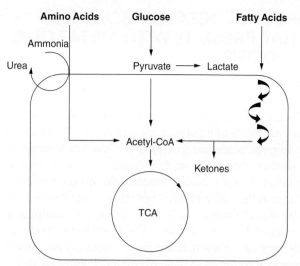

FIGURE 60-2 Basic pathways. Amino acids, carbohydrates, and fatty acids all undergo multiple processes to be converted into energy. The final common pathway is the formation of acetyl-CoA (coenzyme A), which can enter the tricarboxylic acid (TCA) cycle. Hydrogenated nicotinamide adenine dinucleotide (NADH) generated by the TCA cycle can be fed to the electron transport chain to generate adenosine triphosphate (ATP), the main energy source for numerous cellular functions. Defects in amino acid, carbohydrate, or fatty acid metabolism will lead to decreased energy production.

as with blood, urine, cerebrospinal fluid (CSF) cultures in addition to a good cardiovascular examination with 4 extremity blood pressures and echocardiogram should be performed. Even if 1 of these secondary causes is identified, additional testing for an IEM should be considered.

In addition to the MUDPILES list, ketosis is a common cause for an increased AG. Although ketosis can be seen during times of illness, when consuming a ketogenic or very-low-calorie diet, or starvation, it is always pathologic in the neonate. Finally, the major component of this chapter is the discussion of IEMs.

Inborn errors of metabolism are disorders in which a particular enzyme is unable to function appropriately in the breakdown of amino acids, carbohydrates, or fatty acid oxidation (Figure 60-2). The enzyme deficiency often leads to accumulation of substrate and insufficiency of product. The precursors that accumulate in IEMs are often acids or are processed into acids that can act as intoxicating molecules and damage organs, including the liver, pancreas, kidney, heart, skeletal muscle, and brain, either directly or by inhibiting the organ's usual functions, such as ammonia breakdown, or production of energy.

The IEMs that present in the neonatal period include those of the intoxication type, such that they present with decreased feeding and increasing lethargy, which can progress to encephalopathy, seizures, coma, and even death if not treated. One of the major indications of any of these disorders is the presence of metabolic acidosis, especially with an AG because of the accumulation of free acids secondary to the enzyme block. Most of these disorders can be diagnosed by routine metabolic testing (Table 60-2), including plasma amino acid and plasma acylcarnitine profile and urine organic acid analyses.

SPECIFIC DETAILS ABOUT IEMs THAT PRESENT WITH METABOLIC ACIDOSIS

Disorders of Amino Acid Metabolism

Disorders of amino acid metabolism will result in the accumulation of organic acids and are also referred to as organic acidemias (OAs). The OAs are a series of disorders that result in free organic acids detectable in urine. Many of these disorders are on the newborn screen in the United States, but infants can present with symptoms of metabolic acidosis prior to obtaining the results of the screening test. The following sections do not provide an all-inclusive list of disorders but rather the more common of these disorders (Figure 60-3).

Propionic Acidemia

Propionic acidemia (PA) is caused by deficiency of propionyl-coenzyme A carboxylase (PCC), which is a biotin-dependent, mitochondrial enzyme with 2 subunits (α and β).[3] PA is inherited in an autosomal recessive

manner in which mutations in both copies of 1 of the 2 PCC-encoding genes, *PCCA* at 13q32 (α subunit) or *PCCB* at 3q21-22 (β subunit), lead to disease. The incidence is approximately 1 in 100,000 newborns worldwide but is more common in Saudi Arabia and the Amish and Mennonite groups. PCC is necessary for breakdown of valine, odd-chain fatty acids, methionine, isoleucine, and threonine (VOMIT). Patients present with poor feeding, vomiting, dehydration, hypotonia, seizures, and lethargy shortly after birth as well as during times of metabolic decompensation, usually with an intercurrent illness or stress. Significant morbidity and mortality are secondary to hyperammonemia, infection, cardiomyopathy, pancreatitis, and basal ganglial stroke.[2–5]

Laboratory studies in an untreated or metabolically decompensated patient with PA can include evaluation for metabolic acidosis, lactic acidosis, hyperammonemia, ketosis, and hypo- or hyperglycemia. Several cases also presented with pancytopenia, including neutropenia, anemia, and thrombocytopenia. Plasma amino acids show an elevated glycine, which was 1 of the first observations, so PA was initially known as "ketotic hyperglycin(a)emia."[6,7] Urine organic acids

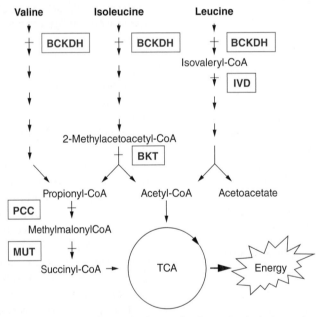

FIGURE 60-3 Detailed pathway of amino acid metabolism. The branched-chain amino acids valine, isoleucine, and leucine share a common enzymatic conversion by branched-chain α-ketoacid dehydrogenase (BCKDH) for the second step of their metabolism; deficiency of BCKDH results in maple syrup urine disease (MSUD). The next step in the leucine pathway is the formation of isovaleryl-CoA (coenzyme A), which is then converted to 3-methyl-crotonyl-CoA by isovaleryl-CoA dehydrogenase (IVD); deficiency of IVD results in isovaleric acidemia. Valine undergoes 5 additional steps, and isoleucine undergoes 4 additional steps prior to the formation of propionyl-CoA. In the isoleucine pathway, just prior to the formation of propionyl-CoA is the conversion of 2-methyl-acetoacetyl-CoA to propionyl-CoA and acetyl-CoA by β-ketothiolase (BKT); deficiency of BKT leads to BKT deficiency. Acetyl-CoA can enter the tricarboxylic acid (TCA) cycle to generate adenosine triphosphate (ATP). Propionyl-CoA is converted to methylmalonyl-CoA by propionyl-CoA carboxylase (PCC); deficiency of PCC leads to propionic acidemia. Methylmalonyl-CoA is converted by methylmalonyl-CoA mutase (MUT) to succinyl-CoA, which can then enter the TCA cycle to generate ATP; deficiency of MUT leads to methylmalonic aciduria.

Table 60-2 Laboratory Tests for Any Patient With a Known or Suspected Inborn Error of Metabolism (IEM)

Venous/arterial blood gas
Glucose
Lactate
Ammonia
Comprehensive Metabolic Panel
Anion gap ($[Na^+] - ([Cl^-] + [HCO_3^-])$)
Complete blood cell count
Blood culture
Plasma amino acids
Plasma acylcarnitine profile
Urinalysis to assess ketones
Urine organic acids
Urine culture

show elevations of 3-hydroxypropionate, propionylglycine, tiglylglycine, and methylcitrate. Carnitine can be deficient because of a secondary carnitine deficiency. Acylcarnitine profile analysis shows elevated propionylcarnitine (C3), which is the basis of detection by expanded newborn screening. Confirmation of diagnosis can be done by sequence analysis of *PCCA* and *PCCB* as well as PCC enzyme activity on blood or fibroblasts. Prenatally, chorionic villi sampling or amniocentesis can be done to probe for known family mutations, PCC activity, or methylcitrate levels for prenatal diagnosis.

Acute management in a severely affected patient with PA focuses on reversal of catabolism and scavenging of toxic metabolites. A complete protocol developed for PA acute management is available in an article by Chapman et al.[4] See Table 60-3 for acute management guidelines and Table 60-4 for discharge planning. Briefly, blood for glucose, electrolytes, ammonia, AG, blood gas, serum urea nitrogen, creatinine, amylase, lipase, and urinalysis for ketones is drawn to determine the level of decompensation. As with most of the intoxication disorders, the initial step of intervention includes the rapid reversal of catabolism, which is often obtained using a 10% dextrose-containing intravenous solution running at least at 6–8 mg glucose/kg/min in a neonate and 20% intralipids (2–3 g/kg/d). Toxic intermediates can be scavenged using levocarnitine (100 mg/kg/d) as well as sodium benzoate/sodium phenylacetate for hyperammonemia prior to confirmation of PA. Infants with severe metabolic acidosis and hyperammonemia do benefit from the rapid reduction of toxic intermediates seen with hemodialysis, extracorporeal membrane oxidation (ECMO), and hemofiltration. Neonates with PA can also have the complication of cardiomyopathy, so an emergent echocardiogram is occasionally useful in the correct setting.

Chronic treatment includes avoidance of catabolism during fasting and focuses on substrate reduction using a low-protein, high-calorie diet providing World Health Organization (WHO) protein requirements and using metabolic partial component formulas such as Prophree® and Propimex1® as examples. Individuals often require carnitine supplementation to assist with elimination of propionic acid by formation of C3 as well as to prevent secondary carnitine deficiency. Although PCC is a biotin-dependent enzyme, only 2 patients have been reported to be responsive so biotin is not usually necessary. Because propionic acid is produced by bacterial colonization of the gastrointestinal tract, treatment with antibiotics such as metronidazole (10–15 mg/kg/d, 7–10 d/mo) has shown benefit. Some children with persistent elevations of ammonia require additional nitrogen scavenging by sodium benzoate.

Individuals diagnosed with PA with symptoms often have a more complicated course, with multiple hospitalizations for metabolic decompensations, especially in early childhood.[8] In addition, long-term studies examining PA patients have illustrated a number of long-term complications, including developmental delay, cardiomyopathy, optic neuropathy, and intellectual disability.[8-12] Recommendations for screening for long-term complications were reviewed by Sutton et al.[10] In general, these include serial screening for known complications and treatment of those complications. In a survey of patient families, approximately 72% of affected individuals had some level of cognitive impairment, 19% had a form of cardiomyopathy with risk with increasing age, 30% had some form of arrhythmia, 18% had a history of pancreatitis at any time, and 18% had a metabolic stroke, with 13% having a movement disorder.[12]

Methylmalonic Acidemia

Methylmalonic acidemia (MMA) describes several disorders in which methylmalonic acid is increased in the urine and blood.[13] These include classical MMA, which results from deficiency of the methylmalonyl-CoA (coenzyme A) mutase enzyme as well as several disorders related to metabolism of vitamin B_{12}, which is a cofactor for mutase, including cobalamin A, B, C, and D deficiencies. Elevations of MMA in the urine as well as mild metabolic acidosis can also be seen in infants of mothers with severe vitamin B_{12} deficiency because the mutase enzyme is vitamin B_{12} dependent. A maternal history of gastric bypass surgery or vegan diet may assist with diagnosing maternal B_{12} deficiency.

Classical MMA is caused by a defect in the enzyme methylmalonyl-CoA mutase (*MUT*) located at 6p21. Its incidence is about 1:80,000 and is the most common IEM that results in the finding of MMA. The infantile form presents with lethargy, vomiting, hypotonia,

Table 60-3 Acute Management Protocol

Stabilization
Intubate and ventilate, if necessary.
Place intravenous lines. Do not use right intrajugular or 1 of the 2 femoral sites (these locations are necessary for hemodialysis). If unable to obtain access, intraosseus and nasogastric tube are acceptable.
Add vasopressors as necessary to maintain blood pressure.
Normal saline fluid bolus can be given. Avoid overhydration and do not delay reversal of catabolism to give normal saline bolus.
Draw laboratory studies mentioned in Table 60-2; do not discard any blood left over after analysis. If the presenting institution cannot run the laboratory tests, transport samples with the patient.

Reversal of Catabolism
Stop all sources of protein (enteral and parenteral nutrition).
Give nonprotein calories in the form of intravenous fluids with minimum 10% dextrose and electrolytes at 120-150 mL/kg/d or goal of 6–8 mg glucose/kg/min.
If intralipids are available and a fatty acid oxidation defect is not suspected, give 2–3 g/kg/d to provide additional calories.
Do not stop calorie delivery for any reason (eg, medications, additional required fluid bolus, or hyperglycemia).
Consider an insulin drip (0.01 units/kg/h). If hypoglycemia occurs, increase dextrose amount or delivery rate.

Other interventions
Start antibiotics after blood cultures are drawn.
If newborn screen results are unknown, call state laboratory to check for results or expedite their processing (normal results do not rule out metabolic disease).
Arrange transport to a metabolic center as soon as there are concerns for metabolic disease or decompensation.
Arrange for and initiate hemodialysis, hemofiltration, or extracorporeal membrane oxygenation (ECMO) if clinical or laboratory evaluations identify ammonia greater than 300 µmol/L, extreme acidosis/electrolyte imbalance, coma, dilated pupils, poor neurological findings, or increased respiratory rate and based on clinical judgment. Do not use peritoneal dialysis.
For hyperammonemia in an undiagnosed patient, consider starting sodium benzoate/sodium phenylacetate (at same doses as for urea cycle defects).
Intravenous carnitine 100 mg/kg/dose 3–4 times daily over a minimum of 30 minutes can be given if urine output is appropriate (or hemofiltration ongoing) and there is no concern for a long-chain fatty acid oxidation defect.
Follow ammonia, electrolyte, and blood gas values at regular intervals. The frequency is dictated by the patient's condition and the speed at which results can be obtained.
Protein should be reintroduced within 24–36 hours of initiation of therapy. Protein must be reintroduced even if patient is on hemodialysis or ECMO.
Consider sedation, ventilation, and chemical paralysis if aggressive management is necessary. If used, continuous electroencephalography (EEG) is helpful to monitor progress.
Transfuse packed red blood cells as necessary based on age, clinical condition, and physician discretion.

Transition from acute to chronic management and discharge planning
Establish home metabolic nutrition support regimen.
Provide gastrostomy tube (G tube) or nasogastric tube (NG tube) placement for enteral feeding.
Medications should be transitioned to oral administration.
Complete studies including echocardiogram, electrocardiogram (ECG), hearing screen, optic fields (if cerebral edema) and dilated ophthalmologic examination according to underlying diagnosis.
Involve physical therapy and occupational therapy and refer to early intervention.
Any parental training needed is completed prior to discharge.

and encephalopathy within hours to the first few weeks after birth is usually not vitamin B_{12} responsive. These individuals usually have undetectable levels of mutase activity and can be referred to as having MMA mut⁰.

Less common is the vitamin B_{12}-responsive (mut⁻) patient with MMA who presents in the first few months or years of life with feeding intolerance, failure to thrive, hypotonia, developmental delay, and occasionally acute decompensation with stress or illness. These individuals usually have decreased but detectable levels of mutase

activity and can be referred to as having MMA mut⁻. Patients with MMA mut⁻ can have genetic changes in 1 of 3 genes, *MUT* or *MMAA*, located at 4q31 and known as cobalamin A disease or *MMAB* located at 12q24 and known as cobalamin B disease.

Infants and children with MMA present with metabolic acidosis, possibly hypoglycemia, often hyperammonemia, and always ketosis. In more specific biochemical testing, plasma amino acids show elevated glycine, plasma acylcarnitine analysis shows increased C3, which

Table 60-4 Discharge instructions

Parental training
  Preparation of metabolic formula with a home gram scale
  G-tube or NG-tube (if present) care
  Lessons in giving all medications
  Instructions on how to use ketosticks
Medications and formula
  Prescriptions for all medications and ketosticks
    Give at least 2 days prior to discharge to have time to fill
  One-week supply of all medications
  List of medications with dosages, times, and reasons for use
  Several cans of metabolic formula
  Paper and electronic copy of diet with list of feeding times
Follow-up
  Emergency room letter
  Emergency contact information for the metabolic physician and clinic
  Appointment date and time for metabolic clinic and other specialists
  Referral to early intervention

is the basis of detection by expanded newborn screening and occasionally methymalonylcarnitine (C4DC). Urine organic acid analysis demonstrates elevations in methylmalonic acid as well as 3-hydroxypropionate, propionylglycine, tiglylglycine, and methylcitrate. Urine and blood show increased ketone bodies and lactate with illness. Hyperammonemia levels in neonates can reach levels similar to those seen in individuals with urea cycle disorders prior to initiation of therapy. Confirmation of the type of MMA can be obtained by mutation analysis of *MUT*, *MMAA*, or *MMAB* genes or complementation studies in fibroblasts.

Acute management in a severely affected patient with MMA is similar to that for PA except for the use of vitamin B_{12} in MMA. All infants with MMA should be treated with hydroxycobalamin 0.5–1 mg per day by intramuscular injections until proven to be unresponsive to B_{12} supplementation. Table 60-3 provides acute management guidelines.

Chronic therapy focuses on substrate reduction using a low-protein, high-calorie diet providing WHO protein requirements and using metabolic partial component formulas, such as Prophree and Propimex1. Levocarnitine should be continued, as should the hydroxycobalamin in those who are vitamin B_{12} responsive. Because the precursor of methylmalonic acid is produced by bacterial colonization of the gastrointestinal tract, treatment with antibiotics such as metronidazole (10–15 mg/kg/d, 7–10 d/mo) has shown benefit. Some children with persistent elevations of ammonia require additional nitrogen scavenging by sodium benzoate.

Even with early diagnosis and treatment, classical MMA has a disappointing outcome. Many children, even with optimal therapy, have intellectual disability, developmental delay, and failure to thrive. Long-term complications include immune and bone marrow suppression, pancreatitis, and metabolic stroke, which usually occurs within the basal ganglia and will lead to a movement disorder. Also significant in the long-term outcome of patients with MMA is the development of tubulointerstitial nephritis, which leads to end-stage renal disease. Finally, combined liver and kidney transplantation is a possibility and is used to address the metabolic dysfunction and end-stage renal disease; however, this does not cure the individual of MMA and leads to its own set of complications.[13]

Isovaleric Acidemia

Isovaleric acidemia is caused by a deficiency of isovaleryl-CoA dehydrogenase, and patients can present with a "sweaty feet" odor. Neonates can become critically ill with metabolic acidosis, hyperammonemia, elevated lactate, ketosis, tachypnea, vomiting, lethargy, bone marrow suppression, seizures, and coma in the acute intermittent form. Others will be identified by newborn screening if available and may not be as metabolically fragile, occasionally remaining asymptomatic in the neonatal period.

Laboratory studies in IVA show an increased level of isovalerylcarnitine (C5) on acylcarnitine profile. Urine organic acids can show abnormal excretion of isovalerylglycine with or without 3-hydroxyisovalerate, 4-hydroxyisovalerate, methylsuccinate, 3-hydroxyisoheptanoate, isovalerylglutamate, isovalerylglucuronide, isovalerylalanine, and isovalerylsarcosine. Plasma amino acids can show an elevation of glycine, and sometimes a slight elevation of alloisoleucine (2–10 μM) will be detected and is typically less than that seen in individuals with maple syrup urine disease (MSUD). Diagnosis is confirmed by DNA analysis of *IVD* located at 15q.[14,15] The common mutation p.A282V (c.932C>T) has been found in several asymptomatic infants identified by newborn screening (NBS) and their healthy, older siblings and so is thought to be related to mild disease. Prenatal testing can be done for future pregnancies by evaluating for the familial mutation or looking for an elevation of isovalerylglycine in amniotic fluid.

Acute management of IVA in those patients who are symptomatic follows a similar approach to that of acute management in PA and MMA. Blood studies for glucose, electrolytes, ammonia, AG, blood gas, serum urea nitrogen, and creatinine; urinalysis for ketones determines the level of decompensation. The initial step of intervention includes the rapid reversal of catabolism and is often obtained using a 10% dextrose-containing intravenous solution running at least at 6–8 mg glucose/kg/min in a neonate and 20% intralipids (2–3 g/kg/d). Toxic intermediates can be scavenged with levocarnitine (100 mg/kg/d) and glycine (150–250 mg/kg/d). Both of these supplements will assist with removal of isovaleric acid by the formation of C5 and isovalerylglycine as well as prevent secondary deficiency of carnitine and glycine.

Chronic treatment should always include carnitine supplementation (100 mg/kg/d) and glycine supplementation (150–250 mg/kg/d). Occasionally, long-term dietary restriction with a combination of natural and medical protein will continue. Patients should avoid aspirin because it competes with glycine and prevents excretion as isovalerylglycine.

Outcome is dependent on whether the initial presentation is adequately treated and the underlying genotype.[14,15] Some may never develop a hyperammonemic or metabolic acidotic crisis based on their phenotype or prompt diagnosis and treatment, and they have exceptional outcomes. Those who have milder disease also have less-severe outcomes and few hospitalizations for metabolic acidosis. However, inadequate and nontimely diagnosis and management can be devastating in a small portion of this population, resulting in brain damage. Triggers for catabolic events are most commonly infectious in origin outside the neonatal period, but a large percentage (21.7%) do not have an apparent cause.[15] Most well-treated individuals will have a normal IQ and decreased risk of metabolic decompensation with age.[15]

Maple Syrup Urine Disease

Infants with MSUD may not have pH disturbance if they present early. MSUD is caused by branched-chain α-ketoacid dehydrogenase (BCKAD) deficiency, which is the first step of metabolism of the branched-chain amino acids leucine, isoleucine, and valine. Elevation in leucine can be brain toxic, so it is a major complication. Accumulation of branched-chain metabolites leads to a maple syrup odor that is best smelled in cerumen as early 12 to 24 hours of life. Neonates can present with ketonuria, irritability, and poor feeding noted at 2 to 3 days of life. If not diagnosed or treated, symptoms will progress to encephalopathy by 4 to 5 days and eventually coma at 7 to 10 days of life. Breast-fed babies typically present a few days later than formula-fed infants because breast milk generally contains less protein.

The incidence is 1:185,000 in the general population but is much more common in the Mennonite population (1:200) and is inherited in an autosomal recessive manner. Diagnosis is confirmed by BCKAD enzyme activity in fibroblasts, lymphocytes, or liver or by mutation analysis of the genes that encode the various subunits of the BCKAD enzyme; *BCKDHA* is located at 19q13.1-q13.2 and encodes the E1α

subunit, *BCKDHB* is located at 6q14 and encodes the E1β subunit, and *DBT* is located at 1p31 and encodes the E2 subunit.

Laboratory testing includes investigation of plasma amino acids with elevations of leucine, isoleucine, and valine. Typically, the level of leucine is most abnormal. Occasionally, isoleucine and valine levels are normal. Alloisoleucine is also noted at levels greater than 5 μmol/L and is typically a much larger value than seen in IVA. Urine organic acids show elevated branch-chain ketoacids, including 2-ketoisocaproic, 2-hydroxyisovaleric, 2-hydroxyisocaproic, 2-hydroxy-3-methylvaleric, and 2-keto-3-methylvaleric acids.

Acute management focuses on adequate reduction of leucine levels. This can be done through hemodialysis (see Table 60-3) or using increased hypertonicity saline solutions.[18]

Chronic therapy includes a low-protein diet with decreased natural protein intake and the addition of synthetic protein. Isoleucine and valine are supplemented at 5–100 mg/kg/d to compete with leucine at receptors and prevent upregulation of receptors because of their deficiency. Levocarnitine at 50 mg/kg/d and thiamine at 50–100 mg/d are also supplemented. Because of the low-protein diet and risk of deficiency Ca, Mg, Zn, Se, folate, and omega 3 (Ω-3) essential fatty acids are monitored.

Leucinosis outside the neonatal period may be from increased catabolism during infection, surgery, injury, and stress. Any episode of leucinosis can lead to cerebral edema and may result in mild-moderate intellectual disability, attention-deficit/hyperactivity disorder in childhood, and anxiety/depression in adulthood. Children can also develop pancreatitis, complicating management. Some patients have successfully undergone liver transplantation and have been able to resume a mostly regular diet.

Intellectual outcomes are dependent on early treatment of the early presentation of MSUD and whether an individual has early-onset or late-onset disease. In general, with earlier treatment of early-onset and in late-onset MSUD, patients have better intellectual outcomes and can have normal IQs.[19,20] Unfortunately, metabolic decompensations that are inadequately treated can result in hyperleucinosis; consequently, brain damage results, so attention should be paid to this type of episode throughout life.

Multiple Carboxylase Deficiency

Multiple carboxylase deficiency (MCD) occurs from a loss of holocarboxylase synthetase (HCS) function. HCS incorporates biotin into 4 carboxylase enzymes and is encoded by *HLCS* at 21q22.1. Patients with MCD have dysfunction of 3 mitochondrial enzymes—pyruvate carboxylase (PC), PCC, and β-methylcrotonyl-CoA carboxylase (MCC)—and the cytosolic enzyme acetyl-CoA carboxylase (ACC) and subsequently present early in infancy with metabolic acidosis. Patients often have feeding and breathing problems, hypotonia, lethargy, and seizures as a neonate and can develop rash and alopecia over time.

The incidence of MCD is about 1:100,000 worldwide and is more common in Samoa and the Faroe Islands, with the common mutations being IVS1015G4A in the Faroe Islands, L237P and 780delG in Japan, and L216R in Samoa.

Laboratory findings include metabolic acidosis and hyperammonemia. Acylcarnitine profile analysis shows increased C3⁻ and C_5OH-carnitine and therefore should be detected with expanded newborn screening. Urine organic acids show increased lactic, 3-hydroxypropionic, 3-hydroxyisovaleric, and methylcitric acids as well as 3-methylcrotonylglycine and tiglylglycine. Because HCS incorporates biotin into other enzymatic pathways, the inability to recycle biotin by a biotinidase deficiency must be ruled out because it can present similarly in older patients.

Prenatal testing is best done by molecular DNA mutation analysis because organic acid analysis (eg, for methylcitrate) on amniotic fluid is unreliable in this disorder, and the role of carboxylase activity on chorionic villus sampling (CVS) or amniocentesis is unclear.

Acute and chronic treatment focus on providing 5–20 mg/d biotin in hopes of increasing the function of HCS and 100 mg/kg/d carnitine as a scavenger of precursors for the resulting dysfunctional enzymes.

No matter the intervention, outcomes are generally poor in this patient population.[16] However, pharmacological doses of biotin can be used with some limited improvement.[16,17] There are some patients who are more biotin responsive.[17]

β-Ketothiolase Deficiency

β-Ketothiolase (BKT) deficiency is a disorder of both ketogenesis and ketolysis. It is inherited in an autosomal recessive manner such that 2 mutations in *ACAT1*, which is located at 11q2.3-23.1, are identified. Historically, individuals have presented at 6–24 months with intermittent and severe ketoacidosis with emesis during intercurrent illness or periods of prolonged fasting. This disorder can be identified with expanded newborn screening; therefore, a neonate may be diagnosed prior to the onset of symptoms.

Laboratory studies include those for the presence of ketones in urine and blood, metabolic acidosis, abnormally low glucose levels, and occasionally hyperammonemia. Plasma amino acids show increased glycine and urine organic acids have increases in 2-methyl-3hydroxybutyrate, tiglylglycine, and 2-methylacetoacetic acid.[21] Note that because of the metabolic defect, patients are unable to generate the usual ketone body acetoacetate. Diagnosis is confirmed using an enzyme assay or molecular analysis.[21]

Present therapy focuses on avoidance of fasting in addition to the use of dextrose-containing intravenous fluids if the patient is unable to tolerate feedings. Because of its role as a precursor, isoleucine is restricted, and metabolic formulas are used. Carnitine supplementation is often necessary. Special care must be used in treatment of acidosis because aggressive alkalinization may lead to hypernatremia.

The spectrum of complications in children is wide, ranging from normal development to basal ganglia changes, intellectual disability, and dystonia. In severe episodes of ketoacidosis, disease can progress to include coma and death. Patients can also have cardiomyopathy, prolonged QT interval, neutropenia, or thrombocytopenia.[21]

Disorders of Carbohydrate Metabolism

The disorders of carbohydrate metabolism and transport have a wide clinical spectrum and may be caused by toxicity, energy deficiency, hypoglycemia, or storage (Figure 60-4).

Pyruvate Carboxylase Deficiency

Pyruvate carboxylase deficiency presents with failure to thrive, developmental delay, seizures, metabolic acidosis, and renal tubular acidosis (RTA). PC is 1 of the biotin-dependent carboxylases and is coded on 11q13.4-q13.5. PC deficiency has an overall incidence of 1:250,000; however, it is much more common in the Algonquin-speaking population in North America. There are 3 major subtypes of PC deficiency: groups A, B, and C.

The severe neonatal form has findings of hepatomegaly, pyramidal tract signs, abnormal movements, and early death. These patients include those with group A disease who are predominately Algonquin-speaking in North America who have a common 1828G>A mutation and group B disease patients whose origin is European, especially those from France, and where there is no common mutation identified. In comparison, group C disease is an intermittent-to-benign form. These patients have normal-to-mild delays in development and episodic metabolic acidosis.[22,23]

Laboratory testing shows increased blood lactate and pyruvate levels and increased ratio of lactate to pyruvate (>20). Ketosis and hyperammonemia may also be observed. Plasma amino acids have increases in alanine, citrulline, and lysine in group B disease only. Diagnosis is made by enzyme activity in fibroblasts. At the time of this book's publication, DNA analysis was only available as a research test.

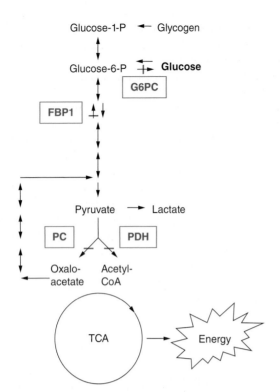

FIGURE 60-4 Detailed pathway of carbohydrate metabolism. Glucose is transported into the cell to undergo metabolism. If it does not need to be used immediately, it will be converted to glycogen through the intermediaries glucose-6-phosphate and glucose-1-phosphate for use at a later point in time. In the reverse reactions, glucose-6-phosphatase (G6PC) will convert glucose-6-phosphate to glucose so that it may enter glycolysis and generate energy. Deficiency of G6PC will result in excessive storage of glycogen as the body is unable to break down glycogen, leading to hypoglycemia and hepatomegaly, the common findings seen in glycogen storage disease type I (GSD I). The majority of the steps between glucose and pyruvate are reversible, although they may require separate enzymatic conversions. In gluconeogenesis, glucose is formed from pyruvate by a series of reactions of which fructose-1,6-bisphosphatase (FBP1) is a critical step. Deficiency of this enzyme will result in hypoglycemia and other symptoms. Pyruvate is mostly formed from glycolysis and can be converted by pyruvate dehydrogenase (PDH) to acetyl-CoA (coenzyme A) to enter the tricarboxylic acid (TCA) cycle and create energy. Pyruvate can also be converted by pyruvate carboxylase (PC) to oxaloacetate, which is necessary for gluconeogenesis and can help to replenish TCA cycle intermediates. Both PDH and PC deficiency result in severe energy deficiency and lactic acidosis.

Patients are treated with biotin at a dose of 10 mg/d. Thiamine and lipoic acid are used occasionally. Supplementation of the tricarboxylic acid intermediates citrate and succinate and the amino acid aspartate may be of benefit. Patients have been treated with liver transplant, and the risk-to-benefit ratio must be considered from patient to patient. Patients should avoid fasting as well as a ketogenic diet.

As stated, outcomes are generally thought to be poor, but some individuals survive to adulthood if mosaicism for the PC mutation is present.[23]

Pyruvate Dehydrogenase Deficiency

Pyruvate dehydrogenase (PDH) has multiple subunits, including *PDHA1* located at Xp22.2-p22.1 and encoding the E1α subunit, *PDHB* located at 3p13-q23 and encoding the E1β subunit, *DLAT* located at 11q23.1 and encoding the E2 subunit, *DLD* located at 7q31–32 and encoding the E3 subunit, and *PDHX* located at 11p13, which is also known as component X and binds to the E3 subunit.

Mutations in *PDHA1* are the most common, and as this is an X-linked condition, males rarely survive infancy. More commonly, it is recognized in female heterozygotes that are variably affected. Two mutations in *DLAT* are the second most common causes of PDH deficiency and are inherited in an autosomal recessive fashion. Patients with 2 mutations in *DLD* will also have MSUD because it also encodes for BCKAD. PDH requires 5 coenzymes to function properly: thiamine, lipoic acid, flavin adenine dinucleotide (FAD), CoA, and nicotinamide adenine dinucleotide (NAD).

There are 2 major presenting phenotypes of PDH deficiency. One phenotype presents with metabolic acidosis caused by lactate, and patients will often have neurologic features, such as a Leigh-like syndrome. The other phenotype presents with developmental delay, regression, seizures, hypotonia, weakness, ataxia, dystonia, spasticity, abnormal eye movements, poor response to visual stimuli, and cerebellar degeneration.

Laboratory testing is consistent with elevations in lactate and pyruvate with a normal lactate-to-pyruvate ratio less than 20 (as opposed to PC deficiency, for which the ratio is elevated). Generally, in PDH deficiency, CSF lactate elevations are much greater than for blood. Urine organic acids can show 2-ketoglutarate, and in patients with mutations in E3, there are elevated branched-chain amino acid metabolites similar to that seen in MSUD. Diagnosis is confirmed by DNA analysis.

Treatment is primarily supportive and includes supplementation of thiamine at a dose of 500–2000 mg/d and a ketogenic (low-carb, high-fat) diet.[24,25]

There is little consistency between genotype and phenotype. In general, outcomes are poor, with high mortality. In 1 study, 29% of the patients studied had normal/borderline or mild intellectual disability, 17% had moderate intellectual disability, and 57% had severe or profound intellectual disability.[24] A majority of surviving patients who could ambulate had ataxia, and there were many with structural brain abnormalities.

Fructose-1,6-Bisphosphatase Deficiency

Fructose-1,6-bisphosphatase (FBP1) deficiency is caused by abnormal function of the hexose bisphosphatase or FBP1, which is encoded at 9q22.2-q22.3. Of patients, 50% will present within the first 4 days of life. An additional 25% present by 6 months of age, and the remainder will typically present between 6 months and 4 years. Affected children will have episodic spells of hyperventilation, apnea, hypoglycemia, ketosis, and lactic acidosis, which can be precipitous and often lethal. Patients also have been described with hepatomegaly despite normal liver enzyme tests, cerebral edema, and seizures. These episodic spells can result from periods of fasting, illness, or stress. Patients do not have emesis after fructose intake and have no aversion to sweets, as opposed to those with hereditary fructose intolerance.[26]

Laboratory studies indicate elevations in lactate and pyruvate. Urine organic acids have elevated glycerol, α-ketoglutarate, lactate, and ketone bodies. The gold standard for diagnosis is enzyme activity in the liver, but occasionally this can be done on leukocytes. DNA analysis is also performed for point mutations, single-nucleotide deletion, or larger deletions.

Treatment is primarily symptomatic, and patients are treated by standard protocols for hypoglycemia and acidosis; typically, fasting is avoided. Fructose and sucrose are limited in their diet as well.[27]

Individuals with FBP1 deficiency typically respond to treatment and will do well if they continue to avoid fasting. Neurological sequelae including seizures, and brain damage can occur in those who have profound episodes of hypoglycemia.

Glycogen Storage Disease Type I

Glycogen storage disease (GSD) type I has an incidence of 1:100,000. Type Ia is caused by dysfunction of glucose-6-phosphatase, encoded by *G6PC* located at 17q21, accounting for about 80% of affected individuals. Type Ib is caused by glucose-6-phosphate translocase, encoded by *SLC37A4,* which is located at 11q23 and accounts for about 20% of patients.

Patients with GSD I present with profound neonatal hypoglycemia, hepatomegaly, renomegaly, and hypoglycemia-related seizures. They can have a doll-like face (fat cheeks, thin limbs, and protuberant belly), short stature, xanthomas, diarrhea, and impaired platelet function, leading to increased risk of bleeding.

Laboratory studies show lactic acidosis, hyperuricemia, and hyperlipidemia. Patients with type Ib disease also have neutropenia. Urine organic acids can have elevations in 2-ketoglutarate. Diagnosis is confirmed by measuring glucose-6-phosphatase activity in liver biopsy tissue or by mutation analysis.

Common mutations in *G6PC* are R38C in the Jewish population, R83H in the Chinese, 378_379dupTA in the Hispanic population, 648G>T in the Asian population, and 79delC, G188R, and Q347X in Caucasians. Common mutations in *SLC37A4* are W118R in the Japanese and 1042_1043delCT or G339C in Caucasians.

Treatment focuses on avoidance of hypoglycemia with frequent meals and cornstarch overnight. Patients should avoid fructose, sucrose, galactose, and lactose and require calcium supplementation. Many need allopurinol to treat hyperuricemia and Neupogen® if neutropenia is present.

Patients are prone to infections, ulcers, osteoporosis, gout, pulmonary hypertension, renal disease, polycystic ovaries, and pancreatitis as well as hepatic adenomas, which can become malignant. Patients do better in terms of adenomas if treated early and hypoglycemia is avoided.[28]

Disorders of Fatty Acid Metabolism

Fatty acid oxidation is required for energy production during times of starvation (Figure 60-5). Defects of fatty acid oxidation typically present with hypoglycemia and hypoketosis and may not have a disturbance in pH. Accumulation of toxic metabolites from these disorders will result in damage to the liver, heart, or skeletal muscle. Maternal history may be significant for HELLP (hemolysis, elevated liver enzymes, and low platelet count) syndrome or AFLP.

Very Long-Chain Acyl-CoA Dehydrogenase Deficiency

Very long-chain acyl-CoA dehydrogenase deficiency (VLCADD) is a deficiency of very long-chain acyl-CoA dehydrogenase, a mitochondrial fatty acid β-oxidation enzyme. VLCADD is inherited in an autosomal recessive manner and is encoded by *ACADVL,* located at 17p13, and has an incidence of 1 in 42,500 to 125,000 newborns. There is a genotype-phenotype correlation such that missense mutations lead to mild disease, and null mutations result in severe disease, making genetic testing beneficial.

Patients with VLCADD can have 1 of 3 different phenotypes. The severe, early-onset form presents with cardiomyopathy and early death. The milder, childhood form has less cardiac involvement and is more likely to cause hypoketotic hypoglycemia. Finally, the more mild adult form has no cardiac involvement and is restricted to muscle involvement with rhabdomyolysis, especially under stress from fasting, infection, or excessive exercise.[29–32]

Cardiovascular presentations include hypertrophic cardiomyopathy, cardiac arrest, and sudden cardiac death. Some patients will have gastrointestinal findings,

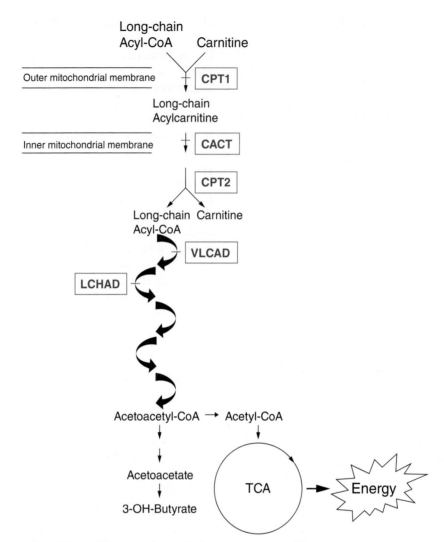

FIGURE 60-5 Detailed pathway of fatty acid metabolism. Oxidation of fatty acids is an important source of energy during times of fasting when glucose is unavailable. The carnitine shuttle facilitates the import of long-chain fatty acids into the mitochondria by several steps. In the outer mitochondrial membrane, carnitine and long-chain fatty acids create a long-chain acylcarnitine by carnitine palmitoyltransferase I (CPT I). This acylcarnitine species is transported through the inner mitochondrial membrane by carnitine/acylcarnitine translocase (CACT), and finally the long-chain acyl-CoA (coenzyme A) species are removed from carnitine so that they may enter fatty acid β-oxidation. Specific enzymes, including very long-chain acyl-CoA dehydrogenase (VLCAD) and long-chain hydroxyacyl-CoA dehydrogenase (LCHAD), shorten the acyl-CoA compounds by 2 carbons, eventually forming acetoacetyl-CoA and acetyl-CoA. Acetyl-CoA can then enter the tricarboxylic acid (TCA) cycle to generate adenosine triphosphate (ATP).

including vomiting, hepatomegaly, hepatic steatosis, or hepatocellular necrosis. Muscle involvement ranges from hypotonia to muscle weakness associated with fasting or infection in children to muscle pain with exercise, stiffness, and rhabdomyolysis with exercise in adolescents and adults. Myopathic episodes can be triggered by exercise, fasting, infection, and cold temperatures.

On laboratory evaluation, patients have nonketotic hypoglycemia. Their acylcarnitine profile can have

elevations of C14:1, C14, C16, C18:1 carnitines. Urine organic acid analysis can show dicarboxylic aciduria. There is decreased plasma carnitine from secondary effects. Some adults will have exercise-induced myoglobinuria. If a patient has symptomatic muscle involvement, the patient will have increased serum creatine kinase (CPK).

Neonates with hypoglycemia are typically treated with intravenous fluids containing at least 10% dextrose.

Carnitine supplementation is controversial; however, low-dose therapy may be necessary to maintain blood free and total carnitine levels within the normal range. During times of increased stress, such as with an intercurrent illness, intravenous fluids containing at least 10% dextrose with electrolytes should be given at 1.5 times the maintenance rate.

Patients are taught to avoid of fasting, and some will require cornstarch at night. In the more severe presentation, dietary intake of long-chain fatty acids is limited, and medium-chain triglyceride (MCT) oil is supplemented. Approximately 30% of total calories and 90% of total fat should be provided by MCT oil, with the remaining 5%–10% fat intake coming from long-chain triglycerides. Some individuals may require supplemental carnitine to maintain their free and total carnitine levels within the normal range.[29-32]

Infants with the severe phenotype are fragile and often prone to recurrent episodes of hypoglycemia, especially with fasting and during times of illness. They may have difficulty tolerating feedings and frequently have gastroesophageal reflux, requiring gastrostomy tubes. They are also at risk for liver failure, with findings of hepatomegaly and elevated transaminases. The phenotype can progress to recurrent episodes of rhabdomyolysis in childhood. Regular monitoring by cardiologists for the cardiovascular manifestations and by a nutritionist to ensure these individuals do not develop an essential fatty acid deficiency from their low-fat diet is recommended.

Long-Chain Acyl-CoA Dehydrogenase Deficiency

The mitochondrial trifunctional protein (MTP) mediates activity of 3 enzymes:L-3-hydroxyacyl-CoA dehydrogenase (LCHAD), 2-enoyl-CoA hydratase (LCEH), and 3-oxoacyl-CoA thiolase (LCKAT). The LCHAD function is the most clinically significant of the 3 enzymes, making LCHAD and MTP deficiency essentially indistinguishable from each other. The trifunctional protein is comprised from the α subunit encoded by *HADHA* and the β subunit encoded by *HADHB*. Both genes are located on 2p23, and LCHAD and MTP deficiency are inherited in an autosomal recessive manner.[30-32]

Patients with LCHAD/MTP deficiency present with fasting-induced hypoketotic hypoglycemia, Reye-like syndrome with liver disease, hypertrophic cardiomyopathy, myopathy, and prior to expanded newborn screening, sudden infant death syndrome (SIDS). They can have a protracted progressive course associated with myopathy, recurrent rhabdomyolysis, and sensorimotor axonal neuropathy. Pigmentary

retinopathy is rare. In general, children with LCHAD deficiency present at a few months of age with liver disease caused by accumulation of fat in the liver. Severely affected children with MTP deficiency present with heart problems in the first few weeks of life. Those with mild MTP deficiency can present at an older age, generally greater than 2 years of age, with myopathy and neurological abnormalities.

Laboratory findings include hypoglycemia and elevated CPK and lactate. Myoglobinuria is often present. An acylcarnitine profile shows elevations of C14-OH, C16-OH, C18-OH, and C18:1-OH carnitines. Urine organic acids may have dicarboxylic and 3-hydroxydicarboxylic aciduria. In fact, TFP seems to be the only fatty acid oxidation defect (FAOD) in which blood lactate is consistently elevated even when the patient is asymptomatic because of the inhibition of PDH by excessive 3-OH-palmitoyl-CoA.[31,32]

Treatment includes avoiding fasting and supplementation of carnitine in small doses but only if needed for secondary carnitine deficiency. Dietary intervention may include the addition of MCT oil and potentially uncooked cornstarch.

Children and adults can have progressive myopathy and recurrent episodes of rhabdomyolysis that may not have an identifiable trigger.

Carnitine-Palmitoyl Transferase I Deficiency

Carnitine-palmitoyl transferase (CPT) I is an outer mitochondrial membrane enzyme that converts acyl-CoA compounds to acylcarnitine analogues. The gene *CPT1A*, predominantly expressed in the liver is located at 11q13. Patients with CPT I deficiency can present with hepatic encephalopathy, hypoketotic hypoglycemia, severe liver failure, and RTA. Mothers carrying infants with CPT I deficiency have been reported to have AFLP.[33,34]

Laboratory studies show an increase in blood free and total carnitine levels, typically around 70–170 μM, with normal being 20–70 μM. An acylcarnitine profile tends to show a decrease in C18 and C18:1 carnitines. Diagnosis can be made by enzyme activity in fibroblasts or mutation analysis. There is a common mutation, P479L, in the Native Alaskan Inuit population.[33,34]

Treatment focuses on avoidance of fasting and hypoglycemia by dextrose-containing intravenous fluids when unable to tolerate feeding and addition of cornstarch and MCT oil to usual daily feeding regimens.[33,34]

Individuals can have normal growth and development in between episodes of hepatic encephalopathy until there is an episode of decompensation

CHAPTER 60

that results in neurological damage. Periodic evaluation of liver transaminases and synthetic function is recommended.

Carnitine-Palmitoyl Transferase II Deficiency and Carnitine/Acylcarnitine Translocase Deficiency

Carnitine/acylcarnitine translocase (CACT) is a transmembrane transporter that transfers acylcarnitines through the mitochondrial membrane. CACT deficiency is inherited in an autosomal recessive manner by mutations in both copies of *SLC25A20* located at 3p21.31. CPT II is a mitochondrial matrix enzyme that is required to reesterify acylcarnitines to acyl-CoA esters and is coded by the gene *CPT2*, which is located at 1p32.

There are several presentations, including the lethal neonatal and severe infantile forms, as well as a milder myopathic form.[34,35] The lethal neonatal and severe infantile forms result in liver failure with hyperammonemia and elevated transaminases, hypoketotic hypoglycemia, cardiomyopathy, arrhythmia, seizures, and early death. The milder form usually presents later in life with muscle pain and weakness that occurs especially during times of exercise. Patients can have rhabdomyolysis with elevations in CPK and myoglobinuria, and these findings tend to occur more commonly in males than in females.

Laboratory studies show decreased blood free and total carnitine and elevations of long-chain acylcarnitine species, particularly C16, C18, and C18:1 carnitines, by acylcarnitine profile analysis. Diagnosis of CACT deficiency can be confirmed by mutation analysis of *SLC25A20*. Diagnosis of CPT II is confirmed by enzyme activity in fibroblasts, whole blood, or muscle or by mutation analysis of *CPT2*. Genotype-phenotype correlations can be made. Lethal mutations are P227L, K414TfsX7, and K642TfsX6. Severe mutations are Y120C, R151Q, N328G, R382K, R503C, Y628S, and R631C. Milder myopathic mutations are S113L, P50H, and K414TfsX7.[34,35]

Treatment includes carnitine supplementation if a secondary carnitine deficiency is identified, adequate hydration with the avoidance of fasting and hypoglycemia, in addition to the use of a high-calorie diet with MCT oil supplementation. Those with myopathic symptoms should take specific care to avoid dehydration, excessive exercise, and fasting. Valproate, ibuprofen, high-dose diazepam, and general anesthesia should be avoided.

Those who present symptomatically as neonates usually have poor outcomes, and death is common. Milder presentations may benefit from treatment,

although sudden death from arrhythmias has been described. Long-term complications can include rhabdomyolysis and liver failure. Routine cardiology evaluation with electrocardiogram and Holter monitoring is recommended; pacemakers should be considered in those identified to have arrhythmias.

FINAL THOUGHTS

To summarize, IEMs are enzyme deficiencies that result from amino acid, carbohydrate, or fatty acid metabolism (Figure 60-2). Most of these disorders can be diagnosed by routine metabolic testing, including plasma amino acid, plasma acylcarnitine profile, and urine organic acid analyses. Table 60-5 provides a summary.

Treatment of the IEMs consists of the basic principle dietary restriction of the offending substrate, such as amino acids or long-chain fats, and supplementation of compounds that can dispose of toxic metabolites, such as carnitine or cofactors that can increase activity of deficient enzymes, including hydroxocobalamin. Whenever a diet is altered from baseline with a medical formula, it is important to supplement with essential amino acids and ensure adequate caloric intake to avoid catabolism and support anabolism. Occasionally, total parenteral nutrition may be necessary, but it must be used with caution.

Outpatient evaluations for individuals with IEMs are numerous and include a physician who deals with metabolics and a nutritionist to monitor biochemistry frequently and adjust diet and supplements for growth, a good pediatrician to monitor growth and development and provide immunizations, in addition to any other specialist required for organ-specific evaluations.

Episodes of decompensation can occur frequently in children with an IEM. Fever, vomiting, diarrhea, infection, and fasting can all be triggers. These episodes can be life threatening, so emergent and aggressive treatment is required. Treatment typically includes reversing catabolism by any means possible, often with extra calories provided from dextrose and lipids when allowed and restriction of the toxic metabolite, such as protein in the OAs.

If a neonate has severely decompensated, is unlikely to be resuscitated, and an IEM is suspected, there are several studies that should be obtained, not only for the purpose of diagnosis but also for genetic counseling, including accurate recurrence risk assessment for the family. These specimens include at a minimum collection of blood, urine, and skin. Table 60-6 provides the entire list.

Table 60-5 Summary of Inborn Errors of Metabolism (IEMs) and Their Findings

IEMs	Enzyme	Gene(s)	Newborn Screen	Plasma Amino Acids	Plasma Acylcarnitines	Urine Organic Acids
Amino Acid Metabolism						
Propionic acidemia	Propionyl-CoA carboxylase	PCCA, PCCB	C3 propionylcarnitine	Glycine	C3 propionylcarnitine	3-Hydroxypropionic, methylcitric acids
Methylmalonic acidemia	Methylmalonyl-CoA mutase	MUT, MMAA, MMAB	C3 propionylcarnitine	Glycine	C3 propionylcarnitine	Methylmalonic, 3-hydroxypropionic, Methylcitric acids
Isovaleric acidemia	Isovaleryl-CoA dehydrogenase	IVD	C5 Isovaleryrlcarnitine	N/A	C5 isovalerylcarnitine	Isovalerylglycine, 3-hydroxyisovaleric acid
Maple syrup urine disease	Branched-chain ketoacid dehydrogenase	BCKDHA, BCKDHB, DBT, DLD	Leucine	Leucine, isoleucine, valine, alloisoleucine	N/A	2-Hydroxyisovaleric, 2-ketoisocaproic acids
Multiple carboxylase deficiency	Holocarboxylase synthetase	HLCS	C3 propionyl- and C5OH hydroxy-isovaleryl-carnitine	Alanine	C3 propionyl- and C5OH hydroxy-isovaleryl-carnitine	Lactic, 3-hydroxy-isovaleric, methylcitric acids, methyl-crotonylglycine
β-Ketothiolase deficiency	β-Ketothiolase	ACAT1	C5OH 2-methyl-3-hydroxybutyrylcarnitine	N/A	C5OH 2-methyl-3-hydroxybutyrylcarnitine and C5:1 tiglylcarnitine	2-Methyl-3-hydroxybutyric and 2-methylacetoacetic acids, tiglylglycine
Carbohydrate Metabolism						
Pyruvate carboxylase deficiency	Pyruvate carboxylase	PC	Citrulline	Citrulline, alanine, lysine, proline	N/A	Lactic, 2-ketoglutaric acids
Pyruvate dehydrogenase deficiency	Pyruvate dehydrogenase	PDHA1, PDHB, DLAT, DLD, PDHX	N/A	Alanine	N/A	Lactic acid
Fructose-1,6-bisphosphatase deficiency	Fructose-1,6-bisphosphatase	FBP1	N/A	N/A	N/A	Lactic, 2-ketoglutaric acids
Glycogen storage disease I	Glucose-6-phosphatase	G6PC	N/A	N/A	N/A	Lactic and uric acids

(Continued)

Table 60-5 Summary of Inborn Errors of Metabolism (IEMs) and Their Findings (*Continued*)

IEMs	Enzyme	Gene(s)	Newborn Screen	Plasma Amino Acids	Plasma Acylcarnitines	Urine Organic Acids
Fatty Acid Metabolism						
Very long-chain acyl-CoA dehydrogenase deficiency	Very long-chain acyl-CoA dehyrdogenase	ACADVL	C14:1 tetradecenoylcarnitine	N/A	C14:1 tetradecenoylcarnitine	Dicarboxylic acids
Long-chain hydroxyacyl-CoA dehydrogenase deficiency	Long-chain hydroxyacyl-CoA dehydrogenase	HADHA, HADHB	C16-OH 3-hydroxyhexadecanoyl- and C18-OH 3-hydroxyoctadecanoyl-carnitine	N/A	C16-OH 3-hydroxyhexadecanoyl- and C18-OH 3-hydroxyoctadecanoyl-carnitine	(Hydroxy)dicarboxylic acids
Carnitine palmitoyltransferase I deficiency	Carnitine palmitoyltransferase I	CPT1A	C0 free carnitine with decreased C16, C18, C18:1	N/A	C0 free carnitine with decreased C16, C18, C18:1	N/A
Carnitine palmitoyltransferase II deficiency	Carnitine palmitoyltransferase II	CPT2	C16 hexadecanoyl-, C18 octadecanoyl- and C18:1 octadecenoyl-carnitine	N/A	C16 hexadecanoyl-, C18 octadecanoyl- and C18:1 octadecenoyl-carnitine	N/A
Carnitine translocase deficiency	Carnitine/acylcarnitine translocase	SCL25A20	C16 hexadecanoyl-, C18 octadecanoyl- and C18:1 octadecenoyl-carnitine	N/A	C16 hexadecanoyl-, C18 octadecanoyl- and C18:1 octadecenoyl-carnitine	N/A

Table 60-6 Perimortem Specimen Collection

1. Whole blood in EDTA (ethylenediaminetetraacetic acid) tube for DNA extraction; stored at room temperature
2. Blood dropped on filter paper card; stored at room temperature
3. Plasma collected in heparinized tube, separated, and deep-frozen
4. Urine collected in sterile container and deep-frozen
5. Skin biopsy for fibroblast culture; must be sterile procedure
6. Liver biopsy; snap-frozen in liquid nitrogen
7. Muscle (heart or skeletal) biopsy; snap-frozen in liquid nitrogen

REFERENCES

1. Tschudy, Arcara MM, Kristin M, eds. *The Harriet Lane Handbook: A Manual for Pediatric House Officers.* 16th ed. Philadelphia, PA: Mosby; 2002.

2. de Baulny HO, Benoist JF, Rigal O, Touati G, Rabier D, Saudubray JM. Methylmalonic and propionic acidaemias: management and outcome. *J Inherit Metab Dis.* 2005;28(3):415–423.

3. Fenton WA, Gravel RA, Rosenblatt DS. Disorders of propionate and methylmalonate metabolism. In: Scriver CR, Sly WS, Childs B, et al, eds. *The Metabolic and Molecular Basis of Inherited Disease.* 8th ed. New York, NY: McGraw-Hill; 2001:2165–2193.

4. Chapman KA, Gropman A, MacLeod E, et al. Acute management of propionic acidemia. *Mol Genet Metab.* 2012;105(1):16–25.

5. Seashore MR. The organic acidemias: an overview. 2001 Jun 27 [Updated 2009 Dec 22]. In: Pagon RA, Adam MP, Ardinger HH, et al., editors. GeneReviews® [Internet]. Seattle (WA): University of Washington, Seattle; 1993-2014. Available from: http://www.ncbi.nlm.nih.gov/books/NBK1134/.

6. Childs B, Nyhan WL. Further observations of a patient with hyperglycinemia. *Pediatrics.* 1964;33:403–412.

7. Childs B, Nyhan WL, Borden M, Bard L, Cooke RE. Idiopathic hyperglycinemia and hyperglycinuria: a new disorder of amino acid metabolism. I. *Pediatrics.* 1961;27:522–538.

8. Grunert SC, Mullerleile S, de SL, et al. Propionic acidemia: neonatal versus selective metabolic screening. *J Inherit Metab Dis.* 2012;35(1):41–49.

9. Pena L, Franks J, Chapman KA, et al. Natural history of propionic acidemia. *Mol Genet Metab.* 2012;105(1):5–9.

10. Sutton VR, Chapman KA, Gropman AL, et al. Chronic management and health supervision of individuals with propionic acidemia. *Mol Genet Metab.* 2012;105(1):26–33.

11. Sass JO, Hofmann M, Skladal D, Mayatepek E, Schwahn B, Sperl W. Propionic acidemia revisited: a workshop report. *Clin Pediatr (Phila).* 2004;43(9):837–843.

12. Pena L, Burton BK. Survey of health status and complications among propionic acidemia patients. *Am J Med Genet A.* 2012;158A(7):1641–1646.

13. Manoli I, Venditti CP. Methylmalonic acidemia. 2005 Aug 16 [Updated 2010 Sep 28]. In: Pagon RA, Adam MP, Ardinger HH, et al., editors. GeneReviews® [Internet]. Seattle (WA): University of Washington, Seattle; 1993-2014. Available from: http://www.ncbi.nlm.nih.gov/books/NBK1231/.

14. Ensenauer R, Vockley J, Willard JM, et al. A common mutation is associated with a mild, potentially asymptomatic phenotype in patients with isovaleric acidemia diagnosed by newborn screening. *Am J Hum Genet.* 2004;75(6):1136–1142.

15. Grunert SC, Wendel U, Lindner M, et al. Clinical and neuro-cognitive outcome in symptomatic isovaleric acidemia. *Orphanet J Rare Dis.* 2012;7:9.

16. Wilson CJ, Myer M, Darlow BA, et al. Severe holocarboxylase synthetase deficiency with incomplete biotin responsiveness resulting in antenatal insult in samoan neonates. *J Pediatr.* 2005;147(1):115–118.

17. Morrone A, Malvagia S, Donati MA, et al. Clinical findings and biochemical and molecular analysis of four patients with holocarboxylase synthetase deficiency. *Am J Med Genet.* 2002;111(1):10–18.

18. Strauss KA, Puffenberger EG, Morton DH. Maple syrup urine disease. 2006 Jan 30 [Updated 2013 May 9]. In: Pagon RA, Adam MP, Ardinger HH, et al., editors. GeneReviews® [Internet]. Seattle (WA): University of Washington, Seattle; 1993-2014. Available from: http://www.ncbi.nlm.nih.gov/books/NBK1319/.

19. le RC, Murphy E, Hallam P, Lilburn M, Orlowska D, Lee P. Neuropsychometric outcome predictors for adults with maple syrup urine disease. *J Inherit Metab Dis.* 2006;29(1):201–202.

20. Morton DH, Strauss KA, Robinson DL, Puffenberger EG, Kelley RI. Diagnosis and treatment of maple syrup disease: a study of 36 patients. *Pediatrics.* 2002;109(6):999–1008.

21. Fukao T, Scriver CR, Kondo N. The clinical phenotype and outcome of mitochondrial acetoacetyl-CoA thiolase deficiency (beta-ketothiolase or T2 deficiency) in 26 enzymatically proved and mutation-defined patients. *Mol Genet Metab.* 2001;72(2):109–114.

22. Wang D, De Vivo D. Pyruvate carboxylase deficiency. 2009 Jun 2 [Updated 2014 Jul 24]. In: Pagon RA, Adam MP, Ardinger HH, et al., editors. GeneReviews® [Internet]. Seattle (WA): University of Washington, Seattle; 1993-2014. Available from: http://www.ncbi.nlm.nih.gov/books/NBK6852/.

23. Wang D, Yang H, De Braganca KC, et al. The molecular basis of pyruvate carboxylase deficiency: mosaicism correlates with prolonged survival. *Mol Genet Metab.* 2008;95(1–2):31–38.

24. Debrosse SD, Okajima K, Zhang S, et al. Spectrum of neurological and survival outcomes in pyruvate dehydrogenase complex (PDC) deficiency: lack of correlation with genotype. *Mol Genet Metab.* 2012;107(3):394–402.

25. Wexler ID, Hemalatha SG, McConnell J, et al. Outcome of pyruvate dehydrogenase deficiency treated with ketogenic diets. Studies in patients with identical mutations. *Neurology.* 1997;49(6):1655–1661.

26. van den Berghe G. Disorders of gluconeogenesis. *J Inherit Metab Dis.* 1996;19(4):470–477.

27. Burlina AB, Poletto M, Shin YS, Zacchello F. Clinical and biochemical observations on three cases of fructose-1,6-diphosphatase deficiency. *J Inherit Metab Dis.* 1990;13(3):263–266.

28. Matern D, Seydewitz HH, Bali D, Lang C, Chen YT. Glycogen storage disease type I: diagnosis and phenotype/genotype correlation. *Eur J Pediatr.* 2002;161(Suppl 1):S10–S19.

29. Leslie ND, Valencia CA, Strauss AW, et al. Very long-chain acyl-coenzyme A dehydrogenase deficiency. 2009 May 28 [Updated 2014 Sep 11]. In: Pagon RA, Adam MP, Ardinger HH, et al., editors. GeneReviews® [Internet]. Seattle (WA): University of Washington, Seattle; 1993-2014. Available from: http://www.ncbi.nlm.nih.gov/books/NBK6816/.

30. Allen SK, Luharia A, Gould CP, Macdonald F, Larkins S, Davison EV. Rapid prenatal diagnosis of common trisomies: discordant results between QF-PCR analysis and karyotype analysis on long-term culture for a case of trisomy 18 detected in CVS. *Prenat Diagn.* 2006;26(12):1160–1167.

31. Spiekerkoetter U, Lindner M, Santer R, et al. Treatment recommendations in long-chain fatty acid oxidation defects: consensus from a workshop. *J Inherit Metab Dis.* 2009;32(4):498–505.

32. Spiekerkoetter U. Mitochondrial fatty acid oxidation disorders: clinical presentation of long-chain fatty acid oxidation defects before and after newborn screening. *J Inherit Metab Dis.* 2010;33(5):527–532.

33. Bennett MJ, Santani AB. Carnitine palmitoyltransferase 1A deficiency. 2005 Jul 27 [Updated 2013 Mar 7]. In: Pagon RA, Adam MP, Ardinger HH, et al., editors. GeneReviews® [Internet]. Seattle (WA): University of Washington, Seattle; 1993-2014. Available from: http://www.ncbi.nlm.nih.gov/books/NBK1527/.

34. Longo N, Amat di San Filippo C, Pasquali M. Disorders of carnitine transport and the carnitine cycle. *Am J Med Genet C Semin Med Genet.* 2006;142C(2):77–85.

35. Wieser T. Carnitine palmitoyltransferase II deficiency. 2004 Aug 27 [Updated 2014 May 15]. In: Pagon RA, Adam MP, Ardinger HH, et al., editors. GeneReviews® [Internet]. Seattle (WA): University of Washington, Seattle; 1993-2014. Available from: http://www.ncbi.nlm.nih.gov/books/NBK1253/.

Congenital Muscular Dystrophies and Congenital Myopathies

Peter B. Kang, Pankaj B. Agrawal, and Alan H. Beggs

BACKGROUND

There are a number of neuromuscular disease categories that cause hypotonia and weakness in infancy. Arranged in order of neuroanatomic localization, these include motor neuron diseases (eg, spinal muscular atrophy), neuropathies (eg, congenital hypomyelinating neuropathies), disorders of the neuromuscular junction (eg, congenital myasthenic syndrome), and muscle diseases. Major categories of muscle disease in infancy include congenital myopathies, congenital muscular dystrophies, congenital myotonic dystrophies, and glycogen storage diseases. Congenital myopathies and congenital muscular dystrophies are the subjects of this chapter.

Muscular dystrophies share in common a set of histopathological findings consistent with muscle degeneration, including excessive fiber size variability, myofiber necrosis, myofiber regeneration and centralized nuclei, and infiltration of connective tissue and fat with rounded fibers. Congenital muscular dystrophies have traditionally been regarded as muscular dystrophies with congenital onset. Many of the protein products of genes implicated in congenital muscular dystrophy are involved directly or indirectly with the structures of the extracellular matrix.

Congenital myopathies have traditionally been defined as a category of myopathies with onset at birth and histopathological findings of structural abnormalities in myofibers rather than the degenerative changes characteristic of congenital muscular dystrophies. The genetic etiologies of many, although not all, cases of congenital muscular dystrophies and congenital myopathies have been characterized. This genetic knowledge has revealed that later-onset variants exist for a number of subtypes. It is also becoming recognized that some muscle diseases of infancy share features of both congenital muscular dystrophy and congenital myopathy.

Many, although not all, congenital muscular dystrophies are associated with structural brain malformations, central nervous system dysfunction, or eye abnormalities, distinguishing them from congenital myopathies, which are rarely associated with these complications. Patterns of weakness and contractures may also help assign subtype classifications in cases of congenital muscular dystrophy.

DIAGNOSIS

The diagnostic evaluation of patients with suspected congenital muscular dystrophy or myopathy may be difficult as there is overlap between the phenotypes of the 2 categories of muscle disease, and other neuromuscular diseases (eg, spinal muscular atrophy) may be included in the differential diagnosis. All of these diseases may be associated with areflexia, hypotonia, and skeletal muscle weakness. Physical examination can help differentiate among these categories. For example, muscle weakness found in the face, extraocular muscles, or both may be suggestive of a congenital myopathy, whereas intact cranial nerves may be more consistent with spinal muscular atrophy. Eye abnormalities may suggest a congenital muscular dystrophy.

Serum creatinine kinase (CPK, also known as CK) levels may be mildly elevated in congenital muscular dystrophy, congenital myopathy, and sometimes even spinal muscular atrophy, although more dramatic elevations are more suggestive of congenital muscular dystrophy. Aldolase is another muscle enzyme that can be measured in serum. The enzymes alanine aminotransferase (ALT), aspartate aminotransferase (AST), and lactate dehydrogenase (LDH) are often measured in serum and are commonly referred to as "liver function tests," but they are also found in small amounts in muscle; thus, it would be more appropriate to refer to them as transaminases. Elevations in the CPK are typically more dramatic than those of the transaminases, and the predicted ratio between them can be calculated mathematically in muscular dystrophies.[1] Because of the more frequent assessments of transaminases for a variety of indications, an increasing number of patients with muscular dystrophy are being identified based on incidental findings of elevations in these enzymes.

If the physical findings and basic laboratory studies do not convincingly point to 1 of these categories, an electromyography (EMG) study may help distinguish between neurogenic and myopathic disorders. If the EMG findings are neurogenic, genetic testing for spinal muscular atrophy will confirm the diagnosis. If the EMG findings are myopathic, a muscle biopsy is often helpful in identifying the specific type of muscle disease that is present and remains critical to the diagnosis in many cases.

Muscle biopsy is a key diagnostic modality for the diagnosis of congenital muscular dystrophies and congenital myopathies. Histological features that suggest the diagnosis of congenital muscular dystrophy include variation in fiber size, rounded fibers, inflammation, degenerating fibers, regenerating fibers, and endomysial connective tissue infiltration. Immunohistochemical stains can detect deficiencies in proteins related to congenital muscular dystrophy, such as merosin and collagen VI. In congenital myopathies, basic histological findings, such as nemaline rods, centralized nuclei, central cores, and fiber sizes, can help assign a case to a particular subtype. Electron microscopy can provide further details on the structural abnormalities and may help assign subtypes to particular cases.

A relatively new diagnostic modality that may be helpful in the diagnosis of congenital muscular dystrophies is muscle ultrasound. Specific patterns of muscle involvement are associated with different subtypes of congenital muscular dystrophy, and such patterns may be detected noninvasively in this manner.

Genetic testing is critical for the diagnosis of many cases of congenital muscular dystrophies and congenital myopathies but must be interpreted in the context of the clinical phenotype for 2 reasons. First, several of the known causative genes are associated with several subtypes of disease; thus, gene mutations alone

may not be sufficient for a subtype-specific diagnosis. Second, despite the major genetic advances in recent years, a significant proportion of patients with either type of disease do not have mutations in any of the known associated genes.

The differential diagnosis for a particular patient often includes several subtypes of congenital muscular dystrophy or congenital myopathy. Outside these entities, the differential diagnosis may include some or all of the diseases discussed in the first paragraph of the chapter. And, in some cases, diseases that are not typically classified as peripheral nervous system disorders may present with such features, most notably Prader-Willi syndrome.

CONGENITAL MUSCULAR DYSTROPHIES

There are 3 major categories of congenital muscular dystrophy, based on the function of the protein products of the implicated genes. In overall descending order of severity, they are the dystroglycanopathies, merosinopathies, and collagenopathies. However, the phenotypic range of each subtype, especially the dystroglycanopathies, has expanded to the point that a significant overlap in severity among the subtypes is now recognized. Dystroglycanopathies encompass both classic phenotypes such as Walker-Warburg syndrome, muscle-eye-brain disease, and Fukuyama congenital muscular dystrophy and newer phenotypes such as fukutin-related protein (FKRP) deficiency and LARGE deficiency. Sometimes, the classic phenotypes overlap with the genes associated with the newer ones; for example, FKRP deficiency has been associated with Walker-Warburg syndrome. Merosin-deficient congenital muscular dystrophy is the only merosinopathy identified to date. The 2 collagenopathies are Ullrich congenital muscular dystrophy and Bethlem myopathy. In addition, rigid spine congenital muscular dystrophy is a rare variant that has been associated with mutations in *SEPN1*.

Biochemically, a number of the proteins involved with congenital muscular dystrophies are directly or indirectly involved with the extracellular matrix. For example, collagen VI and merosin are found primarily in the extracellular matrix. The proteins associated with the dystroglycanopathies are involved with the process of glycosylation of α-dystroglycan, a sarcolemmal membrane protein that connects the subsarcolemmal cytoskeleton with merosin and other components of the extracellular matrix.

Walker-Warburg syndrome is generally regarded as the most severe of the congenital muscular dystrophies and has been described in numerous populations around the world. In addition to the muscular dystrophy manifesting as severe hypotonia and weakness at birth, affected infants also have severe brain malformations that may include cobblestone lissencephaly, agyria, cerebellar hypoplasia, hydrocephalus, and agenesis of the corpus callosum. Functional central nervous system complications such as epilepsy and cognitive delays also occur. Structural eye abnormalities, such as cataracts, microphthalmos, and buphthalmos, are also common. Walker-Warburg syndrome is generally inherited in an autosomal recessive manner, and 5 associated genes have been identified to date: *POMT1*,[2,3] *POMT2*,[4] *POMGnT1*,[5] *FKTN*,[6,7] and *FKRP*.[8] Many affected children do not survive infancy.

Muscle-eye-brain disease, as the name suggests, shares some of the multiorgan system features of Walker-Warburg syndrome, and affected infants usually present at birth with severe, diffuse hypotonia and weakness. It also appears to have a worldwide distribution. In its classic form, muscle-eye-brain disease is associated with a slightly milder phenotype than Walker-Warburg syndrome, but there is significant overlap in severity between the 2 subtypes. The muscle tissue typically demonstrates classic dystrophic features. Structural brain abnormalities such as pachygyria, polymicrogyria, cerebellar malformations, and flattening of brainstem are common; these tend to be less severe than in Walker-Warburg syndrome. Functional central nervous system abnormalities such as epilepsy and cognitive delays frequently occur. Eye abnormalities may include microphthalmos, retinal hypoplasia, and glaucoma. Muscle-eye-brain disease is inherited in an autosomal recessive pattern. Mutations in *POMGnT1* are the most commonly known cause of muscle-eye-brain disease,[9–11] but mutations in *FKRP*[8] and *POMT2*[12,13] have also been described in this disease. Life expectancy is more variable than in Walker-Warburg syndrome. At the more severe end of the spectrum, children may not survive infancy, while at the milder end, a small proportion of children are able to walk at some point in their course.

Fukuyama congenital muscular dystrophy is the most common congenital muscular dystrophy in Japan and also appears to be a common congenital muscular dystrophy in other Asian countries, such as Korea. However, in the rest of the world, it has so far proven to be rare, with scattered reports from other countries. Muscle histology demonstrates typical dystrophic features. Fukuyama congenital muscular dystrophy has many phenotypic similarities with muscle-eye-brain disease. Structural brain malformations may include polymicrogyria, pachygyria, and in some cases even agyria. Cerebellar cysts are a characteristic finding. Epilepsy is common. Eye abnormalities may include cataracts and a range of functional ocular problems. An autosomal recessive retrotransposal insertion in the gene *FKTN* is a founder mutation that is the cause

of most cases of this disease in Japan, and the carrier frequency in that country has been estimated[14] as 1/88. Cardiac and pulmonary complications are common. Affected individuals are sometimes able to walk with support at some point during the course of the disease and typically survive into adolescence or early adulthood.

FKRP deficiency has been associated with cases of congenital muscular dystrophy with dystroglycanopathy that do not meet the definition of Walker-Warburg syndrome.[15] These patients have congenital onset, are not able to walk, and have significant elevations in serum CPK levels. Brain structure and function were preserved in the first series published,[15] but 2 patients with cerebellar cysts and cognitive delays were later reported.[16] Severe restrictive lung disease is common, and cardiac abnormalities have been observed.[15]

LARGE deficiency causes a rare type of congenital muscular dystrophy with dystroglycanopathy.[17] The first reported patient was able to walk during childhood, but then developed motor regression. She had severe cognitive delays, white matter abnormalities in the brain, and elevated serum CPK levels.

Merosinopathy, also known as merosin deficiency and merosin-deficient congenital muscular dystrophy, is a moderately severe congenital muscular dystrophy that is a more common subtype in many populations. It presents with hypotonia and weakness at birth that follows a stable or slowly progressive course. Feeding difficulties in infancy may require nasogastric or gastrostomy tube feeds. Diffuse white matter lesions are characteristic of this disorder, and when found in conjunction with high serum CPK levels, a dystrophic muscle biopsy, or both, are highly suggestive of the diagnosis. Representative histological features from a muscle biopsy are presented in Figure 61-1. Recessive mutations in the extracellular matrix gene *LAMA2* have been found to cause merosinopathy.[18] No other associated genes have been identified to date. Nearly all patients with complete merosin deficiency on muscle biopsy have been found to have mutations in *LAMA2*.[19,20] The rate of *LAMA2* mutation detection appears to be lower when there is partial deficiency of merosin.[21,22] At least transient ambulation has been reported in some patients. Pulmonary complications may be exacerbated by scoliosis, and cardiac complications are common. Life expectancy is variable, depending on the severity of the case and the aggressiveness of supportive interventions.

Most forms of Bethlem myopathy are inherited in an autosomal dominant pattern, with childhood onset, weakness of proximal and extensor muscles, and contractures of multiple joints, including the elbows and heel cords.[23] The collagen genes *COL6A1* and *COL6A2* on chromosome 21q22.3[24] and *COL6A3* on chromosome 2q37[25] have been associated with

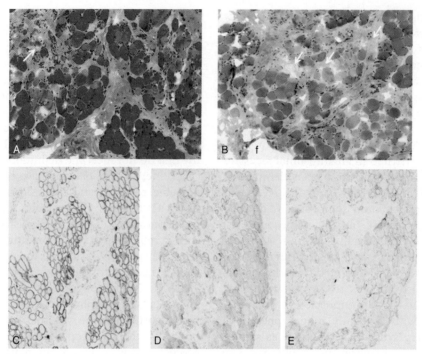

FIGURE 61-1 Representative light microscopic images from a muscle biopsy obtained from a patient with merosin-deficient congenital muscular dystrophy. A, A hematoxylin and eosin section at ×20 magnification demonstrates marked excess variability in fiber size, increased endomysial fibrosis (blue arrow), many atrophic fibers, rounded fibers, increased internalized nuclei, focal necrosis (white arrow), scattered hypertrophic fibers, rare basophilic regenerating fibers (red arrow), and fatty replacement. B, Gomori trichrome stain reveals markedly increased endomysial and perimysial connective tissue (white arrows). C, Dystrophin immunocytochemistry demonstrates intact sarcolemmal labeling. D, Merosin immunocytochemistry using an antibody to the 300-kDa fragment shows patchy partial sarcolemmal staining. E, Merosin immunocytochemistry using an antibody to the 80-kDa fragment shows patchy partial sarcolemmal staining. (Used with permission of Hart G. W. Lidov, MD, PhD.)

Bethlem myopathy. The clinical course is slowly progressive, but many of the patients lose ambulation during adulthood.[26] More recently, compound heterozygous mutations in *COL6A2* have been associated with an autosomal recessive variant of Bethlem myopathy in several patients.[27,28]

Ullrich congenital muscular dystrophy has a characteristic clinical presentation of proximal joint contractures, distal joint laxity, spinal rigidity, and respiratory distress.[29] The disease can be inherited in an autosomal recessive or dominant manner, and causative mutations in the collagen genes *COL6A1*,[30,31] *COL6A2*,[32,33] and *COL6A3*[34] have been identified, the same genes associated with Bethlem myopathy.

Rigid spine congenital muscular dystrophy is characterized by spinal rigidity and respiratory insufficiency; thus, its phenotype overlaps with that of Ullrich congenital muscular dystrophy to some extent.[35] It is caused by mutations in *SEPN1*[36] and *FHL1*.[37]

Other congenital muscular dystrophies have been associated with mutations in *ITGA7*,[38] *DNM2*,[39] *TCAP*,[40] and *CHKB*.[41] More genes are likely to be identified in the future.

CONGENITAL MYOPATHIES

There are 4 major histological categories of congenital myopathy, arranged in descending order of severity of the classical phenotypes: centronuclear myopathy (including X-linked myotubular myopathy), nemaline myopathy, central core disease, and congenital fiber-type disproportion.[42] However, clinical variants have now been described for all these diseases, broadening the range of severity for each, and it is clear that there is considerable phenotypic overlap among these subtypes.[43,44] For example, centronuclear myopathy is typically associated with more severe weakness than nemaline myopathy, but severe cases of nemaline myopathy may be associated with worse outcomes than milder cases of centronuclear myopathy. There are also rare forms of congenital myopathy that do not fall into 1 of the traditional histological categories. These include multiminicore myopathy and other subtypes that are associated with defects in specific muscle proteins, such as actinopathy and desminopathy. The causative genes and clinical features are summarized in Table 61-1.

Table 61-1 Subtypes of Congenital Myopathy With Causative Genes and a Summary of Clinical Features

Disease	Genes	Proteins	Onset	Weakness	Cardiac	Respiratory	Facial	Oculomotor	Prognosis
Centronuclear myopathy, X-linked (myotubular myopathy)	MTM1	Myotubularin	Prenatal – congenital	+++	-	++	+++	+++	Death in infancy, some survive to adulthood
Centronuclear myopathy, classic	BIN1	Amphiphysin 2	Late infancy – early childhood	+	-	++	++	++	Ambulation until adolescence
Centronuclear myopathy, adult	DNM2	Dynamin 2	2nd – 3rd decade	+	-	-	+	+/-	Slowly progressive
Nemaline myopathy, severe (neonatal)	**ACTA1** **NEB** TPM3 **TNNT1**	α-actin Nebulin α-tropomyosin$_{SLOW}$ Troponin T type 1	Birth	+++	-	++	+++	-	Death in neonatal period
Nemaline myopathy, typical (classical)	ACTA1 NEB TPM3 TPM2 CFL2	α-actin Nebulin α-tropomyosin$_{SLOW}$ β-tropomyosin Cofilin 2	1st year	++	+/-	+	+++	-	Many survive to adulthood
Nemaline myopathy, childhood	ACTA1 NEM2 TPM3 KBTBD13	α-actin Nebulin α-tropomyosin$_{SLOW}$ KBTBD13	Pre-pubertal	+	-	-	-	-	Many survive to adulthood
Nemaline myopathy, adult	ACTA1 NEM2	α-actin Nebulin	3rd – 6th decade	+	+	+/-	++	-	Adulthood
Central core, classical	RYR1	Ryanodine receptor	Infancy	+	Rare	-	+	-	Adulthood?
Congenital fiber-type disproportion	ACTA1 SEPN1 TPM3 RYR1	α-actin Selenoprotein α-tropomyosin$_{SLOW}$	1st year	+ to +++	Rare	+ to +++ (30%)	+	+/-	Variable

(Continued)

Table 61-1 Subtypes of Congenital Myopathy With Causative Genes and a Summary of Clinical Features *(Continued)*

Disease	Genes	Proteins	Onset	Weakness	Cardiac	Respiratory	Facial	Oculomotor	Prognosis
Multiminicore disease	SEPN1 RYR1	Selenoprotein Ryanodine receptor	Infancy – to early childhood	++	Rare	++	++	Rare	Variable
Actin myopathy (non-nemaline)	ACTA1	α-actin	Congenital	+++	+	+++	++	?	High mortality
Bethlem myopathy	COL6A1 COL6A2 COL6A3	Collagen type VI α1, α2, α3 chains	1st or 2nd decade	+	–	+	+/–	–	Good
Myofibrillar myopathies	DES CRYAB ZASP FLNC MYOT	Desmin αB-crystallin Z-disk assoc prot Filamin C Myotilin	2nd to 8th decade	+	+	+	–	–	Some patients lose ambulation

Some physical findings may help differentiate among the various classical subtypes. Both facial and extraocular muscle weakness are found in patients with centronuclear myopathy, including myotubular myopathy. Patients with nemaline myopathy tend to have facial weakness without external ophthalmoplegia. Central core disease may or may not be associated with facial weakness, but extraocular muscle strength is usually preserved. Exceptions to these patterns exist, but observations of cranial nerve findings can be helpful in suggesting possible diagnoses.

Centronuclear myopathy, as the name suggests, is characterized by centralized nuclei in a high proportion of myofibers. It should be noted, however, that centralized nuclei in a small number of myofibers are nonspecific findings that suggest muscle regeneration and may in fact be more suggestive of congenital muscular dystrophy than congenital myopathy. Classic centronuclear myopathy is inherited in an autosomal recessive manner and has been associated to date with mutations in *BIN1*[45]; milder variants have been identified that follow an autosomal dominant pattern of inheritance, and mutations in *DNM2* have been associated with this subtype.[46] The protein products amphiphysin 2 and dynamin 2 interact with each other.

X-linked myotubular myopathy is also characterized by centralized nuclei in a high proportion of myofibers; thus, it is now generally regarded as a subtype of centronuclear myopathy. The histological features are reminiscent of fetal myotubes, from which the disease name arises. An example of classic histological features of X-linked myotubular myopathy is illustrated in Figure 61-2A. In contrast to autosomal centronuclear myopathy, myotubular myopathy is inherited in an X-linked recessive manner and tends to have a more severe clinical course than autosomal centronuclear myopathy. Many affected individuals do not survive infancy, although rare cases of survival into adulthood

have been reported. The gene associated with many cases of myotubular myopathy is *MTM1*.[47]

Nemaline myopathy is associated with the very distinct histological finding of nemaline rods on muscle biopsy; these rods are typically seen in clusters that are most easily observed on Gomori trichrome stains (Figure 61-2B) and identified in greater detail on electron microscopy. In contrast to the centralized nuclei in centronuclear myopathy, nemaline rod accumulations are irregular, may be found anywhere in the sarcoplasm, and are often localized near the sarcolemma. Ten genes have been associated with nemaline myopathy to date: *ACTA1*,[48] *CFL2*,[49] *NEB*,[50] *TNNT1*,[51] *TPM2*,[52] *TPM3*,[53] *KBTBD13*,[54,55] *KLHL40*,[73] *KLHL41*,[74] and *LMOD3*.[75]

Central core disease is characterized histologically by well-circumscribed areas of poor oxidative activity that lack mitochondria and are localized at or near the center of type 1 muscle fibers. The cores may be observed best on oxidative histochemical stains, such as succinate dehydrogenase (SDH), nicotinamide dehydrogenase (NADH), or cytochrome *c* oxidase (COX) stains, and may be less apparent on basic hematoxylin and eosin stains or Gomori trichrome stains. Central core disease and isolated malignant hyperthermia are associated with mutations in *RYR1*.[56,57] The phenotypic spectrum of *RYR1* mutations has expanded recently, and these mutations have been described in several other myopathies as well.

Congenital fiber-type disproportion has been a controversial entity, as it is histologically a diagnosis of exclusion. The fiber-type disproportion found in congenital fiber-type disproportion is also found in other congenital myopathies, such as nemaline myopathy. However, congenital fiber-type disproportion is defined by the finding of fiber-type disproportion in the absence of histological markers for those other diseases. Thus, it was previously proposed that this category would eventually disappear. Several genes have been associated with congenital

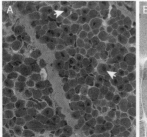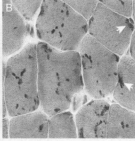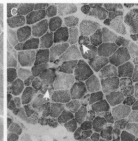

FIGURE 61-2 Representative light microscopic images from muscle biopsies obtained during infancy and early childhood from patients with various forms of congenital myopathy. A, A hematoxylin and eosin stain of a muscle biopsy from a child with X-linked myotubular myopathy. The histology is characterized by an abundance of centralized nuclei, examples of which are indicated by the arrows. B, A modified Gomori trichrome stain illustrates the abundance of nemaline rods (arrows) that are typically found in children with nemaline myopathy. C, Multiple minicores (arrows) are seen on cytochrome oxidase staining of muscle tissue from a child with multiminicore myopathy.

CHAPTER 61

fiber-type disproportion. *TPM3* is probably the most common associated gene, accounting for 20%–25% of cases by 1 estimate.[58] *RYR1* mutations have also been found to be common.[59] Mutations in *ACTA1*[60] and *SEPN1*[61] are relatively rare causes. Mutations in *MYH7*[62] and *TPM2*[63] have been reported in 1 family each.

Multiminicore disease is characterized histologically by minicores, which are areas of myofibrillar disorganization (Figure 61-2C). The disease has been associated with mutations in *SEPN1*[64] and *RYR1*.[65,66]

OVERLAP DISEASES

There are several rare muscle diseases that have histological characteristics of both congenital muscular dystrophy and congenital myopathy. One example is *MEGF10* myopathy, which is associated with early-onset weakness with respiratory distress, scoliosis, and joint contractures. There is a severe phenotype that has been described as early-onset myopathy, areflexia, respiratory distress, and dysphagia (EMARDD),[67] which has been associated primarily with null mutations in *MEGF10*.[68] A milder phenotype has also been described that is associated with missense mutations in *MEGF10*.[69]

PROGNOSIS AND TREATMENTS

The most severe forms of both types of disorders (eg, Walker-Warburg syndrome among congenital muscular dystrophies and X-linked myotubular myopathy among congenital myopathies) are associated with a high mortality rate in infancy. The mild and moderately severe forms are often slowly progressive or static in their clinical courses. Cognition is generally intact in congenital myopathy and the milder forms of congenital muscular dystrophy; thus, many of these children may be able to participate in mainstream classroom settings with the proper physical accommodations. A number of supportive measures may extend the life expectancy and improve the quality of life for affected children.

Pulmonary complications are frequently encountered in both congenital muscular dystrophy and congenital myopathy; thus, management of pulmonary issues is key to maximizing life expectancy and quality of life. The selection of potential pulmonary interventions for children with neuromuscular disorders has become more diverse in recent years with the rising popularity of noninvasive ventilation options. In particular, masks and nasal cannula may be used instead of tracheostomies to deliver pressure support to children, either at night or at all times.

Orthopedic management and physical therapy resources are important in the care of patients with congenital muscular dystrophies and congenital myopathies. Contractures may be managed conservatively with physical therapy and orthotic devices. In severe cases, especially if contractures are interfering with the ability of the child to walk, surgical procedures may help alleviate the problem. If significant scoliosis develops, to the point that respiratory function is threatened, spinal fusion surgery may be beneficial.

Occupational therapy may be helpful if the child needs assistance to manage activities of daily living, including school activities. A speech/language evaluation may help with communication and speech issues. This is especially important if the patient requires significant respiratory support during school hours.

Nutritional guidance can play a key role if swallowing and feeding issues are present. Some of the more severely affected children will benefit from gastrostomy feedings. Even some of the patients with milder disease may have trouble gaining adequate weight and would benefit from nutritional guidance and supplementation.

Cardiac complications have not been strongly associated with congenital myopathy. However, cardiac functional abnormalities have been described on echocardiography in several subtypes of congenital muscular dystrophy,[70] including Fukuyama congenital muscular dystrophy, merosin-deficient congenital muscular dystrophy,[71] *FKRP* congenital muscular dystrophy,[15] and rigid spine syndrome.[72] Given that the incidence of cardiac complications may not be fully recognized in all subtypes of congenital muscular dystrophy, a baseline cardiology evaluation would be reasonable at diagnosis of any congenital muscular dystrophy, and ongoing cardiac surveillance afterward should be guided by the available literature. Cardiac complications should be monitored and treated appropriately.

CONCLUSIONS

Individually, each subtype of congenital muscular dystrophy and congenital myopathy is relatively rare, but in aggregate, these disorders form a substantial proportion of inherited muscle diseases in childhood. Early diagnosis at least of the overall category of disease is important as this information may be useful in guiding prognosis and management, including decisions regarding ongoing pulmonary and nutritional support. Subtype diagnosis, including identification of causative mutations, helps produce even more specific prognoses and paves the way for genetic counseling. Therapeutic interventions are largely supportive at the current time, but these are becoming more sophisticated, especially in the realm of pulmonary management, and thus treatment of these children continues to advance.

REFERENCES

1. McMillan HJ, Gregas M, Darras BT, Kang PB. Serum transaminase levels in boys with Duchenne and Becker muscular dystrophy. *Pediatrics.* 2011;127:e132–e136.
2. Currier SC, Lee CK, Chang BS, et al. Mutations in POMT1 are found in a minority of patients with Walker-Warburg syndrome. *Am J Med Genet A.* 2005;133A:53–57.
3. Beltran-Valero de Bernabe D, Currier S, Steinbrecher A, et al. Mutations in the O-mannosyltransferase gene POMT1 give rise to the severe neuronal migration disorder Walker-Warburg syndrome. *Am J Hum Genet.* 2002;71:1033–1043.
4. van Reeuwijk J, Janssen M, van den Elzen C, et al. POMT2 mutations cause alpha-dystroglycan hypoglycosylation and Walker-Warburg syndrome. *J Med Genet.* 2005;42:907–912.
5. Taniguchi K, Kobayashi K, Saito K, et al. Worldwide distribution and broader clinical spectrum of muscle-eye-brain disease. *Hum Mol Genet.* 2003;12:527–534.
6. Manzini MC, Gleason D, Chang BS, et al. Ethnically diverse causes of Walker-Warburg syndrome (WWS): FCMD mutations are a more common cause of WWS outside of the Middle East. *Hum Mutat.* 2008;29:E231–E241.
7. de Bernabe DB, van Bokhoven H, van Beusekom E, et al. A homozygous nonsense mutation in the fukutin gene causes a Walker-Warburg syndrome phenotype. *J Med Genet.* 2003;40:845–848.
8. Beltran-Valero de Bernabe D, Voit T, Longman C, et al. Mutations in the FKRP gene can cause muscle-eye-brain disease and Walker-Warburg syndrome. *J Med Genet.* 2004;41:e61.
9. Diesen C, Saarinen A, Pihko H, et al. POMGnT1 mutation and phenotypic spectrum in muscle-eye-brain disease. *J Med Genet.* 2004;41:e115.
10. Hehr U, Uyanik G, Gross C, et al. Novel POMGnT1 mutations define broader phenotypic spectrum of muscle-eye-brain disease. *Neurogenetics.* 2007;8:279–288.
11. Yoshida A, Kobayashi K, Manya H, et al. Muscular dystrophy and neuronal migration disorder caused by mutations in a glycosyltransferase, POMGnT1. *Dev Cell.* 2001;1:717–724.
12. Godfrey C, Clement E, Mein R, et al. Refining genotype phenotype correlations in muscular dystrophies with defective glycosylation of dystroglycan. *Brain.* 2007;130:2725–2735.
13. Mercuri E, D'Amico A, Tessa A, et al. POMT2 mutation in a patient with "MEB-like" phenotype. *Neuromuscul Disord.* 2006;16:446–448.
14. Kobayashi K, Nakahori Y, Miyake M, et al. An ancient retrotransposal insertion causes Fukuyama-type congenital muscular dystrophy. *Nature.* 1998;394:388–392.
15. Brockington M, Blake DJ, Prandini P, et al. Mutations in the fukutin-related protein gene (FKRP) cause a form of congenital muscular dystrophy with secondary laminin alpha2 deficiency and abnormal glycosylation of alpha-dystroglycan. *Am J Hum Genet.* 2001;69:1198–1209.
16. Topaloglu H, Brockington M, Yuva Y, et al. FKRP gene mutations cause congenital muscular dystrophy, mental retardation, and cerebellar cysts. *Neurology.* 2003;60:988–992.
17. Longman C, Brockington M, Torelli S, et al. Mutations in the human LARGE gene cause MDC1D, a novel form of congenital muscular dystrophy with severe mental retardation and abnormal glycosylation of alpha-dystroglycan. *Hum Mol Genet.* 2003;12:2853–2861.
18. Helbling-Leclerc A, Zhang X, Topaloglu H, et al. Mutations in the laminin alpha 2-chain gene (LAMA2) cause merosin-deficient congenital muscular dystrophy. *Nat Genet.* 1995;11:216–218.
19. Oliveira J, Santos R, Soares-Silva I, et al. LAMA2 gene analysis in a cohort of 26 congenital muscular dystrophy patients. *Clin Genet.* 2008;74:502–512.
20. Pegoraro E, Marks H, Garcia CA, et al. Laminin alpha2 muscular dystrophy: genotype/phenotype studies of 22 patients. *Neurology.* 1998;51:101–110.
21. Pegoraro E, Mancias P, Swerdlow SH, et al. Congenital muscular dystrophy with primary laminin alpha2 (merosin) deficiency presenting as inflammatory myopathy. *Ann Neurol.* 1996;40:782–791.
22. Tezak Z, Prandini P, Boscaro M, et al. Clinical and molecular study in congenital muscular dystrophy with partial laminin alpha 2 (LAMA2) deficiency. *Hum Mutat.* 2003;21:103–111.
23. Bethlem J, Wijngaarden GK. Benign myopathy, with autosomal dominant inheritance. A report on three pedigrees. *Brain.* 1976;99:91–100.
24. Jobsis GJ, Keizers H, Vreijling JP, et al. Type VI collagen mutations in Bethlem myopathy, an autosomal dominant myopathy with contractures. *Nat Genet.* 1996;14:113–115.
25. Pan TC, Zhang RZ, Pericak-Vance MA, et al. Missense mutation in a von Willebrand factor type A domain of the alpha 3(VI) collagen gene (COL6A3) in a family with Bethlem myopathy. *Hum Mol Genet.* 1998;7:807–812.
26. Jobsis GJ, Boers JM, Barth PG, de Visser M. Bethlem myopathy: a slowly progressive congenital muscular dystrophy with contractures. *Brain.* 1999;122(Pt 4):649–655.
27. Gualandi F, Urciuolo A, Martoni E, et al. Autosomal recessive Bethlem myopathy. *Neurology.* 2009;73:1883–1891.
28. Foley AR, Hu Y, Zou Y, et al. Autosomal recessive inheritance of classic Bethlem myopathy. *Neuromuscul Disord.* 2009;19:813–817.
29. Mercuri E, Yuva Y, Brown SC, et al. Collagen VI involvement in Ullrich syndrome: a clinical, genetic, and immunohistochemical study. *Neurology.* 2002;58:1354–1359.
30. Pan TC, Zhang RZ, Sudano DG, Marie SK, Bonnemann CG, Chu ML. New molecular mechanism for Ullrich congenital muscular dystrophy: a heterozygous in-frame deletion in the COL6A1 gene causes a severe phenotype. *Am J Hum Genet.* 2003;73:355–369.
31. Giusti B, Lucarini L, Pietroni V, et al. Dominant and recessive COL6A1 mutations in Ullrich scleroatonic muscular dystrophy. *Ann Neurol.* 2005;58:400–410.
32. Camacho Vanegas O, Bertini E, Zhang RZ, et al. Ullrich scleroatonic muscular dystrophy is caused by recessive mutations in collagen type VI. *Proc Natl Acad Sci U S A.* 2001;98:7516–7521.
33. Higuchi I, Shiraishi T, Hashiguchi T, et al. Frameshift mutation in the collagen VI gene causes Ullrich's disease. *Ann Neurol.* 2001;50:261–265.
34. Demir E, Sabatelli P, Allamand V, et al. Mutations in COL6A3 cause severe and mild phenotypes of Ullrich congenital muscular dystrophy. *Am J Hum Genet.* 2002;70:1446–1458.
35. Dubowitz V. Rigid spine syndrome: a muscle syndrome in search of a name. *Proc R Soc Med.* 1973;66:219–220.
36. Moghadaszadeh B, Petit N, Jaillard C, et al. Mutations in SEPN1 cause congenital muscular dystrophy with spinal rigidity and restrictive respiratory syndrome. *Nat Genet.* 2001;29:17–18.
37. Shalaby S, Hayashi YK, Goto K, et al. Rigid spine syndrome caused by a novel mutation in four-and-a-half LIM domain 1 gene (FHL1). *Neuromuscul Disord.* 2008;18:959–961.
38. Hayashi YK, Chou FL, Engvall E, et al. Mutations in the integrin alpha7 gene cause congenital myopathy. *Nat Genet.* 1998;19:94–97.
39. Susman RD, Quijano-Roy S, Yang N, et al. Expanding the clinical, pathological and MRI phenotype of DNM2-related centronuclear myopathy. *Neuromuscul Disord.* 2010;20:229–237.
40. Ferreiro A, Mezmezian M, Olive M, et al. Telethonin-deficiency initially presenting as a congenital muscular dystrophy. *Neuromuscul Disord.* 2011;21:433–438.
41. Mitsuhashi S, Ohkuma A, Talim B, et al. A congenital muscular dystrophy with mitochondrial structural abnormalities caused by defective de novo phosphatidylcholine biosynthesis. *Am J Hum Genet.* 2011;88:845–851.
42. Riggs JE, Bodensteiner JB, Schochet SS Jr. Congenital myopathies/dystrophies. *Neurol Clin.* 2003;21:779–794; v–vi.

CHAPTER 61

43. Dubowitz V, Fardeau M. Proceedings of the 27th ENMC sponsored workshop on congenital muscular dystrophy. 22–24 April 1994, The Netherlands. *Neuromuscul Disord.* 1995;5:253–258.

44. Ryan MM, Ilkovski B, Strickland CD, et al. Clinical course correlates poorly with muscle pathology in nemaline myopathy. *Neurology.* 2003;60:665–673.

45. Nicot AS, Toussaint A, Tosch V, et al. Mutations in amphiphysin 2 (BIN1) disrupt interaction with dynamin 2 and cause autosomal recessive centronuclear myopathy. *Nat Genet.* 2007;39:1134–1139.

46. Bitoun M, Maugenre S, Jeannet PY, et al. Mutations in dynamin 2 cause dominant centronuclear myopathy. *Nat Genet.* 2005;37:1207–1209.

47. Laporte J, Hu LJ, Kretz C, et al. A gene mutated in X-linked myotubular myopathy defines a new putative tyrosine phosphatase family conserved in yeast. *Nat Genet.* 1996;13:175–182.

48. Nowak KJ, Wattanasirichaigoon D, Goebel HH, et al. Mutations in the skeletal muscle alpha-actin gene in patients with actin myopathy and nemaline myopathy. *Nat Genet.* 1999;23:208–212.

49. Agrawal PB, Greenleaf RS, Tomczak KK, et al. Nemaline myopathy with minicores caused by mutation of the CFL2 gene encoding the skeletal muscle actin-binding protein, cofilin-2. *Am J Hum Genet.* 2007;80:162–167.

50. Pelin K, Hilpela P, Donner K, et al. Mutations in the nebulin gene associated with autosomal recessive nemaline myopathy. *Proc Natl Acad Sci U S A.* 1999;96:2305–2310.

51. Johnston JJ, Kelley RI, Crawford TO, et al. A novel nemaline myopathy in the Amish caused by a mutation in troponin T1. *Am J Hum Genet.* 2000;67:814–821.

52. Donner K, Ollikainen M, Ridanpaa M, et al. Mutations in the beta-tropomyosin (TPM2) gene—a rare cause of nemaline myopathy. *Neuromuscul Disord.* 2002;12:151–158.

53. Laing NG, Wilton SD, Akkari PA, et al. A mutation in the alpha tropomyosin gene TPM3 associated with autosomal dominant nemaline myopathy. *Nat Genet.* 1995;9:75–79.

54. Gommans IM, Davis M, Saar K, et al. A locus on chromosome 15q for a dominantly inherited nemaline myopathy with core-like lesions. *Brain.* 2003;126:1545–1551.

55. Sambuughin N, Yau KS, Olive M, et al. Dominant mutations in KBTBD13, a member of the BTB/Kelch family, cause nemaline myopathy with cores. *Am J Hum Genet.* 2010;87:842–847.

56. Zhang Y, Chen HS, Khanna VK, et al. A mutation in the human ryanodine receptor gene associated with central core disease. *Nat Genet.* 1993;5:46–50.

57. Quane KA, Healy JM, Keating KE, et al. Mutations in the ryanodine receptor gene in central core disease and malignant hyperthermia. *Nat Genet.* 1993;5:51–55.

58. Clarke NF, Kolski H, Dye DE, et al. Mutations in TPM3 are a common cause of congenital fiber type disproportion. *Ann Neurol.* 2008;63:329–337.

59. Clarke NF, Waddell LB, Cooper ST, et al. Recessive mutations in RYR1 are a common cause of congenital fiber type disproportion. *Hum Mutat.* 2010;31:E1544–E1550.

60. Laing NG, Clarke NF, Dye DE, et al. Actin mutations are one cause of congenital fibre type disproportion. *Ann Neurol.* 2004;56:689–694.

61. Clarke NF, Kidson W, Quijano-Roy S, et al. SEPN1: associated with congenital fiber-type disproportion and insulin resistance. *Ann Neurol.* 2006;59:546–552.

62. Ortolano S, Tarrio R, Blanco-Arias P, et al. A novel MYH7 mutation links congenital fiber type disproportion and myosin storage myopathy. *Neuromuscul Disord.* 2011;21:254–262.

63. Brandis A, Aronica E, Goebel HH. TPM2 mutation. *Neuromuscul Disord.* 2008;18:1005.

64. Ferreiro A, Quijano-Roy S, Pichereau C, et al. Mutations of the selenoprotein N gene, which is implicated in rigid spine muscular dystrophy, cause the classical phenotype of multiminicore disease: reassessing the nosology of early-onset myopathies. *Am J Hum Genet.* 2002;71:739–749.

65. Monnier N, Ferreiro A, Marty I, Labarre-Vila A, Mezin P, Lunardi J. A homozygous splicing mutation causing a depletion of skeletal muscle RYR1 is associated with multi-minicore disease congenital myopathy with ophthalmoplegia. *Hum Mol Genet.* 2003;12:1171–1178.

66. Jungbluth H, Zhou H, Hartley L, et al. Minicore myopathy with ophthalmoplegia caused by mutations in the ryanodine receptor type 1 gene. *Neurology.* 2005;65:1930–1935.

67. Hartley L, Kinali M, Knight R, et al. A congenital myopathy with diaphragmatic weakness not linked to the SMARD1 locus. *Neuromuscul Disord.* 2007;17:174–179.

68. Logan CV, Lucke B, Pottinger C, et al. Mutations in MEGF10, a regulator of satellite cell myogenesis, cause early onset myopathy, areflexia, respiratory distress and dysphagia (EMARDD). *Nat Genet.* 2011;43:1189–1192.

69. Boyden SE, Mahoney LJ, Kawahara G, et al. Mutations in the satellite cell gene MEGF10 cause a recessive congenital myopathy with minicores. *Neurogenetics.* 2012;13:115–124.

70. Finsterer J, Ramaciotti C, Wang CH, et al. Cardiac findings in congenital muscular dystrophies. *Pediatrics.* 2010;126:538–545.

71. Spyrou N, Philpot J, Foale R, Camici PG, Muntoni F. Evidence of left ventricular dysfunction in children with merosin-deficient congenital muscular dystrophy. *Am Heart J.* 1998;136:474–476.

72. Stubgen JP. Rigid spine syndrome: a noninvasive cardiac evaluation. *Pediatr Cardiol.* 2008;29:45–49.

73. Ravenscroft G, Miyatake S, Lehtokari V-L, et al. Mutations in KLHL40 are a frequent cause of severe autosomal-recessive nemaline myopathy. *Am J Hum Genet.* 2013;93:6–18.

74. Gupta VA, Ravenscroft G, Shaheen R, et al. Identification of KLHL41 mutations implicates BTB-Kelch-mediated ubiquination as an alternative pathway to myofibrillar disruption in nemaline myopathy. *Am J Hum Genet.* 2013;93:1108–1117.

75. Yuen M, Sandaradura SA, Dowling JJ, et al. Leiomodin-3 dysfunction results in thin filament disorganization and nemaline myopathy. *J Clin Invest.* 2014;124:4693–4708.

Skeletal Dysplasias

Juliet Taylor and Ravi Savarirayan

INTRODUCTION

Skeletal dysplasias are heritable disorders of bone caused by abnormal development, growth, and maintenance of the human skeleton. They are a heterogeneous group of conditions that vary significantly in clinical severity, ranging from conditions that almost always cause death in utero or soon after to birth, to conditions resulting in short stature and chronic health complications that are not generally life limiting. This chapter presents an approach to the diagnosis and management of the skeletal dysplasias that commonly present in the neonatal period.

EPIDEMIOLOGY

The overall birth prevalence of all types of skeletal dysplasias is estimated to be 2–3 per 10,000 births.[1,2] The 2010 revision of the Nosology and Classification of Genetic Skeletal Disorders recognized 456 different conditions and classified them into different groups by their clinical and radiographic features and molecular pathogenesis.[3] Skeletal dysplasias classified as lethal (those that result in death in utero or early neonatal death) make up about 50%. The most common groups of disorders are osteogenesis imperfecta (various types), disorders related to fibroblast growth factor receptor 3 (FGFR3) disorders (thanatophoric dysplasia and achondroplasia are most common), and type II collagenopathies (achondrogenesis is most common) (see further sections for descriptions of these disorders).[1] Achondroplasia is the most common cause of

disproportionate short stature that is not associated with in utero or early neonatal death. The prevalence of achondroplasia has been estimated at 0.36–0.6 per 10,000 live births (1/27,780–1/16,670 live births).[4]

PATHOGENESIS

Identification of the genes responsible for many of the skeletal dysplasias has led to better understanding of the underlying pathogenesis and emerging treatments of these disorders.

Defects in Local Regulation of Cartilage Growth

Defects in local regulation of cartilage growth include disorders caused by abnormalities in growth factors and their receptors. FGFR3 plays a role in the negative regulation of bone growth by inhibiting cell growth in cartilaginous growth plates. Almost all cases of achondroplasia are caused by 1 of 2 specific gain-of-function mutations in the FGFR3 gene, which result in upregulation of the FGFR3 pathway. The lethal thanatophoric dysplasias (type I and II) are caused by different mutations in the FGFR3 gene.

Defects in Structural Proteins of Cartilage

Defects of structural cartilage proteins such as collagen type I, II, IX, X, and XI and extracellular matrix proteins such as COMP (cartilage oligometric matrix protein)

935

result in various different forms of skeletal dysplasias. Mutations in the gene encoding collagen type II cause the group of disorders known collectively as the type II collagenopathies, which comprise achondrogenesis type II, hypochondrogenesis, spondyloepiphyseal dysplasia congenita (SEDC), Kneist dysplasia, and Stickler syndrome.

Defects in Cartilage Metabolic Pathways

Defects of enzymes, ion channels, and transporters essential for cartilage metabolism and homeostasis have been identified as the cause of other skeletal dysplasias.

TRPV4

The transient receptor potential cation channel, subfamily V, member 4 (TRPV4) gene encodes for a calcium-permeable ion channel, transient receptor potential cation channel subfamily V, member 4. Dominant mutations in this gene result in activation of the channel, leading to increased concentration of calcium within chondrocytes. Mutations in *TRPV4* are the cause of a number of skeletal dysplasias, including lethal and nonlethal metatropic dysplasia, which present prenatally or in the neonatal period and spondylometaphyseal dysplasia Kozlowski type, which presents in childhood.[5] The variable severity of clinical features seen in the *TRPV4* groups of skeletal dysplasias can be correlated with the degree of activation of the channel.[6] Interestingly, other mutations in the *TRPV4* gene can present with an arthritic phenotype predominantly involving the hands and feet.[7]

Diastrophic Dysplastic Sulfate Transporter

The diastrophic dysplastic sulfate transporter (DTDST) gene encodes for a sulfate transporter (*SLC26A2*). Recessive mutations in this gene result in impairment of sulfate transport into the chondrocytes. *DTDST* mutations are the cause of the lethal disorders achondrogenesis IB and atelosteogenesis II, the nonlethal but severe disorder diastrophic dysplasia, and the much milder condition autosomal recessive multiple epiphyseal dysplasia. The variation in the severity of clinical features is correlated with the degree of impairment of transport of sulfate. The more severe phenotypes are caused by null mutations in both alleles of the gene, whereas the milder phenotypes are caused by mutations that only partially impair sulfate transport.[8]

DIFFERENTIAL DIAGNOSIS

Making a diagnosis of a specific skeletal dysplasia is often difficult given the vast number of recognized types. The involvement of physicians with specific skills in skeletal dysplasias, such as clinical geneticists, orthopedic specialists, and pediatric radiologists, is essential when trying to make an accurate diagnosis in the neonatal period.

Based on clinical history and examination, family history, and expert evaluation of radiology (the single most powerful diagnostic tool), it is usually possible to make a diagnosis in the majority of those who present in the neonatal period with a skeletal dysplasia. Molecular testing can provide confirmation of a clinical diagnosis. In some cases, a skeletal dysplasia will be unclassifiable in the neonatal period, but with time, the development of additional clinical or radiographic features will allow a specific diagnosis to be made.

Including all possible diagnoses is beyond the scope of this chapter, so examples of the more commonly occurring conditions are given to illustrate the different presentations in the neonatal period. Key radiographic findings are discussed, but given the complexity of the skeletal changes for each type of dysplasia, it is not possible to provide extensive details of the radiographic findings for each condition

"Lethal" Skeletal Dysplasias

"Lethal" skeletal dysplasias are those that lead to death in utero or shortly after birth because of respiratory insufficiency. They will generally have been detected antenatally because of characteristic ultrasound findings. These conditions are presented first in each section.

Infant With Short Limbs

Thanatophoric Dysplasia (Types 1 and 2)

Thanatophoric dysplasias are characterized by very short limbs, a relatively normal trunk length, and narrow thorax. The head is relatively large, and craniosynostosis (cloverleaf skull deformity) occurs more commonly in type 2. Radiographs show short ribs; narrow thorax; severe flattening of the ossification centers of the vertebral bodies (platyspondyly); short, broad pelvic bones; and short, broad femora, which are bowed in type 1 and straight in type 2. Both types of thanatophoric dysplasia are due to dominant mutations in the fibroblast growth factor receptor 3 (FGFR3) gene. Long-term survival may be possible with invasive respiratory support but is associated with a poor long-term outcome with severe cognitive impairment (often secondary to temporal lobe dysplasia), ventilator dependence, and a final height of 80–90 cm.

Fibrochondrogenesis

Fibrochondrogenesis is an autosomal recessive disorder caused by mutations in the type XI collagen gene. It is characterized by midfacial hypoplasia, short nose with anteverted nares, micrognathia, short limbs, and small thorax. Radiographs show platyspondyly (flattened vertebrae) with ossification defects of the posterior aspects of the vertebrae, short long tubular bones with bulbous metaphyseal ends, and short ribs with cupped ends.

Atelosteogenesis (Types I, II, III)

Type I: Infants have rhizomelic limb shortening, midfacial hypoplasia, short broad hands, and talipes equinovarus. Radiographic changes include distal hypoplasia of humerus and femur; short bowed radius/ulna and fibular hypoplasia; broad short tubular bones; absent ossification of metacarpals and distal/middle phalanges; and hypoplastic vertebrae with coronal clefts of the bodies.

Type III: The facial features in type III are similar to those seen in type I. Multiple joint dislocations of elbows, hips, and knees are present. Hand and feet changes include broad distal phalanges, syndactyly, camptodactyly of fingers and toes, and talipes equinovarus.

Type I and III atelosteogenesis are allelic disorders caused by dominant mutations in filamin B. Long-term survival is possible in type III.

Type II: Clinical features include relative macrocephaly, short trunk, small chest, short limbs with hitchhiker thumbs, sandal gap between first and second toe, and talipes equinovarus. Typical facial features include midfacial hypoplasia, micrognathia, and cleft palate. Type II atelosteogenesis is caused by mutations in the diastrophic dysplasia sulfate transporter (*DTSDT*) gene.

Nonlethal Skeletal Dysplasias

Achondroplasia

Achondroplasia is the most common nonlethal skeletal dysplasia causing disproportionate short stature. The clinical features are well recognized and allow a diagnosis to be made in most infants in the neonatal period. Infants have short limbs with rhizomelic segments relatively shorter than other limb segments (which are also short), relative macrocephaly, kyphosis at the thoracolumbar junctions, "trident" hand configuration, and characteristic facial features that include depressed nasal bridge, mild midfacial hypoplasia, and frontal bossing. It is common to see loose redundant skin folds in the limbs, which reflect normal soft tissue growth over shortened bones. In infancy, the signs on radiographs, which allow confirmation of a clinical diagnosis, include characteristic changes in the pelvis (squared iliac wings, narrow sacrosciatic notches, flat acetabular margins); reduction in the interpediculate distance from the upper to lower lumbar vertebrae (distance normally widens); and a typical area of radiolucency at the proximal femur (Figure 62-1A–1C). Achondroplasia is caused by mutations in the *FGFR3* gene, and in the majority of cases (80%), these are de novo.

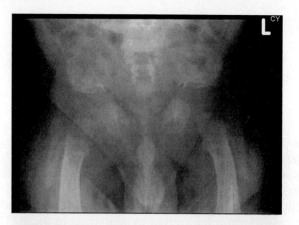
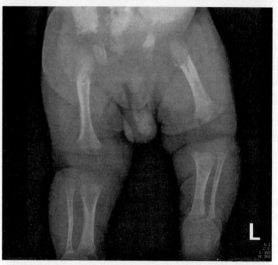
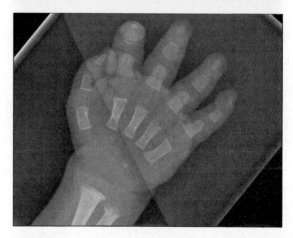

FIGURE 62-1 A, Pelvis radiograph of an infant with achondroplasia. Note reduction in the interpediculate distance from the upper to lower lumbar vertebrae, squared iliac wings, and areas of radiolucency at the proximal femora. **B,** Lower-limb radiograph of an infant with achondroplasia. Note shortening of the long bones with the rhizomelic segments relatively shorter than the other segments and redundant skin folds seen in the soft tissues. **C,** Radiograph of the hand of an infant with achondroplasia. Note short, broad proximal bullet-shaped middle and proximal phalanges and separation of the fingers, giving the "trident" appearance to the hand.

Ellis van Creveld Syndrome (Chondroectodermal Dysplasia)

Ellis van Creveld syndrome (chondroectodermal dysplasia) causes short limbs with progressive shortening of proximal-to-distal segments and short ribs, leading to narrow thorax. Polydactlyly of fingers and often toes is a feature. Ectodermal abnormalities, including hypoplastic nails and dental anomalies (eg, neonatal teeth are also seen). The upper lip is short and connected to the alveolar ridge by multiple frenulae. Structural cardiac abnormalities are present in 50% of infants. This syndrome is an autosomal recessive condition caused by mutations in the *EVC* gene. Parents should be examined as they can display minor dental, hand, and feet anomalies (Weyers acrofacial dysostosis).

Metatropic Dysplasia

Infants with metatropic dysplasia usually have normal length because of their long trunk with short limbs and a narrow chest. A tail-like caudal appendage overlying the sacrum is a common feature. The joints are prominent and often restricted in movement. Radiographs show defective ossification and abnormally shaped vertebral bodies and narrow thorax. A rapidly progressive kyphoscoliosis usually develops in childhood. A lethal form with more severe clinical and radiographic signs also exists. Metatropic dysplasia is caused by dominant mutations in the *TRPV4* gene.[5]

Diastrophic Dysplasia

Clinical features of diastrophic dysplasia include short limbs and short stature at birth, with talipes equinovarus and contractures of other joints present. The thumbs are proximally placed and abducted ("hitchhiker thumb"), and there is an increased gap between the first and second toe. The cystic swellings of the external ears that usually appear within the first 12 weeks of life are pathognomonic for this condition and can ossify. Cleft palate occurs in approximately 50% of cases. In infancy, radiographs show cervical kyphosis; short tubular bones with broad metaphyses; and short, rounded first metacarpals. Diastrophic dysplasia is caused by mutations in the *DTDST* gene and is inherited as an autosomal recessive trait.

Infants With Bowing/Shortening of Bones

Campomelic Dysplasia

A proportion of infants with campomelic dysplasia will die in the early neonatal period because of respiratory insufficiency secondary to pulmonary hypoplasia (small thorax) and larynotracheomalacia from deficient airway cartilage. Some, but not all, long-term survivors have cognitive impairment. The clinical features include bowing of femora and tibia with pretibial skin dimples; micrognathia; dysmorphic facial features (flat nasal bridge, low-set ears, long philtrum); dislocated hips; and talipes equinovarus. In up to 75% of XY males with campomelic dysplasia, the external genitalia are either ambiguous or normal female. This is associated with abnormalities of the internal genitalia, with a mixture of Müllerian and Wolffian duct structures present. The key radiographic findings include bowing of the femur and tibia; hypoplastic scapula; small, bell-shaped thorax; 11 pairs of ribs; hypoplastic vertebrae; and narrow iliac wings. Campomelic dysplasia is an autosomal dominant condition caused by mutations in the *SOX9* gene.

Hypophosphatasia

Two forms of hypophosphatasia are relevant in the neonatal period. The perinatal lethal form is characterized by absence of ossification of the bones of the skull and limbs, leading to the clinical findings of a soft head and short, deformed extremities. Bony spurs ("Bowdler" spurs) of the midshafts of bones may be palpable. The ribs are short and thin, which leads to respiratory insufficiency, and death usually occurs shortly after birth. The infantile form is characterized by symptoms of hypercalcemia (episodic vomiting, failure to thrive, constipation, irritability, and hypotonia). The cranial sutures are widely patent and fontanelles bulging. The long bones are bowed with associated skin dimples. The ends of the long bones and ribs are swollen. The key radiographic findings include delayed and defective ossification of the skull bones, ribs, and long bones. Paradoxically, given the widely open sutures, craniosynostosis can develop, leading to raised intracranial pressure. With supportive treatment, including management of hypercalcemia and respiratory support, infants survive. The laboratory findings for both conditions are identical, with very low/absent alkaline phosphatase, hypercalcemia, elevated plasma pyridoxal 5′ phosphate, and elevated calcium and phosphoethanolamine in the urine. The disorder is caused by deficiency of the tissue nonspecific alkaline phosphatase enzyme because of mutations in the *ALPL* gene and is inherited in an autosomal recessive pattern.

Osteogenesis Imperfecta

There are a number of types of osteogenesis imperfecta, and they are classified according to severity. The perinatal lethal form is classically known as type II, and infants are usually stillborn or die shortly after birth. Infants have small chests; shortened, deformed long bones caused by fractures; and blue sclera. Radiographs show defective ossification and generalized osteopenia of all bones; multiple Wormian bones in the skull; fractures; short, thick ribs with beading representing multiple fractures; and bowed, deformed long bones. Many cases of type II osteogenesis imperfecta are caused by heterozygous mutations in genes coding for type I collagen (*COL1A1*, *COL1A2*). A number of recessive forms have recently been delineated, so a history of consanguinity in parents or recurrence within a sibship should alert clinicians to this possibility given the recurrence risk of 25%.

Infant With Short Limbs and Trunk

Achondrogenesis IA, IB, and II and Hypochondrogenesis

Achondrogenesis IA, IB, and II and hypochondrogenesis make up a group of disorders characterized by short trunk and extremely short limbs with defective ossification of vertebral bodies. Infants commonly develop hydropic changes during pregnancy. Types IA and IB are autosomal recessive conditions caused by heterozygous (dominant) mutations in *TRIP11* and *DTDST* genes, respectively. The long bones in types IA and IB are extremely short and unusually shaped (eg, triangular, round).

Type II achondrogenesis and hypochondrogenesis are caused by mutations in *COL2A1* and are the most severe disorder in the type II collagenopathy family. The facial features typical of this family of disorders include flat midface, micrognathia, and cleft palate. Radiographs show small ovoid vertebrae, which are unossified in the cervical and sacral regions; unossified pubic bones; and hypoplastic ilia. The long bones are short and broad. The clinical and radiographic changes are less severe in hypochondrogenesis, although infants still generally have a poor prognosis due to a constricted chest and consequent respiratory insufficiency.

Nonlethal

Spondyloepiphyseal Dysplasia Congenita

Spondyloepiphyseal dysplasia congenita is a member of the type II collagenopathy family characterized by short trunk and limbs and typical facial features (midfacial hypoplasia, prominent eyes, Pierre Robin sequence) and associated with high-grade myopia (congenital and progressive) and hearing loss. Respiratory difficulties are common in the first year of life and may be associated with cervical spinal instability because of odontoid hypoplasia. The key features on the radiographs in infancy are absence of the ossification centers of the pubic bones and knee epiphyses, cervical vertebral bodies, and delayed ossification of the sacrum. The vertebral bodies of the thoracic and lumbar spine are ovoid with posterior wedging.

Kneist Dysplasia

Kneist dysplasia is another member of the type II collagenopathy family. The condition can be differentiated from SEDC by the presence of prominent joints that have restricted range of motion (contractures). The radiographs show generalized vertebral changes, including platyspondyly and coronal clefts of the bodies; short long bones with expanded metaphyses; and broad, short femoral necks.

Infants With Short Ribs and Polydactyly

Short-Rib (Polydactyly) Syndromes

Short-rib syndromes are a heterogeneous group of disorders characterized by extreme shortening of the ribs. Not all conditions in this group have polydactyly as a feature. All are lethal because of pulmonary hypoplasia. These conditions are autosomal recessive with a risk of recurrence of 1 in 4 (25%).

Asphyxiating Thoracic Dysplasia

Infants with asphyxiating thoracic dysplasia have short limbs and a long, narrow thorax, which causes variable-severity respiratory distress in the neonatal period, but in most cases the respiratory status improves. In later childhood, progressive renal disease and hepatic fibrosis can occur. Radiographically, the ribs appear short and horizontal with irregular costochondral junctions, and there is a trident appearance to the acetabular roofs.

Infants With Multiple Joint Dislocations

Larsen Syndrome

Infants present with multiple congenital joint dislocations, most commonly of the hips, knees, and elbows. The characteristic facial features include a prominent forehead, low nasal bridge, and hypertelorism. Cleft palate occurs in approximately 50% of cases. Changes in the extremities, including forefoot deformities, cylindrical fingers, and broad thumbs, may be seen. A key radiographic sign is the presence of an extra calcaneal ossification center. Larsen syndrome is an autosomal dominant disorder caused by mutations in the *FLNB* gene.

Desbuquois Dysplasia

Infants with Desbuquois dysplasia have short limbs with joint laxity or dislocations and axial deviation of the thumb. Deformities of the feet, such as metatarsus adductus, are common. The key radiographic signs are the characteristic "monkey wrench" appearance of femoral heads and additional ossification centers between the metacarpals and phalanges of the first and second finger. Desbuquois syndrome is an autosomal recessive condition caused by mutations in the *CANT1* gene.

Infants With Joint Contractures

Regarding infants with joint contractures, consider Kneist and Diastrophic dysplasia, described previously in this section.

Infants With Increased Bone Density: Osteopetrosis

There are various forms of osteopetrosis with the infantile ("malignant") form presenting with failure to thrive, anemia, and developmental delay and the finding of increased bone density on radiographs. Sclerosis of the skull base may lead to cranial nerve compression and the development of hydrocephalus. The infantile form is genetically heterogeneous, with mutations in the known genes inherited in an autosomal recessive pattern.[9]

Infants With Fragmented Prenatal Ossification: Chondrodysplasia Punctate

A number of different types of chondrodysplasia punctata are caused by deficiencies in enzymes necessary for peroxisomal biogenesis present in the neonatal period. Infants with the classic type 1 rhizomelic chondrodysplasia punctata have congenital cataracts, rhizomelic shortening of the limbs, and the presence of punctate calcifications in the epiphyseal cartilage of the joints on radiographs. The diagnosis is confirmed biochemically by measuring the concentrations of red blood cell plasminogen, plasma photonic acid, and very long chain fatty acids. Type 1 rhizomelic chondrodysplasia punctata is associated with poor outcome, with severe postnatal growth deficiency and intellectual impairment; survival beyond the first decade of life is unusual. It is caused by mutations in the *PEX7* gene and is inherited in an autosomal recessive pattern. X-linked dominant chondrodyplasia punctata (Conradi-Hünermann) is lethal in males and causes asymmetric findings in females, such as unilateral cataracts, limb shortening, punctate calcifications, alopecia, and ichthyosis. This condition is caused by mutations in the *EBP* gene located on the X chromosome. Intellectual impairment may occur in some children.

Infants With Cleft Palate

Infants with cleft palate or Pierre Robin sequence (micrognathia, glossoptosis, and U-shaped cleft of the palate) should be evaluated for other signs of the type II collagenopathy group of disorders. The skeletal phenotype of SEDC and Kneist dysplasia should be readily apparent in the neonatal period, whereas Stickler syndrome, which is associated with mild spondyloepiphyseal dysplasia with mild short stature and early-onset arthritis, may be missed if not considered. A complete eye examination should be performed by an ophthalmologist to look for ocular manifestations, such as high-grade myopia, abnormalities of the vitreous, and retinal detachment. Audiometry should be performed because of the association with sensorineural hearing loss. Stickler syndrome is genetically heterogeneous, with other forms of the condition caused by mutations in the genes encoding types 9 and 11 collagen. The various types can usually be differentiated on the basis of clinical findings and inheritance pattern.

Table 62-1 indicates the key features of the most common skeletal dysplasias that present in the neonatal period.

DIAGNOSTIC TESTS

The diagnosis of a skeletal dysplasia relies on the synthesis of information obtained from family history, clinical history, physical examination, and radiographic evaluation. The role of molecular genetic testing is primarily for confirmation of a clinical diagnosis rather than a first-line investigation. The single most powerful diagnostic tool remains critical and expert radiographic evaluation.

The process of making a diagnosis often begins in the antenatal period, when the onset of skeletal changes may first be detected. Many of the lethal skeletal dysplasias are associated with increased nuchal translucency on ultrasound at the end of the first trimester. Other signs of a lethal skeletal dysplasia are generally present on ultrasound scans performed early in the second trimester. Indicators of a high probability of lethality include ratio of femur length to abdominal circumference, small bell-shaped thorax, and decreased bone echogenicity.[10] The first signs of achondroplasia are not usually detected until the third trimester of pregnancy, when short long bones and macrocephaly may be seen.

A detailed family history should be obtained, which in some cases will assist with making a diagnosis in the neonate. A family history of short stature, stillborn infants, early-onset arthropathy, and hearing or visual problems should be elicited. The age of the father

Table 62-1 Key Features of the Most Common Skeletal Dysplasias That Present in the Neonatal Period

Disorder Presenting in the Neonatal Period	Group	Key Clinical Features	Genes	Inheritance
Osteogenesis imperfecta: perinatal lethal	Osteogenesis imperfecta group	Short, deformed limbs secondary to fractures, small thorax, blue sclera	COL1A1, COL1A2, CRTAP, LEPRE1, PPIB	AD AR
Thanatophoric dysplasia (I and II) Achondroplasia	FGFR3-chondrodysplasia group	Lethal; very short limbs, narrow chest, relative macrocephaly with or without craniosynostosis, respiratory insufficiency Rhizomelic limb shortening, normal trunk length, relative macrocephaly, frontal bossing, midface hypoplasia, trident hand	FGFR3	AD
Achondrogenesis II Hypochondrogenesis Spondyloepiphyseal dysplasia congenita (SEDC)	Type II collagenopathies	Lethal; short trunk and limbs; small thorax; flat facies, micrognathia, cleft plate Nonlethal; short trunk and limbs; cervical instability because of odontoid hypoplasia; flat facies, prominent eyes, high-grade myopia	COL2A1	AD

Abbreviations: AD, autosomal dominant; AR, autosomal recessive.

may be relevant as spontaneous or de novo autosomal dominant mutations, such as those in the FGFR3 gene causing achondroplasia, are associated with advanced paternal age. A history of consanguinity increases the risk of autosomal recessive skeletal dysplasias.

The pattern of associated anomalies can aid in diagnosis. The type II collagenopathies are typically associated with cleft palate and ocular manifestations such as high-grade myopia and congenital vitreous abnormalities, which can be detected in the neonatal period.

A careful physical examination will provide many clues to the diagnosis. Birth parameters should be plotted on appropriate growth charts to determine whether short stature is present at birth, indicating prenatal onset of short stature. The origin of disproportionate short stature can be determined by determining the ratio of the upper to the lower segment (US:LS) and comparing to normative values. A lower-than-expected US:LS ratio is seen in short-trunk dysplasias, whereas short-limb dysplasias are characterized by a higher-than-expected US:LS ratio. An assessment of which limb segments are shortened should be undertaken, for instance, whether they are rhizomelic (proximal segment), mesomelic (middle segment), or acromelic (distal segment) (Figure 62-2). Some skeletal dsyplasias have characteristic facial features. Macrocephaly with

frontal bossing and midfacial hypoplasia in an infant with rhizomelic limb shortening is highly suggestive of achondroplasia. Infants with type II collagenopathies typically have prominent eyes, midfacial hypoplasia, and Pierre Robin sequence (micrognathia, glossoptosis, cleft palate). The hands and feet can also provide important diagnostic clues. The trident hand appearance is characteristic of achondroplasia. Polydactyly is seen in the short-rib polydactyly group of dysplasias. Abducted or hitchhiker thumbs/great toes are seen in diastrophic dysplasia.

A full ophthalmologic and hearing assessment in infants with a suspected type II collagenopathy can assist with making a specific diagnosis as some changes (eg, congenital vitreous abnormalities) are only seen in certain disorders (eg, Stickler syndrome).

A thorough radiographic evaluation is the most useful diagnostic tool when evaluating an infant with a suspected skeletal dysplasia. In stillborn and liveborn infants less than 6 months of age, anteroposterior and lateral radiographs of the whole body ("babygram"), lateral view of the skull, and anteroposterior (AP) films of both hands should be obtained. In older infants and children, a complete skeletal survey includes individual AP views of the long bones, hands, and feet; AP and lateral views of the lumbar, thoracic, and cervical

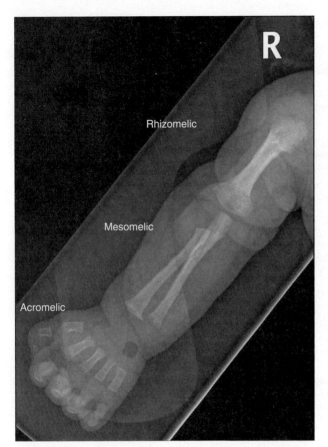

FIGURE 62-2 Radiograph of an upper limb demonstrating rhizomelic (upper), mesomelic (middle), and acromelic (distal) segments.

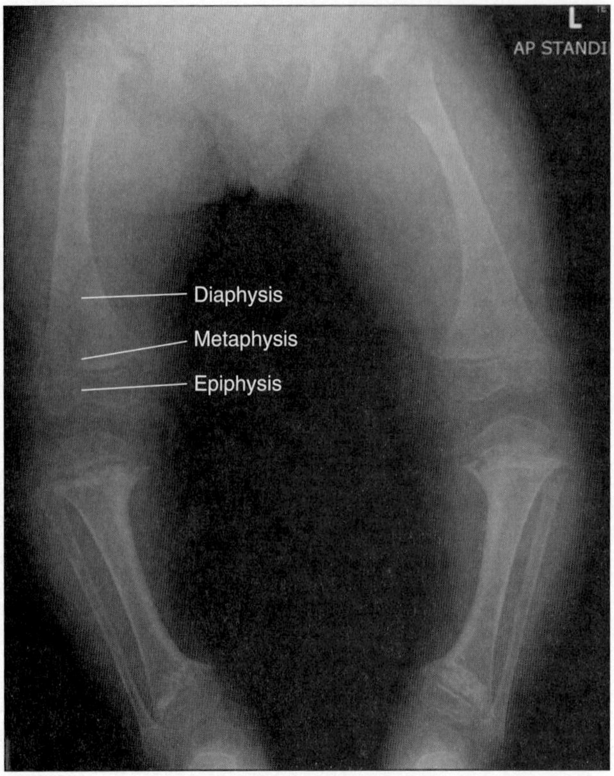

FIGURE 62-3 Radiograph of a lower limb in a child demonstrating the epiphysis, metaphysis, and diaphysis of the distal femur. This child has spondylometaphyseal dysplasia (SMD)-Kozlowski type; note genu varum and prominent metaphyseal changes.

(plus flexion/extension) spine; AP pelvis and chest; and Caldwell, lateral, and Townes views of the skull. Radiographs should be evaluated for the parts of the skeleton that are involved and within each bone the site of abnormality (epiphyseal, metaphyseal, diaphyseal involvement; Figure 62-3); ossification; density; fractures; and any pathognomonic changes (as discussed in the section on differential diagnosis).[11]

Genetic testing is available clinically for most skeletal dysplasias. Genetic testing provides confirmation of a clinical/radiographic diagnosis and should only be undertaken after consultation with a clinical genetics service and appropriate genetic counseling for the family.

MANAGEMENT

The management of a particular skeletal dysplasia depends on the natural history and risk of potential complications for that condition. This section discusses the general principles of management of skeletal dysplasias in the neonatal period and then provides examples of key issues to be considered in the management of several of the more common skeletal dysplasias.

An *accurate* diagnosis is paramount to developing an appropriate management plan for a neonate with a skeletal dysplasia. Careful physical examination and radiographic evaluation as described in the diagnostic test section along with review by a clinical geneticist or other specialist with expertise in the diagnosis and management of skeletal dysplasias should be the priorities in management.

The majority of the lethal skeletal dysplasias will have been detected on antenatal imaging and parents counseled regarding the poor outcome for the neonate because of chest deformity, underlying lung hypoplasia, and respiratory insufficiency. Decisions regarding whether to institute invasive respiratory support in the event of a liveborn infant with a lethal skeletal dysplasia will ideally have been made prior to delivery. In cases that have not been detected prenatally, making a diagnosis in a neonate with respiratory insufficiency caused by an underlying skeletal dysplasia is necessary to guide acute management based on the natural history and expected long-term outcome. A specific diagnosis is also important to enable families to receive accurate genetic counseling regarding risk of recurrence, particularly in the lethal skeletal dysplasias.

Neonates with achondroplasia are at risk of compression of the cervicomedullary spinal cord secondary to a narrow foramen magnum. This can present with central apnea or neurological symptoms/signs such as weakness, hyperreflexia, hypertonia, and clonus. There is a risk (up to 5%) of sudden death in infants with achondroplasia related to cervicomedullary compression.[12] Enlargement of the ventricles is a common finding in infants with achondroplasia, although it is unusual for obstructive hydrocephalus requiring shunting to develop.[13] Recommendations for neuroimaging for baseline assessment and surveillance vary between different countries, so local practices should be followed. Magnetic resonance imaging (MRI) can be performed of the skull bases to obtain dimensions of the foramen magnum, but images should be evaluated by a radiologist familiar with normal measurements for patients with achondroplasia. Indications for cervicomedullary decompression include evidence of neurological compromise in the form of abnormal neurological examination or central sleep apnea and foramen magnum measurement below average for individuals with achondroplasia with evidence of spinal cord compression.[14] Flexion and extension MRI can demonstrate dynamic cervicomedullary cord compression and alterations in cerebrospinal fluid dynamics, which can also result in neurological symptoms and indicate a need for decompression surgery.[15]

Infants with suspected type II collagenopathies should have ophthalmological review for assessment for high-grade myopia and vitreous abnormalities. Audiometry should also be performed as these infants are at risk of sensorineural hearing loss. Infants with SEDC should have cervical x-rays to assess for atlantoaxial instability. Review by a specialist cleft palate team should be arranged for those infants with a cleft palate.

Orthopedic management is required in the neonatal period for infants with joint contractures or joint dislocations.

Infants with dysplasias associated with reduced bone density, such as those with osteogenesis imperfecta, should be assessed by the endocrinology service to determine their suitability for treatments such as bisphosphonates. For infants with the lethal form of infantile hypophosphatasia, enzyme replacement with recombinant tissue nonspecific alkaline phosphatase (TNSALP) is giving promising results.[16]

There are a number of potential therapeutic agents currently under investigation for the treatment of achondroplasia. C-natriuretic peptide (CNP) has been shown to be a potent stimulator of endochondral bone growth.[17] Administration of a CNP analogue via a daily subcutaneous injection has been shown to increase bone growth in a mouse model of achondroplasia.[18] A phase 2 study to evaluate the safety tolerability and efficacy in children aged 5-14 years with achondroplasia is currently ongoing with results expected in late 2015.[19].

Treatment with statins has recently been shown to rescue patient induced pluripotent stem cell models and a mouse model of FGFR3 skeletal dysplasia.[20] A motion sickness medication meclizine increases longitudinal bone growth in fetal and juvenile mice.[21] The results of these initial studies suggest that these medications may potentially be effective for patients with achondroplasia but human trials have not yet been commenced.

A clinical genetics service should be involved with all neonates with suspected skeletal dysplasia to assist with making a diagnosis and providing information and support to the family regarding the diagnosis as well as advice on management in both the acute and long-term periods.

OUTCOME/FOLLOW-UP

The ongoing care of infants and children with skeletal dysplasias needs to be tailored to the medical and orthopedic complications associated with the specific condition as well as the associated psychosocial and architectural implications of a condition associated with significantly short stature. Many centers have established multidisciplinary clinics to provide optimal care to children and families by allowing access to a number of medical and allied health professionals in a single setting.

Guidelines for the health supervisions of children with achondroplasia have been established.[22,23] These guidelines are not universally applicable to every type of skeletal dysplasia, but their general principles serve as a framework when considering the care of a child with a skeletal dysplasia.

There are specific medical complications associated with each of the different skeletal dysplasias. Awareness of these potential complications allows early identification and management should they occur in an infant or child.

As discussed in the section on management, infants with achondroplasia are at risk of serious neurological complications in the form of cervicomedullary spinal cord compression from a narrow foramen magnum or cervical spinal canal and the development of hydrocephalus. At each medical visit, an infant should be evaluated for symptoms and signs of high cervical myelopathy and hydrocephalus (ie, rapidly increasing head circumference, hyperreflexia, muscle weakness, change in behavior, or loss of developmental milestones). Older children and adults are at risk of lumbar spinal cord compression from spinal canal stenosis, which presents with lower-limb pain, sensory symptoms, bladder and bowel dysfunction, and abnormal neurological signs on examination. Infants with skeletal dysplasias such as SEDC and Larsen syndrome are at risk of atlanto-axial instability, so parents should be advised about appropriate head support for infants, and older children should avoid contact sports and other activities with a high risk of cervical spine injury.

Infants and children with achondroplasia are at increased risk of acute and chronic otitis media, and the hearing deficit associated with this may be an explanation for the delay in language development seen in these children. Children should be assessed for the presence of middle ear fluid when unwell with intercurrent respiratory illness, and audiometry should be performed at any stage if there are concerns regarding hearing. Midfacial hypoplasia and narrow airways in infants with achondroplasia may be associated with obstructive sleep apnea. Polysomnography should be performed to identify infants at risk of both obstructive and central apnea (from cervicomedullary cord compression). Infants with skeletal dysplasias associated with a narrow thorax may experience respiratory complications requiring continuous noninvasive respiratory support, such as low-flow oxygen, or intermittent support (eg, for nocturnal continuous positive pressure ventilation or during intercurrent illness).

Orthopedic complications are the most common problem in all children with skeletal dysplasias. The types of complications vary depending on the type of dysplasia. Some complications are present at birth (eg, talipes equinovarus in campomelic dysplasia, multiple joint dislocations in Larsen syndrome), and others are present in late infancy/early childhood as children begin to bear weight (eg, genu varum [bowed legs] in achondroplasia). It is essential that any operative management be performed by orthopedic surgeons experienced with the natural history and expected outcomes of children with underlying skeletal dysplasias. Joint pain is common in older children with skeletal dysplasias and can often be difficult to manage. Obesity is a common problem in older children and adults with achondroplasia and is associated with increased orthopedic complications as well as the primary adverse obesity-related health outcomes.

Children with type II collagenopathies should be reviewed regularly by an ophthalmologist to monitor for complications such as cataracts, glaucoma, and retinal detachment.

The majority of skeletal dysplasias are associated with a normal intellectual outcome. The long-term outcome for adults with skeletal dysplasias is typically good, with most individuals living functional lives, achieving employment, establishing relationships, and having children. Orthopedic complications leading to chronic pain are the most common problems in adults with skeletal dysplasias.[24]

Parents should be made aware of the characteristic pattern of developmental delay seen in infants with achondroplasia. Significant delay in attainment of gross motor skills and in language development is seen compared to infants without achondroplasia.[25,26] Gross motor delay is related to the combined effects of macrocephaly, hypotonia, and joint hypermobility. Language delay may be related to hearing deficit from acute or chronic otitis media.

Infants with conditions such as osteogenesis imperfecta, hypophosphatasia, and osteopetrosis require ongoing follow-up with endocrinology services, which have responsibility for instituting and monitoring therapies such as bisphosphonates.

Growth hormone is generally not indicated in the management of most skeletal dysplasias because of the potential for increasing the rates of orthopedic complications.

All families should be seen by a clinical genetics service to receive genetic counseling, education, and information about the condition and in some centers ongoing coordination of management.

Children with skeletal dysplasias that have a significant impact on predicted adult height need input from occupational therapists to address the architectural consequences as well as provide assistance/alternative strategies to allow children to complete the daily activities that may be difficult with short stature or limb-trunk disproportion.

From the time of diagnosis, it is vital that the psychosocial needs of the family and later the older child are addressed with regard to the adjustment to the diagnosis of a skeletal dysplasia. This can be achieved by specialized medical and social support and referral to patient support and advocacy groups such as SSPA (Short Statured People of Australia), Little People of America (United States), and the United Kingdom's Restricted Growth Association (RGA).

REFERENCES

1. Buck COB, Orioli IM, Castilla EE, Lopez-Camelo JS, Dutra M, Cavalcanti DP. Birth prevalence rates of osteochondrodysplasias (OCD) in South America (SA): an epidemiologic study in a large population. Paper presented at: Proceedings of the 10th Biennial Meeting of the International Skeletal Dysplasia Society; June 2011; Queensland, Australia.

2. Orioli IM, Castilla EE, Barbosa-Netot JG. The birth prevalence rates for the skeletal dysplasias. *J Med Gen.* 1986;23:328–332.

3. Warman ML, Cormier-Daire V, Hall C, et al. Nosology and classification of genetic skeletal disorders: 2010 revision. *Am J Med Genet A.* 2011;155:943–968.

4. Waller DK, Correa A, Vo TM, et al. The population-based prevalence of achondroplasia and thanatophoric dysplasia in selected regions of the US. *Am J Med Genet A.* 2008;146A:2385–2389.

5. Andreucci E, Aftimos S, Alcausin M, et al. *TRPV4* related skeletal dysplasias: a phenotypic spectrum highlighted by clinical, radiographic and molecular studies in 21 new families. *Orphan J Rare Dis.* 2011;6:37.

6. Camacho N, Krakow D, Johnykutty S, et al. Dominant *TRPV4* mutations in nonlethal and lethal metatropic dysplasia. *Am J Med Genet A*. 2010;152A:1169–1177.

7. Lamandé SR, Yuan Y, Gresshoff IL, et al. Mutations in *TRPV4* cause an inherited arthropathy of hands and feet. *Nat Genet*. 2011;43:1142–1146.

8. Karniski LP. Functional expression and cellular distribution of diastrophic dysplasia sulfate transporter (DTDST) gene mutations in HEK cells. *Hum Mol Genet*. 2004;3(19):2165–2171.

9. Stark Z, Savarirayan R. Osteopetrosis. *Orphanet J Rare Dis*. 2009;4:5.

10. Yeh P, Saeed F, Paramasivam G, Wyatt-Ashmead J, Kumar S. Accuracy of prenatal diagnosis and prediction of lethality for fetal skeletal dysplasias. *Prenat Diagn*. 2011;31:515–518.

11. Savarirayan R, Rimoin DL. Skeletal dysplasias. *Adv Pediatr*. 2004;51:209–229.

12. Rimoin DL. Cervicomedullary junction compression in infants with achondroplasia: when to perform neurosurgical decompression. *Am J Hum Genet*. 1995;56:824–827.

13. King JAJ, Vachhrajani S, Drake JM, Rutk JT. Neurosurgical implications of achondroplasia: a review. *J Neurosurg Pediatr*. 2009;4:297–306.

14. Pauli RM, Horton UK, Glinski LP, Reiser CA. Prospective assessment of risks for cervico-medullary junction compression in infants with achondroplasia. *Am J Hum Genet*. 1995;56:732–744.

15. Danielpour M, Wilcox WR, Alanay Y, Pressman BD, Rimoin DL. Dynamic cervicomedullary cord compression and alterations in cerebrospinal fluid dynamics in children with achondroplasia. *J Neurosurg*. 2007;(6 Suppl Pediatr)107:504–507.

16. Yadav MC, Lemire I, Leonard P, et al. Dose response of bone-targeted enzyme replacement for murine hypophosphatasia. *Bone*. 2011;49(2):250–256.

17. Yasoda A, Kitamura H, Fujii T, et al. Systemic administration of C-peptide as a novel therapeutic strategy for skeletal dysplasias. *Endocrinology*. 2009;150:3138–3144.

18. Lorget F, Kaci N, Peng J, et al. BMN 111, a CNP analogue, rescues femur growth and growth plate architecture in a severe model of *FGFR3*-related chondrodysplasia. Paper presented at: Proceedings of the 10th Biennial Meeting of the International Skeletal Dysplasia Society; June 2011; Queensland, Australia.

19. US National Institutes of Health. Clinical trials.gov. Accessed March 2, 2015.

20. Yamashita A, Morioka M, Kishi H, et al. Statin treatment rescues FGFR3 skeletal dysplasia phenotypes. *Nature*. 2014;513(7519):507–511.

21. Matsushita M, Hasegawa S, Kitoh H, et al. Meclozine promotes longitudinal skeletal growth in transgenic mice with achondroplasia carrying a gain-of-function mutation in the FGFR3 gene. *Endocrinology*. 2015;156(2):548–554.

22. Trotter TL, Hall JG. Health supervision for children with achondroplasia. *Pediatrics*. 2005;116:771–783.

23. Wright MJ, Irving MD. Clinical management of achondroplasia. *Arch Dis Child*. 2012;97(2):129–134.

24. Hoover-Fong J, Alade Y, Tunkel D, Yost T, Ain M. Surgical history, pain and function in skeletal dysplasia patients. Presented at: Proceedings of the 10th Biennial Meeting of the International Skeletal Dysplasia Society; June 2011; Queensland, Australia.

25. Ireland PJ, Johnson S, Donaghey S, et al. Developmental milestones in infants and young Australasian children with achondroplasia. *J Dev Behav Pediatr*. 2010;31(1):41–47.

26. Ireland PJ, McGill J, Zankl A, et al. Functional performance in young Australian children with achondroplasia. *Dev Med Child Neurol*. 2011;53:944–950.

63 Developmental Dysplasia of the Hip

Amanda Roof, Thomas Jinguji, Klane White,
Michael Goldberg, and Meghan Imrie

INTRODUCTION FOR THE NEONATOLOGIST

The term *developmental dysplasia of the hip* (DDH) indicates a spectrum of pathologies from stable acetabular dysplasia (femoral head stable in hip socket but socket is shallow) to "located" hips that are unstable (femoral head can be moved in and out of the confines of the acetabulum), to frankly dislocated hips in which there is a complete loss of contact between the femoral head and acetabulum. Congruent reduction and stability of the femoral head are necessary for normal growth and development of the hip joint. The natural history of DDH is variable: Acetabular dysplasia often resolves spontaneously. Unstable or dislocated hips may reduce spontaneously, but some will require treatment to normalize.

Whether dysplastic, dislocatable, or completely dislocated, DDH in the newborn period is pain free and asymptomatic. However, failure to diagnose this entity can have drastic results. In cases that have persistent dysplasia or untreated dislocation, infants have a significantly increased risk of developing precocious arthritis with moderate-to-severe hip pain as young adults.[1,2] This pain can be debilitating. Early detection and treatment of DDH are therefore important in avoiding the devastating sequelae of a late diagnosis. Given the complexity and acuity of patients in the neonatal intensive care unit and the silent nature of this disorder, DDH can easily be overlooked in this patient population. Fortunately, the diagnosis of DDH requires only modest vigilance to detect in the majority of cases.

INCIDENCE AND ETIOLOGY

Developmental dysplasia of the hip occurs in 11.5 of 1000 infants, with 1–2/1000 having frank dislocations.[3,4] Although all children should be screened for DDH by physical examination, there exist particular risk factors for DDH that warrant closer scrutiny. These risk factors include a positive family history (boys, 9.4/1000; girls, 44/1000); breech presentation (boys, 26/1000; girls, 120/1000); and the presence of an unstable hip examination at birth. The left hip alone is affected in 60%, the right hip in 20%, and both hips in 20% of infants.[4]

Despite newborn screening programs, 1 in 5000 children will have a dislocated hip detected at 18 months of age or older.[5] It is important to appreciate that not all dislocated hips are present at birth, and not all hips dislocated at birth are detectable in the newborn period.

Dislocations can be divided into two groups: syndromic and typical. *Syndromic* dislocations are most frequently associated with neuromuscular conditions such as myelodysplasia and arthrogryposis or with dysmorphic syndromes such as Larsen syndrome. These abnormalities probably occur between week 12 and week 18 of gestation.[3] *Typical* dislocations occur in otherwise-healthy infants in the third trimester or postnatal period. Syndromic dislocations are often fixed

947

and nonreducible and require orthopedic referral. The rest of this chapter deals only with typical dislocation.

PHYSICAL FINDINGS

There are no pathognomonic signs of a dislocated hip. The physical examination requires patience on the part of the examiner and a quiet, calm infant/patient. This may be facilitated by having the baby feed from a bottle and dimming the room light. Evaluation for asymmetry of hip movement is an important key to the evaluation for DDH, although asymmetry may not be evident in bilateral dislocations. The presence of asymmetric thigh folds may be indicative of dislocatable hip but is often present in unaffected children and can be seen in up to 20% of normal infants. Asymmetric thigh folds in the absence of other physical examination findings should be considered a nonspecific finding and does not require further imaging or workup. Presence of asymmetric flexed hip abduction is suggestive of a dislocation, as is a *Galeazzi sign* (Figure 63-1). The Galeazzi sign is elicited with the baby placed supine on an examining table so that the pelvis is level, and the hips and knees are flexed to 90°. With the baby's hips in neutral abduction, the examiner determines if the knees are at the same height. If one femur appears shorter, the hip may be dislocated posteriorly. Limited hip abduction in babies older than 12 weeks is the most reliable examination finding suggestive of DDH. Adduction of 30° and abduction of 75° should be possible in most newborns. Hip abduction is performed with the hip in flexion. Side-to-side variations should be noted. Each of these signs, individually or in combination, may serve to increase the index of suspicion of the examiner and lower the threshold for further diagnostic studies or referral to a pediatric orthopedist.

There are two common ways of assessing hip stability in the newborn. The *Ortolani test* (Figure 63-2) is performed, one leg at a time, with the calm newborn supine on the examining table. The index and middle fingers of the examiner are placed along the greater trochanter; the thumb is placed on the medial aspect of the thigh. The pelvis is stabilized by placing the thumb and ring or long finger of the opposite hand on top of both anterior iliac crests simultaneously. Alternatively, the opposite thigh may be held in the same manner as the examined side while the hip is held in abduction. The hip is flexed to 90° and gently abducted while the leg is lifted with the hip in neutral external/internal rotation. A palpable "clunk" is felt as the dislocated femoral head reduces into the acetabulum. This finding is reported as the Ortolani sign (positive result on the Ortolani test).

The *Barlow test* (Figure 63-3) is an attempt to dislocate or subluxate a located but unstable hip. The thigh is held and the pelvis stabilized in the same manner as for the Ortolani test. With the hip in neutral external/internal rotation and at 90° of flexion, the leg is then gently adducted with mild posteriorly directed pressure applied to the knee. A palpable clunk or sensation of marked posterior movement constitutes a positive result. Each hip should be examined separately. High-pitched "clicks" are frequently elicited with hip range of motion. These sounds are most frequently attributed to snapping of the iliotibial band over the greater trochanter and are not associated with dysplasia.[6] To differentiate between a clunk of the Ortolani and Barlow tests and a ligamentous click takes time and experience. With progressive soft tissue contractures, both the Ortolani and Barlow tests become unreliable after 3 months of age, and loss of flexed hip abduction becomes the best indicator.

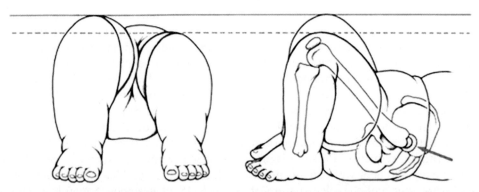

FIGURE 63-1 The Galeazzi sign. The left femur appears shorter than the right. This is an indication that the left hip may be dislocated. (Reproduced with permission from the Merck Manual of Diagnosis and Therapy, edited by Robert Porter. Copyright 2012 by Merck Sharp & Dohme Corp., a subsidiary of Merck & Co, Inc, Whitehouse Station, NJ. Available at http://www.merckmanuals.com/professional/. Accessed December, 2014.)

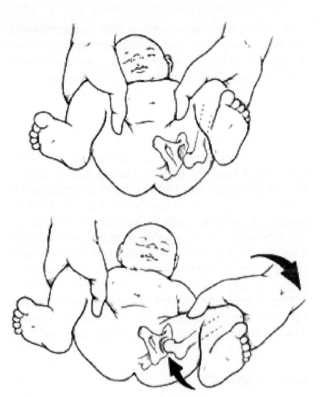

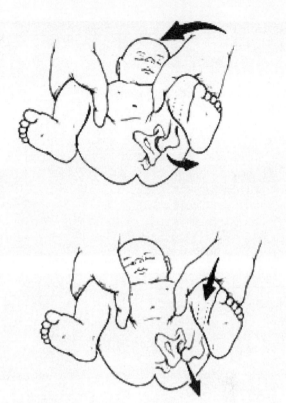

FIGURE 63-2 The Ortolani sign. With the hip flexed to 90° and the leg gently abducted, if the hip is dislocated initially, reduction of the hip with abduction will **produce a palpable clunk.** (Reproduced with permission from Guille JT, Pizzutillo PD, MacEwen GD. Development dysplasia of the hip from birth to six months. *J Am Acad Orthop Surg.* 2000;8(4):232–242.)

FIGURE 63-3 The Barlow sign. The hips are flexed to 90° and adducted. Then, a gentle downward force is placed on the leg. A clunk can be appreciated if the hip is unstable and dislocates posteriorly.

Torticollis and metatarsis adductus are orthopedic conditions that can be associated with developmental hip dysplasia. Appropriate DDH evaluation for an infant with an isolated finding of torticollis or metatarsus adductus is a careful, focused evaluation of the hips. If the hip examination is stable and no risk factors for DDH are noted, no further imaging or evaluation is necessary.

Imaging

Imaging of the immature hip is a valuable adjunct to the physical examination. An anteroposterior (AP) x-ray of the pelvis is difficult to interpret before age 4 to 5 months. The femoral head is composed entirely of cartilage until the secondary center of ossification appears. Before the appearance of the secondary center, ultrasound examination is the method of choice for visualizing the cartilaginous femoral head and acetabulum (Figure 63-4). Static ultrasound images allow visualization of acetabular and femoral head anatomy; complementary dynamic images give information on the stability of the hip joint.[7,8] The primary

limitation of hip ultrasonography is that results are dependent on the experience and skill of the operator, especially when performed on infants within the first 3 weeks of life.[9] For these reasons, ultrasonography is recommended as an adjunct to clinical evaluation rather than as a screening tool.[3] Studies conducted before 4 weeks of life may be useful for confirming equivocal physical examination findings and for monitoring treatment of hips with known dislocations. Clinicians must be aware, however, that ultrasound images in this age group often reveal minor degrees of dysplasia that usually resolve spontaneously and may lead to overtreatment of physiological hip variations. Ultrasonography is the technique of choice for screening infants with risk factors for DDH up to 4 months of age (ideally between 6 and 12 weeks of age) and, again, is useful in following the results of intervention. We primarily utilize α-angle[8] and femoral head coverage (FHC) when evaluating neonatal ultrasounds. Normal FHC should exceed 50% and α-angle should exceed 60° by 3 months of age (Figure 63-5). After 4 months of age, the gold standard remains the AP pelvis radiograph.

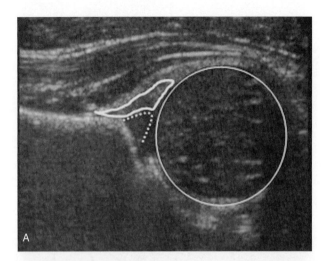

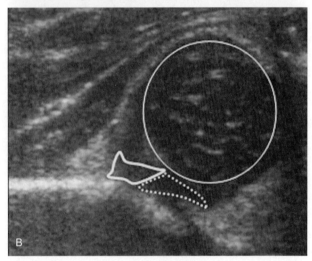

FIGURE 63-4 A, a normal hip ultrasound in which the femoral head (black line) is well seated in the acetabulum (thin white line, femoral head; dotted line, acetabular cartilage; thick line, labrum); B, an abnormal ultrasound of a dislocated hip in which the femoral head is laterally and superiorly displaced and the labrum is blunted.

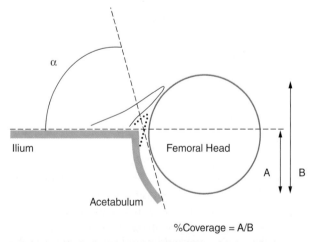

FIGURE 63-5 Schematic of a normal hip ultrasound. Normal values are an α angle of greater than 60° and percentage coverage of over 50% (in a child >12 wks).

Routine ultrasound screening of the stable hip with risk factors (or the hip that stabilizes spontaneously) should be performed at chronologic age rather than corrected age. Breech presentation in the premature infant does not cause the same level of intrauterine constraint and restriction as is the case in term infants. Studies indicate that prematurity reduces the associated risk of DDH in breech presentation. Thus, it is not necessary to correct for gestational age in ultrasound of the hip. A study by Bick et al found that the α angle in preterm infants was higher than in children born at term.[10] This is thought to be because of the morphologic changes in the premature infant. Gardiner found no real difference in α angle for preterm and term infants[11]; however, the β angle was increased for preterm infants, and this was thought to be caused by changes in the hormonal milieu between term and preterm infants.

Hip radiography (x-ray) should probably be performed at corrected age to allow for normal ossification and better visualization of the femoral head.

TREATMENT

All newborns should be screened by physical examination for DDH by a properly trained health care provider (Figure 63-6). Treatment of the premature infant should follow recommendations as determined by chronological age, not adjusted age. Risk factors for DDH include the presence of an unstable hip examination, breech presentation, and a positive family history for DDH. If there are no risk factors, then serial examinations are recommended at well-child visits until the child is an established walker. If during these periodic visits physical findings raise suspicion of DDH or if there is a parental concern of hip disease, referral to a pediatric orthopedist (or other practitioner with expertise in medical and surgical management of newborn hip disease) for age-appropriate imaging and expert physical examination is recommended.

If the baby has positive risk factors, such as breech presentation or positive family history, but a stable hip examination, then age-appropriate imaging is recommended. This can be ultrasonography at 6 weeks or x-ray at 4 months. Ultrasound is considered the study of choice because it allows for earlier intervention. For stable hips with acetabular dysplasia, we recommend treatment of patients in which the ultrasound demonstrates an α angle less than 50° *and* FHC less than 40%. If the ultrasound shows an α angle greater than 50° or FHC above 40%, repeat ultrasound should be obtained in 2–4 weeks. Referral to a pediatric orthopedist should be made if the follow-up ultrasound is abnormal.

When a positive Ortolani or Barlow test is present at birth, this infant should be sent to a pediatric

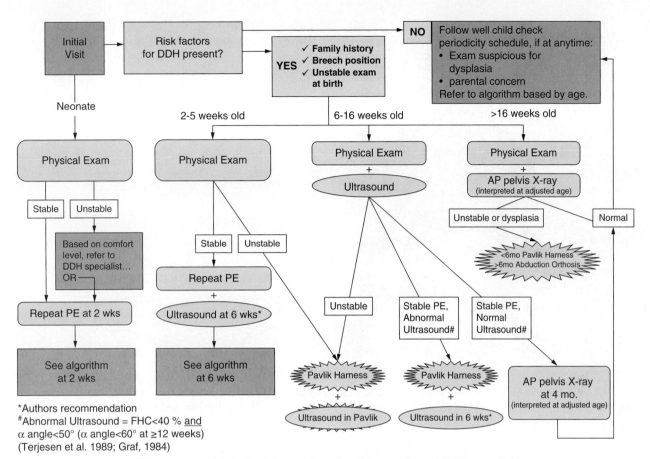

When treatment is indicated consider, referral to experienced DDH specialist

FIGURE 63-6 Recommended algorithm for neonatal screening of developmental dysplasia of the hip (DDH). Indications for ultrasonographic screening include instability on physical examination, family history of DDH, and breech presentation. All ages are chronologic, not adjusted.

orthopedist for confirmatory examination or should be rechecked in 2 weeks based on clinician preference. If the hip remains unstable beyond age 2–4 weeks, the infant should definitely be referred to an orthopedist for management. However, if the positive Ortolani or Barlow test disappears by 2–4 weeks, then age-appropriate imaging (ultrasonography at 6 weeks or x-ray at 4 months) is warranted. Clear communication between providers is encouraged if the practitioner examining the newborn in the hospital is different from the 2-week follow-up examiner.

For children 0 to 6 months of age, DDH is treated with a Pavlik harness. Triple diapering is not an accepted form of treatment of DDH. Treatment of preterm infants should be based on chronologic age, not adjusted age, assuming treatment does not interfere with more critical life supportive care. The Pavlik harness is a dynamic splint that allows the infant to actively move the hips through a sphere of motion that encourages deepening and stabilization of the acetabulum (Figure 63-7). The harness is applied as

soon as possible after the diagnosis of DDH is made. The length of treatment is dependent on age at presentation and improvement on imaging. Progress is judged by serial physical examinations and repeat ultrasonography or radiography in the older patient. In the case of a frankly dislocated hip, treatment is abandoned if no improvement is noted within 4 weeks of harness application. Closed reduction under general anesthesia, usually with arthrographic evaluation and subsequent spica casting, is then attempted at 4 to 5 months of age (adjusted). For a persistently irreducible dislocation, which is unusual in the 0- to 6-month age group, open operative reduction of the hip with subsequent spica casting is undertaken. The success of Pavlik harness treatment is variable and correlates with the severity of the hip dysplasia. Treatment is successful in nearly 100% of stable hips, greater than 90% in dislocatable (Barlow positive) hips, 61%–93% in dislocated but reducible (Ortolani-positive) hips, and as low as 40% in irreducible dislocations.[12-16]

CHAPTER 63

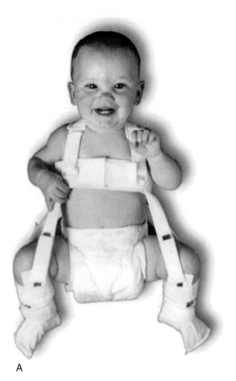
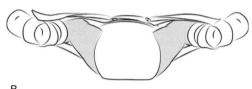

A   B

FIGURE 63-7 Proper fitting of the Pavlik harness is demonstrated. The hips should be held in 90° of flexion and the infant should then sit in a relaxed position of flexion and abduction. Hyper flexion and hyperabduction should be avoided are associated with femoral nerve palsy and femoral head osteonecrosis, respectively.

SUMMARY

Developmental hip dysplasia is a spectrum of disorders. This entity is not uncommon, and it can be seen in about 1 in 100 newborns. All newborns, whether premature or term, should be screened for this condition. In the newborn period and in the neonatal intensive care unit, DDH is usually an asymptomatic condition and can be overlooked when surrounded by other more immediate and life-threatening care issues.

Recognition is critical; performing a careful physical examination, knowledge of DDH risk factors, and obtaining appropriate and timely imaging are needed for this diagnosis. Once the diagnosis is made, treatment of DDH is straightforward and overall successful. Treatment often involves referral to a pediatric orthopedic surgeon.

REFERENCES

1. Cooperman DR, Wallensten R, Stulberg SD. Acetabular dysplasia in the adult. *Clin Orthop.* 1983;175:79.
2. Wedge JH, Wasylenko MJ. The natural history of congenital disease of the hip. *J Bone Joint Surg Br.* 1979;61:334–338.
3. American Academy of Pediatrics (AAP) Subcommittee on Developmental Dysplasia of the Hip, Committee on Quality Improvement. Clinical practice guideline: early detection of developmental dysplasia of the hip. *Pediatrics.* 2000;105:896.
4. Guille JT, Pizzutillo PD, MacEwen GD. Developmental dysplasia of the hip from birth to six months. *J Am Acad Orthop Surg.* 2000;8(4):232–242.
5. Dezateux C, Godward S. Evaluating the national screening programme for congenital dislocation of the hip. *J Med Screen.* 1995;2:200.
6. Bond CD, Hennrikus WL, DellaMaggiore ED. Prospective evaluation of newborn soft-tissue "clicks" with ultrasound. *J Pediatr Orthop.* 1997;17:199.
7. Clarke NM, Harcke HT, McHugh P, et al. Real-time ultrasound in the diagnosis of congenital dislocation and dysplasia of the hip. *J Bone Joint Surg Br.* 1985;67:406.
8. Graf R. Fundamentals of sonographic diagnosis of infant hip dysplasia. *J Pediatr Orthop.* 1984;4:735.
9. Marks DS, Clegg J, al-Chalabi AN. Routine ultrasound screening for neonatal hip instability. Can it abolish late-presenting congenital dislocation of the hip? *J Bone Joint Surg Br.* 1994;76:534–538.
10. Bick U, Muller-Leisse C, Troger J. Ultrasonography of the hip in preterm neonates. *Pediatr Radiol.* 1990;20:331–333.
11. Gardiner HM, Clarke NM, Dunn PM. A sonographic study of the morphology of the preterm neonatal hip. *J Pediatr Orthop.* 1990;10:633.
12. Sucato DJ, Johnston CE, Birch JG, Herring JA, Mack P. Outcome of ultrasonographic hip abnormalities in clinically stable hips. *J Pediatr Orthop.* 1999;19(6):754.
13. Viere RG, Birch JG, Herring JA, Roach JW, Johnston CE. Use of the Pavlik harness in congenital dislocation of the hip. An analysis of failures of treatment. *J Bone Joint Surg Am.* 1990;72:238–244.

14. Hangen DH, Kasser JR, Emans JB, et al. The Pavlik harness and developmental dysplasia of the hip: has ultrasound changed treatment patterns? *J Pediatr Orthop.* 1995;15:729–735.

15. Lerman JA, Emans JB, Millis MB, Share J, Zurakowski D, Kasser JR. Early failure of Pavlik harness treatment for developmental hip dysplasia: clinical and ultrasound predictors. *J Pediatr Orthop.* 2001;21:348–353.

16. Swaroop VT, Mubarak SJ. Difficult-to-treat Ortolani-positive hip Improved success with new treatment protocol. *J Pediatr Orthop.* 2009;29(3):224–230.

CHAPTER 63

Hand, Foot, and Limb Anomalies

Meghan N. Imrie

INTRODUCTION

The orthopedic examination of a newborn can at times be intimidating, even to an experienced pediatric orthopedist; just as children are not small adults, neonates are not small children. A thorough, consistent approach and agreed-on nomenclature can help identify musculoskeletal anomalies that may be present in isolation or may be part of a larger syndrome; treatment may vary from observation to casting or bracing to surgery. Being familiar with the most common diagnoses, their treatments, and anticipated outcomes can help ease parental anxiety and avoid unnecessary delays in treatment or overtreatment. Management of parental expectations is often one of the most important roles we as physicians serve.

PHYSIOLOGIC MUSCULOSKELETAL FINDINGS

Familiarity with the range of musculoskeletal findings in a newborn is important in that the line between physiologic and pathologic can be subtle. Often, severity and flexibility can be clues about whether a finding is normal.

Joint contractures, especially of the elbows, hips, and knees, are normal and slowly resolve over time; absence of these normal contractures may be the sign of an abnormality, such as arthrogryposis or congenital knee dislocation. If the contractures are especially severe and very stiff, that may also be a sign of arthrogryposis. Thumb-in-palm positioning is physiologic at

birth, but lack of resolution over time may be a sign of neurologic abnormality.

Most infants are born with a bowed appearance of the tibia, which, in conjunction with the common external rotation contracture at the hip, gives the legs a "bowlegged" appearance. In fact, most of the apparent bowing is actually caused by internal tibial torsion; when the patella is placed directly forward, the knee will appear neutral to even slightly valgus. With time, the external rotation contracture at the hip and internal tibial torsion resolve so that by toddlerhood, most legs have "straightened out." Abnormal tibial alignment in the neonate includes posteromedial and anterolateral bowing. Posteromedial bowing of the tibia is usually distal and often is associated with calcaneovalgus positioning of the foot; both resolve over time without formal treatment, but posteromedial bowing is associated with an ultimate leg length discrepancy of up to 3–4 cm that parents should be informed of at the outset. Anterolateral bowing can be midshaft or distal and is commonly associated with neurofibromatosis type 1 (NF 1); if anterolateral bowing is found on physical examination, it should be further evaluated by x-ray (Figure 64-1), and the patient should be closely examined for café-au-lait spots, axillary freckling, iris hamartomas, and other manifestations of NF 1. Finally, more nonspecific bowing of the tibia or the femur can be a sign of osteogenesis imperfecta.

Variation in foot alignment is extremely common in newborns and is usually the result of intrauterine packaging. The most common pathologic conditions of the foot include clubfoot and congenital vertical talus (CVT), which are covered further in this chapter.

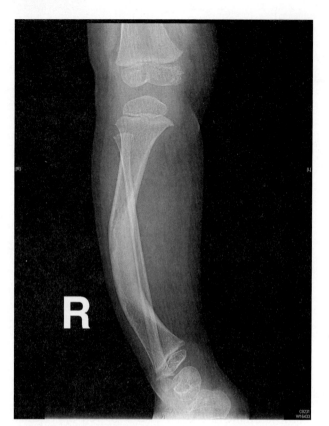

FIGURE 64-1 Radiographic appearance of anterolateral tibial bowing seen in neurofibromatosis type 1.

Findings that are more benign include metatarsus adductus and calcaneovalgus. Metatarsus adductus is characterized by a "bean-shape" to the foot: The lateral border is convex, and the forefoot is adducted on the mid- and hindfoot. Occasionally, the forefoot is slightly supinated as well, and the foot can be confused for a clubfoot. If the hindfoot is normal and the deformity is completely passively correctable, it is likely a metatarsus adductus. As long as it is flexible and actively corrects with eversion of the foot, formal treatment is usually not necessary; spontaneous resolution is expected. If the foot is a little stiffer and the foot can only be passively corrected to neutral, occasionally stretching or casting may be recommended; feet in an extremely small subset do not correct and undergo surgical correction after the age of 4 to 6 years.

Calcaneovalgus is common in newborns and is characterized by extreme dorsiflexion of the entire foot with some component of eversion; the foot can be "plastered against the tibia." It is caused by intrauterine packaging, and its natural history is characterized by reliable resolution, although occasionally stretching exercises will be recommended if it is tight. It is important to distinguish isolated calcaneovalgus from calcaneovalgus associated with a posteromedial bow due to a possible projected leg length discrepancy associated with the latter. The distinguishing feature will be the apex of the deformity, which is in the ankle in the isolated calcaneovalgus foot and in the tibia when associated with posteromedial bowing.

ANOMALY BY ANATOMIC LOCATION

Upper Extremity

Neonatal Brachial Plexus Palsy

Brachial plexus injuries are one of the more common orthopedic conditions presenting in the neonatal setting. The incidence of this condition is thought to be between 0.1% and 0.4% of live births,[1,2] although the incidence has been slightly decreasing in the United States over the last decade.[3] Because the presumed mechanism of injury is a stretch across the brachial plexus, risk is increased by those factors associated with larger infants with wider shoulder girdles and difficult or prolonged labor. Commonly cited risk factors include maternal diabetes; high birth weight (once fetal weight is greater than 3500 g, the shoulder cross-sectional area often exceeds the size of the infant's head); breech position; prolonged second stage of labor; forceps delivery; prior delivery of an infant with a brachial plexopathy; and shoulder dystocia. In the most recent survey of US births, shoulder dystocia had a 100 times increased risk of brachial plexus palsy; birth weight greater than 4500 g and forceps delivery had 14 times and 9 times greater risk, respectively.[3] However, in this study, the majority of patients with neonatal brachial plexus injury had no known risk factors, and other authors have found that although risk factors like maternal diabetes, birth weight greater than 4000 g, and prolonged labor increase the chances of shoulder dystocia, they do not necessarily increase the risk of brachial plexus palsy.[4] In summary, like many orthopedic conditions, certain factors may place patients at increased risk of brachial plexus injury, but most patients presenting with the condition have no known risk factors.

As mentioned, the mechanism of injury is a stretch to the brachial plexus, usually during the process of birth. The amount of stretch needed to cause a permanent or severe neurologic injury is not exactly known. The brachial plexus itself is composed of nerve roots C5 to T1, which branch and combine to become the nerves of the arm and shoulder girdle. The most common nerve roots affected are C5 and C6, also known as Erb palsy, which leads to weakness or absence of shoulder abduction, external rotation, elbow flexion, and wrist extension. This leads to the classic "waiter's tip" position of the upper extremity, so called because the flail arm is held adducted, internally rotated with the elbow extended and the palm turned up, as if the baby were waiting to be slipped a subtle gratuity. C7 may also occasionally be involved. Even less frequent is an injury to the entire plexus (C6 to T1), which affects function of the hand, as does isolated injury to the lower plexus (Klumpke palsy), which results in a clawed appearance of the hand. Lower plexus lesions are thought to be caused by traction on an abducted arm, as when an infant is delivered by being pulled by his or her arm above the head.

In addition to which nerves roots are involved, the level at which they are involved is an important prognostic indicator: The ganglion arises just adjacent to the spinal cord, so that preganglionic lesions are essentially nerve root avulsions directly off the spinal cord and have significantly worse chance for spontaneous motor recovery than postganglionic lesions. The presence of unilateral Horner syndrome, which is characterized by a droopy eyelid with constricted pupil and decreased sweating on one side of the face (ptosis, miosis, and anhydrosis), indicates injury to the sympathetic chain and carries a poor prognosis for spontaneous recovery. Injury to the phrenic nerve, indicated by an elevated hemidiaphragm, and to the long thoracic nerve, indicated by a winged scapula, also raise serious concern about a preganglionic injury.[5]

The typical presentation of an infant with a brachial plexus injury is a flail arm that is noted to have a lack of movement following delivery; when it is noticed depends on the circumstances surrounding the birth and the severity of the palsy. Bilaterality is extremely rare and should raise the possibility of syringomyelia, arthrogryposis, or arachnoid cyst.[6,7] The top 3 differential diagnoses for a nonmoving arm are neonatal brachial plexus injury, fracture (clavicle or humerus), or infection (osteomyelitis or septic arthritis). Less-common possibilities are arthrogrypotic conditions that affect the upper extremities preferentially and intraspinal causes such as syringomyelia or an arachnoid cyst. The perinatal history and physical examination are often all that is needed to make the diagnosis. For example, the history can be helpful in distinguishing infection from a brachial plexus palsy or fracture because in infection the limb was likely normal at birth and subsequently the parents and caregivers may have noticed a progressive or sudden loss of active movement of the arm as the infection manifested. On physical examination, there is no arm movement with Moro reflex testing, whereas in a flail arm caused by infection or fracture, the patient will typically still have some movement with the Moro reflex (the patient is not moving the arm because of pain, not because of a problem with nerve communication to the muscles of the arm—a pseudoparalysis vs a true palsy). It is important to note that a small subset of patients with a fracture may have a concomitant brachial plexus injury, up to 10% of clavicle fractures,[8] so the physical

examination of a patient with neonatal brachial plexus palsy should include palpation of the clavicle and humerus to look for deformity or crepitus indicative of fracture. After a thorough history and physical examination, if there is still a question of the diagnosis, an x-ray can be helpful in finding a fracture, and ultrasound can be helpful in evaluating for a joint effusion in infection or altered anatomy in a transphyseal separation. The physical examination is also helpful in distinguishing arthrogryposis from neonatal brachial plexus palsy; early on, passive range of motion will be normal to near normal in a brachial plexus palsy as it is a relatively recent injury, whereas joint motion will be limited in arthrogrypotic infants.

Many patients with neonatal brachial plexus palsy will improve over time and will not require surgical intervention; the main goal of early treatment is to maintain passive range of motion while waiting for nerve recovery. Occupational therapy should be utilized along with a supervised home stretching program to maintain motion, but initiation is usually deferred for a week or 2 after birth to allow any associated pain to subside. The prevention of joint contractures is of utmost importance. Because the decision to proceed with surgery is based on the degree of motor function recovery, patients should be referred to, and followed by, a surgical specialist early on so that sequential neurologic examinations can be initiated and documented, preferably by the same provider. The rates of spontaneous, complete recovery vary depending on the study and are mentioned[9] as anywhere from 7% to 95%; poor prognostic factors for recovery include total plexopathy, Horner syndrome, and involvement of lower cervical nerve roots.

Surgical treatment consists of early microsurgical reconstruction and later procedures for residual deformities and contractures. Early microsurgical reconstruction is often undertaken at 3 months in patients with global plexopathy and Horner syndrome because of an unfavorable natural history. Otherwise, traditionally, return of antigravity biceps function has been used to help predict recovery and, in its absence, identify patients who will benefit from early surgical intervention. Exactly how long to wait for bicep functional recovery is somewhat controversial; historically, 3 months has been the cutoff as early studies suggested that patients without biceps function by age 3 months eventually gained this function but had poorer shoulder outcomes at 5 years and an increased likelihood of secondary procedures later.[10] Later secondary procedures are targeted toward a patient's residual deficiencies and deformities, most commonly lack of shoulder abduction and internal rotation contracture at the shoulder; they consist of joint releases, tendon transfers, and humeral derotation osteotomies.

Outcomes of patients with neonatal brachial plexus palsy vary widely from complete recovery with normal upper extremity function to profound impairment of the limb. Girth of the affected limb may be smaller, and asymmetry may lead to postural deformities and abnormal gait.[10] Despite all of this, however, children with brachial plexus palsy lead full lives; for example, they participate in sports at the same rate as their peers.[11]

In summary, neonatal brachial plexus palsy incidence appears to be decreasing, potentially because of better understanding of its etiology; however, most patients have no known risk factors. Diagnosis is made by physical examination, and it can be distinguished from other causes of a flail extremity by total lack of movement with reflex testing and normal passive joint motion early on. Initial treatment is supportive and is aimed toward maintaining range of motion; the timing of microsurgical reconstruction is controversial but is generally accepted at age 3 months for those patients who have more severe injuries as evidenced by Horner syndrome or total plexopathy. For the most common presentation, Erb palsy, spontaneous recovery and full return of function can be expected for many patients.

Arm Dysplasias

Longitudinal deficiencies of the upper extremity represent a spectrum of dysplasias and hypoplasias affecting any part of the arm—humerus, radius, ulna, hand, fingers, and thumb—and include phocomelia (proximal longitudinal dysplasias), radial dysplasias (radial club hand), and ulnar dysplasias (ulnar club hand). These are rare deformities, with the more common radial deficiencies occurring in 1 in 30,000 live births and the rarer ulnar deficiencies in 1 in 100,000 births. Thalidomide-related phocomelia is thought to have affected approximately 10,000 living patients worldwide in the 1950s and 1960s.

True isolated phocomelia with a clear intercalary or segmental defect that is otherwise normal above and below the defect with a normal hand is extremely rare; most cases diagnosed as phocomelia in fact represent the proximal extent of a radial or ulnar longitudinal dysplasia[12]; this chapter therefore focuses on these 2 deficiencies. Although they share nomenclature, radial and ulnar longitudinal deficiencies are very different in their associations, presentations, and severity (Table 64-1).

Radial longitudinal deficiency is the more common of the 2 and includes anything from just a slightly hypoplastic thumb on the affected side to a completely absent radius with associated deficiency of the humerus and glenoid. It is frequently bilateral, although often the degree of involvement is asymmetric between sides. When it occurs in isolation, which

Table 64-1 Comparison of Radial and Ulnar Dysplasias

	Radial Deficiency	Ulnar Deficiency
Incidence	1:30,000–50,000	1:100,000
Laterality	Often bilateral, although frequently asymmetric	Usually unilateral
Associated anomalies	Nonmusculoskeletal; ie, Holt-Oram Fanconi's anemia TAR VATER/VACTERL	Musculoskeletal; ie, PFFD DDH Clubfoot Longitudinal deficiency of tibia or fibula
Hand involvement	Either normal or just radial carpals and digits affected	Can involve ulnar, radial, or both sides of hand
Wrist involvement	Frequently unstable	Often abnormal but not clinically unstable
Elbow involvement	Usually not affected	May be stable but frequently unstable or fused
Degree of forearm involvement	Radius often totally absent	Ulna often at least partially present as bone or cartilaginous anlage

Abbreviations: DDH, developmental dysplasia of the hip; PFFD, proximal femoral focal deficiency; TAR, thrombocytopenia-absent radius syndrome; VACTERL, vertebral, anal, cardiac, tracheoesophageal, renal, and limb (association).

is only one-third of the time, it is usually a sporadic mutation with no known pattern of inheritance.[13] More frequently, radial dysplasia is part of a broader syndrome or condition (Table 64-1), many of whose etiology is slightly better understood.

Holt-Oram syndrome is the association of radial dysplasia and cardiac anomalies, most commonly atrial or ventricular septal defects or conduction abnormalities (which may not present until adulthood); although caused by a spontaneous mutation in TXB5 on chromosome 12 most of the time, it is autosomal dominant with complete penetrance. Fanconi anemia is inherited in an autosomal recessive pattern and is the product of defects in 1 of 11 *FANC* genes, which code for proteins in a complex involved in DNA repair; patients must have 2 bad copies to be affected, either homozygous for 1 gene or heterozygous for 2. Ninety percent develop pancytopenia at some point, and patients are at risk for malignancy, especially acute myeloid leukemia.

The etiology of thrombocytopenia-absent radius (TAR) syndrome is not well understood, although in some cases it is autosomal recessive. TAR is characterized by an absent radius (as its name would imply) but a relatively normal-appearing thumb and episodic bleeding that often starts in early infancy; it is confirmed by laboratory tests, which demonstrate abnormalities by one week of life in half of patients and by 4 months in almost all.

Finally, VACTERL (vertebral, anal, cardiac, tracheoesophageal, renal, and limb) or VATER (vertebral, anal, tracheoesophageal, and renal anomalies) association is a sporadic cluster of congenital anomalies, including vertebral anomalies, anal atresia, cardiac malformations, tracheoesophageal fistula, renal anomalies, and limb anomalies (most frequently, radial dysplasia); patients must have at least 3 abnormalities to be diagnosed. Although the exact cause is not known, it is thought to be related to a defect in embryonic mesodermal development. Given the frequent association of radial dysplasia with other serious conditions, patients with any sign of radial longitudinal deficiency, including just a hypoplastic thumb, should be thoroughly evaluated for any cardiac, renal, hematopoietic, or other anomalies.

Management of radial longitudinal deficiency depends on the extent of involvement, bilaterality, and so on. Stretching and splinting that begin in early infancy can be helpful in maintaining soft tissue length; surgical correction is focused on not sacrificing function for cosmesis. A patient with a severe-looking wrist deformity but poor elbow motion may rely on his or her significant radial deviation to get his or her hand to mouth so a centralization procedure that improves the appearance of the arm may take away that crucial hand-to-mouth ability.

Ulnar dysplasias are much less common than radial dysplasias by a factor of 3 or more and do not have the same association with other organ system abnormalities. They are, however, more commonly associated with other musculoskeletal anomalies, such as scoliosis, proximal femoral focal deficiency, and fibular deficiency. The exact cause is unknown but likely occurs during the fourth or fifth week of gestation, earlier than for radial deficiencies. Treatment is focused mainly on the hand, as that is where the most function can be gained. Splinting and stretching may be helpful early for maintaining flexibility and motion.

Digit Anomalies

Anomalies of the fingers and thumb are numerous; this chapter touches on polydactyly, syndactyly, and trigger thumb.

Polydactyly (Figure 64-2) is the most frequent deformity of the pediatric hand and ranges from innocuous floating digits to more challenging, central duplications.

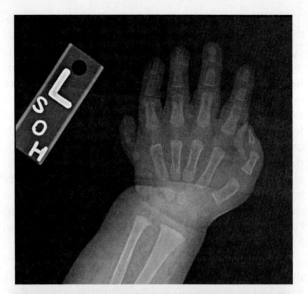
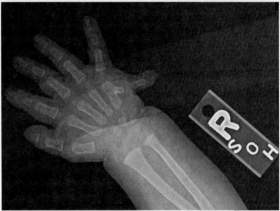

FIGURE 64-2 A and B, Variations in types of postaxial polysyndactyly of the hand.

The inheritance pattern is varied, depending on location and race, with ulnar-sided polydactyly in blacks and central duplications in whites showing a dominant inheritance pattern. Polydactyly in whites is more frequently associated with other anomalies than blacks, whose extra digit is usually isolated. The cause is likely related to abnormalities in the homeobox gene. Treatment of postaxial, or ulnar-sided, duplications is usually fairly straightforward. If there is no skeletal attachment and the stalk is thin, occasionally these can be treated with ligation in the nursery soon after birth, and the extra digit can be allowed to desiccate and autoamputate. However, this can lead to prolonged bleeding from the stump, so it is often prudent to more formally excise the extra digit in the operating room under controlled conditions. The treatment of a duplicated thumb or central duplication is more involved and beyond the scope of this chapter.

Syndactyly of the hand, or webbing of the fingers, occurs in 1 in 2000 live births and is caused by a failure of apoptosis because all hands are initially webbed.

The exact cause of this failure, however, is unknown. Syndactyly can be described as simple (soft tissue connection only) or complete (bony involvement) and partial (not all the way distal) or complete (connected all the way to the tips of the digits). If there is an associated polydactyly or complex coalition, it is called complex syndactyly. Acrosyndactyly is reserved for cases associated with constriction bands, which cause fetal injury and the associated variable deformities. The syndactyly may be isolated or may be associated with any number of syndromes; long-ring-finger involvement is most common. Treatment depends on the extent of deformity and ranges from observation to complex reconstruction; if surgery is to be done, it is best to wait until at least 6 months of age.

Trigger thumb is characterized by an otherwise totally normal thumb whose interphalangeal (IP) joint is locked in flexion; it is developmental, rather than congenital, and parents may describe a period of triggering prior to the IP joint becoming fixed. A fullness in the flexor tendon, called the Notta nodule, is often palpable. Various nonoperative treatments, such as splinting or injection, have been described; surgical release of the A1 pulley, however, is fairly simple and effective and usually is the treatment of choice.

Lower Extremity

Congenital Knee Dislocation

Hyperextension deformity of the knee, which represents a spectrum from true hyperextension to subluxation to dislocation of the femoral-tibial joint, is rare, with an estimated prevalence of 1 in 100,000. It may be an isolated deformity but is often seen as a manifestation of other conditions, such as myelomeningocele, arthrogryposis, or Larsen's syndrome. If it is bilateral, it is most certainly syndromic. It is frequently associated with clubfoot and developmental hip dysplasia, and the presence of a congenital dislocation of the knee (CDK) should prompt evaluation of both hips for instability.

Regardless of whether the deformity is an isolated musculoskeletal finding or part of a larger syndrome, its pathophysiology is related to intrauterine positioning. Once the limb is positioned abnormally, decreased fetal movement, as in arthrogryposis or spina bifida, or hyperlaxity, as in Larsen syndrome, leads to persistence of the deformity. The final result is fibrosis and atrophy of the quadriceps, and the quadriceps tendon is shortened and fibrosed as well.[14] In addition, the patella is often hypoplastic, and the iliotibial band is contracted. The anterior cruciate ligament (ACL) is often incompetent or even absent, especially in bilateral cases or when associated with hyperlaxity syndromes.[15] Some authors believe the absent or deficient ACL is the root cause of the fetal instability and dislocation.[16]

The clinical presentation of a patient with hyperextension deformity of the knee is usually striking—it is not a subtle diagnosis. Physical examination and x-ray can be helpful in classifying the deformity as a simple hyperextension vs a true anterior dislocation. A knee with congenital hyperextension can be flexed beyond neutral, and x-rays will show no anterior translation of the tibia on the distal femur. A congenital knee subluxation usually can be flexed just to neutral, and x-rays show some anterior translation of the tibia on the femur. In the most severe cases, CDKs, the knees cannot be flexed to neutral, and the tibia may displace laterally on the femur when flexion is attempted. X-rays will confirm anterior dislocation of the tibia on the femur (Figure 64-3). Ultrasound can also be helpful in diagnosing and tracking the dislocation and can be used to rule out a distal femoral transphyseal separation, which can have a similar clinical presentation. The differential diagnosis for CDK is limited and includes distal femoral transphyseal separation (diagnosed by ultrasound) and potentially distal femoral or proximal tibial fracture (diagnosed by x-ray).

Management varies and depends on the severity of dislocation and any concomitant diagnoses. The first step is often serial casting, which ideally begins within the first few days of birth. Care must be taken during the stretching and casting process not to create iatrogenic trauma: fracture, distal femoral physeal separation, or plastic deformity of the proximal tibia. Other deformities, such as clubfeet, can be addressed at the same time. Reduction of the joint is followed with x-ray, and if it is not achieved, nonoperative treatment should be modified or even abandoned. Shah et al published results of their "minimally invasive" treatment protocol, consisting of serial casting and mini-open quadriceps tenotomy when concentric reduction and 90° of knee flexion could not be achieved by casting alone. In 16 knees of 8 patients, all of whom had associated neuromuscular diagnoses, only 3 knees were treated with casting alone; the remaining 13 had a mini-open tenotomy. Although 2 developed recurrent deformity,[14] results were excellent in 11, good in 3, and fair in 2. In isolated CDK cases, recurrence is uncommon. For those knees that are not successfully treated by casting, surgical treatment includes lengthening the quadriceps (V-Y quadricepsplasty) with anterior, medial, or lateral capsulotomy as necessary. Texas Scottish Rite Hospital for Children has recently published their surgical technique of femoral shortening with limited arthrotomy and ACL reconstruction if necessary; it compares favorably to the traditional open quadricepsplasty.[17]

Because CDK is so rare, large outcome studies are not available, and most authors are reporting on small series of less than 20 patients with fairly incomplete and subjective outcome data. However, Oetgen et al reported

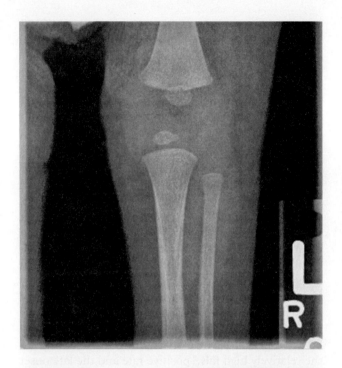

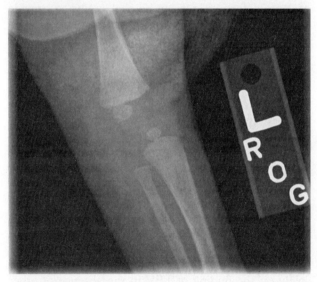

FIGURE 64-3 A and B, Anteroposterior and lateral x-ray of the congenital knee dislocation in a patient with arthrogryposis. Note the anterior translation of the tibia on the femur.

on 7 patients treated surgically; patients were evaluated at an average follow-up of 12 years using validated outcomes measures. Despite 5 of the 7 patients having Larsen syndrome with numerous other musculoskeletal problems, patients scored similarly to normal data on the PODCI (Pediatric Outcomes Data Collection Instrument, a pediatric-specific, patient-reported subjective assessment of overall health, pain, and ability to participate in activities); the only domain in which they

scored lower was sports participation. Most patients had near-normal knee range of motion, but 78% had some knee instability, which did not appear clinically significant. There were no statistically significant differences between the quadricepsplasty and femoral shortening groups.[17]

In conclusion, hyperextension deformity at the knee represents a spectrum of disease from physiologic hyperextension to true CDK. It is frequently seen as part of a larger condition, such as Larsen syndrome, and may be associated with an absent ACL. Treatment includes serial casting, beginning shortly after birth, and frequently surgical realignment and reconstruction. Despite a high rate of residual instability, most patients achieve functional knee range of motion and are able to ambulate without any orthotics.

Clubfoot

Congenital talipes equinovarus (TEV), more commonly known as clubfoot, is one of the most common musculoskeletal anomalies requiring treatment. Its incidence is estimated at 1 to 2 per 1000 live births, with a male-to-female predominance of 2:1. Both feet are affected in 50% of cases.[18] It is frequently idiopathic, but approximately 25%–50% of the time, it is associated with a neuromuscular condition such as myelodysplasia, arthrogryposis, diastrophic dysplasia, and constriction band syndrome, to name a few.[19] Because of the persistent risk of recurrence and inherent differences between the affected and unaffected foot despite successful treatment, the "idiopathic" clubfoot is thought to represent a local, but primary, dysplasia of all tissue of the affected extremity from the knee down.

Despite being described as early as the fourth century BC by Hippocrates, the exact etiology of idiopathic clubfoot is still not entirely known. Numerous theories have been proposed and investigated; they include vascular anomalies, intrauterine factors such as abnormal positioning and amniocentesis, environmental factors such as smoking, abnormal muscle insertions, and genetic factors. To date, no single unifying factor has been identified, and idiopathic clubfoot is most likely multifactorial, against the backdrop of genetic predisposition. Approximately 25% of patients with clubfoot have a family history, and there is a 33% concordance rate in identical twins vs 3% in fraternal twins,[19] so clearly genetic factors play a role. Although the inheritance does not follow any Mendelian inheritance pattern, several genes have been implicated in TEV, and it is currently best explained by the common disease–common variant genetic hypothesis.[20] In this hypothesis, rare genetic variants (single-nucleotide polymorphisms presenting with allele frequency < 5%)

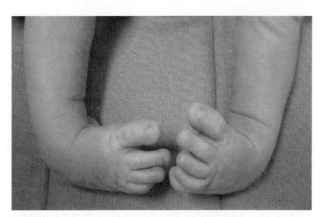

FIGURE 64-4 Classic appearance of clubfoot. Note the cavus, varus, adductus, and equinus.

each confer a moderate risk with higher penetrance.[20] Recently, the PITX1-TBX4 transcriptional pathway has been implicated in TEV[21]; it is a pathway responsible for early limb development and is attractive as an explanation for clubfoot as it is preferentially expressed in the hindlimb over the forelimb.[20]

The diagnosis of clubfoot is based on physical examination (Figure 64-4) and recognition of the 4 components of the deformity, which can be remembered by the mnemonic CAVE: cavus, adductus, varus, and equinus. These terms can be intimidating, as can the deformity. Cavus refers to the forefoot, that the first ray is plantar flexed compared to the rest of the foot and metatarsals, leading to a crease of variable severity on the medial border of the foot. Adductus also refers to the forefoot and the fact that, in TEV, the metatarsals are all "pointing in," or medially directed, so that the lateral border of the foot is "bean shaped." As for varus, this refers to the position of the hind- and midfoot, with the heel turned in and up so that the sole of the baby's foot is often facing up. Finally, equinus also affects the hindfoot and means that, because of a tight Achilles, the foot cannot be brought past neutral in dorsiflexion.

The differential diagnosis for clubfoot includes positional clubfoot, metatarsus adductus, oblique talus, and CVT. In positional clubfoot, at rest, the foot will be similarly positioned plantar flexed and turned in, but it will be completely correctable on examination, and the talar head will not be palpable in the lateral aspect of the foot, as it is in a true clubfoot. Positional clubfoot has a very different natural history in that, once corrected with or (more commonly) without casting, the risk of recurrence is essentially none; the tissues are otherwise normal, a stark difference when compared to TEV. Compared to clubfoot, metatarsus adductus is a deformity only affecting the forefoot and may be passively correctable; the hindfoot and ankle will have a normal position and range of motion. Again, the natural history of untreated metatarsus adductus is

favorable (see previous section in this chapter). CVT, and to a lesser extent oblique talus, will present with a rocker bottom deformity of the foot that dorsiflexes the forefoot and may therefore vaguely resemble the forefoot component of TEV; however, in CVT, there is no coronal plane deviation (meaning no adduction or abduction of the forefoot), and the heel is in calcaneus (dorsiflexed compared to the tibia) as opposed to equinus as in TEV. Finally, the talar head in CVT is palpable in the plantar-medial aspect of the foot rather than dorsolaterally as is the hallmark of a true clubfoot.

As prenatal ultrasound equipment and techniques continue to improve, fetal abnormalities are being increasingly identified before birth, and one of the most commonly diagnosed is clubfoot. Although TEV can be detected by ultrasound as early as 12 weeks, it is more frequently seen on the scan around 20 weeks' estimated gestational age or later; some consider that it can be both a transient and late-onset phenomenon,[22] and false-positive rates vary significantly from 0% to 30%.[23] Specific prenatal counseling is difficult given the relatively high false-positive rate and the late onset of some deformities; it can be challenging to provide accurate information about a fetal clubfoot when some abnormal-looking feet will be normal at birth and some normal-looking feet on 20-week ultrasound will be abnormal at birth.

Glotzbecker et al developed a novel sonographic rating system of mild, moderate, and severe; the authors reported an overall false-positive rate of 19% but found that those feet classified as "mild" on prenatal ultrasound were significantly less likely to have TEV at birth. When those mild cases were excluded,[23] the false-positive rate dropped to 7%. Given the association between clubfeet and more global neuromuscular and chromosomal abnormalities, some authors recommend amniocentesis with karyotyping when TEV is found on prenatal ultrasound[24]; however, other authors recommend against amniocentesis based solely on the finding of TEV in the absence of other indicators based on the low risk of missing major associated malformations.[25]

Treatment has changed significantly since the start of the millennium, with a massive shift from primarily surgical treatment to near-universal adoption of nonoperative techniques. A recent survey of members of the Pediatric Orthopaedic Society of North America (POSNA) found that 93% of respondents treated clubfoot nonoperatively, and that this technique was a departure from how they were trained for 75% of respondents.[26] There are 2 main nonoperative techniques currently used around the world: the French physical therapy method and the Ponseti method. Both are comparably efficacious and fairly labor intensive; the French method is, as one would gather based on its name, used frequently in France. The Ponseti method is used preferentially in North America and is the focus of this discussion.

Until relatively recently, the vast majority of orthopedists treated clubfoot with a (usually unsuccessful) trial of casting followed by extensive surgery consisting of a posteromedial release before the age of 1 year; this was because the results of casting alone had been universally unsuccessful. However, in Iowa, Dr Ignacio Ponseti began successfully treating patients with his casting method in the early 1950s. Although he published promising short- and midterm results in 1963, his method was largely ignored outside the state of Iowa; surgery continued to be considered the "gold standard" until around the turn of this century, when several events brought about a shift in treatment paradigm. In 1995, Cooper and Dietz published the long-term results of patients treated under Ponseti's direction compared to unaffected controls and found that using pain and functional limitation as outcome criteria, 78% of clubfoot patients had good-to-excellent results vs 85% of the control group.[27] These results are much more favorable than the results of surgically treated feet, which are characterized by frequent pain, recurrence, stiffness, over- and undercorrection, leading to activity limitations.[28]

Around the same time period, another group outside Iowa published results using the Ponseti method, showing that it could be successfully applied outside the institution where it was developed; Herzenberg and colleagues reported on their first 34 feet treated by the Ponseti method and compared them to a group of matched controls treated with the "traditional" casting method. They found that only 3% of patients casted by the Ponseti method required extensive open surgery vs 94% in the control group.[29]

Finally, at the end of the 20th century, the Internet was becoming more ubiquitous, and families of patients with clubfeet were going online for information; those not living Iowa were surprised to hear that their child's condition did not necessarily have to be treated by extensive surgery. Ponseti himself credited parents asking their practitioners about his method in helping to spread knowledge and popularity of his technique.[30] The combination of increased visibility of and curiosity about the technique coming from patient families and data showing that the Ponseti method was reproducible by other practitioners and had superior long-term outcomes has led us to where we are today: The Ponseti method is now the preferred method of treatment of idiopathic TEV in North America and is being taught in developing countries all over the world with considerable success.[31] In addition, the method has recently been applied to syndromic clubfoot, such as in constriction band syndrome, arthrogryposis, and myelodysplasia, with good success, although patients often require more casts and have a higher rate of

failure necessitating surgical correction than for idiopathic clubfeet.[32,33]

The Ponseti method consists of a series of long leg casts that are placed weekly; the foot is gently stretched for a short period before each cast is placed (Figure 64-5). Casting can begin any time after birth but does not have to begin immediately; waiting a

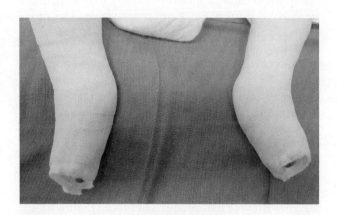

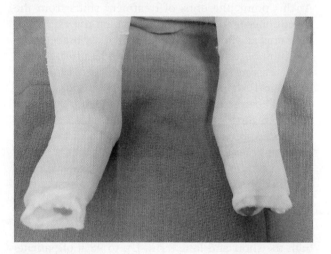

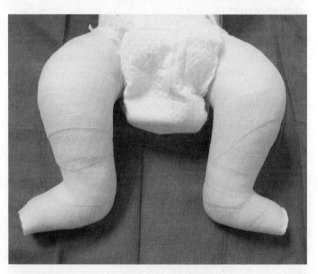

FIGURE 64-5 A, First cast; B, second cast; C, final cast following percutaneous tendoachilles lengthening.

week or even more will not significantly jeopardize a patient's successful outcome. In the case of neonates in the neonatal intensive care unit who may be premature or very small for gestational age or have other comorbidities, having one or both legs casted for weeks at a time may be of significant inconvenience for blood draws, other procedures, positioning, and so on; in these cases, the start of casting may sometimes be delayed until patients are more stable. The order of deformity correction achieved by the technique is cavus, adductus, varus, and equinus (CAVE); the equinus is corrected last and should not be attempted until at least 45°–60° of foot external rotation relative to the tibia can be achieved. The vast majority of patients require a percutaneous Achilles tenotomy (either in office or in the operating room) to achieve full correction. The cast placed immediately following tendon release is usually left for several weeks to allow for healing of the tendon; patients are then transitioned to a foot abduction orthosis (FAO), such as a Denis-Browne bar or Mitchell brace (Figure 64-6). At this point, the onus of treatment shifts from the practitioner who has been performing the casting to the families who must comply with daily brace wear.

Clubfoot recurrence is common, when treated with either casting or surgery, and has been repeatedly linked to FAO noncompliance, with an odds ratio of 183.[34] The brace is usually worn full time for 3 months and then during nighttime and naps until age 3 or 4 years. Approximately one-third of patients treated with the Ponseti method will ultimately need a tibialis anterior tendon transfer to help with dynamic supination that often develops and may cause some patients to walk on the lateral border of their foot.

The outcome of a patient with clubfoot when treated with Ponseti casting is usually quite good in both the short and long term. Up to 98% of patients with idiopathic clubfeet can achieve initial correction with this method, at an average time to correction of 20 days and a recurrence rate of 11%.[35] As previously mentioned, the long-term results are also favorable, with 78% of patients having good-to-excellent results

at an average age of 34 years; in this particular study, 54% of patients participated in sports compared to 40% of controls.[27] In another study, 90% of patients with clubfoot were satisfied with the appearance of their feet.[36]

In summary, congenital TEV, also known as clubfoot, occurs in approximately 0.1% of the population and is most commonly idiopathic. The deformity can be detected on prenatal ultrasound, and the accuracy of this diagnostic modality is improving. At birth, the foot is noted to be in cavus, adductus, varus, and equinus and will not be correctable on physical examination initially. The most widely accepted treatment at this time is the Ponseti method of serial casting, usually begun within the first weeks of birth and consisting of weekly long leg casts, followed by a percutaneous Achilles tenotomy and use of FAO for several years following correction. The vast majority of deformities can be successfully treated this way, and patients maintain their good and excellent results at 30-year follow-up.

Congenital Vertical Talus

Congenital vertical talus is characterized by a rocker bottom deformity of the foot and is much more rare than clubfoot; it is present in approximately 1 in every 10,000 live births. It is isolated in at least half of the cases and associated with neuromuscular or genetic anomalies in the other half. Associated diagnoses are most frequently arthrogryposis and myelomeningocele but also include spinal muscular atrophy, neurofibromatosis, trisomy 13–15 and 18, among others. The exact etiology of CVT is not entirely known but is thought to be related to overpull of the tibialis anterior tendon or intrauterine compression; there may also be a genetic component as 10% of isolated cases appear to be familial, and mutations in the genes associated with early limb development such as *HOXD10* and *GDF5* have recently been implicated.[37]

Congenital vertical talus is a rigid deformity characterized by equinus of the hindfoot with dorsiflexion of the forefoot; the navicular is dorsally dislocated on the plantar-flexed talus, leading to the characteristic rocker bottom deformity. The talar head will be palpable in the plantar-medial aspect of the foot (as opposed to the dorsolateral aspect of the foot seen in clubfoot). The differential diagnosis of CVT includes oblique talus and a calcaneovalgus foot. A true CVT deformity is rigid, and the dislocated navicular will not be reducible onto the plantar-flexed talar head; an oblique talus is an intermediate deformity that looks clinically similar to a vertical talus but will be more flexible, and the navicular will reduce on a maximal plantar flexion lateral x-ray. A calcaneovalgus foot is more flexible still and is characterized by dorsiflexion of the forefoot against the anterior aspect

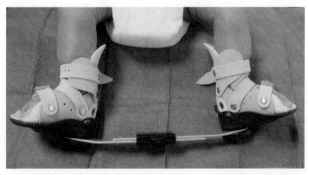

FIGURE 64-6 Foot abduction orthosis (FAO).

of the tibia. Compared to a vertical talus, in addition to being flexible and fully passively correctable, the hindfoot in a calcaneovalgus foot is dorsiflexed rather than plantar flexed; also, the plantar surface of the foot is flat rather than convex. Calcaneovalgus feet are a result of intrauterine packaging, as opposed to manifestations of abnormal tissue, and have a more benign natural history with spontaneous resolution over several months.

Diagnosis of CVT is usually made by physical examination only, although a lateral foot x-ray in neutral and maximal plantar flexion can help distinguish between it and an oblique talus. In a vertical talus, the forefoot will not line up with the talus on maximal plantar flexion, and in an oblique talus, the navicular will reduce and the forefoot will line up with the talus (Figure 64-7). Some authors also recommend genetics evaluation or evaluation of the neuraxis when a CVT is identified because of the relatively high rate of associated anomalies.[38]

Treatment is challenging as these feet are stiff and abnormal. Traditionally, surgery at around 1 year of age consisting of extensive soft tissue releases has been the mainstay of treatment, as it once was for clubfeet. Results can be good but are often complicated by undercorrection, recurrence, and stiffness. More recently, Dobbs et al published on a Ponseti-inspired casting protocol that finishes with percutaneous pinning of the talonavicular joint and tendoachilles lengthening.[37,39] Using this technique, the authors were able to avoid any extensive joint releases, and patients had good postoperative motion. However, 16% of isolated and 20% of syndromic feet had recurrence in their studies.[37,39] Long-term outcomes are difficult to find given the rarity of the condition and associated anomalies; however, midterm studies reported mostly good-to-fair results, with most patients and families satisfied with the appearance and function of their foot.[40]

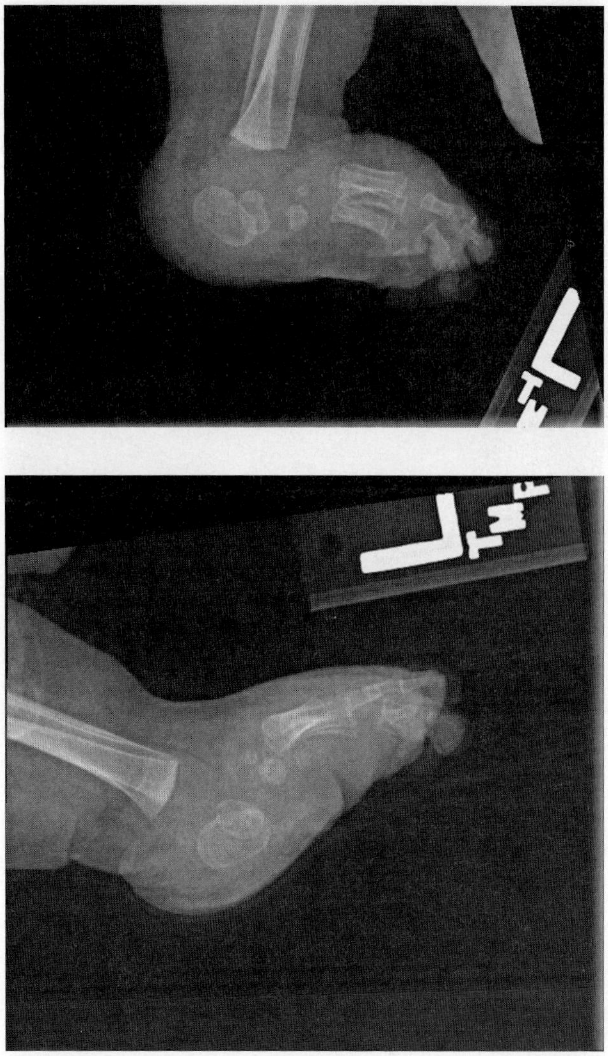

Toe Anomalies

Although there are numerous toe anomalies, this chapter focuses on those that commonly present in the neonatal period: polydactyly, syndactyly, hallux varus, and macrodactyly.

Like polydactyly of the hand, polydactyly of the foot is the most common congenital toe deformity, occurring in more than 1 of every 1000 live births, and it is more common in blacks. It is present bilaterally 50% of the time, and about one-third of cases have a positive family history. It can be preaxial (Figure 64-8), meaning the duplication is medial; postaxial (Figure 64-9), with lateral duplication; or central. Postaxial polydactyly is far more common than preaxial, and central polydactyly is extremely uncommon. Polydactyly can be seen in certain syndromes, such

FIGURE 64-7 A, Lateral of foot with congenital vertical talus; B, lateral of foot with congenital vertical talus in maximal plantar flexion. Note the forefoot remains dorsally positioned to the talus.

as Ellis-van Creveld syndrome, Down syndrome, trisomy 13, and tibial hemimelia, and associated syndromes are more common with preaxial (20%) than postaxial (12%) involvement.[41] Recommended treatment is usually formal surgical excision around the age of 9 to 12 months to help with shoe wear and improve cosmesis. Preaxial polydactyly is often complicated by postoperative progress hallux varus, so care must be taken to appropriately balance the foot during surgery. Otherwise, results are usually good to excellent.[42]

Syndactyly of the foot is also common and is described by the same terms as in syndactyly of the hand: simple or complex (soft tissue or bony involvement), complete or partial (extends all the way distally

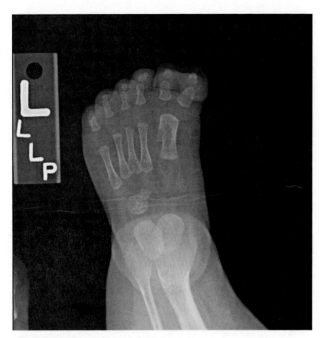

FIGURE 64-8 Preaxial polydactyly.

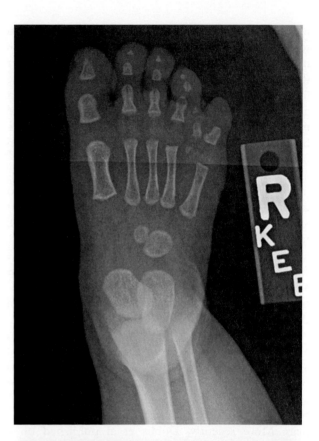

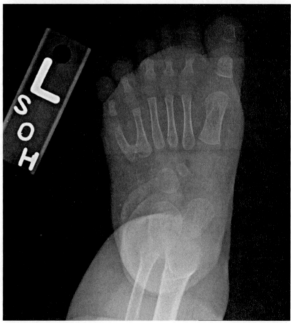

FIGURE 64-9 A and **B,** Two representations of postaxial polydactyly.

or not). Unlike in the hand, function is not negatively impacted by syndactyly; therefore, surgical separation is not advised. Often, the cosmesis of separation is worse than leaving the toes connected (Figure 64-10). If it is complex, and therefore associated with a polydactyly, surgical correction is done to improve shoe wear.

Hallux varus, or medial deviation of the great toe, can occur as an isolated finding with an otherwise-normal first metatarsal, or it may be associated with a longitudinal epiphyseal bracket of the first metatarsal causing medial deviation of the whole first ray. It may also be associated with preaxial polydactyly and, very occasionally, with a larger skeletal dysplasia, such as diastrophic dysplasia. The etiology depends on its associations, and when occurring in isolation, it is caused by a tight, fibrous band running along the medial aspect of the great toe to the base of the first metatarsal. Regardless of the cause, the deviation of the toe makes shoe wear difficult because of the wideness of the forefoot and may worsen over time; therefore, surgical correction is recommended for these reasons and to improve cosmesis.[38]

Macrodactyly is the term used to describe enlargement of one or more of the toes, both bony and soft tissue elements. It can be seen in isolation but can also be part of various other conditions, such as Proteus syndrome, neurofibromatosis, and Klippel-Trénaunay-Weber syndrome. If the entire foot is symmetrically enlarged, treatment is usually nonoperative, and patients can be managed with a larger shoe size on the affected side. Localized gigantism, or enlargement of one or more digits out of proportion to the rest of the foot, is extremely challenging to treat as complications are numerous, and it is nearly

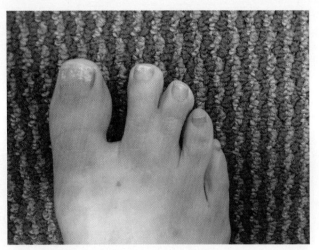

FIGURE 64-10 Appearance of partial simple syndactyly in adulthood.

impossible to satisfactorily and permanently debulk the toes. For a single affected toe, ray resection is often the best option.

REFERENCES

1. Hardy AE. Birth injuries of the brachial plexus: Incidence and prognosis. *J Bone Joint Surg Br.* 1981;63:98–101.
2. Greenwald AG, Schute PC, Shively JL. Brachial plexus birth palsy: a 10-year report on the incidence and prognosis. *J Pediatr Orthop.* 1984;4:689–692.
3. Foad SL, Mehlman CT, Ying J. The epidemiology of neonatal brachial plexus palsy in the United States. *J Bone Joint Surg.* 2008;90:1258–1264.
4. Ouzounian JG, Korst LM, Miller DA, et al. Brachial plexus palsy and shoulder dystocia: obstetric risk factors remain elusive. *Am J Perinatol.* Epub 2012 Aug 16.
5. Waters PM. Obstetric brachial plexus injuries: evaluation and management. *J Am Acad Orthop Surg.* 1997;5:205–214.
6. Cagan E, Sayin R, Dogan M, et al. Bilateral brachial plexus palsy and right Horner syndrome due to congenital cervicothoracic syringomyelia. *Brain Dev.* 2010;32:595–597.
7. Morota N, Sakamoto K, Kobayashi N. Traumatic cervical syringomyelia related to birth injury. *Childs Nerv Syst.* 1992;8:234–236.
8. McBride MT, Hennrikus WL, Malogne TS. Newborn clavicle fractures. *Orthopedics.* 1998;21:317–319.
9. Herring JA. Disorders of the upper extremity. In: Herring JA, ed. *Tachdjian's Pediatric Orthopaedics.* 4th ed. Philadelphia, PA: Saunders Elsevier; 2008:613–626.
10. Hale HB, Bae DS, Waters PM. Current concepts in the management of brachial plexus birth palsy. *J Hand Surg Am.* 2010;35:322–331.
11. Bae DS, Zurakowski D, Avallone N, et al. Sports participation in selected children with brachial plexus birth palsy. *J Pediatr Orthop.* 2009;29:496–503.
12. Herring JA. Disorders of the upper extremity. In: Herring JA, ed. *Tachdjian's Pediatric Orthopaedics.* 4th ed. Philadelphia, PA: Saunders Elsevier; 2008:525–600.
13. Bednar MS, James MA, Light TR. Congenital longitudinal deficiency. *J Hand Surg.* 2009;34A:1739–1747.
14. Shah NR, Limpaphayom N, Dobss MB. A minimally invasive treatment protocol for the congenital dislocation of the knee. *J Pediatr Orthop.* 2009;29:720–725.
15. Herring JA. Disorders of the knee. In: Herring JA, ed. *Tachdjian's Pediatric Orthopaedics.* 4th ed. Philadelphia, PA: Saunders Elsevier; 2008:919–929.
16. Oetgen ME, Walick KS, Tulchin K, et al. Functional results after surgical treatment for congenital knee dislocation. *J Pediatr Orthop.* 2010;30:216–223.
17. Katz MP, Grogono BJ, Soper KC. The etiology and treatment of congenital dislocation of the knee. *J Bone Joint Surg Br.* 1967;49:112–120.
18. Roye DP, Roye BD. Idiopathic congenital talipes equinovarus. *J Am Acad Orthop Surg.* 2002;10:239–248.
19. Dobbs MB, Gurnett CA. Update on clubfoot: etiology and treatment. *Clin Orthop Relat Res.* 2009;467:1146–1153.
20. Dobbs MB, Gurnett CA. Genetics of clubfoot. *J Pediatr Orthop B.* 2012;21:7–9.
21. Alvarado DM, McCall K, Aferal H, et al. Pitx1 haploinsufficiency causes clubfoot in humans and a clubfoot-like phenotype in mice. *Hum Mol Genet.* 2011;20:3943–3952.
22. Keret D, Ezra E, Lokiec F, et al. Efficacy of prenatal ultrasonography in confirmed club foot. *J Bone Joint Surg Br.* 2002;84-B:1015–1019.
23. Glotzbecker MP, Estroff JA, Spencer SA, et al. Prenatlly diagnosed clubfeet: comparing ultrasonographic severity with objective clinical outcomes. *J Pediatr Orthop.* 2010;30:606–611.
24. Shipp TD, Benacerraf BR. The significance of prenatally identified isolated clubfoot: is amniocentesis indicated? *Am J Obstet Gynecol.* 1998;178:600–602.
25. Malone FD, Marino T, Bianchi DW, et al. Isolated clubfoot diagnosed prenatally: is karyotyping indicated? *Obstet Gynecol.* 2000;95:437–440.
26. Zionts LE, Sangiorgio SN, Ebramzadeh E, et al. The current management of idiopathic clubfoot revisited: results of a survey of the POSNA membership. *J Pediatr Orthop.* 2012;32:515–520.
27. Cooper DM, Dietz FR. Treatment of idiopathic clubfoot. A thirty-year follow-up note. *J Bone Joint Surg Am.* 1995;77:1477–1489.
28. Dobbs MD, Nunley R, Schoenecker PL. Long-term follow-up of patients with clubfeet treated with extensive soft-tissue release. *J Bone Joint Surg.* 2006;88:986–996.
29. Herzenberg JE, Radler C, Bor N. Ponseti versus traditional methods of casting for idiopathic clubfoot. *J Pediatr Orthop.* 2002;22:517–521.
30. Morcuende JA, Egbert M, Ponseti IV. The effect of the Internet in the treatment of congenital idiopathic clubfoot. *Iowa Orthop J.* 2003;23:83–86.
31. Tindall AJ, Steinlechner CW, Lavy CB, et al. Results of manipulation of idiopathic clubfoot deformity in Malawi by orthopaedic clinical officers using the Ponseti method: a realistic alternative for the developing world? *J Pediatr Orthop.* 2005;25:627–629.
32. Morcuende JA, Dobbs MB, Frick SL. Results of the Ponseti method in patients with clubfoot associated with arthrogryposis. *Iowa Orthop J.* 2008;28:22–26.
33. Gerlach DJ, Gurnett CA, Limpahayom N, et al. Early results of the Ponseti method for the treatment of clubfoot associated with myelomeningocele. *J Bone Joint Surg Am.* 2009;91:1350–1359.
34. Dobbs MB, Rudzki JR, Purcell DB, et al. Factors predictive of outcome after use of the Ponseti method for the treatment of idiopathic clubfeet. *J Bone Joint Surg Am.* 2004;86:22–27.
35. Morcuende JA, Dolan LA, Dietz FR, et al. Radical reduction in the rate of extensive corrective surgery for clubfoot using the Ponseti method. *Pediatrics.* 2004;113:376–380.
36. Laaveg SJ, Ponseti IV. Long-term results of treatment of congenital club foot. *J Bone Joint Surg Am.* 1980;62:23–31.
37. Chalayon O, Adams A, Dobbs MB. Minimally invasive approach for the treatment of non-isolated congenital vertical talus. *J Bone Joint Surg Am.* 2012;94:e73.

38. Herring JA. Disorders of the foot. In: Herring JA, ed. *Tachdjian's Pediatric Orthopaedics*. 4th ed. Philadelphia, PA: Saunders Elsevier; 2008:1047–1139.

39. Dobbs MB, Purcell DB, Nunley R, et al. Early results of a new method of treatment for idiopathic congenital vertical talus. *J Bone Joint Surg Am*. 2006;88:1192–1200.

40. Kodros SA, Dias LS. Single-stage surgical correction of congenital vertical talus. *J Pediatr Orthop*. 1999;19:42–48.

41. Castilla EE, Lugarinho R, da Graça Dutra M, Salgado LJ. Associated anomalies in individuals with polydactyly. *Am J Med Genet*. 1998:80:459–465.

42. Belthur MV, Linton JL, Barnes DA. The spectrum of preaxial polydactyly of the foot. *J Pediatr Orthop*. 2001;31:435–447.

Part L: Skin

65 Neonatal Bullous Disorders

Phuong T. Khuu and Alfred T. Lane

INTRODUCTION

The development of vesicles, pustules, or bullae on the neonatal skin raises a broad differential, which includes infectious, inflammatory, autoimmune, or hereditary causes. The initial clinical presentation of many of these conditions may appear similar. Thus, it is helpful to identify and categorize based on primary morphologic changes (Table 65-1).

Vesicles are defined as a blister measuring less than 1 cm in size. Blisters larger than 1 cm are termed bullae. Pustules are vesicles with purulent fluid. Vesicles, pustules, and bullae may rapidly rupture, resulting in erosions and ulcerations as the predominant morphology. In other cases, the vesicles and pustules may be miniscule and difficult to discern.

While most of these conditions are benign and transient, there are a few serious, life-threatening conditions that require prompt diagnosis and treatment. Given the broad differential raised by the presence of neonatal blisters, it is helpful to identify the predominant morphology of the eruption and take into account a thorough history and physical.

BENIGN CAUSES OF NEONATAL BLISTERS

Erythema Toxicum Neonatorum

Erythema toxicum neonatorum (ETN) is 1 of the most common transient, benign skin disorders in the neonatal period. It occurs in about 20% of term newborns,[1–4] with some reports[5–8] of frequencies as high as 40%–70%. These erythematous papules and pustules are usually not present at birth but will appear during the first day or 2 of life.[8]

The lesions of ETN are characterized by small papules and pustules overlying an erythematous macule or wheal. The lesions are most frequently found on the trunk and thighs but can also occur on the face and arms.[1] The eruption spares the palms and soles.

The differential diagnosis of ETN includes transient neonatal pustular melanosis (TNPM), miliaria rubra, and eosinophilic pustular folliculitis.

The diagnosis of ETN is usually made clinically. In some instances, confirmation of the diagnosis can be obtained by Wright staining of a pustule, which would show numerous eosinophils.[8,9] Peripheral eosinophilia can be seen in about 15% of patients with ETN, which correlates with the severity of the eruption.[8,10]

No treatment is needed for ETN. Parents can be reassured that the condition is common, benign, asymptomatic, and transient. Lesions resolve spontaneously without sequelae by 2 weeks of age.

Transient Neonatal Pustular Melanosis

Transient neonatal pustular melanosis is a benign idiopathic eruption that is usually present at birth or within the first 1 to 2 days of life.[8] Unlike ETN, TNPM is seen less commonly. It occurs in about 1% to 5% of newborns, with higher incidences in babies of darker pigmentation.[3,4,11]

Affected babies may present with small 1- to 3-mm pustules that quickly rupture, leaving behind small, round collarettes of scale that surround hyperpigmented macules.

Table 65-1 Differential Diagnosis of Neonatal Blistering Diseases

Predominantly Small Vesicles and Pustules		
Benign Transient	**Infectious**	**Other**
Erythema toxicum neonatorum (ETN)	Bacterial folliculitis	Acropustolosis of infancy
Miliaria	Candidiasis	Incontinentia pigmenti
Neonatal acne	Herpes simplex virus	Langerhans cell histiocytosis
Transient neonatal pustular melanosis	Scabies	
	Varicella zoster virus	
Predominantly Large Bulla and Erosions		
Hereditary	**Infectious**	**Other**
Epidermolysis bullosa	Bullous impetigo	Bullous aplasia cutis congenita
Epidermolytic hyperkeratosis	Congenital candidiasis	Langerhans cell histiocytosis
	(exfoliating erythrodermic type)	Neonatal pemphigoid gestationis
	Staphylococcal scalded skin	Neonatal pemphigus vulgaris
	syndrome (SSSS)	Trauma (scalp electrode injury, birth trauma)

In fact, the pustules may be so superficial and fragile that babies may be born with minimal pustules and only exhibit the collarettes of scale and the hyperpigmented macules. The lesions are usually present on the chin, neck, trunk, and thighs. The palms and soles may also be affected.[9]

The differential diagnosis includes ETN, miliaria, acropustulosis of infancy, and bullous impetigo. However, these conditions may be differentiated based on clinical morphology. Unlike ETN, TNPM is usually present at birth and has small pustules with little surrounding erythema and superficial pustules that rupture easily, resulting in small, 1- to 3-mm hyperpigmented macules.[8] The pustules of acropustulosis of infancy are localized to the hands and feet, whereas TNPM lesions can occur anywhere on the body. Miliaria crystallina vesicles are extremely fine and easily rupture without resultant hyperpigmentation.

The diagnosis is made clinically. A Wright stain of the pustule may be performed, which will show many neutrophils and occasional eosinophils.[9]

This is a benign, self-resolving condition, and parents should be reassured that the hyperpigmentation will fade spontaneously with time. No treatment is needed.

Miliaria

Miliaria is a common benign, transient condition that can occur in any age group but can also manifest during the neonatal period. It is estimated to occur in about 9%–13% of newborns.[12–14]

Miliaria is caused by the occlusion of eccrine sweat. Depending on the level of the occlusion that occurs along the sweat ducts, the lesions may range from small clear delicate vesicles to pustules or erythematous papules and nodules. The more common presentation in the neonatal period is miliaria crystallina, which appears as delicate, tiny, clear superficial vesicles, most commonly on the forehead.[14] Miliaria rubra is another common eruption in the neonatal period and presents as small erythematous papules and pustules on the face, neck, and trunk.[14] Plugging of the eccrine sweat duct occurs in the setting of fever, excessive warming, and underneath occlusive dressings.

The differential diagnosis includes ETN, TNPM, congenital candidiasis, and folliculitis.

The diagnosis is made clinically. Often, there is a history of excessive warming. If the diagnosis is uncertain, a skin biopsy may be performed.

Usually, no treatment is needed for miliaria, and parents can be reassured regarding the benign and transient nature of this eruption. Care should be taken to remove any possible triggers, such as occlusive dressings, or minimizing overheating.

Acropustulosis of Infancy

Acropustulosis of infancy is an uncommon condition of unknown etiology that usually presents during infancy but can present at birth or during the first few weeks of life.[15] It is thought that there are 2 forms of acropustulosis of infancy, an idiopathic variant and a postscabetic phenomenon, with the latter more common.[15–17] Postscabetic acropustulosis is thought to occur after severe or prolonged scabies infestations.[18]

Small pruritic vesicles and pustules appear on the palms, soles, dorsal hands and feet. Rarely, atypical forms of this disorder can present with more widespread distribution of the vesicles and pustules. These lesions occur in crops every few weeks (Figure 65-1A, 65-1B).

The diagnosis can be made clinically based on the history and acral distribution of the lesions. A Wright stain of the lesions may also be performed, which

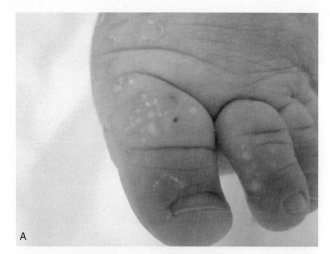

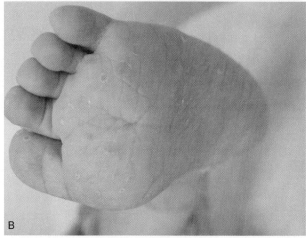

FIGURE 65-1 A and B, Acropustulosis of infancy. Small, 1- to 2-mm vesicles and pustules are symmetrically distributed on both feet. There is a lack of linear burrows noted. B, The collarette of scale is recognized on the sole after the vesicles and pustules rupture.

would show polymorphonuclear neutrophils (PMNs) and some eosinophils. Rarely, skin biopsies may also be performed for diagnostic confirmation. Given that the differential diagnosis includes active scabies infection, it is important to explore this possibility through careful physical examination and performing skin scrapings to look for scabies.[17]

The differential diagnosis includes active scabies infestation, dyshidrotic eczema, and epidermolysis bullosa simplex (EBS).

This condition spontaneously resolves within a few years, usually within 18 to 20 months.[15] To alleviate symptoms, mid- to high-potency topical steroids can be safely and effectively used.[16] If pruritus is causing sleep disruption, oral antihistamines can be taken at bedtime for their sedative effects.[19] Dapsone has been reported to be efficacious, but because of the concerns for side effects, this medication should be used

cautiously and only reserved for severe cases refractory to other treatments.[15]

INFECTIOUS CAUSES OF NEONATAL BLISTERS

Superficial Bacterial Infections

Skin infections caused by *Staphylococcus aureus* can occur during the neonatal period. However, these infections tend to occur within the first few weeks of life and are usually not seen right at birth. More commonly, the infections are superficial and present as impetigo, bullous impetigo, or folliculitis. In some cases, the patient may be severely affected, with bacteremia or staphylococcal scalded skin syndrome. A recent analysis from a teaching institution in India found that impetigo was the most common cause of neonatal vesiculobullous disorders at their hospital, comprising 13.5% of cases. Among these, *S. aureus* was twice as common as group A streptococcus as the etiologic cause.[6] It was reported that among children with impetigo, 87% of cases cultured positive for *S. aureus*.[20]

Impetigo can occur anywhere on the skin. In nonbullous impetigo, the lesions are erythematous plaques with overlying honey-colored crusts. In bullous impetigo, the lesions are either solitary or clustered pustules and bullae (Figure 65-2).

The differential diagnosis includes other infectious causes of pustules and vesicles. The lesions of bullous impetigo tend to be flaccid and filled with pus. These bullae can rupture easily, resulting in a shallow erosion with a collarette of scale. A diagnostic clue suggesting nonbullous impetigo is the appearance of characteristic honey-colored crusts. The lesions are usually

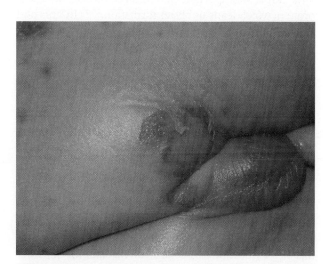

FIGURE 65-2 Bullous impetigo. Bullae that have ruptured result in superficial erosions.

localized or clustered in 1 area, although they may become more widespread.

The diagnosis can be made with Gram stain and culture of the fluid from a pustule.[9] Skin biopsies are rarely needed unless the diagnosis is in question. A bacterial culture is helpful because staphylococcal impetigo is indistinguishable from streptococcal impetigo. Furthermore, a culture will also aid in determining antimicrobial sensitivities of the causative strain of bacteria.[21]

Impetigo can be complicated by cellulitis, bacteremia, and toxin-mediated staphylococcal scalded skin syndrome (SSSS). The bullous form of impetigo, which is thought to be a localized form of SSSS, is especially at risk for rapid progression to systemic infection. Treatment should be initiated promptly. In the case of bullous impetigo, the recommended therapy is with parenteral antibiotics. If the patient does not exhibit any systemic symptoms and once the lesions have started to improve, the patient may finish the course of antibiotics orally.

Staphylococcal Scalded Skin Syndrome

Staphylococcal scalded skin syndrome is a toxin-mediated infection that leads to generalized blistering, erythroderma, and superficial desquamation. It is more commonly seen in the pediatric population. Outbreaks of neonatal SSSS have been reported.[22,23]

Affected babies are usually fussy and may present with generalized erythema and tender skin. There may be honey-colored crusting localized to perioral skin and desquamation especially noticeable around flexural regions (Figure 65-3). A positive Nikolsky sign is seen, which is characterized by gentle rubbing of uninvolved skin to produce a blister.[24] Occasionally, the initial presentation may be a bullous impetigo that rapidly progresses. Exfoliative toxins A and B produced by the *S. aureus* bacteria, target an important epidermal cell-to-cell adhesion protein, which leads to blister formation.[25–27] Infants and young children are most susceptible because of the lack of protective antibodies and immature renal clearance of the toxins.

Other blistering disorders that may be considered in the differential diagnosis include viral exanthem, toxic epidermal necrosis, congenital candidiasis, and bullous congenital ichthyosiform erythroderma. However, clues to the diagnosis of SSSS include the presence of perioral honey-colored crusting and flexural desquamation as well as tender, erythrodermic skin in a very fussy baby.

Often, the diagnosis of SSSS is clinical. This may be supported by the presence of a toxin-producing strain of *S. aureus*, although the clinical usefulness of this has been questioned because of the lack of sensitivity and specificity.[28] Blister formation is secondary to toxins produced by the *S. aureus* at distant colonizing

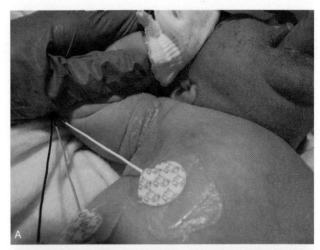

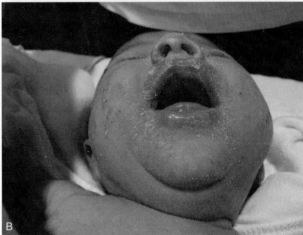

FIGURE 65-3 A and B, Staphylococcal scalded skin syndrome. A, Superficial erosions are noted in the flexural regions. B, Honey-colored crusting is seen in the periorificial regions.

or infective sites. As a result, cultures taken from the bullae are usually negative. High-yield areas for a positive swab culture are from skin around the nose, eyes, mouth, umbilicus, and any area where there is honey-colored crusting.[24] Biopsy can be performed but is rarely required. Histopathology will show an intraepidermal split at or below the granular layer with minimal inflammation.[24]

Management of SSSS is with antistaphylococcal intravenous antibiotics. Exfoliation may continue for 24–48 hours after antibiotics are initiated.[21] Supportive care, including pain control and wound care for the desquamated skin, is the mainstay of therapy. Temperature control and management of fluid and electrolyte balance are necessary if there are widespread erosions.

There is about a 3% mortality for children affected with SSSS.[24] Because the blister formation is superficial, the skin will usually heal within 2–3 weeks without scarring. There are usually no long-term sequelae from the disease.

Herpes Simplex Infection

Herpes simplex virus (HSV) infection during the neonatal period can have significant morbidity and mortality. It is estimated that the incidence of neonatal herpes infection in the United States is 9.6 per 100,000 live births.[29] Neonates can acquire HSV in utero, during delivery, or with postnatal exposure. Congenital HSV infection from in utero exposure is rare and is thought to account for less than 5% of cases.[30] The clinical features of congenital HSV are similar to other TORCH (toxoplasmosis, rubella, cytomegalovirus, HSV) infections. Postnatal infection with HSV is usually caused by contacts with family members or hospital personnel who are shedding HSV. Finally, neonatal HSV is most commonly acquired during delivery through an infected birth canal. There are 3 types of HSV infections in the neonate: disseminated infection; localized infection of the skin, eyes, and mouth (SEM); and central nervous system (CNS) infection. Localized SEM disease is the most common presentation, accounting for 45% of neonatal HSV cases. CNS disease accounts for 30% of cases, and disseminated disease occurs in 25% of cases.[31] The greatest risk for HSV transmission occurs in neonates born to a mother with primary genital herpes infection near the time of delivery, with an estimated risk of about 50%. The risk for HSV transmission in neonates born to a mother with reactivation of HSV infection[31,32] is less than 2%.

Skin disease can present with small 2- to 4-mm vesicles that are usually in clusters. A common site of involvement is on the scalp at the site of fetal scalp monitor electrodes. Babies may present only with systemic symptoms, including features of sepsis or seizures. In 1 study, 7% to 39% of patients did not have skin findings at the time of presentation and did not develop vesicles during their disease course.[33]

The differential diagnosis of neonatal HSV includes other infectious causes, such as varicella (varicella zoster virus, VZV), bullous impetigo, and candidiasis. A rare entity, incontinentia pigmenti (IP), can also present with vesicles, although these are more likely to be in linear configurations along the lines of Blaschko. Localized vesicles or erosions at the site of fetal monitor electrode placement may be mistaken for trauma or on the scalp may be mistaken for aplasia cutis congenita.

In cases with skin findings, rapid diagnosis can be made with a Tzanck smear of epithelial cells from the base of a vesicle,[34] although the sensitivity of this test is about 76%.[35] Cultures should be obtained from the mouth, nasopharynx, conjunctivae, and anal skin. In addition, direct fluorescent antibody and culture should also be obtained from skin vesicles. Skin and conjunctival cultures provide the greatest yield.[31,33] Skin biopsies may be performed, which can confirm the diagnosis and rule out other causes of blistering in the neonate.

Prompt recognition and treatment with intravenous acyclovir can decrease morbidity and mortality. All cases of presumptive neonatal HSV infection require treatment with intravenous acyclovir; topical and oral acyclovir should not be used.[32] Patients with SEM disease are treated for 14 days; those with CNS or disseminated disease are treated for a longer duration.[31]

Neonatal HSV infection can have devastating consequences. Of the 3 patterns of infections, newborns with SEM disease have the best outcome. More than 50% of those with CNS infection may suffer from long-term neurologic abnormalities and developmental problems. Newborns who have disseminated disease have mortality rates of 20%–30% even with treatment.[31,32]

Varicella Infection

Varicella (VZV) infection of the newborn can occur as a result of intrauterine infection or postnatal infection. If newborns develop symptoms of VZV infection during the first 10 to 12 days of life, then the etiology of their infection is through intrauterine exposure. If VZV infection develops after the first 12 days of life, then the most likely etiology is postnatal exposure.[36]

It is estimated that VZV infection occurs in about 1 to 10 per 10,000 pregnancies. When maternal VZV occurs during the first 20 weeks of pregnancy, there is 1%–2% risk for congenital varicella, also known as fetal varicella syndrome, which is characterized by limb abnormalities, scarring in a dermatomal pattern, ocular abnormalities, and CNS abnormalities.[37–40]

When maternal VZV infection occurs around the time of delivery, neonatal varicella can occur because of a lack of maternal antibodies and an immature neonatal immune system.[38] If mothers develop VZV infection 1 week before or 2 days after delivery, the risk for severe disseminated neonatal varicella is about 50%; approximately 20% of these affected infants died.[36]

Affected neonates with varicella infection have a generalized vesicular eruption and may have systemic multiorgan involvement.[41]

The differential diagnosis includes HSV infection, IP, and other causes of generalized vesicular eruption. The diagnosis can be made by obtaining polymerase chain reaction (PCR), direct fluorescence assay (DFA), and viral culture of scraping from a vesicle.[31]

Candidiasis

Congenital cutaneous candidiasis (CCC) is an uncommon condition as a result of utero exposure to *Candida* spp., and fewer than 100 cases have been reported. Although candidal vulvovaginitis occurs in about 20%–25% of pregnant women, fewer than 1% of these will result in infection of the placenta.[42] Risk factors include the presence of a cervical foreign body. Preterm babies are more susceptible to the disease because of an impaired epidermal barrier and immature immune system.

The skin eruption appears during the first few days of life as erythematous papules and pustules, which can evolve to form vesicles and bullae. The palms and soles are usually involved. However, the diaper area is spared, and thrush is usually not seen. In rare cases, there is progression to a more generalized exfoliative erythroderma.[42]

The differential diagnosis includes other blistering disorders, such as impetigo, HSV, ETN, and TNPM. In addition, there is a distinction between CCC, which is rare, and neonatal candidiasis, which is more common. Neonatal candidiasis is acquired during birth through an infected birth canal or postnatally through external exposure. Neonatal candidiasis usually presents as thrush, diaper dermatitis, or perianal dermatitis.

The diagnosis can be made with the presence of spores and pseudohyphae on skin scrapings. Confirmation can be obtained by culture. If the diagnosis is in doubt, a skin biopsy can be performed, which will show fungal elements in the stratum corneum. Premature, low birth weight infants and any infant showing signs of systemic disease should have cultures performed of the skin, blood, urine, and cerebrospinal fluid.[43]

Full-term infants with skin-limited disease who do not have systemic symptoms can be treated with topical antifungals. Any neonate with systemic infection or an exfoliative dermatitis should be treated with systemic antifungal therapy.

In general, full-term infants with CCC that is skin limited follow a benign course with no long-term sequelae; most skin lesions will resolve within 2 weeks. Infants who develop rapid progression toward an exfoliative dermatitis are at risk for the development of systemic infection and have a poor prognosis. Premature infants with birth weights less than 1000 g are most at risk for systemic infection.[42]

INHERITED CAUSES OF BLISTERING

Epidermolysis Bullosa

Epidermolysis bullosa (EB) is a rare inherited skin fragility disorder that is characterized by the formation of blisters and erosions in reaction to minor frictional forces on the skin and mucosa. The incidence of EB is estimated to be 19 per million live births based on data derived from the National EB Registry (NEBR).[44]

Epidermolysis bullosa is now classified into 4 major types, which differ both phenotypically and genotypically. The types of EB are categorized based on the location of the target proteins and the level of the blister split. These 4 main types are EB simplex (EBS), junctional EB (JEB), dystrophic EB (DEB), and Kindler syndrome. EBS is the most common type and is defined by an intraepidermal split. This type of EB is mainly inherited in an autosomal dominant pattern and may have a milder course of disease.[45] The blisters in JEB have a level of skin cleavage through the lamina lucida, which is located at the junction between the epidermis and dermis. JEB is inherited in an autosomal recessive pattern.[46] DEB is characterized by blisters at the level of the sublamina densa of the basement membrane zone. This form of EB can be inherited in an autosomal dominant or recessive pattern, dominant dystrophic EB (DDEB) and recessive dystrophic EB (RDEB), respectively.[47] Finally, Kindler syndrome is a rare autosomal recessive condition that is characterized by skin fragility and photosensitivity.[48,49]

The majority of affected babies present at birth or shortly after birth with erosions and bullae. Blisters may arise in areas prone to frictional trauma or as a result of adhesives placed on the skin (Figure 65-4). The oral mucosa may be involved, causing difficulties with feeding. In some types of EB, babies may have hoarseness and respiratory distress because of tracheolaryngeal involvement. In 1 rare subtype of JEB, there may be associated pyloric atresia. Other complications include poor weight gain, infection, and anemia.

The differential diagnosis of EB includes other blistering disorders. Clues to the diagnosis include the presence of erosions at birth and blister formation at sites that are subjected to frictional trauma, such as areas where monitors and adhesives are placed. Occasionally, babies who have EB are also born with congenital localized absence of skin (Figure 65-5). For the subtypes of EB with autosomal dominant mode of inheritance, there could be a family history of other family members with a blistering disorder.

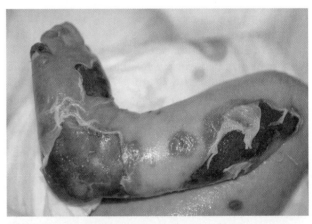

FIGURE 65-4 Epidermolysis bullosa. Bullae and large erosions are seen on the leg of a 5-day-old neonate.

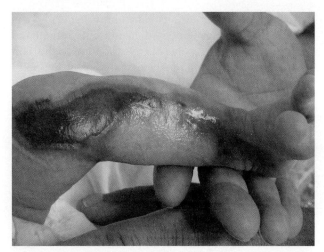

FIGURE 65-5 Epidermolysis bullosa (EB). Occasionally, aplasia cutis congenita is seen in association with EB.

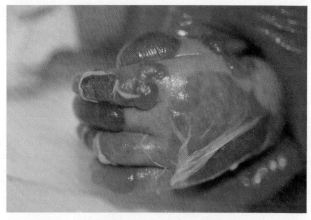

FIGURE 65-6 Epidermolysis bullosa (EB). This neonate has recessive dystrophic EB (RDEB) with large bullae on the fingers. These blisters should be drained with a sterile needle to prevent extension of the blisters.

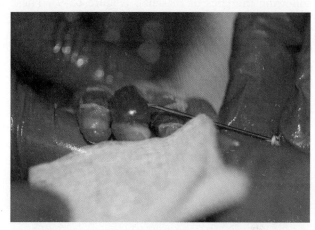

FIGURE 65-7 Epidermolysis bullosa. A large-bore sterile needle is used to gently puncture a hole in the blister. Gauze is then used to help drain the fluid from the blister. The roof of the blister should be left intact to act as a barrier over the erosion.

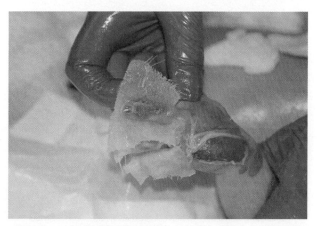

FIGURE 65-8 Epidermolysis bullosa. After the large blisters are drained, each finger should be individually dressed using Vaseline-impregnated gauze.

The diagnosis is made with skin biopsy and genetic mutation analysis. The skin biopsy should be performed on an induced blister and sent for analysis by immunofluorescence and electron microscopy. Once the diagnosis has been established and the type of EB is determined, genetic mutation analysis can be performed.[50]

It is paramount to initiate gentle handling of the baby to prevent further development of blisters. As much as possible, avoid procedures that may further traumatize the skin and mucosa. Adhesives should not be used on the skin, such as tape, monitor leads, skin temperature probes, and oxygen saturation probes. For the oxygen saturation probe, a transparent dressing may be used to line the probe prior to placement on the skin. For intravenous stabilization, special arrangements should be made to avoid the placement of tape directly on the skin. One proposed method is to stabilize the intravenous line using a soft cotton woven dressing or self-adherent compression wrap. There are specialized nonadherent "tapes" designed to be easily removed from fragile skin without traumatizing it. The elastic band of diapers should be cut, and the diapers should be placed loosely. Blisters larger than 1 cm should be drained using sterile needles (Figures 65-6 to 65-8). In patients with a diagnosis of RDEB, dressings should be applied individually to each finger to prevent the development of pseudosyndactyly.

The prognosis varies depending on the subtype of EB. Regardless, parents should be educated that there is no cure for this condition and that this is a lifelong condition of skin fragility. Affected babies with EBS and DDEB tend to have the best prognosis. In a particular subtype of JEB whereby there is absence of a key basement membrane component, affected newborns may die within the first year of life. When there is associated pyloric atresia in patients with JEB, the risk of mortality during the neonatal period is extremely high.

Patients with RDEB may survive beyond the neonatal period, but they suffer from severe and debilitating extracutaneous complications, including esophageal strictures, poor growth, chronic infections, unremitting anemia, and significant pseudosyndactyly.[50,51]

Incontinentia Pigmenti

A rare genodermatosis, IP, is an X-linked dominant disorder affecting the skin, dentition, eyes, and possibly CNS. It is caused by mutations in the nuclear factor kappa B (NF-κB) essential modulator (NEMO) gene and is usually lethal in males. There are 4 stages of the disease: inflammatory (or vesicular), verrucous, hyperpigmented, and atrophic.[52] The skin findings may present at birth or during the first few months of life.

Classically, during the first 2 weeks of life, affected babies present with vesicles in linear configurations following the lines of Blaschko (Figure 65-9). These vesicles may occur on any part of the body, but they usually spare the head and neck. This stage usually lasts for the first few months of life. As the vesicular stage subsides, the skin enters a verrucous stage whereby hyperkeratotic lines and whorls are seen on the trunk and extremities. These hyperkeratotic plaques may or may not correspond to the preceding

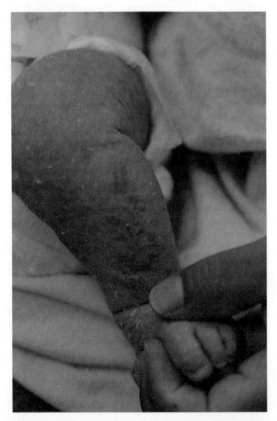

FIGURE 65-9 Incontinentia pigmenti. Erythematous papules and vesicles in a linear distribution on the leg of a female neonate with incontinentia pigmenti.

pattern of vesicular lesions. The third stage is characterized by hyperpigmented linear and reticulated patches that slowly resolve over years. Finally, the skin enters a hypopigmented stage with linear hypopigmented patches and subtle atrophic hairless plaques, which are usually found on the lower extremities.[52]

Other skin manifestations of the disease include alopecia and nail dystrophy. About 50%–70% of affected individuals have abnormal dentition, including dental shape anomalies, delayed dentition, and hypodontia.[53,54] Ocular abnormalities that have been described include avascular areas and fibrovascular proliferations resembling retinopathy of prematurity, cataracts, strabismus, uveitis, and optic nerve atrophy.[55] It is estimated that up to 30% of patients also have CNS abnormalities, including seizures, encephalopathy, and developmental delay.[56,57]

Clues to the diagnosis include the clinical presentation of vesicles patterned in a linear, whorled configuration following lines of Blaschko. Examination of the affected infant's mother may reveal linear hypopigmented patches on the lower extremities. The diagnosis can be made with a skin biopsy. The findings on biopsy vary depending on the stage of the lesion that is biopsied. The most specific histologic findings for the disease can be seen in the inflammatory stage. Genetic testing is also available commercially.

Once a diagnosis of IP is made, patients should have an opthalmological evaluation to assess for ocular abnormalities; serial follow-up is recommended. A thorough neurologic examination should be performed, and any abnormality should prompt referral to neurology. It should be noted that patients who have retinal abnormalities are more likely to have associated CNS involvement, and imaging may be considered in these cases.

OTHER CAUSES OF NEONATAL BLISTERS

Langerhans Cell Histiocytosis

Langerhans cell histiocytosis (LCH) is a heterogeneous group of disorders that can present at any age. Using data from a population-based German Childhood Cancer Registry, the calculated incidence of neonatal LCH, as defined by diagnosis of LCH within the first 28 days of life, is estimated to be 1 to 2 per million.[58] The disease is categorized based on the extent of organ involvement. Patients either have single-system involvement (SS-LCH) or multisystem involvement (MS-LCH). The organs that can be affected by LCH include, in order of frequency, the skin, liver, bone, hematological system, spleen, lymph nodes, lungs, and gastrointestinal tract. By far the most common initial manifestation of LCH is with cutaneous lesions.

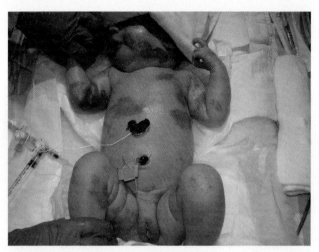

FIGURE 65-10 Erosive Langerhans cell histiocytosis (LCH). Erythematous to purpuric patches, plaques, and shallow erosions are seen on this neonate. Note the stellate ulcer on the right arm. A skin biopsy showed features of LCH.

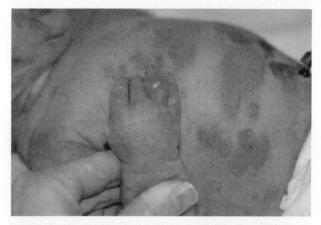

FIGURE 65-11 Neonatal bullous pemphigoid. Tense bullae and vesicles with associated urticarial plaques are seen in this neonate born to a mother who had pemphigoid gestationis.

The clinical cutaneous presentation ranges from red-brown crusted papules to moist, brightly erythematous papules and nodules. In neonates, the lesions may appear vesicular or erosive (Figure 65-10).

The diagnosis of LCH is made by skin biopsy for routine histology and immunohistochemical stains, which characteristically demonstrate histiocytes with reniform nuclei and abundant cytoplasm, which stain with S-100 and CD1a. Once a diagnosis of LCH is made, it is recommended that the following baseline studies be performed to evaluate for extent of disease: complete blood cell count, liver function tests, coagulation studies, chest radiography, skeletal surveys, and urine osmolality tests.[59] If these baseline studies indicate any abnormality, then further diagnostic studies, such as bone marrow biopsy and computed tomographic (CT) scan, should be pursued.[59]

The prognosis for those neonates with SS-LCH is excellent. Spontaneous regression can occur in patients with cutaneous SS-LCH. A recent study suggested that certain morphologic features may indicate greater likelihood of self-regression, including skin lesions that are solitary, with necrosis, and located on the extremities.[60] However, there are also reports of disease progression even in SS-LCH and recurrence of cutaneous SS-LCH even after complete resolution of the skin lesions. Thus, long-term follow-up is indicated for all patients with LCH, even after complete resolution has been achieved.

The management of these patients varies depending on the extent of organ involvement. Those with SS-LCH have excellent long-term survival. For those with cutaneous SS-LCH, there may be spontaneous regression of their disease even in the absence of treatment.

Blistering Caused by Maternal Antibodies

There are several diseases that cause blistering in the mother and subsequently may cause blistering in the newborn infant (Figure 65-11). Based on the history and clinical course of the mother, the physician should be aware of the possibilities of these conditions. Pemphigoid gestationis occurs in about 1 in 20,000 to 50,000 pregnant women, and it may result with blisters or erosions in the infant.[61] Neonatal pemphigus vulgaris can cause blisters in the neonatal period.[62] In 1 study, pemphigus vulgaris occurred in 45% of neonates born to mothers who had pemphigus vulgaris.[63] Only 5% to 10% of infants born to mothers with pemphigoid gestationis are affected with skin lesions.[64]

Each of these diseases is associated with transplacental passage of antibodies to the skin. Pemphigoid gestationis is associated with antibodies to the basement membrane, while pemphigus vulgaris is associated with antibodies to the surface keratinocytes.

The differential is included in the other diseases associated with blisters and erosions in the neonate.

Confirmation of these immunological diseases is usually completed by diagnosis of the condition in the mother. The titer of transplacental antibodies may be too low to be identified in the infant. Examination of a skin biopsy in the infant may show immunological staining in the basement membrane or between the keratinocytes. The staining may identify immunoglobulin (Ig) G or complement (C3). The cutaneous lesions in the infants can be treated with topical lubrication or possibly topical steroids. If the disease becomes severe or secondarily infected, then additional treatment may be necessary.

The maternal antibodies slowly dissipate after delivery, allowing slow resolution the course of the disease. The cutaneous lesions should resolve without scarring.

REFERENCES

1. Monteagudo B, Labandeira J, Cabanillas M, Acevedo A, Toribio J. Prospective study of erythema toxicum neonatorum: epidemiology and predisposing factors. *Pediatr Dermatol.* 2012;29(2):166–168.
2. Kanada KN, Merin MR, Munden A, Friedlander SF. A prospective study of cutaneous findings in newborns in the United States: correlation with race, ethnicity, and gestational status using updated classification and nomenclature. *J Pediatr.* 2012;161:240–245.
3. Moosavi Z, Hosseini T. One-year survey of cutaneous lesions in 1000 consecutive Iranian newborns. *Pediatr Dermatol.* 2006;23:61–63.
4. Rodriguez-Garcia C, Rodriguez C, Sanchez R, et al. Prevalence of cutaneous findings in Spanish neonates and relationships to obstetric and parental factors. *Pediatr Dermatol.* 2012;29:232–233.
5. Zagne V, Fernandes NC. Dermatoses in the first 72 h of life: a clinical and statistical survey. *Indian J Dermatol Venereol Leprol.* 2011;77:470–476.
6. Tarang G, Anupam V. Incidence of vesicobullous and erosive disorders of neonates. *J Dermatol Case Rep.* 2011;5:58–63.
7. Liu C, Feng J, Qu R, et al. Epidemiologic study of the predisposing factors in erythema toxicum neonatorum. *Dermatology.* 2005;210:269–272.
8. Berg FJ, Solomon LM. Erythema neonatorum toxicum. *Arch Dis Child.* 1987;62:327–328.
9. Van Praag MC, Van Rooij RW, Folkers E, Spritzer R, Menke HE, Oranje AP. Diagnosis and treatment of pustular disorders in the neonate. *Pediatr Dermatol.* 1997;14:131–143.
10. Levy HL, Cothran F. Erythema toxicum neonatorum present at birth. *Am J Dis Child.* 1962;103:617–619.
11. Wyre HW Jr, Murphy MO. Transient neonatal pustular melanosis. *Arch Dermatol.* 1979;115:458.
12. Nanda A, Kaur S, Bhakoo ON, Dhall K. Survey of cutaneous lesions in Indian newborns. *Pediatr Dermatol.* 1989;6:39–42.
13. Ferahbas A, Utas S, Akcakus M, Gunes T, Mistik S. Prevalence of cutaneous findings in hospitalized neonates: a prospective observational study. *Pediatr Dermatol.* 2009;26:139–142.
14. Hidano A, Purwoko R, Jitsukawa K. Statistical survey of skin changes in Japanese neonates. *Pediatr Dermatol.* 1986;3:140–144.
15. Kahn G, Rywlin AM. Acropustulosis of infancy. *Arch Dermatol.* 1979;115:831–833.
16. Mancini AJ, Frieden IJ, Paller AS. Infantile acropustulosis revisited: history of scabies and response to topical corticosteroids. *Pediatr Dermatol.* 1998;15:337–341.
17. Elpern DJ. Infantile acropustulosis and antecedent scabies. *J Am Acad Dermatol.* 1984;11:895–896.
18. Good LM, Good TJ, High WA. Infantile acropustulosis in internationally adopted children. *J Am Acad Dermatol.* 2011;65:763–771.
19. Jarratt M, Ramsdell W. Infantile acropustulosis. *Arch Dermatol.* 1979;115:834–836.
20. Darmstadt GL. Oral antibiotic therapy for uncomplicated bacterial skin infections in children. *Pediatr Infect Dis J.* 1997;16:227–240.
21. Ladhani S, Garbash M. Staphylococcal skin infections in children: rational drug therapy recommendations. *Paediatr Drugs.* 2005;7:77–102.
22. Neylon O, O'Connell NH, Slevin B, et al. Neonatal staphylococcal scalded skin syndrome: clinical and outbreak containment review. *Eur J Pediatr.* 2010;169:1503–1509.
23. Curran JP, Al-Salihi FL. Neonatal staphylococcal scalded skin syndrome: massive outbreak due to an unusual phage type. *Pediatrics.* 1980;66:285–290.
24. Shwayder T, Akland T. Neonatal skin barrier: structure, function, and disorders. *Dermatol Ther.* 2005;18:87–103.
25. Amagai M, Yamaguchi T, Hanakawa Y, Nishifuji K, Sugai M, Stanley JR. Staphylococcal exfoliative toxin B specifically cleaves desmoglein 1. *J Investig Dermatol.* 2002;118:845–850.
26. Amagai M, Matsuyoshi N, Wang ZH, Andl C, Stanley JR. Toxin in bullous impetigo and staphylococcal scalded-skin syndrome targets desmoglein 1. Nat Med 2000;6:1275–1277.
27. Hanakawa Y, Schechter NM, Lin C, et al. Molecular mechanisms of blister formation in bullous impetigo and staphylococcal scalded skin syndrome. *J Clin Investig.* 2002;110:53–60.
28. Ladhani S, Robbie S, Chapple DS, Joannou CL, Evans RW. Isolating Staphylococcus aureus from children with suspected staphylococcal scalded skin syndrome is not clinically useful. *Pediatr Infect Dis J.* 2003;22:284–286.
29. Flagg EW, Weinstock H. Incidence of neonatal herpes simplex virus infections in the United States, 2006. *Pediatrics.* 2011;127:e1–e8.
30. Robinson JL, Vaudry WL, Forgie SE, Lee BE. Prevention, recognition and management of neonatal HSV infections. *Expert Rev Anti Infect Ther.* 2012;10:675–685.
31. American Academy of Pediatrics. *Red Book: 2012 Report of the Committee on Infectious Diseases.* 29th ed. Pickering LK, ed. Elk Grove Village, IL: American Academy of Pediatrics; 2012.
32. Corey L, Wald A. Maternal and neonatal herpes simplex virus infections. *New Engl J Med.* 2009;361:1376–1385.
33. Kimberlin DW, Lin CY, Jacobs RF, et al. Natural history of neonatal herpes simplex virus infections in the acyclovir era. *Pediatrics.* 2001;108:223–229.
34. Veien NK, Vestergaard BF. Rapid diagnostic tests for cutaneous eruptions of herpes simplex. *Acta Derm Venereol.* 1978;58:83–85.
35. Ozcan A, Senol M, Saglam H, et al. Comparison of the Tzanck test and polymerase chain reaction in the diagnosis of cutaneous herpes simplex and varicella zoster virus infections. *Int J Dermatol.* 2007;46:1177–1179.
36. Sauerbrei A, Wutzler P. Neonatal varicella. *J Perinatol.* 2001; 21:545–549.
37. Enders G, Miller E, Cradock-Watson J, Bolley I, Ridehalgh M. Consequences of varicella and herpes zoster in pregnancy: prospective study of 1739 cases. *Lancet.* 1994;343:1548–1551.
38. Mandelbrot L. Fetal varicella—diagnosis, management, and outcome. *Prenat Diagn.* 2012;32:511–518.
39. Pastuszak AL, Levy M, Schick B, et al. Outcome after maternal varicella infection in the first 20 weeks of pregnancy. *N Engl J Med.* 1994;330:901–905.
40. Figueroa-Damian R, Arredondo-Garcia JL. Perinatal outcome of pregnancies complicated with varicella infection during the first 20 weeks of gestation. *Am J Perinatol.* 1997;14:411–414.
41. Nathwani D, Maclean A, Conway S, Carrington D. Varicella infections in pregnancy and the newborn. A review prepared for the UK Advisory Group on Chickenpox on behalf of the British Society for the Study of Infection. *J Infect.* 1998;36(Suppl 1):59–71.
42. Darmstadt GL, Dinulos JG, Miller Z. Congenital cutaneous candidiasis: clinical presentation, pathogenesis, and management guidelines. *Pediatrics.* 2000;105:438–444.
43. Tieu KD, Satter EK, Zaleski L, Koehler M. Congenital cutaneous candidiasis in two full-term infants. *Pediatr Dermatol.* 2012;29:507–510.
44. Fine JD. Inherited epidermolysis bullosa. *Orphanet J Rare Dis.* 2010;5:12.
45. Sprecher E. Epidermolysis bullosa simplex. *Dermatol Clin.* 2010;28:23–32.
46. Laimer M, Lanschuetzer CM, Diem A, Bauer JW. Herlitz junctional epidermolysis bullosa. *Dermatol Clin.* 2010;28:55–60.
47. Bruckner-Tuderman L. Dystrophic epidermolysis bullosa: pathogenesis and clinical features. *Dermatol Clin.* 2010;28:107–114.
48. Fine JD, Eady RA, Bauer EA, et al. The classification of inherited epidermolysis bullosa (EB): Report of the Third International

Consensus Meeting on Diagnosis and Classification of EB. *J Am Acad Dermatol*. 2008;58:931–950.

49. Intong LR, Murrell DF. Inherited epidermolysis bullosa: new diagnostic criteria and classification. *Clin Dermatol*. 2012;30:70–77.

50. Murrell DF. Dermatologic Clinics. Epidermolysis bullosa: part II—diagnosis and management. Preface. *Dermatol Clin*. 2010;28:xix.

51. Fine JD, Johnson LB, Weiner M, Suchindran C. Gastrointestinal complications of inherited epidermolysis bullosa: cumulative experience of the National Epidermolysis Bullosa Registry. *J Pediatr Gastroenterol Nutr*. 2008;46:147–158.

52. Bruckner AL. Incontinentia pigmenti: a window to the role of NF-kappaB function. *Semin Cutan Med Surg*. 2004;23:116–124.

53. Minic S, Novotny GE, Trpinac D, Obradovic M. Clinical features of incontinentia pigmenti with emphasis on oral and dental abnormalities. *Clin Oral Investig*. 2006;10:343–347.

54. Minic S, Trpinac D, Gabriel H, Gencik M, Obradovic M. Dental and oral anomalies in incontinentia pigmenti: a systematic review. *Clin Oral Investig*. 2013;17(1):1–8.

55. Holmstrom G, Thoren K. Ocular manifestations of incontinentia pigmenti. *Acta Ophthalmol Scand*. 2000;78:348–353.

56. Meuwissen ME, Mancini GM. Neurological findings in incontinentia pigmenti; a review. *Eur J Med Genet*. 2012;55:323–331.

57. Hsieh DT, Chang T. Incontinentia pigmenti: skin and magnetic resonance imaging findings. *Arch Neurol*. 2011;68:1080.

58. Minkov M, Prosch H, Steiner M, et al. Langerhans cell histiocytosis in neonates. *Pediatr Blood Cancer*. 2005;45:802–807.

59. Broadbent V, Gadner H, Komp DM, Ladisch S. Histiocytosis syndromes in children: II. Approach to the clinical and laboratory evaluation of children with Langerhans cell histiocytosis. Clinical Writing Group of the Histiocyte Society. *Med Pediatr Oncol*. 1989;17:492–495.

60. Battistella M, Fraitag S, Teillac DH, Brousse N, de Prost Y, Bodemer C. Neonatal and early infantile cutaneous langerhans cell histiocytosis: comparison of self-regressive and non-self-regressive forms. *Arch Dermatol*. 2010;146:149–156.

61. Intong LR, Murrell DF. Pemphigoid gestationis: current management. *Dermatol Clin*. 2011;29:621–628.

62. Gushi M, Yamamoto Y, Mine Y, et al. Neonatal pemphigus vulgaris. *J Dermatol*. 2008;35:529–535.

63. Kardos M, Levine D, Gurcan HM, Ahmed RA. Pemphigus vulgaris in pregnancy: analysis of current data on the management and outcomes. *Obstet Gynecol Surv*. 2009;64:739–749.

64. Al-Mutairi N, Sharma AK, Zaki A, El-Adawy E, Al-Sheltawy M, Nour-Eldin O. Maternal and neonatal pemphigoid gestationis. *Clin Exp Dermatol*. 2004;29:202–204.

66 Desquamating and Hyperkeratotic Disorders in the Neonatal Period

Megha M. Tollefson and Latanya T. Benjamin

INTRODUCTION

In the neonatal period, disorders may sometimes present with hyperkeratosis and desquamation of the skin. The differential diagnosis for hyperkeratosis and desquamation in the neonatal period is broad and includes infectious, genetic, inflammatory, immunodeficiency, and metabolic causes. Rarely, these disorders may also present with erythroderma, or generalized skin erythema affecting at least 90% of the body surface.[1] Scaling is a commonly associated symptom of erythroderma. Although the frequency of hyperkeratotic and desquamating disorders in the newborn period is unknown, the incidence of neonatal erythroderma has been estimated[2] to be 0.11%.

These skin changes are nonspecific and do not indicate any particular diagnosis; thus, this constellation of findings may prove to be challenging both diagnostically and therapeutically. Clinical clues and diagnostic testing can be of great importance in reaching a diagnosis. Management can be extremely challenging, as often these neonates are quite ill. Both general management principles and treatments aimed at the specific disorder are vital to the care of these babies. Despite advanced care, the mortality rate[3] in these patients, particularly those with erythroderma, can approach 15%. Factors contributing to this high mortality rate are large ratio of surface area to body mass with subsequent increased transepidermal fluid loss and increased susceptibility to infection.

INFECTIOUS CAUSES

Staphylococcal Scalded Skin Syndrome

Staphylococcal scalded skin syndrome (SSSS), which has also been called pemphigus neonatorum, is a toxin-mediated blistering condition of the skin that primarily affects infants and young children. Neonatal SSSS and outbreaks in neonatal intensive care units are also known to occur.[4] The more localized form of the disease is called bullous impetigo; the more widespread counterpart with generalized involvement is called SSSS.

The initiating staphylococcal infection may start with impetigo that is localized, most commonly in the nares, eyes, or umbilicus in neonates. Toxins produced by the *Staphylococcus aureus* bacteria, exfoliative toxins A and B, are released by the bacteria. These toxins target desmoglein 1, which is a protein vital in epidermal cell-to-cell adhesion.[5] Infants and young children are most susceptible because of a lack of protective antibodies and immature renal clearance of these toxins. Clinical manifestations are that of initial facial and perioral erythema followed by superficial blisters that may progress rapidly to generalized erythroderma and the appearance of "wrinkled" skin. This is often more noticeable around the mouth and in skin folds.[4] Affected infants are usually fussy.

Other disorders that may be considered in the differential diagnosis are few, although it may be mistaken for Kawasaki disease, viral exanthema, drug eruption, or toxic epidermal necrolysis. Many of these do not usually occur in the neonatal period.

Often, SSSS is a clinical diagnosis. Any cultures taken from the bullae are expected to be sterile as blisters are directly caused by the toxin and not the bacteria itself. Biopsy can be performed but is rarely required. Histopathology will show an intraepidermal split above or below the granular layer with minimal inflammation.[5]

Management of SSSS is with antistaphylococcal intravenous antibiotics. Supportive care for pain control, careful handling of the patient's skin, and prevention of secondary infection is often required. Bland emollients such as Aquaphor or white petrolatum should be used to areas of denuded skin. Close attention to fluid balance and body temperature is critical, particularly in the neonatal period.

Overall prognosis for SSSS is quite good. The most common complications are rare and include cellulitis, sepsis, and pneumonia, with a 3% mortality rate.[5] The skin will usually heal rapidly within 2–3 weeks without scarring. Desquamation of the palms and soles can continue for an additional 2–3 weeks after the initial disease. Long-term follow-up is usually not needed.

Congenital Cutaneous Candidiasis

Congenital cutaneous candidiasis is a rare condition. Less than 100 cases have been reported in the literature.[6] Although 20%–25% of pregnancies are complicated by vaginal candidiasis, less than 1% of these will proceed to ascending infections involving the placenta and amnion.[6] Preterm infants are more susceptible to the presence of the disease, with increased risk of disease severity, in large part because of immature keratinization of the skin.

When congenital candidal infection occurs, small erythematous macules, papules, and pustules erupt within the first week of life. These may then become confluent and progress to exfoliative erythroderma.[7] Nail dystrophy may be present.[8] The oral cavity and diaper area can be spared. There can be severe systemic involvement, especially in premature or small-for-gestational-age neonates.

Other infectious skin diseases may present similarly, including SSSS, herpes simplex virus infection, varicella zoster virus infection, and syphilis. Neonatal blistering skin conditions such as epidermolysis bullosa, congenital ichthyosiform erythroderma (CIE), and incontinentia pigmenti may also be considered. Additional benign considerations include neonatal pustular melanosis and miliaria. However, neonatal candidiasis is usually acquired from the birth canal, develops after the first week of life, and tends to involve the intertriginous areas, including the diaper area. Erythroderma is not typical of neonatal candidiasis.

Diagnosis of congenital cutaneous candidiasis can be made at the bedside by demonstrating spores and pseudohyphae on skin scraping of a pustule. Biopsy of the skin may also be performed, demonstrating fungal elements in the stratum corneum, but is often unnecessary.[9]

Any neonate who has signs of systemic candidiasis should be pan cultured. Full-term infants without systemic disease can usually be treated successfully with topical antifungal therapy. Neonates who are preterm and those who are systemically ill will require parenteral antifungal therapy.

Neonates with congenital candidiasis limited to the skin and without systemic symptoms do well with quick resolution of skin findings without sequelae. Neonates with systemic infection have a much more guarded prognosis, particularly those who are less than 1 kg. These infants have a high mortality rate[6] of up to 40%. Otherwise, follow-up is not necessary after the infection is cleared and the skin normalizes.

ICHTHYOSES

Nonsyndromic Ichthyoses

The ichthyoses (Table 66-1) are a heterogeneous group of disorders of abnormal cornification that results in scaly skin. Many of these disorders present in the neonatal period or early childhood. The nonsyndromic ichthyoses are diseases that are primarily limited to the skin and do not have significant systemic involvement.

Self-Healing Collodion Membrane

Rarely, a neonate may be born with a collodion membrane. The condition generally cannot be detected in utero, and diagnosis is therefore usually made at birth. A collodion baby has a "membrane" covering the entire body that is smooth and taut with a shiny surface. The skin is thick and inelastic with frequent contractures of the joints and eversion of the mouth and eyelids. This sign can signify the presence of a significant underlying skin disorder but may also be seen in a neonate who will not go on to develop a skin disorder, thus termed a "self-healing" collodion baby. The presence of a collodion membrane is rare, with approximately 300 cases reported in the literature (Figure 66-1). Approximately 10%–20% of these babies end up with clear skin.[10]

The pathogenesis of the self-healing collodion baby has yet to be fully understood. Several genes, including the transglutaminase 1 (TGM1) gene and *ALOX12B*, have been implicated but not definitively linked.

The differential diagnosis for the underlying cause of a collodion baby also includes the various types of congenital ichthyoses, namely, CIE, lamellar ichthyosis (LI), epidermolytic hyperkeratosis (EHK), and Sjogren-Larsson syndrome (SLS).

Skin biopsy can aid with diagnosis of an underlying congenital ichthyosis; however, no diagnostic tests are

Table 66-1 Ichthyoses

	Harlequin Ichthyosis (HI)	Collodion Membrane (Self-Healing)	Congenital Ichthyosiform Erythroderma (CIE)	Lamellar Ichthyosis (LI)	Epidermolytic Ichthyosis (EI)	X-Linked Ichthyosis (XLI)
Inheritance	Autosomal recessive	Unknown	Autosomal dominant	Autosomal recessive	Autosomal dominant	X-linked recessive
Genetics	ABCA12	Transglutaminase 1 ALOX12B	ALOX12B ALOXE3 TGM1 ABCA12	TGM1	Keratin 1 Keratin 10	STS
Incidence	1 in 1 million	Rare; < 300 reported	1 in 300,000	1 in 300,000 to 500,000	1 in 100,000 to 300,000	1 in 6000
Examination findings	Polygonal hyperkeratotic plaques with fissuring forming an armor-like casing	Collodion baby Ectropion Eclabium Malformed ears Underdeveloped limbs	Erythroderma with fine white scales	Collodion baby Ichthyosis with plate-like scales Ectropion Alopecia Nail dystrophy	Neonatal erythema Blistering Superficial erosions Later develops hyperkeratotic scales	Dark brown, tightly adherent scales Ocular abnormalities Cryptochordism
Location	Diffuse	Diffuse	Generalized	Spares central face and flexural areas	Generalized Flexures and joints typically involved	Scalp Preauricular areas Neck
Diagnosis	Clinical	Clinical ±Skin biopsy	Clinical	Clinical ±Skin biopsy ±Molecular studies	Clinical Skin biopsy ±EM	Clinical ±Skin biopsy ±Genetic testing
Clinical course	Guarded prognosis	Good prognosis Eventual normal skin	Normal life expectancy	Persists throughout life Risk for heat intolerance and heat exhaustion	Lifelong and debilitating Risk for significant odor	Good prognosis Skin may improve with age Increased risk for testicular cancer
Treatment	Supportive care Bland emollient use Oral retinoids	Supportive care	Frequent use of skin emollient	Frequent use of skin emollient Topical keratolytics	Gentle, supportive skin care with bland emollient use	Frequent use of skin emollient Topical keratolytics

Abbreviations: EM, electron microscopy; STS, steroid sulfatase; TGM1, transglutaminase 1.

necessary in diagnosing a self-healing collodion baby. Self-healing collodion baby is a diagnosis that is made with clinical observation.

Collodion babies are at high risk for increased transepidermal water loss, electrolyte imbalance, temperature instability, and infection.[5] Supportive care with specific attention to maintaining hydration and fluid and electrolyte balance, controlling temperature, and vigilance for infection is important. Keratolytic agents should never be used. Light emollients and wet compresses can aid in peeling of the membrane skin. Ophthalmologic care should be sought to manage eversion of the eyelids. Oral retinoids can be considered for severe collodion babies whose shedding is delayed beyond 3 weeks.

Self-healing collodion babies have a good prognosis with essentially normal skin after the neonatal period. Shedding of the collodion membrane is usually complete within 3 weeks but can sometimes take longer.[11] Follow-up is not necessary after skin normalization.

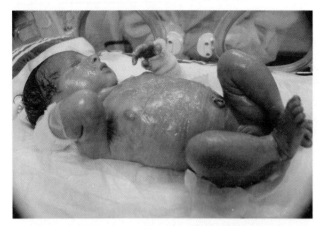

FIGURE 66-1 Self-healing collodion membrane baby. On presentation, collodion membrane is seen with eventual skin desquamation.

Congenital Autosomal Recessive Ichthyosis

Autosomal recessive (AR) ichthyosis is an umbrella term that encompasses CIE, LI, and harlequin ichthyosis (HI).[12]

Congenital Ichthyosiform Erythroderma

Congenital ichthyosiform erythroderma is also a frequent cause of collodion membrane; in fact, nearly 50% of collodion membrane babies go on to develop features consistent with CIE.[11] Although the true incidence of CIE is unknown, it is likely underreported as the features can be mild and subtle in some patients.

The most common mutations involved in the development of CIE are in the *ALOX12B* and *ALOXE3* genes. Also involved, but less commonly, are mutations in tissue TGM1 and ABCA12. At times, a genetic mutation cannot be found. If a collodion membrane is present at birth, on shedding of the membrane, erythroderma with fine white scales in a generalized distribution is noted. If there is no collodion membrane, the erythroderma and fine white scales usually develop in the first few weeks of life. Patients' disease ranges in severity.

Lamellar ichthyosis and other congenital ichthyoses can be considered in the differential diagnosis. Diagnosis is usually made on clinical grounds. Skin biopsy may be minimally helpful as findings are not specific. Genetic testing is usually not indicated but useful.

Hydration of the skin is necessary, with regular bathing followed by a good skin moisturization regimen. Petrolatum-based emollients should be used. There may be increased absorption of ingredients that may be added to moisturizers; thus, caution must be used when selecting an emollient. Referral to the Foundation for Ichthyosis and Related Skin Types (FIRST) can be a helpful resource for families.[13]

The prognosis for patients with CIE may vary depending on phenotype. Minimally affected patients may be able to live as "normal" children, while more severely affected patients will need intensive care of their skin on a daily basis. Life expectancy is normal. Periodic monitoring by a dermatologist may be necessary depending on the severity of disease.

Lamellar Ichthyosis

Lamellar ichthyosis is felt to be on a clinical spectrum with CIE. It has an incidence[12] of 1 in 300,000 to 500,000. Approximately 20% of collodion babies have underlying LI.[11]

Lamellar ichthyosis is most often caused by mutations in TGM1, which encodes an enzyme responsible for the integrity and function of the stratum corneum. Patients with LI have thick plate-like scales covering much of the cutaneous surface, most pronounced on the face and lower legs.[5] Blockage of the eccrine glands by hyperkeratosis of the skin leads to subsequent diminished ability to sweat and resulting heat intolerance and hyperthermia. Scalp alopecia and ectropion of the eyelids are common features. Nail dystrophy can be present.

The scaling of X-linked ichthyosis (XLI) may be similar in appearance but it is seen in males and should not have associated features of alopecia, with ichthyosis usually sparing the central face and flexural areas.

The diagnosis of classical LI is primarily clinical. Biopsy results from skin are nonspecific, and genetic testing is usually not necessary.

Hydration and moisturization of the skin are necessary in all patients. Topical retinoids can be helpful in reducing scaling, as can other keratolytics, but these should not be used in the neonatal period. Low-dose oral retinoids may also be used in some patients as oral retinoids have been shown to upregulate TGM1 activity. Careful attention must be paid to the eyes, with continued corneal lubrication and involvement by ophthalmology.[5] Counseling should be provided to families to educate and prevent heat exhaustion, particularly those that live in hot and humid climates. Referral to FIRST can be helpful for families.[13]

Most patients have significant difficulty with the thickness of scale on their skin and are often limited in their physical activity. There are also significant psychosocial implications and morbidity. Close follow-up with a dermatologist should be maintained.

Harlequin Ichthyosis

Harlequin ichthyosis is the most severe type of AR ichthyosis. It is rare, with an incidence of approximately 1 in 1 million.[13] The disorder is inherited in an AR manner and is caused by mutations in the gene encoding adenosine triphosphate binding cassette transporter

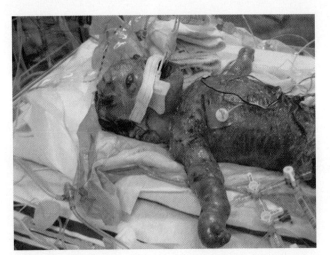

FIGURE 66-2 Harlequin ichthyosis. Severely affected neonate born with extensive fissuring of the cutaneous surface; thick, plate-like scales; ectropion; eclabium; and underdeveloped limbs.

protein ABCA12.[14] Affected neonates present at birth with thick plate-like scales covering the entire body with significant fissuring throughout the cutaneous surface (Figure 66-2). There is frequently associated ectropion and eclabium and sometimes underdevelopment of the nose, ears, and distal limbs.

The differential diagnosis is limited. In the mildest forms, it may be confused with a collodion baby. The diagnosis is made on clinical grounds. Genetic testing is not needed but can be obtained for diagnostic confirmation to exclude other conditions, such as self-healing collodion baby.

Oral retinoids can be started on the first day of life and likely improve prognosis. However, initiation of therapy is individualized depending on the neonate's likelihood for longevity and compatibility with life. A significant amount of supportive care is necessary in the neonatal period, including assistance with ventilation, maintenance of hydration, fluid and electrolyte balance, pain control, and prevention of secondary infection and sepsis. The use of bland emollients is central to skin care. Ophthalmology must be involved closely for management of severe ectropion.

In the past, HI was nearly universally fatal, but with improved supportive care and the use of oral retinoids,[14] survival can approach 50%. Prognosis of affected neonates is still poor, and survivors have lifelong difficulty with CIE-like skin, developmental delay, and visual difficulties.[14,15] Those patients who survive will need lifelong monitoring by a dermatologist and possibly an ophthalmologist.

Epidermolytic Ichthyosis

Epidermolytic ichthyosis (EI) is an autosomal dominant disorder that was previously known as bullous

CIE or EHK. It is a rare disorder and is estimated to have an incidence[16,17] of 1 in 100,000 to 1 in 300,000.

Epidermolytic ichthyosis results from mutations in keratin 1 or keratin 10. Although it is autosomal dominant, half of cases can be new or sporadic mutations.[18] Seventy-one percent of patients have lesions at birth and present with erythema, blistering, and superficial erosions in the newborn period.[16] Beyond the neonatal period, patients develop hyperkeratotic spiny ridges that are easily infected with bacteria. Older patients have a distinct odor.

Ichthyosis bullosa of Siemens is a variant of EHK caused by mutation in keratin 2e. Because keratin 2e is expressed in the upper half of the spinous layer of the epidermis, the blistering is more superficial that seen in EKH. Furthermore, the compensatory hyperkeratosis is less and skin thickening is clinically milder.

Early in the neonatal period, other blistering disorders may also be considered. These include epidermolysis bullosa, SSSS, Omenn syndrome, and toxic epidermal necrolysis.

Epidermolytic ichthyosis is a clinical diagnosis that is usually confirmed by histopathologic analysis. Skin histology is fairly typical and shows hyperkeratosis, separation, and vacuolization in the epidermis. Electron microscopy shows clumping of intermediate filaments within the keratinocytes in the epidermis.

In the neonatal period, children should be handled with care because of skin fragility. The babies should be placed in an isolette with humidified air and temperature control and monitored for dehydration and secondary infection. Skin care should consist of bland with ointment-based moisturizer emollients, nonadherent dressings, and padded wrapping. Referral to support groups such as FIRST should be offered to parents.

Patients with EI may have physical and psychological morbidity because of their skin disease. The odor associated with the hyperkeratotic scale can be significant and debilitating. With diligent wound care, life expectancy may be normal. Patients should be monitored by a dermatologist throughout their lives.

X-Linked Ichthyosis

X-linked ichthyosis is inherited in an X-linked recessive manner. It is the second most common ichthyosis after ichthyosis vulgaris and is estimated to have a frequency of 1 in 6000 male births.[18] It has rarely been reported to occur in female offspring of affected males or female carriers.[19]

X-linked ichthyosis is caused by a mutation in the gene encoding steroid sulfatase (STS), also known as arylsulfatase C. Defects in STS result in compromise of the stratum corneum, which then results in excess scaling. Seventy-five percent of infants with XLI will have skin manifestations within the first week of life. This consists of polygonal translucent scales that develop into large, dark brown, tightly adherent scales primarily on the extensor surfaces and trunk.[20] These scales have a "dirty" appearance. In infancy, the scalp, preauricular areas, and neck are affected. Patients can also have hypohidrosis, ocular abnormalities, and cryptorchidism.

X-linked ichthyosis may have a presentation similar to atopic dermatitis or other ichthyoses, such as ichthyosis vulgaris and LI.

Family history and birth history are important for the diagnosis of XLI. Affected neonates may have male relatives on the mother's side with ichthyosis, low-to-absent levels of estriol may be present on triple screen during pregnancy, and there may be a history of prolonged labor.[21] The diagnosis of XLI can be confirmed with genetic testing of the STS gene. A skin biopsy is usually not helpful as histopathologic changes are nonspecific.[20]

The majority of patients with XLI have disease that is limited to the skin. Skin-directed therapy is aimed at hydration of the skin and reduction of scaling. Soaking baths and bland emollients should be used daily. Topical keratolytics such as lactic acid, salicylic acid, and retinoids can be used as well. Patients with extracutaneous complications such as cryptorchidism or deep corneal opacities should be managed by the appropriate subspecialists. Patients are also at increased risk of testicular cancer and thus families should be instructed on regular testicular self-examinations.

X-linked ichthyosis is a lifelong disease, but skin symptoms generally improve with age. Long-term follow-up with a dermatologist is indicated.

Syndromic Ichthyoses

The syndromic ichthyoses, as opposed to the nonsyndromic ichthyoses, are disorders with multisystem disease where 1 major manifestation is in the skin. Several of the most common syndromic ichthyoses that may present in the neonatal period are discussed here.

Netherton Syndrome

Netherton syndrome is a rare AR disorder. Its estimated frequency is 1 in 50,000 to 1 in 100,000. Eighteen percent of cases with neonatal and infantile erythroderma had Netherton syndrome.[3]

Netherton syndrome is caused by a mutation in the SPINK5 gene that encodes the serine protease inhibitor LEKTI. This results in a compromised skin barrier. At birth, neonates with Netherton syndrome usually present with an exfoliative erythroderma. Individuals with Netherton syndrome who have exfoliative erythroderma at birth can also have failure to thrive, hypernatremia,

hypothermia, and recurrent infections, which may be life-threatening.[22] Many infants will go on to develop characteristic polycyclic and erythematous plaques with double-edged scale, also called ichthyosis linearis circumflexa. Asthma, food allergy, and elevated immunoglobulin (Ig) E level are often seen in patients with Netherton syndrome.

When presenting with erythroderma, other disorders that can cause neonatal erythroderma should be considered. These include generalized seborrheic dermatitis, SSSS, metabolic disorders, and congenital psoriasis.[22,23]

The most specific clinical finding in Netherton syndrome is a hair abnormality called trichorrhexis invaginata. This can be visualized under light microscopy and dermoscopy. This, however, may not be present during the neonatal period, making the diagnosis difficult. Skin biopsy is often nonspecific. Genetic testing for SPINK5 mutations may be done for children suspected to have this disorder.

Extreme caution must be used when applying topical preparations to the skin of patients with Netherton syndrome as transcutaneous absorption is greatly increased. The use of topical tacrolimus is strongly discouraged in these patients because immune-suppressing levels can be reached from topical application alone.

In the neonatal period, intensive medical care, including close attention to hydration, thermoregulation, electrolyte balance, and prevention of infection, is necessary. Regular moisturization is a necessary intervention. Low-dose systemic retinoids may be indicated in some patients. Other systemic symptoms such as infection, growth failure, and allergies must be managed as well. Lifelong follow-up with close attention to the status of the skin barrier is necessary.

Keratitis, Ichthyosis, Deafness Syndrome

Keratitis, ichthyosis, deafness (KID) syndrome is an extremely rare syndrome, with approximately 100 cases reported in the literature. Although it may be inherited in an autosomal dominant manner, most cases are caused by new mutations.

The most common cause of KID syndrome is a missense mutation in connexin 26. These mutations lead to the main features of the disorder: keratitis, ichthyosis, and deafness. Patients with KID syndrome may present with erythroderma at birth that then fades to erythema with hyperkeratotic plaques within days to weeks.[24] There is often alopecia, palmoplantar hyperkeratosis, varying amounts of alopecia, and characteristic facies with deep grooves. Hearing loss is congenital bilateral neurosensory hearing loss; photophobia and vascularizing keratitis usually develop with time. Patients are susceptible to superinfection, particularly with *Candida*.[24]

As KID syndrome has fairly unique defining characteristics, the diagnosis is fairly easy to make. In the neonatal period when the only known manifestation may be erythroderma, other causes of neonatal erythroderma as discussed previously should be considered.

The diagnosis is suggested by the constellation of clinical findings. Histopathology on skin biopsy is nonspecific. Confirmation can be obtained by testing for connexin 26 genetic mutation.

Regular moisturization and use of keratolytics is recommended. Systemic retinoids may be helpful in some severely affected patients. Oral fluconazole has also been reported to be successful in the treatment of candidiasis in patients with KID syndrome.

Patients have lifelong disease and require regular surveillance by various specialties. There can be morbidity and mortality from superinfection and poorly controlled patients. A dermatologist will monitor for the possible development of squamous cell carcinoma and other tumors of the skin. Ophthalmology longitudinal follow-up is also necessary because of vascularizing keratitis.

Trichothiodystrophy

Trichothiodystrophy (TTD) is also known as IBIDS for ichthyosis, brittle hair, intellectual impairment, decreased fertility, and short stature. PIBIDS is also used, where the P stands for photosensitivity. It is inherited in an AR manner and is present worldwide.[18]

Genes that are involved in nucleotide excision repair are responsible for the development of TTD. *ERCC2* and *ERCC3* are most frequently implicated. These mutations lead to the constellation of findings listed , although not all patients have all of the manifestations. Low sulfur content is seen in the hair because of a decrease in sulfur-containing amino acids. Ichthyosiform erythroderma or fine desquamation is noted at birth or in the first few months of life.[25] Newborns may have congenital alopecia and collodion membranes. Diffuse alopecia with fragile hair shafts, intermittent hair loss, nail abnormalities, and dental caries may be observed later in life. Patients may also have associated neurologic, ocular, cardiovascular, skeletal, and other findings. Cryptorchidism may be seen in male patients.

The differential diagnosis of TTD includes other genetic disorders associated with photosensitivity. Xeroderma pigmentosa and Cockayne syndrome may both be considered in the differential diagnosis, although characteristic features of both of these entities are usually seen.

Abnormalities of the hair shaft are paramount to the diagnosis of TTD. With light microscopy, transverse fractures of the hair shafts can be seen. With polarizing microscopy, a characteristic "tiger-tail" pattern of alternating light and dark bands is seen. This pattern

may not be seen in the neonatal period, thus making diagnosis in that age group difficult.

Photoprotection and moisturization are the mainstay of therapy for the skin.

Prognosis and outcome are dependent on the degree of skin and systemic involvement. Infection may lead to mortality early in life.

Sjogren-Larsson Syndrome

Sjogren-Larsson syndrome is a rare disorder that is most common in Sweden, where its prevalence is 0.4 per 100,000 people.[26] It is inherited in an AR manner and presents at birth.[27]

Sjogren-Larsson syndrome is caused by mutations in the fatty aldehyde dehydrogenase gene, which results in interference of epidermal permeability and in the biosynthesis of epidermal lipids. This results in erythema and ichthyosis at birth, followed by thickening of the skin with accentuated skin markings particularly in flexural areas. Skin findings are especially noticeable around the umbilicus and in flexural folds. Individuals are extremely pruritic. Older patients will develop neurological symptoms, specifically spastic diplegia, and will develop perifoveal glistening white dots of the eyes.

Before the appearance of neurologic and ocular symptoms, other ichthyoses such as CIE and other AR ichthyoses, can be considered. DNA-based molecular testing is used to diagnose SLS. Skin biopsy findings are nonspecific. Eye examination findings of glistening perifoveal white dots are supportive of the diagnosis.

Management of SLS requires multidisciplinary care from dermatology, ophthalmology, neurology, and orthopedics specialties. Aggressive physical therapy should be implemented early. Leukotriene inhibitors may be beneficial. Patients are debilitated and have increased risk of mortality. Follow-up from the specialists mentioned should be lifelong.

Conradi-Hünermann-Happle

Conradi-Hünermann-Happle (CHH) is a rare X-linked autosomal dominant disease. There are no published data on its frequency, but it has been estimated at 1 in 200,000.

Most cases of CHH are caused by a mutation in the gene that encodes emopamil-binding protein (EBP). Mutations in EBP cause a severe disturbance in cholesterol biosynthesis, leading to clinical defects. At birth, patients often have significant erythroderma that follows the lines of Blaschko. Within a few months, this usually resolves but leaves behind follicular atrophoderma, pigmentary changes, and scarring alopecia on the scalp. Patients have lifetime ichthyosis on the extremities. Nonskin findings that are also seen include stippled calcification of the bone with various skeletal defects.[12] Other causes of neonatal erythroderma may be considered but should not have involvement primarily in the lines of Blaschko.

Histologic features are often nonspecific, but in the neonatal period may show calcification in follicular keratosis, which is indicative of CHH. Electron microscopy may show cytoplasmic vacuoles of keratinocytes in the epidermis.

Management is similar to that for other causes of neonatal erythroderma.

Skin disease usually improves with age. Erythema resolves after the first few months of life, whereas ichthyosis often persists. Partial alopecia is sometimes the only persisting feature into adulthood. Patients should have close orthopedic follow-up.

PRIMARY IMMUNODEFICIENCY

Primary immunodeficiency syndromes can present with variable skin findings, including erythroderma, in the neonatal period. They account for approximately 30% of all neonatal erythroderma.[2]

Severe Combined Immunodeficiency

Severe combined immunodeficiency (SCID) is a group of heterogeneous immunodeficiency disorders, the most common of which are the X-linked recessive and AR forms. Seventy-five percent of those affected are males.

There are multiple different mutations that cause the clinical phenotype of SCID. Most commonly, mutations in the γ chain of the interleukin 2 receptor are seen, but there are at least 10 other mutations that cause SCID.[28] Patients may present with erythroderma or generalized seborrheic dermatitis. Affected infants may also have failure to thrive, diarrhea, and increased susceptibility to infections in the neonatal period.

Patients may also present with graft-vs-host disease (GVHD). Nearly all neonates with GVHD have underlying T-cell immunodeficiency, many of whom will have SCID. GVHD presents as an asymptomatic generalized eruption caused from engraftment of maternal lymphocytes or from lymphocytes from nonirradiated blood products.

The differential diagnosis includes causes of neonatal erythroderma and other immunodeficiency syndromes, such as Ommen syndrome.

The diagnosis of SCID is made by measuring lymphocyte count and the presence of T lymphocytes. Further classification is achieved with fluorescence-activated cell-sorting analysis and with confirmation through genetic testing. The diagnosis of GVHD is usually made on skin biopsy.

Patients with SCID are quite ill. There should be close surveillance for the development of infection. Without intervention, most individuals will die by the age of 2. Stem cell transplantation is the treatment of choice and can lead to significantly improved survival if done early in life. Lifelong close follow-up is necessary.[29]

Ommen Syndrome

Ommen syndrome is a variant of SCID caused by mutations in the *RAG1* and *RAG2* genes in the majority of cases. It often presents similarly with an exfoliative dermatitis and erythroderma in the setting of eosinophilia and elevated IgE.[30] Alopecia and significant lymphadenopathy may also be present. Lymphocyte count can be misleading in Ommen syndrome as they may have normal-to-high lymphocyte count, but humoral immunity is usually depressed while IgE level is quite high.[30,31] Treatment is similar to that for patients with SCID.

Congenital Psoriasis

Although psoriasis occurs commonly in childhood[32] with an incidence of 40 per 100,000, congenital presentations are quite rare. However, psoriasis is a fairly common underlying reason for erythroderma.

The pathophysiology of the development of psoriasis is still being elucidated, but there is a complex epidermal and immunologic interplay between T lymphocytes and interleukins. This leads to characteristic well-defined erythematous skin lesions with overlying red scale. In the neonatal period, it most commonly presents as erythroderma, seborrheic dermatitis type of eruption, or diaper dermatitis.[33,34]

Other causes of neonatal erythroderma as discussed previously should be considered. Seborrheic and atopic dermatitis may be in the differential diagnosis in the neonatal period.

Psoriasis is usually a clinical diagnosis. Skin biopsy is frequently diagnostic and can be helpful, but similar histopathologic changes can be seen in disorders such as Netherton syndrome and immunodeficiencies in the neonatal period.[23]

Topical corticosteroid medications, vitamin D analogues, and liberal use of emollients are the initial mainstay of therapy for psoriasis in the pediatric population. If erythroderma is present, close attention should be paid to the patient's hydration and calcium status.

Psoriasis is usually a lifelong condition. Patients who present with neonatal erythroderma tend to have more severe disease and a poorer overall prognosis when compared with other patients with psoriasis.

REFERENCES

1. Fraitag S, Bodemer C. Neonatal erythroderma. *Curr Opin Pediatr.* 2010;22:438–444.

2. Sarkar R, Basu S, Sharma RC. Neonatal and infantile erythrodermas. *Arch Dermatol.* 2001;137:822–823.

3. Pruszkowski A, Bodemer C, Fraitag S, Teillac-Hamel D, Amoric JC, de Prost Y. Neonatal and infantile erythrodermas: a retrospective study of 51 patients. *Arch Dermatol.* 2000;136:875–880.

4. Neylon O, O'Connell NH, Slevin B, et al. Neonatal staphylococcal scalded skin syndrome: clinical and outbreak containment review. *Eur J Pediatr.* 2010;169:1503–1509.

5. Shwayder T, Akland T. Neonatal skin barrier: structure, function, and disorders. *Dermatol Ther.* 2005;18:87–103.

6. Darmstadt GL, Dinulos JG, Miller Z. Congenital cutaneous candidiasis: clinical presentation, pathogenesis, and management guidelines. *Pediatrics.* 2000;105:438–444.

7. Hoeger PH, Harper JI. Neonatal erythroderma: differential diagnosis and management of the "red baby". *Arch Dis Child.* 1998;79:186–191.

8. Raval DS, Barton LL, Hansen RC, Kling PJ. Congenital cutaneous candidiasis: case report and review. *Pediatr Dermatol.* 1995;12:355–358.

9. Tieu KD, Satter EK, Zaleski L, Koehler M. Congenital cutaneous candidiasis in two full-term infants. *Pediatr Dermatol.* 2012;29(4):507–510.

10. Theiler M, Mann C, Weibel L. Self-healing collodion baby. *J Pediatr.* 2010;157:169.e1.

11. Van Gysel D, Lijnen RL, Moekti SS, de Laat PC, Oranje AP. Collodion baby: a follow-up study of 17 cases. *J Eur Acad Dermatol Venereol.* 2002;16:472–475.

12. Oji V, Tadini G, Akiyama M, et al. Revised nomenclature and classification of inherited ichthyoses: results of the First Ichthyosis Consensus Conference in Soreze 2009. *J Am Acad Dermatol.* 2010;63:607–641.

13. Oji V, Traupe H. Ichthyosis: clinical manifestations and practical treatment options. *Am J Clin Dermatol.* 2009;10:351–364.

14. Rajpopat S, Moss C, Mellerio J. Harlequin ichthyosis: a review of clinical and molecular findings in 45 cases. *Arch Dermatol.* 2011;147:681–686.

15. Harvey HB, Shaw MG, Morrell DS. Perinatal management of harlequin ichthyosis: a case report and literature review. *J Perinatol.* 2010;30:66–72.

16. Kucharekova M, Mosterd K, Winnepenninckx V, van Geel M, Sommer A, van Steensel MA. Bullous congenital ichthyosiform erythroderma of Brocq. *Int J Dermatol.* 2007;46(Suppl 3):36–38.

17. Irvine AD, McLean WH. Human keratin diseases: the increasing spectrum of disease and subtlety of the phenotype-genotype correlation. *Br J Dermatol.* 1999;140:815–828.

18. DiGiovanna JJ, Robinson-Bostom L. Ichthyosis: etiology, diagnosis, and management. *Am J Clin Dermatol.* 2003;4:81–95.

19. Mevorah B, Frenk E, Muller CR, Ropers HH. X-linked recessive ichthyosis in three sisters: evidence for homozygosity. *Br J Dermatol.* 1981;105:711–717.

20. Fernandes NF, Janniger CK, Schwartz RA. X-linked ichthyosis: an oculocutaneous genodermatosis. *J Am Acad Dermatol.* 2010;62:480–485.

21. Honour JW, Goolamali SK, Taylor NF. Prenatal diagnosis and variable presentation of recessive X-linked ichthyosis. *Br J Dermatol.* 1985;112:423–430.

22. Hausser I, Anton-Lamprecht I. Severe congenital generalized exfoliative erythroderma in newborns and infants: a possible sign of Netherton syndrome. *Pediatr Dermatol.* 1996;13:183–199.

23. Shwayder T, Banerjee S. Netherton syndrome presenting as congenital psoriasis. *Pediatr Dermatol.* 1997;14:473–476.

24. Caceres-Rios H, Tamayo-Sanchez L, Duran-Mckinster C, de la Luz Orozco M, Ruiz-Maldonado R. Keratitis, ichthyosis, and deafness (KID syndrome): review of the literature and proposal of a new terminology. *Pediatr Dermatol.* 1996;13:105–113.

25. Itin PH, Sarasin A, Pittelkow MR. Trichothiodystrophy: update on the sulfur-deficient brittle hair syndromes. *J Am Acad Dermatol.* 2001;44:891–920; quiz 1–4.

26. Liden S, Jagell S. The Sjogren-Larsson syndrome. *Int J Dermatol.* 1984;23:247–253.

27. Vahlquist A, Ganemo A, Pigg M, Virtanen M, Westermark P. The clinical spectrum of congenital ichthyosis in Sweden: a review of 127 cases. *Acta Derm Venereol Suppl (Stockh).* 2003;(213):34–47.

28. Denianke KS, Frieden IJ, Cowan MJ, Williams ML, McCalmont TH. Cutaneous manifestations of maternal engraftment in patients with severe combined immunodeficiency: a clinicopathologic study. *Bone Marrow Transplant.* 2001;28:227–233.

29. Abrams M, Paller A. Genetic immunodeficiency diseases. *Adv Dermatol.* 2007;23:197–229.

30. Villa A, Notarangelo LD, Roifman CM. Omenn syndrome: inflammation in leaky severe combined immunodeficiency. *J Allergy Clin Immunol.* 2008;122:1082–1086.

31. Katugampola RP, Morgan G, Khetan R, Williams N, Blackford S. Omenn's syndrome: lessons from a red baby. *Clin Exp Dermatol.* 2008;33:425–428.

32. Tollefson MM, Crowson CS, McEvoy MT, Maradit Kremers H. Incidence of psoriasis in children: a population-based study. *J Am Acad Dermatol.* 2010;62:979–987.

33. Lehman JS, Rahil AK. Congenital psoriasis: case report and literature review. *Pediatr Dermatol.* 2008;25:332–338.

34. Salleras M, Sanchez-Regana M, Umbert P. Congenital erythrodermic psoriasis: case report and literature review. *Pediatr Dermatol.* 1995;12:231–234.

Section III

Atlas of Management Approach and Procedures

(78) Use of aEEG/NIRS

(79) Workup of Neonatal Stroke

Part C: Heart

(80) Cyanotic Congenital Heart Disease

(81) Management of Congestive Heart Failure

(82) Blood Pressure Support

(83) Patent Ductus Arteriosus Management

(84) Practical Approach to Arrhythmias

Part D: Lungs

(85) Mechanical Ventilation

(86) Chronic Lung Disease

(87) High-Frequency Ventilation

(88) Noninvasive Support of Respiratory Failure

(89) Inhaled Nitric Oxide

(90) Extracorporeal Membrane Oxygenation (ECMO)

Part E: Blood

(91) Anemia

(92) Thrombocytopenia

(93) Polycythemia

(94) Transient Myeloproliferative Disorder

Part F: Gastro-Intestinal

(95) Management of Abdominal Wall Defects

(96) Management of Perforated Necrotizing Enterocolitis

CHAPTER 67

Part A: Fundamentals

67 The Resuscitation of the Newborn With a Difficult Airway

Christopher E. Colby

INTRODUCTION

Successful resuscitation of the newborn nearly always begins with the establishment of a patent airway through which gas exchange will occur. However, the neonatal airway may be compromised by a number of developmental anomalies that make resuscitation challenging. Some of these anomalies are relatively benign and respond to simple maneuvers to achieve an airway. On the other end of the spectrum are other anomalies that may be lethal despite prenatal diagnosis and delivery at a center with advanced airway management capability. In either case, delivery room management will be influenced by the severity of the anomaly and the resulting degree of airway obstruction. Appropriate interventions in the delivery room may range from the placement of an ancillary device to maintain patency of the airway to the coordinated, multidisciplinary surgical intervention while the infant continues to be supported by the placental circulation. This chapter reviews the differential diagnosis of newborn airway obstruction and describes the overall approach to delivery room management of airway anomalies that range from mild to severe.

DIFFERENTIAL DIAGNOSIS

Obstruction of the neonatal airway may occur at many different levels. *Choanal atresia* is an upper airway anomaly that may cause respiratory distress immediately after birth or on initiation of early feeding attempts.[1] Choanal atresia most often is caused by bony obstruction and may affect either 1 or both sides of the nasal passages.[2] Choanal atresia may be isolated or a component of CHARGE association (coloboma, heart defect, atresia choanae [also known as choanal atresia], retarded growth and development, genital abnormality, and ear abnormality).[3] There are other, rarer anatomic obstructive processes at the level of the nose in the neonate, ranging from the solid (glioma, rhabdomyosarcoma, and other tumors) to the cystic (dermoid and epidermoid cysts and meningoencephaloceles).

The development of the jaw and tongue may also influence initial airway management during resuscitation. *Micrognathia* may be seen as an associated finding with other disorders, including trisomies 13 and 18 and Treacher Collins syndrome. *Macroglossia* most commonly presents as part of a constellation of developmental anomalies, as would be the case in Beckwith-Wiedemann syndrome, trisomy 21, and congenital hypothyroidism. However, macroglossia also may represent underlying pathology in the tongue itself (tumor or vascular malformation) or underdevelopment of the mandible or maxillae.[4] The combination of micrognathia, cleft palate, and upper airway obstruction defines the *Pierre Robin sequence.*

The newborn may present with *bilateral congenital paralysis* of the vocal cords. Although this typically does not result in true obstruction of the airway, the neonate may cough recurrently and develop respiratory difficulties with feedings. In congenital vocal cord paralysis, the cords are left in the open position, leaving the neonate potentially unable to protect the airway.[5] Although not a usual cause of airway obstruction, appropriate airway evaluations should be performed.

Likewise, *tracheoesophageal fistula* typically does not cause an anatomical airway obstruction. However, the newborn with associated esophageal atresia will be unable to clear oral secretions, which may pool in the posterior pharynx and cause a viscous obstruction to the airway.

Congenital high airway obstruction syndrome (*CHAOS*) may be diagnosed prenatally as either an isolated finding or associated with other anomalies. The level of the airway obstruction may be supraglottic, glottic, or infraglottic and range from laryngeal to tracheal obstruction. The true incidence of this syndrome is unknown but IS considered rare.[6]

Cystic hygromas are nonmalignant malformations of dilated cystic lymphatic vessels. In the cervical area, they may cause external compression of the larynx or trachea and subsequent obstruction. Chromosomal anomalies, including trisomies 18 and 21, Noonan, and Turner syndromes may be seen in a high percentage of cases.

The most common location for *teratomas* in the neonate is the sacrococcygeal region. However, these tumors may be found in the cervical area and contribute significantly to airway obstruction. The teratomas may have a variety of tissue present, including every embryonal tissue. The malignant potential of these tumors is unclear (Table 67-1).[7]

Prior to Delivery

Many of the diagnoses that result in partial or complete airway obstruction may be identified prenatally, thus allowing for consultation with appropriate personnel who may be involved in the initial resuscitation and care of the newborn.

PARTIAL AIRWAY OBSTRUCTION

Pierre Robin sequence and tracheoesophageal fistula are diagnoses that may be identified prenatally, and consultation with a neonatologist should be considered. During the prenatal consultation, the discussion should include the necessity of airway patency evaluation shortly after birth. If the baby is suspected of having Pierre Robin sequence, it is appropriate to mention that the infant may breathe more reliably in the prone position or may need initial airway support with a nasopharyngeal airway, endotracheal intubation, or placement of a laryngeal mask airway (LMA). The baby with suspected tracheal esophageal fistula likely will require the placement of a suction catheter into the proximal esophageal pouch to assist in clearance of viscous oral secretions.

COMPLETE AIRWAY OBSTRUCTION

If either a large neck mass or congenital high airway obstruction is diagnosed prenatally, referral to a center with expertise in immediate airway management of the fetus is appropriate. Prenatal imaging (ultrasound/magnetic resonance imaging [MRI]) findings that would suggest airway compromise from a cervical teratoma or cystic hygroma would include polyhydramnios (from esophageal compression), tracheal deviation, and a heterogeneous or cystic mass in the anterior cervical region. Prenatal findings consistent with congenital high airway obstruction would include a dilated proximal airway, lung hypertrophy, downward displacement of the diaphragm, ascites, or hydrops. During prenatal consultation, a medical geneticist should be involved to determine if there are associated findings or a syndromic component to the diagnosis. A multidisciplinary team will be needed to determine the optimal method of delivery and the potential need to resuscitate the infant while supported by the placental circulation (ex utero intrapartum treatment, or EXIT).[8]

EQUIPMENT PREPARATION

There should be at least 1 area with close approximation to labor and delivery where neonatal resuscitation occurs. That location should be stocked with all the necessary equipment required to perform a successful

Table 67-1 Causes of Airway Obstruction in the Neonate

Nasal	Choanal atresia Meningoencephalocele Dermoid cyst Epidermoid cyst Mucocele Solid tumor
Mandible	Pierre Robin sequence
Tongue	Macroglossia Beckwith-Wiedemann syndrome Trisomy 21
Neck	Esophageal atresia (mechanical, viscous obstruction from oral secretions) Laryngeal atresia Tracheal atresia Laryngeal webs Subglottic cysts Cystic hygroma Cervical teratoma

Table 67-2 Recommended Neonatal Airway Management Equipment

1. Pulse oximetry and sensor.
2. Positive pressure device either hand bag or T-piece resuscitator. Hand bag resuscitation may be performed with either a flow or self-inflating bag. A self-inflating bag should have an oxygen reservoir.
3. Pressure manometer.
4. Oral airway.
5. Neonatal sized laryngoscope and blades (size 00, 0, and 1).
6. Endotracheal tubes (internal diameter of 2.5, 3.0, 3.5, and 4 mm).
7. Suction catheters ranging in size from 5 to 10 French.
8. Meconium aspirator.
9. Carbon dioxide monitor.
10. Laryngeal mask airway.

resuscitation. For the purposes of this chapter, the focus is on the equipment required to manage the newborn's airway. Prenatally diagnosed airway issues allow for time and organization of materials that may facilitate the ease of resuscitation. *It is an absolute necessity to have immediately available, well-organized airway assistance equipment.* Table 67-2 lists the equipment that may be required for airway support.

TECHNIQUE

Providers taking part in neonatal resuscitation must be proficient in delivering appropriate bag mask ventilation, a skill that is emphasized during Neonatal Resuscitation Program (NRP)[9] training. An improvement in heart rate is a reliable indicator of effective delivery of bag mask ventilation. It is important to learn how to troubleshoot ineffective ventilation, which should be recognized when no improvement in heart rate is seen despite initial positive pressure ventilation attempts. A mnemonic proposed by the NRP for correcting ineffective ventilation is MR.SOPA, described in Table 67-3.

SPECIAL CONSIDERATIONS

Meconium-Stained Amniotic Fluid

The Neonatal Resuscitation Program proposes an algorithm for the resuscitation of the neonate born through meconium-stained amniotic fluid. The algorithm begins with a rapid assessment of the newborn's activity level. *Resuscitative measures for the active, vigorous newborn are different from those for the newborn with respiratory depression.* The current recommendation is that the vigorous baby has the mouth and nose cleared of secretions if any obstruction is suspected and then routine resuscitative measures if necessary. The nonvigorous baby should have both the mouth and trachea suctioned. It is vitally important to monitor the nonvigorous newborn's heart rate during resuscitation. If the infant has prolonged bradycardia during attempts at tracheal suctioning, it is appropriate to consider bag mask ventilation even if the airway has not been fully cleared of meconium.

Partial Airway Obstruction

Choanal Atresia

The baby with bilateral choanal atresia will have labored respirations when the mouth is partially or fully closed. If the diagnosis is suspected based on the inability to pass a suction catheter through the nasal

Table 67-3 Troubleshooting Ineffective Ventilation

Mask	Check to make sure that the mask is the appropriate size and placed above the nose and mouth. The mask should not apply pressure to the eyes as this may induce vagal bradycardia.
Reposition head	The baby should have the head slightly extended in the "sniffing position." Avoid undue flexion or hyperextension.
Suction mouth and nose	Consider the need to suction the upper airway, which may be partially occluded by mucous plugging or blood clots.
Open mouth	It is possible if the baby has sufficient tone in the jaw that the pressure you are delivering is not being transmitted to the lower airways as the mouth is closed. Insert index finger into mouth temporarily and open the mouth of the baby.
Pressure increase	Determining the ideal pressure to target that will result in an improvement in heart rate may require escalation of the initial pressure until a response is seen.
Alternate airway	If bag mask or T-piece resuscitation is ineffective, it may be necessary to consider intubation or placement of a laryngeal mask airway.

passages, placement of an oral airway and monitoring with pulse oximetry are appropriate while waiting for an evaluation from those in otolaryngology.

Pierre Robin Sequence

The neonate with Pierre Robin sequence may present challenges from the perspective of airway patency and maintenance. If the baby is noted to have intermittent obstructive apnea, placing the patient prone while monitored with pulse oximetry may relieve posterior pharyngeal obstruction. It may be necessary to consider an alternate airway if the patient is persistently bradycardic despite attempts at bag mask ventilation. Endotracheal intubation may be considered; however, if anatomically challenging, a size 1.0 laryngeal mask airway may be placed if the patient is greater than 2 kg. A nasopharyngeal airway can also be effective and is achieved by passing a small (2.5F) endotracheal tube through the nose and into the pharynx distal to the base of the tongue.

Macroglossia

Occasionally, the newborn with macroglossia will have a partial airway obstruction. This can be managed effectively with the placement of an oral airway.

Tracheal Esophageal Fistulae

The diagnosis of tracheal esophageal fistula may be made prenatally or shortly after birth. Clinical suspicion of this diagnosis is raised in a newborn with copious oral secretions. The baby may experience intermittent respiratory distress from the resultant inability to clear secretions from the airway. Placement of a suction catheter into the proximal esophageal pouch may be both diagnostic on imaging studies and, when connected to suction, alleviate the pooling of secretions in the pharynx.

Complete Obstruction

If the diagnosis of cystic hygroma, cervical teratoma, or CHAOS was identified prenatally, the time of birth will involve multiple medical and surgical services to establish an airway in the neonate. An EXIT procedure may be planned to achieve an airway while the infant is supported on maternal circulation. Unfortunately, for the neonate with a cystic hygroma, cervical teratoma, or CHAOS that was not identified prenatally, supporting ventilation should be attempted while emergent airway support is requested from the appropriate surgical service.

REFERENCES

1. Dinwiddie R. Congenital upper airway obstruction. *Paediatr Resp Rev.* 2004;4:17–24.
2. Cinnamond MJ. Congenital anomalies of the nose. In: Scott-Brown WE, ed. *Paediatric Otolaryngology.* London, UK: Butterworth; 1987:215–225.
3. Sporik R, Dinwiddie R, Wallis C. Lung involvement in the multisystem CHARGE association. *Eur Res J.* 1997;10: 1354–1355.
4. Vogel JE, Muliken JB, Kaban LB. Macroglossia: a review of the condition and a new classification. *Plas Reconstruct Surg.* 1986;78: 715–723.
5. Dedo DD, Dedo HH. Neurogenic diseases of the larynx. In: Stool E, Alper CM, Arjinan EM, Casselbrant ML, Dohar JE, Yellon E, eds. *Pediatric Otolaryngology.* Philadelphia, PA: Saunders; 2003:1505–1510.
6. Hedrick MH, Ferro MM, Filly RA. Congenital high airway obstruction syndrome (CHAOS): a potential for prenatal treatment. *J Pediatr Surg.* 1992;29:271–274.
7. Pearl RM, Wisnicki, Sinclair G. Metastatic cervical teratoma of infancy. *Plas Reconstr Surg.* 1986;77:469–473.
8. MacKenzie TC, Crombleholme TM, Flake AW. The ex-utero intrapartum treatment. *Curr Opin Pediatr.* 2002;14(4):453–458.
9. American Academy of Pediatrics and American Heart Association; *Neonatal Resuscitation Textbook.* 6th Edition. American Academy of Pediatrics and American Heart Association; 2011.

68 Protocol for Delivery Room Management of Hydrops

Arun Gupta and Henry C. Lee

INTRODUCTION

The transition to breathing for the hydropic infant after birth is a particularly tenuous situation. The delivery room management of hydrops can be a critical period of intervention and a highly intense event with a critically sick infant requiring extensive resuscitation and multiple procedures immediately following delivery.[1] The basic principles for resuscitation of high-risk newborns still apply. However, because of the possibility of pleural effusions and ascites in hydrops, the team must be prepared to perform two additional procedures that are not commonly performed by delivery room personnel: thoracentesis and paracentesis. This chapter outlines the overall approach to delivery room management for hydrops and provides detailed descriptions of these two procedures.

PREPARATION FOR DELIVERY

Prenatal Counseling

Prior to delivery, appropriate counseling of the family may involve discussion of the etiology of hydrops, if known, and the prognosis.[2] In some situations, hydrops may be an end-stage process, and comfort care after delivery may be a reasonable alternative to intensive resuscitation. This decision can be made prior to delivery with informed consent of the parents, allowing them to hold the infant soon after birth and to provide comfort. Prognosis in hydrops is dependent on the etiology, although the etiology may be indeterminate in

about a quarter of cases. The prognosis can be discussed prior to delivery if time is available.

If resuscitation is planned, counseling of the parents should involve explaining the procedures that may be carried out in the delivery room. The delivery room will be a busy and intense environment; thus, preparation of the parents may help to relieve some degree of anxiety.

Delivery Room Staff

The makeup of the resuscitation team may vary by institution. Table 68-1 offers a potential delineation of roles that can be modified depending on availability of specific clinical personnel. The expected duties of clinicians may vary by institution, and this table can serve as a template for developing protocols that are more specific. However, it should be noted that the list of tasks is extensive, and a team consisting of at least 5, and possibly more, members is not an unreasonable expectation for this scenario.

Delivery Room Equipment

The equipment necessary for delivery room management of an infant with hydrops will include the basic equipment necessary for resuscitation of any high-risk infant, including a radiant warmer, and equipment for intubation and airway management. Furthermore, as the likelihood for volume resuscitation and medications may be high, supplies for umbilical line placement should be readily available.

Table 68-1 Roles of Team Members in Delivery Room Management of Hydrops

Team Member	Step 1	Step 2
MD, NNP	Assess infant, manage airway and ventilation	Continued assessment, perform thoracentesis and/or paracentesis as needed
MD, NNP	Assess heart rate, perform chest compressions	Umbilical catheter placement to obtain labs and facilitate medication and volume infusion
RN	Dry infant, help with temperature control measures, apply monitors (pulse oximeter/ECG leads if available), assess breath sounds	Draw up medications and fluids, prepare and assist with other equipment as needed
RT	Assist with airway management	Take over ventilation and airway management
RN	Record resuscitation, help with calling for assistance, and help with drawing up medications, preparing equipment, and so on	
Runner	Take specimens to the laboratory, bring other supplies (including blood, etc) to the delivery room	

Abbreviations: ECG, electrocardiograph; MD, doctor of medicine; NNP, neonatal nurse practitioner; RN, registered nurse; RT, respiratory therapist.

Difficulty with ventilation in hydrops may lead to the need for paracentesis or thoracentesis, and supplies for these procedures should also be prepared. The typical equipment used for these procedures is shown in Figure 68-1. A list of other equipment that may be used in the resuscitation of hydropic infants is provided in Table 68-2.

AIRWAY/BREATHING

As in all neonatal resuscitation, airway and breathing should be the first priority. Assessment and management should generally follow the procedures as described previously. However, there are several special

Table 68-2 Equipment That May Be Used in Delivery Room Management of Infant With Hydrops

Warming equipment
Oxygen saturation probe/pulse oximeter/electrocardiograph monitor
Equipment for intubation/airway management
Equipment for umbilical line placement
Equipment for blood transfusion (if indicated)
Equipment for paracentesis or thoracentesis
Transducing equipment/defibrillator/pacing equipment (if indicated)
Collection containers for laboratory evaluation

considerations that can complicate management of the airway and ventilation in an infant with hydrops.

Edema

There may be a significant amount of soft tissue edema caused by hydrops that can distort both external and internal anatomy.

Congenital Airway Malformation

Congenital Airway Malformation may be a possible etiology of hydrops. Therefore, it is important that a clinician who is skilled in intubation be assigned the task of airway management. A smaller endotracheal tube may be necessary if there is significant edema. If airway abnormalities are expected, involvement of a pediatric otolaryngologist or anesthesiologist in the delivery room may be warranted.

Asphyxia

Asphyxia commonly accompanies hydrops, so meconium may be present at delivery, and intratracheal suctioning may need to be performed in accordance with the Neonatal Resuscitation Program (NRP) guidelines.

Intubation

In contrast to a typical resuscitation, a plan to immediately intubate and start positive pressure ventilation is a reasonable approach because mask ventilation may be ineffective as a result of generalized edema and decreased lung compliance. Typical rules of thumb for determining length of endotracheal tube placement may not be reliable because of distortion of anatomy. Thus, placement of the endotracheal tube should be based on visualization of passage

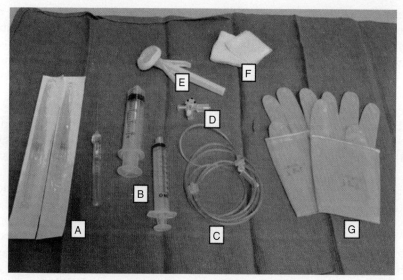

FIGURE 68-1 Supplies needed for paracentesis or thoracentesis: A, 18- to 20-gauge intravenous catheter with stylet; B, syringe(s); C, connection tubing; D, 3-way stopcock; E, sterile prep; F, sterile gauze; G, sterile gloves.

of the tube through the vocal cords or postintubation assessment using end-tidal CO_2 monitors and auscultation.

Ventilator Support

Because there can be significant effusions, higher peak inspiratory pressures may be needed for adequate ventilation due to both the pleural effusions and the possibility of pulmonary hypoplasia. Limiting the use of excessive oxygen has been a growing priority in neonatology. However, if anemia is the cause of hydrops, there may be reduced oxygen-carrying capacity, and increasing the fraction of inspired air (FiO_2) more readily than in other scenarios may be reasonable.

Paracentesis/Thoracentesis

If resuscitation efforts are not effective despite the usual strategies, thoracentesis or paracentesis may be necessary. The steps for these two procedures are outlined in this chapter.

CIRCULATION

Anemia

The need for circulatory support with volume resuscitation and medications is likely in moderate-to-severe hydrops. When fetal anemia is known to be the cause of hydrops, blood for transfusion can be prepared and should be ready in the delivery room. It is best to use O-negative, cytomegalovirus (CMV)-negative, irradiated, packed red blood cells cross-matched against the mother's blood. In any case of hydrops, if blood is not readily available in the delivery room, procedures for quick preparation of blood from the blood bank would be prudent. Personnel should be prepared for umbilical venous catheterization and/or blood transfusion.

Umbilical Vein Catheterization

In an emergency, umbilical vein catheterization is often the quickest method for establishing vascular access. If the etiology of hydrops is known to be anemia and there is evidence of volume depletion, the patient can receive a blood transfusion prior to obtaining laboratory results.

Umbilical Artery Catheterization

If enough personnel and resources are available, umbilical arterial catheterization to facilitate ongoing laboratory collection and blood pressure transduction may be beneficial. It will also allow for quick collection of blood for laboratory evaluation, including obtaining blood gas and hematocrit values. This will also facilitate partial exchange transfusion, which may be ideal in cases of severe anemia without significant volume depletion.

Myocardial Dysfunction

Myocardial dysfunction (including heart block and cardiomyopathy) may be present as the primary cause of hydrops or as a result of pericardial effusions. Although delivery room management may not be able to completely address this dysfunction, quick establishment of vascular access for medications may help to assist in optimal resuscitation. Electrocardiographic (ECG) leads will allow for detecting arrhythmias that may require intervention. Furthermore, ECG leads will help provide continuous assessment of heart rate, particularly if pulse oximetry is difficult to interpret because of subcutaneous edema. If cardiac complications (or need for pericardiocentesis) are anticipated, arrangements should be made to have a pediatric cardiology team (as well as an echocardiogram, defibrillator, or pacing equipment) available at the delivery.

EFFUSIONS

If ventilation is not effective despite intubation and positive pressure ventilation with higher inspiratory pressures, it is possible that pleural or peritoneal effusions may be interfering with ventilation. If this is the case, thoracentesis or paracentesis may be indicated. Deciding which procedure to perform first depends on the history and clinical assessment. If there are known to be large pleural effusions, thoracentesis may be the first step. Based on the relative frequencies of significant effusions in hydrops, paracentesis is often the more likely procedure to be performed first.

Paracentesis

If the abdomen is clearly distended and taut and ventilation is ineffective, paracentesis may be indicated as the first step. The steps for paracentesis are shown in Figure 68-2. The needle should be inserted into the lower right or left abdomen lateral to the rectus muscle to avoid hitting the liver or spleen, which may

be enlarged. When fluid begins to flow through the hub of the needle, the catheter can be gently advanced as the stylet is withdrawn. The catheter can then be connected to the tubing, 3-way stopcock, and syringe. Fluid can be withdrawn with a syringe and collected for laboratory testing.

The purpose of the procedure is not to remove all of the ascites fluid as this may lead to circulatory instability and may ultimately be ineffective. Rather, the goal is to remove a sufficient amount of fluid (approximately 10–20 mL/kg) to assist in easing ventilator management. The amount of fluid to be removed can be based on an assessment of the decrease in abdominal distension/tautness and improvement in clinical status. In addition, usually there is communication between the peritoneal and the pleural spaces, so paracentesis may remove some of the pleural fluid. Once a sufficient amount of fluid has been removed, the catheter can be taped in place and the stopcock turned to the off position to allow later withdrawal of fluid if necessary. If a significant amount of fluid is removed, the tips of previously placed umbilical catheters may move, and their positions should be verified.

Thoracentesis

The steps for thoracentesis are shown in Figure 68-3. The intravenous catheter needle is inserted into the fourth or fifth intercostal space at the midaxillary line and directed posteriorly. To avoid the blood vessels and nerves that run just below the rib, the needle should be inserted just above it. When fluid begins to flow through the hub of the needle, the catheter can be gently advanced as the stylet is withdrawn.

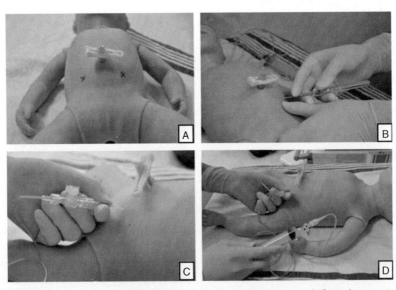

FIGURE 68-2 Steps for paracentesis: A, Location for inserting needle in lower left or lower right abdomen; **B,** insertion of needle in lower left abdomen; **C,** attachment of catheter to stopcock and tubing (after advancement of catheter and removal of stylet); **D,** withdrawal of ascitic fluid into syringe.

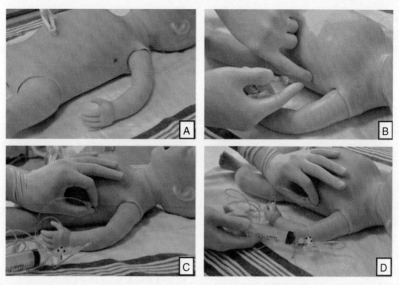

FIGURE 68-3 Steps for thoracentesis: A, Location for inserting needle in fourth or fifth intercostal space; B, insertion of needle at midaxillary line; C, connection of tubing, 3-way stopcock, and syringe to catheter (after advancement of catheter and removal of stylet); D, withdrawal of pleural fluid into syringe.

The catheter can then be connected to the tubing, 3-way stopcock, and syringe. Fluid can be withdrawn with a syringe to alleviate pressure. Note that removal of pleural fluid may not necessarily improve lung function if pulmonary hypoplasia or pulmonary edema is present. If desired, pleural fluid can be collected for laboratory testing, which can include cell count, culture, and estimation of protein content.

Chest Tube

In some cases of hydrops, thoracentesis with a small catheter may not be enough for resuscitation.

Furthermore, because of the high pressures required for resuscitation, pneumothorax may be a potential occurrence. Therefore, preparation for chest tube placement for either fluid removal or pneumothorax may be necessary.

One quick method of chest tube placement utilizes a blunt-tip safety chest tube kit (as illustrated in Figure 68-4). This method is quicker than using a hemostat for dissection into the pleural space and therefore easier to place in the delivery room setting if necessary. First, the fourth or fifth intercostal space at the anterior axillary line is located. The length of chest tube insertion can be estimated by measuring

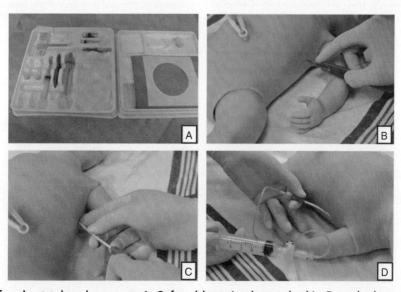

FIGURE 68-4 Steps for chest tube placement: A, Safety blunt-tip chest tube kit; B, scalpel used to make an incision at the fourth or fifth anterior axillary line; C, chest tube with trocar is inserted—anteriorly for pneumothorax, posteriorly for pleural effusion; D, syringe can be used for initial withdrawal of fluid prior to connection to vacuum system.

CHAPTER 68

the distance from the apex of the lung to the insertion site. After sterile preparation of the area, a scalpel is used to make a one-eighth to one-quarter inch incision overlying the space. The safety trocar is pushed into the incision and interspace, palpated above the rib. The trocar can be removed as the chest tube is held firmly in place. The tube is then advanced to the estimated length or approximately 3–4 cm for a term infant.

Pneumothorax

If the indication for the chest tube is a pneumothorax, the tip should be aimed anteriorly toward the second intercostal space so that the tip will lie at the highest point of the infant's chest when lying supine. The tube is then connected to a water-seal vacuum drainage system and secured with suture and dressing.

Pleural Drainage

If the indication for the chest tube is to drain a pleural effusion, the tube can be directed posteriorly. Prior to connection to the vacuum system, a syringe can be used to obtain fluid for laboratory testing if desired. After the infant is stabilized, a chest x-ray should be obtained to confirm proper placement of the chest tube.

OTHER CONSIDERATIONS

Hypothermia

As intense, prolonged resuscitations can often be associated with unintended hypothermia, procedures that allow for relatively easy temperature monitoring and regulation should be implemented. The radiant warmer should be turned on to the maximum heat setting prior to delivery, and if possible, arrangements should be made to optimize the ambient temperature in the delivery room itself. Using a plastic wrap and a chemical warming mattress are other potential considerations. A continuous-temperature probe can be placed to also assist in temperature monitoring and regulation.

Hypoglycemia

Hypoglycemia may often occur soon after birth in infants with hydrops. Thus, glucose measurements should be obtained, and initiating an intravenous dextrose infusion should be considered as soon as feasible.

CONCLUSION

The delivery room management of an infant with hydrops is complex and requires skilled personnel who are appropriately trained in advanced resuscitation techniques. In addition to airway management and circulatory support, the team should be ready to perform additional procedures that may be required in the delivery room, such as thoracentesis and paracentesis. Proper preparation and anticipation of the procedures that may be necessary are essential for optimal resuscitation of an infant with hydrops.

REFERENCES

1. McMahan M, Donovan E. The delivery room resuscitation of the hydropic neonate. *Semin Perinatol.* 1995;19(6):474–482.
2. Santo S, Mansour S, Thilaganathan B, Papageorghiou A, Calvert S, Bhide A. Prenatal diagnosis of non-immune hydrops fetalis: what do we tell the parents? *Prenat Diagn.* 2011;31(2):186–195.

Initial Fluid Management

R. S. Cohen

INTRODUCTION

Background

Maintenance of normal fluid and electrolyte balance for the first few days of life in neonatal intensive care unit (NICU) patients, specifically those who cannot feed orally, is an important part of their management. Indeed, it is a significant and challenging part of NICU admission orders. Neonates initially should be in good fluid and electrolyte balance immediately after birth. Exceptions can and do occur rarely but need to be recognized in a timely fashion. At birth, babies have excess total body water that they need to diurese. Despite this, they generally have normal serum electrolytes, which means that they also have increased total body sodium. Thus, initial salt and water requirements are nil. However, sick neonates in an NICU usually need intravenous access, and some fluid may be needed to keep this patent stable. Furthermore, they often need glucose, calcium, protein, and so on, and if not feeding, intravenous fluids may be needed to provide these items. Thus, the goals of initial fluid management are as follows:

1. Prevent excessive weight loss and dehydration, which can result in hypotension, cell damage, hyperkalemia, and intraventricular hemorrhage (IVH).

2. Allow appropriate diuresis while avoiding salt and water overload, which may be associated with

   pulmonary edema,

   prolonged ductal patency, and

   an increased risk of chronic lung disease.

3. Keep indwelling catheters patent.

4. Provide adequate calcium, glucose, and amino acid (AA) delivery.

5. Initiate enteral nutrition as soon as possible, preferably with maternal milk.

Maternal History

Occasionally, the maternal history can be an indicator of abnormal fluid and electrolyte status in the fetus and neonate. Some examples of maternal indicators of possible abnormal fluid and electrolyte balance include

1. Renal diseases with abnormal electrolytes;

2. Diuretic therapy;

3. Endocrine disorders (eg, diabetes, hypoparathyroidism); or

4. Malnutrition or very abnormal diet.

Fetal Findings

Rarely, there will be fetal evidence of increased risk for hyponatremia in the newborn. Findings on fetal ultrasonography suggestive of renal disease, such as

1. Oligohydramnios;

2. Renal cystic dysplasia;

3. Marked hydronephrosis/hydroureter; or

4. Inability to visualize a fetal bladder, and so on.

Neonatal Examination

Although there are usually no specific physical examination findings diagnostic of fluid and electrolyte imbalances, there can be findings suggestive of abnormal status:

1. Edema/anasarca;

2. Ascites, abdominal/flank masses;

3. Very immature skin (translucent red and shiny) in extremely low gestational age neonate (ELGAN);

4. Skin disorders with open bullæ, cracked skin, and the like; or

5. Open spinal or abdominal wall defect.

Laboratory

In general, the newborn infant, even the very premature patient, does not need serum electrolytes measured immediately after birth. Initially, a neonate's electrolytes and serum urea nitrogen (BUN)/creatinine should reflect the mother's status. Patients with a history or physical findings such as those mentioned may need to have electrolyte panels checked. Note that in the face of normal placental and maternal renal function, a totally anephric neonate will have a normal (ie, maternal) creatinine level at birth.

Differential Diagnosis/Diagnostic Algorithm: This is the same as previously mentioned. Abnormal initial electrolytes, if such values are obtained, usually indicate significant maternal disease, maternal medications, or placental dysfunction.

Exclusions/Contraindications: The major exclusions or contraindication to standard fluid and electrolyte management in the newborn would be underlying significant renal dysfunction and the abnormal findings listed previously.

TREATMENT/PROCEDURE

Consent/Assent/Ethical Considerations

Most units consider peripheral intravenous lines and umbilical catheters to be covered by the general consent for admission to the NICU. However, most consider central venous and peripheral arterial catheters (both percutaneously and surgically inserted) as more invasive and thus requiring separate informed consent for these procedures.

Monitoring for treatment

1. Intake and Output (I&O) must be monitored strictly, especially in the smallest patients.

2. Weights should be charted no less than daily and may need to be checked more frequently in high-risk

situations. For this, the use of bed scales may be beneficial.

3. Glucose should be monitored closely, preferably with bedside "point-of-care" technology to provide rapid data and minimize blood loss. Glucose levels should be checked on admission.

   If the initial glucose value is low, then monitoring should be every half hour until stable on a consistent glucose infusion rate (GIR).

   If within normal range on admission, then follow glucose values every hour until stable on maintenance fluids.

   Thereafter, monitoring can be tapered to every 4 hours and then, if still stable, to daily and with changes in fluid administration.

4. Assuming none of the possible causes of abnormal in utero fluid and electrolyte balance exists, there is no need to check electrolytes immediately after birth. Baseline serum chemistries should be checked at about 12-hours of age and then every 12 hours for the first few days until stable on a consistent fluid regimen with normal renal function.

Initial Parenteral Fluid Management

Begin parenteral fluids for most neonates at the following:

1. For infants larger than 1500 g, provide 60–80 mL/kg daily;

2. For infants 1000–1500 g, provide 80 mL/kg daily;

3. For infants less than 1000 g, provide 100 mL/kg daily.

ELGANs may have immature skin as described previously and thus have markedly increased transepidermal fluid loss; these infants may have much higher fluid to avoid severe hypernatremic dehydration.

1. Starting at 120–150 mL/kg daily may be appropriate for these patients and, depending on their response, may go up to 200 mL/kg daily.

2. Humidified incubators may decrease insensible fluid loss, weight loss, and hypernatremia for these small babies.

Starting fluids should provide an approximate GIR of 4–6 mg/kg per minute (see Figure 69–1). This is usually accomplished with 10% dextrose in water (D10W), except for the ELGANs described previously, for whom much less-concentrated glucose would be appropriate. In general, infants less than about 750 g should start with 5% dextrose in water (D5W).

No sodium or potassium should be added to initial fluids.

Calcium gluconate should be added to avoid hypocalcemia; the target range is 200–400 mg/kg daily. The total may be limited by the resulting concentration of

Step 1:	Convert Dextrose to Glucose Glucose (g) = Dextrose (g) × (10/11)
Step 2:	Calculating Glucose Delivery from Dextrose Concentration & IV Rate (D%)×(10/11)×(mL/kg per day)/(144) = mg/kg per min (D%)×(10/11)×(mL/kg per day)/(100) = g/kg per day

FIGURE 69-1 Calculating glucose infusion rate.

the parenteral solution. Calcium gluconate is irritating to veins, and extravasations can cause significant injury. We try to limit the amount in a peripheral intravenous solution to no more than 100 mg/dL; central venous catheter solutions may go up to 400 mg/dL.

Amino acids should be provided as soon as possible after birth to avoid protein catabolism. Neonates tolerate AA quite well and can start with as much AA as possible, given the limitations of solubility in intravenous solutions. This is usually about 2 g/dL for peripheral and 3 g/dL for central venous line solutions. Because neonates can lose more than 1 g/kg of protein daily if none is provided, AA should be added immediately in the highest concentration allowed.

Management Algorithm

Weight monitoring is needed to avoid excessive loss. Daily weights are adequate for most neonates, but twice-daily weights may be needed for ELGAN patients. Total weight loss should not exceed 10% of birth weight, and recent studies suggested that, with early hyperalimentation, may not need to exceed 6%. Weight should be plotted on appropriate growth curves. Excessive weight loss should result in a 10–20 mL/kg increase in daily intravenous rate.

Electrolyte monitoring should be done twice daily initially and again perhaps more frequently for ELGANs.

1. Hypernatremia must be watched for and responded to rapidly, again by increasing fluid administration by 10–20 mL/kg daily.

2. Hyponatremia in the first days of life almost always means free-water overload and not inadequate sodium intake. Thus, rather than treating this with added sodium in the parenteral solution, further fluid restriction is the best first step.

3. Nonoliguric hyperkalemia is a significant concern in ELGANs. There is some evidence that increased AA administration may minimize this. Nevertheless, do not add potassium to initial intravenous fluids until good urine output and renal function are ensured and then only add slowly with close monitoring of serum levels.

4. The safest and most effective way to provide calcium to infants is via the enteral route. This is

another argument for initiating enteral nutrition as soon as possible.

The GIR should be calculated whenever intravenous lines are changed to avoid the risk of delivering either too much or too little glucose.

1. Too low a GIR can result in hypoglycemia and inadequate growth.

2. Too high a GIR can result in hyperglycemia, osmotic diuresis, increased carbon dioxide production, and liver injury. In general, try to keep the GIR no more than about 12 mg/kg per min.

3. The following are indications to increase fluid administration:

   Excessive weight loss;

   Gastroschisis/omphalocele;

   Immature, sticky, translucent skin;

   Polyuria;

   Hyperglycemia;

   Hypernatremia; and

   Hyperkalemia.

4. Indications for decreasing fluid administration are as follows:

   Asphyxia/cerebral edema;

   Generalized body edema;

   Oliguria (eg, renal failure, syndrome of inappropriate secretion of antidiuretic hormone [SIADH], indomethacin);

   Heart failure or patent ductus arteriosus (PDA);

   Pulmonary edema;

   Excessive weight gain;

   Hyperglycemia; and

   Hyponatremia.

SUGGESTED READINGS

Bell EF, Acarregui MJ. Restricted versus liberal water intake for preventing morbidity and mortality in preterm infants. *Cochrane Database Syst Rev.* 2008;(1):CD000503. doi:10.1002/14651858.CD000503.pub2.

Bhatia J. Fluid and electrolyte management in the very low birth weight neonate. *J Perinatol.* 2006;26(Suppl 1):S19–S21.

Elstgeest LE, Martens SE, Lopriore E, Walther FJ, te Pas AB. Does parenteral nutrition influence electrolyte and fluid balance in preterm infants in the first days after birth? *PLoS One.* 2010;5:e9033. doi:10.1371/journal.pone.0009033.

Friis-Hansen B. Body water compartments in children: changes during growth and related changes in body composition. *Pediatrics.* 1961;28:169–181.

Hartnoll G, Bétrémieux P, Modi N. Randomised controlled trial of postnatal sodium supplementation on oxygen dependency and body weight in 25–30 week gestational age infants. *Arch Dis Child Fetal Neonatal Ed.* 2000;82:F19–F23.

Iacobelli S, Bonsante F, Vintéjoux A, Gouyon J-B. Standardized parenteral nutrition in preterm infants: early impact on fluid and electrolyte balance. *Neonatology.* 2010;98:84–90.

Khan MAG, Upadhyay Am, Chikanna S, Jalswal V. Efficacy of prophylactic intravenous calcium administration in first 5 days of life in high risk neonates to prevent early onset neonatal hypocalcaemia: a randomised controlled trial. *Arch Dis Child Fetal Neonatol.* 2010;95:F462–F463. doi:10.1136/adc.2009.179663.

Kim SM, Lee EY, Chen J, Ringer SA. Improved care and growth outcomes by using hybrid humidified incubators in very preterm infants. *Pediatrics.* 2010;125:e137–e145.

Lorenz JM. Fluid and electrolyte therapy and chronic lung disease. *Curr Opin Pediatr* 2004;16:152–156.

McCallie KM, Lee HC, Mayer O, et al. Improved outcomes with a standardized feeding protocol for very low birth weight infants. *J Perinatol.* 2011;31(Suppl 1):S61–S67.

Stephens BE, Gargus RA, Walden RV, et al. Fluid regimens in the first week of life may increase risk of patent ductus arteriosus in extremely low birth weight infants. *J Perinatol.* 2008;28:123–128.

70 Hyperalimentation and Monitoring

Kevin Pieroni and John Kerner

INTRODUCTION

Nutrition support plays a crucial role in the management of premature neonates. Parenteral nutrition (PN) especially has continued to have an impact on the care of neonates who are unable to ingest sufficient enteral calories and fluids. The use of PN has evolved in the neonatal intensive care unit (NICU) to minimize the metabolic complications that interrupt normal growth. To deliver PN to neonates, those involved in the ordering and delivery of PN need to be educated and trained to ensure safety and standardization.[1] This chapter provides a practical overview to provide optimal nutrition support to neonates in the NICU, keeping in mind the particular conditions and physiology of premature neonates.

INDICATIONS

Parenteral nutrition can be used as the sole source of nutrition and fluids for neonates. There are multiple conditions that can inhibit or limit the use of enteral nutrition. Patients can develop short-bowel syndrome from intestinal atresia, volvulus, or necrotizing enterocolitis. Motility issues can arise from Hirschsprung disease, meconium ileus, ileus as a result of generalized illness, or gastroschisis. Neonates with asphyxia or hypotension with use of vasopressors might not be clinically stable enough for the initiation of enteral nutrition. Preterm neonates on slowly advancing feedings

will also require PN supplementation to obtain substantial calories and fluids until goal feedings have been reached. PN or enteral nutrition should be started within 24 hours after birth.[2-5] More aggressive administration of both glucose and amino acids has led to the use of standard, starter, or "vanilla" total parenteral nutrition (TPN). Many of these solutions come premixed; many institutions still compound the mixture in the hospital pharmacy. These initial solutions usually contain 7.5% to 10% dextrose and 3% amino acids.[6] The goal is to have a glucose infusion rate (GIR) of 6–8 mg/kg/min and amino acid administration of 2 to 3 g/kg/day.

ROUTE OF ADMINISTRATION

Peripheral venous access limits the osmolality of fluids that can be infused through it, which limits dextrose concentration to 12.5%. Increased osmolality that infuses through a peripheral catheter increases the risk of thrombophlebitis, although concomitant infusion of a fat emulsion can reduce venous irritation.[7,8] Central venous access, either through an umbilical venous catheter (UVC) or a peripherally inserted central catheter (PICC) is generally needed. Positioning of these catheters must be confirmed with an x-ray showing the tip terminating at the junction of the superior vena cava and right atrium of the heart. Continuous infusion of heparin 0.5 IU/kg/h has been shown to reduce occlusions of PICC lines in neonates and can be added directly to the PN fluid.[9,10]

PARENTERAL NUTRITION COMPONENTS

Calories

There are many factors that can increase the metabolic demands of neonates, including increased heat loss, small for gestational age (SGA), fever, sepsis, respiratory distress, and the accelerated rate of growth. Neonates who receive a caloric intake as low as 70 kcal/kg/d have demonstrated a positive nitrogen balance. Weight gain can occur with parenteral intake of 80 to 130 kcal/kg/d if there is adequate protein intake. The caloric goal of premature neonates is 100 to 120 kcal/kg/d, and the goal of term neonates is 90–108 kcal/kg/d (Table 70-1).[11] Calorie utilization is maximized if given in balanced allotments of macronutrients. Carbohydrates should be the main source of calories at 40% to 50%, followed by lipids at 30% to 40% and protein at 10%–30% of the caloric intake.[12] Optimal calorie goals aim to sustain appropriate "catchup" growth. Excessive calorie intake must be avoided as this can result in excessive fat deposition in the subcutaneous tissue and liver as well as greater carbon dioxide production, which complicates any underlying respiratory conditions.[13]

Fluids

The nutritional and caloric composition is a particular focus when discussing TPN, but the volume that is delivered is just as crucial (Table 70-1). Premature neonates have increased fluid losses because of radiant warmers, phototherapy, increased skin permeability, and respiratory distress. As a result of these factors, the premature neonate has higher volume needs than the term neonate. If there is fluid restriction, the concentration of nutrients needs to be increased, resulting in high osmolarity and issues with solubility. To help improve tolerance of these high-osmolar solutions, the amino acid–dextrose solution is typically run over 24 hours so the infusion rate can be as low as possible. Fat emulsions are also better tolerated if infused over 18 to 24 hours.

Carbohydrates

For neonates, carbohydrate delivery in PN should begin at approximately 6 to 8 mg/kg/min and be advanced, as tolerated, to a goal of 10 to 14 mg/kg/min.[12] Dextrose is normally started at 10% concentration so that it will deliver a GIR around 7 mg/kg/min if infused at a rate of 100 mL/kg/d. As the GIR is increased, a trace amount of glucosuria is not uncommon, but the GIR may need to be decreased as serum glucose levels are also monitored (Table 70-1). Hyperglycemia in neonates can be associated with complications, including death, infections, visual problems, and intraventricular hemorrhage. The routine use of insulin to help prevent hyperglycemia in premature neonates has not been well established and can be associated with risk,

Table 70-1 Recommendations for Parenteral Nutrition Macronutrients for Neonates[a]

Source	Initiation	Advancement	Goal	Neonate	Blood or Plasma Monitoring
Amino acids	1.5–2 g/kg/d	0.5–1 g/kg/d	2–3 g/kg/d	Term	BUN, ammonia, arterial pH
	2–3 g/kg/d	0.5–1 g/kg/d	3.5–4 g/kg/d	ELBW	
	1 g/kg/d	0.25–0.5 g/kg/d	3–4 g/kg/d	Septic, hypoxic	Lactate
Dextrose	8 mg/kg/min	1–3 mg/kg/min	12–14 mg/kg/min	≥1 kg	Glucose < 150 mg/dL
	6 mg/kg/min	1–3 mg/kg/min	12–14 mg/kg/min	<1 kg	Glucose < 125 mg/dL
Fat	1–2 g/kg/d	0.5–1 g/kg/d	3 g/kg/d	Term	Triglycerides < 200 mg/dL
	0.5–1 g/kg/d	0.25–1 g/kg/d	3 g/kg/d	Preterm	Bilirubin, glucose
	0.5 g/kg/d	0–0.5 g/kg/d	1–2 g/kg/d	Hyperbilirubinemia Sepsis Severe respiratory distress	Bilirubin
Energy			90–108 kcal/kg/d	Term	
			100–120 kcal/kg/d	Preterm	
Fluids			130–150 mL/kg/d	Term	
			130–180 mL/kg/d	Preterm	

Abbreviations: BUN, serum urea nitrogen; ELBW, extremely low birth weight.
[a]Data from ASPEN Board of Directors and the Clinical Guidelines Task Force. Guidelines for the use of parenteral and enteral nutrition in adult and pediatric patients. *APEN J Parenter Enteral Nutr.* 2002;26(1 Suppl):1SA-138SA; and Nash MA. The management of fluid and electrolyte disorders in the neonate. *Clin Perinatol.* 1981;8(2):251-262.

such as lactic acidosis and death.[11,14,15] Continuous insulin infusions at 0.01 to 0.1 units/kg/h may be necessary for managing hyperglycemia in neonates.[12]

Protein

Commercial pediatric amino acid solutions are formulated to result in plasma amino acid profiles that are comparable to breast-fed infants. These formulations contain taurine, tyrosine, histidine, aspartic acid, and glutamic acid and contain less glycine, methionine, and phenylalanine than adult amino acid formulations.[11] Cysteine, a conditionally essential amino acid for neonates, is not added to pediatric amino acid formulations because of its short shelf life. Cysteine hydrochloride can be added to PN fluid at a dose of 40 mg/g of amino acids. Carnitine, required for optimal fatty acid metabolism, is also not added to pediatric amino acid formulations. There have not been any convincing studies to demonstrate that carnitine has any effect on lipid utilization and ketogenesis, although fatty acid oxidation is impaired if the tissue carnitine level falls below 10% of normal.[16] Still, it has become practice to add L-carnitine 2 to 5 mg/kg/d to PN fluids, especially for neonates having difficulty with hypertriglyceridemia.[12] This dose is the same quantity received from breast milk and infant formula.[17] As stated previously, amino acids should be started within the first 24 hours of life and then advanced to the goal (Table 70-1). Newer retrospective data argue for starting amino acids within the first few hours of life.[18]

Fat

Fat constitutes a high-caloric nutrient source in any diet. Fat emulsions are currently available as 10% or 20% soy or soy-safflower oil. The use of 20% emulsion is preferred because it is more calorically dense yet has the same phospholipid concentration, has improved clearance of triglycerides and phospholipids, and has the same osmolarity as the 10% emulsion. These emulsions can prevent essential fatty acid deficiency (EFAD) at a minimum rate of 0.5 to 1 g/kg/d in the presence of adequate energy intake. If a neonate is in an energy-deficient state, then EFAD may not be prevented at this minimal rate because essential fatty acids will be oxidized to meet energy needs. Fat emulsions should be started within 3 days of life to prevent EFAD. Fat emulsions are safe to start within the first 24 hours of life and can be increased to a goal rate (Table 70-1). Fat emulsion delivery at a continuous rate over 24 hours optimizes lipid clearance. The maximum infusion rate should not exceed 0.15 g/kg/h, but this rate may need to be lower in very low birth weight infants or SGA infants. Heparin also stimulates the release of lipoprotein lipase, which may improve lipid clearance.

Jaundice and sepsis are not contraindications for using fat emulsions. There is a theoretic risk that fatty acids can displace bilirubin from albumin, resulting in increased serum unconjugated (free) bilirubin concentration, thus increasing the risk of kernicterus. Fat emulsion given at a rate of 1 to 4 g/kg/d did not show any effect on the bilirubin and albumin levels in neonates.[19] Even with these findings, if the unconjugated bilirubin concentration approaches the level indicating an exchange transfusion, it is recommended that the fat emulsion rate should be decreased to 0.5 to 2 g/kg/d, and the rate should not be advanced until the bilirubin has decreased to 50% of the exchange transfusion level. Serum triglyceride levels can increase in the presence of bacterial sepsis, trauma, and stress and should be monitored. Although the risk of infection increases with the administration of fatty acids, this risk is not reason enough to avoid the use of fat emulsion.[20]

Electrolytes and Minerals

Close monitoring of electrolyte status is essential in neonates as daily adjustments are often necessary with the initiation of PN. The addition of electrolytes to PN may be deferred until the second day of life until regular urine output is ensured. Sodium is usually added once diuresis has begun, and potassium is added once good urine output and normal kidney function are established. Table 70-2 provides reference ranges of electrolyte requirements.

Calcium and phosphorus play a major role in neonatal PN because preterm neonates have not fully mineralized their bones. During the first 2 days of life, PN can contain less than maintenance phosphorus because of the concern of hyperphosphatemia. The maintenance dosing can be found in Table 70-2 but can also be listed as milligrams per liter, in which case it would be dosed at calcium 500 to 600 mg/L and phosphorus 350–500 mg/L of PN. The goal calcium-to-phosphorus ratio is 1.3 to 1.7:1. The difficulty with calcium and phosphorus administration is the concern of solubility. The solubility curves of calcium and phosphorus are multifactorial, but it has been clearly established that the pH of the solution plays a key role, so increasing the amount of amino acids, and possibly adding cysteine, as well as increasing dextrose can help increase the solubility.[21]

Trace Elements

There is no reason to avoid providing trace elements to neonates requiring short-term PN. The concentrations and composition of pediatric formulations are similar. Recommended dosing can be found in Table 70-3. Individual trace element products would need to be used to meet trace element needs because

Table 70-2 Daily Electrolyte and Mineral Dosing Guidelines[a,b]

Electrolytes	Preterm Neonate	Infants/Children	Adolescents and Children > 50 kg
Sodium	2–5 mEq/kg	2–5 mEq/kg	1–2 mEq/kg
Potassium	2–4 mEq/kg	2–4 mEq/kg	1–2 mEq/kg
Calcium	2–4 mEq/kg	0.5–4 mEq/kg	10–20 mEq/d
Phosphorus	1–2 mmol/kg	0.5–2 mmol/kg	10–40 mmol/d
Magnesium	0.3–0.5 mEq/kg	0.3–0.5 mEq/kg	10–30 mmol/d
Acetate	As needed to maintain acid-base balance		
Chloride	As needed to maintain acid-base balance		

[a]Reprinted with permission from Mirtallo et al.[34]
[b]Assumes normal organ function and losses.

commercially available multitrace products would not meet these needs.

Zinc is important in cell growth and development. Additional zinc may be required in cases with elevated urinary and stool zinc excretion.

Copper is an essential component of several key enzymes. Additional copper may be required because of increased biliary losses secondary to a jejunostomy or biliary drain. Copper has been held from PN in patients with cholestasis, but cases of copper deficiency have been reported.[22] If cholestasis develops, copper can be withheld from PN; then, monitoring copper and ceruloplasmin levels is crucial, and copper can be restarted individually if levels become deficient. Some recommend maintaining a dose of 20 µg/kg/d, but others have decreased the rate to only 10 µg/kg/day.[22,23]

Manganese is a component of several enzymes. Manganese deficiency has not been documented, although toxicity has been documented. Individually supplementing manganese should be done with caution, especially because it is already a contaminant of PN solutions. Manganese has been shown on magnetic resonance imaging (MRI) to deposit in the basal ganglia, leading to central nervous system symptoms such as Parkinsonism.

Chromium potentiates the action of insulin and has a key role in glucose, protein, and lipid metabolism. Chromium intake can be decreased in patients with renal impairment. Chromium is also a major contaminant of PN solutions and does not need to be routinely added to PN.

Selenium is a component of glutathione peroxidase. Supplementation is recommended in patients who continue on PN for longer than 30 days; levels should be monitored after that time. The dose should be decreased when renal dysfunction is present.

Multivitamins

See Table 70-4 for recommended dosing of multivitamins.

MONITORING

The guidelines for metabolic monitoring of neonates while on PN are shown in Table 70-5.

Table 70-3 Trace Element Requirement[a,b]

Trace Element	Preterm Neonates < 3 kg (µg/kg/d)	Term Neonates 3–10 kg (µ/kg/d)	Children 10–40 kg (µ/kg/d)	Adolescents > 40 kg (per day)
Zinc	400	50–250	50–125	2–5 mg
Copper	20	20	5–20	200–500 µg
Manganese	1	1	1	40–100 µg
Chromium	0.05–0.2	0.2	0.14–0.2	5–15 µg
Selenium	1.5–2	2	1–2	40–60 µg

[a]Reprinted with permission from Mirtallo et al.[34]
[b]Assumes normal organ function and losses.

Table 70-4 Daily Dose Recommendations for Pediatric Multiple Vitamins[a-c]

Manufacturer		AMA-NAG[d]	
Weight (kg)	Dose (mL)	Weight (kg)	Dose
<1	1.5	<2.5	2 mL/kg
1–3	3.25	>2.5	5 mL
>3	5		

[a]Reprinted with permission from Mirtallo et al.[34]
[b]Assumes normal age-related organ function and normal losses.
[c]Pediatric multiple vitamin formulation (5 mL): A, 2300 IU; D, 400 IU; E, 7 IU; K, 200 μg; C, 80 mg; B_1, 1.2 mg; B_2, 1.4 mg; B_3, 17 mg; B_5, 5 mg; B_6, 1 μg; B_{12}, 1 μg; biotin, 20 μg; folic acid, 140 μg.
[d]American Medical Association Nutrition Advisory Group.

Catheter Occlusion

Central venous catheters used for the administration of PN can become occluded for several reasons. A thrombus or clot is the most common cause of a catheter occlusion. For this reason, it is recommended to add 0.25 to 1 U/L of heparin to the PN solution.[24] If a thrombus is occluding the catheter, then 2 mg/2 mL alteplase can be instilled into the catheter at 110% of the catheter volume and left to dwell in the catheter for 30 minutes. If there is no response, leave in place for 2 hours; if no response, give a second dose, which can dwell up to an additional 2 hours. Lipid deposition can also occlude a catheter. In this case, 70% ethanol can be instilled in the catheter for 1 to 2 hours; the dose is 0.55 mL/kg (to a maximum of 3 mL). Calcium/phosphorus precipitate can be cleared from a catheter using 0.5 mL of 0.1 N hydrochloric acid. Acidic drug precipitate has been cleared with 0.2 to 1 mL of 0.1 N hydrochloric acid, and basic drug precipitate has been cleared from a catheter using 1 mL of 0.1 N sodium hydroxide or 1 mL of 1 mEq/L sodium bicarbonate.[25]

Cholestasis

Neonates are at high risk for developing cholestasis because prematurity, low birth weight, sepsis, and limited enteral intake are all risk factors. PN can increase this risk because manganese, copper, and aluminum can all have hepatotoxic effects. Recent studies suggested that the proinflammatory omega-6 polysaturated fatty acids in plant oil–based lipid emulsions (Intralipid, Liposyn III) and the presence of phytosterols contribute to the development of hepatotoxicity.[26] Once a neonate on PN develops cholestasis, there are multiple strategies that can be implemented to help prevent and treat the cholestasis. The neonate must receive a pediatric amino acid formulation. Ensure that the neonate is not receiving excessive caloric intake. Decrease the fat emulsion to about 1 g/kg/d.

Table 70-5 Guidelines for Metabolic Monitoring During Parenteral Nutrition[a]

Variable to Be Monitored	Initial Period[b]	Later Period[c]
Growth Weight Head circumference Length	Daily Baseline Baseline	Daily Twice weekly Weekly
Intake and output	Every shift	Daily
Glucose reagent strips	1 to 3 times/day	As indicated
Serum electrolytes, urea nitrogen, creatinine	Baseline and every 1 to 3 days	Every 1 to 2 weeks
Serum calcium, magnesium, phosphorus	Baseline and every 2 to 3 days	Every 1 to 2 weeks
Serum triglycerides	Daily during dose increase	Every 1 to 2 weeks
Serum glucose	As needed	As needed
Total and direct bilirubin	Baseline, as needed clinically	Every 1 to 2 weeks
Total protein and albumin	Baseline	Every 2 to 3 weeks
Alanine aminotransferase, aspartate aminotransferase, and alkaline phosphatase	Baseline	Every 2 to 3 weeks
Complete blood cell count	Baseline	Every 2 to 3 weeks
Vitamin and trace mineral status and other specific tests	As indicated	As indicated

[a]Reproduced with permission from Carney et al.[34]
[b]The period before reaching maximum glucose, amino acids, and lipid emulsion or during any period of metabolic instability. This period normally lasts 3 to 4 days.
[c]The period during which the patient is in a metabolic steady state. For clinically stable infants receiving the desired intake of nutrients, the interval between laboratory measurements may be increased beyond these recommendations.

Remove trace elements from the PN solution, while supplementing with zinc and selenium, then monitor copper and manganese serum levels and supplement individually if needed. Starting enteral feedings is the key to stimulate bile flow. Ursodeoxycholic acid 20 to 30 mg/kg/day given enterally is safe and effective and should be started as soon as possible once cholestasis is identified.[27]

CHAPTER 70

Table 70-6 Weaning Parenteral Nutrition (PN)

PN Macronutrients	Enteral Feeding Volume					
	Goal Total PN (Nothing by Mouth)	20 mL/kg/d	40 mL/kg/d	60 mL/kg/d	80 mL/kg/d	100 mL/kg/d
Amino acids (g/kg)	3–3.5	3–3.5	2.5–3	2–2.5	2	0
Lipids (g/kg)	3–3.5	3–3.5	2–2.5	1.5–2	1–1.5	0
Glucose (mg/kg/min)	12–14	~10–12	~8–10	~7–9	5–7	~4–6[a]

[a]Data from Bhatia J, Gates A. Neonatal nutrition handbook, 6th edition. Elk Grove Village, IL: American Academy of Pediatrics, 2006.
[b]Wean PN rate from goal as needed to maintain hydration as enteral feedings advance.

Aluminum

Aluminum has long been known to be a contaminant of PN solutions. Toxicity from aluminum can manifest with neurologic impairment, decreased bone mineralization, microcytic anemia, and cholestasis. Calcium and phosphorus solutions have the most contamination, which puts premature neonates at highest risk because of their high demand for these minerals and poor renal clearance of aluminum by neonates. As a result, the Food and Drug Administration (FDA) mandated specific labeling requirements.[28,29] Many organizations have also developed guidelines to help minimize the risk of aluminum toxicity.[30,31] It has been shown that the FDA regulations cannot be met with the current PN solutions available.[32] To minimize the risk, the PN solutions with the least contamination can be purchased and used by pharmacies.[33]

Weaning Parenteral Nutrition

The ultimate goal of PN is to wean the infant from it and transition to enteral nutrition as quickly and safely as possible. Table 70-6 illustrates a tactic to wean PN as enteral nutrition is gradually increased, yet administer adequate nutrition.

Basic TPN Calculations

Guidelines for calculating GIR and for calculating macronutrient calories are shown in Table 70-7.

Table 70-7 Calculations

Glucose Infusion Rate (GIR)
1. Convert grams of dextrose monohydrate to the equivalent in anhydrous glucose with the correction factor (180/198) based on their molecular weights, which is reduced to (10/11).
2. Formula for GIR mg/kg/min = (D%)(10/11)(# mL/kg/d)(1/144).
3. Formula for GIR g/kg/d = (D%)(10/11)(# mL/kg•d)(1/100).

Calories
1. Carbohydrate calories, either
   a. (Glucose mg/kg/min)(1.44)(3.8 kcal/g) = kcal/kg•d from dextrose, or
   b. (Glucose g/kg/day)(3.8 kcal/g) = kcal/kg/d from dextrose.
2. Protein kcal/kg/d = (grams Amino Acid/kg/d)(4 kcal/g).
3. Lipid calories, either
   a. (grams Lipid/kg/d)(10 kcal/g) = kcal/kg/d from lipid, or
   b. (milliliters 20% Lipid/kg/d)(2 kcal/mL) = kcal/kg/d from lipid.

REFERENCES

1. Board of Directors and Task Force on Parenteral Nutrition Standardization, Kochevar M, Guenter P, et al. A.S.P.E.N. statement on parenteral nutrition standardization. *J Parenter Enteral Nutr.* 2007;31(5):441–448.
2. Ziegler EE, Carlson SJ, Ekhard. Early nutrition of very low birth weight infants. *J Matern Fetal Neonatal Med.* 2009;22(3):191–197.
3. Denne SC, Poindexter BB. Evidence supporting early nutritional support with parenteral amino acid infusion. *Semin Perinatol.* 2007;31(2):56–60.
4. Ziegler EE, Thureen PJ, Carlson SJ. Aggressive nutrition of the very low birthweight infant. *Clin Perinatol.* 2002;29(2):225–244.
5. Wilson DC, Cairns P, Halliday HL, et al. Randomised controlled trial of an aggressive nutritional regimen in sick very low birthweight infants. *Arch Dis Child Fetal Neonatal Ed.* 1997;77(1):F4–F11.
6. Uhing MR, Das UG, Michael. Optimizing growth in the preterm infant. *Clin Perinatol.* 2009;36(1):165–176.
7. Putet G. Lipid metabolism of the micropremie. *Clin Perinatol.* 2000;27(1):57–69.
8. Committee on Nutrition. Nutritional needs of the preterm infant. In Kleinman RE, ed. *Pediatric Nutrition Handbook.* 6th ed. Elk Grove Village, IL: American Academy of Pediatrics; 2009:79–112.
9. Shah PS, Shah VS. Continuous heparin infusion to prevent thrombosis and catheter occlusion in neonates with peripherally

placed percutaneous central venous catheters. *Cochrane Database Syst Rev.* 2008;(2):CD002772.

10. Uslu S, Ozdemir H, Comert S, Bolat F, Nuhoglu A. The effect of low-dose heparin on maintaining peripherally inserted percutaneous central venous catheters in neonates. *J Perinatol.* 2010;30(12):794–799.

11. Koo WWK, McLaughlin K, Saba M. Neonatal intensive care. In: Merritt R, ed. *The A.S.P.E.N. Nutrition Support Practice Manual.* 2nd ed. Silver Spring, MD: American Society for Parenteral and Enteral Nutrition; 2005:301–314.

12. American Society for Parenteral and Enteral Nutrition. Guidelines for the use of parenteral and enteral nutrition in adult and pediatric patients. *J Parenter Enteral Nutr.* 2002;26(1 Suppl):1SA–138SA.

13. Yunis KA, Oh W. Effects of intravenous glucose loading on oxygen consumption, carbon dioxide production, and resting energy expenditure in infants with bronchopulmonary dysplasia. *J Pediatr.* 1989;115(1):127–132.

14. Sinclair JC, Bottino M, Cowett RM. Interventions for prevention of neonatal hyperglycemia in very low birth weight infants. *Cochrane Database Syst Rev.* 2009;(3):CD007615.

15. Decaro MH, Vain NE. Hyperglycaemia in preterm neonates: what to know, what to do. *Early Hum Dev.* 2011;87(Suppl 1): S19–S22.

16. Cairns PA, Stalker DJ. Carnitine supplementation of parenterally fed neonates. *Cochrane Database Syst Rev.* 2000;(4):CD000950.

17. Borum PR. Carnitine in parenteral nutrition. *Gastroenterology.* 2009;137(5, Supplement 1):S129–S134.

18. Valentine CJ, Fernandez S, Rogers LK, et al. Early amino-acid administration improves preterm infant weight. *J Perinatol.* 2009;29(6):428–432.

19. Brans YW, Ritter DA, Kenny JD, et al. Influence of intravenous fat emulsion on serum bilirubin in very low birthweight neonates. *Arch Dis Child.* 1987;62(2):156–160.

20. Greer FR. Nutrition support of the premature infant. In: Baker SS, Baker RD, Davis AM, ed. *Pediatric Nutrition Support.* Sudbury, MA. Jones and Barlett; 2007:383–392.

21. Poole RL, Rupp CA, Kerner JA Jr. Calcium and phosphorus in neonatal parenteral nutrition solutions. *J Parenter Enteral Nutr.* 1983;7(4):358–360.

22. Hurwitz M, Garcia MG, Poole RL, Kerner JA. Copper deficiency during parenteral nutrition: a report of four pediatric cases. *Nutr Clin Pract.* 2004;19(3):305–308.

23. Frem J, Sarson Y, Sternberg T, Cole CR. Copper supplementation in parenteral nutrition of cholestatic infants. *J Pediatr Gastroenterol Nutr.* 2010;50(6):650–654.

24. Carney LN, Nepa A, Cohen SS, et al. Parenteral and enteral nutrition support: determining the best way to feed. In: Corkins MR, ed. *The A.S.P.E.N. Pediatric Nutrition Support Core Curriculum.* Silver Spring, MD: American Society for Parenteral and Enteral Nutrition; 2010:433–447.

25. Kerner JA Jr, Garcia-Careaga MG, Fisher AA, Poole RL. Treatment of catheter occlusion in pediatric patients. *J Parenter Enteral Nutr.* 2006;30(1 Suppl):S73–S81.

26. Fallon EM, Le HD, Puder M. Prevention of parenteral nutrition-associated liver disease: role of omega-3 fish oil. *Curr Opin Organ Transplant.* 2010;15(3):334–340.

27. Guglielmi FW, Regano N, Mazzuoli S, et al. Cholestasis induced by total parenteral nutrition. *Clin Liver Dis.* 2008;12(1):97–110.

28. Food and Drug Administration. Aluminum in large and small volume parenterals used in total parenteral nutrition. *Fed Regist.* 2000;65:4103–4111.

29. Food and Drug Administration. Aluminum in large and small volume parenterals used in total parenteral nutrition; amendment; delay of effective date. *Fed Regist.* 2002;67:70691–70692.

30. The American Society for Parenteral and Enteral Nutrition (A.S.P.E.N.) Aluminum Task Force: Pamela J. Charney, chair. A.S.P.E.N. statement on aluminum in parenteral nutrition solutions. *Nutr Clin Pract.* 2004;19(4):416–417.

31. Committee on Nutrition. Aluminum toxicity in infants and children. *Pediatrics.* 1996;97(3):413–416.

32. Poole RL, Schiff L, Hintz SR, et al. Aluminum content of parenteral nutrition in neonates: measured versus calculated levels. *J Pediatr Gastroenterol Nutr.* 2010;50(2):208–211.

33. Poole RL, Pieroni KP, Gaskari S, et al. Aluminum in pediatric parenteral nutrition products: measured versus labeled content. *J Pediatr Pharmacol Ther.* 2011;16(2):92–97.

34. Mirtallo J, Canada T, Johnson D, et al. Safe practices for parenteral nutrition. *J Parenter Enteral Nutr.* 2004:28(6):S39–S70.

Feeding Protocols for VLBW Infants

71

Katherine McCallie

INDICATION

Clinical Findings

History

The protocols in this chapter are for neonates with very low birth weight (VLBW) (≤1500 g) who are clinically stable for initiation of enteral feedings. The goal is to initiate enteral feedings by day of life 3.

Physical

There should be no congenital gastrointestinal defects precluding enteral feedings.

Exclusions/Contraindications

1. Hemodynamic instability requiring volume resuscitation, dopamine > 5 µg/kg/min, or initiation of hydrocortisone

   a. Feeding should be delayed until hemodynamically stable for 24–48 hours.

   b. Patient may be started on feedings while on hydrocortisone (ie, weaning course of treatment) if the patient is hemodynamically stable.

2. Hemodynamically significant patent ductus arteriosus (PDA) requiring indomethacin treatment or surgical closure: Feeding should be delayed until 24–48 hours after indomethacin course is completed or surgery is completed.

3. Abdominal distension, signs of obstruction, abdominal discoloration consistent with peritonitis, or surgical abdomen

4. Large-volume gastric fluid, discolored (eg, bilious) gastric fluid

5. Sepsis, severe metabolic acidosis, hypoxia-asphyxia: Feeding should be delayed based on clinical evaluation.

PREPARATION

Consent

Per individual units' policies, parental assent or informed consent may need to be obtained for use of banked donor breast milk if maternal breast milk (MBM) is not available.

Monitoring During Treatment

1. Cardiorespiratory and oxygen saturation monitoring is necessary during treatment.

2. Gastric residuals may be measured prior to each feeding per unit policy.

TREATMENT/PROCEDURE

Initiation

Colostrum Administration

1. The change from colostrum to transitional milk is individual. However, as a working definition, milk

obtained from mothers during the first 7 days will be considered colostrum. During this time, fresh colostrum (not previously frozen) may be used.

2. If the infant is ready to begin enteral feedings, colostrum may be administered in trophic feedings given via gavage tube (see the sample feeding volume and advancement schedule).

3. If colostrum is available but the infant is not ready for enteral feedings, colostrum may be administered in the following fashion: Colostrum, 0.5 - 1 mL every 6 hours, may be delivered via syringe into the buccal pouch of the mouth *or* may be delivered via sterile cotton swab to the buccal cavity.

Enteral Feeding Choice

Maternal breast milk is the enteral feeding of choice unless contraindications for its use exist.

1. *Possible* contraindications for MBM use (individual units will have their own policies) are the following:

   a. Infant with galactosemia

   b. Mother with active untreated tuberculosis

   c. Mother receiving diagnostic or therapeutic radioactive isotopes or with exposure to radioactive materials

   d. Mother receiving antimetabolites or chemotherapeutic agents

   e. Mother positive for human immunodeficiency virus (HIV)

   f. Mother with active herpes lesion on breast(s). Milk may be used from unaffected breast.

   g. Mother with varicella determined to be potentially infectious to infant

   h. Mother with human T-cell leukemia virus type 1 (HTLV-1)

2. Breast pumping and hand expression should be initiated within the first 6 hours postpartum.

3. The value of colostrum should be emphasized: Fresh colostrum should be collected and used in the first feedings (see the section on colostrum administration).

4. Lactation consultation should occur, ideally, on the day of delivery or as soon as the mother is available (ie, if the baby has been transferred from another hospital).

If MBM is not available, pasteurized donor human milk is preferable to formula for initiation of feedings in very low birth weight (VLBW) infants.

If formula must be used, a 20-calorie/oz premature infant formula should be used.

Table 71–1 Initiation and Advancement of Enteral Feedings for Very Low Birth Weight (VLBW) Infants

Feeding Day	Total Feed Volume[a]	Feed Frequency
≤1000 g or ≤ 27 + 0/7 Weeks' Gestation		
Day 1	10 mL/kg/d	Divided every 6 hours
Day 2	10 mL/kg/d	Divided every 6 hours
Day 3	10 mL/kg/d	Divided every 6 hours
Day 4	10 mL/kg/d	Divided every 6 hours
Day 5	20 mL/kg/d	Divided every 3 hours
Day 6	20 mL/kg/d	Divided every 3 hours
Day 7	20 mL/kg/d	Divided every 3 hours
Day 8	20 mL/kg/d	Divided every 3 hours
Day 9	40 mL/kg/d	Divided every 3 hours
Day 10	60 mL/kg/d	Divided every 3 hours
Day 11	80 mL/kg/d	Divided every 3 hours
Day 12	100 mL/kg/d	Divided every 3 hours
Day 13	120 mL/kg/d	Divided every 3 hours
Day 14	140 mL/kg/d	Divided every 3 hours
Day 15	160 mL/kg/d	Divided every 3 hours
1001–1500 g or ≤ 31 + 0/7 Weeks' Gestation		
Feeding Day	Total Feed Volume[a]	Feed Frequency
Day 1	20 mL/kg/d	Divided every 3 hours
Day 2	20 mL/kg/d	Divided every 3 hours
Day 3	40 mL/kg/d	Divided every 3 hours
Day 4	40 mL/kg/d	Divided every 3 hours
Day 5	60 mL/kg/d	Divided every 3 hours
Day 6	80 mL/kg/d	Divided every 3 hours
Day 7	100 mL/kg/d	Divided every 3 hours
Day 8	120 mL/kg/d	Divided every 3 hours
Day 9	140 mL/kg/d	Divided every 3 hours
Day 10	160 mL/kg/d	Divided every 3 hours

[a]Round to nearest milliliter.

Sample Feeding Volume and Advancement Schedule

A sample feeding volume and advancement schedule is presented in Table 71-1.

Management

Feeding Intolerance

1. Episodes of feeding intolerance are common for preterm infants with poor peristalsis. Clinical assessment and integration of numerous pieces of

information are required to ascertain the implications and importance of findings.

2. The following are serious signs of clinical problems and important reasons to stop feeding, consistent with possible necrotizing enterocolitis (NEC) or sepsis. The physician should be immediately notified and the patient evaluated.

   a. Abdominal distention, new "visible loops," abdominal discoloration

   b. Worsening clinical status, including hemodynamic or respiratory instability (eg, increasing bradycardia or apnea), poor perfusion, hypo- or hyperglycemia

   c. Bloody stools not associated with anal fissure

   d. Bloody gastric residual or emesis

3. Potentially serious signs of impending or developing problems that should trigger assessment by physician are the following:

   a. *"Bilious" (green or yellow) gastric residuals*: These may be associated with developing clinical problems or may simply indicate a mechanical issue such as the orogastric tube at or beyond the pyloric sphincter.

   b. *"Large-volume" emesis*: In a VLBW infant who has reached 50% of full-volume feedings, a large-volume emesis is considered to be 50% of the last feeding volume. Other factors, such as the color of the emesis, whether emesis is a new finding, changes in feeding regimen, and the clinical status of the infant should be assessed.

   c. *Gastric residuals*: The volume of gastric residual may or may not be indicative of looming problems. Gastric residuals should be evaluated in the context of the overall clinical assessment. Few data exist regarding the "normal" or "safe" volume of gastric residual in a feeding preterm infant.

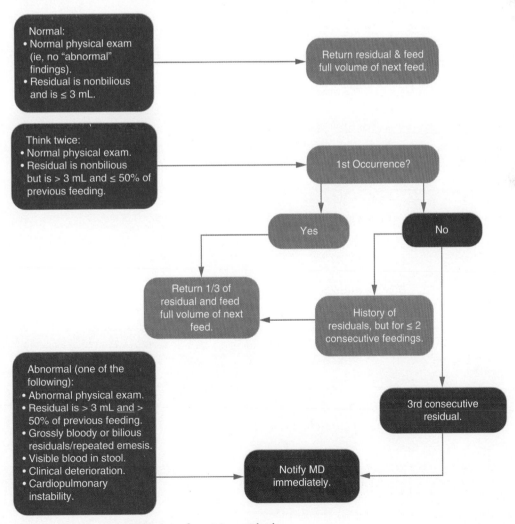

FIGURE 71–1 Algorithm for management of gastric residuals.

Sample Algorithm

A sample algorithm for management of gastric residuals is presented in Figure 71-1.

REFERENCES

Adamkin, DH. *Nutritional Strategies for the Very Low Birthweight Infant.* New York, NY: Cambridge University Press; 2009.

Hanson C, Sundermeier J, Dugick L, Lyden E, Anderson-Berry AL. Implementation, process, and outcomes of nutrition best practices for infants < 1500 g. *Nutr Clin Pract*; 2011;26(5):614–624.

McCallie KR, Lee HC, Mayer O, Cohen RS, Hintz SR, Rhine WD. Improved outcomes with a standardized feeding protocol for very low birth weight infants. *J Perinatol*; 2011;31(Suppl 1): S61–S67.

Morgan J, Young L, McGuire W. Delayed introduction of progressive enteral feeds to prevent necrotising enterocolitis in very low birth weight infants. *Cochrane Database Syst Rev.* 2011;(3):CD001970.

Quigley MA, Henderson G, Anthony MY, McGuire W. Formula milk versus donor breast milk for feeding preterm or low birth weight infants. *Cochrane Database Syst Rev.* 2007;(4):CD002971.

Rodriguez NA, Meier PP, Groer MW, Zeller JM, Engstrom JL, Fogg L. A pilot study to determine the safety and feasibility of oropharyngeal administration of mother's own colostrum to extremely low-birth-weight infants. *Adv Neonatal Care.* 2010;10(4):206–212.

Management of Hypocalcemia

Sejal Shah

DIAGNOSIS/INDICATION

Clinical Background

Disorders of calcium metabolism frequently develop in neonates in the intensive care setting. Hypocalcemia is the most common. Hypocalcemia is defined as serum calcium below 8 mg/dL (ionized calcium < 1.1 mmol/L) in a full-term infant or serum calcium less than 7 mg/dL (ionized calcium < 1 mmol/L) in a preterm infant. The etiology and treatment of hypocalcemia is often determined by the age of onset.

Premature infants are at risk for poor mineral stores because the fetus accrues 80% of its calcium stores in the third trimester.[1] Similar accrual occurs for magnesium and phosphorus stores as well. Fetal parathyroid hormone is secreted in response to maternal calcium levels. After birth, there is a rapid drop in the serum calcium because of the loss of the transplacental infusion of calcium. The sudden removal of this calcium source requires the neonate to rely on endogenous parathyroid hormone production, ingested calcium, renal tubular reabsorption of calcium, and bone calcium stores. There is a physiologic nadir in the serum calcium level that occurs at 24–48 hours of life. In response to the falling calcium levels, there is a rise in the parathyroid hormone level, resulting in an increased serum calcium level. Abnormalities in this physiological response can lead to hypocalcemia in the neonate.

History

Maternal History

Key aspects of the maternal history include a history of gestational diabetes, maternal vitamin D deficiency, and maternal hypercalcemia from hyperparathyroidism or large intake of calcium carbonate in antacids.

Birth History

Key aspects of the birth history include premature gestational age, low birth weight, intrauterine growth restriction/small for gestational age, large for gestational age, and perinatal stress.

Patient History

Key aspects of the patient's history include diuretic use, daily calcium and phosphorus intake, vitamin intake, fat malabsorption, liver dysfunction, renal disease, and use of parenteral nutrition.

Physical Examination

Signs of hypocalcemia include the following:

- irritability,
- jitteriness or tremulousness,
- facial spasms,
- tetany,

- stridor, and
- focal or generalized seizures.

Nonspecific signs of hypocalcemia include

- apnea,
- tachycardia,
- cyanosis,
- emesis, and
- poor feeding.

Note that the Chvostek sign (tapping over the facial nerve at the angle of the jaw, resulting in a twitch of the nose or lips) or Trousseau sign (inflating the blood pressure cuff above systolic pressure for 2 minutes, leading to carpal muscle spasm) are not commonly seen in neonates.

Confirmatory Laboratory Studies

Specific laboratory tests obtained during a period of hypocalcemia will provide important diagnostic information regarding the underlying etiology. The following laboratory tests should be obtained when the infant is hypocalcemic (Table 72-1):

- serum calcium and ionized calcium,
- albumin,
- serum phosphorus,
- serum magnesium,
- intact parathyroid hormone (iPTH),
- urine calcium-to-creatinine ratio, and
- 25-hydroxyvitamin D level and 1,25-dihydroxyvitamin D level for late-onset or chronic hypocalcemia.

If a maternal etiology is suspected in early-onset hypocalcemia, the following are the recommended maternal laboratory tests:

Table 72-1 Key Laboratory Studies for Evaluation of Hypocalcemia

Serum calcium
Ionized calcium
Serum phosphorus
Intact parathyroid hormone
Serum albumin
Magnesium
Urine calcium-to-creatinine ratio
Serum creatinine
25-Hydroxyvitamin D[a]
1,25-Dihydroxyvitamin D

[a]If blood volume is a concern, consider obtaining maternal levels of 25-hydroxyvitamin D to assess neonatal stores.

- serum calcium,
- serum phosphorus,
- iPTH,
- 25-hydroxyvitamin D level.

Additional baseline ancillary tests include

- an electrocardiogram to evaluate for prolongation of the QTc (corrected QT) interval or
- radiographs of the long bones or ribs to look for rachitic changes.

Serum albumin concentrations affect serum calcium concentrations; thus, the serum calcium concentration must be adjusted: Corrected calcium [mg/dL] = Measured total calcium (mg/dL) + 0.8 (Normal serum albumin [g/dL]) − Serum albumin [g/dL]). The amount of ionized calcium is inversely proportional to the serum pH. There is a direct pH effect; alkalosis leads to a lower-than-expected value of ionized calcium for the serum calcium concentration, and acidosis leads to a higher-than-expected ionized calcium value.

Differential Diagnosis/Diagnostic Algorithm

The etiology of neonatal hypocalcemia is classified based on age at presentation: early onset (<72 hours of life) or late onset (> 72 hours of life) (Table 72-2).

Early Onset

Early onset of neonatal hypocalcemia occurs prior to 72 hours of life.

Infant of a Diabetic Mother

The causes of hypocalcemia in an infant of a diabetic mother include

- reduced placental transfer of calcium because of increased maternal urinary excretion of calcium and magnesium;
- decreased neonatal parathyroid hormone secretion;
- elevated calcitonin levels in the first 24–48 hours of life; and
- decreased calcium absorption and decreased calcium intake after birth.

Severe Vitamin D Deficiency

Poor maternal vitamin D stores lead to poor neonatal vitamin D stores, resulting in hypocalcemia in the early newborn period.

Maternal Hyperparathyroidism

Maternal hyperparathyroidism leads to increased transplacental transfer of calcium to the fetus. Higher fetal calcium levels suppress fetal parathyroid hormone

Table 72-2 Differential Diagnosis of Hypocalcemia

	Calcium	Phosphorus	iPTH	Magnesium	Urine Calcium/ Creatinine	25-OH Vitamin D	1,25 (OH)₂ Vitamin D
IDM	↓		↓	↓			
Maternal hyperparathyroidism	↓	↑	↓				
Vitamin D deficiency	↓	↓	↑			↓	
Prematurity	↓	Nl/↓	↓ (relative to Ca)				
Hypoparathyroidism	↓	↑	↓ (relative to calcium)	↓	↑	Nl	↓
Hypercalciuric hypocalcemia	↓	Nl	Nl		Nl/↑		

Abbreviation: iPTH, intact parathyroid hormone.

production, which can persist for several months after birth.

Prematurity

Premature infants have a blunted rise in parathyroid hormone in the first 24–48 hours of life. There is also physiologic resistance at the level of the kidney to phosphate secretion.

Perinatal Stress/Birth Asphyxia

With perinatal stress or birth asphyxia, there is an increased phosphate load from cell injury as well as elevated calcitonin levels, leading to hypocalcemia.

Exchange Transfusion

Citrate, an anticoagulant added to stored blood, complexes with calcium and reduces the amount of ionized calcium, leading to hypocalcemia. Hypocalcemia caused by citrate is not seen usually with small-volume (eg, 10–20 mL/kg) blood transfusions but can be seen with repeated or exchange transfusions because the amount of citrate is significantly higher.

Late Onset

Late onset of neonatal hypocalcemia occurs after 72 hours of life.

Hypoparathyroidism

Hypoparathyroidism results in hypocalcemia and hyperphosphatemia, along with decreased conversion of 25-hydroxyvitamin D to 1,25-dihydroxyvitamin D via the 1-α-hydroxylase enzyme. Hypoparathyroidism may be transient (a few weeks) or prolonged. Transient hypoparathyroidism is caused by a lack of maturity of the parathyroid gland after birth or maternal diabetes mellitus and resolves in the first few weeks of life.

Prolonged hypoparathyroidism can be due to error in embryogenesis of the parathyroid gland, including DiGeorge syndrome (22q11.2 deletion, velocardiofacial syndrome); mitochondrial disorders (eg, Kerns-Sayre syndrome); and calcium-sensing receptor gain-of-function mutations for which the calcium set point at which parathyroid hormone is secreted is lower than normal. Insensitivity or end-organ resistance to parathyroid hormone can lead to clinical hypoparathyroidism in the setting of elevated serum parathyroid hormone concentrations.

Vitamin D Deficiency

Low 25-hydroxyvitamin D concentrations (<20 ng/dL) in neonates can be caused by poor maternal stores that lead to poor vitamin D stores in the infant, infants who are exclusively breast fed without vitamin D supplementation, and more rare causes, including diminished 1-α–hydroxylase activity in the kidney (caused by vitamin D–dependent rickets or renal disease) or loss of function of the vitamin D receptor. Hypocalcemia from vitamin D deficiency can occur without physical or radiographic evidence of rickets.

Hyperphosphatemia

Excessive phosphate intake in evaporated milk or cow's milk formula creates a poorly soluble calcium salt, leading to decreased intestinal absorption of calcium and hypocalcemia.

Hypomagnesemia

Magnesium affects parathyroid hormone secretion and function. Hypomagnesemia can lead to impaired end-organ response to parathyroid hormone and diminished parathyroid hormone release. Hypocalcemia is refractory to calcium replacement therapy in the setting of hypomagnesemia.

Diuretic Therapy

Loop diuretics, such as furosemide, cause hypercalciuria by decreasing the tubular reabsorption of calcium, leading to hypocalcemia and bone demineralization.

TREATMENT

Initiation

Early-onset hypocalcemia in the first 72 hours of life is often asymptomatic, and expectant management is recommended unless the serum calcium is very low (total serum calcium < 6 mg/dL in preterm infant or < 7 mg/dL in term infant) or the neonate is symptomatic. In the symptomatic neonate, 10% calcium gluconate (elemental calcium 9.3 mg/mL) at a dose of 100 mg/kg over 5–10 minutes with continued monitoring of the heart rate and infusion site is recommended. The dose can be repeated if there is no clinical response in 10 minutes (total dose not to exceed 20 mg elemental calcium/kg).[2] After acute treatment is provided, maintenance calcium replacement therapy must be started. Maintenance calcium replacement can be given by adding calcium gluconate to the intravenous solution (50–75 mg elemental calcium/kg/d as a continuous drip or divided dose every 6 hours) or, if enteral feedings are tolerated, as calcium glubionate 50–100 mg elemental calcium/kg/d divided into 4–6 doses. Asymptomatic neonates can be managed by increasing the oral calcium intake using calcium glubionate (50–100 mg elemental calcium/kg/d divided into 4–6 doses) or calcium carbonate in divided doses every 4 to 6 hours and a low phosphorus formula such as Similac PM 60/40⁻ to establish an overall 4:1 ratio of calcium/phosphate intake. Neonates with hypoparathyroidism require treatment with calcitriol to allow absorption of enteral calcium; neonates with vitamin D deficiency rickets require treatment with ergocalciferol or cholecalciferol to restore vitamin D stores. Neonates with concurrent hypomagnesemia require magnesium supplementation to maintain appropriate serum magnesium levels.

Tests to Follow

Serum calcium or ionized calcium levels along with urine calcium and creatinine levels should be followed frequently and treatment modified to maintain eucalcemia (serum calcium in the low-normal range) and prevent hypercalciuria. Serum phosphate levels should also be followed in neonates with hypoparathyroidism. It is important to watch for side effects of treatment, including iatrogenic hypercalcemia, hypercalciuria, nephrocalcinosis, and renal insufficiency. Follow-up radiographs may be appropriate for infants with baseline rachitic changes.

Management Algorithm/Decision Tree

Indications for Discontinuation

Calcium supplementation should be adjusted to maintain eucalcemia and can be decreased when serum calcium concentrations are in the high-normal range to avoid hypercalcemia. Transient hypocalcemia may only require supplementation for a few days or few weeks; cases of prolonged hypocalcemia require many years, even lifelong, calcium replacement therapy. Hypocalcemia caused by diuretic use will resolve when the diuretic dose is sufficiently decreased or stopped, eliminating the need for calcium supplementation.

CONCLUSION/FOLLOW-UP

Aftercare Monitoring

Careful follow-up and monitoring of the neonate with hypocalcemia is required. Parents must be instructed on the signs and symptoms of hypocalcemia and situations in which the infant may be prone to hypocalcemia. Illness resulting in vomiting or diarrhea, poor enteral intake, and inability to tolerate oral calcium supplementation can result in a fall in the serum calcium level, necessitating frequent monitoring of the serum calcium and an increase in calcium supplementation. Neonates who no longer require daily calcium supplementation may be prone to hypocalcemia during illness or other stress (initiation or increase of diuretic therapy) and should have the serum calcium levels followed closely. Neonates with diuretic-induced hypocalcemia may require adjustment in calcium supplementation when doses of diuretics are increased or decreased.

Follow-up Tests

After discharge from neonatal intensive care, continued monitoring of serum calcium and phosphorus levels is required to adjust calcium supplementation. In neonates with vitamin D deficiency, repeat 25-hydroxyvitamin D levels should be obtained after the treatment course of vitamin D is complete. Follow-up radiographs may be appropriate to view resolution of rachitic changes.

Clinical Follow-up

After discharge from the hospital, the neonate should be followed by a pediatric endocrinologist who will monitor serum calcium levels, adjust medication dosage, and monitor growth and development. Certain neonates may require other subspecialty care based on associated medical issues.

Long-Term Outcome/Implications for Patient/Family

Transient hypocalcemia may resolve in a few days to weeks, and continued calcium supplementation is not required. Prolonged hypocalcemia will require long-term monitoring of serum calcium levels as the calcium requirements for infants change as they grow. Infants and children are at risk for hypocalcemia during illness, changes in certain medications (increase in loop diuretic therapy), or decreases in enteral intake, requiring close monitoring of calcium levels during these occasions. Infants with DiGeorge syndrome may have learning disabilities, cardiac disease, or poor growth because of feeding difficulties. These infants should be closely followed with individualized care with an emphasis on multidisciplinary care.

REFERENCES

1. Root AW, Diamon FB. Disorders of mineral homeostasis in the newborn, infant, child, and adolescent. In: Sperling MA, ed. Pediatric Endocrinology. 3rd ed. Philadelphia, PA: Saunders Elsevier; 2008:686–769.
2. Bringhurst FR, Demay MB, Kronenberg HM. Hormones and disorders of mineral metabolism. In: Kronenberg HM, Melmed S, Polonsky KS, Larsen PR, eds. Williams Textbook of Endocrinology. 11th ed. Philadelphia, PA: Saunders Elsevier; 2008:1203–1268.

Management of Hyperkalemia

R. S. Cohen

INDICATION

Management of hyperkalemia involves treatment of elevated serum potassium levels in patients in the neonatal intensive care unit (NICU), particularly those dependent on parenteral fluids.

Clinical Findings

Initially, neonates should be in good fluid and electrolyte balance and thus have normal serum potassium concentrations. Exceptions can and do occur rarely but need to be recognized in a timely fashion.

1. Maternal history suggestive of abnormal fluid and electrolyte status
   a. Renal diseases with abnormal electrolytes
   b. Diuretic therapy
   c. Malnutrition or very abnormal diet
   d. Oligohydramnios
2. Physical findings suggestive of abnormal electrolyte balance
   a. Edema/anasarca
   b. Ascites, abdominal/flank masses
   c. Ambiguous genitalia

Confirmatory/Baseline Tests

The usual neonate, even the very premature patient, does not need serum electrolytes measured immediately after birth. Initially, a neonate's electrolytes and creatinine should reflect the mother's status. Patients with a history or physical findings like those mentioned in the

discussion of clinical findings may need an electrolyte panel early in life. Note that in the face of normal placental and maternal renal function, a totally anephric neonate may have normal (ie, maternal) serum creatinine and potassium levels at birth.

1. Serum electrolytes should be followed closely in all low birth weight (LBW) and sick patients in the NICU. Serum potassium levels in neonates tend to be somewhat higher than in older children and adults and not uncommonly will be in the range of 5 to 6 mEq/L. However, levels greater than 6.5 should be watched closely, and those greater than 7 are associated with poor outcomes.
2. Hyperkalemia results in specific recognizable changes in the electrocardiogram (ECG) in the following progression:
   a. Tall, peaked T waves
   b. Prolonged P-R interval
   c. Widened QRS
   d. Bradycardia with abnormal QRS axis
   e. Ventricular fibrillation

Differential Diagnosis/Diagnostic Algorithm

Hyperkalemia in the neonate can be thought of in 4 categories:

1. Nonoliguric hyperkalemia (NOHK) occurs in the first few days of life in very low birth weight infants in the presence of normal urine output. It is caused by the transfer of potassium from the very high

intracellular concentration (~150 mEq/L) to the relatively low concentration in extracellular fluids. Factors that contribute to this potassium flux include

a. Immaturity of the energy-dependant Na^+-K^+ ion pump, which may be worsened by perinatal hypoxia or hypoglycemia

b. Acidosis resulting in increased H^+-K^+ exchange across cellular membranes

c. Epidemiologic findings associated with NOHK, including

   (1) Birth weight less than 1000 g
   (2) Fetal distress
   (3) Metabolic acidosis
   (4) Hyperglycemia (caused by osmolality and low insulin)
   (5) Polyuric renal failure
   (6) No antenatal steroid treatment

d. Tissue breakdown (eg, hemolysis, necrosis) is a minor contributor[1] to NOHK. Indeed, severe hemolytic disease of the newborn does not commonly result in life-threatening hyperkalemia. Rare situations exist in which tissue breakdown may result in hyperkalemia:

   (1) Tumorlysis (eg, congenital leukemia)
   (2) Rhabdomyolysis from trauma, commonly concomitant with oliguria
   (3) Rapid massive hemolysis (eg, transfusion reaction)

2. Secondary to renal dysfunction: Decreased urine output can result in inappropriate potassium retention commonly seen with renal failure.

3. Secondary to endocrine dysfunction: Disordered renin-aldosterone-angiotensin system function can result in hyperkalemia with or without hyponatremia.

   a. Congenital adrenal hyperplasia (CAH)
   b. Pseudohypoaldosteronism
   c. Hyporeninemic hypoaldosteronism
   d. Massive adrenal hemorrhage

4. Iatrogenic

   a. Administration of too high an intravenous potassium load can overwhelm the limited excretory capabilities of the premature kidney and result in hyperkalemia; for this reason, no potassium is added to the initial intravenous fluids until good renal function and falling serum potassium concentrations are demonstrated.

   b. Factitious hyperkalemia is caused by leakage of intracellular potassium into serum samples during heel sticks.

   c. Drug-induced hyperkalemia can be caused by several drugs used in the NICU, most commonly the following:

      (1) Spironolactone (impairs renal K^+ excretion)

      (2) Angiotensin-converting enzyme (ACE) inhibitors
      (3) Nonsteroidal anti-inflammatory drugs (NSAIDS; eg, indomethacin, Ibuprofen)
      (4) Calcium channel blockers
      (5) β-Blockers
      (6) Succinylcholine
      (7) Digoxin

MANAGEMENT

Workup for Etiology of Hyperkalemia

1. Nonoliguric
   a. Rule out drug related
   b. Rule out factitious (*particularly if heel stick sample*)
   c. Rule out potassium overload: consider nonobvious source (eg, transfused old blood, medications)
   d. Rule out acidosis with arterial blood glass (ABG) examination
   e. Rule out hyperosmolality: electrolytes/glucose/osmolality
   f. Rule out polyuric renal failure: creatinine/serum urea nitrogen (BUN)
   g. History consistent with NOHK

2. Renal dysfunction: usually oliguric but may be polyuric
   a. Elevated creatinine/BUN
   b. Elevated fractional excretion of sodium (FeNa)
   c. Postobstructive diuresis, renal tubular acidosis, and so on

3. Endocrine: lack of aldosterone function in kidney
   a. CAH screen (hydrocortisone, 17-hydroxyProgesterone, etc)
   b. Hypoaldosteronism (aldosterone levels)
   c. Pseudohypoaldosteronism (renin, angiotensin)

Monitoring for Treatment

1. Intake and output (I&O) must be monitored strictly, especially in the smallest patients.

2. Weights should be charted no less than daily and may need to be checked more frequently in high-risk situations. For this, the use of bed scales may be beneficial.

3. Initial laboratory studies should include those for serum electrolytes, BUN/creatinine, calcium, and glucose, and an ABG to assess for acidosis. If there is acidosis, then blood gases will need to be followed, or at least serum electrolytes with bicarbonates, to monitor for metabolic acidosis.

4. Potassium, calcium, and glucose should be monitored closely, preferably with bedside "point-of-care" technology, to provide rapid data and minimize blood loss.

5. Continuous ECG monitoring with diagnostic capabilities to evaluate T waves, rate/rhythm, P-R interval, QRS, and so on should be initiated.

TREATMENT

Figure 73-1 indicates the steps in treatment.

1. Calcium: Calcium treats abnormal ECG (does not lower serum potassium). Note that hypocalcemia may be more common in neonates with NOHK[2] and should be corrected.
   a. Works on myocardial cells to improve membrane potential, but does not lower serum potassium
   b. Dose: 10% calcium gluconate 0.5 mL/kg IV over 5 minutes

2. A glucose/insulin infusion moves potassium from extra- to intracellular space with adenosine triphosphatase (ATPase) pump
   a. Start dextrose infusion first, at 0.5–1.0 g/kg/h, because this will increase endogenous insulin levels.
   b. Once glucose levels increase to over 150 mg/dL, initiate Insulin infusion at 0.1 U/kg/h and adjust per glucose levels.

3. Albuterol inhalation (0.4 mg/kg q 2h by nebulizer) may also be helpful in lowering serum potassium but is less effective than glucose/insulin.[3] This also works via the ATPase pump. It must be used with care in patients with tachyarrhythmias.

4. Cation exchange resins have been used but appear to be less effective and have a significant risk of gastrointestinal injury (eg, perforation, necrotizing enterocolitis [NEC]).[4] They bind about 0.5–1.0 mEq of potassium per gram of resin given.[5]

5. Infusions of saline (10 mL/kg) and furosemide (1 mg/kg) have not been proven effective in altering outcome but may lower serum potassium levels acutely.

6. Sodium bicarbonate (1 mEq/kg IV) increases pH and thus may increase potassium flux from extracellular to intracellular space. Although recommended in cases of acidosis, its efficacy for treating hyperkalemia has not been demonstrated.

FOLLOW-UP

After resolution of the acute hyperkalemic event, ongoing monitoring to detect any relapse is indicated. The type and frequency of monitoring vary with the etiology.

1. NOHK usually is self-limited to the first few days of life.

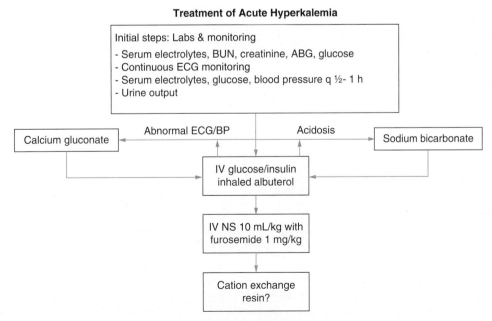

FIGURE 73-1 Treatment of acute hyperkalemia. ABG, arterial blood gas; BP, blood pressure; BUN, serum urea nitrogen; ECG, electrocardiogram; IV, intravenous; NS, normal saline.

2. Renal dysfunction, depending on exact cause and severity, will need ongoing monitoring with nephrology and may need dialysis.

3. Endocrine causes such as CAH are usually ameliorated by proper hormonal manipulation.

4. Iatrogenic causes usually resolve once the cause is corrected.

Neurologic follow-up is indicated for neonates with marked hyperkalemia requiring treatment because this has been associated with neurologic injury.

1. Cranial sonography should be obtained once stable.

2. Follow-up in high-risk infants is recommended.

REFERENCES

1. Mildenberger E, Versmold HT. Pathogenesis and therapy of non-oliguric hyperkalaemia of the premature infant. *Eur J Pediatr.* 2002;161:415–422.

2. Yaseen H. Nonoliguric hyperkalemia in neonates: a case-controlled study. *Am J Perinatol.* 2009;26:185–189.

3. Vemgal P, Ohlsson A. Interventions for non-oliguric hyperkalaemia in preterm neonates. *Cochrane Database Syst Rev.* 2007;(1):CD005257. doi:10.1002/14651858.CD005257.pub2.

4. O'Hare FM, Molloy EJ. What is the best treatment for hyperkalemia in a preterm infant? *Arch Dis Child.* 2008;93:174–176.

5. Masilamani K, van der Voort J. The management of acute hyperkalaemia in neonates and children. *Arch Dis Child.* 2012;97:376–380. doi:10.1136/archdischild-2011-300623.

Management of Hyponatremia

R. S. Cohen

INDICATION

This chapter outlines the treatment of low serum sodium levels in patients in the neonatal intensive care unit (NICU), particularly those dependent on parenteral fluids.

Epidemiology

The reported incidence of a serum sodium below 130 for very low birth weight infants in the NICU varies in the literature from about one-quarter to one-third.

Clinical Findings

Initially, neonates should be in good fluid and electrolyte balance and thus have normal serum sodium concentrations at birth. Exceptions can and do occur rarely but need to be recognized in a timely fashion.

1. Maternal history suggestive of abnormal fluid and electrolyte status
   a. Renal diseases with abnormal electrolytes
   b. Diuretic therapy
   c. Malnutrition or very abnormal diet
   d. Oligohydramnios
2. Physical findings suggestive of abnormal electrolyte balance
   a. Edema/anasarca
   b. Ascites, abdominal/flank masses
   c. Ambiguous genitalia

Laboratory

Usually, the neonate, even the very premature patient, does not need measurement of serum electrolytes immediately after birth. Initially, a neonate's electrolytes and creatinine values should reflect the mother's status. Patients with history or physical findings such as those mentioned may need to have an early evaluation of their electrolyte panel. Note that, in the face of normal placental and maternal renal function, a totally anephric neonate may have normal (ie, maternal) serum creatinine and sodium levels at birth.

1. Serum chemistries. These should be followed closely in all low birth weight (LBW) and sick patients in the NICU.
   a. Serum sodium levels in neonates tend to be somewhat lower than in older children and adults, and not uncommonly, they will be in the range of 130 to 140 mEq/L. However, levels less than 130 mEq/L should be watched closely, and levels less than 120 mEq/L are associated with poor outcomes.
   b. Serum potassium levels may be elevated in several conditions associated with hyponatremia (as discussed in the material that follows) and thus also should be followed.
   c. Serum urea and creatinine are markers for renal dysfunction and should be followed; again, they will be normal initially if placental and maternal renal functions are normal.
2. Urine chemistries. Urine sodium levels generally run below 30 mEq/L. We do not recommend routinely

Fractional excretion of Sodium (FeNa)

FeNa = [Urine Na/Serum Na] ÷ [Urine Creatinine/Serum Creatinine] × 100.

Sodium deficit

Na deficit (mEq) = (Wt in kg) (0.6)(target serum Na* – Serum Na)

*NB: Usually initial correction is to target Na of 125!

Serum Osmolality (Osm)

Osm = 2(Serum Na mEq/L) + (BUN mg/d ÷ 2.8) + (Glucose mg/dL ÷ 18)

FIGURE 74–1 Calculations for the fractional excretion of sodium. BUN, serum urea nitrogen.

following urine chemistries, but they can be useful in determining the etiology of electrolyte abnormalities. Simultaneous urine creatinine determinations also can be useful for calculating the fractional excretion of sodium (FeNa) (see Figure 74-1).

3. Serum and urine osmolality.

4. Weights. Weights need to be checked daily at a minimum. Falling serum sodium with climbing weight suggests fluid retention; falling weight suggests sodium depletion.

Differential Diagnosis/Diagnostic Algorithm

Hyponatremia in the first days of life generally reflects only a few pathophysiologies:

1. Fluid ("free water") overload. As discussed in Chapter 9, neonates are born with excess water that must be excreted. Because they are eunatremic at birth, this means that newborns also have a high total body sodium. However, the neonatal, particularly the premature, kidney has a limited ability to excrete a fluid load in the first few days of life. Thus, very early hyponatremia commonly is a problem of too much water and not too little sodium. Note that the chronic lack of thyroid hormone results in an inability to excrete a water load and thus can cause hyponatremia.

2. Increased sodium losses. Although unusual in the first few days, these can occur later in the NICU stay. Increased sodium losses can be caused by the following:

   a. Renal losses (eg, diuretic therapy)

   b. "Third-space" losses (eg, sepsis, necrotizing enterocolitis [NEC])

   c. Gastrointestinal losses (eg, emesis, large naso-gastric tube drainage)

3. Renal salt wasting. Immature kidneys can have increased obligate sodium losses. A slow decrement in serum sodium over the first week of life in the presence of a normal sodium intake implies increased renal losses. Elevated urinary sodium levels can help confirm this diagnosis.

4. Secondary to renal failure. Decreased renal function can result in oliguria, inappropriate water retention, and decreased reabsorption of sodium. This can result in increased urine sodium losses and excess free water and thus hyponatremia.

5. Disordered renin-aldosterone-angiotensin system function. This can result in salt loss and hyperkalemia, such as from

   a. Congenital adrenal hyperplasia (CAH)

   b. Pseudohypoaldosteronism

   c. Hyporeninemic hypoaldosteronism

   d. Adrenal hemorrhage

   e. Hypertensive-hyponatremia syndrome. This is a rare complication of renovascular hypertension with natriuresis, hypovolemia, and secondary hyperaldosteronism.

6. Inadequate sodium intake. Over time, a low sodium intake can result in hyponatremia. It is important to note that human milk provides a relatively low-sodium diet. This rarely results in severe hyponatremia. Remember that salt depletion results in secondary volume depletion.

7. Factitious hyponatremia. This can be caused by other circulating osmoles (eg, hyperglycemia, contrast agents) or hyperlipidemia.

8. Drug-induced hyponatremia. Several drugs used in the NICU, most commonly diuretics such as furosemide or the combination of hydrochlorothiazide and spironolactone ("Aldactazide"), can result in hyponatremia.

9. Syndrome of inappropriate secretion of antidiuretic hormone (SIADH). This is somewhat unusual in a neonate but may be seen in the presence of raised intracranial pressure or in response to increased intrathoracic pressure.

   a. Nephrogenic SIADH has been described in neonates.

b. Cerebral salt wasting (CSW). This is a poorly understood phenomenon of inappropriate salt and water loss after central nervous system (CNS) injury. Although hyponatremia with elevated urine osmolality may suggest SIADH, by definition CSW results in marked hypovolemia.

10. Hypothyroidism can impair water excretion and thus result in hyponatremia caused by fluid retention.

11. Glucocorticoid deficiency can impair water excretion and thus result in hyponatremia caused by fluid retention.

WORKUP FOR ETIOLOGY OF HYPONATREMIA

Figure 74-2 provides a 4-step algorithm for the workup for the etiology of hyponatremia.

Is It Real?

1. Rule out factitious hyponatremia (particularly if lab sample was drawn from vascular catheter).

2. Rule out hyperosmolality: Electrolytes/glucose/osmolality (eg, every 100 mg/dL increase in serum glucose decreases sodium by about 2.4 mEq/L).

3. Rule out diuretic induced hyponatremia.

Is It Renal Failure?

1. Creatinine/serum urea nitrogen (BUN) and FeNa are elevated (remember that diuretics will increase FeNa).

2. Renal failure usually is oliguric but may be polyuric.

3. If creatinine/BUN are normal but FeNa and urine sodium are elevated, look for causes of salt wasting (eg, renal salt wasting, CSW).

Is It Caused by Excess Free Water?

Neonates need to excrete significant water load in the first few days of life; too much fluid intake results in hypotonic fluid retention and either inadequate weight loss or even weight gain. These patients have no signs of hypovolemia.

1. FeNa and urine sodium are low: Edema is from exogenous fluid overload.

2. Urine osmolality and sodium are elevated: Consider causes of inadequate water diuresis (eg, SIADH, hypothyroidism, glucocorticoid deficiency).

Is It Caused by Low Total Body Sodium?

1. Sodium depletion results in secondary hypovolemia.

2. Excess weight loss, oliguria, and low blood pressure follow.

3. FeNa and urine sodium are low, but the creatinine/BUN may be slightly elevated because of hemoconcentration.

4. Serum potassium concentration usually is normal.

If Hyperkalemic

If hyperkalemia is present, consider renal-aldosterone dysfunction.

1. CAH screen (hydrocortisone, 17-hydroxyprogesterone, etc)

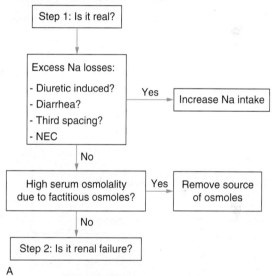

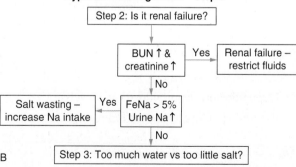

FIGURE 74–2 A 4-step algorithm for the workup for the etiology of hyponatremia. BP, blood pressure; BUN, serum urea nitrogen; FeNa, fractional excretion of sodium; HR, heart rate; NEC, necrotizing enterocolitis; nl, normal; N-SIADH, nephrogenic SIADH; SIADH, syndrome of inappropriate secretion of antidiuretic hormone; Sl, slight wt, weight.

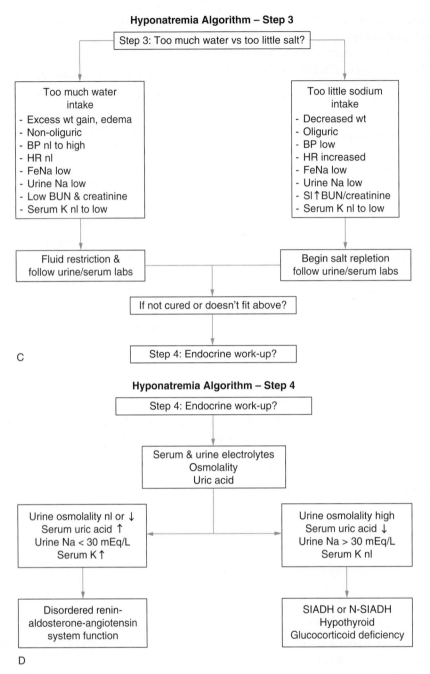

Hyponatremia Algorithm – Step 3

Step 3: Too much water vs too little salt?

Too much water intake
- Excess wt gain, edema
- Non-oliguric
- BP nl to high
- HR nl
- FeNa low
- Urine Na low
- Low BUN & creatinine
- Serum K nl to low

Too little sodium intake
- Decreased wt
- Oliguric
- BP low
- HR increased
- FeNa low
- Urine Na low
- Sl ↑ BUN/creatinine
- Serum K nl to low

Fluid restriction & follow urine/serum labs

Begin salt repletion follow urine/serum labs

If not cured or doesn't fit above?

Step 4: Endocrine work-up?

C

Hyponatremia Algorithm – Step 4

Step 4: Endocrine work-up?

Serum & urine electrolytes
Osmolality
Uric acid

Urine osmolality nl or ↓
Serum uric acid ↑
Urine Na < 30 mEq/L
Serum K ↑

Urine osmolality high
Serum uric acid ↓
Urine Na > 30 mEq/L
Serum K nl

Disordered renin-aldosterone-angiotensin system function

SIADH or N-SIADH
Hypothyroid
Glucocorticoid deficiency

D

FIGURE 74–2 *(Continued)*

2. Hypoaldosteronism (aldosterone levels)

3. Pseudohypoaldosteronism (renin, angiotensin)

Monitoring for Treatment

1. Intake and output (I&O) must be monitored strictly, especially in the smallest patients.

2. Weights should be charted no less than daily and may need to be checked more frequently in high-risk situations. For this, the use of bed scales may be beneficial.

3. Electrolytes, BUN, and creatinine values should be monitored closely, preferably with bedside "point-of-care" technology to provide rapid data and minimize blood loss.

TREATMENT

Fluid Restriction

Decreasing free water intake by approximately 20% will start correcting hyponatremia caused by excess free water that results from either administration of too much fluid or inappropriate water retention (ie, SIADH).

Normal Saline

Normal saline (NS) (0.9%; 154 mEq/L) is usually infused as the first and safest step for replenishing a sodium deficit. An intravenous bolus of NS, 10 mL/kg, will restore both sodium and volume losses and improve hyponatremia caused by hypovolemia or increased sodium losses in the presence of appropriate levels of antidiuretic hormone (ADH); it will not help SIADH.

Hypertonic Saline

Hypertonic saline (3%; 513 mEq/L) is used for severe hyponatremia (sodium < 120 mEq/L) to correct to a target serum sodium of 125 mEq/L over about 12 hours, then correct the rest of the deficit over the next 24 hours (see Figure 74-2 for calculation). The rate of correction should not exceed 0.5 mEq/L per hour.

FOLLOW-UP

1. After resolution of the acute hyponatremic event, ongoing monitoring to detect any relapse is indicated. The type and frequency of monitoring vary with the etiology.

2. Iatrogenic fluid overload should not recur once recognized and appropriate fluid restriction is initiated.

3. Inadequate sodium intake needs to be followed with both serum and urine sodium levels to ensure that sodium intake is greater than ongoing urinary losses.

4. Renal dysfunction, depending on exact cause and severity, will need ongoing monitoring with nephrology and may need dialysis.

5. Endocrine causes such as CAH are usually ameliorated by proper hormonal manipulation but require close follow-up.

6. Neurologic follow-up is indicated for neonates with marked hyponatremia requiring treatment because this has been associated with neurologic injury and hearing loss.

   a. Cranial sonography should be obtained once stable.

   b. Audiology screening should be done prior to discharge.

   c. Follow-up in the high-risk infant is recommended.

SUGGESTED READING

Baraton L, Ancel PY, Flamant C, Orsonneau JL, Darmaun D, Rozé JC. Impact of changes in serum sodium levels on 2-year neurologic outcomes for very preterm neonates. *Pediatrics.* 2009;124:e655–e661. doi:10.1542/peds.2008–3415.

Barnette AR, Myers BJ, Berg CS, Inder TE. Sodium intake and intraventricular hemorrhage in the preterm infant. *Ann Neurol.* 2010;67:817–823.

Daftary AS, Patole SK, Whitehall J. Hypertension-hyponatremia syndrome in neonates: case report and review of literature. *Am J Perinatol.* 1999;16:385–389.

Ertl T, Hadzsiev K, Vincze O, Pytel J, Szabo I, Sulyok E. Hyponatremia and sensorineural hearing loss in preterm infants. *Biol Neonate.* 2001;79:109–112.

Guarner J, Hochman J, Kurbatova E, Mullins R. Study of outcomes associated with hyponatremia and hypernatremia in children. *Pediatr Dev Pathol.* 2011;14:117–123. doi:10.2350/10-06-0858-OA.1

Marcialis MA, Dessi A, Pintus MC, Irmesi R, Fanos V. Neonatal hyponatremia: differential diagnosis and treatment. *J Matern Fetal Neonatal Med.* 2011;24(Suppl 1):75–79.

Rivkees SA. Differentiating appropriate antidiuretic hormone secretion, inappropriate antidiuretic hormone secretion and cerebral salt wasting: the common, uncommon, and misnamed. *Curr Opin Pediatr.* 2008;20:448–452.

75 Management of Transient Hypoglycemia

R. S. Cohen

BACKGROUND

Serum glucose levels (GLU) in the fetus are dependent on transplacental transfer of glucose from the mother and generally reflect maternal levels. Elevated maternal GLU can cause fetal hyperglycemia and increased insulin production by the fetal pancreas, resulting in fetal macrosomia. After separation from the placenta, newborn infants have to maintain their own GLU without maternal assistance. Thus, although usually euglycemic, the newborn could be either hyperglycemic or hypoglycemic depending on the maternal serum glucose and the infant's ability for endocrine autoregulation.

EPIDEMIOLOGY

The exact incidence of transient neonatal hypoglycemia is unknown. Studies using continuous glucose monitoring have suggested that it is more common than previously believed, but the significance of this finding in asymptomatic, otherwise-well babies is unclear. Specific subgroups of neonates have been identified as having significantly increased risk of developing hypoglycemia:

Small-for-gestational-age (SGA) infants

Large-for-gestational-age (LGA) infants

Infant of diabetic mother (IDM)

Infant of gestational diabetic mother (IGDM)

Septic infants

Late preterm infants (LPTIs) born at 34^{+0} to 36^{+6} weeks' gestation

Postdate infants

CLINICAL FINDINGS

1. Maternal history suggestive of abnormal glucose status

   Diabetes mellitus

   Obesity

   Intravenous glucose administration

   Abnormal fetal growth

   Placental abnormalities (eg, too large/small, abruption)

   Fetal intolerance of labor (eg, abnormal tracing, meconium staining)

2. Neonatal findings suggestive of abnormal glucose homeostasis

   Intrauterine growth restriction/SGA

   Macrosomia/LGA

   Jitteriness

   Seizures

   Lethargy/poor feeding

   Apnea

   Unremarkable examination

LABORATORY WORKUP

Screening is recommended as follows only for at-risk infants:

1. IDM and LGA infants: screen for first 24 hours
2. LPTIs and SGA infants: screen for first 12 hours
3. Continue screening hypoglycemic infants until maintaining preprandial GLU 45 mg/dL or more for 2–3 feeding intervals

The definition of neonatal hypoglycemia has been debated, but most recently, the American Academy of Pediatrics (AAP) has defined it as follows:

GLU less than 40 mg/dL *and* symptomatic

GLU less than 25 mg/dL from birth to 4 hours of age after initial feeding

GLU less than 35 mg/dL prior to subsequent feeding from 4 to 24 hours of age

A simplified algorithm for screening is shown in Figure 75-1.

TREATMENT

Enteral

Initial treatment is by enteral nutrition whenever possible if the baby is asymptomatic. See Figure 75-1 for a simplified treatment algorithm for asymptomatic neonates.

Glucose Infusion

If the baby is symptomatic or the GLU remains below 25 mg/dL when checked 1 hour after feeding, then intravenous treatment is needed:

1. Minibolus of 200 mg/kg dextrose (eg, 2 mL/kg of 10% dextrose in water [D10W]), followed by intravenous infusion.
2. Dextrose intravenously at about 5–8 mg/kg per minute (approximately 80–130 mL/kg daily of D10W) adjusted to keep GLU in the range of 40 to 60 mg/dL.
3. Avoid hyperglycemia, which can lead to increased insulin secretion, thus exacerbating the problem.

Once the GLU has stabilized in the appropriate range, the intravenous D10W can be weaned slowly by decreasing the rate by small increments every other feeding while continuing to feed and following GLU prefeeding.

If the patient does not maintain GLU of 45 mg/dL or greater after treatment as outlined or does not tolerate attempts to wean the rate of intravenous D10W, then proceed to work up for persistent hyperglycemia, beginning with obtaining critical laboratory values (see Chapter 105).

FOLLOW-UP

Continue to monitor GLU for screening interval described in Figure 75-1 and previously this chapter.

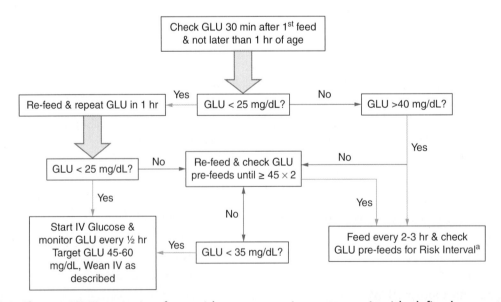

FIGURE 75-1 Glucose (GLU) screening for at-risk asymptomatic neonates. At risk defined as gestational age 34^{+0} to 36^{+6} weeks (late-preterm infants, LPTIs). small for gestional age (SGA); infant of diabetic mother (IDM); large for gestational age (LGA). [a]Risk interval defined as up to 24 hours for LPTIs and SGA infants and up to 12 hours for IDMs and LGA infants. IV, intravenous.

Symptomatic infants are at significant risk of neurologic injury and may be considered for magnetic resonance imaging (MRI) before discharge. They should be followed closely for evidence of developmental delay.

Asymptomatic infants with easily controlled transient hypoglycemia do not require neuroimaging or special developmental follow-up.

SUGGESTED READING

Boluyt N, van Kempen A, Offringa M. Neurodevelopment after neonatal hypoglycemia: a systematic review and design of an optimal future study. *Pediatrics*. 2006;117:2231–2243.

Burns CM, Rutherford MA, Boardman JP, Cowan FM. Patterns of cerebral injury and neurodevelopmental outcomes. *Pediatrics*. 2008;122:65–74.

Committee on Fetus and Newborn. Postnatal glucose homeostasis in late-preterm and term infants. *Pediatrics*. 2011;127:575–579. doi:10.1542/peds.2010-3851.

Harris DL, Battin MR, Weston PJ, Harding JE. Continuous glucose monitoring in newborn babies at risk of hypoglycemia. *J Pediatr*. 2010;157:198–202.

Harris DL, Weston PJ, Harding JE. Incidence of neonatal hypoglycemia in babies identified as at risk. *J Pediatr*. 2012. doi:10.1016/j.jpeds.2012.05.022.

Kerstjens JM, Bocca-Tjeertes IF, de Winter AF, Reijneveld SA, Bos AF. Neonatal morbidities and developmental delay in moderately preterm-born children. *Pediatrics*. 2012;130;e265–e272. doi:10.1542/peds.2012-0079.

Straussman S, Levitsky LL. Neonatal hypoglycemia. *Curr Opin Endocrinol Diabetes Obes*. 2010;17:20–24.

Part B: Brain

(76) # Therapeutic Hypothermia

Arlene Sheehan, Vishnu Priya Akula,
M. Bethany Ball, and Krisa Van Meurs

INDICATION

Randomized clinical trials performed around the world have shown that therapeutic hypothermia reduces death and major neurodevelopmental disability for infants with moderate-to-severe hypoxic ischemic encephalopathy (HIE).[1–7]

Hypothermia is initiated within 6 hours after birth and continued for 72 hours, with a target temperature of 33°C–34°C for whole-body hypothermia and 34°C–35°C for selective head cooling. Eligible infants were 35 weeks or greater gestational age in 2 trials and 36 weeks or greater or 37 weeks or greater in the remaining trials. A recent systemic review and meta-analysis that included 7 large randomized clinical trials and 1214 newborns showed a reduction in the risk of death or major neurodevelopmental disability (risk ratio [RR], 0.76; 95% confidence interval [CI], 0.69–0.84) and an increase in the rate of survival with normal neurological function (RR, 1.63; CI, 1.36–1.95) at age 18 months.[8] The number needed to treat is 7 to prevent 1 case of neonatal death or major disability. Newborns with moderate HIE had a greater reduction in the risk of death or major neuro-developmental disability at age 18 months (RR, 0.67; 95% CI, 0.56–0.81) when compared to those with severe HIE (RR, 0.83; CI, 0.74–0.92). There was no difference in head vs whole-body cooling. Follow-up at 6 to 7 years of age of the National Institute of Child Health and Human Development (NICHD) Neonatal Network trial participants found that death or an IQ score below 70 occurred in 47% of the hypothermia group compared to 62% of the control group ($p = .06$).[9] This result was not statistically significant; however, hypothermia was associated with a lower death rate without an increase in the rate of severe disability in survivors.

Clinical Findings

History

The recognition of moderate or severe HIE requires a detailed obstetric history, including any acute perinatal event, such as a placental abruption, cord events such as prolapse or complete knot, maternal hemorrhage, uterine rupture, prolonged fetal bradycardia, or nonreassuring fetal heart tracings. Other essential criteria include Apgar score of 5 or less at 10 minutes or the continued need for ventilator support initiated at birth and continued for more than 10 minutes.

Physical

A modified Sarnat neurologic examination is performed to determine eligibility for therapeutic hypothermia unless seizures have been observed. Abnormalities must be identified in at least 3 of the following 6 categories: level of consciousness, spontaneous activity, posture, tone, primitive reflexes, and autonomic nervous system (Table 76-1).

Baseline Tests

The laboratory eligibility criteria for therapeutic hypothermia include a pH of 7.0 or less or base deficit of less than 16 mmol/L in an umbilical cord gas or any gas during the first hour after birth. If the pH is between 7.01 and 7.15, base deficit is between 10 and

Table 76-1 Criteria for Defining Moderate and Severe Encephalopathy

Category	Moderate Encephalopathy	Severe Encephalopathy
Level of consciousness	Lethargic	Stupor/coma
Spontaneous activity	Decreased	No activity
Posture	Distal flexion	Decerebrate
Tone	Hypotonia (focal, general)	Flaccid
Primitive reflexes		
Suck	Weak	Absent
Moro	Incomplete	Absent
Autonomic system		
Pupils	Constricted	Skew deviation/dilated/nonreactive to light
Heart rate	Bradycardia	Variable heart rate
Respirations	Periodic breathing	Apnea

15.9 mmol/L, or no blood gas is available, additional criteria are required, including an acute perinatal event *and* 10-minute Apgar score of 5 or less *or* assisted ventilation for 10 or more minutes.

Several of the randomized clinical trials required amplitude-integrated electroencephalography (aEEG) with abnormal background activity for study entry; many centers continue to use this eligibility criterion for therapeutic hypothermia.[1,4,5]

Other baseline laboratory studies performed in this population include a complete blood cell count (CBC), blood culture, C-reactive protein value, coagulation panel, complete metabolic panel, and creatinine kinase, troponin, and lactate values. Conventional EEG, when performed with video recording, helps with identification of infants with clinical and subclinical seizures.

Differential Diagnosis

The following diagnostic categories must be considered when evaluating an encephalopathic infant, particularly in the absence of an acute perinatal event:

- Metabolic disorders
- Sepsis
- Neuromuscular disorders
- Chromosomal disorders and genetic syndromes
- Central nervous system malformations or injury (eg, subdural or subgaleal hemorrhage)

Exclusions

The following are exclusions for treatment:

1. Infants with lethal chromosomal or congenital anomalies are usually excluded.

2. Infants presenting after 6 hours of age are often not cooled as there are few data suggesting benefit. The window for therapeutic hypothermia is not specifically known; however, it is known that neuroprotection is influenced by the timing of therapy.[10,11] The NICHD Neonatal Research Network is currently conducting a trial to evaluate the effect of cooling initiated between 6 and 24 hours of age (http://ClinicalTrials.gov, identifier: NCT00614744).

3. Infants with profound asphyxia are not likely to benefit; however, early identification of these infants is challenging. At this time, no reliable early clinical markers of nonresponse have been identified, and in the absence of this information, therapeutic hypothermia is initiated and later discontinued if other information, such as neurologic examination, EEG, and magnetic resonance imaging (MRI), confirm that the prognosis is poor.

4. The use of therapeutic hypothermia to treat mild HIE is controversial. Two trials unintentionally enrolled newborns with mild HIE.[6,7] Zhou et al found no death or severe disability in the newborns with mild HIE; Jacobs et al reported a sizable rate of death and disability associated with mild HIE.[6,7] The latter study did not use a standardized neurologic assessment tool or formally certify the transport personnel who assessed newborns for eligibility. Misclassification of the level of encephalopathy is potentially responsible for the higher-than-anticipated rates of death and disability.

5. Parental refusal is a cause for exclusion.

PREPARATION

Ethical Considerations and Consent

Neonatal therapeutic hypothermia has been studied in a specific patient population: near-term infants who are less than 6 hours of age and meet strict criteria for moderate-to-severe HIE. Multiple prospective, randomized, controlled trials have shown improved neurodevelopmental outcomes in infants with HIE who are cooled. Based on the results of these studies, it would be unethical to withhold this treatment from near-term infants with moderate-to-severe HIE.[12] Parents must be informed of the availability of this therapy in a timely fashion and offered the option of transfer to another facility if hypothermia is not available at the birth hospital.

The situation becomes less clear if the patient is identified as a candidate for cooling outside the 6-hour window postbirth, if the infant is less than 36 weeks' gestational age, or if the neurologic status does not meet the specific criteria used in randomized clinical trials. Because the complications of hypothermia are few, it could be argued that ethically any patient who might benefit from the therapy should be offered treatment, for instance, the infant who qualifies for treatment but does not arrive at a tertiary facility until 7 hours of age or the infant who qualifies for treatment but is 35 weeks' gestation. Is it ethical to withhold treatment from such patients because they do not meet criteria used in studies? Conversely, is it ethical to treat patients who may not benefit from the therapy? Some centers have chosen only to treat infants who meet the strict criteria followed in the clinical trials; others decide whether to treat on an individual basis. If treatment is offered to infants who do not meet the criteria used in randomized clinical trials, informed parental consent is essential.[12]

Another ethical dilemma encountered by centers that offer hypothermia treatment is the potential for delay in outcome prediction. The early sequelae of HIE present during the 72-hour period in which cooling has been shown to be helpful. Cooling can suppress seizures and alter the EEG pattern, confounding the prediction of poor neurologic outcome based on electrographic evidence. Imaging studies such as computed tomography (CT) or MRI are difficult, if not impossible, to obtain in the cooled infant. Cooled patients are often treated with sedatives or narcotics that alter neurologic status. Discussions about prognosis and decisions about continuation of intensive care are often delayed until after the 72-hour treatment window, by which time the cardiorespiratory status of these patients may have improved to such an extent that discontinuation of support is no longer an option. The result can be prolongation of life in a severely damaged infant, greatly altering the options available to parents.[13] If during the 72-hour treatment period the prognosis for a severely ill infant becomes hopeless, parents should be informed that they may choose to end hypothermia treatment and consider withdrawal of intensive support.[12]

Multiple studies have shown that cooling should begin as soon as possible following a neurologic insult, hence the 6-hour postbirth window used in the clinical trials completed to date. Informed parental consent is mandatory when offering a treatment within the confines of a clinical trial. Obtaining consent within the 6-hour window can be difficult for many reasons and may result in nontreatment because of lack of consent. Because hypothermia is considered by many to be standard of care for moderate-to-severe HIE in the first 6 hours of life, consent is not routinely required. In fact, failure to treat based on lack of consent could be viewed as unethical. Outside a study protocol, treatment should be initiated within the 6-hour window, with the intent of informing the parents and reaching agreement about treatment as soon as possible.[12]

Monitoring for Treatment

Intensive Care Monitoring

Infants with neonatal encephalopathy are at risk for multiorgan failure. These infants should be cared for in a level III neonatal intensive care unit (NICU) that can provide intensive monitoring and cardiorespiratory support, correction of metabolic disturbances, treatment of seizures, access to neuroimaging, and consultation with pediatric neurology.

Laboratory Workup

The CBC with platelet count; coagulation panel; chemistries, including liver enzymes; and lactate should be monitored.

Although no increased risk for bleeding has been seen in the randomized controlled trials of hypothermia therapy, changes in hematologic parameters are evident with cooling. Lower platelet counts, abnormalities of platelet activation and aggregation, and delayed activation of the fibrinolytic system have been reported.

Blood Gas Monitoring

Temperature Correction
Blood gas equipment is calibrated to analyze a sample at a "typical" patient body temperature, generally 37°C. Two of the early trials of hypothermia recommended that blood gases run on cooled patients should be performed on an instrument calibrated to the core temperature.[1,3] In an evaluation of the iStat® instrument (Abbott Point of Care, Princeton, NJ), blood gases from patients cooled to 33.5°C were 15% lower

on the corrected instrument than on the instrument calibrated to 37°C, and pH was 15% higher (Sheehan, personal communication). Failure to monitor ventilation with an instrument calibrated to the appropriate temperature in hypothermic patients can result in nontreatment of hypocarbia and alterations in cerebral blood flow.

Avoidance of Hypocarbia

Pappas et al explored the association of hypocarbia and outcome and concluded that death and disability was increased with longer cumulative exposure to carbon dioxide levels below 35 mm Hg.[14]

Electroencephalography

It is unknown whether seizures result in brain injury or if their presence signifies an underlying brain disorder. It also remains unclear whether treatment of seizures provides neurodevelopmental benefit. Studies have shown an association between neonatal seizures and neurologic deficits.[15,16] Glass et al compared the neurodevelopmental outcomes of infants who had HIE and seizures with those of infants who had HIE alone and found infants with HIE and seizures had more adverse neurologic outcomes.[17] They concluded that clinical neonatal seizures and their treatment are associated with adverse cognitive and neuromotor outcome and speculated that seizures impair the developing brain. The available evidence supports routine EEG or aEEG monitoring of infants who qualify for cooling, as well as treatment with antiepileptics when seizures are detected.

Drug Monitoring

Therapeutic hypothermia may alter the pharmacokinetics and pharmacodynamics of drugs used in critically ill newborns with HIE. Some drugs have reduced clearance, longer elimination half-life, and a smaller volume of distribution when used during cooling, related to the decline in function of the cytochrome P450 enzyme system and other physiologic adaptations to low temperature. Drugs known to be affected by hypothermia include morphine, midazolam, fentanyl, vecuronium, phenytoin, phenobarbital, and gentamicin.[18]

Sedation and Pain Control Considerations

Pain and discomfort can be challenging to assess in cooled newborns as the majority are encephalopathic and do not exhibit the usual indicators of pain. Some cooled infants will demonstrate signs of stress with grimacing, crying, and shivering. Because most patients develop sinus bradycardia while cooled, a heart rate in the normal range may be an indicator of pain. Elevated cortisol levels were reported in cooled animals as compared to normothermic controls.[19] Furthermore, in the same animal model, hypothermia without sedation failed to provide neuroprotection.[19] The authors speculated that inadequate sedation of infants undergoing hypothermia may block the protective effects of hypothermia.

PROCEDURE

Therapeutic hypothermia can be achieved using passive or active cooling methods. The ideal method achieves the desired temperature quickly, maintains that temperature without fluctuation, and avoids over- and undercooling during the initiation and rewarming phases.

Passive cooling is defined as withholding of external heat sources. The isolette or warmer is turned off, and no blankets or clothes are used. The temperature is monitored manually, and heat is provided if the patient becomes too cold. This method of cooling is frequently associated with profound overcooling and great fluctuations in temperature.[20–23]

Active cooling employs devices such as water- or gel-filled mattresses, fans, and gel or water pillows. Active cooling methods may be manual, with adjustments to devices made by the caregiver, or servo controlled, with the patient temperature regulated by an electronic temperature probe with a feedback mechanism to the cooling device. Compared to adults, infant body temperature is more responsive to conductive heating and cooling because of a higher ratio of skin contact area to body mass. Servo-controlled cooling is superior to manually controlled cooling with respect to avoidance of over- and undercooling and fluctuations in core temperature.[24]

Active servo-controlled cooling has been studied in newborns with HIE using several different methods, including selective head cooling, whole-body cooling, and servo-regulated fan. Selective head cooling utilized a servo-regulated, water-filled, fitted cooling cap attached to a heating/cooling unit (Olympic Medical Cool Care System, Olympic Medical, Seattle, WA). It was used in conjunction with a radiant warmer to maintain a core rectal body temperature of 34°C–35°C. Studies of newborns with moderate-to-severe encephalopathy demonstrated a neuroprotective benefit from mild hypothermia achieved with selective head cooling.[1,6] A servo-controlled fan was designed to provide an inexpensive and safe method of delivering whole-body hypothermia to infants with HIE. This technique, which uses a fan directed cephalocaudally over the infant and a radiant warmer to control core temperature, was successful in cooling patients without overshoot or significant temperature variability.[25]

Whole-body cooling with a water-filled blanket system is the most extensively used and studied of the techniques currently available for hypothermia in newborns. The radiant warmer is turned off, and cooling to 33°C–34°C is achieved using a water-filled blanket, esophageal or rectal temperature probe, and servo-controlled heating/cooling unit. The devices available in the United States suitable for use in newborns are the CritiCool® (Mennen Medical, Southampton, PA) and the Blanketrol® system (Cincinnati Sub-Zero, Cincinnati, OH).

Initiation

Whole-Body Cooling Using the Blanketrol System

The Blanketrol II and III are used to control patient temperature through conductive heat transfer. Both devices contain a heater, compressor, circulating pump, and microprocessor board. For initiation and maintenance of hypothermia and for rewarming, the servo-regulated mode is used with the Blanketrol II. The Blanketrol III can be used like the Blanketrol II for maintenance and rewarming in standard servo mode or by utilizing a software program called Gradient Control to minimize fluctuations in water temperature. With either system, an infant-size blanket is placed under the patient and water is continuously circulated between the Blanketrol heater/cooler unit and the blanket. A probe is placed in the esophagus or rectum for servo-regulation of patient temperature. When using the Blanketrol in standard servo mode, a second larger blanket added to the cooling circuit will act as a heat sink and damp patient temperature fluctuations that occur when only the small neonatal-size blanket is used. The current standard of care is to cool to a temperature of 33°C–34°C and maintain this temperature for 72 hours. Rewarming is done slowly, increasing the temperature by 0.5°C per hour. Care should be taken to avoid rapid rewarming and hyperthermia. Patients should be monitored closely as seizures and hypotension can occur during, and in the hours following, rewarming.

Infants Who Are Slow to Rewarm

Many infants will not reach normothermia in the initial 7-hour rewarming period, and some may take up to 24 hours. The Blanketrol system should remain in place with the temperature set to 37°C degrees. The radiant warmer should remain off. The system should be checked to make sure it is functioning properly, and the environment should be checked for drafts. If after 24 hours of rewarming, normothermia has not been achieved, the Blanketrol system can be discontinued and the final warming done slowly using the radiant warmer, being careful not to exceed a warming rate of 0.5°C per hour.

Hypothermia on Extracorporeal Membrane Oxygenation

Selected patients on extracorporeal membrane oxygenation (ECMO) may also meet the criteria for therapeutic hypothermia. All ECMO systems include a heating/cooling device that is used to control blood temperature in the extracorporeal circuit. This can be used to provide therapeutic hypothermia by setting the device to cool the patient to the desired temperature and manually adjusting based on a core temperature reading. The ECMO heater displays fluid temperature (circuit blood temperature), but this reading does not accurately reflect core body temperature and should not be used to servo control cooling during hypothermia treatment. Esophageal or rectal temperatures can be used to monitor the hypothermia patient on ECMO, but care must be taken with use of these probes because of systemic heparinization during extracorporeal bypass.

Hypothermia During Neonatal Transport

Initiation of hypothermia must occur within 6 hours of birth for optimal neuroprotection. The 6-hour window is easily achieved when an infant is born at a level III NICU; however, the majority of the infants in the large randomized trials were outborn and required transport to a setting where therapeutic hypothermia could be provided. In the 3 randomized trials that performed cooling in transport, there were limited data or discussion of the specific implementation, temperature profiles, or outcomes of infants cooled in transport.[2,4,7]

Many cooling centers have chosen to offer cooling during transport by withholding external heat sources (passive cooling) or by using ice/gel packs (active cooling).[26] Despite careful attention to temperature management in transport and the development of clinical protocols, the temperatures achieved during transport are not consistently in the target range (33°C–34°C).[20–22] Until recently there were no portable servo-regulated cooling devices approved by the Food and Drug Administration (FDA) for use during transport in the United States. The Tecotherm Neo (Inspiration Healthcare, LTD, Leicester, UK), a small, portable, servo-regulated cooling device with continuous core temperature monitoring, is now approved for use.

Monitoring

Temperature Monitoring

During cooling, the minimal standard for temperature monitoring is a core temperature measurement every 15 minutes for the first 4 hours, every hour for the next 8 hours, and every 4 hours during the remaining period of hypothermia treatment.[27] The goal of hypothermia treatment is to cool the brain temperature to 33°C–34°C. Because brain temperature cannot be directly monitored at the bedside, esophageal or rectal temperatures are routinely used as surrogates. In a study of patients undergoing deep hypothermia during cardiopulmonary bypass, with brain temperature measured directly with a thermocouple embedded in the cerebral cortex, esophageal temperature was found to be a better approximation of brain temperature than nasopharyngeal, rectal, pulmonary artery, bladder, or axillary measurements.[28] Skin temperature as a proxy for core temperature was studied; a wide discrepancy between skin and rectal temperatures was seen.[22] Landry et al compared simultaneous axillary and rectal temperature measurements and found a wide variability at all stages of cooling.[29]

Overcooling is seen with non–servo-regulated cooling, particularly during transport. It can lead to "cold-injury syndrome," which is associated with body temperature below 34°C and is characterized by increased mortality, sclerema, renal failure, pulmonary hemorrhage, disseminated intravascular coagulation (DIC), hypoglycemia, electrolyte and acid-base disturbance, increased risk of infection, and cardiac complications.[30]

Elevated body temperature may occur during rewarming or after hypothermia is discontinued. It is important to be aware that elevated body temperature has been associated with exacerbation of the brain injury caused by HIE.[31,32] For this reason, it is imperative that patients be rewarmed slowly, no more than 0.5°C hourly, and that body temperature be monitored frequently in the postcooling period.

Positioning

Infants must remain supine. Rolls should be placed under the blanket for nesting, bringing it up around the sides of the infant and under the legs, increasing the surface area in contact with the blanket.

Vital Signs

Heart Rate

Most cooled infants develop benign sinus bradycardia, with heart rates between 60 and 100 beats per minute. Heart rates above 120 beats per minute may be a sign of pain or stress in the cooled infant.

Blood Pressure

Therapeutic hypothermia has not been associated with hypotension. A multicenter, randomized, controlled study showed that mild systemic hypothermia did not affect arterial blood pressure or the need for inotropes or volume in infants with moderate-to-severe encephalopathy.[33]

Skin Integrity

In the cooled infant, perfusion of the skin may be decreased by perinatal asphyxia and further decreased by hypothermia. Cooled patients may exhibit skin changes, including cyanosis, erythema, and sclerema. More rarely, patients may develop subcutaneous fat necrosis, which usually presents several days or even weeks after discontinuation of cooling therapy.[34,35] Skin complications may be lessened by patient positioning, such as tilting side to side to avoid constant pressure on the back during cooling. Avoidance of overcooling may be protective of skin integrity. Filippi et al studied 39 infants cooled with the Blanketrol III system and compared the automatic temperature control mode to the gradient control mode.[36] Two of the 11 infants cooled in the automatic mode developed skin complications consistent with subcutaneous fat necrosis; none of the 28 infants treated with the gradient control mode developed skin complications. The gradient control mode may be superior because of fewer temperature fluctuations.

Hypercalcemia is a potentially lethal complication of subcutaneous fat necrosis.[37] The etiology is uncertain but may involve production of nonrenal $1,25(OH)_2D_3$ from the skin lesions. It may present at the same time as the skin lesions or up to 6 months later. Treatment includes limiting calcium and vitamin D ingestion, hydration, and diuretics. Any infant with the diagnosis of subcutaneous fat necrosis posthypothermia should have serum calcium levels followed regularly in the first 6 months of life.

Exit Strategy

Infants who qualify for hypothermia are often critically ill. Despite intensive care, their condition may deteriorate, and a decision may be made to discontinue support. The timing of this decision should not be affected by a desire to complete the therapeutic hypothermia treatment regimen.

REFERENCES

1. Gluckman PD, Wyatt JS, Azzopardi D, et al. Selective head cooling with mild systemic hypothermia after neonatal encephalopathy: multicentre randomized trial. *Lancet.* 2005; 365(9460):663–670.

2. Eicher DJ, Wagner CL, Katikaneni LP, et al. Moderate hypothermia in neonatal encephalopathy: efficacy outcomes. *Pediatr Neurol.* 2005;32(1):11–17.

3. Shankaran S, Laptook AR, Ehrenkranz RA, et al. Whole body hypothermia for neonates with hypoxic-ischemic encephalopathy. *N Engl J Med.* 2005;353(15):1574–1584.

4. Azzopardi DV, Strohm B, Edwards AD, et al. Moderate hypothermia to treat perinatal asphyxial encephalopathy. *N Engl J Med.* 2009;361(14):1349–1358.

5. Simbruner G, Mittal RA, Rohlmann F, Muche R. Systemic hypothermia after neonatal encephalopathy: outcomes of neo. nEURO.network RCT. *Pediatrics.* 2010;126:e771–e778.

6. Zhou WH, Cheng GQ, Shao XM, et al. Selective head cooling with mild systemic hypothermia after neonatal hypoxic-ischemic encephalopathy: a multicenter randomized controlled trial in China. *J Pediatr.* 2010;157(3):367–372.

7. Jacobs SE, Inder TE, Stewart M, et al. Whole-body hypothermia for term and near term newborns with hypoxic-ischemic encephalopathy: a randomized controlled trial. *Arch Pediatr Adolesc Med.* 2011;165(8);692–700.

8. Tagin MA, Woolcott CG, Vincer MJ, Whyte RK, Stinson DA. Hypothermia for neonatal hypoxic ischemic encephalopathy: an updated systematic review and meta-analysis. *Arch Pediatr Adolesc Med.* 2012;166(6):558–566.

9. Shankaran S, Pappas A, McDonald SA, et al. Childhood outcomes after hypothermia for neonatal encephalopathy. *N Engl J Med.* 2012;366(22):2085–2092.

10. Gunn AJ, Gunn TR, Gunning MI, Williams CE, Gluckman PD. Neuroprotection with prolonged head cooling started before post-ischemic seizures in fetal sheep. *Pediatrics.* 1998;102(5):1098–1106.

11. Gunn AJ, Bennet L, Gunning MI, Gluckman PD, Gunn TR. Cerebral hypothermia is not neuroprotective when started after post-ischemic seizures in fetal sheep. *Pediatr Res.* 1999;46(3):274–280.

12. Wyatt JS. Ethics and hypothermia treatment. *Semin Fetal Neonatal Med.* 2010;15(5):299–304.

13. Shevell M. Ethical perspectives in cooling for term infants with intrapartum asphyxia. *Dev Med Child Neurol.* 2012;54(3):197–199.

14. Pappas A, Shankaran S, Laptook AR, et al. Hypocarbia and adverse outcome in neonatal hypoxic-ischemic encephalopathy. *J Pediatr.* 2011;158(5):752–758.

15. Schmid R, Tandon P, Stafstrom CE, Holmes GL. Effects of neonatal seizures on subsequent seizure-induced brain injury. *Neurology.* 1999;53:1754–1761.

16. Davis A, Hintz SR, Van Meurs KP, et al. Seizures in extremely low birth weight infants are associated with adverse outcome. *J Pediatr.* 2010;157(5):720–725.

17. Glass, HC, Glidden D, Jeremy RJ, Barkovich JA, Ferriero DM, Miller SP. Clinical neonatal seizures are independently associated with outcome in infants at risk for hypoxic-ischemic brain injury. *J Pediatr.* 2009;155(3):318–323.

18. Zanelli S, Buck M, Fairchild K. Physiologic and pharmacologic considerations for hypothermia therapy in neonates. *J Perinatol.* 2011;31(6):377–386.

19. Thoresen M, Satas A, Loberg EM, et al. Twenty-four hours of mild hypothermia in unsedated newborn pigs starting after a severe global hypoxic-ischemic insult is not neuroprotective. *Pediatr Res.* 2001;50(3):405–411.

20. Fairchild K, Sokora D, Scott J, Zanelli S. Therapeutic hypothermia on neonatal transport: 4-year experience in a single NICU. *J Perinatol.* 2010;30:324–329.

21. Hallberg B, Olson L, Bartocci M. Edqvist I, Blennow M. Passive induction of hypothermia during transport of asphyxiated infants: a risk of excessive cooling. *Acta Pediatr.* 2009;98:942–946.

22. Kendall GS, Kapetanakis AK, Ratnavel N, Azzopardi D, Robertson NJ. Passive cooling for initiation of therapeutic hypothermia in neonatal encephalopathy. *Arch Dis Child Fetal Neonatal Ed.* 2010;95:F408–F412.

23. Akula VP, Gould JB, Davis AS, Hackel A, Oehlert J, Van Meurs KP. Therapeutic hypothermia during neonatal transport: Data from the California Perinatal Quality Care Collaborative (CPQCC) and California Perinatal Transport System (CPeTS) for 2010. *J Perinatol.* 2012;33:194–197.

24. Hoque N, Chakkarapani E, Liu X, Thoreson M. A comparison of cooling methods used in therapeutic hypothermia for perinatal asphyxia. *Pediatrics.* 2010;126(1):e124–e130.

25. Horn A, Thompson C, Woods D, et al. Induced hypothermia for infants with hypoxic-ischemic encephalopathy using a servo-controlled fan: an exploratory pilot study. *Pediatrics.* 2009;123(6):e1090–e1098.

26. Akula VP, Davis AS, Gould JB, Van Meurs KP. Therapeutic hypothermia during neonatal transport: current practices in California. *Am J Perinatol.* 2012; 29(05):319–326.

27. Shankaran S. Therapeutic hypothermia for neonatal encephalopathy. *Currt Treat Options Neurol.* 2012;14:608–619.

28. Stone JG, Young WL, Smith CR, Soloman A, Wald N, Ostapkovich N. Do standard monitoring sites reflect true brain temperature when profound hypothermia is rapidly induced and reversed? *Anesthesiology.* 1995;82(195):344–351.

29. Landry MA, Doyle LW, Lee K, Jacobs SE. Axillary temperature measurement during hypothermia treatment for neonatal hypoxic-ischaemic encephalopathy. *Arch Dis Child Fetal Neonatal Ed.* 2012;98(1):F54–F58.

30. Sarkar S, Barks JD. Systemic complications and hypothermia. *Semin Fetal Neo Med.* 2010;15(5):270–275.

31. Battin M, Bennet L, Gunn AJ. Rebound seizures during rewarming *Pediatrics.* 2004;114(5):1369.

32. Laptook A, Tyson J, Shankaran S, et al. Elevated temperature after hypoxic-ischemic encephalopathy: risk factor for adverse outcomes. *Pediatrics.* 2008;122(3):491–499.

33. Battin MR, Thoresen M, Robinson E, Polin RA, Edwards AD, Gunn AJ; Cool Cap Trial Group. Does head cooling with mild systemic hypothermia affect requirement for blood pressure support? *Pediatrics.* 2009;123(3):1031–1036.

34. Strohm B, Hobson A, Brocklehurst P, Edwards AD, Azzopardi D. Case report: subcutaneous fat necrosis after moderate therapeutic hypothermia in neonates. *Pediatrics.* 2011;128(2):e450–e452.

35. Hogeling M, Meddles K, Berk DR, et al. Extensive subcutaneous fat necrosis of the newborn associated with therapeutic hypothermia. *Pediatr Dermatol.* 2012;29(1):59–63.

36. Filippi L, Catarzi S, Padrini L, et al. Strategies for reducing the incidence of skin complications in newborns treated with whole-body hypothermia. *J Matern Fetal Neonatal Med.* 2012;25(10):2115–2121.

37. Akcay A, Akar M, Oncel MY, et al. Hypercalcemia due to subcutaneous fat necrosis in a newborn after total body cooling. *Pediatr Dermatol.* 2012;30(1):120–123.

Seizures and Status Epilepticus

Don Olson

DIAGNOSIS/INDICATION

History

1. Seizure-predisposing conditions in the neonate are, for example,

    Asphyxia

    Prolonged low Apgar scores/resuscitation

    Birth trauma

    Sepsis or central nervous system (CNS) infection

2. Maternal factors

    Diabetes (hypoglycemic infant)

    Fever/chorioamnionitis (sepsis)

    Viral infection (eg, herpes)

    Group B streptococcus carriage

3. Pharmacologically restrained and sedated neonates with "at-risk" conditions

4. Family history of siblings or parents with recognized or suspected genetic conditions predisposing to seizures (eg, benign familial neonatal seizure [BFNS], tuberous sclerosis)

Physical

1. Dysmorphic features or multiple congenital anomalies (suggesting possible cerebral malformation)

2. Seizures most commonly occur as repeated, stereotyped episodes of

    Focal clonic limb jerking

    Tonic limb posturing with or without head and eye deviation

    Subtle phenomena, such as stereotyped chewing, tongue thrusting, bicycling, or swimming movements

    Vital sign changes (eg, apnea, tachycardia, hypo- or hypertension)

Confirmatory/Baseline Tests

1. Initial blood tests

    Glucose

    Electrolytes

    Calcium/magnesium

    Culture

    Complete blood cell count and differential

2. Urine analysis and culture

3. Cerebrospinal fluid

    Cell count and differential

    Glucose (simultaneous serum glucose recommended) and protein

    Bacterial and viral cultures

    Herpes polymerase chain reaction (PCR)

4. Electroencephalogram (EEG) to look for evidence of frequent or continuous seizures, correlate suspicious movements with ictal EEG rhythm, features suggesting focal cortical dysfunction or underlying inborn error of metabolism

5. Neuroimaging

Ultrasound (intraparenchymal hemorrhage, malformation with ventriculomegaly)

Computerized tomography (intraparenchymal and superficial hemorrhage, cerebral malformation, intraparenchymal calcification [congenital infection])

Magnetic resonance imaging (MRI) (cerebral malformation, stroke, hemorrhage, sinovenous thrombosis, vascular malformation)

Further Tests

1. Further blood tests

Amino acids

Arterial lactate, pyruvate, and ammonia levels

Carnitine level and acyl-carnitine profile

Karyotype

Hepatic enzymes

Biotinidase

2. Urine

Organic acids

Purine and pyrimidine metabolites

Sulfites

3. Many other possible diagnostic and screening tests for genetic conditions/inborn errors of metabolism depending on circumstances

Differential Diagnosis/Diagnostic Algorithm

Physical examination: Vigorous stimulation and repositioning are often useful means to try to interrupt suspicious, seizure-like behavior that is, in fact, nonepileptic (eg, benign sleep myoclonus, jitteriness).

EEG testing (as previously described) should help differentiate subtle seizures from nonepileptic behaviors (eg, apnea, tachycardia, oxygen desaturation).

Consider long-term EEG monitoring for less-frequent, stereotyped, seizure-like behavior.

TREATMENT/PROCEDURE

Initiation

Monitor respiratory and cardiac function, oral secretions. Secure vascular access.

Tests to Follow

Correct deranged metabolic conditions: hypoxia, hypoglycemia, hypocalcemia, hypomagnesaemia, hyponatremia.

Once treatment with an antiseizure medication is initiated, follow serum levels of readily measurable drugs (eg, phenobarbital, phenytoin).

Management Algorithm/Decision Tree

Acute treatment with antiseizure medication: Initially consider a single dose of a benzodiazepine:

Lorazepam: 0.05 mg/kg/dose IV (preferred; longer duration of action)

Diazepam: 0.2 mg/kg/dose IV (hard to give, incompatible with most intravenous solutions, may precipitate or adhere to intravenous tubing)

Midazolam: 0.05 mg/kg/dose (very short duration of action)

Persistent clinical or electrograph seizures require longer-term treatment, classically with phenobarbital:

Load: 15–20 mg/kg initially

Initial "target" serum levels are 15–40 µg/mL, with level achieved usually approximately the same as the total loading dose.

Seizure control may require additional doses to achieve serum drug levels of 40–50 µg/mL.

Maintenance: Give 3–4 mg/kg daily, divided every 12 hours; start once the baby demonstrates the ability to metabolize the drug.

Follow levels closely, as once fully "loaded," neonates in the first few days have minimal phenobarbital metabolism and can reach markedly elevated levels; subsequently, the dose may need to increase to 5 mg/kg daily or higher as liver function improves and matures.

For seizures that persist after phenobarbital loading to high therapeutic serum levels, consider loading with additional medications, such as

Fosphenytoin/phenytoin: Load with 15–20 mg/kg (dosing for phenytoin and fosphenytoin is the same, but fosphenytoin is measured as "mgPE," indicating "phenytoin equivalents"). Maintenance is 5–8 mg/kg daily, usually divided every 12 hours.

Levetiracetam: Give 10–15 mg/kg initial dose, titrating to 50 mg/kg daily over 5 days.

If initial antiseizure medications fail, particularly in the absence of definite seizure risk factors, consider

Pyridoxine challenge: Give 100 mg intravenous pyridoxine during EEG monitoring. Caution: This may cause acute respiratory depression.

Folinic acid: Give 2.5 mg twice daily.

Exit Strategy/Weaning/Indications for Discontinuation

For acute seizures following asphyxia, a transient electrolyte derangement, or hypoglycemia, there may be no need for maintenance therapy after a good response to initial loading dose.

For initially difficult-to-control seizures following an acute asphyxia insult, consider early medication weaning if no seizures recur after the first week. There is no "set time" for weaning, but between a week and 3 months may be considered.

For seizures in the setting of a traumatic or hemorrhagic insult, it is reasonable to treat for 3 months and wean medication if there has been no seizure recurrence.

For seizures secondary to congenital structural abnormalities, assess a trial of weaning medication at 3 months.

CONCLUSION/FOLLOW-UP

Aftercare monitoring: Follow-up care should focus on monitoring for recurrent seizures, screening for medication toxicity, and following developmental progress.

Follow-up tests: For children who remain on seizure medications, following serum concentrations of phenobarbital, carbamazepine, and phenytoin is reasonable.

In most cases, a "routine" follow-up EEG will be of little benefit. If there are paroxysmal spells suspicious for seizures, in that case consider an extended monitoring study, such as inpatient or outpatient video EEG.

Clinical follow-up

Obtain a history to look for stereotyped paroxysmal spells that may be seizures, particularly if associated with altered level of consciousness or motor phenomena that cannot be physically interrupted.

Watch for signs of delayed attainment of developmental milestones.

Long-term outcome/implications for patient/family

Neonatal seizures mean there is an increased risk of epilepsy (see chapter).

Parents should be instructed in basic seizure first aid (eg, turn child on his or her side and do not put anything in the mouth; activate emergency services for seizures over 3–5 minutes).

Parents should be instructed to observe seizure precautions (eg, no bathing unattended by an adult).

SUGGESTED READING

Garfinkle J, Shevell MI. Predictors of outcome in term infants with neonatal seizures subsequent to intrapartum asphyxia. *J Child Neurol.* 2011;26(4):453–459.

Glass HC, Pham TN, Danielsen B, et al. Antenatal and intrapartum risk factors for seizures in term newborns: a population-based study, California 1998–2002. *J Pediatr.* 2009;154(1):24–28 e1.

Glass HC, Wirrell E. Controversies in neonatal seizure management. *Child Neurol.* 2009;24:591

Gospe SM. Pyridoxine-dependent seizures. In: Pagon RA, et al, eds. *GeneReviews.* Seattle, WA: University of Washington, Seattle; 1993.

Guerrini R, Aicardi J. Epileptic encephalopathies with myoclonic seizures in infants and children (severe myoclonic epilepsy and myoclonic-astatic epilepsy). *J Clin Neurophysiol.* 2003;20(6):449–461.

Holmes GL. The long-term effects of neonatal seizures. *Clin Perinatol.* 2009;36(4):901–914, vii–viii.

Painter MJ, Scher MS, Stein AD, et al. Phenobarbital compared with phenytoin for the treatment of neonatal seizures. *N Engl J Med.* 1999;341(7):485–489.

Rossi S, Daniele I, Bastrenta P, et al. Early myoclonic encephalopathy and nonketotic hyperglycinemia. *Pediatric Neurol.* 2009;41(5):371–374.

Wusthoff CJ, Kessler SK, Vossough A, et al. Risk of later seizure after perinatal arterial ischemic stroke: a prospective cohort study. *Pediatrics.* 2011;127(6):e1550–e1557.

Use of aEEG/NIRS

Alexis S. Davis and Valerie Y. Chock

AMPLITUDE-INTEGRATED ELECTROENCEPHALOGRAPHY

What Is Amplitude-Integrated Electroencephalography?

Amplitude-integrated electroencephalography (aEEG) is a simplified, bedside EEG device used to continuously monitor brain function. Brain wave activity is recorded from scalp electrodes, and the raw EEG data are processed using a filter to attenuate frequencies less than 2 Hz and greater than 15 Hz, transform the amplitudes into a rectified and time-compressed signal, and display on a semilogarithmic scale in microvolts (μV). This results in patterns that are easily recognizable without formal training in EEG analysis. Interpretation of the aEEG recording includes assessment of the minimum amplitude, maximum amplitude, bandwidth, and the presence of sleep-wake cycles (SWCs) (Figure 78-1).

Indications for aEEG Monitoring

The following are indications for aEEG monitoring:

1. Confirmation of suspected clinical seizures, especially when formal EEG is not available
2. Assessment for subclinical seizures in high-risk infants
3. Continuous monitoring of therapeutic effects of antiepileptic medication

4. Prediction of outcomes in hypoxic ischemic encephalopathy (HIE)
5. Other potential, but not well-studied, uses for aEEG include metabolic encephalopathy, patients on extracorporeal membrane oxygenation (ECMO), assessment of neuromaturation in preterm infants, assessment of posthemorrhagic hydrocephalus, surgical anesthesia, and postoperative recovery

Placement of aEEG

1. Types of electrodes
   a. Hydrogel: disposable electrodes similar to regular electrocardiographic (ECG) electrodes; used in most commercial aEEG devices
   b. Cup-disk: reusable; requires EEG conductive paste
   c. Needle: minimal skin preparation required and achieves low impedances; invasive, with theoretical risk for infection
2. Recording montages: location of electrodes based on the 10–20 international classification system modified for neonates (Figure 78-2)
   a. Single channel: Traditionally, electrodes are positioned at P3 and P4, which is the area overlying the cortical watershed zone in infants with HIE; alternatively, if using the CoolCap® System, electrodes may be modified to Fp1 and Fp2.

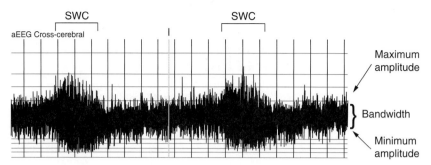

FIGURE 78-1 Determination of the presence of sleep-wake cycles (SWCs). aEEG, amplitude-integrated electroencephalogram.

b. Three channel: Electrodes positioned at C3, P3, C4, P4 create two biparietal channels (C3-P3, C4-P4) and a cross-cerebral channel (P3-P4).

c. All devices require an additional ground electrode, usually placed on the back or forehead. Some devices may also require a reference electrode on the scalp (typically Cz).

d. Other EEG recording systems may utilize additional channels.

3. Skin preparation: When cup-disk or hydrogel electrodes are used, skin should be cleaned and exfoliated prior to application.

4. Data quality: Impedance is continuously measured during the aEEG recording. Impedances greater than 10 kΩ indicate poor electrode contact,

insufficient skin preparation, or electrical interference, and the electrodes should be checked.

Interpretation of aEEG Recordings

1. Background pattern interpretation

   a. Basic background pattern descriptions (Figure 78-3)

      (1) Continuous: minimum amplitude greater than 5 μV and maximum amplitude greater than 10 to 25 μV

      (2) Discontinuous: minimum amplitude less than 5 μV but demonstrating variability; maximum amplitude greater than 10 μV

      (3) Burst suppression: minimum amplitude less than 3–5 μV with minimal variability; bursts greater than 25 μV of variable density

      (4) Low voltage: continuous background with both minimum and maximum amplitudes less than 10 μV

      (5) Inactive/flat: primarily isoelectric tracing with amplitudes less than 5 μV

   b. Term infants with hypoxic-ischemic encephalopathy and prediction of outcome

      (1) Background pattern: Recovery of a normal background pattern (either continuous or discontinuous) within 36–48 hours has been associated with a good outcome.

      (2) Sleep-wake cycles: Shorter time to recovery of SWCs (before 36 hours) is associated with a good outcome. Never developing SWCs is strongly predictive of a poor outcome.

      (3) Recovery of background pattern and SWCs may be delayed for infants treated with hypothermia.

   c. Preterm infants: In healthy preterm infants, the aEEG matures from a discontinuous pattern to a continuous pattern with advancing gestational

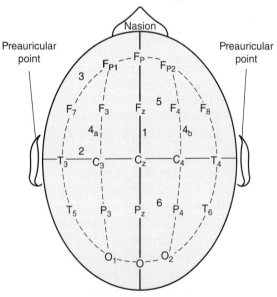

FIGURE 78-2 One-channel amplitude-integrated electroencephalogram (aEEG) typically utilizes the P3-P4 channel. Three-channel aEEG utilizes electrodes at C3, C4, P3, and P4 to create a right-side channel (C4-P4), a left-side channel (C3-P3), and a cross-cerebral channel (P3-P4).

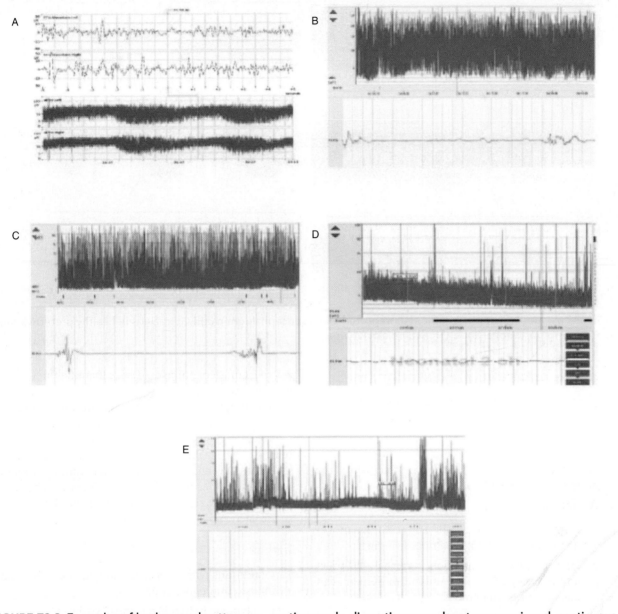

FIGURE 78-3 Examples of background patterns: a, continuous; b, discontinuous; c, burst suppression; d, continuous low voltage; and e, isoelectric/flat tracing. (From Hellstrom et al.[1])

and postmenstrual age (Figure 78-4). In other words, the minimum amplitude increases, the bandwidth and maximum amplitude decrease, and there is interval development of SWCs. Isoelectric and low-voltage patterns have been associated with the development of intraventricular hemorrhage.

2. Seizures

   a. An isolated seizure is reflected by an increase in the minimum amplitude; repetitive seizures appear as a "sawtooth" pattern (see Figure 78-5).

   b. It is important to confirm seizure activity on the raw EEG tracing (see the section on limitations).

3. Sleep-wake cycling

   a. Immature SWCs may begin to appear as early as 25 to 27 weeks' gestational age, as evidenced by sinusoidal fluctuations in the minimum amplitude.

   b. SWCs that are more mature in healthy infants appear between 30 and 34 weeks' gestational age but are often shorter in duration compared to mature SWCs, which emerge at 36–37 weeks' gestational age.

   c. In healthy preterm infants, SWCs may appear at earlier postmenstrual ages than would be expected of a newborn at an equivalent gestational age.

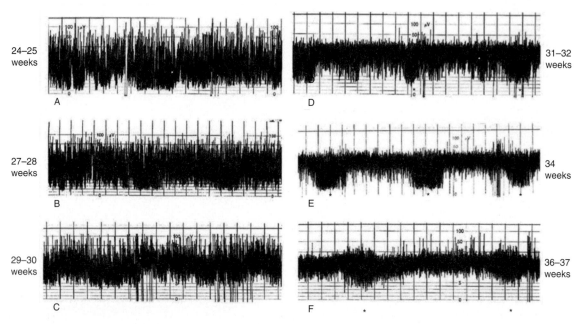

FIGURE 78-4 Representative amplitude-integrated electroencephalogram (aEEG) tracings in healthy preterm infants at advancing gestational ages. (From Burdjalov VF et al.[2])

Limitations of aEEG Monitoring

1. Because of the nature of the time-compressed recording, brief seizures (<30 seconds) may be missed.

2. As only 1 to 3 channels are recorded, seizures or abnormal background activity in the frontal or occipital regions will not be recognized.

3. Artifacts

   a. Mimics of seizures include any repetitive movement, such as burping, patting, swinging.

   b. High-frequency ventilation, external electrical interference, ECG, and muscle movement can falsely elevate amplitudes.

   c. Contact between electrodes (either by physical contact or by a bridge created by paste/moisture) can result in falsely low amplitudes.

   d. Sedative medications may depress the background pattern or inhibit SWCs.

NEAR-INFRARED SPECTROSCOPY

What Is Near-Infrared Spectroscopy?

Near-infrared spectroscopy (NIRS) is a noninvasive technique to continuously monitor regional tissue oxygenation. It has most commonly been used for cerebral oximetry, although monitoring of renal and mesenteric oxygenation are other potential applications. A skin sensor transmits near-infrared light, which penetrates underlying tissues to a depth of 2.5 to 3 cm (depending on device manufacturer). Light is differentially absorbed by oxyhemoglobin and deoxyhemoglobin from the tissue vasculature, and remaining light is then detected by the sensor (see Figure 78-6). A regional tissue oxygen saturation (rSO_2) or a hemoglobin difference (HbD) signal is then calculated based on a weighted average of 20% arterial blood, 75% venous blood, and 5% capillary blood in the underlying tissue. The rSO_2 value reflects a regional balance between tissue oxygen supply and demand.

Indications for NIRS Monitoring

1. Conditions with altered hemodynamic states causing cerebral hypoxemia

   a. Hypoxic ischemic encephalopathy

   b. Congenital heart disease, especially with potentially decreased systemic outflow for perioperative monitoring

   c. Patent ductus arteriosus, particularly after interventions to close the ductus

   d. Prematurity with altered cerebral autoregulation

2. Conditions with altered hemodynamics affecting mesenteric or renal oxygenation

   a. Shock. A drop in somatic oxygenation may be an early potential indicator of low cardiac output before other indicators such as blood pressure, acidosis, and decreased urine output.

   b. Congenital heart disease.

   c. Renal dysfunction.

   d. Necrotizing enterocolitis.

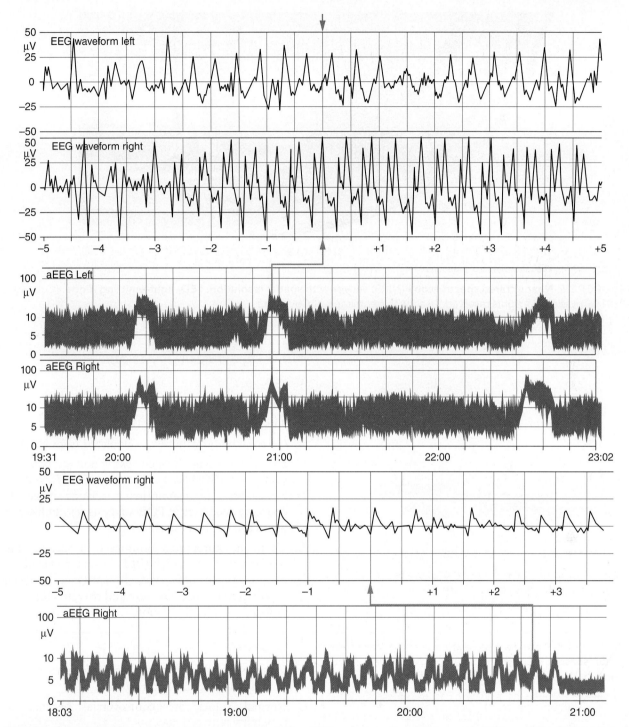

FIGURE 78-5 Examples of repetitive seizure activity. EEG, electroencephalogram; aEEG, amplitude-integrated electroencephalogram.

e. ECMO, to evaluate interventions while on ECMO or to assist with prediction of successful weaning.

3. Other potential applications for NIRS include assessment of intraventricular hemorrhage (IVH), intraoperative management, anesthetic management and with conditions such as anemia, hypoglycemia, seizures, or metabolic disorders.

Placement of NIRS

1. Locations (Figure 78-7)

   a. Cerebral sensor on lateral forehead

   b. Renal sensor on flank

   c. Mesenteric (splanchnic) sensor on abdomen, typically inferior to umbilicus in lower left quadrant

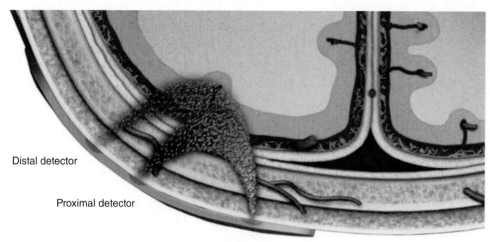

FIGURE 78-6 Near-infrared spectroscopy (NIRS) sensor with spatial resolution. LED, light-emitting diode. (Copyright ©2014 Covidien. All rights reserved. Used with permission of Covidien.)

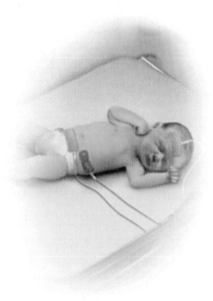

FIGURE 78-7 Placement of near-infrared spectroscopy (NIRS) sensors. (Copyright ©2014 Covidien. All rights reserved. Used with permission of Covidien.)

2. Duration is dependent on manufacturer's recommendations. Evaluate for skin sensitivity, especially if monitoring for longer than 24 hours.

3. Data quality
   a. Right-to-left differences in regional cerebral oxygenation can be up to 10% during periods of unstable systemic arterial oxygenation.
   b. Excessive light may interfere with signal detection.
   c. Adhesion of sensor may interfere with signal detection.

NIRS Measures (Direct and Indirect)

1. rSO_2 (%).
2. HbD signal.
3. Tissue oxygenation index (TOI) (%).
4. Cerebral blood volume as calculated from HbD.
5. Fractional tissue oxygen extraction (FTOE) = $(SaO_2 — rSO_2)/SaO_2$. Elevated FTOE reflects higher oxygen consumption in relation to oxygen delivery; decreased FTOE suggests less utilization of oxygen by the tissues.
6. There are autoregulation measures such as the pressure passivity index (PPI), which is calculated by percentage time with concordance between mean arterial blood pressure and rSO_2 to indicate a pressure passive circulation.

Interpretation of NIRS Data

1. Values are validated using jugular venous saturation measurements (Figure 78-8).
2. Normal values are controversial because of variability between patients.
   a. Cerebral oxygenation
      (1) Term infants: 60%–80% or approximately 30% less than arterial saturation
      (2) Preterm infants
          (a) The cerebral oxygen saturation decreases over the first 1–2 weeks of life in preterm infants less than 34 weeks' gestation.
          (b) Range is typically 70% ± 8% in the first 72 hours of life.
          (c) There is a mean PPI of 20%.

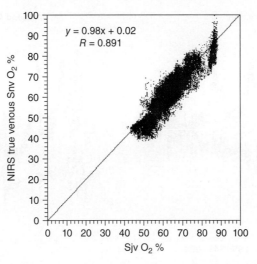

FIGURE 78-8 Validation of cerebral saturation with jugular venous bulb saturation. (From Benni PB et al.[3])

b. Somatic oxygenation

(1) Term infants: typically 5%–15% above cerebral saturations

(2) Preterm infants

(a) Renal oxygen saturations also typically decrease over the first 1–2 weeks of life in preterm infants less than 34 weeks' gestation.

(b) Renal rSO_2 range is typically 80% ± 10% in first week of life.

(c) Mesenteric (abdominal) oxygen saturation values show significant variability and increase with gestational age, ranging from 32% to 66% in the preterm population.

3. Abnormal values and associations with outcomes

a. Cerebral oxygenation

(1) Cardiac surgery absolute levels: Values less than 35%–40% for more than 10 minutes are associated with early postoperative neuropsychological dysfunction, lower developmental quotient scores, EEG changes, intracellular anaerobic metabolism, and histopathologic neuronal injury.

(2) Cardiac surgery changes in rSO_2: Greater than a 20% decrease in rSO_2 is associated with development of seizures, hemiparesis, and adverse neurodevelopmental outcome at 18 months of age.

(3) Hypoxic ischemic encephalopathy: Greater than 50% decrease in FTOE and increased rSO_2 levels are associated with adverse neurodevelopmental outcomes at 1 to 2 years of age. Increased cerebral blood volume predicts death or disability.

b. Somatic oxygenation

(1) A ratio less than 0.75 for splanchnic:cerebral oxygenation has been associated with intestinal ischemia.

(2) Splanchnic (abdominal) saturations are lower in infants with feeding intolerance.

(3) Renal saturations less than 50% for more than 2 hours are associated with higher incidence of acute kidney injury after cardiac surgery.

c. Autoregulation: Loss of autoregulation (Figure 78-9) has been associated with increased mortality and severe IVH and PVL in preterm infants.

Interventions to Improve rSO_2

1. Improve blood pressure

2. Avoid hypocarbia or hypercarbia

3. Correct anemia with a red blood cell transfusion

4. Increase the fraction of inspired oxygen (FiO_2)

5. Minimize metabolic demand (ie, temperature regulation, sedation)

Limitations of NIRS Monitoring

1. The depth of signal penetration limits measurement of deeper tissue structures: For cerebral monitoring, regional oxygenation of cortex and not deeper brain structures is measured.

2. It is better to trend rSO_2 values over time or with interventions in an individual patient rather than compare absolute values of rSO_2 between patients because of the potential for significant variability between patients.

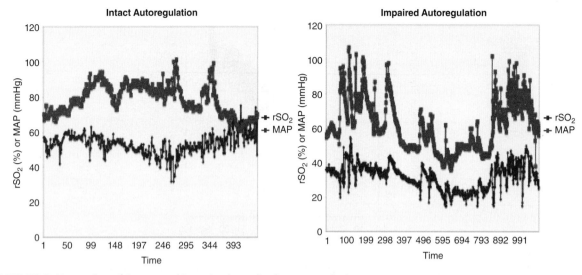

FIGURE 78-9 Examples of intact and impaired cerebral autoregulation.

3. There is a risk of skin sensitivity caused by the sensor adhesive.

4. Interpretation must be made in the context of all factors that influence oxygen extraction and delivery, such as anemia, hypotension, hypocarbia, and metabolic rate.

REFERENCES

1. Hellström-Westas L, Rosén I, deVries LS, et al. Amplitude-integrated EEG classification and interpretation in preterm and term infants. *NeoReviews.* 2006;7(2):e76–e87.
2. Burdjalov VF, Baumgart S, Spitzer AR. Cerebral function monitoring: a new scoring system for the evaluation of brain maturation in neonates. *Pediatrics.* 2003;112(4):855–861.
3. Benni PB, Chen B, Dykes FD, et al. Validation of the CAS neonatal NIRS system by monitoring vv-ECMO patients: preliminary results. *Adv Exp Med Biol.* 2005;566:195–201.

SUGGESTED READING

Cortez J, Gupta M, Amaram A, Pizzino J, et al. Noninvasive evaluation of splanchnic tissue oxygenation using near-infrared spectroscopy in preterm neonates. *J Matern Fetal Neonatal Med.* 2011;24:574–582.

Hellström-Westas L, Rosén I, deVries LS, et al. Amplitude-integrated EEG classification and interpretation in preterm and term infants. *NeoReviews.* 2006;7(2):e76–e87.

Hoffman GM, Ghanayem NS, Tweddell JS. Noninvasive assessment of cardiac output. *Semin Thorac Cardiovasc Surg Pediatr Card Surg Annu.* 2005;8:12–21.

Lemmers PM, Toet M, van Schelven LJ, van Bel F. Cerebral oxygenation and cerebral oxygen extraction in the preterm infant: the impact of respiratory distress syndrome. *Exp Brain Res.* 2006;173:458–467.

McNeill S, Gatenby JC, McElroy S, Engelhardt B. Normal cerebral, renal, and abdominal regional oxygen saturations using near-infrared spectroscopy in preterm infants. *J Perinatol.* 2011;31:51–57.

Petrova A, Mehta R. Near-infrared spectroscopy in the detection of regional tissue oxygenation during hypoxic events in preterm infants undergoing critical care. *Pediatr Crit Care Med.* 2006;7:449–454.

Shah DK, Boylan GB, Rennie JM. Monitoring of seizures in the newborn. *Arch Dis Child Fetal Neonatal Ed.* 2012;97(1): F65–F69. E pub 2010 Aug 5.

Thoresen M, Hellström-Westas L, Liu X, de Vries LS. Effect of hypothermia on amplitude-integrated electroencephalogram in infants with asphyxia. *Pediatrics.* 2010;126(1):e131–e139.

Toet MC, van Rooij LGM, deVries LS. The use of amplitude-integrated electroencephalography for assessing neonatal neurological injury. *Clin Perinatol.* 2008;35:665–678.

Wong FY, Leung TS, Austin T, Wilkinson M, et al. Impaired autoregulation in preterm infants identified by using spatially resolved spectroscopy. *Pediatrics.* 2008;121:e604–e611.

CHAPTER 78

79 Workup of Neonatal Stroke

Alexandra Abrams and Michael R. Jeng

DIAGNOSIS/INDICATION

Definition of Neonatal Stroke

A stroke, in general, is defined as an event that leads to poor blood flow to a localized area of the brain. One of the difficulties in studying strokes in the neonate is that, until recently, there has not been full agreement on the definition of neonatal stroke. Recently, however, the National Institute of Child Health and Human Development and the National Institute of Neurological Disorders and Stroke provided a consensus definition of neonatal stroke as "a group of heterogeneous conditions in which there is a focal disruption of cerebral blood flow secondary to arterial or cerebral venous thrombosis or embolization between 20 weeks of fetal life through 28th post-natal day, and confirmed by neuroimaging or neuropathological studies." Neuroimaging was defined as T2-weighted magnetic resonance imaging (MRI), magnetic resonance angiography (MRA), or diffusion-weighted imaging, as head ultrasounds can miss anterior and posterior lesions and computed tomography (CT) may not detect small or early lesions.[1] However, ultrasounds and CT scans remain commonly used techniques in the evaluation of neonatal stroke. Neuropathological studies included autopsy and detailed evaluation of the placenta. Thus, the definition of neonatal stroke is currently defined by neuroimaging or neuropathologic findings, is either venous or arterial, and is either thrombotic or hemorrhagic. The location and type of stroke, as well as the neonate's clinical status, help guide the workup.

Neonatal stroke is a common clinical event; with an estimated incidence between 1/2300 and 1/5000 live births.[1] The incidence in this age category is second only to the incidence seen in elderly adults. The majority of neonatal strokes are caused by thrombosis of the arteries (70%), with a lower rate of hemorrhagic strokes (20%) and sinus venous thrombosis (10%). There is a slightly increased frequency in males compared to females and in African American infants when compared with Caucasian babies. A majority of these events occur in term infants because of their physiological hypercoagulable state near the time of delivery. As neuroimaging techniques become more sophisticated and the technology becomes more available, neonatal stroke may be more easily diagnosed, and this reported incidence may begin to rise.

Maternal Risk Factors

1. Thrombotic Stroke
   a. Pregnancy results in a relative hypercoagulable state with several plasma proteins affected and increased thrombin generation, putting both mother and baby at increased risk of thrombus.[2] Several publications reported that about half (50%) of mothers of infants diagnosed with a thrombotic stroke were found to have prothrombotic abnormalities.
   b. Chorioamnionitis has also been shown to be associated with increased risk of thrombotic strokes in neonates. A multivariate analysis of a retrospective case control study involving a total of 208 infants found that maternal fever, even

in the absence of an identified infection, had a statistically significant association with perinatal arterial ischemia.[3]

Maternal autoimmune disorders, in particular lupus, can lead to neonatal stroke. The maternally derived autoantibodies can cross the placenta and cause myriad clinical findings in the neonate. In particular, these antibodies can also cause a vasculitis in the neonate, leading to cerebral arterial or venous thrombosis.

  c. Other maternal factors that compromise the placenta, including the use of cocaine, increase the risk of stroke in the prenatal or perinatal periods.

2. Hemorrhagic Stroke

  a. Quantitative platelet disorders can lead to hemorrhagic neonatal stroke and may be related to the mother. The main maternal risk factor for hemorrhagic stroke is a maternal-paternal platelet antigen mismatch leading to neonatal alloimmune thrombocytopenia (NAIT). Because of the risk of subsequent neonatal hemorrhagic stroke in future infants, this is an important diagnosis to make correctly. Prophylactic measures, such as maternal intravenous immune globulin (IVIG) administration, may be effective in preventing thrombocytopenia, and thereby stroke, caused by NAIT.

The mother may also have maternal immune-mediated thrombocytopenia (ITP), which carries less risk than NAIT. In this scenario, the mother's autoantibodies, which are directed at antigens on her own platelets, cross the placenta and then increase the clearance of the infant's platelets, leading to thrombocytopenia and the potential for increased hemorrhagic stroke. Thus, obtaining the mother's platelet count, if available, is often helpful in guiding the workup in neonatal hemorrhagic stroke caused by neonatal thrombocytopenia.

Infant Risk Factors

1. Thrombotic Strokes

  a. The physiology of newborns places them at increased risk for thrombotic strokes. Their physiologically elevated hematocrit, which can be made worse in the setting of twin-twin transfusion, increases the risk of thrombosis. Neonates also have a relatively decreased rate of cerebral blood flow. The patent foramen ovale, always present at birth with variable rate of closure, allows a thrombus entering the right side of the heart to pass to the brain.

  b. Congenital cardiac abnormalities are at risk for developing intracardiac thrombi, and these may embolize to the central nervous system (CNS), leading to arterial stroke. Testing for congenital thrombophilic disorders remains controversial in neonates. Testing for congenital thrombophilias, such as factor V Leiden, prothrombin mutations, hyperhomocysteinemia, and protein C/S and antithrombin deficiencies is often performed, but the utility for screening for these disorders in the neonate with thrombotic strokes, both arterial and sinus venous thrombosis, is controversial. Testing may not influence treatment or ultimate length of treatment. Thus, with the limitations of blood available for diagnostic testing, the clinician should be judicious in ordering these tests and when to begin testing. One recommended test in infants is to look for antiphospholipid antibodies, which may be placentally transferred from the mother, possibly contributing to development of thrombotic stroke.

  c. Any foreign bodies, such as arterial or venous catheters, particularly in the setting of extracorporeal membrane oxygenation (ECMO), increase turbidity of the blood and therefore increase the risk of thrombosis.

  d. Similar to the contribution of infections to hemorrhagic stroke, infections leading to disseminated intravascular coagulation (DIC) may thus also contribute to the development of a thrombotic stroke. Hemorrhagic stroke may also occur because of DIC.

2. Hemorrhagic Strokes

  a. Gestational age is important in the evaluation of hemorrhagic strokes. Typically, there is an increased risk for hemorrhagic stroke with increasing prematurity.[1] Most neonatal intensive care units (NICUs) have standardized screening policies that utilize head ultrasounds to screen for hemorrhagic stroke based on gestational age. The pathophysiology is likely caused by the increased vascular fragility of blood vessels in the premature infant.

  b. Newborns are born physiologically deficient in vitamin K and have a high rate of hemorrhagic strokes (hemorrhagic disease of the newborn) before the use of vitamin K right after delivery. Congenital bleeding diatheses, most commonly such deficiencies in factors 8 or 9 and 13, may lead to hemorrhages as well. Abnormal fibrinogen, both quantitatively and qualitatively, and severe homozygote factor 7 deficiency may also lead to hemorrhagic stroke in the neonate.

Clinical Symptoms and Presenting Features

Neonates who have suffered a stroke often have minimal detectable symptoms. Because of this, the symptoms are often found incidentally in an asymptomatic infant. Subtle clinical findings may include unexplained apnea, hypotonia, or irritability.[1] Many of the deficits caused by stroke, although perhaps easily identifiable in adults, are frequently missed in infants. This may be because developmental milestones, which would reflect asymmetry or loss of function, have not yet been reached. If not detected during the perinatal period, the presenting sign to the clinician may be early preference for a hand (ie, early right handedness) or may be a child who has failed to reach developmental milestones. In combination with a concern for a perinatal neurological event, these children are often given the diagnosis of "presumed perinatal stroke."

Clinical symptoms that are more overt include seizures, which are often the first sign of neonatal stroke. All seizures in the neonatal period should be worked up with neuroimaging. Hemiplegia may also be an overt finding. For unclear reasons, the left middle cerebral artery is the most commonly affected vessel; thus, right hemiplegia is more often observed than left hemiplegia.

Differential Diagnosis

Many other possible diagnoses may mimic the symptoms of a stroke in the neonate. Table 79-1 lists a few diagnostic considerations to take into account and how to differentiate these from either hemorrhagic or thrombotic stroke in the neonate.

CONFIRMATORY/DIAGNOSTIC TESTING

Imaging Studies

Ultrasound

As cranial ultrasounds are easily obtained and do not require sedation, they are often the imaging modality of choice when initially assessing an infant with neurologic symptoms. Numerous studies have assessed the role of ultrasound in diagnosing stroke. Unfortunately, the sensitivity of cranial ultrasound in the acute phase is poor, with studies reporting 30%–68% of strokes being identified by ultrasound.[4-6] These studies also clearly demonstrated that the skill of the ultrasonographer can greatly contribute to their sensitivity. In addition, this technique does not expose the infants to any radiation.

Computed Tomography

Computed tomography may not detect small or early lesions.[7] CT is most likely to miss strokes during the first 24 hours after they occur. However, the scans are generally easy to obtain and fast, but they do expose the infant to radiation. A CT scan is generally not used for diagnosis of neonatal stroke but may be ordered when considering other diagnoses as the cause for workup.

Magnetic Resonance Imaging

If the patient is stable enough to tolerate the duration of the imaging, and the suspicion for stroke is high, then the recommended neuroimaging is T2-weighted

Table 79-1 Differential Diagnosis

Other Conditions	Features of These Disorders
Encephalitis	• More diffuse findings on imaging
Kernicterus	• Significantly elevated bilirubin
Posterior reversible encephalopathy syndrome (PRES)	• Often associated with hypertension (also associated with some antirejection medications) • Magnetic resonance imaging (MRI) generally shows cortico-subcortical areas of T2-weighted hyperintense signal involving the bilateral occipital and parietal lobes with or without the pons
Nonaccidental trauma	Retinal hemorrhages often present if severe enough for significant central nervous system (CNS) symptoms • Other signs of abuse
Mitochondrial disorders	• May have elevated ammonia • Often a diagnosis of exclusion
Malignancy	• CNS malignancy rare at birth and generally visible on imaging • Likewise, paraneoplastic syndromes rare in the neonatal period • Neuroblastoma 4s can lead to fulminant liver failure, leading to encephalopathy, but infant usually has other symptoms and distended abdomen

MRI, MRA, or diffusion-weighted imaging.[1] These techniques also spare the infant from radiation exposure. However, cost, availability, and expertise in reading neuroimages in the neonate may limit these techniques. MRA, may also be obtained at the same time, which permits visualization of the blood vessels of the CNS, allowing for determination of anatomical abnormalities that may have led to the stroke. This technique is the recommended diagnostic examination when suspicion for neonatal stroke is high.

Laboratory Testing

Maternal Risk Factors

1. Sepsis, chorioamnionitis: Blood culture of the mother and full sepsis workup of the infant once imaging confirms a lumbar puncture is safe to perform.

2. Antiphospholipid syndrome: Antiphospholipid antibody, anticardiolipin antibody, and lupus anticoagulant screens may be indicated in a woman who has exhibited the clinical triad suggestive of antiphospholipid syndrome. These symptoms include recurrent miscarriages, thrombotic events, and thrombocytopenia. Any history of maternal autoimmune disease should trigger consideration of testing for these antibodies.

3. Maternal ITP: Maternal thrombocytopenia or history of previous maternal ITP, especially with a history of maternal splenectomy, should raise concern for maternal antiplatelet antibodies having crossed the placenta.

4. Urine toxicology

Congenital Thrombophilia in the Neonate

See Chapter 32 for a discussion of congenital thrombophilia in the newborn.

1. Antithrombin III level
2. Protein C and S activity
3. Factor V Leiden mutation analysis
4. Prothrombin G20210A mutation analysis
5. Homocysteine level or methylene tetrahydrofolate reductase (MTHFR) C677 mutation analysis

TREATMENT CONSIDERATIONS

Thrombotic Stroke

1. Thrombolysis: If a thrombus is felt to be life threatening and there is no significant hemorrhage and

no recent or planned invasive surgery, fibrinolytic therapy can be considered.[8] Although likely with a limited availability for this age group, interventional radiology for mechanical removal and catheter-directed thrombolysis may be considered for serious thromboses. Prior to initiation of thrombolytic therapy, the platelet count should be at least 100,000/µL and the fibrinogen at least 1. Neonates may require supplementation of plasminogen (which is naturally lower in neonates) via FFP. Tissue plasminogen activator (tPA) is generally the drug of choice because it has been most effective toward neonatal thrombosis, with the least risk for hypersensitivity.[8] There have not been any clinical trials to define ideal dosing, but bleeding complications are not infrequent, so the blood bank should be notified and prepared to provide the appropriate products.

2. Anticoagulation and antiplatelet agents: Numerous groups, including the American Heart Association, recommend anticoagulation for neonates only if the following criteria are met: The neonate does not have significant intracranial hemorrhage, there is evidence of thrombus propagation or emboli, or the neonate is found to have a severe prothrombotic state. Based on guidance from the American College of Chest Physicians, the use of anticoagulants depends on the type of stroke and comorbidities.[9] If surgical intervention is a potential, then often standard, unfractionated heparin may be used because this is easily reversible. It is important when administering heparin that antithrombin III levels be checked; they may be physiologically low and require replacement for effective anticoagulation. Antiplatelet agents have not been well studied in this age group for treatment of thrombotic events.

3. Cerebral venous sinus thrombosis (CVST). In neonates with CVST, many may be associated with concomitant hemorrhage around the thrombus, so it is critical to assess for the degree of hemorrhage prior to initiating anticoagulation. In the absence of a significant hemorrhage, low molecular weight heparin (LMWH) is a recommended treatment modality because of its stable delivery, but an optimal dose has not been determined in a controlled study for neonates because renal clearance is likely higher in this age group. Checking for a therapeutic level is important in this age group. CVSTs tend to recanulate quickly in neonates, so if anticoagulation is initiated, reimaging should be performed at 6 weeks; if full recanulation has occurred, anticoagulation can be discontinued. If at 6 weeks thrombosis is still present, the neonate should complete

a 3-month course of LMWH. If a neonate with CVST presents with significant hemorrhage, the infant should be reimaged at 5–7 days to assess for propagation of the thrombus, at which point the degree and direction of propagation will have to be weighed against the degree of hemorrhage in determining whether to begin anticoagulation.

4. Arterial ischemic stroke (AIS). In the absence of evidence of an ongoing source, such as a cardioembolic source, no anticoagulation or aspirin therapy is recommended. If no cause is found, the likelihood of recurrence is low, whereas hemorrhagic conversion is seen.[9]

5. Remove any noncritical indwelling line.

Hemorrhagic Stroke

1. Intracerebral hemorrhage: Platelets should be corrected and maintained at least at 100,000/μL. Prothrombin time (PT) and partial thromboplastin time (PTT) should be checked at least twice daily and corrected with FFP as needed. Vitamin K should be administered if not already given or if there is a defect in vitamin K-dependent coagulation factors. Urgent neurosurgical intervention may be required for drainage or shunting.

2. Neonates who are found to have homozygous protein C deficiency may benefit from protein C replacement. Provide either FFP 10–20 mL/kg every 12 hours or protein C concentrate at 20–60 units/kg until the lesion has resolved.

Supportive Care

Regardless of the cause, brain injury requires standard supportive care. Patients should receive adequate oxygen to maintain normal PaO_2, sodium should be closely followed to minimize cerebral edema, blood pressure should not be allowed to be elevated above or fall below age-appropriate values, and cooling may be useful in decreasing CNS injury during the acute phase.

On the Horizon

Many studies are underway to assess the role of stem cells (cord blood and other sources) in the attenuation of brain injury following neonatal stroke, but significant evidence supporting this therapy has not yet been shown.

REFERENCES

1. Raja T, Nelson K, Ferriero D, Lynch J. Ischemic perinatal stroke: summary of a workshop sponsored by the National Institute of Child Health and Human Development and the National Institute of Neurological Disorders and Stroke. *Pediatrics*. 2007;120(3):609–616.
2. Lynch JK. Epidemiology and classification of perinatal stroke. *Semin Fetal Neonatal Med*. 2009;14(5):245–249.
3. Harteman JG, Groenendaal F, Kwee A, et al. Risk factors for perinatal arterial ischaemic stroke in full-term infants: a case-control study. *Arch Dis Child Fetal Neonatal Ed*. Epub 24 Mar 2012.
4. Bassan H, Feldman HA, Limperopoulos C, et al. Periventricular hemorrhagic infarction: risk factors and neonatal outcome. *Pediatr Neurol*. 2006;35(2):85–92.
5. Cowen F, Mercuri E, Groenendaal F, Bassi L, et al. Does cranial ultrasound imaging identify arterial cerebral infarction in term neonates? *Arch Dis Child Fetal Neonatal Ed*. 2004;90(3):F252–F256.
6. Dzieko D, Wendland M, Derugin N, Ferriero DM, Vexler ZS. Magnetic resonance imaging (MRI) as a translational tool for the study of neonatal stroke. *J Child Neurol*. 2011;26(9):1145–1153.
7. Roelants-van Rign AM, Nikkels PG, Groenendaal F. Neonatal diffusion-weighted MR imaging: relation with histopathology or follow-up MR examination. *Neuropediatrics*. 2001;32(6):286–294.
8. Roach SE, Golomb MR, Adabs R. Management of stroke in infants and children: a scientific statement from a special writing group of the American Heart Association Stroke Council and the Council on Cardiovascular Disease in the young. *Stroke*. 2008;39(9):2644–2691.
9. Manco-Johnson MJ, Grabowski EF, Hellgreen M, et al. Recommendations for tPA thrombolysis in children. On behalf of the Scientific Subcommittee on Perinatal and Pediatric Thrombosis of the Scientific and Standardization Committee of the International Society of Thrombosis and Haemostasis. *Thrombosis and Haemostasis*. 2002;88(1):157–158.
10. Monagle P, Chalmers E, Chan A, et al. Antithrombotic therapy in neonates and children. *Chest*. 2007;133(6):951S.

Part C: Heart

80 Cyanotic Congenital Heart Disease

Gail Wright

BACKGROUND

Epidemiology

Congenital heart defects (CHDs) are the most commonly reported major birth defect. Severe CHDs, the forms requiring early treatment at a cardiac center, have an incidence of approximately 3 per 1000 live births; the majority of these are cyanotic lesions. Although the overall incidence has climbed over the years, perhaps because of improved diagnostic methods such as echocardiography, the incidence of the major cyanotic types has remained fairly stable.

Etiology

The vast majority of CHDs are idiopathic. However, there are many known risk factors and associations.

1. Risk factors include
   a. Maternal diabetes;
   b. Maternal antihypertensive medications;
   c. Maternal retinol/high-dose vitamin A intake;
   d. Maternal lithium treatment (increased risk of Ebstein anomaly); and
   e. Maternal rubella.
2. Genetic causes are numerous, with more added all the time, including
   a. Trisomies;
   b. Williams-Beuren syndrome;

c. DiGeorge velocardiofacial syndrome (deletion 22q11);
   d. Turner and Noonan syndromes;
   e. Alagille syndrome;
   f. CHARGE (coloboma, heart defects, choanal atresia, mental retardation, genitourinary and ear anomalies) association;
   g. Costello syndrome; and others.
3. There are syndromes/sequences without known genetic markers, such as VACTERL (vertebral, anal, cardiac, tracheoesophageal, renal, and limb) association.

EVALUATION AND WORKUP

Pathophysiology

The differential diagnosis of the cyanotic neonate begins with a pathophysiologic question: Is the etiology intrapulmonary shunting, intracardiac shunting, or alveolar hypoventilation (Figure 80-1)?

1. A thorough physical examination (Table 80-1), chest radiograph (Table 80-2), and hyperoxia test can distinguish congenital heart disease from parenchymal lung disease and central nervous system depression as etiologies of central cyanosis (Figure 80-2).
2. Conceptually, the hyperoxia test assesses whether there is a diffusion barrier in the lungs that limits oxygenation or whether there is shunting of deoxygenated blood into the systemic circulation at the cardiac level.

1067

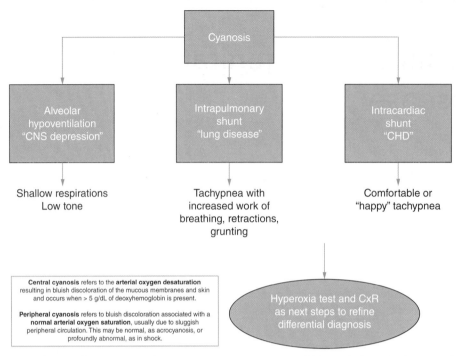

FIGURE 80-1 Causes of central cyanosis in the neonate. CHD, congenital heart defect; CNS, central nervous system; CxR, chest x-ray.

Laboratory Examinations

Concurrently, the differential diagnosis can be narrowed further based on the specific results of the physical examination, chest radiograph, hyperoxia test, and electrocardiogram (Figure 80-3). The degree of mixing of the pulmonary and systemic circulations helps frame the results of these bedside diagnostic tests.

1. Insufficient mixing, resulting in an extremely low PaO_2 (partial pressure of oxygen) on the hyperoxia test;

2. Complete admixture, resulting in a PaO_2 of 40; or

3. Complete admixture with excess pulmonary blood flow, resulting in mild cyanosis not improved with administration of oxygen but PaO_2 greater than 50.

4. Once intracardiac shunting has been confirmed as the etiology of the cyanosis, goal-directed therapies should be initiated.

Electrocardiograms

Electrocardiograms (ECGs) are generally insensitive tests in neonates because the normal findings of right axis deviation and right ventricular hypertrophy mask pathology. However, ECGs, which are easily available

Table 80-1 Physical Exam Pearls for Cyanotic Neonate With Congenital Heart Defect (CHD)

1. Distinguish central vs peripheral cyanosis.
2. The tip of the tongue is a good place to check for central cyanosis; circulation is not sluggish there and not affected by ethnicity.
3. With anemia, central cyanosis will be less prominent, whereas with polycythemia, central cyanosis is apparent at a higher arterial saturation.
4. Differential cyanosis upper vs lower body (examination, pulse oximetry) = right-to-left shunting at patent ductus arteriosus (PDA).
5. Systolic ejection murmur at LUSB suggests obstruction to pulmonary blood flow.
6. Four-extremity blood pressures are essential part of the examination.

Table 80-2 Chest X-ray Pearls for Cyanotic Neonate With Congenital Heart Defect (CHD)

1. "Egg on a string" = narrow mediastinal silhouette = TGA
2. "Boot-shaped heart" = absence of pulmonary artery = ToF
3. Right aortic arch associated with ToF and truncus arteriosus
4. Massive cardiomegaly = Ebstein anomaly
5. Abdominal situs inversus or ambiguous associated with heterotaxy, usually single-ventricle variant, may have associated PA/PS with or without TAPVR

Abbreviations: TAPVR, total anomalous pulmonary venous return; ToF, tetralogy of Fallot.

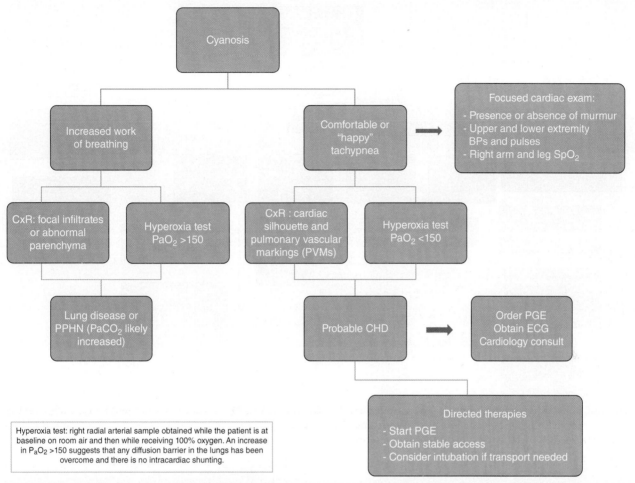

Hyperoxia test: right radial arterial sample obtained while the patient is at baseline on room air and then while receiving 100% oxygen. An increase in P_aO_2 >150 suggests that any diffusion barrier in the lungs has been overcome and there is no intracardiac shunting.

FIGURE 80-2 Etiologies of central cyanosis. BP, blood pressure; CHD, congenital heart defect; CxR, chest x-ray; ECG, electrocardiogram; $PaCO_2$, partial pressure of carbon dioxide; PaO_2, partial pressure of oxygen; PGE, prostaglandin E; PPHN, persistent pulmonary hypertension of the newborn; SpO_2, oxygen saturation as measured by pulse oximetry.

and cheap, are still very useful because, for certain lesions, the ECG findings are so pathognomonic that, in combination with physical examination and hyperoxia test results, they lead to the diagnosis (Figure 80-3 and Table 80-3). This is typically the case for lesions with absent right-side structures, such as pulmonary atresia or tricuspid atresia, which show a paucity of rightward forces on ECG.

TREATMENT

Prostaglandin

The prostaglandin alprostadil should be ordered, stable access obtained, and intubation considered if transport might be needed. Cardiology consultation should be requested, but therapies should *not* be deferred while waiting for the cardiologist.

Insufficient Mixing Lesions

It is crucial to recognize lesions with insufficient mixing because time is of the essence for these

patients. In these cases, so little oxygenated blood makes it to the systemic circulation that anaerobic metabolism occurs. Without emergent intervention, death or injury may ensue within minutes to hours. Transposition of the great arteries with intact atrial septum and obstructed total anomalous pulmonary venous return are the two leading etiologies. Early involvement of an interventional cardiologist and cardiac surgeon facilitates emergent atrial septostomy or surgery as indicated.

Complete Admixture Lesions

The complete admixture defects allow for complete mixing of the deoxygenated systemic venous return and the richly oxygenated pulmonary venous return. The majority of cyanotic congenital heart lesions fall within this broad pathophysiologic category.

1. Transposition of the great arteries, with some mixing at the patent foramen ovale or an atrial septal defect, is by far the most common lesion of all cyanotic CHDs in neonates.

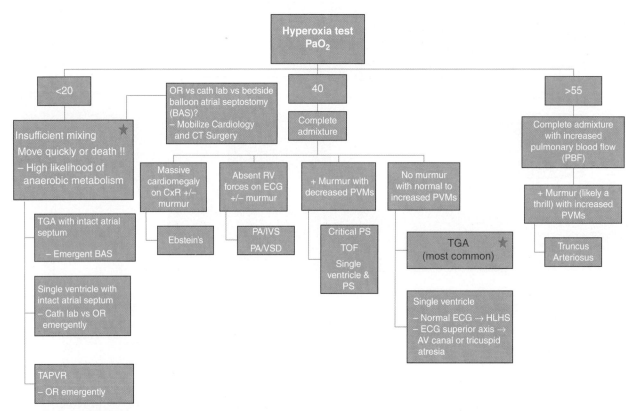

FIGURE 80-3 Differential diagnosis. AV, atrioventricular; CT, computed tomography; CxR, chest x-ray; ECG, electrocardiogram; HLHS, hypoplastic left heart syndrome; OR, operating room; PaO₂, partial pressure of oxygen; RV, right ventricle; TAPVR, total anomalous pulmonary venous return; TOF, tetralogy of Fallot.

2. In lesions with limitation of pulmonary blood flow, there is mechanical obstruction of the right ventricular outflow tract. As a secondary consequence, deoxygenated blood shunts right to left at the atrial or ventricular level, resulting in desaturated blood entering the systemic circulation. The anatomic outflow tract narrowing results in flow disturbance, which causes a murmur audible on physical examination, and there usually are decreased pulmonary vascular markings on chest x-ray. These findings are helpful in the differential diagnosis and suggest tetralogy of Fallot, critical pulmonic stenosis, or a single-ventricle variant with pulmonic stenosis (Figure 80-3 and Table 80-1).

3. The Ebstein anomaly, in which there is an abnormal tricuspid valve with severe tricuspid regurgitation leading to marked cardiomegaly, should be considered when the cardiac silhouette takes up the entire thoracic cavity on chest x-ray.

SUMMARY

With this conceptual framework for cyanotic congenital heart disease and a few easily accessible bedside diagnostic tests, the diagnosis can be reached independently and initiate lifesaving, goal-directed therapy expeditiously. The echocardiogram then provides anatomic detail to guide further management in collaboration with a cardiologist and cardiac surgeon.

Table 80-3 Electrocardiogram (ECG) Pearls for Cyanotic Neonate With Congenital Heart Defect (CHD)

1. RAD and RVH are expected normal patterns that should be present.
2. Any other QRS axis or a paucity of RV forces is *abnormal*.
3. ECGs are insensitive tests in neonates (eg, patients with HLHS do not have half their heart but have normal ECGs for age because they have RAD and RVH). However, certain classic findings, when present, are extremely useful in making a diagnosis.
4. Superior axis + cyanosis = tricuspid atresia.
6. Paucity of RV forces = right heart hypoplasia (pulmonary or tricuspid atresia)
6. Delta waves = WPW + cyanosis = Ebstein anomaly.
7. ST segment changes = ischemia + cyanosis = truncus arteriosus.

Abbreviations: HLHS, hypoplastic left heart syndrome; RV, right ventricle; RVH, right ventricular hypertrophy; WPW, Wolff-Parkinson-White syndrome.

SUGGESTED READING

Alsoufi B, Bennetts J, Verma S, Caldarone CA. New developments in the treatment of hypoplastic left heart syndrome. *Pediatrics*. 2007;119:109–117.

Browning Carmo KA, Barr P, West M, et al. Transporting newborn infants with suspected duct dependent congenital heart disease on low-dose prostaglandin E1 without routine mechanical ventilation. *Arch Dis Child Fetal Neonatal Ed*. 2007;92:F117–F119.

Hoffman JIE, Kaplan S. The incidence of congenital heart disease. *J Am Coll Cardiol*. 2002;39:1890–1900.

Laas E, Lelong N, Thieulin A-C, et al. Preterm birth and congenital heart defects: a population-based study. *Pediatrics*. 2012;130:1–9.

Meckler GD, Lowe C. To intubate or not to intubate? Transporting infants on prostaglandin E1. *Pediatrics*. 2009;123:e25–e30.

Oster ME, Lee KA, Honein MA, et al. Trends in survival among infants with critical congenital heart defects. *Pediatrics*. 2013;131:e1502–e1508.

Pierpont ME, Basson CT, Benson DW Jr, et al. Genetic basis for congenital heart defects: current knowledge. *Circulation*. 2007;115:3015–3038.

Van der Linde D, Konings EEM, Slager MA, et al. Birth prevalence of congenital heart disease worldwide. *J Am Coll Cardiol*. 2011;58:2241–2247.

Williams GD, Cohen RS. Perioperative management of low birth weight infants for open-heart surgery. *Pediatr Anesth*. 2011;21:538–553.

81 Management of Congestive Heart Failure

Seth A. Hollander and Daniel Bernstein

INTRODUCTION

In neonates, congestive heart failure (CHF) secondary to congenital heart lesions predominates, with primary cardiac functional abnormalities (eg, dilated cardiomyopathy, myocarditis) relatively rare. When present, primary myocardial disease is associated with decreased intrinsic cardiac function and cardiac output, leading to tachycardia, diaphoresis, fluid overload, pulmonary congestion (secondary to increased left-sided filling pressures), feeding intolerance, ischemic injury of the brain and other end organs, and eventually death.[1] In contrast, in patients with heart failure secondary to congenital heart disease, several mechanistic pathways and modes of presentation exist. In left ventricular (LV) obstructive lesions (eg, critical aortic stenosis), severely increased afterload depresses apparent cardiac function even if the muscle itself is normal. In severe forms in which subendocardial fibrosis is present, cardiac contractility may be truly reduced. In patients with left-to-right shunts, intrinsic cardiac contractile function is either normal or enhanced, and cardiac output is usually well preserved until the late stages of disease. Increased (and inefficient) cardiac work results in typical heart failure symptoms as described, with end-stage heart failure manifesting as reduced end-organ perfusion secondary to selective vasoconstriction, cardiovascular collapse, and death.

The symptoms of CHF and its root causes must be recognized quickly and appropriate therapy initiated. Strategies for management of CHF in the neonate are largely similar based on whether the etiology is congenital heart disease or a primary myocardial disorder; however, there are some key differences. Thus, management of these patients should always involve consultation with a pediatric cardiologist.

DIAGNOSIS

In the newborn population, the age at presentation can provide clues regarding the most likely etiology (Table 81-1). Signs and symptoms of CHF in the neonate are summarized in Table 81-2. Heart failure, especially that associated with left-sided obstructive lesions, can present dramatically. However, in other conditions, it often presents insidiously. Generalized constitutional symptoms are common, and even with substantially reduced ventricular function, the neonate with CHF may demonstrate little more than failure to thrive, irritability, or unexplained tachycardia. If cardiac output is inadequate, peripheral vasoconstriction, arrhythmia, and deteriorations in laboratory indices of renal and hepatic function may develop. This condition, termed *cardiogenic shock*, requires urgent treatment before irreversible end-organ dysfunction occurs.

MANAGEMENT

Management goals for the neonate with CHF are twofold: (1) restoring normal fluid balance and hemodynamics and (2) addressing the underlying disease. General management strategies are summarized in Figure 81-1.

Table 81-1 Heart Failure Presenting in the Neonate by Age at Presentation

Heart failure that presents at birth:

Persistent pulmonary hypertension of the newborn

Total anomalous pulmonary venous return with obstruction

Ebstein anomaly of the tricuspid valve (large heart and cyanosis)

Myocarditis acquired in utero

Arrhythmias (fetal heart block, supraventricular tachycardia)

Complete heart block secondary to maternal anti-SSA/Ro or anti-SSB/La antibodies

Arterio-venous malformations (AVMs), often cerebral

Lactic acidosis

Sepsis

Heart failure that presents in the first week of life (LV outflow tract obstructions):

Coarctation of the aorta

Critical aortic stenosis

Mitral stenosis (often part of Shone complex)

Left-to-right shunts with LV outflow tract obstruction (eg, VSD plus coarctation)

Primary cardiomyopathies (dilated, hypertrophic, restrictive) in this age group often associated with genetic syndromes or mitochondrial, glycogen storage, or metabolic diseases

Heart failure that presents after the first week of life:

Primary cardiomyopathies (dilated, hypertrophic, restrictive)

Large left-right shunts (VSD, AV septal defect)

Postnatally acquired myocarditis

Abbreviations: AV, atrioventricular; LV, left ventricular; VSD, ventricular septal defect.

Table 81-2 Signs and Symptoms of Congestive Heart Failure in the Neonate

Tachycardia

Irritability

Failure to thrive/poor feeding

Respiratory distress (tachypnea, rales, wheezing, pulmonary edema on chest x-ray)

Fluid overload (edema, ascites, hydrops fetalis)

Cardiomegaly

Cool extremities, pallor, mottled skin

Poor peripheral pulses, narrow pulse pressure

Hepatomegaly, elevated central venous pressure

S3 or S4 gallop, holosystolic murmur consistent with mitral or tricuspid valve regurgitation, other murmurs consistent with specific congenital heart lesions

Restoring Fluid Balance and Hemodynamics

The mainstays of symptomatic treatment of CHF in the neonate are diuretics and inotropic agents. For patients with fluid overload or pulmonary edema, diuretics should be initiated with careful attention to maintaining adequate renal perfusion. The loop diuretic furosemide can be given intermittently (starting dose 1 mg/kg IV given every 6 to 12 hours or 1–2 mg/kg orally given every 6 to 12 hours) or via continuous infusion (starting dose 0.1 mg/kg/h) and should be titrated based on response, with the general goal to achieve euvolemia. Goals of diuresis should be to improve respiratory mechanics, reduce edema/ascites, and improve oral feeding tolerance. For patients who require additional diuretic therapy, the addition of chlorothiazide (2.5–5 mg/kg IV or 5–10 mg/kg orally, generally every 12 hours) often has a synergistic effect. Spironolactone (1 mg/kg orally every 12 hours) can be added to minimize potassium depletion. Overdiuresis leading to prerenal or intrinsic renal failure should be avoided, and meticulous monitoring and correction of electrolyte disturbances are imperative because arrhythmias are generally poorly tolerated in the neonate with impaired ventricular function.

For patients with primary myocardial disease, judicious use of intravenous inotropic agents can improve cardiac output, reverse pathologic perturbations of vasomotor tone, and improve end-organ perfusion. Commonly used inotropes, their indications, and side effect profiles are listed in Table 81-3. Understanding of each agent and its effects on myocardial contraction, heart rate, and peripheral vasomotor tone as well as its side effect profile is imperative for safe administration. Furthermore, inotropic agents must be used with extreme caution in patients with congenital heart disease because they may increase left-to-right shunting and potentiate cardiac ischemia in left-sided obstructive lesions.

Primary Diseases of the Myocardium

Primary myocardial diseases (eg, dilated cardiomyopathy, hypertrophic cardiomyopathy, myocarditis) can manifest at any age, including in the neonatal period. Coincidence with known genetic syndromes or primary mitochondrial, glycogen storage, or metabolic diseases is common. A history of prenatal fever or other signs of infection in the mother may be obtained. If CHF is present, management is aimed at restoring normal fluid balance and hemodynamics, as described previously. For some conditions, disease-specific therapies are available (eg, enzyme replacement in Pompe disease). Myocarditis may resolve spontaneously.

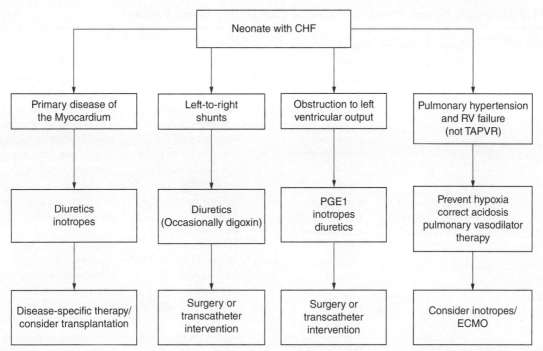

FIGURE 81-1 Cause-specific management of congestive heart failure (CHF) in the neonate. ECMO, extracorporeal membrane oxygenation; PGE1, prostaglandin E₁; RV, right ventricle; TAPVR, total anomalous pulmonary venous return.

However, for the primary dilated cardiomyopathies, cardiac transplantation is often the only definitive cure.

Obstructions to Left Ventricular Output

Patients with lesions that prevent blood from exiting the LV (coarctation of the aorta, aortic stenosis) may be asymptomatic until the ductus arteriosus closes, usually in the first 2–7 days of life, at which point the abrupt increase in LV afterload can lead to impaired systemic perfusion and decreased ventricular function. Mechanical release of the obstruction, via either surgery or transcatheter techniques, is imperative. While arrangements are made for intervention, intravenous infusion of prostaglandin E₁ (alprostadil, PGE₁) (0.01 to 0.1 μg/kg/min IV) can be lifesaving. PGE₁ can be infused through a central venous catheter, peripheral intravenous line, or an arterial line. Common side effects of PGE₁ are hypotension and apnea, and elective intubation at higher doses of PGE₁ may be necessary. When indicated, the adjunct use of an inotropic agent such as dopamine can improve cardiac output; however, vasodilator agents should be avoided as they can reduce coronary perfusion.

Left-to-Right Shunts

Patients with left-to-right shunts (eg, ventricular septal defects) are at risk for pulmonary overcirculation, fluid overload, and heart failure once the pulmonary vascular resistance falls. Patients with left-to-right shunts presenting early in the neonatal period must be evaluated for combined lesions (eg, ventricular septal defect and coarctation) because severe heart failure symptoms from a septal defect alone in the first 2–3 weeks of life would be unusual. Treatment of CHF in this setting includes the use of diuretics (as previously discussed). Digoxin, once the mainstay of treatment in these patients, is now less commonly used, although it can be helpful in reducing tachycardia and diaphoresis. Oxygen must only be used judiciously because its pulmonary vasodilatory properties can increase the left-to-right shunt. Anemia should be corrected to a high-normal hemoglobin level, which can reduce CHF symptoms and facilitate somatic growth. Surgical closure of the defect is ultimately necessary. Pulmonary artery banding, used rarely in the modern area, should still be considered in those patients for whom surgery must be delayed for other reasons.

Abnormalities of Pulmonary Vascular Resistance

Persistent pulmonary hypertension of the newborn (PPHN), bronchopulmonary dysplasia, meconium aspiration, and cardiac diseases that increase left atrial pressure (eg, mitral stenosis) are other common causes of pulmonary hypertension (PH) that present in the first week of life and can lead to increased right

Table 81-3 Inotropic Agents Used in Neonatal Congestive Heart Failure[a]

Class	Name/Common Dosing	Pharmacologic Effect	Indications	Side Effects
Sympathomimetic	Dopamine (5–15 µg/kg/min gtt)	DA1 and DA2 receptors at low doses, β1 (inotropy) at appropriate doses, α1 (vasoconstriction) at higher doses	Systolic dysfunction, hypotension, fluid overload (theoretical improvement in renal improvement via DA receptors at low doses)	Tachycardia, arrhythmia, peripheral vasoconstriction, tissue burn with extravasation,[b] compromised renal blood flow at high doses; may increase risk of infection
	Dobutamine (5–15 µg/kg/min gtt)	Primarily β1 (inotropy), some α1, minimal β2 effect	Systolic dysfunction without hypotension; patients with ischemia or arrhythmic potential	Tachycardia, arrhythmia, peripheral vasoconstriction, tissue burn with extravasation; less tachycardia and arrhythmogenicity than dopamine; may reduce coronary perfusion in left-sided obstructive lesions
	Epinephrine (0.01–0.1 µg/kg/min gtt)	β1 (inotropy) and β2 (vasodilation) at appropriate doses, α1 (vasoconstriction) dominates at higher doses	Should be reserved for patients who require stronger inotropic support than dopamine or dobutamine can provide	Tachycardia, arrhythmia, peripheral vasoconstriction, tissue burn with extravasation, compromised renal blood flow at high doses, elevated blood glucose levels, elevated WBC counts
Phosphodiesterase inhibitor	Milrinone (0.25–1 mcg/kg/min gtt)	Increased cAMP levels lead to increased β2 (vasodilation), α1, and β1 (mild inotropy)	Peripheral vasoconstriction, diastolic dysfunction; increased cAMP levels lead to vasodilation and lusitropy (improved diastolic function), decreased SVR	Hypotension, thrombocytopenia, arrhythmia; should have minimal effect on heart rate; may reduce coronary perfusion in left-sided obstructive lesions
Cardiac glycoside	Digoxin (3–5 µg/kg orally twice daily[c])	Increases in Ca^{2+} influx via activation of $NaCa^{2+}$ pump	Systolic dysfunction, certain arrhythmias, heart rate control	Sinus bradycardia and AV nodal slowing via parasympathetic activation, atrial and ventricular arrhythmias, toxicity if overdosed (especially in the setting of decreased K^+)

Abbreviations: AV, atrioventricular; cAMP, cyclic adenosine monophosphate; DA, dopamine receptor; gtt, continuous intravenous infusion; NE, norepinephrine; SVR, systemic vascular resistance; WBC, white blood cells.
[a]Used with permission of Dr. Stephen Roth.
[b]Inotropic agents should be administered through a central venous line whenever possible. Epinephrine should always be administered through a central venous line.
[c]Digoxin dosing is variable. Its administration should be in consultation with a pediatric cardiologist, especially when administered to premature infants.

ventricular afterload and decreased right ventricular function.[2] However, PH related to left-to-right shunt lesions does not usually present in the neonatal or infant period. PH occurs more frequently in patients with trisomy 21 than in the general population.[3]

Treatment goals are aimed at reducing pulmonary arterial pressure, preventing hypoxia, and correcting acidosis. Intravenous inotropic support can augment right ventricular output, if necessary. Refractory cases may require extracorporeal membrane oxygenation

(ECMO), which has been shown to improve survival.[4] Use of PGE$_1$ to maintain ductal patency in neonates with PH is controversial.

Total anomalous pulmonary venous return (TAPVR) with obstruction is a unique cause of increased pulmonary arterial pressures and is a surgical emergency. If TAPVR is suspected (small heart and whiteout of lung fields on chest x-ray), cardiology and cardiothoracic surgery departments should be consulted immediately and an echocardiogram performed as soon as possible. PGE$_1$ has little role in the management of this lesion, and pulmonary vasodilators are generally contraindicated.

REFERENCES

1. Katz AM. *Heart Failure Pathophysiology, Molecular Biology and Clinical Management*. Philadelphia, PA: Lippincott, Williams, and Wilkins; 2000.
2. Dhillon R. The management of neonatal pulmonary hypertension. *Arch Dis Child Fetal Neonatal Ed*. 2012;97:F223–F228.
3. Cua CL, Blankenship A, North AL, Hayes J, Nelin LD. Increased incidence of idiopathic persistent pulmonary hypertension in Down syndrome neonates. *Pediatr Cardiol*. 2007;28(4):250–254.
4. Hintz SR, Benitz WE, Colby CE, Sheehan AM, Rycus P, Van Meurs KP. Utilization and outcomes of neonatal cardiac extracorporeal life support: 1996–2000. *Pediatr Crit Care Med*. 2005;6(1):33–38.

82 Blood Pressure Support

David M. Axelrod and Stephen J. Roth

GENERAL CONCEPTS

Physiology of Blood Pressure in the Neonate

Neonatal Blood Pressure Support and Physiology of Blood Pressure

Caring for a critically ill neonate often requires the provider to consider the physiology, goals, complications, and pharmacologic methods of increasing a newborn patient's blood pressure. Although various methods and medications are available to increase systemic blood pressure, few human data convincingly support the common practices for blood pressure support in adult intensive care unit, pediatric intensive care unit, or neonatal intensive care unit (NICU).[1–11] This chapter describes the physiology of systemic blood pressure in the neonate, defines the pharmacologic target receptors, and presents the medications most commonly used to raise blood pressure.

Cardiac Output, Systemic Vascular Resistance, and Blood Pressure

Systemic blood pressure is determined by the product of cardiac output and systemic vascular resistance (SVR). Cardiac output is determined by the product of heart rate and stroke volume; stroke volume is determined by the preload, afterload, and contractility of the myocardium. Derangements in any of these parameters can produce hypotension in the neonatal patient. It should be noted, however, that simply increasing the blood pressure may not achieve the desired physiologic effect if the goal is to increase organ blood flow and oxygen delivery. Blood pressure and systemic blood flow are poorly correlated in the newborn,[12,13] reflecting the importance of SVR in the neonate. Importantly, the neonate has unique physiology that must be understood when considering systemic blood pressure. Because of a relatively noncompliant myocardium, neonates are more dependent on heart rate to generate cardiac output than adults.[14–17] Also unique to neonates are the transitional circulation immediately following birth, less-functional cerebral autoregulation mechanisms, the potential state of prematurity, and the ongoing maturation of the myocardium and vascular bed.[18–20]

Defining Neonatal Hypotension

The definition of hypotension in the newborn continues to challenge the clinician. "Mean arterial pressure greater than or equal to gestational age" frequently is touted as a guideline for minimum acceptable blood pressure for a neonate, but few data exist to support this practice.[21–27] Clinicians often use both gestational age and birth weight as guidelines for estimating expected blood pressure in a neonate (Figures 82-1 and 82-2). In principle, the blood pressure must be adequate to deliver oxygen to the tissues and support delivery of nutrients to the organs (most importantly the brain and heart) while removing toxic waste products from cells. The inability to achieve adequate tissue oxygen delivery and waste removal defines neonatal shock. Blood pressure is clearly inadequate if organs are poorly perfused (eg, leading to acute kidney injury or necrotizing enterocolitis [NEC]) or if biochemical markers indicate inadequate perfusion (eg, elevated lactate or base deficit on blood gas analysis).

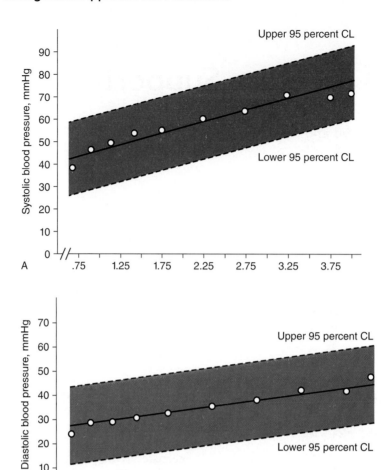

FIGURE 82-1 Linear regression of mean systolic (A) and diastolic (B) blood pressure vs *birth weight* in 329 newborns admitted to the neonatal intensive care unit on day of life 1. CL; confidence limit. (Reproduced with permission from Zubrow et al.[25])

The goal of managing neonatal hypotension should be to maximize oxygen delivery and minimize oxygen consumption, thereby providing the optimal oxygen supply/demand ratio. A detailed discussion of oxygen content, delivery, consumption, and extraction ratio is beyond the scope of this chapter.[18,28] Although defining hypotension is difficult, data in the premature neonate have correlated hypotension with intraventricular hemorrhage, poor neurodevelopmental outcomes, and death, thus highlighting the importance of adequate tissue perfusion in these patients.[1,27,29–34] Further study of neonatal blood pressure and cerebral blood flow using superior vena caval flow measurement or near-infrared spectroscopy (NIRS) may help define what an "adequate" blood pressure is for a given newborn.[26,35]

Differential Diagnosis of Neonatal Hypotension

The differential diagnosis of inadequate tissue perfusion (including "hypotension" and "low-output states")

in the newborn is broad and varies based on the gestational age of the patient. The most common causes of shock and hypotension are hypovolemia (including placental hemorrhage or organ hemorrhage in the perinatal period); infection (sepsis, NEC); extreme prematurity; perinatal asphyxia; severe pulmonary disease (often with pulmonary hypertension); adrenal crisis/insufficiency; large left-to-right shunts (most commonly a large patent ductus arteriosus); and poor cardiac function (because of pump failure, arrhythmias, and obstructive congenital cardiac lesions, among others).[6–9,11,22]

Echocardiography is a noninvasive tool to assess cardiac structure and function in the hypotensive neonate. Cardiac pathology, such as left-sided obstructive lesions, a large patent ductus arteriosus, and poor myocardial contractility, can be delineated by an echocardiogram. These findings may lead the clinician to initiate inotropic agents sooner or modulate blood pressure in other ways when appropriate (eg, initiating prostaglandins in a ductal-dependent lesion such as critical aortic stenosis).

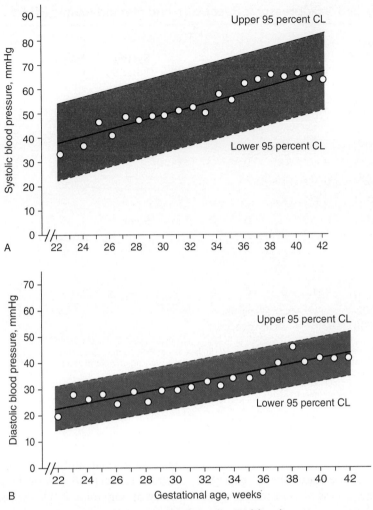

FIGURE 82-2 Linear regression of mean systolic (A) and diastolic (B) blood pressure vs *gestational age* in 329 newborns admitted to the neonatal intensive care unit on day of life 1. (Reproduced with permission from Zubrow et al.[25])

Treatment of hypotension (ie, blood pressure support) necessitates understanding the physiologic abnormality and the primary cause of the patient's abnormal physiology. Maintaining intravascular volume (with saline or albumin infusions) is supported by physiologic principles, but it has not been shown to improve systemic blood flow compared to pharmacologic support.[36,37] However, it is common practice to ensure adequate volume administration before initiating inotropes, and most inotropes and pressors require an adequate preload volume to augment blood pressure effectively. The remainder of this chapter focuses on the principles of pharmacologic management of hypotension.

PHARMACOLOGIC BLOOD PRESSURE SUPPORT

Inotropes and Vasopressors

The mainstays of pharmacologic treatment of neonatal hypotension remain inotropes and vasopressors, with the former defined as agents that increase the force of myocardial contraction and the latter defined as agents that increase blood pressure by constricting the arterial vasculature (ie, increasing SVR).[2,3,9,10,38,39] (Vasodilators may also increase systemic blood flow, but they usually do not increase blood pressure and thus are not discussed here.) Inotropes are classified as sympathomimetics (eg, dopamine), phosphodiesterase inhibitors (eg, milrinone), and cardiac glycosides (eg, digoxin); their mechanism of action is to increase intracellular calcium concentration, thus increasing the force of myocardial contraction. Also frequently used are agents that increase heart rate (chronotropes), improve myocardial relaxation (lusitropes; phosphodiesterase inhibitors), and medications that work by other mechanisms to increase blood pressure (steroids, calcium, thyroid hormone). When initiating inotropes or vasopressors, the clinician must consider methods of monitoring intravascular volume status and the effectiveness of pharmacologic therapy. Blood pressure should be measured by an invasive arterial catheter (peripheral or umbilical) when a patient

Table 82-1 Inotropes and Vasopressors: Receptors and Hemodynamic Effects

	Dose (µg/kg/min)	α_1	β_1	β_2	DA	HR	Systolic Function	Diastolic Function	Myocardial O_2 Demand	SVR	PVR
Inotropes											
Dopamine	1–5	0	+	0	++	↑	Minimal change	—	Minimal change	–/↑	–
Dopamine	6–10	+	++	0	++	↑	↑	—	↑	↑	–/↑
Dopamine	11–20	++	++	0	++	↑	↑	—	↑	↑↑	–/↑
Dobutamine	1–20	0/+	+++	+	0	↑	↑	—	↑	↓	–/↓
Epinephrine	0.01–1	++	+++	++	0	↑	↑↑	—	↑	↑	–/↑
Norepinephrine	0.01–1	+++	++	0	0	↑	Some ↑	—	↑	↑↑	–/↑
Milrinone	0.1–1	None (PDE inhibitor)					↑	Improved	Minimal change	↓	↓
Vasopressors											
Phenylephrine	0.1–2	+++	0	0	0	—	—	—	—	↑↑↑	—
Vasopressin[b]	0.0003–0.008	+	None (stimulates ADH receptor)			—	—	—	—	↑↑↑	?

Abbreviations: ADH, antidiuretic hormone; DA, dopamine receptors; HR, heart rate; PVR, pulmonary vascular resistance; PDE, phosphodiesterase; SVR, systemic vascular resistance. Receptor activity is delineated by 0 (no activity) and by varying degrees of receptor stimulation (graded from + to +++). Hemodynamic effects are delineated by — (no effect), ↑ (increased) or ↓ (decreased).
[a]Data from Saraswati Kache, MD, and UpToDate. Use of Vasopressors and Inotropes, authors Nalaka Gooneratne MD, MSCE and Scott Manaker, MD, PhD.
[b]Vasopressin dosing units are units/kilogram/minute.

requires multiple interventions for the treatment of hypotension. Similarly, volume status should be measured with central venous access to confirm adequate cardiac preload.

Adrenergic Receptor Subtypes

To understand the actions of these medications, it is critical that the provider recall the receptor subtypes which are activated on the cell membrane. The relevant subtypes are the α_1, β_1, and β_2 adrenergic receptors and the dopamine receptors.[9,39–41] The α_1-adrenergic receptors, when activated in vascular walls, promote vasoconstriction; α_1-stimulating medications elevate blood pressure by increasing SVR. The α_1 receptor has also been found in the myocardium, and its activation increases cardiac contractility.[42] Animal data also suggest that receptors in the right ventricle may differ from those in the left ventricle, thus promoting the specific targeting of right ventricular strain in clinical scenarios such as pulmonary hypertension.[43] Activation of β_1-adrenergic receptors promotes increased inotropy and chronotropy (without vasoconstriction); β_1-stimulating medications increase blood pressure by increasing cardiac output. The β_2-adrenergic receptors promote vasodilation in the cardiovascular system and bronchodilation in the lung. Dopamine receptor stimulation promotes dilation of the cardiac,

gastrointestinal, and renal vascular beds via dopamine 1 (DA-1) receptors and of the peripheral vascular bed through dopamine 2 (DA-2) receptors. Stimulation of dopamine receptors can also induce norepinephrine release and act as a vasoconstrictor (see the discussion that follows). A summary of pharmacologic receptor subtype activity, mechanism of action, and hemodynamic effects for the most commonly used inotropes and vasopressors is included (Table 82-1).

SPECIFIC AGENTS FOR BLOOD PRESSURE SUPPORT IN THE NEONATE

The pharmacologic agents for blood pressure support have been studied in human neonates; however, controversy still exists regarding which inotrope or vasopressor is preferred for a given patient. The following is a description of the primary mechanism of action, indications, side effects, and physiologic properties of the most commonly used blood pressure medications. Not described in this chapter are steroids, which have been studied in neonatal septic shock[44–51] and are included in the Surviving Sepsis Campaign and guidelines for the management of pediatric and neonatal septic shock.[52,53]

Dopamine

Dopamine is a drug commonly used in neonates to treat hypotension from a variety of medical or surgical causes (especially postoperative cardiac).[10,11,54,55] Dopamine's effect on blood pressure is mediated via direct stimulation of β_1 receptors on the myocardium along with the indirect effect of increasing norepinephrine, which stimulates α_1 receptors.[56–58] In animal studies, neonatal myocardium has been shown to have more dopamine receptor sensitivity compared to adult myocardium.[59,60]

Frequently discussed is the dose-response curve of dopamine on the cardiovascular system.[55,61] At doses of 1–3 µg/kg/min, the effects are primarily vasodilation of the cerebral, coronary, renal, and gastrointestinal vascular beds via stimulation of DA-1 receptors and dilation of peripheral vascular beds via DA-2 receptors. Doses in the range of 5–15 µg/kg/min are often referred to as "inotropic range" dosing because the stroke volume is increased with less effect on heart rate. As dosing increases in this range, there are increasing β_1 (elevated heart rate) and α_1 (elevated SVR) effects. Above 20 µg/kg/min, dopamine acts mainly on α_1 receptors; it increases inotropy but may compromise blood flow by elevating vascular resistance in the kidney, periphery, and gastrointestinal system, among others.[54,62–65]

Dopamine can cause cardiac dysrhythmias (most commonly sinus tachycardia), vasoconstriction, tissue necrosis with extravasation, and immunosuppression with prolonged use. It has been shown to alter the production of prolactin by the hypothalamus.[55] In select populations, dopamine has been shown to increase oxygen consumption more than oxygen delivery,[66] and it may increase pulmonary artery pressure in premature newborns with a patent ductus arteriosus.[67] Studies in premature and term neonates have compared dopamine to volume administration,[68] dobutamine,[35,65,69–73] epinephrine,[74,75] phosphodiesterase inhibitors,[76,77] and steroids.[78] These data suggest that dopamine augments blood pressure and may increase renal and mesenteric blood flow. However, based on current data, it cannot be recommended for use over other agents.

A large adult study recently compared dopamine to norepinephrine for the treatment of shock; although no difference in mortality was detected, dopamine resulted in significantly more side effects, such as cardiac arrhythmias.[79] These data suggest that dopamine is effective at increasing blood pressure,[11,55,57,62,72,80] but whether it improves mortality, morbidity, or neurodevelopmental outcomes is unclear.[11,13,35,37,81]

Dobutamine

Dobutamine (1–10 µg/kg/min), a synthetic catecholamine, stimulates predominantly β_1 receptors with very little α or β_2 stimulation.[2,3,6,7,10,11] Dobutamine, like dopamine, may exhibit a clinically significant dose-response curve. At doses less than 5 µg/kg/min in children, heart rate does not increase, but cardiac output and blood pressure increase, and left atrial pressure decreases. Heart rate increases at doses greater than 7.5 µg/kg/min.[82] Dobutamine increases inotropy and heart rate and decreases SVR, thus increasing cardiac output and organ blood flow. Decreasing SVR may lower blood pressure; for this reason, dobutamine is mainly used for myocardial dysfunction without severe hypotension. Dobutamine also decreases ventricular filling pressure, pulmonary vascular resistance (PVR), and SVR more effectively than dopamine.[83] Dobutamine does not stimulate norepinephrine release, which also differentiates it from dopamine.

Intestinal perfusion in preterm neonates increases with dobutamine infusion.[62] Data in preterm neonates suggest that dobutamine may be superior to dopamine in increasing systemic blood flow[71,72] (Figures 82-3, 82-4), but conflicting data suggest that dopamine increases blood pressure more effectively.[13,69–71] It remains unclear which inotrope is superior in the premature or term newborn in the NICU,[7,13,71–73] and neurodevelopmental outcomes appear similar after blood pressure support with both agents.[35] Because dobutamine does not stimulate β_2 receptors and has less chronotropic effect, indications for use include patients with systolic dysfunction and normal blood pressure and who are at risk for dysrhythmias. A study in children after cardiopulmonary bypass (CPB), however, revealed little reduction in SVR and significant tachycardia.[84]

Epinephrine

Epinephrine is a potent, endogenously produced adrenergic stimulator that strongly activates the β_1 receptor and moderately activates the β_2 and α_1 receptors. Like dopamine, clinicians use the dose-response curve of epinephrine to affect these 3 receptors. At low doses (0.01–0.1 µg/kg/min), epinephrine increases blood pressure and heart rate by β_1 stimulation, thus increasing cardiac output. The simultaneous α_1 and β_2 receptor stimulation results in little change to SVR at this dose. At higher doses (>0.1 µg/kg/min), epinephrine primarily acts as an α_1-stimulating agent, increasing blood pressure by elevating SVR and increasing inotropy. In the lung, PVR is elevated, and bronchioles are dilated.

Epinephrine is primarily reserved for neonates with extended exposure to CPB with myocardial dysfunction or for patients with medical disease, such as sepsis, that is refractory to 1 inotrope.[2,6,9–11,85] It is also included in the algorithms for neonatal and pediatric resuscitations.[86,87] Epinephrine has been studied in preterm neonates and is effective at increasing blood pressure, although the literature does not support its specific use compared to other inotropes.[3,5,74,75,88]

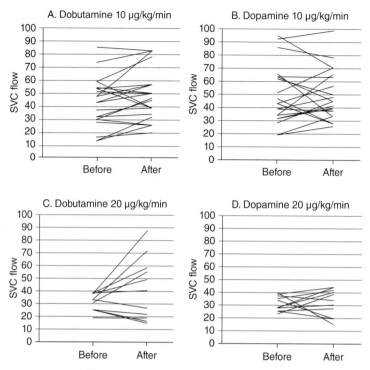

FIGURE 82-3 Superior vena cava (SVC) flow, a surrogate for oxygen delivery to the brain, as measured in neonates receiving dopamine vs dobutamine (each at lower and higher doses). Only higher-dose dobutamine increased SVC flow. (Reproduced with permission from Osborn et al.[72])

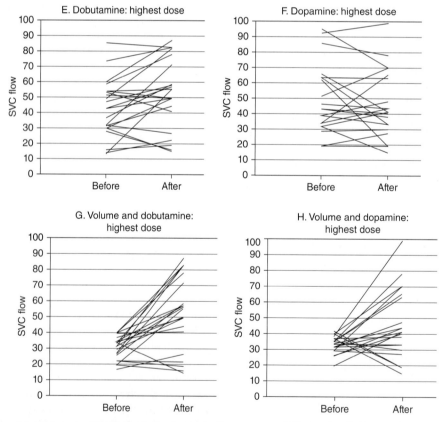

FIGURE 82-4 Superior vena cava (SVC) flow, a surrogate for oxygen delivery to the brain, as measured in neonates receiving dopamine vs dobutamine, each at high doses (E, F) and then with volume administration (G, H). High-dose dopamine and dobutamine increased SVC flow when administered with volume, illustrating the need for adequate volume resuscitation with inotrope administration. (Reproduced with permission from Osborn et al.[72])

The use of epinephrine may be limited by side effects, which occur more commonly than with dobutamine or dopamine. These include tachycardia, ventricular dysrhythmias (especially in those with ischemia), hyperglycemia, lactic acidosis, increasing base deficit, tissue burns (if extravasated), and vasoconstriction, among others.[5,74,88]

Norepinephrine

Norepinephrine (0.01–1 µg/kg/min) is an endogenous catecholamine that stimulates α_1 and β_1 receptors, but unlike epinephrine, it does not have activity on β_2 receptors.[56] Therefore, administration of norepinephrine increases blood pressure by increasing SVR and, to a lesser extent, by increasing cardiac output. The unopposed increase in SVR and lack of β_2-induced vasodilation make norepinephrine the preferred medication for patients with "warm" (septic) shock.[52,53,89] Studies in adults have compared norepinephrine to other inotropes and vasopressors,[3,89,90] and data suggest that norepinephrine may support blood pressure with a more favorable side effect profile compared to dopamine.[79] Its use is limited in neonates and may be affected by concerns for NEC caused by intestinal vasoconstriction.[9]

Phenylephrine

Phenylephrine (0.1–2 µg/kg/min) is a pure α agonist that increases blood pressure by increasing SVR. There is minimal primary effect on inotropy or heart rate; however, vasoconstriction may not necessarily increase systemic blood flow and can result in reflex bradycardia. Phenylephrine has limited use in the NICU population and is reserved for patients in a low-SVR state such as warm septic shock or after anesthetic-induced vasodilation.[91] A special indication for phenylephrine is in the setting of acute pulmonary hypertension, for which it can be used as an adjunct medication to increase SVR and right coronary artery perfusion pressure (when using a sedative and muscle relaxant for intubation, for example). Data from adults suggest it can be detrimental in the management of chronic pulmonary hypertension.[92] Preferentially increasing SVR compared to PVR with phenylephrine is also useful in neonates with tetralogy of Fallot who experience hypercyanotic episodes ("tet spells").[18]

Calcium

The neonatal myocardium handles calcium differently from the adult because of the immature sarcoplasm reticulum in the neonatal cardiac myocyte.[14,93]

Neonates depend more on circulating ionized calcium to enter the cardiac myocyte and stimulate actin-myosin cross-bridge formation and contraction.[16,19,94] For this reason, calcium chloride infusions (2–20 mg/kg/h) have been used to improve cardiac contractility. Ionized calcium levels are monitored with a goal to maintain levels of 1.1–1.3 mmol/L. Notably, excess calcium influx into the cardiac myocytes has been associated with myocyte necrosis and diastolic dysfunction.[95–97] In older children and adults, the mature sarcoplasmic reticulum stores calcium more effectively; exogenous administration of calcium chloride stimulates calcium receptors in the vascular endothelium and acts as a vasopressor.[94] Therefore, in the adult, calcium administration increases SVR and is a pressor agent; in the neonate, it acts as an inotrope. Calcium administration is included in the guidelines for management of pediatric and neonatal septic shock.[52]

Vasopressin

Vasopressin (0.0003–0.008 U/kg/min) is a nonadrenergic agent that stimulates vasopressin receptors and increases blood pressure by elevating SVR. In the adult and pediatric intensive care units, there may be a benefit when added to other inotropes to treat septic shock, although clinical trials have yielded conflicting results.[52,89,90,98,99] Children have decreased arginine vasopressin levels following CPB,[100] and vasopressin administration has been beneficial in hypotensive infants after cardiac surgery.[101,102] Vasopressin has also been used in premature neonates with hypotension refractory to 1 or more inotropes/pressors.[103–106] In patients susceptible to arrhythmias, vasopressin offers the advantage of increasing blood pressure with little chronotropic (β_1) activity. However, in the failing myocardium, chronic vasopressin administration may increase afterload and lead to worsening cardiac performance.

Milrinone

Milrinone (0.1–1 µg/kg/min) is a synthetic phosphodiesterase inhibitor frequently used in patients with cardiac dysfunction, especially in the postoperative setting. By increasing intracellular cyclic AMP (adenosine monophosphate) levels, milrinone increases contractility, vasodilates the systemic and pulmonary vascular beds, and promotes cardiac diastolic relaxation (lusitropy). Because of its primary effects on contractility (increasing inotropy) and dilation of the vascular bed, milrinone is often referred to as an "inodilator." Initial studies in adults revealed a reduction in myocardial oxygen consumption with the use of amrinone, a similar phosphodiesterase inhibitor.[107]

Studies of neonates after cardiac surgery indicated that milrinone attenuated the predictable decrement in cardiac output in the first 24 hours following exposure to CPB[108–111] (Figure 82-5). Comparison of a phosphodiesterase inhibitor (amrinone) vs dopamine and nipride showed that amrinone provided a superior oxygen delivery/consumption ratio and higher cardiac output in neonates after repair of congenital heart defects.[76,77] Neonates with persistent pulmonary hypertension may benefit from milrinone therapy, but there is insufficient evidence to suggest it should be used instead of inhaled nitric oxide.[112,113]

The safety and efficacy of milrinone in preterm neonates has not been established,[114,115] and careful attention to renal clearance is warranted, as milrinone will accumulate in the setting of renal dysfunction.[116] Milrinone has a longer half-life than other inotropes (2–3 hours) and a larger volume of distribution in neonates compared to adults.[117,118] Neonatal clearance of the drug is less than 25% of that in children, indicating that neonates may require lower-dose infusions (eg, 0.25 μg/kg/min) for equal inodilator effect.[117] Important side effects include thrombocytopenia, ventricular dysrhythmias, and abnormal hepatic enzymes.[118]

Thyroid Hormone

Triiodothrionine (T$_3$) has been studied in specific neonatal populations to improve postoperative cardiac output and blood pressure. Neonates recovering from cardiac surgery were administered T$_3$ and exhibited significantly increased blood pressure (with similar cardiac output) compared to placebo.[119] Whether T$_3$ has a role in other models of neonatal shock remains to be determined.

MECHANICAL SUPPORT: EXTRACORPOREAL MEMBRANE OXYGENATION AND VENTRICULAR ASSIST DEVICES

In the setting of continued inadequate oxygen delivery and tissue perfusion despite maximal medical therapy with inotropes or pressors, venoarterial extracorporeal membrane oxygenation (VA ECMO) is a final option to support severe circulatory failure. Ventricular assist devices (VADs) also provide a longer-term option for cardiac support in larger neonates (≥ 3.5 kg) who are candidates for cardiac transplantation. Of the VADs available in 2014 for implantation in pediatric patients, only the Berlin Heart EXCOR® was an appropriate size for neonates. Discussion of these devices is beyond the scope of this chapter, but the clinician should be aware of mechanical support options and contact a referral center with ECMO/VAD capabilities in the setting of persistent shock despite aggressive medical therapy.

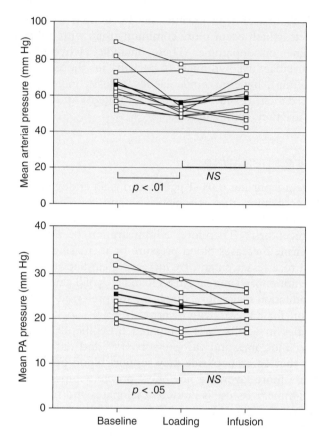

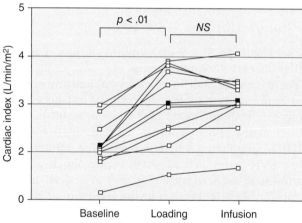

FIGURE 82-5 Systemic and pulmonary arterial (PA) pressures with loading and infusion doses of milrinone. Top: Mean arterial blood pressure decreased after the loading stage but did not decrease further at the infusion stage. Middle: Similar to mean systemic blood pressure, mean PA pressure decreased significantly after the loading dose of milrinone and remained lowered during the infusion stage as well. Bottom: Cardiac index. The baseline cardiac indices increased with the milrinone loading stage and increased slightly more at the infusion stage. The increase in cardiac index and decrease in systemic blood pressure result from a significant decrease in systemic vascular resistance (not shown). (Adapted with permission from Chang et al.[108])

CONCLUSION

Realizing that data regarding outcomes between specific inotropic infusions are limited, the clinician can use the physiologic principles described to support blood pressure with these pharmacologic agents. Further study is needed to understand which inotropes and pressors are most effective at reducing neonatal morbidity and improving outcomes, and continued clinical trials in the neonatal population are essential to an improved understanding of these medications.

REFERENCES

1. Al-Aweel I, Pursley DM, Rubin LP, et al. Variations in prevalence of hypotension, hypertension, and vasopressor use in NICUs. *J Perinatol*. 2001;21(5):272–278.
2. Driscoll DJ. Use of inotropic and chronotropic agents in neonates. *Clin Perinatol*. 1987;14(4):931–949.
3. Havel C, Arrich J, Losert H, et al. Vasopressors for hypotensive shock. *Cochrane Database Syst Rev*. 2011;(5):CD003709.
4. Laughon M, Bose C, Allred E, et al. Factors associated with treatment for hypotension in extremely low gestational age newborns during the first postnatal week. *Pediatrics*. 2007;119(2):273–280.
5. Pellicer A, Bravo M del C, Madero R, et al. Early systemic hypotension and vasopressor support in low birth weight infants: impact on neurodevelopment. *Pediatrics*. 2009;123(5):1369–1376.
6. Schmaltz C. Hypotension and shock in the preterm neonate. *Adv Neonatal Care*. 2009;9(4):156–162.
7. Seri I, Evans J. Controversies in the diagnosis and management of hypotension in the newborn infant. *Curr Opin Pediatr*. 2001;13(2):116–123.
8. Seri I, Noori S. Diagnosis and treatment of neonatal hypotension outside the transitional period. *Early Hum Dev*. 2005;81(5):405–411.
9. Subhedar NV. Treatment of hypotension in newborns. *Semin Neonatol*. 2003;8(6):413–423.
10. Zaritsky A, Chernow B. Use of catecholamines in pediatrics. *J. Pediatr*. 1984;105(3):341–350.
11. Seri I. Inotrope, lusitrope, and pressor use in neonates. *J Perinatol*. 2005;25(Suppl 2):S28–S30.
12. Kluckow M, Evans N. Relationship between blood pressure and cardiac output in preterm infants requiring mechanical ventilation. *J. Pediatr*. 1996;129(4):506–512.
13. Osborn DA, Paradisis M, Evans N. The effect of inotropes on morbidity and mortality in preterm infants with low systemic or organ blood flow. *Cochrane Database Syst Rev*. 2007;(1):CD005090.
14. Fisher DJ, Towbin J. Maturation of the heart. *Clin Perinatol*. 1988;15(3):421–446.
15. Teitel DF, Sidi D, Chin T, et al. Developmental changes in myocardial contractile reserve in the lamb. *Pediatr Res*. 1985;19(9):948–955.
16. Rowland DG, Gutgesell HP. Noninvasive assessment of myocardial contractility, preload, and afterload in healthy newborn infants. *Am J Cardiol*. 1995;75(12):818–821.
17. Anderson PA. Maturation and cardiac contractility. *Cardiol Clin*. 1989;7(2):209–225.
18. Rudolph AM. *Congenital Diseases of the Heart: Clinical-Physiological Considerations*. 3rd ed. New York, NY: Wiley-Blackwell; 2009.
19. Wiegerinck RF, Cojoc A, Zeidenweber CM, et al. Force frequency relationship of the human ventricle increases during early postnatal development. *Pediatr Res*. 2009;65(4):414–419.
20. Munro MJ, Walker AM, Barfield CP. Hypotensive extremely low birth weight infants have reduced cerebral blood flow. *Pediatrics*. 2004;114(6):1591–1596.
21. Hegyi T, Carbone MT, Anwar M, et al. Blood pressure ranges in premature infants. I. The first hours of life. *J Pediatr*. 1994;124(4):627–633.
22. Noori S, Seri I. Pathophysiology of newborn hypotension outside the transitional period. *Early Hum Dev*. 2005;81(5):399–404.
23. Nuntnarumit P, Yang W, Bada-Ellzey HS. Blood pressure measurements in the newborn. *Clin Perinatol*. 1999;26(4):981–996, x.
24. Park MK, Lee DH. Normative arm and calf blood pressure values in the newborn. *Pediatrics*. 1989;83(2):240–243.
25. Zubrow AB, Hulman S, Kushner H, Falkner B. Determinants of blood pressure in infants admitted to neonatal intensive care units: a prospective multicenter study. Philadelphia Neonatal Blood Pressure Study Group. *J Perinatol*. 1995;15(6):470–479.
26. Hunt RW, Evans N, Rieger I, Kluckow M. Low superior vena cava flow and neurodevelopment at 3 years in very preterm infants. *J Pediatr*. 2004;145(5):588–592.
27. Cunningham S, Symon AG, Elton RA, Zhu C, McIntosh N. Intra-arterial blood pressure reference ranges, death and morbidity in very low birthweight infants during the first seven days of life. *Early Hum Dev*. 1999;56(2–3):151–165.
28. Russell JA, Phang PT. The oxygen delivery/consumption controversy. Approaches to management of the critically ill. *Am J Respir Crit Care Med*. 1994;149(2 Pt 1):533–537.
29. Batton B, Zhu X, Fanaroff J, et al. Blood pressure, antihypotensive therapy, and neurodevelopment in extremely preterm infants. *J Pediatr*. 2009;154(3):351–357, 357.e1.
30. Goldstein RF, Thompson RJ, Oehler JM, Brazy JE. Influence of acidosis, hypoxemia, and hypotension on neurodevelopmental outcome in very low birth weight infants. *Pediatrics*. 1995;95(2):238–243.
31. Miall-Allen VM, de Vries LS, Whitelaw AG. Mean arterial blood pressure and neonatal cerebral lesions. *Arch Dis Child*. 1987;62(10):1068–1069.
32. Richard SKY, Hernandez MJ, Yagel SK. Selective reduction of blood flow to white matter during hypotension in newborn dogs: a possible mechanism of periventricular leukomalacia. *Ann Neurol*. 1982;12(5):445–448.
33. Tsuji M, Saul JP, du Plessis A, et al. Cerebral intravascular oxygenation correlates with mean arterial pressure in critically ill premature infants. *Pediatrics*. 2000;106(4):625–632.
34. Watkins AMC, West CR, Cooke RWI. Blood pressure and cerebral haemorrhage and ischaemia in very low birthweight infants. *Early Hum Dev*. 1989;19(2):103–110.
35. Osborn DA, Evans N, Kluckow M, Bowen JR, Rieger I. Low superior vena cava flow and effect of inotropes on neurodevelopment to 3 years in preterm infants. *Pediatrics*. 2007;120(2):372–380.
36. Osborn DA, Evans N. Early volume expansion for prevention of morbidity and mortality in very preterm infants. *Cochrane Database Syst Rev*. 2004;(2):CD002055.
37. Osborn DA, Evans N. Early volume expansion versus inotrope for prevention of morbidity and mortality in very preterm infants. *Cochrane Database Syst Rev*. 2001;(2):CD002056.
38. Keeley SR, Bohn DJ. The use of inotropic and afterload-reducing agents in neonates. *Clin Perinatol*. 1988;15(3):467–489.
39. Barrington KJ. Hypotension and shock in the preterm infant. *Semin Fetal Neonatal Med*. 2008;13(1):16–23.
40. Ahlquist RP. A study of the adrenotropic receptors. *Am J Physiol*. 1948;153(3):586–600.

41. Collins S, Caron MG, Lefkowitz RJ. Regulation of adrenergic receptor responsiveness through modulation of receptor gene expression. *Annu Rev Physiol.* 1991;53:497–508.

42. Woodcock EA, Du X-J, Reichelt ME, Graham RM. Cardiac alpha 1-adrenergic drive in pathological remodelling. *Cardiovasc Res.* 2008;77(3):452–462.

43. Wolff DW, Dang HK, Liu MF, Jeffries WB, Scofield MA. Distribution of alpha1-adrenergic receptor mRNA species in rat heart. *J Cardiovasc Pharmacol.* 1998;32(1):117–122.

44. Baker CFW, Barks JDE, Engmann C, et al. Hydrocortisone administration for the treatment of refractory hypotension in critically ill newborns. *J Perinatol.* 2008;28(6):412–419.

45. Gaissmaier RE, Pohlandt F. Single-dose dexamethasone treatment of hypotension in preterm infants. *J Pediatr.* 1999;134(6):701–705.

46. Higgins S, Friedlich P, Seri I. Hydrocortisone for hypotension and vasopressor dependence in preterm neonates: a meta-analysis. *J Perinatol.* 2010;30(6):373–378.

47. Ng PC, Lee CH, Bnur FL, et al. A double-blind, randomized, controlled study of a "stress dose" of hydrocortisone for rescue treatment of refractory hypotension in preterm infants. *Pediatrics.* 2006;117(2):367–375.

48. Noori S, Friedlich P, Wong P, et al. Hemodynamic changes after low-dosage hydrocortisone administration in vasopressor-treated preterm and term neonates. *Pediatrics.* 2006;118(4):1456–1466.

49. Sasidharan P. Role of corticosteroids in neonatal blood pressure homeostasis. *Clin Perinatol.* 1998;25(3):723–740, xi.

50. Seri I, Tan R, Evans J. Cardiovascular effects of hydrocortisone in preterm infants with pressor-resistant hypotension. *Pediatrics.* 2001;107(5):1070–1074.

51. Seri I. Hydrocortisone and vasopressor-resistant shock in preterm neonates. *Pediatrics.* 2006;117(2):516–518.

52. Brierley J, Carcillo JA, Choong K, et al. Clinical practice parameters for hemodynamic support of pediatric and neonatal septic shock: 2007 update from the American College of Critical Care Medicine. *Crit Care Med.* 2009;37(2):666–688.

53. Dellinger RP, Levy MM, Carlet JM, et al. Surviving Sepsis Campaign: international guidelines for management of severe sepsis and septic shock: 2008. *Crit Care Med.* 2008;36(1):296–327.

54. Seri I, Abbasi S, Wood DC, Gerdes JS. Regional hemodynamic effects of dopamine in the sick preterm neonate. *J Pediatr.* 1998;133(6):728–734.

55. Seri I. Cardiovascular, renal, and endocrine actions of dopamine in neonates and children. *J Pediatr.* 1995;126(3):333–344.

56. Allwood MJ, Cobbold AF, Ginsburg J. Peripheral vascular effects of noradrenaline, isopropylnoradrenaline and dopamine. *Br Med Bull.* 1963;19:132–136.

57. Lundstrøm K, Pryds O, Greisen G. The haemodynamic effects of dopamine and volume expansion in sick preterm infants. *Early Hum Dev.* 2000;57(2):157–163.

58. Seri I. Cardiovascular, renal, and endocrine actions of dopamine in neonates and children. *J Pediatr.* 1995;126(3):333–344.

59. Ding G, Wiegerinck RF, Shen M, et al. Dopamine increases L-type calcium current more in newborn than adult rabbit cardiomyocytes via D_1 and β_2 receptors. *Am J Physiol Heart Circ Physiol.* 2008;294(5):H2327–H2335.

60. Xiao RP, Tomhave ED, Wang DJ, et al. Age-associated reductions in cardiac beta1- and beta2-adrenergic responses without changes in inhibitory G proteins or receptor kinases. *J Clin Invest.* 1998;101(6):1273–1282.

61. Padbury JF, Agata Y, Baylen BG, et al. Pharmacokinetics of dopamine in critically ill newborn infants. *J Pediatr.* 1990;117(3):472–476.

62. Hentschel R, Hensel D, Brune T, Rabe H, Jorch G. Impact on blood pressure and intestinal perfusion of dobutamine or dopamine in hypotensive preterm infants. *Biol Neonate.* 1995;68(5):318–324.

63. Perez CA, Reimer JM, Schreiber MD, Warburton D, Gregory GA. Effect of high-dose dopamine on urine output in newborn infants. *Crit Care Med.* 1986;14(12):1045–1049.

64. Wong FY, Barfield CP, Horne RSC, Walker AM. Dopamine therapy promotes cerebral flow-metabolism coupling in preterm infants. *Intensive Care Med.* 2009;35(10):1777–1782.

65. Osborn DA, Evans N, Kluckow M. Left ventricular contractility in extremely premature infants in the first day and response to inotropes. *Pediatr Res.* 2007;61(3):335–340.

66. Li J, Zhang G, Holtby H, et al. Adverse effects of dopamine on systemic hemodynamic status and oxygen transport in neonates after the Norwood procedure. *J Am Coll Cardiol.* 2006;48(9):1859–1864.

67. Liet J-M, Boscher C, Gras-Leguen C, et al. Dopamine effects on pulmonary artery pressure in hypotensive preterm infants with patent ductus arteriosus. *J Pediatr.* 2002;140(3):373–375.

68. Gill AB, Weindling AM. Randomised controlled trial of plasma protein fraction versus dopamine in hypotensive very low birthweight infants. *Arch Dis Child.* 1993;69(3 Spec No):284–287.

69. Greenough A, Emery EF. Randomized trial comparing dopamine and dobutamine in preterm infants. *Eur J Pediatr.* 1993;152(11):925–927.

70. Klarr JM, Faix RG, Pryce CJ, Bhatt-Mehta V. Randomized, blind trial of dopamine versus dobutamine for treatment of hypotension in preterm infants with respiratory distress syndrome. *J Pediatr.* 1994;125(1):117–122.

71. Subhedar NV, Shaw NJ. Dopamine versus dobutamine for hypotensive preterm infants. *Cochrane Database Syst Rev.* 2003;(3):CD001242.

72. Osborn D, Evans N, Kluckow M. Randomized trial of dobutamine versus dopamine in preterm infants with low systemic blood flow. *J Pediatr.* 2002;140(2):183–191.

73. Ruelas-Orozco G, Vargas-Origel A. Assessment of therapy for arterial hypotension in critically ill preterm infants. *Am J Perinatol.* 2000;17(2):95–99.

74. Valverde E, Pellicer A, Madero R, et al. Dopamine versus epinephrine for cardiovascular support in low birth weight infants: analysis of systemic effects and neonatal clinical outcomes. *Pediatrics.* 2006;117(6):e1213–e1222.

75. Pellicer A, Valverde E, Elorza MD, et al. Cardiovascular support for low birth weight infants and cerebral hemodynamics: a randomized, blinded, clinical trial. *Pediatrics.* 2005;115(6):1501–1512.

76. Laitinen P, Happonen JM, Sairanen H, Peltola K, Rautiainen P. Amrinone versus dopamine and nitroglycerin in neonates after arterial switch operation for transposition of the great arteries. *J Cardiothorac Vasc Anesth.* 1999;13(2):186–190.

77. Laitinen P, Happonen JM, Sairanen H, et al. Amrinone versus dopamine-nitroglycerin after reconstructive surgery for complete atrioventricular septal defect. *J Cardiothorac Vasc Anesth.* 1997;11(7):870–874.

78. Bourchier D, Weston PJ. Randomised trial of dopamine compared with hydrocortisone for the treatment of hypotensive very low birthweight infants. *Arch Dis Child Fetal Neonatal Ed.* 1997;76(3):F174–F178.

79. De Backer D, Biston P, Devriendt J, et al. Comparison of dopamine and norepinephrine in the treatment of shock. *N Engl J Med.* 2010;362(9):779–789.

80. DiSessa TG, Leitner M, Ti CC, et al. The cardiovascular effects of dopamine in the severely asphyxiated neonate. *J Pediatr.* 1981;99(5):772–776.

81. Hunt R, Osborn DA. Dopamine for prevention of morbidity and mortality in term newborn infants with suspected perinatal asphyxia. http://onlinelibrary.wiley.com.laneproxy.stanford.edu/doi/10.1002/14651858.CD003484/abstract. Accessed August 8, 2011.

82. Habib DM, Padbury JF, Anas NG, Perkin RM, Minegar C. Dobutamine pharmacokinetics and pharmacodynamics in

pediatric intensive care patients. *Crit Care Med.* 1992;20(5):
601–608.

83. Loeb HS, Bredakis J, Gunner RM. Superiority of dobutamine over dopamine for augmentation of cardiac output in
patients with chronic low output cardiac failure. *Circulation.*
1977;55(2):375–378.

84. Bohn DJ, Poirier CS, Edmonds JF, Barker GA. Hemodynamic
effects of dobutamine after cardiopulmonary bypass in children. *Crit Care Med.* 1980;8(7):367–371.

85. Moran JL, O'Fathartaigh MS, Peisach AR, Chapman MJ, Lep-
pard P. Epinephrine as an inotropic agent in septic shock: a
dose-profile analysis. *Crit Care Med.* 1993;21(1):70–77.

86. Perlman JM, Wyllie J, Kattwinkel J, et al. Part 11: Neonatal
resuscitation: 2010 International Consensus on Cardiopulmonary Resuscitation and Emergency Cardiovascular Care
Science With Treatment Recommendations. *Circulation.*
2010;122(16 Suppl 2):S516–S538.

87. Kleinman ME, de Caen AR, Chameides L, et al. Part 10: Pediatric basic and advanced life support. *Circulation.* 2010;122
(16 Suppl 2):S466–S515.

88. Heckmann M, Trotter A, Pohlandt F, Lindner W. Epinephrine
treatment of hypotension in very low birthweight infants. *Acta
Paediatr.* 2002;91(5):566–570.

89. Russell JA, Walley KR, Singer J, et al. Vasopressin versus norepinephrine infusion in patients with septic shock. *N Engl J
Med.* 2008;358(9):877–887.

90. Albanèse J, Leone M, Delmas A, Martin C. Terlipressin or
norepinephrine in hyperdynamic septic shock: a prospective,
randomized study. *Crit Care Med.* 2005;33(9):1897–1902.

91. Gregory JS, Bonfiglio MF, Dasta JF, et al. Experience with
phenylephrine as a component of the pharmacologic support
of septic shock. *Crit Care Med.* 1991;19(11):1395–1400.

92. Zamanian RT, Haddad F, Doyle RL, Weinacker AB. Management strategies for patients with pulmonary hypertension in the intensive care unit. *Crit Care Med.* 2007;35(9):
2037–2050.

93. Qu Y, Boutjdir M. Gene expression of SERCA2a and L- and
T-type Ca channels during human heart development. *Pediatr
Res.* 2001;50(5):569–574.

94. Schwartz SM, Duffy JY, Pearl JM, Nelson DP. Cellular and
molecular aspects of myocardial dysfunction. *Crit Care Med.*
2001;29(10 Suppl):S214–S219.

95. Katz AM. Potential deleterious effects of inotropic agents
in the therapy of chronic heart failure. *Circulation.* 1986;73
(3 Pt 2):III184–III190.

96. Katz AM, Lorell BH. Regulation of cardiac contraction and
relaxation. *Circulation.* 2000;102(20 Suppl 4):IV69–IV74.

97. Nakayama H, Chen X, Baines CP, et al. Ca^{2+}- and mitochondrial-
dependent cardiomyocyte necrosis as a primary mediator of heart
failure. *J Clin Investig.* 2007;117:2431–2444.

98. Dünser MW, Mayr AJ, Ulmer H, et al. Arginine vasopressin in
advanced vasodilatory shock: a prospective, randomized, controlled study. *Circulation.* 2003;107(18):2313–2319.

99. Mutlu GM, Factor P. Role of vasopressin in the management
of septic shock. *Intensive Care Med.* 2004;30(7):1276–1291.

100. Morrison WE, Simone S, Conway D, et al. Levels of vasopressin in children undergoing cardiopulmonary bypass. *Cardiol
Young.* 2008;18(2):135–140.

101. Rosenzweig EB, Starc TJ, Chen JM, et al. Intravenous arginine-
vasopressin in children with vasodilatory shock after cardiac
surgery. *Circulation.* 1999;100(19 Suppl):II182–II186.

102. Lechner E, Hofer A, Mair R, et al. Arginine-vasopressin in
neonates with vasodilatory shock after cardiopulmonary
bypass. *Eur J Pediatr.* 2007;166(12):1221–1227.

103. Bidegain M, Greenberg R, Simmons C, et al. Vasopressin for
refractory hypotension in extremely low birth weight infants.
J Pediatr. 2010;157(3):502–504.

104. Ikegami H, Funato M, Tamai H, et al. Low-dose vasopressin
infusion therapy for refractory hypotension in ELBW infants.
Pediatr Int. 2010;52(3):368–373.

105. Meyer S. Vasopressin infusion therapy for refractory hypotension in extremely low birthweight neonates. *Pediatr Int.*
2011;53(2):287.

106. Meyer S, Gottschling S, Baghai A, Wurm D, Gortner L.
Arginine-vasopressin in catecholamine-refractory septic versus
non-septic shock in extremely low birth weight infants with
acute renal injury. *Crit Care.* 2006;10(3):R71.

107. Benotti JR, Grossman W, Braunwald E, Carabello BA. Effects
of amrinone on myocardial energy metabolism and hemodynamics in patients with severe congestive heart failure due to
coronary artery disease. *Circulation.* 1980;62(1):28–34.

108. Chang AC, Atz AM, Wernovsky G, Burke RP, Wessel
DL. Milrinone: systemic and pulmonary hemodynamic
effects in neonates after cardiac surgery. *Crit Care Med.*
1995;23(11):1907–1914.

109. Hoffman TM, Wernovsky G, Atz AM, et al. Prophylactic
intravenous use of milrinone after cardiac operation in pediatrics (PRIMACORP) study. Prophylactic intravenous use of
milrinone after cardiac operation in pediatrics. *Am Heart J.*
2002;143(1):15–21.

110. Hoffman TM, Wernovsky G, Atz AM, et al. Efficacy and safety
of milrinone in preventing low cardiac output syndrome in
infants and children after corrective surgery for congenital
heart disease. *Circulation.* 2003;107(7):996–1002.

111. Wernovsky G, Wypij D, Jonas RA, et al. Postoperative course
and hemodynamic profile after the arterial switch operation in neonates and infants. A comparison of low-flow cardiopulmonary bypass and circulatory arrest. *Circulation.*
1995;92(8):2226–2235.

112. Bassler D, Kreutzer K, McNamara P, Kirpalani H. Milrinone for persistent pulmonary hypertension of the newborn.
Cochrane Database Syst Rev. 2010;(11):CD007802.

113. McNamara PJ, Laique F, Muang-In S, Whyte HE. Milrinone improves oxygenation in neonates with severe persistent pulmonary hypertension of the newborn. *J Crit Care.*
2006;21(2):217–222.

114. Paradisis M, Evans N, Kluckow M, Osborn D, McLachlan AJ.
Pilot study of milrinone for low systemic blood flow in very
preterm infants. *J Pediatr.* 2006;148(3):306–313.

115. Paradisis M, Evans N, Kluckow M, Osborn D. Randomized trial of milrinone versus placebo for prevention of
low systemic blood flow in very preterm infants. *J Pediatr.*
2009;154(2):189–195.

116. Zuppa AF, Nicolson SC, Adamson PC, et al. Population pharmacokinetics of milrinone in neonates with hypoplastic left
heart syndrome undergoing stage I reconstruction. *Anesth
Analg.* 2006;102(4):1062–1069.

117. Bailey JM, Hoffman TM, Wessel DL, et al. A population pharmacokinetic analysis of milrinone in pediatric patients after cardiac
surgery. *J Pharmacokinet Pharmacodyn.* 2004;31(1):43–59.

118. Ramamoorthy C, Anderson GD, Williams GD, Lynn
AM. Pharmacokinetics and side effects of milrinone in
infants and children after open heart surgery. *Anesth Analg.*
1998;86(2):283–289.

119. Mackie AS, Booth KL, Newburger JW, et al. A randomized,
double-blind, placebo-controlled pilot trial of triiodothyronine in neonatal heart surgery. *J Thorac Cardiovasc Surg.*
2005;130(3):810–816.

83 Patent Ductus Arteriosus Management

Valerie Y. Chock and Stacie Rohovit

GENERAL

The patent ductus arteriosus (PDA) is usually functionally closed within 12 hours of life. Anatomic closure normally occurs within 10 days. In the premature infant, closure often will not occur until term.

Left-to-right shunting through the ductus may contribute to increasing pulmonary edema, persistent need for ventilator support, and the development of bronchopulmonary dysplasia (BPD). Decreased systemic perfusion to end organs such as the brain, kidney, and intestines may also occur. These potential complications have traditionally been the motivation to achieve ductal closure.

It remains unclear if treatment of a PDA results in improved long-term outcomes. Recent analyses have shown that treatment of a PDA does *not* reduce the common complications of prematurity, including death, BPD, intraventricular hemorrhage (IVH), or necrotizing enterocolitis (NEC).[1] Risks of medical or surgical closure also exist. Therefore, determination of the hemodynamic significance of the PDA in a particular patient is essential to approaching management strategies until further evidence from clinical studies can be acquired to guide optimal treatment.

DIAGNOSIS

Clinical Signs and Symptoms

Suspect a hemodynamically significant PDA in premature infants when the following exist:

1. A systolic or continuous "grating" murmur heard in the left upper sternal border (LUSB).

2. Bounding pulses (often palmar pulses are palpated).
3. Wide pulse pressure greater than 20 mm Hg with decreased diastolic pressure may be present but has poor diagnostic power in very low birth weight infants.
4. Difficulty weaning from the ventilator (above what is expected for the typical respiratory distress syndrome [RDS] picture); increased arterial partial pressure of carbon dioxide ($PaCO_2$) may be the only finding.
5. Congestive heart failure (CHF), cardiomegaly, and pulmonary edema visible on chest x-ray.
6. Metabolic acidosis from retrograde aortic flow ("ductal steal").
7. Feeding intolerance.
8. Oliguria, rising creatinine levels, from decreased renal perfusion (ductal steal).
9. *Note*: Not uncommonly, a PDA is asymptomatic ("silent ductus") in small, sick premature infants.

Echocardiographic Findings

Confirmation of clinical suspicion is by echocardiogram (echo):

1. Echo characteristics to consider include
   a. Size of the duct,
   b. Direction of blood flow (left to right, bidirectional), and
   c. Evidence of fluid overload (eg, elevated ratio of left atrial to aortic root [La:Ao ratio] or atrial enlargement), and
   d. Evidence of holoretrograde diastolic flow, or
   e. Mitral regurgitation.

2. The echo will only capture a moment in time. As the PDA is dynamic, multiple echo studies may be necessary for clinical correlation.

3. If ductal closure is considered, it is important to rule out a ductal-dependent lesion.

TREATMENT

Conservative Management

In the asymptomatic patient, consider waiting for spontaneous closure with conservative management.

1. Limit the fluid volume to the essential amount necessary to meet estimated needs.
2. Diuretic therapy may be necessary to minimize pulmonary edema.
3. Treat hypotension with pressors until ductal closure is confirmed.
4. Maintain higher positive airway distending pressures to decrease pulmonary overperfusion and edema.
5. Consider blood transfusions to maintain adequate systemic oxygenation.
6. Feedings may need to be limited if significant ductal steal is present.

Medical Closure

1. Indomethacin 0.2 mg/kg/dose every 12–24 hours for 3 doses. Course may be repeated if laboratory values and renal function are stable.
2. Ibuprofen, 10 mg/kg IV followed by 5 mg/kg IV every 24 hours for 3 doses, has a similar efficacy rate but may have less impact on perfusion to kidneys, brain, and intestines. It is more expensive than indomethacin.
3. Pretreatment laboratory studies: creatinine, platelets. Both indomethacin and ibuprofen may impair renal perfusion and decrease platelet function. Some will check laboratory values prior to each dose; others only check before the first dose unless oliguria or bleeding occurs. Neither causes thrombocytopenia.
4. Medical closure contraindications include
    a. Thrombocytopenia (eg, platelets < 100,000),
    b. Renal dysfunction (eg, elevated creatinine, oliguria),
    c. NEC,
    d. Hemorrhage (but not by IVH per se), or
    e. Patient on hydrocortisone (because of the risk of spontaneous intestinal perforation).

5. Closure rate is 65%–75%. Some will reopen, especially with increased intravenous fluid volume. Treatment is less effective after the first 2 weeks of life.
6. Some centers may use ibuprofen instead of indomethacin for PDA closure because of a similar efficacy rate but improved perfusion to kidneys, brain, and intestines.
7. Prophylactic management for PDA: Some centers may use indomethacin prophylactically for preterm infants in the first 24 hours of life at 0.1 mg/kg/dose every 24 hours for 6 doses. This has been shown to reduce the risk of severe IVH and development of PDA but does not improve neurodevelopmental outcomes.

Surgical Management

1. For those for whom medical management is unsuccessful or contraindicated, surgical ligation by an experienced surgery team is indicated. Commonly, this is done in the neonatal intensive care unit to avoid the risks related to transferring the patient to the operating room.
2. Acute complications of surgical ligation include risks of anesthesia, vocal cord paralysis, pneumothorax, myocardial dysfunction, infection, and bleeding.
    a. Patients may need increased ventilator support during the postoperative period.
    b. Left ventricular dysfunction is common, and one should be prepared to provide pressor support postoperatively.
3. Long-term complications may include an increased risk of BPD and neurodevelopmental impairment.
4. In the immediate postoperative period, infants are at higher risk for impaired cerebral autoregulation and would benefit from maintenance of stable cerebral perfusion by close monitoring of systemic blood pressure and avoidance of hypocarbia.[2]

REFERENCES

1. Benitz WE. Treatment of persistent patent ductus arteriosus in preterm infants: time to accept the null hypothesis? *J Perinatol.* 2010;30:241–252.
2. Chock VY, Ramamoorthy C, Van Meurs KP. Cerebral autoregulation in neonates with a hemodynamically significant patent ductus arteriosus. *J Pediatr.* 2012;160:936–942.

CHAPTER 83

84 Practical Approach to Arrhythmias

Anne M. Dubin and Christina Y. Miyake

INTRODUCTION

Tachycardias and bradyarrhythmias are important problems in the neonate. Clear understanding and recognition of these arrhythmias are important for optimal management.

TACHYCARDIA

Tachycardia can be either supraventricular (SVT) or ventricular (VT) in origin.

Atrioventricular Reentrant Tachycardia Including Wolff-Parkinson-White Syndrome

Pathophysiology

Atrioventricular reentrant tachycardia (AVRT) is the most common arrhythmia seen in the neonate. This reentry rhythm utilizes both the atrium and the ventricle and involves normal antegrade conduction across the atrioventricular (AV) node and retrograde conduction via an accessory pathway. This results in a narrow complex SVT, with retrograde p waves usually seen in leads II, III, and aVF and rates of 230–260 bpm (Figure 84-1). About one-third of accessory pathways are able to conduct antegrade as well and give the appearance of preexcitation or Wolff-Parkinson-White (WPW) syndrome on the baseline electrocardiogram (ECG) (Figure 84-2).

Presentation

The infant with neonatal SVT often presents with heart failure symptoms: poor perfusion, hepatosplenomegaly, poor feeding, and tachypnea. The differential for SVT must include infection with a sinus tachycardia.

Diagnosis

The 12-lead ECG will allow for accurate measurement of the heart rate and confirmation of the diagnosis.

Therapy

Acute management of SVT may include vagal maneuvers (ice to the face, rectal stimulation), intravenous adenosine (100–200 µg/kg as a rapid intravenous push), or synchronized cardioversion. Medical therapy consisting of β-blockers (propranolol 2–4 mg/kg/d orally divided four times a day) or digoxin (10 µg/kg/d divided twice daily) is used for chronic management; however, digoxin should not be used if the patient has WPW syndrome.

Follow-up

Neonatal SVT self-resolves in approximately 50% of children during the first year of life. If SVT does not resolve, ablation therapy is a curative procedure that can electively be performed when a child weighs more than 15–20 kg.

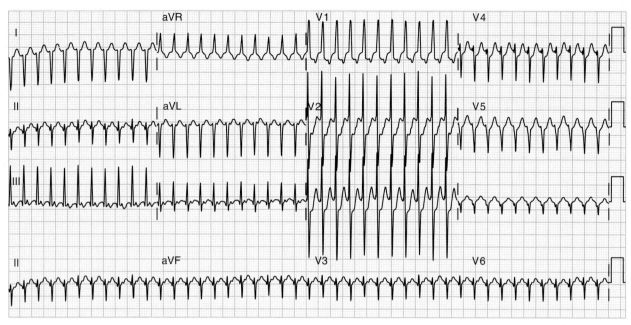

FIGURE 84-1 Electrocardiogram (ECG) of atrioventricular reentrant tachycardia in a 2-day-old. The ECG shows a narrow complex tachycardia at a rate of 280 bpm. Retrograde p waves are visible in leads II, III, and aVF.

Atrial Flutter

Pathophysiology

Atrial flutter is commonly seen in the newborn period. It is caused by a reentry rhythm within the atria. The ECG reveals a sawtooth pattern in the atria, best seen in leads II, III, and aVF, with an atrial rate between 300 and 500 bpm and 2:1 ventricular conduction (Figure 84-3).

Presentation

Atrial flutter in the newborn is usually recognized secondary to fixed tachycardia (ventricular rates usually 200–220 bpm). Over time, infants can develop signs

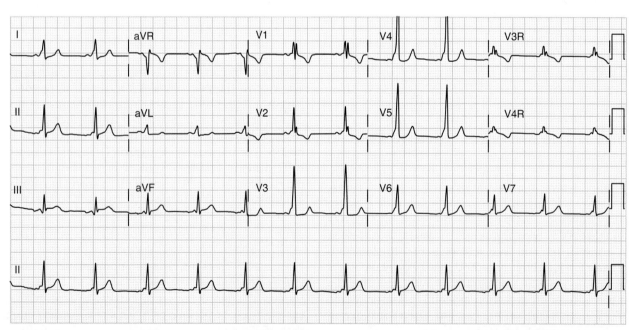

FIGURE 84-2 Electrocardiogram showing Wolff-Parkinson-White syndrome. The patient is in sinus rhythm with a short PR interval and clear delta wave.

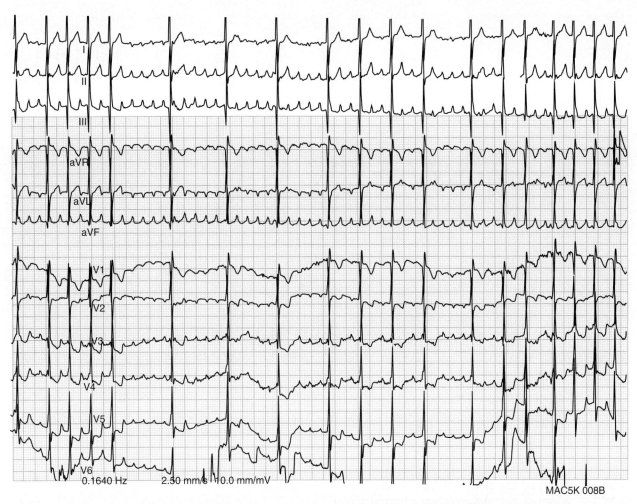

FIGURE 84-3 Electrocardiogram of an infant in atrial flutter who has just received a dose of adenosine. The adenosine blocks conduction throughout the atrioventricular node (AVN), which allows for better visualization of the sawtooth pattern p waves and thus can be a useful aid for diagnosis of the rhythm.

of heart failure, including tachypnea, hepatosplenomegaly, and poor perfusion.

Diagnostics

The 12-lead ECG is important for evaluation of the tachycardia to determine rhythm. An echocardiogram will rule out any structural heart disease.

Treatment

Synchronized cardioversion or transesophageal pacing can terminate the arrhythmia. Digoxin therapy has also been used to medically manage infant atrial flutter.

Follow-up

Atrial flutter of the newborn is usually a self-limited arrhythmia. Recurrence is rare, and medical therapy,

if used, is usually discontinued before the child's first birthday.

Ventricular Tachycardia

Pathophysiology

It is important to always consider VT when faced with wide-complex tachycardia in the neonate. VT is wide complex and may have fusion beats or ventricular-atrial (VA) dissociation, which can differentiate it from SVT with aberrancy (Figure 84-4).

Presentation

Ventricular tachycardia in the newborn will usually have 1 of 2 presentations: either the infant will be completely asymptomatic with the rhythm recognized by chance (accelerated idioventricular rhythm

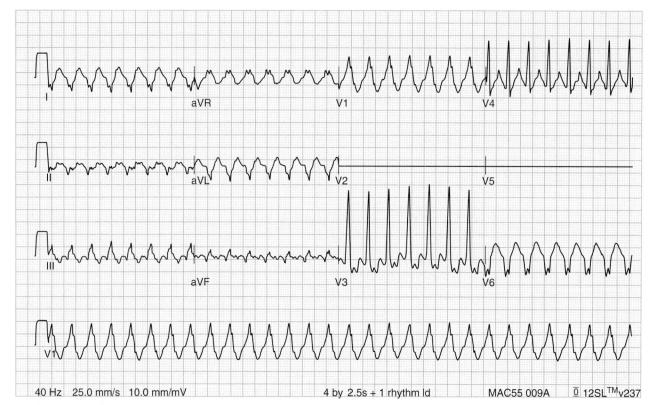

| 40 Hz | 25.0 mm/s | 10.0 mm/mV | | 4 by 2.5s + 1 rhythm ld | | MAC55 009A | $\overline{0}$ 12SL™v237 |

FIGURE 84-4 Electrocardiogram of ventricular tachycardia. The electrocardiogram shows wide-complex tachycardia at a rate of 180 bpm.

CHAPTER 84

in the newborn) or the child will have severe hemodynamic compromise. Accelerated idioventricular rhythm of the newborn is classified as a ventricular rhythm that is not much faster than sinus rhythm. It usually has a left bundle branch block pattern (right ventricular origin), and intermittent sinus rhythm is seen. Children with this condition are asymptomatic. Rapid VT can be seen with metabolic disorders or myocarditis or secondary to intracardiac tumors. Ventricular function is usually poor in these conditions, and the patient often shows signs of cardiovascular collapse (poor perfusion, hepatosplenomegaly, and respiratory distress).

Diagnostics

The 12-lead ECG is necessary when assessing a child for possible VT. VA dissociation and sinus fusion beats may be important clues when trying to differentiate between SVT with aberrancy and VT. The neonate with VT may have only minimal widening of the QRS on 1 lead, and all 12 leads may be necessary to discern wide-complex tachycardia. Echocardiography is necessary to assess ventricular function. Arterial blood gas and lactate levels can help determine level of hemodynamic compromise.

Treatment

The child with accelerated idioventricular rhythm of the newborn does not require therapy. For children with hemodynamically significant VT, emergent direct current cardioversion is indicated. Medical therapy with lidocaine or amiodarone may be helpful to control the rhythm. Hemodynamic support, including inotropes or, in severe cases, extracorporeal membrane oxygenation (ECMO) may be necessary. It is important to address any underlying metabolic disturbances if the VT mechanism is thought to be reversible.

Follow-up

Accelerated idioventricular rhythm of the newborn is a benign entity that usually resolves within the first few months of life. No long-term effects of this rhythm are known. VT prognosis depends on the etiology. In patients thought to have a tumor, the VT usually resolves by 5 years of age. In patients with myocarditis, one-third will progress to cardiomyopathy and may require heart transplantation in the future.

BRADYCARDIAS

Bradycardias usually represent some degree of heart block.

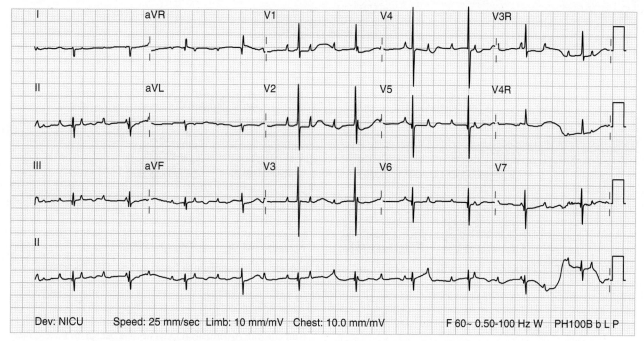

FIGURE 84-5 Electrocardiogram (ECG) of a neonate born to a mother with anti-SSA and anti-SSB antibodies and complete heart block. The ECG shows an atrial rate of 150 bpm and a ventricular rate of 70 bpm.

Pathophysiology

Third-degree heart block is the most important cause of bradycardia in the neonate. It can be recognized in the fetal period on screening fetal ultrasound or echocardiogram and often is related to maternal anti-SSA or anti-SSB antibodies. Complete heart block (CHB) is defined as a complete absence of AV conduction. No relationship between the atrial rate and ventricular rate can be established on ECG (Figure 84-5).

Presentation

The infant with CHB may have a variable presentation depending on ventricular rate and associated heart disease. In the child with the structurally normal heart, ventricular rates greater than 55 bpm are usually well tolerated. In children with ventricular rates less than 55 bpm, there often is hemodynamic compromise, with a high rate of hydrops and fetal demise, especially in association with other heart disease. Children with severe bradycardia and CHB are at risk of development of torsade de pointes and must be closely monitored for such.

Diagnostics

The mainstay of diagnosis is the ECG. It is important to differentiate CHB from an accelerated junctional rhythm. In CHB, the atrial rate is faster than the ventricular rate, and no relationship between the atria and ventricles is seen. A full echocardiogram is important to rule out any structural heart disease and to assess ventricular function. Maternal and neonatal anti-SSA and anti-SSB antibodies may help determine etiology of heart block.

Treatment

Treatment of this condition is dependent on ventricular rate and hemodynamic state. Infants with a heart rate of less than 55 bpm should receive a permanent pacemaker. If the child is showing evidence of hemodynamic compromise, emergent pacemaker placement is indicated, with support of blood pressure and rate via inotropes. If the child has a heart rate greater than 55 bpm, observation is sufficient (Figure 84-6).

Follow-up

Children with heart block and adequate ventricular rates are closely followed in a cardiology clinic, with the majority requiring pacemaker placement prior to adulthood secondary to poor exercise tolerance. Infants who receive pacemakers will require monitoring of the pacemaker every 3–6 months. Pacemakers usually need to be replaced within 3–7 years because of rapid depletion of the battery secondary to the high heart rates needed in the infant.

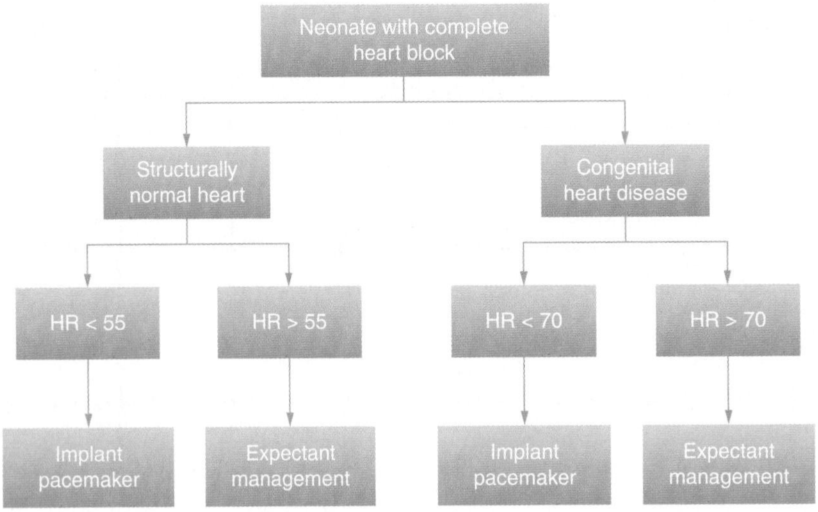

FIGURE 84-6 Flow diagram illustrating management of the newborn with complete heart block. HR, heart rate.

SUGGESTED READING

Buyon JP, Hiebert RM, Copel J, et al. Autoimmune-associated congenital heart block: demographics, mortality morbidity and recurrence rates obtained from a national lupus registry. *J Am Coll Cardiol.* 1998;31:1658–1666.

Garson A Jr, Bink-Boelkens M, Hesslein PS, et al. Atrial flutter in the young: a collaborative study of 380 cases. *J Am Coll Cardiol.* 1986;6:871–878.

Gilljam T, Jaeggi E, Gow RM. Neonatal supraventricular tachycardia: outcomes over a 27-year period at a single institution. *Acta Paediatr.* 2008;97:1035–1039.

Levin MD, Stephens P, Ranel RE, et al. Ventricular tachycardia in infants with structurally normal heart: a benign disorder. *Cardiol Young.* 2010;20:641–647.

Michaelsson M, Engle MA. Congenital complete heart block: an international study of the natural history. *Cardiovasc Clin.* 1972;4:85–101.

Perry JC, Garson A Jr. Supraventricular tachycardia due to Wolff-Parkinson-White syndrome in children: early disappearance and later recurrence. *J Am Coll Cardiol.* 1990;16:1215–1220.

Part D: Lungs

Mechanical Ventilation

Nick Mickas

INDICATION

The goal of mechanical ventilation, as for any respiratory support, is simply to achieve adequate gas exchange to maintain physiologic neutrality. Mechanical ventilation is indicated when noninvasive forms of respiratory support such as nasal continuous positive airway pressure (NCPAP) are inadequate to support the infant's respiratory needs. This may manifest as hypoxia, hypercarbia, or apnea. Far less-common indications for mechanical ventilation include airway anomalies and central or pharmacologically induced apnea. Mechanical ventilation of the neonate can seem intimidating to even the most seasoned practitioner. This chapter provides a systematic approach to management of the ventilated neonate, addressing the basic physiology underlying neonatal pulmonary pathology.

In the neonate, the cause of respiratory distress does not change the mode of support to be employed, with the potential exception of air leak syndromes (pneumothorax, pulmonary interstitial emphysema [PIE]). The majority of neonatal patients requiring respiratory support have either an absolute or a functional deficiency of surfactant. Whether treating an infant with respiratory distress syndrome (true surfactant deficiency) or meconium aspiration or pneumonia (surfactant inactivation), we are faced with a lung with decreased compliance and prone to atelectasis.

Conventional, or tidal, ventilation is the most frequently used mode of respiratory support and is addressed in this chapter. Gas is delivered in positive pressure breaths, with exhalation occurring by the lung's elastic recoil. Simply stated, breath goes in, breath comes out like the tide, hence the term *tidal*. One can think of conventional ventilation in terms of bulk flow gas exchange.

RESPIRATORY PHYSIOLOGY

Before proceeding, it is worth simply reviewing the concept of compliance because this guides the decisions we make. The lung as a unit can be thought of as any other elastic spherical structure and will behave as shown in Figure 85-1.

Although overly simplistic and not entirely correct, the lung can be thought of as a balloon. Blowing up a balloon is something we all have experienced. There is a certain amount of work that must be done to inflate the balloon; often, the initial inflation is the hardest part of blowing it up. The first inflection point of the curve represents this, and we refer to this point of inflation as "opening pressure." This point of the curve can also be thought of as our ideal functional residual capacity (FRC), as at this point we exert the minimal amount of pressure to maintain inflation. Maintaining this pressure will ensure that we avoid collapse and minimize work of breathing because at this point in the curve, additional volume can be achieved with little added pressure. The slope of the curve at any point is lung compliance. As you reach the point of overinflation, the balloon becomes relatively inelastic, and with further inflation, you risk rupture. This is represented by the "overdistention" segment of the curve. Here, a good amount of pressure is needed to achieve any additional volume, and in the case of a lung, this is a dangerous place to be.

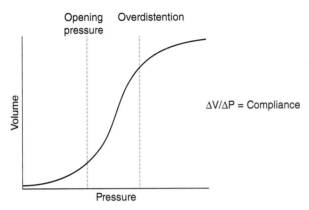

FIGURE 85-1 Pressure/volume curve

All of the recommendations made regarding ventilator manipulations assume that we are functioning in the segment of the compliance curve between our opening pressure and overdistention.

METHOD

Getting Started

When placing a patient on a ventilator, a mode must first be selected. There are 3 simple modes to consider, although each ventilator manufacturer has multiple other "hybrid"-type modes available. It is critical for the practitioner to understand the basics of the mode, most notably what triggers a breath, how size of breath is determined (volume or pressure), and what will happen to the ventilator rate should the patient's respiratory drive change. Other modes not mentioned tend to be some variation of the modes listed. If placing a patient on a mode of ventilation that you are not familiar with, it is essential to take the time with your respiratory therapist to understand exactly what the ventilator is delivering and how it is being triggered to do so. Without understanding this, choosing the proper ventilator change to make is impossible.

1. *Intermittent mandatory ventilation (IMV):* The ventilator divides a minute by the determined rate to set a cycle time and delivers that breath at the start of each cycle. If there is a set rate of 30, the ventilator delivers a breath every 2 seconds like clockwork (60 seconds/30 = 2). The breath is delivered independent of the infant's respiratory cycle.
2. *Synchronized intermittent mandatory ventilation (SIMV):* The ventilator divides a minute by the determined rate to set a cycle time and assists a patient-triggered breath during that cycle. Using the hypothetical rate of 30, the ventilator assists 1 patient breath every 2 seconds for a rate of 30.

Other patient breaths are not supported. If the infant becomes apneic, this mode functions as IMV.
3. *Assist control (A/C):* The ventilator delivers a breath with every patient effort. The set rate essentially becomes an apnea rate. With our hypothetical ventilator rate of 30, if the infant is breathing more than 30 breaths/minute, the infant sets the rate as long as 1 breath is taken every 2 seconds. If the infant becomes apneic, the mode functions as IMV.

Pressure or Volume

Ventilator breaths are limited by either the maximal pressure to be delivered or the volume of the breath to be delivered. The decision regarding which to use is largely institutionally driven, and neither is advocated here. The rationale for "pressure-limited" ventilation is to avoid the damage of excessive pressure on the developing lung, so-called barotrauma. Ventilation at high inspiratory pressures, even for relatively brief periods, has been shown to induce lung injury.[1,2] Institutions using "volume ventilation" do so to avoid excessive volumes and their potential role in the development of chronic lung disease, referred to as *volutrauma*. There is compelling animal data that would suggest that it is volume delivered, rather than pressure, that has an impact on alveolar injury.[3–5] In practice, pressure and volume are not distinct; pressure-limited ventilation is usually volume targeted, and in centers using volume ventilation, there is still attention paid to maximal ventilator pressures.

Anatomy of a Ventilator Breath

For the sake of demonstration, assume we have chosen to place a patient on pressure-limited SIMV at a rate of 30 breaths per minute. Next, we must decide on ventilator settings.

1. Positive end-expiratory pressure (PEEP): This is the base pressure that the ventilator delivers at the end of expiration and maintains as a minimum throughout the respiratory cycle. Looking back at our compliance curve, to stabilize our lung and optimize pressure delivered, the PEEP should be set at what we believe to be our opening pressure to optimize FRC.
2. Peak inspiratory pressure (PIP): This is the maximal pressure to be delivered by the ventilator during the inspiratory phase. PIP should be limited so that exhaled volumes as measured by the ventilator are not excessive. At our own institution, we target 4–6 mL/kg exhaled tidal volumes, using pressure limits.
3. Time: The cycle time can be divided into inspiratory time (i-time or T_i) (Figure 85-2), the duration of inspiration, and the expiratory time (e-time or T_e), the time interval allowed for expiration. These are

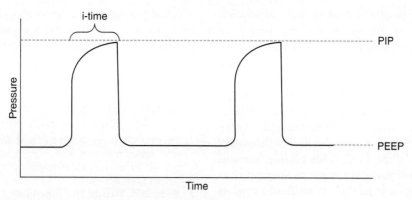

FIGURE 85-2 Parameters of a conventional ventilator breath.

set as absolute time in seconds. Discussion of time constants is far beyond the scope of this conversation, and T_i will be largely institution dependent. It is important to consider the relationship of T_i to the T_e, the inspiratory-to-expiratory (I/E) ratio, to ensure gas is not trapped within the lung. A rule of thumb is that the expiratory phase should be at least twice the inspiratory phase for an I/E ratio of at least 1:2.

MONITORING

In response to a change in patient status, either by pulse oximetry or blood gas sample, ventilator settings may require adjustment. Before making a ventilator change, it is always prudent to ensure that there is not a mechanical problem, and that the airway is patent. When manipulating ventilator settings, it is easiest to consider oxygenation and ventilation as completely separate.

Oxygenation

Oxygenation occurs throughout the respiratory cycle as long as the alveolus is inflated with oxygen-rich gas and that the alveolus is perfused. The more optimally recruited the lung, the more alveoli are available for gas exchange. Looking back at our compliance curve, volume is proportional to pressure. Taking this a step further, the mean airway pressure Paw will dictate the recruited lung volume.

$$Paw = (PIP \times T_i) + (PEEP \times T_e)/Cycle\ time$$

As most of the respiratory cycle is spent in expiration, an increase in PEEP will have a larger impact on Paw than any other ventilator change. That said, an increase in essentially any ventilator parameter would also increase Paw. This can be thought of as the "clockwise approach to oxygenation," in that dialing any dial clockwise will increase oxygenation.

Again, to increase oxygenation, increase Paw. The ventilator changes to consider are the following:

1. Increase PEEP (likely to have largest impact).
2. Increase PIP.
3. Increase T_i.
4. Increase rate.

A couple of points of clarification with oxygenation need to be made: First, an increase in rate will only increase Paw if the T_i remains constant; if the I/E ratio remains constant, changing the rate will not increase the Paw. Marked increases in PEEP may impair pulmonary blood flow, thus negatively impacting oxygenation, or result in gas trapping, thus negatively impacting ventilation.

Ventilation

When considering ventilation, it is worth thinking back to physiology. Carbon dioxide equilibrates rapidly across the alveolus, and further CO_2 removal can only occur with removal of that gas. The equation for alveolar minute ventilation includes factors such as dead space but can be simplified to

$$Minute\ ventilation = Tidal\ volume \times Rate$$

In volume modes, this makes the manipulation of ventilation an easy task: simply increase the ventilator rate or increase the volume of each breath. If using pressure-limited ventilation, referring to our compliance curve:

$$Tidal\ volume \propto Compliance \times \Delta P$$

Therefore,

$$Minute\ ventilation \propto Rate \times \Delta P$$

So, in order of impact, to increase minute ventilation,

1. Increase rate.
2. Increase PIP.
3. Decrease PEEP.

A couple of points of clarification with ventilation are necessary: First, an increase in rate will only have an impact if the rate change has an impact on the ventilator rate. In patient-triggered modes such as A/C, the patient's respiratory rate may far exceed the set ventilator rate, so an increase in set ventilator rate will not change minute ventilation. If considering a decrease in PEEP, proceed with caution. Although decreasing PEEP may increase minute ventilation, it may also lead to derecruitment and instability of the FRC. **This change should only be considered if there is reason to suspect that a patient's ventilation is in the overinflated region of the compliance curve, and close attention must be paid to ensure the status of oxygenation.**

Reviewing once again, to increase

Oxygenation α Paw	Ventilation α Rate × Tidal volume (ΔP)
↑ PEEP	↑ Rate
↑ PIP	↑ PIP
↑ Rate	↓ PEEP (proceed with caution)
↑ T_i	

If a ventilator change is made and the result on the patient is different from what you expect, consideration should be given to where the patient is on the compliance curve. If the FRC is unstable or the lung is overdistended, the rules given may not necessarily hold true. There are also some situations in which the required volumes for effective ventilation are large enough to cause concern. In these cases, high-frequency ventilation may be an alternative to escalating conventional ventilator support because of the risk of volutrauma/barotrauma.

REFERENCES

1. Dreyfuss D, Basset G, Soler P, et al. Intermittent positive pressure hyperventilation with high inflation pressures produce pulmonary microvascular injury in rats. *Am Rev Respir Dis.* 1985;132(4):880–884.
2. Webb HH, Tierney DF. Experimental pulmonary edema due to intermittent positive pressure ventilation with high inflation pressures: protection by positive end expiratory pressure. *Am Rev Respir Dis.* 1974;110(5):556–565.
3. Hernandez LA, Peevy KJ, Moise AA, et al. Chest wall restriction limits high airway pressure-induced lung injury in young rabbits. *J Appl Physiol.* 1989;66(5):2364–2368.
4. Carlton DP, Cummings JJ, Scheerer RG, et al. Lung overexpansion increases microvascular protein permeability in young lambs. *J Appl Physiol.* 1990;69(2):577–583.
5. Dreyfuss D, Soler P, Basset G, et al. High inflation pressure pulmonary edema. Respective effects of high airway pressure, high tidal volume, and positive end expiratory pressure. *Am Rev Respir Dis.* 1988;137(5):1159–1164.
6. Martin RJ, Fanaroff AA, Walsh MC. *Fanaroff and Martin's Neonatal-Perinatal Medicine.* 8th ed. Philadelphia, PA: Mosby/Elsevier; 2006.
7. West JB. *Respiratory Physiology: The Essentials.* 8th ed. Baltimore, MD: Lippincott, Williams and Wilkins; 2008.
8. Polin RA, Fox WW, Abman SH. *Fetal and Neonatal Physiology.* 4th ed. Philadelphia, PA: Elsevier/Saunders; 2011.
9. Goldsmith JP, Karotkin EH. *Assisted Ventilation of the Neonate.* 5th ed. Philadelphia, PA: Saunders; 2011.

86 Chronic Lung Disease

Anne Hilgendorff

DIAGNOSIS AND INDICATION

Clinical Findings

History

The definition of bronchopulmonary dysplasia (BPD) has been modified over the years. The initial description by Northway et al was followed by a definition of BPD that required a history of positive pressure ventilation during the first 2 weeks of life, clinical signs of respiratory compromise, and requirement for supplemental oxygen beyond 28 days of age, in addition to characteristic radiologic abnormalities. The current definition of chronic lung disease (CLD) in the newborn distinguishes between mild, moderate, and severe disease and uses O_2 dependency at 36 weeks' postconceptual age, thereby "correcting" for the degree of immaturity (Table 86-1). The disease is characterized by alveolar arrest and impaired vascular development, which is more significant at lower gestational ages.

Physical

Clinical signs of CLD include evidence of respiratory distress, such as tachypnea, nasal flaring, and use of accessory muscles with intercostal and substernal retractions, grunting, and cyanosis. The decrease in gas exchange surface area leads to impaired gas exchange (ie, hypoxemia with need for supplemental O_2 and alveolar hypoventilation with resultant hypercapnia) as a result of ventilation and perfusion mismatch. The clinical picture can be complicated by increased pulmonary vascular resistance, typically characterized by impaired

responsiveness to inhaled nitric oxide (iNO) and other vasodilators, sometimes progressing to pulmonary hypertension and right heart failure. Biventricular failure is unusual when sufficient oxygenation is maintained, and the development of severe pulmonary hypertension is avoided. Pulmonary function testing in these infants often demonstrates increased airway resistance, hyperreactive airways, and reduced compliance. Infants can present with episodic bronchoconstriction and cyanosis. Increased work of breathing contributes to impaired somatic growth and neurologic development observed in severe cases from an early stage.

Confirmation/Baseline Tests

The diagnosis is defined by the need for supplemental oxygen or ventilator support to maintain oxygen saturation above 85% at 36 weeks' postconceptual age. Blood gas analysis shows an increase in bicarbonate and partial pressure of carbon dioxide (pCO_2), indicating increased ventilation-perfusion mismatch. Continuous pulse oximetry is needed to monitor oxygen saturation and control oxygen supply. Chest radiographic findings include fibrosis/interstitial markings, cystic elements, and hyperinflation starting in the first week of life, with severely affected infants showing cystic changes (Figure 86-1). High-resolution computed tomography (HRCT) demonstrates linear and reticular opacities, areas of architectural distortion, and gas trapping or hyperexpansion. Increased pulmonary vascular resistance can be tested by echocardiography or by right heart catheterization when insufficiency of the tricuspid valve is present. Severe cases can present with cor pulmonale and right heart failure.

Table 86-1 Degrees of Bronchopulmonary Dysplasia[a]

Gestational Age at Birth	<32 Weeks	≥32 Weeks
	FiO$_2$ > 0.21 at day 28	
Mild	FiO$_2$ 0.21 at 36 weeks	FiO$_2$ 0.21 at day 56
Moderate	FiO$_2$ < 0.30 at 36 weeks	FiO$_2$ < 0.30 at day 56
Severe	FiO$_2$ ≥ 0.30 or PPV/CPAP at 36 weeks	FiO$_2$ ≥ 0.30 or PPV/CPAP at day 56

Abbreviations: CPAP, continuous positive airway pressure; FiO$_2$, fraction of inspired oxygen; PPV, positive pressure ventilation.
[a]Adapted with permission from Jobe and Bancalari.[1]

Differential Diagnosis/Diagnostic Algorithm

The absence of the typical history for BPD (eg, extreme prematurity accompanied by mechanical ventilation), a family history of (undiagnosed) pulmonary diseases, or signs of additional malformations should lead to consideration of other differential diagnoses. These include members of the family of interstitial lung diseases (ILDs) in children. Compromised lung function can also be found in association with congenital heart disease, arterial hypertensive vasculopathy, or congenital lymphatic diseases, as well as in chromosomal disorders that result in impaired pulmonary growth. Pulmonary hypoplasia, as seen in congenital diaphragmatic hernia, and surfactant dysfunction disorders should also be included in the differential diagnoses. Rare diseases, including neuroendocrine cell hyperplasia of infancy and pulmonary interstitial glycogenesis, as well as opportunistic infections in potentially immunocompromised patients also need to be considered.

PREPARATION, PRETREATMENT, AND PRE-WORKUP MANAGEMENT

Consent, Assent, and Ethical Considerations

Ethical considerations need to include long-term perspectives in patients at a high risk to develop severe BPD in association with other complications of prematurity, such as intraventricular hemorrhage (IVH), necrotizing enterocolitis (NEC), or severe infections that critically influence pulmonary as well as neurologic long-term outcome.

Monitoring for Treatment, Procedure, and Workup

Treatment monitoring has to include indicating acute and long-term outcome in this patient cohort. Need for supplemental oxygen and oxygenation, days with ventilator support, and lung function parameters define acute treatment response. Survival without BPD, abnormal lung function, clinical signs of pulmonary impairment (eg, hospitalization, infections), or even death characterize long-term therapeutic effectiveness.

Sedation/Pain Control Considerations

Sedation and pain control medication may be needed under long-term ventilation. Their interference with the ability to ventilate and oxygenate as well as their potential impact on neurologic outcome has to be considered.

Laboratory

Tests should include monitoring of gas exchange by arterial blood gas analysis and arterial oxygen saturation (SaO$_2$); monitoring of pH and pCO$_2$ by capillary blood gas analysis; lung function testing to define compliance, airway resistance, and lung volume; as well as chest radiography to exclude atelectasis as a cause of pulmonary problems. Hematocrit and electrolytes, especially while on diuretic therapy, as well as alkaline phosphatase need to be monitored. The assessment of other variables, for example, NT-proBNP may be helpful to indicate pulmonary hypertension but need further validation before routine clinical use.

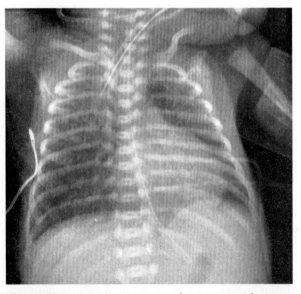

FIGURE 86-1 Anterior posterior chest x-ray with a score of 5; 4 for interstitial shadows in all 4 quadrants, 1 for lung expansion, and 0 for cysts. (Reproduced with permission from Greenough et al.[2])

Cardiac Function

Echocardiography and electrocardiography (ECG) are used to assess cardiac function for possible cor pulmonale.

Measurements

Monitoring of somatic growth 2–3 times per week, including body weight, length, and head circumference, is needed to ensure appropriate growth and to help define adequate calorie intake.

TREATMENT PROCEDURE

Prevention

Administration of antenatal glucocorticoids and surfactant replacement therapy, routinely used in the care of premature infants, have been shown to reduce the risk for BPD. Figure 86-2 summarizes contributing factors. Most treatment strategies aim at preventing their impact in order to minimize further injury of the immature lung, thereby decreasing the risk for BPD.

Infection Management

The presence of severe prenatal infections increases the risk for preterm delivery and BPD development. Postnatally, careful and frequent evaluations to detect early signs of infection, meticulous monitoring of aseptic technique in infant handling, management of ventilator circuits and airway care, as well as early initiation of appropriate antimicrobial treatment of infection are critical issues in helping to reduce the incidence and severity of BPD. Routine use of erythromycin or azithromycin for eradication of *Ureaplasma* or *Chlamydia* species cannot be recommended thus far.

Mechanical Ventilation

The strategy for mechanical ventilation of premature infants should include low positive inspiratory pressure (PIP), relatively short inspiratory times, sufficient positive end-expiratory pressures (PEEP) and low tidal volumes (4–6 mL/kg), which may require higher rates of ventilation to ensure adequate minute volumes. Proper heating and humidification of the inspired gas and caution with endotracheal tube suctioning, which provokes lung collapse, are important considerations for preventing airway injury. Permissive hypercapnia, with $PaCO_2$ as high as 55 or 60 mm Hg as long as the pH was 7.25 or greater, remains controversial and should be applied with caution. Weaning from mechanical ventilation should focus on reducing PIP and tidal volume prior to decreasing the respirator rate to avoid lung overdistension. Cessation of invasive ventilation

should be considered as early as possible to reduce the incidence of supplemental oxygen therapy at 28 days as well as number of days on mechanical ventilation. Following extubation, frequent desaturations caused by apneic episodes and limited pulmonary capacity can be prevented by application of continuous positive airway pressure (CPAP) or noninvasive positive pressure ventilation (NIPPV). Treatment with caffeine should be initiated before extubation to reduce the risk of apnea and to potentially reduce the incidence of BPD.

Oxygen Therapy

Although it is important to reduce the inspired O_2 concentration quickly if the oxygen saturation is greater than 96% or if the PaO_2 is greater than 80 mm Hg, targeting an SpO_2 of 85%–89% in immature babies was associated with slightly increased mortality rates and therefore cannot currently be recommended. Common practice to date is to maintain PaO_2 above 55 mm Hg. SaO_2 needs to be correlated with the PaO_2, and in general SaO_2 should be maintained between 90% and 95% to reach an appropriate PaO_2.

Transfusion

Hematocrit should be maintained at approximately 30%–35% as long as supplemental oxygen is needed.

Nitric Oxide

In case of severe pulmonary hypertension in the early or later course of the disease, iNO can be considered. However, a treatment regimen using iNO as a rescue therapy did not reduce the incidence of BPD. Prophylactic application cannot be recommended to prevent the development of BPD. If applied, iNO treatment has to be performed under close monitoring for potential toxicities of iNO therapy, including interference with normal platelet function. Furthermore, side effects of iNO, including oxidant lung injury and loss of surfactant function resulting from the production of peroxynitrite, as well as long-term neurodevelopmental disability have to be considered prior to the institution of therapy.

Steroids

Treatment with potent anti-inflammatory steroids (eg, dexamethasone) to facilitate weaning from mechanical ventilation is currently contraindicated as it was found to be associated with an increased incidence of cerebral palsy and poor neurologic outcome.[4] Current recommendations are to reserve the use of dexamethasone as a last resort in infants who cannot otherwise be weaned

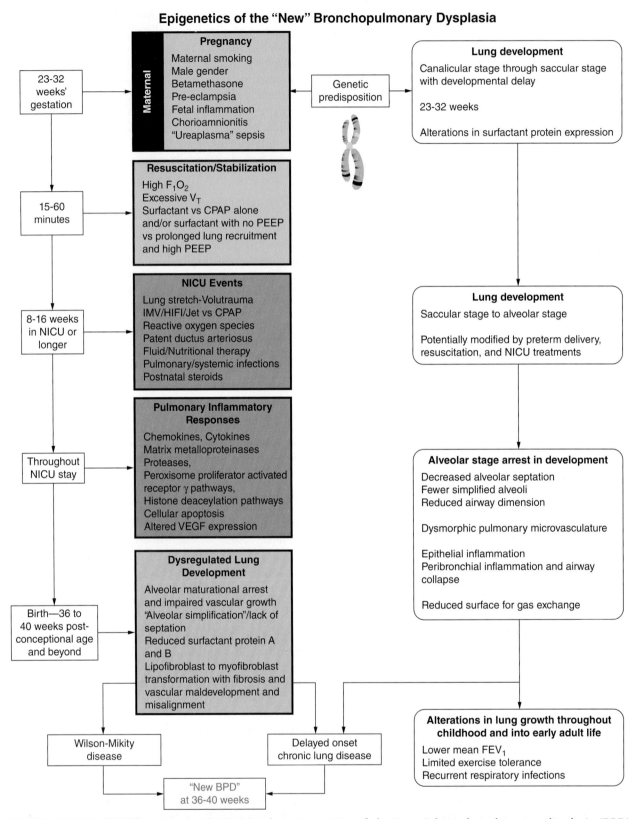

FIGURE 86-2 Multiple factors contributing to the epigenetics of the "new" bronchopulmonary dysplasia (BPD) associated with lung development and gestational and postnatal developmental periods. FIO$_2$, fraction of inspired oxygen; V$_T$, tidal volume; CPAP, continuous positive airway pressure; PEEP, positive end-expiratory pressure; NICU, neonatal intensive care unit; IMV, invasive mechanical ventilation; HIFI, High Frequency Ventilation in Premature Infants study; VEGF, vascular endothelial growth factor; FEV$_1$, forced expiratory volume in 1 second. (Reproduced with permission from Merritt et al.[3])

from mechanical ventilation. In these cases a short, low-dose regimen aimed at increasing the weaning rate in extremely low birth weight infants should be employed. Complications of dexamethasone treatment include glucose intolerance, systemic hypertension, and transient catabolic state. Total neutrophil counts and platelet counts may increase during treatment. Hypertrophic cardiomyopathy sometimes occurs, but is transient, as well as adrenal suppression. Hydrocortisone can be used in the first days of life for fluid-resistant arterial hypotension. Furthermore, short courses of hydrocortisone have been shown to significantly decrease mortality and improve survival of preterm infants with a history of chorioamnionitis without increasing the risk of BPD, suppressing adrenal function, or compromising short-term growth. Such therapy can be preceded by an ACTH (corticotropin) stimulation test (1 μg/kg test dose). Interestingly, however, low cortisol levels were not predictive of adverse long-term outcomes, and high cortisol concentrations, although predictive of short-term adverse outcomes such as IVH and periventricular leukomalacia, did also not predict adverse outcome. Inhaled steroids, as well as bronchodilators, currently cannot be recommended for treatment or prevention of BPD other than in cases of symptomatic bronchoconstriction.

Bronchoscopy

In case of stridor or persistent respiratory distress, vocal cord injury, associated with either patent ductus arteriosus (PDA) ligation or prolonged ventilation, hemangiomas, subglottic stenosis, or other structural problems need to be excluded. Bronchoscopy, or endoscopy with small devices through the nose, can facilitate the diagnosis.

Cardiovascular System

Early closure of the ductus arteriosus, either by pharmacologic intervention or surgical ligation, appears to reduce the risk of pulmonary edema and of severe BPD. However, prophylactic ligation cannot be recommended as this procedure significantly increased the incidence of BPD and mechanical ventilation at 36 weeks.[5–7] Prophylactic administration of cyclooxygenase inhibitors such as indomethacin and ibuprofen is currently not justified as the short-term benefits of these treatments were not associated with any beneficial effect on mortality or neurodevelopmental outcome.

Fluids

Restricting fluid and salt intake to prevent fluid overload and allowing for diuresis and a progressive loss of about 10%–15% body weight in the first week of life has been shown to reduce the risk of BPD. Excessive fluid and heat losses in the first week of life should be minimized, especially in the very immature infant below 26 weeks' gestation, by keeping the infant in a warm, humidified chamber covered with foil. The overall fluid balance—including the insensible loss through evaporation through skin and airways—should be monitored closely, such as by keeping the infant on a bed scale or by measuring body weight at frequent intervals and by keeping accurate records of fluid intake and urine output. In a suitably humidified environment, appropriate initial rates of intravenous fluid intake for the premature infant are 80–90 mL/kg during the first day of life and 160–180 mL/kg on the sixth day of life, with a stepwise increase of 10–20 mL/kg per day. Frequent measurements of serum electrolytes, every 6 hours for the very immature infant and every 12 hours for the infant greater than 26 weeks' gestation, can help guide fluid therapy. Sodium should be withheld from intravenous fluids for at least the first 24 hours and should not be added until there is good diuresis (>2 mL/kg/h) and the weight is at least 5% below birth weight. After the brisk diuresis that usually occurs during the first 3–7 days of life, urine output generally decreases to about 2–4 mL/kg/h, and fluid intake can be adjusted—and should generally not exceed—about 120–150 mL/kg/d.

Diuretics

Diuretics must be used with caution because of their potential complications, which include electrolyte deficiencies (notably of sodium, potassium, and chloride); bone demineralization from urinary calcium loss; nephrocalcinosis; and hearing impairment without benefits on long-term outcome.

1. Furosemide: 1–2 mg/kg every 12 hours or every other day.
2. Hydrochlorothiazide: 1–2 mg/kg/dose every 12 hours.
3. Spironolactone: 1–2 mg/kg/dose every 12 hours.
4. Supplemental KCl (2–5 mEq/kg) or arginine HCl (if serum potassium is high) usually corrects for contraction alkalosis with associated potassium and chloride depletion, usually heralded by a rising serum bicarbonate concentration and a low serum chloride concentration.

Nutrition

Nutritional needs of the infant with BPD depend on environmental conditions. The goal should be a neutral thermal environment, but work of breathing and general metabolism, which may be slightly greater than for infants without BPD, need to be considered. Early delivery of parenteral nutrition, including protein and lipid, through an umbilical catheter or a peripherally placed central venous line is helpful in establishing early positive nitrogen balance and facilitating growth and lung repair. A retrospective analysis revealed that aggressive early parenteral nutrition and receipt of calorie-dense milk improved growth for early low birth weight infants with BPD. Actual recommendations state a protein intake of a minimum 3 g/kg body weight beginning from the second day of life. In orally fed infants, caloric, protein, and mineral needs usually can be met with fortification of mother's breast milk or with premature infant formula with a caloric density of 24–30 kcal/oz. Furthermore, premature infants with BPD require nutritional supplements of calcium and phosphorus, in addition to adequate vitamins, and if they are receiving diuretics, their overall electrolyte balance needs to be monitored closely. Nonetheless, it has to be considered that there are no sufficient studies to date with respect to increased energy intake for infants with BPD.

Vitamins

Retinol (vitamin A) has been shown to decrease the incidence and severity of BPD in extremely premature infants, who are typically deficient in vitamin A. For the smallest infants on ventilatory support, retinol is given intramuscularly at a dose of 5000 IU 3 times/week for a total of 12 injections, which is the regimen that was used in a multicenter, double-blind, randomized, controlled trial.[8] The specific mechanism by which retinol treatment helps to prevent BPD is unclear. However, a recent report found that retinol treatment of mechanically ventilated premature baboons yielded no apparent benefit in terms of either lung physiology or alveolar structure.

Gastroesophageal Reflux

If gastroesophageal reflux is suspected, an esophageal pH study should be done to test for the presence of reflux and possible apnea to establish the severity and frequency of the problem. If significant reflux is documented, drugs that might contribute to the problem should be discontinued, and antireflux medications should be considered.

FOLLOW-UP

Clinical Follow-up

Clinical follow-up should include examination of the following:

1. Cardiac function. Blood pressure measurements, ECG, and echocardiography should be followed for signs of pulmonary hypertension or elevated systemic blood pressure.
2. Lung function. The simplest is by blood gas analysis or oximetry. Pulmonary function testing can be performed in some centers and may help to identify infants in need of inhalation therapy. Some infants require apnea and oxygen saturation monitors in combination with home oxygen therapy.
3. Nutrition. Comprehensive monitoring of somatic growth is needed and should influence the decision regarding cessation of oxygen therapy or ventilatory support.
4. Ophthalmology. As retinopathy of prematurity (ROP) is more common in infants with BPD, frequent consultation with an ophthalmologist needs to be part of the follow-up program.
5. Audiology. As use of ototoxic drugs as well as prematurity increase the risk for sensorineural hearing loss, screening with auditory brainstem responses should be performed at discharge and, if clinically indicated, repeated during the follow-up process.
6. Vaccination. Patients with BPD should receive respiratory syncytial virus (RSV) prophylaxis and be kept up to date on vaccinations to decrease the risks of further lung injury.

Pulmonary Outcome

Preterm infants with BPD may show acute and long-term pulmonary impairment, including oxygen dependency for months or years (Figure 86-3). Infants suffering from BPD have a high readmission rate, with up to 70% requiring a hospital stay and about 30% requiring 3 readmissions in the first 2 years of life and a high rate of infections with RSV. The risk for persistent wheeze and need for chronic pulmonary medication is increased in these patients, with 20%–30% of infants with BPD having symptoms at 6 and 12 months of age; respiratory symptoms remain common at preschool and school age and can persist into adulthood. Lung function testing should include peak oxygen consumption, forced expiratory volume at 1 second (FEV_1), and gas transfer as well as peak workload, breathing frequencies, and tidal volumes and residual capacity. Airway obstruction needs to be considered and can persist into puberty and adulthood. Furthermore, patients with BPD need to be aware of a potential rapid deterioration of lung function. Overall mortality from pulmonary dysfunction or associated cardiovascular problems is estimated at 10%–20% during the first year of life. The risk increases with duration of oxygen exposure and level of ventilatory support. Death is frequently caused by infection. The risk of sudden unexpected death may be increased, but the cause is unclear.

Neurologic Outcome

About 40% of infants with BPD have 1 or more of the following: cerebral palsy, cognitive delay, severe hearing loss, or bilateral blindness at 18 months of age (Table 86-2). Children with severe BPD performed more poorly on IQ tests and language measures at 3 years of age and performance IQ and perceptual organization at age 8 years and thus received special education services

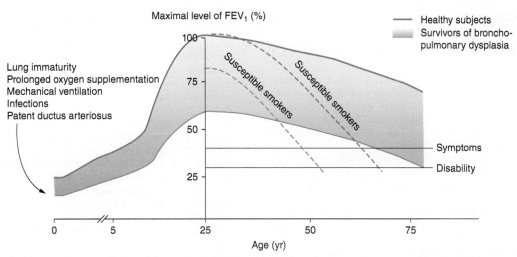

FIGURE 86-3 Theoretical model of changes in forced expiratory volume in 1 second (FEV$_1$ in survivors of broncho-pulmonary dysplasia and healthy subjects according to age. Theoretical curves are shown for the FEV1 in healthy subjects and survivors of bronchopulmonary dysplasia. Survivors of bronchopulmonary dysplasia may have variable airflow limitation from the first years of life, with little evidence of "catch-up" growth in lung function. In some of these patients, FEV$_1$ does not reach the normal maximal value in early adulthood, and the phase of declining FEV$_1$ values starts from a substantially reduced maximal value. Whether the rate of decline with advancing age will parallel that among healthy persons or will be accelerated is not known. The dashed lines represent the potential effect of smoking on the rate of decline of FEV$_1$ in susceptible subjects. Values for FEV$_1$ in the first 3 years of life are extrapolated from measurements of maximal flow at functional residual capacity. (Adapted with permission from Fletcher and Peto.[9])

at a higher rate than did children with mild BPD. Thus, standardized testing procedures for cognitive and motor outcome are mandatory for long-term follow-up.

Growth

Children born at the limit of viability attain poor growth in early childhood, followed by catchup growth to age 11 years, but remain smaller than their term-born peers.[11] Studies in younger infants showed that, despite an improvement in weight compared to

infants with BPD from the last decade, poor growth attainment at birth, 40 weeks, and 20 months corrected age remains a major problem among infants with BPD.[12]

ACKNOWLEDGMENT

This chapter is with acknowledgment to my clinical and scientific mentors as well as to Dr. Antje Brand and Dr. Harald Ehrhardt.

Table 86-2 Univariate Relationships Between Individual Neonatal Morbidities and Outcomes at 18 Months[a]

Neonatal Morbidity		Poor 18-Month Outcome: Death or Neurosensory Impairment[a]			Components of Poor 18-Month Outcome: Death and Individual Impairments, No./Total (%)				
		No./Total (%)	OR (95 % CI)	P Value	Death	CP	MDI <70	Deaf	Blind
BPD	Present	193/409 (47)	2.5 (1.9-3.4)	<.001	28/409 (6.8)	64/381 (17.0)	135/374 (36.0)	13/370 (3.5)	7/377 (1.9)
	Absent	130/501 (26)			6/501 (1.2)	46/494 (9.3)	94/487 (19.0)	7/489 (1.4)	9/491 (1.8)
Brain injury	Present	116/194 (60)	3.7 (2.6-5.2)	<.001	17/194 (8.8)	63/177 (36.0)	73/172 (42.0)	5/172 (2.9)	5/175 (2.9)
	Absent	207/716 (29)			17/716 (2.4)	47/698 (6.7)	156/689 (23.0)	15/687 (2.2)	11/693 (1.6)
Severe ROP	Present	58/89 (65)	3.9 (2.4-6.4)	<.001	9/89 (10.0)	19/80 (24.0)	34/69 (49.0)	3/78 (3.8)	12/80 (15.0)
	Absent	265/821 (32)			25/821 (3.0)	91/795 (12.0)	91/792 (25.0)	17/781 (2.2)	4/788 (0.5)

Abbreviations: BPD, bronchopulmonary dysplasia; CI, confidence interval; CP, cerebral palsy; MDI, Mental Development Index; OR, odds ratio; ROP, retinopathy of prematurity.
[a]The rate of poor outcome in the entire cohort was 323/910 (35%).[10]

REFERENCES

1. Jobe AH, Bancalari E. Bronchopulmonary dysplasia. *Am J Respir Crit Care Med.* 2001;163(7):1723–1729.
2. Greenough A, Thomas M, Dimitriou G, et al. Prediction of outcome from the chest radiograph appearance on day 7 of very prematurely born infants. *Eur J Pediatr.* 2004;163(1):14–18.
3. Merritt TA, Deming DD, Boynton BR. The "new" bronchopulmonary dysplasia: challenges and commentary. *Semin Fetal Neonatal Med.* 2009;14(6):345–357.
4. Doyle LW, Ehrenkranz RA, Halliday HL. Dexamethasone treatment in the first week of life for preventing bronchopulmonary dysplasia in preterm infants: a systematic review. *Neonatology.* 2010;98(3):217–224.
5. Clyman R, Cassady G, Kirklin JK, et al. The role of patent ductus arteriosus ligation in bronchopulmonary dysplasia: reexamining a randomized controlled trial. *J Pediatr.* 2009;154(6):873–876.
6. Walsh MC, Yao Q, Horbar JD, et al. Changes in the use of postnatal steroids for bronchopulmonary dysplasia in 3 large neonatal networks. *Pediatrics.* 2006;118(5):e1328–e1335.
7. Mosalli R, Alfaleh K, Paes B. Role of prophylactic surgical ligation of patent ductus arteriosus in extremely low birth weight infants: systematic review and implications for clinical practice. *Ann Pediatr Cardiol.* 2009;2(2):120–126.
8. Landman J, Sive A, Heese HD, et al. Comparison of enteral and intramuscular vitamin A supplementation in preterm infants. *Early Hum Dev.* 1992;30(2):163–170.
9. Fletcher C, Peto R. The natural history of chronic airflow obstruction. *Br Med J.* 1977;1(6077):1645–1648.
10. Schmidt B, Asztalos EV, Roberts RS, et al. Impact of bronchopulmonary dysplasia, brain injury, and severe retinopathy on the outcome of extremely low-birth-weight infants at 18 months: results from the trial of indomethacin prophylaxis in preterms. *JAMA.* 2003;289(9):1124–1129.
11. Farooqi A, Hagglof B, Sedin G, et al. Growth in 10- to 12-year-old children born at 23 to 25 weeks' gestation in the 1990s: a Swedish national prospective follow-up study. *Pediatrics.* 2006;118(5):e1452–e1465.
12. Madden J, Kobaly K, Minich NM, et al. Improved weight attainment of extremely low-gestational-age infants with bronchopulmonary dysplasia. *J Perinatol.* 2010;30(2):103–111.

SUGGESTED READING

Andreasson B, Lindroth M, Mortensson W, et al. Lung function eight years after neonatal ventilation. *Arch Dis Child.* 1989;64(1):108–113.

Aquino SL, Schechter MS, Chiles C, et al. High-resolution inspiratory and expiratory CT in older children and adults with bronchopulmonary dysplasia. *AJR Am J Roentgenol.* 1999;173(4):963–967.

Aucott SW, Watterberg KL, Shaffer ML, et al. Early cortisol values and long-term outcomes in extremely low birth weight infants. *J Perinatol.* 2010;30(7):484–488.

Ballard HO, Shook LA, Bernard P, et al. Use of azithromycin for the prevention of bronchopulmonary dysplasia in preterm infants: a randomized, double-blind, placebo controlled trial. *Pediatr Pulmonol.* 2011;46(2):111–118.

Barrington KJ, Finer N. Inhaled nitric oxide for respiratory failure in preterm infants. *Cochrane Database Syst Rev.* 2010;(12):CD000509.

Baumgart S. Reduction of oxygen consumption, insensible water loss, and radiant heat demand with use of a plastic blanket for low-birth-weight infants under radiant warmers. *Pediatrics.* 1984;74(6):1022–1028.

Broughton S, Roberts A, Fox G, et al. Prospective study of healthcare utilisation and respiratory morbidity due to RSV infection in prematurely born infants. *Thorax.* 2005;60(12):1039–1044.

Broughton S, Thomas MR, Marston L, et al. Very prematurely born infants wheezing at follow-up: lung function and risk factors. *Arch Dis Child.* 2007;92(9):776–780.

Carlo WA, Finer NN, Walsh MC, et al. Target ranges of oxygen saturation in extremely preterm infants. *N Engl J Med.* 2010;362(21):1959–1969.

Colaizy TT, Morris CD, Lapidus J, et al. Detection of ureaplasma DNA in endotracheal samples is associated with bronchopulmonary dysplasia after adjustment for multiple risk factors. *Pediatr Res.* 2007;61(5 Pt 1):578–583.

Costarino AT Jr, Gruskay JA, Corcoran L, et al. Sodium restriction versus daily maintenance replacement in very low birth weight premature neonates: a randomized, blind therapeutic trial. *J Pediatr.* 1992;120(1):99–106.

Darlow BA, Graham PJ. Vitamin A supplementation to prevent mortality and short and long-term morbidity in very low birthweight infants. *Cochrane Database Syst Rev.* 2007;(4):CD000501.

Deutsch GH, Young LR, Deterding RR, et al. Diffuse lung disease in young children: application of a novel classification scheme. *Am J Respir Crit Care Med.* 2007;176(11):1120–1128.

Doyle LW, Cheung MM, Ford GW, et al. Birth weight < 1501 g and respiratory health at age 14. *Arch Dis Child.* 2001;84(1):40–44.

Doyle LW, Davis PG, Morley CJ, et al. Outcome at 2 years of age of infants from the DART study: a multicenter, international, randomized, controlled trial of low-dose dexamethasone. *Pediatrics.* 2007;119(4):716–721.

Doyle LW, Ehrenkranz RA, Halliday HL. Dexamethasone treatment after the first week of life for bronchopulmonary dysplasia in preterm infants: a systematic review. *Neonatology.* 2010;98(4):289–296.

Doyle LW, Faber B, Callanan C, et al. Bronchopulmonary dysplasia in very low birth weight subjects and lung function in late adolescence. *Pediatrics.* 2006;118(1):108–113.

Fowlie PW, Davis PG, McGuire W. Prophylactic intravenous indomethacin for preventing mortality and morbidity in preterm infants. *Cochrane Database Syst Rev.* 2010;(7):CD000174.

Greenough A, Alexander J, Burgess S, et al. Home oxygen status and rehospitalisation and primary care requirements of infants with chronic lung disease. *Arch Dis Child.* 2002;86(1):40–43.

Greenough A, Alexander J, Burgess S, et al. Preschool healthcare utilisation related to home oxygen status. *Arch Dis Child Fetal Neonatal Ed.* 2006;91(5):F337–F341.

Greenough A, Cox S, Alexander J, et al. Health care utilisation of infants with chronic lung disease, related to hospitalisation for RSV infection. *Arch Dis Child.* 2001;85(6):463–468.

Greenough A, Dimitriou G, Bhat RY, et al. Lung volumes in infants who had mild to moderate bronchopulmonary dysplasia. *Eur J Pediatr.* 2005;164(9):583–586.

Greenough A, Limb E, Marston L, et al. Risk factors for respiratory morbidity in infancy after very premature birth. *Arch Dis Child Fetal Neonatal Ed.* 2005;90(4):F320–F323.

Gross SJ, Iannuzzi DM, Kveselis DA, et al. Effect of preterm birth on pulmonary function at school age: a prospective controlled study. *J Pediatr.* 1998;133(2):188–192.

Hakulinen AL, Heinonen K, Lansimies E, et al. Pulmonary function and respiratory morbidity in school-age children born prematurely and ventilated for neonatal respiratory insufficiency. *Pediatr Pulmonol.* 1990;8(4):226–232.

Hammarlund K, Sedin G, Stromberg B. Transepidermal water loss in newborn infants. VII. Relation to post-natal age in very pre-term and full-term appropriate for gestational age infants. *Acta Paediatr Scand.* 1982;71(3):369–374.

Hammarlund K, Sedin G, Stromberg B. Transepidermal water loss in newborn infants. VIII. Relation to gestational age and post-natal age in appropriate and small for gestational age infants. *Acta Paediatr Scand.* 1983;72(5):721–728.

Hardy P, Clemens F. Stopping a randomized trial early: from protocol to publication. Commentary to Thome at al.: outcome of extremely preterm infants randomized at birth to different PaCO$_2$ targets during the first seven days of life (*Biol Neonate* 2006;90:218–225). *Biol Neonate.* 2006;90(4):226–228.

Hartnoll G, Betremieux P, Modi N. Randomised controlled trial of postnatal sodium supplementation on oxygen dependency and body weight in 25–30 week gestational age infants. *Arch Dis Child Fetal Neonatal Ed.* 2000;82(1):F19–F23.

Hilgendorff A, Reiss I, Gortner L, et al. Impact of airway obstruction on lung function in very preterm infants at term. *Pediatr Crit Care Med.* 2008;9(6):629–635.

Hjalmarson O, Sandberg KL. Lung function at term reflects severity of bronchopulmonary dysplasia. *J Pediatr.* 2005;146(1):86–90.

Howling SJ, Northway WH Jr, Hansell DM, et al. Pulmonary sequelae of bronchopulmonary dysplasia survivors: high-resolution CT findings. *AJR Am J Roentgenol.* 2000;174(5):1323–1326.

Jarreau PH, Fayon M, Baud O, et al. [The use of postnatal corticosteroid therapy in premature infants to prevent or treat bronchopulmonary dysplasia: current situation and recommendations] [in French]. *Arch Pediatr.* 2010;17(10):1480–1487.

Kaempf JW, Campbell B, Brown A, et al. PCO$_2$ and room air saturation values in premature infants at risk for bronchopulmonary dysplasia. *J Perinatol.* 2008;28(1):48–54.

Kasper DC, Mechtler TP, Bohm J, et al. In utero exposure to Ureaplasma spp. is associated with increased rate of bronchopulmonary dysplasia and intraventricular hemorrhage in preterm infants. *J Perinatol Med.* 2011;39(3):331–336.

Kinsella JP, Greenough A, Abman SH. Bronchopulmonary dysplasia. *Lancet.* 2006;367(9520):1421–1431.

Koletzko B, Goulet O, Hunt J, et al. 1. Guidelines on Paediatric Parenteral Nutrition of the European Society of Paediatric Gastroenterology, Hepatology and Nutrition (ESPGHAN) and the European Society for Clinical Nutrition and Metabolism (ESPEN), supported by the European Society of Paediatric Research (ESPR). *J Pediatr Gastroenterol Nutr.* 2005;41(Suppl 2):S1–S87.

Lai NM, Rajadurai SV, Tan KH. Increased energy intake for preterm infants with (or developing) bronchopulmonary dysplasia/chronic lung disease. *Cochrane Database Syst Rev.* 2006;(3):CD005093.

Laughon MM, Smith PB, Bose C. Prevention of bronchopulmonary dysplasia. *Semin Fetal Neonatal Med.* 2009;14(6):374–382.

Lopez E, Mathlouthi J, Lescure S, et al. Capnography in spontaneously breathing preterm infants with bronchopulmonary dysplasia. *Pediatr Pulmonol.* 2011;46(9):896–902.

Marshall DD, Kotelchuck M, Young TE, et al. Risk factors for chronic lung disease in the surfactant era: a North Carolina population-based study of very low birth weight infants. North Carolina Neonatologists Association. *Pediatrics.* 1999;104(6):1345–1350.

Morley CJ, Davis PG, Doyle LW, et al. Nasal CPAP or intubation at birth for very preterm infants. *N Engl J Med.* 2008;358(7):700–708.

Naik AS, Kallapur SG, Bachurski CJ, et al. Effects of ventilation with different positive end-expiratory pressures on cytokine expression in the preterm lamb lung. *Am J Respir Crit Care Med.* 2001;164(3):494–498.

Northway WH Jr, Moss RB, Carlisle KB, et al. Late pulmonary sequelae of bronchopulmonary dysplasia. *N Engl J Med.* 1990;323(26):1793–1799.

Oh W, Poindexter BB, Perritt R, et al. Association between fluid intake and weight loss during the first ten days of life and risk of bronchopulmonary dysplasia in extremely low birth weight infants. *J Pediatr.* 2005;147(6):786–790.

Oppenheim C, Mamou-Mani T, Sayegh N, et al. Bronchopulmonary dysplasia: value of CT in identifying pulmonary sequelae. *AJR Am J Roentgenol.* 1994;163(1):169–172.

Pelkonen AS, Hakulinen AL, Turpeinen M. Bronchial lability and responsiveness in school children born very preterm. *Am J Respir Crit Care Med.* 1997;156(4 Pt 1):1178–1184.

Pierce RA, Joyce B, Officer S, et al. Retinoids increase lung elastin expression but fail to alter morphology or angiogenesis genes in premature ventilated baboons. *Pediatr Res.* 2007;61(6):703–709.

Pohlandt F. Prevention of postnatal bone demineralization in very low-birth-weight infants by individually monitored supplementation with calcium and phosphorus. *Pediatr Res.* 1994;35(1):125–129.

Saugstad OD, Aune D. In search of the optimal oxygen saturation for extremely low birth weight infants: a systematic review and meta-analysis. *Neonatology.* 2011;100(1):1–8.

Saugstad OD, Speer CP, Halliday HL. Oxygen saturation in immature babies: revisited with updated recommendations. *Neonatology.* 2011;100(3):217–218.

Schmidt B, Roberts RS, Davis P, et al. Caffeine therapy for apnea of prematurity. *N Engl J Med.* 2006;354(20):2112–2121.

Schmidt B, Roberts RS, Fanaroff A, et al. Indomethacin prophylaxis, patent ductus arteriosus, and the risk of bronchopulmonary dysplasia: further analyses from the Trial of Indomethacin Prophylaxis in Preterms (TIPP). *J Pediatr.* 2006;148(6):730–734.

Schulze A. Respiratory gas conditioning and humidification. *Clin Perinatol.* 2007;34(1):19–33, v.

Seger N, Soll R. Animal derived surfactant extract for treatment of respiratory distress syndrome. *Cochrane Database Syst Rev.* 2009;(2):CD007836.

Short EJ, Kirchner HL, Asaad GR, et al. Developmental sequelae in preterm infants having a diagnosis of bronchopulmonary dysplasia: analysis using a severity-based classification system. *Arch Pediatr Adolesc Med.* 2007;161(11):1082–1087.

Stefano JL, Abbasi S, Pearlman SA, et al. Closure of the ductus arteriosus with indomethacin in ventilated neonates with respiratory distress syndrome. Effects of pulmonary compliance and ventilation. *Am Rev Respir Dis.* 1991;143(2):236–239.

Steinhorn RH. Neonatal pulmonary hypertension. *Pediatr Crit Care Med.* 2010;11(2 Suppl):S79–S84.

Stewart A, Brion LP, Ambrosio-Perez I. Diuretics acting on the distal renal tubule for preterm infants with (or developing) chronic lung disease. *Cochrane Database Syst Rev.* 2011;(9):CD001817.

Subramanian S, El-Mohandes A, Dhanireddy R, et al. Association of bronchopulmonary dysplasia and hypercarbia in ventilated infants with birth weights of 500–1,499 g. *Matern Child Health J.* 2011;15(Suppl 1):S17–S26.

Sweet DG, Carnielli V, Greisen G, et al. European consensus guidelines on the management of neonatal respiratory distress syndrome in preterm infants—2010 update. *Neonatology.* 2010;97(4):402–417.

Tanney K, Davis J, Halliday HL, et al. Extremely low-dose dexamethasone to facilitate extubation in mechanically ventilated preterm babies. *Neonatology.* 2011;100(3):285–289.

Theile AR, Radmacher PG, Anschutz TW, et al. Nutritional strategies and growth in extremely low birth weight infants with bronchopulmonary dysplasia over the past 10 years. *J Perinatol.* 2012;32(2):117–122.

Thome UH, Carroll W, Wu TJ, et al. Outcome of extremely preterm infants randomized at birth to different PaCO$_2$ targets during the first seven days of life. *Biol Neonate.* 2006;90(4):218–225.

CHAPTER 86

Van Marter LJ, Leviton A, Allred EN, et al. Hydration during the first days of life and the risk of bronchopulmonary dysplasia in low birth weight infants. *J Pediatr.* 1990;116(6):942–949.

Van Marter LJ, Leviton A, Kuban KC, et al. Maternal glucocorticoid therapy and reduced risk of bronchopulmonary dysplasia. *Pediatrics.* 1990;86(3):331–336.

Wada K, Jobe AH, Ikegami M. Tidal volume effects on surfactant treatment responses with the initiation of ventilation in preterm lambs. *J Appl Physiol.* 1997;83(4):1054–1061.

Watterberg KL, Shaffer ML, Mishefske MJ, et al. Growth and neurodevelopmental outcomes after early low-dose hydrocortisone treatment in extremely low birth weight infants. *Pediatrics.* 2007;120(1):40–48.

Welsh L, Kirkby J, Lum S, et al. The EPICure study: maximal exercise and physical activity in school children born extremely preterm. *Thorax.* 2010;65(2):165–172.

Wheeler KI, Klingenberg C, Morley CJ, et al. Volume-targeted versus pressure-limited ventilation for preterm infants: a systematic review and meta-analysis. *Neonatology.* 2011;100(3):219–227.

Yuksel B, Greenough A. Relationship of symptoms to lung function abnormalities in preterm infants at follow-up. *Pediatr Pulmonol.* 1991;11(3):202–206.

Zbar RI, Chen AH, Behrendt DM, et al. Incidence of vocal fold paralysis in infants undergoing ligation of patent ductus arteriosus. *Ann Thorac Surg.* 1996;61(3):814–816.

High-Frequency Ventilation

R. S. Cohen

BACKGROUND

Definition

High-frequency ventilation (HFV) is defined by the following:

1. Ventilator rates generally greater than 120 breaths per minute (bpm) or 2 breaths per second (Hz);
2. Tidal volumes (V_T) less than dead space.

The use of such small tidal volumes generally requires maintaining higher mean airway pressures (Paw) to avoid atelectasis.

For conventional ventilation,

$$\text{Minute ventilation} \propto (V_T) \times (\text{Rate})$$

However, HFV minute ventilation is more dependent on rate:

$$\text{Minute ventilation} \propto (V_T) \times (\text{Rate})^2$$

Types of HFV

High-Frequency Jet Ventilation

High-frequency jet ventilation (HFJV) is a type of HFV that is characterized by the injection of high-velocity gas boluses into the airway over a very short inspiratory time followed by passive expiration. The most common example in US neonatal intensive care units (NICUs) is the Bunnell Jet.

1. The Jet is used in conjunction with a conventional ventilator that requires replacing the endotracheal tube adapter with a special specific adaptor.

2. The conventional ventilator provides positive end-expiratory pressure (PEEP) and allows easy transition between conventional and Jet ventilation.
3. If desired, the conventional ventilator can also provide "sigh" breaths in synchrony with the Jet.

High-Frequency Oscillatory Ventilation

High-frequency oscillatory ventilation (HFOV) uses oscillatory movements of a piston in line with the respiratory gas flow, resulting in active movement of air both during inspiration and during the expiratory phase. The most common example in US NICUs is the Sensormedics 3100A.

1. No conventional ventilator is used with the 3100A.
2. A rigid ventilator circuit is needed to avoid volume loss caused by tubing expansion between the baby and the HFOV.
3. The active expiratory phase allows HFOV to run at somewhat higher frequencies than HFJV and smaller V_T but makes either gas trapping or atelectasis a concern.

INDICATIONS

High-frequency ventilation was originally developed as a "rescue" treatment of pulmonary air leak situations. Subsequent studies indicated it could be useful for rescue of severe pulmonary hypertension and for patients prior to extracorporeal membrane oxygenation (ECMO). Recent trials have demonstrated efficacy for treatment of respiratory distress syndrome (RDS). Studies have shown that inhaled nitric oxide (iNO) may be more effective when used in conjunction with HFV.

Improvements in conventional ventilators and their management have tended to obscure the difference between HFV and conventional ventilation. Nevertheless, many centers still resort to HFV when patients:

1. Have persistent hypoventilation despite increased pressures,
2. Have pulmonary interstitial emphysema (PIE) or pneumothoraces while requiring mechanical ventilation at high pressures,
3. Have persistent hypoxemia on high FiO_2 despite high Paw, or
4. Are approaching criteria for iNO or ECMO.

TRANSITION TO HFV

Table 87-1 offers values for transitioning to HFV. Baseline preparations include the following:

1. Chest x-rays
   a. Determine expansion
   b. Check for interstitial emphysema or pneumothorax
2. Arterial blood gases (ABG)
3. Final conventional settings
4. Nurse, respiratory care practitioner, other practitioners are all prepared and present as rapid adjustments may be needed.

Make sure the HFV device is calibrated and ready to take over respiratory support before discontinuing conventional ventilation.

1. HFOV: Ensure patient is positioned appropriately for rigid circuit.
2. HFJV: Ensure the heater/humidifier is prepared and the endotracheal tube adapter is ready to be changed.

Table 87-1 Transitioning to High-Frequency Ventilation

Setting	HFOV	HFJV
Rate	8–12 Hz (540–720/min)	300–480/min (5–7 Hz)
PEEP	—	Increase by about 2[a]
Paw	Increase by about 2[a]	—
PIP	—	About the same[b]
ΔP	About the same[b]	

Abbreviations: HFJV, high-frequency jet ventilation; HFOV, high-frequency oscillatory ventilation; PEEP, positive end-expiratory pressure; PIP, positive inspiratory pressure.
[a]Not if treating "air leak."
[b]Adjust per jiggle.

The following are the starting settings when converting to HFV:

1. PEEP or Paw:
   a. The tiny V_T used for HFV makes atelectasis a risk.
   b. PEEP or Paw is increased 1–2 cm H_2O above conventional.
   c. Too low a PEEP or Paw increases risk of hyperventilation.
   d. The exception is when treating an "air leak"; in this situation, the PEEP or Paw is generally *not* increased because "degassing" the lung and allowing some atelectasis may be the desired result.
2. Positive inspiratory pressure (PIP) or amplitude (ΔP):
   a. Usually start about the same as conventional
   b. Adjust by watching abdominal "jiggle"
3. Rate or frequency (*f*) is determined mostly by device:
   a. Oscillators generally run in the 8- to 12-Hz range.
   b. Jets generally run in the 360- to 480-bpm range.
4. The second determinant of rate or *f* is patient size:
   a. Size is a major contributor to the time constant (K_T).
   b. Smaller patients have a shorter time constant.
   c. Start smaller patients at higher end of the machine's range.
5. The third determinant of rate or *f* is disease state:
   a. Diseases with low compliance (eg, RDS) have a shorter (K_T) and thus use a rate or *f* at the higher end of the range.
   b. Airways diseases (eg, meconium aspiration syndrome [MAS], PIE) have longer (K_T) and thus do better at the lower end of the rate or *f* range.
   c. As RDS improves and compliance increases, you may need to decrease the rate to avoid gas trapping.
6. The risk of too high a rate or *f* is gas trapping; when in doubt and there is CO_2 retention, consider slowing the rate or *f*.
   a. The oscillator has a fixed I:E ratio of 1:3 and thus a decreased *f*:
      (1) Increases T_i, resulting in a larger V_T.
      (2) Increases T_e, allowing better exhalation.
   b. The Jet has a fixed T_i of 0.02 seconds and thus a decreased rate:
      (1) Decreases I:E ratio, allowing better exhalation
      (2) Does not affect T_i, so usually it does not change the V_T
7. In general, changing the rate or *f* significantly means moving by 1 Hz or by 60 bpm; smaller changes are usually not significant clinically.

ADJUSTING HFV IN CLINICAL USE

Figures 87-1 to 87-4 provide four "laws" for adjusting HFV in clinical use.

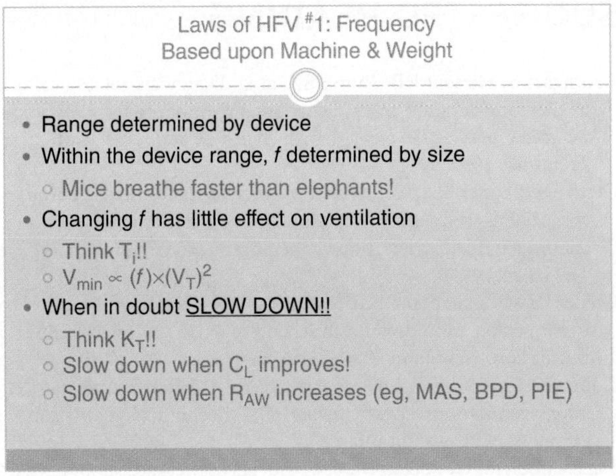

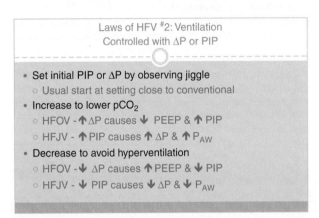

FIGURE 87-1 First law of high-frequency ventilation. BPD, bronchopulmonary dysplasia; HFV, high-frequency ventilation; MAS, meconium aspiration syndrome.

FIGURE 87-2 Second law of high-frequency ventilation. HFJV, high-frequency jet ventilation; HFOV, high-frequency oscillatory ventilation; HFV, high-frequency ventilation; PCO$_2$, partial pressure of carbon dioxide; Paw, mean airway pressure; PEEP, positive end-expiratory pressure; PIP, positive inspiratory pressure.

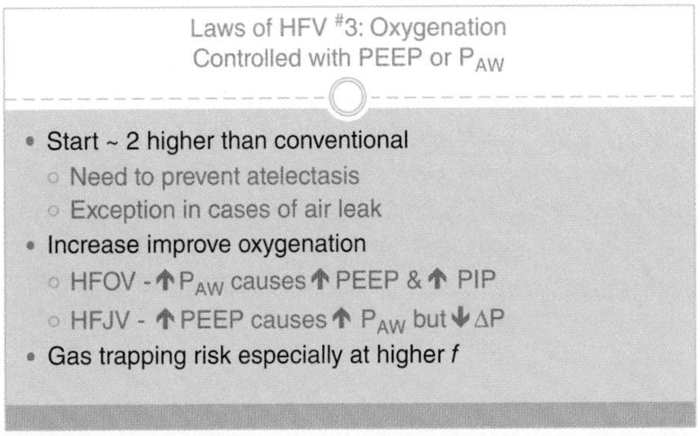

FIGURE 87-3 Third law of high-frequency ventilation. HFJV, high-frequency jet ventilation; HFOV, high-frequency oscillatory ventilation; HFV, high-frequency ventilation; PEEP, positive end-expiratory pressure; PIP, positive inspiratory pressure.

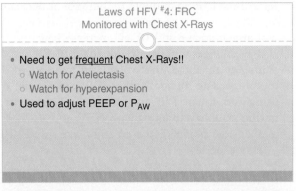

FIGURE 87-4 Fourth law of high-frequency ventilation. FRC, funtional residual capacity; HFV, high-frequency ventilation; PEEP, positive end-expiratory pressure.

Oxygenation

As with any ventilator, the major determinants of oxygenation are FiO$_2$ and Paw. As with all ventilators, Paw is a product of PIP, PEEP, and the I:E ratio.

1. Oscillator
   a. Paw is set directly:
   b. It may be adjusted in increments of 0.5 cm H$_2$O.
   c. Remember that increasing Paw results in not only an increased PIP but also a decrease in PEEP.
   d. Thus, after several increases in Paw, consider increasing ΔP to avoid having a PEEP that is too low.
2. Jet
   a. Paw is measured but not set directly.
   b. Paw with the Jet is generally adjusted by changing PEEP, set on the conventional ventilator but measured on the Jet.
   c. As PEEP is increased, ΔP decreases.
   d. Thus, after several increases in PEEP, consider increasing PIP to maintain adequate ΔP.
3. After significant Paw or PEEP changes, follow-up chest x-ray is needed to monitor for hyperexpansion or atelectasis.

Ventilation

As with any ventilator, the major determinant of PaCO$_2$ is minute ventilation (see previous equation), which is more sensitive to changes in V$_T$ than rate or f with HFV.

1. Oscillator: Adjust ΔP up or down to increase or decrease V$_T$:
   a. Increasing ΔP at a set Paw results in not only increased PIP but also decreased PEEP.
   b. Thus, after several increases in ΔP, consider increasing Paw to avoid having a PEEP that is too low.

CHAPTER 87

2. Jet: Adjust PIP up or down to increase or decrease V_T:
   a. Large increases in PIP will increase Paw.
   b. PIP changes with Jet do not affect PEEP.
3. With *any* machine, the worst way to ventilate is to compensate for too little PEEP (atelectasis) by using too much PIP (volutrauma). Thus, when having trouble ventilating with HFV,
   a. Consider points discussed and make sure PEEP is not too low.
   b. Frequent chest x-rays are needed to assess lung volumes.

TRANSITIONING FROM HFV TO CONVENTIONAL VENTILATION

Some NICUs will extubate directly from HFV. If transition to conventional ventilation is desired, most NICUs have criteria for HFV settings prior to transition:

1. FiO_2 is generally about 40% or less.
2. Paw is generally about 12 cm H_2O or less.
3. Conventional settings can be chosen by reversing the process for choosing initial HFV settings:
   a. Use the same PIP or ΔP and adjust per chest excursion.
   b. PEEP or Paw is about the same as HFV if oxygenating well.
   c. Rate is about 40 bpm.
   d. Check ABG and chest x-ray shortly after transition (15–30 minutes).

SUGGESTED READING

Baumgart S, Hirschl RB, Butler SZ, et al. Diagnosis-related criteria in the consideration of extracorporeal membrane oxygenation in neonates previously treated with high-frequency jet ventilation. *Pediatrics*. 1992;89:491–494.

Clark RH, Yoder BA, Sell MS. Prospective, randomized comparison of high-frequency oscillation and conventional ventilation in candidates for extracorporeal membrane oxygenation. *J Pediatr*. 1994;124:447–454.

Coates EW, Klinepeter ME, O'Shea TM. Neonatal pulmonary hypertension treated with inhaled nitric oxide and high-frequency ventilation. *J Perinatol*. 2008;28:675–679.

Courtney SE, Durand DJ, Asselin JM, et al. High-frequency oscillatory ventilation versus conventional mechanical ventilation for very-low-birth-weight infants. *N Engl J Med*. 2002;347:643–652.

Dani C, Bertini G, Pezzati M, et al. Effects of pressure support ventilation plus volume guarantee vs high-frequency oscillatory ventilation on lung inflammation in preterm infants. *Pediatr Pulmonol*. 2006;41:242–249.

Froese AB, Kinsella JP. High-frequency oscillatory ventilation: lessons from the neonatal/pediatric experience. *Crit Care Med*. 2005;33(Suppl):S115–S121.

Henderson-Smart DJ, De Paoli AG, Clark RH, Bhuta T. High frequency oscillatory ventilation versus conventional ventilation for infants with severe pulmonary dysfunction born at or near term. *Cochrane Database Syst Rev*. 2009;(3):CD002974. doi:10.1002/14651858.CD002974.pub2.

Keszler M, Modanlou HD, Brudno DS, et al. Multicenter controlled clinical trial of high-frequency jet ventilation in preterm infants with uncomplicated respiratory distress syndrome. *Pediatrics*. 1997;100:593–599.

Kinsella JP, Truog WE, Walsh WF, et al. Randomized, multicenter trial of inhaled nitric oxide and high-frequency oscillatory ventilation in severe, persistent pulmonary hypertension of the newborn. *J Pediatr*. 1997;131:55–62.

Plavka R, Dokoupilova M, Pazderova L, et al. High-frequency jet ventilation improves gas exchange in extremely immature infants with evolving chronic lung disease. *Am J Perinatol*. 2006;28:467–472.

88 Noninvasive Support of Respiratory Failure

Jen-Tien Wung and Rakesh Sahni

INTRODUCTION

Despite its clear association with lung injury, mechanical ventilation (MV) continues to be widely practiced in many neonatal intensive care units (NICUs). Recent data suggest that trauma to the respiratory system can be avoided by gentle respiratory support initiated soon after birth. Accordingly, in the past decade there has been increasing interest in using noninvasive respiratory support with nasal continuous positive airway pressure (CPAP) or nasal intermittent positive pressure ventilation (NIPPV) for managing respiratory failure in infants, with the focus to reduce the use of MV and protect the lung. Nasal CPAP therapy has been the mainstay of noninvasive respiratory support. However, the literature reflects conflicting results on the effectiveness of nasal CPAP in infants with respiratory failure because of inconsistencies in the guidelines for CPAP therapy, use of different devices and ventilator modes, and variations in training and levels of experience with nasal CPAP use. Little attention is paid to the best ways of practicing nasal CPAP therapy.

This chapter discusses the physiological effects, indications for use, application aspects, weaning strategies, complications, and controversies of nasal CPAP therapy based on the firsthand personal experience using binasal prongs CPAP for over 3 decades. These management protocols[1] have been practiced successfully in our NICU for nearly 40 years and have been shown to reduce chronic lung disease in preterm infants without increasing morbidity or mortality. They have been increasingly adopted and practiced at many NICUs throughout the world with good results.

We also provide an overview of some of the other types of noninvasive respiratory support strategies used in newborn infants.

NASAL CPAP THERAPY

The mainstay nasal CPAP is a particular form of noninvasive respiratory support that applies positive pressure to the airway of a spontaneously breathing patient throughout the respiratory cycle.

Physiological Effects

1. Increases transpulmonary pressure and functional residual capacity (FRC) and improves lung compliance.
2. Prevents alveolar collapse (atelectrauma), decreases intrapulmonary shunt, and provides progressive alveolar recruitment.
3. Conserves surfactant.
4. Prevents pharyngeal wall collapse.
5. Stabilizes the chest wall and decreases thoracoabdominal asynchrony and work of breathing.[2]
6. Increases airway diameter and splints the airways.
7. Splints the diaphragm.
8. Stimulates lung growth.[3]
9. Bubble CPAP adds high-frequency ventilation[4] and stochastic resonance effects.[5]

Excessive CPAP pressure may lead to serious consequences, such as air leak syndromes and increased dead space ventilation, leading to a rise in $PaCO_2$. Furthermore, high levels of CPAP can increase intrathoracic pressure, resulting in diminished venous return to the heart and reduced cardiac output, decreased pulmonary perfusion, and enhanced ventilation-perfusion mismatch.

Indications for Nasal CPAP Therapy

Evidence has accumulated over the past 4 decades to support the use of nasal CPAP not only to facilitate weaning in intubated infants but also as a primary mode of support in infants with various types of respiratory compromise situations, including the following:

1. Diseases with low FRC, such as respiratory distress syndrome (RDS), transient tachypnea of the newborn, patent ductus arteriosus, pulmonary edema
2. Apnea and bradycardia of prematurity
3. Meconium aspiration syndrome
4. Airway closure disease (eg, bronchiolitis, bronchopulmonary dysplasia [BPD])
5. Tracheomalacia
6. Partial paralysis of diaphragm
7. Respiratory support after extubation

Early initiation of CPAP (preferably before fetal lung fluid is absorbed) in preterm infants helps prevent alveolar collapse by continuously applying positive pressure and allowing these infants to produce endogenous surfactant. Spain and colleagues[6] studied the amount and redistribution of lung surfactant during the perinatal period in rats and concluded that packaging of surfactant may be active immediately postbirth. Within 10 minutes of the initiation of air breathing, small increases in type II cell lamellar body content are observed. By 24 hours, the whole lung and alveolar extracellular pool surfactant lipid increases substantially. In our experience since 1973, early application of nasal CPAP therapy, usually within 5 minutes of life, in spontaneously breathing preterm infants prevents alveolar collapse, allows infants to breathe and produce adequate endogenous surfactant, decreases work of breathing, and helps lower the fraction of inspired oxygen (FiO_2). More than 77% of infants 1250 g or less at birth do not require intubation or surfactant replacement therapy.[7] The extended use of CPAP can also stimulate the growth of the premature lung[3] and further decrease the incidence of BPD. Thus, CPAP is both a corrective and a supportive therapy that help the process of gas exchange while allowing the premature lungs to grow.

CPAP Delivery Devices

A good CPAP delivery system should include a patient system that is easily and rapidly applicable to very low

birth weight (VLBW) infants; is readily removable and reconnectable; causes the least trauma to the infant; is capable of producing stable desired pressure levels; readily accepts humidification and supplementary oxygen at a desired temperature; is associated with low resistance to breathing; offers minimal dead space; is easily understood, maintained, and sterilized; and is safe and cost effective. Given the infrequent use of nonnasal methods of CPAP in current clinical practice, this review focuses exclusively on nasal interfaces and modes of pressure generation utilized in nasal CPAP delivery systems.

Essentially, a CPAP delivery system consists of 3 components:

1. Circuit for continuous flow of inspired gases: Oxygen and compressed air sources provide inspired gases at the desired FiO_2. The flowmeter controls the rate of flow. The minimum flow rate used should be sufficient to prevent rebreathing of carbon dioxide, for instance, usually 2.5 times the infant's minute ventilation. The flow should also compensate for leaks around connectors and the CPAP prongs. Excessive flow through the circuit will generate high pressure against which the infant must exhale. Usually, a flow rate of 5–10 L/min is sufficient in infants. The inspired gases are warmed and humidified prior to delivery to the infant.
2. Nasal interface to connect the CPAP circuit to the infant's airway: Single and binasal tubes/prongs of varying lengths, ending in the nares or nasopharynx, have been used as nasal interfaces. Nasal masks were an early means of applying CPAP to infants. However, they lost popularity because of the difficulty in maintaining an adequate seal and keeping them in place. Nasal cannulas are often used in infants to deliver supplemental oxygen at low flows (<0.5 L/min) with no intention of generating CPAP. Binasal prongs, when first introduced to apply CPAP, were felt to be simple to use, effective, and safe, but they can potentially cause nasal trauma. A number of binasal devices are now in common use, including Hudson prongs[1] and Argyle prongs.[8]

Efforts were directed at designing a nasal interface that would lower work of breathing. The resultant short-pronged binasal devices, currently known as Infant Flow (EME Medical Inc) and Arabella Generators (Hamilton Medical), are structured to allow the jet flow to flip between inspiratory and expiratory routes (coanal effect). They aim to provide sufficient demand flow on inspiration while minimizing expiratory resistance. Work with lung models and a small study on preterm infants with minimal lung disease[9] demonstrated reduced work of breathing when compared with conventional devices. Limited randomized crossover and nonrandomized clinical studies, in preterm infants, have compared the Infant Flow nasal CPAP system with single-prong nasal CPAP. They found no significant difference in short-term measurement of physiological variables. Prongs inserted to the nasopharyngeal level have also been shown to deliver effective CPAP.[10] They received early criticism because they were perceived to be poorly tolerated, difficult to insert, and increased resistance when compared with short nasal tube insertion. Despite these shortcomings, the use of nasopharyngeal tubes became established in clinical practice and featured in several trials that examined both binasal and single forms. In common with nasoendotracheal tubes, nasal CPAP interfaces have the potential to cause nasal excoriation and scarring if inappropriately applied or infrequently monitored.[11]

3. Modes of positive pressure generation in the CPAP circuit: The CPAP pressure is usually provided by varying the resistance to flow in expired tubing. This can be achieved by several techniques. In *variable pressure-flow resistors*, the level of peak end-expiratory pressure (PEEP)/CPAP is directly proportional to the product of the gas flow through the orifice of the expiratory pressure valve and the set resistance of the expiratory valve of the ventilator. The CPAP pressure varies with the infant's respiration. With *threshold resistors*, the CPAP level is determined by the force applied to the surface area of the valve. During *bubble CPAP*, the expiratory limb is vented through an underwater seal. The pressure generated varies with the depth of submersion of expiratory tubing and is independent of the infant's respiration.

Bubble CPAP is appealing because of its simplicity and low cost and has remained in use since first devised in the early 1970s. It has also been suggested that the bubbling creates pressure oscillations in the circuit and helps with removal of carbon dioxide.[4] Using an artificial lung and sheep models, Pillow and colleagues[5] demonstrated that decreasing compliance of the lung increased the magnitude of pressure oscillations in the model lung. These data suggest that use of bubble CPAP in the poorly compliant lung may promote lung volume recruitment (stochastic resonance) and augment the efficiency of gas mixing.

In a more recent study, Pillow and colleagues[12] compared differences in gas exchange physiology and lung injury resulting from treatment of RDS with either bubble or constant-pressure CPAP. In this comparison with ventilator-derived CPAP, bubble CPAP was associated with a higher pH, PaO_2 (arterial partial pressure of oxygen), oxygen uptake, and area under the flow volume curve. In addition, animals placed on bubble CPAP had decreased alveolar protein (a marker of lessened injury) and a lower $PaCO_2$ (arterial partial pressure of carbon dioxide). The better oxygenation and more efficient removal of carbon dioxide are consistent with enhanced patency of peripheral airways and a greater surface area available for exchange.

The modes of pressure generation can be varied independently of nasal interfaces. There are multiple nasal CPAP delivery systems. Not all devices are similar, and success with nasal CPAP may be device specific. Further studies need to focus on the most effective nasal CPAP interface and the best mode of pressure generation for the delivery of nasal CPAP. Unfortunately, most of the CPAP studies do not show the device used. The short binasal curved prongs (Hudson CPAP prongs by Hudson-RCI, Temecula, CA) shown in Figures 88-1 and 88-2 were created for simplicity and minimizing trauma and have been successfully used at Columbia University Medical Center[1] since 1973 in over 20,000 infants.

Application of Nasal CPAP

Initiation

1. Position the infant in supine position with the head elevated about 30°.
2. Place a small neck roll under the infant to prevent flexion of the neck and airway obstruction.

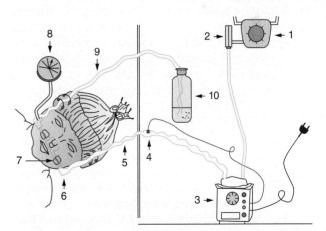

FIGURE 88-1 Nasal prong continuous positive airway pressure (CPAP) delivery system: 1, oxygen blender; 2, flowmeter; 3, heated humidifier; 4, thermometer; 5, proximal connecting tubings (with heating wire inside); 6, nasal CPAP cannula with 2 curved prongs (size 0–5); 7, Velcro to wrap around cannulas to prevent compressing nasal septum; 8, manometer (optional); 9, distal connecting tubings; and 10, bottle containing a solution of 0.25% acetic acid filled to a depth of 7 cm and the distal tubing submerged to a depth of 5 cm to create CPAP 5 cm H_2O.

CHAPTER 88

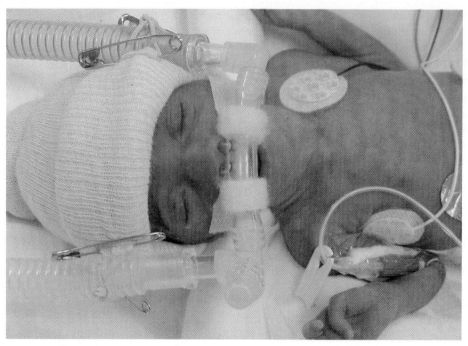

FIGURE 88-2 Nasal CPAP system that was created and has been used at Columbia University Medical Center since 1973.

3. Place a premade hat or stockinet on the infant's head to hold the inspired and expired gas tubing.
4. Choose the desired FiO_2 to keep the PaO_2 in the 50s or O_2 saturation around 90%.
5. Keep the temperature of the inspired gas at 37°C.
6. Adjust the flow rate (5–10 L/min) to provide adequate flow to prevent rebreathing of carbon dioxide, compensate for leakage from tubing connectors and around CPAP prongs, and generate desired CPAP pressure (usually 5 cm H_2O).
7. Insert the distal end of the expiratory tubing into a bottle of liquid (eg, 0.25% acetic acid solution or sterile water) filled to a height of 7 cm. The expiratory tubing is submerged to a depth of 5 cm to create 5 cm H_2O CPAP as long as there is air bubbling out of the solution. A nonintubated infant on nasal CPAP of 5 cm H_2O (with physiological PEEP of 3 cm H_2O) is equivalent to an intubated infant with PEEP of 8 cm H_2O in terms of FRC. For these infants, CPAP levels greater than 5 cm H_2O are not routinely used or recommended as increased gastric distension or mouth leaks and adverse cardiopulmonary effects may occur.
8. Choose the appropriate size nasal cannula.
9. Place the prongs curved side down and direct into nasal cavities.
10. Adjust elbows so the corrugated tubing lies along both sides of the face and head.
11. Secure tubing on both sides of the hat.

Maintenance

1. Monitor infant's vital signs, oxygenation, and activity.
2. Systematically check the CPAP delivery system, inspired gas temperature, and air bubbling out of the solution and empty condensed water in the circuit.
3. Check the position of the CPAP prongs and keep the CPAP cannula off the nasal septum at all times. A snug cap is used to securely hold the tubing in place, and if necessary, self-adhesive Velcro is used to keep the cannula away from the nasal septum to prevent pressure injury.
4. Suction nasal cavities, mouth, pharynx, and stomach every 3–4 h and as needed. If the infant swallows too much air into the stomach, an indwelling orogastric tube is placed and left opened to air, with frequent suctioning to make sure the lumen is patent at all times.
5. Change the infant's position frequently.
6. Change the CPAP circuit once a week.

After the CPAP is properly applied, the infant should breathe more easily, and the respiratory rate and retractions should decrease. The FiO_2 should be adjusted to keep the PaO_2 in the 50s or O_2 saturation around 90%. Infants on nasal CPAP therapy can be fed by nipple, gavage, or continuous tube feeding if they are clinically stable.

Weaning

As the infant's respiratory distress improves, the FiO_2 should be lowered in decrements of 0.02 to 0.05, keeping the CPAP pressure at 5 cm H_2O and maintaining appropriate oxygen saturation. Once the infant is stable on room air CPAP with no respiratory distress and no significant apneas and bradycardia, he or she may be given a trial off CPAP. Failure may occur within minutes of coming off CPAP or as much as 12 to 24 hours later. If the infant is experiencing frequent episodes of apnea and bradycardia or develops respiratory distress while off CPAP, the CPAP should be reintroduced even though the infant may be breathing room air. As long as the infant is still symptomatic (ie, tachypnea, retraction, or apnea and bradycardia), it is important to keep CPAP on for periods long enough to stimulate the growth of premature lung[3] and reduce the incidence of BPD.[7,13] It is better, in terms of length of stay, duration on oxygen, and BPD, to remain on CPAP until successfully and completely weaned. Recently, a multicenter, randomized, controlled trial[14] also showed taking off CPAP with the view to stay off significantly shortens CPAP weaning time, CPAP duration, oxygen duration, BPD, and length of hospitalization in comparison to either cycled on and off CPAP with incremental time off or cycled on and off CPAP but during off periods supported by 2-mm nasal cannula at a flow of 0.5 L/min.

Failure of CPAP

If nasal CPAP of 5 cm H_2O is not sufficient to maintain adequate oxygenation and ventilation, the infant is probably sick enough to be ventilated mechanically. The following conditions are considered CPAP failure, and the infant will require MV:

1. Inability to maintain an appropriate PaO_2/SpO_2 (pulse oximetry) while breathing FiO_2 of 60% or more.
2. Increasing $PaCO_2$ levels (>65 mm Hg).
3. Intractable metabolic acidosis.
4. Severe retractions.
5. Frequent episodes of apnea and bradycardia.

Prior to initiation of MV, it is important to observe the infant's clinical condition. If the blood gas results are not compatible with the clinical appearance, further investigation is needed before abandoning nasal CPAP therapy. For example, the blood gas machine may be malfunctioning or the timing or technique of collecting the blood sample might be faulty. It is also important to rule out the improper application of CPAP, poor fit of the CPAP prongs, nasal obstruction caused by secretions, airway obstruction caused by a flexed neck, gastric distention, or too frequent handling of the unstable infant.

Potential Complications

Complications of CPAP therapy depend on the interface used. With the nasal prong CPAP described,[1] they include the following:

1. Nasal obstruction from secretions or improper application of nasal prongs.
2. Gastric distention from swallowing air, especially in infants on methylxanthines, which tend to decrease intestinal mobility and relax the gastroesophageal sphincter. This can be minimized by using an indwelling orogastric tube.[15]
3. Nasal septum erosion or necrosis, which can essentially be prevented with vigilant care to keep the cannula off the septum. Choose the correct size nasal prongs and make sure the cannula is held securely in place without touching and compressing the nasal septum with the aid of Velcro (Figure 88-2).
4. Fluctuating PaO_2/SpO_2 when the infant breathes with mouth widely open.
5. Pneumothorax usually occurs within the first few days of CPAP use, not after a week. Furthermore, in our experience, pneumothoraces are generally less severe and less frequent in infants on CPAP compared to intubated infants on MV.

Most of these complications are preventable with appropriate training and well-directed unit policies. The majority of the problems with CPAP can be attributed to the use of poor devices, inappropriate use, or a lack of training or experience.

HIGH-FLOW NASAL CANNULA AS AN ALTERNATIVE TO NASAL CPAP

In addition to nasal CPAP, a variety of other noninvasive respiratory support strategies have been introduced with less-intensive scrutiny in recent years. Nasal cannulas delivering high flows of oxygen or air have become a popular form of respiratory support because of relative ease of use. These high-flow nasal cannulas (HFNCs) with flow rates between 2 and 8 L/min are simpler to use and have been shown to be as good as nasal CPAP with Argyle prongs in treating premature infants with apnea and bradycardia.[16] However, others have shown that nasal CPAP is superior to HFNC during support for respiratory compromise.[17] The use of HFNC remains controversial, primarily because of concerns over the unreliable pressure and FiO_2 delivery. With HFNCs, the amount of pressure generated and FiO_2 delivered are related to multiple factors, including the flow rate, the diameter of the cannula, the size of the leak around the nasal cannula, and the degree of mouth opening. The amount of oxygen and pressure delivered at the hypopharyngeal level with HFNC flow rates between 0.5 and 2.0 L/min are extremely variable, and Kubicka et al[18] also warned that there is no safety mechanism to ensure that excessive positive pressures are not generated when HFNCs are used at higher rates of flow.

NASAL INTERMITTENT POSITIVE PRESSURE VENTILATION

Nasal intermittent positive pressure ventilation has been employed to augment nasal CPAP by combining CPAP with superimposed ventilator breaths through nasal prongs or a nasopharyngeal tube. With this mode, intermittently elevated pharyngeal pressures are created that may improve the patency of upper airways and initiate inspiratory reflexes and activate respiratory drive. Studies have shown some success of NIPPV over nasal CPAP in treating preterm infants with apnea,[19] during postextubation care,[20] or as the initial treatment of RDS in infants less than 35 weeks' premature.[21] However, most of the premature infants, even VLBW infants can be treated with nasal CPAP alone.[7,13]

There are concerns that NIPPV requires more nursing care and might cause more gastrointestinal complications because of gastric distention leading to cessation of feedings or perforation. Although these infants are not intubated, air leaks could be a big problem. Often, nasal shields and chin straps are necessary to seal air leaks from the nose and mouth to maintain peak inspiratory pressure above 15 mm Hg. Indwelling orogastric tubes are also required to reduce gastric distension, with frequent suctioning to ensure that the lumen is patent at all times. Furthermore, there are limited guidelines for the clinicians to determine the most effective ventilator settings to utilize this mode, and future studies are needed.

Although NIPPV with most modern ventilators is nonsynchronized, synchronized NIPPV may be advantageous as the positive pressure ventilator inflation is delivered only after initiation of respiratory effort by the infant, when the glottis is likely to be open. Noninvasive neurally adjusted ventilatory assistance (NAVA) with the Servo-i can be used as pressure support. Future studies will need to investigate whether synchronization has an advantage over nonsynchronized ventilation and to compare the effectiveness of modes of synchronization.

CURRENT CONTROVERSIES

Use of Early Nasal CPAP

Previous studies of nasal CPAP use showed conflicting results, including no decrease in the incidence of BPD. The reasons for this difference are related to the variety in experiences, devices used, criteria of CPAP failure among various institutions, and shorter durations of CPAP therapy. However, not a single case report or trial has ever demonstrated increased incidences of BPD, mortality, or long-term disability in association with nasal CPAP therapy when compared to MV. Not all CPAP devices are created equal, and there is a learning curve for nasal CPAP therapy. The importance of clinical experience and a consistent approach to improving the effectiveness of CPAP support over time has been shown by Aly and colleagues.[22] Recently, a large randomized trial, the COIN Trial,[23] demonstrated that early use of nasal CPAP in preterm infants (25–28 weeks' gestation) resulted in a 50% reduction of subsequent intubation, ventilation, and surfactant therapy without reducing the BPD rates. Premature infants frequently have not only RDS, which is the problem during the first few days, but also immature lungs that require catchup growth; CPAP is known to stimulate growth of premature lung.[3] We keep our VLBW infants on CPAP, even on room air CPAP, as long as they are symptomatic (ie, tachypnea, inspiratory retraction, or apnea). We believe that is a main reason we have been able to keep the incidence of BPD below 10% for decades.[7,13,24,25] We believe most studies do not show a significant reduction of BPD because CPAP therapy was discontinued too early to take advantage of stimulation of lung growth.

The Intubate-Surfactant-Extubate Strategy

The intubate-surfactant-extubate (INSURE) strategy includes intubation, administration of prophylactic surfactant, and early extubation.[26] A recent meta-analysis of several small randomized trials evaluating the INSURE approach concluded that this approach was associated with less need for MV, reduced frequency of air leaks, and decreased rates of BPD.[27] However, few of the infants enrolled in these trials were less than 27 weeks' gestation; thus, the benefit of this approach in very immature infants is not as well established. The major objection to the application of the INSURE strategy is the need for tracheal intubation, which is a significant traumatic procedure for an infant. INSURE-associated MV, even for a short period of time, may have consequences. At our institution, 84.6% and 30.2% of VLBW infants at 26 weeks or more and 26 weeks or less of gestation, respectively, were successfully treated with nasal CPAP without intubation or surfactant replacement, and morbidity or mortality is lower in those infants.[7] If we adopted the INSURE strategy, many VLBW infants would have been intubated, given surfactant, and stressed unnecessarily. However, if MV is deemed necessary in this group of infants, surfactant should be given and extubation should be performed as early as possible. Unfortunately, in extremely low birth weight infants (≤26 weeks of gestation), extubation after surfactant therapy is usually not possible because of deterioration from stressful intubation.

SUMMARY

The use of noninvasive respiratory support is contingent on the thorough understanding of the equipment being used and astute assessment of the infant to select the correct respiratory support modality that will result in minimal volu- or barotrauma and reduce the development of BPD. Not all CPAP devices are created equal, and there is a learning curve for nasal CPAP therapy. The more you do it, the easier it will feel, the better your outcomes will be, and the fewer complications you will encounter. Existing literature shows conflicting results with nasal CPAP therapy because of variable guidelines for use, different devices and ventilator modes, and variations in training and experience. More recently, there has been a wealth of experimental and clinical data supporting the effectiveness of using early nasal CPAP therapy for respiratory failure in VLBW infants to reduce the need for intubation and surfactant replacement therapy. Nasal CPAP also facilitates weaning from MV to reduce lung injury.

For preterm infants with immature lungs, prolonged periods of nasal CPAP support, even without oxygen supplementation, enhance lung growth and can potentially reduce the incidence of BPD. NICUs not using nasal CPAP are encouraged to gain training and experience from an experienced center that uses nasal CPAP appropriately and has proven superior respiratory outcomes. Units implementing "best practices" have demonstrated improved patient outcomes.[28,29]

Key strategies for the successful use of nasal CPAP therapy include the following:

1. Choose the right nasal CPAP device.
2. Familiarize caregivers with the device.
3. Learn to use nasal CPAP correctly and troubleshoot.
4. Maintain nasal CPAP with meticulous airway care.
5. Pay attention to details and minimize complications.
6. Gain experience (as there is a learning curve).
7. Initiate nasal CPAP as early as possible (usually in the delivery room) to all infants (no birth weight or gestational age limits) having spontaneous breathing with respiratory distress.
8. Tolerate permissive hypercarbia ($PaCO_2$ 50–65) if oxygenation is adequate.
9. Extend use of nasal CPAP support to enhance the growth of the premature lung.
10. Work as a team.

REFERENCES

1. Wung JT, Driscoll JM, Epstein RA, et al. A new device for CPAP by nasal route. *Crit Care Med.* 1975;3:76–78.
2. Elgellab A, Riou Y, Abbazine A, et al. Effects of nasal continuous positive airway pressure (NCPAP) on breathing pattern in spontaneously breathing premature newborn infants. *Intensive Care Med.* 2001;27:1782–1787.
3. Zhang S, Garbutt V, McBride JT. Strain-induced growth of the immature lung. *J Appl Physiol.* 1996;81:1471–1476.
4. Lee KS, Dunn MS, Fenwick M, Shennan AT. A comparison of underwater bubble continuous positive airway pressure with ventilator-derived continuous positive airway pressure in premature neonates ready for extubation. *Biol Neonate.* 1998;73:69–75.
5. Pillow JJ, Travadi JN. Bubble CPAP: is the noise important? An in vitro study. *Pediatr Res.* 2005;57(6):826–830.
6. Spain CL, Silbajoris R, Young SL. Alterations of surfactant pools in fetal and newborn rat lungs. *Pediatr Res.* 1987;21:5–8.
7. Ammari A, Suri MS, Milisavljevic V, et al. Variables associated with the early failure of nasal CPAP in very low birth weight infants. *J Pediatr.* 2005;147:341–347.
8. Kamper J, Ringsted C. Early treatment of idiopathic respiratory distress syndrome using binasal continuous positive airway pressure. *Acta Paediatr Scand.* 1990;79:581–586.
9. Pandit PB, Courtney SE, Pyon KH, et al. Work of breathing during constant- and variable-flow nasal continuous positive airway pressure in preterm neonates. *Pediatrics.* 2001;108:682–685.
10. Novogroder M, MacKuanying N, Eidelman AI, et al. A simple and efficient method of delivering continuous positive airway pressure. *J Pediatr.* 1973;82:1059–1062.
11. Robertson NJ, McCarthy LS, Hamilton PA, et al. Nasal deformities resulting from flow driver continuous positive airway pressure. *Arch Dis Child Fetal Neonatal Ed.* 1996;75:F209–F212.
12. Pillow JJ, Hillman N, Moss TJ, et al. Bubble continuous positive airway pressure enhances lung volume and gas exchange in preterm lambs. *Am J Respir Crit Care Med.* 2007;176(1):63–69.
13. Sahni R, Ammari A, Suri MS, et al. Is the new definition of bronchopulmonary dysplasia more useful? *J Perinatol.* 2005;25:41–46.
14. Todd DA, Wright A, Broom M, et al. Methods of weaning preterm babies < 30 weeks gestation off CPAP: a multicentre randomized controlled trial. *Arch Dis Child Fetal Neonatal Ed.* 2012;97(4):F236–F240.
15. Jaile JC, Levin T, Wung JT, et al. Benign gaseous distension of the bowel in premature infants treated with nasal CPAP: a study of contributing factors. *AJR.* 1992;158:125–127.
16. Sreenan C, Lemke RP, Hudson-Mason A, et al. High-flow nasal cannulae in the management of apnea of prematurity: a comparison with conventional nasal continuous positive airway pressure. *Pediatrics.* 2001;107:1081–1083.
17. Abdel-Hady H, Shouman B, Aly H. Early weaning from CPAP to high flow nasal cannula in preterm infants is associated with prolonged oxygen requirement: a randomized controlled trial. *Early Hum Dev.* 2011;87:205–208.
18. Kubicka ZJ, Limauro J, Darnall RA. Heated, humidified high-flow nasal cannula therapy: yet another way to deliver continuous positive airway pressure? *Pediatrics.* 2008;121:82–88.
19. Lin CH, Wang ST, Lin YJ, et al. Efficacy of nasal intermittent positive pressure ventilation in treating apnea of prematurity. *Pediatr Pulmonol.* 1998;26:349–353.
20. De Paoli AG, Davis PG, Lemyre B. Nasal continuous positive airway pressure versus nasal intermittent positive pressure ventilation for preterm neonates: a systematic review and meta-analysis. *Acta Paediatr.* 2003;92(1):70–75.
21. Kugelman A, Feferkorn I, Riskin A, et al. Nasal intermittent mandatory ventilation versus nasal continuous positive airway

pressure for respiratory distress syndrome: a randomized, controlled, prospective study. *J Pediatr.* 2007;150:521–526.

22. Aly HZ, Milner JD, Patel K, et al. Does experience with the use of nasal continuous positive airway pressure improve over time in the extremely low birth weight infants? *Pediatrics.* 2004;114:697–702.

23. Morley CJ, et al. COIN trial: nasal CPAP or intubation for very premature infants. *N Engl J Med.* 2008;358:700–708.

24. Avery ME, Tooley WH, Keller JB, et al. Is chronic lung disease in low birth weight infants preventable? A survey of eight centers. *Pediatrics.* 1987;79:26–30.

25. Van Marter LJ, Allerd EN, Pagano M, et al. Do clinical markers of barotrauma and oxygen toxicity explain interhospital variation in rates of chronic lung disease? *Pediatrics.* 2000;105: 1194–1201.

26. Lindner W, Vossbeck S, Hummler H, et al. Delivery room management of extremely low birth weight infants:spontaneous breathing or intubation? *Pediatrics.* 1999;103:961–967.

27. Stevens TP, Harrington EW, Blennow M, et al. Early surfactant administration with brief ventilation vs. selective surfactant and continued mechanical ventilation for preterm infants with or at risk for respiratory distress syndrome. *Cochrane Database Syst Rev.* 2007;(4):CD003063.

28. Birenbaum HJ, Dentry A, Cirelli J, et al. Reduction in the incidence of chronic lung disease in very low birth weight infants: results of a quality improvement process in a tertiary level neonatal intensive care unit. *Pediatrics.* 2009;123:44–50.

29. Levesque BM, Kalish LA, LaPierre J, et al. Impact of implementing 5 potentially better respiratory practices on neonatal outcome and cost. *Pediatrics.* 2011;128:e218–e226.

89 Inhaled Nitric Oxide

Katherine McCallie and Krisa Van Meurs

INDICATION

Clinical Findings

History

This protocol for use of inhaled nitric oxide (iNO) applies to neonates with gestational age 34 weeks or greater on mechanical ventilation with hypoxic respiratory failure. This protocol is *not* intended for any patient on an active research protocol involving nitric oxide or preterm infants less than 34 weeks' gestational age.

Physical

Infants will have an elevated oxygenation index (OI) of 25 or greater on 2 arterial blood gases at least 15 minutes apart.

Confirmatory/Baseline Tests

1. OI =

$$\frac{FiO_2\ (\%) \times MAP\ (mm\ Hg) \times 100}{PaO_2\ (mm\ Hg)}$$

FiO_2: fraction of inspired oxygen (eg, 50% FiO_2 = 0.5)

MAP: mean airway pressure, from ventilator

PaO_2: partial pressure of arterial oxygen, from arterial blood gas (ABG)

2. Echocardiogram

   a. Evaluate for structural heart disease, which may require surgical intervention.

   b. Evaluate for elevated right-sided heart pressures indicating pulmonary hypertension, as indicated by:

      1. Right ventricular or atrial dilation
      2. Interventricular septal bowing
      3. Elevated right atrial pressure as estimated by tricuspid regurgitation

Differential Diagnosis

1. Meconium aspiration syndrome
2. Pneumonia/sepsis
3. Congenital diaphragmatic hernia
4. Pulmonary hypoplasia
5. Surfactant deficiency or surfactant protein deficiency
6. Congenital alveolar dysplasia (alveolar capillary dysplasia)

Exclusions/Contraindications

1. Neonates with congenital heart disease whose condition would be worsened by decreasing pulmonary vascular resistance (eg, total anomalous pulmonary venous return) are excluded.

2. Inhaled nitric oxide has been approved by the Food and Drug Administration (FDA) for the treatment of hypoxic respiratory failure in neonates born after 33 weeks of gestation. In 2010, a panel from the National Institutes of Health (NIH) developed a consensus statement for the use of nitric oxide in premature infants that discourages its routine use in infants less than 34 weeks of gestation.

PREPARATION

Consent

Consent is not necessary to initiate treatment with iNO.

Monitoring During Treatment

1. Pre- and postductal oxygen saturation monitoring
2. Arterial access for blood pressure and ABG monitoring
3. Measurement of methemoglobin (metHb) and nitrogen dioxide (NO_2) levels

Sedation/Pain Control

Treatment with iNO is not inherently painful, but sedation and pain control can be helpful in minimizing spikes in pulmonary blood pressure that can exacerbate hypoxic respiratory failure.

TREATMENT/PROCEDURE

Initiation

See Figure 89-1 for iNO initiation procedure.

Tests to Follow

Methemoglobin and nitrogen dioxide levels are measured within 3 hours after starting iNO, then every 12 hours if the dose is greater than 20 ppm, every 24 hours if the dose is 5–20 ppm, or every 48 hours if the dose is less than 5 ppm.

Management Algorithm

See Figure 89-2 for subsequent management of iNO.

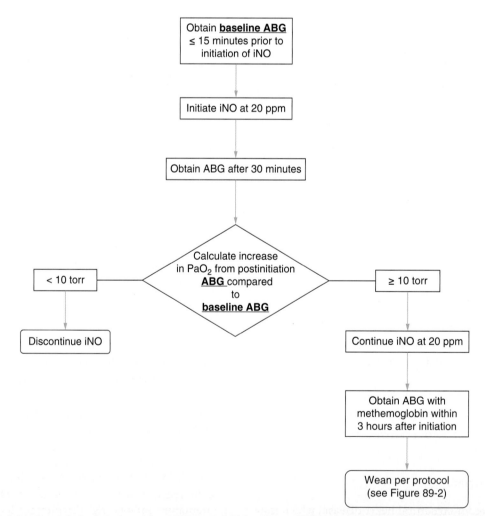

FIGURE 89-1 Initiating inhaled nitric oxide. ABG, arterial blood gas; iNO, inhaled nitric oxide; ppm, parts per million.

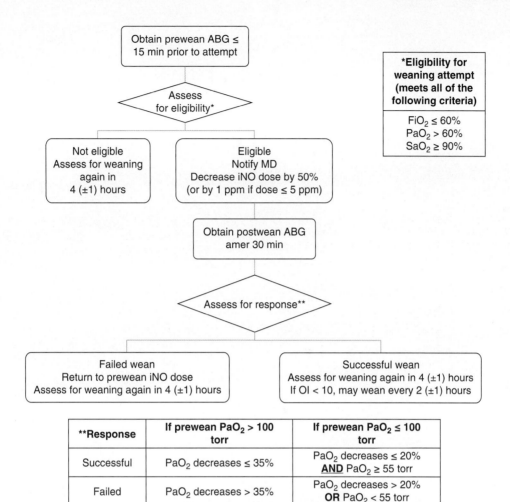

FIGURE 89-2 Weaning inhaled nitric oxide. *Note:* Ventilator settings and FiO$_2$ should not be changed during wean attempts. ABG, arterial blood gas; FiO$_2$, fraction of inspired oxygen; iNO, inhaled nitric oxide; OI, oxygenation index; PaO$_2$, partial pressure of arterial oxygen; ppm, parts per million; SaO$_2$, oxygen saturation.

Monitoring for Toxicity

1. If the NO$_2$ levels are 3 ppm or greater, wean by 50% (or if iNO ≤ 5 ppm, wean by 1 ppm) every 15 minutes until NO$_2$ level is less than 3 ppm.

2. If NO$_2$ levels are greater than 5 ppm, discontinue iNO.

3. If metHb levels are 5% or greater, wean by 50% (or if iNO ≤ 5 ppm, wean by 1 ppm) every 15 minutes until the metHb level is less than 5%.

4. If metHb levels are greater than 10%, discontinue iNO.

CONCLUSION/FOLLOW-UP

During weaning or discontinuation of iNO, monitor for rebound pulmonary hypertension caused by down-regulation of nitric oxide synthase activity and resulting decrease in level of native nitric oxide.

90 Extracorporeal Membrane Oxygenation (ECMO)

Krisa Van Meurs and Alexis Davis

INDICATION

Extracorporeal membrane oxygenation (ECMO) is the use of prolonged extracorporeal circulation and gas exchange via a modified heart-lung machine to provide temporary life support in patients with cardiac or respiratory failure who are refractory to maximum ventilatory and medical management. ECMO allows the lungs to rest and recover while avoiding the damaging effects of aggressive mechanical ventilation, including barotrauma and oxygen toxicity. The first successful use of extracorporeal support in a newborn was reported in 1976 by Dr. Robert Bartlett.[1] Subsequent data suggested that ECMO provided improved survival when compared with historical controls[2,3]; however, only 2 small trials with adaptive designs were performed prior to widespread use of ECMO.[4,5] The UK Collaborative ECMO Trial, published in 1996, confirmed that ECMO significantly reduced mortality when compared with standard medical care (32% vs 59%, relative risk 0.55; 95% confidence interval 0.36–0.80) with improved survival in all diagnostic categories.[6]

The Extracorporeal Life Support Organization (ELSO), established in 1989, maintains a patient registry to collect data from more than 200 ECMO centers around the world. ELSO Registry data as of July 2013 included 27,000 newborns placed on ECMO for respiratory support.[7] Approximately 800 neonatal respiratory cases are performed annually, with a cumulative survival of 75%. Review of the neonatal ELSO Registry data demonstrated ongoing demographic changes. ECMO use for neonatal respiratory failure has declined over the last 2 decades, likely related to the increasing use of high-frequency ventilation (HRV), surfactant replacement, and inhaled nitric oxide (iNO).[8-10] There have also been significant changes in the diagnostic categories of those receiving ECMO. Dramatic decreases in the use of ECMO for respiratory distress syndrome and sepsis/pneumonia have occurred. There has also been a downward trend in the use of ECMO for meconium aspiration syndrome; it is no longer the most common indication for ECMO. In recent years, congenital diaphragmatic hernia (CDH) has become the most common indication for ECMO; however, the survival rate continues to decline for this and the other diagnostic categories. Most ECMO centers are treating fewer patients annually; however, the length of bypass is longer, and survival is lower. These changes challenge ECMO centers to maintain their expertise with a complex technology despite lower patient volumes.

Hypoxemic Respiratory Failure

Hypoxemic respiratory failure (HRF) frequently occurs in association with persistent pulmonary hypertension of the newborn (PPHN). PPHN is characterized by markedly elevated pulmonary vascular resistance and pulmonary arterial pressure, in conjunction with striking pulmonary vasoreactivity. This produces right-to-left shunting at the patent ductus arteriosus (PDA) and patent foramen ovale (PFO). It results in hypoxemia from extrapulmonary shunting, which can be poorly responsive to medical management. PPHN is felt to represent failure of the pulmonary circulation to adapt to postnatal conditions and as such is sometimes called "persistent fetal circulation." The pulmonary vascular bed is abnormal, with extension of the medial smooth muscle layer into the smaller and more peripheral intra-acinar vessels. PPHN can occur in several clinical settings, described next.

Idiopathic

Idiopathic PPHN occurs when there is abnormally constricted pulmonary vasculature without parenchymal lung disease. It has been called "black lung" PPHN because of the lack of pulmonary vascular markings on a chest radiograph.

Parenchymal Lung Disease

Frequently, PPHN accompanies meconium aspiration syndrome, respiratory distress syndrome, sepsis, or pneumonia. In these settings, evidence of PPHN is seen in addition to intrapulmonary shunting from parenchymal lung disease.

Lung Hypoplasia

Lung hypoplasia can be seen with CDH and in infants with premature prolonged rupture of the membranes and long-standing oligohydramnios. In these conditions, lung growth and development are affected, and there is a variable degree of lung hypoplasia. This results in a decrease in the cross-sectional area of the pulmonary vascular bed with subsequent pulmonary hypertension and pulmonary vasoconstriction.

Rare, Fatal Conditions

Respiratory failure and PPHN can be the presenting features in surfactant protein B (SPB) deficiency, alveolar capillary dysplasia (ACD), and lymphangectasia.

Initial Treatment for HRF

1. Identify infants at risk for PPHN. Infants with meconium suctioned from below the cords should be monitored with pulse oximetry following birth.

2. Closely monitor these and other infants at risk for PPHN for signs of respiratory distress and desaturation. Umbilical artery catheter (UAC) placement should be considered earlier in the management of infants at risk of PPHN who have respiratory distress.

3. Promptly treat hypoxemia and acidosis. Hypoxemia and acidosis increase pulmonary vascular resistance and should be promptly addressed.

4. Ensure adequate cardiac output. Maintain a mean arterial pressure greater than 45 mm Hg in a term or near-term infant to lessen the right-to-left shunt. This may be achieved with a combination of either volume boluses or pressors. Central arterial and

venous pressure monitoring are desirable to guide fluid and pressor therapy.

5. Maintain adequate oxygen-carrying capacity by keeping the hematocrit greater than 40. Hematocrits in excess of 50 may result in increased pulmonary vascular resistance.

6. If there is evidence of pulmonary hypertension, either clinically or by echocardiography, then the suggested target arterial blood gas (ABG) values are pH greater than 7.40 and PaO_2 greater than 60. $PaCO_2$ values under 35 can decrease cerebral blood flow and increase the risk for brain injury. Consider use of cerebral near-infrared spectroscopy (NIRS) in this patient population to monitor for cerebral vasoconstriction. HFV may be considered to achieve the blood gas targets mentioned.

7. Minimize unnecessary handling and noise.

8. Ensure appropriate sedation and analgesia. Neuromuscular blockade may be considered if oxygenation remains suboptimal after other therapeutic approaches have been used, although this may exacerbate fluid retention and edema formation.

9. Calculate and follow the oxygenation index (OI) for all infants with oxygen requirement of 60% or greater:

$$OI = (Mean\ airway\ pressure) \times (FiO_2/PaO_2) \times 100$$

Maximal Medical Therapy Alternatives for HRF

High-Frequency Ventilation

High-frequency ventilation is used with the goal of decreasing ventilation-perfusion mismatch and optimizing lung inflation.[11] HFV is generally considered when the OI is greater than 10.

Surfactant Therapy

Surfactant should be considered when the OI is 15 or greater. Infants with lung injury caused by parenchymal disease may have a secondary surfactant deficiency. A masked randomized trial reported a significant reduction in the need for ECMO with surfactant therapy.[12] Subgroup analysis showed the greatest benefit in the group with an OI of 15–22. Consider using a test dose in unstable infants.

Inhaled Nitric Oxide Therapy

Inhaled nitric oxide therapy is a selective pulmonary vasodilator that has been shown in two prospective randomized trials[13,14] to significantly reduce the need for ECMO in newborns with an OI greater than 25. Earlier use of iNO with an OI of 15–25 has been shown to decrease the progression of respiratory failure to an OI greater than 30 ($P = .002$) and to the composite outcome of an OI greater than 30 or ECMO/death ($P = .02$).[15,16]

PRE-ECMO MANAGEMENT

Neonatal ECMO Selection Criteria

Neonatal ECMO selection criteria include the following:

1. Gestational age 34 weeks or greater and weight 2.0 kg or greater.
2. No intracranial hemorrhage greater than grade II.
3. No lethal congenital or chromosomal anomalies.
4. Not greater than 7–10 days of assisted ventilation.
5. No irreversible brain injury.
6. No significant coagulopathy or uncontrolled bleeding.
7. Cardiac or respiratory failure despite maximal medical therapy with a mortality estimated to be approximately 80%. The most commonly used quantitative measurement is an OI greater than 40 on 2 ABG measurements 30 minutes apart.

Pre-ECMO Procedures

Echocardiogram

The echocardiogram is obtained to exclude congenital heart disease, to assess for pulmonary hypertension, and to assess myocardial function, which will help decide whether the infant will receive venovenous (VV) or venoarterial (VA) ECMO. VA ECMO provides complete cardiorespiratory support via 2 catheters in the internal jugular vein and carotid artery; VV ECMO provides respiratory support alone via a single dual-lumen catheter in the internal jugular vein. VV should be considered in all neonates except when double-lumen VV cannulation is not possible, with septic shock refractory to pressor support, or when cardiac instability is significant and cardiac arrest appears imminent.

Cranial Ultrasound

A cranial ultrasound is done to check for significant intracranial hemorrhage, which could extend with systemic heparinization. Intracranial hemorrhage is a risk associated with ECMO and occurs in 5%–10% of patients on ECMO. This occurs most commonly in those of lower gestational age and with other risk factors, such as asphyxia, acidosis, and coagulation abnormalities. If there is a grade I or II bleed, ECMO is still possible, but with lower activated clotting time (ACT) targets and consideration of using aminocaproic acid, an antifibrinolytic agent.

Coagulation Studies

Prothrombin time (PT), partial thromboplastin time (PTT), fibrinogen, platelet count, antithrombin III, and D-dimer should be evaluated for patients considered for ECMO. Any coagulation abnormalities should be corrected prior to ECMO cannulation.

ECMO Consent

As for other surgical procedures, written informed consent with full discussion of the risks, benefits, and alternatives must be obtained from the family prior to initiating ECMO.

Mobilizing the ECMO Team

The ECMO team includes a perfusionist, ECMO nurse, and pediatric/cardiovascular surgeon. The team needs to be given timely notification to be prepared to place the patient on ECMO in a controlled, organized fashion.

Blood Product Needs

A typical neonatal ECMO circuit prime requires 2 units of packed red blood cells (RBCs) and 1 unit of fresh frozen plasma (FFP). Unpacked platelets should be given to the circuit once bypass support has been initiated. Whenever ECMO is performed in the neonatal intensive care unit (NICU), an emergency RBC unit should be readily available.

CARE OF THE NEONATE ON ECMO SUPPORT

ECMO Circuit Considerations

Pump Flow

Oxygenation is regulated by varying the pump flow rate. After cannulation, the pump flow is increased until the infant's oxygen saturation is in the target range (VA > 90%, VV > 85%). Typical pump flow for VA ECMO is 80–120 mL/kg/min. For VV ECMO, the pump flow is usually 100–120 mL/kg/min. On VV bypass, higher pump flows may result in recirculation.

Sweep Gas

Sweep gas is the air/oxygen mixture delivered to the oxygenator. The sweep gas through the oxygenator provides CO_2 removal as well as oxygenation. The sweep gas is typically started at 0.5–1 L/min and adjusted based on the circuit gases. Be cognizant of the minimum and maximum sweep flows for the oxygenator, as this may vary by manufacturer. Too low sweep flow will result in condensation on the membrane and ineffective ventilation; too much sweep flow can lead to membrane rupture and air embolus. If the CO_2 is too low on minimum sweep flow, CO_2 may need to be introduced into the sweep gas flow.[17]

Circuit Emergencies

Circuit emergencies include air in the circuit, clots, circuit rupture, oxygenator failure, and equipment failure. Medical and nursing staff should be trained to manage circuit emergencies through recurring skills workshops and simulation exercises.

Respiratory

Once on ECMO, ventilator settings can be weaned quickly to "rest" settings. Infants previously on HFV are transitioned to conventional ventilation, and iNO can be discontinued. Infants supported with VV ECMO should be weaned more slowly and may require higher rest settings. Daily chest radiographs should be obtained to evaluate cannula positions and to determine lung expansion. Monitoring of tidal volumes on the ventilator can also provide a clue to lung recovery. Infants with persistent atelectasis may benefit from higher positive end-expiratory pressure (PEEP), aerosolized medications, surfactant administration, or bronchoalveolar lavage.

The decision to wean ECMO is based on a daily assessment of the patient's chest radiograph, blood gas data, and lung mechanics. Mixed venous saturation is also a helpful parameter to follow for patients on VA ECMO. The pump flow is weaned slowly, and ABG and saturation values are monitored closely. After tolerating "idling" flow, defined as 10% of the calculated cardiac output or 20 mL/kg/min, for several hours with blood gas values in the normal range, patients are ready for decannulation from extracorporeal support. In VA ECMO, a full "trial off" can be performed routinely or only in circumstances when the patient's stability off bypass is in question. Trialing off involves clamping the arterial and venous cannulae and resuming circuit flow across the bridge. In VV ECMO, a trial off is routinely performed and can be achieved by disconnecting the gas source and capping the egress port of the oxygenator. During the decannulation procedure, ventilator settings are adjusted after the infant is given a short-acting neuromuscular blocking agent and narcotics.

Cardiac

Infants on VA ECMO can usually wean off pressors immediately after initiation of bypass; infants on VV ECMO will wean off more slowly. Cardiac stun, defined as transient decrease in left ventricular shortening fraction by greater than 25%, may be seen early in the VA ECMO run and is associated with higher mortality

after ECMO. Hypertension may occur because of excessive pump flow, particularly in patients on VA ECMO, with pain/agitation, and with fluid overload. This should be managed aggressively to avoid intraventricular hemorrhage as a possible sequela.

Fluids, Electrolytes, and Nutrition

Fluid overload is a common problem for infants on ECMO because of the need for fluid resuscitation prior to cannulation, renal impairment related to illness severity, third spacing caused by sepsis, and sedation and paralysis. The goal is to provide nutrition with adequate calories with the least amount of fluids. Diuretics are often given routinely to infants on ECMO bypass, and electrolytes should be checked frequently; aminophylline and dopamine may also be of benefit to improve diuresis. In the setting of severe renal dysfunction, continuous hemofiltration/dialysis may need to be incorporated into the ECMO circuit.

Hematologic

Transfusion requirements are high in the ECMO setting because of consumption from the circuit and the need for frequent blood sampling. Systemic heparinization is required to avoid clotting in the circuit and oxygenator. Hematocrit, platelet counts, and coagulation panels, including antithrombin III and heparin activity levels, should be checked frequently while infants are on ECMO. Target ranges for ACTs and platelet counts should be individualized based on the infant's clinical status and risk for bleeding.

Neurologic

Patients on ECMO should have close surveillance with daily ultrasound for intracranial hemorrhage or infarcts. Neuromonitoring with NIRS and amplitude-integrated encephalography (EEG) is suggested to monitor cerebral oxygenation and to assess for subclinical seizures. EEG should be ordered if there is concern for clinical seizures. The goal of sedation should be directed toward maintaining patient comfort and avoiding inadvertent decannulation. Excessive sedation and paralysis will exacerbate fluid retention and confound the neurologic assessment.

POST-ECMO MANAGEMENT

Respiratory

In general, patients weaned off ECMO no longer have PPHN physiology. The respiratory care goals should target normal blood gases. After the infant has awakened from the vecuronium and fentanyl given for the decannulation procedure, the ventilator can be weaned. Most patients on ECMO can be extubated within 48–72 hours after ECMO with the exception of infants with CDH, who may still have PPHN, necessitating longer periods of ventilation post-ECMO and weaning of mechanical ventilation that is more gradual.

Fluids, Electrolytes, and Nutrition

The fluid requirements and nutrition will depend on the infant's weight gain over birth weight and urine output. Electrolytes should be checked frequently in the first 48 hours after transitioning off bypass.

Hematologic

Transfusion requirements will be reduced once off bypass. In the immediate decannulation period, platelet count should be maintained at greater than 75,000/μL.

Neurologic

No further head ultrasounds are needed after removal from bypass; however, magnetic resonance imaging (MRI) should be obtained prior to discharge to determine if there is evidence of hemorrhagic or nonhemorrhagic injury.

Follow-up

Patients who receive ECMO should be followed by a high-risk infant follow-up program after discharge. Despite the severity of illness in the newborn period, the medical and neurodevelopmental outcomes are encouraging, with major disability or handicap reported[18] in approximately 15%. Most of the disability is mild-to-moderate cognitive delay. The majority of ECMO survivors are functioning in the normal range, although mean IQ scores are lower than normal. ECMO survivors are at risk for delayed-onset sensorineural hearing loss and should be referred for audiology evaluation. The Joint Committee on Infant Hearing added PPHN and ECMO as risk indicators for hearing loss and recommended audiologic evaluation every 6 months until 3 years of age.[19] Newborns with CDH have growth and medical issues that are more significant following discharge and benefit from multidisciplinary follow-up.

REFERENCES

1. Bartlett RH, Gazzaniga AB, Jefferies MR, Huxtable RF, Haiduc NJ, Fong SW. Extracorporeal membrane oxygenation (ECMO) cardiopulmonary support in infancy. *Am Soc Artif Intern Organs.* 1976;22:80–93.

2. Bartlett RH, Andrews AF, Toomasian JM, Haiduc NJ, Gazzaniga AB. Extracorporeal membrane oxygenation for newborn respiratory failure: forty-five cases. *Surgery.* 1982;92:425–433.

3. Short BL, Miller MK, Anderson KD. Extracorporeal membrane oxygenation in the management of respiratory failure in the newborn. *Clin Perinatol.* 1987;14:737–747.

4. Bartlett RH, Roloff DW, Cornell RG, Andrews AF, Dillon PW, Zwischenberger JB. Extracorporeal circulation in neonatal respiratory failure: a prospective randomized study. *Pediatrics.* 1985;76:479–487.

5. O'Rourke PP, Crone RK, Vacanti JP, et al. Extracorporeal membrane oxygenation and conventional medical therapy in neonates with persistent pulmonary hypertension of the newborn: a prospective randomized study. *Pediatrics.* 1989;84:957–963.

6. UK Collaborative ECMO Trial Group. UK collaborative randomized trial of neonatal extracorporeal membrane oxygenation. *Lancet.* 1996;348:75–82.

7. Neonatal ECMO Registry of the Extracorporeal Life Support Organization (ELSO). Ann Arbor, MI, July 2013. http://www.elso.org/Registry/Statistics/InternationalSummary.aspx.

8. Roy BJ, Rycus P, Conrad SA, Clark RH, for the Extracorporeal Life Support Organization (ELSO) Registry. The changing demographics of neonatal extracorporeal membrane oxygenation patients reported to the Extracorporeal Life Support Organization (ELSO) Registry. *Pediatrics.* 2000;106:1334–1338.

9. Hintz SR, Suttner DM, Sheehan AM, Rhine WD, Van Meurs KP. Deceased use of neonatal extracorporeal membrane oxygenation (ECMO): how new treatment modalities have affected ECMO utilization. *Pediatrics.* 2000;106:1339–1343.

10. Wilson JM, Bower LK, Thompson JE, Fauza DO, Fackler JC. ECMO in evolution: the impact of changing patient demographics and alternative therapies on ECMO. *J Pediatr Surg.* 1996;31: 1116–1123.

11. Kinsella JP, Abman SH. Clinical approaches to the use of high frequency mechanical ventilation in neonatal respiratory failure. *J Perinatol.* 1996;16:S52–S55.

12. Lotze A, Mitchell BR, Bulas DI, Zola EM, Shalwitz RA, Gunkel JH. Multicenter study of surfactant (beractant) use in the treatment of term infants with severe respiratory failure. Survanta in Term Infants Study Group. *J Pediatr.* 1998;132:40–47.

13. Neonatal Inhaled Nitric Oxide Study Group. Inhaled nitric oxide in full-term and nearly full-term infants with hypoxic respiratory failure. *N Engl J Med.* 1997;336:597–604.

14. Clark RH, Kueser TJ, Walker MW, et al. Low dose nitric oxide for persistent pulmonary hypertension of the newborn. *N Engl J Med.* 2000;342:469–474.

15. Konduri GG, Solimano A, Sokol GM, et al for the Neonatal Inhaled Nitric Oxide Study Group. A randomized trial of early versus standard inhaled nitric oxide therapy in term and near-term newborn infants with hypoxic respiratory failure. *Pediatrics.* 2004;113:559–564.

16. Konduri GG, Sokol GM, Van Meurs K, et al for the Neonatal Inhaled Nitric Oxide Study Group. Impact of early surfactant and inhaled nitric oxide therapies on outcomes in term/late preterm neonates with moderate hypoxic respiratory failure. *J Perinatol.* 2013;33(12):944–949. Epub 18 Jul 2013.

17. Short BL, Williams L, eds. *ECMO Specialist Training Manual.* 3rd ed. Ann Arbor, MI: Extracorporeal Life Support Organization; 2010.

18. Glass P, Wagner A, Papero P, et al. Neurodevelopmental status at age five years of neonates treated with extracorporeal membrane oxygenation. *J Pediatr.* 1995;127:447–457.

19. Joint Committee on Infant Hearing, American Academy of Audiology, American Academy of Pediatrics, American Speech-Language-Hearing Association, Directors of Speech and Hearing Programs in State Health and Welfare Agencies. Year 2000 position statement: principles and guidelines for early hearing detection and intervention programs. *Pediatrics.* 2000;106:798–817.

CHAPTER 90

Part E: Blood

91 Anemia

Magali J. Fontaine, Jennifer Andrews, and Alexis Davis

DIFFERENTIAL DIAGNOSIS OF ANEMIA

Figure 91-1 indicates pathways to a diagnosis of anemia.

Blood Loss

1. Maternal factors
   a. Vaginal bleeding
   b. Abruptio placentae
   c. Placenta previa
2. Hemorrhage From the Umbilical Cord
   a. Velamentous insertion
   b. Rupture during delivery
   c. Entanglement/nuchal cord
3. Fetal-fetal transfusion (only in monozygotic multiples)
4. Fetomaternal hemorrhage
   a. Occurs in 30%–50% of pregnancies although usually with clinically insignificant volumes
   b. Incidence increases with preeclampsia, cesarean section, delayed cord clamping
5. Birth trauma: extraction, breech, instrumentation
   a. Intracranial hemorrhages (subdural, subarachnoid, or subependymal bleeding)
   b. Caput succedaneum (common)
   c. Cephalohematoma (largest-volume blood loss)
6. Internal bleeding
   a. Defects in hemostasis

b. Consumption of coagulation factors from disseminated intravascular coagulation (DIC), sepsis
c. Congenital factor deficiency
d. Deficiency of vitamin K-dependent factors (II, VII, IX, X) caused by failure to administer vitamin K after birth or use of antibiotics

Increased Red Blood Cell Destruction/Hemolytic Anemia

Increased red blood cell (RBC) destruction or hemolytic anemia is usually accompanied by reticulocytosis and hyperbilirubinemia.

1. Extrinsic factors
   a. Immune
      1. Isoimmune hemolytic anemia (warm or cold)
      2. Alloimmune hemolytic disease of the newborn (ABO, Rh or minor blood group antigens)
      3. Drug reaction
   b. Nonimmune/infections
      1. Bacterial
      2. Congenital viral infections
2. Intrinsic factors/congenital
   a. RBC structural defects
      1. Hereditary spherocytosis
      2. Hereditary elliptocytosis
      3. Hereditary pyropoikilocytosis
   b. RBC enzyme defects
      1. Glucose-6-phosphate dehydrogenase (G-6-PD) deficiency
      2. Pyruvate kinase deficiency

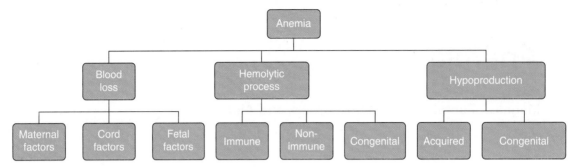

FIGURE 91-1 Underlying causes for neonatal anemia.

c. Hemoglobinopathies
1. Quantitative defects (eg, thalassemias α and β)
2. Qualitative defects (eg, sickle cell syndromes [including hemoglobin SS, SC]), Unstable hemoglobins (>500 variants)

3. Acquired factors

a. Iatrogenic blood loss (eg, from surgery, repeated phlebotomy)

b. Mechanical (eg, extracorporeal membrane oxygenation [ECMO], artificial heart valve)

Hypoproduction

1. Acquired

a. Iron deficiency anemia (supplement in neonates, especially preterm)

b. Vitamin E deficiency (supplement in neonates receiving intravenous nutrition)

c. Aplastic anemia (parvovirus B19)

d. Anemia of prematurity: low reticulocyte count, inadequate response to erythropoietin

e. Infections (eg, rubella, syphilis)

2. Congenital

a. Diamond-Blackfan anemia

b. Fanconi anemia

c. Congenital dyserythropoietic anemias

d. Sideroblastic anemias

e. Congenital leukemia (usually associated with other hematologic abnormalities)

WORKUP

The clinical workup for anemia in the neonate is shown in Figure 91-2.

Primary Workup

1. Hemoglobin
2. RBC indices

a. Microcytic or hypochromic suggest fetomaternal or twin-twin hemorrhage or α-thalassemia.

b. Normocytic or normochromic suggest acute hemorrhage, systemic disease, intrinsic RBC defect, or hypoplastic anemia.

3. Reticulocyte count

a. Elevation suggests antecedent hemorrhage or hemolytic anemia.

b. A low count is seen with hypoplastic anemia.

4. Blood smear looking for

a. Spherocytes (immune-mediated hemolysis or hereditary spherocytosis)

b. Elliptocytes (hereditary elliptocytosis)

c. Pyknocytes (G-6-PD)

d. Schistocytes (consumption coagulopathy)

5. Direct Coombs test: positive in isoimmune or autoimmune hemolysis

Secondary Workup

1. Hypoplastic anemia workup: bone marrow aspiration

2. Congenital viral infection workup

a. Chest x-ray, bone films

b. Cord immunoglobulin (Ig) M levels

c. Viral serologies

d. Urinalysis and cytomegalovirus (CMV) culture

3. DIC and platelet consumption: coagulation workup

a. Platelet count

b. Fibrinogen, fibrin split products

c. Prothrombin time/partial thromboplastin time (PT/PTT), international normalized ratio (INR)

4. Hemorrhagic workup for occult hemorrhage

a. Cranial ultrasound

b. Abdominal ultrasound

5. Intrinsic RBC defects

a. RBC enzyme studies

b. Hemoglobin electrophoresis and high-performance liquid chromatography (HPLC) for globin chain ratios

c. RBC membrane studies

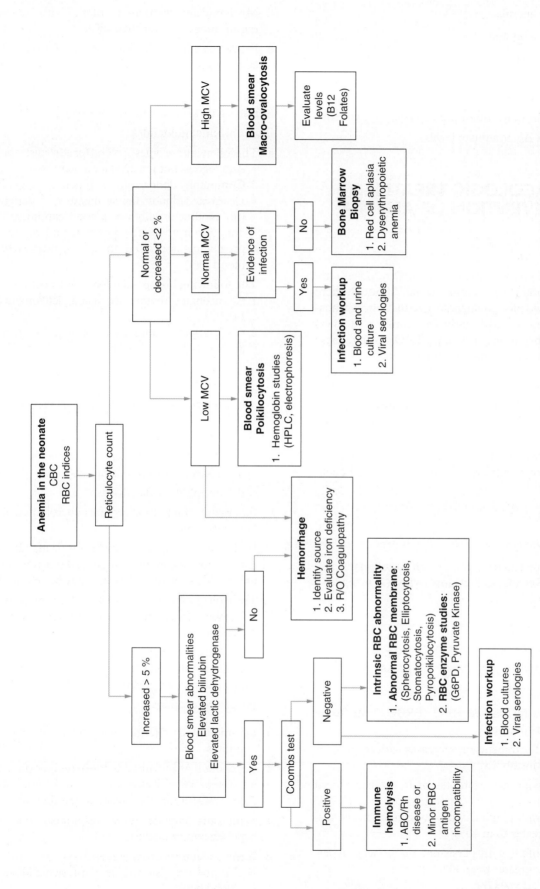

FIGURE 91-2 Clinical workup for anemia in the neonate. CBC, complete blood cell count; HPLC, high-performance liquid chromatography; MCV, mean corpuscular volume; RBC, red blood cells; R/O, rule out.

6. Hemolytic anemia
   a. Free hemoglobin
   b. Haptoglobin
   c. Lactate dehydrogenase (LDH)
   d. Indirect and total bilirubin
   e. Serum iron, iron-binding capacity, transferrin
   f. Vitamin B_{12} and folate levels

PHARMACOLOGIC TREATMENT AND PREVENTION OF ANEMIA

Erythropoietin (EPO)

1. Anemia of prematurity: Use of EPO to offset anemia of prematurity is controversial. Although there is some evidence to suggest a reduction in transfusion exposure with early (beginning < 8 days) and late (beginning > 8 days) EPO dosing, these reductions are of limited clinical benefit. A study from Ohlsson et al. in Cochrane Review also cited a potential increase in the rate of retinopathy of prematurity as a result of EPO administration.

2. Anemia of chronic disease: There is a potential role for EPO administration to infants with chronic renal disease and those undergoing myeloablative chemotherapy, although clear evidence of benefit is lacking.

Iron Supplementation

Dietary ferrous sulfate can be given to infants at risk for anemia. Recommended doses vary (2–6 mg/kg/d elemental iron).

TRANSFUSION GUIDELINES FOR SYMPTOMATIC ANEMIA

1. Indications for packed RBC (PRBC) transfusion are patient specific.
2. The need for transfusion increases with respiratory or cardiac instability.
3. The following are examples of target hematocrit ranges:
   a. Preoperative infant with congenital heart disease: greater than 40%
   b. Term infant with persistent pulmonary hypertension: greater than 40%
   c. Patient on ECMO: greater than 35%–40%

d. Mechanically ventilated infant with oxygen requirement: greater than 25%–30%
e. Premature infant with poor growth, feeding difficulties, or frequent apnea/bradycardia/desaturation events: greater than 20%–30%; still controversial, with trials conflicting regarding outcome with restricted vs liberal transfusion guidelines

4. Blood product guidelines
   a. The following are types of blood for administration:
      1. Autologous: not practical for a neonate
      2. Community donor: most common
      3. Designated donor: family member or designee (nb: mother usually not a good candidate for donation immediately postpartum because of pregnancy-associated anemia or intrapartum blood loss)
   b. The following are specific issues for neonates:
      1. All neonates require irradiated, leukoreduced PRBCs.
      2. CMV-negative units are indicated for infants at increased risk of clinically significant CMV disease:
         a. Premature infants (<35 weeks)
         b. Suspected severe immunodeficiency (eg, DiGeorge, severe combined immunodeficiency [SCID])
         c. Infants born to mothers with human immunodeficiency virus (HIV) infection
         d. Complex cardiac disease
   c. Emergency transfusion requires uncrossmatched, O-negative blood.
   d. In the case of massive transfusion or inability to handle a significant potassium load (eg, renal failure, acidosis), washed PRBCs may be required.
   e. The typical volume transfused is 10–15 mL/kg over 1–4 hours, depending on hemodynamic status of the infant.
   f. Fluid-sensitive patients may require diuretic administration following transfusion, although studies do not support doing this routinely.

5. Transfusion reactions
   a. IgE-mediated allergic reactions are rare in neonates.
   b. Reactions may be caused by the hemolytic process, inflammatory mediators in the blood component being transfused, or bacterial contamination.
   c. Symptoms include fever, respiratory distress, hypotension, or acidosis.
   d. If transfusion reaction is suspected:
      i. Immediately discontinue transfusion and notify blood bank.

ii. The unit may be returned to the blood bank for further testing.

iii. A coombs test may be ordered to rule out a hemolytic transfusion reaction.

FOLLOW-UP

1. Monitor vital signs for evidence of transfusion reaction, fluid overload, and so on.

2. Wait at least 4 hours following transfusion to recheck hemoglobin/hematocrit to allow for adequate mixing.

3. Assess for ongoing losses.

SUGGESTED READING

Aher SM, Ohlsson A . Late erythropoietin for preventing red blood cell transfusion in preterm and/or low birth weight infants. *Cochrane Database Syst Rev.* 2014;4:CD004868.

Arnon S, Dolfin T, Bauer S, et al. Iron supplementation for preterm infants receiving restrictive red blood cell transfusions: reassessment of practice safety. *J Perinatol.* 2010;30:736–740.

Baer VL, Henry E, Lambert DK, et al. Implementing a program to improve compliance with neonatal intensive care unit transfusion guidelines was accompanied by a reduction in transfusion rate: a pre-post analysis within a multihospital health care system. *Transfusion.* 2011;51:264–269.

Bell EF, Strauss RG, Widness JA, et al. Randomized trial of liberal versus restrictive guidelines for red blood cell transfusion in preterm infants. *Pediatrics.* 2005;115:1685–1691.

Galel SA, Fontaine MJ. Hazards of neonatal blood transfusion. *NeoReviews.* 2006;7:e69–e75.

Gibson BE, Todd A, Roberts I, et al. Transfusion guidelines for neonates and older children. *Br J Haematol.* 2004;124:433–453.

Kirpalani H, Whyte RK, Andersen C, et al. The Premature Infants in Need of Transfusion (PINT) study: a randomized, controlled trial of restrictive (low) versus liberal (high) transfusion threshold for extremely low birth weight infants. *J Pediatr.* 2006;149: 301–307.

Litty CA. Neonatal red cell transfusions. *Immunohematology.* 2008;24: 10–14.

Ohlsson A, Aher SM. Early erythropoietin for preventing red blood cell transfusion in preterm and/or low birth weight infants. *Cochrane Database Syst Rev.* 2014;4:CD004863.

Valieva OA, Strandjord TP, Mayock DE, Juul SE. Effects of transfusions in extremely low birth weight infants: a retrospective study. *J Pediatr.* 2009;155:331–337.

Warwood TL, Lambert DK, Henry E, Christensen RD. Very low birth weight infants qualifying for a "late" erythrocyte transfusion: does giving darbepoetin along with the transfusion counteract the transfusion's erythropoietic suppression? *J Perinatol.* 2011;31(Suppl 1): S17–S21.

Thrombocytopenia

Wendy Wong, Clara Lo, and Bert Glader

INTRODUCTION

Thrombocytopenia in neonates is defined as a platelet count of less than 150×10^9/L. The prevalence of thrombocytopenia in healthy term infants is 1%–2%, whereas up to 35% of neonates admitted to intensive care units may have low platelet counts.[1] There are developmental differences in megakaryopoiesis between neonates and older children. Neonatal megakaryocytes are less capable of upregulating platelet production or mounting as high a level of thrombopoietin (Tpo) when compared to adults with the same degree of thrombocytopenia.[2] These developmental differences account for the vulnerability of sick neonates to thrombocytopenia.

The major causes of neonatal thrombocytopenia are increased platelet consumption or decreased platelet production. However, both mechanisms can contribute to thrombocytopenia in any given patient, particularly in sick or premature neonates.

DIAGNOSIS/INDICATION

Clinical Findings: History and Physical

A detailed medical history and physical examination will guide the diagnostic approach to thrombocytopenia. Medical history and complications during pregnancy are important because many maternal factors can cause neonatal thrombocytopenia. Maternal drugs and antibodies that cross the placenta can affect an infant's platelet count. Complications during pregnancy that result in chronic fetal hypoxia or intrauterine growth retardation (IUGR) are frequent causes of early-onset neonatal thrombocytopenia.[3] Causes of chronic fetal hypoxia and IUGR include pregnancy-induced hypertension or diabetes, placental insufficiency, and placental infarction or malformation. Perinatal asphyxia is another common cause of early-onset thrombocytopenia. Family history of chronic thrombocytopenia suggests a hereditary thrombocytopenia or a genetic syndrome associated with low platelet counts; a family history of previous neonatal thrombocytopenia suggests maternal immune-mediated thrombocytopenia.

Physical findings of thrombocytopenia vary with the platelet count and the primary cause of thrombocytopenia. Many neonates are asymptomatic. However, in those who have bleeding manifestations, bruising and petechiae are the most common presenting symptoms, often noted on the face and head secondary to birth trauma. Thrombocytopenia commonly is associated with mucocutaneous bleeding. Bleeding also can occur with trauma following phlebotomy, after intramuscular injections (prophylactic vitamin K or hepatitis vaccine), umbilical stump bleeding, or associated with circumcision. Intra-abdominal bleeding and intracranial hemorrhage (ICH) generally occur only in severe thrombocytopenia (platelet count less than 50×10^9/L). A bulging fontanel, seizures, or other neurologic signs in a thrombocytopenic neonate warrant urgent radiographic evaluation for an intracranial bleed. Sick infants in the intensive care unit also may have bleeding from intravenous sites, surgical sites, or endotracheal tubes.

Confirmatory/Baseline Tests

When a low platelet count is suspected, a complete blood cell count (CBC) with a review of the peripheral blood smear should be done. The diagnostic approach to multilineage cytopenias is different from that for isolated thrombocytopenia. The morphology of platelets as well as red and white blood cells (WBCs) may provide clues to diagnosis. For example, the presence of WBC inclusions and large platelets suggests a hereditary macrothrombocytopenia, and the presence of microangiopathic red blood cell changes will lead to further investigation for disseminated intravascular coagulation (DIC) or other microangiopathic hemolytic processes. Thrombocytopenia is often an incidental finding when a CBC is obtained for assessing other hematologic parameters. In these cases, the primary reason for a CBC may explain the thrombocytopenia (eg, an elevated WBC count in an infant born to mother who has a fever most likely has thrombocytopenia secondary to sepsis). If the clinical picture is not consistent with the degree of thrombocytopenia, the platelet count should be repeated. Spurious thrombocytopenia can be seen with platelet agglutination or platelet satellitism.[4] Both are often associated with ethylenediaminetetraacetic acid (EDTA), the anticoagulant in sample collection tubes. If spurious thrombocytopenia is suspected, review of the peripheral blood smear should provide the accurate count.

Differential Diagnosis/Diagnostic Algorithm

The differential diagnosis for neonatal thrombocytopenia is broad (see Figure 92-1 for a diagnostic algorithm).

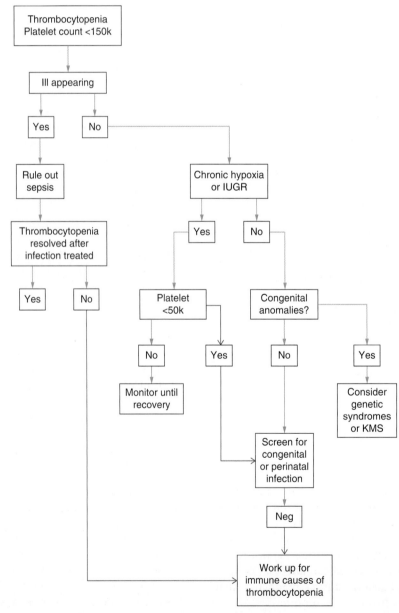

FIGURE 92-1 Diagnostic algorithm. IUGR, intrauterine growth retardation; KMS, Kasabach-Merritt syndrome.

A most useful approach in sorting out the cause is based on the neonate's clinical status. Thrombocytopenic neonates roughly fall into three different groups based on their clinical features (Table 92-1).

ILL-APPEARING PREMATURE INFANTS BORN TO MOTHERS WITH SIGNS OF MEDICAL ILLNESS

Within the group of premature neonates with thrombocytopenia who are ill appearing and born to mothers with pregnancy complications or with other signs of medical illness, the time of onset of thrombocytopenia is useful to further guide the inquiry.

Mild-to-moderate thrombocytopenia (50,000–100,000) developing within the first 72 hours is most likely secondary to maternal/pregnancy-related factors.[3,5] Fetuses exposed to chronic intrauterine hypoxia from a variety of complications as well as fetuses with IUGR are often thrombocytopenic at birth. The pathophysiology for the low platelet count is thought to be related to decreased platelet production, a consequence of reduced megakaryocyte progenitors and inadequate upregulation of Tpo.[2] Often, these neonates also will have neutropenia, nucleated red blood cells (nRBCs), and sometimes polycythemia. These hematologic abnormalities generally are not severe and resolve within the first 2 weeks of life. This group of patients can safely be monitored without additional workup until thrombocytopenia has resolved. However, if thrombocytopenia persists beyond 10 days or becomes severe (less than 50,000), further workup is warranted.

Infections, a frequent cause of thrombocytopenia in both term and preterm infants, should be ruled out in any ill-appearing newborn with low platelet count. Congenital, perinatal, or acquired postnatal infections all are associated with thrombocytopenia.

Bacterial sepsis is the most common cause of late onset of thrombocytopenia, occurring at greater than 72 hours of life.[1,3] Thrombocytopenia secondary to bacterial infection usually develops rapidly and is often severe, particularly in preterm infants. Gram-negative sepsis leads to a most severe thrombocytopenia. DIC frequently complicates neonatal sepsis and is a major mechanism for the low platelet count observed in infections.

Congenital and perinatal viral infections also cause neonatal thrombocytopenia. Cytomegalovirus (CMV) and herpes simplex virus infections are the ones most commonly associated with low platelet counts. Neonates with congenital infections may not be ill appearing but often will have other suggestive clinical

Table 92-1 Differential Diagnosis of the Thrombocytopenic Newborn

Differential diagnosis of neonates with thrombocytopenia who are ill appearing, born prematurely, born to a mother with pregnancy complications and with other signs of medical illness considers the following:
- Pregnancy complications:
  - Chronic hypoxia from placental insufficiency
  - Intrauterine growth retardation
    - Preeclampsia
- Labor and delivery complications:
  - Hypoxia or acidosis after birth trauma
- Infections:
  - Bacterial infections (sepsis)
  - Congenital viral infections (cytomegalovirus, rubella)
  - Disseminated intravascular coagulation (DIC)
- Neonatal complications:
  - Necrotizing enterocolitis (NEC)
  - Thrombosis (DIC, indwelling vascular catheters, extracorporeal membrane oxygenation [ECMO])
  - Exchange transfusions
- Neonatal diseases:
  - Bone marrow disorders (leukemia, neuroblastoma or other solid tumors, storage diseases)

Neonates with thrombocytopenia and physical abnormalities or dysmorphic features:
- Thrombocytopenia with absent radius (TAR) syndrome
- Amegakaryocytic thrombocytopenia and radioulnar synostosis (ATRUS)
- Jacobsen syndrome
- Chromosomal disorders caused by trisomy 13, 18, or 21 and Turner syndrome
- Kasabach-Merritt syndrome

Neonates with thrombocytopenia but who are otherwise healthy appearing with no physical abnormalities or other medical conditions:
- Occult infection
- Immune-mediated thrombocytopenia:
  - Secondary to maternal autoimmune thrombocytopenia (ITP)
  - Neonatal alloimmune thrombocytopenia (NAIT)
- Amegakaryocytic thrombocytopenia
- Hereditary macrothrombocytopenias
- Wiskott-Aldrich syndrome (WAS)
- Bernard-Soulier syndrome

features (ie, microcephaly, seizures, hepatosplenomegaly, intracerebral calcification, or hearing loss).

Many other medical complications seen in the neonatal intensive care unit (NICU) are associated with thrombocytopenia. For example, thrombocytopenia is found in 50% of infants with *necrotizing enterocolitis* (NEC). In the early stage of NEC, the degree of thrombocytopenia correlates with the severity of bowel necrosis.[6] Increasing platelet counts suggest improvement of the disease process. *Thrombosis* causes thrombocytopenia by increased platelet consumption. NICU patients are at high risk for thrombosis because of increased susceptibility to DIC, the use of indwelling vascular catheters, and the use of extracorporeal membrane oxygenation (ECMO). *Exchange transfusions* also can cause thrombocytopenia by dilution.

Less-frequent causes of thrombocytopenia among this group of neonates include bone marrow infiltration diseases such as congenital malignancies (leukemia, neuroblastoma, or other solid tumors) and storage diseases. In these conditions, there usually are other physical findings (hepatomegaly, splenomegaly, and other masses).

THROMBOCYTOPENIA AND PHYSICAL ABNORMALITIES OR DYSMORPHIC FEATURES

Careful examination for congenital anomalies can provide important clues to the diagnosis in neonates with thrombocytopenia. Many chromosomal abnormalities (trisomy 13, 18, or 21 and Turner syndrome) are associated with low platelet counts. Most neonates with Jacobsen syndrome are thrombocytopenic or pancytopenic at birth.[7] Jacobsen syndrome is caused by partial deletion of the long arm of chromosome 11; in addition to thrombocytopenia, there is a high incidence of platelet dysfunction. These patients therefore might have more bleeding manifestation.

Thrombocytopenia with absent radius (TAR) syndrome is a rare autosomal recessive disorder characterized by severe thrombocytopenia present at birth with skeletal abnormalities of the radius.[8] Patients with TAR have radial aplasia, usually bilateral, but thumbs are always present. However, these thumbs are often abnormal (hypoplastic or held in an abnormal position), and there occasionally is also hypoplasia of the humerus and ulnar bones. In addition, cardiac defects, brain anomalies, and dysmorphic facial features are common in patients with TAR. Most infants with TAR present with profound thrombocytopenia (platelet counts often less 10×10^9/L) in the first week after birth. Risks for serious bleeding complications are greatest in the first months after birth. Platelet counts gradually improve over their first year of life and are usually normal after several years.

Amegakaryocytic thrombocytopenia and radioulnar synostosis (ATRUS) is another rare autosomal recessive syndrome with upper limb anomalies and thrombocytopenia. This syndrome is caused by mutations in the *HOXA11* gene, and in contrast to TAR, the thrombocytopenia does not improve.[8]

Children with Fanconi anemia (FA), a congenital bone marrow failure syndrome, can have radial anomalies similar to patients with TAR but those individual's thumbs are always affected. Median age of thrombocytopenia in patients with FA is 7 years old, so it is unlikely to be an issue in the neonatal period.[1]

Kasabach-Merritt syndrome (KMS) is characterized by consumptive coagulopathy (thrombocytopenia, hypofibrinogenemia, elevated fibrin degradation products) with vascular malformations. It was first described in a child with a large capillary hemangioma; however, recent studies have shown that KMS is mainly associated with aggressive vascular tumors such as Kaposiform hemagnioendotheliomas and tufted angioma, not infantile hemangiomas.[9] Local platelet sequestration and activation of coagulation proteins within these vascular tumors lead to shortened platelet survival. Significant thrombocytopenia (below 50×10^9/L) and bleeding complications are common. In 50% of patients, the vascular lesions are notable at birth. These generally are single large lesions in the subcutaneous or deep-tissue compartment, and they are locally invasive. The subcutaneous lesions often are notable on physical examination, but visceral malformations may not be apparent and their presentation may be abdominal distention, organ dysfunction, or high-output cardiac failure.

THROMBOCYTOPENIA IN OTHERWISE HEALTHY-APPEARING NEONATES WITH NO PHYSICAL ABNORMALITIES OR OTHER MEDICAL CONDITIONS

Thrombocytopenia in otherwise-healthy infants is primarily caused by immune-mediated platelet destruction because maternal antibodies have crossed the placenta into the fetal circulation. However, neonates with occult infection may also be well appearing; therefore, infection should always be considered in this clinical setting. Less-common causes of thrombocytopenia in healthy-appearing infants include hereditary thrombocytopenias without dysmorphic features. These include amegakaryocytic thrombocytopenia, hereditary macrothrombocytic disorders, Wiskott-Aldrich syndrome (WAS), and Bernard-Soulier syndrome.

Neonatal thrombocytopenia secondary to maternal idiopathic thrombocytopenia purpura (ITP) is primarily a maternal disorder that secondarily affects the fetus and infant. ITP is a common cause of immune thrombocytopenia during pregnancy and is seen in association with other maternal autoimmune diseases, including systemic lupus erythematosus (SLE), lymphoproliferative disorders, and Graves disease. Maternal antibodies in these disorders are directed against "public" platelet antigens, usually glycoproteins IIb/IIIa and Ib/IX.

The immunoglobulin (Ig) G antibody-coated platelets are cleared by the reticuloendothelial system, causing maternal thrombocytopenia. The fetus is secondarily affected because maternal antibodies cross the placenta and bind to the same public antigens on fetal platelets.

Maternal ITP is the most likely cause of moderate-to-severe thrombocytopenia (platelet counts less than $70 \times 10^9/L$) occurring in otherwise-healthy pregnant women. This is to be distinguished from "gestational benign thrombocytopenia," a common cause of mildly decreased platelet counts (greater than $70 \times 10^9/L$) in otherwise-healthy pregnancies. This gestational thrombocytopenia occurs in asymptomatic women with no history of low platelet counts prior to pregnancy, appears in late gestation, and generally resolves spontaneously after delivery. This is a maternal condition and does not cause thrombocytopenia in neonates.

In mothers with ITP, 10%–15% of their neonates will have transient mild neonatal thrombocytopenia (platelet count less than 100,000) with minimal-to-no bleeding symptoms. The incidence of severe neonatal thrombocytopenia (platelet counts below $50 \times 10^9/L$) and bleeding complications is 3%–5%. In pregnant women with ITP, there is no reliable predictor of the expected degree of neonatal thrombocytopenia except for the magnitude of thrombocytopenia in a previous pregnancy.[10] The diagnosis of secondary autoimmune thrombocytopenia in infants is based on maternal history of ITP and the clinical course of the neonate once other causes of a low platelet count are excluded.

Neonatal alloimmune thrombocytopenia (NAIT) is the platelet equivalent of hemolytic disease of the newborn caused by Rh D incompatibility. It occurs when maternal platelets lack an antigen that the fetus has inherited from the father. Maternal IgG antibodies form against the "foreign" antigen on fetal platelets, cross the placenta, and destroy fetal platelets. In contrast to neonatal autoimmune thrombocytopenia, NAIT can result in very low platelet counts, and affected fetuses and neonates are at high risk for serious bleeding complications. There are no maternal consequences. Unlike Rh hemolytic disease, 50% of NAIT cases occur in the first pregnancy of an at-risk couple.

Neonatal alloimmune thrombocytopenia has been associated with sensitization to several different platelet-specific alloantigens. The most commonly identified antibody in sensitized Caucasian women is anti-human platelet antigen 1a (HPA-1a), accounting for 80%–90% of NAIT cases. Homozygosity for HPA-1b antigen (ie, HPA-1a negative) is seen in about 2% of pregnant women, but not all HPA-1a-negative women become alloimmunized. Sensitization in this population is related to human leukocyte antigen (HLA) type and is more common in women with HLA-B8, HLA-DR3, and HLA-DR52a. In Asians,

NAIT occurs with sensitization to HPA-4. NAIT also occurs with maternal HLA antibodies alone or in combination with HPA antibodies. HLA antibodies, though common, usually do not cause significant thrombocytopenia because other tissues bearing HLA antigens also can absorb these antibodies, thus sparing platelets.

Clinical manifestations of NAIT vary from mild to moderate thrombocytopenia in a healthy-appearing infant to severe thrombocytopenia with bleeding complications. The platelet count commonly falls further during the first week after birth. The most serious complication of NAIT is ICH. It is estimated that ICH occurs in about 10%–20% of affected newborns. Of most importance, more than 25% of these ICH events occur in utero prior to delivery. One should suspect NAIT in any healthy newborn with unexplained severe thrombocytopenia and whose mother has a normal platelet count with no history of ITP or of having had a prior splenectomy for ITP. The workup should include antiplatelet antibody testing of maternal serum; however, sometimes no antibodies are found in presumed NAIT cases. It is for this reason that platelet antigen testing of both parents also is critical in the diagnostic workup. The recurrence rate of NAIT is greater than 75% in subsequent pregnancies, and generally the thrombocytopenic course is more severe in subsequently affected children.

Several genetic disorders are associated with thrombocytopenia at birth, and these conditions may not have other clinical features notable at birth. These genetic conditions include WAS, congenital amegakaryocytic thrombocytopenia (CAMT), hereditary macrothrombocytopenia, and Bernard-Soulier syndrome.

Wiskott-Aldrich syndrome is a rare X-linked disorder characterized by immunodeficiency, eczema, and thrombocytopenia. A unique hematologic feature of this disorder is that platelets are much smaller than normal. This syndrome is caused by mutation of the *WAS* gene on the short arm of chromosome X. Children with WAS have thrombocytopenia, small platelet size at birth, and impaired platelet function. Gastrointestinal (GI) bleeding commonly is seen and may be the presenting sign. Symptoms associated with immune dysregulation (frequent infections, eczema, autoimmune phenomena) generally become more apparent later. The diagnosis is confirmed by determining WAS protein expression by flow cytometry. Bone marrow transplantation is the only curative treatment.

Congenital amegakaryocytic thrombocytopenia is a rare autosomal recessive disorder associated with severe thrombocytopenia. This disorder often presents in infancy with bleeding symptoms (petechiae, mucosal and GI bleeding). Subgroups of children with CAMT also have congenital anomalies (cardiac defects, abnormal facies, microcephaly). Bone marrow examination reveals a paucity of megakaryocytes but is otherwise normal. Thrombocytopenia progresses to pancytopenia in later childhood, and progression to leukemia sometimes occur. Stem cell transplantation is the only curative treatment.

Hereditary macrothrombocytopenias are a group of autosomal dominant disorders caused by mutations in the *MYH9* gene. Collectively, these disorders include May-Hegglin anomaly, Sebastian syndrome, Fechtner syndrome, and Epstein syndrome. They are characterized by mild-to-moderate thrombocytopenia with giant platelets. Neutrophil inclusions (Dohle bodies), nephritis, and deafness are seen in some cases. Usually, these macrothrombocytopenic disorders are not associated with a significant bleeding tendency.

Like hereditary macrothrombocytopenia, mild thrombocytopenia and giant platelets also are seen in *Bernard-Soulier syndrome*. This is a rare autosomal recessive disorder caused by mutations in components of the GP1b/IX/V platelet receptor.[11] Bernard-Soulier patients' platelets are unable to adhere to vascular subendothelium. Because of platelet dysfunction, patients with Bernard-Soulier syndrome will experience bleeding symptoms in excess of their degree of thrombocytopenia.

TREATMENT

Treatment of thrombocytopenic neonates should be guided by the degree of thrombocytopenia and bleeding symptoms. Also important is discovering the most likely diagnosis and the likelihood of bleeding associated with that diagnosis.

Neonates with mild bleeding symptoms and platelet counts greater than 50,000 can be safely monitored without treatment. However, if the infant is experiencing significant bleeding or needs to undergo an invasive procedure or surgery, treatment to increase the platelet count is necessary. In most circumstances, thrombocytopenia can be corrected rapidly by platelet transfusions. Administration of 10–15 mL/kg of platelets can be both a therapeutic and a diagnostic intervention. A more than 50,000 rise in platelet count obtained 30–45 minutes posttransfusion suggests decreased production as the primary cause of the thrombocytopenia, and a lack of an appropriate increase suggests increased platelet destruction.

Since the mid-1990s, there have been no randomized controlled trials addressing the appropriate platelet transfusion threshold in neonates. There are some published guidelines; however, there is no agreed-on threshold.[3,5,12,13] Most guidelines take into account the platelet count and the neonates' clinical condition.

For stable term infants with only mild bleeding symptoms, many consider keeping the platelet count greater than 20,000. For preterm or clinically unstable term infants, it is reasonable to keep the platelet count greater than 30,000 given their increased risk of bleeding. Any neonate with major hemorrhage should be transfused to maintain the platelet count greater than 50,000. In general, infants with platelet counts over 100,000 do not experience increased bleeding. If significant bleeding is noted at this level of thrombocytopenia, other causes of hemorrhage, such as platelet dysfunction or coagulation defects, should be investigated. Platelet transfusions in this group of patients are unlikely to improve the hemorrhagic condition.

For immune-mediated thrombocytopenia (neonatal autoimmune and NAIT), platelet transfusions sometimes do not result in a rise in platelet count because of the presence of maternal antibodies. For neonatal thrombocytopenia secondary to maternal ITP, intravenous immune globulin (IVIG) should be given to those with a platelet count less than 30,000 or who have any bleeding manifestations. A dose of 1 g/kg is safe and effective, with a response rate of 80%–90%. For infants with suspected or known NAIT but no evidence of hemorrhage, IVIG and prophylactic platelet transfusion should be given to term infants with platelet counts less than 30,000 and preterm infants with platelet counts less than 50,000. If HPA antigen mismatch is known, HPA-compatible platelets can be used. However, given that most cases of NAIT are unsuspected and there is a high incidence of bleeding associated with the diagnosis, platelet transfusions should not be delayed while waiting workup or availability of compatible platelets. Random donor platelet transfusions have been shown to produce a significant elevation of the platelet count in most cases of NAIT.[14,15] For infants with ICH or other bleeding symptoms, platelet transfusions should be first-line treatment, with the goal to keep the platelet count greater than 50,000–100,000. Some recommend complementing random platelet transfusions with IVIG (1 g/kg/d for up to 3 days) and intravenous methylprednisolone (1 mg every 8 hours with IVIG).[16] For both of these immune thrombocytopenia conditions, platelet counts fall during the first week of life and therefore needs to be monitored closely until there is consistent recovery to a safe platelet level.

Severe thrombocytopenia seen in consumptive processes such as infection and KMS should improve when the underlying conditions improve with treatment. Because these disease processes often have other coagulopathies, such as low fibrinogen or other factor levels, coagulation studies should be performed and replacement of specific factors given if they are low and the patient is experiencing bleeding.

Thrombocytopenia secondary to medical conditions that cause decreased platelet production, such as genetic syndromes and a marrow infiltrative process, may require regular transfusions to treat or prevent bleeding complications, particularly in those with associated platelet dysfunction such as WAS. In neonates with thrombocytopenia caused by impaired production, platelet transfusions should result in an improvement of platelet count that gradually falls over the next 5–7 days. Lack of an appropriate platelet response to transfusion suggests development of an alloantibody against an antigen on the transfused platelets. This complication is usually not seen in the neonatal period.

FOLLOW-UP

For immune-mediated neonatal thrombocytopenia (NAIT and neonatal thrombocytopenia secondary to maternal ITP), parents need to be counseled regarding the risks and management of future pregnancies. They should be referred to obstetricians specialized in managing high-risk pregnancies. For both conditions, the best predictor for the degree of fetal thrombocytopenia in the future is the disease severity of a previously affected infant in the same family. There are no reliable noninvasive methods for monitoring and managing affected pregnancies. No data support that antenatal treatment of maternal ITP alters the neonatal outcome. On the other hand, for pregnancies with a known history of NAIT and particularly with a history of neonatal ICH, antenatal treatment is critical to prevent serious in utero bleeding. Treatment generally involves weekly IVIG and daily prednisone. The timing and intensity of the treatment are guided by outcome of previously affected fetuses. If there was ICH in utero, treatment is started earlier than when bleeding previously was minimal. In the past, fetal platelet measurements by percutaneous umbilical cord sampling were recommended. However, significant bleeding complications were seen with this procedure. Fetal blood sampling is used much less currently.[16] For fetuses with suspected NAIT, delivery by cesarean section is recommended.

Long-term outcome of neonates with thrombocytopenia depends on the cause of thrombocytopenia and the associated bleeding complications.

Neurocognitive defects and death are seen in children with serious ICH. Infants who have chronic thrombocytopenia caused by genetic syndromes associated with defective thrombopoiesis might be transfusion dependent for life, but in general, platelet transfusions in this group are reserved for major hemorrhage or in preparation for invasive procedures.

REFERENCES

1. Holzhauer S, Zieger B. Diagnosis and management of neonatal thrombocytopenia. *Semin Fetal Neonatal Med.* 2011;16(6):305–310.
2. Sola-Visner M, Sallmon H, Brown R. New insights into the mechanisms of nonimmune thrombocytopenia in neonates. *Semin Perinatol.* 2009;33:43–51.
3. Roberts I, Stanworth S, Murray NA. Thrombocytopenia in the neonate. *Blood Rev.* 2008;22:173–186.
4. Zandecki M, Genevieve F, Gerard J, Godon A. Spurious counts and spurious results on haematology analysers: a review. Part I: platelets. *Int J Lab Hematol.* 2007;29:4–20.
5. Chakravorty S, Roberts I. How I manage neonatal thrombocytopenia. *Br J Haematol.* 2012;156(2):155–162.
6. Kenton AB, O'Donovan D, Cass DL, et al. Severe thrombocytopenia predicts outcome in neonates with necrotizing enterocolitis. *J Perinatol.* 2005;25:14–20.
7. Mattina T, Perrotta CS, Grossfeld P. Jacobsen syndrome. *Orphanet J Rare Dis.* 2009;4:9.
8. Toriello HV. Thrombocytopenia-absent radius syndrome. *Semin Thromb Hemost.* 2011;37(6):707–712.
9. Kelly M. Kasabach-Merritt phenomenon. *Pediatr Clin North Am.* 2010;57(5):1085–1089.
10. Koyama S, Tomimatsu T, Kanagawa T, Kumasawa K, Tsutsui T, Kimura T. Reliable predictors of neonatal immune thrombocytopenia in pregnant women with idiopathic thrombocytopenic purpura. *Am J Hematol.* 2012;87(1):15–21.
11. Handin RI. Inherited platelet disorders. *Hematol Am Soc Hematol Educ Program.* 2005:396–402.
12. Christensen RD. Platelet transfusion in the neonatal intensive care unit: benefits, risks, alternatives. *Neonatology.* 2011;100(3):311–318.
13. Gibson BE, Todd A, Roberts I, et al. Transfusion guidelines for neonates and older children. *Br J Haematol.* 2004;124:433–453.
14. Allen D, Verjee S, Rees S, Murphy MF, Roberts DJ. Platelet transfusion in neonatal alloimmune thrombocytopenia. *Blood.* 2007;109:388–389.
15. Kiefel V, Bassler D, Kroll H, et al. Antigen-positive platelet transfusion in neonatal alloimmune thrombocytopenia (NAIT). *Blood.* 2006;107:3761–3763.
16. Bussel J. Diagnosis and management of the fetus and neonate with alloimmune thrombocytopenia. *J Thromb Haemost.* 2009;7(Suppl 1):253–257.

CHAPTER 92

Polycythemia

Clara Lo and Wendy Wong

INTRODUCTION

The normal hematocrit of a healthy term infant ranges from 45% to 61%. This relatively high red cell mass is an adaptive response to the hypoxic intrauterine environment. Neonatal polycythemia, an abnormal elevation of red cell mass, is most often defined in textbooks as a venous hematocrit of 65% or more. It occurs in 1.5%–4% of healthy live births.[1] Passive erythrocyte transfusion and increased fetal red cell production are 2 major causes for neonatal polycythemia.

Many patients are asymptomatic. When present, signs and symptoms are presumed to be secondary to associated hyperviscosity. Although not all polycythemic blood is hyperviscous, there is an exponential increase in blood viscosity when the hematocrit is 65% or higher, with a correlative decrease in oxygen transport (Figure 93-1). Poor oxygenation and microthrombi formation are believed to result in organ dysfunction in polycythemia. The central nervous, cardiopulmonary, endocrine, and gastrointestinal systems are commonly affected. Treatment of symptomatic polycythemia is partial exchange transfusion (XT). However, criteria for and benefit from this treatment are controversial.

DIAGNOSIS AND INDICATION

Clinical Findings: History and Physical

Causes of polycythemia in neonates can be divided into 2 major categories: passive red blood cell (RBC) transfusion and increased erythropoiesis secondary to intrauterine hypoxia. During delivery, passive placental RBC transfusion can occur from delayed cord clamping or if the infant is held below the level of the introitus. Perinatal asphyxia and maternal oxytocin administration have also been known to increase placental RBC transfer to the fetus.[3] In monochorionic twin pregnancies, twin-twin transfusion results in polycythemia in the recipient, who most commonly is the larger infant.

Increased erythropoiesis can occur in response to intrauterine hypoxia, and result in neonatal polycythemia. This is seen in pregnancies with placental insufficiency, which can result from multiple etiologies (Table 93-1). Increased erythropoiesis is also seen in pregnancies with increased fetal oxygen consumption, including congenital thyrotoxicosis and maternal diabetes.[3]

Polycythemia has been observed in neonates with trisomy 13, 18, and 21, as well as in those with Beckwith-Weidemann syndrome. The cause of polycythemia in patients with these genetic disorders is not known. Infants who are large or small for gestational age are also at risk. A comprehensive list of factors is outlined in Table 93-1.

The American Academy of Pediatrics (AAP) does not recommend routine screening for polycythemia.[4] However, screening should be done in neonates who are at risk or have clinical signs suspicious for polycythemia. Common early signs include plethora, jitteriness, and poor feeding. Tachypnea, abdominal distention, irritability, and lethargy are also common. Hypoglycemia and hypocalcemia are frequently observed endocrine abnormalities, with up to 40% of patients having hypoglycemia. Associated hematologic complications include hyperbilirubinemia and thrombocytopenia. Neonates with polycythemia may also have significantly decreased

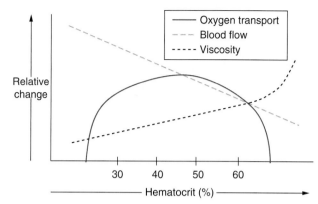

FIGURE 93-1 Effect of hematocrit on blood flow, viscosity, and oxygen transport. (Adapted with permission from Glader.[2])

CHAPTER 93

gastrointestinal blood flow, which places them at risk for necrotizing enterocolitis (NEC). Renal vein thrombosis, proteinuria, and priapism are other rarer symptoms. A more comprehensive list of clinical features is outlined in Table 93-2. It is important to note that these signs and symptoms are not specific for polycythemia, and when present, other causes for these abnormalities should also be investigated.

Baseline and Confirmatory Tests

To accurately diagnose polycythemia, there are 3 major areas that require attention: site of blood draw, timing of draw, and mode of analysis. Capillary blood flow can have significant variability and result in up to 15% higher hemoglobin and hematocrit values compared to venous samples.[1] Therefore, a capillary hematocrit of 65% or greater needs to be confirmed with a venous sample.

The timing of blood draws needs to be noted as hematocrit values peak 2 hours postpartum, at which time values up to 71% may be considered normal.[5] This initial increase in hematocrit is related to movement of fluid from the intravascular to the extravascular space.

After this point, values begin to decrease in response to higher extrauterine ambient oxygen concentrations. Therefore, screening is best done after 6 to 8 hours of life if performed in an asymptomatic infant.[6] Earlier testing may be considered in patients with risk factors for, or clinical signs of, polycythemia. Finally, the method of hematocrit analysis is known to affect values. Spun hematocrits are more accurate and have greater correlation with blood viscosity compared to those analyzed by automated counters. However, most hospitals now use automated hematology counters.

Blood viscosity is thought to be the major culprit for the signs associated with polycythemia. It is affected by more than the red cell mass. Plasma viscosity, erythrocyte aggregation and rigidity, blood vessel diameter, and RBC shear force are other important determinants.[7] A high hematocrit (≥65%) is therefore not always associated with hyperviscosity by blood viscosity studies. Whole-blood viscosity can be measured using a microviscometer at various shear rates. However, because of the limited availability of this tool, viscosity is not routinely measured, and hematocrit remains the surrogate diagnostic marker for hyperviscosity.

Table 93-1 Factors and Conditions Associated With Neonatal Polycythemia

Erythrocyte Transfusion	Increased Fetal Erythropoiesis	Other Fetal Risk Factors

• Delayed cord clamping
• Cord stripping
• Delivery below the level of the introitus
• Twin-twin transfusion
• Maternal-fetal transfusion
• Maternal oxytocin administration
• Perinatal asphyxia
	• Intrauterine growth restriction
	• Maternal diabetes
	• Delivery at high altitudes
	• Congenital thyrotoxicosis
	• Placental insufficiency
	  • Preeclampsia
	  • Gestational hypertension
	  • Chronic/recurrent placental abruption
	  • Maternal cyanotic heart disease
	  • Postdate pregnancy
	  • Maternal smoking
	  • Maternal heavy alcohol intake
		• Trisomy 13, 18, 21
		• Congenital hypothyroidism
		• Congenital adrenal hyperplasia
		• Beckwith-Weidemann syndrome
		• Large for gestational age
		• Small for gestational age

Table 93-2 Clinical Features Associated With Polycythemia and Hyperviscosity

Central nervous system	Hypotonia, jitteriness, irritability, lethargy, seizures, stroke Late effects: motor deficits, lower intelligence quotient scores
Endocrine	Hypoglycemia, hypocalcemia
Cardiopulmonary	Tachypnea, tachycardia, cyanosis, plethora, apnea, pleural effusions, cardiomegaly, pulmonary hypertension, decreased cardiac output
Gastrointestinal	Poor feeding, vomiting, necrotizing enterocolitis, cholestasis/cholelithiasis
Hematologic	Thrombocytopenia, hyperbilirubinemia
Renal	Proteinuria, oliguria, renal vein thrombosis, renal tubular damage
Miscellaneous	Priapism, peripheral gangrene

Diagnostic Algorithm

Screening should be performed in those at risk or in those who have clinical features suspicious for polycythemia. Given the ease of capillary sampling in this population, it is reasonable to screen with a capillary hematocrit. A normal capillary hematocrit at 2 hours of life rules out polycythemia, and no repeat testing is necessary unless the patient becomes symptomatic.[5]

If a capillary sample demonstrates a hematocrit of 65% or greater, a venous sample should be drawn to confirm the finding. Asymptomatic infants with peripheral venous hematocrits between 65% and 70% can be observed without immediate treatment. However, they should be closely monitored for signs associated with polycythemia and hyperviscosity. These include metabolic imbalances such as hypoglycemia and hypocalcemia. In particular, hypoglycemia combined with polycythemia is associated with poorer neurocognitive outcomes.[8,9] Patients should also be monitored for jaundice, and serum bilirubin levels should be drawn if indicated. Lethargy, poor feeding, feeding intolerance, and cardiorespiratory symptoms are other common signs. Dehydration, which can cause hemoconcentration and falsely elevate the hematocrit, needs to be ruled out and treated if present. If the patient remains asymptomatic, a venous hematocrit should be repeated in 12 to 24 hours. Infants who remain asymptomatic by 48 to 72 hours of age will likely remain asymptomatic.

TREATMENT

In asymptomatic patients with a hematocrit of 70% or higher, the management is controversial. Historically, these patients underwent XT to reduce their hematocrit. However, recent studies demonstrated no long-term difference in outcome between patients who did and did not undergo XT treatment.[6,9–11]

If a neonate has a venous hematocrit greater than 65% and has clinical signs associated with polycythemia and hyperviscosity, treatment with partial XT should be considered. The principle of XT is to reduce the hematocrit and blood viscosity while maintaining circulatory volume. The most common technique is through umbilical venous catheterization. Alternate routes may also be used, particularly in cases of omphalitis or difficulties with umbilical vein cannulation. These alternates include umbilical arterial-peripheral venous exchange and peripheral venous exchange.

During XT, withdrawal of blood is performed with concordant volume replacement. The procedure is typically done in 5- to 10-mL aliquots, depending on the neonate's weight and treatment tolerance. Feedings should be held during XT. Vital signs should be continually monitored, with immediate resuscitative measures for any instability. It is also important to closely monitor calcium and glucose levels and to have medical therapy readily available to address disturbances.

Both colloid and crystalloid solutions have been used as replacement fluid for XT. Colloid solutions include fresh frozen plasma (FFP) and 5% albumin. Commonly used crystalloid solutions include isotonic saline and Ringer's lactate. In randomized controlled trials, crystalloid solutions have demonstrated similar decreases in venous hematocrit and hyperviscosity symptoms compared with colloid solutions, without the potential risk of transfusion-associated infections or reactions.[12,13] They are also inexpensive and readily available. Therefore, crystalloids are now the preferred replacement fluid for XT.[12,13]

The equation to calculate the total exchange volume is outlined in Table 93-3. The desired hematocrit is typically 50%–55%, with goals at the lower end of this range in cases of hyperviscosity symptoms that are more significant. As a general rule, the volume of exchanged blood is typically 20 mL/kg.

In the absence of symptoms, initiation of XT is controversial because its potential benefits may be outweighed by its reported complications. Reported complications include NEC, thrombocytopenia, catheter malfunction, hypotension, and sepsis.[14]

Based on these findings, we recommend the following for asymptomatic patients: close monitoring and potential intravenous hydration for hematocrit values between 65% and 70% and consideration of XT for patients whose hematocrit values exceed 70% (Figure 93-2).

Table 93-3 Partial Exchange Transfusion for Neonatal Polycythemia

Preprocedure management	• Evaluate for and manage signs and symptoms (Table 93-2) • Initiate parenteral nutrition, hold feedings • Obtain venous access
Partial exchange transfusion	Formula to calculate total blood exchange volume desired: $$\text{Total exchange volume (mL)} = \frac{\text{Blood volume (mL)}^* \times (\text{Observed Hct\%} - \text{Desired Hct\%})}{\text{Observed Hct\%}}$$ *Blood volume in term neonates estimated to be 80–90 mL/kg; blood volume in preterm neonates estimated to be 90–100 mL/kg. • Desired Hct%: 50%–55% • 5- to 10-mL aliquot concordant volume exchange • Crystalloid volume replacement: isotonic saline, Ringer's lactate
Postprocedure management	• Hold feedings for 2–4 hours after XT completion; monitor for NEC • Monitor fluid status; diurese or volume replace as necessary • Continue supportive care as necessary

Abbreviations: NEC, necrotizing enterocolitis; Hct%, hematocrit%; XT, partial exchange transfusion.

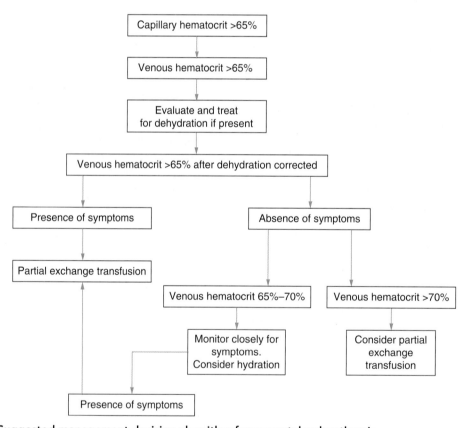

FIGURE 93-2 Suggested management decision algorithm for neonatal polycythemia.

FOLLOW-UP

Aftercare Monitoring

Exchange transfusion through the umbilical vein route is associated with an increased risk of NEC.[9–11] This association is particularly strong when XT is performed with colloid solutions. Therefore, feedings should be withheld for 2 to 4 hours after XT completion, after which time feedings can be slowly initiated and close monitoring should continue.

Monitoring and correction of metabolic disturbances should be continued after cessation of XT until values normalize. Fluid status should also be evaluated, as patients may require diuresis or further volume replacement after XT. Cardiopulmonary symptoms associated with polycythemia should resolve with adequate treatment; however, symptoms may persist until fluid imbalances are corrected.

Long-Term Outcome

Clinical outcome studies revealed measurable benefits following XT. These include improved cardiopulmonary function, renal function, and feeding tolerance.[6,11] However, despite XT, patients with a history of neonatal polycythemia have an increased incidence and risk of late-onset neurodevelopmental delays; this is particularly true for patients with a history of concordant hypoglycemia.[8,9] These delays include motor deficits, lower intelligence quotient scores, and lower achievement scores. Outcome studies have not demonstrated long-term neurodevelopmental benefits from XT.[6,9–11] This finding suggests that neurocognitive late effects are primarily caused by the underlying etiologies rather than the polycythemia itself. This finding also highlights the need for continued neurodevelopmental monitoring and therapy for children with a history of neonatal polycythemia.

REFERENCES

1. Kates EH, Kates JS: Anemia and polycythemia in the newborn. *Pediatr Rev.* 2007;28(1):33–34.
2. Glader BE. Erythrocyte disorders in infancy. In: Taeusch HW, Ballard RA, Avery ME, eds. *Diseases of the Newborn.* 6th ed. Philadelphia, PA: Saunders;1991:822–823.
3. Remon J, Raghavan A, Maheshwari A. Polycythemia in the newborn. *Neoreviews.* 2011;11(1):e20–e28.
4. Committee on Fetus and Newborn. Routine evaluation of blood pressure, hematocrit, and glucose in newborns. *Pediatrics.* 1993;92(3):474–476.
5. Jeevasankar M, Agarwal R, Chawla D, et al. Polycythemia in the Newborn. *Indian J Pediatr.* 2008;75:68–72.
6. Pappas A, Delaney-Black V. Differential diagnosis and management of polycythemia. *Pediatr Clin North Am.* 2004;51:1063–1086.
7. Linderkamp O. Blood viscosity of the neonate. *Neoreviews.* 2004;5(10):e406–e416.
8. Sarkar S, Rosenkrantz TS. Neonatal polycythemia and hyperviscosity. *Semin Fetal Neonatal Med.* 2008;13(4):248–255.
9. Mimouni FB, Merlob P, Dollberg S, et al. Neonatal polycythaemia: critical review and a consensus statement of the Israeli Neonatology Association. *Acta Paediatr.* 2011;100(10):1290–1296. Epub ahead of print.
10. Ozek E, Soll R, Schimmel MS. Partial exchange transfusion to prevent neurodevelopmental disability in infants with polycythemia. *Cochrane Database Syst Rev.* 2010;(1):CD005089.
11. Demsey EM, Barrington K. Short and long term outcomes following partial exchange transfusion in the polycythemic newborn: a systematic review. *Arch Dis Child Fetal Neonatal Ed.* 2006;91(1):F2–F6.
12. Demsey Em, Barrington K. Crystalloid or colloid for partial exchange transfusion in neonatal polycythemia: a systematic review and meta-analysis. *Acta Paediatr.* 2005;94:1650–1655.
13. de Waal KA, Baerts W, Offringa M. Systematic review of the optimal fluid for dilutional exchange transfusion in neonatal polycytaemia. *Arch Dis Child Fetal Neonatal Ed.* 2006;91:F7–F10.
14. Hopewell B, Steiner LA, Ehrenkranz RA, et al. Partial exchange transfusion for polycythemia hyperviscosity syndrome. *Am J Perinatol.* 2011;28(7):557–564.

CHAPTER 93

Transient Myeloproliferative Disorder

Jay Michael S. Balagtas and Norman Lacayo

INTRODUCTION

Transient myeloproliferative disorder (TMD) is a unique clonal proliferation of megakaryocytic precursors that is clinically indistinguishable from congenital leukemia and is seen almost exclusively in neonates with trisomy 21 (Down syndrome).[1] TMD is typically characterized by the presence of leukocytosis and circulating blast cells in the blood of an otherwise healthy-appearing newborn. These blast cells will generally resolve spontaneously by 3–6 months of age without any specific interventions.[2] However, approximately 20% of patients will present with severe hydrops, organomegaly, hepatic fibrosis, and other life-threatening complications, with an associated mortality rate approaching 45% at 3 years.[3]

Because of their clinical heterogeneity, patients with TMD have been classified into 3 distinct groups: high risk, intermediate risk, and low risk[4] (Table 94-1). High-risk patients with TMD (20%) include those with severe life-threatening complications, such as cardiorespiratory compromise, hyperleukocytosis (white blood cells [WBCs] > 100 × 10³/μL) and liver failure (with attendant cholestasis, ascites, or disseminated intravascular coagulation [DIC]). The intermediate-risk patients (40%) include infants with hepatomegaly and hepatic dysfunction but no acute life-threatening complications. Interestingly, although these patients rarely die from acute TMD-related complications, they still have an overall mortality of 23% at 3 years. In contrast, the low-risk patients (40%) experience an 8% overall mortality at 3 years.

Approximately 10%–20% of newborns with Down syndrome with TMD develop acute myeloid leukemia (AML) within the first 2 years of life.[1] This leukemia most commonly takes the form of acute megakaryoblastic leukemia (AMKL) and can be traced to the patient's original TMD by unique genetic markers (ie, GATA1 mutations).[5–7]

CLINICAL FINDINGS

History and Physical

The patient with "classic" TMD is an otherwise healthy-appearing infant with physical characteristics suggestive of trisomy 21 (eg, epicanthal folds, hypotonia, single palmar crease). However, as discussed, patients with higher-risk TMD may present with cardiorespiratory compromise caused by severe hydrops (with concomitant edema, pericardial/pleural effusions, ascites) or marked hepatosplenomegaly. Patients may also present with signs and symptoms of hyperviscosity syndrome secondary to hyperleukocytosis, with attendant thrombotic complications. These symptoms may include respiratory distress, apnea, lethargy, irritability, seizures, or other stroke-like symptoms. More recently, an association with a vesiculopustular rash that typically appears on the face has been reported, although the exact relationship with TMD remains unclear.[8–10] Finally, it should be noted that patients with mosaicism of trisomy 21 may not demonstrate any of the physical characteristics of Down syndrome but may present only with TMD.[11,12] Therefore, the

Table 94-1 Transient Myeloproliferative Disorder (TMD) Risk Groups

	Low-Risk TMD	Intermediate-Risk TMD	High-Risk TMD
Percentage of TMD	40	40	20
Clinical characteristics	No hepatomegaly *OR* hepatomegaly without hepatic dysfunction No life-threatening complications	Hepatomegaly plus evidence of non-life-threatening hepatic dysfunction (ie, significantly elevated AST, ALT, or bilirubin) No life-threatening complications	Cardiorespiratory compromise, edema, pericardial/pleural effusions, hyperleukocytosis, hepatomegaly, life-threatening hepatic dysfunction
Therapy	Observation only	Strongly consider very-low-dose cytarabine therapy	Aggressive supportive care (ie, exchange transfusion or leukopheresis) Very-low-dose cytarabine therapy

Abbreviations: ALT, alanine aminotransferase; AST, aspartate aminotransferase.

presence of proliferating blasts in a neonate without obvious signs of trisomy 21 should prompt consideration of a diagnosis of mosaic trisomy 21.

Laboratory Testing

All infants with either a prenatal diagnosis of or physical characteristics consistent with trisomy 21 should have a screening complete blood cell count (CBC) with differential within the first 24 hours of life. TMD is usually diagnosed by the presence of circulating blast cells on a blood smear in conjunction with leukocytosis, although the range of WBC values can be broad (4.6–259 × 10^3/μL, with a median value of 32.8 × 10^3/μL).[4] Hepatic dysfunction, as evidenced by elevated liver transaminases, bilirubin, or prothrombin time/partial thromboplastin time (PT/PTT), is an important component of risk stratification and can be a potentially life-threatening complication. Tumor lysis laboratory values (potassium, creatinine, phosphate, calcium, lactate dehydrogenase [LDH], uric acid) should also be monitored, especially in patients with markedly elevated WBC counts. Additional laboratory testing is generally not necessary in classic TMD, but flow cytometry and cytogenetics may be required for atypical presentations.

Differential Diagnosis

In an infant presenting with leukocytosis and circulating blast cells, consideration should be given to congenital viral and bacterial infections. Increased bone marrow turnover secondary to a hemolytic process (ie, hemolytic disease of the newborn) may also present similarly. Although the WBC count may be significantly elevated in these cases, circulating blast percentage is generally low and can be helpful in distinguishing these entities from TMD.

Another important diagnosis to consider is that of congenital myeloid leukemia. Like TMD, congenital leukemia presents with leukocytosis and significantly elevated blast percentage, but unlike TMD, it is a progressive disease and does not spontaneously resolve. While hemoglobin and platelet levels in TMD tend not be as depressed as in frank leukemia,[13] TMD and congenital leukemia may be otherwise clinically indistinguishable. Consideration should therefore be given to sending blood or bone marrow aspirate for flow cytometry and cytogenetics. Fortunately, congenital leukemia is a rare entity and differentiation from TMD is possible in most, but not all, cases.

Pretreatment Workup

As previously noted, any infant presenting with physical characteristics suggestive of trisomy 21 should have a CBC with differential and smear within the first 24 hours of life. The finding of circulating blasts with or without leukocytosis should prompt consultation with a pediatric hematologist/oncologist. Subsequent workup, treatment, and follow-up should then be performed with the assistance of a pediatric hematologist/oncologist.

A patient with classic TMD will require little workup beyond serial CBCs and liver transaminase testing, but an atypical patient (ie, phenotypically normal infant or a higher-risk TMD patient) may require flow cytometry and cytogenetic testing to establish a definitive diagnosis. In general, flow cytometry of TMD is positive for the megakaryocytic markers CD41 and CD61, although the M7 (megakaryoblastic) variant of AML may also express these markers. The stem cell marker CD34, with coexpression of CD7, and variable expression of the panmyeloid markers CD13 and CD33 may be present in TMD as well.[14] Cytogenetically, TMD is characterized by few cytogenetic aberrations other than trisomy 21, in contrast to acute leukemias.[13]

SUPPORTIVE MANAGEMENT

Subsequent management of TMD is determined by the infant's clinical stability and risk stratification. Because low-risk TMD patients demonstrate no evidence of life-threatening complications, these patients will typically require only "watchful waiting" with occasional laboratory testing to monitor WBC count, blast percentage, and hepatic function. By definition, intermediate-risk TMD patients will also be clinically stable, with no evidence of life-threatening complications. However, these patients typically do have evidence of hepatomegaly and hepatic dysfunction, with an increased risk of development of hepatic fibrosis and later mortality.[4] Recent evidence suggests that intermediate-risk patients may benefit from early treatment with cytarabine at a very low dose.[2,15,16]

Because high-risk TMD patients may present in an unstable manner (ie, cardiorespiratory compromise, hydrops), initial management of these patients may involve active airway management, fluid resuscitation, vasopressor support, and so on. These interventions are covered elsewhere in this book and are not discussed in detail here. If a patient with TMD presents with hyperleukocytosis (WBC > $100 \times 10^3/\mu L$), the infant will be at risk for tumor lysis syndrome and should be monitored with tumor lysis laboratory studies (see discussion of laboratory testing) and started on allopurinol with intravenous hydration. Rasburicase should be considered if the uric acid level reaches greater than 8 mg/dL. Patients with TMD with hyperleukocytosis are also at risk for hyperviscosity syndrome because of the decreased malleability of the circulating blast cells. Consideration should therefore be given to performing an exchange transfusion or leukopheresis to quickly decrease the WBC count. Cytarabine therapy should then be instituted as soon as possible because there can be a propensity for the WBC count to rapidly "bounce back" to dangerous levels.

TREATMENT

If given early, very-low-dose cytarabine therapy has been shown to significantly reduce mortality associated with hepatic dysfunction and other high-risk features.[2,3,15–17] The most commonly used regimens recommend a dose of 0.4–1.5 mg/kg/dose every 12 hours for 3–12 days. The majority of patients will require only 1 cycle of cytarabine therapy to reduce WBC count or hepatic dysfunction to acceptable levels. A few patients, however, will demonstrate a more limited response and may require additional courses of chemotherapy. The very-low-dose cytarabine regimen itself is well tolerated in our experience, with minimal side effects. Higher-dose regimens do not appear to add any significant benefit and carry the risk of increased toxicity.

CLINICAL FOLLOW-UP

The natural history of low-risk TMD is eventual clearance of circulating blast cells over the course of 3–6 months. This natural history also holds true for successfully treated intermediate-risk and high-risk TMD patients; however, these patients are more likely to also have medical complications (ie, hepatic fibrosis) that may require intensive follow-up care. Regardless of risk stratification, all patients with TMD are at significant risk for the development of AMKL in the first 2 years of life. A number of TMD patients will also develop myelodysplastic syndrome (MDS), which may, or may not, serve as a precursor to full-blown AMKL. At this time, the risk of MDS and AMKL development does not appear to be altered by cytarabine therapy and cannot be reliably predicted based on other prognostic factors. All patients with TMD should therefore receive close follow-up by a pediatric hematologist/oncologist for outpatient monitoring. This will allow early detection of disease and the prompt institution of appropriate chemotherapy.

REFERENCES

1. Zipursky A. Transient leukaemia—a benign form of leukaemia in newborn infants with trisomy 21. *Br J Haematol.* 2003;120(6):930–938.
2. Massey GV, Zipursky A, Chang MN, et al. A prospective study of the natural history of transient leukemia (TL) in neonates with Down syndrome (DS): Children's Oncology Group (COG) study POG-9481. *Blood.* 2006;107(12):4606–4613.
3. Al-Kasim F, Doyle JJ, Massey GV, et al. Incidence and treatment of potentially lethal diseases in transient leukemia of Down syndrome: Pediatric Oncology Group Study. *J Pediatr Hematol Oncol.* 2002;24(1):9–13.
4. Gamis AS, Alonzo TA, Gerbing RB, et al. Natural history of transient myeloproliferative disorder clinically diagnosed in Down syndrome neonates: a report from the Children's Oncology Group Study A2971. *Blood.* 2011;118(26):6752–6759, quiz 6996.
5. Gurbuxani S, Vyas P, Crispino JD. Recent insights into the mechanisms of myeloid leukemogenesis in Down syndrome. *Blood.* 2004;103(2):399–406.
6. Vyas P, Crispino JD. Molecular insights into Down syndrome-associated leukemia. *Curr Opin Pediatr.* 2007;19(1):9–14.
7. Vyas P, Roberts I. Down myeloid disorders: a paradigm for childhood preleukaemia and leukaemia and insights into normal megakaryopoiesis. *Early Hum Dev.* 2006;82(12):767–773.
8. Moriuchi R, Shibaki A, Yasukawa K, et al. Neonatal vesiculopustular eruption of the face: a sign of trisomy 21-associated transient myeloproliferative disorder. *Br J Dermatol.* 2007;156(6):1373–1374.
9. Nornhold E, Li A, Rothman IL, et al. Vesiculopustular eruption associated with transient myeloproliferative disorder. *Cutis.* 2009;83(5):234–236.

10. Piersigilli F, Diociaiuti A, Boldrini R, et al. Vesiculopustular eruption in a neonate with trisomy 21 syndrome as a clue of transient myeloproliferative disorders. *Cutis.* 2010;85(6): 286–288.

11. Hanna MD, Melvin SL, Dow LW, et al. Transient myeloproliferative syndrome in a phenotypically normal infant. *Am J Pediatr Hematol Oncol.* 1985;7(1):79–81.

12. Ridgway D, Benda GI, Magenis E, et al. Transient myeloproliferative disorder of the Down type in the normal newborn. *Am J Dis Child.* 1990;144(10):1117–1119.

13. Hayashi Y, Eguchi M, Sugita K, et al. Cytogenetic findings and clinical features in acute leukemia and transient myeloproliferative disorder in Down's syndrome. *Blood.* 1988;72(1):15–23.

14. Litz CE, Davies S, Brunning RD, et al. Acute leukemia and the transient myeloproliferative disorder associated with Down syndrome: morphologic, immunophenotypic and cytogenetic manifestations. *Leukemia.* 1995;9(9):1432–1439.

15. Klusmann JH, Creutzig U, Zimmermann M, et al. Treatment and prognostic impact of transient leukemia in neonates with Down syndrome. *Blood.* 2008;111(6):2991–2998.

16. Lange B. The management of neoplastic disorders of haematopoiesis in children with Down's syndrome. *Br J Haematol.* 2000;110(3):512–524.

17. Dormann S, Kruger M, Hentschel R, et al. Life-threatening complications of transient abnormal myelopoiesis in neonates with Down syndrome. *Eur J Pediatr.* 2004;163(7):374–377.

CHAPTER 94

95 Management of Abdominal Wall Defects

Zachary Kastenberg and Matias Bruzoni

DIAGNOSIS

Omphalocele and gastroschisis represent the 2 most frequently encountered abdominal wall defects requiring neonatal intensive care. As discussed previously in this book, these defects occur in roughly 1–3 per 10,000 live births. Although the incidence of omphalocele has remained constant in recent years, the incidence of gastroschisis has been increasing for unclear reasons.

Clinical Findings

Omphalocele is associated with advanced maternal age and karyotype abnormalities; gastroschisis is associated with maternal age less than 20, smoking, and use of over-the-counter vasoactive drugs and salicylates during pregnancy.[1–3] In addition, illicit drug abuse and smoking may influence the severity of gastroschisis.[4]

Omphalocele is characterized by the failure of the viscera to return to the abdominal cavity following physiologic midgut herniation during the 10th week of gestation. As a result, the omphalocele is contained within a protective membranous sac composed of amniotic epithelium lined by peritoneum, with the intervening space filled by Wharton's jelly. The stomach, small bowel, colon, and liver are frequently involved. Associated anomalies occur in 50%–70% of infants with omphalocele; cardiac defects are observed in 30%–50%. Karyotype abnormalities occur in 30% of cases, with trisomies 13, 18, and 21 most common.[2]

Gastroschisis, on the other hand, is characterized by prenatal evisceration through a defect in the anterior abdominal wall, almost always located just to the right of the umbilicus. This right-sided predilection is theorized to be caused by abnormal embryonic regression of the right umbilical vein. Importantly, the eviscerated abdominal contents do not have a protective membrane and are in direct contact with the amniotic fluid. The involved intestine is edematous, sometimes foreshortened, and almost always nonrotated. Of neonates with gastroschisis, 7%–10% will have an associated intestinal atresia. Unlike omphalocele, gastroschisis is not associated with karyotype abnormalities.[2]

The effective management of both omphalocele and gastroschisis hinges on early diagnosis and the involvement of appropriately trained staff (trained nurses, neonatologist, and pediatric surgeons). The embryologic and anatomic differences, however, lead to the differences in management depicted in the discussion that follows.

Confirmatory (Diagnostic) Tests

Prenatal Imaging

The sensitivity and specificity of prenatal ultrasound in identifying abdominal wall defects are 60%–75% and 95%, respectively.[5,6] Once a fetus with an abdominal wall defect is identified, directed ultrasounds should be performed to look for associated anomalies and malformations. Fetal magnetic resonance imaging is gaining popularity and is now used as a reflex imaging study if initial ultrasound is suspicious for gastroschisis or omphalocele in many centers.

Laboratory Tests

There is a marked elevation of maternal serum α-fetoprotein (AFP) in cases of gastroschisis; omphalocele tends to have a more modest AFP elevation (7–9 multiples of the mean compared to 4 multiples of the mean, respectively).[7,8] As discussed previously in another chapter, a positive ultrasound or a significant elevation of maternal serum AFP should lead to a discussion regarding possible amniocentesis or chorionic villus sampling to identify significant chromosomal abnormalities.

Differential Diagnosis

Umbilical Hernia

Umbilical hernias are differentiated from gastroschisis and omphalocele by the presence of normal skin overlying the defect. They contain easily reducible omentum or intestine. Repair is not undertaken in the neonatal period unless incarceration is present as nearly 90% of these defects close spontaneously by 3 to 4 years of age.[9]

Prune Belly Syndrome

Prune belly (Eagle-Barrett) syndrome consists of deficiency or absence of abdominal wall musculature; a constellation of ureteral, bladder, and urethral anomalies; and bilateral cryptorchidism. Prune belly syndrome is distinguished from other abdominal wall defects by complete containment of the abdominal viscera within a continuous layer of skin with a normal umbilicus. In most cases, the lack of abdominal musculature does not cause significant functional impairment.

Megacystis-Microcolon

Megacystis-microcolon is a rare congenital anomaly resulting in a massively distended, nonobstructed bladder and a secondary microcolon, often with associated hypoperistalsis and small-bowel malrotation.[10] The components of the abdominal wall are present and intact, but the abdomen is massively dilated secondary to the mass effect of the dilated bladder. Diagnosis is typically made by preoperative ultrasound, and initial treatment consists of transurethral bladder drainage. The underlying etiology is poorly understood, and the condition is generally not survivable as a result of the severely dysfunctional and underdeveloped gastrointestinal tract.

PRETREATMENT

Ethical Considerations

Advances in neonatal intensive care and surgical technique have made both gastroschisis in the absence of abdominal catastrophe and isolated omphalocele

survivable conditions with little to no long-term morbidity. If however, severe associated anomalies are identified on prenatal imaging or if a significant karyotype abnormality exists, the likelihood of long-term survival is dramatically reduced. A discussion with the parents is necessary to explain the possible outcomes and options, including, if appropriate, pregnancy termination.

Monitoring for Treatment/Procedure/Workup

Serial ultrasounds are necessary to identify any significant comorbidities or fetal compromise.

Sedation/Pain Control Considerations

There are different management options with regard to sedation and analgesia during the reduction of these defects. One option is to intubate the neonate and perform the procedure under general anesthesia along with, most of the time, neuromuscular blockade. In the past few years, there has also been a tendency to perform bedside reductions using oral sucrose solutions for comfort and intravenous narcotics for analgesia. Neuromuscular blockade is not mandatory, and the sedation/analgesia conduct has to be tailored to each particular patient, depending on the size and type of defect, as well as the presence of associated anomalies.

TREATMENT

Prenatal

Early diagnosis and referral to a specialized neonatal center is key to the management of congenital abdominal wall defects. Currently, there is no strong evidence to recommend elective cesarean section vs vaginal delivery, or early vs term delivery in neonates with abdominal wall defects.

Postnatal: Management Algorithm

Both gastroschisis and omphalocele present with varying degrees of severity; nonetheless, the presence of a neonatologist and pediatric surgeon should be considered mandatory in all cases whenever possible. Initial stabilization includes immediate placement of an orogastric tube (OGT) to facilitate visceral decompression, intubation to protect the airway when needed, placement of a urethral catheter in cases of distended bladder to increase the space inside the abdominal cavity, and covering of the exposed viscera with a plastic bag and warm saline. Fluid resuscitation should be aggressive and without delay. The exposed viscera cause significant insensitive fluid loss. Initial resuscitation should include a 20-mL/kg crystalloid bolus followed by two-times maintenance, thereafter. Close blood glucose monitoring is also necessary given the high incidence of Beckwith-Wiedemann syndrome in infants with omphalocele.

After stabilization, the surgeon must assess the viability of the exposed structures. If bowel necrosis is present, the management is much more complicated and the surgical strategy has to be tailored to each particular case. These include emergent resections, creation of stomas, tube diversions, and so on. In the absence of necrosis, the decision on whether to perform a primary vs a delayed reduction depends on the type and size of the defect (omphalocele vs gastroschisis) and the reducibility of the eviscerated structures.

Omphalocele requires postnatal karyotype analysis, echocardiography, renal ultrasound, and detailed physical examination to assess for musculoskeletal defects prior to operative intervention. The definitive intervention depends on the size of the omphalocele. Primary closure of small omphaloceles may be carried out in the immediate neonatal period. Giant omphaloceles, however, are managed by allowing epithelialization of the sac with topical application of silver sulfadiazine, serial reductions with a custom-made splint, and elective repair at 6–24 months (Figures 95-1 through 95-4). Ruptured omphaloceles have a poor prognosis and require silo placement with delayed primary closure. A complete management algorithm for omphalocele is depicted in Figure 95-5.

Gastroschisis is much less commonly associated with other congenital malformations and does not require as extensive a preoperative assessment. Protection of the eviscerated structures is paramount to the early management of neonates with this defect. Primary or

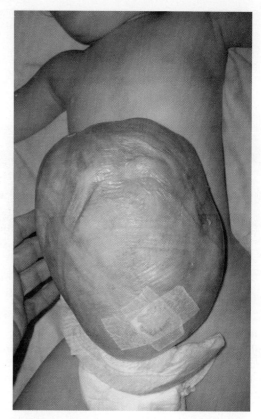

FIGURE 95-2 Giant omphalocele following treatment with silver sulfadiazine. The sac is completely epithelialized.

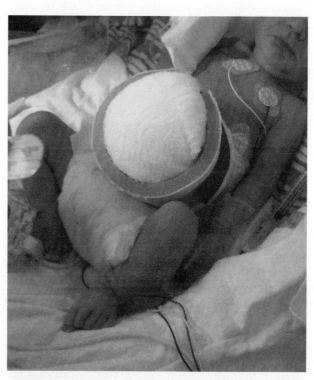

FIGURE 95-3 Custom splint in place overlying an epithelialized omphalocele. Serial tightening of the splint assists reduction of the omphalocele contents.

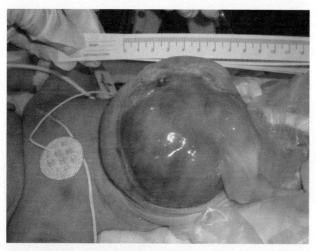

FIGURE 95-1 Giant omphalocele contained within its protective sac. Liver is seen through the sac on the infant's right. The umbilical cord emanates from the apex of the omphalocele.

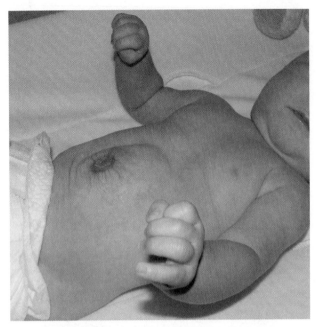

FIGURE 95-4 Completely reduced omphalocele. The umbilicus will continue to heal by secondary intention/contracture. Umbilicoplasty is often undertaken at a later stage depending on the ultimate cosmetic outcome.

delayed reduction of the eviscerated abdominal organs is still controversial, and there is growing evidence to suggest that a nonoperative reduction may be undertaken with comparable outcomes (Figure 95-6).[11-13] Defects with easily reducible contents are typically repaired primarily with either sutured or sutureless repair (Figure 95-6). Large eviscerations require silo placement with a delayed closure (Figures 95-7 through 95-10). A complete management algorithm for gastroschisis is depicted in Figure 95-11.

Postreduction: Aftercare

The management of both omphalocele and gastroschisis following reduction focuses on nutritional balance and early recognition of comorbidities. Most surgeons and neonatologists recommend 48 hours of antibiotics following reduction or establishment of silo protection. Parenteral nutrition is established early in all cases of gastroschisis given the near ubiquity of prolonged ileus and is given selectively in omphalocele if ileus is expected. Orogastric feeds are initiated as OGT output decreases and bowel function returns. Given the extent of the ileus in cases of gastroschisis, workup for stricture/atresia is not undertaken until 6 weeks of life. If oral feedings are not tolerated at 6 weeks, an upper gastrointestinal study with small bowel follow through is obtained, and delayed repair of any stricture or atresia is planned (Table 95-1).

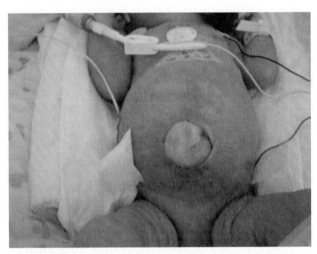

FIGURE 95-6 Primary reduction and sutureless closure of gastroschisis. The defect will close over time by secondary intention.

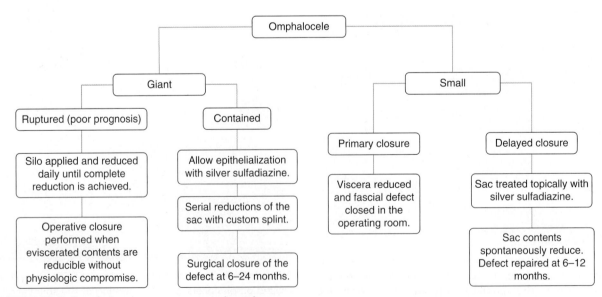

FIGURE 95-5 Omphalocele management algorithm.

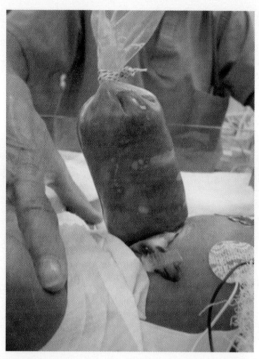

FIGURE 95-7 Silastic silo placement over the eviscerated intestines. Note the characteristic location of the gastroschisis defect to the right of the umbilicus.

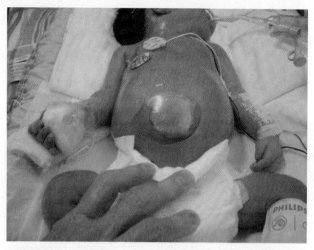

FIGURE 95-9 After complete reduction of the intestine, a sutureless closure is performed, with healing to occur by secondary intention. Alternatively, an operative closure may be performed at this stage.

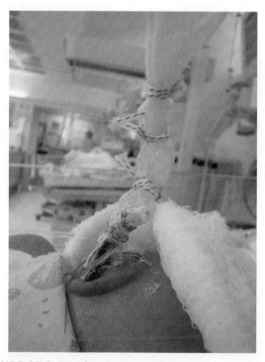

FIGURE 95-8 Serial reductions of the eviscerated intestines by tying off successive segments of the silo.

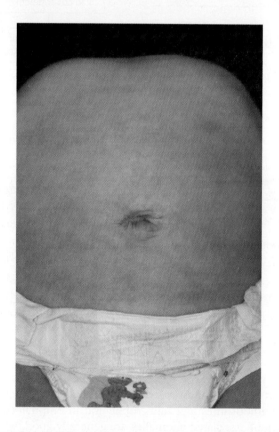

FIGURE 95-10 Outcome in an infant with gastroschisis treated with silo reduction followed by sutureless closure.

CONCLUSION/FOLLOW-UP

Omphalocele and gastroschisis encompass the majority of severe abdominal wall defects encountered in the neonatal period. Prenatal diagnosis, referral to an experienced center, and immediate postnatal

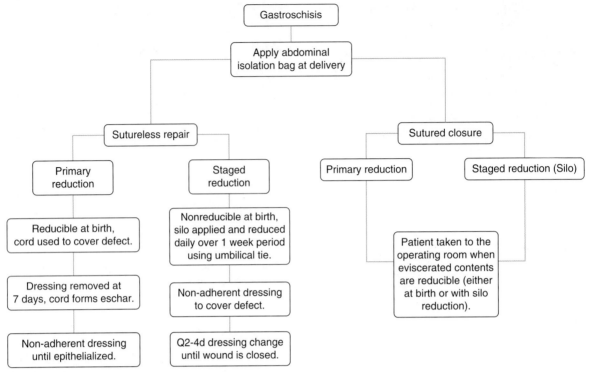

FIGURE 95-11 Gastroschisis management algorithm.

Table 95-1 Typical Postnatal Management of Infants With Omphalocele and Gastroschisis Following Protection of the Eviscerated Organs

	Immediate	Antibiotics	Parenteral Nutrition	Enteral Nutrition	GI Studies
Omphalocele	NPO OGT	48 hrs	If needed	Early on	None required
Gastroschisis	NPO OGT	48 hrs	Yes, ileus expected	As OGT output decreases	UGI with small bowel follow through if not tolerating PO feeds at 6 weeks

Abbreviations: NPO, nothing by mouth; OGT, orogastric tube; UGI, upper gastrointestinal contrast study. The typical postnatal management of these infants focuses on establishment of intravenous access and initiation of parenteral nutrition. The characteristic ileus in cases of gastroschisis is generally longer lasting than that observed in cases of omphalocele. Enteral feeding is started when bowel function returns.

intervention are the key factors to effective management of these conditions. The outcomes in gastroschisis without intestinal catastrophe and in omphalocele without associated anomalies are generally good, with little to no long-term morbidity.

REFERENCES

1. Langer JC. Abdominal wall defects. *World J Surg*. 2003;27(1): 117–124.
2. Ledbetter DJ. Gastroschisis and omphalocele. *Surg Clin North Am*. 2006;86(2):249–260, vii.
3. Mac Bird T, Robbins JM, Druschel C, Cleves MA, Yang S, Hobbs CA. Demographic and environmental risk factors for gastroschisis and omphalocele in the National Birth Defects Prevention Study. *J Pediatr Surg*. 2009;44(8):1546–1551.
4. Weinsheimer RL, Yanchar NL. Impact of maternal substance abuse and smoking on children with gastroschisis. *J Pediatr Surg*. 2008;43(5):879–883.
5. Rankin J, Dillon E, Wright C. Congenital anterior abdominal wall defects in the north of England, 1986–1996: occurrence and outcome. *Prenat Diagn*. 1999;19(7):662–668.
6. Walkinshaw SA, Renwick M, Hebisch G, Hey EN. How good is ultrasound in the detection and evaluation of anterior abdominal wall defects? *Br J Radiol*. 1992;65(772):298–301.
7. Palomaki GE, Hill LE, Knight GJ, Haddow JE, Carpenter M. Second-trimester maternal serum alpha-fetoprotein levels in pregnancies associated with gastroschisis and omphalocele. *Obstet Gynecol*. 1988;71(6 Pt 1):906–909.
8. Saller DN Jr, Canick JA, Palomaki GE, Knight GJ, Haddow JE. Second-trimester maternal serum alpha-fetoprotein, unconjugated

CHAPTER 95

estriol, and hCG levels in pregnancies with ventral wall defects. *Obstet Gynecol*. 1994;84(5):852–855.

9. O'Donnell KA, Glick PL, Caty MG. Pediatric umbilical problems. *Pediatr Clin North Am*. 1998;45(4):791–799.

10. Berdon WE, Baker DH, Blanc WA, Gay B, Santulli TV, Donovan C. Megacystis-microcolon-intestinal hypoperistalsis syndrome: a new cause of intestinal obstruction in the newborn. Report of radiologic findings in five newborn girls. *AJR Am J Roentgenol*. 1976;126(5):957–964.

11. Lansdale N, Hill R, Gull-Zamir S, et al. Staged reduction of gastroschisis using preformed silos: practicalities and problems. *J Pediatr Surg*. 2009;44(11):2126–2129.

12. Riboh J, Abrajano CT, Garber K, et al. Outcomes of sutureless gastroschisis closure. *J Pediatr Surg*. 2009;44(10):1947–1951.

13. Owen A, Marven S, Johnson P, et al. Gastroschisis: a national cohort study to describe contemporary surgical strategies and outcomes. *J Pediatr Surg*. 2010;45(9):1808–1816.

CHAPTER 95

Management of Perforated Necrotizing Enterocolitis

Reed Dimmitt

INTRODUCTION

Necrotizing enterocolitis (NEC) continues to be associated with extreme prematurity, resulting in increased morbidity and mortality. Various studies have reported an incidence of NEC of 14% in infants with a birth weight of 501–750 g and an odds ratio for death of 14 for nonsurgical NEC and 25 for surgical NEC. There remains some controversy regarding the diagnosis of perforated NEC vs spontaneous intestinal perforation, and an ongoing multicenter, randomized, controlled trial is attempting to better define the 2 conditions. Regardless of the etiology, severe inflammation and subsequent necrosis, ischemia, perforation, and peritonitis may result in not only death but also severe neurodevelopmental impairment and intestinal failure (IF).

The 2 common surgical interventions for intestinal perforation are exploratory laparotomy and peritoneal drainage. Several case series and observational studies examined the utility and outcome of both operations. To date, only 2 randomized studies compared the 2 operations, with conflicting results concerning mortality. There is a paucity of data regarding the long-term outcomes of either operation.

This chapter focuses on the dilemma of surgical intervention for intestinal perforation/NEC. This discussion includes preoperative, operative, and postoperative management. In addition, the chapter reviews novel therapies designed to prevent the complications associated with surgical NEC.

PREOPERATIVE MANAGEMENT

It is essential first to determine if a patient actually has perforated NEC. Whenever possible, it is strongly recommended to obtain a pediatric surgical consultation when concerned about perforation. Several clinical scenarios of perforation can present to the caregivers. The first is the presence of free abdominal gas within the peritoneal cavity. A patient may demonstrate a large pneumoperitoneum that is easily appreciated on supine abdominal imaging. Radiographic findings include a large gas bubble or gas surrounding the liver, as well as the so-called football sign by which free abdominal gas highlights the falciform ligament. It can be more difficult to detect when there is less free abdominal gas. In these cases, it is imperative to obtain both supine and left lateral decubitus radiographs. The left lateral decubitus image is preferred to a "cross-table" supine study as the former allows free abdominal gas to migrate between the body wall and the liver and not be confused with a gas-filled loop of intestine. In the absence of free abdominal gas, the determination of intestinal perforation is more challenging.

To date, there are no studies designed to confirm perforation by either radiographic or biomarker methods. There are case reports of clinicians utilizing abdominal paracentesis to detect perforation. This technique is associated with significant complications and should be reserved for patients who require therapeutic paracentesis for severe abdominal distension that is having an impact on ventilation. Often, patients with a "gasless" abdomen or with presumed NEC totalis (extensive NEC involving the entire intestinal tract) may require surgical intervention even with no clinical evidence of perforation.

Once the diagnosis of proven or presumed intestinal perforation is made, the patient needs to be quickly moved to a center where pediatric surgical evaluation can be obtained. Regardless of the location, the ABCs of resuscitation need to be applied. Most patients require tracheal intubation and mechanical ventilation. Establishing arterial catheter monitoring of both ventilation and hemodynamics is desirable. The clinician needs to correct any acid-base imbalance and maintain normal age-appropriate arterial blood pressure. Commonly, there is marked fluid loss into the peritoneal spaces, and patients with NEC and sepsis may become markedly edematous. Resuscitation with large amounts of volume may be necessary to support blood pressure and perfusion of the bowel and kidneys. Maintaining adequate urine output has been associated with improved outcome. It is important to remember that patients with perforated NEC will often deteriorate after their operation, so establishing secure vascular access before the surgery will avoid the potential need for subsequent surgically obtained venous catheters.

Although only 25% of patients with NEC have culture-proven bacteremia, broad-spectrum antibiotics need to be administered. Common initial choices are vancomycin, gram-negative coverage such as an aminoglycoside or piperacillin/tazobactam, and metronidazole as an aerobic bacterial antibiotic. As mentioned, many of these patients have extensive abdominal distention, so placing a large-diameter sump-type orogastric tube with adequate continuous suction will assist in decompression and improve mesenteric perfusion and diaphragmatic excursion.

By developing a long-standing and collegial relationship with pediatric surgeons, the preoperative period can be streamlined. Two major impediments to timely surgical intervention are the availability of an operating room/team and blood products for operation. Many institutions have developed protocols permitting both peritoneal drainage and exploratory laparotomy at the bedside in the neonatal intensive care unit (NICU), thus eliminating the need for an operating room and the time and risk involved in moving the patient. It is important for the nonsurgical clinician to remember that performing a laparotomy requires an entire surgical team and often a pediatric anesthesiologist. Thus, consulting a surgeon early will avoid delays. Last, regardless of surgical procedure choice, cross-matched blood products need to be available prior to any operation.

OPERATIVE MANAGEMENT

Once the decision has been to proceed with surgical intervention, the next step is to determine what type of operation would result in the best outcome. The debate over the preferred operation has a long history and even now is a subject of ongoing clinical research. Prior to 1978, the standard surgical approach for premature infants with perforated NEC was an exploratory laparotomy with resection of diseased intestine. That year, Ein et al reported their experience with a novel surgical intervention in which 5 premature infants underwent peritoneal drainage as a temporizing therapy. The decision to delay laparotomy and default to peritoneal drainage was based on the surgeons' assessment that the patients were too medically unstable to tolerate a definitive operation. In this case series, 3 patients survived and did not require a subsequent laparotomy. The other 2 infants died but were found to have intact intestines at autopsy.

Over the next 20 years, myriad case studies were published comparing primary peritoneal drainage (PPD) to standard laparotomy. Moss et al published a meta-analysis of these studies in 2001. The results of that study demonstrated marked bias in operation choice based on patient birth weight and gestational age, thus making it impossible to determine the best surgical approach. This study was the basis of the first multicenter, randomized, controlled trial comparing patient survival between PPD and laparotomy. The mortality rate in both groups was approximately 35%; thus, the conclusion of the trial was neither operation was superior to the other. A similar study by Rees et al in Europe published in 2008 had similar results, although the authors suggested laparotomy might result in better survival.

At the time of writing, a third multicenter trial funded by the National Institutes of Health was under way, comparing PPD to laparotomy with regard to not only survival but also long-term complications (ie, neurodevelopment and the development of IF).

If the decision is PPD, this operation is usually not performed in the operating room. After adequate sedation, the surgeon surgically places a Penrose drain in the right lower abdominal quadrant through a small incision and secures the drain with a suture. The advantage of PPD is that it avoids a long operation and patient transport. The disadvantages are that the abdomen is not visualized and diseased tissue not resected.

When undergoing laparotomy, the patient receives general anesthesia in the operating room. Once the abdominal cavity is exposed, the surgeon inspects the intestine to determine the site or sites of perforation as well as the extent of necrotic intestine. In some cases, the surgeon is able to resect the affected intestine and perform a primary anastomosis. More often, an enterostomy is created using the proximal portion of the intestine. In some cases, the distal portion of the intestine is used to create a mucous fistula. The fistula promotes drainage and decompression of the distal intestinal tract and can be used for "refeeding" (see postoperative management). If a mucous fistula is not established, the distal intestine is surgically sutured to create a blind pouch. The advantages of a laparotomy are that the surgeon sees the extent of NEC and perforation and any ischemic bowel is removed.

The disadvantages include not only the inherent stress from a large operation but also the quandary about how much intestine to remove. Some patients have obvious demarcation between healthy and diseased intestine, but in others, the line between dead and inflamed/ischemic intestine is unclear. The surgeon can also be presented with a situation where there the entire intestinal tract is necrotic. Historically, in this case no resection is attempted and the patient's abdomen is closed with the anticipation that the infant will receive comfort care and expire. With the advent of novel interventions that are mentioned further in the chapter, some surgeons will resect extensive amounts of intestine in the hope that intestinal rehabilitation or multivisceral transplantation may be possible.

POSTOPERATIVE MANAGEMENT

The postoperative management, both short term and long term, is unique for both surgical approaches. That stated, all patients receive a long course of broad-spectrum antimicrobial therapy. As in the preoperative period, the patients may require escalated ventilator assistance, correction of acidosis (both metabolic and respiratory), multiple transfusions of various blood products, pressor support to maintain adequate hemodynamics, and pain control.

Patients undergoing PPD are closely monitored for worsening clinical parameters. As mentioned, PPD was initially designed as a temporizing operation that evolved into definitive surgical management. Some surgeons will perform a so-called salvage laparotomy soon after PPD if they feel the patient's clinical presentation warrants. More often, the infant is managed with only medical intervention. Most surgeons will wait at least 6 weeks after PPD to assess intestinal integrity. If the patient's abdominal examination normalizes and defecation has resumed, a trial of trophic feedings may be initiated without further intestinal imaging. If, however, there are concerns for an intestinal stricture or other post-NEC complications, contrast imaging is required. The standard decision is to have the patient undergo a contrast enema first as most

NEC-associated strictures occur in the distal bowel. Following passage of the contrast material, the proximal bowel is studied using fluoroscopy to investigate the stomach and duodenum, followed by serial supine radiographs to detect normal passage of contrast material. If there is concern for post-NEC complications, the patient is taken to the operating room for an exploratory laparotomy.

Patients undergoing initial laparotomy have a different postoperative course. The enterostomy is kept moist and observed for signs of necrosis. Once there is passage of intestinal content, an ostomy bag is placed. The nature and volume of ostomy output need to be closely monitored. The mucous fistula, if present, is maintained in a similar manner. Once intestinal function has returned, enteral feedings can be resumed. The location of the enterostomy will dictate enteral feedings based on the volume of output. The surgical teaching for normal output is less than 50 mL/kg/d or 2 mL/kg/h. If there is a proximal enterostomy, there may be a large amount of ostomy output when feedings are resumed. It may be necessary to utilize continuous gavage feedings to prevent "dumping." Human breast milk is the preferred feeding substrate, but patients with a proximal enterostomy or extensive short-bowel may need an elemental formula to allow adequate absorption.

As mentioned, some patients may have a mucous fistula. The fistula can be used to allow enteral feeding advancement. In this technique, the distal intestine is examined using either antegrade or retrograde contrast imaging. If no strictures are present, the contents from the proximal ostomy can be collected into a syringe and infused using a catheter into the distal mucous fistula. This practice has several advantages. By refeeding, the clinician essentially provides a conduit that approximates bowel integrity. Thus, feeding advancement is not limited by the volume of proximal ostomy output but rather by rectal stooling pattern. If the mucous fistula includes a portion of small intestine, it also provides additional absorption of enteral nutrition. In addition, refeeding the distal small intestine promotes the normal enterohepatic circulation and thus prevents cholestasis. Refeeding promotes small intestinal adaptation, which is essential when large amounts of intestine were resected. Last, this technique "primes" the colon for eventual surgical anastomosis by establishing water absorption and a more normal microbiome.

Once the patient is clinically stable and enteral feedings are tolerated, the next decision is when to the patient should undergo intestinal anastomosis. As with PPD, a 6-week waiting period is commonly used before any subsequent operation is performed. Following an anastomosis and return of bowel function, enteral feedings can be resumed.

INTESTINAL REHABILITATION AND INTESTINAL FAILURE-ASSOCIATED LIVER DISEASE

Often, infants who require surgical intervention for perforated NEC develop IF. The current definition of IF is the inability to establish enteral nutrition adequate for reasonable growth without the need for at least some parenteral nutrition. IF is associated with intestinal motility dysfunction, small-bowel bacterial overgrowth, and intestinal failure-associated liver disease (IFALD). Patients with IF may require medications that alter motility, not only to promote normal peristalsis but also to prevent extensive defecation. Some patients with proven or presumed small intestinal bacterial overgrowth respond to a short course of enteral antibiotics followed by a similar course of probiotic therapy.

The etiology of IFALD is likely multifactorial. Ongoing intestinal inflammation and bacterial translocation, lack of enteral feeding with associated cholestasis, and parenteral nutrition have all been thought to contribute to ongoing liver disease. Recently, the amount and composition of the lipid component of parenteral nutrition has been shown to be a major cause of IFALD. One technique to avoid IFALD is lipid restriction. Restricting to 1 g/kg/d or less of a standard omega-6 lipid emulsion has been associated with resolution of IFALD. Even more recently, several centers have reported using a similar dose of reduced omega-3 lipids with even better results. To date, no randomized, controlled trial has compared the 2 lipid preparations for efficacy and safety.

As mentioned, there is often concern regarding the ethical nature of extensive intestinal resection. Although the patient may survive in the short term, the long-term course of patients with short bowel can be difficult. It is important that the clinician understand this when counseling parents about therapeutic options. There are, however, novel therapies that may provide some promise with regard to patients with ultrashort bowel. Many centers have established dedicated multidisciplinary intestinal rehabilitation teams that have been shown to have better outcomes than more traditional caregivers. Bowel-lengthening operations are becoming less complicated and have better results. One such operation is the serial transverse enteroplasty (STEP). This is a simpler operation and can double the length of dilated intestine. Last, the outcomes of multivisceral transplantation have improved over since the mid-2000s, with some centers reporting a 5-year survival of 70%. All of these modalities may provide a degree of hope for parents and caregivers in the face of perforated NEC and extensive necrosis.

SUGGESTED READING

Blakley ML, Tyson JE, Lally KP, et al. Laparotomy versus peritoneal drainage for necrotizing enterocolitis or isolated intestinal perforation in extremely low birth weight infants: outcomes through 18 months adjusted age. *Pediatrics.* 2006;117(4):e680–e687.

Ching YA, Fitzgibbons S, Valim C, et al. Long-term nutritional and clinical outcomes after serial transverse enteroplasty at a single institution. *J Pediatr Surg.* 2009;44(5):939–943.

Hintz SR, Kendrick DE, Stoll BJ, et al. Neurodevelopmental and growth outcomes of extremely low birth weight infants after necrotizing enterocolitis. *Pediatrics.* 2005;115(3):696–703.

Mangus RS, Tector AJ, Kubal CA. Multivisceral transplantation: expanding indications and improving outcomes. *J Gastrointest Surg.* 2013;17(1):179–186.

Moss RL, Dimmitt RA, Barnhart, et al. Laparotomy versus peritoneal drainage for necrotizing enterocolitis and perforation. *N Engl J Med.* 2006;354(21):2225–2234.

Venick RS, Calkins K. The impact of intravenous fish oil emulsions on pediatric intestinal failure-associated liver disease. *Curr Opin Organ Transplant.* 2011;16(3):306–311.

97 Management of Unconjugated Hyperbilirubinemia

Vinod K. Bhutani

INDICATION

Reduction of elevated or increasing unconjugated (indirect) bilirubin levels, measured as total plasma bilirubin (TB) or transcutaneous bilirubin (TcB), is key to the prevention of bilirubin toxicity. Preterm and sick infants are at increased risk for hyperbilirubinemia and its sequelae. Factors that place these populations at risk for hyperbilirubinemia include impaired bilirubin-albumin binding, decreased enteral intake, and decreased gastrointestinal activity, resulting in increased enterohepatic circulation. As a result of biological conditions such as vulnerability of the blood-brain barrier, asphyxia, acidosis, and hypoalbuminemia, neurotoxicity may occur at lower bilirubin levels than for term and healthy infants.

Clinical

Levels of Hyperbilirubinemia

1. Newborns 35 weeks' gestational age (GA) or older
   - Significant hyperbilirubinemia: greater than 95th percentile for age hours
   - Severe hyperbilirubinemia: hour-specific value at which phototherapy is recommended
   - Extreme hyperbilirubinemia: TB greater than 25 mg/dL
2. Newborns less than 35 weeks' GA
   - Significant hyperbilirubinemia: greater than 5 mg/dL (possibly: no consensus opinion)

- Severe hyperbilirubinemia: hour-specific value at which phototherapy is recommended
- Extreme hyperbilirubinemia: TB greater than 20 mg/dL (possibly: no consensus opinion)

Clinical Risk Factors

1. TB greater than 95th percentile for age in hours (≥35 weeks' GA)
2. Neonatal hemolysis (intravascular, extravascular)
3. Male gender
4. Asian race
5. Prematurity (each week)
6. Glucose-6-phosphate dehydrogenase (G-6-PD) deficiency (race/ethnicity: African Americans with jaundice, East Asians, Middle Eastern, and Mediterranean)
7. Maternal diabetes mellitus
8. Suboptimal breast milk intake
9. Early discharge (before age 72 hours)
10. Family history (of jaundice or its treatment)

Clinical Manifestations

Jaundice can be detected by blanching the skin with digital pressure to reveal the underlying skin and subcutaneous tissue color at the forehead, sternum, iliac crest, patella, and malleolus. Jaundice should be assessed whenever the infant's vital signs are measured, but no less than every 8 to 12 hours. The assessment of jaundice must be done in a well-lit room or, preferably, in daylight with ambient sunlight. There is usually a cephalocaudal progression, and sometimes it can fade in and out like a tan. Color varies from lemon yellow to bright orange and sienna. Assessment may be limited by skin pigmentation, plethora, decreased ambient light, and exposure to sun or phototherapy. Absence of jaundice is not an indication of the absence of hyperbilirubinemia; estimating the degree of hyperbilirubinemia can lead to errors, and the absence or severity of jaundice is not predictive of subsequent severe hyperbilirubinemia.

1. *Onset of jaundice* in the first 24 hours of life should be considered a sign of excessive rate of bilirubin rise and indication for emergency bilirubin testing and further evaluation.

2. *Progression of jaundice* is usually seen, with appearance first in the face and progressing caudally to the trunk and extremities, but sometimes it appears and fades similar to a tan.

Testing

1. *TB is measured in plasma* to objectively assess the severity of jaundice. In term and late-preterm infants, this level is plotted on an hour-specific nomogram that identifies risk zones or assessment of clinical risk factors. The hour-specific nomogram provides a more appropriate understanding of the magnitude of hyperbilirubinemia and its projected rate of rise in the contexts of postnatal age in hours and the percentile level as defined for healthy infants.

2. *TcB testing is a noninvasive alternative to TB measurement.* TcB devices are useful screening tools and provide a valid estimate of the TB level, although data are limited.

   a. Measurements in newborns using the new TcB devices are within 2–3 mg/dL of the TB and are useful to screen for or trend TB levels less than 12 mg/dL.

   b. The use of TcB measurements in sick and preterm infants as well as those undergoing phototherapy has not yet been validated.

   c. Confounding effects of skin melanin content among different races and manufacturing consistency among devices are additional limitations.

Differential Diagnosis

Table 97-1 shows the basis for the differential diagnosis.

Table 97-1 Differential Diagnosis

Biological Basis	Clinical Conditions
↑ Bilirubin production	Isoimmunization: Rh, ABO, and minor group incompatibilities RBC enzyme defects: G-6-PD deficiency, pyruvate kinase deficiency, hexokinase deficiency, congenital erythropoietic porphyria, and so on RBC structural defects: hereditary spherocytosis (autosomal dominant; especially if 1 parent has splenomegaly or had splenectomy); hereditary elliptocytosis; infantile pyknocytosis Sepsis: bacterial, viral (eg, CMV), protozoal infestations Extravasted blood: bruising, cephalohematoma, subgaleal bleed, subdural hematoma, hemangiomas Polycythemia
↑ Enterohepatic circulation	Prematurity Starvation Decreased gastrointestinal activity Delayed bacterial colonization of the gut Pyloric stenosis, gastrointestinal immotility or obstruction
↓ Elimination	Crigler-Najjar syndrome (type 1 uridine-glucuronosyl-transferase [UGT]): autosomal recessive, diagnosed by liver biopsy Gilbert syndrome (UGT polymorphisms): neonatal variant often confused as "breast milk jaundice"; sometimes coinherited with G-6-PD deficiency Arias syndrome (type II UGT): autosomal dominant with variable penetrance Transient familial neonatal hyperbilirubinemia (Lucey-Driscoll syndrome): rare, caused by inhibitor of UGT from mother Drugs: such as novobiocin, excessive sedation/paralysis Infant of diabetic mother

Abbreviations: CMV, cytomegalovirus; G-6-PD, glucose-6-phosphate dehydrogenase; RBC, red blood cells.

EVALUATION

Table 97-2 provides information on the clinical evaluation of the jaundiced infant at 35 weeks' gestation and older.

Table 97-2 Clinical Evaluation of the Jaundiced Infant 35 Weeks' Gestation and Older

Indication	Laboratory Assessment/Use of Clinical Tool Kits
Jaundice at age < 24 hours	Measure TcB or TB Assess for neonatal hemolysis
Jaundice excessive for infant's age	Measure TcB or TB
Bilirubin > 40th percentile for age (age 18–60 hours)	Measure TB for TcB > 12 mg/dL Review maternal, birthing, and neonatal history for risk factors Assess GA and risk-related gestational age < 39 weeks Assess for neonatal hemolysis (laboratory tests or ETCOc, if available) Consider G-6-PD quantitative screen Assess phototherapy need (such as BiliTool.org)

Infant receiving phototherapy
TB rising rapidly (such as crossing percentiles)
Unexplained by history and physical examination
	Review results for
	  Blood type and Coombs test, if not obtained with cord blood
	  Complete blood cell count and peripheral smear
	Measure direct or conjugated bilirubin
	Optionally, assay reticulocyte count, G-6-PD, carboxyhemoglobin, or ETCOc (if available)
	Repeat TB in 4–24 hours depending on infant's age and TB level

TB approaching exchange levels Failure of response to phototherapy	Reticulocyte count, G-6-PD, albumin, ETCOc (if available) Blood type and crossmatch for possible exchange transfusion Preparation and consent for possible exchange transfusion Double-check that maximal exposure of light is being delivered (irradiance check, surface area > 80% check, blue light wavelength check)
Elevated direct (or conjugated) bilirubin level	Urinalysis and urine culture Evaluate for sepsis indicated by history and physical examination Review state newborn screen results
Jaundice at age > 2 weeks or a sick infant with jaundice	Total and direct (or conjugated) bilirubin level, G-6-PD (quantitative assay) If direct bilirubin is elevated, evaluate for causes of cholestasis Check results for newborn thyroid and galactosemia screen; review family history of Gilbert disease and confirm results from state newborn screening

Abbreviations: ETCOc, end tidal carbon monoxide, corrected for ambient carbon monoxide; GA, gestational age; G-6-PD, glucose-6-phosphate dehydrogenase; TB, total serum bilirubin; TcB, transcutaneous bilirubin.

TREATMENT STRATEGIES FOR BILIRUBIN REDUCTION

Strategies to rapidly reduce the bilirubin load are described in the 2004 American Academy of Pediatrics Practice Parameters, a recent Technical Report, and an Expert Commentary. Be alert to nonspecific signs of acute bilirubin encephalopathy (ABE), especially in preterm infants. Severely jaundiced babies and symptomatic babies should be admitted directly to the neonatal intensive care unit (NICU).

Interventions for Bilirubin Reduction

Table 97-3 provides the possible interventions for bilirubin reduction.

Table 97-3 Interventions for Bilirubin Reduction

Interventions for Bilirubin Reduction	Choice of Approach
Enteral feedings	Promote breast-feeding as primary preventive strategy
Effective phototherapy	Requires hospitalization
Exchange transfusion	Assess individualized risk-benefit ratio; indicated for clinical signs of acute bilirubin encephalopathy
Chemoprevention	Use of intravenous immunoglobulin (for Rh disease and certain ABO incompatibilities)

Effective Phototherapy

Background Information

The optimal light source is blue-green light with a narrow-range wavelength (such as that provided by light-emitting diodes [LEDs]) that is distributed evenly to 1 plane of the body (and can be increased to both ventral and dorsal planes or even circumferentially) at an irradiance of more than 30 to less than 65 µW/cm² surface area. The effect of light on bilirubin is almost immediate and may not be reflected by measured TB value. The absorption of light by the normal form of bilirubin (4Z,15Z bilirubin), at a peak wavelength of 460 nm, generates transient excited-state bilirubin molecules. These fleeting intermediates can react with oxygen to produce colorless, lower molecular weight products, or they can undergo rearrangement to become structural isomers (lumirubins) or isomers in which the configuration of at least 1 of the 2 Z-configuration double bonds has changed to an E configuration. The plasma from an infant undergoing phototherapy contains several photoisomers, including the predominant 4Z,15E isomer. The photoisomers are less lipophilic than the natural 4Z,15Z form of bilirubin and can be excreted unchanged in the bile without undergoing glucuronidation. Once in bile, the configurational isomers revert spontaneously to the natural bilirubin. Most lumirubins and some photo-oxidation products are excreted in the urine. Bilirubin photoisomer by-products may confound the total bilirubin assay and have an impact on bilirubin's ability to bind to albumin.

Blue lights in the 425- to 475-nm range (Phillips F-20 T12/BB or NeoBlue™) should be easily and rapidly accessible and periodically inspected and maintained to ensure proper functioning. These light sources may be complemented with white halogen lights to cover a wider surface area. Avoid shadows with multiple lights and other interferences for optimal light exposure. Avoid exposure to ultraviolet lights.

Practice Considerations for Optimal Administration of Effective Phototherapy

Table 97-4 discusses practice considerations for the optimal administration of effective phototherapy.

Figure 97-1 provides guidelines for intensive phototherapy in infants older than 35 weeks.

- Use total bilirubin. Do not subtract direct-reacting or conjugated bilirubin.
- Neurotoxicity risk factors are isoimmune hemolytic disease, G-6-PD deficiency, asphyxia, significant

Table 97-4 Optimal Administration of Effective Phototherapy Practice Considerations

Parameters	Specific Interventions	Assessment
Light source (nm)	Blue light spectrum (eg, 460 ± 10 nm)	Use narrow-wavelength spectral range (eg, LED [light-emitting diode] lights)
Light irradiance (dose)	Optimal irradiance (eg, > 30 µW/cm²/nm by 1 or more light source)	Uniformity over the light footprint (5-point test: both shoulders and knees and umbilicus)
Body surface area (BSA; cm²)	Close to the skin surface: 1 surface (about 40% of BSA) or increased to maximally exposed BSA (about 80%)	Expose entire body surface (exclude eye patches and diaper area) for maximal skin area
Response	Ensure efficacy of intervention	Degree of TB decline (1–2 mg/dL/over 3 to 4 hours)
Interruption of therapy	May use intermittent phototherapy (to allow breast-feedings)	After confirmation of adequate response
Duration	Discontinue at desired bilirubin threshold	Serial TB measurements defined by rate of decline

Abbreviation: TB, total plasma bilirubin.

lethargy, temperature instability, sepsis, acidosis, or albumin less than 3.0 g/dL (if measured).
- For well infants at 35 to 37 + 6/7 weeks, TB levels can be adjusted for intervention around the medium risk line. It is an option to intervene at lower TB levels for infants closer to 35 weeks and at higher TB levels for those closer to 37 + 6/7 weeks.
- It is an option to provide conventional phototherapy in the hospital or at home at TB levels 2–3 mg/dL (35–50 mmol/L) below those shown, but home phototherapy should not be used in any infant with risk factors.

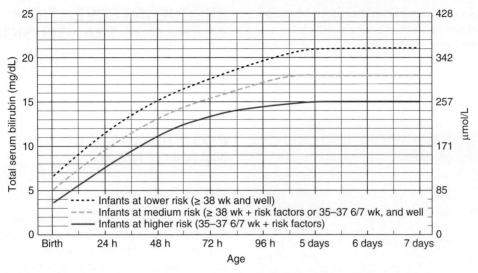

FIGURE 97-1 Guidelines for intensive phototherapy in infants of 35 or more weeks of gestation.

"Crash-Cart" Approach for an Infant Readmitted for Severe Hyperbilirubinemia

1. Assess for ABE (neurologic signs) regardless of the TB level.

2. Check TB/TcB and send labs (stat).

3. Conduct procedures while the infant is under phototherapy lights.

4. Prepare for an exchange transfusion (look for line placement sites).

5. Evaluate for concurrent dehydration (such as hypernatremia): Intravenous infusions will not lower TB levels.

6. Continue enteral feedings to decrease enterohepatic circulation of bilirubin. Breast-feeding can occur with infant (and mother) under phototherapy lights. The baby is unwrapped for skin exposure, and heat lamps may be needed to maintain temperature.

Table 97-5 provides considerations for the crash-cart approach.

Management of Hyperbilirubinemia in Sick and Preterm Infants

The primary strategy of clinical management for sick and preterm infants is prevention. Jaundice should be monitored along with other vital signs. Bilirubin testing should be conducted every 8–12 hours; testing can be decreased to every 12–24 hours during phototherapy, when bilirubin levels are decreasing, or when the infant is beyond 1 week of age. Sick and preterm infants may be at increased risk for an acute rise of bilirubin with concurrent infection or illness, when not receiving anything orally, or as a result of a transfusion or acute hemolysis. Table 97-6 provides operational thresholds for management of hyperbilirubinemia in preterm infants (<35 weeks' GA).

Table 97-5 Considerations for a Crash-Cart Approach

Options	Identify the most effective means to minimize brain damage
Risk	Weigh against the potential risk of ABE vs intervention
Pretreatment	Start total body phototherapy (while procedures are being done) Consider intravenous immune globulin (IVIG) for isoimmunization Consider albumin infusion (1 g/kg) for hypoalbuminemia (<3.4 g/dL)
Procedure	Use isovolume double-volume exchange (170 mL/kg in term, 190 mL/kg in preterm infants)
Duration	May be accomplished within 3–4 hours (consent, labs, lines, and procedures)
Technical problems	Single-volume exchange transfusion may be adequate until technical problems resolved

Abbreviation: ABE, acute bilirubin encephalopathy.

CHAPTER 97

Table 97-6 Operational Thresholds to Manage Hyperbilirubinemia in Preterm Infants (<35 Weeks' Gestational Age [GA])

Stratification by Birth Weight	Operational TB Levels to Initiate Phototherapy	Double Blood Volume Exchange Transfusion (190 mL/kg)
<28 weeks' GA	5–6 mg/dL	11–14 mg/dL
28–29 weeks' GA	6–8 mg/dL	12–14 mg/dL
30–31 weeks' GA	8–10 mg/dL	13–16 mg/dL
32–33 weeks' GA	10–12 mg/dL	15–18 mg/dL
≥34 weeks' GA	12–14 mg/dL	17–19 mg/dL

Abbreviation: TB, total serum bilirubin.
Use the lower range of the listed TB levels for infants at greater risk for bilirubin toxicity, for example, (1) lower gestational age; (2) serum albumin levels below 2.5 g/dL; (3) rapidly rising TB levels, suggesting hemolytic disease; and (4) those who are clinically unstable. When a decision is being made about the initiation of phototherapy or exchange transfusion, infants are considered to be clinically unstable if they have 1 or more of the following conditions: (1) blood pH below 7.15; (2) blood culture positive for sepsis in the prior 24 hours; (3) apnea and bradycardia requiring cardiorespiratory resuscitation (bagging or intubation) during the previous 24 hours; (4) hypotension requiring pressor treatment during the previous 24 hours; and (5) mechanical ventilation at the time of blood sampling.
Recommendations for exchange transfusion apply to infants who are receiving intensive phototherapy to the maximal surface area but whose TB levels continue to increase to the levels listed.

SEQUELAE AND PROGRESSION OF CLINICAL SIGNS OF ABE

Table 97-7 gives the sequelae and progression of clinical signs of ABE.

RESCUE INTERVENTION: EXCHANGE TRANSFUSION

Figure 97-2 provides guidelines for exchange transfusion in infants older than 35 weeks.

POSTDISCHARGE MANAGEMENT

Initial Follow-up

Care for initial follow-up is individualized to assess for rebound hyperbilirubinemia and prolonged unconjugated hyperbilirubinemia (TB > 14 mg/dL) and is based on postnatal age, GA, hemolysis, and etiology of jaundice. Follow-up should include the following

1. Neurologic and neurodevelopmental evaluation at discharge and within 3 months

2. Neuroimaging with magnetic resonance imaging (MRI) at discharge

3. Auditory evoked brainstem responses (ABRs) at discharge and within 3 months.

Long-Term Follow-up

Infants with TB levels greater than 25 mg/dL and those who receive an exchange transfusion should have developmental follow-up through infancy until school age for awkwardness, gait abnormality, failure of fine stereognosis, gaze abnormalities, hearing loss, poor coordination, and exaggerated extrapyramidal reflexes. They may be at risk of subtle posticteric sequelae during infancy and childhood.

Table 97-7 Sequelae and Progression of Clinical Signs of Acute Bilirubin Encephalopathy (ABE)

Severity of Clinical Signs	Mild	Moderate	Severe
Mental status	Sleepy Poor feeding	Lethargic Irritable	Stupor Seizures Coma
Muscle tone	Neck stiffness Mild hyper-/hypotonia	Arching neck retrocollis Arching trunk	Bowing of trunk Opisthotonus
Cry pattern	High pitched	Shrill	Inconsolable

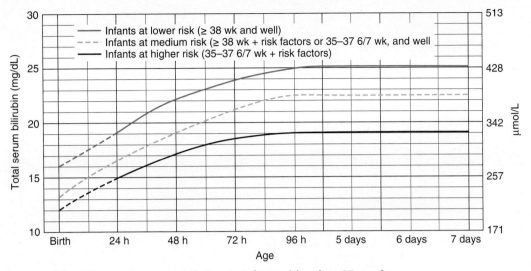

FIGURE 97-2 Guidelines for exchange transfusion in infants older than 35 weeks.

SUGGESTED READING

American Academy of Pediatrics, Subcommittee on Hyperbilirubinemia. Clinical practice guideline: management of hyperbilirubinemia in the newborn infant 35 or more weeks of gestation. *Pediatrics*. 2004;114:297–316.

Bhutani VK, Committee on Fetus and Newborn. Technical report: phototherapy to prevent severe neonatal hyperbilirubinemia in the newborn infant 35 or more weeks of gestation. *Pediatrics*. 2011;128:e1046–e1052.

Bhutani VK, Johnson L, Sivieri EM. Predictive ability of a redischarge hour-specific serum bilirubin for subsequent significant hyperbilirubinemia in healthy-term and near-term newborns. *Pediatrics*. 1999;103:6–14.

Dennery PA, Seidman DS, Stevenson DK. Neonatal hyperbilirubinemia. *N Engl J Med*. 2001;334:581–590.

Kramer LI. Advancement of dermal icterus in the jaundiced newborn. *Am J Dis Child*. 1969;118:454–458.

Maisels MJ, Watchko JF, Bhutani VK, Stevenson DK. An approach to the management of hyperbilirubinemia in the preterm infant < 35 weeks of gestation. *J Perinatol*. Epub June 2012. doi:10.1038/jp.2012.71.

Subcommittee on Hyperbilirubinemia (1 Jul 2004). Management of hyperbilirubinemia in the newborn infant 35 or more weeks of gestation. *Pediatrics*. 114: 297–316.

Maisels MJ, Bhutani VK, Bogen D, Newman TB, Stark AR, Watchko JF. Hyperbilirubinemia in the newborn infant ≥ 35 weeks' gestation: an update with clarifications. *Pediatrics*. 2009;124(4):1193–1198.

98 Management of Conjugated Hyperbilirubinemia (Neonatal Cholestasis)

Vinod K. Bhutani

INDICATION

Jaundice that persists or recurs during the second week of life requires inquiry. Frequently, such jaundice is caused by elevation of the unconjugated, or indirect, bilirubin and is often the result of a benign process. More concerning is jaundice caused by elevation of the conjugated bilirubin fraction. Neonatal cholestasis is caused by an accumulation of biliary substances, such as bilirubin and bile acids, because of impaired canalicular bile flow. Manifestations of conjugated hyperbilirubinemia must be differentiated from unconjugated hyperbilirubinemia because it is more often associated with a specific disease process (Figure 98-1). The medical management of cholestasis is largely supportive because the underlying disease is often untreatable medically. Such treatment addresses complications of chronic cholestasis rather than the underlying cause. These complications include malabsorption, nutritional deficiencies, and pruritus.

Clinical

Levels of Hyperbilirubinemia

1. Direct bilirubin greater than 10% of total bilirubin (TB; < 5 mg/dL)
2. Conjugated bilirubin greater than 1 mg/dL (TB < 5 mg/dL)
3. Direct bilirubin greater than 20% of TB (TB > 5 mg/dL)
4. Conjugated bilirubin greater than 2 mg/dL (TB > 5 mg/dL)

Clinical Risk Factors for Hyperbilirubinemia

The Cholestasis Guideline Committee recommended that any infant noted to be jaundiced at 2 weeks of age be evaluated for cholestasis with measurement of total and direct serum bilirubin.

Clinical Manifestations

1. *Onset of jaundice* after the first weeks of age should be considered abnormal.
2. *Persistence of jaundice* after 2 weeks of age should be considered abnormal.
3. *Association of pale stools or dark urine* should be an alert for cholestasis.

Testing

The most commonly used laboratory determination (the diazo or van den Bergh method) does not specifically measure conjugated bilirubin but reports direct bilirubin. For methodological reasons, the higher the total bilirubin (even if it is all unconjugated) value, the higher the reported direct bilirubin will be. Measurements of direct bilirubin may vary significantly both within and between laboratories.

DIFFERENTIAL DIAGNOSIS

Table 98-1 provides information on the differential diagnosis of conjugated hyperbilirubinemia.

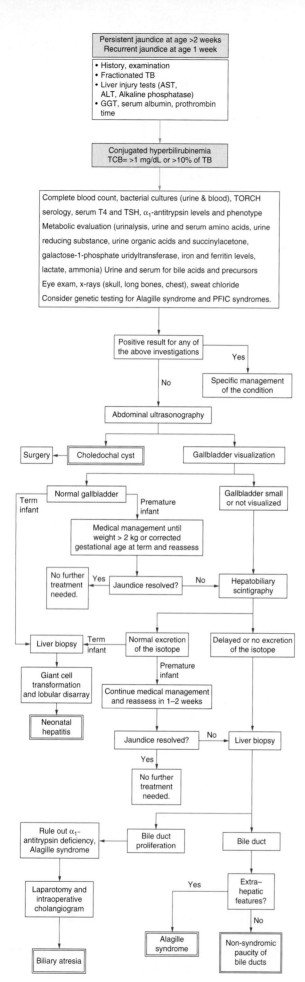

FIGURE 98-1 An approach to a neonatal intensive care unit patient with conjugated hyperbilirubinemia. ALT, alanine transferase; AST, aspartate transferase; GGT, γ-glutamyl transpeptidase; PFIC, progressive familial intrahepatic cholestasis; T$_4$, thyroid hormone, thyroxine; TB, total bilirubin; TCB, transcutaneous bilirubin; TORCH, toxoplasmosis, rubella, cytomegalovirus, herpes simplex virus; TSH, thyroid-stimulating hormone

Table 98-1 Differential Diagnosis of Conjugated Hyperbilirubinemia

Condition	Disorders
Idiopathic	Neonatal hepatitis
Viral infections	Cytomegalovirus Rubella Reovirus 3 Adenovirus Coxsackie virus Human herpes virus 6 Varicella zoster Herpes simplex Parvovirus Hepatitis B and C Human immunodeficiency virus
Bacterial infections	Sepsis Urinary tract infection Syphilis Listeriosis Tuberculosis
Parasitic infections	Toxoplasmosis Malaria
Bile duct anomalies	Biliary atresia Choledochal cyst Alagille syndrome Nonsyndromic bile duct paucity Inspissated bile syndrome Caroli syndrome Choledocholithiasis Neonatal sclerosing cholangitis Spontaneous common bile duct perforation
Metabolic disorders	α_1-Antitrypsin deficiency Galactosemia Glycogen storage disorder type IV Cystic fibrosis Hemochromatosis Tyrosinemia Arginase deficiency Zellweger syndrome Dubin-Johnson syndrome Rotor syndrome Hereditary fructosemia Niemann-Pick disease, type C Gaucher disease Bile acid synthetic disorders Progressive familial intrahepatic cholestasis North American Indian familial cholestasis Aagenaes syndrome X-linked adrenoleukodystrophy
Endocrine-related disorders	Hypothyroidism Hypopituitarism (septo-optic dysplasia)
Chromosomal disorders	Turner syndrome Trisomy 18 Trisomy 21 Trisomy 13 Cat's-eye syndrome Donahue syndrome (leprechaunism)

CHAPTER 98

(Continued)

Table 98-1 Differential Diagnosis of Conjugated Hyperbilirubinemia (*Continued*)

Condition	Disorders
Toxic	Parenteral nutrition Fetal alcohol syndrome Drugs
Vascular	Budd-Chiari syndrome Neonatal asphyxia Congestive heart failure
Neoplasm	Neonatal leukemia Histiocytosis X Neuroblastoma Hepatoblastoma Erythrophagocytic lymphohistiocytosis
Miscellaneous	Neonatal lupus erythematosus Le foie vide (infantile hepatic nonregenerative disorder)

IMMEDIATE ACTION

If total parenteral nutrition (TPN) is prescribed, either wean or discontinue intravenous lipid infusion, especially in preterm infants, until a nutrition plan is developed and individualized.

EVALUATION

Table 98-2 delineates the steps in the evaluation process.

BILIRUBIN FOLLOW-UP

1. Serial TB/direct bilirubin assay for progression of hyperbilirubinemia until levels decline
   a. Newborns 35 weeks or older gestational age (GA)
      - For onset of jaundice: check immediately
      - Persistence: check every 1–2 days until levels plateau or decline
      - Aggressively investigate for etiology
   b. Newborns less than 35 weeks' GA
      - All infants: check levels every day initially
      - Serial follow-up until TB declines: 1–2/week based on rate of TB rise/decline
      - After significant decline: may track clinical resolution of jaundice
2. Serial TB/direct bilirubin assay to track decline of hyperbilirubinemia to levels <1 mg/dL.

MANAGEMENT

Nutritional Goal

The nutritional goal is to discontinue parenteral feedings and transition to full enteral feedings. In infants who are not tolerating full enteral feedings, management includes trophic enteral feedings, making changes to TPN substrates (eg, limiting glucose intake to 15 g/kg/d), supplementation with taurine and glutamine, limiting intake of lipid emulsions, and cycling of the TPN to 12 hours/day.

Medications

Pharmacologic management (see Table 98-3) includes ursodeoxycholic acid to increase bile acid excretion. Cholecystokinin-octapetide and the cholecystokinin analogue ceruletide may prevent cholelithiasis or liver disease in patients receiving TPN by stimulating gallbladder contraction.

Growth Parameters and Nutrition

Growth parameter and nutrition assessment, such as height and weight for age and weight for height, should be closely followed by tracking growth velocity, percentile track, and signs of malabsorption of fats.

Nutrient Choice

Long-chain fatty acids are not well absorbed; this leads to malnutrition and fat-soluble vitamin deficiency.

Table 98-2 Evaluation of Conjugated Hyperbilirubinemia

Steps	Process
Initial investigations Establish cholestasis and determine severity of liver disease	Detailed history and physical examination (include family and pre- and postnatal history, stool color) Fractionated serum bilirubin levels Tests of liver injury (AST, ALT, alkaline phosphatase, GGT) Liver function tests (serum albumin, prothrombin time, serum ammonia, blood glucose)
Detect conditions Require immediate treatment	Complete blood cell count, bacterial cultures (blood and urine) to rule out sepsis Serum T_4 and TSH to rule out hypothyroidism To detect metabolic conditions: urinalysis, urine-reducing substance, urine organic acids, urine and serum amino acids, urine succinylacetone, galactose-1-phosphate uridyl transferase, serum lactate, serum iron and ferritin levels VDRL and viral serologies and cultures
Differentiate Extrahepatic disorders from intrahepatic causes of cholestasis	Ultrasonography Hepatobiliary scintigraphy Percutaneous liver biopsy (histology, electron microscopy, immunohistochemistry) Exploratory laparotomy with intraoperative cholangiogram
Establish Other specific diagnoses	Serum α_1-antitrypsin levels and phenotype Sweat chloride for cystic fibrosis Urine and serum for bile acids and precursors Genetic testing for Alagille syndrome and PFIC syndromes. X-rays of skull and long bones to look for congenital infection, chest x-ray for heart disease, eye examination for posterior embryotoxon or choreoretinitis Bone marrow examination and skin fibroblast culture for storage disorders

Abbreviations: ALT, alanine transferase; AST, aspartate transferase; GGT, γ-glutamyl transpeptidase; PFIC, progressive familial intrahepatic cholestasis; T_4, thyroid hormone, thyroxine; TSH, thyroid-stimulating hormone; VDRL, Venereal Disease Research Laboratory.

Table 98-3 Formulary for Neonatal and Infant Cholestasis

Medication	Dose	Side Effects
Ursodeoxycholic acid	10–30 mg/kg/d	Diarrhea, hepatotoxicity
Rifampin	10 mg/kg/d	Hepatotoxicity, drug interactions
Phenobarbital	3–10 mg/kg/d	Sedative effects, behavioral changes
Cholestyramine	0.25–0.50 g/kg/d	Constipation, steatorrhea, hyperchloremic metabolic acidosis

Medium-chain triglycerides (MCTs) are more readily absorbed and are a better source of fat calories. These infants should be started on a formula containing MCTs such as Enfaport, Pregestimil, or Alimentum. If oral intake is not sufficient, patients may be started on nocturnal enteral feedings. Because of steatorrhea and increased energy expenditure, the caloric intake goal should be 125% of recommended dietary allowance based on ideal body weight.

Vitamins

The intestinal absorption of fat-soluble vitamins (A, D, E, and K) requires the presence of bile acids. Doses of at least 2–4 times the recommended daily allowance are given. Vitamin supplementation (Table 98-4) should continue for 3 months after resolution of jaundice.

Table 98-4 Vitamin Supplementation for Neonatal and Infant Cholestasis

Vitamins	Dose	Side Effects
Vitamin A (Aquasol A®)	5000–25,000 IU/d	Hepatotoxicity, hypercalcemia
Vitamin D: cholecalciferol 25-OH cholecalciferol	2500–5000 IU/d, 3–5 µg/kg/d	Hypercalcemia, nephrocalcinosis
Vitamin K (phytonadione)	2.5–5 mg every other day	None
Vitamin E (Aquasol E®)	50–400 IU/d	Potentiation of coagulopathy
TPGS (d-alpha tocopheryl polyethylene glycol-succinate)	15–25 IU/kg/d	Hyperosmolality
Water-soluble vitamins	Twice the recommended daily allowance	

Neonatal Phototherapy in Cholestasis

The bronze infant syndrome is the dark, grayish-brown discoloration of skin as a complication of phototherapy and may be caused by accumulation of porphyrins and other metabolites. This is generally benign; if there is an urgent need for phototherapy for excessive unconjugated bilirubinemia, direct hyperbilirubinemia should not be an absolute contraindication. However, the products of phototherapy are excreted in bile, and cholestasis can reduce the effectiveness of phototherapy or may impair bilirubin-albumin binding. Furthermore, the potential neurotoxicity of the isomers attributed to conjugated bilirubin and the "bronze pigment" or porphyrins has not been excluded. Importantly, the direct serum bilirubin should not be subtracted from the total serum bilirubin concentration when making decisions about exchange transfusions.

SUGGESTED READING

Best C, Gourley GR, Bhutani VK. Neonatal cholestasis-conjugated hyperbilirubinemia. In: Buonocore G, Bracci R, Weindling M, eds. *Neonatology. A Practical Approach to Neonatal Diseases*. Milan, Italy: Springer-Verlag Italia; 2012:65–68.

Coakley RJ, et al. Alpha1-antitrypsin deficiency: biological answers to clinical questions. *Am J Med Sci*. 2001;321(1):33–41.

Lomas DA, et al. The mechanism of Z alpha 1-antitrypsin accumulation in the liver. *Nature*. 1992;357(6379):605–607.

Moyer V, Freese DK, Whitington PF, Olson AD, Brewer F, Colletti RB, Heyman MB; North American Society for Pediatric Gastroenterology, Hepatology and Nutrition. Guideline for the evaluation of cholestatic jaundice in infants: recommendations of the North American Society for Pediatric Gastroenterology, Hepatology and Nutrition. *J Pediatr Gastroenterol Nutr*. 2004;39(2):115–128.

Suchy FJ. Neonatal cholestasis. *Pediatr Rev*. 2004;25(11):388–396.

Suchy F, Sokol RJ, Balistreri WF, eds. *Liver Disease in Children*. 3rd ed. New York, NY: Cambridge University Press; 2007:1030.

Venigalla S, Gourley GR. Neonatal cholestasis. *Semin Perinatol*. 2004;28(5):348–355.

Walker WA, et al. *Pediatric Gastrointestinal Disease: Pathophysiology, Diagnosis, Management*. 3rd ed. Hamilton, ON, Canada: BC Decker; 2004.

Part G: Genito-Urinary Tract

99 Acute Kidney Injury in Neonates and Infants

Gia Oh and Paul Grimm

DIAGNOSIS/INDICATIONS

Clinical Findings

1. Increasing serum creatinine (Cr)
2. Decreasing urine output to less than 0.5–1 mL/kg/h

History and Physical Examination

Table 99-1 provides information on the history and physical examination.

Additional Workup

1. Check electrolytes, complete blood cell count (CBC)
2. Consider urinalysis, urine sodium, urine urea, urine Cr (FeNa, FeUrea)
3. Consider renal ultrasound (RUS) with Doppler to evaluate structure and blood flow

Diagnostic Algorithm

1. Consider prerenal, intrinsic, postrenal (obstructive) causes of acute kidney injury (AKI)
2. Clues to prerenal AKI
   a. Hypovolemia on examination
   b. Decreased weight
   c. Negative fluid balance
   d. FeNa less than 2.5% or FeUrea less than 35%

$$FeNa = \frac{(Urine\ Na \times Plasma\ Na) \times 100}{(Urine\ Cr \times Plasma\ Cr)}$$

$$FeUrea = \frac{(Urine\ Urea \times Plasma\ Serum\ Urea\ Nitrogen) \times 100}{(Urine\ Cr \times Plasma\ Cr)}$$

3. Clues to intrinsic AKI
   a. Prolonged hypovolemia or hypotension
   b. Exposure to nephrotoxic medication
   c. Presence of clinical conditions associated with AKI
      (1) Sepsis/multiorgan dysfunction syndrome
      (2) Congenital cardiac surgery
      (3) Perinatal asphyxia
      (4) Extracorporeal membrane oxygenation (ECMO)
4. Clues to postrenal (obstructive) AKI
   a. Prenatal history of hydronephrosis/other urologic anomaly
   b. Potter syndrome
   c. Abdominal mass
   d. RUS showing thickened bladder wall, dilated collecting system, hydronephrosis

TREATMENT/MANAGEMENT ALGORITHM

1. Assess fluid status; fluid resuscitate if hypovolemic
2. Ensure blood pressure is adequate for renal perfusion
   a. Volume resuscitation
   b. Vasopressor support if needed

Table 99-1 History and Physical Examination Findings in Neonates/Infants With Acute Kidney Injury (AKI)

Findings	Comments
History	
Prenatal ultrasound (US)	• Oligohydraminios/anhydraminios in obstructive uropathy • Renal hypoplasia, dysplasia, and other structural abnormalities
Perinatal history	• Placenta abruption • Apgar score (perinatal asphyxia) • Twin-twin transfusion
Umbilical artery/vein catheterization?	• Increased risk for renal artery thrombosis/renal vein thrombosis
Exposure to nephrotoxic medications?	• Aminoglycosides, nonsteroidal anti-inflammatory drugs (NSAIDs), other antimicrobials, chemotherapy agents
Physical Examination	
Weight trend	• Volume status
Urine output	• Oliguria usually defined as less than 0.5–1 mL/kg/h
Hypertension	• May suggest hypervolemia, renal artery thrombosis • Coarctation of aorta may cause renal hypoperfusion
Hypotension	• Renal hypoperfusion
Heart murmur	• Large left-to-right shunts may cause renal hypoperfusion
Abdominal examination	• Significant distention may suggest abdominal compartment syndrome or urine ascites causing "pseudo"-AKI (rare). • Tenderness may suggest renal vein thrombosis. • Mass may suggest autosomal recessive polycystic kidney disease (ARPKD)/obstructive AKI.
Potter syndrome	• Pulmonary insufficiency, flattened nasal bridge, low-set ears, joint contractures seen in obstructive uropathy
Gross hematuria	• Renal artery thrombosis, infection, hemorrhage, cortical necrosis

3. Consider urethral Foley catheter placement

   a. Relieves possible obstruction.

   b. Facilitates strict in and out measurement.

   c. Measures intravesical pressure via Foley catheter if there is concern for abdominal compartment syndrome. In children and infants, abdominal compartment syndrome has been described in those with intraabdominal pressures greater than 10–12 mm Hg.

4. Consider acute management therapies for intrinsic AKI

   a. Rasburicase 0.2 mg/kg IV once if serum uric acid greater than 8 mg/dL

   b. Aminophylline 5 mg/kg IV once followed by 1.8 mg/kg IV every 6 hours; Target trough level of 5–7 μg/mL

5. Continue maintenance therapies for intrinsic AKI

   a. Remove nephrotoxic medications

   b. Adjust medication doses for reduced renal clearance

   c. Maintain euvolemia

   (1) Intake should be limited to insensible water loss plus output.

   (2) Consider diuretics (loop diuretic + thiazide) in oliguric patients.

   (a) Furosemide 1–2 mg/kg/dose every 8–24 hours IV or 0.05–0.3 mg/kg/h continuous drip

   (b) Bumetanide 0.01–0.05 mg/kg/dose every 24 to 48 hours or 0.005–0.025 mg/kg/h continuous drip

   (c) Chlorothiazide 1–4 mg/kg/dose IV twice daily (doses up to 20 mg/kg/d have been used)

   (d) Metolazone 0.2 mg/kg orally every 24 hours

   d. Correct electrolyte anomalies

   (1) Hyperkalemia

   (a) Remove potassium from IVF/PN (parenteral nutrition)

   (b) Stabilize cardiac resting potential: Calcium chloride (central line) or calcium gluconate

   (c) Decrease total body potassium: Sodium polystyrene sulfonate (Kayexalate) or furosemide

(d) Decrease extracellular potassium by increasing intracellular shift: sodium bicarbonate (if acidosis is present; correct concomitant hypocalcemia); insulin/dextrose; inhaled β-adrenergic agonist

(e) Consider pretreating then decanting enteral feed (maternal breast milk [MBM] or Similac® PM 60/40) with sodium polystyrene sulfonate

(2) Hyponatremia

    (a) Restrict free water if secondary to fluid retention

    (b) Consider sodium supplementation if increased sodium loss

(3) Hyperphosphatemia: Consider pretreating then decanting enteral feed (MBM or PM 60/40) with phosphate binder such as sevelamer

(4) Metabolic acidosis

    (a) Consider sodium bicarbonate

    (b) Correct concomitant hypocalcemia to prevent acute decrease in ionized calcium

Optimize Nutrition

1. Maternal breast milk is the preferred nutrition in infants with AKI.
2. Renal formula PM 60/40 is given if MBM not available.

3. Concentrate enteral feeding/parenteral feeding and increase caloric density to limit volume.

Consider Renal Replacement Therapy

1. Indications for renal replacement therapy (RRT)

    a. Hyperkalemia or metabolic acidosis not responsive to pharmaceutical interventions

    b. Signs of uremia (pericarditis, bleeding, encephalopathy)

    c. Hypervolemia

    d. Need for increased fluid intake with inadequate ability to increase diuresis accordingly

2. Acute peritoneal dialysis (PD) vs intermittent hemodialysis (IHD) vs continuous renal replacement therapy (CRRT) (Table 99-2)

    a. The choice of modality depends on patient factors and the availability of qualified personnel and local resources.

    b. Patient factors to consider include the following:

        i. hemodynamic stability

        ii. ease of vascular access vs peritoneal access

        iii. comorbidities (ie, congenital diaphragmatic hernia, postabdominal surgery, severe hemorrhage)

        iv. need for rapid correction of the metabolic derangement

Table 99-2 Advantages and Disadvantages of Peritoneal Dialysis (PD), Intermittent Hemodialysis (IHD), and Continuous Renal Replacement Therapy (CRRT) in Neonates/Infants With Acute Kidney Injury (AKI)

	Advantages	Disadvantages
PD	• No vascular access • No anticoagulation needed • Can be used in small infants • Well tolerated in hemodynamically unstable patients	• Slower and less-effective removal of solutes, fluid • Risk of peritonitis • Risk of peritoneal fluid leaks • Additional risks and benefits assessment needed in those with recent abdominal surgery, intra-abdominal complications, massive organomegaly, congenital diaphragmatic hernia (CDH)
IHD	• Rapid solute clearance • Rapid fluid removal	• Requires vascular access • Requires blood prime • Requires anticoagulation • Not tolerated by hemodynamically unstable patients • Difficult to do in small infants
CRRT	• Well tolerated in hemodynamically unstable patients • Can use regional anticoagulation with citrate • Gentler, slower solute and fluid removal	• Requires vascular accesses • Requires blood prime • Clearance of nutrition, medications

3. PD catheters
   a. Acute catheters can be placed using the Seldinger technique.
   b. Surgical catheter insertion by surgeons familiar with PD catheters is preferred.
   c. Tenckhoff catheters are most commonly used in the United States.
   d. Curled catheters are more commonly used and preferred over straight catheters.
   e. Two cuffs are preferred over 1 cuff for tunneled catheters.
   f. The exit site should be point downward, away from the diaper region and away from stomas (Figure 99-1).
4. IHD/CRRT catheters (Table 99-3): Circuit life is less than 20 hours when CRRT is delivered using two 5.0F single-lumen catheters; therefore, this is not recommended.

Ethical Considerations

1. Consensus should be present between the neonatologist, nephrologist, parents, and other members of the multidisciplinary team on the decision to provide or withhold RRT.
2. If such consensus is lacking, the various parties involved in the patient's care need to discuss again the risks and benefits of RRT to reach a consensus.

WEANING RRT

1. Signs of improving renal function include increase in urine output, improvement in metabolic derangements (without increase in delivered dialysis dose), and overall clinical improvement.

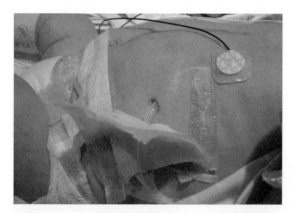

FIGURE 99-1 Surgically placed permanent Tenckhoff peritoneal dialysis (PD) catheter in an infant. Note that the PD exit site is away from the diaper region and downward pointing. A downward-pointing exit site has been associated with lower risk of tunnel infection and peritonitis.

Table 99-3 Intermittent Hemodialysis (IHD)/ Continuous Renal Replacement Therapy (CRRT) Catheters for Neonates/Infants With Acute Kidney Injury (AKI)

Patient Size	Catheter	Insertion Site
Neonate	Dual lumen 7.0F	Internal/external jugular, femoral vein
3–6 kg	Dual lumen 7.0F	Internal/external jugular, femoral vein
6–30 kg >15 kg	Dual lumen 8.0F Dual lumen 9.0F	Internal/external jugular, femoral vein

2. PD can be weaned easily:
   a. Dextrose can be reduced to decrease ultrafiltration.
   b. Number of cycles and fill volume can be reduced to decrease diffusive clearance.
3. CRRT can be weaned in stepwise fashion.
   a. Hourly ultrafiltration rate (patient removal) can be reduced to increase intravascular volume.
   b. Dialysate and convective clearance can be reduced to decrease solute clearance. Weaning the clearance while maintaining the same blood flow may result in increased incidence of citrate lock syndrome when using citrate-based anticoagulation. In this case, a trial of discontinuation of CRRT may be required.
   c. The patient can be given a trial off CRRT.
      (1) Fluid rate should be reduced
      (2) Remove potassium from IVF/PN
      (3) Consider removing/reducing phosphate and magnesium from PN
      (4) Recommend locking the catheter lumens with alteplase to prevent clotting
      (5) Consider "diuretic challenge" with furosemide, chlorothiazide, and aminophylline after the patient has been off CRRT for a few hours
4. IHD can be weaned off easily by skipping increasing number of days between IHD sessions.

FOLLOW-UP

1. AKI and the need for RRT are independent risk factors for increased mortality.
2. At a mean follow-up of 7.5 ± 4.6 years, 9/20 patients (45%) had estimated glomerular filtration rates (GFRs) less than 75 mL/min/1.73 m². Urine protein/creatinine ratio greater than 0.6 and serum Cr greater than 0.6 mg/dL at 1 year of age were predictive of chronic renal insufficiency (univariate analysis).

100 Renal Masses and Urinary Ascites

Aviva E. Weinberg and William A. Kennedy II

RENAL MASSES

Abdominal masses are frequent in the neonate, and nearly two-thirds are renal in origin. Most are benign, representing hydronephrosis, multicystic dysplastic kidney (MCDK), polycystic kidney disease, or congenital mesoblastic nephroma. Less commonly, a flank mass may be caused by a malignant renal lesion, such as a Wilms tumor. The initial diagnosis may be made on prenatal ultrasonography (US), found in an asymptomatic infant on physical palpation, or discovered as a consequence of postnatal imaging performed for hypertension, hematuria, urinary sepsis, or difficult feeding in the new infant.[1] Fetal ultrasonography may demonstrate not only the renal mass but also associated findings, such as oligohydramnios, polyhydramnios, renal cysts, hydronephrosis, and bladder wall thickness, which may aid in developing a more specific diagnosis in the antenatal period.[2] Early recognition of renal masses may allow timely treatment of congenital renal anomalies that would otherwise be missed because of their asymptomatic nature.

The postnatal examination will be the first opportunity to palpate an abdominal mass and evaluate for any associated genitourinary or systemic anomalies. Examination of the external genitalia and lumbosacral region is imperative because malformations of these organ systems are increased in the setting of renal and urinary anomalies. A postnatal abdominal US should be performed to confirm the renal origin of the mass, define whether it is solid or cystic, and better delineate the collecting system anatomy. More specific postnatal imaging, such as voiding cystourethrogram (VCUG),

nuclear medicine renal scans, and magnetic resonance imaging (MRI) will be guided by the suspected diagnosis.

Cystic Masses

Cystic masses of the neonate may include hydronephrosis, MCDK, and autosomal dominant and autosomal recessive polycystic kidney disease. The most common cause of a renal mass in the newborn is hydronephrosis. This may be caused by ureteropelvic junction (UPJ) obstruction, primary megaureter, vesicoureteral reflux (VUR), ureterovesical junction obstruction, or bladder outlet obstruction. Follow-up imaging with repeat renal bladder US and a VCUG should be performed to delineate the etiology of the hydronephrosis. The recommended timing of the first postnatal US has been a controversial subject. It has been posited that an US performed within the initial 24-48 hours of life may underestimate the degree of hydronephrosis because of relative dehydration[3] (Figure 100-1).

Multicystic dysplastic kidney is the second-most-common cause for a cystic renal mass in the newborn. More than 50% of cases are detected antenatally. It is typically a unilateral cystic renal mass, more commonly found in male infants, and is characterized sonographically by numerous noncommunicating cysts separated by dysplastic renal tissue. The contralateral kidney may show compensatory hypertrophy or may be associated with other defects, such as rotation anomalies, VUR, ureteroceles or UPJ obstruction. The prognosis is favorable in cases of solitary, unilateral MCDK, whose

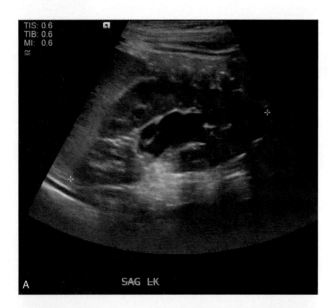

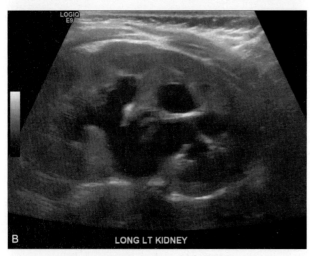

FIGURE 100-1 A, Newborn with left antenatal hydrone-phrosis imaged with ultrasound on day one of life with minimal hydronephrosis (Society for Fetal Urology Grade 1). **B,** Same newborn with left antenatal hydronephrosis imaged with ultrasound at one week of life with moderate hydronephrosis (Society for Fetal Urology Grade 3).

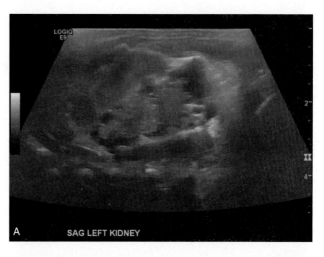

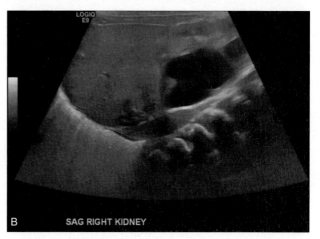

FIGURE 100-2 A, Newborn with left multicystic dys-plastic kidney (MCDK) imaged with ultrasound at birth. **B,** Contralateral right kidney in the same newborn has moderate hydronephrosis which progressed ulti-mately requiring pyeloplasty for a ureteropelvic junction obstruction.

natural history without intervention is typically involu-tion of the affected kidney. Chronic renal insufficiency has been seen in up to 50% of cases if there is contra-lateral genitourinary involvement; therefore, long-term follow-up by a pediatric urologist is mandatory to monitor renal function[4] (Figure 100-2).

Two forms of hereditary cystic disease may be diag-nosed in the setting of an imaged or palpated renal mass in the perinatal and neonatal period. Autosomal recessive polycystic kidney disease (ARPKD), previ-ously called infantile polycystic kidney disease, is a recessively inherited disorder characterized by dilation of the distal tubules and collecting ducts. There is a spectrum of presentation of this condition. Infants are

more likely to present with a history of oligohydram-nios, Potter facies, massively enlarged kidneys, pulmo-nary hypoplasia, and rapid progression to end-stage renal disease.[5] Patients who present later in life more commonly display features of hepatic disease, includ-ing hepatosplenomegaly, hypersplenism, variceal bleeding, cholangitis, and less-severe renal involve-ment. ARPKD can be diagnosed after 24 weeks of ges-tation by fetal US demonstrating markedly enlarged kidneys with increased echogenicity and loss of cor-ticomedullary differentiation, often without discretely visible cysts. Infants may have marked abdominal dis-tention from bilateral renal involvement on physical examination. Molecular genetic testing is only used in the setting of an uncertain diagnosis or during prena-tal diagnosis and counseling.

Autosomal dominant polycystic kidney disease, or adult polycystic kidney disease, has been increasingly diagnosed in neonates and children. It is characterized by cystic dilations in all parts of the nephron. The kidneys are distended with large radiographically detectable cysts. The diagnosis is most commonly made in the pediatric population on the basis of a renal US performed in the setting of a positive family history. It is distinct from the recessive form of the disease in that hepatic, pancreatic, and splenic involvement is rarely observed in childhood, and renal insufficiency does not typically develop until adulthood.[6] Management of these two diseases is largely supportive, with attention to long-term follow-up of renal function.

Solid Renal Masses

Solid renal masses may result from benign causes such as renal vein thrombosis and congenital mesoblastic nephroma or be caused by malignant conditions such as Wilms tumor.

Renal vein thrombosis (RVT) may be suspected in the ill neonate with a classic triad of microscopic or macroscopic hematuria, a palpable flank mass, and thrombocytopenia. It accounts for 10% of cases of venous thrombosis in newborns and is the leading cause of non-catheter-associated venous thrombosis. Risk factors include perinatal asphyxia, maternal diabetes mellitus, prematurity, dehydration, and infection.[7] Sonographic features are notable for diffuse renal enlargement, diffusely or focally increased echogenicity, and perivascular echogenic streaking, with abnormal Doppler flow caused by intravenous thrombus.[8] Treatment is largely supportive care, correction of the underlying etiology, and anticoagulation therapy depending on the extent of the thrombus.

Congenital mesoblastic nephroma is the most frequent cause of a solid renal mass in the neonate. It is a renal mesenchymal tumor whose behavior is typically benign, although it may exhibit local infiltration and rarely distant metastatic spread. It predominates in boys, at a 2:1 ratio. Diagnosis is usually made in the third trimester because of severe polyhydramnios in the setting of a well-defined, unilateral hilar renal mass. Premature delivery occurs in up to 25% of cases.[9] Maternal transport to a tertiary care center is essential for multidisciplinary management by a team of perinatologists, neonatologists, and pediatric surgeons. Postnatal diagnostic evaluation may reveal hematuria, anemia, hypertension, hypercalcemia, and elevated renin levels. US features include a unilateral, well-demarcated solid renal mass with homogeneous echogenicity, often located at the hilum, and involving the renal sinus. Arteriovenous shunts as well as a thin hypoechoic rim with arterial and venous flow may be seen on color Doppler.[10] Differential diagnosis with Wilms tumor is only made by histologic evaluation;

therefore, radical nephrectomy is typically performed within the first weeks of life. Surgical excision is almost always curative (Figure 100-3).

Wilms tumor is the most common neonatal malignancy and the fourth-most-common childhood cancer.

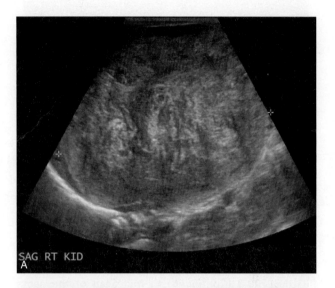

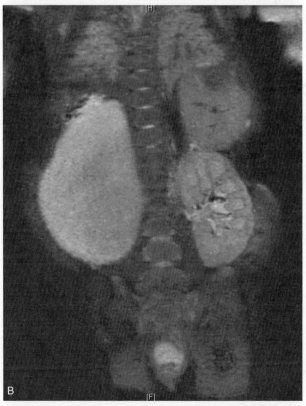

FIGURE 100-3 A, Ultrasound image of large right abdominal mass in a newborn which is isoechoic with the right kidney, characteristic of a congenital mesoblastic nephroma. **B,** MRI Scan of the same newborn demonstrating the right mesoblastic nephroma occupying the right renal fossa and the normal contralateral left kidney.

CHAPTER 100

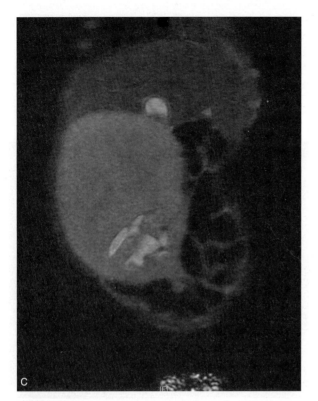

FIGURE 100-3 (*Continued*) C, MRI Scan of the same newborn with right mesoblastic nephroma which demonstrates the functional portion of the right kidney displaced anteriorly and inferiorly by the mass.

It has been rarely documented in the neonate. It may be seen as an isolated tumor or in association with a malformation syndrome such as WAGR (Wilms tumor, aniridia, genitourinary abnormalities, mental retardation), Denys-Drash, and Beckwith-Wiedemann. The physical examination will typically reveal a firm, smooth mass that does not cross the midline. Five percent of cases are bilateral. A variety of associated congenital anomalies, such as aniridia, hemihypertrophy, cryptorchidism, hypospadias, or ambiguous genitalia, may be found.

Laboratory evaluation for Wilms tumor should include a urinalysis, liver function panel, serum calcium, a complete blood cell count, a basic metabolic panel, and coagulation studies. Abdominal US is usually the first-line imaging study, which will demonstrate an encapsulated mass with heterogeneous echogenicity representing fat, necrosis, calcification, or hemorrhage. Contrast computed tomographic (CT) imaging is recommended to further delineate any nodal, pulmonary, or hepatic metastases, renal vein or caval tumor extension, contralateral synchronous tumor, and associated nephrogenic rests.[11] MRI is the most sensitive modality for determination of caval infiltration but requires procedural sedation. Multimodality treatment with radical nephrectomy, neoadjuvant, and adjuvant chemotherapy as well as radiation therapy have resulted in a 5-year survival rate greater than 90%.

URINARY ASCITES

Ascites is defined as the abnormal accumulation of fluid within the peritoneal space, which may be accompanied by symptoms specific to the underlying organ system and etiology. Extravasation of urine into the peritoneal cavity is an uncommon cause of fetal ascites. It is typically caused by a disruption of the urinary tract as a result of increased pressure from an area of obstruction.[12] Renal pelvis, calyx, or forniceal perforation with resultant perinephric urinoma may result from a severe UPJ obstruction, and a bladder rupture may be seen as a consequence of posterior urethral valves (PUVs).[13] Alternative etiologies include difficult umbilical artery catheterization with resultant trauma to the bladder dome and, rarely, complex cloacal malformations that allow for urinary reflux into the genital tract and subsequent peritoneal ascites (Table 100-1). PUVs are the most common cause for fetal urinary ascites, accounting for nearly 70% of cases.[14] The development of urinary ascites, or in some cases a contained perirenal urinoma, is thought to function as a "pop-off mechanism" or "safety valve," which may effectively protect the fetal kidneys from further damage from the high pressure of an obstructed fetal urinary tract.[15]

The initial diagnosis of urinary ascites may be established on a prenatal US or suspected postnatally in an infant with increasing abdominal distention and oliguria, with or without respiratory distress (Figure 100-4). Physical signs of ascites in the newborn include shifting dullness to percussion, a fluid wave, and visible abdominal distention. An increased respiratory rate or frank respiratory distress may be the result of diaphragmatic

Table 100-1 Differential Diagnosis for Fetal Urinary Ascites

Urologic Etiologies of Fetal Urinary Ascites	Clinical Features
• Posterior urethral valves • Collecting system perforation • Spontaneous bladder rupture • Cloacal anomalies • Prune belly syndrome • Neurogenic bladder • Iatrogenic bladder perforation from umbilical artery catheterization	Abdominal distention, fetal distress, respiratory compromise, azotemia, hyperkalemia, hyponatremia, hypochloremia, metabolic acidosis

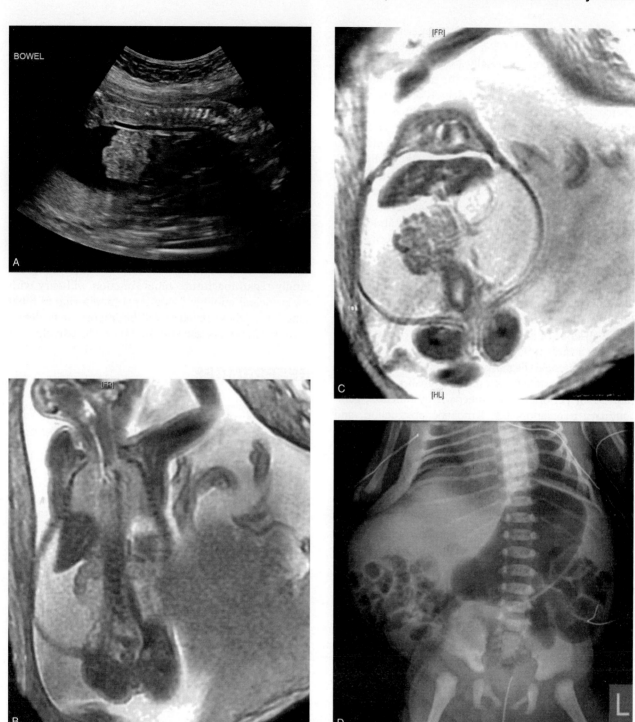

FIGURE 100-4. A, Maternal ultrasound performed at 22 weeks gestation demonstrating fetal abdominal ascites (black region left lateral and inferior) with small bowel (hyperechoic central tissue) floating in fluid. B, Maternal Fetal MRI scan performed at 22 weeks gestation demonstrating fetal abdominal ascites (bright white) surrounding liver edge and the right kidney with hydroureteronephrosis. C, Maternal Fetal MRI scan performed at 22 weeks gestation demonstrating fetal abdominal ascites (bright white) surrounding small bowel and the thickened bladder in fetus with posterior urethral valves. D, Postnatal abdominal X-ray of the same fetus demonstrating classic "ground glass" appearance of abdominal ascites. (Note the abdominal distension and easily visualized small bowel loops.)

elevation from the accumulated intraperitoneal fluid. The liver, spleen, or both may be ballotable. Signs of peritoneal irritation are usually absent.

A postnatal US will confirm the presence of ascites and may reveal the level and degree of urinary tract obstruction. Common US findings might include free fluid in the abdomen, unilateral or bilateral hydronephrosis, renal dysplasia, megaureters, an enlarged thickened bladder wall, or the classic "keyhole sign" caused by a dilated posterior urethra seen with PUVs. Associated findings, such as intra-abdominal testes and abdominal muscular deficiency, may be discovered in cases of prune belly syndrome. A plain abdominal x-ray showing centralization of intestinal contents is highly suggestive of abdominal ascites. The symptom triad of oliguria or anuria, abdominal distention, and azotemia after umbilical artery catheterization should alert the clinician to the possibility of an iatrogenic bladder injury.[16] Spontaneous rupture of the bladder in the absence of any underlying genitourinary abnormality is a rare etiology of urinary ascites.[17]

The differential diagnosis of neonatal ascites includes Rhesus incompatibility, intestinal anomalies with resultant bowel perforation, portohepatic dysfunction, genitourinary tract anomalies, lymphatic obstruction, and infectious, cardiac, and rarely traumatic etiologies.[18] In neonates, ascites usually originates from a biliary, urinary, or lymphatic problem. The combination of postnatal US, laboratory evaluation, and paracentesis will usually isolate the definitive diagnosis.

The laboratory evaluation is critical for delineating that the ascites is urinary in origin. Extravasation of urine into the peritoneum will typically result in an elevated ratio of serum urea nitrogen (BUN) to creatinine, a low ratio of urine to serum creatinine, as well as azotemia, hyperkalemia, hypochloremia, hyponatremia, and metabolic acidosis. Paracentesis should be performed in cases of sepsis, when the diagnosis is still uncertain, and as a therapeutic measure to relieve intra-abdominal pressure in infants with respiratory compromise.[19] An elevated creatinine level in the fluid retrieved on paracentesis is diagnostic for urinary ascites. Further investigation with a VCUG may help identify the level of injury and site of obstruction. The VCUG might reveal urinary extravasation or the presence of PUVs or VUR.

The initial management entails adequate fluid hydration, correction of electrolyte abnormalities, respiratory support if necessary, and antibiotic prophylaxis. Urinary catheter decompression is imperative. Typically, the pediatric urologist will be called for catheter placement, which is usually done with a small feeding tube. In the setting of PUVs, catheter insertion may be difficult, and bedside US can be an excellent modality to document the correct placement. Urologic management may include vesicostomy, cutaneous ureterostomy, pyelostomy, as well as eventual cystoscopy and valve ablation.

With PUV, a diverting vesicostomy is often used as a temporizing measure until the infant has matured enough to undergo definitive valve ablation. Percutaneous drainage of the urinoma or renal ascites is only necessary in the presence of respiratory compromise or intra-abdominal abscess. Upper-tract drainage and primary repair of the perforation site are rarely indicated.

The long-term prognosis is dependent on the underlying urologic anomaly and, most importantly, the degree of bladder outlet obstruction. Cases with a severe degree of bladder outlet obstruction are often accompanied by marked oligohydramnios and lung hypoplasia. Children with PUVs, UPJ obstruction, and neurogenic bladder can have varying degrees of hydronephrosis and resultant renal dysfunction. Because of the heterogeneity of presentation, counseling the family regarding future renal function will vary with the principal etiology. Long-term monitoring of renal function in these patients will be important to detect chronic kidney disease and intervene accordingly.

REFERENCES

1. Pinto E, Guignard JP. Renal masses in the neonate. *Biol Neonate*. 1995;68:175–184.
2. Fernbach SK. Imaging of neonatal renal masses. *Urol Radiol*. 1991;12:214–219.
3. Wiener JS, O'Hara SM. Optimal timing of initial postnatal ultrasonography in newborns with prenatal hydronephrosis. *J Urol*. 2002;168:1826–1829; discussion 1829.
4. Eckoldt F, Woderich R, Smith RD, Heling K-S. Antenatal diagnostic aspects of unilateral multicystic kidney dysplasia-sensitivity, specificity, predictive values, differential diagnoses, associated malformations and consequences. *Fetal Diagn Ther*. 2004;19:163–169.
5. Gunay-Aygun M, Font-Montgomery E, Lukose L, et al. Correlation of kidney function, volume and imaging findings, and PKHD1 mutations in 73 patients with autosomal recessive polycystic kidney disease. *Clin J Am Soc Nephrol*. 2010;5(6):972–984.
6. Fick GM., Duley IT, Johnson AM, Strain JD, Manco-Johnson ML, Gabow PA. The spectrum of autosomal dominant polycystic kidney disease in children. *J Am Soc Nephrol*. 1994;4(9):1654–1660.
7. Brandã LR, Simpson EA, Lau KK. Neonatal renal vein thrombosis. *Semin Fetal Neonatal Med*. 2011;16:323–328.
8. Cremin BJ, Davey H, Oleszczuk-Raszke K. Neonatal renal venous thrombosis: sequential ultrasonic appearances. *Clin Radiol*. 1991;44:52–55.
9. Goldstein I, Shoshani G, Ben-Harus E, Sujov P. Prenatal diagnosis of congenital mesoblastic nephroma. *Ultrasound Obstet Gynecol*. 2002;19:209–211.
10. Kelner M, Droullé P, Didier F, Hoeffel JC. The vascular "ring" sign in mesoblastic nephroma: report of two cases. *Pediatr Radiol*. 2003;33:123–128.
11. Lowe LH, Isuani BH, Heller RM, et al. Pediatric renal masses: Wilm's tumor and beyond. *Radiographics*. 2000;20(6):1585–1603.
12. Oei J, Garvey PA, Rosenberg AR. The diagnosis and management of neonatal urinary ascites. *J Paediatr Child Health*. 2001;37:513–515.
13. Chun KE, Ferguson RS. Neonatal urinary ascites due to unilateral vesicoureteric junction obstruction. *Pediatr Surg Int*. 1997; 12:455–457.

14. Arora P, Seth A, Bagga D, Aneja S, Taluja V. Spontaneous bladder rupture secondary to posterior urethral valves in a neonate. *Indian J Pediatr.* 2001;68:881–882.

15. Adzick NS, Harrison MR, Flake AW, deLorimier AA. Urinary extravasation in the fetus with obstructive uropathy. *J Pediatr Surg.* 1985;20:608–615.

16. Mata JA, Livne PM, Gibbons MD. Urinary ascites: complication of umbilical artery catheterization. *Urology.* 1987;30:375–377.

17. Vasdev N, Coulthard MG, De la hunt MN, Starzyk B, Ognjanovic M, Willetts IE. Neonatal urinary ascites secondary to urinary bladder rupture. *J Pediatr Urol.* 2009;5(2):100–104.

18. Aslam M, DeGrazia M, Gregory MLP. Diagnostic evaluation of neonatal ascites. *Am J Perinatol.* 2007;24:603–609.

19. Griscom NT, Colodny AH, Rosenberg HK, Fliegel CP, Hardy BE. Diagnostic aspects of neonatal ascites: report of 27 cases. *AJR Am J Roentgenol.* 1977;128:961–969.

CHAPTER 100

101 Neonatal Urinary Tract Infections

Curtis J. Clark and William A. Kennedy II

INTRODUCTION

Urinary tract infections (UTI) in the neonate pose a number of difficulties for the clinician. Symptoms are vague and overlap with a variety of other conditions. Accurate diagnosis requires testing of urine, which necessitates invasive techniques in the newborn child. The development of a UTI may be associated with the presence of other factors that increase the likelihood of pyelonephritis and subsequent renal scarring. In addition, significant ambiguity exists within the medical community about when further testing is necessary, which tests to obtain, and the appropriate timing of such testing. With these issues in mind, we address the basic workup and treatment of UTI in the neonate and briefly discuss some current controversies.

DIAGNOSIS

Urinary tract infection occurs in 0.1%–0.4% of infant girls, 0.702% of uncircumcised infant boys, and 0.188% of circumcised infant boys.[1] UTI is more common in premature (2.9%) and very low birth weight (4%–25%) infants in comparison to full-term infants (0.7%).[2] One of the most difficult aspects of UTI in neonates is the lack of any visible signs early in the process. Although adults and older children may experience symptoms such as frequency, urgency, and dysuria at the beginning of a UTI, neonates typically present with a fever or general irritability. The history may include malodorous urine or general fussiness or may consist only

of fever. The presence of a fever without an identified focus in a neonate prompts workup, including a full physical examination and obtaining samples of urine, blood, and cerebrospinal fluid for analysis and culture.[3] Admission to the hospital and initiation of intravenous antibiotics are routine. As in older children, bacteria of enteric origin cause most UTIs, with *Escherichia coli* the most common.[4] Table 101-1 lists some of the most common bacteria causing UTIs in children.

Physical examination in the neonate with a UTI is unlikely to provide any additional information, although the external genitalia should certainly be assessed. The presence of an intact foreskin and degree of physiologic phimosis should be noted in boys, as well as the presence of labial adhesions in girls. These anatomic considerations may complicate the accuracy of urine samples, as well as be potential areas of intervention for prevention of future infections. In addition, evaluation of the lower spine for a sacral dimple should be performed, with ultrasonography of the spine if a deep lesion is identified.

Accurate sampling of urine in neonates requires a sample to be obtained prior to antibiotic administration using either suprapubic aspiration (SPA) or catheterization of the urethra. SPA presents the least opportunity for contamination of a specimen but is the most invasive approach. Briefly, after cleansing the suprapubic area, a fine needle (21 gauge) is passed 1 fingerbreadth above the pubic bone, angling down toward the pelvis while aspirating.[5] The use of ultrasound guidance may increase the accuracy and safety of this procedure.[6] Because of the invasive nature of this approach, informed consent should be obtained

Table 101-1 Common Bacteria Causing Urinary Tract Infections in Children[a]

Escherichia coli (70%–90%)	*Pseudomonas* spp.
Klebsiella spp.	*Enterobacter* spp.
Proteus spp.	*Staphylococcus* spp.
Enterococcus spp.	

[a]Data from Lohr et al.[2]

whenever possible. Urethral catheterization is a less-invasive procedure, although it carries a higher risk of contamination from bacteria in the distal urethra and on the external genitalia, particularly in uncircumcised boys and girls with labial adhesions. Despite employment of sterile technique, the risk of contamination with catheterization leads to a sensitivity of 95% and a specificity of 99% in comparison to SPA.[7] Bagged urine is not appropriate for diagnosis of UTI in the neonate because of the high rate of falsely positive specimens.[8]

Evaluation for leukocyte esterase and the presence of nitrates on a urinalysis should be performed on a fresh specimen, as well as microscopic evaluation for the presence of white blood cells and bacteria. When the presence of leukocyte esterase and nitrates is positive on urinalysis, particularly in the presence of bacteria on microscopy, there is a high probability of a UTI. When urinalysis is suspicious or there is clinical concern for UTI, the urine should be sent for culture and sensitivities. Additional blood work, including a complete blood cell count with differential and C-reactive protein (CRP) value, may be helpful in assessing the neonate's overall condition and the severity of the infection, as well as in monitoring the success of treatment.

TREATMENT

Treatment of a suspected UTI in the neonate should consist of initiation of antibiotic therapy with an age-appropriate intravenous antibiotic after urine is obtained for culture. Despite data suggesting that delay in treatment of UTI may not increase the risk of renal scarring,[9] it is generally accepted that treatment should be initiated as soon as possible to minimize the risk of renal damage. Outpatient therapy for pyelonephritis is well accepted in pediatric literature[10] and has been successfully demonstrated in 1- to 3-month-olds using intravenous antibiotics[11]; however, neonates will invariably require admission to the hospital. Intravenous fluids are initiated to replace losses from fever and decreased oral intake. After obtaining appropriate specimens for culture, empiric intravenous antibiotics are initiated, with later conversion to oral therapy once the offending organism and its antibiotic sensitivities are known.

Oral and intravenous antibiotic choices are limited in this age group because of medicine side effects and neonatal physiology. The initial antibiotic choice should cover bacteria that frequently cause UTI (most commonly *Escherichia coli*, as listed in Table 101-1) and with knowledge of local resistance patterns.[4,12] A cephalosporin (such as ceftriaxone) or a penicillin derivative (ampicillin, etc) is a common empiric choice, with consideration of the addition of an aminoglycoside such as gentamicin to broaden coverage. Table 101-2 lists commonly used empiric intravenous antibiotics. Once oral therapy is initiated, generally after sensitivities are known and the patient is improving, penicillin derivatives and cephalosporins are the most commonly used antibiotics. Trimethoprim-sulfamethoxazole, an antibiotic commonly used to treat UTIs in children, is not appropriate in the first 2–3 months of life, and the same holds true for nitrofurantoin. Furthermore, nitrofurantoin is not an acceptable antibiotic for the febrile infant with a UTI as it does not reach adequate serum/tissue levels, making it an unacceptable choice for pyelonephritis. Ciprofloxacin is approved for use in complicated UTIs in children but is generally reserved for when there are no other oral options.

In its most recent recommendation, the American Academy of Pediatrics (AAP) sought to determine an

Table 101-2 Some Common Parenteral Antibiotics Used for Urinary Tract Infections in Neonates[a]

	Route	0–7 Days Old (Weight > 2 kg)	8–28 Days Old (Weight > 2 kg)	>28 Days Old
Ampicillin	IV, IM	150 mg/kg/d divided every 8 h	200 mg/kg/d divided every 6 h	200 mg/kg/d divided every 6 h
Ceftriaxone	IV, IM	25 mg/kg/d every 24 h	50 mg/kg/d every 24 h	50 mg/kg/d every 24 h
		27–34 Weeks' EGA (Corrected)	**35–42 Weeks' EGA (Corrected)**	**>43 Weeks' EGA (Corrected)**
Gentamicin	IV, IM	2.5 mg/kg/dose every 18 h	2.5 mg/kg/dose every 12 h	2.5 mg/kg/dose every 8 h
Vancomycin	IV	15 mg/kg/dose every 18 h	15 mg/kg/dose every 12 h	15 mg/kg/dose every 8 h

Abbreviation: EGA, estimated gestational age.
[a]Data from Bradley and Sauberan.[24]

optimal duration of antibiotic therapy based on the current literature.[8] Although shorter durations (1–3 days) were inferior in a meta-analysis[14] in 2002, no convincing data were available to determine if a 7-, 10-, or 14-day course is optimal. In clinical practice, more severe infections, particularly those in which blood cultures are positive, cases with abnormal anatomy, and UTIs in the very young, should be treated with a longer course (14 days). The total course should be calculated, including the duration of intravenous and oral antibiotic treatment.

Monitoring after initiation of antibiotics should consist of following urine output, oral intake, and routine vital signs. Adequately treated pyelonephritis often follows a course of intermittent daily fevers with decreasing daily maximum temperature. When improving appropriately and as expected, repeat laboratory tests and a follow-up urine culture are most often unnecessary. When the neonate does not improve as expected, consideration should be given to additional blood work, repeat culture of the urine, and additional imaging.

IMAGING

While there is significant debate regarding imaging for UTIs, renal/bladder ultrasonography (RBUS) is generally agreed on as the first-line imaging. Without any radiation exposure or sedation, ultrasonography allows for assessment of gross bladder abnormalities, hydroureter proximally or distally, renal size, renal blood flow, the presence of hydronephrosis, and the presence of a fluid collection concerning for renal abscess. Ultrasonography is capable of detecting gross abnormalities but is less accurate than nuclear imaging in detecting renal scars or developmental dysplasia.[15] When the patient's clinical condition improves as expected, RBUS can be obtained either at outpatient follow-up or as an inpatient. Severe infections, complicated cases, and those that do not improve appropriately should have the infant imaged as an inpatient.

Significant debate exists about both the need for and timing of additional imaging after UTI. Classically, febrile UTIs prompted workup, including RBUS and voiding cystourethrography (VCUG) to evaluate for vesicoureteral reflux (VUR), the retrograde flow of urine into the upper tracts. This approach is still frequently employed in the neonate after an initial diagnosis of febrile UTI. Additional imaging options include renal scan, utilizing either dimercaptosuccinic acid (DMSA) or Mag3 as the radiotracer, when RBUS or VCUG causes concern for renal scarring or obstruction. In neonates, a low threshold for further imaging remains appropriate, with understanding of the risks related to radiation exposure in this population.

In recent years, the relationship between VUR, UTI, and renal scarring has come under new scrutiny. With the increasing acceptance of the concept that VUR without infection does not cause scarring[16] and increasing skepticism about the value of treatment of VUR, the need to diagnose/treat all VUR has become an ongoing debate. Questions have arisen about whether classic approaches to VUR (continuous antibiotic prophylaxis and surgical correction) prevent new renal scarring. Alternative approaches for workup and imaging have been proposed that center on evaluating for renal scarring as the initial testing ("top-down" approach) and determination of the need for VCUG based on the presence or absence of scarring.[17] Additional factors to be considered in both the "bottom-up and top-down approaches are the relative invasiveness of testing (intravenous administration, catheter insertion); the need for sedation; and the relative radiation dose associated with these tests. However, significant variability can exist in the effective doses of these tests between different institutions and between individual patients. Knowledge of the average effective doses at an institution may help in following the ALARA (as low as reasonably achievable) principle for radiation exposure when deciding on additional testing.[18]

The debate surrounding these issues has led some to propose alternative guidelines for imaging after UTI. These guidelines often delay recommending VCUG and, in some cases, eliminate testing for VUR altogether. When considering these approaches, however, multiple factors must be taken into account, including the severity of the infection, social situation, family history, and presence of abnormalities on RBUS. Because of the ongoing debate, we strongly encourage urologic consultation to discuss the advantages and disadvantages of additional imaging, particularly in the neonatal time period. Two examples of guidelines developed in recent years to help the pediatrician are the National Institute for Health and Clinical Excellence (NICE) guidelines[19] and the recent update of the AAP guidelines for UTI.[8]

In 2007, NICE published guidelines for UTI in children; the guidelines were based on an extensive review of the literature. These recommendations significantly decrease imaging for older children who develop a UTI. In the case of a child less than 6 months old who develops a routine UTI and responds well to treatment, RBUS is the only imaging study recommended. For infants with recurrent or atypical UTIs, the recommendation is for a RBUS and VCUG, with a DMSA renal scan obtained at 4–6 months. UTIs are considered "recurrent" when a child experiences 2 or more episodes of pyelonephritis, an episode of pyelonephritis and an episode of acute cystitis, or 3 or more episodes of cystitis. A UTI is considered "atypical" if any of these criteria are met: The child is seriously ill, has poor urine flow, has an abdominal/bladder mass, has an elevated serum creatinine, has sepsis, fails to respond within 48 hours, has a non-*E. coli* UTI.

In 1999, the AAP published a practice parameter on UTI in children.[20] This guideline was recently updated with the publication in September 2001 of "Urinary Tract Infection: Clinical Practice Guideline for the Diagnosis and Management of the Initial UTI in Febrile Infants and Children 2–24 Months."[8] Based on an extensive review of the literature and expert opinion, this guideline does not address children less than 2 months old because of a lack data. Nonetheless, although not supported by clinical data, application to the neonate with a UTI is worthy of thoughtful consideration and use of appropriate clinical judgment.

The updated guideline recommended RBUS as the initial imaging study. This study can be obtained in a delayed manner when the child responds appropriately to therapy, while inpatient ultrasonography is recommended when the illness is severe or the child is felt to be slow in responding to therapy. DMSA renal scan was not recommended as an initial study as it rarely changes acute clinical management. With growing questions about the effectiveness of VUR treatment (continuous antibiotic prophylaxis, surgery) in preventing renal scarring and about the need to diagnose all VUR, the AAP recommendation was updated to eliminate routine VCUG after initial UTI in those with normal urinary tract anatomy. This recommendation is the subject of debate in the urologic community, and VCUG should be considered, taking into account the overall clinical and social situation. When abnormalities are seen on RBUS or UTIs are complex, then a VCUG is indicated. When UTIs are recurrent, further workup is recommended, likely with VCUG or DMSA renal scanning. Consultation with a pediatric urologist when available to assist in determining the need for further imaging is recommended.

FOLLOW-UP

Once an appropriate course of antibiotics has been completed, no follow-up urine culture is necessary unless symptoms are evident because of the invasiveness of accurate urine testing and the high rate of false-positive cultures with noninvasive acquisition of urine. Follow-up is generally performed in 2–4 weeks, although there is no agreed-on schedule. The NICE guidelines recommended consultation with a specialist when the child is less than 3 months old, with consideration of referral for those older than 3 months. In light of the controversy regarding the need to diagnose VUR, urologic consultation to discuss the pros and cons of further imaging after UTI is appropriate when

pediatric urologic services are available, particularly in the case of infection during the neonatal time period.

Prophylaxis is not indicated after initial UTI without a diagnosis of VUR; however, it may be considered until consultation with a specialist can be obtained, particularly in cases of recurrence, abnormal anatomy, or severe infection. Amoxicillin and cephalexin are the most common antibiotics used for prophylaxis in the neonate, generally with once-a-day dosing at one-quarter of the normal treatment dose. The most recent meta-analysis looking at prophylaxis in children without VUR but with recurrent UTIs showed a small benefit in preventing symptomatic UTIs.[21] When a history of UTI is present, parents should be instructed that a low threshold be used to evaluate for UTI when a fever of unknown origin is present. Circumcision is known to decrease the risk of UTI in infants.[22,23] Whether a UTI alone should be considered an indication to perform circumcision is an area of debate. Consultation with a pediatric urologist should address this issue, taking into account the benefits and risks of circumcision, as well as parental preference, in making a decision. When renal scarring is known to have occurred as a result of pyelonephritis, monitoring for high blood pressure and proteinuria is appropriate.

SUMMARY

Although old paradigms may be changing regarding UTI and VUR in children, the diagnosis and treatment of UTI in the neonate remain relatively stable. UTI should be included in the differential diagnosis for the febrile neonate. Once diagnosed, UTI should be treated promptly and with an adequate course of antibiotics. Ultrasonography is generally agreed on as the first choice in imaging, but the rationale for additional imaging is an area of significant debate. Consultation with a pediatric urologist is recommended when possible. Long-term follow-up should include observation for hypertension and proteinuria in those with a history of significant infection or scarring.

REFERENCES

1. Foxman B. Epidemiology of urinary tract infections: incidence, morbidity, and economic costs. *Am J Med.* 2002;113(1A):5S–13S.
2. Lohr J, Downs S, Schlager T. Genitourinary tract infections. In: Long S, ed. *Principles and Practice of Pediatric Infectious Diseases*, 3rd ed. Philadelphia, PA: Saunders; 2009:339–343.
3. Nield L, Kamat D. Fever without a focus. In: Kliegman R, Stanton B, Geme J, Schor N, Behrman R, eds. *Nelson Textbook of Pediatrics.* 19th ed. 2011. Elsevier/Saunders Philadelphia, PA, pp 896-902. Accessed online October 2011.
4. Ismaili K, Lolin K, Damry N, Alexander M, Lepage P, Hall M. Febrile urinary tract infections in 0- to 3-month old infants: a prospective follow-up study. *J Pediatr.* 2011;158(1):91–94.

5. Barkemeyer B. Suprapubic aspiration of urine in very low birth weight infants. *Pediatrics*. 1994;92:457–459.

6. Buys H, Pead L, Hallett R, Maskell R. Suprapubic aspiration under ultrasound guidance in children with fever of undiagnosed cause. *BMJ*. 1994;308(6930):690–692.

7. Kramer MS, Tange SM, Drummond KN, Millis EL. Urine testing in young febrile children: a risk-benefit analysis. *J Pediatr*. 1994;125(1):6–13.

8. American Academy of Pediatrics, Subcommittee on Urinary Tract Infection. Urinary tract infection: clinical practice guideline for the diagnosis and management of the initial UTI in febrile infants and children 2 to 24 months. *Pediatrics*. 2011;128:595–610.

9. Hewitt I, Zuccheta P, Rigon L, et al. Early treatment of acute pyelonephritis in children fails to reduce renal scarring: data from the Italian renal infection study trials. *Pediatrics*. 2008;122:486–490.

10. Hoberman A, Wald ER, Hickey RW, et al. Oral versus intravenous therapy for urinary tract infections in young febrile children. *Pediatrics*. 1999;104(1):79–86.

11. Doré-Bergeron MJ, Gauthier M, Chevalier I, et al. Urinary tract infections in 1- to 3-month-old infants: ambulatory treatment with intravenous antibiotics. *Pediatrics*. 2009;124:16–22.

12. Shortliffe LD. Infection and inflammation of the pediatric genitourinary tract. In: Wein A, Kavoussi L, Novick A, Partin A, Peters C, eds. *Campbell-Walsh Urology*. 10th ed. 2011. Elsevier/Saunders Philadelphia, PA, pp 3085-3122. Accessed online October 2011.

13. Bradley J, Sauberan J. Antimicrobial agents. In: Long S, ed. *Principles and Practice of Pediatric Infectious Diseases*. Rev. reprint, 3rd ed. Philadelphia, PA: Saunders; 2009:1453–1484.

14. Keren R, Chen E. A meta-analysis of randomized, controlled trials comparing short- and long-course antibiotic therapy for urinary tract infections in children. *Pediatrics*. 2002:109(5):E70-0.

15. Sinha M, Gibson P, Kane T, et al. Accuracy of ultrasonic detection of renal scarring in different centres using DMSA as the gold standard. *Nephrol Dial Transplant*. 2007;22:2213–2216.

16. Ransley PG, Risdon RA, Godley ML. High pressure sterile vesicoureteral reflux and renal scarring: an experimental study in the pig and minipig. In: Hodson CJ, Heptinstall RH, Winberg J, eds. *Reflux Nephropathy Update: 1983*. New York: Karger; 1984:320–343.

17. Hansson S, Dhamey M, Sigström O, et al. Dimercaptosuccinic acid scintigraphy instead of voiding cystourethrography for infants with urinary tract infection. *J Urol*. 2004;172:1071–1074.

18. Routh JC, Lee RS, Chow JS. Radiation dose and screening for vesicoureteral reflux [letter]. *AJR Am J Roentgenol*. 2010;194(2):W243.

19. National Institute for Health and Clinical Excellence. *Urinary Tract Infection in Children: Diagnosis, Treatment, and Long-Term Management: NICE Guideline 54*. London, UK: National Institute for Health and Clinical Excellence; 2007. http://www.nice.org.uk/nicemedia/live/11819/36032/36032.pdf. Accessed October 2011.

20. American Academy of Pediatrics, Committee on Quality Improvement, Subcommittee on Urinary Tract Infection. Practice parameter: the diagnosis, treatment, and evaluation of the initial urinary tract infection in febrile infants and young children. *Pediatrics*. 1999;103(4):843–852.

21. Williams G, Craig JC. Long-term antibiotics for preventing recurrent urinary tract infection in children. *Cochrane Database Syst Rev*. 2011;(3):CD001534.

22. American Academy of Pediatrics, Task Force on Circumcision. Circumcision policy statement. *Pediatrics*. 1999;103:686–693.

23. Singh-Grewal D, Macdessi J, Craig J. Circumcision for the prevention of urinary tract infection in children: a systemic review of randomised trials and observational studies. *Arch Dis Child*. 2005;90:853–858.

24. Bradley J, Sauberan J. Antimicrobial agents. In: Long S, ed. *Principles and Practice of Pediatric Infectious Diseases*, 4th ed. Philadelphia, PA: Elsevier/Saunders; 2012.

102 Disorders of Sexual Development

Rajiv Kumar and Bruce Buckingham

BACKGROUND

Approach

1. Approach the newborn with ambiguous genitalia with sensitivity, avoiding use of ambiguous pronouns.
2. Determine if there is a related life-threatening illness.
3. Activate a multidisciplinary team to help establish a diagnosis and eventually the sex of rearing.

Embryology

1. Humans have bipotential embryologic tissues.
2. Gender is differentiated by an orchestra of expression and interaction of specific genes and gene products.
3. Chromosomes determine gonadal sex, but local factors influence differentiation of the internal and external genital structures.

DIFFERENTIAL DIAGNOSIS

46,XX Disorder of Sex Development (DSD) (Overvirilized Female)

1. There are normal ovaries and Mullerian structures.
2. Masculinization of the external genitalia occurs as a result of in utero exposure to androgens.
3. Congenital adrenal hyperplasia (CAH) is most common and is potentially life threatening.

4. 46,XX with testicular tissue
   a. Anomalous Y-to-X translocation, including the *SRY* gene during meiosis
   b. Ranges from ovotesticular DSD, to some degree of sexual ambiguity, to normal male phenotype

46,XY DSD (Undervirilized Male)

1. Testes present
2. Internal duct system or the external genitalia incompletely masculinized
3. Phenotype is variable and can look like a normal female.
4. Hypospadias, cryptorchidism, penoscrotal transposition, blind vaginal pouch
5. Adrenal blocks potential causes of undervirilization
6. Leydig cell failure or unresponsiveness to hCG and luteinizing hormone (LH)
   a. Decreased testosterone and/or dihydrotestosterone (DHT, seen with 5-alpha reductase deficiency) DHT
   b. No support of Wolffian ducts
   c. No support of external male genitalia
7. Androgen insensitivity syndrome (AIS) or "testicular feminization"
   a. Can be partial
   b. Mutation of the steroid-binding domain of androgen receptor
   c. Testes present, but patient looks like a phenotypic female

8. 5-α-Reductase deficiency

   a. Testosterone cannot be converted to DHT at target tissue.

   b. Patient is a normal male inside, but ambiguous on the outside.

   c. At puberty, testosterone increases significantly and masculinizes the external genitalia; this may be associated with a change in gender identity.

9. Persistent Mullerian duct syndrome

   a. Abnormal anti-Mullerian hormone (AMH; formerly Mullerian Inhibitor Factor or Mullerian Inhibitory Substance) or its receptor occurs.

   b. Patient may look like a phenotypic male.

   c. This diagnosis is often made at the time of inguinal hernia repair or orchiopexy, when internal Mullerian structures (uterus, cervix, Fallopian tubes, upper two-thirds of vagina) are found.

10. Congenital anorchia ("vanishing testes")

    a. Loss of testes before 8 weeks' gestation: female internally and externally with streak gonads

    b. At 8–10 weeks: ambiguous genitalia and variable duct formation

    c. At 12–14 weeks: male phenotype with anorchia

11. Maternal ingestion of progesterone or estrogen or environmental hazards: pesticides, DES (diethylstilbestrol), OCPs (oral contraceptives), and in vitro fertilization (IVF) medicines all implicated

12. Increased incidence of hypospadias in boys born through IVF

Chromosome DSD

1. Klinefelter (XXY) and the 46,XY/47,XXY mosaic: usually not evident until adolescence

2. Turner (XO) and the 45,XO/46,XX mosaic: streak gonads

3. Can also have 46,XX and 46,XY with streak gonads

Ovotesticular DSD (Gonadal Dysgenesis)

1. *SRY* (Sex determinng region Y) gene transposition (complete gonadal dysgenesis)

2. DAX-1 is a nuclear receptor protein that can antagonize *SRY*

3. WT1 (Denys-Drash and WAGR)

4. SOX9 (campomelic dysplasia/lethal skeletal malformation)

5. Swyer syndrome (female inside and out with two dysgenetic gonads in the abdomen)

6. Partial gonadal dysgenesis (risk of gonadoblastoma higher in those with a Y chromosome)

CLINICAL FINDINGS

History

1. Pregnancy: ingestion of exogenous maternal hormones used in assisted reproduction, maternal use of OCP during pregnancy, abnormal prenatal ultrasound, discordance of the fetal karyotype with the genital sonogram, abnormal virilization, or Cushingoid appearance of the child's mother

2. Family history: urologic anomalies, neonatal deaths, precocious puberty, amenorrhea, infertility, consanguinity

Physical

1. Examine in a warm environment, supine in frog-leg position with both legs free (when possible).

2. Are there testes? Check size, location, and texture of both gonads (if palpable).

3. Is uterus palpable? Note phallic size (width and stretched length), position of the urethral meatus, number of perineal orifices.

4. Examine for skin hyperpigmentation, abnormal blood pressure (BP), other physical anomalies.

Laboratory Tests

1. Karyotype (not negated by amniocentesis) and consider fluorescence in situ hybridization (FISH) for SRY (faster than comparative genomic hybridization [CGH])

2. Electrolytes, urine sodium and potassium, and serum 17-OH-progesterone (may need subsequent 11-deoxycortisol and deoxycorticosterone) to screen for CAH

3. Testosterone and DHT (must be drawn in first 24 hours of life, or need to perform hCG stimulation test or wait for minipuberty of infancy between 2-6 months of age): testosterone/DHT ratio greater than 20 suggests 5-α-reductase deficiency

4. AMH and inhibin B to assess the existence of normal testicular tissue

5. Androgen precursors before and after hCG stimulation test (a ratio of testosterone to androstenedione

< 0.8 suggests a 17-beta-hydroxysteroid dehydrogenase deficiency frame).

6. A high follicle-stimulating hormone (FSH) and LH with low testosterone in the first 24 hours or in minipuberty suggests anorchia

Imaging

1. Abdominal/pelvic ultrasound (US) detects intra-abdominal testes 50% of the time. It can also detect gonads in the inguinal regions and assess Mullerian structures.

2. Magnetic resonance imaging (MRI) can detect ectopic gonads and immature testes/ovaries.

3. A genitogram may be used to find the urethral path.

4. Laparoscopy with gonadal biopsies for histologic evaluation may be required.

TREATMENT

1. Assess karyotype (genotypic sex), external reproductive system (phenotypic sex), internal reproductive system, gonadal functionality (potential hormone secretion and fertility), and hormone responsiveness.

2. Treatment should be individualized to each patient. Tertiary care hospital is appropriate through the adult years.

3. A multidisciplinary team is involved: parents; neonatal intensive care unit (NICU) staff; individuals from genetics, endocrinology, urology, obstetrics/gynecology, radiology, psychology, psychiatry; support groups.

4. Focus on open and direct communication with parents, who should participate in gender assignment.

5. Surgery depends on anatomy, functional status, and opinions of the family and medical team.

OTHER DISORDERS OF SEXUAL DIFFERENTIATION

Micropenis

1. Stretched length is less than 2.5 cm in a term male.

2. Girth is equally important.

3. This finding indicates hypopituitarism until proven otherwise.

4. Low FSH and LH indicate low testosterone causing microphallus with or without cryptorchidism.

5. Genital ambiguity is not anticipated with hypogonadotropic hypogonadism.

6. Growth hormone deficiency may result in micropenis.

7. Hypopituitarism can be life threatening (hypocortisolism or hypoglycemia) and may also result in jaundice/increased liver function tests (LFTs).

8. Kallman syndrome is a gonadotropin-releasing hormone (GnRH) deficiency.

Cryptorchidism

1. Of males, 3% of full term infants and 30% of premature infants have cryptorchidism (70% spontaneously descend by 1 year of age).

2. In a "male" infant, bilateral undescended testes can be associated with CAH, hypogonadotropic hypogonadism, an ovotesticaular disorder, anorchia or bilateral undescended testes.

3. Persistent unilateral or bilateral undescended testes is associated with an increased risk of testicular tumor in either the descended or undescended testes.

Neonatal Hypertension

Abanti Chaudhuri and Scott M. Sutherland

INTRODUCTION

Over the past several decades, we have learned much about neonatal hypertension, resulting in an increased awareness in the modern neonatal intensive care unit (NICU). In healthy term infants, hypertension is exceedingly uncommon,[1] with an incidence of approximately 0.2%. In critically ill infants admitted to the NICU, however, the incidence is higher, with reported rates[2-4] ranging from 0.7% to 3.0%. The diagnosis of hypertension in neonates and infants can be challenging because their normal blood pressure (BP) range is dynamic, varying along with a number of factors, including gestational age, postnatal age, and weight. Despite this, a careful diagnostic evaluation should allow determination of the underlying cause of hypertension in most hypertensive neonates. There are numerous treatment options, and treatment decisions should be tailored individually based on the severity of the hypertension and concomitant disease states. Fortunately, in most infants, hypertension resolves over time, although a small number may have persistently elevated BPs throughout childhood.

DEFINING AND DIAGNOSING NEONATAL HYPERTENSION

Normative Neonatal Blood Pressures

One of the greatest challenges when diagnosing hypertension in neonates is the fact that the normative BP range is dynamic. BPs exhibit a variable pattern, and one must consider gestational age at birth, postnatal or postconceptual age, birth weight, and appropriateness of size for gestational age. In general, BP normally increases with increasing gestational and postconceptual age, as well as with increasing birth weight.[5-9] Not surprisingly, a greater rate of increase is seen in preterm and infants small for gestational age, compared to term neonates. Fortunately, several recent studies have provided normative data that greatly facilitate the identification of neonates with elevated BPs.

Zubrow et al defined mean and upper/lower 95% confidence limits for neonatal BPs based on prospective, serial oscillometric BP measurements from 608 neonates admitted to multiple NICUs.[9] On day of life 1, systolic and diastolic BPs correlated strongly with birth weight and gestational age. BP progressively increased after birth, most rapidly during the first 5 days (1.6–2.7 mm Hg/d). This increase continued after the fifth day, albeit at more gradual increments (0.15–0.27 mm Hg/d). Most notably, in a multiple-regression analysis, the primary determinant of BP was postconceptual age (Figure 103-1).

In addition, Pejovic et al examined BPs measured by an oscillometric device in 373 hemodynamically stable premature and term neonates to evaluate the influence of gestational age, postnatal age, birth weight, gender, and sleep state on BP.[8] Systolic and diastolic BPs progressively increased during the first month of life, with BP increasing more rapidly in preterm infants than in full-term infants. BPs on day 1 of life correlated with gestational age and birth weight. Multiple-regression analysis showed that mean BP during the first week and on the 30th day increased with gestational age.

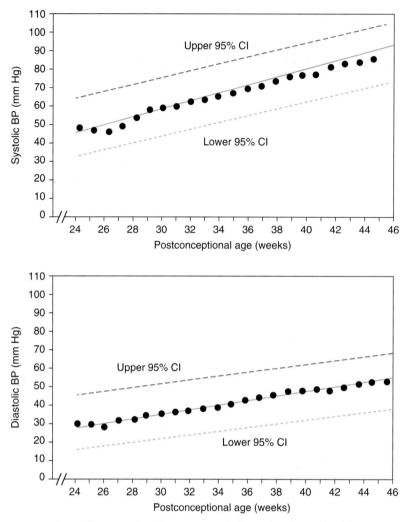

FIGURE 103-1 Linear regression of mean systolic (top) and diastolic (bottom) blood pressures (BPs) by post-conceptual age in weeks, with 95% confidence intervals (upper and lower dashed lines). CI, confidence interval. (Reproduced with permission from Zubrow et al.[9])

Furthermore, BPs were higher in the awake state than in the sleep state.

An Australian prospective study of oscillometric BP measurement in 406 term infants with a mean gestational age of 40 weeks showed no difference in BP on day 1 of life based on birth weight, length, or gestational age.[5] In the first day of life, median systolic, diastolic, and mean arterial BPs were 65 (range 46 to 94), 45 (range 24 to 57), and 48 (range 31 to 63), respectively. BP measurements increased over the 4 successive days, albeit at a slower rate than seen in preterm infant studies, usually by 1–2 mm Hg/d; in addition, this study demonstrated that BPs stabilized earlier in term than in preterm infants.

Finally, Kent and colleagues studied BP measurements using oscillometric methods in 147 nonventilated, stable, premature neonates with gestational age ranging from 28 to 36 weeks. This study demonstrated that the period of rapid BP rise occurred over the first 2–3 weeks in infants born at 28–31 weeks'

gestation but only over the first week in infants born at greater than 32 weeks' gestational age.[7] Premature neonates were noted to stabilize their BP after 14 days of life; thereafter, they had BPs similar to those of age-matched term infants.[5]

These data highlight how challenging it is to establish normative values for neonatal BP, especially in preterm and critically ill infants, because of the effects of gestational age and maturation on BP values.

Diagnostic Criteria

Based on a review of published data, Dionne et al created a reference table of normal BP values after the first 2 weeks of life in infants with postconceptual ages between 26 and 44 weeks[10] (Table 103-1). This table and the data shown in Figure 103-1 are the best currently available tools to identify infants with hypertension. Neonates who have BPs persistently above the 95th percentile should be considered hypertensive.

Table 103-1 Estimated Values for Blood Pressures After 2 Weeks of Age in Infants From 26 to 44 Weeks' Postconceptual Age[a,b]

Postconceptual Age		50th Percentile	95th Percentile	99th Percentile
44 weeks	SBP	88	105	110
	DBP	50	68	73
	MAP	63	80	85
42 weeks	SBP	85	98	102
	DBP	50	65	70
	MAP	62	76	81
40 weeks	SBP	80	95	100
	DBP	50	65	70
	MAP	60	75	80
38 weeks	SBP	77	92	97
	DBP	50	65	70
	MAP	59	74	79
36 weeks	SBP	72	87	92
	DBP	50	65	70
	MAP	57	72	71
34 weeks	SBP	70	85	90
	DBP	40	55	60
	MAP	50	65	70
32 weeks	SBP	68	83	88
	DBP	40	55	60
	MAP	48	62	69
30 weeks	SBP	65	80	85
	DBP	40	55	60
	MAP	48	65	68
28 weeks	SBP	60	75	80
	DBP	38	50	54
	MAP	45	58	63
26 weeks	SBP	55	72	77
	DBP	30	50	56
	MAP	38	57	63

Abbreviations: DBP, diastolic blood pressure; MAP, mean arterial pressure; SBP, systolic blood pressure.
[a]Data from Dionne et al.[10]
[b]The 95th and 99th percentile values serve as a reference to identify infants with persistent hypertension that may require treatment.

The 95th percentile curve in Figure 103-1 and the 95th/99th percentile values shown in Table 103-1 are intended to serve as a reference to identify infants with persistent systolic and diastolic hypertension that may require treatment. The data in Table 103-1 have the added benefit of mean arterial pressure (MAP) data. Some practitioners are more comfortable assessing neonatal BPs using a MAP value. MAP provides an assessment of the overall perfusion pressure, which may help guard against treatment of isolated systolic hypertension in infants with labile BPs.

For older infants, the percentile curves reported by the Second Task Force of the National High BP Education Program (NHBPEP) Working Group (Figure 103-2)[11] remain the most widely available reference values. These curves can be used similarly to those from Figure 103-1.

MEASUREMENT OF BP IN NEONATES

Accurate BP measurement is the crucial first step in the diagnosis of neonatal hypertension. Crying, pain, feeding, and agitation all can increase BP in a neonate.[12] BP is best measured by an oscillometric device, preferably 1.5 hours after feeding or a medical intervention when the infant is sleeping or resting. A critical component of noninvasive BP measurement is the use of an appropriate-size cuff,[13] which is a cuff with an inflatable bladder width that is at least 40% of the arm circumference at a point midway between the olecranon and the acromion. In addition, the cuff bladder length should cover 80%–100% of the circumference of the arm; thereby, the bladder width-to-length ratio should be at least 1:2. Hence, in the term infant with a maximum arm circumference of 10 cm, the usual dimensions of an appropriate-size cuff bladder are 4 cm in width and 8 cm in length.[13] BP usually is measured in an arm because most normative oscillometric data are based on right arm pressures; in addition, leg pressures tend to be higher in children. Because of this, it is important for the medical record to note the site of measurement. After cuff placement, the BP should be measured several minutes after the infant has settled into a calm state. Ideally, 3 successive BP readings should be obtained at 2-minute intervals.

In critically ill neonates, continuous, direct intra-arterial BP measurement through a catheter placed in the aorta or the radial artery is the most accurate technique. Although radial artery systolic BP measurements may be 20% to 30% higher than central values in adults,[14] radial pressures appear to more closely mimic aortic pressures in newborns.[15] Intra-arterial catheters should be discontinued as the neonate clinically improves to avoid possible risk of complications like infection and thrombosis.

ETIOLOGY OF NEONATAL HYPERTENSION

Numerous potential causes of neonatal hypertension have been identified (Table 103-2). However, the most common etiologies are umbilical artery

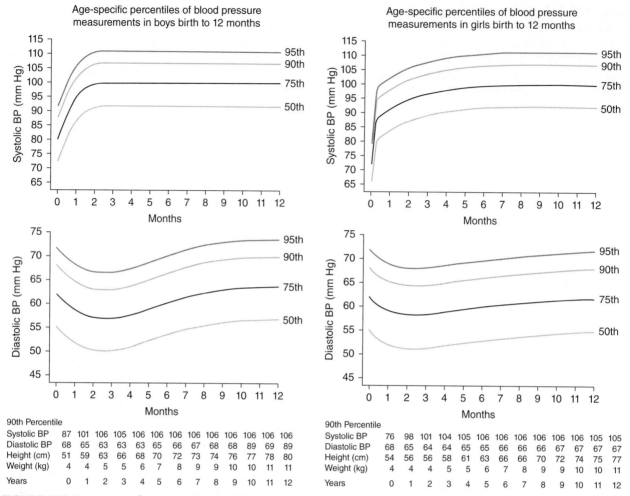

Age-specific percentiles of blood pressure measurements in boys birth to 12 months

Age-specific percentiles of blood pressure measurements in girls birth to 12 months

90th Percentile

Systolic BP	87	101	106	105	106	106	106	106	106	106	106	106	106
Diastolic BP	68	65	63	63	63	65	66	67	68	68	89	69	89
Height (cm)	51	59	63	66	68	70	72	73	74	76	77	78	80
Weight (kg)	4	4	5	5	6	7	8	9	9	10	10	11	11
Years	0	1	2	3	4	5	6	7	8	9	10	11	12

90th Percentile

Systolic BP	76	98	101	104	105	106	106	106	106	106	106	105	105
Diastolic BP	68	65	64	64	65	65	66	66	66	67	67	67	67
Height (cm)	54	56	56	58	61	63	66	66	70	72	74	75	77
Weight (kg)	4	4	5	5	6	7	8	9	9	10	10	11
Years	0	1	2	3	4	5	6	7	8	9	10	11	12

FIGURE 103-2 Age-specific percentiles for blood pressure (BP) in (a) boys and (b) girls during the first 12 months of life. (Reproduced with permission from Report of the Second Task Force on Blood Pressure Control in Children—1987. Task Force on Blood Pressure Control in Children. National Heart, Lung, and Blood Institute, Bethesda, Maryland. Pediatrics. 1987;79(1):1–25.)

catheter-associated thromboembolism, followed by chronic lung disease and renal parenchymal disease. Other common etiologies include fluid overload, medication-related side effects, and inadequate sedation for intubated patients. Although a thorough history and examination, coupled with screening diagnostics, usually allow identification of an etiology, at times no cause can be identified. In such cases, hypertension may be caused by the presence of an undetectable renovascular event. Table 103-2 offers a comprehensive list of possible etiologies; the more common etiologies are discussed next.

Vascular Etiologies

The most common cause of hypertension in neonates is vascular occlusion caused by thromboembolic events related to umbilical artery catheterization.[16] Low-lying catheters are just as likely to be associated with the development of hypertension as "high" catheters[17]; however, a longer duration of catheterization is associated with a higher rate of thrombus formation.[18] Renal vein thrombosis, which classically presents with the triad of gross hematuria, thrombocytopenia, and a palpable renal mass, can also be associated with hypertension. It is often associated with hypercoagulable disorders, such as infants of diabetic mothers or factor V Leiden mutations.[19,20] Aortic coarctation is a potential cause of neonatal hypertension that can be easily identified and treated.[4] Uncommonly, hypertension in neonates may be related to renal artery stenosis or narrowing caused by fibromuscular dysplasia, congenital rubella infection, or mechanical compression from an abdominal mass.[21-23]

Renal Etiologies

Neonates with congenital renal parenchymal abnormalities comprise the next largest group of neonates with hypertension. Autosomal dominant and recessive polycystic kidney disease (PKD) may present in the newborn period with nephromegaly and hypertension.[24]

Table 103-2 Etiology of Neonatal Hypertension

Renovascular
  Thromboembolism (especially with umbilical artery catheterization)
  Renal artery stenosis
  Renal artery compression
  Renal vein thrombosis
  Coarctation of the aorta
  Idiopathic arterial calcification
  Abdominal aortic aneurysm
Renal parenchymal disease
  Polycystic kidney disease (ARPKD/ADPKD)
  Renal dysplasia/hypoplasia
  Multicystic kidney disease
  Obstructive uropathy
  Acute tubular necrosis/cortical necrosis
  Resolving acute kidney injury
  Pyelonephritis
  Nephrocalcinosis
  Tuberous sclerosis
  Hemolytic uremic syndrome
  Interstitial nephritis
Endocrine
  Congenital adrenal hyperplasia
  Hyperaldosteronism
  Hyperthyroidism
Neoplasia
  Wilms tumor
  Neuroblastoma
  Mesoblastic nephroma
  Pheochromocytoma
	Medications/drugs
	  Maternal cocaine exposure
	  Maternal heroin exposure
	  Corticosteroids
	  Theophylline
	  Caffeine
	  Pancuronium
	  Phenylephrine
	  Vitamin D intoxication
	  Adrenergic agents
	Pulmonary
	  Bronchopulmonary dysplasia
	  Pneumothorax
	Neurologic
	  Pain
	  Seizures
	  Inadequate sedation
	  Intracranial hypertension
	  Intraventricular or intracranial hemorrhage
	  Subdural hematoma
	  Familial dysautonomia
	Miscellaneous
	  Monogenic hypertension
	  Hypercalcemia
	  Fluid overload
	  Adrenal hemorrhage
	  Prolonged total parental nutrition administration
	  Closure of an abdominal wall defect
	  Extracorporeal membrane oxygenation
	  Birth asphyxia

Abbreviations: ADPKD, autosomal dominant polycystic kidney disease; ARPKD, autosomal recessive polycystic kidney disease.

In addition, hypertension has been reported in neonates born with unilateral multicystic dysplastic kidneys.[2,25] Urinary obstruction caused by congenital ureteropelvic junction obstruction, posterior urethral valves, or other intra-abdominal masses may be accompanied by hypertension, which is likely mediated by the renin-angiotensin system.[2,26] Less commonly, hypertension can be related to acquired renal parenchymal disease, such as acute kidney injury and resolving acute tubular necrosis, interstitial nephritis, or cortical necrosis; in these situations, the hypertension is usually related to volume overload or hyperreninemia. Hemolytic uremic syndrome is rare but has been described in term and preterm infants,[27] usually accompanied by severe hypertension.

Pulmonary Etiologies

Neonates with bronchopulmonary dysplasia (BPD) are clearly at increased risk for development of systemic hypertension. Commonly, the hypertension may not become manifest until late in the NICU course or even after discharge. Hypertension in these infants correlates with the severity of lung disease and a greater need for diuretics and bronchodilators.[28] Moreover, those who show concurrent nephrocalcinosis are significantly more likely to develop late-onset hypertension.[29] This emphasizes the importance of monitoring for the development of hypertension in "NICU graduates" as 5%–40% of neonates with BPD are hypertensive.[28] The physiology of this association is not completely understood but may be related to increases in sympathetic activity and angiotensin II.[30]

Endocrine Etiologies

Endocrine disorders that can produce hypertension in infancy include congenital adrenal hyperplasia with 11-β-hydroxylase or 17-α-hydroxylase deficiency.[31] Other heritable forms of hypertension, including primary hyperaldosteronism[32] and hyperthyroidism,[33] are rare but important diseases that should be considered in the setting of hypertension and a normal serum renin level.

Drug Causes

Intrauterine and postnatal drug and medication exposures constitute another important category of potential etiologies for neonatal hypertension. Substances ingested during pregnancy such as maternal cocaine or heroin use may lead to significant problems with hypertension in the neonate.[34] Commonly used medications in the NICU, including corticosteroids, bronchodilators, and vasopressors, have been shown to elevate the BP. In addition, high doses of adrenergic agents, prolonged use of pancuronium, or administration of theophylline and caffeine may also raise the BP. Such hypertension typically resolves when the offending agent is discontinued or its dose reduced. For infants receiving prolonged total parenteral nutrition, hypertension may result from salt and water overload or from hypercalcemia caused either directly by excessive calcium intake or indirectly by vitamin A or D intoxication.

Neoplasia

Tumors, including neuroblastoma, Wilms tumor, and mesoblastic nephroma, may present in the neonatal period and produce hypertension, either because of compression of the renal vessels or ureters or because of the production of vasoactive substances, such as catecholamines.[35]

Neurologic Etiologies

Seizures, intracranial hypertension, and pain should be considered in neonates with unexplained hypertension.[36]

Miscellaneous Etiologies

Approximately 50% of neonates requiring extracorporeal membrane oxygenation (ECMO) develop hypertension; this is postulated to be secondary to fluid overload, altered handling of sodium and water, and derangements in atrial baroceptor function.[37] In addition, there is growing evidence that nephrogenesis is impaired in preterm and small-for-gestational-age infants, which makes them more vulnerable to the development of hypertension as well as cardiovascular and renal disease later in life. This further emphasizes the need for routine screening for hypertension as well as proteinuria in the low birth weight preterm infant after discharge from the NICU.[38]

CLINICAL PRESENTATION OF HYPERTENSIVE NEONATES

Most often, hypertension is asymptomatic in neonates and detected on routine vital sign monitoring. Nonspecific signs and symptoms include feeding difficulties, tachypnea, apnea, lethargy, and irritability.

Older infants, who may have been discharged from the NICU, can also present with unexplained irritability or failure to thrive. Severe hypertension can be associated with seizure activity, congestive heart failure, and renal dysfunction.

DIAGNOSTIC APPROACH FOR NEONATAL HYPERTENSION

The diagnosis of hypertension in a neonate begins with a focused history. Close attention should be paid to pertinent prenatal exposures, the neonate's clinical course, concurrent disease processes, and procedures performed (eg, umbilical catheter placement). In addition, the current medication list should be scrutinized for substances that can elevate BP. The physical examination likewise plays an important role. The proper BP measurement technique should be followed to ensure accurate readings, and appropriate cuff size should be confirmed. BP readings should be obtained in all 4 extremities at least once to screen for coarctation of the aorta. The general appearance of the infant should be assessed, with particular attention paid to the presence of any dysmorphic features that may indicate an obvious diagnosis, such as congenital adrenal hyperplasia. A careful cardiac and abdominal examination should be performed. The presence of a flank mass may point the clinician toward a diagnosis of renal vein thrombosis or ureteropelvic junction obstruction; an epigastric bruit may suggest renal artery stenosis.

The next step is the assessment of renal function and examination of urinary findings, both of which may be abnormal in the presence of renal parenchymal disease. Other diagnostic studies, such as the determination of cortisol, renin, aldosterone, or thyroxin levels, should be obtained when there is a pertinent history. Results of plasma renin activity, in particular, must be interpreted with caution. Plasma renin activity is typically high in infancy, particularly in premature infants, and minimal normative data are available. In addition, although renal artery stenosis and thromboembolism are typically considered high-renin states, peripheral plasma renin activity may not be actually be elevated. Conversely, plasma renin may be falsely elevated by medications commonly used in the NICU, such as the methylxanthines, caffeine, and aminophylline. Alternatively, renin and aldosterone levels may be helpful in infants with electrolyte abnormalities, such as hypokalemia, that suggest a potential genetic disorder in tubular sodium handling.[39]

Doppler ultrasound imaging of the genitourinary tract is a relatively inexpensive, noninvasive, and quick study that should be obtained in all hypertensive infants. An accurate renal ultrasound can help uncover potentially correctable causes of hypertension, such as renal venous thrombosis, may detect aortic or renal arterial thrombi, and can identify anatomic renal abnormalities or other congenital renal diseases. For infants with extremely severe BP elevation, if the suspicion of a renal artery abnormality is high, angiography may be necessary. A formal arteriogram utilizing the traditional femoral approach offers the most accurate method of diagnosing renal artery stenosis, particularly given the high incidence of intrarenal branch vessel disease in children with fibromuscular dysplasia. Although theoretically possible in infants, size is obviously a limiting factor. Computed tomography or magnetic resonance angiography will not detect branch stenosis in neonates and should not be ordered. It may be necessary to defer angiography, managing the hypertension medically until the baby is large enough for an arteriogram to be performed safely. Echocardiography is helpful if aortic coarctation is suspected and may identify left ventricular hypertrophy.

TREATMENT OF NEONATAL HYPERTENSION

Treatment of neonatal hypertension should be tailored to the severity of the BP elevation, as well as to the underlying cause of hypertension. Strong evidence regarding the efficacy and safety of different antihypertensive agents in neonates is lacking; however, direct vasodilators, diuretics, angiotensin-converting enzyme (ACE) inhibitors, β-adrenergic blockers, and calcium channel blockers have been used successfully in this population (Table 103-3).

Drug therapy should be considered when the neonate's BP is consistently at the 99th percentile or greater. Of course, treatment should be started earlier if systemic symptoms exist or there is evidence of end-organ damage. However, prior to initiating any antihypertensive therapy, all iatrogenic causes should be assessed and eliminated. This would include inadequate sedation or pain, inotrope administration in excess of need, hypercalcemia, and volume overload.

Neonates with acute severe hypertension, especially those with systemic symptoms, are best treated with a continuous intravenous infusion (Table 103-3); this allows titrating the medication dose more exactly to achieve the desired level of BP control and prevents the frequent BP fluctuations seen with intermittent dosing.[40] Oral agents have variable onset and unpredictable antihypertensive response and hence are not appropriate in these situations. It is imperative to avoid a rapid reduction in BP as it can precipitate cerebral ischemia and hemorrhage; this is particularly problematic in premature infants with immature periventricular circulation.[40] Table 103-3 lists several choices for continuous infusion. Although we prefer to utilize the calcium channel blocker nicardipine[41] in these situations, esmolol,[42] labetalol,[43] and nitroprusside[44] have been used effectively. BP should be monitored continuously, preferably via an indwelling arterial catheter. If this is unavailable, cuff BPs should be repeated frequently (every 10–15 minutes) with an oscillometric device to monitor therapeutic response.

Intermittently administered intravenous agents, such as hydralazine and labetalol, can be used for mild-to-moderate hypertension, particularly in neonates for whom oral therapy is precluded because of the need to allow full gut rest or poor gastrointestinal function. Although available in intravenous form, we discourage the use of enalaprilat because it can cause profound hypotension and prolonged acute kidney injury.

Oral antihypertensive agents (Table 103-3) are best used in stable neonates with more reliable gastric absorption. They are also effective agents in chronically hypertensive neonates when transitioning off an intermittent or continuous antihypertensive medication. Isradipine, a short-acting calcium channel blocker,[45] and amlodipine, a longer-acting calcium channel blocker, are our preferred oral agents. Isradipine is particularly effective when initiating antihypertensive therapy, whereas amlodipine, which has a delayed effect, is a more effective chronic agent that allows the convenience of once- or twice-daily dosing. Both of these medications can be compounded into a 1-mg/mL suspension, which allows dosing in smaller infants. We discourage, however, the use of the rapid-acting oral/sublingual nifedipine because the magnitude of antihypertensive effect is unpredictable.[46] In neonates with chronic lung disease, diuretics may be beneficial in BP control and improve pulmonary function as well.[47] Beta-blockers are relatively contraindicated in the setting of chronic lung disease but can be particularly effective when not contraindicated. It is important to note that propranolol is available as a commercially prepared suspension, which also allows for ease of dosing.

Although much of neonatal hypertension is renin mediated, the use of ACE inhibitors is controversial. Interestingly, captopril is 1 of the few medications for which data exist demonstrating effectiveness in hypertensive neonates. However, all ACE inhibitors have the potential to cause a marked decrement in BP, especially in premature infants.[48] Furthermore, there is some concern that ACE inhibitors may impair the final stages of renal maturation. Thus, we recommend avoiding ACE inhibitors until preterm infants have reached a corrected postconceptual age of 44 weeks.

Surgery is rarely indicated for treatment of neonatal hypertension and is likely to be required infrequently. Aortic coarctation is an excellent example of a hypertensive etiology that is best corrected surgically.[49]

Table 103-3 Antihypertensive Therapeutic Agents

Oral/Topical Antihypertensive Agents			
Agent	**Class**	**Dose**	**Comments**

Isradipine	Ca++ channel blocker	• 0.05–0.15 mg/kg/dose
		  May be given up to 4 times
		  a day
			Onset ~ 30 minutes
			Peak ~ 60–90 minutes

Amlodipine	Ca++ channel blocker	• 0.05–0.3mg/kg/dose
		  Maximum 0.6 g/kg/day
		  May be given daily or twice daily
			Onset ~ 60 minutes
			Peak ~ 6–12 hours

Clonidine patch	Central α₂-agonist	• 1/8–1/4 patch to begin
		  Patch changed every 7 days
			Patch may need to be changed
			  more frequently

Propranolol	β-Blocker	• 0.5–1 mg/kg/dose
		  Maximum 8–10 mg/kg/d
		  May be given up to 3 times daily
			Can titrate based on heart rate
			Avoid with BPD, CLD, CHD,
			  poor cardiac function

Labetalol	α- and β-blocker	• 0.5–1 mg/kg/dose
		  Maximum 10 mg/kg/d
		  May be given 2 or 3 times daily
			Can titrate based on heart rate
			Avoid with BPD, CLD, CHD,
			  poor cardiac function

Hydrochlorothiazide	Thiazide diuretic	• 1–1.5 mg/kg/dose Daily to twice daily	Monitor electrolytes
Chlorothiazide	Thiazide diuretic	• 5–15 mg/kg/dose Up to twice daily	Monitor electrolytes
Spironolactone	Aldosterone antagonist	• 0.5–1.5 mg/kg/dose Up to twice daily	Monitor electrolytes

Captopril	ACE inhibitor	• (<3 months) 0.01–0.5 mg/kg/
		  dose
		  Maximum 2 mg/kg/d
		• (>3 months) 0.15–2 mg/kg/dose
		  Maximum 6 mg/kg/d
		  Up to 3 times daily
			First dose may drop BP
			  precipitously
			Monitor K+ and renal function
			  closely; ARF risk in preterm
			  infants
			Intravenous formulation *not*
			  recommended

Enalapril	ACE inhibitor	• 0.05–0.1 mg/kg/dose Daily to twice daily	
Intravenous Antihypertensive Agents			
Agent	**Class**	**Dose**	**Comments**

Hydralazine	Vasodilator	• 0.1–0.2 mg/kg/dose
		  Up to every 4 hours
			Can cause fluid retention
			If used long term, should be
			  given with a diuretic
			May cause reflex tachycardia

Labetalol	α- and β-blocker	• 0.2–1 mg/kg/dose
		  Every 4–6 hours
			Avoid with BPD, CLD, CHD,
			  poor cardiac function

Continuous Infusion Antihypertensive Agents			
Agent	**Class**	**Dose**	**Comments**
Esmolol	β-Blocker	• 100–500 µg/kg/min	Extremely short acting Avoid with BPD, CLD, CHD, poor cardiac function
Labetalol	α- and β-blocker	• 0.25–3 mg/kg/h	Avoid with BPD, CLD, CHD, poor cardiac function

Nitroprusside	Vasodilator	• 0.5–10 µg/kg/min	Thiocyanate toxicity if used
			  longer than 72 hours or if ARF
			  is present

Nicardipine	Ca++ channel blocker	• 0.5–4 µg/kg/min	Can cause reflex tachycardia

Abbreviations: ACE, angiotensin-converting enzyme; ARF, acute renal failure; BPD, bronchopulmonary dysplasia; CHD, coronary heart disease; CLD, chronic lung disease.

Neonates with urologic abnormalities associated with obstructive uropathy are often hypertensive, and surgical correction (at times preceded by temporary urinary diversion or catheterization) may treat both the abnormality and the hypertension. Many infants with Wilms tumor or neuroblastoma are hypertensive as well. Definitive oncologic treatment of these children usually necessitates surgical removal of the tumor or kidney, which can eliminate the hypertension as well. Neonates with the most severe variants of autosomal recessive PKD are almost always hypertensive. Although the driving force for bilateral nephrectomy is usually gastric compression, abdominal distension, and pulmonary compromise, surgical removal may mitigate the hypertension as well.[50] Although infants with renal artery stenosis may require surgical correction, the procedure can be challenging in small infants, and it may be necessary to manage the infant medically until he or she has grown sufficiently.[51]

OUTCOME OF NEONATAL HYPERTENSION

The long-term prognosis for a hypertensive neonate depends on the underlying etiology of the hypertension; however, overall prognosis is good for most of these infants. For infants with hypertension related to thromboembolism and umbilical artery catheterization, hypertension usually resolves over time.[52] However, it is common for these infants to continue to require antihypertensive therapy at the time of NICU discharge. Thus, it is important to arrange for a reliable oscillometric device for all infants discharged from the NICU on antihypertensive medications. This allows home BP monitoring by the parents, and dosage changes can be made as required. These infants should be followed closely by the pediatric nephrology outpatient clinic, if available.

Many of the children with hypertension related to renal parenchymal disease have persistent hypertension and will need antihypertensive therapy indefinitely.[24] It is also possible for infants with renal vein thrombosis to remain hypertensive, and it has been reported that some of these children will ultimately benefit from removal of the affected kidney.[20,51] In addition, reappearance of hypertension in children who have undergone repair of renal artery stenosis or aortic coarctation should prompt an evaluation for restenosis.

One of the more interesting topics of late is the association between preterm birth, reduced nephron mass, and the development of hypertension in adulthood. The data regarding these associations have been mixed; however, it seems that there is likely a link between prematurity, deregulated glomerulogenesis, and hypertension.[53–56] In 1 of the largest population-based studies,

risk of adult-onset hypertension increased with the severity of the prematurity; patients born between 24 and 28 weeks' gestation, for example, were over 1.9 times more likely to develop hypertension than patients born at term.[53] Furthermore, it seems that this association may be related more to prematurity than low birth weight.[56] Certainly, this will be an area of interest as the large population of "NICU graduates" comes of age.

REFERENCES

1. American Academy of Pediatrics Committee on Fetus and Newborn: routine evaluation of blood pressure, hematocrit, and glucose in newborns. *Pediatrics*. 1993;92(3):474–476.
2. Buchi KF, Siegler RL. Hypertension in the first month of life. *J Hypertens*. 1986;4(5):525–528.
3. Seliem WA, Falk MC, Shadbolt B, Kent AL. Antenatal and postnatal risk factors for neonatal hypertension and infant follow-up. *Pediatr Nephrol*. 2007;22(12):2081–2087.
4. Singh HP, Hurley RM, Myers TF. Neonatal hypertension. Incidence and risk factors. *Am J Hypertens*. 1992;5(2):51–55.
5. Kent AL, Kecskes Z, Shadbolt B, Falk MC. Normative blood pressure data in the early neonatal period. *Pediatr Nephrol*. 2007;22(9):1335–1341.
6. Kent AL, Kecskes Z, Shadbolt B, Falk MC. Blood pressure in the first year of life in healthy infants born at term. *Pediatr Nephrol*. 2007;22(10):1743–1749.
7. Kent AL, Meskell S, Falk MC, Shadbolt B. Normative blood pressure data in non-ventilated premature neonates from 28–36 weeks gestation. *Pediatr Nephrol*. 2009;24(1):141–146.
8. Pejovic B, Peco-Antic A, Marinkovic-Eric J. Blood pressure in non-critically ill preterm and full-term neonates. *Pediatr Nephrol*. 2007;22(2):249–257.
9. Zubrow AB, Hulman S, Kushner H, Falkner B. Determinants of blood pressure in infants admitted to neonatal intensive care units: a prospective multicenter study. Philadelphia Neonatal Blood Pressure Study Group. *J Perinatol*. 1995;15(6):470–479.
10. Dionne JM, Abitbol CL, Flynn JT. Hypertension in infancy: diagnosis, management and outcome. *Pediatr Nephrol*. 2012;27(1):17–32.
11. Report of the Second Task Force on Blood Pressure Control in Children—1987. Task Force on Blood Pressure Control in Children. National Heart, Lung, and Blood Institute, Bethesda, Maryland. *Pediatrics*. 1987;79(1):1–25.
12. Moss AJ, Duffie ER Jr, Emmanouilides G. Blood pressure and vasomotor reflexes in the newborn infant. *Pediatrics*. 1963;32:175–179.
13. The fourth report on the diagnosis, evaluation, and treatment of high blood pressure in children and adolescents. *Pediatrics*. 2004;114(2 Suppl 4th Report):555–576.
14. Pauca AL, Wallenhaupt SL, Kon ND, Tucker WY. Does radial artery pressure accurately reflect aortic pressure? *Chest*. 1992;102(4):1193–1198.
15. Gevers M, Hack WW, Ree EF, Lafeber HN, Westerhof N. Arterial blood pressure wave forms in radial and posterior tibial arteries in critically ill newborn infants. *J Dev Physiol*. 1993;19(4):179–185.
16. Merten DF, Vogel JM, Adelman RD, Goetzman BW, Bogren HG. Renovascular hypertension as a complication of umbilical arterial catheterization. *Radiology*. 1978;126(3):751–757.
17. Barrington KJ. Umbilical artery catheters in the newborn: effects of catheter materials. *Cochrane Database Syst Rev*. 2000;(2):CD000949.

18. Boo NY, Wong NC, Zulkifli SS, Lye MS. Risk factors associated with umbilical vascular catheter-associated thrombosis in newborn infants. *J Paediatr Child Health.* 1999;35(5):460–465.

19. Marks SD, Massicotte MP, Steele BT, Matsell DG, Filler G, Shah PS, et al. Neonatal renal venous thrombosis: clinical outcomes and prevalence of prothrombotic disorders. *J Pediatr.* 2005;146(6):811–816.

20. Mocan H, Beattie TJ, Murphy AV. Renal venous thrombosis in infancy: long-term follow-up. *Pediatr Nephrol.* 1991;5(1):45–49.

21. Tullus K, Brennan E, Hamilton G, Lord R, McLaren CA, Marks SD, et al. Renovascular hypertension in children. *Lancet.* 2008;371(9622):1453–1463.

22. Menser MA, Dorman DC, Reye RD, Reid RR. Renal-artery stenosis in the rubella syndrome. *Lancet.* 1966;1(7441):790–792.

23. Das BB, Recto M, Shoemaker L, Mitchell M, Austin EH. Mid-aortic syndrome presenting as neonatal hypertension. *Pediatr Cardiol.* 2008;29(5):1000–1001.

24. Guay-Woodford LM, Desmond RA. Autosomal recessive polycystic kidney disease: the clinical experience in North America. *Pediatrics.* 2003;111(5 Pt 1):1072–1080.

25. Angermeier KW, Kay R, Levin H. Hypertension as a complication of multicystic dysplastic kidney. *Urology.* 1992;39(1):55–58.

26. Riehle RA, Jr, Vaughan ED, Jr. Renin participation in hypertension associated with unilateral hydronephrosis. *J Urol.* 1981;126(2):243–246.

27. Wilson BJ, Flynn JT. Familial, atypical hemolytic-uremic syndrome in a premature infant. *Pediatr Nephrol.* 1998;12(9):782–784.

28. Anderson AH, Warady BA, Daily DK, Johnson JA, Thomas MK. Systemic hypertension in infants with severe bronchopulmonary dysplasia: associated clinical factors. *Am J Perinatol.* 1993;10(3):190–193.

29. Schell-Feith EA, Kist-van Holthe JE, van der Heijden AJ. Nephrocalcinosis in preterm neonates. *Pediatr Nephrol.* 2010;25(2):221–230.

30. Braren V, West JC, Jr, Boerth RC, Harmon CM. Management of children with hypertension from reflux or obstructive nephropathy. *Urology.* 1988;32(3):228–234.

31. Speiser PW, White PC. Congenital adrenal hyperplasia. *N Engl J Med.* 2003;349(8):776–788.

32. Malagon-Rogers M. Non-glucocorticoid-remediable aldosteronism in an infant with low-renin hypertension. *Pediatr Nephrol.* 2004;19(2):235–236.

33. Schonwetter BS, Libber SM, Jones MD Jr, Park KJ, Plotnick LP. Hypertension in neonatal hyperthyroidism. *Am J Dis Child.* 1983;137(10):954–955.

34. Dube SK, Jhaveri RC, Rosenfeld W, Evans HE, Khan F, Spergel G. Urinary catecholamines, plasma renin activity and blood pressure in newborns: effects of narcotic withdrawal. *Dev Pharmacol Ther.* 1981;3(2):83–87.

35. Weinblatt ME, Heisel MA, Siegel SE. Hypertension in children with neurogenic tumors. *Pediatrics.* 1983;71(6):947–951.

36. Eden OB, Sills JA, Brown JK. Hypertension in acute neurological diseases of childhood. *Dev Med Child Neurol.* 1977;19(4):437–445.

37. Boedy RF, Goldberg AK, Howell CG Jr, Hulse E, Edwards EG, Kanto WP, Jr. Incidence of hypertension in infants on extracorporeal membrane oxygenation. *J Pediatr Surg.* 1990;25(2):258–261.

38. Abitbol CL, Ingelfinger JR. Nephron mass and cardiovascular and renal disease risks. *Semin Nephrol.* 2009;29(4):445–454.

39. Vehaskari VM. Heritable forms of hypertension. *Pediatr Nephrol.* 2009;24(10):1929–1937.

40. Flynn JT, Tullus K. Severe hypertension in children and adolescents: pathophysiology and treatment. *Pediatr Nephrol.* 2009;24(6):1101–1112.

41. Flynn JT, Mottes TA, Brophy PD, Kershaw DB, Smoyer WE, Bunchman TE. Intravenous nicardipine for treatment of severe hypertension in children. *J Pediatr.* 2001;139(1):38–43.

42. Wiest DB, Garner SS, Uber WE, Sade RM. Esmolol for the management of pediatric hypertension after cardiac operations. *J Thorac Cardiovasc Surg.* 1998;115(4):890–897.

43. Thomas CA, Moffett BS, Wagner JL, Mott AR, Feig DI. Safety and efficacy of intravenous labetalol for hypertensive crisis in infants and small children. *Pediatr Crit Care Med.* 2011;12(1):28–32.

44. Benitz WE, Malachowski N, Cohen RS, Stevenson DK, Ariagno RL, Sunshine P. Use of sodium nitroprusside in neonates: efficacy and safety. *J Pediatr.* 1985;106(1):102–110.

45. Flynn JT, Warnick SJ. Isradipine treatment of hypertension in children: a single-center experience. *Pediatr Nephrol.* 2002;17(9):748–753.

46. Flynn JT. Safety of short-acting nifedipine in children with severe hypertension. *Expert Opin Drug Saf.* 2003;2(2):133–139.

47. Engelhardt B, Elliott S, Hazinski TA. Short- and long-term effects of furosemide on lung function in infants with bronchopulmonary dysplasia. *J Pediatr.* 1986;109(6):1034–1039.

48. Tack ED, Perlman JM. Renal failure in sick hypertensive premature infants receiving captopril therapy. *J Pediatr.* 1988;112(5):805–810.

49. Seirafi PA, Warner KG, Geggel RL, Payne DD, Cleveland RJ. Repair of coarctation of the aorta during infancy minimizes the risk of late hypertension. *Ann Thorac Surg.* 1998;66(4):1378–1382.

50. Beaunoyer M, Snehal M, Li L, Concepcion W, Salvatierra O, Sarwal M. Optimizing outcomes for neonatal ARPKD. *Pediatr Transplant.* 2007;11(3):267–271.

51. Kiessling SG, Wadhwa N, Kriss VM, Iocono J, Desai NS. An unusual case of severe therapy-resistant hypertension in a newborn. *Pediatrics.* 2007;119(1):e301–e304.

52. Adelman RD. Long-term follow-up of neonatal renovascular hypertension. *Pediatr Nephrol.* 1987;1(1):35–41.

53. Johansson S, Iliadou A, Bergvall N, Tuvemo T, Norman M, Cnattingius S. Risk of high blood pressure among young men increases with the degree of immaturity at birth. *Circulation.* 2005;112(22):3430–3436.

54. Keijzer Veen M, Finken MJJ, Nauta J, et al. Is blood pressure increased 19 years after intrauterine growth restriction and preterm birth? A prospective follow-up study in The Netherlands. *Pediatrics.* 2005;116(3):725–731.

55. McEniery C, Bolton C, Fawke J, Hennessy E, Stocks J, Wilkinson I, et al. Cardiovascular consequences of extreme prematurity: the EPICure study. *J Hypertens.* 2011;29(7):1367–1373.

56. Rossi P, Tauzin L, Marchand E, Boussuges A, Gaudart J, Frances Y. Respective roles of preterm birth and fetal growth restriction in blood pressure and arterial stiffness in adolescence. *J Adolesc Health.* 2011;48(5):520–522.

Acute Adrenal Insufficiency

Rebecca McEachern and Charlotte M. Boney

EPIDEMIOLOGY

The exact incidence of acute adrenal insufficiency in the neonate is unknown but likely mirrors the incidence of the underlying causes of the adrenal failure. Newborn screening and heightened awareness have resulted in earlier diagnosis of congenital adrenal hyperplasia (CAH) before an acute crisis develops. The incidence of adrenal suppression from pharmacological doses of steroids is likely underestimated, and the exact frequency of adrenal crises in these cases is not known.

PATHOPHYSIOLOGY AND PRESENTATION

An essential component of the normal stress response is the adrenal gland. Cortisol production is increased during stress to maintain hemodynamic stability and glucose homeostasis. In these instances, cortisol prevents hypotension by promoting water and sodium retention, increasing angiotensinogen synthesis in the liver, increasing the vascular reactivity to vasoconstrictors, promoting the enzymatic conversion of norepinephrine to epinephrine, decreasing capillary permeability, and decreasing nitric oxide and other vasodilatory mediators.[1] Cortisol also prevents hypoglycemia by decreasing glucose uptake in the muscle, promoting catabolism of protein and muscle to produce substrates for gluconeogenesis, and increasing expression of gluconeogenic enzymes.[1] Aldosterone is the primary mineralocorticoid produced in the adrenal cortex and exerts effects on the kidney by stimulating reabsorption of sodium and secretion of potassium and hydrogen ions. If an inadequate cortisol response occurs in the face of physiologic stress, the infant will develop an acute adrenal crisis.

Central Adrenal Insufficiency

In infants with central adrenal failure, ACTH (corticotropin) is deficient. ACTH primarily regulates glucocorticoid production and secretion. The renin-aldosterone system is controlled by systemic volume and blood pressure and is unaffected in cases of central adrenal failure; thus, the neonate will not have the severe hyperkalemia or hyponatremia that accompanies mineralocorticoid deficiency. The infant will still be at risk for hypotension, milder hyponatremia, and hypoglycemia.

Primary Adrenal Insufficiency

The adrenal cortex is affected in primary adrenal insufficiency; thus, the neonate may have both cortisol and mineralocorticoid deficiency. These infants are at risk for a salt-wasting adrenal crisis consisting of marked hyperkalemia, hyponatremia, dehydration, and hypotension.

Acute Adrenal Failure or Crisis

In the neonate, adrenal failure can result in complete circulatory collapse and metabolic dysregulation termed an *adrenal crisis*. Other clinical features of acute adrenal failure include severe hyperkalemia and

Table 104-1 Clinical Features of Acute Adrenal Failure

Hypoglycemia
Hyponatremia
Hyperkalemia
Hypotension
Circulatory failure
Apnea
Fever
Vomiting
Jaundice/hyperbilirubinemia
Acidosis

hyponatremia and hypoglycemia, including seizure, hypotension, dehydration, prolonged jaundice, fever, vomiting, and acidosis (Table 104–1). Left untreated, the crisis will progress to shock and death.

DIFFERENTIAL DIAGNOSIS

Any form of adrenal insufficiency, whether from primary or central causes (Table 104-2), can present as acute adrenal failure or crisis. Transient forms of adrenal insufficiency may also present acutely. An infant who has been exposed to prolonged courses of steroids

Table 104-2 Differential Diagnosis of Adrenal Failure

Central or secondary causes
　Suppression from exogenous steroids
　Congenital hypopituitarism
　　Hypoplasia of anterior pituitary
　　Septo-optic dysplasia
　　Mutations in developmental transcription factors
　　　(*PIT-1, PROP-1*)
　Isolated ACTH (corticotropin) deficiency (*TPIT* or
　　POMC mutations)
　Transient adrenal insufficiency
Primary causes
　Congenital adrenal hyperplasia (CAH)
　Adrenal hypoplasia cogenita (*DAX-1* or *SF-1*
　　deletions or mutations)
　Adrenal hemorrhage
　Infection (cytomegalovirus [CMV])
　Medications (interfering with steroid biosynthesis)
　Smith-Lemli-Opitz syndrome
　ACTH resistance
　　Familial GC deficiency (ACTH receptor defect)
　　Triple A or Allgrove syndrome
　Wolman disease
　Adrenoleukodystrophy (rare in infancy)

Abbreviations: DAX-1, double dose adrenal hypoplasia congenital X-linked *Gene* 1; GC, glucocorticoid; PIT-1, pituitary-specific positive transcription factor 1; POMC, pro-opiomelanocortin; PROP-1, prophet of PIT-1; SF-1, steroidogenic factor 1; TPIT, T-box pituitary transcription factor.

is at risk for the development of an adrenal crisis. In these cases, suppression of the hypothalamic-pituitary-adrenal (HPA) axis from exogenous steroids may take several weeks to months to resolve, and if the infant develops an intercurrent illness or undergoes surgery, the infant may not be able to mount the appropriate stress response.[2] In addition, infants exposed to steroids in utero may also have suppression of the HPA axis postnatally. The degree and duration of suppression appear to be related to the dose and duration of antecedent steroid exposure.[2,3] Adrenal hemorrhage in a large infant after traumatic deliveries can present with acute adrenal failure and cardiodynamic instability from blood loss. Infants with known adrenal insufficiency can develop an adrenal crisis if subjected to additional severe stress such as major illness or surgery.[4]

DIAGNOSTIC TESTS

Critical Sample

If an adrenal crisis is suspected, it is prudent to obtain a serum cortisol level prior to empiric treatment. Because significant illness is a stimulus for cortisol secretion, obtaining a cortisol during this time can be informative and is considered a "critical sample." An infant with severe hypoglycemia is also under physiologic stress, and a cortisol obtained while the infant is hypoglycemic is also considered a critical sample. The exact cortisol level during stress has not been definitively determined, but many experts suggest greater than 15 μg/dL reflects an adequate stress response.[2,3] Other adjunct laboratory investigations may include evaluation of electrolytes, blood pH, and glucose level. Renin, aldosterone, and ACTH levels are helpful to determine the presence of a crisis from primary or central adrenal failure.

Cortisol-Binding Globulin Deficiency

Cortisol levels must be interpreted with caution in infants with protein deficiency (eg, severe liver failure) as the total cortisol reflects both free cortisol and cortisol bound to its carrier protein, cortisol-binding globulin (CBG). Deficiency in CBG results in a low total cortisol level but normal free cortisol levels; therefore, under certain conditions, low total cortisol does not necessarily denote cortisol deficiency or inadequate cortisol production.

Stimulation Tests

If the diagnosis of adrenal failure is suspected but the baby is not in immediate danger, investigations that are more specific may be undertaken. The circadian rhythm of cortisol secretion is lacking in neonates; thus, a cortisol level obtained in as much a fasting state as possible can be a first step. An ACTH stimulation test may be indicated if fasting cortisol levels (>15 µg/dL) are not clearly normal. There is some controversy about the indication for a standard dose vs low-dose ACTH stimulation test. A low-dose ACTH stimulation test is sufficient to evaluate most neonates and is more sensitive.[5] The exact dose used for this test varies, but 1 µg/kg appears to be the most discriminating dose.[6] A cortisol level is drawn (in a fasted state if possible), and then synthetic ACTH is given intravenously or intramuscularly and blood for a cortisol level is drawn 30 minutes later. The same considerations of CBG deficiency must be taken in interpreting the results in infants with liver failure or serum albumin levels below 2 g/dL. Extensive studies have not been done to determine the normal response in neonates; thus, the same cutoff values used in older children are commonly used for newborns. An adequate response is achieved if there is an increase of 8–10 µg/dL or if the stimulated cortisol level is greater than 18 µg/dL.

TREATMENT

Steroid Replacement

If adrenal crisis is imminent or occurring, the immediate administration of stress dose steroids is required. Treatment with 50–75 mg/m² of Solu-Cortef should be given intravenously as a loading bolus followed by 100 mg/m²/d divided every 4–6 hours depending on the severity of illness. Solu-Cortef is the preferred steroid formulation for stress because it is a glucocorticoid with sufficient mineralocorticoid activity.

Fluid Replacement

Adequate salt and fluid administration is also required. Replacement of intravascular volume can be achieved with a normal saline bolus of 10 mL/kg, but the bolus may need to be repeated. Continued hydration with normal saline (or half-normal saline if serum sodium and potassium levels are normal) is necessary to replace losses and maintain intravascular volume.

Adjunctive Therapy

Correction of electrolyte abnormalities is achieved with normal saline infusion and may need to be continued in severely hyponatremic or hyperkalemic neonates. Treatment with fluids containing dextrose (10% [D10] or even 25% [D25]) may be needed to prevent or treat hypoglycemia. Treatment of precipitating illness is mandated as well.

OUTCOME AND FOLLOW-UP

Once the acute phase has passed, the infant may be transitioned to maintenance doses of steroids (10 mg/m²/d). Care must be taken to ensure that the neonate is not at risk of further crises. All members of the care team should be alerted that any neonate with a history of high-dose steroid administration will need "stress" doses of steroids should the neonate develop fever, sepsis, respiratory failure, hypoglycemia, or any other significant illness and any surgical procedure involving anesthesia. Neonates with either primary or central adrenal failure will need stress doses, but maintenance doses of Solu-Cortef may not be necessary in neonates with central adrenal insufficiency.

Stress Management Precautions

Once a significant physiologic stress has been identified, doses of 30–50 mg/m²/d divided every 6 hours should be administered until the stress has resolved.[1] If there is severe illness present, 100 mg/m²/d may be needed. Oral doses may be sufficient for some infants. In preparation for procedures or surgery, a dose of 50 mg/m² IV should be given.[1] Major surgery requires a loading dose of 50 mg/m² followed by doses every 4–6 hours for a total dose of 100 mg/m²/d. Stress doses should be continued as long as the infant is deemed to be under physiological stress.

REFERENCES

1. Shulman DI, Palmert MR, Kemp SF. Adrenal insufficiency: still a cause of morbidity and death in children. *Pediatrics.* 2007;119(2):e484–e494.
2. Ford LR, Willi L, Hollis BW, Wright NM, Al FET. Suppression and recovery of the neonatal hypothalamic-pituitary-adrenal axis after prolonged dexamethasone therapy. *J Pediatr.* 1997;131:722–726.
3. Ng PC. Effect of stress on the neonatal hypothalamic-pituitary-adrenal axis in the fetus and newborn. *J Pediatr.* 2011;158 (2 Suppl):e41–e43.
4. Sperling Miller WL, Achermann JC, Fluck CE. The adrenal cortex and its disorders. In: Sperling MA, ed. *Pediatric Endocrinology.* 3rd ed. Philadelphia, PA: Saunders Elsevier; 2008:481–482.
5. Soliman AT, Taman KH, Rizk MM, et al. Circulating adrenocorticotropic hormone (ACTH) and cortisol concentrations in normal, appropriate-for-gestational age newborns versus those with sepsis and respiratory distress: cortisol response to low-dose and standard dose ACTH tests. *Metabolism.* 2004;53(2):209–214.
6. Quintos JB, Boney CM. Transient adrenal insufficiency in the premature newborn. *Curr Opin Endocrinol Diabetes Obesity.* 2010; 17(1):8–12.

CHAPTER 104

Persistent Hypoglycemia and Hyperinsulinemia

Parul Patel

INTRODUCTION

Neonatal hypoglycemia can be transient (see chapter 75 on transient hypoglycemia) or persistent (hyperinsulinism, hypopituitaryism, disorders of gluconeogenesis, glycogenolysis, fatty acid oxidation, or inborn errors of metabolism). Hypoglycemia can be detrimental to the developing central nervous system, resulting in long-term effects. Neonatal hypoglycemia demands urgent diagnosis and treatment.

DIAGNOSIS/INDICATIONS

Definition of Hypoglycemia

Although the definition of persistent hypoglycemia continues to be debated and no consensus or research-based definition is available,[1] many physicians use "operational threshold" levels of less than 45 mg/dL for diagnostic and 70 mg/dL for therapeutic purposes without scientific validation.[2]

Clinical Findings

History

Infants at higher risk of hypoglycemia should have their glucose checked soon postpartum, especially for infants who are small for gestational age (SGA), premature, or large for gestational age (LGA). Additional factors are a maternal history of diabetes during pregnancy (transient hyperinsulinism), history of consanguinity, or history of other children with unexplained deaths or glucose issues. The last 2 may suggest defects in glycogenolysis, gluconeogenesis, or ketogenesis. Timing of hypoglycemia may help differentiate etiology. Symptoms of hypoglycemia in the neonate may include seizures, cyanotic episode, apnea, "respiratory distress," refusal to feed, brief myoclonic jerks, vomiting, somnolence, or subnormal temperature or there may be no overt symptoms. Intravenous glucose infusion rates (GIRs) in excess of 8 mg/kg/min suggest hypoglycemia secondary to hyperinsulinism.

Physical

Large for gestational age; SGA; prematurity; massive hepatomegaly; midline defects (cleft lip/palate, central incisor, holoprosencephaly, or in a male infant, small phallus); macroglossia; hemihypertrophy; or nystagmus should alert the clinician for possible hypoglycemia and its etiology.

Confirmatory/Baseline Labs

If the hypoglycemia is not readily responsive to initial measures (see chapter 75 on transient hypoglycemia), obtain "critical" labs listed in Table 105-1. The blood glucose concentration must be determined immediately using a laboratory enzymatic reaction. Falsely low glucose levels will be reported if there is a delay in processing secondary to metabolism of glucose in the specimen by erythrocytes. A special procedure may be needed for collection of lactic acid or ammonia.

Table 105-1 Critical Laboratory Values to Obtain at Time of Hypoglycemia

Serum glucose
Insulin
Ketones (serum or urine)
Cortisol
Growth hormone
Ammonia
Lactate
Free fatty acids
Urine organic acids
Plasma amino acids
Acylcarnitine profile
IGFBP3

DIFFERENTIAL DIAGNOSIS

Congenital Hyperinsulinism

Congenital hyperinsulinism is the most common cause of persistent hypoglycemia of infancy.[3] For laboratory features consistent with hyperinsulinemic hypoglycemia, see Table 105-2. Genetic etiologies are summarized in Table 105-3.

Mutations of the K_{ATP} Channel

The most common cause of hyperinsulinism is *ABCC8* (SUR-1) or *KCNJ11* (Kir6.2). *Autosomal recessive* (AR) mutations in these genes cause focal (AR in paternal allele or loss of heterozygosity of maternal allele) or diffuse islet cell hyperplasia. Usually, neonates are LGA with severe hypoglycemia after delivery.

Table 105-2 Laboratory Features of Hyperinsulinemic Hypoglycemia

Persistent hypoglycemia (<50 mg/dL)
Insulin (>2 μU/mL)
Serum ketones: β-hydroxybutyrate (<2 mmol/L)
Urine ketones: absent
Low serum free fatty acid (<1.5 mmol/L)
Normal cortisol and growth hormone
Glucagon stimulation test: positive (>30 mg/dL response to 1 mg glucagon)

Frequently, this is diazoxide unresponsive. Autosomal dominant mutations of these genes cause less-severe hypoglycemia that usually is diazoxide responsive.

Glutamate Dehydrogenase

The second most common cause of hyperinsulinism is glutamate dehydrogenase; this causes symptomatic hyperinsulinism with asymptomatic hyperammonemia (HIHA). This usually presents when weaning from breast to cow's milk formula and is a protein- (leucine-) sensitive hypoglycemia. This usually responds well to treatment with diazoxide and diet modification.

Short-Chain 3-Hydroxyacyl-Coenzyme A Dehydrogenase Deficiency

Short-chain 3-hydroxyacyl-coenzyme A (CoA) dehydrogenase deficiency (SCHAD) is a short-chain fatty acid oxidation defect affecting the *HADH* gene; it causes inappropriate insulin release without hyperammonemia. This form of hyperinsulinemia also usually responds to diazoxide.

Table 105-3 Genetic Forms of Hyperinsulinism[a]

Type	Gene	Inheritance	Clinical	Treatment
K_{ATP} channel	*ABCC8* *KCNJ11*	Diffuse: AR Focal: paternally inherited or loss of heterozygosity of maternal allele	Severe hypoglycemia	Pancreatectomy or "conservative" therapy with octreotide and continuous feedings
Dominant K_{ATP} channel	*ABCC8* *KCNJ11*	AD	Milder hypoglycemia	Diazoxide
GDH HI (HIHA)	*GLUD1*	AD	Fasting and postprandial hypoglycemia; less severe than K_{ATP} HI; protein sensitivity; asymptomatic hyperammonemia	Diazoxide
GK HI	GCK	AD	Variable	Diazoxide or pancreatectomy
SCHAD	*HADH*	AR	Mild to severe hypoglycemia; abnormal acylcarnitine profile	Diazoxide

Abbreviations: AD, autosomal dominant; AR, autosomal recessive; GCK, glucokinase; HI, hyperinsulinism; HIHA, symptomatic hyperinsulinism with asymptomatic hyperammonemia; SCHAD, short-chain 3-hydroxyacyl-coenzyme A dehydrogenase deficiency.
[a]Adapted with permission from Kappy et al.[4]

Glucokinase

Glucose sensor mutation lowers glucose set point so lower glucose levels are needed to stop insulin release.

Glycogen Storage Disorders

Glycogen Synthase Deficiency

Glycogen synthase deficiency (glycogen storage disorder [GSD] type 0) is AR with fasting hypoglycemia, postprandial hyperglycemia and increased lactate, and no glycemic response to glucagon. Neonates so affected *do not* have hepatomegaly associated with other forms of GSDs.

Glucose 6-Phosphatase Deficiency

For glucose 6-phosphatase deficiency, GSD type 1a is AR with massive hepatomegaly, fasting hypoglycemia with elevated lactate levels, hyperuricemia, hyperlipidemia, and modestly elevated aspartate aminotransferase/alanine aminotransferase (AST/ALT). Type 1b is similar clinically but with neutropenia (oral lesions, perianal abscess, or chronic enteritis).

Amylo-1,6-Glucosidease Deficiency (Debrancher Deficiency, GSD Type 3)

Amylo-1,6-glucosidease deficiency (debrancher deficiency, GSD type 3) is AR with massive hepatomegaly, fasting hypoglycemia (less severe than GSD type 1), *no* elevation in lactate or uric acid, and elevated AST/ALT. Myopathy and cardiomegaly can be seen in this disorder.

Disorder of Gluconeogenesis: Fructose 1,6-Diphosphatase Deficiency

Fructose 1,6-diphosphatase deficiency is AR with hepatomegaly (secondary to lipid storage), fasting hypoglycemia, hyperketosis, elevated lactic acid, hyperlipidemia, and hyperuricemia.

Disorders of Fatty Acid Oxidation

Fatty acid oxidation disorders include defects of fatty acid and carnitine transport, β-oxidation, electron transport, and ketone production/utilization defects. This group of disorders presents with attacks of hypoketotic hypoglycemia, liver dysfunction, and elevation of urea, ammonia, and uric acid with prolonged fasting.

Inborn Errors of Metabolism

Ketotic hypoglycemia may represent an organic aciduria (propionic, methylmalonic, and isovaleric acidurias) or maple syrup urine disease. These disorders have specific blood or urine findings that facilitate their diagnosis as an inborn error of metabolism.

Other Etiologies of Hypoglycemia

Galactosemia (Galactose 1-Phosphate Uridyl Transferase)

Galactosemia (deficiency of galactose 1-phosphate uridyl transferase) presents with acute decline in multiple organ systems (renal tubular function, liver dysfunction, coagulopathy, neutropenia, or *Escherichia coli* sepsis) after galactose exposure.[5] Any neonate with *E. coli* sepsis should be suspected of having galactosemia.

Pituitary Hormone Deficiency

Pituitary hormone deficiency can be associated with midline defects (cleft lip/palate, septo-optic dysplasia or optic nerve hypoplasia manifested as nystagmus, prolonged jaundice, or in a male neonate, small phallus with or without cryptorchidism).[6] Growth hormone deficiency should be suspected in a male neonate with hypoglycemia and a small phallus. Cortisol deficiency as a result of adrenal disease, such as congenital adrenal hyperplasia, manifests with electrolyte disturbances or ambiguous genitalia rather than hypoglycemia.

Iatrogenic Etiologies

An abrupt discontinuation or disruption of an intravenous dextrose infusion can cause hypoglycemia in the neonate. Hypoglycemia may be a result of an indwelling catheter placed close to the pancreas (eg, umbilical artery catheter near the celiac axis) such that dextrose infusion causes local hyperglycemia and stimulates insulin release.

Signs and symptoms of hypoglycemia can be mimicked by many clinical entities, including sepsis, neurological disorder, malnourishment, hyperviscosity syndrome, or primary cardiac disorder.

Diagnostic Algorithm

Once the critical sample is obtained, the results can be used to help determine the etiology of neonatal hypoglycemia (see Figure 105-1 for a diagnostic algorithm).

TREATMENT

Initiation

Postpartum, it is imperative to initiate early feeding and evaluation of glucose in the neonate if hypoglycemia is suspected given the birth and maternal history. A recent consensus statement proposed that asymptomatic late preterm, term SGA, infant of a diabetic mother, or LGA neonates be screened within the first 12 hours of life.[2] Acute symptomatic hypoglycemia should be treated with a 0.2-g/kg bolus of dextrose

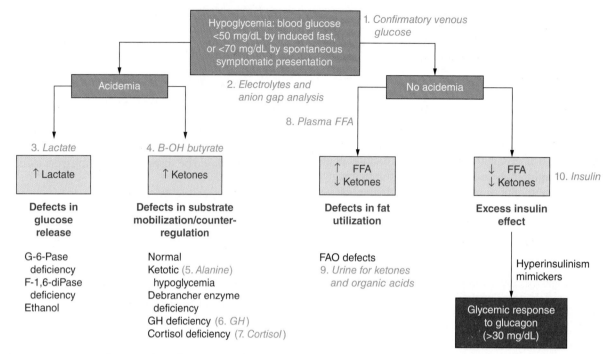

FIGURE 105-1 FAO, fatty acid oxidation; FFA, free fatty acid; GH, growth hormone; G-6-Pase, glucose 6-phosphatase. (Reproduced with permission from Kappy et al.[4])

(2 mL/kg of 10% dextrose in water [D10W]) as initial therapy, after which a dextrose infusion with a GIR of 8 mg/kg/min. Recheck the glucose level 15 minutes later to ensure resolution of hypoglycemia. Some types of persistent hyperglycemia, such as congenital hyperinsulinism, may benefit from starting diazoxide 5–15 mg/kg in divided doses 2 times per day. Often, a thiazide diuretic is started at the same time as diazoxide to help ameliorate edema seen with this medication. Octreotide (5–20 µg/kg divided every 6 hours) can be used in cases of diazoxide resistance for short-term management, but tachyphylaxis and risk of necrotizing enterocolitis (NEC) limit its usefulness. Medical management for congenital hyperinsulinism is the first-line treatment, but if the neonate is not maintaining glucose levels at 70 mg/dL or above, then surgical therapy may be considered (98% pancreatectomy for diffuse disease and focal resection for focal disease).

Testing to Follow-Up

Continue to check glucose levels before feedings, 15 minutes after a glucose bolus, and 15 minutes after a change in the GIR.

Potential Side Effects of Treatment

Regarding potential treatment side effects, diazoxide can cause excessive hair growth, fluid retention, or liver dysfunction. Octreotide can cause diarrhea,

decrease peritoneal blood flow (NEC), and suppress growth hormone and thyroid hormone.

Exit Strategy

The goal of treatment is to protect the brain and maintain euglycemia. Wean the GIR by small increments (10%) for glucose levels of 70 mg/dL or above for 2 readings and reassess glucose levels 15 minutes after weaning. The level of clinically important hypoglycemia is highly debated and still is largely empirical.[2] Once the neonate can safely maintain glucose levels with an appropriate feeding or drug regimen, the family should be instructed how to check glucose levels on a home meter; when to increase the frequency of glucose checks (illness, prolonged fasting time, and symptoms of hypoglycemia); treatment of a low blood glucose (feeding, glucose gel, or if necessary, glucagon); and when to call the pediatric endocrinologist.

CONCLUSION/FOLLOW-UP

Aftercare Monitoring

Close attention must be paid to the neonate at home. Parents and other caretakers must be trained to detect symptoms of hypoglycemia and how to avoid hypoglycemia. For the family, a home glucometer should be provided along with in-hospital teaching regarding its use and parameters for treating an episode of hypoglycemia.

Clinical Follow-Up

After discharge from the neonatal intensive care unit, the neonate should be follow by the pediatrician to monitor growth parameters. The pediatric endocrinologist involved should help manage medication dose adjustment and glucometer downloads, as well as monitor for potential medication side effects. Individuals in other subspecialties may become involved based on the diagnosis of hypoglycemia (individuals working with genetics for familial causes or ophthalmology and neurology for structural defects of the brain causing hypopituitarism).

Neonates with hypoglycemia secondary to congenital hyperinsulinism need to be monitored closely for development of continued hypoglycemia or hyperglycemia as a result of the disease or its treatment. Neonates with genetic causes of hypoglycemia, including disorders of glycogenolysis, gluconeogenesis, and fatty acid oxidation defects, should be started on appropriate treatment and avoid prolonged periods of fasting.

Long-Term Outcomes

Severe psychomotor retardation and epilepsy are more common with neonates with persistent hyperinsulinemic hypoglycemia who underwent surgical rather than medical management.[7] Surgical management with near-total pancreatectomy can lead to persistent hypoglycemia or hyperglycemia.

Despite appropriate treatment of individual causes of hypoglycemia, long-term and progressive neurologic derangement may occur, such as in galactosemia.[8] Although there is no clear evidence that a specific glucose range or duration of hypoglycemia causes brain injury, it is important to avoid long-term effects of the lack of the central nervous system energy source.[9]

REFERENCES

1. Rozance P, Hays WW Jr. Describing hypoglycemia - definition or operational threshold? *Early Hum Dev.* 2010;86(5):275–280.
2. Adamkin DH; Committee on Fetus and Newborn. Postnatal glucose homeostasis in late-preterm and term infants. *Pediatrics.* 2011;127:575–579.
3. Stanley CA. Hypoglycemia in the neonate. *Pediatr Endocrinol Rev.* 2006;4(Suppl 1):76–81.
4. Kappy MS, Allen DB, Geffner ME. *Pediatric Practice: Endocrinology,* 2nd ed. New York, NY: McGraw-Hill Education; 2014.
5. Leslie ND. Insights into the pathogenesis of galactosemia. *Annu Rev Nutr.* 2003;23:59–80.
6. De Leon DD, Stanley CA, Sperling MS. Hypoglycemia in neonates and infants. In: Sperling MA, ed. *Pediatric Endocrinology.* 3rd ed. Philadelphia, PA: Saunders Elsevier; 2008:165–197.
7. Menni F, de Lonlay P, Sevin C. Neurologic outcomes of 90 neonates and infants with persistent hyperinsulinemic hypoglycemia. *Pediatrics.* 2001;107:476–479.
8. Ridel KR, Leslie, ND, Gilbert DL. An updated review of the long-term neurological effects of galactosemia. *Pediatr Neurol.* 2005;33(3):153–161.
9. Hay WW Jr, Raju T, Higgins RD, et al. Knowledge gaps and research needs for understanding and treating neonatal hypoglycemia: workshop report from Eunice Kennedy Shriver National Institute of Child Health and Human Development. *J Pediatr.* 2009;155:612–617.

Neonatal Hyperammonemia

Brendan Lanpher, Marshall Summar, and Mark L. Batshaw

INTRODUCTION

Neonatal hyperammonemia is a feature of many different inborn errors of metabolism that may be individually rare but have about a 1:5000 cumulative incidence.[1,2] It can also be a feature of fulminant liver failure of any cause and of structural anomalies leading to portosystemic shunting. Neonatal hyperammonemia represents a true metabolic emergency as rapid identification and intervention are critical to a positive neurologic outcome. It is essential that neonatal centers have a protocol and plan in place to address these patients. A representative protocol is provided in this chapter (Table 106-1) and details are provided.

TREATMENT PROTOCOL

Hours 0–1: Initial Assessment and Activation of Metabolic Team

Once hyperammonemia is recognized in the neonate, the treating clinician must assess the duration of symptoms; hours 0–1 should involve the initial assessment and activation of the metabolic team. Studies of patients with urea cycle disorders have shown that neurologic and cognitive outcomes are tightly correlated with duration of hyperammonemic coma in the neonate. Diagnosis of hyperammonemia is sometimes delayed; neonates may be initially suspected to have sepsis and are treated with antibiotics for a number

of days before metabolic disorders are considered. In such a patient who has been comatose for greater than 72 hours, consideration should be given to the appropriateness of heroic interventions, as with prolonged hyperammonemia the chances of significant neurologic recovery are small. Withdrawal of care is reasonable in these cases.[3–6]

If the patient has only been symptomatic for a short time, intervention must proceed quickly. Central venous access is critical; this allows frequent laboratory monitoring as well as delivery of medications and dialysis. Antibiotic therapy and evaluation for sepsis are recommended because sepsis is an important consideration in the primary presentation and, if present, may lead to further catabolism. Care should be given to the preservation of potential dialysis access sites. Once critical hyperammonemia is identified, intubation and aggressive sedation are indicated to reduce metabolic activity and catabolism. Initial laboratory assessment may help narrow the differential diagnosis and permit tailoring of specific therapy (Table 106-2). Collected specimens for initial laboratory studies include arterial blood gas, comprehensive metabolic panel, and urinalysis. In addition, specimens for plasma amino acid analysis, urine organic acid analysis, and acylcarnitine profile should all be collected and sent to a regional metabolic center for rapid evaluation.

Immediately after significant hyperammonemia is recognized, patients must be transferred to a metabolic center (if not already at such a center) and a multidisciplinary team must be assembled. This includes individuals from neonatology, metabolic genetics, nephrology,

Table 106-1 Timeline for Management of Hyperammonemia

Hour 0–1
  Arrange transfer to tertiary care center with appropriate facilities and specialists
  Establish central vascular access
    Avoid compromise of potential dialysis sites
  Intubation and airway stabilization
  Sedate aggressively to reduce metabolic demand
  Collect specimens for necessary diagnostic laboratory tests
    Plasma ammonia
    Plasma amino acids
    Urine organic acids
    Plasma acylcarnitine profile
  Assemble multidisciplinary team
    Neonatology
    Metabolic genetics
    Nutrition
    Nephrology
    Surgery
    Nursing
  Alert laboratory team about need for rapid results and frequent assessments
  Alert pharmacy team about need for specialized medications and nutrition
  Intravenous fluids/nutrition
    Stop enteral feeding
    Intravenous fluids
      Maximize glucose infusion rate (10% dextrose in water [D10W] or higher)
      Intralipids (2–3 g/kg/d)
      Goal of 80–120 kcal/kg/d
  Medications
    Urea cycle disorders
      Sodium phenylacetate/sodium benzoate infusion (250 mg/kg of each as initial bolus then as a continuous
        daily infusion)
      Intravenous arginine (200 mg/kg unless AS or AL deficiency suspected, then 400–700 mg/kg) as initial bolus
        then as a continuous daily infusion
      Carbamylglutamate 25 mg/kg/dose every 6 hours (if available)
    Organic acidemias
      Intravenous carnitine (100 mg/kg/dose every 4–6 hours)
      Carbamylglutamate 25 mg/kg/dose every 6 hours (if available)
Hours 1–12
  Begin hemodialysis at maximal flow rates
  Review diagnostic lab results as available
    If essential amino acid deficiency is present, consider reintroducing protein sooner to reverse catabolic state
  Monitor for hypotension
    Common with hemodialysis
    May be exacerbated by arginine infusion (nitric oxide donor)
      May reduce arginine rate if vasodilation/hypotension present
  Monitor for seizures
    Intermittent or continuous EEG; treat if present
Hours 12–48
  Transition from hemodialysis to hemofiltration
    Monitor for rebound hyperammonemia
  Laboratory monitoring
    Electrolytes and ammonia every 6 hours
  Reintroduce protein
    Start with 0.5 g protein/kg/d and titrate upward
    50% of protein goals from essential amino acids
    50% of protein goals from whole protein
    Enteral route preferred

(Continued)

CHAPTER 106

Table 106-1 Timeline for Management of Hyperammonemia (Continued)

Hours 48 and beyond
  Nutrition tailored to specific cause of hyperammonemia
    ~1.5 g protein/kg/d in neonates
    Tailor nutrition to specific inborn error of metabolism
      50% of protein from disease-specific formula
      50% of protein from breast milk or whole-protein formula
    Assess nutritional parameters (growth, plasma amino acids) frequently
  Transition intravenous nutrition and medication to enteral
    Urea cycle disorders: sodium phenylbutyrate 450–600 mg/kg/d
    Organic acidemias: carnitine 100–200 mg/kg/d
    Other medications depending on specific cause
  Assess for neurologic sequelae
    Brain MRI
    EEG
    Developmental assessment
  Consider gastrostomy
    Genetic counseling for family
    Discharge planning
      Emergency protocol given to family
  Ensure home access for medications and nutrition
  Follow up in metabolic clinic

Abbreviations: AS, argininosuccinate synthetase; AL, argininosuccinate lyase; EEG, electroencephalography; MRI, magnetic resonance imaging.

surgery, nutrition, and others (Table 106-3). Every medical facility should have a regional metabolic center to which an affected patient may be transferred to facilitate care. Transport teams caring for neonates with suspected metabolic disorders should carry the intravenous form of sodium phenylacetate/sodium benzoate (Ammonul®), the intravenous form of arginine hydrochloride (10% solution), and 10% dextrose with 77 mEq/L sodium chloride in addition to their routine supplies.[7]

Hours 1–12: Rapid Reversal of Hyperammonemia

The first goal of treatment in hours 1–12 is to physically remove ammonia from the bloodstream. This is best accomplished by hemodialysis, but this takes some hours to organize and begin. While dialysis is being established, intravenous fluids and medications may be administered. Protein-containing feedings should be held initially, but adequate calorie delivery is essential for decreasing catabolism. Intravenous fluids containing a high percentage of dextrose (at least 10%) should be delivered along with Intralipid®. An initial goal of 80–120 kcal/kg/d is reasonable. To be able to administer the amount of glucose needed to reach this goal, administration of insulin is often necessary.

Intravenous medications for hyperammonemia should be started immediately once access is established. If a urea cycle disorder is suspected based on initial clinical and laboratory information, then intravenous sodium phenylacetate and sodium benzoate (Ammonul) should be started immediately. Typically, a bolus dose is given (250 mg/kg of each compound) and then the same dose is given as a continuous infusion over 24 hours. These agents are used in combination to trap nitrogen in excretable forms. Repeated boluses of benzoate/phenylacetate may increase side effects and are generally not thought to further enhance nitrogen clearance. Intravenous arginine is also given to help replenish deficient products of the urea cycle (200 mg/kg/24 h) and as an alternative path for waste nitrogen excretion in suspected argininosuccinate synthetase (AS) and argininosuccinate lyase (AL) deficiency (400–700 mg/kg/24 h). Because arginine is the precursor for nitric oxide production, it is worth considering modification of the arginine dose downward if the patient develops vasodilation and hypotension. If an organic acidemia is suspected (acidosis, ketosis, unusual odors), intravenous carnitine is

Table 106-2 Initial Laboratory Evaluation of Hyperammonemia

Plasma ammonia
Arterial blood gas
Urinalysis
Comprehensive metabolic profile (electrolytes and
  liver function tests)
Lactate
Plasma amino acids
Urine organic acids
Plasma acylcarnitine profile

Table 106-3 Treatment Team and Organization

- Metabolic specialist
  - Coordinate treatment and management
- Intensive care team
  - Assist with physiologic support
  - Provide ventilator management
  - Oversee sedation and pain management
- Nephrologist or dialysis team
  - Manage dialysis
  - Manage renal complications
- Surgical team
  - Place large-bore catheter
  - Perform liver biopsy as necessary
  - Place gastrostomy tube (if indicated)
- Pharmacy staff
  - Formulate nitrogen-scavenging drugs
  - Cross-check dosing orders in complex management
- Laboratory staff
  - Analyze large volume of ammonia samples in acute phase
  - Analyze amino acids and other specialty laboratory tests
- Nursing staff
  - Execute complex and rapidly changing management plan
  - Closely monitor patient for signs of deterioration or change
- Nutritionist
  - Maximize caloric intake with neutral nitrogen balance
  - Educate family in management of complex very-low-protein diet
- Social worker
  - Rapidly identify resources for complex outpatient treatment regimen
  - Work with families in highly stressful clinical situation
- Genetic counselor
  - Educate family in genetics of rare metabolic disease
  - Identify other family members at potential risk (especially important with ornithine transcarbalymase deficieny)
  - Ensure proper samples are obtained for future prenatal testing
  - Contact research/diagnostic centers for genetic testing

indicated (100 mg/kg/dose, 3–4 times daily).[8] Because hyperammonemic patients may have cerebral edema, care should be taken to avoid overhydration. The nitrogen-scavenging drugs are usually administered in a large volume of fluid, which should be taken into consideration, as well as the sodium load from the medication.[7–13]

Hemodialysis is effective at reducing plasma ammonia levels; peritoneal dialysis is ineffective and should not be considered. Ammonia clearance by hemodialysis is dependent on flow rates. Flow rates may be increased by utilizing extracorporeal membrane oxygenation (ECMO) in line with the dialysis equipment. This also helps achieve hemodynamic stability.[14] Complications of hemodialysis include coagulopathy and hypotension.

Hours 12–48: Stabilization and Reversal of Catabolism

Hours 12–48 involve stabilization and reversal of catabolism. Hemodialysis can rapidly reduce plasma ammonia levels but does carry multiple risks. Once ammonia is largely reduced to less than 200 μmol/L, hemodialysis should be transitioned to hemofiltration. This provides a lower rate of ammonia clearance but causes less hemodynamic instability. Rebound hyperammonemia is not uncommon as this transition happens.

Reintroduction of protein (initially 0.5 g/kg/24 h) should occur after approximately 24 hours of restriction, even if hyperammonemia continues. Prolonged protein restriction may lead to increased catabolism of endogenous body protein and worsening hyperammonemia. Nutrition should be tailored to the suspected cause of hyperammonemia. Typically, approximately half of protein needs are provided as essential amino acid mixes (there are specific formulas for many different inborn errors of metabolism), and half is provided as whole protein (typical infant formula or breast milk).[8] Ideally, this should be given enterally through a nasogastric tube, but clinical instability may require parenteral delivery.

Intravenous steroids and valproic acid should be avoided, the former because they may induce catabolism and the latter because it causes secondary urea cycle dysfunction with the same mechanism as in organic acidemias. It should be noted, however, that stress doses of corticosteroids (accompanied by sufficient calories) may be required in these very sick children to avoid catabolism.

During this phase of treatment, careful neurologic monitoring is essential. Cerebral function studies should be conducted to determine the efficacy of treatment and whether continuation is warranted. Electroencephalography (EEG) should be performed to identify evidence of seizure activity. If available, cerebral blood flow as determined by magnetic resonance imaging (MRI) can be used to establish if venous stasis has occurred from cerebral edema. The decision to undertake or continue aggressive treatment is based on baseline neurologic status, duration of the patient's coma, potential for recovery, and of course, parental wishes. Diagnostic samples of DNA, liver, and skin should be obtained if the child dies because they can lead to a definitive diagnosis and aid in family counseling.

Hour 48 and Beyond

As initial hyperammonemia is resolved, the intravenous nutrition and medications should be transitioned to enteral delivery at hour 48 and beyond. For patients with urea cycle disorders, the ammonia scavenger most commonly used is sodium phenylbutyrate (Buphenyl®), an enteral prodrug of phenylacetate. The usual total daily dose of Buphenyl for neonates with urea cycle disorders is 450–600 mg/kg. The medication is to be taken in equally divided amounts with each meal or feeding (ie, 3 to 6 times per day). Citrulline supplementation is recommended for patients diagnosed with a deficiency of N-acetylglutamate synthase, carbamylphosphate synthetase, or ornithine transcarbamylase; the daily recommended intake of citrulline is 0.17 g/kg/d. Arginine supplementation is needed for patients diagnosed with a deficiency of AS and AL; arginine (free base) daily intake is currently recommended at 0.4–0.7 g/kg in AS deficiency (citrullinemia) and as close to 100 mg/kg as possible while maintaining normal arginine levels in patients with AL deficiency (argininosuccinic aciduria, ASA) who also receive phenylbutyrate. For patients with other inborn errors of metabolism, the enteral medication regimen should be tailored to their needs.

Once the patient is stable on enteral nutrition and medications, discharge planning may begin. For patients with inborn errors of metabolism, long-term outcomes are highly dependent on compliance with prescribed medication and nutritional regimen. Permanent gastrostomy access is beneficial because it ensures feeding even when the child is not interested in food or is ill, and it facilitates the delivery of medications (many of which have a noxious taste).

Prior to discharge, the managing team must ensure a home supply of esoteric disease-specific nutritional formula, accurate scales for weighing formula, and medications. Follow-up in the metabolic clinic should be in 1 week or less after discharge to ensure adequate weight gain and stability. Parents should be educated about signs and symptoms of recurrent hyperammonemia and should be counseled to return for emergent evaluation with any concerns. All parents and caregivers should have a copy of an emergency treatment protocol tailored for the specific patient's needs to facilitate rapid and appropriate therapy when presenting to a nonmetabolic emergency facility.[9] For patients with structural anomalies that led to the initial hyperammonemia (ie, portosystemic shunt), surgical correction should prevent further hyperammonemia.

Patients with severe, neonatal-onset, proximal urea cycle defects are prone to frequent, severe, recurrent hyperammonemic crises. Strong consideration should be given to early liver transplantation in these patients.[15,16]

OUTCOME

Outcomes from neonatal hyperammonemia are tightly correlated to duration of symptoms. Those in coma for less than 3 days have far better neurologic and cognitive outcomes than those with comas of longer duration.[3-5] Given the importance of rapid intervention, hyperammonemia must be a consideration for all neonates with suggestive signs and symptoms. Close collaboration between neonatology and the metabolic team can ensure the best-possible outcomes for these critically ill patients.

ACKNOWLEDGMENT

This work was supported by U54HD 061221.

REFERENCES

1. Wilcken B, Wiley V, Hammond J, Carpenter K. Screening newborns for inborn errors of metabolism by tandem mass spectrometry. *N Engl J Med.* 2003;348(23):2304–2312.
2. Tuchman M, Lee B, Lichter-Konecki U, et al. Cross-sectional multicenter study of patients with urea cycle disorders in the United States. *Mol Genet Metab.* 2008;94:397–402.
3. Bachmann C. Outcome and survival of 88 patients with urea cycle disorders: a retrospective evaluation. *Eur J Pediatr.* 2003;162:410–416.
4. Msall M, Batshaw ML, Suss R, Brusilow SW, Mellits ED. Neurologic outcome in children with inborn errors of urea synthesis. Outcome of urea-cycle enzymopathies. *N Engl J Med.* 1984;310:1500–1505.
5. Krivitzky L, Babikian T, Lee HS, Thomas NH, Burk-Paull KL, Batshaw ML. Intellectual, adaptive, and behavioral functioning in children with urea cycle disorders. *Pediatr Res.* 2009;66(1):96–101.
6. Summar ML, Dobbelaere D, Brusilow S, Lee B. Diagnosis, symptoms, frequency and mortality of 260 patients with urea cycle disorders from a 21-year, multicentre study of acute hyperammonaemic episodes. *Acta Paediatr.* 2008;97:1420–1425.
7. Chapman KA, Gropman A, MacLeod E, et al. Acute management of propionic acidemia. *Mol Genet Metab.* 2012;105(1):16–25.
8. Singh RH, Rhead WJ, Smith W, Lee B, King LS, Summar M. Nutritional management of urea cycle disorders. *Crit Care Clin.* 2005;21(4 Suppl):S27–S35.
9. Summar M. Current strategies for the management of neonatal urea cycle disorders. *J Pediatr.* 2001;138(1 Suppl):S30–S39.
10. Matsuda I, Nagata N, Matsuura T. Retrospective survey of urea cycle disorders: part 1. Clinical and laboratory observations of thirty-two Japanese male patients with ornithine transcarbamylase deficiency. *Am J Med Genet.* 1991;38:85–89.
11. Batshaw ML, Brusilow SW. Treatment of hyperammonemic coma caused by inborn errors of urea synthesis. *J Pediatr.* 1980;97(6):893–900.

12. Lanpher BC, Gropman A, Chapman KA, Lichter-Konecki U, Urea Cycle Disorders Consortium, Summar ML. Urea cycle disorders overview.   In: Pagon RA, Bird TD, Dolan CR, Stephens K, Adam MP, eds. *GeneReviews*™. Seattle, WA: University of Washington, Seattle; 1993–2003 Apr 29   [updated 2011 Sep 1].

13. Batshaw ML, MacArthur RB, Tuchman M. Alternative pathway therapy for urea cycle disorders: twenty years later. *J Pediatr.* 2001;138(1 Suppl):S46–S54.

14. Summar M, Pietsch J, Deshpande J, Schulman G. Effective hemodialysis and hemofiltration driven by an extracorporeal membrane oxygenation pump in infants with hyperammonemia. *J Pediatr.* 1996;128(3):379–382.

15. Stevenson T, Millan MT, Wayman K, et al. Long-term outcome following pediatric liver transplantation for metabolic disorders. *Pediatr Transplant.* 2009;14:268–275.

16. Campeau PM, Pivalizza PJ, Miller G, et al. Early orthotopic liver transplantation in urea cycle defects: follow up of a developmental outcome study. *Mol Genet Metab.* 2010;100(Suppl 1):S84–S87.

Initial Management of Metabolic Acidosis

Kristina Cusmano-Ozog and Kimberly Chapman

DIAGNOSIS/INDICATION

Metabolic acidosis in the neonate can have several causes, including increased acid intake from an exogenous source, increased endogenous production of an acid such as seen in an inborn error of metabolism (IEM), inadequate excretion of acid by the kidneys or excessive loss of bicarbonate in urine or stool. Presence or absence of an anion gap (AG) can help to distinguish the underlying etiology. The AG can be calculated using the following equation: $AG = ([Na^+]) - ([Cl^-] + [HCO_3^-])$. A normal AG is typically less than 16 mEq/L.[1] Common anions that result in an elevated AG include lactate and the ketone bodies β-hydroxybutyrate and acetoacetate, as well as the accumulation of the toxic organic acids typically found in individuals with IEMs.

Clinical Findings

Clues that increase the likelihood of identifying an IEM include a family history of consanguinity or history of a neonatal or sibling death. Occasionally, maternal history of acute fatty liver of pregnancy may be solicited.

Infants with IEMs are usually normal at birth. They develop nonspecific findings similar to those for sepsis, such as poor feeding, vomiting, lethargy, hypotonia, hypothermia, seizures, and coma. Infants will try to correct metabolic acidosis by a reflex respiratory alkalosis using hyperventilation and Kussmaul respirations. More severe uncompensated acidosis can decrease peripheral vascular resistance and cardiac ventricular function, leading to hypotension, pulmonary edema, and tissue hypoxia, which will further complicate the picture by increasing lactate production because of hypoxia and poor perfusion.

Confirmatory Tests

The IEMs are enzyme deficiencies that result from amino acid, carbohydrate, or fatty acid metabolism (Figure 107-1). Most of these disorders can be diagnosed by routine metabolic testing (Table 107-1), including plasma amino acid, plasma acylcarnitine profile, and urine organic acid analyses. Please see Table 107-2 for details about IEMs and the specific abnormalities detected by laboratory evaluations.

TREATMENT

Treatment of the metabolic acidosis depends on the cause. Although sodium bicarbonate can be given to improve the pH, it will not treat the underlying cause of the acidosis, especially if the underlying etiology is an IEM. Episodes of decompensation can be life threatening, so emergent and aggressive treatment is required. Treatment typically includes reversing catabolism by any means possible, often with extra calories

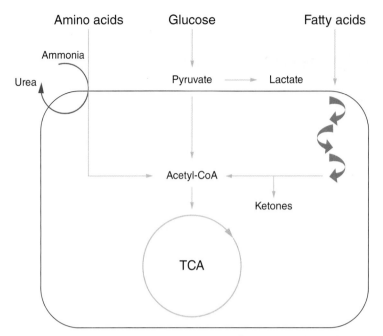

FIGURE 107-1 Basic pathways. Amino acids, carbohydrates, and fatty acids all undergo multiple processes to be converted into energy. The final common pathway is the formation of acetyl-CoA (coenzyme A), which can enter the tricarboxylic acid (TCA) cycle. NADH (nicotinamide adenine dinucleotide, reduced form) generated by the TCA cycle can be fed to the electron transport chain to generate ATP (adenosine triphosphate), the main energy source for numerous cellular functions. Defects in amino acid, carbohydrate, or fatty acid metabolism will lead to decreased energy production.

provided from dextrose and lipids when allowed and restriction of the toxic metabolite, such as protein in the organic acidemias. Please see Table 107-3 for the acute management protocol and Table 107-4 for discharge planning.

Table 107-1 Laboratory Tests for Any Patient With a Known or Suspected Inborn Error of Metabolism

Venous/arterial blood gas
Glucose
Lactate
Ammonia
Comprehensive metabolic panel
Anion gap ($[Na^+] - ([Cl^-] + [HCO_3^-])$)
Complete blood cell count
Blood culture
Plasma amino acids
Plasma acylcarnitine profile
Urinalysis to assess ketones
Urine organic acids
Urine culture

CONCLUSION/FOLLOW-UP

Episodes of decompensation can occur frequently in children with an IEM. Fever, vomiting, diarrhea, infection, and fasting can all be triggers. These episodes can be life threatening, so emergent and aggressive treatment is required.

Treatment of the IEMs is lifelong and consists of dietary restriction of the offending substrate, such as amino acids or long-chain fats, and supplementation of compounds that can dispose of toxic metabolites (eg, carnitine) or cofactors that can increase activity of deficient enzymes (eg, hydroxocobalamin or thiamine). Whenever a diet is altered from baseline with a medical formula, it is important to supplement with essential amino acids and ensure adequate caloric intake to avoid catabolism and support anabolism. Occasionally, total parenteral nutrition may be necessary, but it must be used with caution.

Outpatient evaluations for individuals with IEMs are numerous and include a physician and nutritionist who practice metabolic medicine to frequently

Table 107-2 Summary of Inborn Errors of Metabolism (IEMs) and Their Findings

IEM	Enzyme	Gene(s)	Newborn Screen	Plasma Amino Acids	Plasma Acylcarnitines	Urine Organic Acids
Amino Acid Metabolism						
Propionic acidemia	Propionyl CoA carboxylase	PCCA, PCCB	C3 propionylcarnitine	Glycine	C3 propionylcarnitine	3-Hydroxypropionic and methylcitric acids
Methylmalonic acidemia	Methylmalonyl CoA mutase	MUT, MMAA, MMAB	C3 propionylcarnitine	Glycine	C3 propionylcarnitine	Methylmalonic, 3-hydroxypropionic, and methylcitric acids
Isovaleric acidemia	Isovaleryl CoA dehydrogenase	IVD	C5 isovalerylcarnitine	N/A	C5 isovalerylcarnitine	Isovalerylglycine, 3-hydroxyisovaleric acid
Maple syrup urine disease	Branched-chain keto-acid dehydrogenase	BCKDHA, BCKDHB, DBT, DLD	Leucine	Leucine, isoleucine, valine, allo-isoleucine	N/A	2-Hydroxyisovaleric, 2-ketoisocaproic acids
Multiple carboxylase deficiency	Holocarboxylase synthetase	HLCS	C3 propionyl- and C5OH hydroxy-isovaleryl-carnitine	Alanine	C3 propionyl- and C5OH hydroxy-isovaleryl-carnitine	Lactic, 3-hydroxyisovaleric, methylcitric acids, methylcrotonylglycine
β-Ketothiolase deficiency	β-Ketothiolase	ACAT1	C5OH 2-methyl-3-hydroxybutyrylcarnitine	N/A	C5OH 2-methyl-3-hydroxybutyrylcarnitine and C5:1 tiglylcarnitine	2-Methyl-3-hydroxybutyric and 2-methylacetoacetic acids, tiglylglycine
Carbohydrate Metabolism						
Pyruvate carboxylase deficiency	Pyruvate carboxylase	PC	Citrulline	Citrulline, alanine, lysine, proline	N/A	Lactic, 2-ketoglutaric acids
Pyruvate dehydrogenase deficiency	Pyruvate dehydrogenase	PDHA1, PDHB, DLAT, DLD, PDHX	N/A	Alanine	N/A	Lactic acid
Fructose-1,6-bisphosphatase deficiency	Fructose-1,6-bisphosphatase	FBP1	N/A	N/A	N/A	Lactic, 2-ketoglutaric acids
Glycogen storage disease I	Glucose-6-phosphatase	G6PC, SLC37A4	N/A	N/A	N/A	Lactic and uric acids

(Continued)

Table 107-2 Summary of Inborn Errors of Metabolism (IEMs) and Their Findings (Continued)

IEM	Enzyme	Gene(s)	Newborn Screen	Plasma Amino Acids	Plasma Acylcarnitines	Urine Organic Acids
Fatty Acid Metabolism						
Very long-chain acyl-CoA dehydrogenase deficiency	Very long-chain acyl-CoA dehydrogenase	ACADVL	C14:1 tetradecenoylcarnitine	N/A	C14:1 tetradecenoylcarnitine	Dicarboxylic acids
Long-chain hydroxyacyl-CoA dehydrogenase deficiency	Long-chain hydroxyacyl-CoA dehydrogenase	HADHA, HADHB	C16-OH 3-hydroxyhexadecanoyl- and C18-OH 3-hydroxyoctadecanoyl-carnitine	N/A	C16-OH 3-hydroxyhexadecanoyl- and C18-OH 3-hydroxyoctadecanoyl-carnitine	(Hydroxy)dicarboxylic acids
Carnitine palmitoyltransferase I deficiency	Carnitine palmitoyltransferase I	CPT1A	C0 free carnitine with decreased C16, C18, C18:1	N/A	C0 Free Carnitine with decreased C16, C18, C18:1	N/A
Carnitine palmitoyltransferase II deficiency	Carnitine palmitoyltransferase II	CPT2	C16 hexadecanoyl-, C18 octadecanoyl-, and C18:1 octadecenoyl-carnitine	N/A	C16 hexadecanoyl-, C18 octadecanoyl-, and C18:1 octadecenoyl-carnitine	N/A
Carnitine translocase deficiency	Carnitine:acylcarnitine translocase	SCL25A20	C16 hexadecanoyl-, C18 octadecanoyl- and C18:1 octadecenoyl-carnitine	N/A	C16 hexadecanoyl-, C18 octadecanoyl-, and C18:1 octadecenoyl-carnitine	N/A

Abbreviations: ACAT1, acetyl-CoA acetyltransferase 1; ACADVL, acyl-CoA dehydrogenase, very long chain; PCCA, propionyl CoA carboxylase, alpha polypeptide; BCKDHA, branched chain keto acid dehydrogenase E1, alpha polypeptide; BCKDHB, branched chain keto acid dehydrogenase E1, beta polypeptide; CPT2, carnitine palmitoyltransferase 1A (liver); CPT1A, carnitine palmitoyltransferase 2; DBT, dihydrolipoamide branched chain transacylase E2; DLAT, dihydrolipoamide S-acetyltransferase; DLD, dihydrolipoamide dehydrogenase; FBP1, fructose-1,6-bisphosphatase 1; HADHA, hydroxyacyl-CoA dehydrogenase/3-ketoacyl-CoA thiolase/enoyl-CoA hydratase (trifunctional protein), alpha subunit; G6PC glucose-6-phosphatase, catalytic subunit; HADHB, hydroxyacyl-CoA dehydrogenase/3-ketoacyl-CoA thiolase/enoyl-CoA hydratase (trifunctional protein), HLCS holocarboxylase synthetase (biotin-(propionyl-CoA-carboxylase (ATP-hydrolysing)) ligase); beta subunitIVD, isovaleryl-CoA dehydrogenase; MMAA, methylmalonic aciduria (cobalamin deficiency) cblA type; MMAB, methylmalonic aciduria (cobalamin deficiency) cblB type; MUT, methylmalonyl CoA mutase; PC, pyruvate carboxylase; PCCB, propionyl CoA carboxylase, beta polypeptide; PDHA1, pyruvate dehydrogenase (lipoamide) alpha 1; PDHB, pyruvate dehydrogenase (lipoamide) beta; PDHX pyruvate dehydrogenase complex, component X; SLC37A4 solute carrier family 37 (glucose-6-phosphate transporter), member 4; SCL25A20 solute carrier family 25 (carnitine/acylcarnitine translocase), member 20

Table 107-3 Acute Management Protocol

A. Stabilization
1. Intubate and ventilate, if necessary.
2. Place intravenous lines. Do not use right intrajugular or 1 of the 2 femoral sites (these locations are necessary for hemodialysis). If unable to obtain access, intraosseus and nasogastric tube are acceptable.
3. Add vasopressors as necessary to maintain blood pressure.
4. Normal saline fluid bolus can be given. Avoid overhydration and do not delay reversal of catabolism to give a normal saline bolus.
5. Draw laboratory studies mentioned in Table 107-2; do not discard any blood remaining after analysis. If the presenting institution cannot run the laboratory tests, transport samples with the patient.

B. Reversal of catabolism
1. Stop all sources of protein (enteral and parenteral nutrition).
2. Give nonprotein calories in the form of intravenous fluids with minimum 10% dextrose and electrolytes at 120–150 mL/kg/d or goal of 6—8 mg glucose/kg/min.
3. If intralipids are available and a fatty acid oxidation defect is not suspected, give 2—3 g/kg/d to provide additional calories.
4. Do not stop calorie delivery for any reason (eg, medications, additional required fluid bolus, or hyperglycemia).
5. Consider an insulin drip (0.01 U/kg/h). If hypoglycemia occurs, increase dextrose amount or delivery rate.

C. Other interventions
1. Start antibiotics after blood cultures are drawn.
2. If newborn screen results are unknown, call state laboratory to check for results or expedite their processing (normal results do not rule out metabolic disease).
3. Arrange transport to a metabolic center as soon as there are concerns for metabolic disease or decompensation.
4. Arrange for and initiate hemodialysis, hemofiltration, or extracorporeal membrane oxygenation (ECMO) if clinical or laboratory evaluations identify ammonia greater than 300 µmol/L, extreme acidosis/electrolyte imbalance, coma, dilated pupils, poor neurological findings, or increased respiratory rate and based on clinical judgment. Do not use peritoneal dialysis.
5. For hyperammonemia in an undiagnosed patient, consider starting sodium benzoate/sodium phenylacetate (at same doses as urea cycle defects).
6. Intravenous carnitine at 100 mg/kg/dose 3—4 times daily over a minimum of 30 minutes can be given if urine output is appropriate (or hemofiltration ongoing) and there is no concern for a long-chain fatty acid oxidation defect.
7. Follow ammonia, electrolyte, and blood gas values at regular intervals. The frequency is dictated by the patient's condition and the speed at which results can be obtained.
8. Protein should be reintroduced within 24—36 hours of initiation of therapy. Protein must be reintroduced even if patient is on hemodialysis or ECMO.
9. Consider sedation, ventilation, and chemical paralysis if aggressive management is necessary. If used, continuous electroencephalography (EEG) is helpful for monitoring progress.
10. Transfuse packed red blood cells as necessary based on age, clinical condition, and physician discretion.

Table 107-4 Discharge Planning

A. Parental training
1. Preparation of metabolic formula with their home gram scale
2. Gastrostomy tube or nasogastric care (if present)
3. Lessons in giving all medications
4. Instructions on how to use ketosticks (if needed)

B. Medications and formula
1. Prescriptions for all medications and ketosticks; Provide at least 2 days prior to discharge to have time to fill
2. Provide 1-week supply of all medications
3. Provide list of medications with dosages, times, and reasons for use
4. Provide several cans of metabolic formula
5. Provide paper and electronic copy of diet with list of feeding times

C. Follow-up
1. Emergency room letter
2. Emergency contact information for the metabolic medicine physician and clinic
3. Appointment date and time for metabolic clinic and other specialists
4. Referral to early intervention

CHAPTER 107

monitor biochemistry and adjust diet and supplements for growth, a pediatrician to monitor growth and development and provide immunizations, in addition to any other specialist who may be required for organ-specific evaluations.

REFERENCE

1. Tschudy, Megan M. Arcara, Kristin M., eds. The Harriet Lane Handbook: A Manual For Pediatric House Officers. Philadelphia, PA: Mosby Elsevier, 2012. Print.

CHAPTER 107

108 Common Chromosomal Trisomies 21, 18, and 13

Yael Wilnai and Melanie Manning

INTRODUCTION

Chromosome abnormalities account for a significant portion of genetic disease and are important causes of congenital malformations and pregnancy loss. Cytogenetic disorders are found in nearly 1% of live births; thus, performing a karyotype on a newborn with multiple congenital anomalies can provide valuable information with respect to management questions and prognosis counseling. Chromosome analysis is indicated as a diagnostic procedure in a number of different general clinical situations, such as problems with early growth, development, stillbirth, and neonatal death. For infants in the neonatal period, performing a chromosome analysis may be considered if any of the following features are demonstrated:

- Abnormal growth parameters
- At least 1 major malformation
- 2 or more minor anomalies
- Abnormal neurologic findings

The most common chromosome abnormalities a care provider is likely to encounter in the newborn nursery are trisomies for chromosomes 21, 18, and 13. It is important to be able to recognize characteristic features of these conditions in order to initiate the most appropriate evaluations. For children who have had the diagnosis made prenatally, a formal copy of the chromosome report should be obtained. This report allows the clinician to confirm the diagnosis, review the results with the family, and add the formal diagnosis to the child's medical record. If the results

of prenatal testing are not available, a blood sample can be obtained for postnatal cytogenetic analysis to confirm the diagnosis and rule out a chromosome translocation.

TRISOMY 21 (DOWN SYNDROME)

Introduction

Down syndrome (DS) is the most common autosomal trisomy seen in live births. Incidence is estimated to be 1/600–1/800. The facial appearance of individuals with DS is characteristic and can be the first noticeable sign on physical examination to suggest this diagnosis. Other minor anomalies (eg, small ears, single transverse palmar crease, increased sandal gap), hypotonia, and malformations of other body systems (most importantly the cardiovascular and gastrointestinal systems) can be appreciated in the newborn period. DS is also associated with developmental delay/cognitive impairment, hearing loss, eye anomalies, thyroid dysfunction, atlantoaxial instability, and transient myeloproliferative disorder (TMD)/leukemia.

Diagnosis

Clinical Findings

History
The first step in evaluating a newborn infant suspected of having trisomy 21 is a careful review of the family history and prenatal information, including prenatal screening, chromosome studies done via amniocentesis

or chorionic villi sampling (CVS), or any other genetic testing performed. Previous children born with trisomy 21, developmental differences, or pregnancies that ended in miscarriage may be significant clues that a family may carry a balanced translocation that predisposes them to having children with trisomy 21.

Physical Examination

A physical examination is the most sensitive test in the first 24 hours of life to diagnose trisomy 21 in an infant. If the clinician feels that enough criteria are present on physical examination, then a blood sample should be sent for chromosome evaluation. The clinician should alert the laboratory and request rapid results.

Common physical features are the following:

- Hypotonia
- Small brachycephalic head with large fontanelle
- Epicanthal folds
- Flat nasal bridge/flattened midface
- Upward-slanting palpebral fissures
- Small mouth, small ears with overfolded pinnae
- Redundant nuchal folds
- Single transverse palmar crease
- Brachydactyly, short fifth finger with clinodactyly
- Wide space, often with a deep fissure, between the first and second toes ("sandal gap")
- Hypoplastic nipples/breast buds

Confirmatory Testing

Routine blood karyotype may be ordered STAT. If the patient's mother has had prenatal testing, amniocentesis or CVS that identified trisomy 21, there is no need to repeat testing. High-resolution chromosome analysis is not indicated. Comparative genomic hybridization (CGH) is not an appropriate first-line test to rule out a trisomy.

Differential Diagnosis

Sometimes, features of trisomy 21 can be subtle, depending on factors such as the clinical status and ethnic background. A chromosome analysis will rule out common aneuploidies as well as major structural anomalies that can present with overlapping signs and symptoms to trisomy 21. Consultation by a medical genetics specialist may provide additional insight into additional disorders (eg, single gene) to consider.

Treatment

Ethical Considerations

Although overall survival for children with DS may be reduced in the first 5 years of life when compared to the general pediatric population (likely from heart

defects, respiratory infections), withholding care to a newborn with this diagnosis is not appropriate. Thus, evaluation for associated medical issues is important prior to discharge.

Initiation

There are a number of medical issues common to trisomy 21 that present in the newborn period. Surveillance for these problems is warranted.

Associated medical issues in the newborn period are the following:

- Congenital heart defect (50%): Endocardial cushion defects are the most common.
- Gastrointestinal atresias (12%).
- Thyroid disease (15%).
- Atlantoaxial instability (1%–2%).
- TMD. TMD is an uncontrolled proliferation of myeloblasts occurring only in infants with DS. The majority of infants present from birth to 2–3 weeks of life with elevated white blood cell counts and blasts, very rarely with anemia or thrombocytopenia. The incidence of TMD in DS is around 10%. Most cases of TMD are asymptomatic, with spontaneous resolution by 3 months of age. However, 20% of cases progress to life-threatening organomegaly, hepatic fibrosis, liver failure, or cardiopulmonary disease (caused by blast infiltration).
- Approximately 30% of all cases develop acute megakaryoblastic leukemia between the ages of 1 and 4 years. If TMD is diagnosed in a neonate with DS, the infant should be followed closely by hematology.
- Hirschsprung disease (<1%).

Tests/Evaluations

Evaluation for the common associated medical conditions includes the following:

- Complete blood cell count (CBC) with differential (will detect polycythemia, leukemoid reaction)
- Echocardiogram
- Intestinal obstruction monitoring
- Hearing screen (routine, prior to discharge)
- Newborn screen (will detect congenital hypothyroidism)
- Genetics consult at earliest convenience

Conclusion/Follow-up

Discharge Planning

When formulating the discharge plans for a patient with trisomy 21, a comprehensive team approach is appropriate.

The following are general recommendations:

- Referral for specialty follow-up (eg, cardiology, gastrointestinal [GI], endocrinology, ear-nose-throat [ENT], hematology/oncology) as appropriate
- RSV (respiratory syncytial virus) prophylaxis (if appropriate)
- Cervical spine precautions
- Referral to early intervention programs
- Hearing screen (if abnormal, arrange for outpatient follow-up)
- Parent resources: national DS support groups, local support groups

Clinical Follow-up

Follow-up recommendations are dictated by issues identified in the nursery (eg, cardiology if heart defect is diagnosed). However, the family should be counseled regarding other common medical and developmental problems that can be seen over time and for which the primary care physician should monitor.

Associated medical issues presenting after newborn period include

- Cognitive impairment (100%)
- Hearing loss (75%)
- Otitis media (50%–75%)
- Obstructive sleep apnea (50%–75%)
- Eye disease (60%)
- Thyroid disease (15%)
- Seizures (6%–8%)
- Hip dislocation (6%)
- Atlantoaxial instability (1%–2%)
- Leukemia (<1%)

Long-Term Outcome/Implications for Patient/Family

1. *Early intervention*: Evidence shows that enrollment in early intervention programs providing physical, occupational, and speech therapies are beneficial for helping patients with DS meet their maximum developmental potential. Referral to local programs should be part of the discharge plan.
2. *Genetic counseling*: Families should receive basic counseling regarding the type of DS their baby has and the chance for recurrence within the family.
   - Of trisomy 21 cases, 95% are caused by nondisjunction resulting in 3 separate copies of chromosome 21.
   - Robertsonian translocations between chromosome 21 and another acrocentric chromosome (usually chromosome 14) cause 3%–4% of cases. Approximately three-quarters of these unbalanced translocations are de novo, and

approximately one-quarter are the result of familial translocations.

- Chromosomal mosaicism causes 1%–2% of cases. Mosaic trisomy 21 is also not inherited. It occurs as a random event during cell division early in embryonic development. As a result, some of the body's cells have the usual 2 copies of chromosome 21, and other cells have 3 copies of this chromosome. Mosaic trisomy 21 has been reported in a few patients with a clinical picture that varies between a normal phenotype and that of classical trisomy 21 according to the number of trisomic cells present in the tissues.
- Recurrence risks for having another child with DS (or another similar type of chromosome abnormality) are cited as 1% or mother's age-related risk, whichever is higher.

Summary

The proper management and health supervision of children with trisomy 21 are critical to ensure the best possible outcomes for these special patients. Families will be empowered by receiving anticipatory support and guidance, understanding the special issues that may affect their children, and recognizing the resources available.

TRISOMY 18 (EDWARDS SYNDROME)

Introduction

Trisomy 18 is the second-most-common autosomal trisomy in newborns. Birth prevalence is approximately 1 in 3000 to 1 in 8000. The pattern in trisomy 18 includes a recognizable constellation of major and minor anomalies, a predisposition to increased neonatal and infant mortality, and significant developmental and motor disability in surviving older children. This is a severely handicapping condition, and the rate of early death is high. Life span of the majority of patients is less than 1 year.

Diagnosis

Clinical Findings

History

The first step in evaluating a newborn infant suspected of having trisomy 18 is a careful review of the family history and prenatal information, including prenatal screening, chromosome studies done via amniocentesis or CVS, or any other genetic testing that was performed. Previous children born with trisomy 18 or pregnancies that ended in miscarriage may be significant clues that a family may carry a balanced translocation that predisposes them to having children with trisomy 18.

Physical Examination

If the clinician feels that enough characteristic features are present on physical examination, then a blood sample should be sent for chromosome evaluation. The clinician should alert the laboratory and request rapid results.

The following are common physical features:

- Intrauterine growth retardation (IUGR)
- Clenched hands, overriding fingers (second and fifth fingers over third and fourth fingers)
- Nail hypoplasia
- Short sternum
- Rocker-bottom feet
- Prominent occiput, narrow bifrontal diameter
- Micrognathia
- Inverted triangular face
- Small pelvis, limited hip abduction

Additional physical features include

- Radial limb defect
- Short hallux
- Single palmar crease
- Low-set, malformed ears
- Microcephaly
- High arched palate, cleft lip and palate
- Short palpebral fissures, microphthalmia
- Webbed neck
- Polyhydramnios/oligohydramnios
- Single umbilical artery
- Hypospadias
- Cryptorchidism
- Imperforate anus

Confirmatory Testing

Routine blood karyotyping may be ordered STAT. If the patient's mother has had prenatal testing, amniocentesis or CVS that identified trisomy 18, there is no need to repeat testing.

High-resolution chromosome analysis is not indicated. CGH is not an appropriate first-line test to rule out trisomy 18.

Differential Diagnosis

The anomaly pattern of trisomy 18 is quite discrete and, in its totality, is rarely confused with other conditions. The most common disorder with overlapping features comprises the heterogeneous group of fetal akinesia sequence, distal arthrogryposis, or CHARGE (coloboma, heart defect, atresia choanae [also known as choanal atresia], retarded growth and development, genital abnormality, and ear abnormality) syndrome. A chromosome analysis will rule out common aneuploidies as well as major structural anomalies that can present with overlapping signs and symptoms to trisomy 18. Consultation by a medical genetics specialist may provide additional insight into other disorders (eg, single gene) to consider.

Treatment

Ethical Considerations

After the etiology has been determined, the health care team will need to discuss the diagnosis and prognosis with the parents. Ethical issues regarding aggressive therapies, surgeries, and life-prolonging measures need to be addressed.

Prolonged survival (in some cases into adulthood) has been reported, mainly in cases involving mosaic or partial trisomy (resulting from translocation). The majority of nonmosaic patients develop only limited autonomy, with absence of speech and ambulation. Almost all of these children function in the severe-to-profound developmentally handicapped range. If surgery would be considered for major anomalies, the wisdom of pursuing aggressive treatment should be discussed with the family. Occasionally, it may be necessary to consult the hospital ethics committee.

Initiation

There are multiple life-threatening medical issues common to trisomy 18 that present in the immediate neonatal period. Surveillance for these problems is warranted.

The following are associated medical issues in the newborn period:

- Cardiac defects (ventricular septal defect [VSD], patent ductus arteriosus [PDA], atrial septal defect [ASD], pulmonary hypertension [PHT], double outlet right ventricle [DORV], polyvalvular disease)
- Brain anomalies (cerebellar hypoplasia, brain edema, enlarged cisterna magna, choroid plexus cysts, hydrocephalus)
- Tracheoesophageal fistula, esophageal atresia
- Omphalocele
- Myelomeningocele
- Renal anomalies

Tests/Evaluations

Evaluation for the common associated medical conditions consists of the following:

- At birth, initial management concerns focus on obtaining cytogenetic confirmation of the suspected chromosomal abnormality.
  - Head ultrasound (US)
  - Echocardiography
- Management is supportive only. Surgical treatment of the malformations does little to improve the poor prognosis associated with this syndrome: 90% of infants die within the first year of life from cardiac, renal, or neurological complications or from repeated infections.

Conclusion/Follow-up

Discharge Planning

For infants who survive the neonatal period, planning for hospital discharge should focus on patient and family support services. Social work coordinators can assist with identifying community support services (eg, hospice) geared to a patient with complicated medical issues. Discussions regarding issues such as Do Not Resuscitate orders should be initiated prior to discharge.

When formulating the discharge plans for a patient with trisomy 18, a comprehensive team approach is appropriate.

Referral should be considered to

- Support groups (local, national)
- Hospice
- Early intervention services if applicable

Clinical Follow-up

Follow-up recommendations are dictated by issues identified in the nursery and the family wishes.

Associated medical issues later in life include severe intellectual disability and repeated infections.

Long-Term Outcome/Implications for Patient/Family

Most patients with trisomy 18 will die in the first few weeks of life; the most common causes of death are cardiopulmonary arrest, congenital heart disease, and pneumonia. It is important to recognize that a small but notable percentage will survive the first year. This means that trisomy 18 is not absolutely fatal. This information is important to health care personnel who care for patients with trisomy 18. However, the management of such a baby remains a challenging medical and ethical issue.

Genetic Counseling

Almost all cases of trisomy 18 are sporadic and are usually caused by maternal nondisjunction. Recurrence is uncommon. Advanced maternal age is a risk factor.

Mosaic trisomy 18 is also not inherited. It occurs as a random event during cell division early in embryonic development. As a result, some of the body's cells have the usual 2 copies of chromosome 18, and other cells have 3 copies of this chromosome. This is a rare cause of trisomy 18, with occurrence of less than 5%.

A minority of the cases are the result of an unbalanced translocation. Thus, chromosome analysis to look for an unbalanced translocation is imperative even when the clinical diagnosis is fairly straightforward so that accurate recurrence risks can be provided. Translocation trisomy 18 can be inherited if the parent carries a balanced translocation.

The risk of recurrence in families of an index case with trisomy 18 is around 1%. However, in families in which trisomy 18 is caused by translocation, the recurrence risk may be higher if a parent is a carrier of a balanced translocation.

Summary

Trisomy 18 involves a high mortality rate; however, 5%–8% of infants survive the newborn period. Ongoing support and care by professionals are crucial to a family whose child has a serious medical condition. Families will be empowered by receiving anticipatory support and guidance, understanding the special issues that may affect their children, and recognizing the resources available.

TRISOMY 13 (PATAU SYNDROME)

Introduction

Trisomy 13 (Patau syndrome) is the least common of the 3 frequently seen trisomies, with an incidence ranging from 1 in 12,500 to 1 in 21,000. Trisomy 13 syndrome presents as an obvious pattern of multiple congenital anomalies. The combination of orofacial clefts, microphthalmia/anophthalmia, cutis aplasia, abdominal wall defects, and postaxial polydactyly of the limbs allows for recognition by the clinician.

Diagnosis

Clinical Findings

History

The first step in evaluating a newborn infant suspected of having trisomy 13 is a careful review of the family history and prenatal information, including prenatal screening, chromosome studies done via amniocentesis or CVS, or any other genetic testing that was performed. Previous children born with trisomy 13 or pregnancies that ended in miscarriage, polyhydramnios, or oligohydramnios may be significant clues that a family may carry a balanced translocation that predisposes them to having children with trisomy 13.

Physical Examination

If the clinician feels that enough characteristic features are present on physical examination, then a blood sample should be sent for chromosome evaluation. The clinician should alert the laboratory and request rapid results.

The following are common physical features:

- IUGR
- Hypotonia and hyporeactivity, apneic spells
- Postaxial polydactyly; hyperconvex, narrow fingernails
- Microcephaly, sloping forehead
- Wide sagittal sutures and fontanelle
- Hypo- or hypertelorism
- Arrhinencephaly or nasal malformations
- Orofacial clefts
- Low-set ears with abnormal helices
- Capillary hemangiomas of the forehead
- Cutis aplasia, other scalp defects in the parietooccipital area
- Micro-/anophthalmia, coloboma
- Prominence of the nasal bridge and tip

Confirmatory Testing

Routine blood karyotyping may be ordered STAT. If the patient's mother has had prenatal testing, amniocentesis or CVS that identified trisomy 13, there is no need to repeat testing. High-resolution chromosome analysis is not indicated. CGH is not an appropriate first-line test to rule out trisomy 13.

Differential Diagnosis

The cardinal features of trisomy 13 include a number of manifestations that are seen in various multiple congenital anomaly conditions. However, the pattern in total is distinctive and usually allows for straightforward diagnosis. In the differential are Meckel-Gruber syndrome, holoprosencephaly-polydactyly syndrome, and Smith-Lemli-Opitz syndrome. A chromosome analysis will rule out common aneuploidies as well as major structural anomalies that can present with overlapping signs and symptoms to trisomy 13. Consultation by a medical genetics specialist may provide additional insight into other disorders (eg, single gene) to consider.

Treatment

Ethical Considerations

- After the etiology has been determined, the health care team will need to discuss the diagnosis and prognosis with the parents. Ethical issues regarding

aggressive therapies, surgeries, and life-prolonging measures need to be addressed.

- Prolonged survival (in some cases into adulthood) has been rarely reported, mainly in cases involving mosaicism. The majority of nonmosaic patients develop only limited autonomy, with absence of speech and ambulation. Almost all of these children function in the severe-to-profound developmentally handicapped range.
- If surgery would be considered for major anomalies, the wisdom of pursuing aggressive treatment should be discussed with the family. Occasionally, it may be necessary to consult the hospital ethics committee.

Initiation

There are multiple life-threatening medical issues common to trisomy 13 that present in the immediate neonatal period. Surveillance for these problems is warranted.

The following are associated medical issues in the newborn period:

- Brain malformation (holoprosencephaly, including incomplete development of the forebrain and olfactory and optic nerves)
- Meningomyelocele
- Cardiac defects, most often VSD, ASD, PDA, and dextrocardia
- Urogenital malformations, including cryptorchidism, abnormal scrotum, bicornuate uterus
- Renal anomalies, including polycystic kidneys, hydronephrosis, and hydroureter

Tests/Evaluations

- At birth, initial management concerns focus on obtaining cytogenetic confirmation of the suspected chromosomal abnormality.
- After the etiology has been determined, the health care team will need to discuss the diagnosis and prognosis with the parents. Ethical issues regarding aggressive therapies, surgeries, and life-prolonging measures need to be addressed.
- Evaluation for the common associated medical conditions includes the following:
  - Echocardiogram
  - Brain imaging
  - Renal US
  - Genetics consult
- Management is supportive only. Surgical treatment of the malformations does little to improve the poor prognosis associated with this syndrome: 90% of infants die within the first year of life from cardiac, renal, or neurological complications or from repeated infections.

Conclusion/Follow-up

Discharge Planning

For infants who survive the neonatal period, planning for hospital discharge should focus on patient and family support services. Social work coordinators can assist with identifying community support services (eg, hospice) geared to a patient with complicated medical issues. Discussions regarding issues such as Do Not Resuscitate orders should be initiated prior to discharge.

When formulating the discharge plans for a patient with trisomy 13, a comprehensive team approach is appropriate.

Referral should be considered to

- Support groups (local, national)
- Hospice
- Early intervention services if applicable

Clinical Follow-up

Follow-up recommendations are dictated by issues identified in the nursery and the family wishes.

Associated medical issues later in life include severe intellectual disability and repeated infections.

Long-Term Outcome/Implications for Patient/Family

Most patients with trisomy 13 will die in the first few weeks of life; the most common causes of death are cardiopulmonary arrest, congenital heart disease, and pneumonia. It is important to recognize that a small but notable percentage will survive the first year. This means that trisomy 13 is not absolutely fatal. This information is important to health care personnel who care for patients with trisomy 13. However, the management of such a baby remains a challenging medical and ethical issue.

Genetic Counseling

- Freestanding trisomy 13 is found in around 75% of cases and is caused by nondisjunction of maternal origin (meiosis II error) in about 90% of cases.
- In 20% of cases, trisomy 13 is associated with a Robertsonian translocation in which the supernumerary chromosome 13 becomes attached to another acrocentric chromosome (chromosomes 13, 14, 15, 21, or 22). In rare cases, the syndrome is caused by reciprocal translocation between chromosome 13 and a nonacrocentric chromosome.
- Mosaic trisomy 13 has been reported in a few patients with a clinical picture that varies between a normal phenotype and that of classical trisomy 13 according to the number of trisomic cells present in the tissues.
- The risk of recurrence of trisomy 13 in families of an index case with trisomy 13 is around 1%. However, in families in which trisomy 13 is associated with translocation (Robertsonian or balanced), the risk of recurrence is higher if a parent is a carrier of a balanced translocation.

Summary

Trisomy 13 involves a high mortality rate; however, 10% of infants survive past the newborn period. Ongoing support and care by professionals are crucial to a family whose child has a serious medical condition. Families will be empowered by receiving anticipatory support and guidance, understanding the special issues that may affect their children, and recognizing the resources available.

SUGGESTED READING

Baty BJ, Blackburn BL, Carey JC. Natural history of trisomy 18 and trisomy 13: I. Growth, physical assessment, medical histories, survival, and recurrence risk. *Am J Med Genet.* 1994;49(2):175–188.

Baty BJ, Jorde LB, Blackburn BL, Carey JC. Natural history of trisomy 18 and trisomy 13: II. Psychomotor development. *Am J Med Genet.* 1994;49(2):189–194.

Bull MJ, Committee on Genetics. Health supervision for children with Down syndrome. *Pediatrics.* 2011;128:393–406. doi:10.1542/peds.2011-1605.

Cassidy SB, Allanson JE. *Management of Genetic Syndromes.* 3rd ed. Hoboken, NJ: John Wiley-Blackwell; 2005.

Janvier A, Farlow B, Wilfond BS. The experience of families with children with trisomy 13 and 18 in social networks. *Pediatrics.* 2012;130:293–298.

Matthews AL. Chromosomal abnormalities: trisomy 18, trisomy 13, and microdeletions. *J Perinat Neonatal Nurs.* 1999;13:59–75.

Rios A, Furdon SA, Adams D, Clark DA. Recognizing the clinical features of trisomy 13 syndrome. *Adv Neonatal Care.* 2004; 4:332–343.

Roizen NJ, Patterson D. Down's syndrome. *Lancet.* 2003; 361:1281–1289.

Common Dysmorphic Syndromes

Neda Zadeh

INTRODUCTION

Numerous genetic conditions are evident and diagnosable during the neonatal period because of a specific pattern of clinical features often present on infant physical examination. This chapter reviews several of the more frequently observed genetic dysmorphic conditions neonatal practitioners are most likely to encounter in a newborn (apart from the common trisomies that are addressed separately in this textbook), which include: Turner syndrome (TS), 22q11.2 deletion syndrome, CHARGE (coloboma, heart defect, atresia choanae [also known as choanal atresia], retarded growth and development, genital abnormality, and ear abnormality) syndrome, and VACTERL (vertebral, anal, cardiac, tracheoesophageal, renal, and limb) association.

As several genetic syndromes and 1 association are discussed in this chapter, it is reasonable to define both entities. The term *syndrome* derives from the Greek and means "concurrence" or "along with, together." Thus, a genetic syndrome refers to a pattern of congenital anomalies that can be explained by a common genetic or developmental cause. Syndromes often include developmental abnormalities and increased risk of recurrence in families. An *association* is a collection of physical findings and is considered a nonrandom occurrence; it is known not be a polytypic defect, sequence, or syndrome.[1] Associations are generally not associated with an increased risk of recurrence.[1]

Identification of a specific genetic diagnosis during the immediate newborn period is helpful for appropriate medical management, as well as to provide the infant's family with prognostic information and accurate recurrence risk information.

CLINICAL GENETICS EVALUATION

Physical examination of the neonate is essential in providing diagnostic accuracy as well as focusing differential diagnoses. The genetic dysmorphology evaluation is a careful physical examination of the infant in a head-to-toe manner, taking note of any facial or body asymmetries, malformations, or deformations that may be present externally. This also involves measuring and plotting the growth parameters (length, weight, and head circumference) on appropriate curves for gestational age, such that entities of microcephaly or microsomia are not neglected.

The neonatal head is evaluated by assessing the head shape, size of the anterior and posterior fontanelles, and cranial sutures. Close attention is paid to possible sutural ridging or unusual head shape that is distinct from transient postnatal vertex molding. Careful evaluation of the scalp is performed to uncover lesions such as cutis aplasia congenita or unusual hair patterning that may indicate an underlying cerebral malformation. Facial asymmetry or cranial nerve palsy is best visualized while the infant is crying. Presence of facial asymmetry is often seen in association with syndromes such as CHARGE or 22q11.2 deletion syndrome and thus is of significant diagnostic value.

Evaluation of the eyes with an ophthalmoscope is warranted such that red reflexes can be visualized and irides can be closely examined for the presence of colobomas, which tend to be located inferonasally. Certain ophthalmic anomalies, such as iris Brushfield spots (observed in Down syndrome), retinal coloboma, optic nerve hypoplasia, and abnormal retinal pigmentation are not easily visualized by this methodology and require formal ophthalmology evaluation for detection.

Ears are analyzed for any unusual appearance of the concha, ear positioning, presence of preauricular pits or tags, or malformations such as microtia. The palate and lips are visualized for evidence of clefting, with close attention paid to the uvula to assess if there is a bifid formation or circumferential zona pellucida that could indicate a submucous cleft palate. An infant with frequent nasal regurgitation of feedings may have a submucous cleft or velopharyngeal insufficiency.

Nuchal skin redundancy with a low posterior hairline may be present in association with certain chromosome abnormalities, single-gene disorders, or in infants with complex congenital cardiac defects. If nuchal webbing is noted, close evaluation for limb edema indicating in utero lymphatic obstruction is also helpful diagnostically.

Examination of the limbs, hands, fingers, feet, toes, and palmar and plantar creases provides further insight as well as careful consideration for syndactyly, polydactyly, joint contractures, and limb positioning. Knowledge of a cardiac murmur, abdominal wall defects, hepatosplenomegaly, genitourinary anomalies, sacral dimple, or neural tube defects are essential and will guide the genetic diagnostic workup appropriately.

COMMON DYSMOPRHIC SYNDROMES

Turner Syndrome

Turner syndrome is a genetic condition caused by absence of all (monosomy) or part (partial monosomy) of the second X chromosome; thus, it only affects females. This multisystemic disorder has variable phenotypic severity, and in milder cases, this diagnosis may be overlooked during infancy, without detection until childhood or adolescence once short stature and pubertal delay are recognized.[2]

Turner syndrome has a birth prevalence of 1 in 2000 to 5000 female live births; however, the majority of 45,X concept uses spontaneously abort during the first trimester of pregnancy. TS-affected fetuses that survive into the second trimester are often recognized to have increased nuchal fold and lymphedema on prenatal ultrasound.[3] At birth, affected neonates may present with a constellation of features of a variable phenotypic spectrum. Congenital cardiac defects may often be the sole manifesting feature. Abnormalities of the left outflow tract, such as bicuspid aortic valve, and coarctation of the aorta are

commonly observed. Nuchal webbing, low posterior hairline, residual edema of the dorsum of the hands and plantar surfaces of the feet, and a shield-shaped chest with widely spaced nipples may be identified via careful newborn physical examination. The severity of these findings tends to depend on the degree of in utero lymphedema during embryologic development. Thus, mildly affected females may be diagnostically challenging.

A number of different diagnostic tests can be performed on the female infant suspected to have TS: chromosome analysis from peripheral blood; echocardiogram to evaluate for congenital cardiac defects; and renal ultrasound to look for structural anomalies of the kidney or abnormalities of the renal collecting system.[3] Furthermore, careful hip examination for congenital hip dysplasia and newborn hearing screen prior to discharge are recommended (Table 109-1).

Structural chromosome abnormalities such as isochromosome X, ring X, as well as deletions of a portion of the short arm (Xp) or long arm (Xq) have also been reported in females with TS.[2] A smaller percentage of females may exhibit mosaicism (45,X/46,XX or 45,X/46,XY). Presence of Y chromosome material warrants prophylactic gonadectomy secondary to increased risk for gonadoblastoma or dysgerminoma.[2] This illustrates the importance of chromosome analysis not only for confirmation of the diagnosis, but also to aid in further medical management and accuracy of recurrence risk in cases with structural rearrangements.

22q11.2 Deletion Syndrome

The 22q11.2 deletion syndrome is an autosomal dominant condition considered to be 1 of the most common microdeletion syndromes, with a prevalence of 1 in approximately 2000–4000 live births. This syndrome is also known in the medical literature as velocardiofacial syndrome, as well as DiGeorge syndrome in the subset of patients possessing both the microdeletion and immune deficiency. The microdeletion consists of a very small region, often undetectable by routine karyotype, and involves the 22q11.2 region of the long arm of chromosome 22. This disorder has a wide spectrum of clinical findings; a vast number of congenital anomalies have been observed in association with this condition.

More than 35 genes are present within the 22q11.2 critical region. Haploinsufficiency of this locus can cause malformation of the fourth branchial artery, which is a precursor for the right ventricle and cardiac outflow tract formation during embryogenesis.[4] Furthermore, malformation of the third and fourth branchial pouches may compromise development of the parathyroid, thymus, and craniofacial structures in the fetus.

Table 109-1 Diagnostic Testing for Genetic Dysmorphic Conditions Encountered in the Neonatal Period

Condition	Diagnostic Testing	Additional Studies/Imaging
Turner syndrome	Chromosome analysis	Echocardiogram
		Renal ultrasound
		Evaluate for hip dysplasia
22q11.2 Deletion syndrome	FISH for 22q11.2 microdeletion	Echocardiogram
		Renal ultrasound
		Immune workup
		T-cell subsets or flow cytometry
		Serum calcium level
		Hearing screen
CHARGE syndrome	CT of the temporal bones	Ophthalmology evaluation
	CHD7 full gene sequencing	Echocardiogram
		Renal ultrasound
VACTERL association	Diagnosis of exclusion	Spine and extremity films
		Renal ultrasound
		Ophthalmology evaluation
		Echocardiogram
		Evaluate for tracheoesophageal fistula

Abbreviations: CHARGE, coloboma, heart defect, atresia choanae (also known as choanal atresia), retarded growth and development, genital abnormality, and ear abnormality; CT, computed tomography; FISH, fluorescence in situ hybridization; VACTERL, vertebral, anal, cardiac, tracheoesophageal, renal, and limb.

Knowledge of malformations of certain embryologic structures in the affected fetus facilitates our understanding of common clinical features observed in this condition. Cardiac anomalies, palatal abnormality, thymic and parathyroid hypoplasia/aplasia, and craniofacial anomalies are typically observed. Conotruncal cardiac anomalies, such as tetralogy of Fallot, interrupted aortic arch, truncus arteriosus, and ventricular septal defects, are commonly seen. Cleft palate, submucous cleft palate, velopharyngeal incompetence, or hypotonia of velopharyngeal musculature may cause feeding difficulties, such as severe dysphagia and reflux during infancy.[10]

Certain blood cell counts and chemistries may also be abnormal. Immunodeficiency (reduced T-cell count) and hypocalcemia may be present secondary to hypoplasia or aplasia of the thymus and parathyroid glands, respectively. Hypocalcemia is typically most evident and serious during the neonatal period and tends to normalize with age. However, hypocalcemia may recur later in childhood, especially during illness or puberty.

Craniofacial anomalies are variable in appearance and severity and may include hooded eyelids; ocular hypertelorism; ear abnormalities (overfolded or squared off helices, cupped protuberant ears, associated pits or tags); and asymmetric crying facies. In the absence of a congenital cardiac defect or the presence of minimal or atypical phenotype, diagnosis during infancy may not be made.[1] Table 109-1 lists the appropriate workup for an infant suspected to have this condition.

Fluorescence in situ hybridization (FISH) for the 22q11.2 region on peripheral blood metaphases is the gold standard diagnostic test (Figure 109-1). Of note,

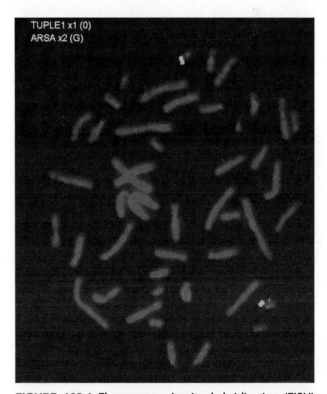

FIGURE 109-1 Fluorescence in situ hybridization (FISH) positive for 22q11.2 microdeletion. This image represents a peripheral blood metaphase cell with FISH for the 22q11.2 microdeletion. Only 1 orange signal for the TUPLE1 probe (specific for the DiGeorge region) is noted, indicating deletion of the q11.2 region on 1 chromosome 22. There are 2 green control probe signals, indicating that 2 chromosome 22s are present. This patient has a confirmed 22q11.2 microdeletion, consistent with 22q11.2 deletion syndrome. (Used with permission of Touran M. Zadeh, MD, Genetics Center, Orange, California.)

comparative genomic hybridization (array CGH) is also capable of detecting this particular microdeletion. In infants, a thorough physical examination, echocardiogram, and measurement of serum calcium level are warranted if a diagnosis of 22q11.2 deletion syndrome is suspected. Immunodeficiency workup may be initialized once FISH confirmation of the diagnosis is made. Ninety percent of 22q11.2 deletion syndrome cases are de novo occurrences; however, it is generally recommended that both parents of a patient with 22q11.2 deletion syndrome be tested as well to provide the most accurate information on risk of recurrence.

CHARGE Syndrome

CHARGE Syndrome is 1 of the most common multiple-anomaly conditions that may be encountered by neonatologists and clinicians. CHARGE is an acronym for the cardinal features typically observed in association with this condition: **c**oloboma, congenital **h**eart defects, choanal **a**tresia, **r**etardation of growth and development, **g**enital abnormalities, **e**ar abnormalities and deafness. This is an autosomal dominant condition, with most cases arising in a de novo manner (ie, unaffected parents). Neonates with CHARGE may have life-threatening complications, especially if more than 1 of these 3 features is present: bilateral choanal atresia, tracheoesophageal fistula, or cyanotic congenital cardiac defect.[5,9]

Neonates with CHARGE syndrome may have normal growth parameters at birth, with observation of decreased linear growth by late infancy. The inability to pass a nasogastric tube during the immediate newborn period should alert the clinician to the presence of choanal atresia, and the possibility of CHARGE syndrome must be considered.[1] The clinical examination can thus be refocused to the heart, eyes, and other potentially involved organ systems accordingly. Imaging of the nasal passages via computed tomography (CT) is helpful in elucidating the quality of blockage. Bilateral choanal atresia is considered a medical emergency requiring surgical intervention.

As CHARGE syndrome affects multiple organ systems, further evaluation of the eyes, heart, and genitourinary system is warranted. Colobomas are present in up to 90% of patients with this condition and may be located in the iris or retinas (affecting the optic nerve or macula). Thus, a formal dilated ophthalmologic evaluation is necessary. Cardiac defects, predominantly conotruncal anomalies, are present in 75%–85% of infants with CHARGE syndrome. Genitourinary anomalies consisting of microphallus, hypospadias, and cryptorchidism in males and hypoplasia of the external female genitalia may be present.[5] In addition, affected females may have atresia of the uterus, cervix, and vagina in a minority of cases.[1] Renal abnormalities, including duplex kidneys, renal agenesis/hypoplasia, and vesicoureteral reflux (VUR), have been reported in up to 40% of infants with CHARGE syndrome.

A consistent feature in approximately 90% of infants with CHARGE syndrome is abnormalities of the semicircular canals.[5] This finding is more specific and accurate than the currently available molecular genetic testing, which involves full gene sequencing of the *CHD7* gene (with only a 60% mutation detection rate). Thus, if CHARGE syndrome is suspected, a CT scan of the temporal bones to look for middle and inner ear bony defects is diagnostically more sensitive and valuable than molecular genetic testing from blood. Furthermore, external ear anomalies may be asymmetric and present as short, protruding, lop or cup-shaped, and simple helices with hypoplastic lobules.[1]

As this is a variable condition, a clinical diagnosis of CHARGE syndrome may be challenging and is dependent on the method in which affected neonates are ascertained. Definite CHARGE syndrome is considered if neonates have the following 4 features: ocular coloboma, choanal atresia/stenosis, cranial nerve dysfunction, and a characteristic CHARGE-appearing ear and inner ear anomalies. Probable/possible CHARGE syndrome is suspected if the neonate has 2 major characteristics as just listed and several minor characteristics (genital hypoplasia, cardiovascular anomalies, orofacial cleft, tracheoesophageal fistula, or distinctive facial features).[5] If CHARGE is suspected, a genetic evaluation is warranted as well as an appropriate evaluation of the previously mentioned organ systems (Table 109-1) to provide the family with the most accurate diagnosis as well as risk of recurrence.

VACTERL Association

In contrast to the other syndromes mentioned in this chapter, VACTERL is an association without an identifiable molecular cause. Another name for this condition is VATER association, which is an acronym for the multisystemic features typically observed: **v**ertebral defects, **a**nal atresia, **t**rach**e**oesophageal fistula with esophageal atresia, and **r**adial and **r**enal dysplasia. The CL has been added more recently to include **c**ardiac and **l**imb defects (as observed in VACTERL). Both VACTERL association and CHARGE syndrome may have overlapping phenotypic features. However, careful physical examination and workup can usually distinguish between these 2 distinct entities.

Neonates with VACTERL do not have dysmorphic features or abnormalities in linear growth. Furthermore, neurocognitive impairment is also not typically observed in patients with VACTERL.[6] A careful physical examination and appropriate imaging modalities are appropriate assessment tools. Vertebral defects can be visualized on anterior-posterior and lateral complete spine radiographs; anomalies include hemivertebrae, segmentation defects, absent vertebrae, and sacral dysgenesis.[6] Anal atresia or stenosis requires immediate surgical intervention, and a range of cardiac anomalies have been described. Renal agenesis, reflux, and ureteropelvic junction (UPJ) obstruction can be observed on ultrasound imaging.

Limb defects tend to involve the upper more than the lower extremities, with radial bones more affected than ulnar bones. Thumb anomalies, including thumb aplasia or hypoplasia, rudimentary thumbs, and preaxial polydactyly, have all been reported.[1] The upper extremity findings can be similar to that observed in Fanconi anemia and Townes-Brocks syndrome and several other genetic conditions.[6]

Fanconi anemia is a genetic condition that can present with multiple physical anomalies during the neonatal period. Most commonly observed manifestations include thumb anomalies and multisystemic involvement, including the eyes, kidneys and urinary tract, ears, and heart, along with hypogonadism and developmental delay. Bone marrow failure is not usually present until 6 to 8 years of age.[7] Townes-Brocks is characterized by a clinical triad of features consisting of abnormal-appearing ears, imperforate anus, and thumb anomalies.[8] These 2 genetic syndromes have an increased risk of recurrence compared to an association, which is generally sporadic in nature.

For diagnostic purposes, x-rays of the upper extremities may be helpful, along with echocardiogram, renal ultrasound, spine films, and ophthalmology evaluation if VACTERL is being considered (Table 109-1). Chromosome breakage studies may be pursued to ensure that a diagnosis of Fanconi anemia is not overlooked. Furthermore, molecular genetic testing for Townes-Brocks syndrome is available clinically with a good mutation detection rate.[1]

VACTERL association is considered a diagnosis of exclusion that should not be made until 1 year of age. Thus, appropriate genetic workup for other syndromes with similar clinical features is necessary prior to assigning this diagnosis.

CONCLUSION

Knowledge of common dysmorphic genetic conditions that often present during the neonatal period is helpful in appropriate medical management and prognosis. Distinction between an isolated malformation, association, or a genetic syndrome also provides further information for the family as well as a more accurate recurrence risk. A genetics evaluation should be considered in any newborn with multiple congenital anomalies.[1]

REFERENCES

1. Kaplan J, Hudgins L. Neonatal presentations of CHARGE syndrome and VATER/VACTERL association. *NeoReviews.* 2008;9:e299–e304.
2. Loscalzo M. Turner syndrome. *Pediatr Rev.* 2008;29(7):219–227.
3. Frias JL, Davenport ML. American Academy of Pediatrics clinical report on health supervision for children with Turner syndrome. *Pediatrics.* 2003;111(3):692–702.
4. Kobrynski LJ, Sullivan KE. Velocardiofacial syndrome, DiGeorge syndrome: the chromosome 2211.2 deletion syndrome. *Lancet.* 2007;370:1443–1452.
5. Oley CA. Charge syndrome. In: Cassidy SB, Allanson JE, eds. *Management of Genetic Syndromes.* 3rd ed. Hoboken, NJ: Wiley-Blackwell; 2010:157–168.
6. Solomon BD. VACTERL/VATER association. *Orphanet J Rare Dis.* 2010;6:56.
7. Alter B, Kupfer G. Fanconi anemia. In: *GeneReviews.* 2011. http://www.genetests.org.
8. Kohlhase J. Townes-Brocks syndrome. In: *GeneReviews.* 2007. http://www.genetests.org.
9. Lalani SR, Hefner MA, Belmont JW, Davenport SLH. CHARGE syndrome. In: *GeneReviews.* 2009. http://www.genetests.org.
10. McDonald-McGinn DM, Emanuel BS, Zackai EH. 22q11.2 deletion syndrome. In: *GeneReviews.* 2005. http://www.genetests.org.

Part J: Immune System

Neonatal Neutropenia

Christopher H. Hsu and Michael R. Jeng

INTRODUCTION: NEUTROPENIA

The neutrophil is a myeloid-derived white blood cell important in combating bacterial and fungal infections. For a more detailed discussion of neutrophil development and immunologic function, refer to chapters 49 and 51. Most neutrophil abnormalities in the neonate involve quantitative disorders of the neutrophil, with the vast majority of clinical issues involving decreased neutrophil counts or neutropenia. Neutropenia is defined as an absolute neutrophil count (ANC) less than 1500/mm³. In a newborn, there can be many causes, some acquired with expected resolution, such as increased utilization of neutrophils with low marrow reserve or failures of production or release from the bone marrow, or there can be congenital causes, which are expected to be lifelong. The patient may have different clinical presentations depending on the etiology. Because of the low neutrophil reserve (capacity to produce neutrophils) in the bone marrow, the neonate is especially prone to development of neutropenia. Differentiating the etiology of neutropenia in an infant is therefore dependent on thorough knowledge of the maternal (both pregnancy and delivery) and neonatal history, as well as the physical examination of the infant, in conjunction with appropriate laboratory tests.

INITIAL CLINICAL APPROACH

Because the severity and the cause of neutropenia may often be fatal in this patient population and because of the limitations of blood volume available for laboratory testing, a prompt but logical approach to the workup is essential. A thorough history can indicate if immediate assessment is necessary. Information, such as appropriate prenatal care, maternal medications, difficulties during pregnancy, fetal vital signs, complications during delivery, and Apgar scores should be included in the initial assessment. The past medical histories of parents and family members, in particular infections, early childhood deaths, or specific diagnoses, may suggest a congenital cause of neutropenia. In addition to assessment of the infant for possible sepsis, particular attention should be made to specific physical findings related to the different causes of neutropenia, such as splenomegaly, skin lesions, and physical anomalies. For example, infants with neonatal lupus may have neutropenia but often will have a rash and splenomegaly. Patients with congenital bone marrow failure syndromes may exhibit abnormal thumbs, be small for gestational age or have a low birth weight, or exhibit a classical facies/congenital abnormalities. Thus, the family history and the appearance of the infant, toxic vs nontoxic, will help narrow the differential diagnosis and thus guide the diagnostic tests and management.

Initial baseline diagnostic tests recommended include a complete blood cell count (CBC) with differential, calculation of the ANC (see Figure 110-1), chemistry, blood cultures, and chest x-ray. Abnormalities detected during physical examination, such as skeletal anomalies and enlarged spleen, warrant further imaging. If the degree of acuity has been thoroughly considered, management may occur depending on the differential diagnosis.

$$\text{ANC (cells/mm}^3) = (S + B) \times \text{wbc (cells/mm}^3)$$

FIGURE 110-1

Sepsis

In general, a newborn who is neutropenic should be always assessed and empirically treated for sepsis. A nontoxic infant with normal vital signs and physical examination, however, does not exclude the diagnosis of sepsis. Thus, all neutropenic patients should be considered septic initially.

Toxic Infants

For ill-appearing infants, a full course of antibiotics and workup for fever in the neonate should be performed (see chapters 51 and 52). Granulocyte colony-stimulating factor (G-CSF), a hormone involved in neutrophil development, may be given to boost the neutrophil count if clinically indicated. With appropriate management, the neutropenia should improve over time if caused by infection. If the clinical situation improves and the neutropenia persists, then further workup is indicated. Initially, it is often impossible to determine if a patient who presents with sepsis and neutropenia developed the infection as a result of neutropenia or if the neutropenia is caused by the sepsis. Thus, treatment and observation of the ANC are required. There is no consensus regarding the period of observation. Because newborns have a low neutrophil reserve, the period of neutropenia recovery after an infection may be longer than in older patients. We suggest beginning a workup if there is no resolution after a 3- to 4-week period.

Nontoxic Infants

If the infant is nontoxic appearing, after a short period of empiric antibiotics and the infant is deemed nonseptic, then consideration of other causes of neutropenia should be considered. It is appropriate to repeat the CBC with differential to confirm persistence of neutropenia and to document the ANC trend. It is not unusual for neutrophil count to decrease in the second or third week of life when lymphocyte maturation predominates.[1] In addition, 50% of premature infants with birth weights less than 2 kg possess ANC below 1500 at birth, and pregnancies complicated by preeclampsia are at risk for neutropenic newborns.[2,3] The neutrophil count gradually normalizes in the majority of premature patients. Ethnicity is another factor to consider. Individuals of African and Jewish decent tend to have lower neutrophil counts at birth.[4] For example, the ANC of Africa American children on average[5] is between 1000 and 1400.

PERSISTENT NEUTROPENIA

If the neutropenia persists or if the neutrophil count is severe (less than 500), then a workup is indicated. The differential diagnosis can be divided into acquired and congenital causes. Reviewing the maternal and family history and determining if previous children or the mother developed neutropenia during pregnancy are initially important, as they may help to suggest an etiology. For example, if there is any suggestion of premature rupture of membranes or maternal fevers, this history may suggest an infectious cause. A maternal history of autoimmune neutropenia, or autoimmune disease, may suggest an alloimmune process in the infant. Finally, if a known family history of chronic neutropenia or severe recurrent infections is obtained, especially if the affected members are children, this may suggest a genetic etiology. Thus, a special effort to take a careful and relevant history should be made.

Acquired Neutropenia

Infections

Infection should always be first on the differential of a neonate with persistent neutropenia. More specifically, congenital infections (namely, toxoplasmosis, rubella, cytomegalovirus, herpes simplex virus, as well as syphilis, hepatitis B, and human immunodeficiency virus [HIV]) should be considered. To our knowledge, there are no published data indicating a particular organism is more commonly associated with isolated neutropenia. Thus, the more likely scenario is neutropenia preceding an infection; however, it is often difficult to discern whether neutropenia led to the infection or is the result of a response to an infection because of low reserves in the neonate. Nonetheless, the patient should be broadly protected with antibiotics based on the patient's level of neutropenia and the institution's guidelines until an infection is empirically treated.

Neonatal Isoimmune/Alloimmune Neutropenia

Neonatal isoimmune/alloimmune neutropenia (NAIN) is an acquired cause of isolated neutropenia and is unique to the neonate. NAIN is a rare condition mediated by transplacental maternal immunoglobulin (Ig) G granulocyte-specific antibodies developed against paternally inherited fetal neutrophil antigens.[6,7] This may also occur if the mother carries the diagnosis of autoimmune neutropenia, in which the mother's autoantibodies cross the placenta. The clinical picture for both of these processes is similar. The incidence of NAIN is approximately less than 1% of all births, and the clinical features of NAIN are varied, mostly presenting incidentally without symptoms or as isolated skin infections. Only on rare occasions this may be associated with life-threatening sepsis.[8]

Diagnosis requires demonstration of antineutrophil antibodies found in 50% of presumed cases.[6] Prophylactic antibiotics are not recommended. *Staphylococcus aureus*, *β-hemolytic streptococci*, or *Escherichia coli* are the infections most often encountered in these infants, presenting as omphalitis, skin infections, or fetomaternal infections.[7] G-CSF is the first-line treatment of NAIN with the goal of increasing ANC to greater than 500/mm³. This condition typically lasts between the first and third month of life but can last up to 6 months.[8] If NAIN is found in an infant, documentation of its occurrence in the mother's pregnancy records should be completed as subsequent pregnancies are also at risk.

Neonatal Lupus

Neonatal lupus is a rare autoimmune disease with a wide array of presentations, from isolated neutropenia to severely affected infants, with symptoms such as cutaneous skin rash, cardiomyopathy, hepatobiliary disease, and pancytopenia.[9] The facial rash may or may not be present at birth but will usually appear at a few days or weeks of life before spontaneous resolution.[10] Although thrombocytopenia or anemia is more commonly observed, isolated neutropenia has been reported.[11,12] The standard for diagnosis is the immunodiffusion assay for antibodies Ro, La, and U_1RNP.[9] Ro/La autoantibodies, which are produced by the mother, cross the placenta and thus affect the infants as an alloimmunization.[12] Systemic steroids are the mainstay of treatment of this condition. As the alloantibodies are cleared from their system, the infants should improve over time. However, these neonates are at increased risk of other autoimmune diseases later in life, such as rheumatoid arthritis, Hashimoto thyroiditis, and type 1 diabetes mellitus.[9]

Congenital Neutropenia

Severe Congenital Neutropenia

Severe congenital neutropenia (SCN) (see Table 110-1) is a heterogeneous disease; neonates present with ANC less than 500 and are at increased risk of life-threatening infections in the first 6 months of life. The most common infections affect lungs, skin, and deep tissue with an absence of pus.[13] Broad-spectrum antibiotics are indicated in these neonates. Examination of the bone marrow exhibits promyelocytic/myeloid stage arrest.[14] It occurs as both a sporadic and autosomal dominant disorder, with multiple genes identified, and confirmation of this condition is by detection of gene mutations, the most common being neutrophil elastase, encoded by the *ELA2* gene, a serine protease

Table 110-1 Common Causes of Congenital Neutropenia and Their Associated Genes

Disease/Syndrome	Gene
Severe congenital neutropenia	*ELA2, CSF3R, Gfl1*
Kostmann syndrome	*HAX1*
Cyclic neutropenia	*ELA2*
Schwachman-Diamond syndrome	*SBDS*
Glycogen storage disease Ib	*SLC37A4*

produced at the promyelocytic stage and stored in primary granules of mature neutrophils.[8,15,16] Over 50 different mutations have been identified in the *ELA2* gene of SCN and patients with cyclic neutropenia (CN) (see the following discussion of CN), and all have been monoallelic. The pathogenesis of *ELA2*-mediated neutropenia is believed to occur through an inadequate cellular response to unfolded proteins leading to activation of proaptotic genes and apoptosis.[14,15]

Another cause of SCN has been identified in *CSF3R*, which codes for the G-CSF receptor important in the proliferation, differentiation, activation, and survival of mature neutrophils and neutrophil precursors.[17] These patients appear to have an increased risk of developing myelodysplastic syndrome (MDS) and acute myeloid leukemia (AML). Furthermore, a small subset of these patients has mutations in the external domain of the receptor, which confers resistance to G-CSF.[18]

Other genes identified as a cause of SCN in rare cases include the Wiskott-Aldrich syndrome (*WAS*) and *Gfl1* genes. *WAS* normally encodes a regulatory protein for actin polymerization important in cellular locomotion and receptor localization.[13] Mutations of this gene are inherited in an X-linked manner and are associated with increased apoptosis of myeloid progenitors. *Gfl1* encodes a zinc finger transcriptional repressor and is inherited in a sporadic fashion.[19]

The first-line treatment of SCN is the subcutaneous administration of G-CSF; however, despite the success of G-CSF in increasing the ANC, these patients may still be at risk of infections. Furthermore, 10% of patients are unresponsive to G-CSF.[15] Included among these patients are neonates with *CSF3R* mutations in the external domain. Patients unresponsive to G-CSF are often considered for hematopoietic stem cell transplantation (HSCT) as a future cure.

Kostmann Syndrome

Kostmann syndrome is a subset of SCN (see previous SCN discussion this chapter) representing 15% of patients with SCN.[13] The neutropenia is more severe in these individuals, often with ANC below 200.[20]

These neonates are therefore at high risk for infections, and broad antibiotic coverage is indicated. The clinical presentation may range from isolated severe neutropenia to epilepsy and developmental delay. The bone marrow, like in SCN, will reflect maturation arrest at the promyelocytic stage. Detection of the gene mutation confirms the diagnosis. Unlike the other SCN mutations, Kostmann syndrome is autosomal recessive, with mutations in *HAX1* that normally code for a mitochondrial membrane protein.[21] Mutations increase apoptosis of neutrophils. G-CSF is the first-line treatment, although many of these patients with Kostmann syndrome are unresponsive; HSCT is an option for them.

Cyclic Neutropenia

Suspicion for CN may present in a child less than 1 year of age, although most commonly it is diagnosed later in life. CN presents with recurrent fever about every 3 weeks or recurrent episodes of pharyngitis, gingivitis, mouth ulcers, lymphadenopathy, or cellulitis.[22] Acute peritonitis manifesting as ileus or septic shock has also been reported but is rare.[22] Mortality also is a rare occurrence. Typically, the neutrophil count in CN oscillates with 21-day periodicity, with the ANC nadir reaching 200/mm^3 for 3 to 5 days and then increasing to below 2000/mm^3 until the next neutropenic period.[22,23] Diagnosis can be made by serial ANC measurements over several weeks, or by *ELA2* gene analysis.

Like some types of SCN (see previous SCN discussion), CN is autosomal dominant, with mutations localized to *ELA2* but in different exons compared to SCN.[16] Over 90% of patients with CN can have the diagnosis confirmed with mutation analysis of *ELA2*. These infants develop normally and do not have increased risk for malignancy; however, oral ulcers and dental hygiene difficulties appear to be recurrent problems. G-CSF is the first-line treatment; it improves symptoms by increasing the amplitude of the neutrophil oscillations as well as shortening the duration of the periodicity.[22] The recurrence of fevers and ulcers is also reduced with treatment. Generally, patients are treated only for symptomatic relief, and unlike patients with Kostmann syndrome, all patients with CN respond to G-CSF.

Schwachman-Diamond Syndrome

Schwachman-Diamond syndrome (SDS) is an autosomal recessive condition presenting in infants as a combination of skeletal abnormalities, exocrine pancreatic dysfunction, and bone marrow dysfunction, which often begins as neutropenia but eventually progresses to bone marrow failure in all cell lineages.[24] The defect is found in the Schwachman-Bodian-Diamond syndrome (*SBDS*) gene, which is involved in regulation of ribosomal RNA.[25] These neonates are also at increased risk of developing MDS or AML. Initial treatment requires replacement of the pancreatic enzymes and G-CSF if the patient is neutropenic with active infection. It should be noted that patients with SDS may have waxing and waning neutrophil counts; ultimately, patients who fail treatment or progress to bone marrow failure are candidates for HSCT.

Glycogen Storage Disease Ib

Glycogen storage disease Ib is an autosomal recessive disorder associated with intermittent neutropenia, defects in neutrophil respiratory burst chemotaxis, calcium flux, and hepatomegaly.[24,26] The genetic defect occurs in the glucose 6-phosphatase translocase (*SLC37A4*) enzyme, and patients are dependent on dietary carbohydrates to maintain euglycemia. Otherwise, they progress to hypoglycemia and lactic acidosis, which may lead to coma or seizures.[27] Neutrophils also undergo apoptosis as a result of the genetic defect. These patients are susceptible to recurrent infections of the skin, perirectal areas, and urinary tracts.[27] The treatment of this condition is G-CSF, especially if persistent infections, severe neutropenia, and gastrointestinal symptoms are problematic; however, patients should be monitored for splenomegaly, which has been noted as a side effect among these patients receiving G-CSF.[27]

REFERENCES

1. Kyono W, Coates TD. A practical approach to neutrophil disorders. *Pediatr Clin North Am.* 2002;49(5):929–971, viii.
2. Handin RI, Lux SE, Stossel TP. *Blood: Principles and Practice of Hematology.* 2nd ed. Philadelphia, PA: Lippincott Williams & Wilkins; 2003:xii.
3. Sharma G, et al. Maternal and neonatal characteristics associated with neonatal neutropenia in hypertensive pregnancies. *Am J Perinatol.* 2009;26(9):683–689.
4. Haddy TB, Rana SR, Castro O. Benign ethnic neutropenia: what is a normal absolute neutrophil count? *J Lab Clin Med.* 1999;133(1):15–22.
5. Caramihai E, et al. Leukocyte count differences in healthy white and black children 1 to 5 years of age. *J Pediatr.* 1975;86(2): 252–254.
6. Gramatges MM, et al. Neonatal alloimmune thrombocytopenia and neutropenia associated with maternal human leukocyte antigen antibodies. *Pediatr Blood Cancer.* 2009;53(1):97–99.
7. Desenfants A, et al. Intravenous immunoglobulins for neonatal alloimmune neutropenia refractory to recombinant human granulocyte colony-stimulating factor. *Am J Perinatol.* 2011;28(6): 461–466.
8. Wiedl C, Walter AW. Granulocyte colony stimulating factor in neonatal alloimmune neutropenia: a possible association with induced thrombocytopenia. *Pediatr Blood Cancer.* 2010;54(7): 1014–1016.

9. Lee LA. Neonatal lupus: clinical features and management. *Paediatr Drugs*. 2004;6(2):71–78.

10. Weston WL, Morelli JG, Lee LA. The clinical spectrum of anti-Ro-positive cutaneous neonatal lupus erythematosus. *J Am Acad Dermatol*. 1999;40(5 Pt 1):675–681.

11. Kanagasegar S, et al. Neonatal lupus manifests as isolated neutropenia and mildly abnormal liver functions. *J Rheumatol*. 2002;29(1):187–191.

12. Neiman AR, et al. Cutaneous manifestations of neonatal lupus without heart block: characteristics of mothers and children enrolled in a national registry. *J Pediatr*. 2000;137(5):674–680.

13. Boztug K, Klein C. Genetic etiologies of severe congenital neutropenia. *Curr Opin Pediatr*. 2011;23(1):21–26.

14. Berliner N. Lessons from congenital neutropenia: 50 years of progress in understanding myelopoiesis. *Blood*. 2008;111(12):5427–5432.

15. Ward AC, Dale DC. Genetic and molecular diagnosis of severe congenital neutropenia. *Curr Opin Hematol*. 2009;16(1):9–13.

16. Horwitz M, et al. Mutations in ELA2, encoding neutrophil elastase, define a 21-day biological clock in cyclic haematopoiesis. *Nat Genet*. 1999;23(4):433–436.

17. Germeshausen M, Ballmaier M, Welte K. Incidence of CSF3R mutations in severe congenital neutropenia and relevance for leukemogenesis: results of a long-term survey. *Blood*. 2007;109(1):93–99.

18. Sinha S, et al. Deletional mutation of the external domain of the human granulocyte colony-stimulating factor receptor in a patient with severe chronic neutropenia refractory to granulocyte colony-stimulating factor. *J Pediatr Hematol Oncol*. 2003;25(10):791–796.

19. Hock H, Orkin SH. Zinc-finger transcription factor Gfi-1: versatile regulator of lymphocytes, neutrophils and hematopoietic stem cells. *Curr Opin Hematol*. 2006;13(1):1–6.

20. Carlsson G, et al. Kostmann syndrome or infantile genetic agranulocytosis, part two: understanding the underlying genetic defects in severe congenital neutropenia. *Acta Paediatr*. 2007;96(6):813–819.

21. Klein C, et al. HAX1 deficiency causes autosomal recessive severe congenital neutropenia (Kostmann disease). *Nat Genet*. 2007;39(1):86–92.

22. Dale DC, Bolyard AA, Aprikyan A. Cyclic neutropenia. *Semin Hematol*. 2002;39(2):89–94.

23. Dale DC, et al. Mutations in the gene encoding neutrophil elastase in congenital and cyclic neutropenia. *Blood*. 2000;96(7):2317–2322.

24. Rivers A, Slayton WB. Congenital cytopenias and bone marrow failure syndromes. *Semin Perinatol*. 2009;33(1):20–28.

25. Ganapathi KA, et al. The human Shwachman-Diamond syndrome protein, SBDS, associates with ribosomal RNA. *Blood*. 2007;110(5):1458–1465.

26. Kannourakis G. Glycogen storage disease. *Semin Hematol*. 2002;39(2):103–106.

27. Calderwood S, et al. Recombinant human granulocyte colony-stimulating factor therapy for patients with neutropenia and/or neutrophil dysfunction secondary to glycogen storage disease type 1b. *Blood*. 2001;97(2):376–382.

Severe Combined Immunodeficiency (SCID)

Jennifer Jenks and Kari Nadeau

BACKGROUND

Severe combined immunodeficiency (SCID) is a fatal primary immune condition characterized by the absence of both humoral and cellular immunity with severe lymphopenia. Patients with SCID have reduced numbers and function of both T and B lymphocytes (and in some cases, natural killer [NK] cells) and hypogammaglobulinemia. If left untreated, babies with SCID most often die within 1 to 2 years of life because of severe, recurrent infections.

Since SCID was initially described over 50 years ago, 15 specific genetic mutations that contribute to disease development have been identified. The most common type is X-linked SCID (SCID-X1), which accounts for approximately 46% of cases in the United States (Figure 111-1). SCID can also be inherited as an autosomal recessive disease that results from deficiencies in adenosine deaminase (ADA), Janus kinase 3 (*JAK3*), interleukin 7 receptor α chain (*IL7R*), recombination activating genes (*RAG1* or *RAG2*), Artemis gene, CD45, and others (Table 111-1).

PATHOPHYSIOLOGY

X-Linked Recessive SCID

The most prevalent form of SCID, SCID-X1, is characterized by the absence of T and NK lymphocytes and by nonfunctional B lymphocytes. Its defect is mapped to the Xq13 region, and the faulty gene is identified as *IL2RG*, which encodes the γc chain shared by 6 cytokine receptors that are critical for maintaining immune homeostasis: interleukins (ILs) 2, 4, 7, 9, 15, and 21.

Although SCID-X1 patients lack T- and B-cell function and have low numbers of T or NK cells, they produce normal or elevated numbers of B cells. These B cells are inherently nonfunctional because they fail to produce immunoglobulin even after bone marrow transplantation and restoration of T-cell function. Similarly, NK cells that are present have low-to-absent cell function, and after bone marrow transplantation in patients with SCID-X1, NK-cell generation fails to persist.

Autosomal Recessive SCID Caused by Adenosine Deaminase Deficiency

About half of those affected with autosomal recessive SCID have ADA deficiency, found in about 16% of the total SCID population.[1] ADA deficiency was the first identified molecular cause of SCID and involves mutation or deletion of the gene encoding ADA on chromosome 20q13-ter. Because accumulation of ADA substrates or metabolites is toxic to T, B, and NK cells, infants with ADA deficiency have more profound lymphopenia than patients with other types of SCID, with mean absolute lymphocyte counts of less than $500/mm^3$. A unique symptom to patients with ADA SCID includes multiple skeletal abnormalities of chondro-osseous dysplasia, which occur primarily at the costochondral junctions.

In addition to general SCID treatment and bone marrow transplantation, ADA-deficient patients may undergo enzyme replacement therapy with polyethylene

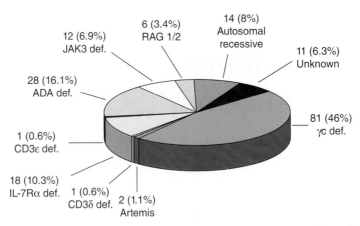

FIGURE 111-1 The relative frequencies of particular genetic mutations were evaluated in 174 consecutive cases of human severe combined immunodeficiency (SCID) evaluated at Duke University over 30 years. The most common type is X-linked SCID, which disables common gamma (γc) signaling. ADA, adenosine deaminase; *JAK3*, Janus kinase 3; *IL7R*, interleukin 7 receptor α chain; *RAG1* or *RAG2*, recombination activating genes 1 or 2. (Reproduced with permission from Buckley.[1])

glycol-modified bovine ADA (PEG-ADA). Although this treatment has achieved success in restoring immunocompetence, bone marrow transplantation is still more effective. Therefore, if bone marrow transplantation is being considered, PEG-AGA therapy should not be initiated because it will enable the patient to produce a graft-vs-host response.

Autosomal Recessive SCID Caused by Janus Kinase 3 Deficiency

Mutations in the γ-chain/JAK3 signaling pathway produce symptoms and lymphopenia similar to those in SCID-X1 patients. JAK3 enables T-cell maturation and differentiation, and the common γ chain is also a receptor of IL-15, a key growth factor for NK cells. Consequently, patients with JAK3 deficiency are depleted of T and NK cells. Antibody production by B cells is still severely impaired because of lack of T-cell interaction.

Furthermore, because mutations in JAK3 abrogate signaling through the same cytokine receptors affected by IL2RG mutations, even after successful bone marrow transplantation and correction of T-cell function, JAK3-deficient SCID infants often fail to develop normal B-cell function, much like SCID-X1 patients. Similarly, production of NK cells after transplantation is impaired.

Autosomal Recessive SCID Caused by Interleukin 7 Receptor α-Chain Deficiency

The third most common autosomal recessive form of SCID is IL7R deficiency. Patients with mutations in IL7R lack B- and T-cell function, although they maintain normal NK-cell function. Absence of the α chain of the IL-7 receptor prevents JAK3 from moderating T-cell

proliferation and differentiation, as in JAK3-deficient SCID patients. However, because the γc pathway is preserved, NK-cell development is unaffected.

Autosomal Recessive SCID Caused by Recombinase-Activating Gene Deficiencies

One form of SCID results from mutations or deletions in *RAG1* or *RAG2*. This condition is also known as Swiss-type agammaglobulinemia because it was originally described in Swiss infants who suffered from fatal infections associated with severe lymphopenia. In this form of SCID, infants are deficient in RAG1 and RAG2 proteins, which are necessary to initiate V(D)J recombination in T and B lymphocytes. Thus, T and B cells are absent, but NK populations and function are normal, as are nonlymphoid hematopoietic cell lineages.

Omenn Syndrome

A type of SCID involving mutations in *RAG1* or *RAG2* genes, Omenn syndrome is characterized by the development shortly after birth of erythroderma and desquamation, diarrhea, hepatosplenomegaly, and hypereosinophilia. Patients also exhibit elevated serum immunoglobulin E (IgE) levels caused by circulating, activated, and antigen-stimulated T helper 2 (Th2) cells that produce cytokines mediating eosinophilia and elevated IgE levels.

DIAGNOSIS

During their first weeks of life, babies are protected by their mothers' antibodies. Consequently, most neonates with SCID do not exhibit symptoms of lymphopenia and appear healthy at birth and for several weeks. Given a

Table 111-1 Classification of Severe Combined Immunodeficiency (SCID)

Lymphocyte Profile						
T Cells	B Cells	Natural Killer (NK) Cells	Disease	Genetic Mutation	Inheritance	Chromosome Band
–	–	–	Adenosine deaminase deficiency	Adenosine deaminase (*ADA*)	AR	20q13.2-q13.11
–	–	–	Reticular digenesis	*AK2*	AR	1q35
–	–	+	Artemis gene deficiency	Artemis gene (*DCLRE1C*)	AR	10p13
–	–	+	Omenn syndrome	*RAG1 or RAG2*	AR	11p13.41
–	–	+	DNA protein kinase catalytic subunit (DNA-PKcs)	*PRKDC*	AR	8q11
–	+	–	X-linked SCID	Common γ chain receptor (*IL-2Rγ*)	XL	Xq13.1
–	+	–	JAK3 deficiency	*JAK3*	AR	19q13.1
–	+	+	Interleukin (IL) 7 α-chain receptor deficiency	Interleukin (IL) 7 α-chain receptor (CD127)	AR	5p13
–	+	+	CD3 deficiency	CD3δ, CD3ε, or CD Z	AR	11q23
–	+	+	Actin-regulating protein coronin 1A (CORO1A) deficiency	*CORO1A*	AR	16p11
CD45⁻	+	+	CD45 deficiency	CD45 tyrosine phosphatase (*PTPRC*)	AR	1q31
CD4⁺	+	+	ZAP70 kinase deficiency	*ZAP70* tyrosine kinase	AR	2q12
CD8⁺	+	+	p56lck deficiency	p56lck	AR	1p35
CD8⁺	B⁺DR	+	Major histocompatibility complex (MHC) II deficiency	*RFXAP*	AR	13q13.3
				CIITA	AR	16p13
				RFXANK	AR	19p13
				RFX5	AR	1q21

Abbreviations: AR, autosomal recessive; XL, X linked.
Numerous genetic mutations contributing to X-linked and autosomal recessive SCID have been identified in humans. They have differential effects on T-, B-, and NK-cell populations and functions.

patient's medical history, physicians who want to examine a neonate for SCID should assess blood absolute lymphocyte counts through lymphocyte cell surface staining and enumeration by flow cytometry and lymphocyte functional tests. The normal range for the cord blood absolute lymphocyte count is 2000 to 11,000/mm³. For neonates with values below 2500/mm³, physicians should arrange for further T-cell phenotypic and functional studies.

Unfortunately, most cases of SCID are not diagnosed until 6 to 7 months of age, when patients start to present with recurrent infections and failure to thrive. At this age, the normal absolute lymphocyte count is much higher, with a mean of 7500/mm³ and a lower limit of normal 4000/mm³. Serum immunoglobulin concentrations are very low to absent, and on immunization, no specific antibody formation occurs. A chest radiograph or ultrasound also reveals that the thymus is often undetected or very small (less than 1 g) and lacks lymphocytes and Hassall corpuscles. The thymus often fails to descend from the neck and lacks corticomedullary distinction. Lymph nodes, spleen, tonsils, adenoids, Peyer patches, and other peripheral lymphoid tissues may also be atrophied and depleted of lymphocytes. However, thymic epithelium is normal, and these tiny thymuses support the maturation of stem cells into normal T cells.

New methods to assess SCID in the prenatal environment and in newborns are under way. Sequencing fetal DNA is a viable but highly cost-inhibitive tool, and because SCID is rare, occurring in 1 of 100,000 births in the United States, prenatal testing of a baby without family history is typically unwarranted. On the other hand, several US states are performing pilot studies to diagnose SCID in newborns through the use of T-cell receptor excision circles (TRECs). Despite these pilot programs, standard testing for SCID is not currently available in newborns because of the diversity of the genetic defects.

DISEASE PHENOTYPE AND COMPLICATIONS

While failure to thrive may be an initial presenting symptom of SCID, repeated severe infections by bacteria, disseminated viruses, fungi, protozoa, and live vaccines (live, attenuated organisms) are the most life-threatening symptoms of SCID and warrant immediate care. In particular, candidal bacterial infections of the oropharynx, esophagus, and skin are common early manifestations. Infections with rotavirus can be persistent and may spread to extraintestinal sites. Respiratory synctial virus infections commonly result in T-cell pneumonia. Varicella, herpes, measles, and adenoviruses can result in progressive, ultimately fatal, infections. Furthermore, patients are susceptible to typically innocuous opportunistic infections, such as *Pneumocystis carinii* or cytomegalovirus, which can lead to chronic, progressive pneumonitis. Patients with SCID should never be vaccinated with live viral vaccines, including that of measles or the mycobacterium bacillus Calmette-Guerin (BCG), as they are almost always fatal.

Other symptoms include chronic diarrhea, otitis, sepsis, cutaneous infections, and slow growth.

THERAPY AND PROGNOSIS

Conventional care for patients with SCID involves avoidance of infection and meticulous skin and mucosal hygienic care. Doctors should beware of signs of sepsis and pulmonary infections, and any sign of fever requires a detailed search for infectious agents. To boost patient immunity, empiric broad-spectrum antibiotics and immunoglobulin infusions may be used, especially prophylactic treatment with antiviral agents against *Pneumocystis*. Intravenous immunoglobulin (IVIG) replacement may also be an ancillary treatment. However, none of these treatments is curative, and to resolve SCID, patients will need to undergo bone marrow transplantation before 1 or 2 years of age.

Bone Marrow Transplantation

Currently, the only definitive treatment of SCID is bone marrow transplantation. Even IVIG to restore humoral immunity fails to halt worsening disease progression. Without bone marrow transplantation from an HLA-identical or haploidentical donor (usually a relative), death usually occurs before the patient's first birthday and almost invariably before the second. On the other hand,[2] transplantation in the first 3.5 months of life increases survival of patients with SCID to over 97%. Therefore, early diagnosis is essential to restoring cell numbers and function. Recent studies suggested that the thymic education of the transplanted allogeneic stem cells is most effective in very young infants. Thymic output appears to occur sooner and to a greater degree in infants transplanted in the neonatal period than in those transplanted after that time. Currently, more than 400 patients with SCID survive worldwide as a result of successful bone marrow transplantation.[3]

Viral-Mediated Gene Therapy

More recently, gene therapy has been attempted as an alternative to bone marrow transplantation. In 1990, viral-mediated transduction of the missing gene to hematopoietic stem cells was first tested in ADA SCID. Most of these trials were unsuccessful. However, in 1999, retroviral gene transfer was used to successfully transduce γc complementary DNA (cDNA) into the autologous marrow cells of 10 infants with SCID-X1. This therapy fully corrected their T- and NK-cell defects, enabling patients with SCID to develop functional immune systems.

Unfortunately, these trials ended abruptly 3 years later when it was discovered that 3 of 9 patients in a trial had developed a leukemic-like process. These patients exhibited insertial oncogenesis in which the γc cDNA integrated into the infants' DNA in the LMO2 (LIM domain only 2 [rhombotin-like 1]) proto-oncogene promoter. Aberrant transcription and expression of LMO2 triggered deregulated premalignant cell proliferation with unexpected frequency. As of 2010, 4 of the 9 patients had developed leukemias, including 1 death.[4] Work is now focusing on correcting the gene without triggering an oncogene. Trials of gene therapy for ADA SCID appear promising and have not resulted in any cases of leukemia, perhaps because ADA SCID does not involve the γc gene, which may be oncogenic when expressed by a retrovirus.

Gene therapy still holds much promise for the treatment of SCID and other genetically determined immunodeficiency diseases for which the molecular bases are known. Since 1999, gene therapy has restored the immune systems of at least 17 children with ADA SCID and SCID-X1.[5]

REFERENCES

1. Buckley JH. The multiple causes of human SCID. *J Clin Invest.* 2004;114(10):1409–1411.
2. Brown L, Xu-Bayford J, Allwood Z, et al. Neonatal diagnosis of severe combined immunodeficiency leads to significantly improved survival outcome: the case for newborn screening. *Blood.* 2011;117(11):3243–3246.
3. Antoine C, Müller S, Cant A, et al. Long-term survival and transplantation of haemopoietic stem cells for immunodeficiencies: report of the European experience 1968–99. *Lancet.* 2003;361(9357):553–560.
4. Hacein-Bey-Abina S, Hauer J, Lim A, et al. Efficacy of gene therapy for X-linked severe combined immunodeficiency. *N Engl J Med.* 2010;363(4):355–364.
5. Buckley RH. Combined immunodeficiency diseases. In: McMillan JA, Feigin RD, DeAngelis C, Jones MD, eds. *Oski's Pediatrics: Principles and Practice.* 4th ed. Philadelphia, PA: Lippincott Williams & Wilkins; 2006:2469–2475

T-Cell Dysfunction

Amanda Jacobson and Kari Nadeau

NEONATAL T-CELL FUNCTION

T cells are major effector cells of the adaptive immune response from influencing antibody production to maintaining tolerance. The defining marker of the T cell is the T-cell receptor (TCR), and 2 distinct T-cell subsets have been characterized based on the structure of the TCR: TCRα/β and TCR$\gamma\delta$. The specificity of the TCRα/β T-cell repertoire is established during fetal development of the thymus, which develops at week 6 of gestation. Immature thymic cells develop from fetal liver cells and, after birth, from hematopoetic stem cells (HSCS) in the bone marrow. T cells develop from common lymphoid progenitor cells derived from HSCs within the thymus and undergo stages of differentiation, expressing 1 or both of the cytodifferentiation (CD) antigens CD4 and CD8. T cells expressing the α/β TCR are divided into various subsets based on surface CD antigens and function. CD4$^+$ T cells, or helper T cells (T$_H$), make up approximately 70% of T cells in the peripheral blood. T$_H$ cells recognize foreign antigens processed and presented in major histocompatibility complex (MHC) class II molecules and can be divided into additional subsets. T$_H$1 CD4$^+$ T cells produce interferon gamma (IFN-γ) and IL-2, favor antibody class switching to immunoglobulin (Ig) G2, and mediate protection against intracellular pathogens. T$_H$2 CD4$^+$ T cells produce IL-4, IL-13, and IL-5, favor class switching to IgG1 and IgE, and participate in atopic diseases and immunity against parasites. More recently, additional subsets of CD4$^+$ T cells have been described that have effector functions against extracellular microbes: T$_H$9 cells produce the anti-inflammatory cytokine IL-10 and are involved in the host defense against nematodes, whereas T$_H$17 cells secrete IL-17, IL-21, and IL-22 and promote protective immunity against extracellular bacteria and fungi at mucosal surfaces. CD8$^+$ cytotoxic T lymphocytes (CTLs) recognize endogenous proteins bound to MHC class I molecules, such as viral and tumor antigens, and mediate cytotoxicity by lysing altered or nonself cells. A third class of T cells (typically CD4$^+$) with immune suppressive function are denoted as regulatory T cells (T$_{reg}$) and can be identified (albeit with some exception) by the expression of the transcription facto FOXP3 (forkhead box P3). T$_{reg}$ cells are produced directly from the thymus (natural T$_{reg}$) or induced within the periphery (induced T$_{reg}$) and play major roles in mediating chronic inflammation, allergic disease, and autoimmunity.[1]

T-cell dysfunction in neonates has implications for a variety of responses and disease states. Infants are more susceptible to infectious agents, and according to the World Health Organization (WHO) estimates, approximately 2.5 million infants under the age of 1 die annually of infection. Infants are also less responsive to vaccination. In vaccinated infants, immunity wanes around 6–9 months after vaccination, and multiple booster shots are needed to maintain immunological memory.[2] Historically, the function of neonatal T cells has been considered impaired, mainly attributed to immaturity of the neonatal immune response. Neonatal antigen-presenting cells produce lower amounts of IL-12, required for IFN-γ responses. The overall bias of the neonatal immune response toward T$_H$2 leads to delayed production of proinflammatory

Table 112-1 Neonatal T-Cell Responses to Vaccines and Infectious Disease

Infectious Agent	T-Cell Responses[a]	
Bordetella pertussis	T_H1 response	
Human cytomegalovirus	Mature CD8 T-cell response, defective CD4 T-cell response	
Human immunodeficiency virus	Mature CD8 T-cell response, defective CD4 T-cell response	
Herpes simplex virus 1 and 2	Delayed IFN-γ and TNF-α response, defective CD4+ T-cell response	
Trypanosma cruzi	Mature CD8 T-cell response, defective CD4+ T-cell response	
Vaccine		Doses Given < 12 Months of Age[b]
Hepatitis B	Predominantly T_H2 response, decreased IFN-γ response	3
Measles, mumps, rubella	Low T_H1 response	1 (≥ 12 months)
Mycobacterium bovis BCG[c]	Mature T_H1 response	
Inactivated poliovirus	Low T_H1 response, decreased IFN-γ response	3
Diptheria, tetanus, pertussis	Mature T_H1 response by 2 months of age	3
Haemophilus influenza type b	Weak memory T-cell response	2–3
Pneumococcal	Low T_H1 response, decreased IFN-γ response	3

Abbreviations: IFN, interferon; TNF, tumor necrosis factor.
[a]As compared to adult.
[b]As recommended by the Center for Disease Control in 2010 (http://www.cdc.gov).
[c]Generally only recommended for use in areas with a high prevalence of tuberculosis.

cytokines and IL-2 and subsequent delayed effective CD8+ CTLs until several months after birth. The T_H2 dominance during early life also influences the class of IgG antibodies, leading to a predominance of IgG1 and IgG3 and low production of IgG2. However, in certain instances, such as BCG vaccination, a proper T_H1 response is mounted in neonates. Thus, baseline normal neonatal adaptive responses range from nonresponsiveness to adult-level T-cell responses (Table 112-1). Genetic defects in neonatal T-cell function tend to increase susceptibility of the already-vulnerable newborn to disease (Table 112-2). Because optimal B-cell function requires T-cell help, a T-cell defect typically results in a B-cell deficiency as well (considered combined immunodeficiencies, such as Wiskott-Alrich syndrome [WAS]). Newborns with primary immunodeficiencies most commonly present with increased cases of infection; however, diagnosing the disease with known characteristics prior to infection is the goal and will typically lead to a better outcome for the patient.

CONGENITAL T-CELL IMMUNODEFICIENCIES

DiGeorge Syndrome

DiGeorge syndrome,[3] or 22q11.2 deletion syndrome, is caused by the deletion affecting the long arm of chromosome 22. It is a genetic recessive immunodeficiency

(in rare cases autosomal dominant) usually inherited from the mother. DiGeorge syndrome has occurred in both males and females and has an estimated prevalence of 1:4000. Some cases of DiGeorge and velocardiofacial syndromes have defects in other chromosomes, notably a deletion in chromosome region 10p14. There is considerable variability in the phenotype, and severity is based on the extent of the microdeletion. Individuals with DiGeorge syndrome may suffer from congenital heart defects, palatal abnormalities, hypocalcemia caused by hypoparathyroidism, distinctive craniofacial features, renal anomalies, and thymic hyplasia.[4] Additional clinical findings associated with the disease and useful evaluations following diagnosis with DiGeorge/22q11.2 deletion syndrome are summarized in Table 112-3.

T-cell immunodeficiency in DiGeorge syndrome is attributed to failure of development of the thymus, and patients may be mildly to severely lymphopenic based on the degree of thymic deficiency. Laboratory evaluation typically reveals normal-to-decreased numbers of T lymphocytes with absent-to-normal T-cell function and normal B-cell function.[5] Serum immunoglobulin levels tend to be within normal limits. However, in the rare patient, B-lymphocyte function and antibody production may be abnormal as well. A defect in the delayed-type hypersensitivity is observed by the failure of affected patients to develop a positive skin test to candidin. Because of defects in cell-mediated immunity, patients are highly susceptible to opportunistic infections and to graft-vs-host disease (GVHD) from nonirradiated blood transfusions.

Table 112-2 Inherited T-Cell Immunodeficiencies and Disease

Syndrome/Disease	T-Cell Dysfunction	Chromosome	Altered Protein
ZAP70 deficiency	CD8 lymphocytopenia	2q12	ZAP70
DiGeorge syndrome	Absent T-cell function	22q11.2 10p13	TBX1 and other
Wiskott-Aldrich syndrome	Dysfunctional B- and T-cell iterations	Xp11.23	WASP
IPEX	Decreased regulatory T-cell function	Xp11.2-q13.3	FOXP3
Nezelof syndrome	Absent T-cell function	?	CD44?
NTED	Overactive TSST-1-specific T cells	?	?

Abbreviations: FOXP3, forkhead box P3; IPEX, immune dysregulation, polyendocrinopathy, enteropathy, X-linked; NTED, neonatal toxic shock syndrome-like exanthematous disease; TBX1, T-box 1; WASP, Wiskott-Aldrich syndrome protein; ZAP70, zeta-chain-associated protein.
aNot all cases are caused by genetic abnormalities.

Diagnosis of individuals with DiGeorge syndrome is confirmed for the microdeletion on chromosome 22 via fluorescence in situ hybridization (FISH) chromosomal analysis.[6] The 2 probes commercially available for 22q11.2 FISH analysis are TUPLE1 and N25. Fewer than 5% of individuals with clinical symptoms of the 22q11.2 deletion syndrome have normal routine cytogenetic studies and negative FISH testing.

Table 112-3 Clinical Characteristics and Diagnosis of DiGeorge/22q11.2 Deletion Syndrome

Common Clinical Features	DiGeorge Syndrome Work-up	Less-Frequent Clinical Features
Congenital heart disease	Echocardiogram	Severe dysphagia
Palatal abnormalities	Speech therapy	Growth hormone deficiency
Hypocalcemia	Calcium, phosphorus, PTH, creatinine	Autoimmune disease
Immune deficiency	Immunoglobulin levels, B and T cell subtypes	Neoplasms
Learning difficulties	Psychiatric and cognitive assessment	–
Characteristic facial features	–	–
Lymphopenia	CBC with differential	–
Renal anomalies	Ultrasound	–
Absence of Thymic gland	Chest x-ray to identify thoracic vertebral abnormalities	–

Fetuses at increased risk may be evaluated between 18 and 22 weeks' gestation by high-resolution ultrasound examination for palatal and other associated anomalies, by echocardiography for cardiac anomalies, or by chromosomal analysis of fetal cells obtained through amniocentesis.

Treatment of the 22q11.2 deletion/DiGeorge syndrome is based on the severity of the disease and may require surgery for cardiac defects and vitamin D, calcium, or parathyroid hormone replacement to correct hypocalcemia and treat seizures. Most infants have a mild-to-moderate deficit in T-cell function that often improves with age and do not suffer from recurrent infections in adulthood. For patients with the complete form of the syndrome with absent T-cell immunity (<0.2%), thymic grafts have been used successfully. Human leukocyte antigen (HLA)-identical bone marrow transplants have been successful at developing T-cell function in these patients, but this treatment cannot correct the thymic defect. Of note, prior to giving live vaccines, T-cell numbers and function should be assessed, if not done earlier, to prevent vaccine-related side effects.

Wiskott-Aldrich Syndrome

Wiskott-Aldrich syndrome is an X-linked recessive immunodeficiency disease caused by mutations in the gene that produces the Wiskott-Aldrich syndrome protein (WASP). Various mutations in the WASP gene have been identified in patients with WAS, each affected family typically carrying its own characteristic mutation. If the mutation interferes completely with the ability to produce the WASP, the patient has the classic and more severe form of WAS. Alternatively, if the mutation only results in lower production of WASP, a milder form of the disorder may result. WAS is characterized by defective interactions between B and T cells, resulting in decreased cell-mediated immunity. Patients with classic WAS present with thrombocytopenia, eczema, and recurrent infection. Common infections are typically caused by pneumococcal bacteria, resulting in pneumonia, meningitis, or sepsis, but may involve all classes of microorganisms. The initial clinical manifestations of WAS may be present soon after birth or develop in the first year of life, with prolonged bleeding from the circumcision site, bloody diarrhea, or excessive bruising. Survival to adulthood is rare; infection, vasculitis, and bleeding are major causes of death.

Diagnosis of WAS should be considered in any male presenting with unusual bleeding and bruises, congenital thrombocytopenia, and small platelets. Patients with WAS have alterations in the humoral response with increased IgA and IgE levels and diminished IgM levels. Patients usually have diminished antibody responses to polysaccharide antigens. Assessment of blood lymphocytes demonstrates a slight reduction of T-cell numbers and response to mitogens. Diagnosis of WAS is confirmed by demonstrating a decrease or absence of the WASP in blood cells or by the presence of a mutation within the WASP gene.

Because WAS is inherited as a X-linked disorder, only boys are affected, and there may be brothers or maternal uncles with similar findings. It is possible that the family history may be negative if the disease is caused by occurrence of a new mutation. Prenatal DNA diagnosis of WAS can be performed by amniocentesis or chronic villus sampling.

Treatment of WAS symptoms include iron supplementation for anemia, prophylactic administration of immunoglobulin replacement for bacterial infections, and steroid creams to control areas of chronic inflammation caused by eczema. HLA-identical sibling bone marrow transplantation (BMT) have been successful at correcting the platelet and immunologic abnormalities and is the treatment of choice for boys with significant clinical findings of WAS.[7] Matched unrelated donor transplantations have shown promise, especially if they are performed while the patient is under the age of 5 and prior to acquiring a severe viral infection or cancer. In some cases, cord blood stem cells have been successfully used for immune reconstitution and correction of platelet abnormalities.

Immune Dysregulation, Polyendocrinopathy, Enteropathy, X-Linked Syndrome

Immune dysregulation, polyendocrinopathy, enteropathy, X-linked (IPEX) syndrome is associated with mutations that abrogate expression of functional FOXP3 protein that results in defective development of $CD4^+CD25^+ T_{reg}$ and subsequent severe dysregulation of the immune system. In rare cases, IPEX could be the result of regulatory or conditional mutations

outside FOXP3 coding regions, resulting in reduction in FOXP3 messenger RNA (mRNA) expression. IPEX syndrome is inherited in an X-linked manner and typically affects males, whereas females remain asymptomatic. This syndrome is extremely rare, with fewer than 150 affected individuals identified worldwide.

Usually, IPEX syndrome presents in the first few months of life with eczema dermatitis, watery diarrhea, and endocrinopathy.[8] Possible other symptoms include cachexia, growth retardation caused by autoimmune enteropathy, and chronic inflammation with excessive cytokine production. Patients with IPEX may also present with hypothyroidism, Coombs-positive anemia, autoimmune neutropenia, and recurrent infection. Several cases have also demonstrated renal insufficiency, arthritis, and ulcerative colitis. Finally, patients with IPEX tend to be immunocompromised as a result of the defect in immunoregulation, resulting in severe infectious complications and sepsis.

Conventional $CD4^+$ and $CD8^+$ T cells numbers and function in vitro appear normal. Typically, patients with IPEX syndrome have elevated levels of serum IgE and, in some cases, IgA. Histopathology shows the absence of normal mucosa of the small bowel and colon with diffuse infiltration of inflammatory cells in the lamina propria. Definitive diagnosis is based on clinical features and DNA analysis of mutations in the *FOXP3* gene. Analysis of peripheral blood by flow cytometry will show decreased numbers of FOXP3-expressing T cells in patients with IPEX syndrome.

Without treatment, IPEX syndrome is fatal within the first 2 years of life because of sepsis or failure to thrive. Immunosuppressive therapy and BMT have shown efficacy for IPEX syndrome.[9] Immunosuppressive medications, such as cyclosporin A, tacrolimus, methotrexate, infliximab, and rituzimab, are only partially effective and limited by toxicity. Prophylactic antibiotic therapy for patients with autoimmune neutropenia or recurrent infections can be used to prevent secondary complications. Patients with IPEX syndrome should undergo periodic evaluation of complete blood cell count, glucose tolerance, thyroid function, kidney function, and liver function for evidence of autoimmune disease.

Neonatal Toxic Shock Syndrome-like Exanthematous Disease

Neonatal toxic shock syndrome-like exanthematous disease (NTED) is caused by overactivation of toxic shock syndrome toxin 1 (TSST-1) reactive T cells. Patients develop systemic exanthema, fever, mildly elevated serum C-reactive protein values, and thrombocytopenia. The disease is induced when patients are colonized with methicillin-resistant *Staphylococcus aureus* (MRSA) that produces TSST-1, which has superantigenic activity. To date, there is no genetic link to the disease. Transfer of maternal anti-TSST-1 IgG through the placenta is effective in protecting against the development of NTED.

Nezelof Syndrome

Nezelof syndrome (NS) is an extremely rare immune deficiency disorder affecting both male and female siblings, indicating that it may be transmitted as an autosomal recessive genetic disorder. NS is caused by thymic hypoplasia and is characterized by absent T-cell function and deficient B-cell function with fairly normal immunoglobulin levels, but little-to-no specific antibody production. Patients with NS present with recurrent pneumonia, otitis media, chronic fungal infections, upper respiratory tract infections, and diarrhea. The lymph nodes and tonsils may be enlarged or absent in infants with the disease.

Definitive diagnosis of the disease includes defective B-cell and T-cell immunity despite a normal number of circulating B cells, a moderate-to-high rise in the number of T cells, a deficiency or an increase in 1 or more classes of immunoglobulins, a non-reactive Schick test after DPT (diphtheria and tetanus toxoids and pertussis) immunization, a reduced or an absent antibody reaction after specific antigen immunization, no thymus shadow on a chest x-ray film, and a decrease in the number of lymphocytes in the blood.

Initial supportive treatment may include immunoglobulin injections and prophylactic use of antibiotics. T-cell function can be temporarily restored by injection of thymosin or fetal thymus transplant. Major histocompatibility-matched BMT is a possible treatment, but the effectiveness is not well documented.

Zeta-Chain-Associated Protein Deficiency

Zeta-chain-associated protein (ZAP70) deficiency is a rare autosomal recessive T-cell immunodeficiency that is caused by mutations in the ZAP70 gene on chromosome 2 at position q12, within the kinase domain, that encodes ZAP70. ZAP70 is a non-src family protein tyrosine kinase important in TCR signaling and has an essential role in positive and negative selection in the thymus. The deficiency results in a selective absence of CD8$^+$ T cells and normal or elevated numbers of circulating CD4$^+$ T cells. In vitro, CD4$^+$ T cells do not respond to mitogens or allogeneic cells. The thymus tends to have normal architecture with normal levels of differentiating CD4/CD8-double-positive thymocytes. Serum immunoglobulin concentrations in patients may be normal, low, or elevated, with normal or elevated B-cell numbers. The condition presents during infancy with severe, recurrent, frequently fatal infection.[10]

ACQUIRED T-CELL IMMUNODEFICIENCIES

Human Immunodeficiency Virus

Human immunodeficiency virus (HIV) is the virus that causes acquired immunodeficiency syndrome (AIDS). This retrovirus has a tropism for human CD4$^+$ T cells, bone-marrow-derived dendritic cells, megakaryocytes, cells of monocyte-macrophage lineage, and the macrophage-microglial and endothelial cells of the central nervous system. A characteristic depletion of CD4$^+$ cell numbers is observed in HIV infections, after which there is a continuous but variable rate of decline of CD4 T cells. Because CD4$^+$ T cells play a pivotal role in many immunoregulatory functions, the loss in these cells is responsible for a reduction in their helper-inducer function and a decrease in other T-cell, B-cell, and monocyte activities, resulting in wide-ranging functional defects in cellular and humoral immunity. Immune dysregulation and innate immune activation are features of HIV disease.

Perinatal transmission may occur in utero, at the time of delivery, or via breast-feeding. Infants infected perinatally usually are asymptomatic during the first few months of life, and size and physical features are not different from uninfected neonates. The level of viremia rises steeply, reaching a peak at age 1–2 months. Infants have a gradual decline in plasma viremia that extends beyond 2 years. Infants generally have plasma virus levels 10 times higher than those in adults.

Identification of the infected infant relies on identification of the infected mother, followed by careful clinical and laboratory monitoring of the infant throughout the first year of life. Diagnostic laboratory tests include serial HIV antibody testing (ie, enzyme-linked immunosorbent assay [ELISA] and immunoblot); serial P24 antigen testing; HIV culture; immunoglobulin levels; T-cell numbers and subsets (see Table 112-4), and 1 or more other diagnostic techniques (eg, polymerase chain reaction [PCR], HIV-IgA, immunoblot assay). Of note, maternal HIV-specific IgG is passively transferred across the placenta and may persist in infants until 18 months of age; thus, for infants under the age of 18 months, the viral PCR assay is preferred over HIV antibody testing. The goal for neonatal HIV infection is to diagnose infection before the onset of severe opportunistic infection.

There is currently no cure for HIV infection, and it is managed with antiretroviral (ARV) therapy drugs. Didanosine, lamivudine, stavudine, zidovudine, and nevirapine are used to treat infants under 3 months of age. Common side effects of ARV therapy include nausea, vomiting, diarrhea, headache, and malaise. The success of ARV therapy is measured by the suppression of HIV replication (as measured by plasma viral

Table 112-4 CD4 Lymphocyte Count Analysis for AIDS Diagnosis in Infants

	CD⁴⁺ T Cells/µL	% of Total Lymphocytes
No evidence of suppression	>1500	>25%
Moderate suppression	750–1499	15%–24%
Severe suppression	<750	<15%

Abbreviation: AIDS, acquired immunodeficiency syndrome.

load) and maintenance of CD4⁺ T-cell counts with the least amount of drug toxicity. The treatment paradigm changes frequently; therefore, prior to initiating treatment, expert consultation should be obtained.

Human T-Cell Leukemia Virus Type 1

Human T-cell leukemia virus type 1 is a retrovirus that infects CD4⁺ T cells and produces adult T-cell leukemia (ATL) and tropical spastic paraparesis, also called HTLV-1-associated myelopathy (HAM). HTLV-1 may also play a role in infective dermatitis, arthritis, uveitis, and Sjögren syndrome. Generally, only T cells are productively infected, but infection of B cells and other cell types is occasionally detected. As HTLV-1 infection results in latent carriage of integrated provirus, does not contain an oncogene, and does not insert into a unique site within the genome, most infected cells do not express viral gene products. The virus

can be transmitted vertically from mothers to infants. Maternal anti-HTLV-1 antibodies inhibit milk-borne infections of HTLV-1 in early life. However, neonatal infection with HTLV-1 is preventable through short-term breast-feeding (<3 months) or bottle feeding. Modes of prevention of ATL and HAM have not been described.

CHRONIC MUCOCUTANEOUS CANDIDIASIS

Chronic mucocutaneous candidiasis (CMC) is an infection of the skin, mucous membranes, and nails by *Candida albicans* and is associated with defective T-cell-mediated immunity that is specific to *Candida*. The T cells of patients with CMC fail to produce cytokines essential for anti-*Candida* cell-mediated immunity. This defect can be caused by an inherited deficiency or have no genetic basis (Table 112-5). In several patients, gene sequencing identified mutations in signal transducer and activator of transcription (STAT) 1, leading to defective immune responses in T_H1 and T_H17 T cells.[11] CMC can also severely affect patients with STAT3 deficiency and lack of IL-17- and IL-22-producing T cells. B-cell function is normal; thus, anti-*Candida* antibodies can be identified in patients.

Neonatal candidiasis presents 3–7 days after birth with oral thrush and diaper dermatitis. More extensive scaling of skin lesions and thickened nails and red, swollen periungual tissues can follow these infections.

Table 112-5 Classification of Infant Patients With Chronic Mucocutaneous Candidiasis (CMC)

Type	Gene Defect	Onset	Clinical Features	Associated Disorders	Noncandidal Infections
Familial CMC	Autosomal recessive	<2 years	Oral candidiasis	No endocrinopathies	Yes
Autoimmune polyendocrinopathy-candidiasis-ectodermal dystrophy syndrome	Autosomal recessive, mutations in the *AIRE* gene	<5 years Endocrine abnormalities between 10 and 15 years of age	Oral and diaper area candidiasis Endocrinopathies and autoimmune disorders	Hypoparathyroidism, hypoadrenalism, thyroid disease, hepatitis, malabsorption, primary hypogonadism, pernicious anemia, alopecia areata	Yes
Chronic localized candidiasis	No known genetic basis	<5 years	Thick, adherent candidal crusts on the scalp and face, oral candidiasis	None	Yes
CMC with keratitis	Autosomal dominant	Early childhood	Candidiasis of the oral cavity, diaper area	Keratoconjunctivitis, alopecia, endocrine abnormalities	Yes

Chronic mucocutaneous candidiasis may be classified based on its association with other conditions. The condition without endocrinopathy is typically not associated with autoimmune disorders; inheritance may be autosomal recessive or dominant. Chronic mucocutaneous candidiasis with endocrinopathy may occur as part of autoimmune polyendocrinopathy syndrome type 1, also known as APECED, or may also be observed in patients with other conditions, such as hyperimmunoglobulin IgE syndrome and HIV infection. Persistent and refractory candidal infections must be distinguished from the more common treatment-responsive overgrowth of *Candida* that occurs in the setting of systemic antibiotic therapy, local/systemic corticosteroid treatment, or hyperglycemia in persons with diabetes mellitus.

Chronic mucocutaneous candidiasis is not associated with a high degree of mortality because disseminated invasive candidal infections are rare. However, patients with APECED have significant morbidity from endocrinopathies or other autoimmune diseases associated with this condition. Orally and topically administered antifungal agents improve the condition of patients with CMC. Fluconazole and itraconazole are available as suspensions and can be used in pediatric populations. Of note, these drugs inhibit the cytochrome P-450 system, and treatment may alter catabolism of other drugs, such as coumadin; immunosuppressive drugs (tacrolimus, cyclosporin A); antimycobacterial drugs (rifampin); and anti-HIV protease inhibitors.[12] In autoimmune disorders, reconstitution of the cell-mediated immune response with leukocyte transfer from healthy, related donors has proven beneficial.

Acute Lymphoblastic Leukemia

Acute leukemias make up a group of lymphopoietic stem cell disorders that are characterized by clonal expansion of immature lymphohematopoietic cells in the bone marrow. Lymphoblasts that are unable to differentiate accumulate in the bone marrow and suppress normal hemopoietic cells. Chromosomal abnormalities have been found in most cases of acute lymphoblastic leukemia (ALL).[13] Around 20% of ALLs are of the T-cell type; the remaining are mainly of the B-cell type. Finally, ALL occurs more frequently among children than myeloid leukemias, reaching a peak at 3–4 years of age.

Patients with ALL develop a normochromic, normocytic anemia and may develop weakness, pallor, and malaise. In most cases, patients develop bleeding secondary to thrombocytopenia. Granulocytopenia is also common in patients with ALL and results in increased bacterial infections. Patients also experience bone pain and generalized lymphadenopathy.

Diagnosis of ALL is accomplished by demonstrating lymphoblasts in the bone marrow. Lymphoblasts can also be detected in peripheral blood and are usually accompanied by an elevated leukocyte count. A normal or decreased leukocyte count may appear in patients without peripheral blood lymphoblasts. The age at onset and initial total leukocyte count are valuable for prognosis. Allogeneic stem cell transplantation is only performed in cases with very high-risk ALL features.[14] Aggressive nonablative chemotherapy has been successful in driving complete remission and is the treatment of choice for children with ALL.[15]

REFERENCES

1. Campbell DJ, Koch MA. Phenotypical and functional specialization of FOXP3+ regulatory T cells. *Nat Rev Immunol.* 2011;11(2):119–130.
2. PrabhuDas M, Adkins B, Gans H, et al. Challenges in infant immunity: implications for responses to infection and vaccines. *Nat Immunol.* 2011;12(3):189–194.
3. Driscoll DA, Budarf ML, Emanuel BS. A genetic etiology for DiGeorge syndrome: consistent deletions and microdeletions of 22q11. *Am J Hum Genet.* 1992;50:924–933.
4. McDonald-McGinn DM, Gripp KW, Kirschner RE, et al. Craniosynostosis: another feature of the 22q11.2 deletion syndrome. *Am J Med Genet A.* 2005;136A:358–362.
5. Sullivan KE. The clinical, immunological, and molecular spectrum of chromosome 22q11.2 deletion syndrome and DiGeorge syndrome. *Curr Opin Allergy Clin Immunol.* 2004;4:505–512.
6. Desmaze C, Scambler P, Prieur M, et al. Routine diagnosis of DiGeorge syndrome by fluorescent in situ hybridization. *Hum Genet.* 1993;90:663–665.
7. Mullen CA, Anderson KD, Blaese RM. Splenectomy and/or bone marrow transplantation in the management of the Wiskott-Aldrich syndrome: long-term follow-up of 62 cases. *Blood.* 1993;82:2961–2966.
8. Powell BR, Buist NR, Stenzel P. An X-linked syndrome of diarrhea, polyendocrinopathy, and fatal infection in infancy. *J Pediatr.* 1982;100:731–737.
9. Wildin RS, Smyk-Pearson S, Filipovich AH. Clinical and molecular features of the immunodysregulation, polyendocrinopathy, enteropathy, X linked (IPEX) syndrome. *J Med Genet.* 2002;39:537–545.
10. DeAngelis C, Feigin RD, McMillan JA, et al. *Oski's Pediatrics: Principles And Practice.* 3rd ed. Philadelphia, PA: Lippincott Williams & Wilkins; 1999.
11. van de Veerdonk FL, Plantinga TS, Hoischen A, et al. STAT1 mutations in autosomal dominant chronic mucocutaneous candidiasis. *N Engl J Med.* 2011;365(1):54–61.
12. Kirkpatrick CH. Chronic mucocutaneous candidiasis. *Pediatr Infect Dis J.* 2001;20:197–206.
13. Bloomfield CD, Lindquist LL, Arthur D, et al. Chromosomal abnormalities in acute lymphoblastic leukemia. *Cancer Res.* 1981;41:4838–4843.
14. Balduzzi A, Valsecchi MG, Uderzo C, et al. Chemotherapy versus allogeneic transplantation for very-high-risk childhood acute lymphoblastic leukaemia in first complete remission: comparison by genetic randomisation in an international prospective study. *Lancet.* 2005;366:635–642.
15. Ribera JM, Oriol A. Acute lymphoblastic leukemia in adolescents and young adults. *Hematol Oncol Clin North Am.* 2009;23:1033–1042, vi.

Early-Onset Sepsis

Valencia P. Walker and Vladana Milisavljevic

EVALUATION

Septic neonates can have dramatic clinical presentations characterized by respiratory failure, persistent pulmonary hypertension of the newborn (PPHN), disseminated intravascular coagulation (DIC), hypotension, or multiorgan failure. More challenging for health care providers, however, are more commonly encountered patients with subtle and nonspecific signs and symptoms or risk factors for sepsis. Considering the deleterious consequences of a missed or delayed diagnosis, a high index of suspicion is warranted when undertaking evaluation of neonates for potential sepsis.

Maternal History

Careful history is essential for determining key risk factors associated with early-onset sepsis (EOS). Clinicians should confirm the following:

1. Maternal group B streptococci (GBS) status.

2. Use of GBS-specific intrapartum antibiotic prophylaxis vs broad-spectrum intrapartum antibiotic use.

3. Duration of time between rupture of membranes and birth.

4. Length of time of intrapartum antibiotic administration (>4 hours).

5. Intrapartum maternal fever.

6. Gestational age of the newborn.

Labor and Delivery

The clinical presentation of a septic infant can start as early as labor and delivery. Signs and symptoms may include the following:

1. Intrapartum fetal tachycardia.

2. Meconium staining of amniotic fluid.[1]

3. Low Apgar scores (newborns with an Apgar score ≤ 6 at 5 minutes had a 36-fold higher likelihood of sepsis than those with Apgar scores ≥ 7).[2]

Clinical Signs and Physical Findings

After birth, clinical signs of sepsis present in a range from nonspecific and subtle to severe multisystem dysfunction. More commonly presenting signs include the following:

1. Neurological: Temperature instability (fever or hypothermia, with fever more common in term newborns and hypothermia more likely in preterm neonates[3]); apnea; lethargy or irritability; hypotonia; weak cry; poor suck; seizures.

2. Respiratory: Tachypnea; respiratory distress (flaring, grunting, retractions, or decreased breath sounds); and pulmonary hemorrhage.

3. Cardiovascular: Tachycardia or bradycardia; cyanosis; hypotension; prolonged capillary refill time; mottled appearance; cool and clammy skin.

4. Hematological: Jaundice, petechiae, purpura, and pallor.

5. Gastrointestinal: Abdominal distension, feeding intolerance, emesis, diarrhea, bloody stools, and hepatomegaly.

6. Renal: Oliguria, anuria.

Diagnostic Tests/Laboratory Testing

Several tests are almost universally obtained for the evaluation of EOS; others are still limited by the lack of evidence to support widespread use:

1. Blood culture: This remains the gold standard for diagnosis of EOS. Although there is a considerably high incidence of false-negative cultures[4,5] obtained from neonates, a culture absent of bacterial growth at 36–48 hours from a newborn with no other signs of EOS is reassuring. One small prospective cohort study has also examined utilizing cord blood for blood culture sampling in asymptomatic term newborns evaluated for sepsis based on the presence of risk factors.[6] The authors concluded it may be a reasonable consideration, but additional studies are needed before a practice recommendation can be made. For those neonates who fail to demonstrate improvement after initiating empiric antibiotic therapy, repeating blood cultures is recommended, with expansion to other sites (cerebrospinal fluid [CSF], respiratory, and urine). If the initial blood culture is positive, blood culture(s) should be repeated 24 hours after antibiotics were initiated.[5]

2. CSF culture/studies: Meningitis in the newborn can be difficult to diagnose clinically. Although the decision to perform a lumbar puncture (LP) remains controversial, guidelines have been provided by the American Academy of Pediatrics (AAP) Committee on Fetus and Newborn for obtaining LP and CSF studies in a clinically unstable newborn or a newborn with a positive blood culture.[7] Consideration for "holding" CSF stored in the laboratory in case additional studies are later needed should always be included in the discussion for performing the procedure. Serial LPs in the absence of an initial positive culture are not recommended because they are unlikely to yield additional benefit that outweighs potential risks and complications.

3. Complete blood cell count (CBC) with (manual) differential count: A CBC is the most readily available and commonly utilized test for EOS. It is typically done as a screening tool between 2 and 12 hours of life. However, values may range widely and be influenced by the timing of the sample acquisition. Serial studies at 6-, 12-, or 24-hour intervals are useful and, in conjunction with other laboratory results and clinical findings, can be recommended to influence the decision to discontinue antibiotic

therapy.[8,9] In sick neonates, thrombocytopenia is frequently observed, but it has no consistent predictive value. For a subset of patients, development of (worsening) thrombocytopenia may signal progression to septic shock or invasive gram-negative or fungal infection (premature infants).

4. Immature neutrophils (band cells + myelocytes + metamyelocytes) to total neutrophils ratio (I/T) 70.20 warrants a greater level of suspicion for EOS, especially in conjunction with other abnormal findings.[10] Values less than 0.2 are usually considered within normal limits. An I:T ratio that "normalizes" within 24–48 hours, particularly in an otherwise-asymptomatic infant, can be considered a reassuring laboratory finding.

5. C-reactive protein (CRP): As an acute phase reactant, any inflammatory condition can elevate CRP. However, abnormally elevated CRPs obtained serially after birth can support a diagnosis of EOS. Furthermore, serial CRP values within normal range, particularly in the absence of other signs of EOS, may provide reassurance for discontinuing empiric antibiotic therapy.[11] Serial CRP values are used by some centers to guide duration of empiric antibiotic therapy. Such protocols typically require at least two CRP levels, obtained 24 hours apart, with results below the laboratory's designated cutoff to identify infants unlikely to be infected.[12,13] We would caution against using this as a singular approach because there are still many unanswered questions about the value of CRP in managing neonatal sepsis. Research is ongoing and includes the intriguing possibility for point-of-care testing.[14]

6. Neutrophil CD64: Neutrophils have been shown to express CD64 when activated. Several studies have found CD64 determination to have high sensitivity and specificity for the determination of EOS when an appropriate cutoff value is selected. Advantages include small blood volume for sampling and rapid results. It is also considered advantageous when used in conjunction with CRP testing for EOS laboratory evaluations.[15–17]

7. Blood gas monitoring: Patients with sepsis often have metabolic or respiratory acidosis, hypoxemia (especially in PPHN), and hypercarbia. Frequent blood gas monitoring can alert the clinician to acute changes in the patient's status that warrant urgent intervention. Arterial blood gas sampling is preferred for its accuracy.

8. Imaging studies: Imaging is helpful when respiratory symptoms predominate (chest x-ray) or there is a concern for intracranial bleeding as a complication of sepsis (cranial ultrasound). An echocardiogram is useful for ruling out congenital cardiac

disease, assessing myocardial dysfunction, or determining the presence and severity of PPHN.

9. Electroencephalogram (EEG): For infants with an abnormal neurological status, including persistent lethargy, hypotonia, and seizure activity, in addition to a LP, an EEG evaluation in consultation with pediatric neurology may be warranted because neonates may have significant subclinical seizure activity requiring anticonvulsant therapy.

Differential Diagnosis/Diagnostic Algorithms

The differential diagnosis for EOS is broad (Table 113-1). However, given that EOS can mimic the presentation of other severe diagnoses, it is important to keep a complete differential in mind when evaluating a

Table 113-1 Differential Diagnostic Considerations for Early-Onset Sepsis

Cause of Sepsis	Diagnostic Consideration Examples
Nonbacterial infections	Viral: HSV, CMV, enterovirus, etc Fungal: Candidiasis (increased risk in preterm infants) Parasitic: Congenital toxoplasmosis Spirochetal: Congenital syphilis
Nonhematological bacterial infections	Congenital pneumonia, UTI (associated with GU malformations), osteomyelitis, myocarditis, septic arthritis
Hypoxic ischemic encephalopathy Perinatal/neonatal asphyxia	Associated with multiorgan dysfunction
Inborn errors of metabolism Metabolic derangements	Galactosemia, glycogen storage diseases, fatty acid oxidation defects Hypoglycemia
Congenital heart disease	HLHS, TAPVR, TGV, pulmonary atresia
Respiratory disease	RDS (particularly in IDMs), TTN, PPHN, meconium aspiration syndrome, CDH
Gastrointestinal emergencies	NEC, malrotation with volvulus
Hemolytic disease of the newborn	Severe Rh/ABO Incompatibility

Abbreviations: CDH, congenital diaphragmatic hernia; CMV, cytomegalovirus; GU, genitourinary; HLHS, hypoplastic left heart syndrome; HSV, herpes simplex virus; IDM, infant of diabetic mother; NEC, necrotizing enterocolitis; RDS, respiratory distress syndrome; TAPVR, total anomalous pulmonary venous return; TGV, transposition of great vessels; TTN, transient tachypnea of the newborn; UTI, urinary tract infection.

newborn. Figure 113-1 represents a diagnostic algorithm for EOS.

MANAGEMENT

When presented with an acutely ill neonate, it is important to promptly administer appropriate supportive measures and initiate clinical investigations into the cause. Management includes broad-spectrum antibiotics as well as supportive therapy. Asymptomatic newborns with risk factors for infection should be carefully monitored for early signs and symptoms of sepsis. For symptomatic infants, full cardiopulmonary monitoring is crucial as a neonate's clinical condition can deteriorate rapidly.

Antibiotic Therapy for EOS

In suspected sepsis, the initial antibiotic therapy is empirical, targeted against the most likely EOS pathogens. Antibiotics need to be initiated as soon as possible, preferably after cultures have been obtained. Once a pathogen is identified, antibiotic therapy should be adjusted and ideally narrowed based on the susceptibilities of the organism(s). Decisions for duration of therapy will be dictated by the source and type of organism(s) isolated as well as the clinical course.

Recommended Empiric Antibiotic Therapy for EOS

The antibiotics recommended for the neonate with suspected EOS are ampicillin and gentamicin.[18] These antibiotics have the additional benefit of intramuscular (IM) or intravenous (IV) administration. A National Institute of Child Health and Human Development (NICHD) network study and other reports have shown the efficacy of this combination.[19,20] Our recommendation is to start meningitic doses of ampicillin if the suspicion for meningitis is strong enough to warrant an LP in the evaluation process, even if the patient is not symptomatic. This also applies to the critically sick infant when the LP is deferred. If treatment is continued longer than 48 hours, meningitis was excluded, and the clinical status is improving, ampicillin can be changed to nonmeningitic dosing.

Use of Third-Generation Cephalosporins/ Alternative Antibiotics for Empiric Therapy

An alternative regimen of ampicillin and a third-generation cephalosporin (eg, cefotaxime, ceftriaxone) is not more effective than ampicillin and gentamicin.

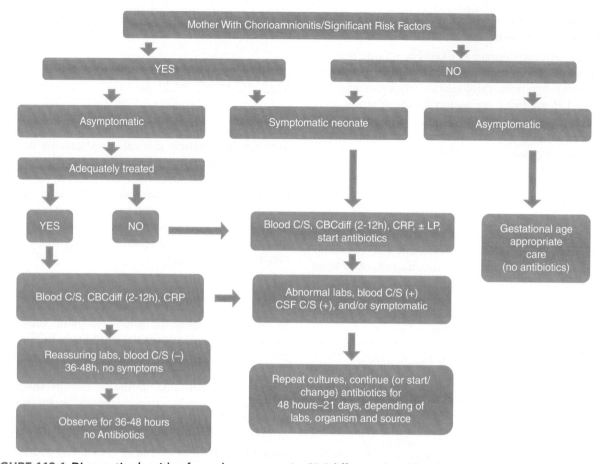

FIGURE 113-1 Diagnostic algorithm for early-onset sepsis. CBCdiff, complete blood cell count with differential; CRP, C-reactive protein; C/S, culture and sensitivity; CSF, cerebrospinal fluid.

Routine use of cefotaxime is discouraged because of the emergence of cephalosporin-resistant bacterial strains (eg, *Enterobacter cloacae*, *Klebsiella*, and *Serratia* species).[18] A large study found that in patients receiving ampicillin, the concurrent use of cefotaxime during the first 3 days after birth was associated with an increased risk of death, compared with patients treated with ampicillin and concurrent use of gentamicin.[21] Third-generation cephalosporins have also been linked to invasive candidiasis infections in extremely premature neonates. Ceftriaxone administration is completely avoided in infants less than 28 days old because of several adverse effects, including hyperbilirubinemia as a result of displacement from albumin and cardiovascular collapse from coadministration with calcium-containing intravenous solutions.[22] Increasingly, piperacillin/tazobactam (Zosyn) is being utilized as a single agent or added to an aminoglycoside for empiric antibiotic therapy in neonatal sepsis.[23,24]

Supportive Therapy

The main goal of supportive therapy is to increase delivery of substrates to meet tissue demand that has been compromised during a septic episode. Necessary therapies may involve the following:

1. Respiratory support: Provide oxygen and, if respiratory distress is present, provide adequate support (from nasal cannula to endotracheal intubation and mechanical ventilation).

2. Volume/fluid/blood pressure support: Initiate rapid fluid resuscitation with crystalloid or colloid parenteral solutions as needed to correct circulatory derangements. An adequate circulating blood volume is necessary to maintain right ventricular filling and cardiac output. However, repeated bolus administration of crystalloid and colloid solutions will not provide additional benefit. Correcting underlying vascular derangements, such as peripheral vasodilation, must be promptly addressed through the use of pressor support (dopamine, dobutamine, epinephrine, etc).

3. Correction of metabolic abnormalities (hypoglycemia, hypocalcemia, etc): Management of fluid and electrolytes is extremely important. Metabolic and respiratory acidosis require timely correction. When glucose abnormalities are present

(hypo- or hyperglycemia), they can be important diagnostic evidence and contributors to neonatal morbidity and mortality,[25] therefore, judicious correction is necessary.

4. DIC: Evidence of abnormal blood clotting should be corrected with transfusions and drugs. However, reversal of DIC often poses considerable challenges despite repletion with blood products. It is important to remember that reversal will not occur until the underlying cause or organism has been effectively treated. Use of factor VII has not been investigated sufficiently to recommend administration to septic neonates in DIC.

5. Provide thermoregulatory support: Hypothermia is a frequent finding in neonatal sepsis. When present, patients' temperature is artificially controlled, and the ability to wean thermoregulatory support should be monitored.

6. Inhaled nitric oxide (iNO): In patients with severe hypoxic respiratory failure unable to maintain the arterial pressure of oxygen (PaO_2) greater than 80 mm Hg despite maximal respiratory support or in a ventilated patient with a significant (>50%) O_2 requirement and echocardiographic evidence of pulmonary artery pressures close to or above systemic pressure, especially if there is evidence of poor cardiac output, iNO may provide some benefit. The appropriate starting dose is 20 ppm. Increasing to levels above 20 ppm has no additional positive impact and increases the likelihood of adverse effects, including methemoglobinemia.

7. Extracorporeal membrane oxygenation (ECMO): Consider this modality if other means of respiratory and cardiovascular support fail to be sufficient. For centers without ECMO support, transfer to a neonatal intensive care unit (NICU) with a higher level of care should be considered and initiated early.

8. Monitoring of renal function: This is particularly important for patients treated with nephrotoxic medications, including aminoglycosides (eg, gentamicin) and vancomycin. Renal injury is typically acute and reversible. However, intravenous fluids and medication administration should be reviewed daily and tailored to the level of renal function present.

9. Sedation/pain control considerations: Measures to provide comfort with procedures (LP, blood draws, etc) should be provided. Newborns do not necessarily need sedation or pain control for ventilator management. However, those patients who are difficult to ventilate/oxygenate because of agitation may benefit from adequate sedation.

Continuous infusion with benzodiazepines (eg, midazolam) should be avoided given concerns for adverse neurodevelopmental outcomes. Recognition of rapid tolerance development/neonatal abstinence syndrome is important as patients recover from sepsis, so timely weaning off continuous analgesic infusions when they are used as a part of clinical management should be initiated as soon as appropriate.

10. Alternative treatment options: Routine use of adjunctive immunotherapeutics, such as white cell transfusions, intravenous immunoglobulin, granulocyte and granulocyte-macrophage colony-stimulating factor administration, activated protein C and lactoferrin, is not recommended as studies have failed to demonstrate an improvement in outcomes for neonatal sepsis.[26]

Indications for Discontinuation of Antibiotic Therapy

By far, the greatest controversy in neonatal sepsis involves the decision to discontinue empiric antibiotic therapy. There is appropriate concern for the adverse effects of prolonged antibiotic therapy in the setting of sterile cultures, as retrospective cohort studies have indicated an increased risk for morbidity and mortality.[27,28] Recent studies have attempted to create predictive models that go beyond assessing infants who are "at risk" or "not at risk" and consider timing of laboratory findings in addition to clinical acumen for determining duration of antibiotic therapy.[11] Unfortunately, current studies are still inadequate and unable to provide final guidance on appropriate testing and timing of testing to cover the range of circumstances necessitating initiation of empiric antibiotic therapy.

Consent/Ethical Considerations

For newborns who require admission to the NICU, appropriate consents from parents or guardians will be necessary. Ethical considerations for investigations and treatment in cases of extreme prematurity or suspected genetic syndromes with known mortality should be undertaken with the family as soon as feasible, ideally before the infant's clinical deterioration.

CONCLUSION/FOLLOW-UP

Aftercare Monitoring

Neonates with resolution of their septic episode should demonstrate the ability to maintain their temperature without thermoregulatory assistance and consume adequate nutrition for growth by oral feeding unless secondary diagnoses preclude the ability to attain these milestones.

Follow-up Tests

For neonates with additional morbidities associated with sepsis, additional evaluation should be performed prior to discharge. This may include repeating head ultrasound, chest x-ray (determine resolution of pneumothorax but not resolution of pneumonia as those findings lag behind evidence of clinical improvement), echocardiogram to assess myocardial function/contractility, or cultures to demonstrate clearance of infection. Patients should be examined carefully for evidence of thrombus formation as well as any evidence of persistent neurological deficits that would necessitate outpatient follow-up in consultation with appropriate subspecialists. Because of potential ototoxicity associated with certain infections and as a recognized side effect of aminoglycoside use, hearing screening should be performed prior to discharge.

Clinical Follow-up

For patients with severe sepsis/septic shock (pressor support, ECMO support, etc), follow-up in 3 to 6 months after discharge with a neonatal/developmental specialist is warranted. Continued follow-up through the first 3 years of life, including regular neurodevelopmental assessments, is also recommended. Should evidence of developmental delay manifest, prompt referral to appropriate services (speech therapy, occupational therapy, physical therapy, etc) is important.

Long-Term Outcome/Implications for Patient/Family

Multiple confounders exist that significantly hamper the ability to definitively predict long-term outcomes for neonates diagnosed with sepsis. The extremely premature infants who had sepsis have a higher incidence of cerebral palsy as compared to those who did not have sepsis during their NICU stay.[29,30] Similarly, infants with bacterial sepsis associated with meningitis have worse neurodevelopmental outcomes, as well as patients who required ECMO support.

REFERENCES

1. Escobar GJ, Li DK, Armstrong MA, et al. Neonatal sepsis workups in infants ≥ 2000 grams at birth: a population-based study. *Pediatrics.* 2000;106(2 Pt 1):256–263.
2. Soman M, Green B, Daling J. Risk factors for early neonatal sepsis. *Am J Epidemiol.* 1985;121(5):712–719.
3. Osborn LM, Bolus R. Temperature and fever in the full-term newborn. *J Fam Pract.* 1985;20(3):261–264.
4. Connell TG, Rele M, Cowley D, Buttery JP, Curtis N. How reliable is a negative blood culture result? Volume of blood submitted for culture in routine practice in a children's hospital. *Pediatrics.* 2007;119(5):891–896.
5. Sarkar S, Bhagat I, Wiswell TE, Spitzer AR. Role of multiple site blood cultures to document the clearance of bacteremia in neonates. *J Perinatol.* 2007;27(2):101–102.
6. Hansen A, Forbes P, Buck R. Potential substitution of cord blood for infant blood in the neonatal sepsis evaluation. *Biol Neonate.* 2005;88(1):12–18.
7. Polin RA; Committee on Fetus and Newborn. Management of neonates with suspected or proven early-onset bacterial sepsis. *Pediatrics.* 2012;129(5):1006–1015.
8. Murphy K, Weiner J. Use of leukocyte counts in evaluation of early-onset neonatal sepsis. *Pediatr Infect Dis J.* 2012;31(1):16–19.
9. Ng PC. Diagnostic markers of infection in neonates. *Arch Dis Child Fetal Neonatal Ed.* 2004;89(3):F229–F235.
10. Hornik CP, Benjamin DK, Becker KC, et al. Use of the complete blood cell count in early-onset neonatal sepsis. *Pediatr Infect Dis J.* 2012;31(8):799–802.
11. Cotten CM, Smith PB. Duration of empirical antibiotic therapy for infants suspected of early-onset sepsis. *Curr Opin Pediatr.* 2013;25(2):167–171.
12. Hengst JM. The role of C-reactive protein in the evaluation and management of infants with suspected sepsis. *Adv Neonatal Care.* 2003;3(1):3–13.
13. McWilliams S, Riordan A. How to use: C-reactive protein. *Arch Dis Child Educ Pract Ed.* 2010;95(2):55–58.
14. Diar HA, Nakwa FL, Thomas R, Libhaber EN, Velaphi S. Evaluating the QuikRead C-reactive protein test as a point-of-care test. *Paediatr Int Child Health.* 2012;32(1):35–42.
15. Streimish I, Bizzarro M, Northrup V, et al. Neutrophil CD64 as a diagnostic marker in neonatal sepsis. *Pediatr Infect Dis J.* 2012;31(7):777–781.
16. Dilli D, Oğuz ŞS, Dilmen U, Köker MY, Kizilgün M. Predictive values of neutrophil CD64 expression compared with interleukin-6 and C-reactive protein in early diagnosis of neonatal sepsis. *J Clin Lab Anal.* 2010;24(6):363–370.
17. Standage SW, Wong HR. Biomarkers for pediatric sepsis and septic shock. *Expert Rev Anti Infect Ther.* 2011;9(1):71–79.
18. American Academy of Pediatrics. In: Pickering LK, Baker CJ, Kimberlin DW, Long SS, eds. *Red Book: 2009 Report of the Committee on Infectious Diseases.* 28th ed. Elk Grove Village, IL: American Academy of Pediatrics; 2009;293, 629.
19. Maayan-Metzger A, Barzilai A, Keller N, Kuint J. Are the "good old" antibiotics still appropriate for early-onset neonatal sepsis? A 10 year survey. *Isr Med Assoc J.* 2009;11:138–142.
20. Muller-Pebody B, Johnson AP, Heath PT, et al. Empirical treatment of neonatal sepsis: are the current guidelines adequate? *Arch Dis Child Fetal Neonatal Ed.* 2011;96:F4–F8.
21. Clark RH, Bloom BT, Spitzer AR, Gerstmann DR. Empiric use of ampicillin and cefotaxime, compared with ampicillin and gentamicin, for neonates at risk for sepsis is associated with an increased risk of neonatal death. *Pediatrics.* 2006;117:67–74.
22. Bradley JS, Wassel RT, Lee L, Nambiar S. Intravenous ceftriaxone and calcium in the neonate: assessing the risk for cardiopulmonary adverse events. *Pediatrics.* 2009;123(4):e609–e613.
23. Chong E, Reynolds J, Shaw J, et al. Results of a two-center, before and after study of piperacillin-tazobactam versus ampicillin and gentamicin as empiric therapy for suspected sepsis at birth in neonates < 1500 g. *J Perinatol.* 2013;33(7):529–532.
24. Wolf MF, Simon A. The use of piperacillin-tazobactam in neonatal and paediatric patients. *Expert Opin Drug Metab Toxicol.* 2009;5(1):57–69.

25. Kermorvant-Duchemin E, Laborie S, Rabilloud M, Lapillonne A, Claris O. Outcome and prognostic factors in neonates with septic shock. *Pediatr Crit Care Med.* 2008;9(2):186–191.

26. Tarnow-Mordi W, Isaacs D, Dutta S. Adjunctive immunologic interventions in neonatal sepsis. *Clin Perinatol.* 2010;37(2):481–499.

27. Cotten CM, Taylor S, Stoll B. NICHD Neonatal Research Network. Prolonged duration of initial empirical antibiotic treatment is associated with increased rates of necrotizing enterocolitis and death for extremely low birth weight infants. *Pediatrics.* 2009;123:58–66.

28. Bizzarro MJ, Dembry LM, Baltimore RS, Gallagher PG. Changing patterns in neonatal *Escherichia coli* sepsis and ampicillin resistance in the era of intrapartum antibiotic prophylaxis. *Pediatrics.* 2008;121:689–696.

29. Schlapbach LJ, Aebischer M, Adams M, et al. Swiss Neonatal Network and Follow-Up Group. Impact of sepsis on neurodevelopmental outcome in a Swiss National Cohort of extremely premature infants. *Pediatrics.* 2011;128(2):e348–e357.

30. Alshaikh B, Yusuf K, Sauve R. Neurodevelopmental outcomes of very low birthweight infants with neonatal sepsis: systematic review and meta-analysis. *J Perinatol.* 2013;33(7):558–564.

114 Health Care-Associated Infections

Valencia P. Walker and Vladana Milisavljevic

EVALUATION

Health care-associated infection (HCAI), also referred to as nosocomial or hospital acquired, is an infection that a patient acquires and (a) becomes evident 48 hours or more after admission, (b) was not present or incubating at the time of admission to the hospital, and (c) develops while the patient is receiving treatment of other conditions. Neonates admitted to the neonatal intensive care unit (NICU) frequently contract HCAIs[1] and may present with a wide range of symptoms, including fulminant sepsis, particularly late-onset sepsis (LOS). A significant number of HCAIs are preventable, even in the high-risk and vulnerable NICU population. Therefore, any discussion of HCAI management must also emphasize the role of preventive measures (refer to chapter 53).

Risk Factors

Recognition of risk factors for HCAIs is important when evaluating an acutely ill/decompensating patient for a possible HCAI.

1. Patient related: These risk factors are strongly influenced by the gestational age or weight at birth.[2] With decreasing gestational age and birth weight, the more likely it is that an HCAI can occur as there is an underdeveloped immune response, increased hospital length of stay, severity of illness, exposure to NICU-related risk factors (see next item), and development of chronic and exacerbating medical conditions such as chronic lung disease (CLD) or necrotizing enterocolitis (NEC).

2. NICU related: These risk factors include the following:
   a. indwelling intravascular or transmucosal catheters,
   b. mechanical ventilation,
   c. total parenteral nutrition (TPN) and intralipids,
   d. broad-spectrum antibiotic therapy,
   e. treatment with histamine$_2$ receptor antagonists (H$_2$ blockers),
   f. steroid administration, and
   g. exposure to the endemic microbial flora of the NICU environment as well as its health care workers.[3-5]

Clinical Signs and Symptoms

The clinical presentation can range from nonspecific and subtle to severe, multisystem organ dysfunction. Common presenting findings are the following:

1. Neurological:
   a. temperature instability (fever or hypothermia);
   b. apnea (unrelated to/distinct from apnea of prematurity);
   c. lethargy or irritability, hypotonia, poor suck; and
   d. seizures.

2. Respiratory:
   a. Tachypnea;
   b. grunting, flaring, retracting, or decreased breath sounds;
   c. worsening gas exchange by blood gas, increased oxygen requirement, pulse oximetry, etc;
   d. change in chest x-ray findings, and

e. new onset or change in character of sputum and increased respiratory secretions and suctioning requirements (for ventilated patients).

3. Cardiovascular:
   a. tachycardia or bradycardia;
   b. arrhythmia;
   c. cyanosis; and
   d. hypotension, prolonged capillary refill time, mottled appearance, cool and clammy skin.

4. Hematological:
   a. leukopenia or leukocytosis,
   b. anemia, and
   c. thrombocytopenia,

5. Skin:
   a. jaundice,
   b. petechiae,
   c. purpura, and
   d. pallor or cyanosis.

6. Gastrointestinal:
   a. abdominal distension, feeding intolerance, emesis;
   b. diarrhea or bloody stools; and
   c. ileus or absent bowel sounds.

7. Renal:
   a. oliguria or anuria and
   b. pyuria or malodorous urine.

Diagnostic Tests/Laboratory Testing

Testing should always include consideration of the patient's risk factors for HCAIs with the caveat that not all "positive" cultures signify the presence of an infection (warranting treatment). Clinicians should also follow available diagnostic guidelines where available (see chapter 53).

1. Blood cultures: At least 1 mL of blood is recommended for each culture.
   a. Draw from all intravascular catheters **and** a peripheral source.
   b. Fungal cultures should also be considered, particularly in extremely low birth weight (ELBW) infants who are at greater risk for invasive fungal infections.
   c. Repeat cultures and expand to other potential sources (urine, CSF, etc.) if no clinical improvement is seen after initiating empiric antibiotic therapy.
   d. If the blood culture is positive, blood cultures from all lines and a peripheral source should be repeated at least every 24 hours after antibiotics/antifungals are initiated until cultures become negative.
   e. For persistently positive cultures caused by an intravascular or indwelling device, removal is necessary.

f. Sending additional cultures of a removed device (eg, catheter tip) rarely aids management in the setting of known positive blood cultures.[6]

2. Cerebrospinal fluid (CSF) culture/analysis: Meningitis in a sick NICU patient can be difficult to diagnose. In a 2004 study by Stoll et al, approximately one-third of patients with meningitis did not have evidence of sepsis.[7] Further complicating the issue are those patients with posthemorrhagic hydrocephalus who have had placement of either a ventricular reservoir or a shunt because they are at increased risk for infection.[8] A decision to evaluate CSF (via either lumbar puncture [LP] or sampling of a reservoir/shunt) should be made prior to initiating empiric antibiotic therapy. The treatment should not be postponed in an ill neonate who is too unstable for CSF evaluation. CSF studies to be obtained include Gram stain, cell count with differential, evaluation of protein and glucose concentrations, and CSF culture(s). However, only the CSF culture is the gold standard for diagnosis.[9] Additional potentially useful diagnostic studies include the following:
   a. CSF lactate: There are reference ranges available for CSF lactate in neonates[10]; however, we are unaware of studies specific to neonates suspected of CSF infection, so any results obtained should be interpreted with caution. Studies involving use of CSF lactate in pediatric patients are available.[11,12]
   b. Polymerase chain reaction (PCR) analysis: This is an excellent test for rapid diagnosis, particularly when viral infection is strongly suspected.[13] It is currently the standard for identification of herpes simplex virus (HSV) and enterovirus in CSF. PCR analysis has good sensitivity and specificity; however, if blood is present in the CSF, results should be cautiously interpreted.

3. Tracheal culture/analysis: Consideration for ventilator-associated pneumonia (VAP) is an important part of the evaluation for an HCAI. When presenting signs or symptoms are consistent with respiratory tract infection, culture and studies are recommended but should be interpreted with caution. Identifying an organism can indicate a pathogen but may just represent colonization. Tracheitis is a diagnostic possibility that may require treatment, but studies are limited in their ability to differentiate it from pneumonia. Gram stains demonstrating the presence of polymorphonuclear leukocytes (PMNs) with bacteria or fungi support the use of empiric therapy but cannot dictate targeted therapy or duration of treatment.[14] Viral studies (respiratory syncytial virus (RSV), metapneumovirus, influenza, enterovirus,

rhinovirus, etc) are important as viral nosocomial infections do occur.[15] Testing (including PCR analysis) for pertussis, mycoplasma, and ureaplasma may also be considered.

4. Urine culture/studies: Compared to early-onset sepsis, the incidence of urinary tract infections (UTIs) is higher in neonates experiencing prolonged hospitalization.[16,17] Premature neonates are particularly susceptible.[18] The presence of an indwelling (Foley) catheter increases the likelihood of a UTI. For diagnosis, urinalysis plus bacterial cultures are recommended. Obtaining fungal cultures is encouraged as clinically indicated.

5. Viral cultures/studies: As previously mentioned, viral studies are important (CSF, blood, urine, nasopharyngeal and tracheal aspirates, skin swabs) because viruses can cause NICU-related HCAIs. PCR analysis is a valuable and rapid diagnostic tool for diagnosing viral infections and can aid in management decisions while awaiting culture results.

6. Complete blood cell count (CBC) with (manual) differential count: A CBC is readily available and frequently obtained from patients hospitalized in the NICU. Results can be trended and used to support or rule out a diagnosis of infection.
   a. Platelets: In sick neonates, thrombocytopenia is frequently observed, but it has no consistent predictive value. Development of new-onset thrombocytopenia (>30% decline from prior baseline value), however, may signal progression to septic shock or invasive gram-negative bacterial or fungal infection.[19]
   b. White blood cells: Either leukocytosis or leukocytopenia heightens a clinician's concern for infection.
   c. Immature/total (I:T) neutrophil ratio: This is calculated as a secondary data point from the differential of the CBC by dividing the total immature neutrophil forms by the total immature plus mature neutrophils. Values less than 0.2 are usually considered within normal limits and not indicative of the presence of an infection.[20] Higher I:T ratios support a diagnosis of infection, especially in conjunction with other abnormal clinical signs and symptoms. An I:T ratio as an isolated index, however, lacks sensitivity and specificity for determining the presence of HCAIs.
   d. Eosinophils: Eosinophilia is also associated with infection in sick infants,[21,22] although there is still debate on the timing of its appearance and potential correlation with other inflammatory conditions (eg, CLD).[23] For more information on the use of the CBC, please see chapter 128.

7. C-reactive protein (CRP): Elevated CRPs obtained serially in conjunction with clinical concern for infection can support a diagnosis of HCAI associated with late-onset sepsis. A clinician should exercise caution when utilizing this test result as a singular index to confirm evidence of infection because there are still many unanswered questions about the value of CRP in managing neonatal sepsis. However, diagnostic accuracy may be improved when used in combination with laboratory indices such as the white blood cell count, I:T ratio, or CD64 count.[24,25] Research into improved application of CRP values is ongoing and includes the intriguing possibility for point-of-care testing.[26]

8. Neutrophil CD64 (nCD64): Neutrophils have been shown to express CD64 when activated. Several studies have found nCD64 determination to have high sensitivity and specificity for the determination of infections when an appropriate cutoff value is selected.[27] Advantages to its use include small blood volume for sampling and rapid results. It is also considered particularly advantageous when used in conjunction with CRP testing for laboratory evaluations of sepsis.[28–30]

9. Other inflammatory markers: Measurements of interleukin (IL) 6, IL-8, tumor necrosis factor α (TNF-α), procalcitonin,[31,32] Neutrophil gelatinase-associated lipocalin (NGAL), and hepcidin[33] have all been examined as additional values providing more accurate diagnosis of infection/sepsis. No robust studies definitively demonstrated that these are superior to current testing modalities. Because there are insufficient data to guide their use for identifying HCAIs in sick neonates, no recommendations are currently made.

10. Blood gas monitoring: Unexplained metabolic acidosis can often indicate infection, and respiratory acidosis, hypoxemia, and hypercarbia may point to new-onset pneumonia or systemic infection. In a sick patient, blood gas monitoring can alert the clinician to acute changes in the patient's status that warrant urgent intervention. Arterial blood gas (ABG) sampling is preferred for its accuracy, although venous or capillary samples may suffice.

11. Imaging studies: Imaging is helpful when respiratory (chest x-ray) or gastrointestinal (abdominal x-ray or ultrasound) symptoms predominate. There may also be concern for intracranial bleeding as a complication of sepsis (cranial ultrasound). An echocardiogram is useful for ruling out worsening cardiac disease (patent ductus arteriosus, persistent pulmonary hypertension of the newborn [PPHN], myocardial dysfunction, etc). Serial imaging is often required.

Table 114-1 Differential Diagnostic Considerations for Health Care-Associated Infections in Neonates

Late-onset sepsis due to perinatally-acquired infection	Late-onset GBS disease, HSV infection
Gastrointestinal emergencies	NEC, malrotation with volvulus
Acute decompensation of chronic/prior disease	CLD, post-NEC stricture, congenital heart disease etc.
Inborn errors of metabolism	Galactosemia, glycogen storage diseases, fatty acid oxidation defects
Iatrogenic	Medication errors

Type of Infection Example Considerations
Abbreviations: CLD, chronic lung disease; GBS, group B streptococci; HSV, herpes simplex virus; NEC, necrotizing enterocolitis.

12. Electroencephalography (EEG): The presence of seizures in premature and sick infants can challenge the clinician caring for NICU patients because seizures can be subclinical or atypical. In addition to a LP, an EEG evaluation in consultation with a pediatric neurologist may be warranted, as neonates can have significant subclinical seizure activity requiring initiation of anticonvulsant therapy to manage the seizures.

Differential Diagnosis/Diagnostic Algorithms

The differential diagnostic list is not extensive for HCAIs, but they can mimic the presentation of other severe diagnoses, including late-onset sepsis associated with perinatally acquired infections (Table 114-1).

MANAGEMENT

Asymptomatic neonates in the NICU with risk factors for HCAI may unexpectedly and rapidly develop symptoms and signs of infection/sepsis. Hence, these patients warrant vigilant monitoring for evidence of developing issues. Once symptomatic, prompt initiation of broad-spectrum antimicrobials and supportive therapy, and clinical investigations into the cause, are critical as a neonate's clinical condition can deteriorate rapidly.

Antibiotic Therapy for HCAIs

When an HCAI is suspected, the initial antibiotic therapy is empirical but targeted against the most likely pathogens. As such, the choice of initial antibiotic therapy may also be guided by previous microorganisms isolated from the patient, as well as the patterns of antibiotic resistance in pathogens causing infections in the patient's NICU. Empiric therapy needs to be initiated promptly, but preferably after cultures have been obtained. If a likely pathogen (not colonizer or contaminant) is identified, then therapy should be tailored and ideally narrowed based on the susceptibilities of the organism(s). Decisions for duration of therapy will be dictated by the source and type of organism(s) isolated as well as the patient's overall clinical course.

1. Intravascular catheter-associated bloodstream infection (CABSI): For infants with suspected CABSI, vancomycin and gentamicin should be initiated to provide empiric coverage for coagulase-negative staphylococci, *Staphylococcus aureus*, and gram-negative bacteria. Linezolid may also be appropriate in units with *Staphylococcus capitis* infections and/or Vancomycin-resistant enterococci.

2. Gram-negative sepsis: In a patient with severe acute deterioration likely caused by a gram-negative organism (eg, *Serratia*, *Enterobacter*, *Klebsiella*, or *Pseudomonas*), double gram-negative coverage may be indicated. For example, both a β-lactam antimicrobial agent (eg, ampicillin or piperacillin-tazobactam) and an aminoglycoside should be initiated in a patient with severe and acute decompensation consistent with gram-negative sepsis. Infections caused by extended-spectrum β-lactamase-producing organisms (or hyperproduction of β-lactamase) need to be treated with meropenem and should be considered in patients with poor response to therapies, even while awaiting susceptibility reports.

3. Anaerobic infection: If there is suspicion that infection can be caused by anaerobic bacteria found in the gastrointestinal tract (eg, necrotizing enterocolitis), clindamycin, metronidazole, or another appropriate antibiotic should be added to the regimen.

4. Consideration of antifungal and antiviral empiric therapy should also be stressed when risk factors are present, particularly when there is a lack of reasonable improvement after initiating broad-spectrum empiric antibiotic therapy.

Supportive Therapy

The main goal of supportive therapy is to increase delivery of substrates to meet tissue demand that has been compromised during an HCAI and prevent recurrent infections. Necessary therapies may involve the following:

1. Remove indwelling intravascular/transmucosal devices: As mentioned, any discussion of HCAIs

includes consideration for their prevention. Indwelling foreign bodies are frequently associated with biofilm production. The formation of biofilm can complicate treatment of an HCAI and impede the clearance of pathogenic organisms, as evidenced by repeatedly positive cultures despite appropriate therapeutic interventions. Removal of indwelling foreign bodies typically facilitates successful eradication of the infection.

2. Administer Oxygen: If necessary (eg, worsening respiratory distress persists), provide adequate support (from nasal cannula to endotracheal intubation and mechanical ventilation).

3. Volume, fluid, and blood pressure support: Initiate rapid fluid resuscitation with crystalloid or colloid parenteral solutions as needed to correct circulatory derangements. An adequate circulating blood volume is necessary to maintain right ventricular filling and cardiac output. However, repeated bolus administration will not provide additional benefit. Correcting underlying vascular compromise, such as peripheral vasodilation and decreased cardiac output, must be promptly addressed through the use of pressor support (dopamine, dobutamine, epinephrine, etc).

4. Treat refractory hypotension/use of corticosteroids: For patients with refractory hypotension, septic shock, or acute adrenal insufficiency not responsive to volume and pressors, the use of hydrocortisone has been reported to have some efficacy in correcting severe hypotension.[34] Short-term adverse effects appear minimal, but many questions remain about long-term consequences. Randomized trials are lacking.

5. Correct metabolic abnormalities (hypoglycemia, hyperkalemia, hypocalcemia, etc): Management of fluid and electrolytes is extremely important. Both metabolic and respiratory acidosis require timely correction.

6. Provide thermoregulatory support: Temperature instability may frequently occur with HCAI and neonatal sepsis. When hypothermia is present, a patient's temperature is artificially regulated. If hyperthermia/fever occurs, pharmacologic cooling measures are appropriate (Nonpharmacologic interventions may also provide benefit.).

7. Reverse disseminated intravascular coagulopathy (DIC): Evidence of abnormal blood clotting should be corrected with transfusions and drugs. However, reversal of DIC often poses considerable challenges despite repletion with blood products. It is important to remember that reversal will not occur until the underlying cause has been effectively treated. Use of factor VII has not been investigated sufficiently to recommend administration to neonates in DIC, although off-label use is anecdotally reported and described in the literature.[35,36]

8. Start inhaled Nitric Oxide (iNO) Therapy: Use of iNO is recommended in infants older than 34 weeks' gestational age[37] with severe hypoxic respiratory failure and inability to maintain the arterial pressure of oxygen (PaO_2) above 80 mm Hg despite maximal respiratory support (in premature infants 34 weeks or less it has equivocal effects on pulmonary outcomes, survival, and neurodevelopmental outcomes). It may also provide support to ventilated infants with a significant (>50%) O_2 requirement and echocardiographic evidence of pulmonary artery pressures close to or above systemic pressure, especially if there is evidence of poor cardiac output. The appropriate starting dose is 20 ppm. Concentrations greater than 20 ppm have no additional positive impact and increase the likelihood of adverse effects, including methemoglobinemia.

9. Initiate extracorporeal membrane oxygenation (ECMO): Consider this modality in neonates older than 34 weeks or 2.5 kg if other means of respiratory and cardiovascular support fail and the patient has a reversible condition. For centers without ECMO support, transfer to a NICU with a higher level of care should be considered and initiated early to optimize the likelihood of a positive outcome for the patient. Long-term follow-up of ECMO survivors demonstrated concerns over neurodevelopmental outcomes, so ethical considerations are important in making the decision to proceed with ECMO support.

10. Monitor renal function closely: This is particularly important for patients treated with nephrotoxic medications, including aminoglycosides (eg, gentamicin) and vancomycin. Renal injury is typically acute and reversible. However, intravenous fluids and medication administration should be reviewed daily and tailored to the level of renal function present. Although typically reversible, infants with confirmed UTI may warrant later follow-up to reassess renal function[18] and genitourinary anatomy. Consultation with pediatric nephrology and/or urology may assist in determining the necessity of additional post-UTI evaluations.

11. Sedation/pain control considerations: Measures to provide comfort with procedures (LP, blood draws, etc) should be undertaken. Neonates do not necessarily require sedation or pain control for ventilator management. However, those patients with PPHN who are difficult to ventilate or oxygenate because of agitation will benefit from adequate sedation. Continuous infusion with benzodiazepines (eg, midazolam)

CHAPTER 114

should be avoided given concerns for adverse neurodevelopmental outcomes. Recognition of rapid tolerance development or neonatal abstinence syndrome is important. Patients already receiving continuous analgesic infusions may require a significantly higher basal infusion rate during an acute episode of HACI. However, as patients recover, timely weaning off or to previous baselines should be initiated as soon as appropriate.

12. Alternative treatment options: Routine use of adjunctive immunotherapeutics, such as white cell transfusions, intravenous immunoglobulin, granulocyte and granulocyte-macrophage colony-stimulating factor administration, activated protein C,[38] pentoxyphylline, and lactoferrin are not recommended as studies were either insufficient to draw adequate conclusions or simply failed to demonstrate an improvement in outcomes for serious infections in neonates.

Prevention

Any discussion regarding the evaluation and management of HCAIs must emphasize prevention, and there are multiple areas to address. Proper hand hygiene and stringent techniques for the handling of invasive catheters yield high-impact results (reductions in HCAIs). The use of prophylactic antifungal therapy continues to be debated and is beyond the scope of this discussion. Please see chapter 53 for additional details on prevention of HCAIs.

Consent/Ethical Considerations

Public disclosure of adverse events and specific disclosure to patients and family members is quickly becoming a legal requirement in many states. Ethically, physicians are expected to discuss adverse events with their patients or patients' families. Given that HCAIs are mostly preventable and inextricably tied to hospital admission, clinicians must consider the legal and ethical ramifications of HCAIs.

CONCLUSION/FOLLOW-UP

Aftercare Monitoring

Neonates with resolution of their HCAI episode should ideally return to their prior baseline or a higher baseline function unless secondary diagnoses or associated complications of the HCAI preclude the ability to attain these goals.

Follow-up Tests

For neonates with additional morbidities associated with HCAIs, additional evaluations should be performed prior to discharge. These may include repeat head ultrasound, brain magnetic resonance imaging (MRI), chest x-ray (determine baseline evidence of CLD at discharge), echocardiography to assess myocardial function/contractility, and cultures to demonstrate clearance of infection (if discharge < 72 hours after resolution of HCAI). Patients should be examined carefully for evidence of thrombus formation as well as for any evidence of persistent neurological deficits that would necessitate outpatient follow-up in consultation with appropriate subspecialists. Because of the potential ototoxicity associated with certain infections and as a recognized side effect of aminoglycoside use, hearing screening has to be performed prior to discharge.

Clinical Follow-up

Neonatal patients with HCAIs were typically sicker and have longer lengths of stay during their hospitalization period. Given that they are considered fragile and at risk, follow-up appointments in 3 to 6 months after discharge with a neonatal/developmental specialist are warranted. Continued follow-up through the first 3 years of life, including regular neurodevelopmental assessments, is also recommended. Should evidence of developmental delay manifest, prompt referral to appropriate services (speech therapy, occupational therapy, physical therapy, etc) is important.

Long-Term Outcome/Implications for Patient/Family

Multiple confounders can significantly hamper the ability to definitively predict long-term outcomes for neonates diagnosed with the infections. The extremely premature infants who had sepsis have a higher incidence of cerebral palsy as compared to those who did not have sepsis during their NICU stay.[39,40] Similarly, infants with bacterial sepsis associated with meningitis have worse neurodevelopmental outcomes, as well as patients that required ECMO support.

REFERENCES

1. Sohn AH, Garrett DO, Sinkowitz-Cochran RL, et al. Pediatric Prevention Network. Prevalence of nosocomial infections in neonatal intensive care unit patients: results from the first national point-prevalence survey. *J Pediatr.* 2001;139(6):821–827.

2. Baltimore RS. Neonatal nosocomial infections. *Semin Perinatol.* 1998;22(1):25–32.

3. Goldmann DA, Durbin WA Jr, Freeman J. Nosocomial infections in a neonatal intensive care unit. *J Infect Dis.* 1981;144(5):449–459.

4. van Ogtrop ML, van Zoeren-Grobben D, Verbakel-Salomons EM, van Boven CP. *Serratia marcescens* infections in neonatal departments: description of an outbreak and review of the literature. *J Hosp Infect.* 1997;36(2):95–103.

5. Edwards JR, Peterson KD, Mu Y, et al. National Healthcare Safety Network (NHSN) report: data summary for 2006 through 2008, issued December 2009. *Am J Infect Control.* 2009;37(10):783–805.

6. Flynn L, Zimmerman LH, Rose A, et al. Vascular catheter tip cultures for suspected catheter-related blood stream infection in the intensive care unit: a tradition whose time has passed. *Surg Infect (Larchmt).* 2012;13(4):245–249.

7. Stoll BJ, Hansen N, Fanaroff AA, et al. To tap or not to tap: high likelihood of meningitis without sepsis among very low birth weight infants. *Pediatrics.* 2004;113:1181.

8. Bruinsma N, Stobberingh EE, Herpers MJ, et al. Subcutaneous ventricular catheter reservoir and ventriculoperitoneal drain-related infections in preterm infants and young children. *Clin Microbiol Infect.* 2000;6(4):202–206.

9. Garges HP, Moody MA, Cotten CM, et al. Neonatal meningitis: what is the correlation among cerebrospinal fluid cultures, blood cultures, and cerebrospinal fluid parameters. *Pediatrics.* 2006;117(4):1094–1100.

10. Leen WG, Willemsen MA, Wevers RA, Verbeek MM. Cerebrospinal fluid glucose and lactate: age-specific reference values and implications for clinical practice. *PLoS One.* 2012;7(8):e427–e445.

11. Eross J, Silink M, Dorman D. Cerebrospinal fluid lactic acidosis in bacterial meningitis. *Arch Dis Child.* 1981;56(9):692–698.

12. Magner M, Szentiványi K, Svandová I, et al. Elevated CSF-lactate is a reliable marker of mitochondrial disorders in children even after brief seizures. *Eur J Paediatr Neurol.* 2011;15(2):101–108.

13. Kimberlin D. Herpes simplex virus, meningitis and encephalitis in neonates. *Herpes.* 2004;11(Suppl 2):65A–76A.

14. O'Horo JC, Thompson D, Safdar N. Is the Gram stain useful in the microbiologic diagnosis of VAP? A meta-analysis. *Clin Infect Dis.* 2012;55(4):551–561.

15. Bennett NJ, Tabarani CM, Bartholoma NM, et al. Unrecognized viral respiratory tract infections in premature infants during their birth hospitalization: a prospective surveillance study in two neonatal intensive care units. *J Pediatr.* 2012;161(5):814–818.

16. Tamim MM, Alesseh H, Aziz H. Analysis of the efficacy of urine culture as part of sepsis evaluation in the premature infant. *Pediatr Infect Dis J.* 2003;22(9):805–808.

17. Samayam P, Ravi Chander B. Study of urinary tract infection and bacteriuria in neonatal sepsis. *Indian J Pediatr.* 2012;79(8):1033–1036.

18. Biyikli NK, Alpay H, Ozek E, Akman I, Bilgen H. Neonatal urinary tract infections: analysis of the patients and recurrences. *Pediatr Int.* 2004;46(1):21–25.

19. Rastogi S, Olmez I, Bhutada A, Rastogi D. Drop in platelet counts in extremely preterm neonates and its association with clinical outcomes. *J Pediatr Hematol Oncol.* 2011;33(8):580–584.

20. Hornik CP, Benjamin DK, Becker KC, et al. Use of the complete blood cell count in early-onset neonatal sepsis. *Pediatr Infect Dis J.* 2012;31(8):799–802.

21. Patel L, Garvey B, Arnon S, Roberts IA. Eosinophilia in newborn infants. *Acta Paediatr.* 1994;83(8):797–801.

22. Juul SE, Haynes JW, McPherson RJ. Evaluation of eosinophilia in hospitalized preterm infants. *J Perinatol.* 2005;25(3):182–188.

23. Yen JM, Lin CH, Yang MM, et al. Eosinophilia in very low birth weight infants. *Pediatr Neonatol.* 2010;51(2):116–123.

24. Dilli D, Oğuz ŞS, Dilmen U, Köker MY, Kizilgun M. Predictive values of neutrophil CD64 expression compared with interleukin-6 and C-reactive protein in early diagnosis of neonatal sepsis. *J Clin Lab Anal.* 2010;24(6):363–370.

25. Hotoura E, Giapros V, Kostoula A, Spyrou P, Andronikou S. Pre-inflammatory mediators and lymphocyte subpopulations in preterm neonates with sepsis. *Inflammation.* 2012;35(3):1094–1101.

26. Diar HA, Nakwa FL, Thomas R, Libhaber EN, Velaphi S. Evaluating the QuikRead C-reactive protein test as a point-of-care test. *Paediatr Int Child Health.* 2012;32(1):35–42.

27. Soni S, Wadhwa N, Kumar R, et al. Evaluation of CD64 expression on neutrophils as an early indicator of neonatal sepsis. *Pediatr Infect Dis J.* 2013;32(1):e33–e37.

28. Ng PC, Li K, Wong RP, et al. Neutrophil CD64 expression: a sensitive diagnostic marker for late-onset nosocomial infection in very low birthweight infants. *Pediatr Res.* 2002;51(3):296–303.

29. Standage SW, Wong HR. Biomarkers for pediatric sepsis and septic shock. *Expert Rev Anti Infect Ther.* 2011;9(1):71–79.

30. Streimish I, Bizzarro M, Northrup V, et al. Neutrophil CD64 as a diagnostic marker in neonatal sepsis. *Pediatr Infect Dis J.* 2012;31(7):777–781.

31. Kocabaş E, Sarikçioğlu A, Aksaray N, et al. Role of procalcitonin, C-reactive protein, interleukin-6, interleukin-8 and tumor necrosis factor-alpha in the diagnosis of neonatal sepsis. *Turk J Pediatr.* 2007;49(1):7–20.

32. Bohnhorst B, Lange M, Bartels DB, et al. Procalcitonin and valuable clinical symptoms in the early detection of neonatal late-onset bacterial infection. *Acta Paediatr.* 2012;101(1):19–25.

33. Wu TW, Tabangin M, Kusano R, et al. The utility of serum hepcidin as a biomarker for late-onset neonatal sepsis. *J Pediatr.* 2013;162(1):67–71.

34. Watterberg K. Evidence-based neonatal pharmacotherapy: postnatal corticosteroids. *Clin Perinatol.* 2012;39(1):47–59.

35. Veldman A, Josef J, Fischer D, Volk WR. A prospective pilot study of prophylactic treatment of preterm neonates with recombinant activated factor VII during the first 72 hours of life. *Pediatr Crit Care Med.* 2006;7(1):34–39.

36. Fischer D, Schloesser R, Buxmann H, Veldman A. Recombinant activated factor VII as a hemostatic agent in very low birth weight preterms with gastrointestinal hemorrhage and disseminated intravascular coagulation. *J Pediatr Hematol Oncol.* 2008;30(5):337–342.

37. Cole FS, Alleyne C, Barks JD, et al. NIH Consensus Development Conference statement: inhaled nitric-oxide therapy for premature infants. *Pediatrics.* 2011;127(2):363–369.

38. Martí-Carvajal AJ, Solà I, Lathyris D, Cardona AF. Human recombinant activated protein C for severe sepsis. *Cochrane Database Syst Rev.* 2012;3:CD004388.

39. Schlapbach LJ, Aebischer M, Adams M, et al. Swiss Neonatal Network and Follow-Up Group. Impact of sepsis on neurodevelopmental outcome in a Swiss National Cohort of extremely premature infants. *Pediatrics.* 2011;128(2):e348–e357.

40. Alshaikh B, Yusuf K, Sauve R. Neurodevelopmental outcomes of very low birthweight infants with neonatal sepsis: systematic review and meta-analysis. *J Perinatol.* 2013;33(7):558–564.

CHAPTER 114

115 Methicillin-Resistant *Staphylococcus aureus* (MRSA) Infection

Kareem Shehab and Kathleen Gutierrez

THE ORGANISM

Staphylococci are aerobic or facultative anaerobic gram-positive cocci in clusters or, less often, chains, pairs, or tetrads. *Staphylococcus aureus* produces coagulase. Staphylococci that do not produce coagulase are reported as coagulase-negative staphylococci (CONS) and include *S. epidermidis*, *S. lugdenensis*, *S. haemolyticus*, and *S. saprophyticus*. Both *S. aureus* and certain species of CONS can cause serious infection in the newborn period. This chapter deals only with infections caused by *S. aureus*.

Staphylococcus aureus became resistant to penicillin shortly after penicillin was introduced in the 1940s by producing penicillinase, which inactivates the β-lactam ring in penicillin. Penicillinase-stable β-lactam antibiotics (methicillin, nafcillin, and oxacillin) were developed to overcome this resistance. However, in 1961, a strain of methicillin-resistant *S. aureus* (MRSA) was identified that was resistant to these newer β-lactam antibiotics.[1] Methicillin resistance occurs as a result of a modified drug target, penicillin-binding protein (PBP2a), encoded by the *mecA* gene[2] on a staphylococcal cassette chromosome (SCC*mec* types I–V).[3] SCC*mec* types II–III typically carry multiple resistance determinants. SCC*mec* types IV–V carry fewer resistance determinants but may be associated with virulence factors such as Panton-Valentine leucocidin (PVL).

Initially, most strains of MRSA were health care or hospital associated (HA-MRSA) and were SCC*mec* types I–III. Now, MRSA can be acquired in the community (CA-MRSA) and colonizes or infects patients who have neither been hospitalized nor had recent access to health care. CA-MRSA is associated with SCC*mec* types IV and V. CA-MRSA tends to be susceptible to more antibiotics compared to HA-MRSA. However, resistance patterns are variable, depending on which strains are circulating in a community.

EPIDEMIOLOGY

Staphylococcus aureus has a propensity to colonize the anterior nares, and many studies evaluating colonization rely on nasal cultures.[4] In infants, other body sites are likely to be colonized, including the throat, umbilicus, skin (groin and axillae), vagina, and rectum.[5–7] Approximately 25%–50% of the population is colonized with *S. aureus*, either methicillin-sensitive strains (MSSA) or MRSA.[8–10] Colonization with MSSA is more common than with MRSA. Children are more likely to be colonized than adults. Some patients are never colonized, some only intermittently, and some persistently. The rate of MRSA colonization in the United States is reported to be low (<2%)[8] but varies depending on the population studied. For example, the following holds:

- Newborns: Fewer than 1% to 40% (colonization rates higher during neonatal intensive care unit [NICU] outbreaks)[11–14]
- Healthy children less than 5 years old: Fewer than 1%–6.7%[15, 16]
- Pregnant women: Fewer than 1%–10% (anogenital cultures)[17–20]
  - There are conflicting reports regarding the association of MRSA genital colonization and group B streptococcus genital colonization.[20]

- Homeless in San Francisco: 2.8%
- Veterinarians: 6.5%[21]
- Pediatric patients in Texas: 22%[22]

It is common for infants to become colonized with *S. aureus* after exposure to their mothers, other family members and friends, or hospital and home environmental surfaces. In most cases, colonization occurs after discharge from the nursery.[23] Transmission of MRSA is reported through the following:

- Infected breast milk and colonized caregivers to neonates[24]
- Health care workers to neonates[25]
- NICU patients to health care workers and their families[26]
- Interinstitutional transfer of MRSA from one nursery to another[27]

Neonatal colonization with *S. aureus* increases with age. Most infants are unlikely to be colonized in the first 3 days of life.[11, 28] Transmission of MRSA from mother to infant during delivery is rare but reported (proven when isolates are matched by pulsed field gel electrophoresis).[23] Most infants colonized with MSSA or MRSA do not develop infection. However, in some studies, 4%–26% of MRSA-colonized infants developed MRSA infection.[11, 12, 28] Risk factors for developing infection with MRSA in the newborn period include[12, 13, 29–35]

- MRSA chorioamnionitis
- Prematurity or very low birth weight
- Cesarean section
- Presence of a central venous or umbilical catheter
- Previous antibiotic use
- Prolonged hospitalization
- Surgical procedures
- Male gender (independent of circumcision)
- Circumcision

Colonization with MRSA clears over time in most infants without specific topical or oral antibiotics for eradication.[11]

Key Point

- In some circumstances, the type of *S. aureus* (MSSA or MRSA) isolated from the anterior nares does not predict the type of *S. aureus* causing infection (eg, MSSA is isolated from the nose but MRSA is isolated from the site of infection or vice versa).[36]

CLINICAL FINDINGS:

MRSA Colonization: Colonized infants are asymptomatic.

MRSA Infection: Clinical features of infection are indistinguishable from those caused by MSSA. Infection with MRSA typically presents after the first week of life[32] but may be present shortly after delivery or a few weeks after discharge from the nursery.

Skin and soft tissue infections (SSTIs): SSTIs comprise most neonatal MRSA infections.

- Superficial skin infection lesions are typical of those seen with *S. aureus* (eg, impetigo) and may be pustular or bullous in appearance.
- Lesions may be present anywhere, but in newborns are often in the diaper area.
- MRSA may cause cellulitis, mastitis, or omphalitis.

MRSA conjunctivitis: MRSA is an increasingly common cause of neonatal bacterial conjunctivitis.[30]

Bacteremia:

- *Staphylococcus aureus* rarely causes early-onset neonatal sepsis.
- Approximately 8% of cases of late-onset sepsis (after 72 hours of life) in low birth weight infants are caused by *S. aureus*.[37, 38]
- Infants with MRSA bacteremia are younger at presentation than those with MSSA bacteremia (mean age at diagnosis 23 vs 32 days).[39]
- Blood cultures may be persistently positive, especially if catheters are not removed immediately.
- Failure to remove a central catheter in less than 4 days has been associated with complicated MRSA disease.[40]

Endocarditis: MRSA endocarditis has been reported in infants and has a high mortality.[40] Premature infants and those with congenital heart disease are most often affected.

Bone and Joint Infections: MRSA bone and joint infections commonly involve multiple foci and are associated with deep vein thromboses with septic embolization to the lungs.

Respiratory: Though MRSA may colonize the respiratory tract or endotracheal tube in asymptomatic infants, it can cause pneumonia, empyema, and lung abscess.[41]

Deep Abscess: Deep abscesses involving the liver and retropharynx have been reported in infants.[42;43]

Central Nervous System Infection:

- Meningitis or brain abscesses are rare but reported, including one case report of an extremely premature infant who succumbed to multiple brain abscesses caused by MRSA.[44]

- Some infants with MRSA bacteremia have a cerebrospinal fluid (CSF) pleocytosis with negative CSF cultures.[31]
- MRSA may cause ventriculoperitoneal shunt infections.

Urinary Tract Infections: These may be seen in infants with bacteremia and disseminated MRSA infection.[45]

Coinfections: Serious coinfections with MRSA and other pathogens have been reported. Infection with MRSA and influenza virus has resulted in serious illness and death.[46,47] MRSA infection occurs in conjunction with other respiratory pathogens such as respiratory synctial virus (RSV), parainfluenza virus, adenovirus, and enteroviruses.[41] *Staphylococcus aureus* (including MRSA) has been isolated from vesiculopustular skin lesions in addition to herpes simplex virus (HSV) in patients with neonatal HSV infection.

DIAGNOSIS

Screening the Asymptomatic Infant

- There are currently no formal consensus guidelines regarding optimal screening procedures for asymptomatic infants for MRSA colonization.[48]
- Many nurseries screen all infants at the time of admission to the hospital. Some screen periodically thereafter until the baby is discharged home. Samples may either be sent for culture (results available within 2–3 days) or *mecA* PCR (results available within 1 day).
- Caregivers of infants who screen positive for MRSA should receive education regarding MRSA.[49] The Centers for Disease Control and Prevention website has educational material for parents regarding MRSA colonization and infection (http://www.cdc.gov/mrsa/index.html).
- Estimated sensitivity of screening for identifying colonized infants[12,50]:
  - Nares: 71%
  - Umbilicus: 60%
  - Skin: 40%
  - Rectum: 21%–60%
  - Nares plus umbilicus: >90%

Evaluation of MRSA in the Symptomatic Infant

- **Physical Examination:** Perform a complete physical examination with particular attention to numbers of venous or arterial catheters, evidence of catheter exit site or tunnel infection, eye discharge, skin lesions, respiratory distress, areas of cellulitis, joint or limb swelling, or failure to move an extremity.

- **Laboratory Testing and Imaging:** Laboratories identify MRSA by determining oxacillin or methicillin resistance by disk diffusion broth microdilution techniques. Larger laboratories may have the technology to identify the *mecA* gene by PCR.[51] Other techniques to differentiate MSSA from MRSA include minilatex agglutination, colorimetric immunoassay methodology, and fluorescence screening.[52]

Evaluation of Specific MRSA Conditions

- Superficial skin infection in a well-appearing healthy infant:
  - Obtain a Gram stain and bacterial culture of pus from skin lesions with full susceptibility testing.
  - Consider testing for HSV and varicella zoster virus (VZV) by direct fluorescent antibody testing, viral culture, or HSV/VZV PCR if lesions are suspicious for HSV or varicella.
- Any infant with signs of sepsis or systemic infection: Perform a full sepsis evaluation, including
  - Lumbar puncture for glucose and protein, complete blood cell count (CBC) with differential, Gram stain, and cultures
  - Blood cultures
  - Urine culture (suprapubic or straight catheterization)
  - C-reactive protein
  - A chest radiograph may show consolidation, pleural effusion, or lung abscess.
  - Echocardiogram should be obtained if blood cultures are positive for *S. aureus* for more than 2–3 days and in patients with congenital heart disease.
  - Plain radiographs of bone can indicate suspected osteomyelitis. Magnetic resonance imaging (MRI) is helpful if feasible. Consider technetium bone scan because multifocal osteomyelitis is seen frequently in neonates.
  - Computed tomography or MRI of the brain should be performed if the patient has clinical or laboratory evidence of central nervous system disease.
  - Abdominal ultrasound can be used to identify liver abscesses, particularly if the patient has had an umbilical catheter in place.[43]

Key Point

- If cultures are positive for MRSA, attention must be paid to the minimum inhibitory concentration (MIC) of the isolate. For organisms with MICs greater than 2 µg/mL to vancomycin or patients who have a poor response to vancomycin, an alternative drug to vancomycin should be considered.

CHAPTER 115

TREATMENT[53]

Key Points

- Methicillin-resistant *S. aureus* is resistant to all penicillins and all first- through fourth-generation cephalosporins.

Vancomycin is recommended as the initial empiric therapy for suspected neonatal MRSA infections pending susceptibility results. Vancomycin trough levels of 15–20 µg/mL are recommended for adults with MRSA infection.[53] Data in neonates and children are limited, but for serious infections, these trough levels may be considered.

Clindamycin can be used empirically if local susceptibility patterns show that less than 10% of isolates are resistant to clindamycin by the D test. Check your hospital antibiogram. Clindamycin can be used for most infections except endovascular or central nervous system infections if the isolate is susceptible.

Linezolid may be considered, except in cases of endovascular infection. Studies evaluating the use of linezolid in neonates with serious MRSA infections are limited. If linezolid is used for a prolonged period (>2 weeks), follow CBC and differential, electrolytes, lactic acid, and liver function studies to assess for toxicity.

Trimethoprim-sulfamethoxazole is not recommended for use in infants less than 2 months of age.

- Colonized asymptomatic infants: No treatment is necessary.
- Uncomplicated superficial skin infection in a healthy term infant:
  - Topical 2% mupirocin
  - Education of caregivers regarding MRSA, including information about the signs and symptoms of invasive disease and guidance concerning measures to prevent the spread of infection in the home.
- SSTI including abscess and cellulitis in well-appearing, afebrile infant:
  - Incision and drainage of abscess
  - No antimicrobial therapy or give an appropriate oral antibiotic. Oral antibiotic choices:
    - Clindamycin is used if susceptible; or
    - Trimethoprim-sulfamethoxazole can be given to infants older than 2 months.
    - Linezolid can be used in select circumstances, but it is costly and associated with bone marrow suppression when used for more than 2 or 3 weeks.
- Extensive SSTI, ill appearing, with temperature instability, prematurity, extremely low birth weight, or immunocompromised:
  - Parenteral therapy with vancomycin or clindamycin (if local rate of resistance is < 10%) can be

used at least until improvement is noted and bacteremia ruled out.
  - If infection is severe, surgical consultation, vancomycin *plus* naficillin with or without other antimicrobials (for gram-negative and anaerobic coverage) are used until culture results are known. The optimal duration of therapy for SSTI is unknown. Courses range from 5 to 14 days and are guided by clinical response.
- MRSA conjunctivitis:
  - Treat with ophthalmic drops (eg, Polytrim®)
  - Consider oral therapy if infection recurs or does not respond to treatment
- Ill-appearing infant with no focal findings who has been hospitalized for several days:
  - Empiric therapy: intravenous vancomycin plus cefotaxime with or without aminoglycoside pending culture results
- Documented MRSA bacteremia:
  - Intravenous vancomycin. Follow vancomcyin levels and consider aiming for trough levels between 15 and 20 µg/mL. Monitor renal function and CBC with differential. If the organism is MSSA, do not use vancomycin. Nafcillin or a first-generation cephalosporin remain drugs of choice for MSSA infection.
  - Intravenous clindamycin (if susceptible) may be considered for non-endovascular bacteremia provided cultures clear immediately.[53]
  - Intravenous linezolid may be considered for nonendovascular bacteremia.
  - Remove all central lines.
  - Continue to obtain blood cultures until negative; MRSA bacteremia may be prolonged.
  - Assess daily for foci of disseminated infection.
  - Treat for a minimum of 14 days (longer if evidence of disseminated infection is present).
- MRSA endovascular infection (endocarditis)[54]:
  - Intravenous vancomycin. Adjunctive therapy with rifampin and gentamicin may be considered after consultation with a pediatric infectious disease specialist.
  - MRSA isolates with a vancomycin MIC of 2 µg/mL or greater by broth microdilution are associated with treatment failures, despite appearing susceptible in vitro. Consultation with an infectious disease specialist in such cases is recommended.
  - Clindamycin and linezolid are bacteriostatic drugs and should not be used as sole treatment of endovascular infections.
  - Echocardiograms should be obtained on all children with congenital heart disease or bacteremia lasting more than 2 or 3 days.
  - The minimum duration of therapy is 6 weeks.
  - A patient with endocarditis must be managed in conjunction with a cardiology specialist.

Infants with *S. aureus* endocarditis are at risk for acute heart failure, dehiscence of a valve, myocardial abscesses, and embolic events.

- MRSA pneumonia:
  - If empyema is present, it should be drained surgically.
  - Antibiotic choices are vancomycin, clindamycin, or linezolid.
- MRSA bone or joint infection[55]:
  - Osteomyelitis:
    - Surgical debridement of infected bone and contiguous soft tissue or muscle abscesses should be performed.
    - Antibiotic choices are intravenous vancomycin, clindamycin, or linezolid.
    - Minimum duration of therapy is 4–6 weeks.
    - A substantial number of cases of osteomyelitis also involve the adjacent joint and multiple bones.
  - Septic arthritis:
    - Drainage or debridement of the joint space should be performed.
    - Antibiotic choices are the same as for osteomyelitis.
    - Duration of therapy is a minimum of 3–4 weeks if bone involvement has been ruled out.
- MRSA central nervous system infections:
  - Meningitis:
    - Intravenous vancomycin may be given for 2 weeks with or without rifampin.
    - Intravenous linezolid may also be considered.
    - If a ventricular shunt is present, it must be removed.
    - Consider head imaging to rule out focal abscess.
  - Brain, subdural, or epidural abscess:
    - Neurosurgical consultation should be provided for abscess drainage.
    - Intravenous vancomycin is given for 4–6 weeks with or without rifampin.
    - Intravenous linezolid may also be considered.

OUTCOMES

Mortality, duration of hospitalization, and neurodevelopmental impairment for infants with MRSA bacteremia are similar to those with MSSA bacteremia.[56] Duration of positive blood cultures is often prolonged.

INFECTION CONTROL

- Excellent hand hygiene is key in preventing nosocomial spread of MRSA.[57] One study showed a negative correlation between the amount of alcohol gel used and prevalence of MRSA colonization in a neonatal intensive care nursery.[58] Hands that are visibly soiled should be washed with soap and water.
- Infants colonized or infected with MRSA should be placed in contact isolation for the duration of hospitalization and subsequent hospitalizations.[59]
- Infants with MRSA pneumonia should receive droplet precautions.
- Other strategies used to prevent or halt outbreaks of MRSA infections in newborn nurseries include[51, 60, 61]
  - Application of 1% chlorhexidine powder, triple dye, or iodophor to the umbilical stump.
  - Prevention of nursery overcrowding or understaffing.
  - Cohorting of colonized or infected babies and caregivers.
  - Use of mupiricin or other antibiotics has not been consistently shown to eradicate colonization.
- An infant who received treatment of MRSA infection and recovers will often remain colonized despite a prolonged course of intravenous or oral therapy.

MATERNAL MRSA INFECTON AND BREASTFEEDING

- A recent review discussed in detail the safety of antibiotics prescribed to lactating mothers with MRSA infections who breast-feed.[62]
- Detailed, up-to-date information regarding safety of drugs used by lactating mothers (to the infant) is available through the United States National Library of Medicine Toxicology Data Network (see LactMed at http://toxnet.nlm.nih.gov/cgi-bin/sis/htmlgen?LACT).
- In general, only low concentrations of antibiotics are found in breast milk. Anticipated adverse events include alteration of infant bowel flora. Caution is recommended if the mother is receiving trimethoprim-sulfamethoxazole and the infant has glucose-6-phosphate dehydrogenase deficiency, is premature or ill, or has hyperbilirubinemia.[63]
- The mother with MRSA mastitis may continue to breast-feed her infant unless the infant is premature or seriously ill.

REFERENCES

1. Jevons M. "Celbenin"-resistant Staphylococci. *BMJ*. 1961: 124–125.
2. Chambers HF, Hartman BJ, Tomasz A. Increased amounts of a novel penicillin-binding protein in a strain of methicillin-resistant *Staphylococcus aureus* exposed to nafcillin. *J Clin Invest*. 1985;76(1):325–331.
3. Deurenberg RH, et al. The molecular evolution of methicillin-resistant *Staphylococcus aureus*. *Clin Microbiol Infect*. 2007;13(3): 222–235.
4. Kluytmans J, van Belkum A, Verbrugh H. Nasal carriage of *Staphylococcus aureus*: epidemiology, underlying mechanisms, and associated risks. *Clin Microbiol Rev*. 1997;10(3):505–520.

5. Andrews JI, et al. Screening for *Staphylococcus aureus* carriage in pregnancy: usefulness of novel sampling and culture strategies. *Am J Obstet Gynecol.* 2009;201(4):396 e1–5.

6. Bizzarro MJ, Gallagher PG. Antibiotic-resistant organisms in the neonatal intensive care unit. *Semin Perinatol.* 2007;31(1):26–32.

7. Faden H, et al. Clinical and molecular characteristics of staphylococcal skin abscesses in children. *J Pediatr.* 2007;151(6):700–703.

8. Gorwitz RJ, et al. Changes in the prevalence of nasal colonization with *Staphylococcus aureus* in the United States, 2001–2004. *J Infect Dis.* 2008;197(9):1226–1234.

9. Kuehnert MJ, et al. Prevalence of *Staphylococcus aureus* nasal colonization in the United States, 2001–2002. *J Infect Dis.* 2006;193(2):172–179.

10. Nakamura MM, et al. Prevalence of methicillin-resistant *Staphylococcus aureus* nasal carriage in the community pediatric population. *Pediatr Infect Dis J.* 2002;21(10):917–922.

11. Gregory ML, Eichenwald EC, Puopolo KM. Seven-year experience with a surveillance program to reduce methicillin-resistant *Staphylococcus aureus* colonization in a neonatal intensive care unit. *Pediatrics.* 2009;123(5):e790–e796.

12. Huang YC, et al. Methicillin-resistant *Staphylococcus aureus* colonization and its association with infection among infants hospitalized in neonatal intensive care units. *Pediatrics.* 2006;118(2):469–474.

13. Maraqa NF, et al. Prevalence of and risk factors for methicillin-resistant *Staphylococcus aureus* colonization and infection among infants at a level III neonatal intensive care unit. *Am J Infect Control.* 2011;39(1):35–41.

14. Murillo JL, Cohen M, Kreiswirth B. Results of nasal screening for methicillin-resistant *Staphylococcus aureus* during a neonatal intensive care unit outbreak. *Am J Perinatol.* 2010;27(1):79–81.

15. Cheng Immergluck L, et al. Prevalence of *Streptococcus pneumoniae* and *Staphylococcus aureus* nasopharyngeal colonization in healthy children in the United States. *Epidemiol Infect.* 2004;132(2):159–166.

16. Miller MB, et al. Prevalence and risk factor analysis for methicillin-resistant *Staphylococcus aureus* nasal colonization in children attending child care centers. *J Clin Microbiol.* 2011;49(3):1041–1047.

17. Andrews WW, et al. Genital tract methicillin-resistant *Staphylococcus aureus*: risk of vertical transmission in pregnant women. *Obstet Gynecol.* 2008;111(1):113–118.

18. Creech CB, et al. Frequency of detection of methicillin-resistant *Staphylococcus aureus* from rectovaginal swabs in pregnant women. *Am J Infect Control.* 2010;38(1):72–74.

19. Reusch M, et al. Prevalence of MRSA colonization in peripartum mothers and their newborn infants. *Scand J Infect Dis.* 2008;40(8):667–671.

20. Chen KT, et al. Prevalence of methicillin-sensitive and methicillin-resistant *Staphylococcus aureus* in pregnant women. *Obstet Gynecol.* 2006;108(3 Pt 1):482–487.

21. Hanselman BA, et al. Methicillin-resistant *Staphylococcus aureus* colonization in veterinary personnel. *Emerg Infect Dis.* 2006;12(12):1933–1938.

22. Alfaro C, et al. Prevalence of methicillin-resistant *Staphylococcus aureus* nasal carriage in patients admitted to Driscoll Children's Hospital. *Pediatr Infect Dis J.* 2006;25(5):459–461.

23. Pinter DM, et al. Maternal-infant perinatal transmission of methicillin-resistant and methicillin-sensitive *Staphylococcus aureus*, *Am J Perinatol.* 2009;26(2):145–151.

24. David MD, et al. Community-associated methicillin-resistant *Staphylococcus aureus*: nosocomial transmission in a neonatal unit. *J Hosp Infect.* 2006;64(3):244–250.

25. Mean M, et al. A neonatal specialist with recurrent methicillin-resistant *Staphylococcus aureus* (MRSA) carriage implicated in the transmission of MRSA to newborns. *Infect Control Hosp Epidemiol.* 2007;28(5):625–628.

26. McAdams RM, et al. Spread of methicillin-resistant *Staphylococcus aureus* USA300 in a neonatal intensive care unit. *Pediatr Int.* 2008;50(6):810–815.

27. McDonald JR, et al. Methicillin-resistant *Staphylococcus aureus* outbreak in an intensive care nursery: potential for interinstitutional spread. *Pediatr Infect Dis J.* 2007;26(8):678–683.

28. Kim YH, et al. Clinical outcomes in methicillin-resistant *Staphylococcus aureus*-colonized neonates in the neonatal intensive care unit. *Neonatology.* 2007;91(4):241–247.

29. Pimentel JD, Meier FA, Samuel LP. Chorioamnionitis and neonatal sepsis from community-associated MRSA. *Emerg Infect Dis.* 2009;15(12):2069–2071.

30. Lessa FC, et al. Trends in incidence of late-onset methicillin-resistant *Staphylococcus aureus* infection in neonatal intensive care units: data from the National Nosocomial Infections Surveillance System, 1995–2004; *Pediatr Infect Dis J.* 2009;28(7):577–581.

31. Fortunov RM, et al. Evaluation and treatment of community-acquired *Staphylococcus aureus* infections in term and late-preterm previously healthy neonates. *Pediatrics.* 2007;120(5):937–945.

32. James L, et al. Methicillin-resistant *Staphylococcus aureus* infections among healthy full-term newborns. *Arch Dis Child Fetal Neonatal Ed,* 2008;93(1):F40–F44.

33. Sakaki H, et al. An investigation of the risk factors for infection with methicillin-resistant *Staphylococcus aureus* among patients in a neonatal intensive care unit. *Am J Infect Control.* 2009;37(7):580–586.

34. Nguyen DM, et al. Risk factors for neonatal methicillin-resistant *Staphylococcus aureus* infection in a well-infant nursery. *Infect Control Hosp Epidemiol.* 2007;28(4):406–411.

35. Van Howe RS, Robson WL. The possible role of circumcision in newborn outbreaks of community-associated methicillin-resistant *Staphylococcus aureus,* *Clin Pediatr (Phila),* 2007;46(4):356–358.

36. Chen AE, et al. Discordance between *Staphylococcus aureus* nasal colonization and skin infections in children. *Pediatr Infect Dis J.* 2009;28(3):244–246.

37. Carey AJ, Saiman L, Polin RA. Hospital-acquired infections in the NICU: epidemiology for the new millennium. *Clin Perinatol.* 2008;35(1):223–249, x.

38. Stoll BJ, et al. Late-onset sepsis in very low birth weight neonates: the experience of the NICHD Neonatal Research Network. *Pediatrics.* 2002;110(2 Pt 1):285–291.

39. Carey AJ, et al. The epidemiology of methicillin-susceptible and methicillin-resistant *Staphylococcus aureus* in a neonatal intensive care unit, 2000–2007. *J Perinatol.* 2010;30(2):135–139.

40. Carrillo-Marquez MA, et al. Clinical and molecular epidemiology of *Staphylococcus aureus* catheter-related bacteremia in children. *Pediatr Infect Dis J.* 2010;29(5):410–414.

41. Carrillo-Marquez MA, et al. *Staphylococcus aureus* pneumonia in children in the era of community-acquired methicillin-resistance at Texas Children's Hospital. *Pediatr Infect Dis J.* 2011;30(7):545–550.

42. Fleisch AF, et al. Methicillin-resistant *Staphylococcus aureus* as a cause of extensive retropharyngeal abscess in two infants. *Pediatr Infect Dis J.* 2007;26(12):1161–1163.

43. Simeunovic E, et al. Liver abscess in neonates. *Pediatr Surg Int.* 2009;25(2):153–156.

44. Woodlief RS, Markowitz JE. Unrecognized invasive infection in a neonate colonized with methicillin-resistant *Staphylococcus aureus,* *J Pediatr.* 2009;155(6):943–943 e1.

45. Nambiar S, Herwaldt LA, Singh N. Outbreak of invasive disease caused by methicillin-resistant *Staphylococcus aureus* in neonates and prevalence in the neonatal intensive care unit. *Pediatr Crit Care Med.* 2003;4(2):220–226.

46. Finelli L, et al. Influenza-associated pediatric mortality in the United States: increase of *Staphylococcus aureus* coinfection. *Pediatrics.* 2008;122(4):805–811.

47. Reed C, et al. Infection with community-onset *Staphylococcus aureus* and influenza virus in hospitalized children. *Pediatr Infect Dis J.* 2009;28(7):572–576.

48. Milstone AM, et al. Identification and eradication of methicillin-resistant *Staphylococcus aureus* colonization in the neonatal intensive care unit: results of a national survey. *Infect Control Hosp Epidemiol.* 2010;31(7):766–768.

49. Sengupta A, et al. Knowledge, awareness, and attitudes regarding methicillin-resistant *Staphylococcus aureus* among caregivers of hospitalized children. *J Pediatr.* 2011;158(3):416–421.

50. Rosenthal A, et al. Optimal surveillance culture sites for detection of methicillin-resistant *Staphylococcus aureus* in newborns. *J Clin Microbiol.* 2006;44(11):4234–4236.

51. Song X, et al. A stepwise approach to control an outbreak and ongoing transmission of methicillin-resistant *Staphylococcus aureus* in a neonatal intensive care unit. *Am J Infect Control.* 2010;38(8):607–611.

52. Long CB, Madan RP, Herold BC. Diagnosis and management of community-associated MRSA infections in children. *Expert Rev Anti Infect Ther.* 2010;8(2):183–195.

53. Liu C, et al. Clinical practice guidelines by the infectious diseases society of america for the treatment of methicillin-resistant *Staphylococcus aureus* infections in adults and children. *Clin Infect Dis,* 2011;52(3):e18–e55.

54. Baddour LM, et al. Infective endocarditis: diagnosis, antimicrobial therapy, and management of complications: a statement for healthcare professionals from the Committee on Rheumatic Fever, Endocarditis, and Kawasaki Disease, Council on Cardiovascular Disease in the Young, and the Councils on Clinical Cardiology, Stroke, and Cardiovascular Surgery and Anesthesia, American Heart Association: endorsed by the Infectious Diseases Society of America. *Circulation.* 2005;111(23):e394–e434.

55. Saphyakhajon P, et al. Empiric antibiotic therapy for acute osteoarticular infections with suspected methicillin-resistant *Staphylococcus aureus* or *Kingella, Pediatr Infect Dis J.* 2008;27(8):765–767.

56. Cohen-Wolkowiez M, et al. Mortality and neurodevelopmental outcome after *Staphylococcus aureus* bacteremia in infants. *Pediatr Infect Dis J.* 2007;26(12):1159–1161.

57. Lepelletier D, et al. Eradication of methicillin-resistant *Staphylococcus aureus* in a neonatal intensive care unit: which measures for which success? *Am J Infect Control.* 2009;37(3):195–200.

58. Sakamoto F, et al. Increased use of alcohol-based hand sanitizers and successful eradication of methicillin-resistant *Staphylococcus aureus* from a neonatal intensive care unit: a multivariate time series analysis. *Am J Infect Control.* 2010;38(7):529–534.

59. Staphylococcal infections. In: Pickering LK, Baker CJ, Kimberlin DW, Long SS, eds. *Redbook: 2012 Report of the Committee on Infectious Diseases,* 29th ed. Elk Grove Village, IL: American Academy of Pediatrics; 2012:653.

60. Milstone AM, et al. Role of decolonization in a comprehensive strategy to reduce methicillin-resistant *Staphylococcus aureus* infections in the neonatal intensive care unit: an observational cohort study. *Infect Control Hosp Epidemiol.* 2010;31(5):558–560.

61. Laing IA, Gibb AP, McCallum A. Controlling an outbreak of MRSA in the neonatal unit: a steep learning curve. *Arch Dis Child Fetal Neonatal Ed.* 2009;94(4):F307–F310.

62. Mitrano JA, Spooner LM, and Belliveau P. Excretion of antimicrobials used to treat methicillin-resistant *Staphylococcus aureus* infections during lactation: safety in breastfeeding infants. *Pharmacotherapy,* 2009;29(9):1103–1109.

63. LactMed. Home page. http://toxnet.nlm.nih.gov/cgi-bin/sis/htmlgen?LACT

Diagnosis of Congenital Toxoplasmosis

Rima McLeod, Daniel Lee, Fatima Clouser, and Kenneth Boyer

INTRODUCTION

Abundant and convincing evidence demonstrates that medicines block transmission of *Toxoplasma gondii* from the pregnant woman to her fetus, kill tachyzoites, reduce or eliminate parasite burden, reduce or eliminate eye disease, reduce or eliminate brain disease, reduce severity of disease, eliminate meningitis, treat meningoencephalitis, and lower immune markers of infection.[1–4] Earlier, there was some controversy in the literature (discussed in Reference 4), but currently, review of data from in vitro and experimental animal studies, attention to older publications of studies that were performed meticulously (reviewed in References 1–4), and several recent studies have clarified the efficacy and benefits of proper, early, and rapid diagnosis and medical treatment.[5,6] The recent data demonstrate how important it is to establish such diagnosis and treatment as the standard for medical care to prevent the loss of productive lives to this disease. The time when the acute infection is diagnosed and treated is critical.[1–5] The earlier the infection is treated, the better the outcomes will be for fetus, infant, and congenitally infected person.[5,6] For this reason, the focus of this chapter is to make clear how diagnosis and treatment of the fetus and infant can be optimized and how this is carried out practically.

PREVENTION WITH EDUCATION DURING GESTATION

The approach to diagnose, prevent, and treat infections of the fetus is summarized in Tables 116-1 to 116-8 and Figures 116-1 to 116-4. The pregnant woman with acute acquired *T. gondii* infection and the mother of a congenitally infected infant may have retinal disease caused by the parasite and should have a retinal examination. Simple instructions concerning avoiding means of acquisition of the parasite provide an opportunity to prevent some fetal infections in the pregnant woman. An educational pamphlet is provided in Chapter 57, Figure 57-3. This may be downloaded from the Internet without charge or copyright (http://www.toxoplasmosis.org/pamphlet.pdf) so it can be provided to pregnant patients or those considering becoming pregnant. However, environmental contamination by oocysts is common and often unrecognized. Risk cannot be eliminated entirely by education. Infection may occur in persons with no recognized risk factors.

GESTATIONAL SCREENING: DIAGNOSIS, PREVENTION, AND TREATMENT OF THE ACUTELY INFECTED PREGNANT WOMAN AND FETUS

Figure 116-1 and Figure 57-23 in Chapter 57 summarizes an approach used universally in France, where it successfully detects seroconversion during gestation to prevent transmission to the fetus and to identify infection in the fetus. This allows treatment without delay. In this approach,[1–21] currently utilized in some of the best obstetrical practices in the United States, serologic screening for *T. gondii* specific antibody to immunoglobulin G (IgG) and immunoglobulin M (IgM) is performed once a month during gestation for all pregnant women who are seronegative and is initiated by the 11th week of gestation. Ideally, such screening

Table 116-1 Guidelines for Treatment of *Toxoplasma gondii* Infection in the Pregnant Woman and Congenital *Toxoplasma* Infection in the Fetus, Infant, and Older Children[a]

Infection	Medication	Dosage	Duration of Therapy
In pregnant women infected during gestation:			
First 18 weeks of gestation or until term if fetus found not to be infected by amniocentesis at 18 weeks or clinical findings	Spiramycin[b]	1 g every 8 hours without food	Until fetal infection is documented or if it is excluded at 18 weeks of gestation until term
If fetal infection confirmed after week 18 of gestation and in all women infected after week 24	Pyrimethamine[c] plus	Loading dose: 50 mg each 12 hours for 2 days; beginning on day 3, give 50 mg/d	Until term[d]
	Sulfadiazine plus	Loading dose: 75 mg/kg; beginning with next dose, 50 mg/kg each 12 hours (maximum 4 g per day)	Until term[d]
	Leucovorin (folinic acid)[c]	10–20 mg daily[e]	During and for 1 week after pyrimethamine therapy discontinued
Congenital *T. gondii* infection in infant[e]	Pyrimethamine[c,e] plus	Loading dose: 1 mg/kg each 12 hours for 2 days; beginning on day 3, give 1 mg/kg/d for 2 or 6 months,[e] then give this dose every Monday, Wednesday, Friday[e]	1 year[f]
	Sulfadiazine[f] plus	50 mg/kg each 12 hours	1 year[f]
	Leucovorin[c]	10 mg 3 times weekly = > daily	During and for 1 week after pyrimethamine therapy
	Corticosteroids[g] (prednisone) have been used when CSF protein is ≥ 1 g/dL and when active chorioretinitis threatens vision	0.5 mg/kg each 12 hours	Corticosteroids continued until resolution of elevated (≥1 g/dL) CSF protein level or active chorioretinitis that threatens vision
Active chorioretinitis in older children	Pyrimethamine[c] plus	Loading dose: 1 mg/kg each 12 hours (maximum 50 mg) for 2 days; beginning on day 3, maintenance, 1 mg/kg/d (maximum 25 mg in young children, 50 mg in older persons)	Usually 1–2 weeks beyond the time that signs and symptoms have resolved
	Sulfadiazine[f] plus	Loading dose: 75 mg/kg; beginning 12 hours later, maintenance, 50 mg/kg every 12 hours	Usually 1–2 weeks beyond the time that signs and symptoms have resolved
	Leucovorin[c]	10–20 mg 3 times weekly[c], = > daily	During and for 1 week after pyrimethamine therapy

(Continued)

Table 116-1 Guidelines for Treatment of *Toxoplasma gondii* Infection in the Pregnant Woman and Congenital *Toxoplasma* Infection in the Fetus, Infant, and Older Children[a] (*Continued*)

Infection	Medication	Dosage	Duration of Therapy
	Corticosteroids[f] (prednisone)	1 mg/kg/d, divided twice daily; maximum 40 mg per day followed by rapid taper	Steroids are continued until inflammation subsides (usually 1–2 weeks) and then tapered rapidly

Abbreviation: CSF, cerebrospinal fluid; PCR, polymerase chain reaction.

[a]Table and caption from Remington et al,[2] with permission.

[b]In the United States, available only on request from the US Food and Drug Administration (call 301-443-5680), and with this approval by the physician's request to Aventis (908-231-3365).

[c]Adjusted for granulocytopenia; complete blood cell counts, including platelets, should be monitored each Monday and Thursday.

[d]Subsequent treatment of the infant is the same as that described under treatment of congenital infection. When the diagnosis of infection in the fetus is established earlier, we suggest that sulfadiazine be used alone until after the first trimester, at which time pyrimethamine should be added to the regimen. The decision about when to begin pyrimethamine/sulfadiazine/leucovorin for the pregnant woman is based on an assessment of the risk of fetal infection, incidence of false-positive and false-negative results of amniocentesis with PCR assay, and risks associated with medicines. When infection of the mother is acquired between 22 and 29 weeks of gestation, the incidence of transmission exceeds 50%. With maternal acquisition of infection after 31 weeks of gestation, incidence of transmission exceeds 60%, and manifestations of infection are in general less severe. When infection is acquired between 21 and 29 weeks of gestation, management varies. After 24 weeks of gestation, we recommend that amniocentesis be performed and that pyrimethamine /leucovorin/sulfadiazine be used instead of spiramycin. In France, standard of care (until late in gestation) is to wait 4 weeks from the estimated time maternal infection is acquired until amniocentesis to allow sufficient time for transmission to occur. This is to ensure diagnosis is accurate. Amniocentesis is not performed before 17 to 18 weeks of gestation. In some instances, when maternal infection is acquired between 12 and 16 weeks of gestation or after the 21st week of gestation, pyrimethamine and sulfadiazine treatment is initiated regardless of the amniotic fluid PCR result. When this approach is used, a delay in amniocentesis when maternal infection is acquired between 12 and 16 weeks and after 21 weeks of gestation would not be logical.

[e]Both regimens appear to be feasible and relatively safe. The optimal duration of therapy is unknown for infants and children, especially those with AIDS.

[f]Alternative medicines for patients with atopy or severe intolerance of sulfonamides have included pyrimethamine and leucovorin with clindamycin, or azithromycin, or atovaquone, with standard dosages as recommended according to weight.

[g]Corticosteroids should be used only in conjunction with pyrimethamine, sulfadiazine, and leucovorin treatment and should be continued until signs of inflammation (high CSF protein, ≥ 1 g/DL) or active chorioretinitis that threatens vision have subsided; dosage can then be tapered and the steroids discontinued.

Table 116-2 Samples Obtained in Delivery Room

Sample	Storage	Shipping	Use
I. 200 g from the insertion cord on the fetal side or whole placenta (approximately 14 cm × 3 cm × 3 cm = 100 g)	• Store sterilely in a sterile saline (*no formalin or other preservative; do not freeze*). • Penicillin (100 U/mL) and streptomycin (100 μg/mL) may be added. • Keep placenta cool (*not frozen*) with ice bag or preferably cold packs.	• Ship immediately by overnight delivery service • The US Reference Laboratory address: Research Institute Palo Alto Medical Foundation Attn: Toxoplasma Serology Laboratory Ames Building 795 El Camino Real Palo Alto, CA 94301 (650) 853-4828 • For shipping to France, please contact: Herve Pelloux HPelloux@chu-grenoble.fr	For subinoculation into mice and PCR
II. 10–20 mL amniotic fluid, if available	• Keep cold (*not frozen*) and ship with sample A as described previously. • Each sample for PCR should be placed in a separate sealed bag to prevent cross-contamination.	To be centrifuged by reference laboratory	For PCR of pellet and subinoculation if clinically indicated; not needed if diagnosis confirmed earlier or essential if unavailable

Abbreviation: PCR, polymerase chain reaction.

This includes placenta to be sent to a reference laboratory for (I) subinoculation into mice and (II) PCR; amniotic fluid, if available.

Table 116-3 Samples Obtained From Infant Subsequent to Delivery

Site	Sample	Use/Instructions
I. Processed and analyzed at the delivering hospital (Use pediatric tubes and minimum volume)	1. Peripheral blood	CBC with differential and platelet count
	2. Serum	• Total IgM, IgG, IgA, albumin • SGPT, SGOT, total and direct bilirubin, creatine
	3. Urine	Urinalysis
	4. Cerebrospinal fluid	• Cell count, glucose protein, and total IgG • Hold 0.5 mL frozen cerebrospinal fluid for quantitative IgG if needed later to calculate antibody load
II. Sent to the Palo Alto Medical Foundation[a]	1. Sterile infant whole peripheral blood, 2.0 mL	• This is peripheral blood (ie, not umbilical cord blood). • Place in **two** purple-top 1-mL tubes. • This is for PCR and subinoculation of buffy coat.
	2. Serum, 1 mL (also send clot underlying serum)	• Serum is for *Toxoplasma* baby panel: Sabin Feldman dye test, IgM ISAGA, IgA ELISA. • Clot is for subinoculation.
	3.a. Cerebrospinal fluid, 0.5 mL 3.b. Cerebrospinal fluid, 1.0 mL	a. *Toxoplasma gondii*-specific IgG (dye test) and IgM ELISA b. PCR
	4. Urine, 5 mL	For PCR (not essential; investigational; might be useful)

Abbreviations: CBC, complete blood cell count; ELISA, enzyme-linked immunosorbent assay; Ig, immunoglobulin; ISAGA, immunosorbent agglutination assay; PCR, polymerase chain reaction; SGOT, aspartate aminotransferase; SGPT, alanine aminotransferase.
[a]Samples should be kept cold (*not frozen*). If physician wishes to discuss results with Toxoplasmosis Center physicians, include permission form for the Palo Alto Medical Foundation (PAMF) to release serologic and isolation results to the Toxoplasmosis Research Institute and Center/Dr. McLeod. Note that these may be stored and shipped with 200 g to whole placenta from the cord insertion area on the fetal side (Table 116-1, I).

Table 116-4 Samples Obtained From Mother Subsequent to Delivery

Site	Sample	Use/Instructions
Sent to the Palo Alto Medical Foundation[a]	2 mL maternal serum	For immunoglobulin (Ig) G in parallel with infant IgG test and can be used for IgM and IgA if clinically indicated

[a]Samples should be kept cold (*not frozen*). If physician wishes to discuss results with Toxoplasmosis Center physicians, include permission form for the Palo Alto Medical Foundation (PAMF) to release serologic and isolation results to the Toxoplasmosis Research Institute and Center/Dr. McLeod. Note that these may be stored and shipped with 200 g to whole placenta from the cord insertion area on the fetal side (Table 116-1, I).

Table 116-5 Examinations and Evaluations of Baby Following Birth

Examination/Evaluation	Details
General examination	
Pediatric ophthalmologist	
Pediatric neurologist	
CT scan of the brain	• Baby should not be sedated and may be gently swaddled. • This examination is done without contrast. • Examines for ventricular size and brain calcifications.
Auditory acoustic emissions or brainstem auditory evoked response (BAER); hearing test	

would, and sometimes does, begin immediately before or early in gestation at the time pregnancy is noted, even when this is earlier than 11 weeks' gestation. Screening is continued monthly through the time the infant is born and is performed at birth and when the infant is 1 month old to detect infections acquired late in gestation. This approach presents the opportunity to confirm when a pregnant woman seroconverts (ie, newly develops specific IgG antibody to *T. gondii*). This is done so that acute acquired infection can be proven by more specialized testing. In the United States, this specialized testing is performed in a reference laboratory (Table 116-7). This then enables the physician to prevent transmission from the newly infected pregnant woman to her fetus through treatment of the mother with spiramycin early in gestation (Table 116-1). Fetal ultrasounds are obtained every 2 weeks until term for mothers who seroconvert. It is then possible to diagnose infection in the fetus by ultrasound or amniocentesis. It enables treatment of the infected fetus when

Table 116-6 Amounts, Handling, and Shipping of Samples (Currently Available Tests in United States or France Reference Laboratories)

Test	Reason	Sample	Preferred (Minimum Amount)	Store/Ship	Additional Comments
Dye test IgG	To establish infection[a]	Serum	0.25 mL (0.15 mL)	Cool[b]	
Direct agglutination IgG	To date infection to ≥ 12–16 weeks	Serum	0.25 mL	Cool	
IgM ELISA	Older child and adult	Serum	0.25 mL	Cool	
IgM ISAGA	Newborn Infant	Serum	0.25 mL	Cool	Only for babies < 6 months
IgA ELISA		Serum	0.25 mL	Cool	
IgE ELISA	May be useful to diagnose acute infection in pregnant woman	Serum	0.25 mL	Cool	Limited clinical use
AC/HS	Pregnant woman	Serum	0.25 mL (0.10 mL)	Cool	For pregnant women
Avidity	Pregnant woman	Serum	0.30 mL (0.25 mL)	Cool	For pregnant women
Subinoculation[c]	To isolate parasite	Buffy coat	1-mL purple-top (EDTA) tube	Cool	Do *not* freeze
		Clot	Underlying serum (0.75–1 mL)	Cool	Do *not* freeze
		Amniotic fluid	Unspun 10–20 mL	Cool	Do *not* freeze
		Placenta	200 g[d]	Cool	Do *not* freeze
		Other tissue	1 g (minimum)	Cool	Do *not* freeze
PCR	To identify parasite DNA in sample	Buffy coat	1-mL purple-top (EDTA) tube	Cool	Do *not* freeze
		Amniotic fluid	Unspun 10–20 mL	Cool	Do *not* freeze
		Placenta	25–50 mg	Cool	Do *not* freeze
		CSF	1 mL	Cool or frozen[e]	
		Other tissue	25–50 mg	Cool or frozen	
		Urine	5 mL sediment	Frozen	Investigational. Usefulness undetermined.

Abbreviations: CSF, cerebrospinal fluid; EDTA, ethylenediaminetetraacetic acid; ELISA, enzyme-linked immunosorbent assay; Ig, immunoglobulin; PCR, polymerase chain reaction.
Commercially available tests that are reliable when performed in accredited hospital laboratories: Tg IgG; Avidity.
[a]Potentially useful in each clinical setting.
[b]Cool = Use ice packs. Do *not* freeze subinoculation samples or EDTA tubes.
[c]Subinoculation = Samples for subinoculation must be shipped promptly by overnight courier and received in laboratory within 72 hours of collection.
[d]Amounts differ depending on reference laboratory performing this procedure.
[e]Frozen = −20°C or less. Note: Only for PCR, *not* placenta. Placenta must not be frozen.

Table 116-7 Contact Information for Reference Laboratories and Programs[a]

Palo Alto Medical Foundation, reference laboratory for serology, isolation, and PCR assay (United States)	650-853-4828; http://www.pamf.org/serology/
Reference laboratory for placenta subinoculation, PCR (Europe)	HPelloux@chu-grenoble.fr
FDA for IND number to obtain spiramycin for treatment of a pregnant woman (United States)	301-827-2335
FDA Public Health Advisory	301-594-3060
Spiramycin (Aventis) for treatment of a pregnant woman (United States)	908-231-3365
Congenital Toxoplasmosis Study Group (United States)	773-834-4131 toxoplasmosis.org toxoplasmosis@surgery.bsd.uchicago.edu
Educational pamphlet/March of Dimes (United States): "Prevention of Congenital Toxoplasmosis"	312-435-4007
Educational pamphlet: "Congenital Toxoplasmosis: The Hidden Threat"	1-800-323-9100
Educational pamphlet: "Toxoplasmosis," NIH publication No. 83-308	301-496-5717; http://www.niaid.nih.gov
Information concerning AIDS and congenital toxoplasmosis (United States)	305-243-6522
Educational information on the Internet	http://www.toxoplasmosis.org
NMS Laboratories, for pyrimethamine and sulfadiazine levels	866-522-2206

[a]Reproduced with permission from Remington et al.[54]
Abbreviations: FDA, US Food and Drug Administration; IND, Investigational New Drug; NIH, National Institutes of Health; PCR, polymerase chain reaction.

Table 116-8 Calculations of Antibody Load

Test	Equation	Comment
Serum antibody load[a]	$$\text{Serum Ab Load} = \frac{(\text{Reciprocal Dye Test Sensitivity})}{\text{Quantitative IgG (mg/dL)}}$$	Follow each month to observe disappearance of maternal passively transferred antibody and for the infant to make his or her own total IgG (mg/dL) without making specific antibody to *Toxoplasma gondii* to exclude diagnosis of congenital toxoplasmosis. This is used when the diagnosis is highly unlikely, but this is not absolutely certain, and a decision not to treat the infant has been made. Please see text in Chapter 57.
CSF-to-serum antibody load ratio[b]	$$\text{CSF-to-Serum Ab Load Ratio} = \frac{\dfrac{\text{CSF (Reciprocal Dye Test Sensitivity)}}{\text{Quantitative IgG (mg/dL)}}}{\text{Serum Ab Load}}$$	A value of 4 or greater is considered consistent with local antibody production.

Abbreviations: Ab, antibody; CSF, cerebrospinal fluid; Ig, immunoglobulin.
[a]Obtain at birth and monthly for untreated infant to exclude *T. gondii* infection as infant loses mother's passively transferred *T. gondii* IgG (half-life = 30 days). See Figure 116-7 for varying patterns of antibody production by infant.
[b]This method has been utilized to determine whether there is local antibody production in CSF indicative of active central nervous system infection.[55]

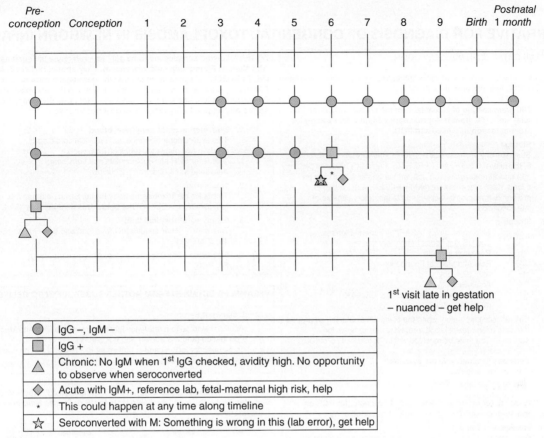

FIGURE 116-1 Algorithm for screening for acquisition of primary *Toxoplasma* infection during gestation. Ig, immunoglobulin.

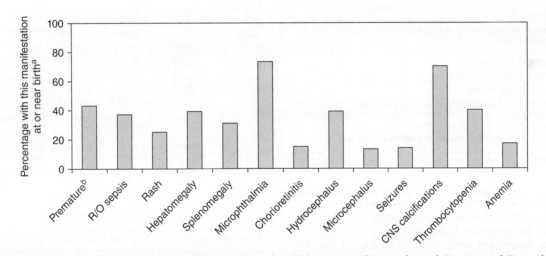

FIGURE 116-2 Manifestations at presentation, National Collaborative Chicago-based Congenital Toxoplasmosis Study (NCCCTS; 1981–2009). [a]Infants diagnosed with congenital toxoplasmosis in the newborn period and referred to the NCCCTS in the first year of life. [b]Less than 37 weeks' gestation. CNS, central nervous system; R/O, rule out.

diagnosed by amniocentesis with polymerase chain reaction (PCR) testing of the amniotic fluid for *T. gondii* DNA or via ultrasound. The infected fetus can then be treated by treatment of the mother with pyrimethamine and sulfadiazine (with leucovorin, folinic acid). Clindamycin, clarithromycin, and azithromycin are second-line medicines used for pregnant women with significant hypersensitivity to sulfadiazine, but there are no data concerning their efficacy. Treatment of the infant continues after birth as described in Chapter 57 and here (Table 116-1; Figure 116-4).

A

NARRATIVE FOR DIAGNOSIS OF CONGENITAL TOXOPLAMOSIS IN NEWBORN INFANT

I) SAMPLES OBTAINED IN DELIVERY ROOM

This includes: Placenta to go to reference laboratory for A-subinoculation into mice and B-PCR. Amniotic fluid, if available

A. **200 gram sample of placenta from the cord insertion area on the fetal side (100 gram is approximately 14cm x 3cm x 3cm) for subinoculation into mice and PCR.**

1. **Storage**
   Store sterilely in sterile saline (NO FORMALIN OR OTHER PRESERVATIVE, DO NOT FREEZE). Penicillin (100 units per mL) and Streptomycin (100 μgm/mL) or gentamicin should be added. Keep placenta cool (NOT FROZEN) with ice bag or preferably frozen cold packs. Send to laboratory capable of subinoculation.

2. **Shipping**
   Ship immediately (ASAP) by Federal Express.
   The US Reference Laboratory Address:
   Research Institute
   Palo Alto Medical Foundation
   Attn: Serology
   Ames Building
   795 El Camino Real Palo Alto, CA 94301
   (650) 853-4828

   Call receiving laboratory when the placenta is obtained so proper handling upon receipt is assured. Note that samples for subinoculation must be received within 72 hours of collection.

   European Laboratory, where available:
   Contact Herve Pelloux
   HPelloux@chu-grenoble.fr

B. **10-20 mL (or more) amniotic fluid, if available (for PCR of pellet and subinoculation). Not essential if obtained early.**

1. **Storage and shipping**
   Keep cold (NOT FROZEN) and ship with sample I(A) as described above.
   Each sample for PCR should be placed in a separate sealed bag to prevent cross-contamination.
   To be centrifuged by Reference Laboratory.

II) CLINICAL EXAMINATIONS AND EVALUATIONS OF BABY FOLLOWING BIRTH

A. General Examination

B. Pediatric Ophthalmologist

C. Pediatric Neurologist

D. CT scan of the brain. Baby should not be sedated and may be gently swaddled. This examination is done without contrast. Examine for ventricular size and brain calcifications.

E. Auditory Acoustic Emissions or BAER (hearing test).

III) SAMPLES OBTAINED FROM INFANT SUBSEQUENT TO DELIVERY AT DELIVERING HOSPITAL

The following samples and tests are obtained for the newborn infant and processed and analyzed at the delivering hospital.

1. CBC with differential and platelet count
2. Serum: total IgM, IgG, IgA, albumin
3. Serum: SGPT, SGOT, total and direct bilirubin, creatinine
4. Urinalysis
5. Lumbar puncture
   a) Cerebrospinal fluid: cell count, glucose protein and total IgG.
   b) Please note that an additional 0.5 mL is to be collected for IgG and IgM specific for *T. gondii* to be sent to a reference lab such as Palo Alto Medical Foundation as described below in "IV) 3."
   c) If available, hold 1.5 mL frozen cerebrospinal fluid for quantitative IgG if needed later to calculate antibody load (0.5 mL) and pcr (1.0 mL). Place 0.5 mL and 1.0 mL in separate tubes.

IV) The following samples are to be sent to a reference lab such as Palo Alto Medical Foundation (address above). They should be kept cold (NOT FROZEN). Remember to include the permission form for the PAMF to release serologic and isolation results to the Toxoplasmosis Research Institute and Center / Dr.McLeod. Note that these may be stored and shipped with sample I(A) described above.

1. **2 mL sterile infant peripheral blood**
   This is peripheral blood (i.e. not umbilical cord blood).
   Place in two purple top tubes of 1 mL each.
   This is for PCR and subinoculation of buffy coat.
   Also send sterile clot from "2" below.

2. **1mL serum**
   This is for the Toxoplasma Baby Panel: Sabin Feldman Dye test, IgM ISAGA, IgA ELISA. **Clot below this sample. See "IV) 1."**

3. **0.5 mL cerebrospinal fluid**
   This is for T.gondii specific IgG (dye test) and IgM ELISA. (See "III) 5" above.)

4. **5 cc urine - Investigational. Not proven sensitivity.**
   For PCR.

V) SAMPLES OBTAINED FROM MOTHER SUBSEQUENT TO DELIVERY

2 mL Maternal Serum

Adult panel to go to a reference laboratory such as Palo Alto Medical Foundation (address above) with **I) A** and **IV)**.
To be used for IgG in parallel with infant IgG test and cab ne used for IgM and IgA if clinically indicated.

VI) Amounts, Handling, and Shipping of *T. gondii*-specific Tests and Samples Table. Currently available tests in US or France Reference Laboratories.

Test	Sample	Preferred (Min. Amount)	Store/Ship	Additional Comments
Dye Test IgG	Serum[a]	0.25 mL (0.15 mL)	Cool[b]	
Direct Agglutination IgG	Serum	0.25 mL	Cool	
IgM ELISA	Serum	0.25 mL	Cool	
IgM ISAGA	Serum	0.25 mL	Cool	Only for babies<6 months
IgA ELISA	Serum	0.25 mL	Cool	
IgE ELISA	Serum	0.25 mL	Cool	Limited clinical use
AC/HS	Serum	0.25 mL (0.10 mL)	Cool	For pregnant woman
Avidity	Serum	0.30 mL (0.25 mL)	Cool	For pregnant woman
Subinoculation[c]	Buffy coat	1 mL purple top (EDTA) tube	Cool	Do NOT freeze
	Clot	1 mL (from same red top tube as whole blood)	Cool	Do NOT freeze
	Placenta	200 g[c]	Cool	Do NOT freeze
	Other tissue	1 g (minimum)	Cool	Do NOT freeze
PCR	Buffy coat	1 mL purple top (EDTA) tube	Cool	Do NOT freeze
	Amniotic fluid	Unspun 10-20 cc	Cool	Do NOT freeze
	Placenta	Same 200 g as above	Cool	Do NOT freeze
	CSF	0.5-1 mL	Cool or frozen[e]	
	Other tissue	25-50 mg	Cool or frozen	
	Urine	Sediment from 5 cc	Cool or frozen	

[a] From peripheral blood. Do NOT use umbilical cord blood.
[b] Cool = Use ice packs. Do NOT freeze subinoculation samples or EDTA tubes.
[c] Subinoculation = Samples for subinoculation must be shipped promptly by overnight courier and received in laboratory within 72 hours of collection.
[d] Amounts differ depending on reference laboratory performing this procedure.
[e] Frozen = ≤ -20° C. Note: only for PCR; NOT placenta, clot, or buffy coat. Placenta must NOT be frozen.
Commercially available tests that are reliable when performed in accredited hospital laboratories: Tg IgG; Avidity.

FIGURE 116-3 A, Approach for tests to diagnose congenital toxoplasmosis in the newborn infant.

B

For newborns and infants less than 6 months of age

☑ *Toxoplasma* Infant Panel (IgG [Dye test]), IgM ISAGA, IgA ELISA) *on serum (0.75 mL minimum)*

Tests to consider according to history and clinical manifestations

☑ PCR (see PCR specimen requirements)
  ☑ Solid tissues (specimen type) _____*Placenta (same sample as below)*_____
  ☑ Whole blood, other body fluids (specimen type) *a) Buffy coat*
    _____*b) Amniotic fluid (if available)*_____

Other Test Options for Newborn Infants

Individual Tests

☑ IgG (Dye Test) – *CSF (0.25 mL)*
☑ IgM ELISA – *CSF (0.25 mL)*
☐ IgA ELISA
☐ PCR (see PCR specimen requirements)
  ☐ Solid tissues (specimen type) _____
  ☐ Whole blood, other body fluids (specimen type) _____
☑ Isolation of *T. gondii* (specimen type)_____ *a) Placenta (200 grams)*
    b) Buffy coat (1 mL purple top tube)
    c) Clot (underlying sample sent for serum above (from 1.5–2.0 mL whole peripheral infant blood)

Test for Mother at Birth (serum)

Individual Tests

☑ IgG (Dye Test)
☑ IgM ELISA
☑ IgA ELISA
☐ Other

C

Testing for Newborn Infant

Serum
  ☑ IgG (Dye Test)[a]
  ☑ IgM ISAGA[a]
  ☑ IgA ELISA[a]

Buffy Coat
  ☑ PCR[a]
  ☑ Isolation[a]

CSF
  ☑ IgG[a], IgM ELISA[a]
  ☑ PCR[a]

Placenta
  ☑ PCR[a]
  ☑ Isolation[a]

Follow-Up of Infant for Antibody Load

Serum
  ☑ IgG (Dye Test)[a] two-fold, parallel with last sample

Testing for Pregnant Woman[b]

Serum
  ☑ IgG (Dye Test)[a]
  ☑ IgM ELISA[a]
  ☑ IgA ELISA[a]
  ☑ AC/HS[a]
  ☑ Avidity[a]

B, Completion of typical order form from reference laboratory for serologic tests for diagnosis of congenital toxoplasmosis. C, Tests for diagnosis of congenital toxoplasmosis by sample. [a] Test specific for *Toxoplasma gondii*. [b] When immunoglobulin (Ig) G is positive in local hospital laboratory. AC/HS, differential agglutination; ASAP, as soon as possible; BAER, brainstem auditory evoked response; CBC, complete blood cell count; CSF, cerebrospinal fluid; CT, computed tomography; EDTA, ethylenediaminetetraacetic acid; ELISA, enzyme-linked immunosorbent assay; ISAGA, immunosorbent agglutination assay; PAMF, Palo Alto Medical Foundation; PCR, polymerase chain reaction; SGOT, aspartate aminotransferase; SGPT, alanine aminotransferase; Tg IgG, *T. Gondii* IgG.

BIRTH: PLACENTA SAMPLES OBTAINED IN THE DELIVERY ROOM

Table 116-2 outlines how the placenta should be processed in the delivery room and afterward.[2]

CLINICAL EVALUATION OF THE INFANT

Clinical evaluation of the infant is summarized in Table 116-5. Figures 116-2 and 57-8 and Tables 57-4 to 57-8 include common manifestations of this infection,[1–45] which should lead to prompt diagnostic evaluation. This highlights the importance of recognition by neonatologists and others caring for such an infant that these findings are manifestations of congenital toxoplasmosis. Details of diagnostic evaluation of the infant to exclude or establish manifestations of this disease are in Tables 116-2 to 116-6 along with some comments about evaluation of the mother and other family members.[2,40,42–47] The tables and figures in Chapter 57 also differently illustrate manifestations of this infection and diagnostic approaches.

A

Oral Suspension Formulations for Pyrimethamine and Sulfadiazine

Pyrimethamine: 2 mg/mL suspension

1. Crush FOUR 25 mg pyrimethamine tablets in a mortar to a fine powder
2. Add 10 cc of syrup vehicle.
3. Transfer mixture to an amber bottle.
4. Rinse mortar with 10 cc of sterile water and transfer.
5. Add enough of the syrup vehicle to q.s. to 50 mL final volume
6. Shake very well until this is a fine suspension
7. Label and give a 7 day expiration.
8. Store refrigerated

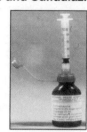

Sulfadiazine: 100 mg/mL suspension

1. Crush TEN 500 mg sulfadiazine tablets in a mortar to a fine powder.
2. Add enough sterile water to make a smooth paste.
3. Slowly triturate the syrup vehicle close to the final volume of 50 mL.
4. Transfer the suspension to a larger amber bottle.
5. Add sufficient syrup vehicle to q.s. to 50 mL final volume.
6. Shake well.
7. Label and give a 7 day expiration.
8. Store refrigerated.

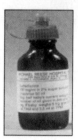

B

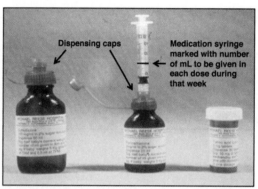

Dispensing caps

Medication syringe marked with number of mL to be given in each dose during that week

Weigh Baby Each Week. Increase Medications Accordingly.		
Sample Label:	**Sample Label:**	**Sample Label:**
Medication: Sulfadiazine	Pyrimethamine	Folinic acid (Calcium leukovorin)
Concentration: 100 mg/mL*	2 mg/mLª	5 mg tablets
Dispense: 50 mL	25 mL	30 tablets
Dosage: Sig: ½ baby's current weight equals number of milliliters given in AM and PM e.g. if baby weighs 5 kg, give 2.5 mL at 7 AM and 2.5 mL 7 PM	Sig: ½ baby's current weight in kg equals number of mLs given once each day. e.g. if baby weighs 5 kg, give 2.5 mL daily	Sig: 10 mg (2 tablets) on Monday, Wednesday, and Friday. Crush and give with formula or apple juice in one dosage.

FIGURE 116-4 A, Method of compounding oral suspension formulations for pyrimethamine and sulfadiazine. **B,** Method of administering medications used to treat congenital toxoplasmosis. ªSuspended in 2% sugar solution. Suspension at usual concentration must be made up each week. Store refrigerated. First loading dose for 2 days is 1 mg/kg twice daily. Third-day dose is 1 mg/kg/d. With in utero treatment, no loading dose postnatally is used. q.s., quantity sufficient. (A, reproduced with permission from Remington et al[2]; B, reproduced with permission from McAuley et al[24].)

SAMPLE AMOUNTS NEEDED FOR SPECIALIZED TESTING AND USEFUL CONTACT INFORMATION

One of the areas of confusion sometimes is which samples and how much of them should be obtained for particular tests. Therefore, Tables 116-2 to 116-4 and 116-6 provide this information. Table 116-7 provides contact information helpful for diagnosis and treatment and

counseling pregnant women and their families and families for whom this diagnosis is suspected or proven.

ANTIBODY LOAD IN SERUM AND CEREBROSPINAL FLUID

In certain circumstances (eg, birth of an infant who is completely normal with a low likelihood of transmission from an acutely infected mother, had negative amniotic fluid PCR for *T. gondii* infection in a reference laboratory, and had no manifestations at birth consistent with infection), a decision is made with the parents not to treat the infant but rather to follow serum antibody load. This is measured as shown in Tables 116-8 and 57-25 (Chapter 57). In this case, a physician monitors the measurement of IgG antibody specific for *T. gondii* each month. Serum is diluted 2-fold in parallel with the previous month's sample and sensitivity of the dye test noted. Passively transferred maternal *T. gondii*-specific IgG will fall by 50% because the half-life of IgG is 30 days. At the same time, the physician monitors that and when the infant begins making his or her own IgG (quantitative immunoglobulin milligrams per deciliter measured in the local hospital's laboratory; also see discussion in Chapter 57).

A similar equation can be used to calculate antibody load in cerebrospinal fluid (CSF) to demonstrate local production of antibody to *T. gondii* due to active brain infection. This is used only when the dye test titer is less than 1:1024 (~300 IU usually). A ratio of antibody produced in CSF of 4 or greater is considered indicative of local antibody production (Tables 116-4 and 57-25 [Chapter 57]).

GUIDELINES FOR TREATMENT OF GESTATIONAL AND CONGENITAL TOXOPLASMOSIS

Table 116-1 provides guidelines for the treatment of the fetus, newborn infant, and child with congenital toxoplasmosis.[2] A method for preparation of medicines and their administration[2] is shown in Figure 116-4. In the unusual circumstance of an infant too sick to be able to utilize pyrimethamine and sulfadiazine by mouth or by feeding tube, intravenous administration of trimethoprim/sulfamethoxazole with clindamycin has been an alternate, but less-satisfactory, approach. Active choriodal neovascular membranes have been treated effectively with intraocular injection of $\propto$ vascular endothelial growth factor ($\propto$-VEGF[33]; LUCENTIS®) in conjunction with *anti-T. Gondii* medicines (Figure 57-22). This has also been safely used to treat retinopathy of prematurity in infants.[48]

TOXICITIES OF MEDICINES

The major toxicity encountered in treatment of the fetus is reversible neutropenia.[24,26] Hypersensitivity to sulfadiazine appears to be much less often encountered as a serious complication in the pregnant woman and infant than in older children and adults.[49] In the infant with congenital toxoplasmosis, the major toxicity of the medicines used to treat toxoplasmosis is

reversible neutropenia. Most children maintain neutrophil counts of about $1000/mL^3$ ($800–1200/mL^3$) during the year of treatment. Concomitant viral infections can result in diminution of the neutrophil count. This is managed by withholding pyrimethamine if absolute neutrophil count (ANC) falls to between 500 and 700. Both pyrimethamine and sulfadiazine are withheld if the ANC is less than 500. Leucovorin is increased to 15–20 mg/day these cases. Leucovorin is always continued for 1 week after discontinuing pyrimethamine because of the relatively long half-life of pyrimethamine (60–90 hours). Granulocyte colony-stimulating factor (G-CSF) has been used to maintain normal neutrophil counts when substantial neutropenia has been a recurrent or refractory problem. Teeth are gently cleaned with a soft pediatric toothbrush or washcloth to prevent development of dental carries due to the sugar suspension agent for the medicines. Three to four months after discontinuing treatment, commonly there is a rebound (elevation) in antibody titer of *T. gondii*-specific IgG, IgM, or IgA, usually without any recognized symptomology.[24,26]

OUTCOMES AND PROGNOSIS

Medical and adjunctive treatment, such as prompt correction of hydrocephalus with ventriculoperitoneal shunt procedures, improves the prognosis.[1–6,10,11,15,21,26–28,30,50,51] The earlier treatment is initiated, the better the prognosis will be.[5,6] This infection, even when it causes hydrocephalus, is treated as expectant for excellent outcomes. Outcomes may be good, although this does not always occur.[1–6,10,11,15,21,23,26–28,30,50–52] It is not possible to predict with certainty when outcomes will be favorable. There can be remarkable expansion and growth of cortical mantle with ventricular peritoneal shunting. Third ventriculostomies were found to fail often in this disease,[16] presumably because of the associated inflammatory process, and thus are not used. When CSF protein is high, lavage of ventricles prior to placement of the shunt to prevent occlusion of the shunt has been used successfully. Figure 57-10 shows this improved prognosis as well as some of the problems that may occur. Brain calcifications often resolve or diminish in size with treatment in the first year of life.[52]

COMPARISON OF CONGENITAL TOXOPLASMOSIS AT BIRTH IN FRANCE, AUSTRIA, GERMANY, AND THE UNITED STATES

Prenatal and postnatal treatment improve outcomes at birth and later in life.[1–6,10,11,15,21,23,26–28,30,50–52] The more rapidly treatment is initiated to stop destruction of

CHAPTER 116

Table 116-9 Ocular and Intracranial Lesions in Treated Infants With Congenital Toxoplasmosis in European Countries With Systematic Prenatal Screening and Treatment Programs for Toxoplasmosis During Gestation[a]

Cohort Region	Recruitment Period	Infected Live-born Children	Clinical Manifestations		
			Any	Ocular Lesions	Intracranial Lesions
France					
Nice	1996–2000	15	1	1	0
Grenoble	1996–2000	6	2	1	1
Lyon	1996–2000	43	10	9	3
Marseille	1996–2000	20	2	2	0
Nice	1996–2000	8	4	2	2
Paris	1996–2000	65	8	8	1
Reims	1996–2000	8	2	2	0
Toulouse	1996–2000	22	3	2	1
Austria	1992–1995	33	3	3	2
	1996–2000	24	5	5	2
Italy					
Naples	1996–2000	11	3	3	3
Milan	1996–2000	4	0	0	0
Slovenia					
Ljubljana	1996	3	3	0	0
Total (%)		262	43 (16.4)	38 (14.5)	15 (5.7)

[a]Adapted with permission from Systematic Review on Congenital Toxoplasmosis Study Group et al.[56] Table from Olariu et al.[45]

the fetus and infant's eyes and to stop brain and systemic infection, the better the outcome will be. This empirical observation is supported by in vitro data and studies with experimental animals. The latter studies demonstrated that medicines used to treat the infection are effective in vitro and in vivo in killing the active tachyzoite that destroys tissue. A contrast of outcomes in France with those in the United States is informative.[1,45] Table 116-9 and Figure 116-2 shows this contrast.[45] In France, there is serologic screening monthly during gestation (Figure 116-1). This facilitates prompt diagnosis and treatment of the fetus without delay. In the United States, screening rarely occurs, and when it does, it may often be performed only once or twice in a more random manner, with consequent delays in treatment.[1,45]

ANALYSIS OF COST-MINIMIZING STRATEGIES IN PERSPECTIVE

Because exposures often are unrecognized (Tables 57-1 and 57-2 and Figure 57-3),[25,29,44] although education about risk factors can help to reduce acquisition of

infection during gestation, serologic screening with prompt diagnosis and treatment or a vaccine are the only means that could almost entirely successfully prevent this disease and the suffering it causes.[3] A vaccine is needed but has not yet been developed for human use. Serologic screening and treatment in gestation and in infancy are predicted to be cost minimizing.[3] This is with the wide range of incidences of infection likely to occur in a variety of populations throughout the world (Figure 57-4).[3,53] Medicines that eliminate cysts and active infection would greatly facilitate treatment and improve outcomes, but are not available.

In 1990, Desmonts from France wrote the following:[57]

"There is a parasite, Toxoplasma, which is harmless for you but which can cause severe impairment in your child if you become infected during pregnancy. You will notice nothing but we could tell you now if you are immune; if you are not, we can monitor you during pregnancy. If you become infected we can detect the infection in your infant even if he looks normal; we can even detect it in utero and treat without delay. Yet we will do nothing, since all this is too expensive. But do not worry. Perhaps you are immune—and if you are not, you will

probably escape infection when pregnant. If the worst does happen your fetus might still escape. And if your infant is severely impaired, there is no risk in having another baby because you will now be immune. Nevertheless, try not to get infected. Eat well-cooked meat and wash your hands. Good luck."

Neonatologists can help improve care by recognizing manifestations promptly at birth and considering and testing for congenital toxoplasmosis in their patients to prevent some sequelae (Figure 116-2).

In 2011, we[45] noted the following:

Congenital toxoplasmosis continues to be a tragedy for parents and children in the United States. Decades ago some countries responded to the challenge by implementing national programs for systematic serologic screening of all pregnant women. Others did so by performing routine serologic screening in all newborns. Yet, despite the fact that all studies performed in the United States continue to reveal that congenitally infected children are born severely affected each year, a national program or policy to address the threat of this disease is currently lacking.

We now have practical means to prevent and treat this infection that were outlined here. They can be easily implemented by obstetricians, perinatologists, neonatologists, and pediatricians. This will prevent suffering and loss of life, sight, cognition, motor function, and seizures from this disease. This can be accomplished by prompt diagnosis and treatment as presented in Chapter 57 and this chapter. This appears to be not only feasible but also likely cost minimizing.

ACKNOWLEDGMENTS

This work was supported by the National Institutes of Health (NIH), National Institute of Allergy and Infectious Diseases (NIAID) R01 AI027530-21 and gifts from the Mann and Cornwell, Taub, Cussen-Kapnick, Rooney-Alden, Engel, Pritzker, Harris, Zucker, Samuel, and Mussilami families and NIH U01 5 U01 AI077887-05 and 2R01AI027530-18A2. We thank those families and physicians who have worked with us to help us learn more about how to diagnose, manage, and treat this disease and those who have taught us about it, especially George Desmonts, Jacques Couvreur, Philippe Thulliez, and Jack Remington.

This chapter is especially in honor of Dana, Chad, Dani Jo, Elena, Graham, Grant, Joshua, Lucky, Margaret, Miguel, Nicky, Robbie, Roxanne, and many others and their families who understand with special poignancy Edward Young's statement "who would not give a trifle to prevent what they would give a thousand worlds to cure."

REFERENCES

1. McLeod R, Kieffer F, Sautter M, Hosten T, Pelloux H. Why prevent, diagnose and treat congenital toxoplasmosis? *Mem Inst Oswaldo Cruz.* 2009;104:320–344.
2. Remington JS, McLeod R, Thulliez, P, Desmonts G. *Toxoplasmosis.* In: Remington J, Klein J, eds. *Infectious Diseases of the Fetus and Newborn Infant.* 7th ed. Philadelphia, PA: Saunders; 2011;918–1040.
3. Stillwaggon E, Carrier CS, Sautter M, McLeod R. Maternal serologic screening to prevent congenital toxoplasmosis: a decision-analytic economic model. *PLoS Negl Trop Dis.* 2011; 5(9):e1333.
4. Thulliez P. Commentary: efficacy of prenatal treatment for toxoplasmosis: a possibility that cannot be ruled out. *Int J Epidemiol.* 2001;30(6):1315–1316.
5. Kieffer F, Wallon M, Garcia P, et al. Risk factors for retinochoroiditis during the first 2 years of life in infants with treated congenital toxoplasmosis. *Pediatr Infect Dis J.* 2008;27(1):27–32.
6. Cortina-Borja M, Tan HK, Wallon M, et al. Prenatal treatment for serious neurological sequelae of congenital toxoplasmosis: an observational prospective cohort study. *PLoS Med.* 2010;7(10):1–11.
7. Couvreur J, Desmonts G, Thulliez P. Prophylaxis of congenital toxoplasmosis: effects of spiramycin on placental infection. *J Antimicrob Chemother.* 1988;22:193–200.
8. Daffos F, Forestier F, Capella-Pavlovsky M, et al. Prenatal management of 746 pregnancies at risk for congenital toxoplasmosis. *N Engl J Med.* 1988;318:271–275.
9. Hohlfeld P, Daffos F, Thulliez P, et al. Fetal toxoplasmosis: outcome of pregnancy and infant follow-up after in utero treatment. *J Pediatr.* 1989;115(5 Pt 1):765–769.
10. Foulon W, Naessens A, Derde MP. Evaluation of the possibilities for preventing congenital toxoplasmosis. *Am J Perinatol.* 1994;11:57–62.
11. Foulon W, Villena I, Stray-Pedersen B, et al. Treatment of toxoplasmosis during pregnancy: a multicenter study of impact on fetal transmission and children's sequelae at age 1 year. *Am J Obstet Gynecol.* 1999;180:410–415.
12. Romand S, Chosson M, Franck J, et al. Usefulness of quantitative polymerase chain reaction in amniotic fluid as early prognostic marker of fetal infection with *Toxoplasma gondii. Am J Obstet Gynecol.* 2004;190:797–802.
13. Villena I, Ancelle T, Delmas C, et al. Congenital toxoplasmosis in France in 2007: first results from a national surveillance system. *Euro Surveill.* 2010;15:pii-19600.
14. Wallon M, Franck J, Thulliez P, et al. Accuracy of real-time polymerase chain reaction for *Toxoplasma gondii* in amniotic fluid. *Obstet Gynecol.* 2010;115:727–733.
15. Peyron F, Garweg JG, Wallon M, et al. Long-term impact of treated congenital toxoplasmosis on quality of life and visual performance. *Pediatr Infect Dis J.* 2011;30(7):597–600.
16. Renier D, Sainte-Rose C, Pierre-Kahn A, Hirsch JF. Prenatal hydrocephalus: outcome and prognosis. *Childs Nerv Syst.* 1988; 4(4):213–222.
17. Montoya JG, Remington JS. Management of *Toxoplasma gondii* infection during pregnancy. *Clin Infect Dis.* 2008;47(4):554–566.
18. Berrebi A, Bardou M, Bessieres M, et al. Outcome for children infected with congenital toxoplasmosis in the first trimester and with normal ultrasound findings: a study of 36 cases. *Eur J Obstet Gynaecol Reprod Biol.* 2007;135:53–57.
19. Forestier F. Fetal disease, prenatal diagnosis and practical measures. *Presse Med.* 1991;1448–1454.
20. Hohlfeld P, Daffos F, Costa J-M, et al. Prenatal diagnosis of congenital toxoplasmosis with a polymerase-chain-reaction test on amniotic fluid. *N Engl J Med.* 1994;331(11):695–699.

21. Brezin AP, Thulliez P, Couvreur J, et al. Ophthalmic outcome after prenatal and postnatal treatment of congenital toxoplasmosis. *Am J Ophthalmol* 2003;138:779–784.

22. Delair E, Latkany P, Noble AG, et al. Clinical manifestations of ocular toxoplasmosis. *Ocul Immunol Inflamm.* 2011;19(2):91–102.

23. Swisher CN, Boyer K, McLeod R, the Toxoplasmosis Study Group. Congenital toxoplasmosis. *Semin Pediatr Neurol.* 1994; 1(1):4–25.

24. McAuley J, Boyer KM, Patel D, et al. Early and longitudinal evaluations of treated infants and children and untreated historical patients with congenital toxoplasmosis: the Chicago collaborative treatment trial. *Clin Infect Dis.* 1994;18:38–72.

25. Boyer KM, Holfels E, Roizen N, et al. Risk factors for *Toxoplasma gondii* infection in mothers of infants with congenital toxoplasmosis: implications for prenatal management and screening. *Am J Obstet Gynecol.* 2005;192:564–571.

26. McLeod R, Boyer K, Karrison T, et al. Outcome of treatment for congenital toxoplasmosis, 1981–2004: the national collaborative Chicago-based, congenital toxoplasmosis study. *Clin Infect Dis.* 2006;42(10):1383–1394.

27. Phan L, Kasza K, Jalbrzikowski J, et al. Longitudinal study of new eye lesions in treated congenital toxoplasmosis. *Ophthalmology.* 2008;115.

28. Phan L, Kasza K, Jalbrzikowski J, et al. Longitudinal study of new eye lesions in children with toxoplasmosis who were not treated during the first year of life. *Am J Ophthalmol.* 2008;146(3): 375–384.

29. Boyer K, Hill D, Mui E, et al. Unrecognized ingestion of *Toxoplasma gondii* oocysts leads to congenital toxoplasmosis and causes epidemics in North America. *Clin Infect Dis.* 2011; 53(11):1081.

30. McLeod R, Boyer KM, Lee D, et al. Prematurity and severity associate with *T. gondii* alleles (NCCCTS, 1981–2009). 2012; 54(11):1595–1605.

31. McLeod R, Mack DG, Boyer K, et al. Phenotypes and functions of lymphocytes in congenital toxoplasmosis. *J Lab Clin Med.* 1990;116(5):623–635.

32. Witola WH, Liu SR, Montpetit A, Welti R, Hypolite M, Roth M, McLeod R. ALOX12 in human toxoplasmosis. *Infection and Immunity,* 2014;82(7):2670–2679. doi:10.1128/IAI.01505-13.

33. Benevento JD, Jager RD, Noble AG, et al. Toxoplasmosis-associated neovascular lesions treated successfully with ranibizumab and antiparasitic therapy. *Arch Ophthalmol.* 2008;126:1152–1156.

34. Kodjikian L, Wallon M, Fleury M, et al. Ocular manifestations in congenital toxoplasmosis. *Graefes Arch Clin Exp Ophthalmol.* 2006;244:14–21.

35. Wallon M, Kodjikian L, Binquet C, et al. Long-term ocular prognosis in 327 children with congenital toxoplasmosis. *Pediatrics.* 2004;113:1567–1572.

36. Guerina NG, Hsu HW, Meissner HC, et al. Neonatal serologic screening and early treatment for congenital *Toxoplasma gondii* infection. *N Engl J Med.* 1994;330:1858–1863.

37. Burrowes D, Boyer K, Swisher CN, et al. Spinal cord lesions in congenital toxoplasmosis demonstrated with neuroimaging, including their successful treatment in an adult. *J Neuroparasitol.* 2012;3(2012): pii: 235533.

38. Jamieson SE, de Roubaix LA, Cortina-Borja M, et al. Genetic and epigenetic factors at COL2A1 and ABCA4 influence clinical outcome in congenital toxoplasmosis. *PLoS One.* 2008;3(6):e2285.

39. McLeod R, Beem MO, and Estes RG. Lymphocyte allergy specific to *Toxoplasma gondii* antigens in a baby with congenital toxoplasmosis. *J Clin Lab Immunol.* 1985;17:149–153.

40. McLeod R, Mack D, Foss R, et al. Levels of pyrimethamine in sera and cerebrospinal and ventricular fluids from infants treated for congenital toxoplasmosis. *Antimicrob Agents Chemother.* 1992; 36:1040–1048.

41. Mets M, Holfels E, Boyer KM, et al. Eye manifestations of congenital toxoplasmosis. *Am J Ophthalmol.* 1996;122:309–324.

42. McLeod R, Boyer K, Roizen N, et al. The child with congenital toxoplasmosis. *Curr Clin Top Infect Dis.* 2000:189–207.

43. Noble, AG, Latkany, P, Kusmierczyk, et al. Chorioretinal lesions in mothers of children with congenital toxoplasmosis in the National Collaborative Chicago-based, Congenital Toxoplasmosis Study. *Sci Med.* 2010;20(1):20–26.

44. Hill D, Coss C, Dubey JP, et al. Identification of a sporozoite-specific antigen from *Toxoplasma gondii. J Parasitol.* 2011; 97(2):328–337.

45. Olariu T, Remington S, McLeod R, Alam A, Montoya J. Severe congenital toxoplasmosis in the United States: clinical and serologic findings in untreated infants. *Pediatr Infect Dis J.* 2011; 30(12):1056–1061.

46. Montoya JG. Laboratory diagnosis of *Toxoplasma gondii* infection and toxoplasmosis. *J Infect Dis.* 2002;185(Suppl 1):S73–S82.

47. Remington JS, Desmonts G. Congenital toxoplasmosis. In: Remington JS, Klein JO, eds. *Infectious Diseases of the Fetus and Newborn Infant.* Philadelphia, PA: Saunders; 1976:297–299.

48. Capone A Jr. Treatment of neovascularization in infants with retinopathy of prematurity with anti-VEGF: vitreous surgery for retinopathy of prematurity. Paper presented at annual meeting of the American Academy of Ophthalmology; November 13, 2006, Las Vegas, NV.

49. McLeod R, Khan AR, Noble GA, et al. Severe sulfadiazine hypersensitivity in a child with reactivated congenital toxoplasmic chorioretinitis. *Pediatr Infect Dis J.* 2006;25(3):270–272.

50. Roizen N, Swisher CN, Stein MA, et al. Neurologic and developmental outcome in treated congenital toxoplasmosis. *Pediatrics.* 1995:95:11–20.

51. Roizen N, Kasza K, Karrison T, et al. Impact of visual impairment on measures of cognitive function for children with congenital toxoplasmosis: implications for compensatory intervention strategies. *Pediatrics.* 2006:118:e379–e390.

52. Patel DV, Holfels EM, Vogel NP, et al. Resolution of intracranial calcifications in infants with treated congenital toxoplasmosis. *Radiology.* 1996:199:433–440.

53. Papoz L, Simondon F, Saurin W, Sarmini H. A simple model relevant to toxoplasmosis applied to epidemiologic results in France. *Am J Epidemiol.* 1986:154–161.

54. Remington JS, McLeod R, Thulliez P, Desmonts G. Toxoplasmosis. In: Remington JS, Klein JO, eds. *Infectious Diseases of the Fetus and Newborn Infant.* 7th ed. Philadelphia, PA: Elsevier Saunders; 2011.

55. Couvreur J, Desmonts G. [Late evolutive outbreaks of congenital toxoplasmosis]. *Cah Coll Med Hop Paris.* 1964; 115:752–758. French.

56. Systematic Review on Congenital Toxoplasmosis (SYROCOT) Study Group, Thiébaut R, Leproust S, Chêne G, Gilbert R. Effectiveness of prenatal treatment for congenital toxoplasmosis: a meta-analysis of individual patients' data. *Lancet.* 2007;369 (9556):115–122.

57. Georges Desmonts J, Dupouy-Camet S, Lavareda De Souza ME, Bougnoux L, Mandelbrot C, Hennequin M, Dommergues R, Benarous C. Tourte-Schaefer. Preventing congenital toxoplasmosis. *The Lancet.* 1990;336(8721):1018. http://dx.doi.org/10.1016/0140-6736(90)92485-Z

Infant of HIV-Positive Mother

Avinash K. Shetty, Fatima Clouser, and Yvonne A. Maldonado

INTRODUCTION

Perinatal transmission rates in the United States are at historic lows (<2%) because of the availability of effective interventions to prevent perinatal human immunodeficiency virus (HIV) transmission.[1] However, transmission does occur in a small number of infants, primarily because of missed prevention opportunities.[2, 3] The neonatologist plays a vital role in the prevention of perinatal HIV transmission in early identification of HIV-exposed newborns born to infected mothers who were not tested for HIV during pregnancy and in administering antiretroviral (ARV) prophylaxis to HIV-exposed infants as early as possible after birth.[4,5] The primary care physician, in conjunction with a pediatric infectious disease specialist, must ensure appropriate follow-up to confirm or exclude the diagnosis of HIV infection in early infancy and provide ongoing counseling, support, and anticipatory guidance[6] (Table 117-1). A comprehensive review of recommendations for evaluation and treatment of the HIV-exposed infant has been published by the American Academy of Pediatrics (AAP) and other experts.[4,5,7,8] This chapter discusses the clinical evaluation, laboratory testing, and treatment of HIV-exposed infants, incorporating the recently updated Public Health Service guidelines with a focus on prevention of perinatal HIV transmission.[5,6]

DIAGNOSIS/INDICATION

Universal prenatal HIV testing is the gateway to access effective antepartum, intrapartum, and postpartum interventions to prevent perinatal HIV transmission. All pregnant women must be routinely tested for HIV ("opt-out" approach) regardless of potential risk factors.[9] Repeat testing during the third trimester of pregnancy is recommended for certain high-risk populations to identify new infections.[9] HIV-negative women should receive counseling to maintain HIV-negative status during pregnancy and thereafter. In contrast, women with acute or recent HIV infection must be linked to care and receive a potent combination ARV drug regimen as soon as possible, with the goal of achieving viral load to undetectable levels and preventing perinatal HIV transmission.[5] Scheduled cesarean delivery at 38 weeks' gestation is recommended for HIV-positive women who have received ARV agents but have viral load greater than 1000 copies/mL near delivery.[5] Care of the HIV-exposed infant must then focus on reducing the risk of transmission with ARV prophylaxis.

If maternal HIV infection status is unknown at the time of delivery or repeat testing during the third trimester has not been done in certain high-risk women as recommended, rapid HIV testing of the mother or infant is recommended as soon as possible after delivery with immediate initiation of ARV prophylaxis if

Table 117-1 Clinical Care of Infants Exposed to Human Immunodeficiency Virus (HIV)

History and physical examination
Infant ARV prophylaxis
Avoidance of breast-feeding
- Infant formula
Determination of HIV status
- Virologic testing at 14–21 days, 1–2 months, and 4–6 months of age
- HIV antibody testing at 12–18 months (for infants in whom serial virologic tests are negative in early infancy) to document HIV seroreversion and definitively exclude infection[a]
PCP prophylaxis
- TMP-SMX from 6 weeks and continued until HIV infection is presumptively or definitively excluded
Psychosocial support to mother and other caregivers
Comprehensive well-baby care
- Immunizations
- Growth and development monitoring
- Anticipatory guidance

Abbreviations: ARV, antiretroviral prophylaxis; PCP, *Pneumocystis jiroveci* pneumonia; TMP-SMX, trimethoprim-sulfamethoxazole.
[a]Expert recommendation. from references 5 and 14.

the rapid test is positive.[5] Western blot testing must be done as soon as possible to confirm positive rapid HIV antibody test on the mother or infant, but infant ARV prophylaxis must not be delayed while waiting for the confirmatory results. ARV prophylaxis can be discontinued if the confirmatory test result is negative.[5]

Clinical Findings

History

The initial assessment of the HIV-exposed infant begins in the delivery room. Prenatal history is critical in the routine evaluation and management of HIV-exposed infants. Identification of perinatal HIV exposure is the first step involved in the delivery of optimal care to the HIV-exposed infant.[6] In most cases, the diagnosis of maternal HIV infection would have been established during the antenatal period. Medical and obstetrical history should be reviewed to determine if the risk of perinatal HIV transmission is high or low depending on whether the mother received effective interventions. Details about maternal HIV diagnosis (viral load, CD4 T-lymphocyte cell count, genotypic drug resistance testing); ARV drug regimen (timing of initiation and compliance); and maternal clinical status must be elicited.[6,8] Maternal history should include history of sexually transmitted infections (such as syphilis, hepatitis B, or herpes simplex virus) or coinfections such as tuberculosis (TB), toxoplasmosis, or hepatitis C.

Infants exposed to 1 or several of these pathogens should undergo further evaluation. In addition, history should include obstetric details (including duration of ruptured membranes, mode of delivery), use of invasive intrapartum monitoring, birth weight, and gestational age.[6]

Physical Examination

Infants with perinatally acquired HIV infection are often asymptomatic, and physical examination is usually normal in the neonatal period.[10] The common features of HIV infection in early infancy are lymphadenopathy, hepatomegaly, and splenomegaly, often noted at around 3 months of age.[10] Other commonly encountered findings in the first year of life include failure to thrive and neurodevelopmental delay.[10,11] HIV-exposed infants must be closely monitored for signs and symptoms of early HIV infection before definitive virologic tests become available.[6]

Baseline Tests

A complete blood cell count (CBC) with differential should be obtained on HIV-exposed infants before initiating ARV prophylaxis.[5] Some experts recommend virologic testing (HIV DNA or RNA polymerase chain reaction [PCR] assay) at birth for diagnosis of intrauterine HIV infection, especially in HIV-infected women who have suboptimal viral suppression during pregnancy or near delivery or there is a concern about infant follow-up.[5]

TREATMENT

Neonatal ARV Prophylaxis

All HIV-exposed infants must receive ARV prophylaxis as soon as possible after birth, preferably at 6–12 hours of life, to reduce the risk of perinatal HIV transmission (Table 117-2).[5] When the mother has received combination ARV therapy (ART) during pregnancy, neonatal zidovudine (ZDV) at gestational age-appropriate dosing for 6 weeks is the recommended ARV prophylaxis regimen of choice.

When the mother has not received antepartum ARV during pregnancy, combination ARV prophylaxis, including ZDV for 6 weeks plus 3 doses of nevirapine (NVP) during the first week of life (birth, 48 hours, and 96 hours of life), is recommended for HIV-exposed infant (Tables 117-2 and 117-3).[5,12] In these scenarios, a pediatric HIV specialist should be consulted and mothers should be counseled regarding the potential benefits and risks of combination ARV prophylaxis. In premature infants, only ZDV and NVP are recommended for ARV prophylaxis

Table 117-2 Antiretroviral Interventions to Prevent Perinatal Human Immunodeficiency Virus (HIV) Transmission[a]

Maternal Regimen	
Antepartum	Combination ARV[b] (include oral ZDV 200 mg 3 times per day or 300 mg 2 times per day as part of maternal ARV regimen)
Intrapartum	ZDV 2 mg/kg IV during the first hour, followed by continuous infusion of 1 mg/kg/h until delivery
Neonatal Prophylaxisc	
ZDV Prophylaxis for Infants Whose Mothers Have Received Antepartum/Intrapartum ARV[d]	
≥35 weeks' gestation	Oral ZDV 4 mg/kg (or 3 mg/kg IV) 2 times per day until 6 weeks of age
≥30 to less than 36 weeks' gestation	Oral ZDV 2 mg/kg (or 1.5 mg/kg IV) 2 times per day for the first 2 weeks of age followed by 3 mg/kg orally (or 2.3 mg/kg IV) 2 times per day for the next 4 weeks of life
<30 weeks' gestation	Oral ZDV 2 mg/kg (or 1.5 mg/kg IV) 2 times per day for the first 4 weeks of age followed by 3 mg/kg orally (or 2.3 mg/kg IV) 2 times per day for the next 2 weeks of life
Combination ARV Prophylaxis for Infants Whose Mothers Have Not Received Antepartum ARV[d]	
>35 weeks' gestation	Oral ZDV 4 mg/kg 2 times per day until 6 weeks of age *plus* oral NVP 8 mg/dose (birth weight 1.5–2 kg) or 12 mg/dose (birth weight > 2 kg) given as a 3-dose regimen[e]

Abbreviations: ARV, antiretroviral prophylaxis; NVP, nevirapine; ZDV, zidovudine.
[a]Data from references 4, 5, and 12.
[b]For maternal treatment or perinatal HIV prevention prophylaxis.
[c]ARV prophylaxis must begin as soon after birth as possible and preferably within 6–12 hours of delivery. If infant unable to tolerate oral ZDV, intravenous administration is recommended.
[d]Data from references 5 and 12.
[e]NVP dosing regimen: dose 1: birth to 48 hours; dose 2: 48 hours after first; and dose 3: 96 hours after second.

because data on pharmacokinetic, dosing, and safety of alternative ARV drugs are lacking. Infant ARV prophylaxis initiated after 48 hours of birth is not effective.[13]

Physicians can contact the Perinatal HIV/AIDS (acquired immunodeficiency syndrome) Hotline (1-888-448-8765) and seek free clinical consultation services on all issues related to perinatal HIV, including infant care.[5] Social services should be involved before the mother and baby are discharged from the hospital to ensure compliance regarding follow-up visits. Newborns should be discharged with a supply of oral ZDV syrup.

Table 117-3 Indications for Combination Antiretroviral (ARV) Prophylaxis to Infants Exposed to Human Immunodefiency Virus[a]

HIV-positive mothers who have not received antepartum and intrapartum ARV drugs
HIV-positive mothers who have only received intrapartum ARV drugs
HIV-positive mothers who received antepartum and intrapartum ARV drugs but have not achieved optimal viral suppression at delivery
Mothers infected with ARV drug-resistant virus

[a]Data from the Panel on Treatment of HIV-Infected Pregnant Women and Prevention of Perinatal Transmission.[5]

Tests

Laboratory Testing

A repeat CBC is recommended at 4 weeks of age after starting infant ZDV prophylaxis to monitor for potential hematologic toxicity (anemia and neutropenia).[3] Anemia is the most frequently encountered adverse event related to ZDV. If there is evidence of hematologic adverse events in infants receiving ARV prophylaxis, a pediatric infectious disease specialist must be consulted to guide decisions regarding early discontinuation of prophylaxis.[5] Serum lactate level measurements are not routinely recommended but may be indicated if an infant experiences severe clinical symptoms of unknown etiology, especially neurologic symptoms.[5] In addition to CBC, some experts recommend serum chemistry and liver function tests at birth and when HIV PCR testing is done in infants exposed to combination ARV drug regimes during pregnancy or during the neonatal period.[5]

Infant HIV Testing

Virologic tests (HIV DNA or RNA assays) are needed for early infant HIV diagnosis and should be performed at 14–21 days of life, at 1–2 months of age, and at 4–6 months of age (Figure 117-1).[5] An infant is diagnosed with HIV infection if 2 separate blood samples test positive for HIV DNA or RNA PCR.[14] HIV

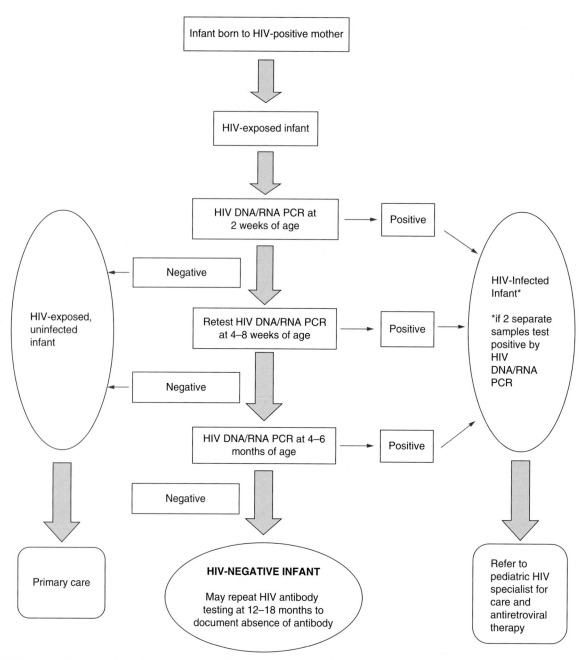

FIGURE 117-1 Diagnostic evaluation of the infant exposed to human immunodeficiency virus. PCR, polymerase chain reaction.

DNA PCR is the preferred virologic test for detection of subtype B HIV virus, the predominant viral subtype prevalent in the United States. For suspected non-subtype B virus detection, HIV RNA PCR should be used for early infant diagnosis.

Infection with HIV can be *presumptively excluded* in non-breast-feeding HIV-exposed children younger than 18 months of age with 2 or more negative virologic tests at age greater than 14 days and at greater than 1 month.[5] HIV infection can be *definitively excluded* in non-breast-feeding HIV-exposed children younger than 18 months of age with 2 or more negative virologic

tests at age greater than 1 month and at more than 4 months.[5] In children with 2 negative virologic tests, many experts confirm HIV-negative status by documenting a negative HIV antibody test result at 12 to 18 months of age ("seroreversion").[5,14] Documentation of negative HIV serology at age 18 months is recommended when non-subtype B HIV is suspected based on maternal origins.[4,5]

For any positive HIV DNA PCR result, the infant should be retested immediately for confirmatory PCR testing. If infection is confirmed by 2 positive virologic tests, ARV prophylaxis must be discontinued and a pediatric infectious disease consultation should be requested for confirming the diagnosis and initiation of combination ART if the infant is found to be HIV infected.[15]

Pneumocystis jiroveci Pneumonia Prophylaxis

Starting at 6 weeks of age after completion of an infant ARV prophylaxis regimen, all HIV-exposed infants with indeterminate HIV status should receive trimethoprim-sulfamethoxazole (TMP-SMX) to prevent *Pneumocystis jiroveci* pneumonia (PCP).[5,16] HIV-infected infants are at high risk of developing PCP between 3 and 6 months of life, which can result in high mortality.[17] Prophylaxis for PCP need not be initiated or can be stopped when infant HIV infection is presumptively or definitely excluded.

Infant Feeding

Mothers who are HIV infected should be advised not to breast-feed their infants in the United States because infant formulas are safe and readily available.[4,5,8] Postnatal transmission of HIV is prevented by complete avoidance of breast-feeding.[4,5,8] In addition, physicians must ask mothers about premastication of foods for infant feeding, counsel HIV-infected caregivers to avoid this practice, and discuss safe feeding options.[5,18]

FOLLOW-UP

Figure 117-1 provides a diagram outlining the initial evaluation and the necessary follow-up tests for an asymptomatic infant born to an HIV-positive mother, as recommended by the AAP.[8,14,19]

Online resources are available for physicians and other health care workers involved in perinatal HIV prevention programs (Table 117-4). In addition, postpartum follow-up care for HIV-positive mothers must

Table 117-4 Postpartum Care of HIV-Positive Mother

HIV specialty care (to make decisions regarding continuing ART postpartum)
Case management and other supportive services (to promote adherence to ART)
Family planning services and contraceptive counseling
Mental health services if indicated
Substance abuse treatment if indicated
Routine primary care

Abbreviations: ART, antiretroviral therapy; HIV, human immunodeficiency virus.

Table 117-5 Selected Online Resources for Perinatal HIV Prevention

Agency	Website Address
Department of Health and Human Services (DHHS)	http://aidsinfo.nih.gov /guidelines
American Academy of Pediatrics (AAP)	http://www.aap.org
Red Book	http://redbook.solutions .aap.org/Redbook.aspx
Antiretroviral Pregnancy Registry (APR)	http://APRegistry.com
Perinatal HIV/AIDS	http://nccc.ucsf.edu /clinician-consultation /perinatal-hiv-aids/
AIDS Education and Training Center (ATEC)	http://www.aidsetc.org
World Health Organization (WHO)	http://www.who.int

be carefully planned at discharge using a multidisciplinary approach. Several issues must be addressed, including contraceptive counseling, decisions regarding continuing ART postpartum, psychosocial support, and prompt linkage to HIV care and treatment of women diagnosed with HIV during labor (Table 117-5).

Long-Term Follow-up of HIV-Exposed Infants

The long-term carcinogenic effect of ARV drug (especially nucleoside analogue) exposure during the in utero/neonatal period is unknown. Therefore, HIV-exposed infants must be closely followed into adulthood. In addition, ARV-exposed neonates who develop significant organ, especially neurologic or cardiac, disease may need evaluation for mitochondrial dysfunction.[5]

Provision of Counseling and Psychosocial Support

Mothers infected with HIVs often face multiple physical, emotional, and social issues, including coping with the diagnosis, HIV illness or death in other family members, lack of health care, financial challenges, substance abuse, depression, and fear of loss of existing support and services. Mothers must be informed about the serial infant HIV-testing schedule during follow-up visits and informed about the delay in the definite exclusion of HIV infection status for the first several months of life.

Counseling, education, and support for mothers and other caregivers is critical and should include a discussion of all issues in the management of the HIV-exposed infant, including education and counseling regarding adherence to prescribed ARV prophylaxis to prevent perinatal HIV transmission and the administration of TMP-SMX prophylaxis to prevent PCP if indicated, avoidance of breast-feeding, infection control measures, schedule of follow-up visits, importance of maintaining confidentiality of test results, and planning for future child care if the parents are seriously ill from HIV/AIDS.[8, 20] Recommendations on the care of HIV-exposed infants in foster care have previously been published.[21] HIV-exposed and HIV-infected infants should not be excluded from day care.[22]

HIV Testing of Family Members

Testing for HIV should be offered to the infant's father and all siblings. Because perinatally acquired HIV-infected children may remain asymptomatic for several years, all siblings should be tested regardless of age.[8]

Anticipatory Guidance and Primary Care for HIV-Exposed Infants

Age-appropriate anticipatory guidance must be provided to all HIV-exposed infants, similar to the guidance provided for non-HIV-exposed infants. In addition, mothers and caregivers of HIV-exposed infants must receive anticipatory guidance around all components of care for the HIV-exposed infant.[6] Mothers must be counseled at every follow-up visit to completely avoid breast-feeding and against premastication of food for older infants.[4] In addition, HIV education related to modes of transmission must be provided to mothers and other caregivers, stressing the fact that touching, hugging, or kissing their infants is safe.[6]

Immunizations

Infants exposed to HIV should receive all routine childhood immunizations, including hepatitis B vaccine, inactivated polio vaccine, diphtheria and tetanus toxoids and acellular pertussis vaccine, *Haemophilus influenza* type b vaccine, pneumococcal conjugate vaccine, and *Rotavirus* vaccine.[4] If infant HIV infection is confirmed, then recommendations for the HIV infected must be followed. Readers are referred to the 2012 edition of the *Red Book* for guidance regarding immunization practices in HIV-infected children.[4]

CONCLUSION

In conclusion, management of the infant born to an HIV-positive mother must take into considerations several unique aspects specific to these infants,

including avoidance of breast-feeding, timely initiation of optimal ARV prophylaxis, serial HIV PCR testing within the first 4 months of life to determine infant HIV status, careful monitoring for toxicity related to ARV prophylaxis and clinical signs and symptoms of HIV infection, appropriate anticipatory guidance, and ongoing education and counseling of parents. Care of the HIV-exposed infant warrants a close partnership between the neonatologist, primary care pediatrician, and the pediatric infectious disease specialist.

REFERENCES

1. Cooper ER, Charurat M, Mofenson LM, et al. Combination anti-retroviral strategies for treatment of pregnant HIV-infected women and prevention of perinatal HIV-1 transmission. *J Acquir Immune Defic Syndr*. 2002;29(5):484–494.
2. Peters V, Liu K, Dominiguez K, et al. Missed opportunities for perinatal HIV prevention among HIV-exposed infants born 1996–2000, pediatric spectrum of HIV disease cohort. *Pediatrics*. 2003;111(5):1186–1191.
3. Centers for Disease Control and Prevention. *HIV/AIDS Surveillance Report 2009*; Vol. 21. http://www.cdc.gov/hiv/surveillance/resources/reports/2009report/#commentary. Published February 2001. Accessed July 29, 2012.
4. American Academy of Pediatrics. Human immunodeficiency virus infection. In: Pickering LK, Baker CJ, Kimberlin DW, Long SS, eds. *Red Book*, 28th ed. Elk Grove Village, IL: American Academy of Pediatrics; 2012:418–437.
5. Panel on Treatment of HIV-Infected Pregnant Women and Prevention of Perinatal Transmission. Recommendations for use of antiretroviral drugs in pregnant HIV-1 infected women for maternal health and interventions to reduce HIV-1 transmission. December 2011:1–117. http://aidsinfo.nih.gov/guidelines. Accessed July 29, 2012.
6. Robinson LG, Fernandez AD. Clinical care of the exposed infants of HIV-infected mothers. *Clin Perinatol*. 2010;37(4):863–872.
7. American Academy of Pediatrics Committee on Pediatric AIDS. HIV testing and prophylaxis to prevent mother-to-child transmission in the United States. *Pediatrics*. 2008;122(5):1127–1134.
8. King SM. American Academy of Pediatrics Committee on Pediatric AIDS; American Academy of Pediatrics Infectious Diseases and Immunization Committee. Evaluation and treatment of the human immunodeficiency virus-1-exposed infant. *Pediatrics*. 2004;114(2):497–505.
9. Branson BM, Handsfield HH, Lampe MA, et al. Revised recommendations for HIV testing of adults, adolescents, and pregnant women in health care settings. *MMWR Recomm Rep*. 2006;55(RR-14):1–17.
10. Galli L, de Martino M, Tovo P, et al. Onset of clinical signs in children with HIV-1 perinatal infection. *AIDS*. 1995;9:455–461.
11. Newell ML, Peckham C, Dunn D, et al. Natural history of vertically-acquired human immunodeficiency virus-1 infection. The European Collaborative Study. *Pediatrics*. 1994;94:815–819.
12. Nielsen-Saines K, Watts DH, Veloso VG, et al. Three postpartum antiretroviral regimens to prevent intrapartum HIV infection. *N Engl J Med*. 2012;366(25):2368–2379.
13. Wade NA, Birkhead GS, Warren BL, et al. Abbreviated regimens of zidovudine prophylaxis and perinatal transmission of the human immunodeficiency virus. *N Engl J Med*. 1998;339(20):1409–1414.
14. Havens PL, Mofenson LM. American Academy of Pediatrics, Committee on Pediatric AIDS. HIV testing and prophylaxis to

prevent mother-to-child transmission in the United States. *Pediatrics.* 2008;122(5):1127–1134.

15. King SM; American Academy of Pediatrics, Committee on Pediatric AIDS. Evaluation and treatment of the human immunodeficiency virus-1-exposed infant. *Pediatrics.* 2004;114(2):497–505.

16. Simonds RJ, Oxtoby MJ, Caldwell MB, et al. *Pneumocystis carinii* pneumonia among US children with perinatally acquired HIV infection. *JAMA,* 1993;270(4):470–473.

17. Mofenson LM, Brady MT, Danner ST, et al. Guidelines for prevention and treatment of opportunistic infections among HIV-exposed and HIV-infected children. Recommendations from CDC, the National Institutes of Health, the HIV Medicine Association of the Infectious Diseases Society of America, the Pediatric Infectious Disease Society, and the American Academy of Pediatrics. *MMWR Recomm Rep.* 2009;58(RR-11):1–166.

18. Ivy W 3rd, Dominguez KL, Rakhmanina NY, et al. Premastication as a route of pediatric HIV transmission: case-control and cross-sectional investigations. *J Acquir Immune Defic Syndr.* 2012;59(2):207–212.

19. Camacho-Gonzalez AF, Ross AC, Chakraborty R. The clinical care of the HIV-1 infected infant. *Clin Perinatol.* 2010;37(4): 873–885.

20. American Academy of Pediatrics, Committee on Pediatric AIDS. Planning for children whose parents are dying of HIV/AIDS. *Pediatrics* 1999;103(2):509–511.

21. American Academy of Pediatrics, Committee on Pediatric AIDS. Identification and care of HIV-exposed and HIV-infected infants, children, and adolescents in foster care. *Pediatrics,* 2000;106(1 Pt 1): 149–153.

22. American Academy of Pediatrics, Committee on Pediatric AIDS and Committee on Infectious Diseases. Issues related to human immunodeficiency virus transmission in schools, child care, medical settings, the home, and community. *Pediatrics.* 1999;104(2 Pt 1):318–324.

Evaluation of Hypotonia

Jin S. Hahn

DEFINITIONS

Muscle tone is the resistance of muscle to passive stretch. Hypotonia is a decreased tone in the limbs, trunk, or other skeletal muscles. With hypotonia, there is decreased resistance to passive movement across a joint.

INTRODUCTION

Hypotonia in a newborn may be caused by a wide variety of conditions. It can occur if there are abnormalities in the peripheral neuromuscular system, the central nervous system (CNS), or both. The severity may vary widely depending on the underlying cause.

HISTORY

A careful history of the pregnancy, labor, and delivery is important in determining possible congenital conditions or antenatal injury. The onset and the quality of fetal movements should be noted. Lack of fetal movements may suggest a myopathy. A history of unusual hyperextension of the neck in utero or breach delivery may suggest a spinal cord injury. Polyhydramnios suggests a fetal swallowing dysfunction, which may be an indicator of brainstem dysgenesis.

A family history of genetic or neuromuscular disorders and mental retardation is critical. A family history of disorders such as myasthenia gravis,

muscular dystrophies, or myotonic dystrophies can be useful in determining the etiology of hypotonia in the newborn infant.

The delivery method and course are also important to explore for possible injury to the brain and spinal cord or for hypoxic-ischemic brain injury. Hypoxic-ischemic encephalopathy is 1 of the most common causes of hypotonia in the neonatal intensive care unit intensive care unit.

The gestational age of the infant at delivery is important because most premature infants will display hypotonia. Postterm infants may also have various reasons for being hypotonic.

The neonatal course is also important for determining the temporal nature of the disorder and determining if there are any acquired conditions. Transient hypotonia is common in disorders such as hypermagnesemia (caused by maternal administration of intravenous magnesium) and transient myasthenia of newborns. Neuromuscular disorders and genetic syndromes will have effects on tone that are more lasting.

PHYSICAL EXAMINATION

A careful general and neurologic examination of the newborn may provide clues to the etiology. The general examination should focus on dysmorphic features that could be associated with genetic syndromes (eg, Down syndrome, Prader-Willi syndrome); size and shape of the head; neck and back examination (for any evidence of spinal dysraphisms); extremities (for limb

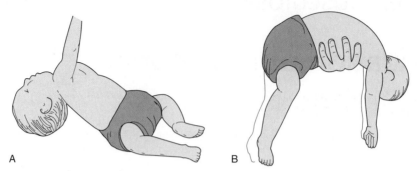

FIGURE 118-1 A, Hypotonic infant pulled into sitting position demonstrates poor head control with lag and lack of flexion of the arm. **B,** Hypotonic infant supported ventrally in horizontal position demonstrates limbs and head that hang limply. (Reproduced with permission from Dunn and Epstein.[1])

dysgenesis and joint contractures); and organomegaly for storage diseases (eg, Zellweger syndrome).

Hypotonia is assessed by passive range of motion of muscles across joints and functional tests such as the "traction response" test. The infant is pulled by arms from a supine position to a "sitting" position while assessing tone in the shoulder muscle and neck. If the infant has significant hypotonia, there will be a head lag (extension) and poor resistance in the upper limbs (Figure 118-1). The ventral suspension maneuver is also useful to determine the tone in the trunk (Figure 118-1).

The neurologic examination should be focused on eliciting clinical findings of an upper motor neuron vs a peripheral dysfunction. Table 118-1 provides some of the key neurologic examination findings depending on the localization of the dysfunction.

The presence of fasciculations, often most easily detectable on the tongue, would suggest a peripheral nerve or motor neuron disorder. The motor neurons may be located in the anterior horn of the spinal cord or in the brainstem nuclei that control bulbar musculature. The absence of deep tendon reflexes would suggest a peripheral neuropathy or anterior horn cell (AHC) disorder. Preservation of cognitive function in the setting of profound weakness suggests a peripheral process.

Initially, the newborns with upper motor dysfunction have normal deep tendon reflexes and hypotonia. Hyperreflexia and spasticity, hallmarks of upper motor neuron disorders, emerge after the newborn period.

ETIOLOGY

Localization and Differential Diagnosis

Hypotonia can occur if there are abnormalities in the muscle, neuromuscular junction (NMJ), axon/myelin sheath of peripheral nerve, AHCs, long tracts of the spinal cord, and the CNS (Figure 118-2). Table 118-2 provides various etiologies categorized by neurological

Table 118-1 Physical Examination Findings and Localization

	Central	Anterior Horn	Nerve	Neuromuscular Junction	Muscle
Strength	Normal	Generalized weakness	Weakness distal > proximal	Weakness in face, eyes, bulbar musculature	Weakness proximal > distal
Deep tendon reflexes	Normal or increased	Decreased or absent	Decreased or absent	Normal	Decreased
Fasciculations	Absent	Present	±	Absent	Absent
Other	Seizures Dysmorphic features	Alert mental status		Examine the mother	Examine the mother

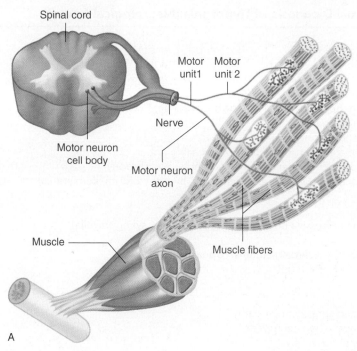

FIGURE 118-2 The motor unit is composed of the anterior horn cell, peripheral nerve, neuromuscular junction, and muscle.

localization. Hypotonia may also occur outside the nervous system and the motor unit. Table 118-3 provides various nonneurological etiologies.

Central Hypotonia

A history of perinatal depression and signs of neonatal encephalopathy point to possible hypoxic-ischemic brain injury as a cause of hypotonia. Intracranial hemorrhage or strokes may also cause seizures along with hypotonia. Drug administration, such as benzodiazepines, will cause hypotonia along with depressed mental status.

The presence of hypotonia with lack of muscle weakness and normal creatine kinase (CK) favors the central type of hypotonia owing to a defect in the CNS. Hundreds of different genetic syndromes with chromosomal or gene defects can cause hypotonia. Common genetic disorders include Down syndrome, Prader-Willi-Angelman syndrome, and William syndrome.[3] The presence of severe epilepsy in the setting of hypotonia may suggest gray matter disorders, such as Rett syndrome in females and *MECP2* duplication syndrome in males.

Infants with Zellweger syndrome have profound hypotonia along with dysmorphic facial features (flattened facial profile and broad nasal bridge), large anterior fontanelle, feeding difficulties, congenital cataracts, chondrodysplasia punctata, and seizures.

Peripheral Hypotonia

Hypotonia associated with true weakness (ie, inability or diminished ability to move limbs against gravity) is suggestive of a peripheral cause of hypotonia. A peripheral cause implies a dysfunction in the motor unit, which includes the AHC (lower motor neuron), peripheral nerves, NMJ, and the muscle (Figure 118-2). Table 118-4 provides a detailed differential diagnosis.

Spinal muscular atrophy (SMA) type 1 (Werdnig-Hoffman disease) is a more common cause of peripheral hypotonia. Infants usually develop hypotonia, progressive proximal weakness, areflexia, tongue fasciculations, and mild contractures. A form that presents prenatally also exists in which hypotonia and arthrogryposis multiplex congenita are present at birth.

Infants with congenital myotonic dystrophy present with severe weakness, facial diplegia, and respiratory distress. In neonates with severe forms, there is maternal transmission, and the mother usually has a milder form. Examination of the mother for myopathic face, grip myotonia, or percussion myotonia is key to the diagnosis in the infants.

Congenital muscular dystrophies are a heterogeneous group of disorders that have varied presentations but often include proximal weakness and contractures. The most common type is merosin-deficient (laminin α2) congenital muscular dystrophy. The second most common form is Ullrich congenital muscular dystrophy.[4]

Table 118-2 Differential Diagnosis of Hypotonia (Neurological Cause)

- **Central**
  - Central nervous system
    » Hypoxic-ischemic encephalopathy
    » Intracranial hemorrhage
    » Chromosomal or gene abnormalities (Down syndrome, Prader-Willi syndrome, Angelman syndrome, William syndrome)
    » Cerebral malformations
    » Infections (sepsis, meningoencephalitis, TORCH, HIV)
    » Peroxisomal disorders (Zellweger, neonatal adrenoleukodystrophy)
    » Toxic/metabolic encephalopathy (benzodiazepine, hypothyroidism, kernicterus)
  - Spinal cord
    » Birth trauma
    » Spinal cord dysraphisms (spina bifida, myelomeningocele, syringomyelia)
  - Anterior horn cell
    » Spinal muscular atrophy (Werdnig-Hoffman disease)
  - Benign familial hypotonia
- **Peripheral**
  - Peripheral nerve
    » Hereditary motor and sensory neuropathy
    » Congenital hypomyelination neuropathy
    » Infantile neuroaxonal dystrophy
    » Familial dysautonomia
    » Guillain-Barré syndrome
  - Neuromuscular junction
    » Myasthenic syndromes
      • Transient neonatal myasthenia
      • Congenital myasthenia syndromes (channelopathies)
      • Familial infantile myasthenia
    » Infantile botulism
    » Magnesium toxicity
  - Muscle
    » Structurally specific congenital myopathies
      • Nemaline (rod) myopathy
      • Central core myopathy
      • Myotubular myopathy
      • Congenital fiber-type disproportion
    » Muscular dystrophies
      • Myotonic dystrophy
      • Infantile fascioscapulohumeral dystrophy
      • Congenital muscular dystrophies (including merosin deficiency)
    » Myopathies with biochemical cause
      • Glycogen storage diseases (Pompe disease)
      • Lipid myopathies
      • Mitochondrial myopathies
      • Carnitine palmitoyltransferase deficiency type 2 (neonatal lethal form)
- **Combined central and peripheral**
  - Dystroglycanopathies
    » Walker-Warburg syndrome
    » Fukuyama type congenital muscular dystrophy
    » Muscle-eye-brain disease
  - Congenital disorders of glycosylation
  - Canavan disease
  - Mitochondrial encephalomyopathies
  - Congenital Pelizaeus-Merzbacher disease

Table 118-3 Nonneurological Causes of Hypotonic Newborns

Hypothyroidism
Amino acid abnormalities
Mucopolysaccharide abnormalities
Metabolic acidosis
Congenital laxity of ligaments: Ehlers-Danlos syndrome, Marfan syndrome
Cyanotic congenital heart disease
Maternal deprivation

EVALUATION

An algorithm for approaching a newborn with hypotonia and weakness caused by a disorder of the motor unit is shown in Figure 118-3. Table 118-4 provides a list of tests depending on the localization. By following the algorithm, tests can be done in a logical sequential order, thus reducing the costs and time to reach a diagnosis. Other findings on the examination or imaging studies may point to a specific diagnosis (Table 118-5).

Laboratory Tests

Unless the etiology of the hypotonia is known, all infants should have a CK test. Other routine laboratory tests include those for thyroid-stimulating hormone (TSH), free T4 (levorotatory thyroxine), liver function test, or ammonia. For metabolic disorders, tests to consider include those for lactate, pyruvate, urine organic acids, plasma amino acids, acylcarnitine profile, isoelectric focusing or serum ferritin glycosylation (for congenital disorders of glycosylation), and cerebrospinal fluid (CSF) neurotransmitter studies.

Very long-chain fatty acids should be analyzed when peroxisomal disorders are suspected.

Imaging

Magnetic resonance imaging (MRI) of the brain is useful for detecting acute changes (eg, diffusion restriction associated with hypoxic-ischemic brain injury, intracranial hemorrhage, underlying cerebral malformation, and white matter changes). T2 hyperintensities of white matter are seen in congenital muscular dystrophy (such as merosin deficiency). Type II (cobblestone) lissencephalies are seen in the dystroglycanopathies.

Electrophysiology Tests

Nerve conduction studies (NCS) and electromyography (EMG) can be useful adjuncts for detecting disorders of peripheral nerves, NMJ, and muscle. A peripheral neuropathy with abnormal myelination may show marked conduction slowing on NCS. Low-amplitude brief compound muscle action potentials point to a myopathy. Repetitive nerve stimulation tests can help detect defects of transmission in the NMJ. However, in our experience, NCS and EMG studies in newborns are often technically challenging and difficult to interpret. The use of molecular genetic testing and histochemical studies of muscle/nerve biopsies have reduced our dependence on electrophysiology tests.

Muscle and Nerve Biopsy

If molecular tests are negative and the electrophysiologic studies suggest a neuropathy or myopathy, a

Table 118-4 Workup and Localization

CNS	AHC	Nerve	NMJ	Muscle
HUS	Molecular genetics	EMG/NCS	EMG/NCS	CK
CT head	EMG/NCS	Nerve biopsy	Anti-Ach antibodies	EMG/NCS
MRI	Muscle biopsy	Molecular genetics	Neostigmine challenge	Muscle biopsy
EEG			*Clostridium botulinum* toxin	Molecular genetics
Karyotype			assay in stool	
Molecular genetics				
TORCH screen				
Metabolic workup				

Abbreviations: CK, creatine kinase; CNS, central nervous system; CT, computed tomography; EEG, electroencephalography; EMG, electromyography; HUS, Head ultrasound; MRI, magnetic resonance imaging; NCS, nerve conduction studies; NMJ, neuromuscular junction; TORCH, toxoplasmosis, rubella, cytomegalovirus, herpes simplex virus.

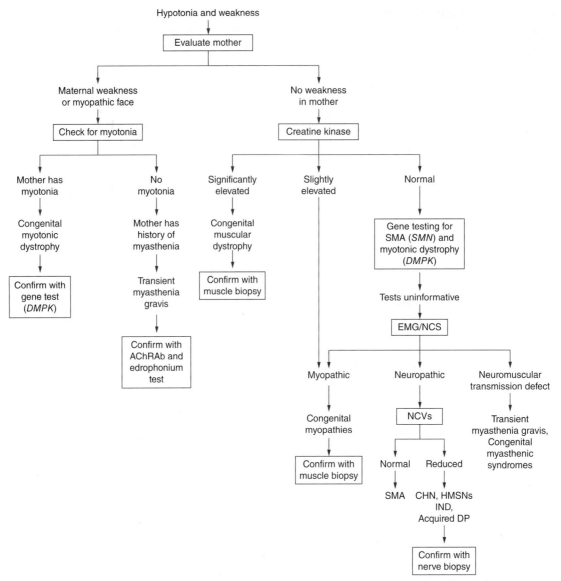

FIGURE 118-3 An algorithm for approaching a newborn with hypotonia and weakness attributable to a disorder of the motor unit (peripheral cause). The motor unit includes the anterior horn cell, peripheral nerve, neuromuscular junction, and muscle. Central causes of hypotonia and weakness are not considered in this diagram. AChRAb, acetylcholine receptor antibody; CHN, congenital hypomyelination neuropathy; DP, demyelinating polyneuropathy; EMG/NCS, electromyography/nerve conduction studies; HMSNs, hereditary motor and sensory neuropathy; IND, infantile neuronal degeneration; NCV, nerve conduction velocity; SMA, spinal muscular atrophy. (Modified with permission from Hahn et al.[2])

muscle/nerve biopsy may be required to establish the diagnosis. The samples should be evaluated by a neuropathology laboratory with expertise in pediatric neuromuscular disorders.

Genetic Tests

For newborns suspected of having a central form of hypotonia, a high-resolution karyotype, array comparative genomic hybridization (CGH), or single-nucleotide polymorphism array is a must. Array CGH will detect duplication and deletion syndromes such as William syndrome and *MECP2* syndromes. Other studies depend on the index of suspicion for various disorders (eg, fluorescence in situ hybridization [FISH] and methylation tests for Prader-Willi/Angelman syndrome). An updated list of available tests for genetic disorders can be found at the GeneTests website (http://www.genetests.org).

Table 118-5 Findings Pointing to Specific Causes of Hypotonia

Findings	Diseases for Consideration
Hepatosplenomegaly	Storage disorders, congenital infections
Renal cysts, high forehead, wide fontanelle	Zellweger syndrome (peroxisome/leukodystrophy)
Hepatomegaly, retinitis pigmentosa	Neonatal adrenoleukodystrophy
Congenital cataracts, glaucoma	Oculocerebrorenal (Lowe) syndrome
Abnormal odor	Metabolic disorders (multiple carboxylase deficiency)
Hypopigmentation, undescended testes	Prader-Willi syndrome
Examination of the mother	Myotonic dystrophy, myasthenia gravis
Arthrogryposis (fixation of joints at birth)	Congenital muscular dystrophy
Abnormal white matter T2 signal intensity on MRI	Congenital muscular dystrophy (laminin α2 or merosin deficiency)
Lissencephaly on MRI	Dystroglycanopathies
Hypertrophic cardiomyopathy on ECHO, shortened P-R interval on ECG	Pompe disease

Abbreviations: ECG, electrocardiogram; ECHO, echocardiogram; MRI, magnetic resonance imaging.

When faced with a newborn with extreme hypotonia and weakness, molecular tests will be useful for certain diagnoses (eg, *SMN* test for SMA; *DMPK* test for congenital myotonic dystrophy; and *POMT* and *FKRP* for dystroglycanopathies).

TREATMENT AND MANAGEMENT

Treatment and management of patients with hypotonia are dependent on the etiology. For all types, proper supportive care, such as dealing with feeding issues, is important. Certain metabolic/genetic diseases may have specific treatments (such as Pompe disease). Patients with peripheral disorders, such as SMA and congenital mypopathies or dystrophies should be referred to a neuromuscular program. Physical and occupational therapy may improve the tone and motor development.

REFERENCES

1. Dunn DW, Epstein LG. *Decision Making in Child Neurology*, Philadelphia, PA: Decker; 1987.
2. Hahn JS, Henry M, Hudgins L, Madan A. Congenital hypomyelination neuropathy in a newborn infant: Unusual cause of diaphragmatic and vocal cord paralyses. *Pediatrics*. 2001:108(5):e95.
3. Lisi EC, Cohn RD. Genetic evaluation of the pediatric patient with hypotonia: perspective from a hypotonia specialty clinic and review of the literature. *Dev Med Child Neurol*. 2011;53:586–599.
4. Sparks SE, Escolar DM. Congenital muscular dystrophies. *Handb Clin Neurol*. 2011;101:47–79.

CHAPTER 118

119 Evaluation of Short-Limbed Infants

Anna-Kaisa Niemi and Louanne Hudgins

INTRODUCTION

Evaluation of a newborn with short limbs is often an urgent challenge for the pediatrician and the neonatologist because of the importance of recognizing lethal neonatal skeletal dysplasias, the ability to provide adequate medical management in nonlethal neonatal skeletal dysplasias, and the ability to provide adequate prognostic information to the family during the stages of the initial evaluation. Sometimes, the diagnosis is evident based on physical examination of the newborn, but more often combined information from prenatal ultrasounds, physical examination of the newborn, and skeletal radiographs and other imaging studies is needed to establish a definitive diagnosis.

The evaluation and initial treatment of the neonate who has short limbs and a suspected skeletal disorder require a multidisciplinary approach, usually the expertise of a neonatologist, a medical geneticist, and a radiologist. Other specialty services are involved depending on the associated findings, and these experts typically include otorhinolaryngology, plastic surgery, orthopedic surgery, ophthalmology, as well as neurosurgery services.

Molecular genetic studies are available for some of the more common disorders and can be used to confirm the diagnosis and to provide for a prenatal diagnosis in the future pregnancies of the family, if desired. There are currently more than 400 recognized genetic skeletal disorders, which can be divided into several groups based on molecular, biochemical, or radiographic criteria.[1] The molecular etiology is known for approximately 300 of these genetic skeletal disorders,[1] providing an opportunity to establish a specific diagnosis and provide accurate prognostic information for the family.

In addition to genetic etiologies of short limbs in newborns, there are nongenetic causes, such as fetal warfarin exposure, which mimics the skeletal phenotype of chondrodysplasia punctatas,[2,3] and maternal diabetes, which has been associated with asymmetric shortening of femoral bones because of proximal focal femoral hypoplasia.[4,5] These nongenetic etiologies are important to recognize to be able to provide accurate information regarding recurrence risk and, in cases of a teratogen exposure, to be able to prevent recurrence in future pregnancies.

PRENATAL ULTRASOUND IN THE EVALUATION AND DIAGNOSIS OF A FETUS WITH SHORT LONG BONES

Because many skeletal disorders begin to manifest in fetal development, a suspicion of a congenital skeletal disorder will often be raised during an ultrasonographic evaluation of a fetus in the second trimester. The clavicle, mandible, ileum, scapulae, and long bones ossify by 12 weeks of gestation; the metacarpals and metatarsals by 12 to 16 weeks; and the talus and calcaneus around 22–24 weeks, and epiphyseal ossification centers are seen on radiographs around 20 weeks of gestation.[6] Some short-limbed skeletal disorders have characteristic findings that can lead to an accurate diagnosis on a prenatal ultrasonographic examination (Table 119-1).[7–9] Early diagnosis of a fetal skeletal disorder during the prenatal period allows time for genetic counseling, may

Table 119-1 Prenatal Ultrasound Findings and Associated Conditions in a Fetus With a Short-Limbed or Bent-Bone Skeletal Disorder[7–9,a]

Ultrasound Finding	Associated Conditions
Absent/hypoplastic/small scapulae	Campomelic dysplasia Cleidocranial dysplasia
Bowing of long bones	Achondrogenesis (types IA, IB) Antley-Bixler syndrome[b] Atelosteogenesis (types I–III) Campomelic dysplasia (tibiae and fibulae) Diastrophic dysplasia Focal femoral hypoplasia (maternal diabetes) Hypophosphatasia Short-rib polydactyly syndromes (I–IV) Stuve-Wiedemann syndrome Thanatophoric dysplasia (type I)
Cloverleaf skull/craniosynostosis	Antley-Bixler syndrome[a] Thanatophoric dysplasia (type II)
Equinovarus (clubfeet)	Achondrogenesis (types IA, IB, II) Atelosteogenesis (types I–III) Campomelic dysplasia Diastrophic dysplasia Hypophosphatasia Osteogenesis imperfecta (types II, III) Short-rib polydactyly syndromes (I–IV) Thanatophoric dysplasia (types I, II)
Fractures of long bones	Hypophosphatasia Osteogenesis imperfecta type II
Hitchhiker thumbs	Atelosteogenesis type I Diastrophic dysplasia (most common) Otopalatodigital syndrome type 2
Nasal flattening/hypoplasia of nasal bone	Achondrogenesis (type II) Thanatophoric dysplasia (type II) Warfarin exposure
Hyperechogenic cartilaginous bone (premature calcification)	Chondrodysplasia punctatas Warfarin exposure
Micrognathia	Achondrogenesis (type II) Campomelic dysplasia Chondrodysplasia punctatas Diastrophic dysplasia Short-rib polydactyly syndrome (type II, Majewski)
Polydactyly	Asphyxiating thoracic dysplasia (Jeune syndrome) Chondroectodermal dysplasia (Ellis-van Creveld) Short-rib polydactyly syndromes (I–IV)
Poor mineralization of the calvarium	Achondrogenesis IA Cleidocranial dysplasia Hypophosphatasia Osteogenesis imperfecta type II
Poor mineralization of the vertebrae	Achondrogenesis (types IA, IB, II) Atelosteogenesis (types I–III) Thanatophoric dysplasia (types I, II)

(Continued)

Table 119-1 Prenatal Ultrasound Findings and Associated Conditions in a Fetus With a Short-Limbed or Bent-Bone Skeletal Disorder[7-9,a] (Continued)

Ultrasound Finding	Associated Conditions
Thoracic hypoplasia (severe)[c]	Achondrogenesis (types IA, IB, II) Asphyxiating thoracic dysplasia (Jeune syndrome) Atelosteogenesis (types I–III) Hypochondrogenesis Short-rib polydactyly syndromes Thanatophoric dysplasia (types I, II)

[a]Adapted with permission from Krakow D, Lachman RS, Rimoin DL. Guidelines for the prenatal diagnosis of fetal skeletal dysplasias. ACMG Practice Guidelines. *Genet Med.* 2009;11:127–133.
[b]Skeletal features in Antley-Bixler syndrome include contractures and femoral bowing but typically not severe shortening of the limbs.[23]
[c]A narrow thorax is also present in campomelic dysplasia, cleidocranial dysplasia, and diastrophic dysplasia, but thoracic hypoplasia is typically not severe enough to cause respiratory compromise and death.

allow for reproductive options for the couple, and helps medical providers plan postnatal care.

Prenatally, it is important to distinguish between lethal and nonlethal skeletal disorders. Approximately 99% of fetuses with a skeletal dysplasia can have the dysplasia correctly classified as either lethal or nonlethal via prenatal ultrasonography (US).[9] Lethality in congenital skeletal disorders is typically related to lung hypoplasia secondary to a narrow thoracic cavity.[9,10] Among the nonlethal forms, it is important to diagnose the specific type of skeletal disorder to allow planning for postnatal care. The diagnostic accuracy by prenatal US is the highest among the two most common skeletal dysplasias: thanatophoric dysplasia (TD) and osteogenesis imperfecta (OI).[9] Given that respiratory compromise is often a life-threatening possibility in many fetal skeletal dysplasias that present with short long bones in a neonate, in the case of a suspicion of such a skeletal disorder, the delivery should be planned for a center that has expertise to manage respiratory difficulties in

a newborn. This expertise typically includes otorhino-laryngology and anesthesiology teams. Other postnatal evaluations and care can also be optimized in a tertiary care center, such as orthopedic (hand and foot deformities), neurosurgical (cervical spine abnormalities), and plastic surgery (cleft palate) evaluations.

FINDINGS ON POSTNATAL PHYSICAL EXAMINATION OF A NEONATE WITH SHORT LONG BONES

A careful physical examination to look for other major and minor anomalies should be performed in any newborn with short limbs. Findings on physical examination not only may provide diagnostic clues (Table 119-2) but also aid in the initial assessment for the need of medical management and further evaluations by expert teams,

Table 119-2 Findings on the Initial Physical Examination of a Newborn With Short Limbs That May Provide Diagnostic Clues[a]

Finding on Clinical Examination	Associated Conditions
Ambiguous genitalia	Campomelic dysplasia
Cataracts	Chondrodysplasia punctatas
Cleft lip or palate	Atelosteogenesis type 2 Campomelic dysplasia Diastrophic dysplasia Short-rib polydactyly syndromes
Dental abnormalities • Dentinogenesis imperfecta • Natal teeth • Supernumerary teeth	Osteogenesis imperfecta Chondroectodermal dysplasia (Ellis-van Creveld) Cleidocranial dysplasia
Earlobe abnormalities	Diastrophic dysplasia ("cauliflower ear")

(Continued)

Table 119-2 Findings on the Initial Physical Examination of a Newborn With Short Limbs That May Provide Diagnostic Clues[a] (*Continued*)

Finding on Clinical Examination	Associated Conditions
Equinovarus (clubfeet)	Achondrogenesis (types IA, IB, II) Atelosteogenesis (types I–III) Campomelic dysplasia Diastrophic dysplasia Hypophosphatasia Osteogenesis imperfecta (types II, III) Short-rib polydactyly syndromes (types I–IV) Thanatophoric dysplasia (types I, II)
Frontal bossing/macrocephaly	Achondroplasia Hypochondroplasia
Gingival frenulae	Asphyxiating thoracic dysplasia (Jeune syndrome) Chondroectodermal dysplasia (Ellis-van Creveld)
Hitchhiker thumbs	Atelosteogenesis type II Diastrophic dysplasia (most common) Otopalatodigital syndrome type 2
Hypoplastic nails	Chondroectodermal dysplasia (Ellis-van Creveld) Chondrodysplasia punctata (brachytelephalangic)
Ichtyosiform skin	Chondrodysplasia punctatas
Large fontanelles/wide sutures	Achondrogenesis Cleidocranial dysplasia Hypophosphatasia
Micrognathia	Achondrogenesis (type II) Campomelic dysplasia Chondrodysplasia punctatas Cleidocranial dysplasia Diastrophic dysplasia Short-rib polydactyly syndrome (type II)
Nasal flattening/hypoplasia of nasal bone	Achondrogenesis (type II) Thanatophoric dysplasia (type II) Warfarin exposure
Polydactyly	Asphyxiating thoracic dysplasia (Jeune syndrome) Chondroectodermal dysplasia (Ellis-van Creveld) Short-rib polydactyly syndromes (types I–IV)
Type of shortening of limbs: acromelic Asymmetric Mesomelic	Asphyxiating thoracic dysplasia (Jeune syndrome) Chondroectodermal dysplasia (Ellis-van Creveld)
Micromelic Rhizomelic	Chondrodysplasia punctata (Conradi-Hunermann) Campomelic dysplasia Achondrogenesis Hypochondrogenesis Spondyloepiphyseal dysplasia congenita Achondroplasia Atelosteogenesis Chondrodysplasia punctata (recessive type) Thanatophoric dysplasia

[a]Note that some of the findings may also be evident in prenatal ultrasonographic evaluation (Table 119-1).

such as in the case of a cleft palate. Initial physical examination also guides the need for further imaging studies in the evaluation of a newborn with short limbs. For example, a finding of polydactyly in an infant who has short limbs should prompt a physician to evaluate carefully for cardiac (chondroectodermal dysplasia) or renal (cystic dysplastic kidneys in short-rib polydactyly syndromes) anomalies (Tables 119-2 to 119-4).

Table 119-3 Radiographic Findings on Skeletal X-ray Study in Infants With Short Limbs

Radiographic Finding	Associated Conditions
Bowing of long bones	Achondrogenesis (types IA, IB) Atelosteogenesis (types I–III) Campomelic dysplasia (tibiae and fibulae) Diastrophic dysplasia Focal femoral hypoplasia (maternal diabetes) Hypophosphatasia Short-rib polydactyly syndromes (I–IV) Stuve-Wiedemann syndrome Thanatophoric dysplasia (type I)
Clavicles: hypoplastic	Cleidocranial dysplasia
Fractures	Hypophosphatasia Osteogenesis imperfecta
Increased bone density	Osteopetrosis
Narrowing of interpedicular distance caudally	Achondroplasia Diastrophic dysplasia Thanatophoric dysplasia
Pelvis: characteristic findings on x-ray	Achondrogenesis (wide symphysis pubis) Achondroplasia (flat acetabular angles, narrow sacroiliac notches, hypoplastic iliae) Cleidocranial dysplasia (wide symphysis pubis) Spondyloepiphyseal dysplasia congenital (wide symphysis pubis, flat acetabular angles, flared iliac crests) Thanatophoric dysplasia (hypoplastic iliae)
Ribs: beaded	Achondrogenesis Osteogenesis imperfecta
Ribs: short	Asphyxiating thoracic dysplasia (Jeune) Thanatophoric dysplasia
Scapulae: hypoplastic	Campomelic dysplasia
Scoliosis/cervical kyphosis	Campomelic dysplasia Diastrophic dysplasia
Short, wide long bones (crumpled)	Osteogenesis imperfecta (reflects fractures)
Stippled epiphyses/punctate cartilage calcifications	Chondrodysplasia punctatas Spondylo-meta-epiphyseal dysplasia (SMED) short limb-hand type (extremely rare) Warfarin exposure
Undermineralization of skeleton	Achondrogenesis Hypophosphatasia Osteogenesis imperfecta
Vertebrae: coronal clefts	Chondrodysplasia punctata (recessive)
Vertebrae: dysplastic	Hypochondrogenesis Spondyloepiphyseal dysplasia congenita

There are four main patterns of limb shortening that may be suggestive of a specific skeletal disorder: rhizomelic, mesomelic, acromelic, and micromelic shortening (Table 119-2). Rhizomelic shortening affects the proximal segment of limbs (femur and humerus) and is typical, for example, of autosomal recessive chondrodysplasia punctata.[3] In mesomelic shortening, the middle segments of limbs (radius, ulna, tibia, and fibula) are affected. Shortening and bowing of tibiae and fibulae are typical of campomelic dysplasia (CD).[11] Acromelic shortening affects the distal segment of limbs (hands and feet). In micromelic shortening, all part of the limbs are shortened.

Table 119-4 Findings on Other Imaging Studies or Evaluations in Newborns With Short Limbs

Imaging Study Finding	Associated Conditions
Basilar impression/brainstem compression	Achondroplasia/hypochondroplasia Chondrodysplasia punctata (recessive) Osteogenesis imperfecta Thanatophoric dysplasia
Central nervous system abnormalities	Thanatophoric dysplasia
Congenital heart defect	Chondroectodermal dysplasia (Ellis-van Creveld)
Hearing loss (C, conductive; SN, sensorineural)	Osteogenesis imperfecta (C, SN)
Polycystic dysplastic kidneys	Short-rib polydactyly syndromes

POSTNATAL SKELETAL RADIOGRAPHS AND OTHER IMAGING STUDIES IN THE DIAGNOSIS OF A NEONATE WITH SHORT LONG BONES

Skeletal radiographic images play a critical role in defining the characteristic skeletal features present in many skeletal disorders (Table 119-3).[12,13] A skeletal survey consisting of frontal and lateral views of the thoracic and lumbar spines; lateral views of the cervical spine and skull; and anteroposterior views of the pelvis, chest, long bones, and hands should be obtained. Some skeletal dysplasias are associated with abnormalities in other organ systems; these can be evaluated for by the means of imaging studies (Table 119-4). Physical examination and the suspicion of a specific skeletal disorder should guide the choice of imaging studies in the diagnostic workup of a newborn with short limbs.

SELECTED COMMON OR SEVERE SKELETAL DYSPLASIAS PRESENTING IN A NEONATE WITH SHORT LONG BONES

Achondroplasia

Achondroplasia is an autosomal dominant condition (OMIM [Online Mendelian Inheritance in Man] 100800) caused by specific mutations in the *FGFR3* gene, with 99% of the mutations occurring in a single nucleotide, the most common change being c.1138G>A

(p.Gly380Arg) in 98% of cases.[14] It is the most common form of short-limb skeletal dysplasia. Achondroplasia is characterized by rhizomelic shortening of the limbs, characteristic facies with frontal bossing and midfacial hypoplasia, exaggerated lumbar lordosis, limitation of elbow extension, genu varum, brachydactyly, and trident appearance of the hands. In infancy, hypotonia is typical, and motor milestones are often delayed. Intelligence and life span are usually normal, although craniocervical junction compression increases the risk of death in infancy. Around 80% of individuals with achondroplasia have parents with normal stature and have achondroplasia as the result of a de novo mutation. If both parents have achondroplasia, the risk to their offspring of having a homozygous lethal achondroplasia is 25%.

Campomelic Dysplasia

Campomelic dysplasia is an autosomal dominant skeletal dysplasia (OMIM 114290) caused by mutations in the *SOX9* gene.[11] It is characterized by distinctive facies, Pierre Robin sequence with cleft palate, shortening and bowing of long bones, club feet, laryngotracheomalacia, and ambiguous genitalia or normal female external genitalia in individuals with a 46,XY karyotype. Many die in the neonatal period from respiratory compromise caused by airway instability or cervical spine instability.[11] Problems in long-term survivors include short stature, cervical spine instability with cord compression, progressive scoliosis, and hearing impairment. CD is usually caused by de novo mutations with a low recurrence risk, but recurrence in siblings because of somatic mosaicism has been described.[15] Thus, careful genetic counseling is recommended.

Diastrophic Dysplasia

Diastrophic dysplasia (DTD) is an autosomal recessive, nonlethal, but progressive skeletal dysplasia (OMIM 222600) caused by mutations in the *SLC26A2* gene.[16] DTD is characterized by shortening of long bones, proximally placed radially deviated thumbs ("hitchhiker thumb"), broad first toes, metatarsus adductus, talipes equinovarus, kyphoscoliosis, and an acquired, characteristic earlobe abnormality also referred to as "cauliflower ear." Other features often present in newborns with DTD include micrognathia, cleft palate (30%), and respiratory issues caused by deficient tracheal cartilage.[16] Mortality during the neonatal period is 25% because of respiratory issues. Most individuals have normal intelligence and, apart from skeletal issues, are in good health.

Osteogenesis Imperfecta Type II

Osteogenesis imperfecta (OI) (OMIM 166210) is a mostly autosomal dominant group of disorders characterized by fractures with minimal/absent trauma, dentinogenesis imperfecta, and often hearing loss and is caused by mutations in *COL1A1* and *COL1A2*.[17] The clinical features are a continuum ranging from perinatal lethality to nearly asymptomatic individuals with a normal life span and a mild predisposition to fractures.[17] OI type II is a perinatal lethal form with multiple rib fractures; minimal skull mineralization; small, beaded ribs (pathognomonic); platyspondyly; compression of long bones (broad, crumpled, bent femurs); severely short stature; and dark blue sclerae. Some fetuses die in utero; more typically, infants die in the immediate neonatal period: 60% die on the first day and 80% within the first week because of respiratory difficulties related to the small thorax, rib fractures, or flail chest because of lack of stable ribs. Survival beyond 1 year is exceedingly rare and involves intensive support, such as continuous assisted ventilation.[17,18]

Thanatophoric Dysplasia

Thanatophoric dysplasia (OMIM 187600 and 187601) is a usually perinatally lethal skeletal dysplasia caused by mutations in the *FGFR3* gene.[19,20] TD is divided into type I with short limbs, bowed femurs, and, uncommonly, cloverleaf skull deformity; type II is characterized by short limbs, straight femurs, and a uniform presence of moderate-to-severe cloverleaf skull deformity.[20] Other features common to both types include polyhydramnios, short ribs, narrow thorax, macrocephaly, distinctive facial features, brachydactyly, hypotonia, and redundant skin folds along the limbs and characteristic "French telephone receiver" femurs that can be detected prenatally. Most infants die of respiratory insufficiency shortly after birth. Some children have survived into childhood with aggressive ventilator support, and rare long-term survivors have been reported.

SUMMARY

A thorough systematic approach in evaluating a newborn with short limbs combines information from prenatal US evaluations (Table 119-1), physical examination of the newborn (Table 119-2), as well as skeletal radiographs (Table 119-3) and other postnatal imaging studies and evaluations (Table 119-4). Assessment for respiratory compromise secondary to lung hypoplasia or tracheobronchomalacia is of primary concern given that respiratory issues are a common cause of neonatal mortality in infants with skeletal dysplasia. After ensuring respiratory status, the rest of the physical examination should be conducted in a systematical manner along with other evaluations. Because of a large number of recognized congenital genetic skeletal disorders,[1] many of which are extremely rare or do

Table 119-5 Inheritance Pattern and Causative Gene of Selected Most Common or Severe Skeletal Dysplasias That Cause Short Limbs in Infants[a]

Inheritance Pattern	Gene	Condition
Autosomal dominant (de novo)	COL2A1	Achondrogenesis type II Hypochondrogenesis
	FGFR3	Achondroplasia Hypochondroplasia Thanatophoric dysplasia
	RUNX2	Cleidocranial dysplasia
	SOX9	Campomelic dysplasia
Autosomal recessive	AGPS	Chondrodysplasia punctata: rhizomelic type 3
	ALPL	Hypophosphatasia
	COL1A2	Osteogenesis imperfecta type II (can also be dominant)
	DTSD (SLC26A2)	Achondrogenesis type IB Atelosteogenesis type II Diastrophic dysplasia
	DHPAT	Chondrodysplasia punctata: rhizomelic type 2
	EVC1	Chondroectodermal dysplasia (Ellis-van Creveld)
	IFT80 and DYNCH2H1	Asphyxiating thoracic dysplasia (Jeune) Short-rib polydactyly syndrome type 1/3 (Saldino-Noonan)
	LIFR	Stüve-Wiedemann syndrome
	PEX7	Chondrodysplasia punctata: rhizomelic type 1
	NEK1	Short-rib polydactyly syndrome type 2 (Majewski)
	TRIP11	Achondrogenesis type IA
X linked	ARSE	Chondrodysplasia punctata (XL recessive)
	EBP	Chondrodysplasia punctata (Conradi-Hunermann, XL dominant)

[a]For a comprehensive list of currently known genetic skeletal disorders and associated genes see Warman et al. "Nosology and Classification of Genetic Skeletal Disorders: 2010 Revision."[1]

not present primarily with short limbs in a newborn, the reader is encouraged to seek further information from other resources as well[1,8,12,13,21,22] and to consult a genetics specialist, especially if the clinical picture does not fit with the common or severe skeletal disorders presented in this chapter. Establishing a definitive diagnosis as early as possible is vital for provision of appropriate medical management to the infant as well as prognostic information to the family and genetic counseling regarding recurrence risk (Table 119-5).

REFERENCES

1. Warman ML, Cormier-Daire V, Hall C, et al. Nosology and classification of genetic skeletal disorders: 2010 revision. *Am J Med Genet A,* 2011;155A(5):943–968.

2. Braverman NE, Bober M, Brunetti-Pierri N, Oswald GL. Chondrodysplasia punctata 1, X-linked recessive. In: Pagon RA, Adam MP, Ardinger HH, et al, eds. *GeneReviews* [Internet]. Seattle, WA: University of Washington, Seattle; 1997–2011. http://www.genetests.org. April 22, 2008. Updated November 3, 2011. Accessed August 16, 2012.

3. Braverman NE, Moser AB, Steinberg SJ. Updated March 2, 2010. Rhizomelic chondrodysplasia punctata type 1. In: Pagon RA, Adam MP, Ardinger HH, et al, eds. *GeneReviews* [Internet]. Seattle, WA: University of Washington, Seattle; 1997–2011. http://www.genetests.org. November 16, 2001. Updated March 2, 2010. Accessed October 2, 2011.

4. Hinson RM, Miller RC, Macri CJ. Femoral hypoplasia and maternal diabetes: consider femoral hypoplasia/unusual facies syndrome. *Am J Perinatol.* 1996;7:433–436.

5. Figueroa C, Plasencia W, Eguiluz I, et al. Prenatal diagnosis and tridimensional ultrasound features of bilateral femoral hypoplasia–unusual facies syndrome. *J Matern Fetal Neonatal Med.* 2009;10:936–939.

6. Olsen BR, Reginato AM, Wang W. Bone development. *Annu Rev Cell Dev Biol.* 2000;16:191–220.

7. Krakow D, Alanay Y, Rimoin LP, et al. Evaluation of prenatal-onset osteochondrodysplasias by ultrasonography: a retrospective and prospective analysis. *Am J Med Genet A.* 2008;146A: 1917–1924.

8. Krakow D, Lachman RS, Rimoin DL. Guidelines for the prenatal diagnosis of fetal skeletal dysplasias. *Genet Med.* 2009;11:127–133.

9. Schramm T, Gloning KP, Minderer S, et al. Prenatal sonographic diagnosis of skeletal dysplasias. *Ultrasound Obstet Gynecol.* 2009;34:160–170.

10. Yeh P, Saeed F, Paramasivam G, Wyatt-Ashmead J, Kumar S. Accuracy of prenatal diagnosis and prediction of lethality for fetal skeletal dysplasias. *Prenat Diagn.* 2011;31:515–518.

11. Unger S, Scherer G, Superti-Furga A. Updated July 31, 2008. Campomelic dysplasia. In: Pagon RA, Adam MP, Ardinger HH, et al, eds. *GeneReviews* [Internet]. Seattle, WA: University of Washington, Seattle; 1997–2011. http://www.genetests .org. July 31, 2008. Updated July 31, 2008. Accessed August 16, 2012.

12. Macpherson RI, Pai GS. Evaluation of newborns with skeletal dysplasias. *Indian J Pediatr.* 2000;67(12):907–913.

13. Alanay Y, Krakow D, Rimoin D, Lachman RS. Angulated femurs and the skeletal dysplasias: experience of the International Skeletal Dysplasia Registry (1988–2006). *Am J Med Genet Part A.* 2007;143A:1159–1168.

14. Pauli R. Achondroplasia. In: Pagon RA, Adam MP, Ardinger HH, et al, eds. *GeneReviews* [Internet]. Seattle, WA: University of Washington, Seattle; 1997–2011. http://www.genetests. org. October 12, 1998. Updated February 16, 2012. Accessed August 16, 2012.

15. Smyk M, Obersztyn E, Nowakowska B, et al. Recurrent *SOX9* deletion campomelic dysplasia due to somatic mosaicism in the father. *Am J Med Genet.* 2007;143A:866–870.

16. Bonafé L, Mittaz-Crettol L, Ballhausen D, Superti-Fuga A. Diastrophic dysplasia. In: Pagon RA, Adam MP, Ardinger HH, et al, eds. *GeneReviews* [Internet]. Seattle, WA: University of Washington, Seattle; 1997–2011. http://www.genetests. org. November 15, 2004. Updated June 12, 2007. Accessed October 2, 2011.

17. Steiner R, Pepin MG, Byers PH. Osteogenesis imperfecta. In: Pagon RA, Adam MP, Ardinger HH, et al, eds. *GeneReviews* [Internet]. Seattle, WA: University of Washington, Seattle; 1997–2011. http://www.genetests.org. Updated January 28, 2005. Accessed August 16, 2012.

18. Byers PH, Tsipouras P, Bonadio JF, Starman BJ, Schwartz RC. Perinatal lethal osteogenesis imperfecta (OI type II): a biochemically heterogeneous disorder usually due to new mutations in the genes for type I collagen. *Am J Hum Genet.* 1988;42:237–248.

19. Bellus GA, Spector EB, Speiser PW, et al. Distinct missense mutations of the *FGFR3* lys650 codon modulate receptor kinase activation and the severity of the skeletal dysplasia phenotype. *Am J Hum Genet.* 2000;67:1411–1421.

20. Karczeski B, Cutting GR. Thanatophoric dysplasia. In: Pagon RA, Adam MP, Ardinger HH, et al, eds. *GeneReviews* [Internet]. Seattle, WA: University of Washington, Seattle; 1997–2011. http://www.genetests.org. May 25, 2004. Updated September 30, 2008. Accessed Aug 16, 2012.

21. Rimoin DL, Cohn D, Krakow D, Wilcox W, Lachman RS, Alanay Y. The skeletal dysplasias: clinical-molecular correlations. *Ann NY Acad Sci.* 2007;1117:302–309.

22. Swarr DT, Sutton VR. Skeletal dysplasias in the newborn: diagnostic evaluation and developmental genetics. *Neoreviews.* 2010;11: e290–e305.

23. McGlaughlin KL, Witherow H, Dunaway DJ, David DJ, Anderson PJ. Spectrum of Antley-Bixler syndrome. *J Craniofac Surg.* 2010;21:1560–1564.

120 Differential and Management of Limb Anomalies

Meghan N. Imrie

EVALUATION AND TREATMENT OF THE FLAIL UPPER EXTREMITY

The differential diagnosis for a flail, or nonmoving, upper extremity is fairly short and includes neonatal brachial plexus palsy (NBPP), fracture, distal humeral transphyseal separation, and bone or joint infection. The history and physical are usually adequate to make the diagnosis, although imaging and laboratory examinations can help.

Clinical Findings

History should focus on the infant's delivery and perinatal events. Both brachial plexus palsy and fractures sustained during birth are associated with difficult deliveries, shoulder dystocia, and larger infants; it is important to remember that a patient may have a fracture concomitant with a brachial plexus palsy. For both NBPP and fracture, the lack of movement will have been present since birth as opposed to a patient with infection, who likely had a period, however short, of normal movement of the limb with subsequent pseudoparalysis developing over time. If an infant sustained a fracture after the neonatal period, he or she will also have had a period of normal movement of the limb. Infections may be characterized by increased fussiness or other general manifestations of malaise, but frequently the pseudoparalytic limb may be the only finding.

The physical examination should focus on inspection for any erythema or swelling, which can be seen not only in infection but also in fractures and transphyseal separations, and palpation for any crepitus, which

would suggest fracture. Pain with palpation or movement of the limb would be seen in fracture, transphyseal separation, and infection but not in NBPP. In addition, reflex testing should be done. Because fractures, transphyseal separations, and infections are painful, the lack of movement of the limb is because of pain inhibition rather than true paralysis. Therefore, on physical examination, any movement with reflex testing (eg, Moro) is supportive of infection or fracture; patients with NBPP will have no movement, even with reflex testing, because of a true paralysis of the limb. Occasionally, patients with arthrogryposis that affects the upper extremities preferentially will have a similar "waiter's tip" appearance as NBPP; the difference will be that, early on, patients with brachial plexus palsy will have normal passive range of motion, whereas arthrogrypotic patients will be stiff from the very beginning. In addition, NBPP is almost universally unilateral, whereas arthrogryposis will affect both upper extremities, although involvement may be asymmetric.

Confirmatory Tests

In brachial plexus palsy, x-ray and ultrasound evaluations will be negative (unless the infant has an associated fracture) and are not routinely ordered because the diagnosis can usually be made by history and physical alone. However, imaging, including x-rays and ultrasound, can be helpful in distinguishing between trauma (fracture or transphyseal separation) and infection. Evaluation should include x-rays of the clavicle and arm; fractures will most likely be of the clavicle or humeral shaft. If the elbow looks dislocated on x-ray, it is most likely a transphyseal separation;

in a neonate, the elbow joint is completely cartilaginous and therefore difficult to see on plain x-ray. True elbow dislocations do not really occur in neonates, but fractures through the growth plate of the distal humerus, or transphyseal separations, do. The displacement of the nonossified epiphysis will look like a dislocation on x-ray; the diagnosis can be made based on the knowledge that transphyseal separation is much more likely than an elbow dislocation and can be confirmed by ultrasonography, which will show the normally articulated joint but separated physis. X-ray findings may be absent or variable in infections; joints, especially the shoulder (or the hip in the lower extremity), may appear subluxed because of a purulent fluid collection. In addition, if the infection has been present long enough, bony changes from ongoing osteomyelitis may be seen (Figure 120-1). Ultrasound can be helpful to evaluate for any joint effusion, which would

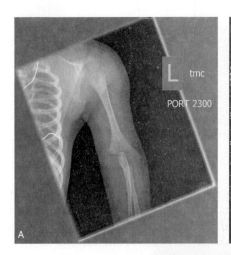
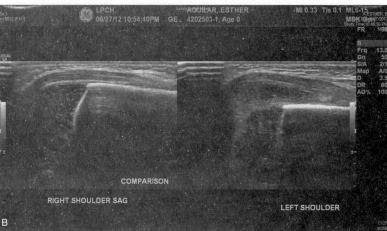
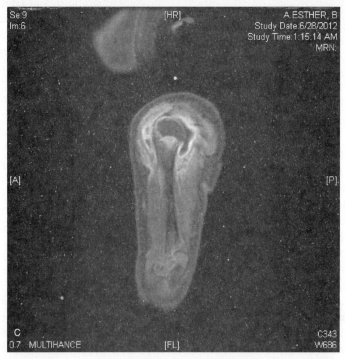

FIGURE 120-1 A, Anteroposterior x-ray of left shoulder in 3-week-old with 2-day history of decreased movement of left arm; **B,** ultrasound of affected and unaffected side demonstrating fluid collection concerning for septic arthritis; **C,** magnetic resonance imaging (MRI) confirming septic arthritis and associated osteomyelitis.

be suggestive of infection; occasionally, magnetic resonance imaging (MRI) is used to fully characterize the extent of the infection. It is not routinely used to make the diagnosis in a flail extremity. Laboratory studies are not routinely helpful in ruling out an infection because white blood cell counts and erythrocyte sedimentation rate (ESR) can be unreliable in neonates.[1] The C-reactive protein (CRP) value is more helpful; if it is normal, it has a 95% negative predictive value for infection.[2] All laboratory values should be normal in NBPP, fracture, and transphyseal separation; however, they may also be normal in neonatal infection.

Treatment

Treatment depends on the cause of the flail extremity. If the patient is diagnosed with brachial plexus palsy based on history and physical examination, initial treatment is stretching of the arm, which begins usually 1 week after birth; the goal is maintenance of range of motion while the patient's neurologic function recovers. Fracture and transphyseal separation treatment is usually supportive. Given the almost-infinite bony remodeling capability of the neonate, fractures usually do not need to be reduced or realigned as any angulation will resolve over time. It is incredibly difficult to splint or cast the upper extremity of a neonate—immobilization to make the infant more comfortable can be achieved with pinning the sleeve to the shirt or with a custom-made stockinette sling. Fractures and transphyseal separations heal incredibly rapidly in infants, and usually patients are asymptomatic within 2–3 weeks of a clavicular or humeral shaft fracture. Treatment of osteomyelitis or septic arthritis varies widely, and the details that go into decision making are beyond the scope of this chapter. In general, however, osteomyelitis is more frequently initially treated with antibiotics; septic arthritis may more commonly be treated with surgery because of the chondrotoxicity associated with bacterial joint infections. It is important to remember that many physes are intra-articular in neonates, so osteomyelitis can rapidly spread to an adjoining joint. A high index of suspicion is required when evaluating and treating bone and joint infections in neonates.

Follow-up

Patients with brachial plexus palsy should be referred to a specialist fairly early because further treatment decisions are based on the degree of motor recovery, so sequential examinations will need to be performed and documented, preferably by the same practitioner. A neonate who sustains a fracture or transphyseal separation at birth should be followed by an orthopedist until fracture healing at about 4–6 weeks, and often with 1 or 2 more visits after that to ensure complete

restoration of function and motion. Of note, a fracture or, specifically, a transphyseal separation sustained in an infant after he or she has gone home from the hospital should raise the possibility of nonaccidental trauma, and appropriate evaluation and investigation should be undertaken.[3] Patients with neonatal infection should be followed longitudinally by an orthopaedist as many of these patients go on to develop growth arrest or epiphyseal abnormalities that need later treatment.[1]

EVALUATION AND TREATMENT OF HYPEREXTENSION DEFORMITY OF THE KNEE

Clinical Findings

There are few things quite as dramatic as a severe congenital knee dislocation (CDK). That being said, hyperextension of the knee may be the manifestation of a CDK, or it may be a transphyseal separation of the distal femur or fracture of the distal femur. The clinical history can be helpful in determining the etiology; a CDK should not be painful, while a distal femoral physeal separation or fracture may be, and parents may note the baby does not move the affected leg normally in these circumstances. More important, CDK is often associated with a broader syndrome, such as Larsen syndrome, arthrogryposis, or myelomeningocele; therefore, a thorough physical examination looking at other joints, the facies, and the neuroaxis in these patients is crucial in identifying any underlying, unifying diagnosis.

Confirmatory Tests

Plain x-ray can be helpful in identifying a fracture or distal femoral physeal separation as the cause of hyperextension about the knee. Because the distal femoral epiphysis may still be nonossified at the time of birth depending on the gestational age of the patient, ultrasound is helpful in differentiating a true knee dislocation from a transphyseal separation based on the location of the displacement (femoral-tibial joint in CDK vs distal femoral physis in transphyseal separation) (Figures 120-2 and 120-3).

Treatment

Treatment of distal femur fracture or physeal separation, like treatment of traumatic upper extremity injuries, is supportive, using either a splint or Pavlik harness to maintain stability and decrease pain. These injuries usually heal rapidly, and infants usually are immobilized only for a few weeks.

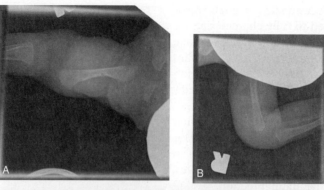

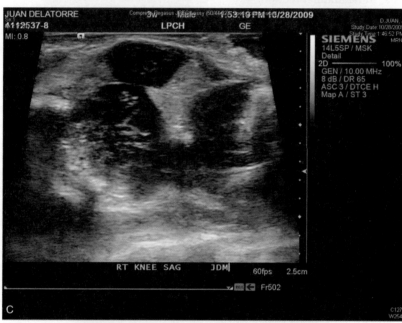

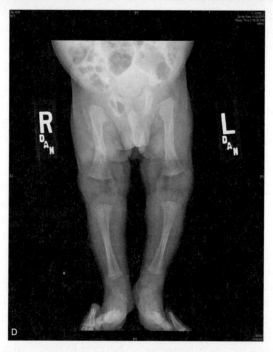

FIGURE 120-2 A and B, Anteroposterior (AP) and lateral view of what appeared clinically to be a dislocated knee in an infant born at 29 weeks. C, Ultrasound confirming congruent knee joint but physeal fracture-separation (left of figure); D, x-rays 3 weeks later showing complete physeal fracture healing with early remodeling; E and F, AP and lateral x-rays 2 years later showing near-normal-appearing distal femurs.

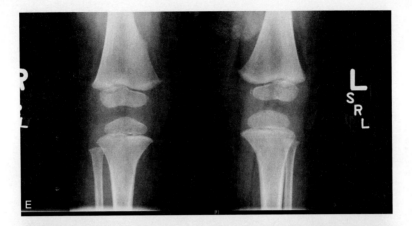

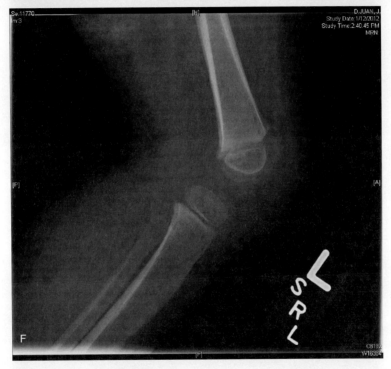

FIGURE 120-2 (*Continued*)

Treatment of a CDK, regardless if it is idiopathic or syndrome related, is initially serial casting. This is often started within a few days of birth and may be done in the intensive care setting if the patient will be hospitalized for more than 1 to 2 weeks. Each casting session starts with gentle traction on the tibia with anterior translation of the distal femur; the cast is then placed from the groin to the toes, correcting any concomitant foot deformities at the same time, with focus on anterior translation of the distal femur before flexion of the knee joint. The process should be gentle to avoid iatrogenic injury to the physis or metaphyseal bone. It should therefore be painless, and analgesic medications or sedation should not be necessary. The cast is usually changed weekly, and periodic x-rays are taken to track the reduction of the femoral-tibial joint; if the joint is not reducing, nonoperative treatment should be abandoned and surgical correction planned for when the patient is older (before age 2 years, preferably).

Follow-up

For fractures or transphyseal separations, follow-up until radiographic union is recommended, with most patients followed until they begin walking to ensure complete recovery. Patients with CDKs will need close follow-up with an orthopedist either to begin or to continue casting and for ongoing treatment of any associated anomalies (clubfoot, congenital vertical

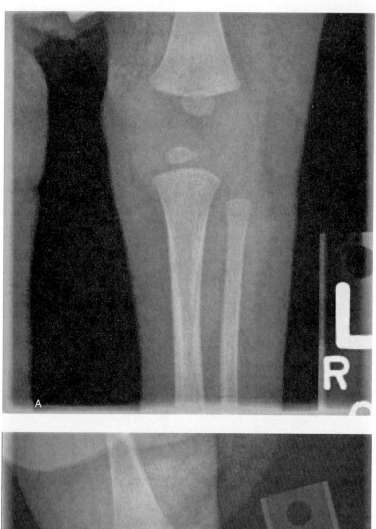

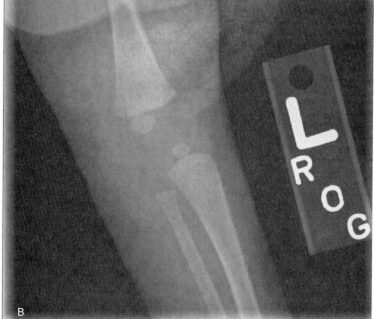

FIGURE 120-3 A and B, Anteroposterior and lateral x-rays of congenital knee dislocation in a newborn with arthrogryposis.

talus, etc); many patients will need some surgical intervention in the future to achieve full, concentric reduction of the knee joint. All patients should be followed as they grow to see if the knee instability commonly associated with CDK is clinically significant and warrants any treatment.

EVALUATION AND TREATMENT OF NEONATAL FOOT DEFORMITIES

Clinical Findings

Foot deformities, especially clubfeet, may sometimes be identified prenatally by ultrasound; otherwise, the diagnosis of foot deformities is based almost entirely on the physical examination. Congenital talipes equinovarus (TEV), or clubfoot (Figure 120-4), is characterized by deformities affecting the forefoot, midfoot, and hindfoot and can be remembered using the mnemonic CAVE: *Cavus* describes the plantar flexion of the first ray, resulting in the crease seen on the medial border of the foot. *Adductus* describes the "curving in" of the forefoot and convex lateral border of the foot. *Varus* describes the medial tilt of the hindfoot, which rotates the plantar aspect of the foot so that it is pointing medially or even upward in severe cases. *Equinus* describes the plantar flexion of the hindfoot, resulting in the crease seen in the posterior aspect of the ankle. The talar head can be palpated on the dorsolateral of the foot, and the foot is usually somewhat stiff and cannot be fully passively correctable. Positional clubfoot will look fairly similar but will be fully passively correctable at birth, and the talar head will be in its normal position along the medial foot. Congenital vertical talus (CVT) is characterized by a rocker-bottom shape to the bottom of the foot, with the hindfoot in equinus and the forefoot significantly dorsiflexed. The talar head will be palpable in the plantar medial head of the foot. Again, the deformity will be stiff and not fully correctable. Calcaneovalgus feet can have a somewhat similar appearance to CVT, but the heel will be dorsiflexed in addition to the forefoot, the plantar surface will be straight rather than convex like the rocker-bottom foot of CVT, and the talar head will not be palpable in the plantar surface. Metatarsus adductus affects only the forefoot and is characterized by a convex lateral border, giving the foot a "bean shape" appearance. It is most commonly flexible and correctable past neutral at birth.

Both TEV and CVT can be associated with other syndromes, specifically myelomeningocele, arthrogryposis, and Larsen syndrome, so a complete history and physical should be done with particular attention paid to findings seen in those diagnoses.

Confirmatory Tests

There is little benefit to diagnostic tests, such as imaging or laboratory tests, in foot deformities because the diagnosis can be made on physical examination alone. The exception is in distinguishing between congenital vertical talus and oblique talus. In the evaluation of a rocker-bottom deformity of the foot, lateral x-rays at neutral and in maximal plantar flexion should be done; if the forefoot lines up with the talus on the plantar flexion x-ray, the patient has an oblique talus, which is a less-severe and more easily correctable deformity. If the forefoot remains dorsally dislocated on the talus, the patient has a congenital vertical talus, which is more difficult to treat (Figure 120-5).

Treatment

Treatment of both TEV and CVT starts with casting. Clubfoot is now routinely treated with the Ponseti casting method, which consists of weekly casting, usually for 4–6 weeks, followed by percutaneous tendoachilles lengthening in most to correct residual equinus; all patients then wear a foot abduction orthosis full time initially and for nighttime and naps until age 3 or 4 years (or until the patient learns how to take the brace off). Casting is ideally started within the first few weeks of life; however, comparable results can be achieved even if casting is not started until several months of age.[4] For this reason, many practitioners prefer to start casting on an outpatient basis, in a controlled clinic environment, rather than in the newborn nursery or, in particular, in the neonatal intensive care unit setting, where respirators, lines, and warmers can make appropriate stretching and cast application difficult. Each casting session is the same, starting with gentle stretching and manipulation of the foot, followed by application of a long leg cast in either plaster or soft cast material. The casts are usually changed weekly, and most patients require from 4 to 6 casts.[5]

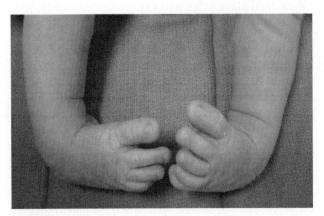

FIGURE 120-4 Classic appearance of clubfoot.

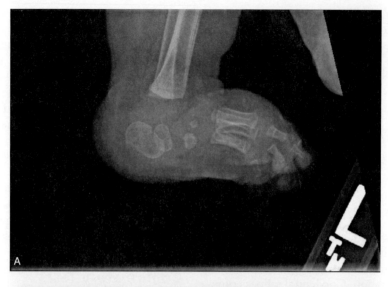

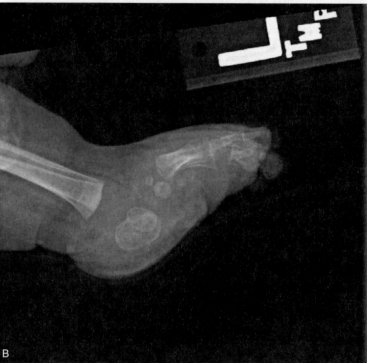

FIGURE 120-5 A and B, Neutral lateral and maximal plantar flexion in patient with congenital vertical talus. Note the forefoot remains dorsally located compared to the talus in the maximal plantar flexion x-ray.

Once the foot achieves at least 45°–60° external rotation, dorsiflexion is assessed. If at least 10° of dorsiflexion can be achieved, no Achilles tendon lengthening is needed, and the patient is transitioned to a foot abduction orthosis (FAO). Most of the time, however, the equinus cannot be corrected, and the patient undergoes a percutaneous Achilles tenotomy (TAL) and final cast placement, either in the clinic setting with local anesthetic or lidocaine cream or in the operating room with a light anesthetic. Members of the Pediatric Orthopaedic Society of North America

(POSNA) reported that patients receive their percutaneous TAL under local anesthesia 40% of the time, under general anesthesia 45% of the time, and under conscious sedation 7% of the time.[5] Most patients need only oral acetaminophen postoperatively for 1 or 2 days. The last cast usually stays on for 3 weeks, and then the patient is transitioned into a FAO, of which there are several types. Families are instructed to use the FAO full time, preferably at least 23 hours per day, for at least 3 months and up to when the patient begins to pull to stand; families are then instructed to use the brace during nighttime and naps until age 3 or 4 years. Recurrence is directly linked to FAO noncompliance, so the importance of correct brace wear cannot be overemphasized.

The schedule and technique of casting in congenital vertical talus is fairly similar to Ponseti casting of clubfoot, but nonoperative treatment is less universally successful, and patients more frequently require moderate-to-extensive soft tissue surgery before walking age. Even those patients whose deformity is successfully treated with casting require percutaneous pinning of the talonavicular joint and TAL in the operating room as part of the casting protocol described by Dobbs and colleagues.[6] Those patients who fail casting usually undergo extensive surgical correction between the ages of 6–12 months.

Calcaneovalgus and mild metatarsus adductus usually do not need any formal treatment as the natural history of these physiologic foot "deformities" is one of resolution. Stretching of the feet can be taught to parents to be done at every diaper change. The direction of the stretch should be in the opposite direction of the deformity (ie, plantar flexion and inversion for calcaneovalgus and forefoot abduction for metatarsus adductus). Occasionally, bracing or serial casting will be done in stiffer feet, especially in the case of metatarsus adductus that can only be passively corrected to, or not fully to, neutral. For stiffer feet with metatarsus adductus, surgery is occasionally required if the deformity is not responsive to casting.

Follow-up

Patients undergoing Ponseti casting for clubfoot are seen in clinic weekly during the casting process and then usually every 3 months until walking age, at which time visits are extended to every 3–6 months until age 3 or 4 years. Once patients reach that age, recurrence is much less likely, so visits become annual or even less frequent. Patients with congenital vertical talus are similarly followed closely during the casting process, with visits continuing at greater intervals as patients continue to grow; follow-up usually continues until adulthood so that any recurrences or late complications can be addressed. Calcaneovalgus feet require no specialist follow-up as long as they are resolving and are not associated with posteromedial bowing of the tibia; if a patient has concomitant tibial bowing, he or she should be followed until skeletal maturity so that any associated leg length discrepancy can be treated (usually by epiphysiodesis a few years before skeletal growth stops). Otherwise, there are no long-term sequelae of calcaneovalgus deformities. Patients with mild metatarsus adductus have a similarly benign natural history and need no formal follow-up with an orthopedist. However, if the foot is not correctable or the deformity is not resolving by 8 months, patients should be followed by a specialist to ensure no casting or bracing should be instituted.

REFERENCES

1. Sankar WN, Weiss J, Skaggs DL. Orthopaedic conditions in the newborn. *J Am Acad Orthop Surg.* 2009;17:112–122.
2. Laborada G, Rego M, Jain A, et al. Diagnostic value of cytokines and C-reactive protein in the first 24 hours of neonatal sepsis. *Am J Perinatol.* 2000;20:491–501.
3. DeLee JC, Wilkins KE, Rogers LF, et al. Fracture-separation of the distal humeral epiphysis. *J Bone Joint Surg Am.* 1980;62;46–51.
4. Yagmurlu MF, Ermis MN, Adkeniz HE, et al. Ponseti management of clubfoot after walking age. *Pediatr Int.* 2011;53:85–89.
5. Zionts LE, Sangiorgio SN, Ebramzadeh E, et al. The current management of idiopathic clubfoot revisited: results of a survey of the POSNA membership. *J Pediatr Orthop.* 2012;32:515–520.
6. Dobbs MB, Purcell DB, Nunley R, et al. Early results of a new method of treatment for idiopathic congenital vertical talus. *J Bone Joint Surg Am.* 2006;88:1192–1200.

121 Acute Management of Blistering Infants

Thomas J. McIntee and Anna L. Bruckner

INTRODUCTION

The management of neonates with blistering requires a disciplined approach that includes a broad differential diagnosis of common and rare disorders. For the purposes of this chapter, *blistering* is broadly defined as primary fluid-filled lesions, such as vesicles, bullae, and pustules, as well as resultant secondary lesions, such as erosions (see Figure 121-1). Blistering lesions are not uncommon in the neonate, and although the majority of etiologies are relatively benign, the rare, life-threatening subset requires that thorough evaluations be considered for all affected neonates.

Over 40 different neonatal disorders can present with bullous or erosive skin changes.[1] A useful diagnostic algorithm divides these conditions into infectious and noninfectious etiologies, with the latter further divided based on localized or generalized distribution, followed by predominant lesion morphology (see Figure 121-2).[2,3] A thorough history, including the prenatal and neonatal course, and physical examination will direct the initial evaluation and treatment. The maternal history should include maternal and family history of skin and mucous membrane disease, prenatal care, maternal serologies, maternal illness, and delivery course (including delivery method and duration of rupture of membranes). If the maternal history is positive for skin or mucous membrane disease, maternal examination is indicated. Neonatal history should include gestation, symptoms of illness, prior procedures, medications, feeding history, neurologic status, and vital sign instability. Skin and mucous membrane evaluation should note lesion distribution, configuration, and morphology. Evaluation of other organ systems may be warranted as indicated (see Table 121-1).[1,2]

The overall goals of management for any neonate with blistering should be to make an accurate and timely diagnosis, halt or minimize the development of new lesions, promote skin healing, treat infection, attend to the infant's overall well-being (including pain control), and support the family through the evaluation and treatment.

INFECTIOUS ETIOLOGIES

Because of their potentially life-threatening nature, viral, bacterial, and fungal disease should be considered first. Table 121-2 reviews the typical presentation, cutaneous manifestations, evaluation, and treatment of these disorders; the more common and significant infections are discussed here. Multiple diagnoses are typically considered simultaneously, and broad antimicrobial coverage is warranted until infectious etiologies are excluded or confirmed, thereby narrowing treatment.[2,4,5]

Herpes Simplex Virus and Varicella Zoster Virus

Clinical Findings

The presentation of neonatal herpes simplex virus (HSV) and varicella zoster virus (VZV) infection will be affected by the timing of maternal infection. For HSV, a maternal history of primary or recurrent genital herpes

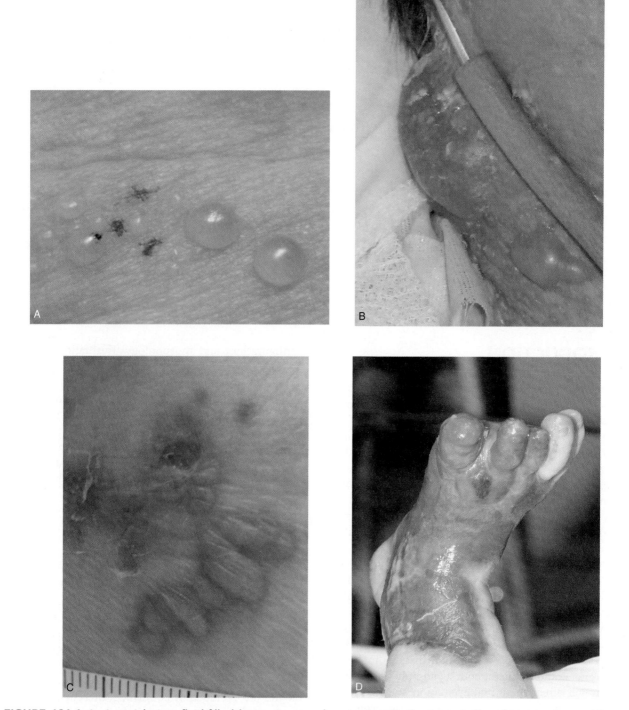

FIGURE 121-1 A, A vesicle is a fluid-filled lesion 1 cm or less in size; B, the term *bulla* refers to a larger blister. Vesiculopustules (C) and pustules are filled with purulent fluid. Note the cloudy-to-white appearance of these lesions. D, Erosions result from loss of the epidermis and are often secondary to prior bullous lesions. This neonate with epidermolysis bullosa has a large congenital erosion.

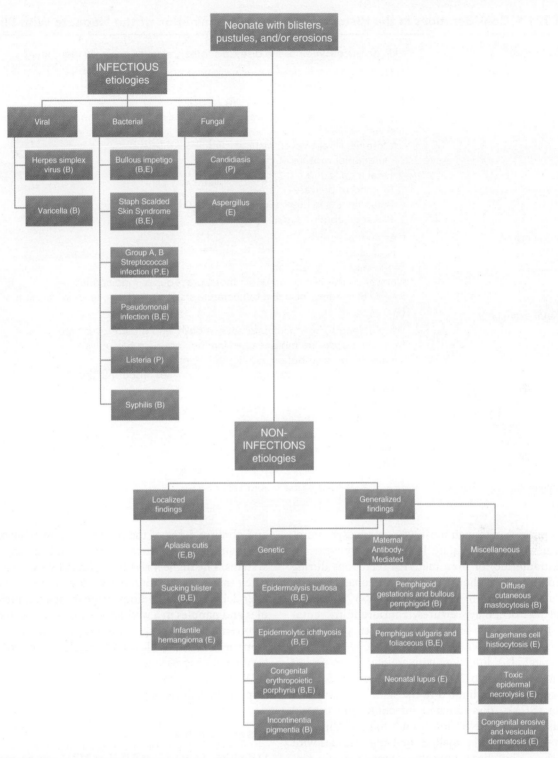

FIGURE 121-2 A diagnostic flowchart for neonates with bullous and erosive lesions, based on the predominant lesion morphology: B, blisters; P, pustules, E, erosions.

Table 121-1 Considerations in the History and Physical Examination of the Neonate With Blisters

Family history	Skin or mucous membrane disease in other relatives or family members

Maternal and prenatal history	History of maternal skin or mucous membrane disease
	Prenatal care and course
	Maternal serologies (eg, HIV, VDRL, rubella)
	Maternal illness, skin eruption, medications, procedures in the peripartum period
	Delivery course
	    Maternal illness, fever, rash
	    Duration of rupture of membranes
	    Fetal monitoring
	    Method of delivery
	    Fetal distress in utero (eg, meconium staining)
	    Placental abnormalities

Neonatal history	Gestational age Apgar scores Birth weight for gestation Nursery course, including prior illness, procedures, medications Review of systems, including temperature stability, alertness, feeding, respiratory drive

Neonatal examination	Vital signs
	Weight, length, head circumference at birth, and growth over time
	Skin and mucous membrane examination, including hair, nails
	    Note lesion distribution, configuration, morphology
	Evaluation of other organ systems for anomalies, abnormalities
	    Ocular
	    Lymph nodes
	    Hepatosplenomegaly
	    Genital
	    Musculoskeletal
	    Neurologic

Abbreviations: HIV, human immunodeficiency virus; VDRL, Venereal Disease Research Laboratory test.

may be positive, although most women are asymptomatic. A newborn can acquire HSV either transplacentally (intrauterine) or from maternal secretions during the birth process or shortly thereafter (neonatal).

Neonatal signs of intrauterine HSV infection include microcephaly, seizures, chorioretinitis, cutaneous blisters, scar formation, large erosions, and absence of skin as seen in aplasia cutis congenita.

Neonatal HSV infection, with an incubation period ranging from days to 3–4 weeks, presents in 3 clinical patterns: disease limited to the skin, eyes, and oral mucosa (SEM); disseminated infection; and central nervous system (CNS) infection.[6] Skin findings of neonatal HSV include small, 2- to 4-mm vesicles with an erythematous base, typically arranged in clusters and concentrated on either the presenting portion of the infant or areas of damaged skin integrity. Lesions may spread locally and progress to erosions or shallow ulcerations. Skin lesions are present in the majority of disseminated and CNS infections.[6]

Intrauterine VZV infection (fetal varicella syndrome) is exceedingly rare and presents with cutaneous ulceration and scarring in a dermatomal pattern as well as underlying tissue hypoplasia, low birth weight,

and abnormalities of the neurologic, musculoskeletal, ophthalmologic, gastrointestinal, and genitourinary systems. The highest risk for neonatal VZV infection is when maternal infection occurs 5 days prior to 2 days after delivery. Skin findings range from a few pink macules and papules in a well-appearing neonate to diffuse involvement with progressive crops of small erythematous macules, papules, and vesicles with peripheral erythema, progressing to necrotic crust. Disseminated VZV infection can be complicated by pneumonitis, respiratory failure, hepatitis, and encephalitis.[4,7]

Diagnostic Tests

Definitive diagnosis of HSV or VZV can be made by confirming the presence of virus in skin lesions, using direct fluorescent antibodies (DFA), polymerase chain reaction (PCR), or viral culture. The highest yield for these studies comes from infected keratinocytes. An intact blister should be unroofed, and the base of the lesion (not blister fluid) should be firmly swabbed or scraped. DFA slides are prepared by scraping the blister base with a number 15 scalpel blade and spreading the material onto DFA slide wells. Viral PCR and

Table 121-2 Neonatal Skin Infections Presenting With Vesiculopustules, Bullae, and Erosions

Disease	Presentation	Lesion Morphology/ Location	Diagnostic Tests	Initial Therapy
Bullous impetigo	First weeks of life Term, well appearing Nosocomial outbreaks	Isolated, fragile, nontender bullae Face, trunk, neck, axillae, groin, and extremities	Gram stain and culture	Topical or oral penicillinase resistant β-lactam or cephalosporin
Staphylococcal scalded skin syndrome (SSSS)	First weeks of life Term Ill-appearing	Descending erythema; fragile, flaccid, tender bullae with progression to erosions; + Nikolsky Flexural distribution on shoulders, buttocks, skin folds, hands, feet	Cultures of blood, nasopharynx, conjunctiva, umbilicus; lesional skin cultures often negative	IV β-lactam antistaphylococcal antibiotics and protein-synthesis-inhibiting antibiotic; monitor fluid status and electrolytes; emollients and nonadherent dressings Pain control
Pseudomonal skin infection	First week of life Ill-appearing ±VLBW Indwelling lines High mortality	Hemorrhagic pustules or bullae ± ecthyma gangrenosum Anogenital, axillae, face, and extremities	Gram stain and culture, blood culture, skin biopsy	IV antipseudomonal penicillin and aminoglycoside
Group A *Strep*	First weeks of life	Pustules, honey-colored crusts Moist umbilical stump	Gram stain and culture Systemic infection	Initial treatment similar to SSSS regimen
Group B *Strep*	Birth–first weeks	Vesicles, erosions, honey-colored crusts	Gram stain and culture Systemic infection	IV ampicillin + gentamicin: synergistic
Listeria	Birth	Hemorrhagic pustules/ petechiae Generalized	Gram stain and culture Systemic infection	IV ampicillin/ gentamicin
Haemophilus influenza	Birth–first week	Vesicles and crusted areas	Gram stain and culture Systemic infection	IV cefotaxime/ ceftriaxone or ampicillin/ chloramphenicol
Neonatal herpes simplex	Birth–first few weeks SGA ± microcephaly Ill-appearing One-third with CNS involvement	Grouped vesicles or punched-out ulcers on scalp, face, buttocks—peripartum HSV Absent skin/diffuse bullae and erosions, including acral sites in intrauterine HSV	Tzanck prep, viral DFA, PCR and culture, serology Potential systemic infection	IV acyclovir 60 mg/ kg/d divided into 3 doses every 8 hours
Congenital and neonatal varicella	Birth or within first 2 weeks SGA, ± ill-appearing, ± limb, ocular, neurologic anomalies	Hemorrhagic vesiculobullae with neonatal VZV, widespread erosions and scarring with congenital VZV; diffuse involvement ± dermatomal distribution	Tzanck prep, viral DFA, PCR, and culture, serology	Supportive care IV acyclovir 60 mg/ kg/d divided into 3 doses every 8 hours in severe disease VZIG for infant if maternal disease 5 days prior to 2 days after delivery

(Continued)

CHAPTER 121

Table 121-2 Neonatal Skin Infections Presenting With Vesiculopustules, Bullae, and Erosions (*Continued*)

Disease	Presentation	Lesion Morphology/Location	Diagnostic Tests	Initial Therapy
Congenital and neonatal candidiasis	First week of life, ± VLBW, ± ill-appearing	Vesiculobullae or diffuse erythematous, erosive, scaling dermatitis; intertriginous or diffuse with acral involvement	KOH prep, *Candida* antigen assay, systemic culture, ± histopathology and skin culture	Topical for superficial disease IV amphotericin B/fluconazole; infectious disease consult; remove infected vascular/peritoneal catheters
Aspergillus	First week–month, VLBW, ill-appearing, high mortality	Grouped pustules ± necrotic eschar; any site—perineum/anogenital	Systemic/skin culture, antigen assay, skin biopsy and culture	IV antifungal (amphotericin) ± surgical debridement
Congenital syphilis	Birth–first few months ±SGA, ± ill-appearing (two-thirds without symptoms), HSM	Hemorrhagic vesiculobullae: periorificial, anogenital, trunk, extremities Desquamation and erosions-acral sites	Treponemal serology, dark field microscopy lesional fluid	IM/IV penicillin G

Abbreviations: CNS, central nervous system; DFA, direct fluorescent antibodies; HSM, hepatosplenomegaly; HSV, herpes simplex virus; IM, intramuscular; IV, intravenous; PCR, polymerase chain reaction; SGA, small for gestational age; VLBW, very low birth weight; VZIG, varicalla zoster immune globulin; VZV, varicella zoster virus.

culture specimens are obtained by rubbing the specimen swab firmly on the blister base. Viral PCR or culture should also be submitted from other mucosal sites, including the conjunctiva, nasopharynx, oral mucosa, and anal mucosa. A single swab may be used, obtaining the sample in a cephalad-to-caudad direction.[4,8]

Treatment

In addition to supportive care, treatment is intravenous acyclovir with duration dependent on disease severity. For HSV, standard recommendations are 60 mg/kg/d divided every 8 hours and given 14 days for SEM and 21 days for disseminated or CNS disease.[4,9,10] Prolonged courses of oral acyclovir postdischarge have been shown to improve neurologic outcome in neonatal HSV infection.[11] In addition to acyclovir, varicella immune globulin, if available, is indicated for infants with neonatal varicella.[4,12]

Staphylococcal Scalded Skin Syndrome and Bullous Impetigo

Clinical Findings

Staphylococcal scalded skin syndrome (SSSS) and bullous impetigo result from exfoliative toxins

produced by *Staphylococcus aureus*. SSSS is a systemic infection with hematogenous spread of the toxin, presenting with acute onset of toxicity, lethargy, vital sign instability, irritability, and poor feeding. Skin signs are erythema with minimal crust around the ocular, nasal, oral, and umbilical sites that progress to diffuse erythroderma and superficial flaccid bullae and erosions. Erythema and bullae are most prominent in skin folds. A positive Nikolsky sign may be produced by applying lateral traction on the skin, resulting in sloughing of the superficial epidermis.[13]

Bullous impetigo is a localized infection and presents as discrete yellow vesiculopustules that progress to cloudy, nontender, flaccid bullae with an erythematous rim. Lesions easily rupture, producing superficial, shiny, erosions with occasional crust. Infants with bullous impetigo are not systemically ill.[13]

Diagnostic Tests

Although SSSS is a clinical diagnosis, laboratory confirmation of *S. aureus* is helpful for both SSSS and bullous impetigo. Swabs for Gram stain and bacterial culture must be obtained from the primary pyogenic site.[4] Blood and urine cultures may rarely be positive. Skin biopsy (although rarely needed) differentiates SSSS from toxic epidermal necrolysis and exfoliative graft-vs-host disease and shows a cleavage plane below the stratum corneum with minimal inflammation.

Treatment

Until antimicrobial sensitivities are known, SSSS treatment should include intravenous antistaphylococcal antibiotics (vancomycin ± synthetic penicillin ± clindamycin), pain control, attention to fluid and electrolyte status, and skin care with petrolatum-based emollients and nonadherent dressings.[4,13-15] Antibiotic therapy should be narrowed when antimicrobial sensitivities are known. The recommended duration of antibiotic therapy is 10–14 days for skin-limited disease.[4] Skin erosions heal rapidly and without scarring once exfoliative toxin production has stopped.

Bullous impetigo may be treated with topical or oral antistaphylococcal antibiotics depending on disease extent.[4,15]

Fungal Disease: Candidiasis and Aspergillus Infection

Clinical Findings

Neonatal candidiasis presents either as localized cutaneous disease or as systemic infection in the critically ill infant. Infections may be acquired in utero (typically presenting in the first days of life) or after birth. Maternal history of vaginal candidiasis, prolonged rupture of membranes, and gynecologic foreign body are risk factors for congenital candidiasis. Otherwise-healthy term infants typically present with diffuse erythematous papules that progress to pustules and eventual desquamation. In contrast, premature and very low birth weight (VLBW) infants are likely to have more significant cutaneous disease (widespread erythema and erosions) and be systemically ill. Additional risk factors for systemic candidiasis are total parenteral nutrition and long-term antibiotics with central intravenous access.[16,17]

Aspergillus should also be considered in the ill-appearing neonate with pustular, erosive, and necrotic skin lesions, especially in premature and VLBW infants. Localized skin changes often present in areas of trauma (eg, intravenous catheter site), whereas disseminated infection presents in systemically ill infants, often on prolonged antibiotic therapy, with grouped pustules that rapidly progress to necrotic ulceration.[17]

Diagnostic Tests

Skin lesions can be examined rapidly for fungal elements using a potassium hydroxide (KOH) preparation. For this test, a vesicle or pustule is scraped with a number 15 scalpel blade and the collected debris is smeared onto a glass slide. A 10%–20% KOH solution and a coverslip are applied, and the slide is examined for hyphae, pseudohyphae, and spores. Vesicopustule fluid can be also submitted for fungal culture (although several days to weeks are often needed to grow fungus in culture). Skin biopsy for histology and tissue culture is another means to confirm the diagnosis, particularly of invasive fungal infection.[4,16,17]

Treatment

Localized candidiasis is easily treated with topical nystatin or an imidazole antifungal preparation; more severe or invasive disease requires intravenous antifungal therapy and removal of all infected foreign bodies, such as vascular and peritoneal catheters.[12] Surgical debridement of necrotic tissue and systemic antifungal therapy are required for *Aspergillus* infection.[16,17]

NONINFECTIOUS ETIOLOGIES

After infectious etiologies have been excluded, evaluation should focus on noninfectious etiologies, many of which are primary skin diseases. The predominant morphology and distribution of the lesions are useful in narrowing the differential diagnosis and directing therapy (see Figure 121-2).

Localized blisters are typically the result of trauma. Sucking blisters are limited in number and found on the distal arms or hands. The primary lesion of aplasia cutis is typically an erosion or ulcer, but bullous forms can occur, particularly on the scalp.[18]

Generalized blistering or erosive diseases are often caused by genetic etiologies. Transient and benign disorders such as erythema toxicum (more pustular than bullous) and miliaria are usually diagnosed clinically, but exuberant or atypical cases can be challenging. Consultation with a pediatric dermatologist is often helpful in guiding the evaluation and management of neonates with generalized blistering and erosions.

Epidermolysis Bullosa

Clinical Findings

Epidermolysis bullosa (EB) may present at birth with absence of skin, typically on the extremities. In addition, blisters and erosions develop hours to days after birth in areas of friction or trauma. Depending on the degree of skin fragility present, affected areas may include skin traumatized during birthing, adhesive tape removal, minor procedures, or routine care such as diapering. Mucosal surfaces, especially the oral mucosa, can also be involved.

Diagnostic Tests

Skin biopsy is necessary to confirm the diagnosis of EB. Consulting a pediatric dermatologist or dermatologist experienced with EB is advised. Routine histology can be used to exclude other etiologies of blistering and erosions. Classifying the specific EB type and subtype requires immunofluorescence microscopy (IFM) and transmission electron microscopy (TEM) studies performed on biopsies of an induced blister. An uninvolved area on the flank or proximal upper or lower extremity is selected, and a blister is induced by rubbing the skin with a pencil eraser in a twisting motion for several seconds. Genetic mutation analysis can be used to confirm the diagnosis but should be guided by the results of IFM and TEM studies.[19,20]

Treatment

General guidelines for wound care management are discussed in Table 121-3. Nontraumatic handling should be instituted, and materials that cause skin trauma, such as adhesives, should be avoided. Wounds should be inspected, cleansed, and dressed daily to every other day with nonadherent dressings. In addition, nutrition needs to be supported, often with supplementation, to provide adequate calories for wound healing and overall growth. Pain should be assessed and treated.[19,21] The Dystrophic Epidermolysis Bullosa Research Association (DebRA) provides support for affected patients and their families. Parents can be referred to their website (http://www.debra.org) for information.

Epidermolytic Ichthyosis

Clinical Findings

Epidermolytic ichthyosis (EI; formerly called epidermolytic hyperkeratosis) presents at or after birth with blisters and erosions. Varying degrees of underlying skin redness are also seen. Later in infancy, the

Table 121-3 Principles of Wound Care Management for the Neonate With Blistering

New Lesion Prevention	Existing Lesion Management	Pain Management	Infection Control

• Minimize handling
• Cushion pressure points
• Use artificial sheepskin or soft bedding base
• Avoid adhesive tape, bandages, electrode adhesives; may apply monitors with nonadherent bandage wrap
• Apply pulse oximeter over transparent silicone dressing (eg, Mepitel[a]) and adhere with Mepitac[a] or nonadhesive bandage wrap
• IV catheters: adhere with Mepitac tape or with nonadherent bandage wrap
• Cotton, comfortable infant clothing
• Daily skin inspection
• Saline presoak adherent bandages for 15–20 minutes prior to removal
	• If Inherited bullous disorder suspected, lance existing bullae at dependent base with sterile needle (21–23 gauge)
	  • May require multiple punctures
	  • Fluid should drain freely; do not apply pressure
	• Do not remove blister roof as it is a natural bandage
	• Apply petrolatum to prevent wound desiccation
	• Cover wounds with nonadherent contact dressings
	  • Silicone dressings recommended
	    • Mepitel, for example, as base dressing
	    • May apply top dressing (eg, Mepilex[a])
	• May use petrolatum-impregnated dressing or Telfa[b] dressings if silicone dressings are not unavailable
	• Ensure adequate nutritional support and anemia treatment
		• Pretreat wound care events
		  • Acetaminophen 30 minutes prior to procedure
		  • Narcotic analgesics
		  • Oral sucrose
		Consider feeding prior to wound care
			• Aseptic technique for dressing changes
			• Clean wound prior to dressing application
			• Culture suspected infected lesions
			• Judicious use of topical/systemic anti-infectives
			  • Avoid use of sensitizing topical antibiotics: neomycin, bacitracin

Abbreviation: IV, intravenous.
[a]Mölnlycke Health Care, Gothenberg, Sweden.
[b]Kendall (Covidien), Dublin, Ireland.

morphology changes to excessive scale and hyperkeratosis. In the neonatal period, these findings can mimic EB, SSSS, and blistering caused by immunoglobulin (Ig) G-mediated immunobullous disease in the mother.[22]

Diagnostic Tests

In the absence of a family history of EI (autosomal dominant inheritance), skin biopsy for routine histology establishes the diagnosis. Histology demonstrates hyperkeratosis with pronounced keratohyaline granules and epidermal lysis. Genetic analysis for mutations in the genes encoding keratin 1 and 10 is confirmatory. The Foundation for Ichthyosis and Related Skin Types (FIRST; http://www.firstskinfoundation.org) is an excellent resource for parents.

Treatment

Neonates with EI have an abnormal skin barrier, predisposing them to dehydration and electrolyte abnormalities. In addition to fluid and electrolyte support, close attention to nutrition and surveillance for secondary infection is important. Gentle handling and frequent application of a bland emollient such as petroleum jelly or Aquaphor ointment is indicated. Bandaging can make erosive lesions worse in EI and should be discontinued if this is the case.[23]

Incontinentia Pigmenti

Clinical Findings

Incontinentia pigmenti (IP) presents in females as linear groups of vesicles and papules along the lines of Blaschko of embryonic ectodermal migration. This disorder is X linked dominant and typically is lethal in males. The verrucous, hyperpigmented, and hypopigmented changes of IP occur outside the neonatal period. Neurologic, developmental, ocular, and dental abnormalities can be seen in IP, although their frequency is likely overrepresented in the literature.

Diagnostic Tests

The distribution of the vesicular lesions along the lines of Blaschko is characteristic. Skin biopsy for routine histology shows an inflammatory process rich in eosinophils. Genetic testing for mutations in the *IKBKG* gene is confirmatory.

Treatment

The vesicular skin lesions resolve over several weeks and require simple skin care, such as emollients and wound care if erosions are present. Neonates with

suspected IP should have a complete ophthalmologic examination, and if eye disease is seen, neurologic evaluation is indicated as well.

Neonatal Immune-Mediated Bullous Disorders

Clinical Findings

Neonates born to mothers with IgG-mediated immunobullous disease can develop blisters and erosions caused by transplacental passage of the pathologic antibodies. In neonates born to mothers with pemphigoid gestationis and bullous pemphigoid, tense bullae are the primary lesions.[24-26] Neonatal pemphigus (vulgaris or foliaceus) manifests with fragile bullae and superficial erosions.[25,26]

Diagnostic Tests

A maternal history of bullous skin disease is typically sufficient to make a clinical diagnosis. If the diagnosis is not clear, the edge of a lesion can be biopsied for histology, and perilesional skin can be biopsied for immunofluorescence studies.

Treatment

The neonate's skin lesions gradually resolve as the maternal antibodies are degraded. In mild cases, supportive treatment with meticulous wound care and proper nutrition is sufficient. In more severe cases, topical or oral steroids may be needed until the disease begins to wane.[27]

Diffuse Cutaneous Mastocytosis

Clinical Findings

Diffuse cutaneous mastocytosis (DCM) is a rare form of mastocytosis caused by generalized infiltration of the skin with mast cells. The skin has an indurated, leathery appearance, and degranulation of the mast cells produces diffuse erythema and bullae. Systemic symptoms of flushing, tachycardia, pruritus, diarrhea, and bronchospasm may be seen with flares caused by skin friction, warm temperatures, or medications. A positive Darier sign (elicitation of erythema and wheals after rubbing of the skin) is supportive of the diagnosis.

Diagnostic Tests

Skin biopsy for histology shows an abundance of mast cells. Serum histamine and tryptase levels can be used to screen for systemic disease, and additional studies may be indicated depending on other symptoms.[28,29]

Treatment

Oral antihistamines and topical or systemic steroids are the mainstay of symptom control. Disease limited to the skin caries a good prognosis and tends to improve over time.[28,29]

Congenital Erythropoietic Porphyria

Clinical Findings

The porphyrias are inherited disorders caused by enzyme defects in the heme synthesis pathway. Although rare, congenital erythropoietic porphyria (CEP) may present in the neonatal period after exposure to ambient lighting, phototherapy, or sunlight. Vesicles, bullae, and skin fragility occur in areas exposed to light; covered areas, such as the diaper area, appear normal. Phototherapy is a typical trigger that brings the condition to attention. Extracutaneous manifestations of CEP in the neonatal period include reddish color urine that fluoresces with a Wood's lamp, profound hemolytic anemia, splenomegaly, photophobia, and keratoconjunctivitis. The differential diagnosis of photosensitive blistering in neonates includes CEP, transient neonatal porphyrinemia, hepatoerythropoietic porphyria, erythropoietic protoporphyria, Kindler syndrome, and xeroderma pigmentosum (XP).[30,31]

Diagnostic Tests

Urine, stool, plasma, and erythrocytes should be sent for porphyrin analysis.

Treatment

Ultraviolet filters should be applied to procedure, overhead, and phototherapy lights. Broad-spectrum sunscreen and protective clothing can be worn by the neonate. Red cell transfusion may be required to treat hemolytic anemia and suppress the heme production pathway. Multidisciplinary consultation is recommended.[30,31]

REFERENCES

1. Friden IJ. The dermatologist in the newborn nursery: approach to the neonate with blisters, pustules, erosions, and ulcerations. *Curr Prob Dermatol.* 1992;4(4):123–168.
2. Ahmad RS, O'Regan GM, Bruckner AL. Blisters and erosions in the neonate. *NeoReviews.* 2011;12(8):e1–e9.
3. Antaya RJ, Robinson DM. Blisters and pustules in the newborn. *Pediatr Ann.* 2010;39(10):635–645.
4. Pickering LK, Baker CJ, Kimberlin DW, Long SS, eds. *American Academy of Pediatrics Red Book: 2012 Report of the Committee on Infectious Diseases,* Elk Grove Village, IL: American Academy of Pediatrics; 2012.
5. Shah SS, Aronson PL, Mohamad Z, Lorch SA. Delayed acyclovir therapy and death among neonates with herpes simplex virus infection. *Pediatrics.* 2011;128(6):1153–1160.
6. Corey L, Wald A. Maternal and neonatal herpes simplex virus infections. *N Engl J Med.* 2009;361(14):1376–1385.
7. Lamont RF, Sobel JD, Carrington D, et al. Varicella-zoster virus (chickenpox) infection in pregnancy. *BJOG.* 2011;118 (10):1155–1162.
8. Wolfert SI, de Jong EP, Vossen AC, et al. Diagnostic and therapeutic management for suspected neonatal herpes simplex virus infection. *J Clin Virol.* 2011;51(1):8–11.
9. James SH, Whitley RJ. Treatment of herpes simplex virus infections in pediatric patients: current status and future needs. *Clin Pharmacol Ther.* 2010;88(5):720–724.
10. Kimberlin DW, Baley J; Committee on Infectious Diseases; Committee on Fetus and Newborn. Guidance on management of asymptomatic neonates born to women with active genital herpes lesions. *Pediatrics.* 2013;131(2):e635–e646. Epub 2013 Jan 28.
11. Kimberlin DW, Whitley RJ, Wan W, et al; National Institute of Allergy and Infectious Diseases Collaborative Antiviral Study Group. Oral acyclovir suppression and neurodevelopment after neonatal herpes. *N Engl J Med.* 2011;365(14):1284–1292.
12. Pan ES, Cole FS, Weintrub PS. Viral infections of the fetus and newborn. In: Taeusch HW, Ballard RA, Gleason CA, eds. *Avery's Diseases of the Newborn,* 8th ed. Philadelphia, PA: Elsevier; 2005:506.
13. Patel GK, Finlay AY. Staphylococcal scalded skin syndrome—diagnosis and management. *Am J Clin Dermatol.* 2003;4(3):165–175.
14. Kapoor V, Travadi J, Braye S. Staphylococcal scalded skin syndrome in an extremely premature neonate: a case report with a brief review of literature. *J Paediatr Child Health.* 2008;44(6):374–376.
15. Ladhani S, Garbash M. Staphylococcal skin infections in children: rational drug therapy recommendations. *Paediatr Drugs.* 2005;7(2):77–102.
16. Smolinski KN, Shah SS, Honig PJ, Yan AC. Neonatal cutaneous fungal infections. *Curr Opin Pediatr.* 2005;17(4):486–493.
17. Darmstadt GL, Dinulos JG, Miller Z. Congenital cutaneous candidiasis: clinical presentation, pathogenesis, and management guidelines. *Pediatrics.* 2000;105(2):438–444.
18. Colon-Fontanez F, Friedlander SF, Newbury R, et al. Bullous aplasia cutis congenital. *J Am Acad Dermatol.* 2003;48 (5 Suppl):S95–S98.
19. Sawamura D, Nakano H, Matsuzaki Y. Overview of epidermolysis bullosa. *J Dermatol.* 2010;37:214–219.
20. Fine JD, Eady RA, Bauer JW, et al. The classification of inherited epidermolysis bullosa (EB): report of the Third International Consensus Meeting on Diagnosis and Classification of EB. *J Am Acad Dermatol.* 2008;58(6):931–950.
21. Lara-Corrales I, Arbuckle A, Sarinehbaf S, et al. Principles of wound care in patients with epidermolysis bullosa. *Pediatr Dermatol.* 2010;27:229–237.
22. Cheng S, Moss C, Upton CJ, Levell NJ. Bullous congenital ichthyosiform erythroderma clinically resembling neonatal staphylococcal scalded skin syndrome. *Clin Exp Dermatol.* 2009;34(6):747–748.
23. DiGiovanna JJ, Robinson-Bostom L. Ichthyosis: etiology, diagnosis, and management. *Am J Clin Dermatol.* 2003;4(2):81–95.
24. Al-Mutairi N, Sharma AK, Zaki A, El-Adawy E, Al-Sheltawy M, Nour-Eldin O. Maternal and neonatal pemphigoid gestationis. *Clin Exp Dermatol.* 2004;29(2):202–204.
25. Panko J, Florell SR, Hadley J, Zone J, Leiferman K, Vanderhooft S. Neonatal pemphigus in an infant born to a mother with serologic evidence of both pemphigus vulgaris and gestational pemphigoid. *J Am Acad Dermatol.* 2009;60(6):1057–1062.

26. Lorente Lavirgen AI, Bernabeu-Wittel J, Dominguez-Cruz J, Conejo-Mir J. Neonatal pemphigus foliaceus. *J Pediatr.* 2012;161(4):768.

27. Hirsch R, Anderson J, Weinberg JM, et al. Neonatal pemphigus foliaceus. *J Am Acad Dermatol.* 2003;49:S187–S189.

28. Koga H, Kokubo T, Akaishi M, et al. Neonatal onset diffuse cutaneous mastocytosis: a case report and review of the literature. *Pediatr Dermatol.* 2011;28(5):542–546.

29. Kleewein K, Lang R, Diem A, et al. Diffuse cutaneous mastocytosis masquerading as epidermolysis bullosa. *Pediatr Dermatol.* 2011;28(6):720–725.

30. Hogeling M, Nakano T, Dvorak CC, Maguiness S, Frieden IJ. Severe neonatal congenital erythropoietic porphyria. *Pediatr Dermatol.* 2011;28(4):416–420.

31. McMahon P, Yan A. Picture of the month (erythropoietic protoporphyria). *Arch Pediatr Adolesc Med.* 2008;162(7):689–690.

122 Care of the Newborn With Ichthyosis

Jonathan A. Dyer and Mary Williams

ICHTHYOSIS/MENDELIAN DISORDERS OF CORNIFICATION

Clinical Findings

Dermatologic dogma suggests differentiation of Mendelian disorders of cornification (MeDOC) subtypes is difficult in the neonatal period. However, neonates with MeDOC may often be classified into specific clinical groups that can guide initial workup and treatment[1]:

1. Exuberant vernix (EV): Affected infants are born with a thickened white covering resembling excessive vernix caseosa. They do not have a collodion membrane.

2. Collodion baby (CB): Affected infants are born encased in a taught, clear, shiny membrane of variable thickness. Fissures may develop, and constriction of limbs or digits may occur. Ectropion or eclabium are often noted along with ear abnormalities. Restriction of movement and occasionally breathing may be noted.

3. Harlequin fetus (HF)/Harlequin ichthyosis (HI): Affected infants are born with grossly distorted features caused by thick plate-like scales with deep fissures and pronounced ectropion/eclabium. Movement and breathing may be highly restricted.

4. Ichthyosiform erythroderma (IE): These infants are born as "red, scaly babies" with diffuse erythema and skin peeling.

5. Bullous ichthyosis (BI): Affected infants exhibit blistering of the skin in the newborn period, and the blistering can be diffuse and severe. The ichthyosis may be mild or subtle in the neonatal period but accentuates with time.

6. Other: Some disorders of cornification show few, if any, skin changes in the newborn period. These include the most common form of MeDOC, ichthyosis vulgaris (IV), as well as the second most common form, recessive X-linked ichthyosis (RXLI).

Confirmatory/Baseline Tests

The following are confirmatory/baseline tests (ie, laboratory tests, radiologic examinations, electroencephalography [EEG], etc) for the specific clinical groups:

1. EV: Sensorineural hearing testing (after clearing the auditory canals of keratotic debris) is mandatory in the newborn period. Infants with ichthyosis prematurity syndrome (IPS) may raise concern prior to birth because of abnormal opacity of the amniotic fluid detected on prenatal ultrasound.[2] This may occur in other forms of EV but is not as clearly described. In patients with suspected keratitis, ichthyosis, deafness (KID) syndrome, close monitoring for systemic infection is paramount.[3] If epidermolytic ichthyosis (EI) is suspected, skin biopsy can be confirmatory.[4]

2. CB: Baseline lab evaluation is performed to screen for hemoconcentration/electrolyte abnormalities. Follow-up lab frequency is determined by clinical severity and the presence/absence of abnormalities on initial screening.[5]

3. HF: If intervention is employed, meticulous monitoring for electrolyte abnormalities and systemic infection is paramount.[6] Affected infants may be detected with high-resolution ultrasound in the prenatal period.[7]

4. IE: Close monitoring is needed for electrolyte abnormalities (especially) and infection. There is a high risk of hypernatremic dehydration, especially in conditions such as Netherton syndrome (NS).[8]

5. BI: Monitor for electrolyte abnormalities/infection. Skin biopsy can be confirmatory in this subtype of MeDOC and can differentiate patients with EI from those with epidermolysis bullosa (EB).[9]

6. Other: Male infants with RXLI may be detected in the prenatal period because of abnormally low estriol levels on the standard triple-screen test during pregnancy.[10]

Differential Diagnosis/Diagnostic Algorithm

Figure 122-1 provides an algorithm for differential diagnosis.

1. EV: Several forms of MeDOC may present with this phenotype. Congenital deafness favors KID syndrome. Normal hearing in a premature infant with polyhydramnios and abnormal amniotic fluid favors IPS. Patients with ABCA12 mutations as well as those with EI may exhibit this neonatal phenotype. Although not clearly reported in the literature, ichthyosis follicularis-atrichia-photophobia (IFAP) syndrome could present with this phenotype.

2. CB: Numerous forms of MeDOC have been reported presenting as CB in the neonatal period. Most commonly, these are autosomal recessive (AR) MeDOC (see Table 122-1).[5]

3. HF: The differential is limited. Most are caused by severe truncating mutations in ABCA12. Neu-Laxova syndrome may have a severe phenotype similar to HF but also exhibits a variety of dysmorphic features and is typically lethal in the newborn period. Restrictive dermopathy may resemble HF, but fissuring is typically less.

4. IE: A variety of AR MeDOC may exhibit IE if a full collodion membrane does not develop. NS may exhibit neonatal IE. In addition, congenital reticular ichthyosiform erythroderma (CRIE), peeling skin disease, and males with X-linked recessive (XLR) ectodermal dysplasia can present with IE in the neonatal period.[11]

5. BI: Neonatal blistering can resemble EB; skin biopsy can aid differentiation.

Exclusions/Contraindications

With all forms of MeDOC, care must be taken in terms of agents or devices that contact the skin. Despite the appearance of peeling or thick skin in these patients, the cutaneous barrier is impaired, and topical agents applied to the skin are more readily absorbed than in patients with normal skin. In addition, the skin can in some cases be more fragile than normal. Adhesives or monitoring pads must be applied and removed carefully.

PREPARATION, PRETREATMENT, AND PREWORKUP MANAGEMENT

Consent, Assent, and Ethical Considerations

The most important ethical considerations in MeDOC involve infants born with HI. The severity of the condition and historically high mortality rates mandate careful discussions with parents to determine how aggressively treatment should be pursued. Importantly, survival of infants born as HF appears to be improving, likely because of interventions and monitoring that are more aggressive in the modern era. Those infants with HI who survive the neonatal period go on to have a severe ichthyosiform erythroderma as children and young adults. Morbidity from this is relatively high. These considerations must be discussed extensively with parents and ideally with an expert in MeDOC.[6,12]

Monitoring for Treatment, Procedure, and Workup

The most important ongoing monitoring in the neonatal period for these infants is for electrolyte abnormalities and evidence of systemic infections. Some conditions, such as KID syndrome, CB, and HF, are associated with an increased risk for rapidly progressive sepsis.[1]

Sedation/Pain Control Considerations

Pain control considerations are similar to those for normal infants except in HF. Infants with HI may perform better in the neonatal period with institution of systemic pain control as the widespread skin fissuring is painful and often leads to restricted inspiration and decreased respiratory effort.[6] Similar consideration may be necessary in more severely affected CB and possibly in severe cases of EI. Importantly, skin emolliation with ointment-based emollient may also improve skin discomfort and respiratory effort.

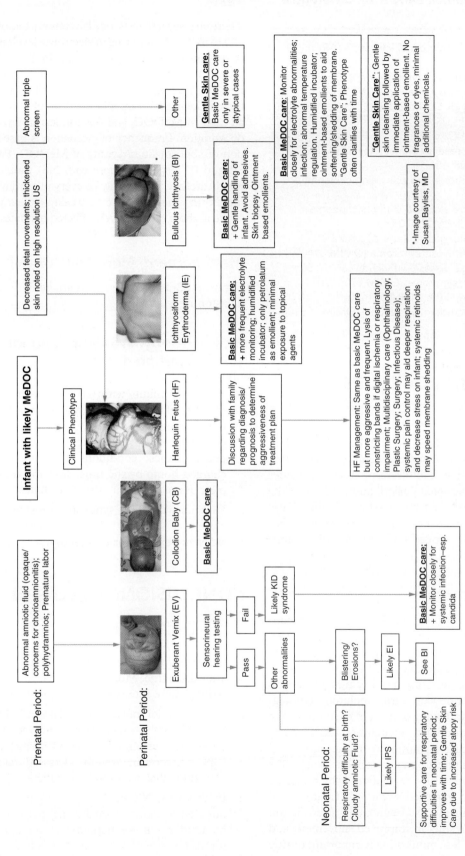

FIGURE 122-1 Differential diagnosis algorithm. EI, epidermolytic ichthyosis; IPS, ichthyosis prematurity syndrome; KID, keratitis, ichthyosis, deafness; MeDOC, Mendelian disorders of cornification; US, ultrasound.

Table 122-1 Collodion Baby (CB): Differential Diagnosis:

Autosomal recessive congenital ichthyosis (ARCI): 60%–70%

Congenital ichthyosiform erythroderma (CIE; Online Mendelian Inheritance in Man® [OMIM] 242100)

Lamellar ichthyosis (LI; OMIM 242300)

Self-healing congenital ichthyosis/self-healing collodion baby (SHCB): 10%

Type 2 Gaucher disease (perinatal lethal Gaucher disease; OMIM 608013)

Ichthyosis, hypotrichosis, and sclerosing cholangitis syndrome (IHSC)

Ichthyosis follicularis, alopecia, and photophobia syndrome (IFAP; OMIM 308205)

Elongation of very long chain fatty acids-like 4 (ELOVL4) neuroichthyosis syndrome (OMIM 614457)

Neutral lipid storage disease with ichthyosis (NLSD; Chanarin Dorfman syndrome; OMIM 275630)

Trichothiodystrophy (TTD; OMIM 601675)

XLR hypohidrotic ectodermal dysplasia (OMIM 305100)

TREATMENT/PROCEDURE

Initiation

Most patients with MeDOC will be diagnosed at birth because of the obvious cutaneous abnormalities. Infants with IPS may exhibit respiratory difficulties in the immediate perinatal period, and if possible, the resuscitation team should be prepared for this. Basic MeDOC care is begun immediately. In cases of HI, basic supportive care typically begins while discussions with the family occur.

"Basic MeDOC Care"

All neonates with suspected MeDOC should be managed cautiously in the immediate neonatal period. Baseline lab testing, including monitoring of electrolytes, should be performed, with follow-up testing determined by subtype. Close monitoring for infection is paramount. "Gentle skin care," including emolliation, is important, and many or most of the more severe infants require humidified incubators (32°C–34°C with 50%–70% relative humidity) in the early neonatal period to minimize transcutaneous water loss and to ensure temperature regulation (which can be difficult because of impaired sweating). Treatment of the skin with ointment-based emollients (petrolatum /Aquaphor) often results in improved movement and respiratory effort. Close monitoring is important during this early period.[1,5]

Tests

There are several tests (ie, laboratory, radiology, EEG, etc) to follow: Monitoring of electrolyte levels is important in the immediate neonatal period. In general, the more severe the MeDOC is, the more likely abnormalities are to develop. Although affected infants exhibit thickened skin, there is increased transepidermal water loss (TEWL) in all cases of MeDOC, and this can lead to hypernatremic dehydration. Frequency of evaluation is based on detection of abnormalities/severity of MeDOC. Patients with HI and IE (especially those with NS) should be monitored carefully. Initial daily or every other day electrolyte monitoring may decrease to weekly or less if levels are stable in these most severely affected neonates.[1,5]

Management Algorithm/Decision Tree

Figure 122-1 provides a management algorithm/decision tree.

Exit Strategy, Weaning, and Indications for Discontinuation

1. For those infants with CB or HF, shedding of the majority of the skin scales typically marks the transition between the relatively high-risk early neonatal period and the somewhat lower-risk maintenance phase of these conditions. They are typically discharged home by the time shedding is nearly complete, if not earlier, if otherwise clinically stable.

2. Patients with KID syndrome must be monitored closely after discharge, with parents educated on signs and symptoms of infection.[1,5]

CONCLUSION/FOLLOW-UP

Aftercare Monitoring

1. Gentle skin care regimens are continued at home after discharge. More severe forms of MeDOC will require more intensive and frequent care.

2. Monitoring for infection, especially in KID syndrome but also in the more severe MeDOC subtypes, is important. Care must be taken regarding topical agents applied to the skin given the increased transcutaneous absorption that occurs in these patients.

3. Infants with NS are at great risk for transcutaneous absorption, and ideally only petrolatum should be used on these patients unless closely monitored. The use of aggressive keratolytics is typically avoided in the immediate neonatal period.[1]

Follow-up Tests

There is a need for follow-up tests (ie, laboratory, radiology, EEG, etc); for instance, electrolytes may be monitored periodically for several months.[1,5]

Clinical Follow-up

For clinical follow-up (physical findings to look for, clinic appointments, etc), on discharge follow-up with a primary care provider and pediatric dermatologist/dermatologist is recommended. In patients with physical limitation from their ichthyosis, physical therapy may be helpful. Other interventions are based on individual sequelae. These patients have an increased risk of skin infection (bacterial, fungal, viral). Also in the neonatal period, monitoring of growth and hydration is important.

Long-Term Outcome/Implications for Patient/Family

1. Long-term outcome varies by individual diagnosis. Historically, determination of a specific diagnosis during the neonatal period has been difficult. However, advances in genetic testing and understanding of MeDOC often lead to much more rapid diagnosis than in the past. Although conditions such as IPS and HI are usually rapidly identifiable, for CB it may take months or even years for the final phenotype to manifest. Supportive care based on the principles outlined is important during that time.[1,5]

2. The Foundation for Ichthyosis and Related Skin Types (FIRST) is a patient support organization for patients and their families with MeDOC. It can be an excellent source of information for patients, families, and their providers. Importantly, FIRST also provides consultation with experts in the field of ichthyosis for providers caring for such patients. This organization can be reached via its website (http://www.firstskinfoundation.org).

REFERENCES

1. Dyer JA, Spraker M, Williams M. Care of the newborn with ichthyosis. *Dermatol Ther.* 2013;26(1):1–15.
2. Blaas H, Salvesen K, Khnykin D, Jahnsen F, Eik-Nes S. Prenatal sonographic assessment and perinatal course of ichthyosis prematurity syndrome. *Ultrasound Obstet Gynecol.* 2012;29(4):473–477.
3. Coggshall K, Farsani T, Ruben B, et al. Keratitis, ichthyosis, and deafness syndrome: a review of infectious and neoplastic complications. *J Am Acad Dermatol.* 2013;69(1):127–134.
4. Oji V, Tadini G, Akiyama M, et al. Revised nomenclature and classification of inherited ichthyoses: results of the First Ichthyosis Consensus Conference in Soreze 2009. *J Am Acad Dermatol.* 2010;63(4):607–641.
5. Prado R, Ellis LZ, Gamble R, Funk T, Arbuckle HA, Bruckner AL. Collodion baby: an update with a focus on practical management. *J Am Acad Dermatol.* 2012;67(6):1362–1374.
6. Harvey HB, Shaw MG, Morrell DS. Perinatal management of harlequin ichthyosis: a case report and literature review. *J Perinatol.* 2010;30(1):66–72.
7. Basgul AY, Kavak ZN, Guducu N, Durukan B, Isci H. Prenatal diagnosis of congenital harlequin ichthyosis with 2D, 3D, and 4D ultrasonography. *Clin Exp Obstet Gynecol.* 2011;38(3):283–285.
8. Pruszkowski A, Bodemer C, Fraitag S, Teillac-Hamel D, Amoric JC, De PY. Neonatal and infantile erythrodermas: a retrospective study of 51 patients. *Arch Dermatol.* 2000;136(7):875–880.
9. Ross R, DiGiovanna JJ, Capaldi L, Argenyi Z, Fleckman P, Robinson-Bostom L. Histopathologic characterization of epidermolytic hyperkeratosis: a systematic review of histology from the National Registry for Ichthyosis and Related Skin Disorders. *J Am Acad Dermatol.* 2008;59(1):86–90.
10. Oji V, Traupe H. Ichthyosis: clinical manifestations and practical treatment options. *Am J Clin Dermatol.* 2009;10(6):351–364.
11. Fraitag S, Bodemer C. Neonatal erythroderma. *Curr Opin Pediatr.* 2010;22(4):438–444.
12. Rajpopat S, Moss C, Mellerio J, et al. Harlequin ichthyosis: a review of clinical and molecular findings in 45 cases. *Arch Dermatol.* 2011;147(6):681–686.

Index

Page references followed by *f* indicate figures; page references followed by *t* indicate tables.